MW01493918

Women's Healthcare in
ADVANCED PRACTICE
NURSING

Ivy M. Alexander, PhD, APRN, ANP-BC, FAANP, FAAN, is clinical professor of nursing and medicine and director of the Adult-Gerontology Primary Care Nurse Practitioner Program at the University of Connecticut (UConn). Her clinical, scholarly, and research interests are in midlife women's healthcare and increasing access to primary care for underserved populations. She has worked extensively with menopause and osteoporosis management and has published and presented widely regarding these subject areas, including two books, which have been translated into Spanish, Greek, and Italian. She has been principal investigator on studies evaluating women's relationships with their primary care providers; Black women's perceptions of menopause, midlife health risks, and self-management techniques used to manage menopause symptoms and reduce health risks; and osteoporosis risks and management. She has served as Project Director for multiple Health Resources & Services Administration–funded programs supporting education and training of primary care nurse practitioners for underserved populations. She has consulted for national and international companies to develop educational programs, conduct research, and provide focused clinician education programs.

Versie Johnson-Mallard, PhD, APRN, WHNP-BC, FAANP, FAAN, Robert Wood Johnson Nurse Faculty Scholar alumna, is a National Certification Corporation board–certified women's health nurse practitioner, faculty, and dean at Kent State University College of Nursing. Scientific discovery and funding were with the Robert Wood Johnson Foundation, Department of Health and Human Services Office on Women's Health, National Institute of Nursing Research (NINR), and National Cancer Institute (NCI) under the National Institutes of Health (NIH). Sexual and reproductive health clinical inquiry was the impetus to advance scientific knowledge about innovative educational interventions designed to promote reproductive health and cancer prevention among young adults. Dr. Johnson-Mallard's board service, clinical interest, research, and publications are in the areas of women's health, sexual and reproductive health promotion, human papillomavirus (HPV)/cancer screening/prevention/vaccination, and behavior change in response to sex, race, and culturally appropriate educational interventions. Dr. Johnson-Mallard provides consultation to partners who share interest in the development of education material, clinical guidelines, and policy around reproductive health and cancer prevention.

Elizabeth A. Kostas-Polston, PhD, APRN, WHNP-BC, FAANP, FAAN, is a U.S. Air Force Veteran; associate professor of nursing at the Daniel K. Inouye Graduate School of Nursing at the Uniformed Services University of the Health Sciences, Bethesda, MD; a board-certified women's health nurse practitioner at Holy Cross Hospital, Germantown, Maryland; and a Robert Wood Johnson Foundation Nurse Faculty Scholar alumna. She received her bachelor of science in nursing from Arizona State University, a master of science in nursing with specialization in women's health (obstetrics, gynecology, and primary care of women) from the University of Florida, and a doctor of philosophy from Loyola University Chicago. Over the last 38 years, her clinical practice, scholarly activities, and leadership have impacted women's health—both within and outside of the U.S. Department of Defense. In her research role, Dr. Kostas-Polston's innovative scholarship is focused on enhancing military women's health and warfare capability through the development of innovative technologies designed to support and maintain urogenital health and operational readiness. She also works to effectively translate new knowledge to inform novel approaches to health promotion and infectious disease prevention in our nation's female warfighters when serving in austere environments across the globe. She has received funding from the National Institutes of Health (NIH)/National Institute of Nursing Research (NINR); the Department of Defense (DoD); the Robert Wood Johnson Foundation; Sigma Theta Tau International (STTI) Nursing Honor Society; and the Faye G. Abdellah Center for Military and Federal Health Research Endowment. The primary aim of Dr. Kostas-Polston's clinical practice is to improve the health of women across the life space and their families. Toward this end, she works with others interested in the development of health promotion and disease-prevention strategies, evidence-based clinical guidelines, and health policy. She is a Fellow and the Immediate Past-Chair of the American Academy of Nursing's Women's Health Expert Panel.

Joyce D. Cappiello, PhD, APRN, FNP-BC, FAANP, is an associate professor emerita of nursing at the University of New Hampshire, where she taught family nurse practitioner and prelicensure nursing students. Her approach to education is through case-based and inquiry-based learning. She was a coeditor and case writer for *A Day in the Office: Case Studies in Primary Care* (2017), and authored numerous cases and simulations for the classroom, objective structured clinical examination (OCSE) evaluation, and statewide Area Health Education Center (AHEC) projects. Her clinical, research and scholarly interests explore how nursing education ensures that graduates can provide expert sexual and reproductive healthcare. Her research promulgated core educational competencies for sexual and reproductive healthcare and early pregnancy decision-making. During her career, she provided prenatal care at an FQHC and comprehensive reproductive healthcare to men and women at a nonprofit feminist health center. Her most recent international research includes collaboration with Australian nursing educators and Kenyan activists working to improve the reproductive health of adolescents postpandemic.

Heather S. Hubbard, DNP, APRN, WHNP-BC, CNE, is a board-certified women's health nurse practitioner; military officer; and instructor at Bradley University Department of Nursing. She has worked extensively to advance maternal health policy through leadership roles within the Defense Health Agency and as the DoD representative for the U.S. Surgeon General's Maternal Health Working Group.

Women's Healthcare in
ADVANCED PRACTICE
NURSING

THIRD EDITION

EDITORS

Ivy M. Alexander, PhD, APRN, ANP-BC, FAANP, FAAN
Versie Johnson-Mallard, PhD, APRN, WHNP-BC, FAANP, FAAN
Elizabeth A. Kostas-Polston, PhD, APRN, WHNP-BC, FAANP, FAAN
Joyce D. Cappiello, PhD, APRN, FNP-BC, FAANP
Heather S. Hubbard, DNP, APRN, WHNP-BC, CNE

EDITORS EMERITAE

Catherine Ingram Fogel
Nancy Fugate Woods

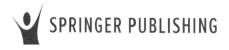
SPRINGER PUBLISHING

Copyright © 2024 Springer Publishing Company, LLC
All rights reserved.

Chapters 8, 16, 17, 21, 22, 24, 28, 32, 37, 38, and 39: The views expressed in these chapters are those of the author(s) and do not reflect the official policy or position of the Department of Defense or the U.S. Government.

First Springer Publishing edition 978-0-8261-9001-7, 2017
No part of this publication may be reproduced, stored in a retrieval system, or transmitted in any form or by any means, electronic, mechanical, photocopying, recording, or otherwise, without the prior permission of Springer Publishing Company, LLC, or authorization through payment of the appropriate fees to the Copyright Clearance Center, Inc., 222 Rosewood Drive, Danvers, MA 01923, 978-750-8400, fax 978-646-8600, info@copyright.com or at www.copyright.com.

Springer Publishing Company, LLC
connect.springerpub.com

Acquisitions Editor: Elizabeth Nieginski
Content Development Editor: Lucia Gunzel
Production Manager: Kris Parrish
Compositor: Amnet

ISBN: 978-0-8261-6721-7
ebook ISBN: 978-0-8261-6722-4
DOI: 10.1891/9780826167224

SUPPLEMENTS:

A robust set of instructor resources designed to supplement this text is located at **http://connect.springerpub.com/content/book/978-0-8261-6722-4.** Qualifying instructors may request access by emailing **textbook@springerpub.com.**

Instructor Materials:
LMS Common Course Cartridge (All Instructor Resources) ISBN: 978-0-8261-6723-1
Instructor Case Studies ISBN: 978-0-8261-6774-3
Instructor Text Bank ISBN: 978-0-8261-6776-7
Instructor PowerPoints ISBN: 978-0-8261-6775-0
Image Bank ISBN: 978-0-8261-6777-4
Mapping to AACN Essentials ISBN: 978-0-8261-6719-4
Transition Guide to the Third Edition ISBN: 978-0-8261-6724-8

23 24 25 26 / 5 4 3 2 1

The author and the publisher of this Work have made every effort to use sources believed to be reliable to provide information that is accurate and compatible with the standards generally accepted at the time of publication. Because medical science is continually advancing, our knowledge base continues to expand. Therefore, as new information becomes available, changes in procedures become necessary. We recommend that the reader always consult current research and specific institutional policies before performing any clinical procedure or delivering any medication. The author and publisher shall not be liable for any special, consequential, or exemplary damages resulting, in whole or in part, from the readers' use of, or reliance on, the information contained in this book. The publisher has no responsibility for the persistence or accuracy of URLs for external or third-party Internet websites referred to in this publication and does not guarantee that any content on such websites is, or will remain, accurate or appropriate.

Library of Congress Cataloging-in-Publication Data

Names: Alexander, Ivy M., editor. | Johnson-Mallard, Versie, editor. |
 Kostas-Polston, Elizabeth A., editor. | Cappiello, Joyce D., editor. |
 Hubbard, Heather S., editor.
Title: Women's healthcare in advanced practice nursing / Ivy M. Alexander,
 Versie Johnson-Mallard, Elizabeth A. Kostas-Polson, Joyce D. Cappiello, Heather S. Hubbard, editors.
Other titles: Women's health care in advanced practice nursing
Description: Third edition. | New York, NY : Springer Publishing Company,
 [2024] | Preceded by Women's health care in advanced practice nursing /
 Ivy M. Alexander, Versie Johnson-Mallard, Elizabeth A. Kostas-Polston,
 Catherine Ingram Fogel, Nancy Fugate Woods, editors. Second edition.
 2017. | Includes bibliographical references and index.
Identifiers: LCCN 2023027812 (print) | LCCN 2023027813 (ebook) | ISBN
 9780826167217 (paperback) | ISBN 9780826167224 (ebook)
Subjects: MESH: Women's Health Services | Nursing Care | Women's Health |
 Advanced Practice Nursing | Health Promotion
Classification: LCC RT42 (print) | LCC RT42 (ebook) | NLM WA 309.1 | DDC
 613/.04244--dc23/eng/20230717
LC record available at https://lccn.loc.gov/2023027812
LC ebook record available at https://lccn.loc.gov/2023027813

Contact sales@springerpub.com to receive discount rates on bulk purchases.

Publisher's Note: **New and used products purchased from third-party sellers are not guaranteed for quality, authenticity, or access to any included digital components.**

Printed in the United States of America.

The editors dedicate this book to the clinicians who provide excellent, individualized care to women and people of minoritized genders.

CONTENTS

PART III Managing Symptoms and Health Considerations

CONTRIBUTORS

Sharon M. Adams, DNP, CNM, ARNP
Clinical Assistant Professor, University of Florida, College of Nursing, Gainesville, Florida

Ivy M. Alexander, PhD, APRN, ANP-BC, FAANP, FAAN
Clinical Professor; Director, Adult-Gerontology Primary Care Nurse Practitioner Program; University of Connecticut School of Nursing, Storrs, Connecticut

Molly Altman, PhD, CNM, MPH, FACNM
Assistant Professor; Child, Family, and Population Health Nursing; University of Washington School of Nursing, Seattle, Washington

Angela Frederick Amar, PhD, RN, FAAN
Professor and Dean, University of Nevada, Las Vegas, Las Vegas, Nevada

Deborah Antai-Otong, RN, MS, APRN, PMHCNS-BC, FAAN
Psychiatric Mental Health and Behavioral Consultant, Dallas, Texas

Leslie L. Balcazar de Martinez, DNP, MSN, BSN*
Women's Health Nurse Practitioner/Certified Nurse Midwife, U.S. Air Force

Zahra Amirkhanzadeh Barandouzi, PhD
Postdoctoral Fellow, Nell Hodgson Woodruff School of Nursing, Emory University, Atlanta, Georgia

Richard S. Bercik, MD
Associate Professor, Department of Obstetrics, Gynecology, and Reproductive Sciences, Yale School of Medicine; Urogynecology and Reconstructive Pelvic Surgeon, Ob/Gyn Department, Yale Medicine; New Haven, Connecticut

Lana J. Bernat, DNP, CNM, CPHQ*
Lieutenant Colonel, U.S. Army Nurse Corps, Falls Church, Virginia

Tara Fernandez Bertulfo, DNP, RN, WHNP, CNE
Clinical Associate Professor, Georgia Baptist College of Nursing, Mercer University, Atlanta, Georgia

Sandra Biolo, APRN, ANP BC
Cardiology Lead Advanced Practice Provider, Western CT Medical Group, Danbury, Connecticut

Maureen B. Boardman, MSN, FNP-C, FAANP
Clinical Assistant Professor of Community and Family Medicine, Dartmouth, Geisel School of Medicine, Hanover, New Hampshire

Kristin A. Bott, DNP, APRN, ACNP-BC
Assistant Professor, Director, AGACNP Program, University of Connecticut School of Nursing, Storrs, Connecticut

Christine Alexandra Bottone, MS, DNP, APRN, NP-C
University of Connecticut, Storrs, Connecticut; CLAIM, LLC (Clinical Associates in Medicine), Farmington, Connecticut

Sandra J. Janashak Cadena, PhD, APRN, FAAN
Professor, Nursing and Medicine/Public Health, Universidad el Bosque, Bogota, Colombia, South America; Professor, Nursing, Universidad Autónoma de Bucaramanga, Bucaramanga, Colombia, South America

Joyce D. Cappiello, PhD, FNP-BC, FAANP
Associate Professor of Nursing, Emerita, University of New Hampshire, Durham, New Hampshire

Rasheeta Chandler, PhD, RN, FNP-BC, FAANP, FAAN
Associate Professor, Emory University, Nell Hodgson Woodruff School of Nursing, Atlanta, Georgia; Adjunct Professor, Morehouse School of Medicine, Department of Community Health and Preventive Medicine, Atlanta, Georgia; Visiting Professor, Center for AIDS Prevention Studies University of California, San Francisco

JiWon Choi, PhD, RN
Associate Adjunct Professor, Department of Social and Behavioral Sciences, Institute for Health and Aging, University of California, San Francisco, California

Cheryl L. Cooke, PhD, DNP, PMHNP-BC
Owner, CookeTherapy PLLC, Edmonds, Washington

Annesley W. Copeland, MD, FACS
Core Surgery Clerkship Director and Clinical Professor, The Department of Surgery at Uniformed Services University of the Health Sciences and the Walter Reed National Military Medical Center, Bethesda, Maryland

Rachel Cox, MSN, RNC-OB, C-EFM*
Flight Commander, Family Birthing Center, Keesler Air Force Base, Mississippi

Kim Curry, PhD, FNP-C, FAANP
Editor in Chief, Journal of the American Association of Nurse Practitioners, Gainesville, Florida

Maria Cutrali, APRN, ANP-BC, CHFN, CCRN, BSN
Nuvance Health Medical Practices – Cardiology, Danbury, Connecticut

Debbie T. Devine, PhD, APRN, FNP
Clinical Assistant Professor, University of Florida College of Nursing, Gainesville, Florida

---

*The views expressed are the contributor's own and do not reflect the official policy or position of the Department of Defense or the U.S. Government.

Christine DiLeone, PhD, RN
Assistant Professor, University of Connecticut School of Nursing, Storrs, Connecticut

Rebeccah Dindinger, CNS, DNP, RNC-OB, IBCLC
Maternal Infant Clinical Nurse Specialist, Center for Nursing Science and Clinical Inquiry, Landstuhl Regional Medical Center, Landstuhl, Germany

Meghan Eagen-Torkko, PhD, CNM, ARNP, FACNM
Associate Professor and Director of Nursing, School of Nursing and Health Studies, University of Washington Bothell, Bothell, Washington

Jody Early, PhD, MS, MCHES
Professor, School of Nursing and Health Studies, University of Washington Bothell, Bothell, Washington

Lauren Eddy, DNP, APRN, FNP-BC
Adjunct Clinical Professor, Family Nurse Practitioner Program; University of Connecticut School of Nursing, Storrs, Connecticut

Lisa L. Ferguson, DNP, APRN, WHNP-BC, CNE
Clinical Assistant Professor, College of Nursing, University of Florida, Gainesville, Florida

Kady Frye, BSN, RNC-OB, C-EFM
Clinical Nurse, Labor and Delivery, RAF Lakenheath, Brandon, Suffolk, England

Lynn Gaddis, DNP, APRN, FNP-BC
Assistant Professor, College of Nursing, Kent State University, Kent, Ohio

Brittany Jessica Hannigan, DNP, CNM
Chief of Midwifery Services, OB/GYN Clinic, Landstuhl Regional Medical Center, Landstuhl, Germany

Tracie Harrison, RN, PhD, FAAN, FGSA
Professor, Sun Endowed Chair in Geriatrics/Gerontology, College of Nursing, The University of Arkansas Medical Sciences, Little Rock, Arkansas

Heather S. Hubbard, DNP, APRN, WHNP-BC, CNE*
U.S. Air Force Military Officer and Instructor, Department of Nursing, Bradley University, Peoria, Illinois

Shavondra Huggins, DNP, CNS, WHNP-BC, FNP-C, APRN, CNE
Clinical Assistant Professor, University of Florida, College of Nursing, Gainesville, Florida

Heather Hutchins-Wiese, PhD, RD
Professor, Dietetics and Human Nutrition Programs; Faculty Affiliate Aging Studies Program; Eastern Michigan University, Ypsilanti, Michigan

Annette Jakubisin-Konicki, PhD, APRN, ANP-BC, FNP-BC, FAANP, FAAN
Clinical Professor; Interim Associate Dean for Graduate Studies; Director, Family Nurse Practitioner Program; University of Connecticut School of Nursing, Storrs, Connecticut

Naomi Jay, RN, NP, PhD, FAAN
Women's Health Nurse Practitioner, UCSF Anal Neoplasia Clinic, Research and Education (ANCRE) Center, San Francisco, California

Versie Johnson-Mallard, PhD, RN, APRN, FAANP, FAAN
Dean, Professor, and Henderson Endowed Chair, College of Nursing, Kent State University, Kent, Ohio

Daniela LaRosa Karanda, MS, APRN, FNP-BC
Nurse Practitioner, Hartford Healthcare Medical Group, Hebron, Connecticut

Heather C. Katz, DNP, MSN, WHNP-BC, RN
Senior Health Management Consultant

Rubby Koomson, MSN, APRN, FNP-C
Instructor, University of Connecticut, School of Nursing, Storrs, Connecticut

Elizabeth A. Kostas-Polston, PhD, APRN, WHNP-BC, FAANP, FAAN
Tenured Associate Professor, and Deputy Director, PhD in Nursing Science Program, Daniel K. Inouye Graduate School of Nursing; Uniformed Services University of the Health Sciences; Robert Wood Johnson Foundation Nurse Faculty Scholar Alumna; Women's Health Nurse Practitioner; American Academy of Nursing Women's Health Expert Panel, Past-Chair; Bethesda, Maryland

Cynthia A. Kuehner, DNP, FNP-BC, NEA-BC*
Rear Admiral, U.S. Navy

Crystal Chapman Lambert, PhD, CRNP, FNP-BC, ACRN, FAAN
Associate Professor, School of Nursing; Family, Community and Health Systems, The University of Alabama at Birmingham; Birmingham, Alabama

Lynda Lee Lapan, MSN, APRN, FNP-BC, AOCNP
Nurse Practitioner, Champlain Valley Hematology Oncology, Colchester, Vermont

Alyssa Davis Larsen, CNM, DNP
Certified Nurse-Midwife, OB/GYN, RAF Lakenheath, Brandon, Suffolk, England

Eldora Lazaroff, DNP, RN, CNP-BC
Professor, College of Nursing, Kent State University, Kent, Ohio

Necole Leland, DNP, RN, PNP, CPN
Assistant Professor in Residence, University of Nevada, Las Vegas, Las Vegas, Nevada

Nathan Levitt, FNP-BC, MSN, BSN, RN, MA
Director of LGBTQ and Gender Justice Learning, Yale School of Nursing, Orange, Connecticut

Carolyn Levy, MSN, CPNP-PC, IBCLC
Doctoral Candidate, School of Nursing, University of Connecticut, Storrs, Connecticut; Pediatric Nurse Practitioner, Lactation Consultant, Children's Medical Group, Hamden, Connecticut

Jenna LoGiudice, PhD, CNM, RN, FACNM
Associate Professor, Midwifery DNP Program Director, Egan School of Nursing and Health Studies, Fairfield University, Fairfield, Connecticut

Monica A. Lutgendorf, MD, FACOG, CAPT, MC, USN*
Maternal-Fetal Medicine Physician, Chair and Associate Professor, Department of Gynecologic Surgery and Obstetrics, Uniformed Services University of the Health Sciences, Bethesda, Maryland

---

*The views expressed are the contributor's own and do not reflect the official policy or position of the Department of Defense or the U.S. Government.

Shalini Manchanda, MD

Professor of Clinical Medicine, Indiana University School of Medicine, Section of Pulmonary, Critical Care, Sleep and Occupational Medicine, Indianapolis, Indiana

Sarah E. Martin, DNP, APRN, CNM, WHNP-BC*

Lt. Colonel, U.S. Air Force; Advanced Practice Registered Nurse; Certified Nurse Midwife; Women's Health Nurse Practitioner; Oakwood, Ohio

Kenya Massey, MSW, LSW, LCSW

Doctoral Student, Department of Sociology, University of Missouri, Columbia, Missouri

Elizabeth Mayerson, DNP, RN, APRN, FNP-BC, CNE

Assistant Clinical Professor, University of Connecticut School of Nursing, University of Connecticut School of Medicine, Storrs, Connecticut

Megan R. Mays, DNP, WHNP-BC

Atrius Health, Boston, Massachusetts

Regina A. McClure, WHNP-BC, BSN, RN

Women's Health Nurse Practitioner, Fort Worth, Texas

Selina A. Mohammed, PhD, MPH, MSN, RN

Professor and Associate Dean, School of Nursing and Health Studies, University of Washington Bothell, Bothell, Washington

Kristi Rae Norcross, DNP, CNM*

U.S. Air Force Certified Nurse Midwife Retired, Landstuhl Regional Medical Center, CNSCI and Women's Health Clinic, Landstuhl, Germany

Rachel Oldani Bender, MSN, WHNP-BC

Mercy Hospital Saint Louis, Department of OBGYN, St, Louis, Missouri

Julie L. Otte, PhD, RN, FAAN

Associate Professor, Indiana University School of Nursing, Indianapolis, Indiana

Jessica L. Palozie, DNP, APRN, ACNP-BC, CNE

Assistant Clinical Professor of Nursing, University of Connecticut, Storrs, Connecticut

Richard M. Prior, DNP, FNP-BC, FAANP

University of Cincinnati College of Nursing, Cincinnati, Ohio

Cherrilyn F. Richmond, MS, WHNP(BC)

Clinical Instructor/Lecturer, Department of Obstetrics, Gynecology, and Reproductive Sciences, Yale School of Medicine; Women's Health Nurse Practitioner, Urogynecology and Re-constructive Pelvic Surgery, Yale Medicine; New Haven, Connecticut

Susan Salazar, PhD, MSN, CNM, WHNP

Assistant Professor, University of South Florida, College of Medicine/ Family Practice, Tampa, Florida

Jacqlyn C. Sanchez, WHNP, DNP*

Major, Primary Care Flight Commander, USAF, Spangdahlem AB, Germany

Susan M. Seibold-Simpson, PhD, MPH, RN, FNP

Adjunct Faculty, School of Nursing, State University of New York at Delhi, Delhi, New York

Traci Sharkey-Wells, CNP, CDCES

Diabetes Management Team, Center for Thyroid Diseases and Endocrinology, Parma Heights, Ohio

Kim Shaughnessy-Granger, DNP, CNM, FACHE, FACNM, FAAN*

Captain, Nurse Corps, U.S. Navy, Vienna, Virginia

Stephanie N. Shivers, DNP, CNM*

Officer in Charge, Obstetrics and Gynecology Clinic, Landstuhl Regional Medical Center, Landstuhl, Germany

Katherine Simmonds, PhD, MPH, RN, WHNP-BC

Clinical Professor, Roux Institute/Bouve College of Health Sciences, Northeastern University, Portland, Maine

Anna G. Small, CNM, MSN, JD, CHC

Senior Vice President and Chief Compliance Officer, Nemours Children's Health, Jacksonville, Florida

Amanda M. Swan, MSN, WHNP-BC

Owner, Swan Integrative Health and Wellness LLC, Glastonbury, Connecticut

Gretchen E. Szymanski, CNM, WHNP-BC*

U.S. Air Force, OB/GYN Department, Landstuhl Regional Medical Center, Landstuhl, Germany

Diana Taylor, PhD, RNP, FAAN

Professor Emerita, School of Nursing, University of California, San Francisco, San Francisco, California

Janiece L. Taylor, RN, PhD, FAAN

Assistant Professor, School of Nursing, Johns Hopkins University, Baltimore, Maryland

Joanne Thanavaro, DNP, RN, AGPCNP-BC, AGACNP-BC, DCC, FAANP

Professor of Nursing, Associate Dean of Graduate Nursing Education, Director of Advanced Practice Nursing and DNP programs, Coleman/Chaifetz Entrepreneurship Fellow, Trudy Busch Valentine School of Nursing, Saint Louis University, St. Louis, Missouri

Kathryn S. Tierney, MSN. APRN, FNP-BC, FAANP

Medical Director, Middlesex Health Center for Gender Medicine and Wellness; Nurse Practitioner, Middlesex Health Multispecialty Group - Endocrinology; Middletown, Connecticut

Kara Vignati, AGPCNP-BC

Advanced Practice Registered Nurse, Starling Physicians, Wethersfield, Connecticut

Justin M. Waryold, DNP, RN, ANP-C, ACNP-BC, GS-C, CNE, FAANP

Assistant Professor, SUNY Upstate Medical University, College of Nursing, Syracuse, New York

Timothy G. Whiting, MPH/CPH, MBA, BSN-RN

Arlington, Virginia

Brookes Williams, MSN, FNP, AG-ACNP*

Commander, Nurse Corps, U.S. Navy

Catherine Takacs Witkop, MD, PhD, MPH*

Colonel (Ret), U.S. Air Force, MD; Associate Dean for Medical Education, Professor, Preventive Medicine and Gynecologic Surgery and Obstetrics, Uniformed Services University, School of Medicine, Bethesda, Maryland

---

*The views expressed are the contributor's own and do not reflect the official policy or position of the Department of Defense or the U.S. Government.

Matthew Witkovic, DNP
Adjunct Clinical Professor, School of Nursing, University of
Connecticut, Storrs, Connecticut

Danielle Wright, MD
Assistant Professor, Gynecologic Surgery and Obstetrics, Uniformed
Services University of the Health Sciences, Bethesda, Maryland

Jennifer Wright, MSN, APRN
Dartmouth Hitchcock Medical Center, Neurology, Headache Clinic,
Lebanon, New Hampshire

Jenny Yung, MS, APRN, FNP-C
Nurse Practitioner, Community Health Center, Inc., New Britain,
Connecticut

FOREWORD

If you picked up this new third edition of *Women's Health Care in Advanced Practice Nursing* to put yourself on the leading edge of contemporary, equitable, diverse, and inclusive care for women, you have done the right thing. After reading it, I am certain you will keep it nearby, especially if you are an advanced practice registered nurse (APRN) or other provider who delivers, aspires to deliver, or wants to influence superlative healthcare for women—at any age and at any stage. Building on the superb foundation of the second edition, important updates warrant perusing this one even if you prized the last edition. Throughout the text and pertinent to today's growing sensitivity to the effects on health of personal implicit bias and system structural bias, you will see enhanced attention to the diversity of women by sex and gender variation (SGV) groups (e.g., women who identify as nonbinary, lesbian, bisexual, or transgender, or who identify as other than completely heterosexual). This is in recognition of evidence that compared to cisgender heterosexual counterparts, women in SGV groups have preexisting vulnerabilities and environmental risks, showing excess prevalence of certain chronic and mental health conditions, greater engagement with health-jeopardizing behaviors (e.g., hazardous alcohol, drug, and tobacco use), and are exposed to excess stressors and experiencing culturally incongruent and insensitive healthcare.

This edition remains visionary, leading, and timely. As I noted for the second edition, the foundational editors are long-standing women's health icons in our field of nursing (Catherine Ingram Fogel and Nancy Fugate Woods). Fogel and Woods conceived of the first version in the early 1980s, a time in women's health when the biomedicine dominance made it narrowly defined (it was mostly about the reproductive phase), and the study of women's health lacked popularity and certainly was not comprehensive. The editors parted from the typical biomedical approach and articulated a framework to speak directly to us in nursing, focusing on what I call *health ecology* (women within their environments or what some refer to as the *context of their lives*). Part I will immerse you in this frame. Already started but accelerated by the recent SARS COVID-19 pandemic, attention to a national disease prevention strategy grows. Part II continues to encompass well-versed current perspectives on preventive care (and health promotion care) for women across the life span. Based on knowing that women most often initiate healthcare for bothersome symptoms associated with chronic physical or emotional conditions, reproductive (pregnancy)

or sexual health–related conditions, and the consequences of violence, Part III covers the most prominent women's health issues open to health restoration though astute APRN clinical practice.

You can be assured that the editors of this book represent the "best in class" for conveying contemporary and futuristic perspectives. The foundational editors (Fogel and Woods) with their early grasp on what would come to be a widespread emphasis on women and their health added much influential discovery and practice scholarship to the field. Cognizant of coalescing ever-burgeoning knowledge to influence ever-expansive clinical practice, added to the editorial team were expert APRN scholars Ivy M. Alexander, Versie Johnson-Mallard, and Elizabeth A. Kostas-Polston. As an adult nurse practitioner clinician scholar, Ivy M. Alexander has focused on midlife women's health and healthcare, especially menopause and osteoporosis. In her scholarly emphases as a women's health nurse practitioner, Versie Johnson-Mallard, sheds new light on women's sexual and reproductive health, including human papillomavirus (HPV)/cancer screening and prevention and behavioral change in response to culturally appropriate educational interventions. In the laboratory as well as the clinic, Elizabeth A. Kostas-Polston, a women's health nurse practitioner, addresses health promotion and disease prevention strategies focused on sexual and reproductive health and HPV-related cancer prevention. With this third edition, two additional scholars in women's health expand the editorial team. Joyce D. Cappiello expands the focus on education related to sexual and reproductive health and early pregnancy decision-making. Importantly, Heather S. Hubbard rounds out the team with her expertise in maternal health.

You can have confidence that the whole editor/author team comprises remarkably knowledgeable "thought leaders" who are powerfully enthusiastic about women's health and evolving access to equitable, inclusive, and culturally congruent healthcare for all women. Indicative of such is their engagement in calling attention to missing links within the national women's health research and clinical services policy agendas. For example, the editors and several contributing authors to this book have participated, as I do, in the Women's Health Expert Panel of the American Academy of Nursing. It is made up of peer-nominated/elected scholars from academia and healthcare practice focused on shaping superior policy for effective healthcare delivery and clinical practice. Collectively, this group has published and spoken out publicly on what is crucial to the health of women, critiqued written exposés that were missing a nursing voice, and recently summarized policy agenda considerations stemming from SARS COVID-19 pandemic effects on women's health.

By now you have gathered that it is my honor to urge you to read this *forward-looking* third edition. We continue to see APRNs bringing a comprehensive approach to primary and collaborative specialty care. No group is better positioned to model the elements brought forward by this book than women's health APRNs. So, whether you are an ardent advocate for, thinking about becoming, on the path to becoming, or are an APRN in women's health, this book should be your provocative and affirming handbook—an accelerant for helping ensure that you are an influential women's health provider, scholar, leader, policy maker, and spokesperson.

Joan L. Shaver, PhD, RN, FAAN
Professor and Dean Emerita
University of Arizona College of Nursing
Tucson, Arizona

We support an individual's right to autonomy in decision-making about their health based on the personal context of their lives, including but not limited to early pregnancy decision-making and gender affirmation. We believe that individuals have the right to high value, equitable, and unbiased care. In this third edition of *Women's Healthcare in Advanced Practice Nursing*, we attempt to make high value, equitable, and unbiased care more evident than in prior editions. While the number of women included in research studies is increasing, we remain limited in our ability to accurately address perspectives and needs for minoritized gender persons because of the lack of research that focuses on, includes, or even identifies transgender and nonbinary persons. Throughout the book we have attempted to use inclusive language while remaining true to research findings, which are translated into evidence-based practice. In many instances, this means we use the terms *woman, women, she, her*, and *hers* because that usage reflects the data that are available. We purposefully use *they, them, theirs, patient, person*, etc. whenever possible.

Women's health has been defined from a variety of perspectives. Women themselves and those who identify as transgender, nonbinary, and queer describe what it means to be healthy. Often their descriptions allude to experiencing the absence of illness or symptoms but more often to being able to perform their roles, and self-identify their gender, and having the mental wellness capacity to respond to stress and strain.

This textbook originated in the 1970s as Catherine Ingram Fogel and Nancy Fugate Woods recognized the need for resources for nurses, advanced practice nurses, and nursing students who were interested in the emerging science and healthcare needs of women. The textbook was revised, updated, and renamed to remain current and address timely issues in 1995, 2008, and 2019. The current edition of *Women's Healthcare in Advanced Practice Nursing* continues the women-centered focus of previous editions and has been expanded to include, as fully as possible, minoritized gender, nonbinary, transgender, and racialized persons, and confront prejudice in healthcare.

Over the past decades, nursing scholars have studied women's health through the lenses of feminist theory, nursing theory, and more recently through critical race theories, postcolonial theories, and womanist theory. In this relatively short period of history—propelled by a fusion of the U.S. feminist movement, a global pandemic, women's health being politicized, and the popular health movement—scholars redefined *women's health* as more than women's reproductive health. *Women's health* grew to be understood to include a holistic view of what it means to be a healthy woman. Indeed, women's health as a discipline was transformed from gynecology to "Gyn Ecology," an understanding of women's health in the context of everyday life. An ecologic perspective considers the multiple environments in which women live their lives, including influences of society, culture, institutions, community, families, and mental and physical health. Taking the lead from patients, clinicians and researchers alike redefined being healthy as the processes of attaining, regaining, and retaining mental and physical health. Moreover, it became more fully appreciated that an individual's health at one part of the life span influences health later in life.

This holistic perspective placed women at the center of clinical services as well as research, focusing on their individual health in the context of their sex and their lives and their communities. Frameworks for understanding women's health shaped by research and clinical scholarship are expanding to include transgender and nonbinary persons. Scholars challenge investigators to consider the intersectionality of a person's identities and their health. One's gender, a social construct, is only one component of who one is: sex (biology), race (social construct), ethnicity, social class, sexual orientation, gender identity, and disability/ableness all intersect in influencing one's definition of health. And yet, one's gender identity is important and must be respected for what it is for that person. Additionally, frameworks prompted by globalization reinforce the need to use many different lenses in viewing the health of each person around the world. Efforts to integrate women's health literature across disciplines has enlarged the perspectives with which communities of nurse scholars and clinicians have come to view women and their health, and provide a solid foundation for doing the same with transgender and nonbinary persons.

Over recent decades, we have also seen dramatic changes in advanced practice nursing. Advanced practice nurses now are an essential part of the healthcare workforce, providing increased access to primary and specialty care. As educational programs transition, the push for educating advanced practice nurses about unique healthcare problems, various models of care, and individualized approaches to providing evidence-based care appropriate for all patients has escalated.

Part I, Lives and Health for Women and Minoritized Gender Persons, views health as inextricably linked to the context in which an individual lives their life, making it impossible to understand health without appreciating the challenges and opportunities they face in everyday living. Understanding lived experiences has become key to understanding their well-being and opportunities for health. In Part I, we consider health for individuals within a population, while appreciating lived experiences. This perspective is limited due to the lack of diversity in research and evidence-based data available. Considerations for vulnerable populations, working as caregivers and being healthcare providers, are explored. The emergence of clinical scholarship of women's health, in contrast to gynecology and obstetrics, gave rise to the need to transform women's health research as well as models of care and health policy. Refocusing to person-centric and person-sensitive models of care has been influential in shaping the delivery of services in a variety of healthcare settings.

Part II, Health Promotion and Prevention, calls attention to the significance of health promotion and prevention, reflected both in one's own self-care as well as the delivery of professional services. Viewed through the lenses introduced in Part I, health for a person is recognized as a multidimensional experience, much of which is managed by the person, with support from health professionals. What a person does to stay healthy has been studied by numerous disciplines. Those who assume the role of health agent for their families often demonstrate a high level of interest in health-related information. Many justify not attending to their own health due to their need to care for their families. They may manage their own and family members' illnesses, and simultaneously provide illness-related care to their children, partners, and parents. Health-promotion advice may be sought from professionals to help sort out valid information and recommendations about staying healthy. In Part II, we trace experiences of health and health promotion in young, midlife, and older people as a foundation for understanding wellness and health. Given the lack of focused research, we extrapolate on this to attempt to understand needs for other minoritized gender persons. The emergence of the emphasis on wellness visits prompts us to consider: What is physical health? What is mental health? How does one attain and maintain optimal health? Health practices span nutrition, exercise/activity, and sleep, each of which demonstrably shapes our health. In an era of personalized healthcare, we examine the influence of the "omics" sciences as foundational to understanding emerging approaches to healthcare delivery. Simultaneously, we consider contextual implications for health and healthcare related to roles in society such as family role, employment role, and, importantly, social perspective of the person and their identified gender. Sexual health, including special considerations for women, lesbians, transgender, bisexual, nonbinary, and questioning persons, and life-stage warrant special consideration for intersection with healthcare access, quality, and choice.

Part III, Managing Symptoms and Health Considerations, includes multiple healthcare problems that advanced practice nurses address. In addition to underscoring the importance of listening, validating, and respecting every patient, Part III includes current information about identifying and managing healthcare needs ranging from cardiovascular and endocrine disorders, sexual and reproductive healthcare, menopause, osteoporosis, human papillomavirus, mental health problems, chronic illness, and many more. Some topics are specific to persons with ovaries and a uterus, while many others are not. All are considered from the unique presentation and perspective of the person experiencing it.

Several online resources are available for each chapter. Case studies provide real-world application of the materials. Test bank review questions reflect the most salient points of content. Sources for additional information, such as websites and apps for smartphones, are provided. Additionally, PowerPoint slides are available for each chapter and may be used as instructional aids or for content review. Supplemental material is available to qualified instructors by emailing Springer Publishing Company at textbook@springerpub.com.

IVY M. ALEXANDER
VERSIE JOHNSON-MALLARD
ELIZABETH A. KOSTAS-POLSTON
JOYCE D. CAPPIELLO
HEATHER S. HUBBARD

ACKNOWLEDGMENTS

The editors gratefully acknowledge the outstanding work of the many current and past contributing authors and emeritus editors whose excellence in research and patient care delivery has enriched this book. We acknowledge the assistance of Springer Publishing Company staff, especially Elizabeth Nieginski, VP and Publisher, Nursing; Lucia Gunzel, Senior Content Development Editor; and Kris Parrish, Senior Production Manager; as well as Vinodhini Kumarasamy, Compositor for this edition and Project Manager at Amnet.

SPRINGER PUBLISHING CONNECT™ RESOURCES

 A robust set of instructor resources designed to supplement this text is located at **http://connect.springerpub.com/content/book/978-0-8261-6722-4**. Qualifying instructors may request access by emailing **textbook@springerpub.com.**

INSTRUCTOR RESOURCES

- **LMS Common Cartridge—All Instructor Resources**
- **Case Studies**
- **Test Bank Questions**
- **PowerPoint Slides**
- **Image Bank**
- **Mapping to AACN Essentials: Core Competencies for Professional Nursing Education**
- **Transition Guide: Second Edition to Third Edition**

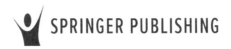

PART I

Lives and Health for Women and Minoritized Gender Persons

CHAPTER 1

Women and Their Health*

SHARON M. ADAMS, SHAVONDRA HUGGINS, AND VERSIE JOHNSON-MALLARD

Women's health can be viewed from a multiplicity of perspectives. Women, themselves, are articulate in their descriptions of what it means to be healthy. The World Health Organization's (WHO's) definition of health is "a state of complete physical, mental, and social well-being and not merely the absence of disease or infirmity" (1946, para.1).

Melnyk and Fineout-Overholt (2019) define the evidence-based practice (EBP) approach to health and wellness as clinical decision-making that integrates the most relevant research evidence, one's own clinical experience, and client preferences and values. Including client's values in clinical decision-making recognizes the influence that client values and beliefs have on health and wellness outcomes of care and situates EBP within the client's cultural context (Connor et al., 2023; Melnyk & Fineout-Overholt, 2019).

Women's health is inextricably linked to the context in which women live their lives, making it impossible to understand women's health without an appreciation of women's lived experiences in the family unit, community, and work. This approach is key to understanding their chances for health and well-being.

The 21st century witnessed a remarkable change in our understanding of women's health and saw extraordinary improvements in the health and well-being of women in the United States resulting from an increase in access to care, research, policy, and innovative approaches to healthcare. Our understanding of women's health and unique challenges—informed by research that extends from genomic molecular events to behavioral, psychological, societal, and economic phenomena—continues as one of the most exciting challenges of scientific inquiry and political inquiry. Despite the progress, the health of women in the United States remains subject to wide disparities. Health disparities is a term used to describe inequalities in health, social, political, economic, and environmental resources that adversely affect communities that are socially and/or economically disadvantaged (Brabeman, 2018; Centers for Disease Control and Prevention [CDC], n.d.-a). Disparities among women are thought to result from a complex interaction among biological factors, environment, socioeconomic

factors, and health behaviors. Social determinants of health are included in contributing to disparities and are considered nonbiological factors that have profound influences on health (Brown & Homan, 2023; Lowdermilk et al., 2020; WHO, 2008). It is important to note that health disparity is not just health difference, but rather a difference that is plausibly avoidable and impacts individuals from communities that are socially, politically, and/or economically disadvantaged, such as people who are lesbian, gay, bisexual, transgender, queer (LGBTQ), immigrant, poor, disabled, and/or of color (Brabeman, 2018). An understanding of women's health issues, if it is to be truly comprehensive, must consider such factors and trends.

The first section of this chapter describes selected sociodemographic characteristics of women in the United States. Some of the most notable of these characteristics at the beginning of the 21st century are the changing educational status of women and racial/ethnic populations. The second section presents selected measures of health status. These include mortality, morbidity, and healthcare access and utilization. Next, we discuss the complicated interplay between the steadily changing scientific knowledge regarding the areas of biology and environment. We conclude with an exploration of the future directions for women's health, including global health trends.

SOCIAL CONTEXT FOR WOMEN'S HEALTH

In 2021, the U.S. population of women was estimated at 167.5 million, with women outnumbering men at 3.8 million to 2.2 million at the age of 85 years and older (U.S. Census Bureau, n.d.-b). Who are these women and how healthy are they? To understand the health of women in the U.S. social context, we present the most recently available data on selected social characteristics of women, with a focus on the changing population demographics. Differences in the life circumstances of women are influenced through several pathways, many of which are not yet understood. Considering the health of

*This chapter is a revision of the chapter that appeared in the second edition of this textbook, coauthored with Nancy Fugate Woods, and we thank her for her original contribution.

women within their broad sociostructural environment is important in light of race/ethnicity and socioeconomic status, all of which have an impact on women's health. Gender differences in some aspects of health status are presented when the differences are remarkable. Notably, data regarding women's health are limited and often are not available by important demographic characteristics. Race/ethnic variation is discussed when the data sources are available. We recognize the limitations of reporting demographics such as race and ethnicity, because definitions vary over time, and data are inconsistently available for small but growing populations. Furthermore, reporting can obscure the diversity within and among subgroups of women. For example, the Asian/Pacific Islanders category includes more than 25 heterogeneous groups, and no distinction is made in terms of their immigration status. The category "Black" includes African Americans whose families have lived in the United States for generations as well as more recent immigrants such as refugees from war-torn countries such as Somalia. In addition, Hispanic origin is separated by the Census Bureau as an ethnicity not a race. In 2021, about 42 million Americans chose two or more racial categories when asked about their race (American Immigration Council, 2020; Kerns-D'Amore et al., 2023). Also, because detailed racial/ethnic information is frequently unavailable, and because socioeconomic status and cultures of ethnic and racial groups may vary dramatically with important health consequences, racial labeling may mask notable health differences and thus should be considered with caution. Finally, given the strong association between socioeconomic status as measured by family income, poverty threshold, or level of education and the health of women, differences are also noted when data permit.

Growth

In 2019, single race non-Hispanic population was about 40 million. Among the U.S. Black population, both multiracial and Hispanic numbers have grown since 2000 (Pew Research Center, 2023). America is becoming a more racially diverse country. The social demographics of multiracial Americans in the United States are steadily growing as a whole. As of 2019, most multiracial Black people in the United States were members of Generation Z (Gen Z; born between 1997 and 2012) or younger, reflecting their youth (Pew Research Center, 2021). Per the U.S. Census Bureau, Gen Z makes up 20.66% of the population and they are said to be the most racially and ethnically diverse. However, millennials (born between 1981 and 1996) still make up the largest generational population at 72.19 million as of 2021 (Duffin, 2022).

In 2020, the total female population was racially and ethnically diverse and was composed of White (76.3%); Black or African American (13.4%); Hispanic or Latinx (18.5%); Asian (5.9%), Pacific Islander (0.2%); and American Indian and Alaska Native (1.3%; Kerns-D'Amore et al., 2023). Population growth rates remain higher among the Hispanic population than among White non-Hispanic or Black subgroups since last noted in 2015. In fact, by the year 2060, population projections indicate that Hispanic (27.5%), Black (15.0%), American Indian (1.4%), Asian (9.1%), and two or more (6.2%) will constitute 59.2% of the total population (Vespa et al., 2020). By the year 2030, racial ethnic minority youth, age 18 years and younger, will be 53% shifting to 59% by 2045 (U.S. Census Bureau, 2020). In 2021, the general fertility rate was 56.6 births per 1,000 women age 15 to 44, the first increase in the rate since 2014 (Hamilton et al., 2022).

Immigration

The United States is largely a nation of immigrants, and the immigrant population is increasing. In 2020, there were 86 million immigrants in the United States, which made up 26% of the population (Kerns-D'Amore, 2023; U. S. Department of Homeland Security, n.d.). There are more than 23.2 million female immigrants in the United States today, outnumbering men. Since 2018, foreign women make up 51.8% of the total foreign-born population (American Immigration Council, 2020). Among the immigrant population, 23.26% were born in Mexico, 5.43% in India, 5.34% in China, 5.22% in the Philippines, 3.11% in Vietnam, 3.07% in El Salvador, 2.93% in Cuba, 2.86% in Dominican Republic, 2.64% in Korea, 1.97% in Colombia, and 44.17% from other areas of the world (American Immigration Council, 2020). The continuing influx of immigrants contributes to growing racial/ethnic diversity in the U.S. population.

Regardless of the country of origin, most immigrants confront challenges such as linguistic differences and changes in financial status on arriving in the United States. The process of immigration can affect health status and behaviors adversely through disruption of social networks; new exposure to racial and class-based discrimination; differential adverse environmental exposures; and adjustment to new language, culture, and values. For example, rates of obesity, smoking, alcohol, and illicit drug use tend to increase among Mexicans who immigrate to the United States.

Linguistic Differences

The United States is not known for being multilinguistic, leading to marked linguistic challenges for some, but not all, immigrant populations. For example, among foreign-born Blacks, most of whom are from island nations such as the Dominican Republic, Haiti, Jamaica, and Trinidad, English proficiency is common. In contrast, more traditional Hispanic immigrants often have limited English proficiency. Similarly, Asian/Pacific Islander women, who emigrate from more than 20 countries, may speak one of more than 1,000 different languages. When immigrant women enter healthcare organizations, their level of English proficiency combined with the healthcare provider's potential lack of linguistic and cultural competence can lead to the underutilization of healthcare services and unintended adverse health outcomes. Linguistic differences may play a role in family dynamics and social, educational, and employment opportunities for immigrants.

Educational Attainment

Educational attainment is one of the most important influences on economic well-being among women and has a profound impact on women's health. Graduating from high school and college significantly improves women's health and well-being by increasing economic security and providing the literacy skills necessary to navigate the healthcare system. Conversely, lacking a high school diploma may cause women to have lower earnings and greater difficulty in obtaining healthcare; in addition, they are more likely to engage in substance abuse and suffer from other adverse health consequences. Although the U.S. overall trends reflect a more educated population, significant differences in educational attainment persist with regard to gender and race/ethnicity. Persons with less than a high school education have death rates at least double the rates of those with education beyond high school. Nonetheless, the educational attainment of women indicates a dramatic improvement for a group that has historically been less educated, and these differences have been decreasing in recent years.

Almost one third (31.7%) of immigrant women age 25 and older had a bachelor's degree or more education in 2018, compared to 33.6% of native-born women and 32.4% of foreign-born men. Immigrant women had a higher percentage of bachelor's degrees or higher compared to their male counterparts in five out of 10 of the top origin countries for female immigrants. Women's progress in educational attainment has been striking over the years. The share of immigrant women with a bachelor's degree or higher education increased from 27.5% in 2012 to 31.7% in 2018. The share of native-born women with a comparable level of education also increased from 29.4% in 2012 to 33.6% in 2018 (American Immigration Council, 2020).

Women have earned more bachelor's degrees than men since 1982, more master's degrees than men since 1987, and more doctorate degrees than men since 2006 (Catalyst, 2022). Despite the narrowing in educational attainment between women and men, persistent differences among racial/ethnic groups may contribute to restricted employment opportunities and decreased financial solvency for less educated women. The educational attainment of foreign-born women in 2018 varied widely according to country of origin. Among the top 10 origin countries for female immigrants, the highest percentage of immigrant women with a bachelor's degree or more education came from India (76.3%), Philippines (51.6%), and Korea (51.1%). At the other end of the spectrum was Mexico and El Salvador (both at 7.9%), and the Dominican Republic (16.8%). Racial/ethnic disparities in education are evident (American Immigration Council, 2020).

Veteran Status

In 1973, the end of the draft and transition to the All-Volunteer Force (AVF) marked a dramatic increase in women's opportunity to serve in the military. This had a huge impact on why women account for an increasing proportion of veterans of the U.S. Armed Forces. In 2020, 1.7 million women were veterans of the Armed Forces. They accounted 9% of the total veteran population and 2% of the total adult female population, and 82% of all female veterans were of working age (18–64 years old), compared with 79.7% of nonveteran women. More than 78% of these women are under the age of 45, with 23% being Black/non-Hispanic and 12% Hispanic. Also, for this same age group, a higher percentage of veterans generally have completed some form of college education compared to nonveteran women (Arsitio & Gutierrez, 2023; Betancourt et al., 2023; Brady & Keller, 2023). Continuous

changes in the military roles of women as well as their multiple deployments and blurring of combat and noncombat operations suggest that the needs of these women may differ greatly from those of women veterans from previous eras. Women veterans are younger than their male counterparts, with 21% younger than 35 years compared with 7% of male veterans, and women account for a much smaller proportion of veterans older than 65 years (45% for men, 16% for women; Eichler, 2022; Holliday et al., 2023). The poverty rate is higher than for male veterans; 10% of women veterans live below the poverty level versus 16% of male veterans (Cohen et al., 2022). Military sexual trauma (MST), sexual assault, and/or severe and threatening sexual harassment occurring during military service have been identified in 15% of women and 7% of men. MST, along with deployment to war zones and combat exposure, increases the risk of posttraumatic stress disorder (PTSD), depression, and substance abuse. Efforts to provide gender-sensitive care for women veterans are discussed in Chapter 3, Women and Healthcare.

Employment

The proportion of women to men in the workforce has changed from previous generations. In 2019, 57.4% of all women participated in the labor force compared to 69.2% of men. From 1970 to 2019, the proportion of women in the labor force holding college degrees ages 25 to 64 quadrupled, yet the proportion of men holding college degrees barely doubled over the same time frame (U.S. Bureau of Labor Statistics, 2021). Although women hold more college degrees, their pay is still less compared to men. Women in the United States earned approximately 82 cents for every dollar earned by men; women of color earn even less. Compared to every dollar earned by White men, Asian women earned 81 cents, Native Hawaiian and other Pacific Islander women earned 63 cents, Black women earned 63 cents, Latinas earn 55 cents, and Native American women earn 60 cents (U.S. Bureau of Labor Statistics, 2021).

Employment can have beneficial or negative effects on the well-being of women. The highest percentage of women in the labor workforce by age is 25 to 54 years. Estimates from the U.S. Bureau of Labor Statistics (2021) are that 76% are age 25 to 54 years, 59.6% are 55 to 64 years, and 16.4% are 65 years and older. The labor force participation rates of women have been increasing across age groups, except among young and older women. Women 16 years and older account for 51.5% of those employed in management, professional, and related occupations (U.S. Bureau of Labor Statistics, 2023). The number of women working full time or with children (or combination of both) have increased their participation in the labor force considerably.

The increase in the percentages of women with children and two-parent families who are employed outside the home highlights the importance of child care issues and support systems for women faced with multiple responsibilities.

The United States is one of the few industrialized countries that does not provide paid maternity leave and health benefits guaranteed by law. Although the 1993 Family and Medical Leave Act (FMLA) guarantees unpaid leave to workers in businesses with 50 or more employees, the FMLA disproportionately excludes low-wage workers who often work in smaller businesses. Prior to March 2010, women who were eligible for FMLA may have opted not to take it due to their plan to breastfeed. However, on March 23, 2010, the Fair Law Standard Act (FLSA) was amended by the Patient Protection and Affordability Act requiring employers to allow a place and time for a breastfeeding parent to express milk from their breast as well as a place for storage (U.S. Department of Labor, n.d.). Per the 2018 FMLA Employee Survey, although men need and take leave for the same reasons as women, women seem (a) to need leave more, yet a higher percentage forgo taking leave when needed and (b) take longer leaves since maternity leave is three times longer than paternity leave on average. Compared to men, the financial loss for women taking FMLA leave is greater. This is not only due to longer leave time, but also due to being a single household, earning lower pay, or facing career penalties for taking leave (Brown et al., 2020). In 1996, the United States dramatically altered its welfare program with the passage of the Personal Responsibility and Work Opportunity Reconciliation Act (PRWORA), which ended federal administration of welfare and replaced it with block grants to the states. This cash assistance program, known as Temporary Aid to Needy Families (TANF), imposes lifetime limits on benefits, more stringent work requirements, and a host of behavioral mandates (Balbus, 2022; Cheng & Lo, 2022; Fusaro & Gerwirtz, 2022). Overall, most women report that they did not receive paid sick leave, paid vacation, or health benefits. The working conditions faced by mothers who had been on welfare previously are worse in part because of their significant lower levels of education, which increases the likelihood of their having to work in poorer conditions, including part-time positions that lack benefits (Brown, 2022; Lleras, 2008; Park & Choi, 2023). Women in the workforce were impacted by COVID-19 because women make up a huge portion of those working in areas considered essential such as healthcare and education (Laughlin & Wisniewski, 2021).

Economic Status

Between 2019 and 2020, poverty rates increased for married couple families and families with a female householder. The poverty rates for married couple families increased from 4.0% in 2019 to 4.7% in 2020. For families with a female householder, the rate increased from 22.2% in 2019 to 23.4% in 2020. The poverty rate for families with a male householder was 11.4% in 2020 (not much difference from 2019; Shrider et al., 2021).

Poverty is most prevalent among the Hispanic and Black ethnic groups, representing 36% living in poverty. The Black ethnic group represent 19.5%. Hispanics are close behind at 17.1%, while white non-Hispanic rates were at 8.1% in 2021 (Creamer et al., 2022; Table 1.1). In 2021, poverty rates in the United States among women under the age of 18 represent 17%, women 18 to 24 represent 21.55%, women 25 to 34 represent 14.75%, women 35 to 44 represent 12.64%, women 45 to 54 represent 10.08%, women 55 to 64 represent 11.45%, women 65 to 74 represent 10.25%, and women 75 years and over represent 13.51% (Statista, n.d.).

Poverty status is related to age. Regardless of race/ethnicity, women 45 to 54, 55 to 64, and 65 to 74 years of age are less likely to experience poverty than those age 18 to 44 years. Women 75 years and over experienced an increase of poverty rate (12.54%). Clearly, poverty status does not discriminate. A person's status can change based on gender, ethnicity,

TABLE 1.1 Persons Below Poverty Level, by Selected Ethnic Groups in the United States, 2021

RACE/ETHNICITY	POVERTY RATE (%)
White	10
Black	19.5
Asian	8.1
Hispanic or Latino	17.1
White, non-Hispanic	8.2

Source: Adapted from Statista Research Department. (2022, September 30). Poverty rate in the United States by ethnic group 2021. https://www.statista.com/statistics/200476/us-poverty-rate-by-ethnic-group

age, educational attainment, or health hazards, specifically the COVID-19 pandemic. Before the most recent recession, caused by COVID-19 pandemic, the median household income was $67,521 in 2020, a decrease of 2.9% from 2019 median of $69,560, the first statistically significant decline in household median increase since 2011 (Shrider et al., 2021).

Household Composition

Dramatic changes in family formation and marriage patterns have occurred since the mid-1960s, especially with the legalization of same-sex marriages in all 50 states as of June 26, 2015. This focus represents the family diversity growing within the United States, married or not. As of 2021, there were roughly 710,000 same-sex married couple households and 500,000 households with same-sex unmarried partners cohabiting (Borelli, 2023; Scherer, 2022; Pathak & Dev, 2023). There has also been a significant increase in the percentage of people, over the age of 15, who have never been married from 23% in 1950 to 34% in 2021. Living arrangements for young adults (ages 18–24) differ greatly now compared to before as well; they represent approximately 58% of population still living within a parent home (U.S. Census Bureau, 2021).

Caregivers

In addition to contributing solely or significantly to their family's income through employment, many women are the main caregivers of children and aging parents for their families. Given that women disproportionately carry the responsibility for family caregiving, they may struggle to meet the demands of both work and family care. Caregiving for women is discussed in detail in Chapter 18, Health Considerations for Women Caregivers.

Reproductive Trends

FERTILITY

The general fertility rate for the United States relates the number of births to the number of women of childbearing age. In 2021, the overall fertility rate was 56.3 per 1,000 women of childbearing age (Martin et al., 2022), which is a decrease from 68.7 per 1,000 women in 2008 (Hamilton et al., 2010) The U.S. fertility rate hit a record low in 2020, just as it did in 2019 and 2018. Although the COVID-19 pandemic seems to have accelerated this decline, the drop has been underway for years. The overall trend in declining birth rates, however, are largely due to women's changing roles, employment shifts, and advances in reproductive health. After WWII, the United States saw rapid change in gender roles with the expansion of women's education and entry into the labor force as previously discussed (McPhail et al., 2023; Toosi & Morisi, 2017).

BIRTH RATES FOR TEENAGERS

The drop in U.S. birth rates for teenagers was first noted after 2007, dropping 7% annually. The teen birth rate has declined to a new low each year since. In 2020, the teen birth rate was 15.4 births for every 1,000 females age 15 to 19, down 8% from 2019 and down 73% from the 1991 peak of 61.8% (U.S. Department of Health & Human Services [DHHS], 2022).

SINGLE-PARENT CHILDBEARING

After rising 13-fold from 1940 through 1990, the rate of increase in nonmarital childbearing slowed during the 1990s. The birthrate among unmarried women in 2007 and 2008 peaked at 51.8% per 1,000 unmarried women aged 15 to 44 years and declined to 37.8 in 2021 (Osterman et al., 2023). There were 158,043 births to females age 15 to 19, which accounted for less than 5% of births in 2020, and given the age of these mothers, in 2020 nine of every 10 (91.7%) of these births occurred outside marriage (Office of Population Affairs, n.d.). The percentage of unintended pregnancies has dropped to 45% in 2011 from 51% in 2008. The rates are higher among low-income and non-Hispanic Black women. Several goals were set by *Healthy People 2030* to improve

planned pregnancy: (1) offering full range of long-acting contraceptives and (2) enhanced education on correct and consistent use of contraceptives (CDC, n.d.-i).

HEALTH STATUS INDICATORS

Health status indicators, one of the simplest ways to understand health status across populations, include using data on mortality, morbidity, and access to and utilization of health services. The following health status indicators are selected primarily based on whether they had a marked impact on women's quality of life, functioning, or well-being; affected a large proportion of women or a subgroup of women; or reflected an important emerging health issue. When data are available and differences for key health conditions are notable, we provide prevalence or incidence estimates based on race/ethnicity and gender. Moreover, given the strong relationship between health and income, which is especially important for women who represent most of the poor in the United States, we report health measures by socioeconomic differences.

Life Expectancy

Life expectancy is a key indicator of health status worldwide, and mortality rate is the measure of the number of deaths per unit of the population. Due to COVID-19, life expectancy decreased more among Hispanic and non-Hispanic Black people than non-Hispanic White people in the United States in 2020 (Figure 1.1). The life expectancy of U.S. women has

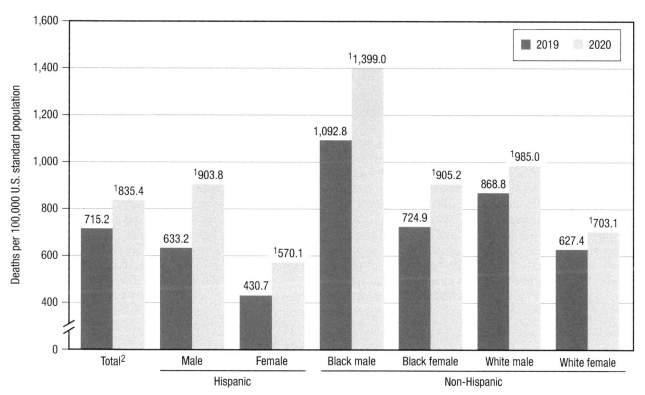

FIGURE 1.1 Age-adjusted death rates, by sex and race and ethnicity: United States, 2019 and 2020.
Source: Reproduced from Murphy, S. L, Kochanek, K. D, Xu, J., & Arias, E. (2021). Mortality in the United States, 2020 *(NCHS Data Brief No. 427). National Center for Health Statistics. https://doi .org/10.15620/cdc:112079*

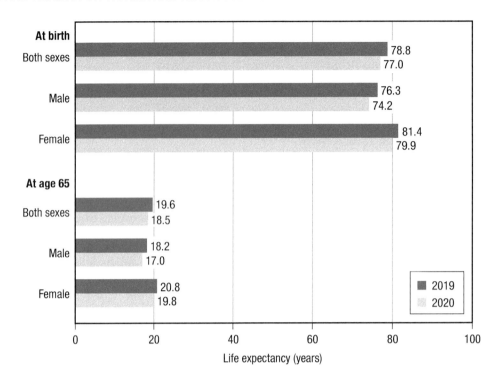

FIGURE 1.2 Life expectancy at birth and age 65, by sex: United States, 2019 and 2020.
Source: Reproduced from Murphy, S. L, Kochanek, K. D, Xu, J., & Arias, E. (2021). Mortality in the United States, 2020 (NCHS Data Brief No. 427). National Center for Health Statistics. https://doi .org/10.15620/cdc:112079

nearly doubled since the turn of the 21st century, from 48 years in 1900 to a record high of 81.4 years in 2019, compared to 76.3 years for men (Figure 1.2; Murphy et al., 2021). Overall, women are expected to outlive men by an average of 5 to 6 years, and this varies by race/ethnicity.

Hispanic women had the longest life expectancy (82.4 years), outliving non-Hispanic Black women (75.7 years) and non-Hispanic White women (80.2 years) in 2020 (Arias et al., 2021). Compared to 2021, Hispanic women's life expectancy decreased to 81 years, non-Hispanic Black women decreased to 74.8 years, and non-Hispanic White women decreased to 79.2 years (Arias et al., 2022).

However, by age 65 years these differences narrow, and life expectancy becomes more similar for White and Black women. Although life expectancy has increased since 1960 for both women and men, women's life expectancy increased by 20.5 years versus 19.8 years in men (average life expectancy is 75.1 years for women vs. 70.6 years for men; WorldData.info, n.d.).

Although the United States has one of the highest healthcare expenditures as a percentage of gross domestic product than other developed countries, the life expectancy for women is lower in the United States than in several other developed countries (Table 1.2; WorldData.info, 2020), specifically Canada.

Causes of Death

In the 21st century, significant progress was made toward increasing the years of life for most Americans, regardless of race/ethnicity or gender. Americans live longer than ever before. Presently, the chronic conditions of heart disease, cancer, COVID-19, and unintentional injuries account for more than half of U.S. deaths and are the leading causes of death for both men and women (Xu et al., 2022). As of 2019, the COVID-19 pandemic began to disrupt the lives of many people around the world. This unexpected pandemic made the top 10 leading causes of death in the United States, ranking No. 3 within 1 year (Figure 1.3).

Although women have a longer life expectancy than men, they do not necessarily live those extra years in good physical and mental health. In 2017, Mississippi and West Virginia remained in the top five states with the highest death rates in the United States. Alabama, Kentucky, and Oklahoma were among the other three. Hawaii remained in the top five having the lowest death rates with New York, Connecticut, California, and Minnesota (Xu, 2019). As a nation we are doing well, but data support that a few states remain burdened with health status indicators of high mortality rates for men and women, calling for unique and targeted systems interventions.

HIV death rates are declining globally, in both men and women, falling below the most common causes of death such as heart disease, liver disease, respiratory conditions, stroke, cancers, and Alzheimer disease as of 2016 (Murphy et al., 2021; WHO, 2020; see HIV section later in chapter). Leading causes of death vary by age, with unintentional injury the leading cause of death for women 25 to 44 years of age and the third leading cause for 45- to 65-year-olds. Suicide and homicide are the fourth and fifth most common causes for 25- to 44-year-olds, and pregnancy complications account for the ninth leading cause of death for this age group. Cancer, heart disease, and chronic lower respiratory disease are the top three causes of death for women 65 to 84 years old, but this shifts to heart disease, Alzheimer disease, and cancer beyond age 85; in both groups stroke is a close fourth (Table 1.3; Heron, 2021).

TABLE 1.2 Life Expectancy at Birth for Selected Countries: Men and Women, 2020

COUNTRY	MEN: LIFE EXPECTANCY (YEARS)	WOMEN: LIFE EXPECTANCY (YEARS)	RANK
Hong Kong	82.9	88	1
Japan	81.6	87.7	4
Spain	79.7	85.1	19
France	79.2	85.3	23
Switzerland	81.1	85.2	8
Australia	81.2	85.3	7
Israel	80.7	84.8	11
Sweden	80.7	84.2	10
Canada	79.7	83.9	18
Greece	78.6	83.7	29
Ireland	80.4	84.1	13
Denmark	79.6	83.6	20
Costa Rica	76.8	81.9	35
Puerto Rico	73.6	82.6	50
United States	74.5	80.2	47
China	75.3	81.1	39
Thailand	75	83.7	43
El Salvador	66.4	75.4	96
South Africa	62.2	68	106
India	68.6	71.8	82
Haiti	61.1	67.1	110
Afghanistan	59.9	65.4	113
Congo	57.8	61.7	120
Somalia	54	58.1	121
Chad	51.2	54.4	123

Source: Data from WorldData.info. (2020). Life expectancy for men and women. https://www.worlddata.info/life-expectancy.php#by-population

Morbidity

Morbidity is a generic measure that assesses the quantity of health in a given population and is easy to interpret and compare across populations and time. The incidence of specific outcomes such as injuries, chronic conditions, mental illness, and activity limitations are summary measures of morbidity, which are presented in this section.

INJURIES

In 2020, 200,955 deaths from unintentional injuries were reported. Unintentional injuries included falls contributing 42,114, motor vehicle accidents (MVA) contributing 40,698, and poisoning contributing 87,404 (CDC, 2020). Male burden of mortality (7.6%) was higher than female (4.4%), ranking as

the third leading cause of death for men and sixth leading cause of death for women (Heron, 2021). Approximately one third of age-adjusted deaths are due to unintentional injuries. Ages 1 to 9 (31%), ages 10 to 24 (38.1%), and ages 25 to 44 (34.2%) make up the one third age-adjusted population. However, by age 45+ unintentional injuries barely make up one tenth of age-adjusted deaths. By ages 45 to 64 (9%) and ages 65 and over (2.9%) a dramatic decrease in the percentage of deaths caused by unintentional injuries is obvious (Figure 1.4; Heron, 2021).

VIOLENCE AGAINST WOMEN

Violence against women is a global issue that goes beyond mortality and injuries, carrying a high burden of morbidity and health illnesses (WHO, n.d.). Violence is a term that encompasses a broad range of maltreatment against women and

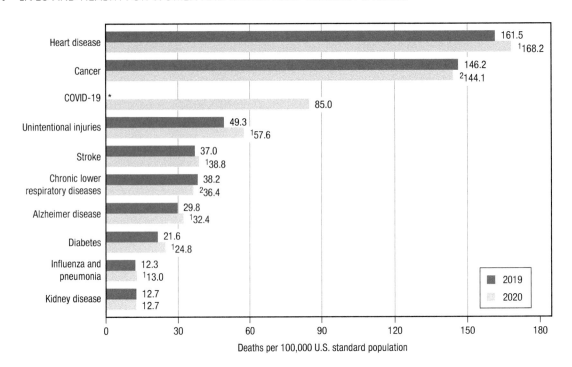

FIGURE 1.3 Age-adjusted death rates for the 10 leading causes of death in 2020: United States, 2019 and 2020.
Source: Reproduced from Murphy, S. L, Kochanek, K. D, Xu, J., & Arias, E. (2021). Mortality in the United States, 2020 (NCHS Data Brief No. 427). National Center for Health Statistics. *https://doi .org/10.15620/cdc:112079*

TABLE 1.3 Leading Causes of Death in Females, All Races and Origins—United States, 2017

RANK	TOTAL (%)	1–19 YEARS (%)	20–44 YEARS (%)	45–64 YEARS (%)	65–84 YEARS (%)	85+ YEARS (%)
1	Heart disease (21.8)	Unintentional injury (32.7)	Unintentional injury (30)	Cancer (34.2)	Cancer (27)	Heart disease (27.7)
2	Cancer (20.5)	Cancer (11)	Cancer (16)	Heart disease (16.3)	Heart disease (19.9)	Alzheimer disease (10.9)
3	Chronic lower respiratory disease (6.2)	Suicide (10.3)	Heart disease (9)	Unintentional injury (6.9)	Chronic lower respiratory disease (8.9)	Cancer (9.9)
4	Stroke (6.2)	Homicide (7.4)	Suicide (7.6)	Chronic lower respiratory disease (5.3)	Stroke (5.8)	Stroke (8.1)
5	Alzheimer disease (6.1)	Birth defects (6.4)	Homicide (3.8)	Diabetes (3.8)	Alzheimer disease (4.4)	Chronic lower respiratory disease (4.9)
6	Unintentional injury (4.3)	Heart disease (3.4)	Chronic liver disease (2.9)	Stroke (3.6)	Diabetes (3.3)	Flu and pneumonia (2.7)
7	Diabetes (2.7)	Flu and pneumonia (2)	Diabetes (2.4)	Liver disease (3.5)	Unintentional injury (2.3)	Unintentional injury (2.6)
8	Flu and pneumonia (2.2)	Stroke (1.4)	Stroke (2)	Suicide (2)	Kidney disease (2.1)	Hypertension (1.9)
9	Kidney disease (1.8)	Chronic lower respiratory disease (1.2)	Pregnancy complications (1.9)	Septicemia (1.8)	Flu and pneumonia (2)	Diabetes (1.8)
10	Septicemia (1.6)	Benign neoplasm (1)	Septicemia (1.2)	Kidney disease (1.6)	Septicemia (1.8)	Kidney disease (1.7)

Source: Adapted from Heron, M. (2021). Deaths: Leading causes for 2018. National Vital Statistics Report, 70(4). https://doi.org/10.15620/cdc:104186.

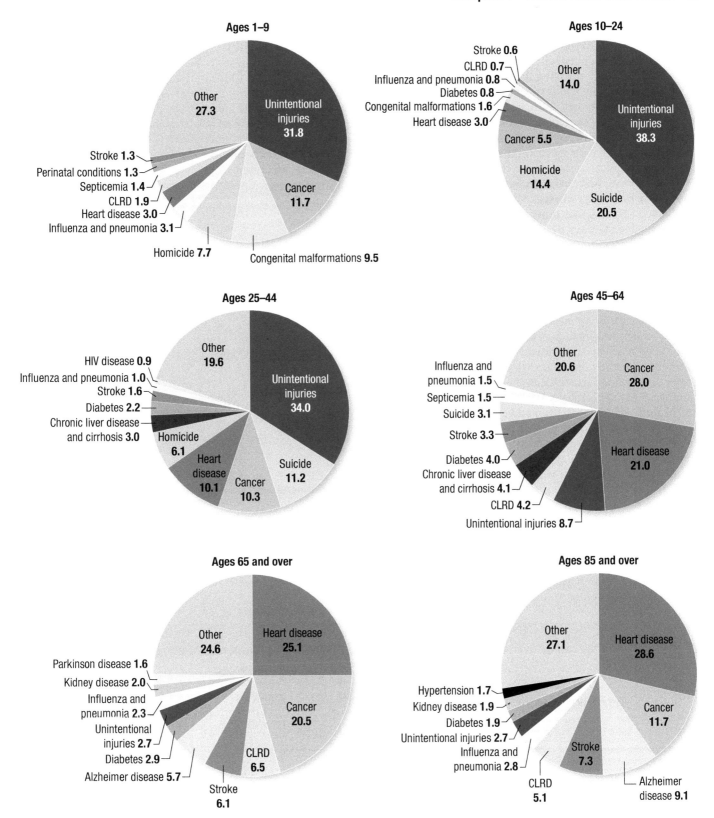

FIGURE 1.4 Percent distribution of the 10 leading causes of death by age group: United States 2019.
Source: Reproduced from Heron, M. (2021). Deaths: Leading causes for 2019. National Vital Statistics Report, 70(4), 11. *https://www.cdc.gov/nchs/data/nvsr/nvsr70/nvsr70-04-508.pdf*

men. As per the United Nations, violence against women is defined as "any act of gender-based violence that results in, or is likely to result in, physical, sexual or psychological harm or suffering to women, including threats of such acts, coercion or arbitrary deprivation of liberty, whether occurring in public or in private life" (1994, p. 3). Intimate partner violence (IPV) and sexual violence (SV) are common forms of violence against women. IPV (the most common form of violence experienced by women) is behavior by an intimate partner or ex-partner that causes physical, sexual, or psychological harm, including physical aggression, sexual coercion, psychological abuse, and controlling behaviors; whereas SV is "any sexual act, attempt to obtain a sexual act, or other act directed against a person's sexuality using coercion, by any person regardless of their relationship to the victim, in any setting" (WHO, n.d.). Per the National Intimate Partner and Sexual Violence Survey (NISVS) of 2010, SV includes five types: rape, being made to penetrate someone else, sexual coercion, unwanted sexual contact, and noncontact unwanted sexual experiences.

Violence against women is a broad term that can include IPV, SV, trafficking, femicide, acid attacks, genital mutilation, and forced marriages. Worldwide, women ages 15 to 49 represent 35% of the population who has reported physical or sexual IPV or nonpartner SV in their lifetime; and out of that number, 30% is specifically IPV (WHO, n.d.). In the United States alone, 35.6% of women and 28.5% of men have experienced some form of IPV. This percentage is likely higher in IPV because the woman usually knows the partner and therefore is comfortable enough to be somewhere alone with them. This is also true for women who are trafficked.

Violence against women, specifically rape, does not discriminate due to a person's age (Figure 1.5), race/ethnicity (Table 1.4), or sexual orientation (Table 1.5). Although the age range of 18 to 24 represents the highest percentage of women rape victims at 37.4%, girls age 10 and younger still represent an alarming 12.3%. Approximately 22% of Black women, 18.8% of non-Hispanic women, 14.6% of Hispanic

women, 26.9% American Indian/Alaska Native, and 33.5% of multiracial non-Hispanic women have reported rape in their lifetime (SDG, Injuries & Violence, 2018).

Approximately 13.1% of lesbian women, 46.1% of bisexual women, and 17.4% of heterosexual women have been raped at some point in their lifetime. The percentages for other sexual violence acts in lesbian, bisexual, and heterosexual women are even higher (Walters et al., 2013). Globally, approximately 38% of murders are committed by intimate partners (WHO, 2021b).

There are many risk factors associated with violence against women. Some factors are shared among IPV and SV,

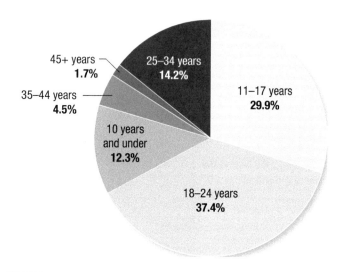

FIGURE 1.5 Age at time of first completed rape victimization in lifetime among female victims.
Source: Reproduced from Black, M. C., Basile, K. C., Breiding, M. J., Smith, S. G., Walters, M. L., Merrick, M. T., Chen, J., & Stevens, M. R. (2011). The National Intimate Partner and Sexual Violence Survey (NISVS): 2010 summary report. National Center for Injury Prevention and Control, Centers for Disease Control and Prevention. https://www.cdc.gov/violenceprevention/pdf/nisvs_report2010-a.pdf

TABLE 1.4 Lifetime Prevalence of Sexual Violence by Race/Ethnicity—U.S. Women

| | HISPANIC | NON-HISPANIC | | | | |
		BLACK	WHITE	ASIAN OR PACIFIC ISLANDER	AMERICAN INDIAN OR ALASKA NATIVE	MULTIRACIAL
Rape Weighted % Estimated Number of Victims	14.6 2,202,000	22.0 3,186,000	18.8 15,225,000	*	26.9 234,000	33.5 452,000
Other sexual violence Weighted % Estimated Number of Victims	36.1 5,442,000	41.0 5,967,000	47.6 38,632,000	29.5 1,673,000	49.0 424,000	58.0 786,000

*Estimate is not reported.
Source: Reproduced from Black, M. C., Basile, K. C., Breiding, M. J., Smith, S. G., Walters, M. L., Merrick, M. T., Chen, J., & Stevens, M. R. (2011). The National Intimate Partner and Sexual Violence Survey (NISVS): 2010 summary report. National Center for Injury Prevention and Control, Centers for Disease Control and Prevention. https://www.cdc.gov/violenceprevention/pdf/nisvs_report2010-a.pdf

TABLE 1.5 Lifetime Prevalence of Sexual Violence by Any Perpetrator by Sexual Orientation—U.S. Women

	LESBIAN		BISEXUAL		HETEROSEXUAL	
	WEIGHTED %	ESTIMATED NUMBER OF VICTIMS	WEIGHTED %	ESTIMATED NUMBER OF VICTIMS	WEIGHTED %	ESTIMATED NUMBER OF VICTIMS
Rape	13.1	214,000	46.1	1,528,000	17.4	19,049,000
Completed forced penetration	*	*	36.5	1,209,000	11.4	12,490,000
Attempted forced penetration	*	*	*	*	5.1	5,590,000
Complete alcohol/drug facilitated penetration	*	*	24.4	810,000	7.6	8,263,000
Other sexual violence	46.4	756,000	74.9	2,482,000	43.3	47,325,000
Sexual coercion	*	*	29.6	981,000	12.4	13,523,000
Unwanted sexual contact	32.3	526,000	58.0	1,922,000	25.9	28,352,000
Noncontact unwanted sexual experiences	37.8	616,000	62.9	2,085,000	32.4	35,422,000

Note: Estimated numbers have been rounded to the nearest thousand.
*Estimate is not reported.
Source: Reproduced from Walters, M. L., Chen J., & Breiding, M. J. (2013). The National Intimate Partner and Sexual Violence Survey (NISVS): 2010 findings on victimization by sexual orientation. National Center for Injury Prevention and Control, Centers for Disease Control and Prevention. https://www.cdc.gov/violenceprevention/pdf/nisvs_sofindings.pdf

while others are specific to each (Table 1.6). Shared factors include history of family violence, history of alcohol and/or drug abuse, lower educational levels, community norms, and gender inequality. Sadly, forms of emergencies, including epidemics and pandemics, tend to increase the amount of violence against women cases. Specifically, the COVID-19 pandemic has exacerbated violence against women, while also limiting access to services.

A women's health can be negatively affected by violence. Health consequences may include, yet are not limited to, death (by homicide or suicide), obstetric issues (unintended pregnancy; late, little, or no prenatal care), gynecologic issues, sexually transmitted infections (STIs), and psychological issues (depression, posttraumatic stress, anxiety, eating disorders, sleeping disorders, suicide ideations/attempts). Children can be affected negatively by violence against women, specifically IPV, as higher rates of infant and child mortality and morbidity have been associated. Children known to have grown up in families with history of violence may suffer from psychological and/or emotional disturbances. Unfortunately, these disturbances have been associated with being an abuser or victim of violence later in life (WHO, 2021b).

Although these data indicate the high prevalence of the problem, reporting of violence against women remains inconsistent. Although some experts believe that studies overestimate the extent of violence against women, others believe that there is underestimation. To date, few national studies report on women who are immigrants, homeless, disabled, in the military, or in other institutionalized situations, which may be populations at significantly greater

TABLE 1.6 Risk Factors Associated With Violence Against Women

ASSOCIATED RISK FACTORS	IPV	SV
Past history of exposure to violence	X	
Marital discord and dissatisfaction	X	
Difficulties in communicating between partners	X	
Male controlling behaviors toward partners	X	
Beliefs in family honor and sexual purity		X
Ideologies of male sexual entitlement		X
Weak legal sanctions for sexual violence		X

IPV, intimate partner violence; SV, sexual violence.
Source: Adapted from World Health Organization. (2021, March 9). Violence against women. http://www.who.int/news-room/fact-sheets/detail/violence-against-women

risk of violence against women. Accurate history taking and overall assessment of girls and women is crucial in the effort to identify and report violence against women, while also providing appropriate care.

EMERGING INFECTIONS

Infectious diseases continue to affect all people, regardless of gender, age, ethnic background, lifestyle, and socioeconomic status. They cause suffering and death and impose an enormous financial burden in the United States. Many infectious diseases have been conquered by modern interventions such as vaccines and antibiotics. New diseases are constantly emerging, including Zika, Ebola, severe acute respiratory syndrome, Lyme disease, hantavirus pulmonary syndrome, and the recent COVID-19; others reemerge in drug-resistant forms, including malaria, tuberculosis, and bacterial pneumonias. Among women, populations of particular concern include pregnant women, immigrants, and refugees. For example, if a pregnant woman acquires an infection, it can increase the infant's risk of preterm delivery, low birth weight, long-term disability, or death. Although many of these adverse birth outcomes could be prevented by prenatal care, access to and utilization of prenatal care are disparate by race/ethnicity and socioeconomic status. For example, infants born to American Indian and Black women have the highest neonatal death rates because of infectious diseases than any other group (Ely & Driscoll, 2021).

CORONAVIRUS

Coronaviruses are important human and animal pathogens. In December 2019, a cluster of cases of pneumonia of unknown cause began to emerge in Wuhan, China. On December 31, 2019, a novel coronavirus was identified as the cause of this cluster of pneumonia cases in Wuhan, a city in the Hubei Province of China. It rapidly spread, resulting in an epidemic throughout China, followed by a global pandemic. In February 2020, WHO designated the disease COVID-19, which stands for coronavirus disease 2019. The virus that causes COVID-19 is designated severe acute respiratory syndrome coronavirus 2 (SARS-CoV-2); previously it was referred to as 2019-nCoV (Rasmussen et al., 2020).

Globally, COVID-19 confirmed cases evolved from the initial case count of 189,000 on March 17, 2019 to 300 million confirmed cases in 2022. The reported case counts underestimated the overall burden of COVID-19, as only a fraction of acute cases were diagnosed and reported (CDC, 2022a). Direct person-to-person respiratory transmission was considered the primary means of transmission of coronavirus 2019. It was transmitted through close-range contact (within 6 feet) via respiratory particles with talking, coughing, or sneezing and at longer distances, particularly in enclosed, poorly ventilated spaces. The period of infection begins prior to development of symptoms and is highest in the early stages of illness when the viral RNA levels from upper respiratory specimens are the highest. Transmission rates are highest in household and congregate settings, but social and work gatherings increase transmission rates as well (CDC, n.d.-d; Zou et al., 2020).

Like all viruses, COVID-19 evolves into different variants of concern over time. The Delta variant was first identified in India in December 2020 and had been the most prevalent, highly transmissible variant worldwide until emergence of the Omicron variant in November 2021 in South Africa. Infection with the Delta variant was associated with a higher risk of severe disease and hospitalization, but emerging data on the clinical impact of Omicron suggest that Omicron has a replication advantage over the Delta variant and evades infection and vaccine-induced humoral immunity to a greater extent than prior variants. Omicron appears to be associated with less severe disease than other variants (Iuliano et al., 2022).

Measures to prevent the spread of COVID-19 have evolved since discovery of the disease and include masking, social distancing, diligent handwashing, respiratory hygiene (covering the cough and sneeze), adequate ventilation of indoor spaces, cleaning frequently touched objects and surfaces, vaccines (Table 1.7), serial testing, self-isolation with symptoms and positive testing, and monoclonal antibody preexposure and postexposure (CDC, 2022a).

TABLE 1.7 Different COVID-19 Vaccines in the United States; January 21, 2022

PFIZER–BIONTECH	MODERNA	JOHNSON & JOHNSON'S JANSSEN
Ages recommended 5+ years old	**Ages recommended** 18+ years old	**Ages recommended** 18+ years old
Primary series 2 doses Given 3 weeks (21 days) apart	**Primary series** 2 doses Given 4 weeks (28 days) apart	**Primary series** 1 dose
Booster dose Everyone ages 18 years and older should get a booster dose of either Pfizer-BioNTech or Moderna (COVID-19 vaccines) 5 months after the last dose in their primary series. Teens 12–17 years old should get a Pfizer-BioNTech COVID-19 vaccine booster 5 months after the last dose in their primary series.	**Booster dose** Everyone ages 18 years and older should get a booster dose of either Pfizer-BioNTech or Moderna (COVID-19 vaccines) 5 months after the last dose in their primary series.	**Booster dose** Everyone ages 18 years and older should get a booster dose of either Pfizer-BioNTech or Moderna (mRNA COVID-19 vaccines) at least 2 months after the first dose of J&J/Janssen COVID-19 vaccine. You may get J&J/Janssen in some situations.
When fully vaccinated 2 weeks after 2nd dose	**When fully vaccinated** 2 weeks after 2nd dose	**When fully vaccinated** 2 weeks after 1st dose

Source: Adapted from Adu, P., Poopola, T., Medvedev, O. N., Collings, S., Mbinta, J., Aspin, C., & Simpson, C. R. (2023). Implications for COVID-19 vaccine uptake: A systematic review. Journal of Infection and Public Health, 16(3), 441–466. https://doi.org/ 10.1016/j.jiph.2023.01.020; Centers for Disease Control & Prevention. (n.d.). Stay up to date with COVID-19 vaccines. Retrieved August 13, 2023 from https://www.cdc.gov/coronavirus/2019-ncov/vaccines/stay-up-to-date.html#recommendations; Khoury, D. S., Docken, S. S., Subbarao, K., Kent, S. J., Davenport, M. P., & Cromer, D. (2023). Predicting the efficacy of variant-modified COVID-19 vaccine boosters. Nature Medicine, 29(3), 574–578

Burden of Disease Associated with COVID-19

The COVID-19 pandemic has changed access to healthcare worldwide, and these changes may have long-term consequences for those diagnosed with cancer. Screening for cancer, STIs, pregnancy, and IPV may have been delayed, leading to patients getting diagnosed and managed later and not having the same outcomes pre-COVID. COVID also disrupted treatment plans and altered patient outcomes. Telemedicine use improved during COVID and increased ability to connect with patients remotely and provided another opportunity for access to healthcare while decreasing risk of COVID exposure. Telemedicine increased access to experts who may not have been accessible in person at this time as well.

Children faced disruption in their daily routines with quarantines, social isolation, and education via Zoom with increased rates of anxiety, depression, and eating disorders. Children were impacted by the pandemic both physically and mentally with long-term sequelae. By 2021, a greater than 30% increase in mental health presentations to the EDs with children having high levels of suicidal ideation, aggression with self-harm, higher rates of substance abuse, and more instances of eating disorders were noted. Vaccines have been slowly approved by the FDA for use in specific age groups and are an important measure in primary prevention. In the United States, COVID vaccines are available to people by groups, ages 5 to 11, ages 12 to 17, and ages 18 and older. Pfizer Biotech is approved for ages 5 to 17 with Johnson & Johnson's Janssen, Pfizer-BioNTech, and Moderna for ages 18 and older (CDC, 2022b).

One particularly rare and serious side effect of COVID-19 is multisystem inflammatory system in children (MIS-C). Almost all children who have contracted MIS-C have been unvaccinated. A child who has been vaccinated but later gets sick is much less likely to become sick enough to be hospitalized or die. Some of the side effects of COVID-19 can affect children for years. It is estimated that over 140,000 children in the United States have lost one parent to COVID-19.

Case counts of pregnant women with COVID-19 were analyzed from 1/22/2020 to 7/25/2022 with 225,656 total cases, 306 total deaths, and 34,693 total hospitalized (CDC, 2022a). Currently research is underway regarding long-term effects of COVID-19 with lingering symptoms, and long-term effects of PTSD, anxiety, depression, suicide, and IPV. COVID-19 impacted how prenatal care was delivered and birth locations due to restrictions on support people and family with limitations on the presence or number of support people present during labor and birth. Many were separated from their newborns and were limited in options for pharmacologic and nonpharmacologic pain relief during labor. The 2019 pandemic helped highlight existing health system weaknesses and revealed a need for health system corrections redefining normal functioning.

ZIKA VIRUS

The Zika virus has a potential impact on sexual and reproductive health of women in the United States. Brazil and Colombia were first to report instances of Zika in the United States. Zika was first isolated in Uganda. Zika, named for a forest in Uganda, is a single-stranded RNA virus. The Zika virus is common in areas of Africa, Asia, and Pacific Islands (CDC, 2016; Foy et al., 2011). Dissemination of accurate and current information is critical to prevent panic and myths.

A single-stranded RNA virus, Zika, was first isolated in 1947 from a monkey in the Zika forest (CDC, 2016; Foy et al., 2011). The Zika virus has been isolated in sperm, urine, and blood (CDC, 2016). It is spread primarily by mosquito bite, and transmitted by pregnant women to fetus, through blood and sexual contact. The illness is usually mild with symptoms lasting for several days to a week (CDC, 2016; Foy et al., 2011). Common symptoms are fever, rash, joint pain, and conjunctivitis. There is no specific antiviral agent; treatment consists of symptom management (e.g., rest, fluids, analgesics, and antipyretics; Foy et al., 2011). Healthcare providers are encouraged to report suspected cases to their state or local health departments to facilitate diagnosis and mitigate the risk of local transmission.

Birth defects such as microcephaly, seizure, intellectual difficulty, and developmental delays have resulted in the babies of women affected during pregnancy. Close monitoring for growth and development is the current management of such infants. Prevention is the primary way of combating the spread of the virus by avoidance of mosquito bites, postponement of travel to areas with Zika, and avoidance of exposure to the virus before, during, and after conception.

HUMAN PAPILLOMAVIRUS

Human papillomavirus (HPV) is the most common sexually transmitted infection (STI). It is so common that most sexually active people will acquire the virus within a lifetime. Approximately 150 types of HPV strain have been identified with 40 infecting the genital area. Currently more than 42 million Americans are infected with HPV and it is estimated that roughly 13 million Americans will become infected yearly (Boersma & Black, 2020).

The only HPV vaccine available in the United States since 2016 is Gardasil-9. Gardasil-9 protects against nine HPV types including 6, 11, 16, and 18. HPV types 6 and 11 (low risk) cause >90% of genital warts, while HPV types 16 and 18 (high risk) contribute to 66% of cervical cancers. Routine vaccination is recommended at ages 11 or 12 years yet may start as early as age 9 years. The recommended cutoff age is 26 years, yet some adults ages 27 to 45 years may benefit from the vaccination, which should be discussed with their healthcare professional (Boersma & Black, 2020).

Generally, when people talk about HPV, the focus is on women, but HPV affects men as well. More than half of men who are sexually active in the United States will have HPV at some time in their lives. About 1% of sexually active men in the United States have genital warts at any one time. The 400 men who get HPV-related cancer of the penis, 1,500 men who get HPV-related cancer of the anus, and 5,600 men who get cancers of the oropharynx (back of the throat) have been exposed to a high-risk strain of HPV (Boersma & Black, 2020). The HPV can remain dormant for months or years before showing signs and symptoms. Low-risk strains of HPV can cause genital warts in both men and women. Genital warts are the first symptom seen in low-risk HPV strains. However, high-risk HPV rarely causes initial symptoms. Genital warts appear as small bumps in the genital area or around the anus. They can be small or large, raised or flat, and even shaped like cauliflower. Pregnant women with genital warts should be counseled concerning the low risk for warts on the larynx (recurrent respiratory papillomatosis) in their infants or children.

In 90% of HPV infections the virus is self-limiting, without any clinical symptoms, and usually resolves on its own within 2 years, therefore a person does not realize they are a carrier prior to passing it along. This contributes to the rapid infection rates and highlights the importance of safe sex practice discussions during office visits, no matter the chief complaint (Boersma & Black, 2020; CDC, n.d.-d). However, when the virus is persistent, lasting longer than 6 to 8 months, or when it is joined by other HPV genotypes, there is a greater likelihood of developing cervical cancer precursor cells or an invasive epithelial lesion. HPV is a major etiologic factor in the development of benign cervical papilloma as well as cervical cancer. Ten percent of HPV cases become persistent and cause more severe health problems ranging from genital warts to cervical cancer. Ninety percent of all cervical cancer cases are caused by a high-risk type of HPV (see Chapter 32, Human Papillomavirus).

HUMAN IMMUNODEFICIENCY VIRUS

HIV death rates are declining globally, in both men and women, falling below most common causes of death such as heart disease, liver disease, respiratory conditions, stroke, cancers, and Alzheimer disease as of 2016 (WHO, 2019). HIV incidence has decreased by 73% from the highest number of infections (130,400) in 1984 and 1985 to 34,800 in 2019. Most infections continue to be attributed to male with male sexual contact (63% in 1981 and 66% in 2019). Over time the proportion of HIV infections have increased among Black people from 29% in 1981 to 41% in 2019 and among Hispanic/Latinx persons (from 16% in 1981 to 29% in 2019).

The CDC (n.d.-g) estimated at the end of 2019 that 1.2 million people had HIV in the United States. In 2020, 30,635 people received a new HIV diagnosis (Table 1.8). In 2020, the age range with the highest number of diagnoses was 25 to 29 years (6,103), with 30 to 34 years (5,233) and 20 to 24 years (4,867) a close second and third (CDC, n.d.-g). As it relates to

race/ethnicity, the annual diagnosis per 1,000 persons most dramatically persists among Black (15,340) and Hispanic women (10,502) while White women (9,018) closely trail. All other race/ethnicity groups listed were less than 1,000 diagnosis per year (CDC, n.d.-e). This is an obvious contribution to the healthcare disparity gap issue.

CHRONIC CONDITIONS

Six in 10 adults in the United States have a chronic disease and four in 10 adults have two or more conditions. Chronic conditions are often debilitating and contribute significantly to key causes of death among women. Chronic diseases are defined broadly as conditions that last 1 year or more and require ongoing medical attention or limit activities of daily living (ADLs) or both. There is a complex and long-term interplay between chronic conditions and health across a woman's life span. Although women live longer than men, women also experience greater morbidity at younger ages and utilize health services at higher rates than men. The nation's $4.1 trillion in annual healthcare costs are driven by three specific chronic conditions: heart disease, cancer, and diabetes (CDC, n.d.-h). As women progress from childbearing ages through menopause and to postmenopause years, the prevalence of chronic conditions increases, with an associated shift to conditions linked to environmental factors.

Overall, the pattern and magnitude of chronic conditions vary markedly by gender. Women were more likely to report arthritis, cataracts, orthopedic impairment, goiter or thyroid disease, diabetes, hypertension, varicose veins, chronic bronchitis, asthma, and chronic sinusitis; men were more likely to report visual impairment, hearing impairment, and heart disease.

Chronic diseases such as heart disease, cancer, chronic lung disease, stroke, Alzheimer disease, diabetes, and chronic kidney disease occurs disproportionately among poor women. Based on National Health Interview Survey (NHIS) data, low income was correlated with the occurrence of diabetes, asthma, hypertension, and thyroid disease (National Center for Health Statistics [NCHS], 2021). Additionally, the differences in chronic conditions by racial/ethnic populations can differ dramatically. For example, American Indians/Alaska Natives were three times more likely to have had diabetes and end-stage renal disease than Asians/Pacific Islanders and six times more likely to have had these conditions than Whites. Blacks were twice as likely as Asians/Pacific Islanders to have diabetes and end-stage renal disease and four times more likely to have these conditions than Whites (American Immigration Council, 2020).

Pain conditions are also common in women, especially low back pain and migraine or severe headache. Arthritis is the most common cause of disability among U.S. adults. Although osteoarthritis is the most common, types of arthritis that primarily affect women are lupus, fibromyalgia, and rheumatoid arthritis. Cancers can be a chronic condition with persistent pain and should not be excluded from this section. In the United States in 2018 there were close to 1.8 million new cancer cases resulting in approximately 600,000 deaths (Figure 1.6).

Arthritis is more common among women than among men (23.5% vs. 18.1%) and increases with age (Figure 1.7). Arthritis affects more adults who are inactive (23.6%) compared to active (18.1%) and is more common in adults with fair/poor health (40.5%) in comparison to excellent/very

TABLE 1.8 New HIV Diagnoses Among Adults and Adolescents in the United States and Dependent Areas by Race/Ethnicity, 2020

RACE OR ETHNICITY	NUMBER OF DIAGNOSES
American Indian/Alaska Native	200
Asian	635
Black/African American	12,827
Hispanic/Latinx	7,999
Native Hawaiian and other Pacific Islander	65
White	7,831
Multiracial	792

Source: Reproduced from Centers for Disease Control and Prevention. (n.d.). HIV: Statistics overview. U.S. Department of Health and Human Services. Retrieved March 31, 2023, from https://www.cdc.gov/hiv/statistics/overview/index.html

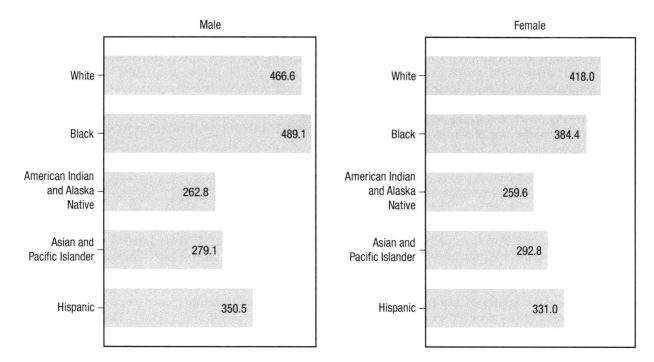

FIGURE 1.6 Rate (per 100,000 people) of all types of new cancers by sex and race and ethnicity.
Source: Data from U.S. Cancer Statistics Working Group. (2021). U.S. Cancer Statistics Data Vi-sualizations Tool, based on 2020 submission data (1999–2018). U.S. Department of Health and Human Services, Centers for Disease Control and Prevention and National Cancer Institute. https://www.cdc.gov/cancer/dataviz

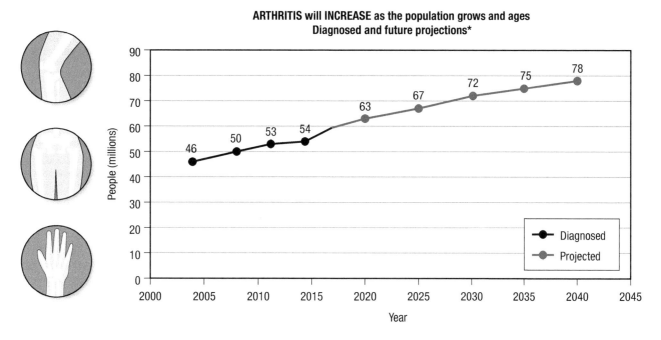

FIGURE 1.7 National arthritis prevalence projections.
Source: Reproduced from Centers for Disease Control and Prevention. (n.d.). Arthritis: National statis-tics. U.S. Department of Health and Human Services. Retrieved February 16, 2023, from https://www .cdc.gov/arthritis/data_statistics/national-statistics.html

good health (15.4%). Arthritis diagnoses are expected to in-crease in the coming decades, suggesting an estimated 78.4 million adults age 18 or older will have arthritis by 2040 and 34.6 million of the adults will report the arthritis affecting their ADLs. Out of the 78.4 million, two thirds of the popula-tion are expected to be women (CDC, n.d.-c).

Vision loss and hearing loss are both sources of disabili-ty for women. Trouble seeing affects approximately 10% of women, whereas hearing difficulty or deafness affects ap-proximately 1.5% (NCHS, 2014b).

Heart disease and stroke are the first and third most common causes of death for women in the United States.

Although much attention has focused on the diagnosis and treatment of women with heart disease, an important aspect to understand is the disability associated with these two diseases. Both heart disease and stroke are associated with increasing age, but like other diseases, these vary with socioeconomic status and race/ethnicity. Although similar proportions of non-Hispanic Black and White women experience heart disease, a higher proportion of non-Hispanic American Indian/Alaska Native and non-Hispanic multiracial women experience heart disease. Stroke incidence increases with age; the lifetime risk for women age 55 to 75 is one in five in the United States. Hispanic and non-Hispanic Black women are more likely to suffer from a stroke than non-Hispanic White women. As a healthcare provider, it is important to know prevention is key, as four in five strokes are preventable.

Chronic obstructive pulmonary disease (COPD) also is an important source of chronic illness and disability for women, as well as the fourth leading cause of death among U.S. women age 18 years and older. Approximately 6% of women report having COPD and its prevalence increases with age (11% of women age 65–74 years and 10.4% of women age 75 and older). COPD varies with race/ethnicity and poverty level. It is most common among non-Hispanic American Indian/Alaska Natives (8.6%) and non-Hispanic women of multiple races (9.9%), followed by non-Hispanic White women (7%), non-Hispanic Black women (6%), Hispanic women (4.9%), and non-Hispanic Asian women (2.6%). Women living with incomes less than 100% of the poverty level are twice as likely to report COPD as those with an income of 400% of the poverty level (10% vs. 4.6%; U.S. Cancer Statistics Working Group, 2021).

Hypertension is common among women, with 17.6% of women age 20 to 44, 55.8% of women age 45 to 64, 74.3% of women age 65 to 74, and 86% of women age 75 and over having been diagnosed with high blood pressure. There is a trend showing that hypertension increases with age. Racial/ethnic variation is evident; more than 55% of non-Hispanic Black women and 45.1% of Hispanic or Latina women have hypertension compared with 37% of non-Hispanic Whites. As of 2015–2018 data, the percentage of Asian women has also surpassed non-Hispanic Whites at 42.8% (NCHS, 2021).

Osteoporosis is more prevalent among women than men and increases with age. Approximately 18.8% of women have been diagnosed with osteoporosis who are over the age of 50 versus 4.2% in men. One in four women 65 years and older reports having been diagnosed. Non-Hispanic White and Mexican American women 65 years and older were more likely to have been diagnosed with osteoporosis than non-Hispanic Black women. Risk of bone fractures among older women is often associated with osteoporosis and may lead to disability or even death (CDC, 2021).

In 2017–2018 the prevalence of obesity in the United States was 42.4% which is an increase from 30.5% back in 1999–2000. Obesity is now considered a *costly* chronic disease contributing to an annual medical cost of nearly $173 billion in 2019. Obesity is associated with increased risk of numerous diseases, including hypertension, type 2 diabetes, cardiovascular and liver diseases, arthritis, some types of cancer, and reproductive health risks. There is little racial/ethnic variation in being underweight, but approximately 41.4% of non-Hispanic white adults are considered obese (body mass index [BMI], >30) compared with 49.9% of non-Hispanic Black adults and 45.6% Hispanic adults, and 16.1% of non-Hispanic Asian adults. Obesity prevalence is at minimum 40% among all age groups (20 to 39 years, 40 to 59 years, and 60 and older; CDC, n.d.-b).

REPRODUCTIVE AND GYNECOLOGIC CONDITIONS

Both reproductive and gynecologic conditions affect a considerable proportion of women. Dysmenorrhea and vulvodynia cause discomfort that interferes with some women's normal activities, but other conditions, such as endometriosis, uterine fibroids (leiomyomas), and ovarian cysts, affect fertility and reproductive functioning. Infertility is estimated to affect 10% of all U.S. women 15 to 44 years of age (CDC, n.d.-j). Endometriosis affects approximately 10% of girls and reproductive-age women (WHO, 2023b), and uterine fibroids are the most common (more than 3 million cases annually) benign tumors among women, especially those in childbearing ages (CDC, n.d.-e). The prevalence increases with age in both; however, uterine fibroids are usually detected in 80% of women by the age of 50 (De La Cruz & Buchanan, 2017). Racial/ethnic differences are noteworthy, with 12.3% of non-Hispanic Black women, 5.6% of white women, and 4.2% of Hispanic women experiencing uterine fibroids. Non-Hispanic white women are most likely to experience endometriosis (6.9%) compared with 3.4% of Black and 3.9% of Hispanic women. These two conditions are most often responsible for hysterectomy. Uterine fibroids account for 39% of all hysterectomies within the US annually (De La Cruz & Buchanan, 2017). In addition to endometriosis and uterine fibroids, age, obesity, and polycystic ovary syndrome are associated with infertility.

MENTAL ILLNESS

Mental illnesses affect women and men differently. Scientists are only beginning to understand the contribution of various biological and psychosocial factors to mental health and mental illness in both women and men. Research on women's health—which has grown substantially in the last 30 years—helps to clarify the risk and protective factors for mental disorders in women and to improve women's mental health treatment outcomes.

Depressive disorders include major depression, postpartum depression, dysthymic disorder (a less severe but more chronic form of depression), and bipolar disorder (manic-depressive illness). Globally, 280 million people (5%) have depression (WHO, 2023a). Within the United States in 2019, 18.5% of adults had some form of depressive symptoms (whether mild, moderate, or severe) within the previous 2 weeks (Figure 1.8). Of that percentage, 2.8% experienced severe, 4.2% experienced moderate, and 11.5% experienced mild symptoms (Villarroel & Terlizzi, 2020). Notably, at its worst, depression can lead to suicide.

Although depression is not the only mental illness that affects women more often than men, it is significant because of its common occurrence, recurrence, and effects on functioning (WHO, 2023a). Trying to become pregnant, pregnancy loss, being pregnant, and giving birth increase risk for depression in women. The prevalence of depressive symptoms also

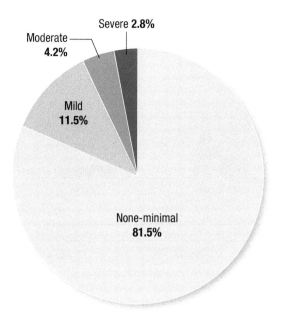

FIGURE 1.8 Percent distribution of severity of depression symptoms in the past 2 weeks among adults age 18 and over: United States, 2019.
Source: Reproduced from Villarroel, M. A., & Terlizzi, E. P. (2020). Symptoms of depression among adults: United States, 2019 (NCHS Data Brief No. 379). National Center for Health Statistics. https:// cdc.gov/nchs/data/databriefs/db379-H.pdf

varies with age groups and race/ethnicity (Figure 1.9). Hispanic, non-Hispanic White, and non-Hispanic Black women were most likely to report depressive symptoms during the past 2 weeks. Non-Hispanic Asian women were the least likely to experience any form of depression compared to other ethnic groups. Age influences the prevalence of depressive symptoms and severity as those in the younger age range (18–29 years) experience a higher percentage of mild symptoms, and there is a significant decrease in moderate and severe symptoms (Villarroel & Terlizzi, 2020). The important influences of income, education, and marital status, as well as age and race/ethnicity, need to be considered in studies of depression.

The main risk factor for developing Alzheimer disease—a dementing brain disorder that leads to the loss of mental and physical functioning and eventually to death—is increased age. Although the number of new cases of Alzheimer disease is similar in older adult women and men, the number of existing cases is twice as high among women as among men, with women older than 65 years constituting 3.2 million diagnosed cases. Alzheimer disease death rates increased between 2000 and 2010 by about 40%, from 141.2 to 196.9 deaths per 100,000 people. The greater prevalence and mortality among women appear to be related to their longevity rather than to an increased sex-specific disease risk (DHHS, 2013).

The chronic stress often associated with caregiving for someone with dementia can contribute to mental health problems for the caregiver (see Chapter 18, Health Considerations for Women Caregivers). Because women in general are at greater risk of depression than men, and as caregivers are much more likely to suffer from depression than the average person, women caregivers of people with Alzheimer disease may be particularly vulnerable to depression.

Mental issues such as schizophrenia, depression, bipolar disorders, Alzheimer disease, and obsessive-compulsive disorders affect nearly one in five Americans each year. Nearly 70% of adults with a diagnosed mental disorder do not receive treatment. Among all areas of healthcare, the mental health field is beset by disparities in the availability of and access to services occurring by means of financial barriers and stigmatization (Reeves et al., 2011).

WOMEN'S PERCEPTION OF THEIR HEALTH AND LIMITATIONS IN FUNCTIONING

Many women who experience chronic illness, whether mental or physical, also experience limitation of activity related to their conditions. About 17% of women report limitations related to chronic illness: Nearly 10% report fair or poor health, by their own assessment and self-assessed health status, that leads to severe psychological distress, and 3.7% report serious psychological distress (NCHS, 2021).

ACTIVITY LIMITATIONS

Women's quality of life is affected by their ability to carry out daily activities at work, at home, and in the community. Adverse health effects all aspects of women's lives, particularly their ability to engage in daily activities. Activity limitation caused by a physical, mental, or emotional health problem is a broad measure of health functioning for women. Women were nearly twice as likely as men to report activity limitation in 2011 to 2012 (17% compared with 9%). Activity limitation caused by chronic conditions such as arthritis was substantially higher among women.

Healthcare Access and Utilization

In the first half of 2022, 8.36% (27.4 million) of people all ages were uninsured and 12.1% of people age 18 to 64 were uninsured (Figure 1.10; Cohen & Cha, 2022). Women in the United States obtain healthcare services through a variety of sources. Numerous factors, including affordability and availability of services and information about how and why it is important to access and utilize such services, affect their access to these services. Given the consolidation of the healthcare system, the shift to managed care, and decreased public funding of healthcare and health-related programs, the changes in healthcare delivery have serious implications for women's healthcare utilization. Although women commonly enter the healthcare delivery system for pregnancy prevention or pregnancy-related services, these reproductive health services are typically provided separately from other aspects of women's healthcare. Health services organizations for women include private- and public-sector groups. For women, the fragmentation of care, lack of coordination of services, and discontinuities in the healthcare delivery system contribute to higher costs to individual women and both deficiencies and excesses in care.

Access to healthcare is important for preventive care and for prompt treatment of illness and injuries. Indicators of healthcare access and utilization include use of preventive services, outpatient care, and inpatient care, and access to these varies by health insurance status, poverty status, and race/ethnicity (Figure 1.11). Hispanic adults were less likely to have health insurance coverage. Women's access to healthcare services is seriously compromised by inadequate health insurance, and

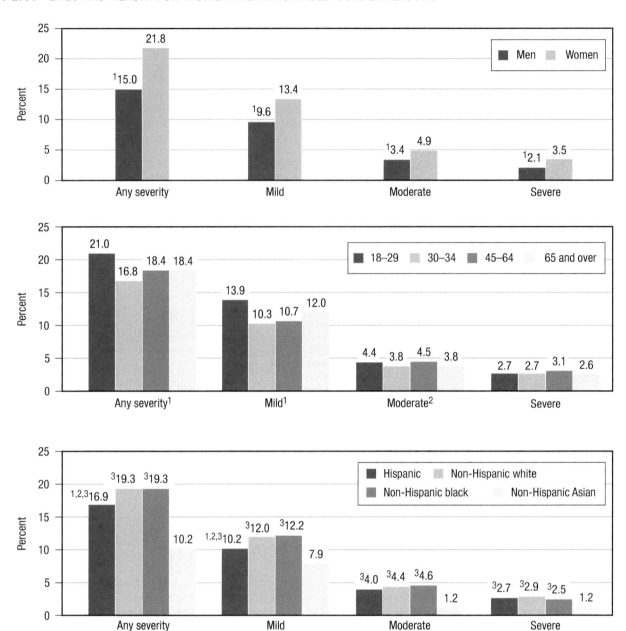

FIGURE 1.9 Depressive symptoms across age groups and race/ethnicity.
Source: Reproduced from Villarroel, M. A., & Terlizzi, E. P. (2020). Symptoms of depression among adults: United States, 2019 *(NCHS Data Brief No. 379). National Center for Health Statistics. https://cdc.gov/nchs/data/databriefs/db379-H.pdf*

women without health insurance generally cannot obtain appropriate healthcare. Although little is known about how women obtain basic healthcare in the United States, national survey data report that women are more likely than men to have a usual source of care, have more outpatient visits, have more hospital stays (even excluding maternity stays), use home health services, and use nursing homes (Table 1.9).

PUBLICLY FUNDED HEALTH PROGRAMS

In 2021, 21.7% of adults age 18 to 64 and 44.3% of children age 0 to 17 had publicly funded healthcare coverage (Cohen et al., 2022). The two major publicly funded health programs are Medicare and Medicaid. Medicare is funded by the federal government and reimburses older adults and those who

are disabled for their healthcare. Medicaid is funded jointly by federal and state governments to provide healthcare for the poor. Although Medicaid eligibility and benefits vary by state, Medicare and Medicaid healthcare utilization and costs often vary dramatically by state. Medicare spending grew 8.4% to $900.8 billion in 2021 while Medicaid spending grew 9.2% to $734 billion (Centers for Medicare & Medicaid Services, 2023). Women are more likely to qualify for Medicaid given their disproportionate share of poverty. The Patient Protection and Affordable Care Act promises to have dramatic effects on women's access to healthcare as well as to a variety of preventive services. See Chapter 3, Women and Healthcare, for a more detailed discussion of this coverage for women.

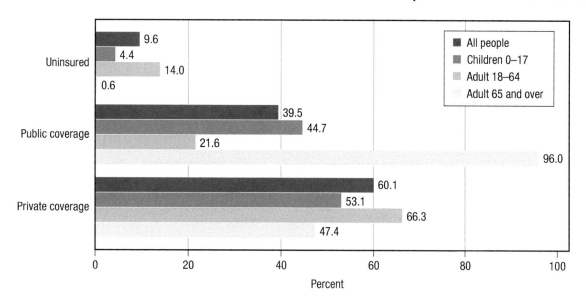

FIGURE 1.10 Percentage of people who were uninsured or had public or private coverage, by age group: United States, January–June 2022.
Source: Reproduced from Cohen, R. A., & Cha, A. E. (2022, December). Health insurance coverage: Early release of estimates from the National Health Interview Survey, January–June 2022. *U.S. Department of Health and Human Services, Centers for Disease Control and Prevention, National Center for Health Statistics. https://www.cdc.gov/nchs/data/nhis/earlyrelease/insur202111.pdf*

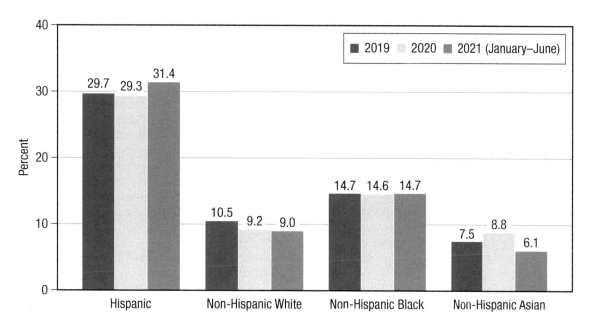

FIGURE 1.11 Percentage of adults age 18 to 64 who were uninsured, by race and ethnicity and year: United States, January–June 2022.
Source: Reproduced from Cohen, R. A., Terlizzi, E. P., Cha, A. E., & Martinez, M. E. (2021). Health insurance coverage: Early release of estimates form the National Health Interview Survey, 2020. *National Center for Health Statistics, National Health Interview Survey Early Release Program. https://www.cdc.gov/nchs/data/nhis/earlyrelease/insur202108-508.pdf*

PRIVATELY FUNDED HEALTHCARE

Approximately 64% of U.S. women younger than 65 years have some form of private health insurance (Cohen & Cha, 2022), most of which is obtained through the workplace. As the health insurance marketplace continues to rapidly change as new types of managed care products emerge, the share of an employee's total compensation for health insurance and the use of traditional fee-for-service medical care continues to decline markedly. Approximately 30% of women had public insurance and 8% were uninsured (Table 1.9). Health insurance coverage varies by race/ethnicity, with non-Hispanic whites having coverage (76.7%), but less than 50% of non-Hispanic Blacks and Hispanics (49.7 and 44.7%, respectively) having coverage. Although women and men report

TABLE 1.9　Women and Men Health Insurance Status: January–June 2022

AGE GROUP (FEMALE)	UNINSURED (%)	PUBLIC COVERAGE (%)	PRIVATE COVERAGE (%)
Under 65	7.9	30.2	63.9
18–64	9.5	25.0	67.5
0–17	3.3	45.0	53.9
AGE GROUP (MALE)	UNINSURED (%)	PUBLIC COVERAGE (%)	PRIVATE COVERAGE (%)
Under 65	12.0	25.0	65.1
18–64	14.8	18.5	68.7
0–17	4.6	42.0	55.7

Source: Adapted from Cohen, R. A., & Cha, A. E. (2022, December). Health insurance coverage: Early release of estimates from the National Health Interview Survey, January–June 2022. U.S. Department of Health and Human Services, Centers for Disease Control and Prevention, National Center for Health Statistics. https://www.cdc.gov/nchs/data/nhis/earlyrelease/insur202212.pdf

similar levels of enrollment for private insurance, enrollment varies significantly by race/ethnicity and poverty status (Cohen & Cha, 2022).

HEALTHCARE PAYMENT AND EXPENDITURES

Major sources of payment for healthcare in the United States include the government and employers. The United States continues to spend more on healthcare than any other industrialized country, and health spending is increasing rapidly (Cohen & Cha, 2022). The expenditures for prescription drugs increased more rapidly than any other type of health expenditure. The United States continues to spend a larger proportion of its gross national product on healthcare than any other major industrialized country. Much of U.S. healthcare spending is directed to care for chronic diseases and conditions that reflect the aging population.

PREVENTION SERVICES

The use of prevention services has substantial positive effects on the long-term health status of women. The use of several different types of preventive services has been increasing; however, disparities in their use according to income and by race/ethnicity persist among all persons.

The importance of promoting wellness and preventing illness among women involves screening for conditions such as breast, cervical, and colorectal cancer. Regular mammographic screening for women age 50 years and older is effective in reducing deaths from breast cancer. In 2013, approximately 65% of women age 65 years and older had had a mammogram within the previous 2 years. Among those 40 years and older, the proportion of women receiving mammograms was 64% or greater for all racial/ethnic groups except multiracial women. The proportion of women receiving mammograms was higher among those with greater levels of education (53% for those who had not completed high school) and much lower (36%) for women who were uninsured than for those with private insurance (74%) or Medicaid (64%). The percentage of women 18 to 44 years of age and 45 to 64 years was relatively high (80% and 77%, respectively), but the proportion older than 65 years dropped to 47%, consistent with changing guidelines about screening. Women who reported having Pap tests within the previous 3 years differed by race/ethnicity. The reported prevalence was as follows: non-Hispanic Black women, 78%; non-Hispanic White women, 73%; Hispanic women, 74%; American Indian/Alaskan Native women, 73%; and Asian women, 68%.

Finally, colorectal cancer is the third leading cause of cancer-related deaths among women after lung and breast cancer. Early detection and treatment can substantially reduce the risks associated with colorectal cancer for people age 50 years and older. Other preventive strategies relevant to women include the HPV vaccine to prevent cervical cancer, anal cancer, and genital warts The preventive care provisions of the Patient Protection and Affordable Care Act should improve access to these preventive services by expanding health insurance access and requiring new plans to cover U.S. Preventive Services Task Force (USPSTF)–recommended preventive services and well-woman visits without copayments required (DHHS, 2013).

OUTPATIENT CARE

Important changes in the delivery of healthcare in the United States are driven in large part by the need to contain rising costs. One significant change has been a decline in the use of inpatient services and an increase in outpatient services such as outpatient surgery and hospice care. From 2009 to 2011, nearly 87% of women had a usual source of care, a place where they could go when sick, such as an office for health professionals or health center, but not an ED. More than 90% of women who have private or public insurance coverage had a usual source of care compared with only 56% who were uninsured. In addition to varying health insurance coverage, having access to a usual source of care varies with race/ethnicity. Nearly 89% of non-Hispanic White women, 85% of non-Hispanic Black women, 85% of American Indian/Alaska Natives, 85.7% of Asians, 85% of Native Hawaiian/Pacific Islanders, and 82% of multiracial women but only 78.6% of Hispanics reported a usual source of care (DHHS, 2013). Having a usual source of care is more commonly experienced by older women who are most likely to have health insurance;

nearly 97% of those older than 65 years had a usual source of care compared with nearly 79% of women 18 to 34 years of age (DHHS, 2013).

Although women frequently enter the healthcare delivery system with reproductive health concerns, they seldom can benefit from primary care that is comprehensive and coordinated. Regardless of the type of provider or reason for accessing care, women's healthcare delivery in the United States remains fragmented. An estimated 80% of women report that they have a usual source of care, which is predominately in physician offices. Among physician providers, family practitioners, general internists, and OB/GYNs provide most basic healthcare to women; however, women may rely on multiple providers (DHHS, 2013). For example, 33% of women age 18 years and older reported seeing an OB/GYN and an additional primary care provider for their regular care. Women who used two or more physicians for regular care were more likely to be younger, have private insurance, and have higher income than women who used only one physician. Also, these women were more likely to have more annual visits and to receive more clinical preventive services. Among women who relied on only one physician, 39% reported using a family practitioner or an internist, 16% used an OB/GYN, 3% used a specialist, and 10% had no regular physician. Finally, despite estimates that more than 100,000 APRNs deliver primary healthcare, less than 2% of women report using nonphysician providers as a regular source of care.

Women made much of their healthcare visits to physicians' offices, with the number increasing as women aged. A similar pattern with age was found for EDs, with the latter especially pronounced for women 75 years and older (Table 1.10).

In 2007, an estimated 1,459,000 women received home healthcare, with 31% of patients younger than 65 years. Of the remainder of women patients, 18% were 65 to 74 years, 29% 75 to 84 years, and 22% older than 85 years (DHHS, 2013).

TABLE 1.10 Women's Visits to Physician Offices and Emergency Departments, 2018: Per 100 Persons

AGE	PHYSICIAN OFFICES	EMERGENCY DEPARTMENTS
Younger than 15 years	165.6	41.4
15–24 years	189.3	48.8
25–44 years	263.9	47.4
45–64 years	346.5	37.8
65–74 years	508.9	35.8
75 and over	617.0	62.2

Sources: Data from National Center for Health Statistics. (2021, September 30). National Ambulatory Medical Care Survey: 2018 national summary tables. U.S. Department of Health and Human Services, Centers for Disease Control and Prevention. https://www .cdc.gov/nchs/data/ahcd/namcs_summary/2018-namcs-web-tables-508.pdf; National Center for Health Statistics. (2021, May 17). National Hospital Ambulatory Medical Care Survey: 2018 emergency department summary tables. U.S. Department of Health and Human Services, Centers for Disease Control and Prevention. https://www.cdc.gov /nchs/data/nhamcs/web_tables/2018-ed-web-tables-508.pdf

In addition, 1,045,100 women received hospice care during that same year in the United States. *Hospice care* is defined as a program of palliative and supportive care services that provides physical, psychological, social, and spiritual care for dying persons, their families, and loved ones. Of the patients enrolled in hospice care, 17% were younger than 65 years, with the remainder accounting for hospice care divided among those 65 to 74 years (15%), 75 to 84 years (29%), and 85 years and older (38%). There is a striking increase in the use of each service as women age. The most common admission diagnoses for home healthcare include malignant neoplasms; diabetes; diseases of the nervous system and sense organs and circulatory, respiratory, and musculoskeletal systems; decubitus ulcers; and fractures. Primary admission diagnoses for hospice care include malignant neoplasms and diseases of the heart and respiratory system.

The proportion of women living in nursing homes is also noteworthy. More than 1,061,000 women resided in nursing homes during 2007, with only 6.4 per 100,000 younger than 65 years of age. Of women 65 to 74 years of age, 98 per 100,000 resided in nursing homes, and of those 75 to 84 years old about 423 per 100,000 resided in nursing homes, increasing after age 85 years to 1,651 per 100,000 (Cohen et al., 2021; Miller et al., 2023; Ne'eman et al., 2022). Differences in marital status between older women and men are reflected in both their living arrangements, such as in a nursing home, and in their relationship to their informal caregivers. Women tend to care for their spouses or partners, and as they age, they find themselves living alone (about 30%). Although most men were cared for by a spouse, lived with family members, and had a primary caregiver with whom they lived, women were more likely to live alone or with nonfamily members. Notably, the primary caregiver of most women was a relative other than a spouse—most often a child or child-in-law.

As more people live to the oldest ages and because the incidence of many debilitating illnesses such as diabetes, dementia, and osteoporosis increases with age, the number of older nursing home residents will continue to grow and issues surrounding long-term care will become increasingly important. The majority of nursing home residents were White, widowed, and functionally dependent women. The leading admission diagnoses for older nursing home residents (both men and women) were diseases of the circulatory system, followed by mental disorders.

INPATIENT CARE

Hospitalization is dependent not only on a woman's medical condition, but also on her ability to access and use ambulatory healthcare. Delaying or not receiving timely and appropriate care for chronic conditions and other health problems may lead to the development of more serious health conditions that require hospitalization. Utilization of inpatient services has declined, as has the number of beds in community hospitals. The National Hospital Discharge Survey is the principal source of national data on the characteristics of patients discharged from nonfederal short-stay hospitals.

Hospital costs are the highest of any type of healthcare service. For example, in 2010, mean healthcare expenses of women older than 18 years who had an expense were greatest for hospital inpatient services at $15,792 per person, compared with home health services at $5,066, hospital outpatient services at $2,529, and office-based services at $1,645. Prescription medications cost women an average of $1,617 per person and ED services cost $1,461 on average. Dental services cost an average of $677 per woman (DHHS, 2013). The average cost of total healthcare services per woman was $6,066 in 2010. Women paid approximately 14.4% of these expenses out of pocket. When they are hospitalized, women have shorter average lengths of stay than men (4.5 vs. 5.5 days in 2010), but the pattern of diagnoses and procedures varied between women and men in large part because of hospitalizations for pregnancy-related causes (including deliveries and diagnoses associated with pregnancy). For women younger than 18 years of age, pneumonia, asthma, injuries, and fractures account for the major reasons for hospitalization. For women 18 to 44 years, HIV infection, childbirth, alcohol and drug problems, serious mental illness, diseases of the heart, intervertebral disc disorders, injuries, and fractures constitute major reasons for hospitalization. For women 45 to 64 years, major reasons for hospitalization are cancer, diabetes, alcohol and drug problems, diseases of the heart, stroke, pneumonia, injuries, and fractures. For those 65 to 74 years old, major causes of hospitalization are cancer, diabetes, serious mental illness, disease of the heart, stroke, pneumonia, osteoarthritis, injuries, and hip fracture. For those 75 years and older, primary causes of hospitalization include cancer, diabetes, serious mental illness, diseases of the heart, stroke, pneumonia, osteoarthritis, injuries, and hip fracture.

ORAL CARE

Dental healthcare is essential for oral health and for the prevention and treatment of tooth decay and infection. As of 2021, there were 201,927 professional active dentists in the United States. There are 60.84 dentists per 100,000 U.S. population (American Dental Association, 2022). The percentage of adults age 18 and over who had a dental visit in 2020 was 63.0% compared to 85.9% of children ages 2 to 17. Between 2015 and 2018, women (23.5%) had fewer untreated dental caries than men (28.4%), which suggests women were more likely than men to have a dental visit (American Immigration Council, 2020). Dental visits were more common among women with household incomes 400% of the poverty level (82%) compared with women with incomes less than 100% of the poverty level (42.6%). Cost represents a significant barrier for women in accessing dental care. Only 20% of adults have dental insurance. In 2011, 16% of women did not obtain needed care because they could not afford it. The rate for women not getting needed care was greater for women with public insurance (23%) and for those who were uninsured (36%; Shrider et al., 2021).

Health Behaviors

All people engage in behaviors that are either helpful or harmful to themselves and others, with consequences to their health and well-being that will have both immediate and long-term effects. Many of these patterns of behavior are associated with morbidity and mortality. Exercising, not smoking, not using drugs, drinking alcohol in moderation, and good nutrition can improve or maintain women's general health and well-being and can also reduce the risk of selected morbidities and the consequences of such morbidities.

PHYSICAL ACTIVITY

The 1996 Surgeon General's report on physical activity and health reported that three quarters of U.S. adults exercise during their leisure time (DHHS, 1996). Despite the implementation of the Title IX, Education Amendments of 1972, which provides for equal opportunity for women in school sporting activities, one third of women report no leisure-time physical activity. Women's multiple roles in the workplace and at home compete with leisure-time physical activity. The *2008 Physical Activity Guidelines for Americans* (DHHS, 2008) recommends that adults should engage in at least 2.5 hours of moderate-intensity or 1.25 hours of vigorous-intensity aerobic activity (e.g., jogging) per week or a combination of both plus muscle-strengthening activities on at least 2 days per week (see Chapter 14, Healthy Practices: Physical Activity). According to Behavioral Risk Factor Surveillance System (BRFSS) 2019 data, in the United States, the crude prevalence among adults age 18 and older who reported meeting recommendations for weekly aerobic activity was 50.7% (Bennie et al., 2019; Fluetsch et al., 2019). Women were a lot less likely to meet muscle-strengthening activity recommendations compared with aerobic activity (19.8% vs. 43.9%). Physical activity varied with education and race/ethnicity. Some unintended adverse health consequences can result from physical activity. For example, exercise undertaken incorrectly can lead to musculoskeletal injuries and metabolic abnormalities. Also, excessive exercise among girls during puberty can result in the female athlete triad: disordered eating, amenorrhea, and osteoporosis (see Chapter 14, Healthy Practices: Physical Activity).

NUTRITION

Given the established relationship between nutrition and health, many health promotion behavior changes are nutrition related. The nutritional status of adult women is the culmination of nutrient intake, metabolism, and utilization over their life span. Although the link between nutrition and good health is established (see Chapter 13, Nutrition for Women), women's eating patterns are affected by numerous societal factors that reflect the cultural and socioeconomic landscape of the 21st century. These factors include increased employment outside the home, consumption of convenience foods, meals eaten away from home, single woman–headed households, and tobacco use. For many reasons such as professional fulfillment, economic necessity, and TANF, women of all age groups are employed and thus burdened by the multiple responsibilities of employment, child care, and home management, which leaves minimal time and energy to prepare well-balanced, home-cooked meals for themselves and their families. According to BRFSS 2019 data, in the United States, the crude prevalence among adults age 18 and older who reported consuming fruit less than once per day was 39.1% (CDC, 2021). Because nutrition is a modifiable factor for numerous chronic diseases, the *Healthy People 2030* nutritional initiative includes objectives that concern weight gain, obesity, dietary intake, and nutrients (folate, calcium, and iron), which directly impact women's health. In 2015–2019, only one in 10 adults met recommendations for fruit and vegetable intake. From 2007 to 2010, 43% of women reported that they had consumed fast food. On average, those who did consumed about 25% of their total daily calories from these items. Fast food consumption declined with age, such that 59% of women age 18 to 24 years consumed fast food compared with 22.9% of women age 65 years and older. More than half of non-Hispanic Black women consumed fast food (55.5%), followed by 47.8% of Mexican American women and 41.4% of non-Hispanic White women. Consumption of sugar-sweetened beverages varied with household income, with 60% of women with incomes less than 200% of the poverty level compared with 36.3% of women with incomes of 400% of the poverty level. Sugar-drink consumption ranged from 43% among non-Hispanic White women to 66.1% of non-Hispanic Black women (DHHS, 2013).

Federal programs of the U.S. Department of Agriculture provide help to low-income families in obtaining food. The Supplemental Nutrition Assistance Program (SNAP), formerly the Federal Food Stamp Program, provides benefits for purchasing foods to individuals and families with incomes usually below 130% of the poverty level. In 2011, SNAP served a record high of 44.1 million people per month, about one in seven Americans. Among households that relied on SNAP, 5.1 million (24.5%) were female-headed households with children. They accounted for 52% of all SNAP households with children. In addition, the Special Supplemental Nutrition Program for Women, Infants, and Children (WIC) also serves low-income women and families by providing supplementary nutritious foods, nutrition education, breastfeeding support, and referrals to health and social services. In 2012, WIC served nearly 2.1 million pregnant women and mothers, accounting for 23.5% of WIC participation. In addition, more than 75% of the 8.9 million individuals receiving WIC benefits were infants and children.

Food security, always having access to enough food for an active, healthy life, is becoming a more prevalent issue in the United States. Households with low food security have multiple food access issues, but little if any reduced food intake. Those with very low food security have reduced food intake and disrupted eating patterns. In 2011, nearly 18 million households experienced food insecurity for one or more members at some point in the year. Very low food security increased from 5.4% to 5.7% in 2011, returning to levels seen in 2008 and 2009 during the recession. Food security varies with household composition. Women and men living alone had similar rates of food insecurity (15%), but female-headed households with children and no spouse were more likely than male-headed households with no spouse to experience food insecurity (36.8% vs. 24.9%).

SUBSTANCE ABUSE

Substance abuse may have a profound impact on the current and future health of women. Women who use illicit substances are more likely to have poor nutrition and serious morbidity and to die from drug overdose, suicide, and violence. Use of selected substances in the past month among persons 12 and older was 11.7% in 2018 with drug overdose deaths from using any opioid per 100,000 population was 20.8% (CDC,

2023; Mattson et al., 2021). Rates of substance use and choice of substance vary by gender, age, race/ethnicity, educational attainment, and poverty status.

Federal law defines illicit drugs as marijuana, cocaine, heroin, hallucinogens, stimulants, inhalants, and nonmedical use of prescription-type psychotherapeutic drugs, such as pain medications, and sedatives. The number of poisoning deaths, most of which are drug related, has increased, including those tracked to use of prescription pain medications, and have surpassed MVA as the leading cause of fatal injury in the United States. From 2009 to 2011, 6.7% of women (vs. 11% of men) age 18 years and older used an illicit drug within the previous month. Most commonly used were marijuana (4.9% for women) and psychotherapeutic drugs (nonmedical use, 2.3%). Less than 1% of women used cocaine, heroin, hallucinogens, or inhalants. Among women, 17% of those 18 to 25 years of age reported using an illicit drug during the previous month compared with less than 5% of women 50 years and older. Non-Hispanic Asian women and Hispanic women were less likely than women of other racial/ethnic groups to report using illicit drugs in the previous month. Illicit drug use was more common among non-Hispanic women of multiple races (9%) and non-Hispanic White women (97.5%) than among non-Hispanic Black women (6.7%; DHHS, 2013).

Although women are more likely than men to be lifetime abstainers, women appear to suffer more severe consequences than men do after shorter duration of less alcohol intake. From 2009 to 2011, 21% of women reported consuming four or more drinks on a single occasion over the course of about 2 hours (binge drinking) and 7.3% reported heavy drinking (consuming on average more than one drink per day). Drinking patterns are related to both household income and age and race/ethnicity. At incomes of 200% of the poverty level, women and men were equally likely to drink heavily (8.2%), and binge drinking tended to increase with income. Nearly 38% of women age 18 to 25 years reported binge drinking in the previous month compared with 6.2% of those 65 years and older. Heavy drinking was also more common among young women (11.4%) and decreased to less than 7% of women age 35 years and older. Binge drinking ranged from 9% among non-Hispanic Asian women to about 25% of non-Hispanic White and native Hawaiian/other Pacific Islander women (DHHS, 2013).

Cigarette smoking is the major preventable cause of death among adult women and leads to an increased risk of cancer, heart disease, stroke, reproductive health problems, and pulmonary conditions. Once women start smoking, they continue to smoke for several reasons, including nicotine addiction, stress management, struggles against depression, and weight management. Women are less likely to report smoking than men (11.0% vs. 14.1%; CDC, n.d.-f).

In 2021, the prevalence of smoking was highest among American Indian women (20.9%) and lowest among non-Hispanic Asian women (7.2%; Table 1.11). Notably, the prevalence of smoking was lower among more education (4.0% of those with graduate degree) versus 21.6% of those with no diploma (Table 1.12). Smoking cessation is an important way to reduce the risk of poor health. The proportions of adults who quit smoking vary with education attainment.

TABLE 1.11 Percentage of Persons Age 18 Years and Older Who Reported Cigarette Use "Every Day" or "Some Days" at Time of Survey and Reported Smoking at Least 100 Cigarettes During Their Lifetime, by Race/Ethnicity, 2020

BY RACE/ETHNICITY	PERCENTAGE
White, non-Hispanic	13.3%
Black, non-Hispanic	14.4%
Asian, non-Hispanic	8.0%
American Indian/Alaska Native, non-Hispanic	27.1%
Hispanic	8.0%
Other, non-Hispanic	19.5%

Source: Adapted from Centers for Disease Control and Prevention. (n.d.). Current cigarette smoking among adults in the United States. U.S. Department of Health and Human Services. Retrieved February 16, 2023, from https://www.cdc.gov/tobacco/data_statistics/fact_sheets/adult_data/cig_smoking/index.htm

TABLE 1.12 Percentage of Persons Age 25 Years and Older Who Reported Cigarette Use, by Education, 2020

BY EDUCATION (ADULTS AGE >/25 YRS)	PERCENTAGE
0–12 (no diploma)	21.5%
GED	32.0%
High school diploma	17.6%
Some college, no degree	14.4%
Associate degree (academic or technical/vocational)	12.7%
Undergraduate degree (bachelor's)	5.6%
Graduate degree (master's, doctoral or professional)	3.5%

Source: Adapted from Centers for Disease Control and Prevention. (n.d.). Current cigarette smoking among adults in the United States. U.S. Department of Health and Human Services. Retrieved February 16, 2023, from https://www.cdc.gov/tobacco/data_statistics/fact_sheets/adult_data/cig_smoking/index.htm

Overall, the profile of health-promoting behaviors for women shows that activity levels decrease with age and that only about 20% of young adult women engage in regular physical activity that meets guidelines for aerobic and muscle-strengthening activity. Fat and carbohydrate intake remains relatively stable at 50% and 33%, respectively, across the life span, but total number of kilocalories taken in decreases with age (National Institute of Diabetes and Digestive and Kidney Diseases, 2021).

Changing Women's Health

BIOLOGICAL AND ENVIRONMENTAL FACTORS

The last decade of the 21st century was a time of significant advances in women's health. Prompted by the feminist movement of the 1960s and 1970s, increasing attention to women's health brought changes in health services, such as freestanding birth centers, development of academic coursework in women's health for professionals and the public, and advances in research about women's health. Each of these changes foreshadows enhanced possibilities for women's health during the 21st century. The consequences of advanced understanding of women's health through research may be the most dramatic in the decades ahead.

THE HUMAN GENOME

Research focused on the human genome has revealed new understandings about sex differences that may have profound implications on health of the nation. Not only have new insights about sex differences in the genetic bases for phenotypic differences between men and women revolutionized this field, but also some genetic discoveries have been made that may drive health consequences for women. Being male or female is linked to differences in health and illness, and these differences are influenced by genetic, physiologic, environmental, and experiential factors (Farrell, 2022). Although in many instances sex differences can be traced to the effects of reproductive hormones, hormones are no longer a universal explanation for these differences. Research on understanding the human genome has provided a basis for learning about the molecular and cellular mechanisms that underlie sex-specific differences in phenotype. Many of these new understandings warrant further investigation (Allen et al., 2021). Sexual genotype (XX in females and XY in males) has effects far beyond elaboration of reproductive hormones. Genes on sex chromosomes can be expressed differently in females and males. Single or double copies of the genes, meiotic effects, X-chromosome inactivation, and genetic imprinting are a few of the phenomena involved. X-chromosome inactivation is the random silencing of one or the other X chromosome that takes place during early embryonic development. X-chromosome inactivation, which occurs about the time of implantation, is a unique biochemical process in that it occurs only in females. Females inherit a paternally imprinted X chromosome, unlike males, who inherit only a maternally imprinted X chromosome. A subset of genes on the X chromosome may escape inactivation. As a result, females can get double doses of certain genes. The Y chromosome has a host of actively transcribed genes that are expressed throughout the male body but are absent from the female body (Abashishvili et al., 2022).

Although the new biological discoveries are important to the understanding of women's health, it remains important to recall that these sex differences are not the same as gender differences. Sex differences refer to differences that are biologically driven, whereas gender refers to differences that are socially influenced: self-representation as male or female and social responses to one's phenotype. There are many differences between males and females in basic cellular biochemistries that can affect health, and many do not arise only because of hormonal differences between the sexes. Research is in progress on the functions and effects of X-chromosome– and Y-chromosome–linked genes in somatic as well as germ cells. Mechanisms of influence of genetic sex differences in biological organization (cell, organ, organ system, and organism), effects of genes versus the effects of hormones, and sex differences across the life span remain to be fully understood.

ENVIRONMENTS FOR WOMEN'S HEALTH

The effects of women's environmental exposures on their health have gained scientific attention (Garcia et al., 2021; Haynes et al., 2017). As a basis for its work, the Federal Interagency Working Group on Women's Health and the Environment of the DHHS defined environment to include the home, school, indoor and outdoor workplaces, public and private facilities and outdoor spaces, and healthcare services and recreational settings. Women's health can be affected by the products women use in these settings as well as by contact with physical, chemical, and biological toxicants in air, water, soil, food, and other organisms. In addition, early life exposures of mothers and children, substances ingested, and economic circumstances can influence health. There are multiple mechanisms by which environmental exposures can influence public health through the life stages of women and their children (Bolte et al., 2022). For example, environmental chemicals may increase or decrease signaling molecules by mimicking or blocking effector molecule signals that disrupt signal pathways.

How populations differ in their susceptibility and how susceptibility changes over time may be explained in part by focusing on the intersection of genetic and environmental influences—for example, understanding how environmental agents with estrogenic-like activity interact with genes. Study of endocrine disruptors and their potentially adverse health effects could contribute significantly to improving women's health through curtailment of environmental exposures. In addition, studies of genetic susceptibility to environmental exposures—for example, the *NATZ* gene, which determines slow acetylation among smokers and its effect on breast cancer—may help reduce risk if these biological indicators become readily available to women.

Finally, as we have come to appreciate the disparities in health experienced by many populations of women, we are understanding and addressing the utility of the concept of gender disparities. Health disparities exist when there are differences in the incidence, prevalence, mortality, and burden of disease and other adverse health outcomes when compared with the general population. Sociocultural environments form the context for women's lives and have profound effects on their health and that of future generations. The critical intersection of gender, race/ethnicity, class, and age shapes the environments that influence women's chances for health. Consequently, it is difficult to attribute gender disparities in health to biology, environments, physiology, or human experience. The intersection of gender with other characteristics often determines the following for women:

- Exposures to toxins
- Social relations such as those linked to low social and economic status

- Racism
- Sexism
- Heterosexism
- Stress
- Tobacco/alcohol/other substance use

Sociocultural as well as physical and toxic environments thus form the context for women's lives and have profound effects on their health and that of future generations (Bolte et al., 2022). It is therefore critical to consider women's health from an integrative perspective and to move beyond research describing the nature of women's health problems to that which engages women in the study of solutions to their health problems (Meleis et al., 2016). Likewise, it is critical to consider both the individual experience of health, providers of healthcare to women, as well as the community's health. A multilevel approach to health is important to institute the kinds of programs that are likely to be successful in improving women's chances for improved and sustained health.

GLOBALIZATION

A final important factor influencing women's health is globalization. As economic forces move women into a global economy, some would point out that the world continues to be an unsafe place for girls and women. Meleis (2005) and Meleis et al. (2016) asserted that the gender divide compromises the safety of women. Women are at risk for violence, rape, trafficking, and abuse. Their mortality and injury rates reflect the limited definition of the nature and type of work they do. Conditions expose them to infections such as HIV/AIDS, pregnancy and birthing cycles, and unsafe abortions owing to the inadequacy and inaccessibility of health services. Meleis urges providers and recipients of services to enhance safe womanhood, not just safe motherhood by addressing health risks associated with women's work, marriage, violence, reproductive rules, and access to resources (Meleis et al., 2016). The education of young girls sets their horizons by determining their options for work. How work is defined limits consideration of the nature, burden of double and triple shifts, and hazards of work that are not currently considered in the economic and labor statistics or health studies. Marriage defines many women and obligates them to provide services and resources to husbands and families, as well as shoulder the burdens of multiple roles. Battering and abuse of girls and women, trafficking, and access to income through sex work all put women at great health risk, including for HIV/AIDS. Wars and terrorism increase women's chances of rape. Pregnancy, birth, and motherhood also escalate the risk of poor health for women. Finally, healthcare services that are fragmented, inaccessible, and focused on disease rather than prevention and health promotion become a source of overload for women. The invisibility of women's healthcare issues on national and international agendas intensifies the risk for women.

Meleis proposes that a fundamental change is necessary in the conceptual framework for women's health. She recommends using a human rights framework that is guided by a focus on women's life situations and experiences as a starting point for considering health. Stigma, exploitation, and oppression are key concepts in understanding women's health. Second, she urges redefinition of women's work from employment to a multidimensional framework that includes the amount of energy, activity, and space occupied; the amount and quality of time; the resources for their work; and the results, values, and meaning of their work. Third, she recommends development of policies that acknowledge women's perspectives, experiences, and life context, as well as give women a platform and advocacy to have their voices heard in the policy arena. Finally, Meleis recommends that societies consider women the center of the family and the community, expecting them to be the agents for continuity of values, gatekeepers, integrators, and guardians of social capital. This implies placing women's health at the forefront of foreign policy and international consciousness in war and peace. (This discussion is continued in Chapter 3, Women and Healthcare.)

THE FUTURE DIRECTIONS OF WOMEN'S HEALTH

Notable advances have been achieved in the scope and depth of women's health and healthcare research in the last century. However, major challenges continue to emerge; these challenges are influenced by socioeconomic and environmental trends; racism, agism, genetic, hormonal, and biological determinants; globalization; and other social issues. Future and emerging issues for women's health in the next century need to address the effects of demographic and sociocultural change on women's health and focus on the impact of such changes on the healthcare system and the ability of women to access appropriate high-quality, equity care. The need to broaden research topics and to consider populations that have been inadequately studied is essential. In general, although healthcare providers are committed to doing everything possible to promote women's health, the range of clinical and public health interventions is often limited, access to healthcare is inequitable, and the research evidence specific to women remains incomplete. Therefore, when considering future directions in research, one should ask whether study results will advance the ability to improve women's health and whether healthcare providers are being educated adequately to promote women's health!

REFERENCES

References for this chapter are online and available at https://connect.springerpub.com/content/book/978-0-8261-6722-4/part/part01/chapter/ch01

CHAPTER 2

Women and Healthcare Workforce: Caregivers and Consumers

Meghan Eagen-Torkko, Diana Taylor, and Molly Altman

WOMEN AND HEALTHCARE IN THE UNITED STATES

Women in the United States have a dual relationship with healthcare, as the majority of the healthcare workforce and as recipients/consumers of that healthcare. The relationships between women and healthcare are further complicated by racism, ableism, homo/transphobia, and ageism that different women experience in very different ways. While it can be said that women's healthcare, like women's experiences in the other spheres of our lives, is impacted by institutional misogyny and sexism, Black, Indigenous, and other people of color (BIPOC); disabled people; lesbian, gay, transgender, bisexual, queer, intersex, and other sexual and gender diverse people such as asexual persons (LGBTQI+);[1] and older people also are affected by racism and other systems of oppression in complex and competing ways. The intersectional nature of oppressions means that we should be very cautious as clinicians and as researchers at Udrawing conclusions about patients and best care practices when those conclusions are not centered in the lived expertise of the people most affected. Much of what we know, or believe we know, about women and healthcare in the United States is drawn from the experiences of White, straight, cisgender, nondisabled women, and may not reflect the realities of healthcare for BIPOC and others. For example, when discussing options for pregnancy-related care, providers will "package" that information differently for BIPOC women than for White women (Altman et al., 2019), which in turn calls into question the adequacy of informed consent for that care. It is critical when examining healthcare for women to also be critical of whose experiences are being centered in the discussion and who is considered the "norm."

In this chapter, we examine the dual role of women in healthcare. As members of the healthcare workforce, women represent the majority of employees, but are disproportionately concentrated in roles with less power and compensation within the larger healthcare workforce. As healthcare consumers, women are more likely to utilize care, particularly during the childbearing years when men of the same age are much less likely to access care, but also experience the negative impacts of sexism while accessing that care. For example, women are much more likely than men to die of cardiac arrest caused by a myocardial infarction, but not because they are more likely to experience that cardiac arrest. Rather, the "classic" signs of cardiovascular disease are much less common in women than in men, leading many women not to seek care, and women are less likely to have their symptoms treated aggressively if they do go to an ED (Aggarwal et al., 2018; Yu et al., 2019). As both workforce members and as consumers, women experience negative aspects of the healthcare system disproportionately to their representation in the general population and within healthcare. Healthcare systems, which could not survive without the labor and expertise of women, will need to evolve in the coming decades to meet the needs of not only their women consumers but also their women workers.

That evolution has begun to incorporate more emphasis on population health needs (gender- and age-focused health, mental health, sexual and reproductive health, for example) as well as the workforce to care for these populations (e.g., women's health, public health, behavioral health). The Patient Protection and Affordable Care Act (ACA, 2010; Health

---

[1] In a 2020 National Academy of Sciences, Engineering, and Medicine (NASEM) report, the phrase *sexual and gender diverse* (SGD) is recommended to describe individuals who identify as lesbian, gay, bisexual, transgender, queer, intersex, or nonbinary, or who exhibit attractions and behaviors that do not align with heterosexual or traditional gender norms (Patterson et al., 2020).

Resources and Services Administration [HRSA], 2021a) incentivized community health for the first time in healthcare regulation and reimbursement, and while the initial promise of the ACA has somewhat faded following a number of Supreme Court decisions that limited some provisions, the SARS-CoV-2 (COVID-19) pandemic that began in January 2020 has spotlighted the need for improved public and community health systems, workforce, and funding. As discussed later in the chapter, healthcare initially began as a community-based system, and professionalization throughout the 19th and 20th centuries moved that system out of the communities where it originated. With a renewed interest in vaccination, infectious disease monitoring, and the role that public and community health workers (CHWs) play in the health of individuals and communities, the potential exists for a more powerful role for both public and community health, and for community-based health workers, both formal and informal. Historically, those workers have been women, and women are likely to reclaim some of that role given the prevalence of women in both the healthcare workforce and consumer base.

One of the challenges of healthcare as we move into a postpandemic, post-ACA era is that we are inheriting a mishmash of healthcare specialties, providers, and foci. In contrast to the United Kingdom's National Health System (discussed later), healthcare for women, trans men, nonbinary people, and other gender diverse populations is fractured between sexual and reproductive healthcare (SRH), which is often delivered via obstetrician-gynecologists (OB/GYN, a surgical specialty), and non-SRH services, including cardiovascular/metabolic assessments, which may be delivered via family practice physicians, internists, or other providers, who may or may not also manage SRH. Confusingly, SRH providers often also deliver non-SRH services such as routine glucose checks, lipid panels, and other screenings. To add yet another layer of difficulty, the U.S. system often divides people first by body system (reproductive, pulmonary, neurology), and then may later subspecialize (urogynecology) by gender, or the gender subspecialization may come first (women's health). Finally, specialties are highly inconsistent in how they define gender (some use a social-personal definition, while others use body parts, which can be traumatic or harmful for gender diverse people to experience). These inconsistencies and specialty-physician focused systems are in stark contrast to the more common model seen in the United Kingdom and other countries where nurses, midwives, and generalist physicians are prioritized within an organized system of primary healthcare that includes both personal (individual) and public (community or region) care. In this model of care, core services are delivered in the home or within neighborhood clinics, or by local public health districts, which is a model much closer to the community-based one the United States previously had than our current illness/specialty-focused care, delivered in centralized healthcare systems that may or may not be familiar with the community of its patients.

There are many challenges that women in the healthcare system face, as patients and as caregivers, and while the U.S. model of primary/secondary/tertiary care is not the sole cause of these, the fractured nature of U.S. healthcare necessarily overemphasizes SRH potentially at the cost of holistic care, since people with uteri must often routinely interact with the healthcare system (for contraception, routine cervical and breast cancer screenings, and sexually transmitted infection [STI] screening and treatment), but may find that their experience of that healthcare system is limited to SRH services. The U.S. specialty-care model likewise limits utilization of public health work in primary prevention and health improvement since such work is incongruent with the diagnosis-treatment norms of this system. Finally, because of the gendered nature of many specialties, people who do not fall into the category of cisgender women may be excluded or harmed by this model of care. As we discuss the existing systems, we need to actively consider how we can adapt or replace those parts of the systems that may be harmful or unnecessarily costly or inefficient.

Note on language used: While many healthcare workers do not identify with the gender binary, the bulk of available data collected does use binary male/female categories. This limits our ability to directly address the issues facing trans and gender diverse healthcare workers in this chapter. The use of "women" is intended not to exclude trans and gender diverse healthcare workers, who may experience discrimination and harm related to their gender identity and their role as healthcare workers, but instead to (a) acknowledge the impacts of sexism and patriarchy on healthcare workers who present as women and make up the large majority of healthcare workers, and (b) reflect the current state of the research. It is our expectation that for the next revision of this text, there will be more information available about the experiences specific to trans and gender diverse healthcare workers.

Likewise, healthcare of trans men and nonbinary people often falls under the purview of "women's health," and we acknowledge the limitations of this terminology. In contrast, trans women's gender is often ignored in favor of current anatomy, particularly if they have not had gender-affirming surgery, and they may be excluded from "women's health" despite their gender. In addition, "women's healthcare" encompasses the whole person, and not solely gynecology/reproductive health. While we do focus on reproductive healthcare as significant in the experience of women in the United States, we reaffirm that women are not defined by our anatomy, and that women's health is a holistic rather than specialty concept.

The U.S. Bureau of Labor Statistics (BLS) collects ethnicity data as Hispanic/non-Hispanic. While Latino/Latina/Latinx are terms more often used by individuals in the United States to reflect ethnicity/identity, they are not synonymous with Hispanic, and therefore cannot be substituted. In this chapter, we use the language used by the BLS in its data, while recognizing that there is difficulty in extrapolating these findings to people who may identify as Latino/Latina/Latinx/Latine. It is our hope that governmental data collection will be reconsidered in future with input from community members.

HEALTHCARE WORKFORCE: GLOBAL AND IN THE UNITED STATES

According to the World Health Organization (WHO), the definition of the health workforce includes "all people engaged in actions whose primary intent is to enhance health" and improve population health outcomes (WHO, 2008, 2016). This includes physicians, nurses, and midwives, but also laboratory technicians, public health professionals, CHWs, pharmacists, and all other support workers whose main function relates to delivering preventive, promotive, or curative health services (WHO, 2016).

National and global efforts to achieve the health targets set by the United Nations (UN) are thwarted in many countries by shortages of health staff, their often-inequitable distribution, and gaps in their capacity and performance. The UN 2030 Agenda for Sustainable Development Goals (SDG) expands the Millennium Development Goals (2000–2015) relevant to health workforce and women's health: SDG 4—Ensure inclusive and equitable quality education and promote lifelong learning opportunities for all; SDG 5—Achieve gender equality and empower all women and girls. Although low- and middle-income countries face the most severe challenges in ensuring a sufficient, fit-for-purpose and fit-to-practice health workforce, countries at all levels of socioeconomic development face the challenge of how to sustain the human capital required to guarantee universal access and universal health coverage (including the elimination of preventable maternal and child deaths and unsafe abortion; UN, 2015).

According to the WHO Global Health Workforce Alliance, a global deficit of over 12 million skilled health professionals (midwives, nurses, and physicians) is estimated by 2035 and implies the need to rethink the traditional models of education, deployment, and remuneration of the health workforce; long-term system-building; comprehensive labor market engagement; and essential data systems (WHO, 2014b).

In 2013, WHO recommended that health begins with health workers and their empowerment (voice, rights, responsibilities), which play a central role in developing and implementing sustainable strategies toward universal health coverage and the improvement of health services and population health outcomes. Some of the common challenges across all countries include current and future shortages of some categories of health workers; replacement of an aging health workforce; the insufficient use of advanced practitioners, midwives, and nurses in many settings; and the difficulty attracting and retaining workers without enabling environments (WHO, 2014b, 2016).

The delivery of health services is one of the largest and fastest growing industries in the United States, with about 22 million workers (U.S. Census Bureau,[2] 2019) either in the health sector or in health occupations employment outside the health sector, accounting for more than 14% of the total U.S. workforce. (Indeed, even the use of the word "industry" demonstrates the problem with our fragmented health service delivery system that expands and contracts based on profit and corporate decisions, and reflects the difference between the United States and global definitions.) About 44% of all healthcare jobs are in hospitals (32%) and offices of healthcare practitioners, and one third are in nursing homes (14%) or other ambulatory or personal care facilities (U.S. Census Bureau, 2019). Of the 15 million healthcare practitioners,

technicians, and support personnel, in 2020, RNs (21%) were the single largest health occupation, followed by nursing assistants (9%), personal care aides (9%), and home health aides (4%; BLS, 2023). Despite the size and anticipated growth of the healthcare workforce, there are significant disparities within that workforce. In the United States, women are 80% of the direct-provision healthcare workforce and 86% of the nursing workforce (BLS, 2023), but men are overrepresented in roles of leadership in healthcare relative to the proportion of nurses (B. W. Smith et al., 2021). Although people of color represent 40% of the total U.S. population (U.S. Census Bureau, 2021a), over 50% of workers in almost every health occupation except personal, psychiatric, nursing, and home health aides are White (HRSA, 2017b). While the racial/ethnic proportion of counselors, social workers, laboratory technicians, and licensed practical nurses come the closest to equity in the U.S. population (37%–40% BIPOC), only 24% of 18 professional categories are filled by those who are BIPOC (HRSA, 2017b). Furthermore, women of color are overrepresented relative to their workforce proportion in lower-paying support work like home health aides, where they experience both less economic stability and increased risk of injury and interpersonal violence (Dill et al., 2020).

Rapid changes in economic, demographic, and healthcare system factors are driving reform in the U.S. health workforce. There are imbalances among geographic and functional health workforce shortages, healthcare reform, and development of healthcare workers to meet the population and health service needs. These health workforce imbalances intersect with continuing systems of oppression and inequities across gender, race, and economic status. Given these changes and inequities, the future healthcare workforce will be increasingly female, young, racially/ethnically diverse, not U.S. born, at or below the poverty level, and less educated. This has implications for relative power and safety of the BIPOC healthcare workforce and demonstrates a need for systems-level protections for healthcare workers in these roles.

In addition to the long-standing issues of equity in the U.S. healthcare workforce, the SARS-CoV-2 pandemic (COVID-19) has both exacerbated and created workforce issues (Khan et al., 2021). Now in its third year as of this writing, the pandemic increased the intended departure of healthcare workers from the bedside (Labrague & de Los Santos, 2021), worsened the mental and physical health of those who remained (Hennein et al., 2021; Shaukat et al., 2020; Sim, 2020), and created a profound relational rupture between workers and institutions, workers and patients, and workers and the public (Eagen-Torkko et al., 2021). Recovery from that rupture will require focused attention from every level of government, as well as from healthcare systems.

In this chapter, we provide an overview of the current U.S. healthcare workforce; trends for the future; and critical drivers, disparities, and challenges to ensure an adequate supply and distribution of well-prepared health workers to meet the nation's healthcare needs. Since women dominate the current and future healthcare workforce, we focus on how gender, and

---

[2] The data from the U.S. Census Bureau's 2019 American Community Survey (ACS) are more up to date than the Health Resources and Services Administration (HRSA) total workforce data analysis of the ACS Public Use Microdata Sample (PUMS) 2011–2015 data (HRSA, 2017a).

other elements that intersect with gender, shapes, strengthens, and empowers women as the primary healthcare workforce to meet current and future population and health service needs.

U.S. HEALTH WORKFORCE: OCCUPATIONS AND PROVIDERS

Definitions of *healthcare providers* (people and places) are rooted in history; their evolution is shaped by social, economic, and political forces. Historically, healthcare was provided by community members who trained in informal or formal apprenticeships, or by family members of the person needing care. The "professionalization" of both nursing and medicine that occurred in the United States in the 19th century, along with the rapid expansion of regulation of both healthcare practice and education, profoundly changed both who were healthcare providers and how they practiced (Matthews, 2012). Medical and nursing education reflected the segregation and exclusion of Black, Indigenous, and people of color (BIPOC) common to many professions, and this gatekeeping led to a healthcare workforce that reflected racist and sexist norms, rather than the communities served by that workforce (Jeffries, 2020). The informal/unlicensed healthcare workforce (home health workers, etc.) continues to represent more diversity in race and class, but with an increasing loss of power, income, and authority.

With the rapid and massive changes in the U.S. healthcare system, badly needed system redesign is occurring along with a redefinition of healthcare workers' roles. These changes are influenced by multiple determinants: the form of government involvement, definitions of health, social values, costs, society's expectations for the healthcare system, the privatization of health delivery systems, and the political power of various stakeholders. Research increasingly supports the need for culturally congruent care, including care providers who reflect the patients they care for, as essential to improving health disparities (Marcelin et al., 2019; Williams et al., 2016). Understanding the historical exclusion of BIPOC and other marginalized groups (whether by religion, sexual orientation/gender identity, or disability, for example) is foundational to creating lasting and meaningful change to the current systems.

The term *healthcare provider* here refers to people who provide care to patients and the settings or systems in which health services are provided. More than 100,000 establishments make up the health services industry with four gen-

eral segments (American Hospital Association [AHA], 2022; Centers for Disease Control and Prevention [CDC], n.d.-a, n.d.-b, n.d.-c, n.d.-e)[3]:

- Hospitals (public and private; AHA, 2022)
- Nursing and personal care facilities (excluding residential, mental health, substance abuse, and other residential care facilities; CDC, n.d.-c)
- Home healthcare (CDC, n.d.-b)
- Ambulatory care settings (excluding home healthcare, but including medical and diagnostic laboratories, offices and clinics of doctors of medicine, offices and clinics of dentists, offices and clinics of other health practitioners [chiropractors, optometrists, podiatrists, occupational/physical therapists, psychologists, speech/hearing therapists, nutritionists, and alternative medicine practitioners], outpatient care centers [kidney dialysis centers, substance use disorder (SUD) treatment clinics, mental health centers, and rehabilitation centers], medical and diagnostic laboratories, and other ambulatory health services [ambulance and helicopter transport services, blood and organ banks, pacemaker monitoring services, and nonhospital surgical centers]; CDC, n.d.-a)

Among the U.S. working-age population, the federal government defines the health workforce as the "occupations [that] include all healthcare providers with direct patient care and support responsibilities" (U.S. Department of Health and Human Services [DHHS], n.d., "Strategies"). This definition is inclusive of workforce occupations defined within the U.S. Department of Labor (DOL), Bureau of Labor Statistics Standard Occupational Classification (SOC) system.[4] The BLS Occupational Employment Statistics categories/groupings, updated most recently by the 2018 SOC system (BLS, 2018), represents the majority of health workforce occupations.[5] The SOC is used by federal statistical agencies to classify workers into occupational categories for the purpose of data collection and analysis, with cross-references with the U.S. BLS (fastest growing occupations), the BLS Occupational Employment Statistics (employment and wage estimates), and the U.S. Census Bureau's American Community Survey (ACS; current demographic data).[6] In addition to the U.S. BLS, the National Center for Health Workforce Analysis (NCHWA), a unit of the HRSA of the DHHS, uses these labor and census data to estimate the current and future supply and demand for U.S.

---

[3] More detailed information on the work settings can be found on the U.S. Census Bureau website: www.census.gov/eos/www/naics.

[4] Variation in definitions reflects the changes in standards and measurement. The BLS estimates occupational employment statistics every 2 years using the classifications developed by the SOC system. However, the SOC is revised about every 10 years, although an update was published in 2018.

[5] These occupational categories have limitations. Before 2010, for example, registered nursing made no distinction between nurse practitioners, nurse midwives, and RNs. The nursing aides, orderlies, and attendants occupational category also includes multiple job titles, levels of training, and certifications and were separated into separate job categories in 2010. Some job titles in a healthcare setting may not necessarily reflect similar Occupational Employment Statistics (OES) occupational classifications, which may cause some problems in reporting. For example, confusion may result from the differences in defining a home health aide as any individual providing services in the home or as one who completes home health aide certification requirements (https://www.bls.gov/soc/2018/soc_2018_manual.pdf).

[6] For more detailed information on the data sources, definitions, methods, and SOC categories, see HRSA (2017a). See also the U.S. Census Bureau website: www.census.gov/eos/www/naics.

health workers in order to produce a health workforce of sufficient size and skill to meet the nation's healthcare needs (HRSA, 2018a, 2018b, 2020).

The NCHWA regularly publishes a summary of data on the size and characteristics of U.S. health occupations based on the U.S. government's SOC system.[7] The most recent summary in *The U.S. Health Workforce Chartbook,* published in September 2018, is based on U.S. Census Bureau data from the ACS Public Use Microdata Sample (PUMS) 2011–2015 (HRSA, 2018b). *The U.S. Health Workforce Chartbook* estimates the total number of individuals in the occupation or occupational grouping, the percentage of women, the percentage of health workers older than age 55, and the highest and lowest number of workers per 100,000 in the working-age population across the 50 states. HRSA's Health Workforce Simulation Model (HWSM) uses a microsimulation approach to link multiple data elements that incorporate behavioral as well as structural changes impacting workforce supply and demand, including population needs for health provider occupations (e.g., women's health, behavioral health, and primary care providers; HRSA, 2021b).

In The *U.S. Health Workforce Chartbook*, health occupation titles are grouped into four categories for ease of reporting (HRSA, 2018b): Part I comprises clinicians (physicians; physician assistants [PAs]; RNs including nurse anesthetists (CRNAs), nurse-midwives (CNMs), and nurse practitioners (NPs); LPN/LVNs; pharmacists; and oral health professions, including dentists, dental hygienists, and dental assistants). Part II includes additional clinician categories (chiropractors, veterinarians, and vision health professionals, including optometrists and dispensing opticians) and occupations concerned with healthcare administration duties (medical/health service managers and medical secretaries). Part III reports on health-related technologists and technicians as well as aides and assistants; and Part IV describes behavioral (psychologists, counselors, and social workers) and allied health (physical therapists and assistant/aides, dietitians/nutritionists, occupational therapists, respiratory therapists [RTs], speech-language pathologists, and massage therapists) occupations. While the grouping of occupations makes the data easier to report and analyze, it must be regarded with some caution, as it eludes the degree to which healthcare functions on a teamwork model, as incentivized by aspects of the ACA, and the reality that the roles of each profession often overlap in any given patient's care.

In the reports from the Census Bureau's 2019 ACS, there were 22 million workers in the healthcare industry, which represents approximately 14% of the U.S. workforce (Laughlin et al., 2021). In the HRSA's *The U.S. Health Workforce Chartbook*, the largest health occupations or groupings were RNs (approximately 3,067,000); nursing, psychiatric, and home health aides (2,845,000); behavioral/allied health practitioners (2,219,000); personal care aides (1,649,000); phy-

sicians (961,000); medical assistants and other healthcare support occupations (1,249,000); and LPN/LVNs (852,000). Almost half of the 34 occupations or occupational groupings (HRSA, 2018a) are greater than 75% female, with dental hygienists, medical secretaries, and speech-language pathologists being more than 95% female (HRSA, 2018a). There are significant variations in age across occupations, from dentists and psychologists (more than 35% being older than 55 years) to emergency medical technicians and paramedics, dental assistants, and physical therapist assistants and aides (fewer than 10% being older than 55 years). More recent data show a significant change in health workforce expansion. The finding that 30% of health workforce left their jobs or were laid off in 2021—driven largely by the pandemic, insufficient pay or opportunities, and burnout—has implications for the entire healthcare system, both in the short term as the country struggles to overcome the COVID-19 pandemic and beyond as the U.S. population continues to age (Galvin, 2021).

WOMEN IN THE U.S. WORKFORCE

In 2020, women were 51.6% of the total U.S. paid labor force, and 57.4% of U.S. women are now in the labor force (BLS, 2020a, 2020b; DOL, 2010a, 2020b). Despite equal opportunity laws, women have not achieved parity with men's earnings, and many continue to be crowded into female "employment ghettos" such as factories and hospitals. BIPOC women often experience the intersection of both racism and sexism in the workforce; in 2019, Hispanic women were paid 55.4% of the earnings of White non-Hispanic men, and Black women were paid 63.0% of the earnings of White non-Hispanic men (DOL, 2020a).

The SARS-CoV-2 pandemic that began in early 2020 profoundly changed workforce participation for women in and out of healthcare (Albanesi & Kim, 2021; Landivar et al., 2020). With the closure of many segments of the service economy for pandemic control, women were disproportionately impacted by the economic stressors of the pandemic, and the closure of schools and day care centers overwhelmingly impacted women's ability to return to work when those sectors reopened, as well as to continue working at jobs that had not been interrupted (Collins et al., 2021). Because women are so disproportionately represented in healthcare, and because as essential workers healthcare providers continued employment throughout the pandemic, the emotional and logistical burden of providing healthcare in a pandemic fell largely on women. As the immediate and delayed effects of chronic understaffing, workplace trauma, and persistent stress ripple through the healthcare system, healthcare workers—who are largely women—are leaving or considering leaving their roles, which has implications for future workforce fitness and capacity (Labrague & de Los Santos, 2021).

---

[7] The National Center for Health Workforce Analysis (NCHWA; bhw.hrsa.gov/data-research/review-health-workforce-research), which is the data and statistics unit of the DHHS/HRSA, provides data resources for county, state, national, and global workforce estimation and analysis. In addition, the NCHWA develops the national infrastructure for workforce data management, supports state governments and organizations to improve workforce data, and supports state/regional health workforce research centers through a grant program.

The paid civilian workforce in the United States includes over 152 million people, of whom just under half (71 million) are women (BLS, 2021a). The official data underestimate the work performed by people in the informal economy, who do not appear in most employment data, particularly the estimated 11 million undocumented residents (Budiman, 2020), who contribute an estimated $5 trillion to the economy over 10 years (Edwards & Ortega, 2017). Using paid employment as the delineation of the workforce also omits the people whose unpaid labor enables the paid workforce, such as parents who work from home, those providing kinship care, volunteers, and others, who are disproportionately women. Therefore, any discussion of women in the paid workforce must also acknowledge the limitations of that definition, and the role that unpaid labor plays in enabling paid labor.

Paid labor is also disproportionately concentrated in traditional "women's work" (e.g., social work, nursing, teaching, administrative support). In 2018, 88.9% of nurses,[8] 96% of dental hygienists, 81.9% of social workers, 86.7% of special education teachers, and 70.9% of office support workers were women (BLS, 2021a). Women represent the majority of people with at least a bachelor's degree in the workforce, but a significant pay gap persists in almost every occupation (American Association of University Women [AAUW], 2021). In 2018, White women working full-time were paid 79% of what White men were paid, and this gap worsened for BIPOC and older women (AAUW, 2021; see Table 2.1).

The gender-based wage gap in the United States is more significant than in nearly every other peer nation (AAUW, 2021), and while education is often seen as a path to better employment, the wage gap persists at every educational level in the United States (BLS, 2021c). For BIPOC women, the pay gap persists across education levels (AAUW, 2021; Bleiweiser et al., 2021).

Across the world, women provide the majority of paid and unpaid healthcare but earn less than men. In a study of 104 countries (Boniol et al., 2019), women represent around 70% of the health workforce, but earn on average 28% less than men. Occupational segregation (10%) and working hours (7%) can explain most of this gap, but even when considering "equal work" an "equal pay" gap of 11% remains. The trend of increasing participation of women in highly paid occupations is predicted to narrow this gap by 4% in the coming 20 years. In the United States, women are overrepresented in the health workforce compared with the total population. Although men represent a larger proportion of the overall U.S. working-age population, women represent the majority of workers in 29 of 34 health occupations, accounting for more than 80% of workers in nearly half (15 of 34) of these occupations (HRSA, 2018a). Although women are making significant advances in the traditionally "male" occupations of medicine, dentistry, pharmacy, and some highly technical health occupations, they continue to far outnumber men in the traditionally "female" health occupations: nurse, occupational and physical therapist, dietitian/nutritionist, dental assistant/dental hygienist, nursing assistant, and health aide/technician.

In general, the majority of the pay gap between men and women in health occupations widens in the highest paying occupations such as medicine and dentistry. For example, women physicians and surgeons earn 75% of what their male counterparts earn, even after controlling for age, race, hours, and education (Whaley et al., 2021). However, the gender pay gap is narrower for women primary care physicians, who are paid at least 90% of men's median annual salary for 10 of 13 internal medicine specialties (Wang et al., 2021). Except for dental hygienists who have no gender pay inequity, male dentists make 26% more, male nurses make 15% more, and male pharmacists make 6% more than their female counterparts (Trapani & Jacobs, 2020). This disparity persists when considering leadership and administration roles in nursing, which are disproportionately filled by men. The gender pay gap narrows but still exists in the lower paid health occupations such as LPNs (11%) and health support workers (10% for nursing and home health aides). And numbers don't tell the whole story. Since women (many of whom are mothers and family breadwinners) are the majority of the healthcare workforce wage gaps compound the problem. When women aren't paid fairly, families suffer, and the American economy suffers.

Overall, the healthcare workforce is more racially diverse than the U.S. population and has increased in racial/ethnic diversity over the past decade. In 2022, the racial distribution in the United States was 59.3% non-Hispanic Whites; 13.6% Black/African American; 18.9% Hispanic; 6.1% Asian/Pacific Islander; and 1.3% American Indian/Alaskan Native but 2.9% of the U.S. population is multiracial (U.S. Census Bureau, 2022. By 2060, these proportions will shift quite dramatically, as there will no longer be any clear racial/ethnic majority because the BIPOC population is projected to rise to 56% of the total population in 2060, compared with 38% in 2014. Less than 45% will be non-Hispanic white; 13% Black/African American; 29% Hispanic origin; almost 10% Asian/Pacific Islander; and less than 1% American Indian, Eskimo, and Aleut (U.S. Census Bureau, 2022). More than half of the nation's children are part of a minority race/ethnic group. This proportion is expected to continue to grow so that by 2060, just 36% of all children (people younger than 18 years) will be single-race non-Hispanic White, compared with 52% today. By 2060, the nation's foreign-born population would reach nearly 19% of the total population, increased from 13% in 2014 (U.S. Census Bureau, 2022).

The statistics presented in Table 2.2 illustrate the racial and ethnic characteristics of selected healthcare occupations.[6] In 2015, 70% of pharmacists, 67% of physicians, 73% of RNs, and 75% of dentists were White (non-Hispanic) compared with 77% White (non-Hispanic) in the U.S. working-age population and 60% in the U.S. population (in 2021; HRSA, 2018a;

---

[8] Depending on the data source (BLS, 2020a, 2020b; HRSA, 2017a, 2017b; U.S. Census Bureau, 2023; U.S. Census Current Population Survey, 2021) the population of nurses may include RNs, LPNs/LVNs, and APRNs. For example, the 2020 CPS data estimated the RN population as 86% women compared to 90% women in their 2015 report (U.S. Census Bureau, 2015). The HRSA's *The Health Workforce Chartbook* (using 2015 data) reports RNs as 90.3% female, CNMs and NPs as 91.8% female, CRNAs as 57.7% women, and LPN/LVNs as 90.6% female (HRSA, 2018b).

U.S. Census Bureau, 2021). Overall, White and Asian workers are more represented among the occupations found within the health diagnosing and treating practitioners subcategory —occupations that often require many years of education or training and are both better-paid than in the U.S. working-age population altogether. Conversely, Hispanic workers of any race, Black/African American, American Indians/Alaska Natives, Pacific Islanders, and individuals reporting multiple or other race are, in general, far more underrepresented in this subcategory. However, Asians are underrepresented in two occupations—APRNs (4%) and speech-language pathologists (2%).

Among the health technologists and technicians subcategory, Black workers have the largest representation (25%) among LPNs, nearly twice their representation in the overall U.S. workforce. However, Hispanic workers are underrepresented in all occupations in this subcategory. Similar to the health technical occupations, there is varying racial/ethnic representation among all the healthcare support occupations—occupations that generally require fewer years of education or training. For example, Black workers have their highest proportion among nursing, psychiatric, and home health aides (32%), whereas Hispanic workers have their highest representation among medical (26%) and dental assistants (23%), both of which are a greater proportion than in the overall national workforce. In addition, multiple races, American Indians/Alaska Natives, and Pacific Islander workers have the largest proportion (2.2%, 1.1%, and 0.5%, respectively) among personal care aides (personal care and service occupation). Conversely, White healthcare workers have their lowest representation among nursing, psychiatric, and home health aides (47%; DHHS, 2017).

The trends in racial/ethnic diversity vary considerably by occupation, reflecting the historical racism of healthcare systems in the United States, as well as current structural oppressions (Yearby, 2021). Black non-Hispanic healthcare workers had the largest gain in share of the overall health workforce (16.9% in 2004 to 18.2% in 2013), which is a larger increase compared with the U.S. population trends (14.0% in 2004 to 14.8% in 2013). While Latinx healthcare workers gained representation in the healthcare workforce (8.5% in 2004 to 10.9% in 2013), it was at a slightly slower rate compared with the U.S. population (14.2% in 2004 to 17.1% in 2014; Salsberg et al., 2021; Snyder et al., 2019). These trends do not reflect the racial and ethnic identities of members of all groups within the healthcare workforce, and the higher paid, more powerful positions within the healthcare hierarchy remain disproportionately White and non-Hispanic.

In a more recent 2019 study of Black, Hispanic, and Native American healthcare workers, weighted data from the 2019 ACS were used to compare the diversity of 10 healthcare occupations (APRNs, dentists, occupational therapists [OTs], pharmacists, physical therapists [PTs], PAs, physicians, RNs, RTs, and speech-language pathologists) with the diversity of the U.S. working-age population, and 2019 data from the Integrated Postsecondary Education Data System (IPEDS) were used to compare the diversity of graduates with that of the U.S. population of graduation age (Salsberg et al., 2021). Among the 10 professions assessed, the mean diversity index for Black people was 0.54 in the current workforce and in the educational pipeline (where a value of 1.0 indicates equal representation of Blacks in the current workforce or pipeline). The diversity index for the current healthcare workforce was lower than 0.50 in nine of 10 professions (all except respiratory therapy) for Hispanic health workers. For Black and Native American health workers, the diversity index for the current healthcare workforce was lower than 0.50 in five of 10 occupations (dentist, pharmacist, physician, OT, and PT). Notably, there is near equity for Black RNs and RTs in the healthcare workforce. In contrast, among graduates of programs leading to the 10 occupations reviewed, the proportion of Black individuals ranged from 3.0% for PAs to 14.2% for APRNs. The proportion of Hispanic graduates of programs leading to the 10 occupations reviewed ranged from 6.5% for pharmacists to 19% for RTs, but significantly less than 21.3% of Hispanics in the U.S. population (aged 20–35 years).

The occupations listed in Tables 2.1 and 2.2 are not all those on which information is available, but they provide a good representation and clear picture of the continued effects of racism and sexism in paid healthcare roles. In Table 2.1, the occupations are listed for women in selected health occupations for 2015, 2019, and 2021, depending on the data source (BLS, 2020a, 2020b, 2021d; HRSA, 2017b)[9] and compared with 1995 data. Notably, the large numbers of nursing aides and medical assistants, of which approximately 90% or more are women, account for the majority of women in all healthcare occupations. Clearly, women, particularly women of color, are clustered in jobs and occupations that are lower in pay, lower in status, and less autonomous than the jobs of most men in the healthcare field (BLS, 2020a; Doyal, 1995; HRSA, 2017b). This concentration in low-power roles also limits the ability of women, particularly BIPOC women, to change the systems that harm them as healthcare workers and harm their clients.

The healthcare industry has seen constant job growth over the past two decades, even during the 2008 economic recession, when healthcare added 428,000 jobs and the rest of the economy lost 7.5 million jobs (Frogner et al., 2015; Wood, 2011). Healthcare employment is expected to rise, in large part because of the growing elderly population that typically requires more healthcare services, as well as the implementation of the ACA of 2010 (Cuckler et al., 2013). Recent projections from the HRSA expect the majority of the increase in primary care demand will be caused by demographics and the remaining 20% will be caused by changes in demand under the ACA (HRSA, 2017a). These projections, however, predate the SARS-Cov-2/COVID-19 pandemic, which seems to be significantly changing the workforce capacity, and potentially the distribution.

---

[9] For the national perspective, the primary source of national data on the racial and ethnic mix of the healthcare workforce is the American Community Survey (ACS), which is an annual nationally representative household survey conducted by the U.S. Census Bureau. Data on the diversity of the pipeline of workers are available through the Integrated Postsecondary Education Data System (IPEDS) for those in occupations requiring at least a postsecondary award; however, data are not available for those with less than a postsecondary award.

TABLE 2.1 Women Workers in Selected Health Occupations, United States, 1995 and 2015–2020[a,b]

HEALTH OCCUPATION	WORKERS (IN 1,000s)	WOMEN (%)[c]		>55 YEARS OLD (%)	AVERAGE WAGE, FULL-TIME WORKERS[d]		
		1995[e]	2015[f]		ALL	WOMEN	MEN
Total employed, age 16 or older[g]	159,825	46.1	46.9	50.3[h]	791	719	871
RNs	3,327.2	93.1	86.7[i]	25.5	1,305	1,274	1,437
APRNs[j]	280[g]	–	85.1	26.2[k]	1,955[l]	1,903	–
LPNs	894	95.4	90.2	26.1	921	918	–
Physicians	980	24.4	33.7[g]	31.0	2,418	2,418	2,647
Physician assistants	165[g]	53.2	64.4[g]	14.2	1,884	1,885	–
Pharmacists	352[g]	36.2	57.8[g]	24.2	2,019	2,087	2,010
Dentists	167[g]	13.4	38.7[g]	38.2	2,492	–	–
Dental hygienists	207[g]	99.4	95.0[g]	18.2	1,269	1,264	–
Physical therapists	235	70.2	70.8	14.0	1,527	1,478	1,551
Emergency medical technicians/paramedics	225.9	–	31.5	7.4	1,288	–	1,352
Clinical laboratory technicians	393.2	71.7	73.6	24.4	1,352	1,140	1,280
Aides: nursing, psychiatric, home health	2,846	89.4[m]	87.2	19.8	626	615	740
Medical assistants	571	–	92.4	9.9	676	668	980
Dental assistants	347.7	98.5	94.6	10.2	665	653	–

[a]Bureau of Labor Statistics. (2020). *Labor force statistics from the current population survey.* https://www.bls.gov/cps/tables.htm#annual
[b]Health Resources and Services Administration. (2018). *The U.S. health workforce chartbook—In brief.* U.S. Department of Health and Human Services. https://bhw.hrsa.gov/sites/default/files/bureau-health-workforce/data-research/hrsa-us-health-workforce-chartbook-in-brief.pdf
[c]Bureau of Labor Statistics. (2021). *Current population survey, health occupations by gender.* http://www.bls.gov/cps/cpsaat11.htm
[d]Bureau of Labor Statistics. (2021). *Current population survey, health occupations by average wage (full-time workers).* http://www.bls.gov/cps/cpsaat39.htm
[e]Bureau of Labor Statistics. (1995). *Current population survey, health occupations by gender.* http://www.bls.gov/cps/aa1995/aat11.txt
[f]Bureau of Labor Statistics. (2019). *Current population survey: Women in the labor force.* Report 1092. https://www.bls.gov/opub/reports/womens-databook/2020/home.htm
[g]Health Resources and Services Administration. (2017). *Sex, race, and ethnic diversity of U.S. health occupations (2011–2015): Technical documentation.* https://bhw.hrsa.gov/sites/default/files/bureau-health-workforce/data-research/diversity-us-health-occupations.pdf
[h]Fry, R. (2021). *Amid the pandemic, a rising share of older U.S. adults are now retired.* Pew Research Center. https://pewrsr.ch/3BL5DIj
[i]2020 Current Population Survey data compared to 90% of women RNs in 2015.
[j]Includes nurse anesthetists (CRNAs), nurse-midwives (CNMs), and nurse practitioners (NPs), but full data available for NPs.
[k]31% of CRNAs were older than 55 years in 2015.
[l]Wage data available only for NPs.
[m]Nursing aides, orderlies, and attendants included in 1995 data.

Workforce supply and capacity are also cyclical. The total number of individuals working in a profession is affected both by capacity (those trained and authorized to provide services in question) and by actual supply (qualified individuals who want to work). As provider shortages become apparent, educational programs expand, producing more graduates, and legal scopes of practice may grant broader practice authority to some professions in underserved areas. (This deficit-model approach to healthcare scope is problematic and is discussed later.) At the same time, practice models shift to integrate new workers into care delivery, effectively expanding capacity. Efforts to increase capacity may coincide with economic trends producing higher-than-anticipated numbers of individuals wanting to work. Evidence of the cyclical nature of workforce supply is the recent undersupply followed by oversupply of nurses and pharmacists (Buerhaus et al., 2009; Zavadski,

2014). However, unusual events can disrupt the accustomed cycles; for example, the SARS-CoV-2/COVID-19 pandemic amplified existing demands on the healthcare workforce, and increased workforce departures while simultaneously increasing rates of mental health issues, moral injury, and burnout among healthcare workers (Pereira-Sanchez et al., 2020; Sriharan et al., 2021; Stone et al., 2021). Shortages can be created not only by a lack of providers to fill roles, but also by trauma-driven loss of capacity of those providers to perform at peak ability (Marvaldi et al., 2021), and the challenge of the healthcare system during the recovery from the pandemic will be to address the harms experienced by healthcare providers during it.

One approach to address this current shortage taken by California's HealthImpact policy and research center is to focus on six opportunities to grow the nursing workforce. The strategies range from introducing K12 students to nursing

TABLE 2.2 Racial and Ethnic Diversity (%) of Workers in Selected Health Occupations, United States, 2015–2021 (Numbers in Thousands)[a,b]

HEALTH OCCUPATION	WHITE (NON-HISPANIC)	HISPANIC OR LATINX	BLACK/AFRICAN AMERICAN (NON-HISPANIC)	ASIAN (NON-HISPANIC)	AMERICAN INDIAN AND ALASKA NATIVE	NATIVE HAWAIIAN AND OTHER PACIFIC ISLANDER	MULTIPLE/OTHER RACE (NON-HISPANIC)
Total U.S. workforce[c]	77.0	18.0	13.0	6.0	1.0	0.5	2.0
U.S. population[d]	60.1	18.5	12.2	5.6	0.7	0.2	2.8
RNs	73.5	5.7	10.4	8.4	0.4	0.1	1.5
APRNs[e]	84.0	4.5	5.7	4.1	0.2	–	1.3
LPNs	60.8	9.4	23.1	4.0	0.7	0.1	1.9
Physicians	67.0	6.3	4.8	19.6	0.1	0.0	2.1
Physician assistants	72.7	10.0	7.1	7.3	0.6	–	2.2
Pharmacists	70.4	3.7	5.9	17.9	0.2	–	1.8
Dentists	74.8	6.1	3.0	14.3	0.1	–	1.7
Dental hygienists	83.4	7.5	3.1	4.2	0.2	–	1.5
Physical therapists	77.8	4.8	4.4	11.1	0.2	0.1	1.6
Emergency medical technician/paramedic	78.9	10.3	6.3	1.9	0.6	0.1	1.9
Clinical laboratory technologists	62.0	9.4	13.7	11.8	0.5	0.2	2.2
Aides: nursing, psychiatric, home health	46.8	13.7	32.0	4.0	0.8	0.2	2.1
Medical assistants	53.6	26.1	13.4	4.2	0.5	0.3	1.9
Dental assistants	81.1	22.5	8.8	6.9	1.0	–	2.2

[a]Health Resources and Services Administration. (2017). Sex, race, and ethnic diversity of U.S. health occupations (2011–2015): Technical documentation. U.S. Department of Health and Human Services. https://bhw.hrsa.gov/sites/default/files/bureau-health-workforce/data-research/diversity-us-health-occupations.pdf
[b]Bureau of Labor Statistics. (2021). Labor force characteristics by race and ethnicity. Report 1095. https://www.bls.gov/opub/reports/race-and-ethnicity/2020/home.htm
[c]Bureau of Labor Statistics. (2021). Employment status of the civilian noninstitutional population by age, sex, and race. https://www.bls.gov/cps/cpsaat05.htm
[d]U.S. Census Bureau. (2021). Quick facts 2020. https://www.census.gov/quickfacts/fact/table/US/PST045221
[e]Includes nurse anesthetists, midwives and nurse practitioners.

as a career, to improving skills in the existing nursing workforce (including transitions from unlicensed roles to licensed roles, as well as LPN-RN and RN-APRN), and improving retention and well-being among practicing nurses (Chan et al., 2021). This collection of strategies targets inflow of potential nurses, growth of the current workforce, and mitigating future workforce loss from trauma and/or burnout and can serve as a model for the multilevel approaches needed to address the complex issue of nursing workforce capacity. Other strategies to address workforce issues include expansion of the role of palliative care nurses, improving seamless transitions between secondary and postsecondary education, and increased funding for nurses and nursing students (Rosa et al., 2020). The troubled Public Service Loan Forgiveness Program, for example, which forgives up to 85% of federal loans in exchange for 10 years of work in nonprofit or government organizations, could be better leveraged to relieve the heavy loan burden of many healthcare providers, as could other loan forgiveness programs for healthcare education at the state and federal levels. These programs have the added benefit of encouraging practice in underserved communities and locations but may also contribute to a lack of investment in the community by healthcare providers who see them as a short-term commitment rather than a career choice. Critical assessment of both intended and unintended sequelae of policy approaches to reducing workforce shortage is essential to avoid reinforcing inequities in an effort to improve them.

Healthcare occupations in the 21st century will have more women in them and will be more ethnically diverse than they are today in terms of the number and proportion of women occupying jobs in the health workforce. Trends in availability, accessibility, acceptability, and quality as well as other implications of gender and ethnic diversity among the health workforce will be explored further.

Historical Perspectives

In prehistoric eras, both men and women shared the activities of healing—herbs and roots were gathered and dispensed to those who were ailing. However, records suggest that gender divisions began even during these early times. Women tended to fulfill the caregiver and midwifery role, and men tended to be medicine givers (Dock & Stewart, 1938). Religion and medicine were united very early, with the role of religious leader and healer often merged into a single powerful entity. Nuns, who were considered immune to the moral pollution of nudity that otherwise threatened women's virtue, frequently served as nurses. In the United States, enslaved women and their descendants served as midwives and nurses to communities, both Black and White, and their knowledge and skill were critical to the safety and survival of large segments of the colonialist Americas, as did their descendents (Suarez, 2020). Although the majority of physicians have been men, since the 19th century, nurses in the United States and Europe have been almost exclusively women[10] (Choy, 2003; D'Antonio, 2010).

During the 19th century, few women received a formal education, and relatively few were formally employed outside the home, although working-class women have always contributed economically and pragmatically to their families'

survival. Middle-class, largely White women in the 1800s were struggling to define a role for themselves in society through the women's suffrage movement of the 1840s, as well as through the early women's health organizations of the time (Ehrenreich & English, 1973). Beginning in the mid-1800s, Florence Nightingale and other nursing reformers leveraged the accepted gender roles of the era to argue that the role of trained nurse allowed women to harness their innately feminine caring traits and contribute meaningfully to society (Reverby, 1987a). These nursing reformers, however, did not extend the role of professional nurse to all women, instead choosing to emphasize the role of White, largely middle-class women to legitimize a role previously filled by women considered unfit for marriage, whether by vows of chastity or, conversely, by a history of sex work or other moral suspicion. The goal of nurse reformers was to consolidate and legitimate the power of professional nurses within the healthcare system, rather than to ensure inclusion of diverse communities. Women who sought education as physicians also appealed to social beliefs about women's attributes, balancing what historian Regina Morantz-Sanchez has called "sympathy and science" (Morantz-Sanchez, 1985). During this critical period of transition in U.S. medical history, urbanization, immigration, and the growth of hospitals led to a gradual replacement of family members as caregivers to reliance on professional nurses and physicians (Rosenberg, 1995).

The landmark Flexner Report, released in 1910, set forth new and more "scientific" standards for medical education (e.g., increasing the number of years of education required of medical school applicants). The report consolidated and formalized ideals that had already been circulating among medical (White, upper-class) "elites," and it resulted in the closure of many schools that had previously educated women and Black physicians. As standards of entry were tightened and the American Medical Association (AMA) and state medical organizations gained more power over the medical profession, it became more difficult for women, Jewish people, and BIPOC to access medical education (Starr, 1982). The number of women in the medical profession continued to decrease through the 1950s, but in the 1960s and beyond, the second-wave feminist movement, affirmative action programs, and women's own determination led women to seek higher education, particularly in the traditionally male medical careers, which may have also implicitly reflected the devaluation of nursing and other traditionally "female" healthcare roles. In an effort to establish authority as physicians, many women opted to distance themselves from other female healthcare providers, including nurses, which resulted in a limitation of the power sheer numbers might have otherwise been expected to bestow.

With better healthcare workforce data and private–public partnerships, the Institute of Medicine (IOM) has led a number of reports that challenge the Flexnerian paradigm in which the focus has been on degrees and specialized training rather than on aligning population needs with healthcare worker training and entry into practice. This is an evident attempt to bring U.S. healthcare more in line with the remainder of the world, including WHO, and has significant support in academia and advocacy work, although possibly less in policy implementation and durable policy changes. The IOM 2021 report, *The Future of Nursing: Charting a Path to Health Equity* thoroughly revised the priorities of the 2011 IOM *Future of Nursing* report to focus on social determinants of health, improving the resilience of the nursing workforce, and emphasizing the need for both financial support for and direct input from nurses in a wide variety of settings (Wakefield et al., 2021). However, the limited change in nursing roles in the decade between these two watershed reports suggests that despite the repeated calls for nurses and nursing to be centered in the U.S. healthcare system, and to play a role more analogous to that in many other countries, nursing remains stymied by regulatory and institutional barriers to full scope care. Because repeated analyses identified nurses and nursing as key healthcare roles for the transition to a more community-based and comprehensive health system, and because the vast majority of nurses are women, careful examination of nurses and nursing are essential to understanding women in the healthcare workforce. And finally, we highlight health workforce analysis that aligns population needs with workforce availability, accessibility, and quality in new reports on primary care, women's health, behavioral and public health workforce, as well as SRH workforce capacity-building.[10]

In this section, we focus intentionally on nursing for two reasons: Nurses are the largest single category of healthcare providers in the United States, and the overwhelming majority of nurses (86%) are women (CPS, 2020). Additionally, nursing has a complex history in the United States and globally: while nursing as a profession has a long history of systematic data collection and analysis, as well as some of the earliest work in infection control and public health, that professionalization often occurred at the cost of BIPOC communities and healthcare workers. The formalization of nursing and midwifery pathways in the United States explicitly excluded BIPOC from these pathways and prioritized the health of White Americans. Mary Breckinridge, for example, who is often lauded as having brought midwifery and public health nursing to Appalachia, did so in an explicit effort to improve the health and fertility of White residents in the region (American College of Nurse-Midwives [ACNM], 2021a). Nurse-midwifery programs that admitted Black applicants, such as at the HBCU Tuskegee University, were short-lived as governmental support for them waned (Dawley & Walsh, 2016). At the same time, regulatory changes excluded the Black grand midwives of the American South, who had largely trained in an apprentice model, and the effects of this exclusion persist to this day: of the nearly 6,500 members of the ACNM in 2019, 92% identify as White (ACNM, 2021a).

Despite its troubled past and present, nursing has the potential to guide the changes in healthcare that are badly needed. As a holistic discipline that includes function and meaning, as well as pathology, in the assessment and care of patients, nursing at its best seeks to improve health in ways

that are meaningful to the individual, within their particular context. This is central to addressing the needs identified by the 2019 IOM report, the 2010 ACA, and the more recent public health crisis of COVID-19. Nurses serve clients in communities, in homes, in schools, and in other settings, as well as in inpatient settings, and because of this have an opportunity for a different perspective on health and healthcare. Next, we examine some of the specific issues affecting nursing, as well as opportunities for the future.

Nursing's Roles in Providing HealthCare: RNS and APRNS

Nurses make up the single largest health profession in the United States (HRSA, 2017a). There were 3.3 million RNs, 280,000 APRNs, and 894,000 LPNs working in the field of nursing between 2015 and 2020 (BLS, 2020a; HRSA NCHWA, 2017). They perform a variety of patient care duties and are critical to the delivery of healthcare services across a wide array of settings, including schools, ambulatory care clinics, hospitals, nursing homes, public health programs, hospice, and home health agencies. Distinctions are made among different types of nurses according to their education, role, and the level of autonomy in practice. LPNs typically receive training for a year beyond high school and, after passing the national NCLEX-PN' exam, become licensed to work in patient care. LPNs provide a variety of direct care services, including administration of medication, taking of medical histories, recording of symptoms and vital signs, and other tasks as delegated by RNs, physicians, and other healthcare providers. RNs may have a bachelor's degree in nursing, a 2-year associate degree in nursing, or a diploma from an approved nursing program and must also pass a national exam, the NCLEX-RN', before they are licensed to practice.

The scope of RN responsibilities is more complex and independent than that of LPNs. RNs provide a wide array of direct care services such as complex health assessments, care planning and coordination, administration of treatments, disease prevention, patient education, and health promotion for individuals, families, and communities. RNs may choose to obtain advanced clinical education and training to become an APRN, defined by four titles—certified nurse-midwife (CNM), certified registered nurse anesthetist (CRNA), clinical nurse specialist (CNS), and NP. APRNs usually have a master's degree, although doctoral-level education is becoming the norm, and are certified to practice in a clinical specialty area.

The changes to healthcare funding and structures that accompanied the 2010 ACA recognized some of the overlooked roles nurses play in the healthcare system (particularly in community health and care coordination) but did not change some of the important aspects of funding and reimbursement

---

[10] Although the workforce necessary to care for an aging and institutionalized population is critically important, we have not included such data here. Since nurses, nursing assistants, and other health support occupations provide the majority of care to these populations, the discussion of the primary care, women's health, behavioral health, and public health workforce overlap with the care to geriatric and long-term care populations. Please refer to Building Geriatric Workforce Enhancement Program at www.hrsa.gov/grants/find-funding/hrsa-19-008 for a more thorough discussion.

that impact nursing. In particular, the ACA did not mandate reimbursement parity for APRNs with physicians and did not change the 1983 Centers for Medicaid & Medicare Services regulations that prohibit reimbursement for nursing care in the inpatient setting (American Nurses Association, 2017). These regulatory decisions have impacts on the financial aspects of nursing in the healthcare setting and on the roles nurses play in those settings.

About 445,000 RNs (16%) and 166,000 LPNs (24%) live in rural areas. The per capita distribution of RNs varies substantially across states (Rural Health Information Hub, 2020), with fewer RNs per 100,000 population working in the West and Southwest states (e.g., Washington, California, Idaho, Nevada, New Mexico, Oklahoma, Texas, Utah, Wyoming) and more RNs per 100,000 population working in the Northeast and Midwest states (e.g., Delaware, Iowa, Maine, Massachusetts, Montana, Nebraska, North/South Dakota, Pennsylvania). The nursing workforce grew substantially in the past decade, with the number of RNs growing by more than 500,000 (24%) and LPNs by more than 90,000 (16%) and outpaced growth in the U.S. population. Despite this, BLS projections for the next decade predict a shortage of nursing staff, in part due to the demographics of the nursing workforce and the U.S. population as a whole.

The average RN is portrayed as a White, married, middle-aged mother working full-time in a hospital, and many assumptions about the workforce and RN scope of practice are derived from this "typical" RN. However, over the past decade, RNs and LPNs are becoming more diverse. The proportion of BIPOC RNs increased from 20% to 27%, a 25% increase, and the proportion of men in the RN workforce increased to almost 14%, a 29% increase. Owing to growth in new entrants, the absolute number of RNs younger than 30 has increased. However, with one third of the nursing workforce older than 50 years of age, the mean age of RNs has increased during the past decade, which has implications for workforce capacity as these RNs reach retirement age (HRSA, 2018c; HRSA, NCHWA, 2017). Currently, more than half of the RN workforce (55%) holds a bachelor's or higher degree.

The annual median wage for a RN (not APRN) was $75,330 in 2020 (BLS, 2020b). The highest paid 10% of RNs made more than $116,230, whereas the bottom 10% earned less than $53,410. The states with the highest RN employment levels also have the highest average wages, ranging from California ($120,560), New York ($89,760), Texas ($76,800), Pennsylvania ($74,170), and Florida ($69,510). The top-paying states for RNs are concentrated in the West and Northeast regions, with annual wages ranging from $96,230 (Oregon), $96,250 (Massachusetts), and $95,250 (Alaska) to $104,830 (Hawaii) and $120,560 (California). Although annual earnings of RNs are above average for all healthcare workers (approximately $41,132; HRSA, 2017a), they are markedly lower than physician, dentist, and pharmacist earnings (see Table 2.1) and below those for physical therapists and laboratory technicians (HRSA, 2017a).

Work settings for nurses are changing as the Baby Boomer generation ages and requires more care, healthcare continues to shift to community settings (driven in part by ACA-incentivized care coordination efforts), and population-based nursing care gains ground in systems. One of the important

changes in health professions over the past 50 years has been the development of advanced practice nursing and the autonomous APRN roles of CNM, CNS, CRNA, and NP. APRNs are prepared by education and certification to assess, diagnose, and manage patient problems; order tests; and prescribe medications. However, many states (27) limit APRN practice by requiring formal physician supervision or collaboration to practice (American Association of Nurse Practitioners [AANP], 2022). In the other states, APRNs practice independently, often in low-resource settings such as rural areas and low-income urban areas. As with RNs, boards of nursing (BONs) in each state license and regulate the practice of APRNs (National Council of State Boards of Nursing [NCSBN], n.d.). The majority of APRNs (55%) are employed in physician/other practitioner offices and outpatient care centers, with less than one third of NPs (26%), CNMs (29%), and CRNAs (30%) employed directly by hospitals (BLS, 2021b).

Depending on the data source, APRNs represent approximately 9% of the national RN population. Although the number of employed APRNs have been estimated at approximately 280,000, according to the U.S. government (BLS, 2020a) in 2020, there were 246,700 employed NPs, 8,100 CNMs, and 45,200 CRNAs (Bureau of Labor Statistics, 2021e). As CNSs are not recognized by statute in all states, neither the BLS nor the HRSA provides regular reports; the National Sample Survey of Registered Nurses (NSSRN) estimated that there were nearly 60,000 CNSs in 2010 (National Association of Clinical Nurse Specialists [NACNS], 2020).

According to 2015 data (HRSA, 2017b), demographic characteristics among the three groups of nurses in advanced practice are similar in terms of race (85% non-Hispanic White) but differ on gender and age. The CNM and NP groups are predominantly female (92%), whereas the CRNA group is nearly half men (44%). Of note, CRNAs are paid significantly more than other APRNs (median salary approached $185,000 in 2020, compared to $112,000 for NPs and CNMs; BLS, 2020b). APRNs are less diverse than the RN population, with 4.5% Hispanic and 6% Black/African American APRNs, although Black nurses are slightly more likely than White nurses to hold a graduate degree in nursing (Smiley et al., 2018). This disparity suggests that racism, access to employment, and factors other than education play a role in the lack of diversity among APRNs. It is particularly striking among CNMs, where almost nine out of 10 midwives are White, but almost half of their patients are BIPOC (CDC, 2021). This failure to reflect the communities many APRNs serve is troubling, given the research on the benefits of culturally congruent care, and will need to be a focus of nursing in the next decade and beyond.

APRNs are often considered to be a lower-cost solution to a shortage of primary care providers, and many regulatory changes reflect this deficit-model framing. The need for primary care providers is well documented, particularly given the increased demands on these providers to manage care under many provisions of the ACA, and nurses in many states have been successful in arguing that independent APRN practice mitigates this shortage. Within the NP workforce, nearly half were working in primary care practices or facilities, frequently in high-need, low-resource settings such as federally qualified health centers (FQHCs), public health centers, Indian Health Services locations, and other relatively low-paid locations. The focus on APRNs as a cost-effective response to a provider shortage is problematic because it reinforces a healthcare hierarchy in which physicians are seen as the "gold standard" and because it makes nursing regulations vulnerable to changes in market forces rather than reflective of the research supporting APRNs as safe and effective providers. Additionally, it strengthens the fractured U.S. service model by focusing on who is providing care, rather than what care is being provided, and seeking to improve that care.

The geographic distribution of APRNs varies due to multiple factors, including local practice statutes, demand, income potential. In particular, there are significant differences in permissible scope of practice for APRNs that reflect the political power and will of physician groups in a state rather than the educational preparation and national scope of practice of APRNs. Western states are most likely to have full independent practice for APRNs, with California, a state with a robust and powerful medical association, a stark outlier. In 22 states, APRNs are required to have supervisory or collaborative formal relationships with physicians, despite decades of data supporting the safety of independent practice for APRNs (AANP, 2021). States that have independent practice may have a required supervisory period for newly licensed APRNs, despite a lack of evidence for this model. In states that have independent practice licensure for APRNs, a frequent rationale given for this is the lack of access to physicians for many low-resource communities, including rural and urban areas. However, this scarcity model of licensure posits a hierarchical relationship between physicians and APRNs and reinforces the role of APRN as a next-best or stopgap measure in shortage situations, rather than as an expert provider capable of independent care and weakens the position of APRNs to continue care delivery if the existing shortage of primary care physicians eases, for example.

The 2008 economic recession resulted in a temporary RN surplus because of deferred retirements and enrollment/graduation surges in nursing programs (McMenamin, 2013). However, as noted above, the SARS-CoV-2/COVID-19 pandemic that began in late 2019 has negatively affected that surplus by increasing temporary or permanent departures from the healthcare workforce, as well as increasing demand on the healthcare system, particularly in acute care settings.

Employment of CRNAs, CNMs, and NPs is expected to grow 45% from 2020 to 2030, much faster than the average for all occupations. Growth will occur because of an increase in the demand for healthcare services. Several factors, including ACA legislation and the resulting newly insured, an increased emphasis on preventive care, and the large, aging Baby Boomer population, will contribute to this demand. APRN reimbursement is also often lower than that of physicians for the same billed visits, which may lead insurance companies to encourage APRN use as a lower-cost option for care; this, of course, does not benefit the APRN, although it may benefit the insurer. The safety and efficacy of APRN care is well documented (e.g., Norton et al., 2016; Traczynski & Udalova, 2018), as is improved patient relationships and medication adherence compared to physician care (e.g., Leach et al., 2018; Muench et al., 2021; van Dusseldorp et al.,

2021). With the IOM- and ACA-driven shift to an emphasis on preventive and primary care, as well as health education and risk reduction, APRNs are well positioned to fill the need for primary care services (BLS, 2021e).

WOMEN AS PATIENTS

As discussed earlier in the chapter, women have a long history as healthcare providers—and, of course, as healthcare consumers. Because of the healthcare needs specific to sexual and reproductive healthcare (SRH)—in particular, contraception and pregnancy—cisgender women are frequent consumers of healthcare at an earlier age than are most men, and because of the role many women play in family logistics, are a powerful factor in healthcare utilization for their families as well (Zimmerman & Hill, 1999). However, this familiarity with the healthcare system does not necessarily translate to better health outcomes, as women 18 to 64 years old are more likely to experience disability and report fair or poor health status than are men ([NASEM, 2018a). Additionally, women are more likely to live in poverty than are men, which is a powerful predictor of health status, and more likely not to fill needed prescriptions due to cost (NASEM, 2018a). Finally, women are subject to morbidity and mortality risks specific to reproductive health and—more acutely—the politicization of reproductive healthcare. In this section, we examine some key aspects of women's healthcare and health outcomes to illustrate how systemic issues like racism and misogyny impact the health of women in the United States.

Pregnancy and Abortion

The capacity to become pregnant is not limited to women (trans men and nonbinary people with uteri can also become pregnant, and people without uteri cannot, regardless of gender), but so many aspects of pregnancy as it relates to health are intimately connected to misogyny and assumptions about women's lives that discussions of the impacts of pregnancy and the healthcare system center on women. Pregnancy—its desirability, its acceptability, its health impacts—is also deeply connected to racism, classism, and ableism in the United States, and the disparate outcomes for pregnancy on health reflect these systemic issues. In this section, we examine a few of the factors affecting the health of women in relation to the capacity for pregnancy.

Pregnancy is an extremely common experience for women in the United States. Approximately 5.6 million pregnancies occur annually in the United States, with approximately 60% of these ending in a birth (Maddow-Zimet & Kost, 2021). Of the 3.8 million births each year, 90% are attended by physicians, and 99% occur in hospitals (ACNM, 2016; Gregory et al., 2021). This is significantly different from the United Kingdom, where 54% of births are by midwives (Stephenson, 2016), and from the Netherlands, where 16% of births occur at home (Sandall, 2015).

While common, pregnancy is also not without risk, particularly in the United States. In 2017, 19 women died for each

100,000 live births in the United States, compared to eight in France, five in Ireland, and two in Norway (United Nations Population Fund [UNFP], 2021). The primary causes of maternal mortality in the United States were cardiovascular disease, hemorrhage, infection, and cardiomyopathy (CDC, n.d.-d). Mortality rates in 2019 varied sharply by state, from 11.2/100K in California to 37.7/100K in Kentucky, reflecting in many cases the strength of the social and health safety net available in a given state (BLS, 2021b).

Racism, however, remains the largest factor in maternal mortality in the United States; while 14.1 White women die for every 100,000 live births, 39.9 Black women die for every 100,000 live births (CDC, n.d.-d). The differences persist across income, education, and geographic location (Hill et al., 2022; Scott et al., 2019). The proposed causes for these disparities are many, and include chronic stress related to racism (Kramer et al., 2019), social factors like limited access to healthcare (or limited access to respectful, culturally congruent healthcare; Muse, 2018), and failure of providers to listen to Black women and families during the childbearing year (Wishart et al., 2021). The racial disparities in birth outcomes in the United States is an anomaly among peer nations, which strongly argues against an inherent physiologic cause for the mortality rates, and its persistence over socioeconomic status makes a single explanation like lower income or education levels unlikely. For Black women in the United States, pregnancy represents risk in a way that is less true for White women in the United States.

For the nearly 3 million pregnancies each year that do not end in a birth, there is another series of issues. Spontaneous pregnancy loss (miscarriage) is extremely common and affects perhaps one in five recognized pregnancies (Linnakaari et al., 2019). While the vast majority of miscarriages occur without complications, possible outcomes include infection, hemorrhage, and, increasingly, scrutiny about whether the miscarriage was truly spontaneous. As abortion care becomes increasingly difficult to access, and legal strategies to limit it pivot more toward the pregnant person and away from the provider, miscarriages are likely to become more scrutinized and possibly criminalized, as they have been broadly in other countries and in some places in the United States (Weigel et al., 2020).

In contrast to birth, abortion in the United States since 1973's *Roe v. Wade* decision legalizing abortion has been extraordinarily safe. A 2012 analysis found a nearly 14-fold increase in mortality rate for birth compared to abortion in the United States, which is consistent with safety data from other settings with legal abortion (Raymond & Grimes, 2012). A 2018 NASEM analysis argued that "it [the committee] should consider how abortion's unique regulatory environment relates to the safety and quality of abortion care" (NASEM, 2018b, p. 6). This regulatory environment has included a ban on federal funding (including Medicaid, Indian Health Services, and federal employee health coverage) for abortion care since 1976; a progressively more restrictive series of laws requiring, among other things, providers to "counsel" people seeking abortion that abortion causes mental illness and breast cancer, despite no research supporting this claim; and targeted regulations of abortion providers (TRAP laws) that included a requirement that an outpatient abortion clinic meet the requirements of a standalone surgical center, even though procedural abortions do not meet the definition of surgery and are extraordinarily

low risk. The Dobbs decision states the federal constitution does not confer a right to abortion and the authority to regulate abortion belongs to the states. Thirteen states had "trigger laws" with the intend to ban abortion if the Supreme Court struck down a federal right to abortion. Other states have attempted to or passed abortion restrictions or bans (Kaiser Family Foundation [KFF], 2022). Since the Dobbs decision, states that have banned or restricted abortion services have experienced higher rates of maternal and infant mortality, especially among women of color; greater racial inequities across their health care systems; fewer maternity care providers; and more maternity care "deserts" (Declercq et al., 2022; Supreme Court of the United States, 2022).

ALIGNING POPULATION NEEDS WITH HEALTH WORKFORCE AVAILABILITY, ACCESSIBILITY, AND CAPACITY: A FOCUS ON POPULATION NEEDS—NOW AND FUTURE

Until recently, most health workforce projections focused on supply and demand of health worker occupations, without acknowledging that individuals work in teams across clinical settings and with a variety of populations. In an attempt to evaluate adequacy of the health workforce to deliver care to specific populations or in specific settings, the NCHWA has estimated projections of supply, demand, and supply adequacy for Women's Health Service Providers (HRSA, 2021c; National Center for Health Workforce Analysis [NCHWA], 2016), and Behavioral Health Providers (HRSA, 2018a, 2019; SAMHSA, 2019). And in keeping with the global model of population needs built on a foundation of primary healthcare (personal healthcare and public health services), the WHO framework for an SRH workforce is described here.

Primary Care Workforce

The IOM Committee on Primary Care (IOM, 1996) defined primary care as the provision of integrated, accessible healthcare services by clinicians who are accountable for addressing a large majority of personal healthcare needs, developing a sustained partnership with patients, and practicing in the context of family and community. The primary care clinician workforce includes physicians, NPs, PAs, and nurse-midwives (CNMs). This definition is distinguished from the WHO term *primary healthcare,* which combines personal health services and population-based, public health services (WHO, 2008, 2014a). Primary healthcare (coordination of patient care across settings, specialties, and populations) results in better health outcomes, reduced health disparities and lower spending, including on avoidable ED visits and hospital care. Primary care services include *health promotion, disease prevention, health maintenance, counseling, patient education, diagnosis, and treatment of acute and chronic illnesses* in a variety of healthcare settings (e.g., office, inpatient, long-term care, home care, schools, telehealth) for individuals and families across the lifespan and of diverse sexualities and genders.

Recent evidence suggests that the current primary care team includes a generalist physician (family or internal medicine), a nurse (RN, LVN), an NP or PA, and about 25% of teams include a clinical pharmacist, a behavioral specialist, or a social worker (AAN 2016; Bodenheimer et al., 2015; Flinter et al., 2018; Jabbarpour et al., 2020; Mason, 2016; Smolowitz et al., 2015). An important team member in primary healthcare systems outside the United States, CHWs have been underutilized in primary care teams in the United States (Hartzler et al., 2018). In an analysis of 30 studies, CHWs play important roles in clinical services, community resource connections, and health education and coaching through multiple functions (i.e., care coordination, health coaching, social support, health assessment, resource linking, case management, medication management, remote care, follow-up, administration, health education, and literacy support) with potential to improve health outcomes and primary care access (Hartzler et al., 2018).

The adequacy of the future primary care workforce, as defined by availability, accessibility, acceptability, and quality, to meet the needs of people in the United States has been partially estimated by HRSA (2020a). In 2018, there were approximately 256,220 full-time equivalent primary care physicians and almost 100,000 full-time NPs (64,490) and PAs (33,400) working in primary care (HRSA, 2020a). By 2030, HRSA projects a 6% to 13% increase in supply of family and general internal physicians and a 2% to 8% decrease in geriatric and pediatric physicians and a 13% to 50% increase in demand for all primary care physicians. Since the supply and demand for primary care providers varies across states and regions, HRSA projects that by 2030, the adequacy of future supply of family physicians will range from 46% to 178%. However, if nurses and NPs (along with PAs) are able to practice to the full extent of their practice ability and authority, the adequacy of the primary care workforce in 2030 could achieve 90% capacity overall (Bosse et al., 2017; HRSA, 2021d). The extent to which the national supply of primary care providers will come close to meeting the national demand in 2030 depends on several factors—effective and efficient use of team-based care, expansion of health insurance coverage under full implementation of the ACA and state Medicaid, health professional regulatory reform, and the implementation of programs and policies to address the maldistribution and diversity of the primary care workforce.

Public Health Workforce

Public health is a broad field, encompassing the protection and promotion of the public's health domestically and globally. The complexity of the U.S. public health infrastructure, which spans 50 state health departments, 2,800 local health departments, and 300 regional and district offices, complicates workforce analysis (Association of State and Territorial Health Officials, 2020). In addition, much of public health has historically been funded through categorical (or vertical) financing streams for specific politically acceptable programs, disease areas, and initiatives, such as communicable disease control, family planning, and maternal and pediatric healthcare (IOM, 2012). In addition, the U.S. federal government plays a large role in the public health

system in the country. It surveys the population's health status and health needs, sets policies and standards, passes laws and regulations, supports biomedical and health services research, helps finance and sometimes delivers personal health services, provides technical assistance and resources to state and local health systems, provides protection against international health threats, and supports international efforts toward global health. The federal government does all these mainly through two delegated powers: the power to regulate interstate commerce and the power to tax and spend for the general welfare. The federal government's regulatory activities, such as labeling hazardous substances, are based in the power to regulate interstate commerce. Its service-oriented programs, such as the cleanup of hazardous substances or financing personal health services through Medicaid and Medicare programs, are based in its power to tax and spend for the general welfare (IOM, 1988). At present, the main federal unit with responsibility for public health is the U.S. Public Health Service in the DHHS. The second major unit is the Health Care Financing Administration, also in the DHHS. Primary care/personal health services differ from public or community health in that public health deals with health from the perspective of populations, not individuals. The clinical healthcare provider—a doctor, nurse, or dentist—helps with personal healthcare issues, or how a condition or disorder affects you individually. The public health approach is different. Public health focuses on the whole neighborhood (or city, county, state, etc.) and determines how many people have a particular disease or problem and what's putting them at risk. Then, public health professionals work out how to reduce those exposures and cut down on the number of new cases. In effect, the "patient" in public health is the entire community.

Public health is also concerned with whether the people with a problem have access to health professionals and are getting good care. If public health does its job, then the whole neighborhood, community, and society are healthier (American Public Health Association [APHA], 2021). Public health professionals try to prevent problems from happening or recurring through implementing educational programs, recommending policies, administering services, and conducting research—in contrast to clinical professionals like doctors and nurses, who focus primarily on treating individuals after they become sick or injured. Public health also works to limit health disparities. A large part of public health is promoting healthcare equity, quality, and accessibility. The U.S. public health system once had a history of robust funding and function, until the advent of Reaganomics in the 1980s drastically cut funding for many integrated social, nutritional, and health services, including community-based services for women, children, families, and vulnerable populations, and has never recovered the lost ground. It was particularly poor timing considering the advent of the HIV pandemic, and the failure of adequate public health systems in the United States may have contributed to its progression both in the United States and abroad. Without that funding, public health systems became increasingly reliant on single-focus programs and short-term funding streams from all levels of government, which significantly weakened the ability of these systems to lead sustained health improvement and workforce.

The public health workforce consists of public health nurses and physicians, dentists, nutritionists, health educators, epidemiologists, sanitarians, public health technicians/engineers, CHWs, scientists, and public health administrators as well as state and local health commissioners. Over the past decade alone, the public health workforce has shrunk by more than 15% (Castrucci & Valdes Lupi 2020). By some estimates, the U.S. public health workforce will need to grow by 80% to provide a minimum set of health services in the country today.

Decades of underinvestment has undermined the public health workforce. Because the "patient" in public health is by definition a broad entity rather than a single individual with a heart-tugging story of illness, cutting public health funding in times of economic distress carries relatively little political risk. With diminished funding, state and local health departments have not been able to attract, recruit, and retain the number of professionals with skills needed to respond to health threats. With shrinking numbers and reduced capacity, workforce development has fallen behind across public health, resulting in several challenges, including (1) lagging skills among workers due to changes in technology, (2) a lack of systems and data to assess and monitor workforce needs, and (3) hiring barriers that exist at federal, state, and local levels. The COVID-19 pandemic highlights the consequences of this underinvestment and the critical need for a strong and diverse public health workforce.

Increased funding recently distributed to the CDC secondary to the COVID-19 pandemic—from the Public Health and Social Services Emergency Fund, American Rescue Plan, and others—expands resources for new and expanded workforce development activities (Division of Scientific Education and Professional Development [DSEPD], 2021). With this funding, state and local public health departments have a unique opportunity to invest in the public health workforce to achieve improved availability, accessibility, and quality. A recent report suggests focusing on six workforce development strategies: reassess capabilities and roles, share resources and engage partners, overhaul the recruitment process, invest in employees, cultivate strong leaders, and promote diversity and inclusion (Kumar et al., 2022). Although these strategies can be considered necessary for any part of the health workforce, they are imperative to building capacity in the public health system and its workforce.

Women's Health Workforce[11]

Although all people share many healthcare needs, women also experience unique healthcare challenges and can face an array of gender-based health disparities. A group of healthcare professionals, traditionally referred to as "women's health providers," typically delivers obstetrics, gynecology, and other preventive and reproductive care services predominantly or solely to cisgender women, and has acquired specialized credentials in the field of women's health. Women's health providers may also offer these same health services to individuals who do not identify as female, although this can be problematic for these individuals as they are literally required to misgender themselves to receive care. (Trans women may experience the opposite problem and find themselves excluded from women's health based on anatomy rather than gender.)

When studied as a group, this cadre of providers often includes OB/GYN physicians, CNMs/certified midwives (CMs),[12] and NPs and PAs specialized in women's health—and hence, these provider types are the focus of a recent HRSA report. Along with family medicine physicians who provide women's healthcare, these professionals have been the focus of two reports on these women's health service providers from the NCHWA (2016, 2021b). The 2021 HRSA report presents projections of supply, demand, and supply adequacy for OB/GYNs, CNM/CMs, NPs, and PAs through 2030. The projections are at the national level by metropolitan/nonmetropolitan areas for all four professions and at the state level for OB/GYNs. The contribution of family medicine physicians in the delivery of women's health services is included. The provider types included in the reports have distinct training paths yet share certain components of their scopes of practice (NCHWA, 2016). Projections extrapolate current national care use and delivery patterns to the future population, accounting for variables including geographic and temporal variation in demographics, lifestyle risk factors, and disease prevalence, which all could affect the future demand for women's health services. This scenario facilitates evaluation of whether the future supply of women's health services providers will be sufficient to maintain current levels of care. However, the inadequacy of the current care levels is evidenced by significant access-to-care issues and substandard health outcomes (MacDorman et al., 2016; DHHS, 2020). This report was finalized in the midst of the COVID-19 pandemic, and the full implications of the pandemic on both short-term and long-term supply and demand for women's health services providers remain uncertain (American College of Obstetricians and Gynecologists [ACOG], 2015). As noted above, trans and gender diverse people may have difficulty accessing needed care, and data are not currently collected on providers who include trans and gender diverse clients in their practice scope.

Findings from HRSA's 2021 HWSM indicate that the nation is training an insufficient number of new OB/GYNs to offset field attrition, while demand for OB/GYN services is growing. At the same time, rapid growth in supply of CNM/CMs and women's health NPs and PAs is projected, which may partially alleviate the growing shortfall of OB/GYNs. CNM/CMs, NPs, and PAs can provide services related to uncomplicated pregnancy and childbirth and can treat many common gynecologic conditions. However, a more relevant

---

[11] Women's health refers to the influence of sex and gender on health, illness, disability, and disease status across the lifespan. For data on workforce projections see data.hrsa.gov/topics/health-workforce/workforce-projections#top.

[12] Because of the widely varying legal status and scope of certified professional midwives (CPMs) and others who are not certified by the American Midwifery Certification Board (AMCB), it is difficult to assess the role of these providers in the national healthcare workforce. This is not a reflection on the care they provide or the important role they play in the care of pregnant people in many jurisdictions.

question may be why the United States relies so heavily on obstetrics, a surgical specialty, for most of women's healthcare. Is there truly a shortage of OB/GYNs, or are the assumptions about the best providers to care for women to blame? The declining OB/GYN specialist physician supply may mean that OB/GYN efforts could increasingly focus on high-risk pregnancies, the management of complex gynecologic conditions, and surgical procedures, which is both an appropriate use of their advanced expertise in pathology and more reflective of the role they take in most other wealthy nations, which, overwhelmingly, have better pregnancy outcomes than does the United States.

Substantial barriers to care prevent many women from receiving the healthcare they need. For example, women from underrepresented racial-ethnic groups tend to use fewer indicated services than their non-Hispanic White counterparts (Child Trends, 2018). Women without health insurance also use fewer women's health services than their insured peers. Addressing differences in healthcare access, strengthening health insurance access, and dismantling racial-ethnic disparity-related barriers may result in a total demand for women's health services much higher than current levels. Additionally, access does not explain the crisis in Black perinatal mortality, which has multiple structural contributions, including racism in housing, education, employment, and daily life, in addition to access issues (Crear-Perry et al., 2021). Addressing this public health crisis will require not only improved access, but also reconceptualizing health delivery away from simple provider availability to address the determinants of health that occur long before the client arrives at the provider office. This in turn will need to drive a shift away from specialty providers to an increasing use of public health nurses and CHWs.

Although geographic maldistribution exists, primary care providers (e.g., family physicians, NPs, and PAs) are likely to contribute to alleviating the increased women's healthcare service demand, especially in nonmetropolitan areas. Women's unique health needs extend well beyond just anatomy-specific reproductive health services, and primary care clinicians play a critical role in closing the many health disparities that women face. Primary care clinicians also deliver many sexual and reproductive health services, which include, among other services, the provision of birth control, cervical cancer screening, prenatal care, and the management of chronic conditions during pregnancy. Furthermore, some family medicine physicians are trained to deliver obstetric care. CNMs and women's health NPs are classified as primary care providers for these populations as well, which OB/GYNs are not. Again, given the need for holistic care for women's health, a pivot away from specialist surgeons to primary care providers of all varieties is logical.

This holistic change will also create opportunities to decouple women's healthcare from SRH, and to decrease the exclusivity of gendered healthcare. Because trans men and trans women, as well as nonbinary people of varying gender presentation, can experience gender-based harm and discrimination both in healthcare and in the larger society, their health needs may reflect not only anatomic health needs (Pap smear for some trans men, for example), but also potentially the effects of misogyny that are shared with cisgender women, albeit in different ways (e.g., sexual violence, wage gaps).

Rather than focusing on "women's health" as a category of care, there is the need to evolve care that acknowledges the impacts of patriarchy and misogyny on people who are not cisgender men, and includes people based on needs, rather than gatekeeping by gender identity. One recent approach to this has come unexpectedly from the ACNM, which in 2021 expanded the midwifery scope of practice to include people of all genders seeking midwifery care (ACNM, 2021b). Although that care will differ depending on anatomic needs, an inclusive approach to gender ensures that people are able to access and benefit from midwifery-model care, which includes awareness of gender politics and power in the United States, and the effects of this on health.

As the healthcare system evolves in response to the growing need for women's health services, through demographic and geographic shifts, with the uptake of new technologies, and with delivery system and reimbursement reforms, each health provider's role and its implications on future availability, acceptability, and accessibility for women's health providers may change. For example, for states that allow greater practice autonomy in care delivery by CNMs, NPs, and PAs (fewer regulatory limitations on scope of practice), the HWSM might underestimate demand for these occupations while overestimating demand for OB/GYNs—and vice versa for states that offer less practice autonomy for these occupations. Although the HWSM projects that the growth in CNM, NP, and PA supply will exceed growth in demand based on current care delivery patterns, there might not be a "surplus" of these providers. Rather, the rapid growth in supply of these providers may have the following implications: (a) Some care historically provided by OB/GYNs could shift to these providers helping alleviate the projected growing shortfall of OB/GYNs. (b) These providers can help increase the comprehensiveness of women's health services provided. (c) These providers can help increase access to services by populations that currently underutilize services, including LGBTQI+ people. In 2018, the annual number of CNM, NP, and PA graduates was relatively high, presumably in response to both a projected shortage of OB/GYNs, a perceived increase in future demand, and reimbursement incentives that encourage provision of team-based care and all team providers working at the top of their licenses. That is, dynamic market forces work to mitigate this gap. Furthermore, the supply estimations and projections for women's health PAs are based on those PAs self-identifying as working in women's health. Commonly, PAs are educated as generalists for their flexibility to change roles based on where they find interest or employment, with up to 8% of PAs changing practice specialties annually (Smith, 2017). As such, new entrant numbers for any given year or number of PAs continuing to practice in women's health in any year are somewhat fluid, and more easily adaptable to market conditions than, for example, physician specialties.

The HWSM assumes that the baseline number of healthcare providers choosing to practice in women's health will continue at the same rate. The growth in demand for women's health services as currently defined, in an era of low birth rates, is growing at a slower rate than demand for other specialties that primarily serve older patient populations and that are projected to experience faster growth in demand. The level of demand for services can have an effect on specialty choice for new healthcare workers, along with numerous other factors (Yang et al., 2019). And future technological innovations (including self-collected human papillomavirus [HPV] screening in place of routine Pap smears, currently under investigation), shifts in the uptake of team-based care, and other coming trends in delivery of women's health services (e.g., movement toward over-the-counter access to contraception) will likely affect provider supply and demand in 2030, and thus may not be fully captured in the workforce projections, outside of their current effect in the baseline study year (2018). The increased use of telemedicine in prenatal care necessitated by the COVID-19 pandemic may continue after the pandemic and may help improve care for those who have difficulties accessing in-person care, although there are potential implications for people who are otherwise not connected to community resources except through prenatal visits (Altman et al., 2021; Fryer et al., 2020).

Finally, this report was prepared during the COVID-19 pandemic. While it is too early to find accurate data about the types, magnitudes, or duration of the pandemic's effects on these projections, the dynamics created by the pandemic suggest there will be some considerable effects on the supply, demand, and delivery of women's healthcare. Evidence from the literature suggests that preventive and routine care, needed treatments, and regular screenings were and are still being missed during the pandemic (1) because of social distancing and quarantining protocols, (2) out of fear of visiting medical facilities during the pandemic, and (3) due to the economic fallout from the pandemic, which is disproportionately impacting women (Glionna, 2020). As a result, the mix of care required until these trends resolve likely will shift toward more later stage treatments to address the issues unaddressed at earlier stages. On the supply side, the drop in business from this delayed care could have long-term implications for the viability of some practices and facilities providing women's healthcare services (AHA, 2020; Rubin, 2020).

SRH Workforce—Integrating Population Needs With Primary Care and Public Health

As mentioned earlier, the global model of primary healthcare provides services to women and men across the lifespan, with emphasis on gender diversity and health equity within an integrated system of primary care and public health. The WHO definition and conceptualization of SRH goes beyond the specialties of obstetrics, gynecology, women's health, and maternal child healthcare to include the sexual and reproductive health of men and women throughout their life cycle, and adolescents of both sexes, and it is closely associated with sociocultural factors, gender diversity and the respect and protection of human rights.

At the 2005 World Summit, the United Nations adopted a resolution that all countries should strive to achieve universal access to SRH by 2015 calling on all national healthcare systems to increase their delivery of SRH services by a workforce that has adequate knowledge, skill, and appropriate attitudes to provide competent SRH (UN, 2005; WHO, 2010). In 2009, WHO also conducted an intercountry survey to identify SRH provision across clinician type, setting, and degree of SRH integration into primary healthcare.[13] A summary of services by CHW, nurse, midwife (these are separate roles in most countries globally), and doctor across six WHO regions and across seven areas of service provision is published by WHO in *The Role of Primary Health-Care Providers in Sexual and Reproductive Health* (WHO, 2011a) followed by a set of core SRH competencies for interprofessional primary healthcare providers with the intent that these would be further adapted by individual countries to fit their unique national contexts (WHO, 2011b). Significantly, WHO identified SRH, including access to abortion, as included under essential health services that must continue in pandemic conditions (WHO, 2020), which emphasizes the value that public health places on SRH.

According to WHO, an expanded definition and conceptualization of SRH is central to the specification of SRH standards and competencies for population health workforce capacity building. SRH extends before and beyond the years of reproduction, and services should be part of the existing healthcare system and delivered as a collection of integrated services that address the full range of SRH needs.[14] The WHO 13 core competencies "reflect the attitudes, tasks, knowledge and skills that health personnel in primary health care need to protect, promote and provide SRH in the community" (WHO, 2011a, p. 1) and apply to all frontline healthcare providers, including nurses, midwives, NPs, PAs, physicians, and CHWs (WHO, 2011a, 2011b).

Current and future shortages of skilled health professionals are especially critical in regions of the world that also have a high burden of unsafe abortion and related sexual and reproductive morbidity and mortality. Additionally, most countries, including many high-income ones, have subnational disparities in the availability of a skilled health workforce, with shortages being particularly high in rural areas or within the public sector. The United Kingdom's National Health Service is an exemplar of SRH workforce capacity building that builds on the WHO framework demonstrating improved health outcomes.

In the United Kingdom, SRH is provided to adults and adolescents within a coordinated system of primary care and public health services and focuses on three areas: (1) The patient experience—ensuring that patients have access to a full choice of contraceptive methods (including abortion) and can see a competent healthcare professional to discuss

---

[13] SRH components: antenatal, childbirth, newborn, family planning/infertility, abortion, sexual/reproductive tract infections (STI/RTI), violence/cancer screening, and sexual health promotion/education.
[14] The WHO SRH concept consists of six components: (1) improving antenatal, perinatal, postpartum and neonatal care; (2) providing high-quality services for family planning, including infertility services; (3) eliminating unsafe abortion; (4) combatting sexually transmitted infection (STI), including HIV, reproductive tract infections (RTIs), cervical cancer, and other morbidities; (5) promoting sexual health; and (6) increasing workforce capacity and program development.

the full range of unintended pregnancy prevention options available to them without fear of harassment or stigma; (2) a well-trained workforce—assuring an optimum provider skill mix to cater for a wide population demand; and (3) the importance of integration—establishing clear referral pathways between services so that care can be integrated around the needs of the individual, not institutional or professional silos. Primary care and public health practitioners have a pivotal role to play in promoting high-quality SRH (Faculty of Sexual and Reproductive Healthcare [FSRH], 2015). In addition, SRH education, training, and certification have been established for RNs, APRNs, midwives, and nonspecialist physicians working in the United Kingdom. The National Health Service builds on general prevention, public health, and primary care competencies by the Royal College of Nursing (RCN), the Royal College of Obstetricians and Gynecologists (RCOG), and the FSRH (FSRH, 2012; RCN, 2009; Wilkinson & Halfnight, 2013). Currently, FSRH offers several competency-based training pathways for a variety of clinicians (FSRH, 2012). In this rational system, curriculum and training processes are coordinated across 10 components using a combination of teaching-learning and evaluation modalities for all categories of frontline primary healthcare providers in the UK national health system (FSRH, 2012).[15]

In the United States, most SRH services are provided in a fragmented health system, (Levi et al., 2013) and increasing the capacity of U.S. clinicians to provide high-quality SRH for all Americans has been declared an urgent public health priority (APHA, 2015). With likely shortages of primary care clinicians including OB/GYN physicians, a shrinking proportion of primary care clinicians prepared to provide women's health, and even fewer health professionals providing services in public health, community clinics, and family planning, there is a need to consider the overall SRH workforce policy options.

The ACA's (2010) focus on primary care and prevention creates an obvious framework for building capacity. In order to improve SRH workforce availability, accessibility, and quality; the areas for immediate action require development and implementation of new ways to prepare future clinicians and frontline health workers, the further development of the existing primary care workforce, the incorporation of SRH into new models of healthcare delivery and reimbursement, and the leveraging of existing professional expertise to improve SRH delivery (Nothnagle et al., 2013). A 2012 study by the RAND Corporation is the first U.S. report focusing on the SRH workforce with analysis of supply and utilization combined with proposals for policy intervention (Auerbach et al., 2012). The impact of the evolving healthcare delivery system and expanding health insurance coverage is analyzed, which offers an opportunity to integrate the currently "siloed" system and bring it closer to the comprehensive system of SRH services integrated across public health and primary care that WHO recommends. The findings and rec-

ommendations are relevant to all providers of SRH services as recommended by WHO. Short and intermediate policy options and interventions spanning education, federal/state policy, and emerging models of care delivery have the potential not only to close expected supply-demand gaps in the SRH workforce but to improve the quality and efficiency of SRH service delivery, expand the provider base delivering SRH services, and better integrate these services with other parts of the healthcare system.

There are multiple challenges preventing integration of SRH information into health professions education. Some of the limitations to engaging the entire healthcare team in SRH lie with inadequate preparation at the prelicensure level, the lack of graduate and postgraduate clinical training opportunities, a failure to recognize the potential distinctive contributions of all healthcare professionals, including physicians and pharmacists, as well as political interference with the provision of SRH. The majority of providers of SRH clinical care are not physicians; they are nurses, NPs, CNM/CMs, PAs, pharmacists, as well as allied and unlicensed health workers, yet there are barriers to universal access to all of these providers, which further limits efforts to reduce unintended pregnancy and sexually transmitted infections and improve SRH promotion. These challenges have been further complicated by political challenges to government involvement in the delivery of SRH, especially the lack of adequate federal funding for unintended pregnancy prevention as well as state restrictions on abortion services. Regardless of the ultimate outcome of this political interference, preparation of and support for providers in all settings to deliver high-quality SRH remain important.

In response to SRH workforce challenges and increased demand for SRH services in the United States, an interprofessional group of SRH experts from a wide range of educational, clinical, and policy backgrounds convened to develop a shared agenda to address SRH workforce issues (Nothnagle et al., 2013). At the outset, the participants agreed on fundamental tenets of SRH: comprehensive SRH that includes care of women and men throughout the life cycle with emphasis on adolescents, gender diversity, and health equity; evidence-based prevention and management of unintended pregnancy, including abortion care; public health prevention models to address health disparities; and team-based, interprofessional models of care. Vulnerable populations have historically had limited access to SRH; therefore, strategies to improve access to care for all underlie all recommendations (Cappiello & Nothnagle, 2013).

As the U.S. health system pivots to focus on primary care and prevention, the need for competencies and pathways to ensure that primary care providers are able to provide quality SRH has emerged (Simmonds et al., 2017). Building on efforts spearheaded by the SRH Workforce Initiative and the WHO SRH workforce competencies, studies were conducted to identify and refine core competencies in SRH for primary

---

[15] Competency-based education, training, and certification in the specialty of SRH includes competencies in 10 areas: Basic SRH services/skills; contraception; unplanned pregnancy care; women's health/common gynecology; assessment of specialty gynecology problems; pregnancy care; genitourinary conditions of men; sexual health promotion; public health, ethical, legal competencies; leadership, management, technology, audit competencies.

care providers in the United States (Cappiello et al., 2016). The 26 core competencies encompass professional ethics and reproductive justice (RJ), collaboration, SRH services and conditions affecting SRH to inform education and training across professions, as well as to fill the gap between an established standard of care necessary to meet patient needs and the outcomes of that care. Of note, in contrast to the WHO and FSRH competencies, RJ is referenced in this U.S.-focused set. In addition, competency-based educational modules have been developed for all health professional students to improve their understanding, clarify their values, and learn of ways to integrate best practices for unintended pregnancy prevention and care into clinic settings (Hewitt & Cappiello, 2015). Each module is based on essential unintended pregnancy prevention and care competencies to help students improve competency and hone their skills in defined areas—professional ethics, pregnancy options counseling, postpartum/postabortion contraception, public health, quality and safety, and global health.

Behavioral Health Workforce

According to the 2019 National Survey on Drug Use and Health (NSDUH), 80% of individuals with a SUD do not get needed care; 57% of those with mental illness also do not get needed care and fully one-third of those living with serious mental illness do not get the care they need (Substance Abuse and Mental Health Services Administration [SAMHSA], 2020a). Given the SAMHSA mission to reduce the impact of mental illness and substance misuse on America's communities, ensuring that individuals with mental illness and SUDs have access to evidence-based high-quality care is a critical focus. A major factor in achieving this goal is addressing the availability, accessibility, and quality of the behavioral health workforce.

In a 2020 report by SAMHSA (2020b), the behavioral health workforce[16] functions in a wide range of prevention, healthcare, and social service settings. These settings include prevention programs, community-based programs, inpatient treatment programs, primary care delivery systems, EDs, criminal justice systems, schools, or higher education institutions. This workforce includes, but is not limited to, psychiatrists, psychologists, social workers, advanced practice psychiatric nurses, marriage and family therapists, certified prevention specialists, addiction counselors, mental health/professional counselors, psychiatric rehabilitation specialists, psychiatric aides and technicians, paraprofessionals in psychiatric rehabilitation and addiction recovery fields (e.g., case managers, homeless outreach specialists, and parent aides), peer support specialists, and recovery coaches.

The identified number of behavioral health providers needed in the United States in this report are based on conservative estimates of those requiring access to mental health and SUD services. This report shows the stark contrast between providers that are currently available versus what is needed to address the mental health issues faced by millions of Americans. The goal of this report is to provide information on evidence-based models of care for those with serious mental illness and SUDs and practitioner numbers needed to meet the behavioral health needs of the American people, and to offer a foundation on which a model for a mental health system that will address these needs can be established.

Although the field is growing due to increases in insurance coverage for mental health and SUD services and the rising rate of military veterans seeking behavioral health services, serious workforce shortages exist for health professionals and paraprofessionals across the United States. The NSDUH has consistently shown that the majority of those in need of treatment for mental illness and SUDs are not served. This yearly public health surveillance instrument also showed that in 2018 there were 57.8 million Americans with mental illness and/or SUDs, while in 2019 this number increased to 61.2 million. These findings underscore the urgent need to address the over 4 million provider shortage for behavioral health services in America.

The nation's mental health and SUD providers are essential because mental illness and SUDs are key factors in disability, mortality, and healthcare costs. As the opioid crisis continues, HRSA is analyzing the size and distribution of the behavioral health workforce, both today and in future years (HRSA, 2018b). The national-level supply and demand for select behavioral occupations (psychiatrist, psychiatric NP and PA, psychologist, social worker, addiction counselor, marriage and family therapist, mental health counselor, and school counselor) are projected from 2017 through 2030 using HRSA's HWSM.

Nationally, two of the nine behavioral health occupations estimated in this report (psychiatrists and addiction counselors) are projected to experience shortages in supply by 2030, if there are no changes in behavioral healthcare utilization from today. If current supply and utilization patterns for behavioral health professionals remain the same throughout the forecast period, seven occupations (NPs, PAs, psychologists, social workers, marriage and family therapists, mental health counselors, and school counselors) will be adequate or may potentially experience an oversupply at the national level. Between 2017 and 2030, the total supply of all psychiatrists is projected to decline as retirements exceed new entrants. Rapid growth in supply of psychiatric NPs and psychiatric PAs may help blunt the shortfall of psychiatrists, but will not fully offset it. In 2030, the supply of these three types of providers will not be sufficient to provide any higher level of care than the national average in 2017, which does not fully meet need. Modeling results suggest that if current trends continue, the overall national supply of social workers will grow rapidly and through 2030 should be more than sufficient to meet demand. However, the role of social workers in care delivery continues to evolve. To the extent that the nation relies greatly on social workers in a patient-centered medical home model that better integrates behavioral health and primary

---

[16] Behavioral healthcare includes care that addresses any behavioral problem, including mental health and substance abuse conditions, stress-linked physical symptoms, patient activation, and health behaviors. https://data.hrsa.gov/topics/health-workforce/workforce-projections#top

care, the increase in demand for social workers could be substantially higher than the projections in this report.

The ability of Americans to access appropriate treatment and community recovery resources is critical to improving the overall population health of our citizens and reducing the impact of mental illness and SUDs on individuals, families, and communities. The discussion of the behavioral health workforce should also take into account the important role of peers in the treatment and the recovery process. Recently, there has been an emergence of recovery support centers or "recovery cafes" that encourage peers to support those in treatment. Recovery support centers may also provide critical services for individuals in recovery such as food, social support, access to housing, recovery education, and referrals to more specialized services. In order to ensure that clients remain in treatment and can fully engage in productive activities, peer support should be a critical part of the behavioral health team and represent a major workforce need.

To support anticipated demands, the SAMHSA-HRSA Center for Integrated Health Solutions (HRSA-CIHS) is at the forefront of helping the behavioral health workforce implement and use new and evolving practices and technologies to better address the needs of people with mental health and substance use conditions (SAMHSA, 2021). The HRSA-CIHS also provides guidelines on how to provide culturally relevant services via the SAMHSA Office of Behavioral Health Equity (SAMHSA, 2020c). And, in 2020, the expansion of telemedicine has broadened access to Medicare telehealth services so that people can receive a wider range of services from their providers without having to travel to a healthcare facility including specialty care (Centers for Medicare & Medicaid Services [CMS], 2020). The expansion of telemedicine may facilitate access to treatment with fewer barriers related to both transportation and stigma, thereby facilitating treatment services for substance use and mental health conditions.

HEALTHCARE WORKFORCE DRIVERS AND DISPARITIES: INTERSECTIONS OF GENDER, RACE/ETHNICITY, ECONOMIC STATUS, AND POPULATION NEEDS

The healthcare system is undergoing major change, which has direct implications for the healthcare workforce. We are moving from acute care treatment to ambulatory care focused on the prevention of chronic disease. With innovations in technology and communications, the professional hierarchy will need to flatten to utilize a diverse healthcare team focused on consumers and cost-effectiveness. Legislative and demographic drivers include ACA expansion and population growth that is increasingly diverse combined with an aging population. The maldistribution of primary care providers—both by type of reimbursement accepted and geographic location—appears to be a more significant problem than overall shortage. The ambulatory care sector will see the largest gain in jobs, mostly because there will be growth in home healthcare and its workers have the lowest level of education

and wages. Given these trends and projections, the healthcare workforce will be increasingly even more female, younger, racially/ethnically diverse, and non-U.S. born, with low income and low education.

Challenges Facing the Healthcare Workforce

These trends point to the challenges of a mismatch across growing populations, a lack of workforce capacity, workforce shortages, and the need to develop healthcare workers. The corporatization of healthcare appears to negatively affect the nursing workforce as well. For example, a third of all nurses are unhappy with their current job, but satisfied with their career choice (George Washington University School of Business [GWU], 2021). If career choice is not a problem and current jobs frequently are, there exists a mismatch between the career and the work, not the career and the carer. This an important distinction with implications for regulation of the healthcare industry, the increasing monopolization in many markets, and public policy going forward. It will also need to factor in decisions made about recovery from the current pandemic and preparation for the next public health crisis.

Challenges of the future concern staff shortages, unmet educational needs, maldistribution of services and providers, and imbalances across gender and racial diversity. Each of these is affected by multiple systems and will require multifaceted approaches to address, which is difficult within a healthcare model that often seems to be less a system and more a collection of disconnected individuals. These changes will also include shifting from a mindset of who is available to do something to what is needed to be done; overcoming long-standing convictions about who can and should do what; redesigning education and training so that incumbent healthcare workers are equipped with the skills needed to improve equity, quality, and safety; and investing in short- and long-term strategies to cultivate the necessary human capital to overcome shortages and develop a diverse healthcare workforce that represents U.S. society, that is fairly compensated, and that does not discriminate against either clients or each other.

Although this chapter focuses primarily on disparities associated with gender and race, much of the impact of these inequities also apply across other population dimensions. Marked differences in the intersecting social determinants, such as poverty, low socioeconomic status (SES), and lack of access to care, exist along racial/ethnic lines and have been shown to contribute to poor health outcomes (De Lew & Sommers, 2022; MacDorman & Mathews, 2011; Sondik et al., 2010) historically linked to exclusion or discrimination. Again, however, it is important to view social determinants of health not as immutable facts or characteristics of risk, but rather as concrete outcomes of the larger systems of oppression (racism, sexism, ableism, etc.) that are built into society. Addressing health disparities requires addressing the systems that have created those disparities in the first place, both within healthcare and in the larger communities. Contrary to articulating gender, race, and class as distinct social categories, intersectionality (a theory developed by U.S. Black feminists, who challenged the notion of a universal gendered experience) postulates that these systems of oppression are mutually constituted and work together to produce inequality (Davis, 1981; Collins, 1990; Schulz & Mullings, 2006). This has begun a shift away from a focus on the individual characteristic to the systems that differentially value that characteristic; from race to racism as the salient fact, for example (Williams & Rucker, 2000). Individuals as workers are shaped simultaneously by race-, class-, and gender-based systems of hierarchy as well as by ability/disability, sexual orientation, and age. Moreover, ecosocial theory integrates the body, mind, and society in understanding the health impact of social conditions and structural inequities, as well as the ways that gender, race, and culture become interwoven in life (Hammarström et al., 2014).

Though the status for women in the workforce has improved over the past several decades, many women, particularly Black women and other women of color, still struggle for equality in many occupations. Despite high levels of education (women are earning postsecondary degrees at a faster rate than men are), and strong representation in professional and technical occupations, women still face a persistent wage and earnings gap. Although a number of factors may influence the differences in earnings between men and women in the aggregate (such as higher numbers of women in lower-paying occupations), the wage gap continues even within individual occupations. Women are also more likely than men to leave and then reenter the workforce if they have children, which may affect accrued seniority or promotions, yet even this is insufficient to explain the entire persistent gap (Department for Professional Employees [DPE], 2015).

Structural racism and its effects on health is central to every facet of American life: education (Noguera & Alicea, 2020), housing (Krieger et al., 2020), employment (Gemelas et al., 2021), reproduction (Roberts, 1999), legal status (Perreira & Pedroza, 2019), chronic stress and trauma (Walters et al., 2011), institutionalized violence and the carceral state (Hayes, Sufrin, and Perritt, 2020), and healthcare (Mateo & Williams, 2021). Racism has an adverse impact on the healthcare environment and on those receiving healthcare services, but it also impacts health outcomes before an individual ever reaches the healthcare system and reduces the potential for healthcare systems to improve those outcomes once they do. Nor are healthcare workers immune to the experience of racism, sexism, or other oppressions from their colleagues and affiliated institutions.

Racism exists in healthcare on an individual level (an attitude of a provider toward a client, for example) and on a systems level (healthcare research, for example; Jones, 2000), and has complex interactions with other aspects of identity, including gender (Crenshaw, 1989). In the healthcare arena, healthcare providers may be victims as well as perpetrators of sexism, racism, and other systems of discrimination and oppression. Selective mistreatment undermines the work experiences of individuals who are identified with groups that are the targets of discriminatory behaviors. Although discrimination occurs on multiple levels—job, housing, and education inequities—it is complicated for women and BIPOC, and multiply complicated for BIPOC women. Classism, racism, and gender inequalities intersect to create structural violence, whereby unequal opportunity and marginalization persist for many in the health workforce (Rhodes et al., 2012).

Gender Discrimination and Sexism

Gender discrimination has been defined as any distinction, exclusion, or restriction made on the basis of socially constructed gender roles and norms that prevents a person from enjoying full human rights (WHO, 2001). While this definition also includes trans and gender diverse individuals, it is usually applied to the experiences of cisgender women and is discussed here as such. Gender discrimination can take many forms, overt and covert, such as wage discrimination, occupational gender segregation, sexual harassment, or conduct that creates an intimidating, hostile, or humiliating school or work environment. Gender discrimination can also be less overt, such as the exclusion of informal or home health workers from protective labor legislation (e.g., overtime payment requirements), reassigning pregnant workers on the basis of their pregnant status, or informally penalizing workers for using paid time off to care for family members—all of which disproportionately impact women workers.

How gender discrimination has affected women in healthcare has been explored by a number of scholars (Ashley, 1976; Cleland, 1971; Doyal, 1995; Hochschild, 1983; Reverby, 1987a, 1987b; Tijdens et al., 2013; Weaver & Garrett, 1983). Most historians attribute the discrepancy in compensation between men and women in the health occupations to gender discrimination and to lack of social value on caring work (Reverby, 1987b). Ashley (1976) described the discriminatory attitudes toward women that institutionalized their servitude in hospitals and points out the far-reaching effects of sexism on the quality and delivery of healthcare in U.S. hospitals. Hochschild (1983) linked the work of "caring" with occupational activities and economics. In a classic study of women service workers, she described how women are expected to sell their "emotional labor"—to pretend to have positive feelings they are not experiencing and to deny their negative responses in order to make others feel they are being cared for in a safe environment (Hochschild, 1983). This often results in "emotional dissonance"—core stress in which the task of managing an estrangement between self and feeling and between self and behavior. Although women in jobs with the greatest responsibility reported the most stress, it was those with the least say over their working lives who suffered the worst effects. Hochschild (1983) also reported that this experience leads to burnout and a loss of self as feelings and emotions became dulled as a defense against an intolerable situation. Subsequent studies have found that women workers with the least autonomy, job status, or control in their work suffered from physical and emotional disorders resulting in significant economic impact (Doyal, 1995; Hochschild, 1983).

Marini (1989) first described wage gaps in segregated occupations: The more an occupation is female-identified, the lower the wages for that occupation. A more recent study (Tijdens et al., 2013) found that "female" tasks and skills are devalued in the labor market, supporting the links among occupational segregation/composition, gender–wage gap, and discrimination. Moreover, even when women choose the same jobs as men, the wage gap persists. For example, male surgeons earn almost 40% more per week than their female counterparts. In real terms, this means that in 2015, a female surgeon earned $756 less per week than her male colleague, which added up to nearly $40,000 over the course of 1 year (Baxter, 2015). Research on nurses found that they experienced moral distress associated with perceived poor ethical climate, such as the dissonance between a lack of respect for colleagues or patients and the nurse's perceived lack of decision-making power (Lamiani et al., 2015). This sense of moral distress was amplified during the SARS-CoV-2/COVID-19 pandemic (Silverman et al., 2021), and is associated with long-term mental health impacts (Lake et al., 2021).

Racism and Xenophobia

Racial/ethnic disparities and discrimination in healthcare occur in the context of broader historical and contemporary social, structural, and economic inequality, with evidence of persistent racial/ethnic discrimination in many sectors of American life. Black, Hispanic/Latinx, American Indian, and Pacific Islander communities, and some Asian American subgroups, are disproportionately represented in the lower socioeconomic ranks, in lower-quality schools, and in poorer-paying jobs (Nelson, 2002). These disparities can be traced to many factors, including historical patterns of legalized segregation, structural racism, and discrimination. Although some institutionalized discrimination and harm have been removed from the official legal systems of the United States, their impacts remain, as does the fallout from a lifetime of experiencing racism-related stress and/or trauma. The effects of racism persist even when SES is controlled for in analyses, which suggests that health outcomes previously ascribed solely to differences in education and income require closer analysis to repair. For example, Black women with university degrees have 1.6 times the risk of perinatal mortality than White women without a high school diploma (Petersen et al., 2019). Examples like these make it clear that health disparities cannot be simply explained by differences in income or education, or even access to care.

Indeed, in addition to the structural racism encountered in daily life, healthcare may not in fact be as good at caring for BIPOC patients and may instead create a new source of harm. Reviews of hundreds of studies conducted in different parts of the country indicate significant differences in healthcare received by persons of different racial/ethnic backgrounds. Differential treatment and access to care in most studies could not be explained by such factors as SES, insurance coverage, stage or severity of disease, comorbidities, type and availability of healthcare services, and patient preferences (e.g., Prather et al., 2018; Schut, 2021; A. C. Smith et al., 2021). Despite efforts to address diversity of the healthcare workforce over the past 30 years, entrenched structural inequities exist in healthcare professional education and within healthcare institutions (e.g., Bell, 2021; Coleman, 2020; Legha et al., 2021; Romano, 2018). Although institutions focus on promoting cultural competence within the health professional workforce, power, White supremacy, and racism/antiracism are not systematically addressed either in education or in practice. Current evidence suggests that if institutionalized racism is addressed by healthcare systems (including education programs), other levels of racism, such as internalized and personally mediated racism, will resolve or have a reduced impact (Altman et al., 2021; Jones, 2000; O'Connor et al., 2019; Taylor, 2021). However, this requires healthcare systems, including educational systems for providers, to accept responsibility for actively combating that racism. The evidence that systems are doing so in an effective way is to date scanty.

Most of the healthcare workforce data on racial discrimination comes from health professions literature on physicians and nurses, who also are less diverse and relatively more powerful than members of other occupational groups, such as home health workers and nursing assistants. Because of the intersections of classism and racism, impacts of racism are likely to be felt even more strongly among workers in these occupations. Even for physicians and nurses, discrimination is a common experience, but via different routes. A recent qualitative study of Black physicians, nurses, and technicians found that relative power in an organization made a difference in how the respondents experienced workplace racism, with physicians noting few instances of individual racism but significant organizational racism, technicians reporting the opposite, and nurses in the middle (Wingfield & Chavez, 2020).

One early national study, conducted in 1993 and 1994 among female physicians, found that approximately 60% of BIPOC respondents reported racial/ethnic discrimination at work (Palepu et al., 1998). Despite significant promises made by governmental agencies and healthcare organizations, there is little evidence that the experiences of BIPOC healthcare workers have changed substantially since this early work. The proportion of physicians who reported that they had experienced racial/ethnic discrimination "sometimes, often, or very often" during their medical career was substantial among BIPOC physicians (71% of Black, 45% of Asian, 63% of "other" race, and 27% of Hispanic/Latinx, compared with 7% of white physicians, all $p < .05$). Similarly, the proportion of BIPOC physicians who reported that they experienced discrimination in their current work setting was substantial (59% of Black, 39% of Asian, 35% of "other" race, 24% of Hispanic/Latinx, and 21% of White physicians; Nunez-Smith et al., 2009). A recent review of studies from 2006 to 2016 found substantial evidence for racism experienced by healthcare providers in a variety of roles that was experienced in ways ranging from microaggressions to stymied career progressions to direct instances of explicit discrimination (Snyder & Schwartz, 2019).

Although explicit recognized race bias is relatively rare among health professionals, an unconscious preference for Whites compared with Blacks is commonly found on tests of implicit bias (Chapman et al., 2013). Implicit racial bias has been implicated in the failure to achieve greater inclusion of Black students in medical education; the percentage of Black men among all medical school graduates has declined over the past 20 years (Ansell & McDonald, 2015). Although nurses are an historically oppressed group, the profession as a whole, like physicians, has not adequately addressed their complicity in the relative silence on race and the role they have in perpetuating racial healthcare disparities (Hall & Fields, 2013). Allen (2006), for example, writes of nursing education as a factory perpetuating racial inequities and White privilege. This is congruent with nursing's continuing veneration of Nightingale and others who actively promoted White supremacist norms as foundational "mothers" of the profession.

Institutional racism at the level of healthcare systems and health professions training is a critically important factor in maintaining discriminary practices. The institutional climate for discrimination in education and healthcare systems is influenced by several elements of the institutional context, including the degree of structural diversity; the historical legacy of inclusion or exclusion of students, clinicians, and faculty of color; the psychological climate (i.e., perceptions of the degree of racial tension and discrimination on campus or institution); and the behavioral dimension (i.e., the quality and quantity of interactions across diverse groups and diversity-related education; e.g., Campbell et al., 2020; Lim et al., 2021; Payne et al., 2020; Ro & Villarreal, 2021; Thurman et al., 2019; Waite & Nardi, 2019).

In a 2004 IOM report (Smedley et al., 2004), a review of the evidence indicated that reducing discrimination and bias among the healthcare workforce and service is associated with improved access to care for racial/ethnic minority patients, greater patient choice and satisfaction, better patient–provider communication, and better educational experiences for health professionals, students, and practitioners. Efforts to increase the proportions of people of color in healthcare professions have met with limited success and have been hampered by gross inequalities in educational opportunity for students of different racial/ethnic groups as well as the overwhelming whiteness of nursing faculty and the racism that students of color encounter (Bonini & Matias, 2021; White et al., 2020). The costs associated with health professions training also may pose a significant barrier for many students of color. Tuition and other educational costs have climbed steadily along with increasing student debt, whereas sources of grant aid have decreased, as in all other areas of education.

Racial discrimination in the job market continues to persist (Emmons & Noeth, 2015). Higher education has not leveled the playing field in terms of occupational success or wage gaps. White and Asian college graduates do much better than their counterparts without college, whereas Latinx and Black graduates do worse comparatively. The unemployment rate for Black workers has consistently been twice as high as the rate for white workers even among college graduates. Black and Latinx workers at all educational levels, including those with college and advanced degrees, earn less than their white counterparts; this means lower lifetime earnings, less ability to save, and less likelihood to receive help from family for education costs. This disparity, coupled with historical housing discrimination, also limits the ability to accumulate generational wealth, which in turn limits the opportunities available to children and grandchildren.

Encouraging, however, are the emerging advocacy efforts, as well as sustainable antiracist action, within the health professions. Recently, health professional leaders have called on their communities to advocate against the implicit bias among professionals that is adversely affecting the health of all marginalized populations and Black patients in particular. Mary Bassett, New York City health commissioner, suggests that healthcare professionals should be accountable for battling the racism that contributes to poor health (Bassett, 2015). Nursing professors Joanne Hall and Becky Fields have called on White nurses to talk to other White nurses about how marginalizing racial disparities are perpetuated in nursing practices, the development of knowledge, and education (Hall & Fields, 2013). In response to the killings of unarmed Black men, a national student-led campaign (White Coats 4 Black Lives) was initiated to call attention to biases among health professionals in learning environments and in administrative decision-making that leads to disparities in the medical community and, ultimately, the health of people (Charles et al., 2015). Mandated action within educational institutions to make real and sustained change includes faculty and staff workshops (e.g., undoing racism workshops in school of nursing), top leadership commitment,[17] institutionally certified mission statements, and institutional maintenance and support for the antiracist efforts (Schroeder & DiAngelo, 2010).

FUTURE DIRECTIONS: WHAT IS BEING DONE AND WHAT SHOULD BE DONE

Developing and maintaining a healthcare workforce that meets the needs of the population and the health service system requires multiple approaches based on a framework to overcome existing and potential challenges. To overcome health workforce challenges, WHO applies a conceptual framework for considering four critical dimensions of human resources for health—availability, accessibility, acceptability, and quality—based on evidence from 36 low-, middle- and high-income countries (WHO, 2014a).

- **Availability:** The sufficient supply of health workers, with the relevant competencies and skill mix that corresponds to the health needs of the population
- **Accessibility:** The equitable distribution of health workers in terms of travel time and transport (spatial), opening hours and corresponding workforce attendance (temporal), the infrastructure's attributes (physical – such as disabled-friendly buildings), referral mechanisms (organizational), and the direct and indirect cost of services, both formal and informal (financial)
- **Acceptability:** The characteristics and ability of the workforce to treat all people with dignity, create trust and enable or promote demand for services; may take different forms such as a same-sex provider or a provider who understands and speaks one's language and whose behavior is respectful according to age, religion, social and cultural values
- **Quality:** The competencies, skills, knowledge, and behavior of the health worker as assessed according to professional norms (or other guiding standards) and as perceived by users

---

[17] Nancy Woods used her power position as dean of the School of Nursing to end the silence surrounding institutional racism at the University of Washington School of Nursing with a public apology. Her action paved the way for continuing antiracist work in the school and the university (Schroeder & DiAngelo, 2010, p. 254).

Even though all four dimensions are equally important, there is a logical sequence in addressing them. Without sufficient availability, accessibility to health workers cannot be guaranteed; and even if availability and accessibility are adequate, without acceptability, the population may not use health services; finally, when the quality of health workers is inadequate, the effects on services in terms of improving health outcomes will be suboptimal. In addition, multiple approaches to overcome health workforce challenges include policy and organizational reforms and private–public partnerships that create good jobs for all workers while addressing diversity and discrimination, working in teams, and empowering women.

A growing body of literature indicates that many healthcare workforce problems have been focusing on the "hardware" issues (i.e., infrastructure, technology, economics) but not on the "software" issues of healthcare systems (i.e., human and social aspects). In attempts to reform health systems, the "economic reductionism and technocratic structuralism" fail to take into account the everyday organizational reality of what goes on inside healthcare delivery systems. Healthcare workers are not simply robots, nor are they angels who have only the best interest of the patients at heart, but they are thinking, reflexive people who internalize and perpetuate the social norms of the societies in which they live and work (Govender & Penn-Kekana, 2008).

Until recently, little has been done to change health professions or healthcare worker enactment of these norms and biases or to include workers as change agents in education or healthcare delivery. Furthermore, little attention has focused on the dynamic between healthcare workers and the healthcare delivery system. In the current market-driven system, healthcare workers are treated as problems (liabilities and expenses) rather than as part of a solution (critical and participatory resources). This is particularly true of the hospital-based health workforce, like inpatient nurses, whose labor and expertise are not billable, and is therefore entered on the deficit side of the healthcare ledger. The usual business approach of focusing on supply and demand fails to capture one of the fundamental problems that healthcare workers and professionals face today—the environment of care. Underpinning these healthcare workforce changes are the shifts in the larger work environment that limit economic mobility and liveable wages. Stable jobs are being replaced with quasi-formal employment, freelancing, and mixed-earning strategies (e.g., a home health aide who drives for Uber or contracts through TaskRabbit), which lack basic benefits such as health insurance, dental and vision care, paid vacation, paid sick leave, or paid paternal leave (Carlton, 2015).

And while the pandemic has challenged every part of the health workforce environment, few have been more impacted than the nursing workforce. The trauma and moral distress of the past 2 years have exacerbated workforce vulnerabilities, but also provide a unique opportunity to accelerate changes (e.g., technology-enabled care models) and make bold investments in what the future health workforce could look like. Health systems, higher education institutions, the public sector, and others have recognized this critical need and have a time-sensitive opportunity to recommit to the support and development of the nursing workforce and ensure all health workers are set up for future success (Berlin et al., 2021).

Private–Public Investments and Policy Reforms

Beginning in 2010, the federal government started to address some of the needs for investment in the healthcare workforce and creating policy levers for sustainable change. Despite years-long political attacks on the ACA after its passage (former President Donald Trump repeatedly promised to eliminate the ACA wholesale, although he failed at this goal), those changes have made significant differences in numbers of uninsured Americans as well as some early steps to address glaring health disparities. One such example is the 2021 Black Maternal Health Momnibus Act, which was introduced by Representative Lauren Underwood (D-IL), an RN, and which was incorporated into President Biden's 2021 Build Back Better bill. The intent of the act was to address significant racial disparities of U.S. perinatal outcomes, using proposed interventions such as diversification of the perinatal workforce, funding community-based organizations, and innovative perinatal reimbursement models, among others (U.S. Congress, 2021–2022). At the time of this writing, the act has passed the House with bipartisan support, but remains stalled in the U.S. Senate along partisan lines.

Increasing and modernizing the healthcare workforce is a major goal of the ACA, which included critical funding for new as well as existing efforts to diversify the nation's healthcare workforce through academic programs, mentoring, and employment opportunities (ACA, 2010). Although, the ACA encountered partisan challenges to its full development, the law contains dozens of provisions related to healthcare workforce issues, including strengthening of primary care through payment reform, academic and financial assistance programs, and examination of the changing role of frontline healthcare workers such as NPs, who are increasingly providing primary care to medically underserved communities.

The politicization of all government health programs increased after the 2016 presidential election and congressional control by lawmakers in the President's party, which resulted in in massive changes in goals, programs, and funding of the DHHS, especially the CDC, USPHS, and workforce development under HRSA. This continued deconstruction and disinvestment in public health became extremely clear with the start of the COVID-19 pandemic, when contact tracing, adequate infectious disease response, and access for public health workers to basic supplies like personal protective equipment (PPE) foundered and potentially lost an opportunity to limit the spread of the pandemic (Woolhandler et al., 2021). During the remainder of the Trump administration's term in office, public health funding and response remained disjointed and limited, and was marked by political attacks on public health officials like National Institute of Health (NIH) director Dr. Anthony Fauci and others who advocated for a vigorous response from the federal government (Collier, 2017; Galea, 2017).

Beginning in January 2021, the Biden administration has shown a markedly different approach to the pandemic but has not yet funded public health to its needed levels (Hanlon & Roque, 2021). The most harmful aspects of the Trump administration are unlikely to be direct results of its attacks on the ACA, or decreased funding for public health, or even the domestic gag order placed on Title X funding, since these are relatively straightforward policy issues to address. The more complex and far-reaching results of the Trump administration policies are likely to stem from the increased pollution that followed the dismantling of environmental regulations, many lifetime appointments to the federal bench (including three Supreme Court Justices), and the promotion of nativism, xenophobia, and violence that peaked in the January 6, 2021 insurrection at the U.S. Capitol Building (Woolhandler et al., 2021). Recent Supreme Court decisions with the new court confirm the disregard of public health issues (Supreme Court of the United States, 2022; West Virginia v. Environmental Protection Agency, 2022).

One approach to limited governmental support has been to seek support from private funding sources. Partnerships between the federal government and private philanthropy have expanded healthcare workforce development, especially HRSA partnerships with the Robert Wood Johnson Foundation (RWJF; interprofessional education/practice, diversity, nursing workforce; RWJF, 2015), the John A. Hartford Foundation (geriatric workforce), and the Josiah Macy Jr. Foundation (primary care workforce). As the largest philanthropy dedicated to health and healthcare in the United States, the RWJF has been the leader of a number of important initiatives to strengthen the healthcare workforce and support the preparation of a diverse and well-trained leadership and workforce to meet the nation's current and future healthcare needs (Ladden & Maher, 2014). For example, leadership programs prepare healthcare professionals for success in a complex and changing health environment and enable them to lead systemic change (www.rwjf.org). Specific RWJF workforce initiatives aim to identify and develop innovations and policies to develop the dental, medical, nursing, and public health workforce in order to improve health systems. For example, the Primary Care Team: Learning From Effective Ambulatory Practices (PCT-LEAP; https://improvingprimarycare.org/) initiative was established to identify changes in policy, workforce, culture, education, and training related to primary care that can improve the way practices function. The program studied 30 high-functioning primary care practices to learn what they do to maximize the contributions of healthcare professionals and other staff.

In addition, the RWJF has advanced women in the health workforce through a decade of investment to strengthen the nursing workforce. Many of the RWJF's nursing programs support recommendations from the IOM's report, *The Future of Nursing: Leading Change, Advancing Health* (2011), which provides a blueprint for transforming the nursing profession to improve healthcare and meet the needs of diverse populations. These recommendations are being implemented through *The Future of Nursing: Campaign for Action*, a collaboration between RWJF and AARP. Through 51 Action Coalitions in every state and Washington, D.C., the *Campaign* works with policy makers, healthcare professionals, educators, and business leaders to respond to the country's increasing demand for safe, high-quality, and effective healthcare. (Campaign for Action, n.d.). However, Woolhandler et al. (2021) caution us against overreliance on private industry, or even philanthropy, in the case of government inaction or failure: "For health care, overreliance on the private sector raises costs and distorts priorities, government must be a doer, not

just a funder–e.g., directly providing health coverage and engaging in drug development rather than paying private firms to carry out such functions" (p. 744). Philanthropy cannot replace the obligation of government to ensure the safety and health of the nation, and a crucial advocacy role for nurses and others is to ensure government fulfills its responsibilities. Reclamation and expansion of the U.S. government's role in delivering health and social services in a coordinated system led by teams of public health professionals (then slowly deconstructed over the past 40 years) must be a priority.

This priority comes with a caveat, however. One important role of advocacy is to act as a brake on systems or policies that may be harmful or oppressive, and the U.S. government has a long history of public health policies that were precisely that. From the elimination of Black midwives and exclusion from health professions schools, to the Tuskegee experiment (which was performed under the auspices of the U.S. Public Health Service), to eugenics laws that legalized involuntary sterilization of disabled people and people convicted of crimes, there have been many instances in which the government did not act in the interests of the public. Less egregious examples, like the prioritization of family planning services over holistic SRH, the CDC's campaign to reduce neural tube defects by instructing all people with uteri to consider themselves "pre-pregnant," and the focus on sexually transmitted infection and disease in LGBTQI+ people all speak to the need to hold the government responsible to deliver care and programs that not only do not violate human rights, but also accomplish the stated goals of improved population health.

Improving Health Workforce Diversity

The 2020 release of the IOM's *The Future of Nursing 2020–2030* took a markedly different approach to nursing workforce issues than did the 2010 report. The explicit focus of the 2021 *Future of Nursing* report was on diversity and equity in healthcare as an approach to improving population health, in contrast to the earlier report's focus on individual nurse preparation for practice (Wakefield et al., 2021). Where the 2010 report advocated for increased levels of education in nursing and expanded scope for RNs and APRNs on a national level, the 2021 report prioritizes the role of nurses in addressing social determinants of health, particularly in changes of program delivery and reimbursement models (Wakefield et al., 2021). While expanded scope of practice/full scope of practice remains a recommendation, the report considers it a means to the end of improved health equity rather than a nursing-specific benefit. Two other significant recommendations that point to a different course for nursing going forward include a recommendation that all nursing programs substantively prepare nurses to address social determinants of health, and that educational and healthcare systems consider ways to support and promote well-being for nurses (Wakefield et al., 2021). Taken together, these recommendations are much more closely aligned with public health models of care such as the U.K. model than they are with the traditional U.S. fee-for-service fragmented healthcare delivery, and if they are fulfilled will have an exciting impact on the capacity of the healthcare system to improve health for populations, particularly those who have been most harmed by the current systems in place. Given the resistance that large-scale changes to the healthcare system have encountered, it is unlikely that the ambitious 2030 timeline will be met, but this nonetheless represents a significant course correction for healthcare. Given that nurses are the largest group of healthcare providers, the adoption of these recommendations in even a partial or limited way will be expected to have a profound effect on U.S. healthcare and its delivery.

One of the common factors in the Momnibus Act, the ACA, and the *Future of Nursing* report is the need to address social determinants of health as well as individual health status in order to improve population health. As health equity research consistently demonstrates, racial and cultural congruence between providers and clients is key to improving outcomes (Hai et al., 2021; Jetty et al., 2021; Schim et al., 2007; Shen et al., 2018). One of the ongoing challenges of the healthcare system has been recruitment and retention of a diverse workforce. BIPOC healthcare providers report experiencing racism in their prelicensure programs (Romano, 2018), in postgraduate training programs (Vinekar, 2022), and as practicing providers (Byers et al., 2021). LGBTQI+ providers likewise report experiencing trans/homophobia in the same settings (Eliason et al., 2011; Lu et al., 2020; Samuels et al., 2021).

Most attempts at improving healthcare workforce diversity have focused on pipeline efforts to hire workers, without necessarily addressing retention of those workers, who may join an organization with high hopes only to encounter racism, homo/transphobia, ableism, and/or sexism. This is not unique to healthcare, and we can take lessons from other industries in seeking to solve them. In the decades since Congress passed the Civil Rights Act of 1964, corporations have experimented with dozens of diversity measures such as diversity training, diversity performance evaluations for managers, affinity networks, mentoring programs, diversity councils, and diversity managers. In a 2007 report of a study of 829 companies, companies that gave diversity councils or diversity managers responsibility for recruiting and retaining more women and BIPOC people into good jobs or created formal mentoring programs typically demonstrated significant increases in the diversity of managers (Dobbin et al., 2007).[18] In the past decade, evidence has emerged to show a growing emphasis on diversity, equity, and inclusion (DEI) on the experiences of women and the state of work more broadly. What ultimately drives organizational health and performance is not just women's representation in companies but also the company's inclusive culture—the way in which all colleagues are equally accepted, respected, and engaged in the business, regardless of gender or other characteristics. The challenge ahead lies in achieving this, and that requires sustained, multiyear, organization-wide change efforts, changing mind-sets, and transforming performance models—a whole ecosystem (McKinsey & Company, 2017).

Tackling racism and discrimination—both personally and in the workplace—is daunting and often viewed as divisive. Renewed efforts are needed to reform healthcare institutions—to hire, promote, train, and retain staff of diverse backgrounds to fully represent the diversity of the populations served (Budig et al., 2019; Dill et al., 2020). Retention has proved to be one of the most difficult parts of diversifying the healthcare workforce and reflects the unwillingness of systems to change structural aspects of racism that harm employees after hire. Engaging the assets and knowledge from communities of color and heeding their beliefs and perspectives, as well as hiring staff from within these communities, will help identify and promote effective policies (Bassett, 2015). Community-based work is congruent with the ACA and IOM priorities for healthcare but must be truly community-driven and -centered, rather than externally devised. Hall and Fields (2013) advocate for "positive profiling" to address and prevent racial health disparities and inequities. They suggest nurses can use evidence to remove barriers to care and implement strategies to avoid the potential for implicit racism that results in delays in care, reduced referrals, or suboptimal treatment.

Although more research is needed to examine the effects of racism, alone and in combination with other forms of social injustice (e.g., class, gender, sexual identity), it is also critical for White professionals to lead discussions among themselves and with their students about the history of power, bias, and racism in the United States and within the healthcare workforce, as well as the current existence of these structural inequalities. As so eloquently stated by Dr. Martin Luther King, Jr. more than 50 years ago, "In the end, we will remember not the words of our enemies, but the silence of our friends; and there comes a time when silence is betrayal" (King, 1957). However, the recent backlash against teaching what opponents term critical race theory (although CRT is a context-specific concept to explain systematic racism developed by Black scholars [Crenshaw et al., 1995], and not how the term is politicized) may limit the ability of faculty to do so in some jurisdictions going forward. This will further increase the need to critically examine and name racism and other inequities in professional spheres if it cannot be done in educational settings.

White professionals must themselves grapple with processes that lead to worsening conditions faced by many people of color, specifically impoverishment, segregation, incarceration, environmental threats, and related health consequences. Recognizing and discussing discrimination is an important first step; using counter-stereotypical exemplars and strategies to override biases must be part of the conversa-

---

[18] Much less effective are diversity training sessions, diversity performance evaluations for managers, and affinity groups for women and minorities. In the average workplace, networking programs lead to only slight increases in pay for white women and decreases for Black men. Although these groups give people a place to share their experiences, they often bring together people on the lowest rungs of the corporate ladder. They may not put people in touch with what they need to know or whom they need to know in order to move up (Campaign for Action, 2014). Mentoring programs, by contrast, appear to help women and other marginalized groups. They show positive effects for Black women, Latinxs, and Asians. Moreover, in industries with many highly educated workers who are eligible for management jobs, they also help white women and Black men.

tion (Stone & Ajayi, 2013; Vedantam, 2013). Recognizing the structural and systemic nature of racism and other oppressions is key to effectively disrupting them, as is commitment to antiracism as an actionable and specific process rather than as an individual attitude. Finally, White healthcare workers must actively seek to avoid the "white savior" mentality that can infantilize and disempower BIPOC colleagues and clients while reinforcing existing lines of power in healthcare, and instead look to BIPOC communities and leaders for ways to support work that has been ongoing in these communities (Budig et al., 2019; Dill et al., 2020).

New health workforce policies require cultural and moral shifts within healthcare organizations regarding their role in perpetuating structural racism within their own workforce that disproportionately undermines the health and well-being of BIPOC people. Such actions will require visionary leadership from CEOs and boards and likely will require incentives through the federal health financing programs such as the CMMS. For example, there is an emerging debate regarding the future structure and value of Graduate Medical Education (GME) indirect and direct payments from CMMS to teaching hospitals. One option for incentivizing this shift by academic medical centers is reforming GME payments to cover some of the costs of this shift. CMMS has supported Accountable Communities for Health (ACH) as an alternative health workforce funding method. CMMS could use the ACH program to pilot these changes in GME funding and evaluate their impact on health through the CMMS Innovation Center.

Advocacy is considered one of the central roles for nurses and other healthcare providers, which includes both advocacy for individual clients and advocacy for communities and increased justice. In terms of broader advocacy, healthcare professionals have an obligation to, for example, participate in health justice groups and nonviolent demonstrations, or to work in other ways to improve the determinants of health in their communities. Some may write editorials or lead forums and teach-ins; engage their politicians to demand change in law, policy, and practice; and work within and across the health professions to advocate for equality. As healthcare professionals, we must break the silences in whatever way we can. According to Ross (2012)—RJ feminist—we all have a role to play in seeking and building a movement against oppression in which every human being is included, and equality is a milestone in the process.

There are historical and recent examples of feminist thinking, racial politics, and the role of racial majorities and minorities in contesting racism and sexism and in demanding civil rights, voting rights, equal employment, and educational opportunities (Higginbotham, 1993; Roberts & Jesudason, 2014; Ross, 2012; Ross & Solinger, 2017). One of the most powerful movements for change in sexual and reproductive health, RJ is a human rights framework developed by Black women activists in 1994 (Ross & Solinger, 2017). It argues that reproduction must be paired with justice and situated within an understanding of the historical and contemporary complexities of the lives of Black and other people of color. RJ advocates for the right to bear children, not to bear children, and to raise those children within a just world, and in doing so, it turns traditional reproductive rights and reproductive

health conceptualizations of reproduction upside down. This radical revisioning of health and justice is a powerful model for how other aspects of health and justice can be reimagined and provides some key guideposts for change going forward. Perhaps most essentially, RJ is the work of Black women, and leadership and ownership of this work must remain with Black women. Advocacy and a desire to improve health cannot be justification for co-optation of the work of others, although that work can certainly inspire and guide future community-led change. Advocacy is central to the professional roles of healthcare workers, and doing that advocacy in ways that center the voices and decisions of marginalized people can be uncomfortable, but necessary to caring for the health of individuals, communities, and ultimately ourselves.

Institutional and Workplace Policies That Make a Difference for All Women

Women and BIPOC workers are themselves changing the work environment and culture and creating a more humane work life. With more women in the workforce, industries outside healthcare are recognizing the value of women's skills and expertise, as well as the socialization that many women experience which prioritizes communication and collaboration. The research does not support the idea that women are inherently better at relational work, but rather that women are often socialized to see such work as intrinsic to their gender role and thus may develop stronger skills in this work. These skills can be well placed to address some of the outstanding challenges in healthcare. Women workers, managers, and professionals have demonstrated skills related to attention to detail, sensitive listening, and empathetic responses, as well as an ability to motivate, organize, and direct others, because these "soft skills" are valued and incentivized in women. As traditional corporations are decentralizing and building staff networks based on teams of equals, they have found that women are often skilled at constructing and maintaining these networks. Women also may gravitate to companies that offer flexible work arrangements in order to balance work and family, and this in turn influences the number of such options available in the market. However, it is important to be cautious about assuming or expecting such skills from women solely because of their gender, and to recognize that one of the reasons women may value job flexibility to balance work–life needs is because we are failing as a society to provide adequate supports for those needs, and because men as a group do comparatively little caretaking and household management, even when both partners work.

The healthcare industry can take lessons from other business sectors that value a diverse, productive, and healthy workforce. Several studies have suggested that organizations that develop women perform better than those that do not. Since 2007 (Devillard et al., 2012), the consulting firm McKinsey & Company has released research reports, titled *Women Matter*, about gender diversity and corporate performance. The first report, *Women Matter 1* (McKinsey & Company, 2007), demonstrated a correlation between a company's performance and the proportion of women serving on its executive board. In McKinsey's *Women Matter 2010* report (Devillard et al., 2012; McKinsey & Company, 2017), companies showed that gender diversity was best supported within an ecosystem consisting of management commitment (executive champion with established targets for gender diversity), women's development programs (skills development and networks to master corporate codes and raise ambitions/profiles), and a set of enablers (human resource policies/processes, family/personal support mechanisms, indicators to track improvements). At the same time, institutions need to be mindful of the double burden of this kind of emotional labor on clinicians, particularly nurses and BIPOC women in the lowest paid health occupations, for whom the expectations as frontline workers, clinicians, and nurturers can be overwhelming (Vinson & Underman, 2020).

Some health systems have focused on improving the work environment, finding that shared governance and shared leadership creates a more satisfying work environment when that shared governance is genuine and has the potential to create real ownership of the work environment (Cheung & Aiken, 2006; Goldstein et al., 2021). This in itself may not improve equity, however, if the shared governance model acts to reinforce hierarchies or in group/out group dynamics. Other important attributes and policies of healthcare services that foster diversity and inclusion include participatory management, enhanced communication, adequate staffing, and investment in the development of nurses and staff. Each of these approaches—in theory—moves away from the capitalist model of labor and toward a more equitable model of collaboration to meet the needs of patients, staff, and the healthcare organization. Such a model could represent a sea change in how healthcare organizations work, and improve the efficacy of their work, but require genuine sharing of power among team members, rather than simply good intentions. While company-wide policies are an important component to achieve diversity, equity, and inclusion, evidence suggests that organizational systems, leaders, and peers/teammates are essential to shaping inclusion for employees (Goldstein et al., 2021).

Some disturbing evidence is surfacing from a study of women in the workforce during the COVID-19 pandemic. According to a 2021 report on U.S. women's workforce (McKinsey & Company & Lean In, 2021), even a year and a half into the COVID-19 pandemic, women made important gains in representation, and especially in senior leadership. But as the pandemic continues to take a toll, women are now significantly more burned out—and increasingly more so than men. There is also a disconnect between companies' growing commitment to racial equity and the lack of improvement we see in the day-to-day experiences of women of color. Women of color face similar types and relative frequencies of microaggressions as they did 2 years ago—and they remain far more likely than white women to be on the receiving end of disrespectful and "othering" behavior. And while more white employees see themselves as allies to women of color, they are no more likely than last year to speak out against discrimination, mentor or sponsor women of color, or take other actions to advocate for them.

A look at what nurses most want from health systems after a year of working during a pandemic provides some insights to health organization change. In a 2021 survey of 400 frontline nurses across workplace settings during COVID-19, investigators found four recommendations for improving

the workforce and the workplace (Berlin et al., 2020). First, nurses want their employers to make workforce health and well-being a part of the organization. For example, recognition (appreciation and economic rewards commensurate with their value), communication, and breaks to recharge are paramount. Also important are increased availability and accessibility of resources (e.g., mental health resources). Next in importance, nurses want an increase in workforce flexibility. COVID-19 accelerated the introduction of scheduling and staffing approaches to create additional flexibility in workforce deployment, and nurses were largely enthusiastic. Next, nurses want to be a part of the solution to reimagine health delivery models. Organizations may consider how to leverage digital tools and adapt care models based on client and employee preferences. For example, some employers may continue (or expand) clinician use of telemedicine platforms, allowing nurses to work remotely more often. And nurses want developing or expanding care models that allow RNs and APRNs to work to their full authority and skill. Finally, organizations should strengthen talent pipelines and build skills for the future. Demand for talent is increasing, and skill sets and capabilities required are shifting. Organizations will need to reskill in some areas, as well as bolster their recruiting pipeline for clinical roles—in some cases leaning on new partners or professional development pathways.

Some policy makers suggest that the health system is a core institution and argue that it should be seen as a space in which to begin to challenge gender and racial norms that have a negative impact on the nature of healthcare workers and clients (Dill et al., 2020; Govender & Penn-Kekana, 2008). While some medical centers have developed strategies to indirectly mitigate the impact of social determinants of health among their own patients by assessing patients' needs and linking patients' needs to community resources, few medical centers have made public commitments to directly addressing the social determinants of health among their own lowest paid employees (i.e., by paying living wages and implementing career ladders). This investment in human capital as opposed to investment in physical and marketing capital (e.g., luxurious hospital atriums, hospital building expansions/renovations, and vertical and/or horizontal healthcare acquisitions and mergers), could ultimately improve the BIPOC diversity within higher wage positions. Many healthcare systems compete for small pools of BIPOC candidates for physician, nursing, technical, and leadership positions rather than advancing the careers of their own BIPOC employees, and by doing so, ultimately increasing the pool of qualified, well-trained BIPOC people within high pay positions.

Interventions recommended to redress gender biases and discrimination in the healthcare system call for action on multiple levels, such as integrating examinations of sexism and racism into healthcare institutions and healthcare worker training and education. This examination must also include issues affecting LGBTQI+ people, since patriarchy, assumptions about gender roles, and heterosexism contribute to both sexism and to homo/transphobia. A first step in eliminating gender bias in the workplace is to understand it. For example, in one large company, they found that in the promotion process, women were judged by their performance, whereas men were judged on their potential. This same gender bias existed in recruitment; recruiters were much more critical of female than male candidates (Devillard et al., 2012). More importantly, healthcare organizations can address gender and racial inequity by raising wages and creating advancement opportunities for workers in direct care and reproductive[19] occupations (Budig et al., 2019; Dill et al., 2020; Duffy, 2007).

In order to reward and retain highly trained staff, many healthcare systems are offering career development as part of their practice change model, providing career ladders with promotions both within and beyond the job category, wage increases, quality bonuses, educational reimbursement, and other nonsalary incentives. Career ladders that make meaningful change within an organization identify pathways or tracks for workers' advancement with pathways that help workers identify a training program and credential that leads to career advancement and upward mobility. Nursing career ladders consistently provide substantial upward mobility for workers in the lower levels of the nursing hierarchy, such as nursing assistants. Healthcare organizations should also support access to higher education by partnering with community colleges to create tuition remission arrangements, onsite classes, and flexible scheduling to accommodate coursework. Workforce development programs that do not reward workers for their time and effort or that make false promises of career advancement are exploitive of low-level workers and risk increasing worker burnout and turnover. Furthermore, the use of career ladders in healthcare organizations cannot address the systemic and chronic devaluation of BIPOC women's labor in the healthcare sector without promoting the well-being of the communities they serve by working to improve the jobs that they provide for workers at all educational levels, including those at the lowest levels. Career development for frontline workers may provide a broader benefit, enabling local healthcare organizations to serve as "economic engines" for the communities they serve, providing not only culturally competent healthcare to clients, but also economic opportunity and upward mobility to the healthcare workers who often originate from those same communities.

In addition to advancement policies, increasing wages in direct care and reproductive occupations are essential to health workforce availability, quality, and equity (International Labour Organization [ILO], 2018). Evidence is mounting about hard work and dismissal compensation received by these workers, especially in the context of COVID-19 (Newman, 2019; Rockwood, 2020). Wages have a direct impact on workers' households and communities. A recent research study found that about 50% of Black and Latina female direct care workers earn less than $15 per hour, and only 10% have employer-based health insurance coverage; increasing the minimum wage to $15 for these low-wage BIPOC women would result in a reduction of household poverty rates among female healthcare workers by up to 27% (Himmelstein & Venkataramani, 2019). Furthermore, increasing wages may benefit healthcare organizations because minimum wage increases have been linked to reductions in injuries and illnesses and decreased worker turnover, with no impact on nursing home profits.

Awareness of structural sexism and assumptions about gender should be a key aspect of both initial and continuing education and organization culture, as well as increased acceptance of a variety of gender performance/expression options. Learning awareness of the gender dynamics that exist has an impact on how and when men and women seek care and how they talk about their symptoms in interactions with healthcare workers but does not require that there be a single acceptable model for "men" or "women." Understanding gender dynamics does not preclude improving acceptance for people who may "do gender" in a way that is unexpected or less common.

Policies that make it easier for women to have children and stay employed can make a difference. One study suggests that a lack of "family-friendly" policies, such as paid leave and a right to work part-time, have contributed to nearly 30% of the decline in female labor force participation (Blau & Kahn, 2013; Goldfarb, 2014). Because working less than full-time has been found to be a risky career move—shown by a number of studies that fewer part-time workers advance in their careers—companies are institutionalizing flexible working options (Devillard et al., 2012). However, men and women may not be exercising these options at the same rate, which may increase, rather than decrease, the gender gap (Perry-Jenkins & Gerstel, 2020). Research suggests that the gender gap in pay would be considerably reduced and might vanish altogether if companies did not have an incentive to disproportionately reward individuals who labored long hours and worked particular hours. Goldin (2014) recommends that a solution for reducing the gender pay gap is workplace flexibility in terms of hours and location. However, these adaptive responses do not address the underlying assumptions about who is responsible for the emotional and physical labor of family/personal work (Perry-Jenkins & Gerstel, 2020), and may reinforce these assumptions if they better enable them to continue.

As the COVID-19 pandemic has demonstrated, women's participation in the workforce is dependent on the existence of reliable child care and education options during a work shift. Since March 2020, women's participation in the workforce decreased significantly compared to men, which is largely attributed to the loss of reliable child care, disproportionate employment in high-loss industries like food service and retail sales, the shift to virtual K-12 education, and the need to facilitate children's education when in a virtual setting (Alon et al., 2020; Stevenson, 2020). These impacts illustrate the need for a social commitment to establish and maintain the kinds of infrastructure—high-quality child care, education, and family leave—that other peer nations have utilized for decades. The pandemic did not create a failing system of family supports, but it uncovered the lack of infrastructure that will allow women full participation in noncaretaking roles. In the postpandemic era, we have a choice about which path we want to take.

---

[19] The concept of reproductive labor is central to an analysis of gender inequality, including understanding the devaluation of cleaning, cooking, child care, and other "women's work" in the paid labor force. This term highlights the challenges to understanding occupational segregation and the devaluation of reproductive labor in a way that analyzes gender and race-ethnicity in an intersectional way and integrates cultural and structural explanations of occupational degradation (Duffy, 2007).

Anticipating women's career needs and planning for them can encourage women to return to work after maternity leave or take on the challenge of a promotion. Identifying women of high potential with the aim of getting them further along in their career paths before they have children has been instituted by some companies because more senior women tend to be more likely to return to work; however, this model may reify a false choice between high achievement and parenting that, in the end, men are not asked to make. Instead, institutions can choose to invest in employees regardless of their personal or family situations. Institutional strategies for recruiting women and other marginalized groups into healthcare careers means starting early, which can include educating young people about opportunities in high school and offering summer internships, establishing low barrier "pipelines" into healthcare and advancement within healthcare, and understanding what supports enable people to enter the profession and thrive in it. These efforts must also consciously address the intersectional effects of racism, sexism, classism, ableism, and homo/transphobia in order to ensure that their benefits do not only accrue to a specific subset of women.

Focusing on gender diversity and disrupting sexism in the healthcare workforce does not mean seeking the end of cisgender men. Human development is not a zero-sum equation in which there are winners and losers. Rather, improving equity in the workplace increases the justice and humanity inherent in that workplace, which can be beneficial for all workers regardless of gender. Men are often currently disincentivized to take advantage of programs such as onsite child care, career planning, and flextime options because of assumptions about gender roles and norms (Chung, 2019; Karu & Tremblay, 2018), but what might a more flexible model look like? Can an institution's culture be modified to promote the wellness and wholeness of its employees, regardless of that employee's gender? If not, how can we expect to improve health for the people we care for?

SUMMARY

Healthcare has been and will continue in the near future to be women's work, and this work cannot be separated from women's lives. Although the increasing numbers of women doctors, dentists, and pharmacists receive a lot of attention and praise for "making it in a man's world," the majority of paid and unpaid healthcare providers are women, with BIPOC women disproportionately concentrated in low-paying, high-risk work with less compensation and little power. Federal and institutional policies may support diversity in the healthcare workforce, with an emphasis on collaboration and team-based care advanced by new technologies, if they are enacted in ways that maximize their potential for equity. The challenge to healthcare systems and employers lies in their ability to empower the workforce, create equitable solutions for workers and for clients, and to find paths for posttraumatic growth following the Covid-19 pandemic. The challenge for women healthcare providers will be to participate in the evolving definitions of what their contributions should produce versus the historical traditions of professional authority. Person-centered caregiving, working in teams, and long-term problem-solving provide the basis for real solutions to the current healthcare dilemmas, including workplace solutions to institutional gender bias and racial discrimination at all levels of the healthcare workforce.

ACKNOWLEDGMENT

We recognize our colleagues who made significant and thoughtful contributions to the first and second editions of this chapter. First, Dr. Carol Leppa contributed as the lead author in the first edition of *History of Women's Health Nurses*. And in the second edition, we acknowledge Lisa Stern, NP, MS, a PhD candidate in the history of health sciences, for her update of the women's health professional history; Dr. Monica McLemore and Dr. Candace Burton for their contribution to the section on intersectionality of discrimination of healthcare providers (both individuals and institutions); and Kim Hildebrandt-Cardozo, CNM, MS, for her critical review of the history and current status of women as healthcare providers.

REFERENCES

References for this chapter are online and available at https://connect.springerpub.com/content/book/978-0-8261-6722-4/part/part01/chapter/ch02

CHAPTER 3

Women and Healthcare*

KIM CURRY AND VERSIE JOHNSON-MALLARD

Improved women's healthcare has been accomplished based on science, policy developed by women for women, and the support of stakeholders for women's health and healthcare. Women have successfully pushed for a redefinition of women's health that transcends the boundaries of reproductive healthcare and incorporates a life-span view that accommodates their health from the perinatal period to the end of life. Women have reconfigured the delivery of women's healthcare by challenging existing systems to replace fragmentation with integration and coordination of healthcare services. Women have services unique for females such as birthing centers, menopause clinics, and transgender care.

Among a long list of aspirations for enhancing women's healthcare, the following are significant (Schiebinger, 2003):

- The greater conceptual clarity of sex, gender, and related concepts has prompted health professionals to demonstrate growing recognition of the importance of gender awareness as essential to avoiding bias and racism in the delivery of services, as well as educating future health professionals and conducting research.
- Healthcare professionals are prepared to provide comprehensive healthcare using gender-sensitive models that span lives of females.
- Researchers design studies in collaboration, analyze changes in women's health data and compare them to health data for men and other male and female vertebrate animals, seek new methodologies and methods to optimize the inclusion of heterogeneous populations of women, and translate their findings directly to clinical and public health practice and for women, themselves.
- The analysis of problems women face in obtaining appropriate, gender-sensitive healthcare has prompted policy changes to promote access to comprehensive, coordinated, integrated women's healthcare that is associated with higher levels of satisfaction, higher rates of use of preventive services, and reduced morbidity and mortality.

- Global research efforts have underscored the importance of gender and race inequality as experienced in many countries and its relationship to patterns of morbidity and mortality and provided evidence to propel changes to promote women's health and enhance the care women receive while ensuring equity.
- Around the world women's contributions to health and healthcare in their countries are valued, compensated, counted, and accounted for in the gross domestic product.

  ○ Countries are accountable to women in providing gender-appropriate and equitable care.
  ○ In the United States, researchers and legal experts have joined in advocating for removing politics from reproductive healthcare and practice, embracing policies promoting equity in access and care for all women (Agénor et al., 2022).

In this chapter we:

1. Examine concepts of sex and gender as a basis for considering gender-sensitive healthcare.
2. Review sexism and gender, racism, and bias as they have existed in U.S. healthcare, education of health professionals, and research.
3. Explore advances in the education of healthcare professionals to provide women's healthcare.
4. Analyze changes in women's health research to guide care (translation).
5. Propose a gender-sensitive approach to healthcare for women, including integration for sexual and reproductive health (SRH) in primary care and life-span approaches.
6. Analyze policy challenges within our existing healthcare "systems" in the United States, including progress and promise of healthcare reform and the Patient Protection and Affordable Care Act (ACA, 2010).
7. Consider a global view of women and healthcare.

---

*This chapter is a revision of the chapter that appeared in the second edition of this textbook, coauthored with Nancy Fugate Woods, Ellen F. Olshansky, and Deborah Ward, and we thank them for their original contribution.

SEX, GENDER, AND HEALTHCARE FOR WOMEN

The definition and differentiation of *sex* and *gender* have been important contributions to the study of women's health and healthcare. Since the second wave of feminism in 1960s and 1970s in the United States, we have seen acknowledgment of the importance of understanding sex and gender, as both are related to health. During most of the 20th century, *sex* was used to guide research about men and women irrespective of the focus of the work being either biological or sociocultural. Contemporary theory and research about sex and gender have revised the thinking of many health professionals about what it means to be female (sex) and what being a woman means within the context of our society (gender).

In documents about women's healthcare and research, sex has been viewed as biologically determined, based on chromosomal patterns and the effects of sex hormones on reproductive organ development. Scientists formulating the National Institutes of Health (NIH) early agenda for research on women's health (U.S. Public Health Service [USPHS], 1992) distinguished between the biological definitions of *male* and *female* based on chromosomal sex and introduced the consideration of gender. Scientific interest in chromosomal and biological elements of sex has been fueled by genomics research (Wizemann & Pardue, 2001).

Definitions of *sex* have emanated from biomedicine and more recent developments in gender-specific medicine, whereas social scientists have defined *gender* as a social category that includes changing definitions of appropriate roles, division of labor, economic power, and political influence. When seen as static differences, both sex and gender have been viewed through dualistic lenses through which *sex* became defined as male or female based on the reproductive organs and functions and *gender* was viewed as a person's representation of self as male or female, rooted in biology and shaped by one's environment, experience, and socialization. The limitations of these definitions may preclude a view of the interplay of sex and gender that allows for the influence of the body and of culture and history, as they simultaneously influence health and behavior. In addition, scholars have emphasized the importance of analyzing gender in relation to other power structures such as class, race/ethnicity, and sexuality (Hammarström et al., 2014).

Concepts of sex and gender continue to be revised as the binaries of male and female are being reexamined to accommodate the human experience of both sex and gender. An analysis of sex, gender, intersectionality, embodiment, gender equality, and gender equity examined their importance to health research (Agénor et al., 2022; Hammarström et al., 2014). Hammarström et al. propose that sex, in interaction with gender, offers the potential for the analysis of sex as a continuum with various options that include X and Y chromosomes, hormonal levels, and internal and external genitalia, and also opens up the possibility to view sex and gender as integration of body–mind–context. These considerations can be viewed not only at the level of the individual, but also at the level of social structures in which gender relations are integrated, including labor markets and the healthcare system.

Hammarström et al. (2014) include the concepts of intersectionality and embodiment to further expand our thinking about sex and gender. Intersectionality is grounded in assumptions of heterogeneity within groups of women and men, prompting recognition that individuals are defined by multiple intersecting dimensions. Women simultaneously have a gender, class, ethnicity, ability/disability, sexual orientation, and age. The addition of these dimensions to gender further guides consideration of equality and equity, denoting populations whose risk for discrimination and bias is unique (Hammarström et al., 2014). Embodiment focuses on how one's body interacts with environments. Body–mind is viewed holistically, in contrast to the split between body and mind, in which the lived body functions as mind–body–world. Social embodiment prompts consideration of social processes and gender relations as they relate to health. Moreover, ecosocial theory integrates the body, mind, and society in understanding the health impact of social conditions, how sex and gender become interwoven in life.

Gender equality and gender equity aid analysis of the distribution of opportunities, resources, and responsibilities between women and men. Equality concerns equal rights, or the absence of gendered discrimination, and gender equity concerns the needs of the genders. Notions of sameness-difference reflect concerns about equality, whereas fairness reflects concerns about equity, concepts important to understanding policy. Do policies advocate equality, the absence of discrimination, and gender equity as meeting the needs of both women and men?

Krieger's (2003) tutorial "Genders, Sexes, and Health: What Are the Connections—and Why Does It Matter?" pointed out that gender relations can influence the expression and the interpretation of biological traits and that sex-linked biological characteristics can contribute to or amplify gender differentials in health. Krieger also includes a definition of *sexism* as inequitable gender relationships and references it to institutional and interpersonal practices by which dominant gender groups accrue privilege by subordinating other gender groups and justify these practices via ideologies of innate superiority, difference, or deviance (Krieger, 2003). Based on clear definitions of sex and gender, Krieger (2003) provides instructive case examples of the differential roles of gender relations and sex-linked biology on health outcomes. As an example, gender relations can be a determinant of men versus women using physical violence against intimate partners (gender relations affect exposure to intimate partner violence) at the same time that sex-linked biology affects exposure (sex as a determinant of muscle strength and stamina and body size). Thus, the health outcome of a lethal assault is related to the greater physical strength and size of men and the gender-related skills and training in inflicting and warding off attack.

Current thinking in healthcare admonishes health professionals to uncouple sex and gender in an effort to establish "gender equal" healthcare. Bachmann and Mussman (2015) consider the marginalization of the transgender community and advocate for a redefinition of what constitutes "normal" male and female. Agénor et al. point out research that indicates sexual preference is not binary, with bisexuality being reported as a sexual option, and that neither sexual preferences nor gender identity are binaries and that gender minority research in the United States is needed to repeal harmful laws and advance social justice (Agénor et al., 2022). These concepts are discussed further in Chapter 20, Primary Care of Lesbian, Gay, and Bisexual Individuals, and Chapter 25, Caring for the Transgender and Gender Nonbinary Patient.

Sex and gender have different and multifaceted influences on health and healthcare, and both have played a role in shaping federal policy. In 1985 an important and still relevant Task Force Report on Women's Health set in motion a series of events that included the development of the Office of Research on Women's Health (ORWH) at the NIH in 1990, development of the first NIH Research Agenda on Women's Health in 1991, and establishment of the Centers of Excellence (CoEs) for Women's Health Care in 1996. Although this body of work clearly focused on both sex and gender, the USPHS Task Force Report offered an early definition of women's health as focusing on health problems specific to women, more common or more serious in women, having distinct causes or manifestations in women, having different treatment or outcomes in women, and having high morbidity and/or mortality rates in women (USPHS Task Force on Women's Health Issues, 1985). The Task Force also recommended that both biomedical and behavioral research should be expanded to ensure emphasis on these areas. Consequences of the Task Force's efforts included three objectives for the ORWH: ensuring that issues pertaining to women were adequately addressed (diseases, disorders, and conditions unique to, more prevalent among, or far more serious in women for which there are different risk factors or interventions for women than for men); ensuring appropriate participation in clinical research, especially clinical trials; and fostering increased involvement of women in biomedical research, emphasizing their decision-making roles in clinical medicine and research. The inclusion of women in NIH-funded health research was required, and this inclusion criterion has since been extended to minorities (underrepresented ethnic groups). In the early reports that emanated from USPHS and NIH, sex and gender were sometimes used interchangeably, but in documents dating from the 2001 Institute of Medicine (IOM) report *Exploring the Biological Contributions to Human Health: Does Sex Matter?* clear distinction was made more frequently between sex and gender (Wizemann & Pardue, 2001).

SEX AND GENDER DIFFERENCES, GENDER BIAS, AND HEALTHCARE

The social and health sciences literature provides evidence of the complex influences of sex and gender in delivering personal health services, educating health professionals, and researching women's health. Investigators have found evidence of sex and gender differences and bias in diagnosis, treatment, prescription of medications, and hospitalization. This body of work contributed important understanding about practices that need to be corrected in the interest of gender equality and gender equity. As noted in Chapter 1, Women and Their Health, women and men experience many common types of health problems, but there are health problems that are unique to women or are much more prevalent

among women than men. Thus, based on research one would anticipate sex differences in the incidence and prevalence of health problems. Gender differences also would arise from the ways in which women and men are socialized. Sex and gender bias occurs in situations in which differences are attributed to women and men that result in one sex or gender receiving care that is unequal or inequitable and not based on clinical research (Streed et al., 2021). Some examples of the complexity of sex and gender differences and bias in healthcare are explored in the following sections.

Mental Health and Mental Illness

Classic studies (Aslin, 1977; Broverman et al., 1970) demonstrated that women judged to behave in gender-appropriate ways were also judged to be psychologically less healthy than men and that the gender of a therapist can influence expectations about women's mental health (see Chapter 12, Mental Health, for further discussion). Assumptions about one sex (female) as inherently less healthy mentally introduced bias into the judgments of actual health. Current work on women's mental health supports that good mental health is essential. Good mental health includes avoiding long-term stress and taking active steps to incorporating rest and sleep.

Gender has been associated with mental health and illness because of sex and gender differences in the presentation and prevalence of various types of mental illnesses and the assumptions about gender underlying ways in which women and men are diagnosed with mental illness. The American Psychiatric Association (APA, 2013) notes that the prevalence of psychiatric disorders varies between men and women. Also mental health can present in different ways and is affected by hormones throughout a woman's lifetime. Women demonstrate higher rates than men of many mental health disorders: mood, anxiety, eating, sleep, personality, somatoform, dissociative, obsessive-compulsive spectrum, and impulse control, as well as late-onset schizophrenia with prominent mood symptoms and dementia of the Alzheimer type (APA, 2013). There is greater prevalence of depression among women. A variety of explanations have been proposed to account for these differences. Some propose that gender role socialization encourages girls and women to express symptoms and discourages these behaviors in boys and men. Others attribute gender differences in mental health to the tendency of women to internalize and men to externalize symptoms/disorders. Still others implicate the more stressful nature of girls' and women's lives, including adverse early experiences of abuse, as well as gender stereotypes about women's and men's mental health. Of note, Black women experience gendered racism, which is harmful to their mental health (Jones et al., 2022).

A study of gendered mental disorders examined masculine and feminine stereotypes about mental disorders and their relationship to stigma. Boysen et al. (2014) found that people held gendered stereotypes about mental disorders, with a masculine stereotype consisting of externalizing disorders such as antisocial personality and substance use and a feminine stereotype of internalizing disorders such as anxiety and mood. The masculine disorders and symptoms elicited more stigma than feminine disorders. Whether men and women fall into gender-neutral diagnostic categories because of gender-neutral evaluations or are guided into gender-biased diagnoses as a result of gender-biased evaluations by health professionals is an important question that continues to be studied.

The intricate interweaving of socially constructed definitions of gender and their relation to diagnostic taxonomies is also illustrated by the continuing controversies surrounding various diagnoses in revisions of the *Diagnostic and Statistical Manual of Mental Disorders* (*DSM*), the standardized diagnostic manual that forms the basis for diagnosis and treatment, not to mention billing and data collection. Investigations of premenstrual dysphoric disorder (PMDD) illustrate the controversies over a menstruation-related mood disorder and their potential consequences on women's health (Zachar & Kendler, 2014; Zachar et al., 2022). Proposals to include PMDD as a diagnosis in the *DSM* (3rd rev. ed.; *DSM-III-R;* and 4th ed.; *DSM-IV;* APA, 1987, 1994) prompted an intense debate, but PMDD was included in the following *DSM* (5th ed.; *DSM-5;* APA, 2013) without significant objection. Concerns about stigmatizing a normal part of women's menstrual cycles had justified not including PMDD in the *DSM-III-R.* Instead of including it in the manual, the APA included a section labeled "late luteal phase dysphoric disorder" (LLPDD) in an appendix. *DSM-IV* retained the diagnosis in the appendix but changed the label from LLPDD to PMDD. In 2013, the APA included PMDD as a diagnosis in *DSM-5.*

A number of factors encouraging the inclusion of PMDD in the *DSM-5* include potential economic effects, social–political consequences, ethical concerns, conservative attitudes, and peer pressure. A recent interview study of mental health clinicians involved in the consideration of PMDD inclusion in the *DSM-IV* revealed several elements of their decision processes that guided their thinking. Reasons given for including PMDD in the main *DSM-IV* included agreement on PMDD symptoms and their time course, recognition of benefits of treatment, and the use of a biomedical model for understanding psychiatric disorders. Those who favored deleting PMDD from *DSM-IV* raised issues such as the likelihood of false-positive diagnosis of PMDD, questionable diagnostic validity of the psychological symptoms, and the belief that premenstrual syndrome (PMS) and PMDD were embedded in cultural assumptions about gender roles. Feminist values and negative social consequences were additional reasons for deleting PMDD from *DSM-IV.* Reference was made to the earlier diagnosis of hysteria and the likelihood of PMDD being used against women or masking the real reasons for women's anger and distress. Another issue was the conviction that the diagnosis of PMDD was being advocated by pharmaceutical manufacturers who stood to profit from sales of medications.

Reasons given for retaining PMDD in the *DSM-IV* appendix included philosophical ideas regarding the nature of disorders: PMDD was seen as an exacerbation of an existing condition, but not a mood disorder because of the inclusion of many somatic symptoms, such as bloating. Some expressed opinions that higher standards of evidence should be available to support the inclusion of PMDD in the *DSM,* weighed with the risk of having a diagnosis that could be used against women. Peer pressure may have been a factor for some of the

participants in the *DSM-IV* decision process (Zachar et al., 2022; Zachar & Kendler, 2014).

Of interest is the fact that the *DSM-5* revision attracted controversies over several decisions but not over PMDD. Several reasons were offered for the lack of debate, including generational changes among feminists who objected to *DSM-IV* decisions and availability of additional research on the validity and treatment of PMDD. At the same time, there were concerns about sexism influencing these decisions, as reflected in a failure to recognize that women's distress was related to cultural roles and powerlessness (Zachar et al., 2022; Zachar & Kendler, 2014).

In the same time frame that Zachar and Kendler (2014) published their investigation, Browne (2015) asked if PMDD was really a disorder. She asserted that PMDD was a socially constructed disorder that pathologizes understandable anger and distress that women experience. Moreover, she notes that PMDD is culture-bound, not a universal syndrome; for example, it is not commonly reported in Asia. Browne argued that PMDD symptoms are caused not by a mental disorder but instead by one's environment and that such distress should be recognized without being defined as a pathology. Browne recommended a feminist solution: changing attitudes toward women's suffering instead of pathologizing women's anger and distress.

These two sets of analyses of PMDD as a diagnosis illustrate the underlying processes by which a contested diagnosis gains acceptance despite consideration of evidence that it is socially constructed. Moreover, these analyses raise important questions about motivations that drive professional decisions to identify new diagnoses. Are health professionals induced to create new diagnoses in the interest of helping women who experience distress? In advancing the position of all women in society? In the interest of gender equality? Gender equity? To what extent was gender disparity or gender bias involved in these deliberations?

Medical Diagnosis and Treatment

The history of women's medical diagnosis is similarly rife with now-discredited categories such as hysteria (Leavitt, 1984). Indeed, there is evidence that links the gender of patients to the type of diagnosis health professionals assign to them. Whether these differences are attributable to health professionals' gender stereotypes or bias or to gender differences in the presentation of symptoms and associated prevalence of disease is challenging to interpret.

Heart disease is the leading cause of death for U.S. women, yet diagnosing and treating cardiac events in women remain fraught with challenges. One challenge in the diagnosis of cardiac events is the differences in symptoms women and men report. Instead of the classic chest pain reported by men, women often report different types of symptoms. In one study of women and men in a myocardial infarction (MI) registry, women were more likely to complain of pain in the left shoulder/arm/hand, throat/jaw, upper abdomen and between the shoulder blades; vomiting and nausea; dyspnea; fear of death; and dizziness. Moreover, women were more likely to report more than four symptoms. There were no significant differences in the reporting of chest pain, feelings of pressure or tightness, diaphoresis, pain in the right shoulder/arm/hand, and syncope. Although women and men did not differ in reports of the chief acute MI symptoms (chest pain, feelings of tightness or pressure, and diaphoresis), women were more likely to report additional symptoms (Fang et al., 2019). Gender differences in symptom reporting by women must be known to prevent delays in getting emergency care by first responders and other members of the health team.

Findings illustrate the complexity of gender effects in the presentation of symptoms as well as in the management and health outcomes; female gender is associated with higher in-hospital mortality rate (Fang et al., 2019). Suggested hypotheses to account for increased female mortality from MI include more serious comorbidity, longer times to revascularization, and use of less optimal reperfusion strategies. Significant differences between women's and men's experiences before reaching the hospital include a smaller proportion of women using the emergency medical ambulance service and less direct access to the cardiac catheterization lab in case of angioplasty. The average time of ischemia was longer for female than male patients, with delayed treatment at all stages, including time from pain onset to calling for help, call to hospital door time, and door to balloon or thrombus aspiration time. Lower rates of some reperfusion techniques in women were apparent. In-hospital morbidity and mortality rates were higher in women, and hospital stay was longer. The mortality rate for women was twice that for men and affected primarily women younger than 69 years. Evidence of excess mortality in the hospital for women remained even after adjustments were made for characteristics of the patients and time to revascularization and the revascularization technique used.

These results present several dilemmas for interpretation: Were the deaths attributable to differences in time to seeking care? Did women call for help later than men after experiencing chest pain? If so, why did women call later? Did they not associate their symptoms with MI? Were women diagnosed less accurately in the absence of ST-segment elevation? Did women receive different treatment? Why did they have less access to the cardiac catheterization lab? Did those who did not survive die from a different disease process (e.g., rupture of the coronary artery plaque that immediately occluded their arteries vs. a more gradual development of plaque that gradually reduced coronary artery blood flow)? How much of the excess mortality was attributable to sex differences in the disease process versus gender difference in the response to chest pain or other symptoms? And how much was due to gender, race, and ethnic bias in treatment?

Pharmacotherapy

Sex and gender differences appear to influence the prescription of medications and ambulator care. During ambulatory care visits 22% of women reported at least two chronic conditions compared to 19% of men; depression was reported more frequently between ages of 45 and 64 years for both genders with depression screening occurring equally between males and females.

Women appear to experience more medication-related adverse reactions, and if they are the targets of over-the-counter drug advertising and physician recommendations for over-the-counter drugs, it could be speculated that clinicians' expectations and market forces might be powerful determinants of the care women receive. Might male physicians (and other male prescribers) embrace certain expectations about women's behavior and adjustment and tend to determine that women are more in need of medications, for example, than their equally troubled but more reticent men patients? Do women request medication more than men, and if so, why? It is not known what the U.S. population of women has as a baseline standard of demand and need for care, apart from the products and services eagerly sold to them. As Ruiz and Verbrugge (1997) stated:

> We know little about how men and women voluntarily adopt some risk behaviours and risk exposures, their different perceptions of symptoms and expression of complaints, how their milieux of social support affect health and health behaviour, and their behavioral strategies for treating and adjusting to health problems. (p. 106)

The conditions that lead women more than men to use medicaments of all kinds await full explication. The historical development of women as herbalists clearly arose from their role as family nurse and healer (Ehrenreich & English, 1973). An argument can be made that faith in pharmaceutical therapy is a logical association with what has been called women's culture—a culture of connection and mutual aid rather than the individualism associated with male culture. Under this theoretical construct, women would be more likely to use drugs of all kinds—from diet pills to megavitamins—whereas men are more apt to be socialized to ignore or endure symptoms such as low energy, despondency, or overeating.

Women's physiology is increasingly thought to play a role in treatment. Sex differences in the pharmacokinetics of antidepressants may be influenced by female sex hormones and oral contraceptives. In a review of sex differences in response to antidepressant pharmacotherapy, Damoiseaux et al. (2014) explored evidence for differences in pharmacokinetic properties, including absorption, distribution, metabolism, and excretion of medications, in women and men. Recent research indicates that sex hormones may influence all pharmacokinetic processes (Beierle et al., 1999; Mauvais-Jarvis et al., 2021). Women experience variation in hormone levels throughout their life span, potentially influencing their response to antidepressants as well as occurrence of adverse events. Depression symptoms have been associated with deficiencies in norepinephrine, dopamine, and/or serotonin, and the presentation of symptoms in women includes a greater tendency to experience negative emotions. Because women and men appear to react differently to antidepressant therapy, these differences may be because of pharmacokinetic differences that may be attributable to sex hormone effects, and thus differences may occur in relation to the menstrual cycle, with use of oral contraceptives, and at other times of hormonal shifts such as the menopausal transition. Because estrogen modulates the neurotransmitters (norepinephrine, serotonin, and dopamine) related to depression, sex differences in the effects of psychotropic drugs affecting these neurotransmitters are not surprising. There are several sex differences in pharmacokinetic processes that include absorption and bioavailability, distribution, metabolism, and excretion. One possible example is the effect of progesterone on prolonging the gut transit time of drugs, providing greater opportunity for absorption of medications. Another is the influence of the cytochrome P450 (CYP) enzymes. Women have higher CYP3A4 activity and the CYP enzymes play a major role in the metabolism of antidepressants. CYP enzymes are modulated by estradiol. Physiologic variation during the menstrual cycle has multiple potential effects on pharmacokinetics, with multiple possible consequences for psychotherapeutic drugs prescribed for depression. For example, increasing the metabolism of antidepressant substrates may result in a lower plasma concentration and possibly lower efficacy, requiring an increase in the dose of the medication. This is of consequence in pregnant women given that clinical trials frequently exclude pregnant women. The sex differences in response to antidepressants discussed here alert clinicians to the possibility that sex-linked biology (e.g., hormonal influences) plays an important role in modulating the effects of these medications and requires careful consideration of appropriate dosage of them.

Surgery

The famous historical study by Wennberg demonstrated a national pattern of extreme variability in physician practice patterns (Wennberg & Cooper, 1999). This variability is influenced by factors such as the practice patterns of regional peers, style and location of medical school training, and penetration by specialty practice. Patient gender has also been found to influence rates and types of surgery.

Gynecology was one of the first specialty areas to fall under the scrutiny of women's healthcare analysts. As of 1980, the hysterectomy had become the most frequently performed major operation for women of reproductive years. At that time, the American College of Obstetricians and Gynecologists estimated that 15% of hysterectomies were performed to remove cancer, 30% to remove noncancerous fibroids, 35% for pelvic relaxation or prolapse, and 20% for sterilization (Scully, 1980). A hysterectomy should not be performed as an elective procedure or when more conservative treatment will suffice, and yet it was estimated that one third of hysterectomies and half of cesarean sections performed in the United States were unnecessary (Seaman, 1972). More recent evidence continues to demonstrate that nonclinical factors (physician characteristics such as background, training, experience, and practice style) play a statistically significant role in this surgical decision.

Cardiology and cardiovascular surgery exemplify another specialty practice arena studied for its utilization by gender. Although the risk of developing coronary artery disease has increased for women and decreased for men since 1950, women were less likely than men to be referred promptly for cardiac surgical consultation (Schwartz et al., 1997). The studies are still mixed in 2022 on referral, treatment, and rehabilitation in women (Mamataz et al., 2022; Verghese et al., 2022). Women and Black patients continue to appear to be significantly less likely to be referred for cardiac catheterization than men and White patients (Verghese et al., 2022). Black women were least likely of all groups to be referred.

The authors concluded that, after careful controls were applied, race and patient gender independently influenced the management of chest pain. The lower rates of referral for cardiac catheterization found in this study illustrate the importance of intersectionality of gender and race that creates unique levels of risk for women.

WOMEN'S HEALTH SCHOLARSHIP AND RESEARCH

Historical Perspectives

The transition in thinking about women's health has been dramatic, given that early efforts to redefine women's health began to emerge in the 1960s and 1970s, an era punctuated by the Title X Family Planning Program, the landmark U.S. Supreme Court decision *Roe v. Wade* (1973) protecting women's rights to choose whether or not to continue a pregnancy, and establishment of women's self-help clinics such as the Los Angeles Feminist Women's Health Center and the Boston Women's Health Book Collective (1973; Ruzek, 1978; Weissman, 1998).

Women's health scholarship, including theory and research, began to flourish in the 1970s in the wake of the resurgence of a women's health movement that focused on demystifying women's health and enhancing women's access to appropriate healthcare. One important element of this scholarship was a broad vision of women's health that transcended the limits of reproductive health and emphasized an integrated, holistic view inclusive of women's bodies, as well as their minds and emotions, in place of a fragmented view of women's health (reproductive/nonreproductive, body/mind) and focused more broadly on health and well-being, not only diseases of women (McBride & McBride, 1991). In 1989, just 3 years after the National Institute of Nursing Research was established, the first Center for Women's Health Research was funded at the University of Washington. Nursing was quick to embrace the new view of women's health. Academic programs such as the Women's Health and Healing Program at the University of California, San Francisco, School of Nursing and the development of a Women's Health Program at the University of Illinois, Chicago (Dan, 1994; Ruzek et al., 1997), led to the development of other academic programs focusing on women.

Transitions in Women's Health Scholarship

Transitions in scholarly works about women's health have been apparent. Scholars have incorporated new frameworks for studying women and employed new methodologies and methods. Novel conceptualization of women's health put women at the center of inquiry, integrated feminist theory, incorporated theoretical models of health and illness specific to women, and emphasized the importance of context in studying health from a holistic perspective, incorporating consideration of person–environment relationships and social determinants of health. Integrating biological, psychosocial, and cultural dimensions of health and emphasizing life transitions as the focus of nursing scholarship represent significant transitions (Andrist & MacPherson, 2001; Taylor & Woods, 2001). Noteworthy was the attention given to the social context of women's lives that drew scholars' attention to the consideration of racism, sexism, classism, and heterosexism (Taylor et al., 1997; Taylor & Woods, 1996).

Women's health scholars looked past empiricist methodology, and integrated interpretive, naturalistic methodologies as well as critical methodology, marking a body of emergent scholarship in nursing in the 1980s. This work emphasized the development of knowledge for and with women instead of about women; new knowledge was seen as a tool of empowerment and liberation (Andrist & MacPherson, 2001). Changing methodologies prompted investigators to engage in reflexivity, considering the impact of their relationships with the women who participated in their studies, cocreating new knowledge. Investigators were encouraged to think of themselves as situated knowers whose positions influenced what they were able to see and know. In 2000, a review of nursing research related to women's health revealed contributions in a variety of areas, including parenting, employment, caregiving, disparities in health experienced by lesbians, menstrual cycle, menopause, stress, fatigue, sleep, violence against women, and women's decision-making related to their health (Taylor & Woods, 2001). These topics reflected everyday concerns of women, many of them neglected before the 1980s.

Over the past 3 decades there have been important transitions in the scholarship of women's health. Among these are a transition from topics that were sex or gender ignorant or that assumed male as the norm to research topics grounded in the understanding of the relationship of women's lives to their health. Central among society's assumptions regarding women is the inherent otherness of women; in this context, normal, positive physiologic functions were seen as pathologic. For example, many menstrual cycle studies conducted before the 1980s were designed to detect the problems women experience because they menstruate (e.g., a hypothesized propensity for illness, violent crimes, or accidents). The new scholarship emphasized understanding menstruation as normative, seeking to learn from women about their lived experiences.

Federal Support for Women's Health Research

In 1985, the USPHS Task Force on Women's Health Issues published a two-volume report in which members recommended expanding biomedical and behavioral research that would include the study of conditions uniquely relevant to women across the life span, more prevalent among women than among men, or in which risk factors were different for women versus men, as well as treatment approaches that differed for women versus men (USPHS Task Force on Women's Health Issues, 1985). In 1986, the NIH Advisory Committee on Women's Health recommended that investigators include women in research, especially in clinical trials; justify exclusion of women from research when appropriate; and evaluate gender differences in their findings. Because of a slow response to these recommendations, the Congressional Caucus

for Women's Issues drafted the Women's Health Equity Act of 1990, which set in motion a series of events that included a Government Accounting Office study of expenditures of NIH funds on women's health research and the eventual establishment of the ORWH at the NIH in 1990. The ORWH was directed to ensure women's health issues were adequately addressed, especially those unique to women, including those for which risk factors differed from those for men, and those for which approaches to care differed. The inclusion of women in clinical trials and the engagement of women as investigators in biomedical research were also part of the original mission (USPHS, 1992). In 1991, the landmark Women's Health Initiative Study was initiated, and Dr. Bernadine Healey, the first woman NIH director, was appointed.

In 1991, the ORWH convened a Task Force on Opportunities for Research on Women's Health that developed research recommendations focusing on women's health (USPHS, 1992). This volume included a life-span view of women's health, and panelists considered science as it intersected with topics such as reproductive biology, early developmental biology, aging processes, cardiovascular function and disease, malignancy, and immune function and infectious disease. A significant contribution of this agenda was the panelists' ability to transcend the boundaries of the disease-focused institutes of NIH and focus on both reproductive and nonreproductive health issues important to women. This agenda has since been updated for the 21st century (USPHS, 1999) and again in 2010 (ORWH, 2010).

The 1999 Agenda for Research on Women's Health, including seven volumes, reflected important efforts at promoting a new level of intellectual vigor in addressing women's health (see ORWH at orwh.od.nih.gov and USPHS, 1999). The 1999 agenda grew from an inclusive process in which women's health advocates as well as scientists participated in regional and national meetings and heard public testimony. Explicit consideration of various groups of women representing America's ethnic groups and those living with disabilities enriched the agenda-setting process. The final reports reflected the deliberations and recommendations from these hearings and assessed the current status of research on women's health. Gaps in knowledge, sex and gender differences that may influence women's health, and factors that affect health of women from various populations were topics of discussion. Enhancing prevention, diagnosis, and treatment was an explicit focus of discussion, as was the development of strategies to improve the health status of women regardless of race/ethnicity, age, or other characteristics. In addition, career issues for women scientists were addressed in the report.

Research topics spanned a wide range of health issues. Among these were disorders and consequences of alcohol, tobacco, and other drug use; behavioral and social science aspects of women's health; bone and musculoskeletal disorders; cancer; cardiovascular diseases; digestive diseases; immunity and autoimmune diseases; infectious diseases and emerging infections; mental disorders; neuroscience; oral health; pharmacologic issues; reproductive health; and urologic and kidney conditions. Chapters also address the use of sex and gender to define and characterize differences between men and women. A special consideration was research design for studies of women, addressing special populations of women, racial/ethnic and cultural diversity, and multidisciplinary perspectives. Although promising, the 1999 agenda gave little emphasis to the health consequences of poverty in women, the power differential between men and women that influences health, and the gendered allocation of work in U.S. society. Moreover, the global perspective needed to examine the consequences of economic development and social policy on women's health was missing (Woods, 2000).

One special initiative of the ORWH has been the development and funding of the Specialized Centers of Research (SCORs). This innovative interdisciplinary research program focuses on sex differences and major medical conditions affecting women. SCORs support research integrating basic, clinical, and translational research approaches to incorporating a sex and gender focus. Eleven SCOR awards are co-funded by the ORWH and the National Institute on Aging, National Institute of Arthritis and Musculoskeletal and Skin Diseases, Eunice Kennedy Shriver National Institute of Child Health and Human Development, National Institute of Diabetes and Digestive and Kidney Diseases, National Institute on Drug Abuse, National Institute of Mental Health, and U.S. Food and Drug Administration (FDA). Some of the topics addressed by the SCORs include addiction and health, substance abuse relapse, fetal antecedents to sex differences in depression, irritable bowel syndrome and interstitial cystitis, pelvic floor disorders, molecular and epidemiologic factors and urinary tract infections, gender-sensitive treatment for tobacco dependence, neurovisceral sciences and pain, sex differences in musculoskeletal disorders, intrauterine environment and polycystic ovary syndrome, vascular dysfunction, and cognitive decline (National Institutes of Health [US], Office of Extramural Research, NIH Outreach Notebook Committee, & NIH Tracking/Inclusion Committee, 2002).

The Building Interdisciplinary Research Careers in Women's Health (BIRCWH) is a mentored career development program that aims to increase the number of women's health and sex differences investigators. This program contributes to the development of future scientists in women's health and sex differences and is already revealing best practices in interdisciplinary mentoring for research careers (Domino et al., 2011; Guise et al., 2012).

A 2001 IOM report *Exploring the Biological Contributions to Human Health: Does Sex Matter?* (Wizemann & Pardue, 2001) alerted scientists to the fact that biological sex differences were important, but often ignored in research, especially research using animals or cells/tissues. Nearly a decade later, Zucker and Beery (2010) reaffirmed the finding that consideration of sex difference in cellular and animal studies is not yet the norm. A recently issued NIH notice focuses on the consideration of sex as a biological variable in NIH-funded research, stipulating that sex as a biological variable will be factored into research designs, analyses, and reporting in vertebrate animal and human studies, to be effective in 2016 (NIH, 2015).

The year 2010 was a watershed year for women's health research, marked by the publication of the ORWH report "Moving into the Future with New Dimensions and Strategies: A Vision for 2020 for Women's Health" (ORWH, 2010) and the IOM report *Women's Health Research: Progress, Pitfalls, and Promise* (IOM, 2010). The updated ORWH research agenda included six new goals to address contemporary issues:

1. Increase sex differences research in basic sciences studies.
2. Incorporate findings of sex and gender differences in the design and applications of new technologies, medical devices, and therapeutic drugs.
3. Actualize personalized prevention, diagnostics, and therapeutics for girls and women.
4. Create strategic alliances and partnerships to maximize the domestic and global impact of women's health research.
5. Develop and implement new communication and social networking technologies to increase the understanding and appreciation of women's health and wellness research.
6. Employ innovative strategies to build a well-trained, diverse, and vigorous women's health research workforce.

In the same year, the IOM of the National Academy of Sciences (IOM, 2010) published the report *Women's Health Research: Progress, Pitfalls, and Promise.* The IOM committee was charged with "examining what research on women's health has revealed; how that research has been communicated to providers, women, the public, and others; and identify gaps in those areas" (p. 2). The committee was directed to identify examples of successful dissemination of findings, paying particular attention to how the communication influenced women's use of care and preventive services, and to make recommendations where appropriate.

The IOM committee focused on health conditions that were specific to women, more common or more serious in women, had distinct causes or manifestations in women, had different outcomes or treatments for women, or had high morbidity and/or mortality rates in women. Seven recommendations from the IOM committee included:

1. U.S. government agencies and other relevant organizations sustain/strengthen focus on women's health, including research spectrum of genetic, behavioral, and social determinants of health and change over lifetimes.
2. The NIH, the Agency for Healthcare Research and Quality, and the Centers for Disease Control and Prevention develop targeted initiatives to increase research on populations of women with highest risks and burdens of disease.
3. Research on women emphasizes promotion of wellness and quality of life; conditions that have high morbidity and affect quality of life; development of better measures or metrics to compare health condition effects, interventions, and treatments; end points to include quality of life outcomes (functional status or functionality, mobility, and pain) in addition to mortality.
4. Cross-institute initiatives in the NIH support research on common determinants and risk factors that underlie multiple diseases and on interventions to decrease the occurrence or progression of diseases in women—urge NIH ORWH and Office of Behavioral and Social Sciences Research collaboration.
5. Government and other funding agencies ensure adequate research participation by women, analysis of data by sex, and reporting of sex-stratified analyses.

6. Research emphasis should be on how to translate research findings into practice and public health policies rapidly and at practitioner and overall public health systems levels.

7. U.S. Department of Health and Human Services (DHHS) appoint a task force to develop evidence-based strategies to communicate and market to women health messages based on research results.

Both the ORWH and the IOM reports emphasized understanding the determinants of health, especially sex and gender differences, as well as life-span considerations. Compared with the ORWH report, the IOM report emphasized the importance of social and environmental determinants of health. The IOM committee commented on scientific progress in understanding conditions affecting women, study of vulnerable groups of women, and use of appropriate research methods. Both reports emphasized the importance of accelerating the translation of research findings into practice and policy implications and communicating with women about their health.

The IOM committee (IOM, 2010) judged research on the following set of conditions to have made major progress: breast cancer, cervical cancer, and cardiovascular disease. Conditions that had some progress included depression, osteoporosis, and HIV/AIDS. Conditions judged to have little scientific progress included unintended pregnancy, maternal morbidity/mortality, autoimmune diseases, alcohol and drug addiction, lung cancer, gynecologic cancers other than cervical cancer, nonmalignant gynecologic disorders, and Alzheimer disease.

Shaver et al. (2013) offered comments relative to both the 2010 ORWH research agenda and the 2010 IOM report on *Women's Health Research*. Their recommendations included:

1. Expanding the development and testing of gender-sensitive interventions—this requires giving voice to women's experiences and perspectives, incorporating complexities and diversities of women's experiences, integrating reflexivity in research, and promoting empowerment and emancipation. Gender-sensitive interventions affirm gender equity by considering needs and preferences of genders and do not privilege the experiences of either gender. Gender-tailored or gender-specific interventions are designed for one gender based on differences and preferences (Im & Meleis, 2001). Women-specific interventions are grounded in the reality of women's lives, unique responsibilities, and biology as exemplified by the SUCCESS program for smoking cessation for pregnant women (Albrecht et al., 2011; Li & Froelicher, 2010).

2. Attending to the intersectionality of gender with other health determinants—essential to the translation of research findings to services. Women simultaneously are Black, Hispanic, poor, heterosexual, and living with disabilities (Hankivsky et al., 2007; Kazanjian & Hankivsky, 2008).

3. Rebalancing emphasis on behavioral, integrative, and pharmacologic therapeutics—requires emphasis on nonpharmacologic therapies such as lifestyle modification. The integration of biological aspects of appetite regulation and metabolism, as well as behavioral, social,

psychological, physical environments of everyday living (such as oppressive social and built environments, understanding obesity) exemplifies this rebalancing.

4. Increasing the study of underemphasized conditions disproportionately affecting women (e.g., functional or stress-related disorders). Examples include studies of osteoporosis and incontinence as they develop over the course of the life span.

5. Enhancing scientific attention to unintended pregnancies and sexually transmitted infections (STIs)—requires attention to the dynamics that promote unintended pregnancy as well as combined, multimodal interventions aimed at prevention, such as providing education about and access to contraceptives, slowing rates of sexual initiation, and enhancing condom use (Jemmott & Jemmott, 1992; Jemmott et al., 2007, 2008). Supporting women in coercive relationships to choose contraception and avoid unprotected sex is an important component (Teitelman et al., 2011).

6. Expanding investigations of prevention and treatment consequences of violence against women—includes study of life-span consequences of violence for girls and women as well as outcomes of military sexual trauma (MST) for women in the military (Yano et al., 2011). The interrelationship of STIs, violence, and unintended pregnancy is an important consideration.

7. Increasing studies of effective technologies and their use to support women as they age and in their caregiving roles—includes adapting communication technologies to detect health problems and provide real-time feedback of health information.

8. Accelerating testing of the models for translating research findings directly to the public—can include using communication technologies to convey health information to women and requiring investigators to develop communication and dissemination plans for their studies (Shaver et al., 2013).

Many have advocated for a reformulation of science, clear views of women's experiences through lenses ground by women. This could include qualitative methods of analysis that are reaching new levels of rigor and reproducibility. It could include the interpretation of biological uniqueness as a sign of health rather than deviance or illness. And reformulated science could include designing research *for* rather than *on* women, with liberating rather than oppressive results (Woods, 1992). Simply adding a cohort of women to a study designed to illuminate issues grounded in thinking about men or increasing the proportion of women researchers in a male-dominated field will not solve the problem of advancing a more complete understanding of women's health.

In 2019, the NIH developed a 5-year plan, the Trans-NIH Strategic Plan for Women's Health Research, to address specific goals for research related to women's health. The plan includes:

- Advancing rigorous research that is relevant to the health of women
- Developing methods and leveraging data sources to consider sex and gender influences that enhance research for the health of women

- Enhancing dissemination and implementation of evidence to improve the health of women
- Promoting training and careers to develop a well-trained, diverse, and robust workforce to advance science for the health of women
- Improving evaluation of research that is relevant to the health of women

This plan follows the NIH policy of factoring sex as a biological variable into research and is part of the effort by NIH to promote rigorous and transparent research in all areas of science.

Research Policy and Funding

As women's health research agendas for the nation have changed, so have policies to support new visions for women's health research. The NIH Revitalization Act of 1993 mandated that the NIH establish guidelines for including women and minorities in clinical research (NIH, 1994). Starting in 1995, all NIH-sponsored research had to comply with those guidelines, which mandated that women and minorities be included in the research; that cost could not preclude such inclusion; and that outreach, recruitment, and retention efforts would be supported (National Institutes of Health [US], Office of Extramural Research, NIH Outreach Notebook Committee, & NIH Tracking/Inclusion Committee, 2002). The peer review process exerts at least an indirect influence on women's health research. The Center for Scientific Review of the NIH, which sets guidelines and policy for research review, now explicitly includes gender, ethnicity, and geographic distribution among its principles for reviewer selection (Center for Scientific Review, 2002).

The FDA (n.d.) has had an Office of Women's Health since 1994. The office has dispersed over $35 million in funds to researchers, including studies on safe labeling, guidance for industry on product development, communications about FDA-regulated products used by pregnant women, and regulatory decisions about products used by women. In addition, the FDA has addressed diversity of clinical trial populations to be more inclusive of women, among other underrepresented groups. Updated guidelines for eligibility criteria and enrollment include:

- Inclusive trial practices
- Enrollment of participants who reflect the characteristics of clinically relevant populations with regard to age, sex, race, and ethnicity
- Inclusion of women in clinical trials in adequate numbers to allow for analysis by sex, for example, by avoiding unjustified exclusion based on sex and taking other actions to promote inclusion
- Expectations for making trial participation less burdensome and more convenient (FDA, 2020)

Of note, the research efforts of the largest single group of healthcare professionals—nurses—were not organizationally included in the NIH until 1986, when the National Center for Nursing Research was established. One of the smallest of the institutes, the nursing center received some $144 million in the 2016 budget, compared with much larger budgets for institutes focusing on prevalent diseases in the United States (www.nih.gov).

Funding for training new investigators in women's health has been established by NIH's ORWH via the BIRCWH program, as well as for programs for nascent scientists among high school girls and women already established in biomedical careers but who encounter barriers that limit their advancement. In addition, the ORWH has funded SCORs described earlier. The picture for funding healthcare research relevant to women has improved, but careful observers should bear in mind the continued disproportion and not forget the baseline from which it started and that funds are limited given multiple competing priorities.

Women are not the only group who may be underrepresented or even mistreated in research studies, but women's unique needs deserve special attention and consideration from prospective researchers. Sechrest (1975) was an early reporter on the coercion that can be applied to ensure women's participation in research projects. She noted that early research on oral contraceptives took advantage of relatively uninformed and low-resource Puerto Rican women who had few options for avoiding pregnancy. More recently, Critchley and colleagues (2020) surveyed studies on menstruation and found underrepresentation in research but that menstrual health and hygiene are gaining momentum, raising awareness that is leading to popular movements to address menstruation-related barriers facing girls in schools and "menstrual equity" movements in higher-income countries.

Financial incentives or provision of free medical care for women and their children may also be irresistible elements in recruiting. Continuing examination of ethics related to women's health research is warranted. Some agencies are becoming more attuned to potential ethical problems related to women's participation in health-related research. One example of this is the FDA (n.d.) Office of Women's Health Research, with goals including tracking the participation of women and special populations in clinical studies and improving subset analyses based on patient demographics.

SEX AND GENDER CONTENT IN HEALTH PROFESSIONS CURRICULA

Historical Perspectives

Analyses of professional education materials, as well as influential advertising directed toward health professionals, demonstrate a history of continuing sex and gender bias. Early work revealed inaccurate information in medical texts concerning subjects such as the strength of women's sexual drives, the roles of the vagina and clitoris in orgasm, and the incidence and prevalence of female sexual dysfunction (Scully & Bart, 1973). One text portrayed women as inherently sick and asserted that the feminine core consisted of masochism, passivity, and narcissism. At the same time, the text advised physicians to counsel their women patients to simulate orgasms if they were not orgasmic with their husbands.

Naomi Wolf, in her 1997 book *Promiscuities* on sexual coming-of-age, provided the lecture we never had on the clitoris. Recognized by medical writers throughout time, the clitoris was well described in 1559 by the Italian anatomist Realdo Columbo. But when sexual purity and ill health for women were popularized, and as the home and family were separated into their own private spheres in the 19th century, information on this sexual organ, along with cognizance of female sexual desire, was suppressed (Wolf, 1997). Wolf argues that Freud was hardly the first authority to examine and misunderstand the clitoris, and she reminds readers that generations of social critics suggested that close attention to female anatomy and physiology could improve intimate relationships. The authors of *A New View of a Woman's Body* (Federation of Feminist Women's Health Centers, 1991) examined the basic research on the anatomy and physiology of the clitoris and have clarified the role of the clitoris as a vital sexual organ whose existence was often omitted from medical texts.

Textbooks and advertisements aimed at gynecologists have reinforced the status and intellectual asymmetry between patients and doctors (Fisher, 1986). "By controlling women and their reproductive capacities," wrote Fisher, "medical domination functioned to sustain male domination" (p. 160). A newer generation of critic suggests that both texts and advertisements have moved away from portraying women as inferior and victim and instead are portraying women as invincible to illness and especially age, so long as they make the right choices about their behavior and the medical goods and services they purchase (Kaufert & Lock, 1997). "Health is the new virtue for women as they age… [I]f she allows her body to deteriorate, then she becomes unworthy, undeserving of support" (Kaufert & Lock, 1997, p. 86). Being characterized as invincible is not much of an improvement over being characterized as a victim, when both stereotypes prevent development of healthcare providers and systems that respond to women's complex and various needs.

Progress in Health Professional Education

Some improvements in care for women have been brought about by national initiatives, such as the establishment of women's health offices in various federal agencies (USPHS, NIH, and FDA) and women's health services at the Veterans Administration (VA). Nonetheless, evidence suggests that the progress in enhancing health professionals' education in women's health and healthcare has been slow and incremental.

Efforts to change the capacity of the healthcare workforce to deliver comprehensive women's healthcare have attempted to reduce fragmentation in service delivery by assembling teams and creating structures such as Women's Health Centers to deliver care. In 1996, the USPHS funded the creation of CoEs in Women's Health at multiple sites in the United States. These had important missions that involved creating new models of care for women, educating health professionals in these models, supporting interdisciplinary clinical research, and mentoring. These are described in more detail in our discussion, Toward Gender-Sensitive Healthcare.

Essential to improving the capacity for delivering comprehensive women's healthcare is the education of health professionals in ways that expose students to:

- Curricula that include current knowledge about women's health based on research on sex and gender differences, among other topics
- Practitioner role models who exhibit sensitivity to and awareness of women's health issues
- Models of service delivery that are gender sensitive and comprehensive
- Organizations that reflect positive values about women and their contributions to the health professions as well as to the larger society
- Faculty with expertise in comprehensive women's health and healthcare and commitment to advancing comprehensive care for women (Writing Group of the 1996 American Academy of Nursing Expert Panel on Women's Health, 1997)

Slow integration of gender-specific information in professional curricula can be attributed to faculty's lack of awareness of scientific evidence, lesser value placed on this information, bloated curricula that already exceed reasonable amounts of content, and resistance to curricular change by those who struggle to maintain areas of knowledge they value more highly.

A recommended strategy for fostering health professions' education about women's health and healthcare includes promoting faculty development in women's health; comprehensive healthcare for women through continuing professional education (including nursing, medicine, pharmacy, etc.) offers the opportunity to integrate updated scientific information, as exemplified in the DHHS Office on Women's Health (OWH) professional education materials. Another option is assessment of specific competencies of faculty and credentialing through specialty board examination in practice disciplines (e.g., nursing and medicine), which afford opportunity to evaluate what providers know. Certification by examination in areas of expertise, such as the North America Menopause Society Menopause Practitioner Examination is one example of a postgraduate certification of expertise (see www.menopause.org). Other strategies include use of interdisciplinary and interprofessional team teaching, introduction of standardized patients demonstrating complex women's health issues, and incorporation of comprehensive and current scientific resources through online libraries accessible across educational institutions and practice settings in which students are placed. Finally, creating and maintaining an audit of exemplary clinical practicum sites (e.g., the CoEs in women's healthcare) provide a rich resource for educational programs.

Wood et al. (2011) urged efforts to "improve women's health and basic sex differences educational curricula for trainees and continuing education for practitioners for all members of today's new interdisciplinary health care teams" (p. 102) and specified the inclusion of nurses, nurse practitioners, physician assistants, dentists, health psychologists, dietitians, and physical therapists as well as physicians (p. 102). Because research is ultimately connected to the preparation of health professionals and in turn to the quality of care provided, the use of tax dollars to prioritize opportunities for research on sex differences and women's health, as well as cross-disciplinary research ensuring communication of findings to current and future health professionals, merits high priority.

The DHHS et al. report on women's health curricula (2013) summarized the deliberations of expert panels on interprofessional education focusing on women's health curricula. Among the expert panel recommendations are those related to:

- Conceptual approaches to women's health content and key content areas for collaboration
- Assessment of institutional readiness for integrating women's health education
- Creation of collaborative opportunities in women's health
- Teaching of recommendations for interprofessional education in women's health

A proposed conceptual framework for interprofessional women's health education is organized by three theoretical perspectives and five major content areas. The three theoretical perspectives are related to the social determinants of health, life-span approach, and cultural considerations. Social determinants of health were identified as central in understanding health inequities, access to care, and environmental and social contexts shaping well-being. The Commission on the Social Determinants of Health (2008) from the World Health Organization (WHO) provided an elaboration of individual (race/ethnicity, socioeconomic status, and gender) and contextual (immediate surroundings, environmental conditions, workplace dangers, and larger cultural patterns, including gender norms) characteristics. Among these are gender inequality, access to care, and experiences related to poverty. Life-span approaches encourage consideration of a woman's current context, role, and life demands, as well as an appreciation for the cumulative experiences affecting her health from the pregnancy experiences of one's mother through one's old age. (Osteoporosis is not a disease of old age but one of cumulative bone health across the life course.) Cultural considerations, as defined in this report, include points of intersection of gender, race/ethnicity, nativity, sexual identity, and sexual orientation, among other characteristics. Intersectionality is a theoretical approach foundational to understanding the diversity of women's health experiences.

The five key content areas proposed for interprofessional curricula include role of the health professional, biological considerations, selected conditions, behavioral health, and wellness and prevention. Table 3.1 includes common content areas across the health professions identified by the Health Resources and Services Administration (HRSA) panel. This report also includes strategies for promoting collaboration across health professions and several teaching recommendations for interprofessional education in women's health.

The implementation of curricular recommendations, such as those in the DHHS et al. report on women's health curricula (2013), focuses on the challenges for faculty. Essential to this transformative effort will be faculty development efforts that infuse both theoretical perspectives of

women's health and research findings about women's health and healthcare.

In addition to HRSA, the ORWH at the NIH has funded Career Development awards, the BIRCWH that were created to promote fellowship training for medical residents and postdoctoral trainees in other disciplines. These programs have enlarged the capacity for preparing investigators for team science and were discussed earlier in this chapter (Domino et al., 2011; Guise et al., 2012).

In recent years, concerns have been raised about the intersection of politics and healthcare provider education. These controversies have impacted women's health provider training. In particular, polarization has occurred around contraception and abortion services. In response to multiple reports of interference, the Women's Health Expert Panel of the American Academy of Nursing issued a position statement decrying political interference in SRH research and health professional education (Taylor et al., 2017). In the position statement, the authors report several instances in which state governments enacted restrictions on lawful SRH services and extended these restrictions to the training of healthcare providers in delivery of these services, including clinical placements in certain facilities. The authors also cited academic administrators as other sources of restrictions on research and education in SRH and noted that the Academy "supports the principles and practices of academic freedom in general, and specifically, as they apply to SRH research and health professional education" (Taylor et al., 2017 p. 347).

Moving Toward the Future

The movement forward in recognizing the special health needs of women accelerated in the late 20th century. This led to enhanced interest in women's health as a field of study. This in turn has developed into a sex- and gender-based medicine (SGBM) movement (Rojek & Jenkins, 2016). The scientific foundations laid in women's health and gender studies need further incorporation into the curricula of health professionals, but there has been some progress toward integration of SGBM concepts (Rojek & Jenkins, 2016).

Johns Hopkins University has established a global women's health fellowship program. The 2-year program integrates clinical training and global health with a focus on women's healthcare in low resource areas. The program pairs an OB/GYN physician with an APRN for collaborative interprofessional learning and research (Johns Hopkins University, n.d.).

The American Academy of Family Physicians (AAFP) has developed an updated curriculum for family medicine physicians specific to women's health and gynecologic care. The curriculum includes a comprehensive list of competencies, knowledge, and skills to master. The authors recognize that "family physicians must be trained to care for women throughout the life cycle and must appreciate challenges such as adolescence, sexuality, family planning, balance of family life and career, and aging within the female patient's culture. Health promotion—including screening, counseling, and vaccination—is a foundation of family medicine. For the majority of their reproductive lives, most women try to prevent pregnancy, so we highlight this aspect of care" (AAFP, 2018).

TABLE 3.1 Common Content Areas in Women's Health Across the Health Professions

AREA	SAMPLE TOPICS
Role of the health professional	Ethics
	Knowledge of other health professions
	Gender in provider–patient communication
	Patient-centered decision-making
	Interprofessional education
Biological considerations	Age
	Sex
	Genetics
	Hormonal influences
	Pharmacokinetics and pharmacodynamics
Selected conditions	Autoimmune disorders
	Cardiovascular disease
	Endocrine disorders
	Endometriosis
	Infectious disease, especially HIV infection
	Pregnancy and breastfeeding, especially medications taken during pregnancy and periodontal health in pregnancy
	Metabolic disorders
	Musculoskeletal health
	Neurologic conditions
Behavioral and mental health	Anxiety/stress
	Depression/bipolar disorders
	Domestic/intimate partner violence
	Eating behaviors/disorders
	Sexual behavior
	Substance abuse
	Traumatic experiences
Wellness and prevention	Access to care
	Environmental health
	Exercise physiology
	Hormonal transitions
	Nutrition
	Oral health
	Reproductive choice, family planning, and obstetrics
	Preventive health screening and immunizations
	Work–family balance

Source: U.S. Department of Health and Human Services, Health Resources and Services Administration, & Office of Women's Health. (2013). Women's health curricula: Final report on expert panel recommendations for interprofessional collaborations across the health professions *(p. 14). U.S. Department of Health and Human Services.*

Within nurse practitioner (NP) education, women's health nurse practitioners (WHNPs) are already one of the six focus areas of education. WHNPs are attuned to the movement toward the clinical doctorate as the entry level degree for NPs. While recognizing that master's programs fully prepare specialists as advanced nurse practitioners in women's health, the National Association of Nurse Practitioners in Women's Health (NPWH) as an organization has endorsed the NP doctorate degree (DNP) to provide advanced competencies and interprofessional education to add to existing skills. Specific to WHNPs, the national NPWH organization has called for the DNP curriculum for the WHNP population focus to incorporate the WHNP Guidelines for Practice and Education (NPWH, 2016).

HEALTHCARE FOR WOMEN: NEW MODELS

A notable shift in healthcare over the past few decades has been from a monopolistically physician-centered and traditionally authoritarian manner of delivering personal health services to a pluralistic array of clinicians, healers, and approaches to cure and care. Moving over time from word of mouth to the telephone book, and more recently the internet, services as diverse as acupuncture and music therapy are entering the everyday consumer vocabulary. At the end of the 20th century, mainstream clinical groups were surprised and even shocked to learn that more visits are paid to alternative than to mainstream clinicians (Eisenberg et al., 1998). At the end of the 20th century, women used alternative therapies more than men (49% vs. 38%); higher income persons and those with college education were more likely to use alternative therapies, but the national use of at least one alternative treatment was 42%, a significant increase from 34% in 1990 (Eisenberg et al., 1999). An expansion in women's use of complementary and alternative healthcare resources was noted, especially in the wake of the findings from the Women's Health Initiative Study. Newton et al. (2002) surveyed women in the Group Health Cooperative plan, learning that 76.1% used any of the therapies, 43.1% used stress management, 37.0% used over-the-counter alternative remedies, 31.6% used chiropractic therapy, 29.5% used massage therapy, 22.9% used dietary soy, 10.4% used acupuncture, 9.4% used naturopathic or homeopathic therapies, and 4.6% used herbalists. Among women who used these therapies, 89% to 100% found them to be somewhat or very helpful (Newton et al., 2002).

The lure of $12+ billion in consumer buying power alone has been enough to bring window dressing and even some fundamental change to healthcare service delivery. Although the evolution of some models of women's personal healthcare delivery has been the result of humanistic movements within some of the professions, women themselves have had a profound influence on the structure of personal health services. In some instances, such as the increasing use of midwives, traditional modes of healthcare, often culturally linked, have come into wider use (Paine et al., 1999). In other instances, women have created new kinds of services, such as self-help clinics, caregiver support teams, and resource groups on the internet. In some cases, professionals appropriated women's efforts, creating modified forms of personal health services that remain firmly under the control of professionals (e.g., the development and promotion of home-like birthing rooms in hospitals).

Healthcare settings such as self-help clinics arose from the women's health movement, which Marieskind (1975) described as a grass-roots organization dating from about 1970. Drawing parallels to the popular health movement of the mid-19th century, Marieskind saw modern interest in women's health linked to activism for political gains for women. Just as the popular health movement was associated with gaining the vote for women, the 20th century's women's health movement was linked to a progressive, feminist political and economic agenda (Leavitt, 1984). Ruzek (1978) and Marieskind (1975) reported some common features of women's health movement organizations: reduction in hierarchy, changes in the profit-making orientation, increased use of lay workers, involvement of clients in their own care, and commitment to a feminist ideology.

Morgen and Julier (1991) revisited a sample of organizations arising from the women's health movement to document development and change over the decades since the late 1960s. They mailed questionnaires to 144 women's health clinics, advocacy groups, and education organizations. The authors reported that a significant number of questionnaires were returned, indicating that the organization was no longer in existence (the actual number was not reported). Three quarters of the responding organizations described themselves as focused on prevention or self-care; two thirds identified themselves as ideologically feminist. Commitment to low-income and minority women was high; most of the organizations served poor and minority women either in excess of or in direct proportion to the percentage of low-income and minority women in their communities. These characteristics conform to much of the original expressed intent of the women's health movement. In contrast to the organizational mission, the organizational structures have tended to change over the decades, from egalitarian staff models (e.g., in some women's health clinics, pay was equal for all workers) to more traditional ranking of workers and from consensus decision-making to hierarchical authority. Staff hiring, training, and development continue to reflect feminist principles such as diversity and group solidarity. This study suggests that the women's health movement continues to influence the delivery of health services and that, not without struggle, alternatives to the health business-as-usual continue their work.

TOWARD GENDER-SENSITIVE HEALTHCARE

Women's healthcare has been described as a "patchwork quilt with gaps" (Clancy & Massion, 1992), reflecting the fragmentation of care that women have experienced, and the lack of some health resources women need. Sadly, that model remains prevalent in many healthcare systems. Nonetheless, many have pursued answers to the question: What could gender-sensitive healthcare look like? Leaders in women's healthcare have been exploring new models to deliver healthcare that would be informed by theoretical and conceptual advances related to sex and gender and healthcare reform efforts, in general. Critics of contemporary healthcare for women, as well as those concerned with improved healthcare for men, have advocated gender-sensitive healthcare. Recommendations to enhance gender sensitivity have emphasized understanding existing gender differences and incorporating these into services. Moreover, some advocates for holistic healthcare emphasize the importance of integration of the concept of intersectionality in healthcare, which warrants consideration of factors such as social class, ethnicity, and sexual orientation in addition to gender.

In a recent study of efforts to bring gender sensitivity into healthcare practice, Celik et al. (2011) identified opportunities and barriers at the health professional, organizational, and national levels. For health professionals, barriers included gender-sensitive medical curricula and on-the-job training in workplaces. Opportunities and barriers at the organizational level related to organizational culture and infrastructure in which balance/imbalance between men and women healthcare professionals shape the consideration of gender with respect to the health professionals as well as patients. Protocols and guidelines used in organizations codify strategies for diagnoses and treatments but may not be based on gender-specific evidence. Finally, policy at organizational as well as national levels is influential in building a gender-sensitive healthcare system. Such considerations could include the incorporation of efforts to tailor care to local populations, reflecting the realities of everyday life. Celik et al. (2011) advocate mainstreaming gender in ways that reorganize, improve, develop, and evaluate policy in ways that support gender equality perspectives. They note that gender-sensitive healthcare will require changing systems and structures as well as enhancing the understanding and skills of health professionals.

Each of these efforts has the attendant risks of reproducing the gendered approaches to healthcare that reinforce gender stereotypes and biases. Gender-neutral or gender-ignorant care is not the goal, but the use of gender-specific theory is evolving to transform care in ways that do not privilege male versus female experiences but do promote gender equity (Im & Meleis, 2001). Gender-tailored or gender-specific interventions are those designed for one gender, reflecting gender as a major factor influencing health. Attention to gender in the scholarship guiding healthcare as well as the education of health professionals will remain critical in the delivery of gender-sensitive healthcare for women.

Centers of Excellence in Women's Health

In an effort to model excellence in women's healthcare, in 1996 the DHHS OWH established the first National Centers of Excellence in Women's Health. By 2009, 18 centers had been developed and designated as part of the national CoEs in Women's Health by the OWH of the DHHS. Seed money funded development of model clinical services for women. Core characteristics of the CoEs included comprehensive, women-friendly, women-focused, women-relevant, integrated multidisciplinary care (Milliken et al., 2001). These centers were envisioned as women-centered sites where primary care would be integrated with reproductive healthcare and prevention/screening efforts, welcoming to women, sources of health education and information and referrals, and capable of delivering comprehensive care across the life span. Desirable features were highly visible women providers and staff, atmosphere and environment not threatening or inappropriate to women, and availability of information of particular interest to women. Some of the specific services provided included age-appropriate preventive health services and screening, family planning, gynecologic care, obstetric care, and care for menopause, mental health issues, breast cancer, osteoporosis, and incontinence. Some centers were established as providing "one-stop shopping," meaning that all services were provided under a single roof/site, whereas others developed as centers without walls. Women's preferences supported both models; for example, some preferred the decentralized without-walls model, as it offered them more choice of providers and more privacy.

Some additional contributions of the CoEs included informational and referral, educational and referral, services of health professionals representing a variety of disciplines, but these are never fully described nor are their contributions to care (Milliken et al., 2001). Some centers contributed culturally appropriate patient education materials and resources in multiple languages to promote informed decision-making. CoEs intended to offer flexible scheduling to accommodate multiple demands in women's lives (e.g., as family caregivers, employed workers) and incorporated expanded hours of operation, community-based sites, transportation assistance, and translation services.

Centers were "sold" to academic health centers based on their ability to develop downstream revenues, serving as magnets for women and their families as patients. Much less attractive to these academic health centers were the transformative approach to care and contributions to the educational mission of the institutions. Although many examples are offered of contributions to medical education, there is no mention of the education of the other health professions associated with CoEs (Fife, 2003).

Unique aspects of these CoEs were the integration of research, education, and clinical care in the centers and provision of care for a more diverse population than those receiving care at other women's health centers across the nation (Weisman et al., 1995; Weisman & Squires, 2000). Indeed, the populations cared for by the CoEs included a larger proportion of women of color and more postreproductive age women than in comparison sites (Killien et al., 2000; Mazure et al., 2000; Weisman & Squires, 2000). Although the translation of research to care is implied in many of the reports of the CoEs, this terminology was not characteristic.

The CoEs included outreach efforts in their development and found that among the most successful were those that involved existing community groups committed to women's health in their planning (Fife et al., 2001). Among their efforts were partnering with other community groups dedicated to women's health, participation in existing grass-roots efforts within the community, and CoE-initiated efforts. Elements of education and healthcare were involved in most efforts. Some examples of community groups were state departments of health, local Native American organizations, minority health coalitions, groups addressing domestic violence, and health alliances. Grass-roots community programs include city and county health departments' efforts to work with women's groups/populations, and CoE-initiated programs that could be delivered to community groups, such as smoking cessation, sponsorship of a day-long conference on women's health, educational materials for teens, and collaborative mobile breast cancer screening programs with a fully equipped outreach Care-a-Van staffed with bilingual volunteers. Partnership with the YWCA, malls, churches, community centers, domestic violence shelters, food banks, retirement communities and nursing homes, non-English speaking communities, housing assistance/homeless shelters, and community events represented some of multiple efforts to bring health information and screening to communities (Fife et al., 2001).

In addition, the CoEs were committed to incorporating the needs of racial/ethnic minority populations into newer care paradigms (Jackson et al., 2001). Jackson et al. (2001) pointed out that an ideal model of healthcare for women of color would consider providers of care, content and process of care, and the healthcare system in which the model operates. They point out that care providers should reflect the diversity of the populations they serve. Absent that diversity, providers need knowledge, attitudes, and skills to provide culturally appropriate care to all women, especially underrepresented ethnic groups. As members of multidisciplinary teams (they name the many health disciplines needed), health professionals together collaborate to address complicated social and healthcare needs of women of color. Content and process of care for women of color should reflect the higher burden of illness, poorer health outcomes, and greater prevalence of risk factors for chronic diseases than other women experience. Life-span approaches for women from adolescence to old age and the integration of prevention, primary care, chronic disease care, reproductive health, and complex psychosocial issues and mental health are needed. Some of the unique services needed include comprehensive risk assessment, community outreach, case management (vs. care or resource management), interpreter services, and health education. Case managers were recommended to bridge women of color and healthcare institutions and links to community resources. Strategies that include providing transportation, locating facilities in nontraditional settings, and extending operating hours stretch the typical use of resources in academic health centers. Commitment to diversity and social justice will be tested by institutions that take this mission seriously. Creative partnerships with institutions in the community in which the center is located are essential to serving specific populations of women whose vulnerability makes their access to care especially challenging. Some of the centers offered courses focusing on health topics for African American or Hispanic women, and others offered classes to medical students, staff, graduate students in nursing, university employees, and to community volunteers.

Some of the challenges to these centers in academic health centers included the marginalization of faculty who practiced in the center; because of requirements of practice panel size and hours available in the clinical setting, many providers in these settings were not those in senior academic appointments who were also teaching students and leading research efforts. The metrics for evaluating productivity also pressed providers and given the practice patterns of women providers who often are sought out by patients for their ability to communicate about their concerns, providers were at risk of being penalized for "lack of productivity." The publications of the CoEs use the cover term *medicine* as they describe the centers and their contributions, obscuring the roles of other health professions in the development of these centers. Consequently, it is impossible to evaluate the impact of all healthcare professions and their contributions, nor is it possible to track interprofessional practice and education in these centers. Sadly, these centers did not foresee the integration of APRNs into the mix of providers that is needed to care adequately for women.

The CoEs represented a new model for women's healthcare in academic health centers that united women's health research, teaching, clinical care, public education and outreach, and career advancement for women in the health sciences (largely focused on medicine vs. other health professions). Based on their first 3 years of experience, Gwinner et al. (2000) suggested that this model required transformation from the fragmented set of activities in academic health centers to an integrated system focused around the goal of advancing women's health. Institutional commitment, dedicated professionals, and ability to build on existing resources and bring added value to their institutions were important components.

In an effort to determine whether these new CoEs were truly making different contributions to women's healthcare, Weisman and Squires (2000) compared the first 12 national CoEs in Women's Heath designated by the DHHS OWH with 56 hospital-based primary care women's health centers that had been identified in the only source of nationally representative data on primary care women's health centers (the 1994 National Survey of Women's Health Centers). Although their analyses revealed similarities of some organizational and clinical attributes of the hospital-based programs that preceded the CoEs, the CoEs demonstrated integration of clinical services with research and medical training in women's health and delivery of services to a more diverse population of women.

In addition to providing some unique features for women, the CoE staff also contributed to the evaluation of healthcare provided in the centers. Anderson et al. (2001) conducted a qualitative analysis of women's satisfaction with primary care using a panel of focus groups in the National CoE in Women's Health program. Seeking patients' perspectives in an effort to evaluate women's satisfaction with primary care delivered in the CoEs, focus groups of ethnically diverse women (*N* = 137) were conducted nationwide on women's experiences and attributes of healthcare that they valued. Women revealed holistic concepts of their health, including physical, mental, and emotional dimensions. Women's general view on their healthcare spanned general, psychological/mental health, social support, roles, reproductive health, childbirth, alternative medicine, and prevention. Dimensions of primary healthcare important to women included access, office staff service and courtesy, privacy and respect, empathy and empowerment by healthcare providers, provider skills, care coordination, and environment. Examples of these are given in Table 3.2.

TABLE 3.2 Dimensions of Primary Healthcare Important to Women Receiving Care at National Centers of Excellence in Women's Health

DIMENSIONS	EXAMPLES
Access	Importance of barriers and supports to using the healthcare system, e.g., health insurance, understanding how system works
Office staff	Service and courtesy of staff, including receptionist and clerks
Privacy	Respect reflected by securing information and records, privacy when disclosing sensitive information, not feeling "diminished" during examination
Empathy and empowerment	Healthcare provider skills including awareness and acknowledgment of patients, sensitivity, caring attitude, courtesy, communication skills, comfort level, and patient trust
Provider skills	Technical skills including knowledge, training, experience
Care coordination	Follow-up, including test results and referrals
Environment	Environment including waiting room, exam room, privacy, gowns provided, room temperature, seating décor, music

Source: Anderson, R. T., Barbara, A. M., Weisman, C., Scholle, S. H., Binko, J., Schneider, T., Freund, K., & Gwinner, V. (2001). A qualitative analysis of women's satisfaction with the primary care from a panel of focus groups in the National Centers of Excellence in Women's Health. Journal of Women's Health, 10, 637–647. https://doi.org/10.1089/15246090152563515

The outcomes led to the creation of a woman-focused healthcare satisfaction instrument to be used to assess and improve healthcare delivery (Anderson et al., 2001, 2007; Scholle et al., 2000, 2004). The Primary Care Satisfaction Survey for Women (PCSSW; Scholle et al., 2004) included three dimensions: communication, administration and office procedures (processes), and comprehensiveness. Communication included items such as the professionals' ability to explain things clearly, answer questions in sensitive and caring ways, and take what women said seriously. Care processes (labeled administrative and office procedures) included courtesy of staff, flexible scheduling, provision of privacy, and offers of chances to talk to professionals while dressed (clothes on). Comprehensiveness included items related to care over the previous 12 months, including professional knowledge of women's health issues, interest in mental and emotional health of the woman, healthcare fitting life stage, and chances to get gynecologic and general healthcare. The complete scale with individual items is included in Scholle et al. (2004, Table 5, p. 44).

Evaluation of the quality of primary care services provided in 15 of the National CoEs in Women's Health in 2001 incorporated self-reported clinical preventive services and patient satisfaction as indicators of quality of care. Data from more than 3,000 women served by CoE programs were surveyed and compared with quality-of-care benchmarks from national and local community surveys, including the 1998 Commonwealth Fund Survey of Women's Health, a community sample of women living within a geographic catchment area for three CoEs, and a sample of more than 70,000 women from the 1999 Consumer Assessment of Health Plans Study of commercial managed care plans. Women in the CoEs were more satisfied with their care and had received more screening tests and counseling services than those in the benchmark studies. The largest effects of CoEs among primary care services were for physical breast examination, mammogram for women 50 and older, and counseling for smoking, domestic violence, and STIs (Anderson et al., 2002).

The evaluation of women's satisfaction with their ongoing primary healthcare services engaged 1,021 women attending primary care visits with at least one prior visit to the sites (Michigan, Pittsburgh, and Wake Forest) before and immediately after visits. Women were asked about their satisfaction with their visit and healthcare over the past 12 months. Women's general health, site continuity, and fulfillment of their expectations for care were linked to global ratings of satisfaction through effects on communication, care coordination, and office staff and administration. Care coordination and continuity mediated ratings of care over the past year but day-of-visit ratings were mediated by communication.

The success of these comprehensive clinical programs rested with the support of the leaders of the academic health centers who understood the importance of multidisciplinary programs to the clinical care of women and the education they provided to future providers of women's healthcare (Milliken et al., 2001). An inquiry to HRSA regarding the CoEs indicated that the OWH no longer certified the centers.

Gender-Sensitive Care in the Veterans Health Administration

Efforts in the U.S. Veterans Health Administration, the largest integrated healthcare system in the country, have increasingly focused on delivery of gender-sensitive comprehensive primary care to women veterans. Implementation of the Patient Aligned Care Team (PACT) initiative to deliver primary care to veterans supports efforts to improve access, continuity, coordination, and comprehensiveness of care that is driven by patients and is patient centered. In a recent examination of how the PACT initiative influences ability to meet the needs of special populations, in particular women veterans, Yano et al. (2014) explored challenges for women veterans in obtaining healthcare and efforts by the VA to provide comprehensive primary care for women. PACT services to provide comprehensive primary care for women veterans are designed to be patient centered, accessible, continuous, coordinating, and delivered in the setting of team-based care. Gender-sensitive comprehensive primary care for women veterans includes providing complete primary care and care coordination by a single primary care provider at one site in a longitudinal relationship to fulfill all primary care needs, including care for acute and chronic illnesses, gender-specific primary care, preventive services, mental health services (e.g., for depression), and coordination of care. Three approved comprehensive primary care clinic models for women veterans have been identified:

Model 1: General primary care clinic with one or more designated women's health providers colocated mental healthcare, efficient referral to specialty gynecology care

Model 2: Designated women's healthcare providers deliver primary care in separate but shared space with readily available or colocated gynecologic and mental healthcare

Model 3: Women's health center with separate, exclusive-use space with a separate entrance, comprising designated women's health providers, with colocated specialty gynecologic, mental health and social work services, and other subspecialty services (e.g., breast care) in the same location

These three models are being implemented with varying degrees of completeness.

The availability of designated women's healthcare providers proficient and interested in providing primary care for women veterans in all VA primary care clinics and comprehensive planning for women's health to increase women veterans' quality of care are also included in the expectations for gender-sensitive comprehensive primary care for women veterans. In addition, ensuring safety, dignity, sensitivity to gender-specific needs through ensuring privacy and respecting security needs constitutes an important part of the environment. Using state-of-the-art healthcare equipment and technology (e.g., for breast imaging and osteoporosis screening) is another expectation, as is the availability of women chaperones for gender-specific exams. Despite these policy changes, challenges remain for women in accessing team care in women's clinics, and designated women's health providers, privacy arrangements, and female chaperones are not universally available. Nonetheless, the VA effort to specify definitions and expectations of gender-sensitive comprehensive primary care for women veterans is a significant contribution to advancing women's healthcare.

An expert panel of clinicians and social scientists with expertise in women's health, primary care, and mental health rated the importance of tailoring more than 100 aspects of care derived from the IOM definition of comprehensive care and sex-sensitive (gender-sensitive) care as a guide to what aspects of care should be tailored to women veterans (deKleijn et al., 2015). The panel rated more than half of the aspects of care as very to extremely important to tailor to women veterans. Fourteen priority recommendations focused on the importance of design and delivery of services sensitive to trauma histories, adapting to women's preferences and

information needs, and sex (gender) awareness and cultural transformation in each aspect of VA operations. Several domains of gender-sensitive comprehensive care were outlined from the first contact, subsequent care, coordination of referrals, healthcare workforce orientation and training, quality-improvement activities and capacity, gender-specific care (e.g., female reproductive health), gender awareness (clinical understanding and systems of care features), and gender sensitivity. Of note were the definitions guiding these domains, in particular:

Gender awareness: Clinical understanding and system of care features ensuring achievement of competencies and processes related to guideline-concordant care for women as well as attention to conditions that are more prevalent in women, present differently, and should be managed differently than those of men

Gender sensitivity: Attributes of care reflecting relational and other preferences (e.g., communication style, same-gender clinician, and privacy/safety needs)

Gender-specific care: Female reproductive healthcare (e.g., menopause care and breast and cervical cancer screening)

Consideration of these elements gave priority to delivering reproductive health services tailored to the needs of women veterans, especially gender-specific examinations and management of pelvic and abdominal pain experienced by women with trauma histories; ensuring privacy, safety, dignity, and security of the healthcare environments; increasing tailoring of care for posttraumatic stress disorder (PTSD), MST, and other forms of sexual violence; tailoring mental healthcare delivery (e.g., depression and anxiety); implementing employee orientation, training, and education on gender-sensitive comprehensive care; tailoring assessments and screening practices (e.g., breast and cervical cancer and MST screening); tailoring behavioral health interventions (e.g., smoking cessation and addiction treatment); and increasing gender awareness and sensitivity of all VA employees as well as other veterans. In addition, other priorities included retaining women veterans in care by ensuring that continuity of care is with their preferred provider; ensuring practice guidelines, electronic record reminders, and templates are reflective of gender; promoting the use of tailored information letters and adapting the website and call centers to reflect women veterans' preferences and information needs; enhancing marketing and education initiatives to promote the awareness of gender-sensitive comprehensive care in VA settings; tailoring debriefing sessions during military discharge processes to consider women's information and clinical care needs; and tailoring care coordination and navigation between VA and non-VA care (deKleijn et al., 2015).

Despite national efforts to improve women's health services within the Veterans Health Administration, women veterans still underutilize VA healthcare. A recent assessment indicated that nearly 20% had delayed healthcare or an unmet need, with younger women experiencing more difficulty in accessing care. Of those who delayed or did not get healthcare, barriers included unaffordable healthcare, inability to take time off from work, and transportation difficulties. In addition, being uninsured, not knowing about VA care, having perceptions that VA providers were not gender-sensitive, and having a history of MST predicted delaying or not seeking care (Washington, Bean-Mayberry, Mitchell et al., 2011; Washington, Bean-Mayberry, Riopelle et al., 2011). Military service era was influential in women's healthcare delivery preferences, with Vietnam era to present veterans using more women's health and mental healthcare and World War II– and Korean War–era women veterans using more specialty care. Operation Enduring Freedom (OEF), Operation Iraqi Freedom (OIF), and Operation New Dawn (OND) veterans made more healthcare visits than women of earlier military eras. Healthcare delivery concerns include location convenience for Vietnam and earlier veterans and cost for the first Gulf War and OEF/OIF/OND veterans. Women of all military service eras rated colocation of gynecology with general healthcare as important. Ensuring access to specialty services close to home for veterans and access to mental healthcare reinforce the needs for the integration and coordination of primary care, reproductive health, and mental healthcare and for the provision of care close to where veterans live (Washington et al., 2013). The VA recommends designated providers for women in primary care clinics or women's health centers as optimal models for women's primary care. Healthcare ratings obtained from VA users in a National Survey of Women Veterans indicated that gender-related satisfaction, gender appropriateness of care, and perceptions of VA provider skills were greater in sites adopting these changes. Establishing these optimal care models at sites around the nation is recommended to improve women veterans' experiences with VA care (Washington, Bean-Mayberry, Riopelle et al., 2011). Indeed, the VA roadmap for delivering gender-sensitive comprehensive care for women may serve well as a model for civilian healthcare settings.

The VA model of care is one that initiated with concerns about veteran health and integrated PACT as an approach to primary care. Gender was not at the center of this model initially but was integrated into the care model while retaining the special concerns about veterans' health. This model exemplifies some elements of intersectionality as discussed by Hankivsky (2012), who alerts us to the possibility of creating additional inequities when using gender as the central point of consideration of health inequities. The importance of considering gender-based inequities as inseparable from other dimensions of women's places in the social structure (e.g., class, race/ethnicity, sexual orientation, immigration, and ability) will be important for further development of gender-sensitive models of healthcare. As Havkinsky points out, although gender may be a logical starting place for such considerations, centering sex and gender may prevent or limit the opportunities to learn about other factors affecting life chances, opportunities, and health. Continuing to ask whether gender is the most salient factor as one analyzes the needs and issues of populations will be foundational to identifying important implications of intersectionality. Systematically adopting and applying intersectionality— as Hankivsky (2012) defines it, a "framework for improving understandings of and responses to the complexities

of people's lives and experiences"—are worthy aspirational goals for those envisioning models of gender-sensitive healthcare.

When both the CoEs and the VA women's health centers were evaluated using comparable key informant surveys, all served urban areas and most had academic partnerships. DHHS CoEs had three times the average caseload as VA centers. Preventive cancer screening and general reproductive services were available at all centers, but DHHS centers offered extensive reproductive services on-site more frequently and VA centers had on-site mental healthcare more frequently. Although these centers share similar missions and have comparable organization, education, and clinical services, they offered on-site services that differed in relation to the needs of their respective populations (Bean-Mayberry et al., 2007).

Integration of Sexual and Reproductive Health Into Primary Care

Another noteworthy effort has been the proposed integration of SRH care into primary care. A continuing challenge for women accessing comprehensive services has been the fragmentation of SRH—and men face similar challenges (Berg et al., 2014; Berg, Taylor et al., 2013). In the United States, SRH services are not integrated within a primary healthcare system of public health and primary care services. Moreover, U.S. national health goals to reduce unintended pregnancies and STIs have not been achieved (DHHS, 2000). Two models that could facilitate a coordinated system of sexual and reproductive services within a public and private primary care system in the United States are the WHO (2011) model of SRH services, including standards and provider competencies, and the United Kingdom (UK) model of community SRH standards and clinical competencies within the Royal College of Nursing (2009).

The WHO view of SRH extends beyond maternal–child healthcare and includes the reproductive health of women and men throughout their life cycles, as well as adolescents. SRH encompasses periods before and beyond reproductive years and is closely associated with sociocultural factors, gender roles, health equity, and respect and protection of human rights. SRH services are envisioned as delivered as a collection of integrated services addressing the full range of SRH needs and must be a part of the existing healthcare system, coordinating with public health and primary healthcare and reflecting human rights. WHO recommended a set of core competencies to achieve universal access to integrated SRH within a primary healthcare system. These are regarded as a minimum package of SRH care all should be able to access regardless of social, physical, and mental status; sex; age; religion; and country.

Thirteen competencies are grouped into four domains:

Domain 1: Fundamental basis of competencies builds on SRH provider's knowledge of ethics, human rights; knowledge, behaviors, and attitudes for providing high-quality SRH care include ethical/technical foundation for SRH delivery; considerations of human rights, social values of equity, solidarity, and social participation

Doman 2: Leadership and management competencies—enabling others and effectively managing primary healthcare teams to provide quality SRH services

Domain 3: General SRH competencies for healthcare providers—community, health education, counseling, assessment, referral

Domain 4: Clinical competencies for SRH provision, including high-quality family planning care; spacing pregnancies; infertility problems; STI and reproductive tract infection (RTI) care; screening/treatment referral for RTIs; comprehensive abortion care; antenatal care; intrapartum care; postnatal care for women/neonates

The UK model is a coordinated system of SRH education, training, and certification for RNs, nurses with advanced training, nurse practitioners, midwives, and nonspecialist physicians working in the National Health Service. Competency-based education, training, and certification in 10 areas have been developed and are foundational to this practice:

1. Basic SRH services/skill, such as assessment by history and physical exam; problem assessment, risk assessment, and triage; effective communication across cultures, gender, life span, and sexual health; knowledge of basic counseling techniques; empowerment of individuals to make informed decisions; coordination/follow-up/referral; time management; urogynecology lab/specimen preparation; pregnancy testing and counseling; sexual/physical violence prevention

2. Contraception, including knowledge of methods of fertility control and family planning for men and women across the life span, people with disabilities, women after abortion, and difficult-to-reach groups; communication of, patient decision-making regarding, and provision and management of fertility control and contraceptive choices; counseling for and management of complex medical/social needs related to contraception and contraceptive requirements and complications resulting from contraceptive failure

3. Unplanned pregnancy care/abortion, including pregnancy diagnostics, pregnancy options counseling and coordination, preabortion and postabortion care for early and later term abortion, medication abortion provision, and aspiration abortion provision by uterine aspiration procedures

4. Women's health/gynecology, such as diagnosis and management of common gynecologic problems; menstrual function/disorders across the life span and basic gynecologic ultrasound exams; managing simple pediatric/adolescent gynecology disorders (e.g., menstrual disorders, fibroids, amenorrhea, nonmenstrual bleeding, congenital abnormalities of the genital tract, and puberty)

5. Assessment of and comanagement of specialty gynecologic problems, such as subfertility problems, infertility diagnostics, gynecologic oncology problems, urogynecology and pelvic floor problems

6. Pregnancy, including diagnosis and management of early pregnancy care and referral, comprehensive antenatal care, labor and delivery/intrapartum care, diagnosis and management of postpartum care and problems for women and/or neonates

7. Genitourinary conditions in men (GUM) including assessment, counseling, referral, coordination of care; performing, collecting, interpreting lab tests; diagnosing/managing GUM, including noncomplicated STIs/RTIs, balanitis/urethritis, infertility, and life-span issues

8. Sexual health promotion, including sexual and self-health promotion for women and men; assessing sexual problems with sexual history taking/diagnostics; assessing, managing, or referring for sexual assault testing

9. Public health, ethics, and legal competencies, including knowledge of laws regarding family planning, abortion, HIV, violence against women and sexual violence, sex work, and sexuality (sexual orientation and gender identity); healthcare providers' legal/ethical obligations; element of SRH services and national guidelines, and economic impact and cost of healthcare options/treatments/prevention

10. Leadership, management, and information technology (IT)/audit competencies, including enabling others or effectively managing teams providing SRH services; knowing national and local SRH policies, standards, and protocols; improving SRH program implementation through evidence and use of technology (Kasliwal et al., 2011; Royal College of Nursing, 2009)

These models of gender-sensitive care attempt to address the need for comprehensive, coordinated, integrated services for women, providing an alternative to the fragmentation of SRH care and primary care or primary healthcare services. Cappiello and Nothnagle (2013) advocate for a vision in which all women and men in the United States receive high-quality, evidence-based sexual and reproductive care through policy changes that make interprofessional education and training on SRH a priority at federal and state levels (Nothnagle et al., 2013).

Gender-Sensitive Counseling and Therapy Models for Women

Another important contribution to women's healthcare has been the development of mental health counseling and psychotherapy models tailored to women. One form of gender-sensitive healthcare is relational-cultural therapy (RCT), a form of therapy developed by Jean Baker Miller and her colleagues that recognized and emphasized the central role of relationships as being growth fostering. Several decades ago, in the 1970s, a group of feminist women therapists came together to discuss new ways of understanding psychological growth. The initial group of women consisted of Jean Baker Miller, Irene Stiver, Judith Jordan, Janet Surrey, and Alexandra Kaplan. Miller wrote a groundbreaking book in 1976 with a second edition published in 1986, titled *Toward a New Psychology of Women* (Miller, 1986). This now classic book provides the basic concepts of relational-cultural theory, which is the foundation for RCT. This section of this chapter describes the basic concepts of RCT, followed by a description of the RCT approach that incorporates these basic concepts.

Concepts of Relational-Cultural Theory

At the Stone Center at Wellesley College, a group of women and others studied prevailing theories of psychological development and recognized that these prevailing theories did not explain much of women's experiences (Gilligan, 1982; Gilligan et al., 1991a, 1991b; Jordan, 1997; Jordan et al., 1991; Miller & Stiver, 1997). The prevailing psychological theories emphasized the importance of separation and individuation as one attains autonomy, which reflects psychological health. Although the scholars at the Stone Center recognized and embraced the importance of a person having agency and a sense of self, they also strongly believed in the need for healthy relationships in order for a person to grow in a psychologically healthy way.

This new approach to understanding women's psychological development was initially referred to as *self-in-relation* theory because it seemed to adequately reflect the notion that individuals develop in relationship to others in their lives. Over time, however, as these feminist scholars continued to study and to learn from one another, they rejected the term *self* and instead shifted their emphasis to relationships and incorporated cultural diversity in an effort to move beyond only the experiences of middle-class White women (who composed this initial group of scholars). They modified how they labeled their theory and began to refer to it as *relational-cultural theory*. Perspectives from women of color, from lesbian women, and from men were actively integrated into the developing theory (Bergman & Surrey, 1997; Coll et al., 1997; Eldridge et al., 1997; Rosen, 1997; Tatum, 1997; Turner, 1997; Walker & Rosen, 2004). This approach does not reject the notion of individuation, but it moderates such separateness with connectedness, contributing to a more complex and insightful understanding of adult development, both male and female. "In short, the goal is not for the individual to grow out of relationships, but to grow into them. As the relationships grow, so grows the individual" (Miller & Stiver, 1997, p. 22).

Of great significance is that relational-cultural theory embraces the social context or social determinants of health in recognizing factors that affect psychological growth. The presence of racism, poverty, and lack of access to healthcare are all examples of social determinants of health that must be understood and addressed in order to foster psychological growth. More recently, scholars at the Stone Center have incorporated current understanding of brain science into relational-cultural theory and RCT. Amy Banks (2006) has written about how neurobiological aspects contribute to interpersonal connections.

Several key factors compose relational-cultural theory. These factors are not mutually exclusive. It is important that they are understood from a holistic perspective in which each factor influences and is influenced by the others.

MUTUALITY

Mutuality refers to the notion of persons experiencing situations together in a simultaneous way. It is important to note that no two persons experience situations in exactly the same way; the key point in mutuality is that experiences do not occur in isolation. Instead, mutuality is characterized by a situation in which two or more persons experience something together, allowing them to share with one another their individual experiences. In this way, each person can better understand the experiences of the others.

AUTHENTICITY

Authenticity is a key concept of healthy relationships and actually reflects the notion that healthy individuals do need a strong sense of self (thus not totally negating the concept of individuation). This concept goes further than simply knowing oneself and having a sense of oneself. Authenticity includes a comfort level in which a person feels safe to share one's authentic, genuine self with others in the relationship.

RECIPROCITY

Similar to mutuality, *reciprocity* refers to a sense of experiencing something together. Different from mutuality, reciprocity emphasizes and highlights the back-and-forth nature of a relationship as opposed to the simultaneity. Similar to mutuality, reciprocity emphasizes the importance of individuals within relationships working together, leading to the understanding of one another as they share back and forth.

EMPATHY

Sharing experiences together and being able to feel what another feels (of course, recognizing that one can never absolutely feel what another is feeling) are key to empathy. *Empathy* describes the process of another person having a sense of sharing experiences of others and being able to express this sense by communicating with and relating to the other person.

CONNECTEDNESS

Connectedness is actually what happens as a result of healthy, growth-fostering relationships. Healthy individuals do not live and function in isolation from others, but instead involve a sense of being a part of another person, whether that be sharing certain ideas and values or sharing certain feelings. Belenky et al. (1997) emphasized connectedness in relation to ways of knowing, with direct reference to women and how women come to know and make meaning of phenomena in their lives. Knowing, making meaning, and developing healthy psychological selves occur within the context of connected relationships with others.

Jean Baker Miller and her colleagues (2012) not only developed what they believed were key concepts that defined healthy relationships, but they also identified what occurs as a result of healthy relationships. These results are referred to as the "five good things" and are as follows: (1) zest or well-being, (2) ability and motivation to take action, (3) increased knowledge of self and others, (4) increased sense of worth, and (5) a desire for more connection beyond the current one.

Zest is a sense of well-being that comes from being in a healthy relationship. Both persons in the relationship experience a feeling of energy and passion and feeling that there is a purpose in one's life.

Ability and motivation to take action is the sense of wanting to make constructive changes and having purpose in life. There is a feeling that one can, indeed, be effective in making such constructive changes.

Increased knowledge of self and others refers to the ability to be self-reflective and to also understand the other, to empathize with the other person in the relationship. Such increased knowledge allows for creating and maintaining authenticity within a relationship.

Increased sense of self-worth is a feeling of being worthwhile, of having a place and voice in the world. It is similar to what might be termed in traditional psychology as *increased self-esteem*. It allows one to feel motivated to take action and be able to do so because it is a sense that one does have the wherewithal to be an active member of a group, a community, and a society.

A desire for more connection reflects one's continuing desire for ongoing relationships, particularly recognizing the growth-fostering capacity that comes from healthy human connection. This ongoing desire allows greater connection and continuing growth.

Relational-Cultural Therapy

Judith Jordan aptly describes the guiding foundation, based in relational-cultural theory, for doing RCT. She states that relational-cultural therapists focus on decreasing isolation, increasing one's capacity for self-empathy as well as empathy for others, and appreciating the importance of context and limiting cultural/relational images. Jordan emphasizes that this approach to therapy is guided by an attitude and quality of mutual engagement rather than on any specific intervention techniques (Jordan, 2010).

The relational-cultural therapist works within connections and disconnections. This means that the therapist themself must be aware of any disconnection they are feeling and must stay present in connection with the patient. The relational-cultural therapist also works with empathy. In this case, the therapist must be self-reflective about their own feelings that are being aroused in the therapeutic situation. The patient must be aware of the therapist's genuine empathic response(s). This is an example of how a therapeutic relationship, which in many ways is a microcosm of all relationships, is growth fostering for both the patient and the therapist. The therapist also works with relational images. In this case, both the therapist and the patient work together through mutual empathy to deconstruct past relational images that are painful and that limit healthy psychological growth. It is important that the therapist be responsive to the patient in an authentic way, which in turn encourages the patient to feel comfortable and safe to present their authentic self to the therapist. In being responsive, the therapist does not put forth an image of being the authority figure but rather creates a context in the therapeutic relationship in which the therapist is truly authentic and present. Jordan (2010) notes that a judicious use of emotional transparency will help the patient understand their own authentic self

and will be comfortable to be authentic in relationships. The therapist must also be aware of and share with the patient the importance and power of the social context. As discussed earlier in this section, the *social context* refers to the social determinants of health, such as racism, poverty, and lack of access to healthcare.

The process of RCT involves a complex approach that, paradoxically, is not complex at all. It is simply being in relationship with the patient. However, being in relationship is not simple at all. Thus, adding to this paradox, this therapeutic approach is most complex as it embraces an authentic involvement in the relationship and in the world itself. Jordan describes how therapists must understand and embrace uncertainty and must live with uncertainty, acknowledging that we all live in an uncertain world. The therapeutic process involves being with the patient in all the complexities this relationship entails.

The efficacy of RCT has been demonstrated in a few studies. Frey (2013) reported on the application of this therapy in June 2004 at the Jean Baker Miller Training Institute. A study conducted by Oakley et al. (2004) used an RCT approach that was time limited and guided by a manual. After collecting and analyzing data at five time points in addition to pretreatment and posttreatment, they found improvement in several outcomes' measures, including depression and anxiety, as well as maintenance of these improved outcomes at 3 months and 6 months follow-up. Frey also reported on a study by Tantillo and Sanftner (2003) that compared cognitive behavioral therapy with RCT in a population of women with bulimia. All outcomes, including binge eating and vomiting, were equivalent in both groups, except that the women in the RCT group perceived greater mutuality.

Considerations Related to Risks Associated With Gender-Sensitive Models

The past decades have seen increasing the recognition of biological differences between the sexes and efforts to reduce inappropriate care for women. Increasingly, healthcare professionals are advised to integrate knowledge of sex and gender differences into treatment plans. Communication in the delivery of healthcare provides opportunity for creating gender-sensitive encounters, yet evidence suggests that communication also reproduces gender differences. Healthcare conversations reproduce stereotypical communication styles that reinforce gender bias, convey different attitudes toward treatments for women and men, and convey information that result in gender bias and unequal care. Gender-sensitive care has been proposed as health professionals using competencies in perceiving existing gender differences and incorporating these into treatment. This approach may also run the risk of interjecting preconceived and unconscious assumptions about gender in ways that lead to stereotypical thinking and communication with patients.

A 2014 analysis of discourse contained in tape-recorded conversations between patients and health professionals revealed different approaches used by female and male patients and health professionals in clinical interactions related to atrial fibrillation (Hedegaard et al., 2014). Women usually used emotional-oriented statements (e.g., referencing feeling unusual) in describing their health problems, and male patients used performance-oriented statements (e.g., referencing inability to swim the usual distance). Health professionals tended to acknowledge concern for female patients and provide reassurance but downplayed male patients' statements and confirmed their descriptions of performance. Hedegaard et al. concluded that female patients were constructed as fragile and males as competent through gender-stereotypical communication. In an effort to provide gender-sensitive healthcare, it is possible that assumptions about sex and gender differences in health problems and their manifestations reinforce stereotypes about gender in a context in which the intent is the opposite. The use of open-ended statements or questions by health professionals instead of leading questions that reinforce gender stereotypes allowed conversations to be less influenced by gender stereotypes. Moreover, reflection on the social construction of gender may also prompt awareness of ways in which stereotypes shape healthcare communications and compromise the equality of treatment.

NATIONAL POLICY AND WOMEN'S HEALTHCARE

Women have unique healthcare needs that impact the amount of care needed and the expense of that care. Among these are women's more complex reproductive healthcare needs, their experience of greater chronic disease rates, gender differences in responses to conditions such as cardiovascular disease, longer life span, and consequent higher levels of spending when compared with men (Zephyrin et al., 2020). Specific issues related to healthcare insurance for women include gaps in insurance coverage and difficulty accessing healthcare that are attributable to making workforce transitions, being employed in part-time jobs without employee health insurance benefits, and being insured as a dependent. Each of these places women at risk for being unable to obtain needed care. In addition to these factors is the disproportionate number of women who live in poverty including those who are among the working poor, unable to afford healthcare and insurance.

The Patient Protection and Affordable Care Act

The ACA was enacted into federal law in 2010 and is the most complex and far-reaching healthcare legislation since the passage of Medicaid and Medicare in 1965. The ACA is paid for through a variety of taxes on individuals and businesses, as well as tax penalties for those who do not purchase health insurance as required under the act (Congressional Budget Office, 2014). Its goals are to increase the number of people with access to health insurance, improve the affordability of health insurance and healthcare services, and improve quality of care (Armstrong, 2015). Anticipated benefits for women include improved access to health insurance coverage, expanded scope of benefits covered by plans, and reduced cost sharing for some services. Although most provisions are not gender specific, the Women's Health Amendment (Section 2713 to Public Health Service Act) mandates coverage for FDA-approved contraceptives, sterilization procedures, and patient education and counseling for women with reproductive capacity, as prescribed by a healthcare provider (Coverage of Certain Preventive Services, 2015).

Women have had access to health insurance coverage before the ACA. Private sector coverage is most often provided through employment-based plans, and public sector sources include Medicare, Medicaid, and state Children's Health Insurance Program (CHIP). Both Medicaid and CHIP provide assistance funded by taxpayers without payment from the recipient. A major barrier to insurance coverage is cost. Despite premium payments, women have often experienced limited coverage of services such as prescription contraceptives and maternity care, which may be excluded services under some plans. Coverage of preventive benefits varied greatly before the ACA under both private and public plans.

Provisions of the ACA expand access to health insurance. These include coverage of adult children up to age 26 years on parents' plans, Medicaid expansion to cover more of the population by raising the income threshold for eligibility, establishing state- or federal-based exchanges or marketplaces that offer individuals options to purchase private insurance that are coupled with tax credits or subsidies for low-income individuals, and supporting policies that include guaranteed issue, prohibition of preexisting conditions, underwriting changes, and individual mandate (Armstrong, 2015). Women with incomes below 133% of the poverty level, including those without children, will be able to access Medicaid coverage in many states. The Medicaid expansion enables coverage for women between the ages of 19 and 64 years, a critical period for women's health.

The ACA expands the scope of benefits covered in insurance plans in significant ways. Plans sold on public and private exchanges are to include essential health benefits, including ambulatory patient services; emergency services; hospitalization; maternity and newborn care; mental health and substance use disorder (SUD) services, including behavioral health treatment; prescription drugs; rehabilitative and habilitative services and devices; laboratory services; preventive and wellness services; and chronic disease management and pediatric services, including oral and vision care. Maternity and newborn care benefits (prenatal care, labor and delivery, and postpartum care services) and preventive and wellness service benefits are of particular relevance to women.

In addition to the reproductive health provisions, the mental health/SUD services are noteworthy for women. A combination of the Mental Health Parity and Addiction Equity Act and the ACA will extend overall health insurance coverage and the scope of coverage to include mental health and substance abuse benefits (Frank et al., 2014). The essential health benefit requirements governing basic coverage include mental health and substance use services. In addition, Medicaid expansion will cover approximately 65% of newly covered people with mental health disorders and SUDs, and single, childless adults will be eligible for Medicaid, including many who have severe and persistent mental disorders and live in extreme poverty, experience unstable housing, and have co-occurring SUDs. Behavioral health parity means that these services will be covered at parity with medical–surgical coverage. Although this represents transformative change in mental health and SUD services, there remain important areas not covered, including assertive community treatment (ACT), supported employment, supported housing, and long-term residential services. Nonetheless, coverage of mental health and SUD services and parity with medical–surgical care represents significant advancements in health insurance that will serve women well (Beronoio et al., 2014; Chin et al., 2014).

An IOM Committee on Clinical Preventive Services for Women (IOM, 2011) focused on closing the gaps in existing preventive services for women. This committee defined preventive health services to include medications, procedures, devices, tests, education, and counseling that had been shown to improve well-being and/or decrease the likelihood of disease or conditions or to delay them. The committee reviewed the preventive services recommended by the U.S. Preventive Services Task Force (USPSTF) for women as highly effective, considered the Bright Futures recommendations for girls and adolescents, and recommended eight additional services for inclusion for no-cost coverage (IOM, 2011). See recommended clinical preventive services for women in Table 3.3 and additional recommended services in Table 3.4.

The Women's Health Amendment of the ACA (section 2713 to the Public Health Service Act) specifies additional services to be covered without cost sharing as recommended by the IOM (2011). These included well-woman visits; screening for gestational diabetes; human papillomavirus DNA testing; counseling for STIs; counseling and screening for HIV; contraceptive methods and counseling; breastfeeding support, supplies, and counseling; and screening and counseling for interpersonal and domestic violence.

TABLE 3.3 NAM Committee on Clinical Preventive Services Recommendations for Inclusion in Well-Woman Visits Under the Patient Protection and Affordable Care Act

PREVENTION/HEALTH PROMOTION	SCREENING	COUNSELING AND INTERVENTIONS
Pregnancy related	Anemia Bacteriuria *Chlamydia* Hepatitis B Syphilis Rh incompatibility PPD Suicide History of CVD-related conditions in pregnancy Prenatal care	Breastfeeding Tobacco use Prenatal care
Cancer	*BRCA* gene Breast cancer Cervical cancer Colorectal cancer	*BRCA* gene Breast cancer chemoprevention
Chronic illness	BP Diabetes Lipid levels Metabolic syndrome Osteoporosis	Osteoporosis
Substance use		Alcohol misuse Tobacco use Tobacco use interventions
Healthy behaviors	Eating behaviors Obesity Physical activity levels Preconception care	Healthy diet Obesity Referrals for interventions Preconception care Folic acid supplementation
STIs	*Chlamydia* <25 years old CT/GC screen >25 years old in high-risk communities GC HIV Syphilis	All STIs counseling for high-risk teens, adults
Mental health	Depression—adolescents, adults	

BP, blood pressure; CT/GC, chlamydia trachomatis/gonococcus; CVD, cardiovascular disease; GC, gonococcus; IOM, Institute of Medicine; NAM, National Academy of Medicine; PPD, postpartum depression; STIs, sexually transmitted infections.
Source: Institute of Medicine. (2011). Clinical preventive services for women: Closing the gaps. *National Academies Press; National Academies of Sciences, Engineering, and Medicine. (2022).* Closing evidence gaps in clinical prevention. *The National Academies Press. https://doi.org/10.17226/26351; National Academies of Sciences, Engineering, and Medicine. (2016).* Improving the health of women in the United States: Workshop summary. *The National Academies Press. https://doi.org/10.17226/23441*

TABLE 3.4 Additional Services Recommended by the IOM Committee on Preventive Services for Women

SERVICE	FOR WHOM AND WHEN
Screening for gestational diabetes	Pregnant women: 24–28 weeks; first prenatal visit for pregnant women at high risk for diabetes
Human papillomavirus testing—addition of high-risk human papillomavirus DNA testing in addition to cytology testing in those with normal cytology results	Women—30 years of age and no more frequently than every 3 years
Counseling for STIs	Sexually active women—annually
Counseling and screening for HIV	Sexually active women—annually
Contraceptive methods (full range of FDA-approved methods, sterilization) with patient education and counseling	Women with reproductive capacity—not specified
Breastfeeding support, supplies, and counseling; comprehensive lactation support and counseling and costs of renting breastfeeding equipment by a trained provider to ensure successful initiation and duration of breastfeeding	All pregnant women and those in postpartum period—during pregnancy and postpartum
Screening and counseling for interpersonal and domestic violence: involves elicitation of information about current and past violence and abuse in culturally sensitive and supportive manner to address current concerns of safety and other current or future health problems	Women and adolescents—timing not specified
Well-woman visits for recommended preventive services including preconception and prenatal care	Adult women—at least one well-woman preventive care visit annually; several visits may be needed to obtain all necessary recommended preventive services depending on health status, health needs, and other risk factors

FDA, U.S. Food and Drug Administration; IOM, Institute of Medicine; STIs, sexually transmitted infections.
Source: Institute of Medicine. (2011). Clinical preventive services for women: Closing the gaps. *National Academies Press.*

The ACA codified the establishment of an Office on Women's Health in major federal agencies, including the Department of Health and Human Services, the Centers for Disease Control and Prevention, the FDA, the HRSA, and the Agency for Healthcare Research and Quality. These offices establish visible points of accountability for women's health across several federal agencies. Prior to the ACA, the OWH was established within the DHHS in 1991 and has long served a coordinating role in addressing women's health issues through advancing policies, education, and programmatic support (OWH, 2018).

Access to at least one annual well-woman visit to obtain recommended preventive services was included in the ACA provisions. More than a single visit may be necessary to complete all preventive screening. Breastfeeding support was also a provision of the ACA, which includes coverage of comprehensive lactation support and counseling, costs of renting or purchasing breastfeeding equipment such as pumps, and workplace requirements to provide time and space for mothers to express milk until the infant is 1 year old.

Another important set of benefits that will improve access for women and girls includes the availability of certified nurse midwives and OB-GYNs regarded as primary care providers; immunization, including the human papillomavirus (HPV) vaccine for women and girls younger than 26 years; allowance of low-income new mothers and newborns to maintain Medicaid coverage beyond the postpartum period; increased support for the reimbursement of certified nurse midwives, birth attendants, and free-standing birth centers; postpartum depression education support services; maternal, infant, and early childhood home visiting programs; and expanded workplace breastfeeding support services. Allowing states to extend eligibility for family planning services to those with incomes below 185% of the poverty level without federal permit process; funding to states to provide evidence-based sex education to reduce teen pregnancy rates and STI incidence; and changes to Medicare to reduce out-of-pocket costs for medications and preventive services are additional provisions.

The ACA has had far-reaching impact on women's health, but there are a number of exceptions made to coverage, such as those seen with accommodation of religious institutions and provisions of contraceptive benefits. The American Academy of Nursing Expert Panel on Women's Health (Berg, Taylor et al., 2013) recommended further elaboration beyond the prevention recommendations in the IOM report and the *National Prevention Strategy* report. These include:

Comprehensive healthcare delivery approaches for preventive services for women

Gender-sensitive and life-span prevention services coordinated in a primary healthcare system of primary care and public health

Preconception healthcare as a model of integrative prevention practice

Integration of primary, secondary, and tertiary prevention guidelines in practice

Development and maintenance of a competent workforce to implement prevention services and meet national health goals (Berg, Taylor et al., 2013)

The American Academy of Nursing Expert Panel on Women's Health endorsed the IOM (2011) clinical preventive services for women and strategies for prevention in the *National Prevention Strategies* report. They also advocate the adoption of prevention guidelines that are evidence based; gender sensitive; culturally appropriate; and inclusive of gay, lesbian, and intergender groups. Other areas include mobilizing health professionals to address national health goals and the integration of essential competencies for primary and secondary prevention and clinical management of SRH into professional practice curricula, as well as focusing service improvements on social and structural determinants of preventive services (National Prevention Council, 2011).

In 2018, the American College of Physicians published a position paper on national women's health policy. The paper was intended to address a variety of challenges facing women who are seeking healthcare and included seven specific recommendations intended to address these challenges, with a goal of ensuring a healthcare system that supports the needs of women and their families throughout their life spans. These recommendations addressed:

1. Training for all clinicians in health issues of particular relevance to the population of women
2. Ensuring access to affordable healthcare coverage that includes evidence-based care
3. Reproductive decision-making rights, including contraception and whether or not to continue a pregnancy, and opposition to government restrictions that would erode or abrogate a woman's right to continue or discontinue a pregnancy
4. Opposition to regulations that limit access to comprehensive reproductive healthcare by putting medically unnecessary restrictions on healthcare professionals or facilities
5. Support for universal access to family and medical leave policies including a minimum period of 6 weeks' paid leave
6. Availability of effective screening tools for physicians or healthcare professionals treating survivors of intimate partner or sexual violence
7. Support of efforts to improve the representation of women's health in clinical research (Daniel & Erickson, 2018)

Challenges for the future include those related to the burgeoning population of older women. Gaps in coverage and high out-of-pocket expenses on long-term services continue to affect older women disproportionately. The ACA included several proposed changes in Medicare affecting benefits for older women. Among these provisions were those that would decrease out-of-pocket costs for drugs and preventive services, an annual personalized health plan, and risk assessment; no cost sharing for mammograms, Pap smears, and bone density testing; and some assistance with long-term care costs through voluntary insurance programs. Many of these benefits were included in the Community Living Assistance Services and Supports (CLASS) Act that was intended to include a national voluntary long-term care insurance program that would make it possible for people to purchase government-sponsored insurance during their working years so that if they became unable to care for themselves, they would have access to a cash benefit to purchase services delivered either at home or in a care facility. This act would have begun shifting the financing of long-term care services from a means-tested Medicaid program to an insurance-based system that would be supported by voluntary private contributions (Gleckman, 2011). Unfortunately, analysis of the CLASS program determined that it was not financially viable, and it was withdrawn from the ACA (Appleby & Carey, 2011). In the United States challenges remain to develop funding for services that older adults will need, in particular women. Other countries (e.g., the Netherlands and Japan) offer comprehensive models of long-term care insurance programs funded by local, regional, and federal taxes.

The strong focus on hospital care covered by Medicare has been well established, but rules related to Medicare claims are becoming more stringent about the use of hospital-based services. Coverage of preventive services, such as Pap smears and mammography, came late (1990 and 1991, respectively) in Medicare's history and required a 20% coinsurance payment, leaving women with significant out-of-pocket expenses. The ACA's inclusion of recommended clinical preventive services was significantly broadened by the elimination of cost sharing for highly effective preventive services as recommended by the USPSTF and a personalized health plan with an annual comprehensive risk assessment (well-woman visit). Drug coverage for older women has also been improved under Medicare Part D, and the low-income subsidy of premium and cost-sharing subsidies for beneficiaries have been a significant benefit for women. What remains problematic for older adults today is the array of needed care that is not covered: hearing aids, eyeglasses, dental care, extended nursing home stays, or personal care needs. Required copayments also contribute to high out-of-pocket costs for women whose incomes are marginal.

Medicaid coverage provides assistance to an estimated 17% of older women who have Medicare coverage: Dual coverage affords many of these women glasses, vision care, dental care, and hearing aids (dependent on the state of residence), offsetting costs for the poorest of low-income older women. Because women constitute a disproportionate share of those residing in nursing homes and residential care communities, they experience a much greater need than do men for services that Medicare does *not* cover, putting women living in poverty at increased risk for low access to the services they need most.

Unpaid and informal caregivers are also predominantly women, and they, too, are not well served by Medicare in its current form. Lack of coverage for services for family members needing care leaves many of the caregivers at financial risk, as they may need to depart from the paid workforce to provide care. Thus, an intergenerational disadvantage may be accrued by families in which an older woman requires long-term care services in the United States (Salganicoff, 2015). The United States continues to struggle with finding solutions to the affordability of healthcare through expanding medical insurance plans in the existing healthcare system versus reassessing the system and removing entrenched barriers to competition that would lower costs and make healthcare more affordable for all citizens.

GLOBAL POLICY AND WOMEN'S HEALTHCARE

The early decades of the 21st century have been a period of dramatic changes in our consciousness of global issues and globalization. Health and healthcare have become global issues, as illustrated by the rapid transmission of infectious diseases across international borders, along with the exchange of innovations in healthcare technology, healthcare personnel, health information, and international collaboration in health professionals' education and research. This rapid change in perspectives has challenged countries around the globe to examine diverse perspectives about health and healthcare.

In 2000, the United Nations (UN), the world's largest intergovernmental organization, established Millennium Development Goals (MDGs) to be achieved by 2015. These included two goals directly related to global women's health and healthcare. The third goal, promoting gender equality and empowering women, had a specific target of eliminating gender disparity in primary and secondary education, preferably by 2005, and in all levels of education, no later than 2015. In 2015, the UN reported that "the developing countries as a whole have achieved the target to eliminate gender disparity in primary, secondary and tertiary education" but also that "women continue to experience significant gaps in terms of poverty, labour market and wages, as well as participation in private and public decision-making" (UN, 2015).

The fifth goal, improve maternal health, had two specific targets: reducing by three-quarters, between 1990 and 2015, the maternal mortality rate, and achieving universal access to reproductive health by 2015. In 2015, findings included "since 1990, the maternal mortality ratio has been cut nearly in half, and most of the reduction occurred since 2000." Monitoring of this goal also revealed that "more than 71 per cent of births were assisted by skilled health personnel globally in 2014, an increase from 59 per cent in 1990" (UN, 2015).

In a review of progress toward the 2015 MDGs, Meleis (2015) acknowledged the progress in achieving the reduction of maternal and infant mortality rates and increasing primary education for girls but identifies four major barriers that slow progress in meeting the goals for achieving optimal well-being for women. First is the narrow definition of women's health, often taken to be synonymous with reproductive health, as measured by maternal and infant mortality rates, and the limited access to healthcare for prenatal and postnatal care and/or family planning services. A life cycle and lifestyle approach that transcends the limits of the reproductive years is needed. Women manage multiple dimensions of health for themselves and their families as well as work inside and outside their homes. Discrimination and gender inequity in compensation challenge women. Moreover, women's longevity may leave them without resources for support as they age and face noncommunicable diseases.

A second barrier is a lack of a coherent theoretical framework for planning and implementing women's health programs, many of which focus on diseases and the reproductive system. Programs that do not accommodate women's multiple roles and the relationship to their environments, social, chemical, and physical, leave women exposed to health-damaging forces that ultimately limit health and development goals. Meleis (2015) recommends that three major concepts frame women's healthcare programs: equity and equitable care, women's roles, and enabling and empowering environments.

The narrow focus of health professionals' education constitutes another barrier. The narrow definition of women's health and lack of consideration of the needs of girls and older women do not prepare health professionals to care accountably for women. Issues that put women at risk for illness and compromised quality of life should be central to a curriculum that also provides integrated interprofessional education and interdisciplinary research programs that reflect gender and sex differences.

The UN used the MDGs as guidance for its initiatives until 2015, when the goals were replaced with Sustainable Development Goals (SDGs). The SDGs consist of 17 goals addressing poverty, hunger, the environment, health, and climate change, among others. Within the third goal, Good Health and Wellbeing, there are indicators specific to maternal health. The fifth goal, Achieve Gender Equality and Empower All Girls, contains nine target areas encompassing human trafficking, forced marriage, and unpaid domestic work, among many others. The UN is promoting a decade of action toward these goals with a target date of 2030.

Recognizing the importance of girls and women in the world, the *Lancet*, an internationally influential medical journal, commissioned "Women and health: The key to sustainable development," a report on the complex relations between women and health in our rapidly changing world. The Commission on Women and Health reported that worldwide priorities in women's health have been changing from a narrow emphasis on maternal and child health to a broader framework of SRH and a more encompassing concept of women's health using a life-span framework spanning fetal life to old age (Langer et al., 2015). The Commission examined the roles of women as both users and providers of healthcare. Providing that they remain healthy throughout life, experience gender equality, and are enabled, empowered, and valued in their societies as caregivers, women make contributions to their own health and that of their families and communities as well as to sustainable development. The Commission recommended the establishment of a women's health movement to address the ethical and public health imperatives of improving women's health; 5 years later, the *Lancet* commissioned a report on gender and global health (Hawkes et al., 2020). The purpose of this commission was to address ongoing neglect in consideration of gender in global health. Commissioners planned a 3-year time frame to identify solutions to achieve gender equity.

Around the globe, there are few gender-sensitive policies enabling women to integrate social, biological, and occupational roles and function to their full capacity. However, a number of countries do offer taxpayer-subsidized parental leave, often to both parents, following childbirth or adoption. In the United States, the Federal Employee Paid Leave Act (FEPLA) was enacted in October 2020, providing certain workers with up to 12 weeks of paid leave following childbirth or adoption (Department of Commerce, Office of Human Resources Management, 2020).

To further address global issues impacting women's health, the International Council on Women's Health Issues (ICOWHI) was formed in 1983. It is a multinational nonprofit organization with a goal of "promoting health, health care, and well-being of women throughout the world through participation, empowerment, advocacy, education, and research" (ICOWHI, n.d., para. 1). There are three specific ICOWHI goals related to women's healthcare:

- Increase the impact of members (individually and collectively) through improving the health and well-being of women internationally
- Contribute to reducing violence and its impact on vulnerable women across their life span in health and illness
- Develop worldwide partnerships and coalitions for the purpose of decreasing risks affecting the health and well-being of women

Inequity for women is reflected in the continuation of cultural practices including child marriage and servitude and limited educational opportunities for girls. Laws prohibiting human trafficking, female genital mutilation, female infanticide, and gender-selective abortion are necessary, as are policies for reporting, educating, preventing, and punishing sexual harassment, abuse, and slavery of women. Laws supportive of education of girls and women and women's decisions about pregnancy and family size are needed in many countries.

REFERENCES

References for this chapter are online and available at https://connect.springerpub.com/content/book/978-0-8261-6722-4/part/part01/chapter/ch03

CHAPTER 4

Oppression, Racism, Income Inequity, and Women's Health Outcomes

Kenya Massey, Jody Early, Cheryl L. Cooke, and Selina A. Mohammed

Nursing has a long history of providing care to oppressed populations who experience disproportionate rates of disease, morbidity, and mortality. Buerhaus et al. (2015) report that in a sample of 1,914 nurse practitioners and physicians whose practices are in primary care, nurse practitioners are more likely to care for racially/ethnically diverse patients and patients who are uninsured. In this chapter, we discuss how social determinants of health, particularly racism, contribute to a cascading series of problems that influence poor health outcomes for women. We also discuss how the concept of oppression is a fundamental cause of health inequality, offer a brief overview of the use of the term *oppression* rather than *vulnerability*, and provide examples of how systems of oppression perpetuate health inequities. Additionally, we provide a discussion on how providers can work more effectively with clients who have experienced systemic racism as well as other forms of oppression. We conclude with the importance of advocacy in nursing professional preparation and practice to design solutions that support "health for all" and equity and equality in women's healthcare (World Health Organization [WHO], 1999).

SOCIAL DETERMINANTS OF HEALTH AND ROOT CAUSES OF HEALTH DISPARITIES

The social determinants of health are the social and material contexts in which people live, learn, work, and play (Robert Wood Johnson Foundation [RWJF], 2014). Diverse populations of women experience the effects of the social determinants of health in unique ways. The outcome of these determinants for oppressed populations is often captured by the term *health inequities*.

In recognition of the relationship between living conditions and health, and the acknowledgment that these living conditions are often caused by societal injustices, the phrase *health inequities* reflects the move from the systematic health differences adversely affecting oppressed groups to a term that more explicitly links identified health differences to deeply rooted social, political, environmental, and economic injustices (Braveman, 2014; Braveman et al., 2011; Falk-Rafael, & Betker, 2012; National Collaborating Centre for Determinants of Health, 2014; Ranji et al., 2021). In order to understand the needs of individuals and groups who experience oppression, and the forces that put them at greater risk for adverse health conditions, we need to understand the structural and fundamental root causes for oppression, which are deeply embedded in racism. Current medical pedagogy fails to address and educate providers on the systemic effects of racism and how this impacts healthcare and medicine (Tsai et al., 2021). Critical race theory (CRT) in public health can help investigate and alleviate root causes of health-based racial inequities (Ford & Airhihenbuwa, 2010). The basic tenet of CRT is that race is a social construct, and that racism is not an individual problem but a problem that is imbedded structurally in systems that impact all areas of individuals' lives (e.g., legal, educational, economic, and political systems). A CRT approach encourages healthcare professionals to look beyond individual risk factors to examining the types of structural inequalities that perpetuate oppression in health and healthcare services (Tsai et al., 2021).

THE IMPACT OF RACISM

Racism and other systems of oppression are deeply embedded in U.S. society. Race is a social construct, not a biological one (Dominguez, 2008; Krieger, 2003). According to the

American Association of Physical Anthropologists (1996), "There is great genetic diversity in all human populations. Pure races, in the sense of genetically homogenous populations, do not exist in the human species today, nor is there any evidence that they have ever existed in the past" (p. 569). As socially constructed, individuals are understood in terms of racial/ethnic groups through self-identification and as others see that individual. Race can be used as a marker that allows for identifying, separating, and then marginalizing populations, often to their detriment. The term *racism* refers to an organized system categorizing groups of people into "races" in order to distribute goods and resources based on this social ranking (Bonilla-Silva, 1996). *Prejudice* can be defined as "learned prejudgment" about individuals from social groups to which we do not belong (Sensoy & DiAngelo, 2012, p. 28). Discrimination is acting on those prejudgments, to the detriment of nondominant groups (Sensoy & DiAngelo, 2012, 2017). Racism and discrimination need to be understood in terms of their structural effects. For example, racist and oppressive acts and behaviors and discriminatory policies within institutionalized social systems, such as education, healthcare, and economic settings, contribute to the long-term damage that low-income earners, people of color, and sexual minorities experience. Therefore, racism must be understood as systemic and as a population-level problem rather than as beliefs or behaviors acted out by problematic people on select individuals or groups (Cooke et al., 2014).

Racism, as we speak of it here, contributes to who experiences oppression. In this chapter we use the term *oppression* instead of *vulnerable*. In healthcare, we usually talk about populations in terms of their vulnerability. However, in this chapter, we use the term *oppression* because *vulnerability* underemphasizes the multidimensional processes that cause unequal distributions of material, cultural, social, and political resources. Furthermore, characterization of susceptibility and vulnerability can be perceived as disempowering, blaming, and deflective of root causes that increase risk (National Collaborating Centre for Determinants of Health, 2014). We use the language of oppression to signify how a group's worth can be relegated within social hierarchies from a central position to that of a lower or subordinate position within society. The effects of oppression diminish the social or political impact an individual or a group can exercise to their benefit within society.

Within the same framework, racism is a fundamental cause of health inequities (Phelan & Link, 2015). In this chapter, we continue our focus on racism as perpetuating oppressive structures and policies within the healthcare system and by those who work in it. Therefore, examining race and racism is essential in understanding patterns of disparity and inequality (Omi & Winant, 2015).

RESOURCE ALLOCATION AND THE UTILITY OF FUNDAMENTAL CAUSE THEORY

To better understand the impact of racism and oppression on health outcomes, we present a discussion on how resource allocation can negatively affect health outcomes. Link and Phelan (1995) describe fundamental cause theory:

A fundamental social cause of disease involves resources that determine the extent to which people are able to avoid risks for morbidity and mortality. Because resources are important determinants of risk factors, fundamental causes are linked to multiple disease outcomes through multiple risk-factor mechanisms. (p. 88)

Fundamental cause theory describes how flexible resources are used in a broad variety of events and how those with better resources have better outcomes (Link & Phelan, 1995; Phelan & Link, 2015). Fundamental cause theory also provides an explanation for disease persistence over time and asserts that social conditions are a root cause of health inequality (Link & Phelan, 1995). Phelan and Link (2015) posit that "systemic racism embodies a set of flexible resources that advantage whites" (p. 315). Examples of flexible resources include nonoccupational power and prestige, beneficial social connections, and freedom, which allow full autonomy over one's life and circumstances. Racism contributes to a lack of these resources for oppressed groups, making it a fundamental cause of health inequalities. Racism as a root cause of health inequities is related to multiple disease outcomes in a variety of ways including, but not limited to, stress and discrimination, neighborhood effects, and medical care (Phelan & Link, 2015; Williams et al., 2019). As such, racism is a poignant social determinant of health. According to Healthy People 2030, social determinants of health are the conditions in which people are born, live, and function that affect quality of life and well-being (Office of Disease Prevention and Health Promotion, 2021). Additionally, Milner et al. (2020) posit that understanding the varied contemporary forms of racism are essential to understanding the effects of the recent COVID-19 (i.e., SARS-Co-V-2) pandemic in communities of color. Therefore, it is fundamental to understand racism's history in the context of social determinants of health and the factors that perpetuate it, in order to dismantle racism and other forms of oppression. In nursing and other health professions, further education focused on addressing racism and oppression is needed to create a more equitable and just healthcare environment.

Groups and populations that experience oppression are more likely to experience stress and anxiety as well as negative health outcomes (Bambra et al., 2020; Phelan & Link, 2015). Women of color, sexual minorities, low-income earners, women with low health literacy, homeless women, substance-using women, immigrants and refugees, and women with physical and/or mental disabilities are examples of socially oppressed and underserved populations. However, it is important to note that these diverse populations experience the impacts of oppression differently from one another. An example of this can be demonstrated with income inequity and unemployment. Black women may face the effects of historical racism when attempting to find employment, which can amplify their experience with income inequality. This compounding effect is a result of overlapping and interdependent systems of discrimination referred to as *intersectionality*. Intersectionality is an analytical framework for understanding how aspects of a person's social and political identities combine to create different modes of discrimination and privilege. The term was coined by Kimberlé Williams Crenshaw in 1989 (Cooper, 2016). Looking at women's health through the lens of intersectionality will help to identify fundamental causes of health inequities and how the effects of oppression, discrimination, and/or racism can negatively impact women's health status.

INTERSECTIONALITY AS A LENS IN WOMEN'S HEALTH

Women experience the effects of the social determinants of health in unique ways, and the COVID-19 pandemic provides clear examples of this. Health inequities that existed prior to the pandemic were magnified, especially for women of color. For example, according to the 2021 Kaiser Family Foundation's (KFF) Women's Health Survey (Ranji et al., 2021), a larger share of women of color, and those from lower income groups, had to quit their jobs as well as take on additional caregiving responsibilities.

Many women have been on the front lines of the COVID-19 emergency, as essential workers, mothers, and caregivers. Lack of paid leave, family caregiving responsibilities, more traditional gender roles, and health concerns have placed many of the burdens of the pandemic squarely on the shoulders of women, and more specifically women of color. Results from a national survey revealed that nearly 1 in 10 women (8%) reported quitting their job for a reason related to COVID-19 and that more women (11%) who quit their jobs were younger, Black or Latina, uninsured, or low-income, and had attained less than a bachelor's degree (Ranji et al., 2021). For example, 17% of low-income women had to quit a job for a COVID-related reason, compared to 5% with higher incomes (Ranji et al., 2021).

The KFF 2021 report also revealed that the share of women who reported leaving a job was significantly higher among single mothers (17%) compared to those who were married or had partners (9%). Single mothers may face the double jeopardy of not having a partner to assist with child care or another source of income. Working outside the home during the pandemic was more common among women who were younger, had lower educational attainment, lived in rural areas, and reported lower incomes. For example, more than half of Hispanic/Latina women (53%) compared to 45% of White women indicated they worked outside their home. Conversely, half of Asian women workers (51%) reported working from home. Geography was also a factor: More than half of women residing in rural areas (58%) report working outside the home, compared to 44% of women in urban communities (Ranji et al., 2021).

In addition to income and geographic effects, gender inequality and negative health outcomes are also associated with caregiving and domestic labor (Guerrina et al., 2021). As a result of gendered work and the type of work that women do in healthcare, women are more often exposed to COVID-19 and at a much higher viral load than men (Penfold & Magee, 2020). We do not yet know the long-term health consequences of this level of exposure. Women make up a smaller percentage of the severe COVID-19 cases presenting in hospitals (Penfold & Magee, 2020), yet seem more likely to suffer from long-COVID-19 (Sudre et al., 2021). When looking at the

health data by race, women of color are more likely to experience morbidity and mortality because of the disadvantages and discrimination they face (Bambra et al., 2020). A systematic review of the published literature on COVID-19 revealed that women of color had an increased risk of infection with COVID-19 compared to White individuals (Pan et al., 2020). Within this review, 12 studies reported worse clinical outcomes, including ICU admission and death. It is interesting to note that very few analyses have drawn the link between comorbidities associated with pandemics and social factors (e.g., gender, class, and racism). The wealth of data collected during this pandemic are helping to identify the shortcomings of the U.S. economic, political, and healthcare systems as well as underscore the role of gender inequity and other social determinants on health outcomes.

INCOME INEQUALITY AS ASOCIAL DETERMINANT OF HEALTH

Income inequality is deeply connected to poor physical and mental health (Burns, 2015; Marmot, 2015), and gender and income inequality are strongly correlated. The U.S. wage gap statistic that often receives the most public attention is the overall ratio of women's to men's earnings among full-time, year-round workers—just 83 cents for women for every $1 earned by men in 2020 (Bleiweis, 2020). However, this statistic provides an incomplete picture because it treats women as a monolith and obscures the vastly different economic realities experienced by many women of color. The intersection of race, ethnicity, and gender has compounding effects, and these effects most often exacerbate and widen the wage gap (Hegewisch & Mefferd, 2021). According to data from the National Women's Law Center (NWLC) and the American Association for University Women (AAUW), for every dollar earned by men in 2020, Asian American and Pacific Islander (AAPI) women earned 87 cents, Black women earned 63 cents, Native/Indigenous women earned 60 cents, and Latina/Hispanic women earned 50 cents (Buchholz, 2021). Nearly half of women in the low-wage workforce are women of color, and one third of all low-wage earners are mothers, with 40% of them having family incomes below the poverty level. Many women are working multiple and/or temporary jobs in order to meet their family's economic needs.

Low levels of wealth are associated with poor health and poor health outcomes (Hajat et al., 2011), and net worth has been significantly associated with poor/fair health status between and within racial and ethnic groups (Pollack et al., 2013). Thinking about each of these conditions separately and through the lens of different populations of women may provide a greater understanding of the intricacies of how lower social status, health burden, and income disparity all contribute to poorer health outcomes. Women of color continue to experience the most severe gender wage gap in the United States, a reality that reflects the effects of intersecting racial, ethnic, and gender biases that threaten the economic security of them and their families. Three major drivers of the gender wage gap for women of color include jobs worked, hours worked, and discrimination (Hegewisch & Mefferd, 2021).

From a global perspective, women are overrepresented in low-paid, precarious sectors, such as retail, tourism, and food services (Oxfam International, 2021). These are sectors that have been hardest hit by the COVID-19 pandemic. Across South Asia, sub-Saharan Africa, and Latin America, the majority of women work in informal employment. Women also make up roughly 70% of the world's health and social care workforce—essential but often poorly paid jobs that put them at greater risk for disease and injury. Natural disasters, war, and pandemics place an added toll on women's income and women's health. Women and girls are generally earning less, saving less, and holding insecure jobs or living close to poverty (United Nations, 2020). The COVID-19 crisis cost women around the world at least $800 billion in lost income in 2020, which is equivalent to more than the combined gross domestic product (GDP) of 98 countries (Oxfam International, 2021).

Across the globe, women have been more likely than men to drop out of the workforce or reduce their hours during the COVID-19 pandemic, largely due to caregiving responsibilities. Even before the virus struck, women and girls put in 12.5 billion hours of unpaid care work each and every day—a contribution to the global economy of *at least $10.8 trillion a year*, which is more than three times the size of the global tech industry (Oxfam International, 2021).

A by-product of income inequity is food insecurity, an issue that affects the health of low-income women and their families and may be considered a risk factor for type 2 diabetes and other health problems (Seligman et al., 2007, 2012). Acute changes in income are related to the severity of food insecurity in some low-income families (Loopstra & Tarasuk, 2013). In a sample of low-income patients from King County, Washington, food insecurity has been linked to depression, poor diabetes control, and poor medication adherence (Silverman et al., 2015). In low-income earners, some women with diabetes not only experienced issues with food insecurity but also had transportation problems and, at times, lacked the functional ability to put healthy food on the table (Cuesta-Briand et al., 2011).

The depth and breadth of income inequality provides a lens through which the provider can see the trade-offs that many patients are forced to make in an effort to meet the basic needs of maintaining food and shelter. The lack of transportation can also limit how a woman participates in her care. An appreciation for the complexities that income inequality adds to a woman's living situation also allows providers to better understand how poor adherence and/or nonadherence to medical treatment or clinic follow-up may occur with this population and also why women in this situation may deem healthcare a lower priority.

Women who are low-income earners are often dealing with workplace problems that can affect their ability to prioritize healthcare needs. Although women have steadily increased their presence in work that takes place outside the home, they can often be found working in low-paying jobs that leave them vulnerable to workplace discrimination; lack of access to paid sick days, paid leave, or fair work schedules; challenges with finding high-quality child care; and lack of access to workplace-provided health insurance, retirement benefits, or comprehensive reproductive health services (Ben-Ishai et al., 2014; Entmacher et al., 2014).

Low income is associated with a persistent cycle of inadequate access to quality food, poorer access to housing, threats to personal safety, lack of access to care, and financial stress (Cunningham, 2018). Each of these issues magnify the health risks for this group. Many of these women end up working multiple jobs and working in harsh work environments. They experience issues such as lack of high-quality, affordable child care because of volatile and nonstandard work schedules and inconsistent paychecks (e.g., instability in work hours causes a lack of stability in earned income), which add additional stressors to these women's lives (Watson & Swanberg, 2011).

All these issues affect the amount of time that low-income women can dedicate to their own self-care. These women are challenged with meeting basic needs versus focusing on health goals. These issues are compounded by the fact that women who suffer from income inequities cannot afford to engage in costly health-promotion behaviors (e.g., gym memberships and yoga classes) and may live in neighborhoods where these amenities do not exist. In addition, physical activity may be further hindered by problems in the built environment, such as lack of sidewalks and a lack of street lighting (DeGuzman et al., 2013).

DISCUSSION

In this chapter, we have described how the social determinants of health and the multiple positionalities of most women in society can contribute to racism and oppression, and how this contributes to income inequality resulting in poor health outcomes for women. As a first step in improving women's health, provider self-reflection must occur. Educators and providers must reflect on their own biases and how they participate in maintaining the structural status quo. By understanding their own behavior, they are better equipped to stop the reproduction of actions that contribute to oppressive healthcare environments.

Other suggestions for improving women's health include designing and implementing social and economic policies through a multifocal equity lens and updating curriculum in nursing programs that are based on antiracist/antioppressive principles. The removal of barriers that prevent the full involvement of women in economic activities, equal pay and equal opportunities, economic and labor reforms, financing for women entrepreneurs, and mechanisms to promote women's self-employment are essential (United Nations, 2020). Such economic responses would need to occur in both the public and private spheres.

Recognizing the many risk factors of oppression is key to providing support and useful interventions to improve women's health. Providers need to view each health encounter as an opportunity to assess women for problems associated with oppression, racism, and other social determinants of health. Additionally, it is important to consider the ways these social determinants of health interact specifically with each client. Once the context in which a woman's health is shaped and maintained has been identified, appropriate resources must be located and offered. For instance, helping women connect with agencies to assist with applications for programs that provide low-income housing and temporary assistance for needy families (i.e., financial support) may be important to improving their quality of life. Food security issues can be addressed through federal programs such as the Women, Infants, and Children (WIC) program, local food banks, and an assessment of school meal programs for children.

Racial and ethnic discrimination must also be addressed, particularly if the provider hopes to better understand the health of women and sexual minorities of color. Understanding the burden of health risks that exists for women of color allows the provider to more closely follow the client and offer a higher level of support. For example, a major predictive risk factor for preterm birth in the United States is being Black. These women are at risk for low-birth-weight babies, preterm labor, and child mortality before first birthdays (Giurgescu et al., 2011). Differences in stressful life events, differences in socioeconomic status (SES), and exposure to racial discrimination and unfair treatment all have an effect on the racial differences in health outcomes, stress, and health (Schulz et al., 2000). Having a sense of the challenges faced by Black women in everyday life allows the provider to work with the client to manage the impact of problems such as implicit bias, microaggressions (e.g., "daily slights"), and overt racism (Burrow & Hill, 2012; Carter, 2007; Jernigan & Daniel, 2011).

Another way that health providers can improve their understanding of the lives of oppressed women is by learning the histories of the populations for which they are caring. The experiences of women of color, immigrant women, women with disabilities, and rural women often provide a nontraditional view of life in the United States that may be unfamiliar to providers, who often have a higher SES and full access to healthcare services, and who may not experience racial or ethnic discrimination in their daily lives. Sometimes, this history can be transmitted by working with these populations in nonprofessional situations such as volunteering in oppressed communities, participating on health services boards, and attending community functions outside a provider's own community.

Exploring diverse topics in patient education can be a way to increase the level of trust between a provider and an oppressed woman. Discussing health topics specific to these clients allows the client to see that the provider is not only interested in the present health problems but has a more global sense of the woman's world and overall well-being. Being available to women as a topic expert allows the client and their community to broaden their understandings of health. It also aids the community in building capacity through an increased access to health education and health systems knowledge.

FUTURE DIRECTIONS: A FOCUS ON SOCIAL JUSTICE

On a broader level, providers can be involved in patient advocacy and social justice. Providers who engage in advocacy can use their roles to support and champion the rights and interests of their clients (Zolnierek, 2012). This advocacy needs to occur in both the individual and the social realms. Because many root causes and drivers of health outcomes stem from social determinants, advocating for a change in social realms and fighting for social justice are imperative to the holistic provision of care. According to Thompson (2014), *social justice* may be defined as:

(a) interventions focused on social, political, economic, and environmental factors that systematically disadvantage individuals and groups; and (b) intervening in the effects of power, race, gender, and class where these and other structural relations intersect to create avoidable disparities and inequities in health for individuals, groups, or communities. (p. E18)

Thus, social justice involves examining the ways that patterns of privileges and disadvantage are created and sustained in society and challenging them.

Changing the educational system is critical to changing how clinicians understand how social histories can affect client health. To facilitate this understanding, academic institutions are well positioned to use antiracist pedagogy as a starting point in curriculum development. Antiracist pedagogy includes embedding a shared language about the historical context of racism in the United States. To accomplish this, faculty members can use nontraditional teaching components such as nonfiction books to facilitate the understanding of structural racism on public health. Additionally, faculty members can have students engage in antiracist case- and community-based projects to enhance real-world health equity skills. Antiracist-embedded curriculum that provides a foundational understanding of the structural nature of racism can foster systemic change in societal behaviors and practices (Rosario et al., 2022).

Clinicians are in a prime position to advocate for the health of their clients and for social justice. Several nursing and health organizations have charged clinicians to engage in social advocacy and social justice. For example, WHO has emphasized the critical role that clinicians have in achieving health equity through social justice (WHO & United Nations Children's Fund, 2020). Viewing the pursuit of health equity as the ethical and moral responsibility of all nurses, the American Association of Colleges of Nursing (AACN) has developed core competencies used for professional nursing education as described in the *Essentials* document that nursing schools use to meet accreditation guidelines. The requirement of social justice advocacy in the education of all levels of nursing is evident in this document (AACN, 2021).

Providers' knowledge of the social determinants of health and participation in activities that promote policy change can significantly improve the lives of their clients. Voting, awareness of changes in healthcare policy and financing, lobbying activities directed toward issues that affect health and healthcare, and civic engagement are crucial to eliminating health inequities. Partnerships among clients, providers, communities, and legislative bodies can create lasting and positive change in the healthcare system.

ADDITIONAL CHAPTER RESOURCES

Websites

SOCIAL DETERMINANTS OF HEALTH: HEALTHY PEOPLE 2030

https://health.gov/healthypeople/objectives-and-data/social-determinants-health

Healthy People 2030, U.S. Department of Health and Human Services, Office of Disease Prevention and Health Promotion.

LIFE EXPECTANCY BY ZIP CODE BY THE ROBERT WOOD JOHNSON FOUNDATION

https://www.rwjf.org/en/library/interactives/whereyouliveaffectshowlongyoulive.html

The latest estimates of life expectancy reveal differences down to the census tract level. Use the Life Expectancy tool by the Robert Wood Johnson Foundation to explore how life expectancy in America differs by area and resources.

RACIAL EQUITY TOOLS

https://www.racialequitytools.org

Racial Equity Tools is designed to support individuals and groups working to achieve racial equity. It offers **tools**, **research**, **tips**, **curricula**, and ideas for people who want to increase their understanding and to help those working for **racial justice at every level**.

Articles

Kuehnert, P., Fawcett, J., DePriest, K., Chinn, P., Cousin, L., Ervin, N., Flanagan, J., Fry-Bowers, E., Killion, C., Maliski, S., Maughan, E. D., Meade, C., Murray, T., Schenk, B., & Waite, R. (2022, January/February). Defining the social determinants of health for nursing action to achieve health equity: A con-sensus paper from the American Academy of Nursing. *Nursing Outlook, 70*(1), 10–27. https://doi.org/10.1016/j.outlook.2021.08.003

Williams, D. R., Lawrence, J. A., & Davis, B. A. (2019). Racism and health: Evidence and needed research. *Annual Review of Public Health, 40*, 105–125. https://doi.org/10.1146/annurev-publhealth-040218-043750

Resource Guides or Textbooks

Ford, C., Griffith, D., Bruce, M., & Gilbert, K. (2019). *Racism: Science and tools for the public health professional.* APHA Press.https://doi.org/10.2105/9780875533049

Kabir, M., & Hasnat, A. (2022). *Intersectionality resource guide and toolkit: An intersectional approach to leave no one behind.* UN Women, United Nations Entity for Gender Equality and the Empowerment of Women. https://www.unwomen.org/sites/default/files/2022-01/Intersectionality-resource-guide-and-toolkit-en.pdf

REFERENCES

References for this chapter are online and available at https://connect.springerpub.com/content/book/978-0-8261-6722-4/part/part01/chapter/ch04

CHAPTER 5

Legal Issues in Women's Healthcare

ANNA G. SMALL

The unique facets of women's sexual and reproductive healthcare are complemented and complicated by legal issues. The legal system, like the healthcare system, can be challenging to navigate, and healthcare consumers, providers, and institutions may become overwhelmed when the two intersect. This chapter provides an overview of key legal issues in women's healthcare so that the reader can navigate the complicated intersection of law and healthcare.

SOCIOCULTURAL CONTEXT

A provider of women's healthcare should have an understanding for the societal and legal context in which care is provided. At one time, in the not-so-distant past, access to contraception was seriously limited for most American women. Birth control was illegal in most states; therefore, women experienced significant challenges when trying to make choices concerning their fertility. The conversation became: Do married couples, extending to unmarried couples, have the right to decide whether to use contraception while engaging in private acts?

Contraception and a Right to Privacy

Into the 1960s, the state of Connecticut prohibited the use of any drug, medicinal article, or instrument for the purpose of preventing conception (*Griswold v. Connecticut*, 1965). Despite this, Planned Parenthood opened a contraceptive clinic in New Haven, Connecticut, and began to provide birth control to married women. Estelle Griswold, who was the executive director of the clinic, and Dr. Buxton, the medical director of the clinic, were arrested and charged with a misdemeanor related to their work. They appealed their convictions and challenged the validity of the law prohibiting contraception. They were ultimately able to convince the U.S.

Supreme Court that the law violated married couples' right to privacy (*Griswold v. Connecticut*, 1965).

The Supreme Court held that married couples had the right to decide whether to use contraception while engaging in private acts. To rule otherwise would be to invade marital privacy. The Court's opinion was significant for two reasons. First, it permitted at least married women to obtain contraception. Second, it established that the right to privacy is a fundamental right even though it is not specifically mentioned in the U.S. Constitution; the right to privacy is in the penumbras of the Constitution. The establishment of privacy as a fundamental right has been the justification for the findings of many courts since that time.

A few years after the landmark case in Connecticut, a Massachusetts case came before the Supreme Court and extended the right to privacy related to contraceptive choice to unmarried women (*Eisenstadt v. Baird*, 1972). The Court held that it was irrational to permit married women the right to use contraception but not to permit unmarried women the same right. Using the equal protection clause of the U.S. Constitution, the Court established that unmarried couples have the same right to contraception as married couples (*Eisenstadt v. Baird*, 1972).

This right to privacy first articulated by the Court in *Griswold* has been relied on by many courts since that time. Citing a right to privacy, the Supreme Court struck down a law prohibiting the distribution of birth control to women younger than 16 years (*Carey v. Population Services*, 1977). In *Moore v. City of East Cleveland* (1977), it struck down a law prohibiting extended families from living in a single household. In *Roe v. Wade* (1973) the Supreme Court struck down a law prohibiting abortion, and in *Loving v. Virginia* (1967), it struck down a law prohibiting interracial marriage. In *Lawrence v. Texas* (2003), the Court struck down laws that attempted to limit consenting adults' right to engage in homosexual sex. All of the decisions in these cases acknowledged that, based on the facts presented, an individual's right to privacy trumps the state's interest in proscribing the behavior in question.

DISCUSSION

The Supreme Court's decisions such as *Griswold* have significance to women's healthcare because it began to establish a woman's right to control her own fertility, but it also established a "zone of privacy" in which the state has no right to interfere. These concepts have since been extended to permit unmarried women to obtain birth control, live with the relatives they choose, and marry whomever they want. These concepts have also been used to support the rights of couples to engage in same-sex sexual relationships.

Right to Contraception Today

Most American women take access to contraception for granted. It is interesting to note that the average American woman desires two children and spends approximately 3 years of her life pregnant, in the postpartum period, or trying to get pregnant and, consequently, three quarters of her reproductive life trying not to get pregnant (Guttmacher Institute, 2019b). It is no surprise that access to and funding for contraception is a critical issue in women's health. It is estimated that every year, half of all pregnancies in the United States are unintended (Guttmacher Institute, 2019b) and that, by age 45, 1 in 4 women have had an abortion (Guttmacher Institute, 2019a). The data indicates that women who undergo abortions span all races, ethnicities, religions, ages, and socioeconomic status; 94% percent of women having an abortion identified as heterosexual, 4% as bisexual, 0.3% as lesbian, and 1% as "something else" (Guttmacher Institute, 2019a).

In 2010, $2.37 billion was spent on contraception, 75% of which were Medicaid dollars (Guttmacher Institute, 2019b). The Patient Protection and Affordable Care Act (ACA) contains a "contraceptive mandate," which means that private insurance plans (most often provided through employers) must cover, without copay or coinsurance, all forms of contraception approved by the U.S. Food and Drug Administration, including sterilization procedures (Guttmacher Institute, 2021).

There have been legal challenges to this contraceptive mandate, with various employers arguing that they have moral or religious objections to providing contraception to women through employer-sponsored plans. Hobby Lobby, a chain of hobby and craft stores owned by a single extended family, challenged the contraceptive mandate and argued that it violated the family's evangelical Christian beliefs. The case was heard by the Supreme Court, and a closely divided Court opined that it was a violation of the Religious Freedom Restoration Act to require certain closely held corporations to comply with the rules promulgated by the U.S. Department of Health and Human Services (DHHS) intended to implement the contraceptive mandate (*Burwell v. Hobby Lobby Stores, Inc.*, 2014).

The result of the *Hobby Lobby* decision is that women who work for employers who are closely held corporations and who have a religious or moral objection to the contraceptive mandate could have no access to contraception like their counterparts who work for other organizations. After the *Hobby Lobby* decision was issued, the DHHS promulgated rules that prevent the expansion of the Supreme Court's decision to companies that are not closely held. In addition,

the rules provide access to contraception for those women who work for the closely held corporations with objections (Planned Parenthood Action Fund, n.d.). Contraception and other preventive health services will be available to female employees of qualified objecting organizations at no cost to the organization or the women and the cost is shifted to insurers (Cooper & Goodstein, 2012).

Women's Access to Legal Abortion

Abortion, in one form or another, has always been available to women who have had unwanted pregnancies. Before approximately 1880, abortion was unregulated in the United States. Slowly the individual states began to make abortion illegal with limited exceptions. Of course, women still obtained abortions, but because of the illegal nature of these abortions, they were frequently unsafe or even self-induced (Baker, 2022).

In 1970, Jane Roe brought suit challenging the constitutionality of the Texas law prohibiting abortion except in cases where the life of the mother was endangered (*Roe v. Wade*, 1973). Roe stated that she was pregnant and unmarried and wanted to end her pregnancy in an abortion but was prohibited from doing so in violation of her constitutional right to privacy. The Supreme Court found that there was a right to privacy granted by the U.S. Constitution that was not explicit, but rather found in the penumbras of the Constitution. By this, the Court meant that the right to privacy and the freedom to make decisions around reproductive rights is found between the lines or implied in the Constitution.

The Court felt, however, that a woman's right to get an abortion is not unlimited. The states have a compelling interest in imposing certain restrictions on abortion. The Court opined that a "State may properly assert important interests in safeguarding health, in maintaining medical standards, and in protecting potential life" (*Roe v. Wade*, 1973, p. 154). Thus, states have the right to restrict and regulate abortion in the second trimester in "ways that are reasonably related to maternal health" (*Roe v. Wade*, 1973, p. 164). After viability, "the State in promoting its interest in the potentiality of human life may, if it chooses, regulate, and even proscribe, abortion except where it is necessary, in appropriate medical judgment, for the preservation of the life or health of the mother" (*Roe v. Wade*, 1973, p. 114).

In the early 1970s, viability was considered to occur at approximately 28 weeks of gestation, which corresponds to the beginning of the third trimester of pregnancy. Although the Supreme Court's written opinion in *Roe v. Wade* acknowledges a woman's right to choose and a woman's right to privacy, it also acknowledges the right of physicians to make these decisions with their patients. The Court stated that during the first trimester, "the abortion decision and its effectuation must be left to the medical judgment of the pregnant woman's attending physician" (p. 163). Additionally, the Court wrote:

> The decision vindicates the right of the physician to administer medical treatment according to his professional judgment up to the points where important state interests provide compelling justifications for intervention. Up to those points, the abortion decision in all its aspects

is inherently, and primarily, a medical decision, and basic responsibility for it must rest with the physician. (*Roe v. Wade*, 1973, pp. 165–166)

Although the Court did protect a woman's right to choose, it also showed deference to physicians' medical decision-making and acknowledged that its decision affected not only the rights of women, but also the rights of physicians to treat their patients as they see fit, preserving the significance of the physician–patient relationship.

Also of interest is that the Supreme Court declined to opine on the definition of personhood or when life begins. Justice Harry Blackmun wrote that since the members of the fields of medicine and philosophy were unable to agree on when life begins, it is a topic the judiciary is not competent to tackle (*Roe v. Wade*, 1973, p. 159).

The decision in *Roe v. Wade* is significant to women's healthcare because it has been the law for more than 40 years and women have had the right to choose abortion, with some restrictions, for close to half a century. The decision also has substantial legal significance because the Court protected a right that is not found explicitly stated in the Constitution and with that implied right invalidated laws about abortion in almost every state. Many scholars look at *Roe v. Wade* as having triggered renewed interest in the roll of the courts in interpreting the Constitution.

Progeny of *Roe v. Wade*

Roe v. Wade has not permanently resolved the abortion debate, but rather, it has been followed by a significant number of legal cases that have attempted to limit the rights to abortion recognized by the Court. In legal parlance, the cases that come after a landmark case and refine the landmark decision are known as *progeny*. Over time, the Supreme Court has been called on to determine whether states have the right to impose certain restrictions on a woman's right to have an abortion. The Court has upheld some restrictions and struck down others, including those in the following list:

- A husband has no right to interfere in a decision regarding abortion when the decision was made between the wife and her physician. States may not require spousal notification or consent before abortion (*Planned Parenthood of Central Missouri v. Danforth*, 1976; *Stenberg v. Carhart*, 2000).
- States may not prohibit specific procedures used for abortion (e.g., saline amniocentesis and partial birth–abortion; *Planned Parenthood of Central Missouri v. Danforth*, 1976). However, after the federal Partial-Birth Abortion Ban Act of 2003 passed, the Supreme Court upheld its constitutionality and the ban on specific abortion procedures included therein (*Gonzalez v. Carhart*, 2006).
- States may not require that all abortions be performed in hospitals (*City of Akron v. Akron Center for Reproductive Rights*, 1983; *Doe v. Bolton*, 1973; *Planned Parenthood Association of Kansas City, Missouri, Inc. v. Ashcroft*, 1983).
- States may require that all second trimester abortions be performed either in a licensed outpatient clinic or a hospital (*Simopoulos v. Virginia*, 1983).

- Statutes requiring parental notification and consent have been struck down if there is no adequate provision for a judicial bypass. A judicial bypass provides a minor with the procedural option of going to court, generally before a probate judge, and seeking an order that she does not need to notify her parents or that she does not require their consent. Generally, the minor must show that she is mature enough to make the decision about having an abortion or that it is not in her best interest to notify or seek permission from her guardian (*Bellotti v. Baird*, 1979; *City of Akron v. Akron Center for Reproductive Rights*, 1983; *Danforth*, 1976; *Hodgson v. Minnesota*, 1990).
- States may impose parental notification and consent requirements on minors when there is an adequate judicial bypass option (*Hodgson v. Minnesota*, 1990; *Ohio v. Akron Center for Reproductive Health*, 1990; *Planned Parenthood v. Casey*, 1992).
- States are not required to make public funds available to pay for abortions (*Harris v. McRae*, 1980; *Maher v. Roe*, 1977).
- States may impose a reasonable waiting period before an abortion is performed (24- to 48-hour waiting period is considered reasonable; *Planned Parenthood v. Casey*, 1992).
- The Supreme Court has declined to hear cases that are challenges to states' laws requiring the performance and explanation of an ultrasound before an abortion (Liptak, 2015).

On the eve of *Roe v. Wade*'s 50th anniversary, the Supreme Court overturned it and *Casey* in an opinion issued on June 24, 2022 (*Dobbs v. Jackson Women's Health Organization*, 2022). The ramifications of the Court's opinion in *Dobbs v. Jackson Women's Health Organization* are still being analyzed; however, they are likely to be significant.

Dobbs originated as a challenge to a 2018 Mississippi law, the Gestational Age Act, which prohibited most abortions after 15 weeks' gestation, even in cases of rape and incest. The law was challenged and made its way over the next few years up to the Supreme Court to oral arguments in December 2021. In an unprecedented development, the draft opinion of the Supreme Court was leaked to the press in May 2022 (Gerstein & Ward, 2022). After 2 months of protests and extensive media coverage, the Supreme Court issued its official opinion on June 24, 2022. The Court opined:

The Constitution does not prohibit the citizens of each State from regulating or prohibiting abortion. Roe and Casey arrogated that authority. We now overrule those decisions and return that authority to the people and their elected representatives. (*Dobbs v. Jackson Women's Health Organization*, 2022, p. 79)

The Court's opinion in *Dobbs* allows individual states the right to limit, prohibit, and criminalize abortion.

In the few years leading up to *Dobbs*, a small number of states passed laws that are collectively known as "heartbeat" laws (Rabin, 2021). These laws prohibit abortion after cardiac activity can be detected by ultrasound, which occurs at approximately 6 weeks of gestation. The laws in Georgia, Mississippi, Kentucky, and Ohio were not being enforced because they were tied up in legal challenges, but the legal landscape changed sufficiently with *Dobbs* to resolve most of these challenges. A law that went into effect on September 1, 2021 in Texas is a type of heartbeat law but was permitted to remain in effect while legal challenges continued in the courts (Rabin, 2021).

The Texas law is unique in that is not enforced by the state or law enforcement but creates a private right of action for citizens. Citizens may sue abortion providers and anyone who aids or abets a woman in her effort to obtain an abortion (McCammon, 2021). A successful lawsuit would lead to an award of $10,000 to the individual bringing the suit.

Opponents of the Texas law have expressed concern about the law's impact. They argue that it has a disparate impact on Hispanic women, low-income women, immigrant women, and teens (Gamboa, 2022). Adrienne Mansanares, CEO of Planned Parenthood of the Rocky Mountains, shares that since the Texas law was enacted, her locations are seeing more women from Texas and these women are coming at later term in their pregnancies since they have to arrange for travel, child care for other children, and the increased expense. She stated, "This is not about White women of means. They are going to get an abortion, they always have. This is about keeping communities of color in poverty" (Gamboa, 2022).

Abortion providers challenged the Texas law, but the court did not prevent the law from going into effect during the legal proceedings. The case has been elevated to the Supreme Court, which remanded it to the Texas appeals court for further consideration. In her dissent to the Supreme Court's Order, Justice Sonia Sotomayor, who is Latina, wrote: "The Court's order is stunning. Presented with an application to enjoin a flagrantly unconstitutional law engineered to prohibit women from exercising their constitutional rights and evade judicial scrutiny, a majority of Justices have opted to bury their heads in the sand" (*Whole Women's Health v. Jackson*, 2021). However, with the change in the law post-*Dobbs*, Justice Sotomayor's statement that the law is flagrantly unconstitutional may no longer be correct.

To date, women in some states still have a legal right to choose abortion. In other states, restrictions remain, or new ones are being enacted. Due to the unique nature of the enforcement of the laws, similar to the law in Texas discussed here, every heathcare provider should be aware of the laws in the state in which they practice. These restrictions are designed to prevent even out-of-state providers who engage in telehealth from providing abortion-related care to the states' citizens. Any provider who decides to offer services related to abortion should make sure they are informed about which laws may affect them and the ramifications of running afoul of the law.

REPRODUCTIVE TECHNOLOGY

Advances in technology and science now permit conception in situations when women were previously unable to conceive. Although the use of these technologies and techniques can be miraculous to a woman who desires a child, the path to motherhood can be fraught with unanticipated legal issues.

In Vitro Fertilization

In vitro fertilization (IVF) was invented to assist couples who were unable to conceive through traditional biological methods. Louise Joy Brown is considered to have been the first baby born alive as a result of IVF (James, 2013). Her parents, British citizens, had been trying to conceive a child for 9 years but were unable to do so through traditional methods because of her mother's blocked fallopian tubes. In 2010, one of the physicians who developed the IVF technique was awarded the Nobel Prize in Physiology or Medicine for his work. Although IVF brought joy to the Brown family and to millions of other families around the world, some have been critical of the use of IVF because of some of the unintended consequences (James, 2013).

One use of IVF is to permit the screening of certain genetic attributes. Preimplantation genetic testing can be used for a number of reasons that are generally accepted. These include when one or both partners has a history of inheritable genetic disorders, one or both partners is a carrier of a chromosomal abnormality, the mother is of advanced maternal age, or the mother has a history of recurrent miscarriages. In these cases, preimplantation screening can be used to prevent the implantation of an embryo with a devastating condition.

There are, however, a number of preimplantation screening practices that many people find more questionable (Hens et al., 2012). Social sex selection is generally disfavored, as is the practice of creating "savior siblings." Although many consider it acceptable to screen for inheritable conditions, which would be devastating to the newborn, selecting against embryos with genes correlated with late-onset and nonfatal conditions is more problematic. Opponents argue that it is a slippery slope to designer children. The selection for purely cosmetic traits (e.g., eye color, hair color, and skin complexion) is generally considered unethical. In addition, advocates for the rights of the disabled argue that it is inappropriate to value certain lives over the lives of those with specific disabilities (Hens et al., 2012).

OWNERSHIP OF UNUSED EMBRYOS

During the IVF process, a larger number of embryos are created than will be implanted in order to avoid repeating the arduous harvesting process if the initial IVF procedure is unsuccessful. In general, no more than two or possibly three embryos are implanted in order to avoid the health risks of high-level multiples to both woman and fetuses. The embryos that are not immediately implanted are cryo-frozen. Some couples use these additional embryos if no embryos implant, and others use them for subsequent pregnancies. However, commonly there are embryos that remain, and debate has arisen as to what should be done with the embryos.

IVF has furthered the discussion of when life begins. The discussion is, at this point, an ethical and moral one that is not regulated. Courts have generally shied away from a legal determination of when life begins. As the Supreme Court stated:

We need not resolve the difficult question of when life begins. When those trained in the respective disciplines of medicine, philosophy, and theology are unable to arrive at any consensus, the judiciary, at this point in the development of man's knowledge, is not in a position to speculate as to the answer. (*Roe v. Wade*, 1973, p. 159)

What courts have been forced to address is the ownership of the embryos and even the resultant children. In *Rogers v. Fasano*, a couple conceived twins through IVF. However, when the twins were born, they were clearly of different racial origins. Genetic testing was done and it became clear that the fertility clinic made a mistake and implanted one of the Fasanos' embryos and one from an unrelated African American couple (*Rogers v. Fasano*, 2000). A custody battle for the African American child ensued. The court "returned" the African American child to its biological parents and did not grant the Fasanos any visitation because it held that despite Mrs. Fasano acting as an unintentional surrogate, she had no legal right to the resultant child. The court discussed the issue of whether the embryos were persons or property.

In a highly publicized case, two celebrities engaged in a court battle over the right to use embryos after the couple's relationship ended. Nick Loeb publicly discussed the case of ownership of the two embryos created with his former fiancée Sofía Vergara when he published an opinion piece in the *New York Times* (Loeb, 2015). The couple created two female embryos, and Mr. Loeb filed suit in California seeking permission to have the embryos implanted in a surrogate and then have full custody of the resultant children. Ms. Vergara objected and apparently wanted to leave the embryos frozen indefinitely (*Doe v. Doe*, 2014). The California court never reached a decision over that case, because Mr. Loeb dismissed the case and then filed suit in Louisiana on behalf of the embryos and established a trust for the embryos, which he named Emma and Isabella (*Loeb v. Vergara*, 2021). In 2017, Ms. Vergara filed suit in Superior Court, Los Angeles County, seeking a declaratory judgment to enforce the parties' original agreement about the embryos and a permanent injunction to prevent Mr. Loeb from taking action to bring the embryos to term without her express written consent (*Loeb v. Vergara*, 2021).

The case Mr. Loeb brought in Louisiana presented unique and novel issues of law around the custody of pre-embryos and theoretical children. The court declined to address those issues and focused instead on whether Louisiana was an appropriate venue for the case (*Loeb v. Vergara*, 2021). In the original case in California, Mr. Loeb sought to have the court determine that an agreement he and Ms. Vergara signed, which stated that neither party would use the embryos without the other's consent, is invalid (*Doe v. Doe*, 2014). In Louisiana, Mr. Loeb alleged that the embryos were living children under Louisiana law, and he sought full custody. The court ultimately dismissed the case due to other legal procedural matters (*Loeb v. Vergara*, 2021).

Ultimately, Ms. Vergara's suit against Mr. Loeb in California was successful and the matter was legally resolved in early 2021 (Mauch, 2021). That court granted Ms. Vergara's permanent injunction, which prevents Mr. Loeb from using the embryos without Ms. Vergara's consent because the court determined their original written agreement with the assistive reproductive technology company prohibited either party from using the embryos without the other's consent. While this battle over the embryos was highly public and followed with interest since the parties were celebrities, it ultimately

did not resolve some of the more unique issues of law related to the potential parents' property rights in the embryos or the potential personhood of the embryos themselves.

Some legal scholars have argued that couples who voluntarily agree to have their gametes made into embryos no longer have a property right in the genetic information contained in the gamete. Thus, an individual whose genetic information is contained in an embryo intended, or at one time intended, to be implanted via IVF cannot prevent the implantation by arguing that they do not want to have a genetically related child brought into the world. Like gamete donation, or in unprotected intercourse, once the embryo has formed, property rights in the donor's genetic material is altered (Chan & Quigley, 2007).

Surrogacy Agreements

Some couples turn to surrogacy in order to reproduce. In such an arrangement, there are two women whose healthcare and legal rights may be at issue: the surrogate and the woman seeking to have a child. In addition, the woman seeking to have a child may have a partner, male or female, whose legal rights may be at issue. Finally, surrogates may be used by same-sex male couples seeking to have a child, in which case the only woman whose legal rights are at issue is the surrogate. A surrogate arrangement may involve a variety of combinations of egg and sperm, making the legal issues even more confounding. A couple seeking to have a child may use their own egg and sperm and have the embryo implanted in a surrogate, or the couple may use a donor egg, donor sperm, or a donor embryo. The couple seeking a child may be any combination of gender or race, their legal relationship status may vary, and single individuals may also seek to have a child without a partner. Due to all these variations, it is difficult to generalize about surrogacy arrangements.

Furthermore, surrogacy has been dealt with in a variety of ways by the states. Some states are considered "friendly" to surrogacy and others are not (American Surrogacy, 2022). What types of surrogacy arrangements are permitted will vary by state and the legal methodology to establish parenthood will also vary. It is critical that any party to a surrogacy arrangement seek the advice and counsel of an attorney specializing in these arrangements.

One of the first legal cases that arose out of a surrogacy arrangement was *In re Baby M* (1988), when a married couple, William and Elizabeth Stern, contracted with Mary Beth Whitehead for Ms. Whitehead to serve as a surrogate. William's sperm was used to artificially inseminate Ms. Whitehead, so the resultant embryo had half its genetic material from William and half from Ms. Whitehead. Such arrangements are now known as *traditional surrogacy* (Field, 2014). In these arrangements, the surrogate contributes half the genetic material for the baby and carries the baby to term, is compensated for her expenses and efforts, and then agrees to give up her parental rights to the couple contracting for the surrogacy (Field, 2014).

The conflict arose when Baby M was born and Ms. Whitehead refused to give up the child to the Sterns. As the biological father, it was clear that Mr. Stern had at least as much right to the child as Ms. Whitehead. And although the parties had entered into a contract that set forth their arrangement, the New Jersey Supreme Court held the contract was void as a matter of public policy and used the "best interests of the child" standard to determine child custody (*In re Baby M*, 1988). In addition, the court stated the contract was illegal under New Jersey law, which prohibited the exchange of money in connection with adoptions. The court held that Ms. Whitehead was the legal mother of the child and Mr. Stern was the legal father of the child. Ultimately, the court case became a custody battle between Ms. Whitehead and Mr. Stern similar to any child custody case. The court is supposed to consider what custody arrangement is in the best interests of the child and in the case of Baby M, the court held that Mr. Stern should have full custody (*In re Baby M*, 1988).

Since the heart-wrenching case of Baby M, the use of surrogates has grown. Many states have passed laws that govern these arrangements and set forth permissible terms of a surrogacy contract. The legislative intent is to protect the rights of the surrogate as well as the party or parties seeking to have a child. A surrogacy contract is a complicated contract, and a healthcare provider would be wise to encourage the parties to seek legal advice and counsel. Generally, a legal surrogacy contract will include provisions that permit the healthcare and basic expenses of the surrogate to be paid by the party seeking to have a baby. It is prohibited, however, to pay a fee to the surrogate for her services. This is intended to prevent surrogacy from becoming an industry, particularly because of the potential abuse of women, which has been reported to occur in some parts of the world (Chan & Quigley, 2007).

With the development of reproductive technology, many surrogacy arrangements are now "gestational surrogacies," in which the surrogate mother has no genetic tie to the resultant child (Field, 2014). These arrangements involve the use of donor eggs, and the courts have analyzed these arrangements in a different manner. One court determined that the birth mother had no parental rights to the resultant child when she had contributed no genetic material to the child. "It is not the role of the judiciary to inhibit the use of reproductive technology when the legislature has not seen fit to do so" (*Johnson v. Calvert*, 1993, p. 787).

Not all states have followed the precedent established by the California court in *Johnson v. Calvert*. Some continue to hold surrogacy contracts void as a matter of public policy and therefore unenforceable. Others have enacted legislation that sets forth the terms and conditions of a valid surrogacy contract. Some states distinguish between traditional and gestational surrogacy, and others distinguish between altruistic surrogacy and compensated surrogacy (Field, 2014). The state of New Jersey, the location of the seminal Baby M case, passed the New Jersey Gestational Carrier Agreement Act in 2018 (N. J. Stat. Ann., 2018). The act sets forth the rights of gestational surrogates, specifies appropriate terms of surrogacy contracts, and establishes a process whereby intended parents obtain a prebirth order (PBO) in order to establish their legal parenthood.

As an example, Florida has legislated surrogacy contracts and requires that the intended parents be married, at least one of the intended parents donate genetic material to the fetus, and a physician has certified that the woman is unable to carry a child to term. The surrogate may not be compensated, but her reasonable expenses may be paid, and she can be required to adhere to medical advice about her prenatal health. Once the birth occurs, the intended parents must petition the court to ensure that their parental rights to the child are established and that the terms of the contract were in compliance with the law (Fla. Stat. § 742.15, 2020). Married same-sex couples may take advantage of gestational surrogacy under the same terms as opposite-sex married couples (Phillips, 2016).

Some states are surrogacy "friendly" and do not place the same restrictions or requirements on surrogacy arrangements. California, like New Jersey, permits the intended parents to obtain a court order before the child's birth, which sets forth that the intended parents are the parents on the birth of the child (Field, 2014). Currently, the surrogacy "friendly" states are California, Connecticut, Delaware, Maine, New Hampshire, Nevada, Oregon, Rhode Island, Washington, and the District of Columbia (American Surrogacy, 2022). New York and Michigan are considered the least surrogacy friendly states (American Surrogacy, 2022). Despite the legal disfavor of surrogacy in New York, the surrogacy business is thriving, with many couples seeking surrogacy arrangements and multiple agencies set up to match intended parents and surrogates (Conklin, 2013). The contracts regarding the surrogacy are simply executed and carried out in other jurisdictions. Of course, the legal disfavor of the contracts becomes a problem only when the parties no longer agree with the original terms of the contract or some other conflict arises.

Gestational surrogacy is the type that is most commonly practiced today and surrogates are often brought together with couples seeking a surrogate through private agencies, which charge various fees. In addition, if the surrogacy arrangement involves the use of donor eggs, additional parties and expenses are involved (Field, 2014).

The legal rights to a child who is born through the use of reproductive technology is a novel issue for courts to address. Courts have had to address the issue of biological versus legal parenthood. Historically, a woman who bore a child was considered the biological and legal mother. If the woman was married at the time of the birth, the husband was the putative father of the child and was thus considered the legal and biological father (*Michael H. v. Gerald D.*, 1989). With the discovery of DNA and the ability to determine scientifically which man is the biological father of the child, courts have more frequently turned to science to determine paternity rights. However, advancing technologies, which permit the use of donor sperm and donor eggs, further complicate courts' determinations. Biological parenthood may be irrelevant to legal parenthood with, at least in some cases, the biological parents not even desiring parental rights.

Women who serve as surrogates may do so of their free will either out of monetary or altruistic motivation. However, that does not mean that all women who serve as surrogates do so because they want to. Serving as a surrogate can prove to be a profitable way for women to use their bodies without engaging in prostitution or selling their children (Conklin, 2013). Particularly in international surrogacy arrangements, women may feel that it is one of few routes to financial stability. And when the contract goes awry, they may have little, if any, recourse.

DRUG USE IN PREGNANCY

As discussed earlier, courts have yet to weigh in on when life begins, but there has been a long line of cases that deals with a woman's right to make decisions during pregnancy when those decisions may be adverse to the interests of the fetus. Prenatal drug use is associated with poor neonatal outcomes and perinatal complications including low birth weight, prematurity, placental abruption, and stillbirth (Hulsey, 2005). Consequently, states have passed laws that permit prenatal testing without consent and laws that are designed to penalize women who engage in prenatal drug use.

There are 24 states that consider substance abuse during pregnancy to be child abuse, and 25 states require healthcare providers to report pregnant women if the provider suspects substance abuse. In contrast, 19 states have created or support substance use treatment centers for pregnant women (Guttmacher Institute, 2023).

In 1996, South Carolina was the first state that prosecuted a woman for illegal drug use in pregnancy on the grounds that it constituted child abuse (Hulsey, 2005). Women were tested for drug use, without consent, in a public hospital in South Carolina. Women who tested positive were arrested, were incarcerated, and faced a prison term of up to 10 years. Several of the women who were arrested under the South Carolina law challenged the law, and the case was ultimately heard by the U.S. Supreme Court, which held that particular law unconstitutional (*Ferguson v. City of Charleston*, 2001). South Carolina continues to have laws that penalize women who use illegal drugs during pregnancy and in 2001 convicted Regina McKnight, whose fetus was stillborn after she used cocaine, of murder. Ms. McKnight was sentenced to 12 years in prison despite having three other minor children. Her sentence was overturned by the South Carolina Supreme Court in 2008 when it ruled that Ms. McKnight did not get a fair trial (Drug Policy Alliance, 2008). A prior appeal of Ms. McKnight failed when the South Carolina Supreme Court held that a pregnant woman who intentionally heightens the risk of a stillbirth could be found guilty of homicide because of her "extreme indifference to human life" (Drug Policy Alliance, 2008).

Alabama has also been aggressive about removing children from a mother's custody when there is evidence of drug use. The children are often placed with a family member or in foster care under a safety plan that can last for years (Martin, 2015). One woman was evaluated by healthcare providers during her postpartum hospitalization and evaluated by social services once she went home with the baby. Social services and her physician felt there was no risk to the baby, but within a few weeks she was arrested and charged with a felony punishable with up to 10 years in prison. Alabama has the country's toughest law on prenatal drug use and this woman was alleged to have violated the law when she admitted to taking two, unprescribed, one-half doses of Valium during the last weeks of her pregnancy. The Alabama law can charge a woman with chemical endangerment of her fetus from the earliest weeks of her pregnancy and even if the baby is born completely healthy. A woman charged with a violation of the law not only faces prison time if convicted, but also faces losing custody of her other children (Martin, 2015).

The goal of the laws making drug use during pregnancy a felony has been articulated as forcing women into treatment, not to necessarily incarcerate women or force children into the foster care system. However, critics of the laws state that treating drug addiction as a crime rather than as a disease makes women avoid prenatal care and can interrupt the bonding of a newborn with its mother at a time when the mother and infant are at their most vulnerable (Martin, 2015). Opponents of the laws argue that healthcare providers should treat all women with compassion and support and avoid stigmatizing women who use drugs (Eggertson, 2013). Loretta Finnegan, MD, a former medical adviser to the Office of Research on Women's Health of the National Institutes of Health, advises using prenatal care as an opportunity to help women with addiction issues and to promote long-lasting meaningful change in the life of a woman and her child. Opponents further urge assisting women during prenatal care with continuing support and assistance into the future in order to effect change (Eggertson, 2013).

Recent research suggests that programs that impose penalties on women who engage in substance use while pregnant are not successful in decreasing substance use (Faherty et al., 2019). In fact, researchers found increased rates of neonatal abstinence syndrome (NAS) in neonates in the years after punitive policies were enacted. The authors of the study suggest that policy makers may wish to expand their efforts instead at primary prevention of substance use.

LEGAL ISSUES IN DOMESTIC VIOLENCE

Intimate partner violence and other forms of domestic violence are at epidemic proportions in the United States and around the world. One in four women experiences domestic violence in her lifetime (National Coalition Against Domestic Violence [NCADV], 2020). Domestic violence against women affects all types of women in all socioeconomic groups. One in three heterosexual women, two in five lesbian women, and three in five bisexual women will experience rape, physical violence or stalking by an intimate partner (Safe Horizons, 2022). Of these women, one in five requires medical care as a result of their experience (NCADV, 2020). Any women's healthcare provider must be attuned to the methods for screening for domestic violence and assist their patients who are victims. However, men are victims of domestic violence and the incidence of male victims may be underreported. In the United States, there are an estimated 10 million total cases of domestic violence annually (NCADV, 2020).

A woman's healthcare provider must be familiar with the social service resources available to aid victims of domestic violence and must also have an understanding of some of the legal issues that surround domestic violence. Domestic violence has significant physical and mental health ramifications; 56% of women who experience any partner violence are diagnosed with a psychiatric disorder. A total of 29% of all women who attempt suicide were battered, 37% of battered women have symptoms of depression, 46% have symptoms of anxiety disorder, and 45% experience posttraumatic stress disorder. Additionally, 37% of women's ED visits are the result of domestic violence (American Bar Association, 2016). Only 34% of those injured in intimate partner violence receive treatment for their injuries (NCADV, 2020).

The problems with assisting victims of domestic violence are well documented in the psychosocial literature on the topic. There are a number of ways in which the legal system can support such victims, and there are also challenges within this system. It is often overwhelming to a victim to initiate contact with law enforcement, but it is critical to the success of the legal system to obtain a timely and comprehensive police report. Victims are often reluctant to bring law enforcement into the case for a multitude of reasons, but without law enforcement involvement, the perpetrator may not be stopped until it is too late (National Coalition Against Domestic Violence, n.d.). Three of four female homicide victims are killed by a husband or a lover, often with no prior report to law enforcement (CNN, 2022).

Women who are victims of domestic violence may experience long-term health risks as well. According to a study done by the Centers for Disease Control and Prevention (CDC), female victims are 80% more likely to suffer a stroke, 70% more likely to have heart disease, 70% more likely to become heavy drinkers, and 60% more likely to become asthmatic than women who are not (Black, 2008). Under the ACA, annual domestic violence screenings are a mandated preventive service (Culp-Ressler, 2013).

Women may not feel supported by law enforcement or the criminal justice system. Not only is it emotionally trying to involve law enforcement, but in many states domestic battery without permanent injury is only a misdemeanor charge. Women may also be faced with the prospect of losing financial support if their abusive partner is arrested, jailed, or charged (National Coalition Against Domestic Violence, n.d.). Whether or not charges are filed against a perpetrator is determined by the state and not the victim. A state may be less likely to bring charges if the victim is uncooperative and the victim may request leniency for the perpetrator, but the victim cannot unilaterally "dismiss the charges." Cerulli et al. (2015) state that, within the criminal justice system, there are a number of options for those accused of domestic violence. Many jurisdictions have diversion programs for first-time offenders. These programs are similar to probation, and the accused must regularly meet with an officer of the state, attend various classes designed to reduce the incidence of domestic violence, participate in community service, pay court costs, and perhaps pass random drug or alcohol testing. If the accused completes the diversion program successfully, the state agrees to drop the charges.

For those who are not first-time offenders, the accused can enter a plea of guilty or nolo contendere (no contest) in exchange for probation or some other reduction in penalty. The terms of probation are generally similar to those of a diversion program. The difference is that if the accused successfully completes the probation, the charges are not dismissed and if he fails to complete the probation or does not comply with the terms, he may be incarcerated.

Some accused will opt to exercise their rights to a trial. Although anyone accused of a crime in the United States is innocent until proven guilty and has a right to a speedy trial, many accused will waive their right to a speedy trial in order to mount a more comprehensive defense. This may cause the case to drag on for many months, which can be an additional stressor for the victim. The victim will be called to testify at trial, which can be an extremely traumatic experience for her, and she may also be concerned if her children or other relatives were witnesses to the violence and are called to trial. Anyone who receives a subpoena compelling them to testify at trial must comply with the subpoena or face being in contempt of court.

Another way the legal systems attempts to assist victims of domestic violence is through domestic violence injunctions (Nichols, 2013). These are court orders that may be obtained by the victim and order the accused to stay away from the victim as well as generally her place of work and her home. They can be obtained based solely on the accusations of the victim, with no proof required, but these are temporary injunctions, which are effective for a matter of days or weeks when there will be a hearing in front of a judge where both victim and perpetrator have the right to appear and testify. These proceedings are also in open court and thus are open to the public. The judge may decide whether to make the injunction permanent or dissolve the injunction. Although the injunction may be made "permanent," it is not indefinite, but for a specific period of time, generally no more than a year.

Some jurisdictions have legal services whereby injunctions can be obtained any day of the week, and there may be volunteers to assist a woman with the paperwork involved. Navigating the judicial system in order to obtain an injunction may be overwhelming, and the victim may need significant support. This support is often available through social services such as women's shelters and other support groups. However, a healthcare provider should be familiar with what is available so that the victim can be pointed in the right direction.

A woman may have additional legal issues to contend with. She may need to obtain a divorce and negotiate child custody issues, including timesharing and child support. She may have lost her only means of financial support and, because of the psychological effects of domestic violence, may have difficulty making her way through the legal system.

FUTURE DIRECTIONS

Improving women's access to care has historically been disproportionately affected by a lack of access to healthcare and this is in part because of underinsurance or a lack of insurance coverage. The ACA, signed into law on March 23, 2010, by President Barak Obama, has increased Americans' access to care (Blumenthal et al., 2015). A provision of the law provides for subsidies for Americans purchasing insurance through the Health Care Marketplace and 87% of those using the Marketplace qualify for governmental subsidies. Additionally, a total of 10.8 million Americans have enrolled in Medicaid since ACA's enactment (Blumenthal et al., 2015).

Women benefit from the ACA in very specific ways. Before enactment of all of the ACA provisions, in 2012 a 25-year-old woman could expect to pay 81% more for the same insurance policy offered to her male counterpart

(DHHS 2015). Additionally, women were more likely to be insured as dependents and therefore more vulnerable to loss of coverage. The ACA provisions make insurance more accessible to women regardless of their status as a dependent. Women are now more likely to be covered and more likely to have better coverage than they did before the ACA (DHHS, 2015). Even women with Medicare are now able to benefit from various preventive services without having to pay any cost sharing.

The ACA is not the first attempt at expanding coverage for women. Breast and cervical cancers are the leading cancers among women and various government initiatives have been established to increase women's access to screening and treatment for these cancers. Low-income and minority women are at risk for increased mortality and morbidity as well as at risk for not having adequate access to care once screening results are positive (Rosenbaum, 2012). In 1990, Congress established the National Breast and Cervical Cancer Early Detection Program. The program provides grants to states to increase access to breast and cervical cancer screenings for at-risk women. The problem for women participating in the program is that once they have a positive screening test, access to further diagnostic tests and treatment may be unavailable or prohibitively expensive. As a result, in 2000 Congress enacted the Breast and Cervical Cancer Prevention and Treatment Act, which was designed to increase access to follow-up care and treatment by permitting states to establish an optional Medicaid program to cover women regardless of income (Rosenbaum, 2012). The ACA ensures that these same women cannot be denied a policy on the private market because of a previous positive screen or treatment through public programs (Rosenbaum, 2012).

States have the ability to opt out of the expanding Medicaid coverage and this "coverage gap" affects hundreds of thousands of women (Norris, 2023). As of early 2022, 38 states and the District of Columbia have expanded access to Medicaid (Norris, n.d.). Women in expansion states are more likely to have greater access to breast and cervical cancer screening and treatment than those in nonexpansion states (Sabik et al., 2015). Women with health insurance are twice as likely to receive breast and cervical cancer screening and therefore are much more likely to receive timely and appropriate treatment (Sabik et al., 2015).

CONCLUSION

A healthcare provider's advocacy for a woman includes assisting her to navigate the intersection of healthcare and the law. There are experts in healthcare law and the provider should be knowledgeable enough to make appropriate referrals to these experts to assist women in their times of legal need.

REFERENCES

References for this chapter are online and available at https://connect.springerpub.comcom/content/book/978-0-8261-6722-4/part/part01/chapter/ch05

CHAPTER 6

Seeing the Whole: Feminist Theory as a Model for Patient Care

Meghan Eagen-Torkko, Selina A. Mohammed, and Cheryl L. Cooke

INTRODUCTION

In the United States, women's health providers are not providing care for just "American" women; they are caring for women and other minoritized genders from disparate countries and living situations. Having a framework that guides understanding of the complexities of women's experiences worldwide provides a broader foundation within which to understand the health needs of these populations. In this chapter, we explore how feminism can guide our thinking about women and how we view and respond to their healthcare needs. We begin with a discussion of feminism, including feminist theory and inquiry, as background against which to consider concepts central to nursing practice with women. We also examine how knowledge of these theories can be useful in understanding the economic, political, and social situations that contribute to poor health outcomes. Finally, we conclude with a case study and apply feminist theory to illuminate ways of supporting gender minoritized populations in attaining optimal health when developing a treatment plan.

Note on language: *Women's health* has been used to describe comprehensive care of women for many years; however, in the past the term has been used exclusively to refer to the care of cisgender women. This is problematic, because many aspects of healthcare for nonbinary, trans, and other gender diverse people are encompassed in "women's health." Using the term to include only cisgender women excludes trans men, for example, from care they may need. Likewise, defining *women's health* exclusively by the anatomy of the person in question will often exclude trans women from that care. In both cases, the use of the term *women's health* requires some people to misgender themselves or be misgendered by their providers to seek healthcare. In both cases, this is harmful to the health of gender diverse people (e.g., Baldwin et al.,

2018). A solution proposed is use of *sexual and reproductive healthcare* (although this does not encompass the nonreproductive healthcare of women and nonbinary people) or a new term yet to be determined.

However, there are relevant aspects to the use of "women's health" in the context of a feminist discussion of healthcare. First, and possibly most centrally, misogyny, homophobia, and transphobia are all deeply gendered oppressions that affect people seen as divergent from the straight, cisgender male "norm." Although these affect people in different ways depending on their gender identity, sexual orientation, and gender expression, they all have at their center a devaluation and disregard for people who are not straight cisgender men. Additionally, as discussed later, racism, xenophobia, ableism, and classism also affect how women and others experience health and healthcare. The use of *women's health* in this chapter is not intended to exclude trans, nonbinary, and other gender diverse people, but rather to acknowledge the role that misogyny plays in health for all those seen as "other," and to examine the ways in which feminism and feminist theory can positively affect that health.

WHY FEMINISM IS AN IMPORTANT CONSIDERATION WHEN PROVIDING HEALTHCARE SERVICES

The word *feminism* invokes a variety of responses reflecting confusion and lack of awareness of the large body of feminist theory. It is not uncommon to find people of all genders who insist they are not "feminists" yet who advocate feminist agendas. For some, feminism conveys threatening images of a social order in which everything is different from the status quo. For others, feminism describes a situation where gender identity is understood as a notion that imparts equity in political, economic, and social rights. Many definitions of feminism include not only equality for all, but improving the circumstances that underpin inequities, as well as those that maintain cycles of discrimination.

DiEmanuele (2013) suggests that feminist theory is important "because, like any study of injustice, it exposes the illogical format of the arguments that support prejudice and discrimination. Furthermore, it provides a point of reason—and thus, understanding—for those who are unaffected" (p. 1). This is precisely the challenge that provokes anxiety and rejection of any social movement that seeks to disrupt the existing social order; this is not specific to feminism. However, the relative success of second-wave feminism's focus on economic and employment changes has led many women—particularly heterosexual White cisgender women, who were the primary beneficiaries of this work—to declare feminism unnecessary, or worse, outdated.

In recent years, the role of "feminism" has been challenged in ways that seem focused on dismantling the forward movement in many areas of women's issues, gender identity, and democratic equality. Language that was once used to support the ideals of inclusion and achievement for women and other traditionally marginalized groups is now being appropriated and used to fragment and dismantle groups that have traditionally promoted human rights for one another. For example, from the 1990s until his death in 2021, a neoconservative talk-show host consistently referred to feminists as "feminazis" (Merriam-Webster, n.d.), which was followed by websites where young women post pictures with handwritten explanations of why they do not need feminism (e.g., womenagainstfeminism.tumblr.com). Prominent cultural tropes of feminism as antifamily and disrespectful of women who choose traditional roles have pushed aside feminism as a movement for equity for all women, aided by the rise of evangelical churches whose adherents promote a model of submission-based "Biblical womanhood" as essential to a moral life (Murray, 2021). Feminism was famously described by one evangelical as "[a] socialist, anti-family political movement that encourages women to leave their husbands, kill their children, practice witchcraft, destroy capitalism and become lesbians" (The Associated Press, 1992). This narrative is less a difference of opinion and more an active propaganda effort to create fear and discomfort about a concept that may not be well understood.

Fear-based reactions to our struggle for equality must be met head-on, making it essential to continue to explore how gender is experienced and enacted, and how our understandings of it may interfere with achieving optimal health for racial and gender minoritized populations. For example, losses based on both racial and gender group identity continue to contribute to the struggles in pay equity and health disparities (Correa-de-Araujo & Clancy, 2006; Goldberg Dey & Hill, 2007; Ligh et al., 2020; Marrero et al., 2021). They also contribute to losses in freedom for women and gendered "Others" that have occurred because of globalization, as well as active policy efforts to limit access to care for sexual and reproductive health and for gender-affirming care for trans and other gender diverse people. Whether direct or indirect, intentional or ancillary, these losses have impacts on the health of women and minoritized gender diverse persons.

The concept of "othering" or marking groups as "other" than dominant involves power differentials in society that serve to privilege members of dominant society (e.g., men, White people, wealthy people) and marginalize others (e.g., minoritized persons such as women; gender and sexually diverse persons; Black, Indigenous, and persons of color [BIPOC]; people living in poverty). This concept describes unequal power relationships between advocates and people who are advocated for, and calls into question who has the right to speak for whom. One of the weaknesses of the second-wave feminist movement of the 1970s, for example, was its overlooking of the voices of BIPOC, low-income people, disabled people, and queer[1] people about their own lives in favor of a largely White middle-class straight cisgender narrative and priorities. This failure not only marginalized many Black and queer activists and scholars, for example, it limited the capacity of feminism to address the unchallenged underlying structures of oppression, including racism and colonialism. The intersections between racism, classism, sexism, and homo/transphobia, as well as ableism, are only recently being recognized and included in analyses of gender oppressions.

This chapter contains historical citations and material from the late 1700s through current times to represent the breadth and depth of thought in feminist theory. We briefly explore several prominent feminist theories and concepts that may be considered as supportive of gender-specific healthcare. Just as there is no single theory that describes health, there is no single definition of feminist theory that covers all situations or gender groups. Feminists are interested in a wide range of concerns influenced by the particular philosophical, cultural, political, and economic perspectives, from which we view, interact within, interpret, and represent our worlds. As feminist theory is varied and is updated in response to political, social, economic, and environmental changes in our world, we can better understand its history by examining it in "waves" and seeing how these changes built one upon another, both affected by and affecting historical change in society.

The first wave of U.S. feminism is classically thought of as the events surrounding women's suffrage (mid-1800s to early 20th century), which coincided with the profound social changes of the Industrial Revolution, the abolition of slavery in the United States (and subsequent reactionary Jim Crow laws), and the concentration of wealth of the Gilded Age. Relevant for healthcare, it also coincided with the centralization of power in allopathic medicine, the marginalization of midwives, and the explosion of "blue laws" banning abortion, contraception, and obscenity (described famously by Supreme Court Justice Potter as "I can't define it, but I know

---

[1] The use of "queer" is intentional here. While the word has been frequently used as a slur, the reclamation as an identity by many LGBTQ+ people has been followed by a growing body of scholarship in queerness as not only a sexual orientation/gender identity, but also as an active challenge to systems of power.

it when I see it," *obscenity* is generally used to refer to scatological or sexual topics not for public discussion) or even discussions of these (Reagan, 1997). Significantly, the first wave ended around the First World War, which represented both a profound disruption of the social order and a movement toward progressive policies that came to fruition with the New Deal policies of the 1930s.

The second wave of feminism in the United States began around the late 1960s and centered on organizing women and using feminism as a resource for seeking equality in social organizations. This centered on economic and educational access to existing systems, rather than a wholesale disruption of these, and while the benefits of this movement were felt by (cisgender) women as a whole, White middle-class straight women disproportionately benefited from that centering. This wave of feminism focused on legal status (legalization of abortion with 1973's *Roe v. Wade* decision is an excellent example) without necessarily adequately addressing access and equity (*Roe* was followed immediately by the Hyde Amendment, which barred the use of federal funds for abortion care and limited access to the ostensible right for low-income pregnant people [Adashi & Occhiogrosso, 2017]). As the progressive policies of the New Deal were followed by the Red Scare of the 1950s and World War II Rosie the Riveters were told to return home in the 1950s, second-wave feminism was followed by a backlash against positions of increased equity, including, surprisingly, a movement against the proposed Equal Rights Amendment to the U.S. Constitution that was led by Phyllis Schlafly, among other women. Reaganomics and other conservative social policies that followed in the 1980s disproportionately affected women and children, and specifically harmed LGBTQ+ people, particularly LGBTQ+ BIPOC, as was seen in the early years of the HIV epidemic.

Feminism's third wave, occurring now, responds to several theoretical problems from its second wave, including a focus on narratives and making space for multiple voices and perspectives, and seeks a nonjudgmental and inclusive approach in an effort to build political coalitions (Evans, 2015; Snyder, 2008). Third-wave feminism is committed to increasing the understanding and integration of feminist perspectives from the perspective of gendered identities, low-resource countries, in the presence of globalization and a globalized world economy, as well as within the post- and neocolonial worlds. The borders of these waves are varied, permeable, and debated, but their historical significance is important to understanding how the social views and situations of women and other minoritized gender persons change over time. As with all the previous waves, we can anticipate a backlash proportional to the anxiety it provokes in existing systems of power, and indeed, we are seeing this now (Flood et al., 2021). If history can be relied on for guidance, it is that we can expect both this backlash, and a fourth wave of feminism.

ORIGINS OF FEMINIST THEORY

Feminist thought has emerged from a variety of philosophical traditions, including liberal Marxist, psychoanalytic, socialist, existentialist, postmodern, and postcolonial philosophies.

In this chapter, we provide an overview of several traditions of feminist philosophical thought. It must be noted that the philosophical traditions upon which much of feminist thought are based have disciplinary uses in other areas. For example, Marxist thought is a philosophical tradition that is often used in understanding economic theory; however, it is also useful in understanding the history and subjugation of women in society. The categories that follow should be considered as a broad guide that underscores the differences in feminist theory, which in many ways reflects the differences in individuals and groups.

Perspectives in Feminist Theory

LIBERAL FEMINISM

Liberal feminists advocate gender justice, with gender equality replacing the politics of exclusion (Tong, 1998). Liberal feminism is exemplified in works such as Mary Wollstonecraft's *A Vindication of the Rights of Woman* (1796) and John Stuart Mill's *On the Subjection of Women* (1878). Liberal feminism often draws on and works within the framework of liberal political theory. The work of the National Organization of Women, in support of equal rights for women, reflects contemporary liberal feminism. Central to the beliefs of liberal feminists is the assumption that women's subordination is rooted in customary and legal constraints blocking women's entrance to and/or success in the so-called public world. Because society has viewed women as less than men, women have been excluded from many arenas of public life. Liberal feminism seeks to expose these injustices and to develop strategies for enhancing the position of women in society. These strategies will necessarily disproportionately benefit women with the most power in other identities, since the focus of liberal feminism is on equality, not equity. (It is not coincidental that Wollstonecraft was a White Englishwoman raised in an initially financially stable family, while Mill was the child of English privilege and later served in Parliament.) In liberal feminism, the assumption is that gender is the relevant variable, because in its development there simply were no other variables considered. While liberal feminism has since been influenced by the development of other feminist philosophies, these limitations remain.

MARXIST AND SOCIALIST FEMINISM

Marxist feminists, exemplified in some works by Angela Davis (1981, 1989), Catharine MacKinnon (1989), and Iris Young (1990), believe it is impossible for anyone, especially a woman, to obtain genuine equal opportunity in a class society where wealth is produced by many people for a powerful few. Marx and Engels were influential voices whose work explored the capitalist economic philosophy that underwrites most of Western political and economic thought and action. Marxist philosophy is also a factor influencing feminist responses to the subjugation of women worldwide. Tracing their works to Engels, Marxist feminists assert that women's oppression originates in introduction of private property. Beasley (1999) concurs, suggesting that sexual oppression is a form of class oppression. To eradicate sexual oppression, Marxist feminists advocate replacing capitalism with a socialist system.

In this new system, the means of production would belong to everyone, and women would no longer be economically dependent on men (Beasley, 1999; Tong, 1998). However, this philosophy assumes that class struggle is the "important" struggle, and that men and women of similar social class have similar challenges and advantages. It also fails to account for the existence of continued sexism and gendered violence in economic systems that largely abolished private ownership of property (the former Union of Soviet Socialist Republics [USSR], Mao-era People's Republic of China). The counterargument is that these actual countries are imperfect examples of socialist/Marxist systems, and in a more perfect example neither sexism nor gendered violence would exist.

RADICAL FEMINISM

Radical feminists, as exemplified by Mary Daly (1978), Andrea Dworkin (1974, 1976), Gena Corea (1986), and Shulamith Firestone (1970), believe the patriarchal system oppresses women. They advocate that a system characterized by power, dominance, hierarchy, and competition cannot be reformed, but must be eradicated. Radical feminist thought suggests that institutions that produce and reproduce hierarchy and dominance, especially the family, the church, and the academy (academic institutions), need to be replaced to achieve equality. Some radical feminists question the concept of "natural order" in which men are "manly" and women "womanly," with a goal of overcoming whatever negative effects this thinking about biology as destiny has had on women and men. Radical feminists assert that biology, gender (masculinity, femininity), and sexuality (heterosexuality and homosexuality are some forms) are sources of women's oppression (Weedon, 1997). Many radical feminists focus on ways in which gender and sexuality have been used to subordinate women to men. They support reproductive rights as a means of enhancing women's choices; however, the philosophy stops short of addressing issues of access, as well as reproductive rights separate from abortion and contraception. Notably, the majority of radical feminist theorists are White financially stable cisgender women, which limits the ability of the philosophy to address the lived experiences of people who do not fall into those categories. The focus on binary gender identity under radical feminism also has led in some cases to the rejection of trans women as "real women," or of the lived experiences of gender diverse people as relevant to feminism or women (e.g., "trans exclusionary radical feminism"), which is troubling in the context of the antitrans backlash currently occurring in the United States (Murib, 2020).

PSYCHOANALYTIC THEORY AND FEMINISM

Psychoanalytic feminist theorists believe that the centrality of sexuality arises out of Freudian theory and concepts, such as the Oedipus complex. Chodorow (1978, 1989, 1994) and Dinnerstein (1976, 1988) exemplify early psychoanalytic, primarily Freudian feminist thought. Central to their work is the assumption that the root of women's oppression is embedded deeply within their psyche. These theorists recommend dual parenting and dual participation in the work force as means to solve women's oppression. A group of prominent French (and Bulgarian-French, in the case of Kristeva) feminist theorists includes Hélène Cixous (1975, 1991), Luce Irigaray (1974, 1977),

and Julia Kristeva (1982, 1995), whose work is conducted in critique of Freudian psychoanalysis. These women challenge the theoretical perspectives of Jacques Lacan, a psychoanalyst whose work furthered that of Freud. Theory presented by the "French feminists" is often conceptualized from both a psychoanalytic and poststructuralist position (discussed next), and focuses on explorations of subjectivity and agency, abjection, and psychosexual identity formation (Weedon, 1997).

POSTMODERNISM AND FEMINIST THEORY

Postmodernism is expressed in feminist theory as a series of theoretical perspectives that view language as constructing our understanding and uses of gender. Much of what is known as postmodern work is conducted from a poststructuralist perspective, a philosophical perspective that heavily relies on the work of Michel Foucault, a French philosopher whose work critiqued how power and knowledge are constructed and reified. Feminist writings from a poststructuralist perspective critique the ideas of essentialism, the use of power in social relations, and how, using language and power, knowledge about the world is produced and legitimated (Butler, 1993, 2000; Weedon, 1997). These orientations involve no single standpoint, rather several perspectives help to account for the experiences of difference, an aspect of feminist theory that has been recently approached from postmodern and/or poststructuralist perspectives.

EXPERIENCES OF WOMEN OF COLOR, WOMANIST TRADITIONS, AND FEMINIST THEORY

The voices and experiences of women of color are increasingly finding a place within feminist theory. Writers using postmodern, poststructuralist, and critical race theories enable this by calling out the use of metanarratives to describe the lives of women of color as essentially similar to those of White women. For example, as noted by hooks (1999a, 2000), the experiences of Black women are not interchangeable with those of White women. Works by and about Black women center the experiences of Black women in a way that profoundly challenges the status quo, of both racism and sexism (Collins, 1989, 2000; Crenshaw, 1995; Davis, 1981, 1989; Dill, 1983, 1987; Gillespie, 1984; Gordon-Bradshaw, 1987; Herman, 1984; hooks, 1984, 1997, 1999a; Lorde, 1984a, 1988; Parmar, 1991; Smith, 1982). These challenges represent both a deep critique of existing systems of power and a potential roadmap for gender equity going forward, because they do not rely on the existing systems of power for their own legitimacy. Audre Lorde, a Black lesbian scholar and activist, famously said, "The master's tools will never dismantle the master's house" (Lorde, 1984b). This is a key question to consider in feminist theory: Can philosophies that maintain or ignore systems of power other than gender ever create lasting change?

The novelist Alice Walker (1983) was first to use the term "womanist," where she describes a theory of feminism that explores and advances the issues of Black women in the U.S. context (Taylor, 1998, 2002, 2004, 2005). Womanist traditions offer a feminist theoretical perspective that seeks to encompass the "uniqueness of African American women's experiences" accentuating the similarities and *differences* between African American women's experiences and those of women from other ethnic and racial groups (Banks-Wallace, 2000, p. 36). Lorde similarly argued:

Advocating the mere tolerance of difference between women is the grossest reformism. It is a total denial of the creative function of difference in our lives. Difference must be not merely tolerated, but seen as a fund of necessary polarities between which our creativity can spark like a dialectic. Only then does the necessity for interdependency become unthreatening. Only within that interdependency of difference strengths, acknowledged and equal, can the power to seek new ways of being in the world generate, as well as the courage and sustenance to act where there are no charters. (Lorde, 1984b)

In this model, failure to recognize and center diversity of experiences automatically limits the ability to find creative and lasting solutions.

In the United States, Latinxs are a rapidly growing demographic, representing just under 20% of the population (U.S. Census Bureau, 2021). This change in national demographics presents an opportunity for the voices of Latinx feminists to emerge and advocate for improvement in healthcare resource allocation, work conditions, and immigration rights. Works about Latinxs or Chicanxs provide insight into the challenges for women from a burgeoning ethnic minority who experience unique physical, political, and health-related concerns (Anzaldua, 1999; Apodaca, 1977; Chavez et al., 1986; del Portillo, 1987; Ginorio & Reno, 1985; Hurtado, 1989, 1996; Kelly et al., 2006; Moraga, 1983, 1997; Moraga & Anzaldua, 1983; Sanchez, 1984; Sanchez-Ayendez, 1989; Segura, 1989). The recent increase in state-sponsored harm of Latinx families and communities tied to immigration policies has disproportionately affected the health and safety of Latinxs (Doshi et al., 2022; Fleming et al., 2019), and the recent SARS-CoV-2/COVID-19 pandemic drastically increased risks to Latinx pregnant people, more so than other racial/ethnic identities (Goldfarb et al., 2020). While Latinxs in the United States are by no means a monolithic group, the burdens of racism and xenophobia are often extended without consideration for individual situations, and thus carry risks that are specific to Latinxs.

Writing about and by Asian Americans, Pacific Islanders, South Asian women, Native American/First Nations is a growing and important area of feminist thought that has been overlooked or intentionally marginalized by White feminism (e.g., Chow, 1987; Im & Meleis, 2001; Johnson et al., 2004; Neufeld et al., 2002; Tsutakawa, 1988; Visweswaran, 1994; Woods et al., 1994). Witt (1984), Hale (1985), and Pirner (2005) provide powerful accounts of issues central to women's lives, illustrating points of difference that may help account for health experiences. Their health issues must be understood within the context of traditional family life and hierarchies, and within a multigenerational context, since many of these women are first- and second-generation immigrants to the United States. Another important area to consider includes their current work situations and histories, as many of these women engage in unseen labor (e.g., housekeepers, farm workers) and in work that exposes them to potential physical and environmental hazards and economic disparities that can complicate their efforts to achieve optimal health.

QUEER THEORY

Queer theory is part of a resistance movement that describes feminism from lesbian, gay, bisexual, transgender, and queer (LGBTQ) perspectives with an emphasis of "affinity and solidarity over identity" (Marcus, 2005). Queer theory provides an opportunity for understanding gender, offering a lens through which lesbian, gay, and transgender people understand and interpret their lives within a heteronormativity (Butler, 1993, 2000; Jagose, 1996). As clinicians, we want to avoid language that is disparaging of individuals or groups, but the use of the term *queer* is taken up as an umbrella term in scholarly and activist contexts "for a coalition of culturally marginal sexual self-identification" LGBTQ studies and theories (Jagose, 1996, p. 1). (This does not, however, mean that *queer* is a universally accepted term for individuals who are LGBTQ+, nor is it a term that is open for use by outsiders as a descriptor.) Queer theory calls on us to question how our discomfort with difference can be directed to work for the good of an often-marginalized group.

Using queer theory as a framework for understanding the health challenges of LGBTQ groups, we begin to understand how social identity operates in ways that amplify health issues. For example, lesbians of childbearing years may be struggling with infertility and have difficulty finding a provider who understand infertility issues in lesbians, or may be denied coverage for assisted reproductive treatments on the grounds that they have not met the common requirement of 1 year of unprotected heterosexual sex to receive "infertility" treatments. Cisgender women who have sex with cisgender women are less likely to been screened for cervical cancer (Saunders et al., 2021), which may make them disproportionately likely to develop cervical cancer (Robinson et al., 2017). LGBTQ+ teens are approximately twice as likely to experience an unintended pregnancy compared to straight cisgender teens (Charlton et al., 2018). Most research on sexually transmitted infections (STIs) has focused on men having sex with men, with relatively little on lesbians and/or bisexual cisgender women, and trans and nonbinary health is only now beginning to be explored in contexts other than risk-based assessments of mental health and STI risk. Because of the limits of the research base, and because LGBTQ+ patients and researchers are often marginalized by existing health systems and funding mechanisms, it is critical to seek out health research that not only focuses on LGBTQ+ populations, but is done by researchers with lived experience or community advisory input.

ECOFEMINISM AND FEMINIST LIBERATION THEOLOGY

Less prominent but equally important are feminist theoretical traditions from ecofeminism and feminist liberation theology. Ecofeminism provides a space for feminists to consider the conditions of women within the context of the environment and nature (Griffin, 1978; Haraway, 1989; Sturgeon, 1997). Feminist liberation theologies (Christian, mujerista, and some womanist traditions) provide a theoretical framework for women to use religious and spiritual traditions to enhance their understandings of women's subjugation and oppression (Fulkerson, 1994; Harrison, 1985; Isasi-Diaz, 1993; Isasi-Diaz & Tarango, 1992; Tigert, 2001). With the emergence of ecofeminism, feminist liberation theologies and queer theory, issues of the ecological, racialized, and gendered experiences of women, communities of color, and LGBTQ+ communities are gaining theoretical prominence and becoming increasingly legitimized in health and academic communities.

POSTCOLONIAL AND TRANSNATIONAL FEMINIST THEORIES

Postcolonial theory calls into question the history of colonial dominance of the West over other geographic regions and people. As the overarching framework for feminist theory, transnational feminist theory adds support to the notion of the need for multiple forms of feminism in a postcolonial world (Scott et al., 1997). Postcolonial theory has initiated discussions about how Western ideas are transmitted into non-Westernized regions and the effects of this transmission, including loss of native languages and traditions, and the Westernization of social structures and institutions. Postcolonial theory offers an opportunity to think and develop strategies that resist contemporary forms of Western colonialism that "undermine and sabotage the self-determining aspirations" of citizens in independent states (Yeatman, 1994, p. 9). In our transglobal environment, the ideals of postcolonialism and transnational feminist theories and movements have become increasingly important.

Postcolonial theory questions the transfer of Western economic strategies and knowledge into more traditional economic systems, often to the economic benefit of the West (sometimes referred to as "the North" in opposition to countries in the Southern hemisphere). While Western technologies and economic strategies have been useful in some ways to some populations, the effects of these technologies have been detrimental to the social structures, environments, and health of many populations. Another use for postcolonial theory is its provision of a theoretical frame for feminists to critique the effects of transnationalism on the lives of women and children. Finally, recent literature describes nursing itself as a colonized profession (McGibbon et al., 2014) and calls for increasing counternarratives that resist subjugation and oppression within the profession.

Issues for women's health providers to consider include the use of child labor and its effects on the family structure, the health effects of transnationalism, and the transfer of health technologies to populations that may not have the infrastructure to support their effective use. Understanding a country's political economy and how it affects the availability of health and social services is another important topic that drives improvement or deterioration of a population's health outcomes. Postcolonial theories and transnational feminism allow nurses to move between local and global ideas, placing the individual within a more globally oriented response to women's health. In doing so, nurses can work beside women in non-Western countries to deal with the effects of transnationalism, such as inadequate infrastructures, economic and social power, and the subsequent health effects that are accentuated under these conditions.

INTERSECTIONALITY

Collins (2000) describes intersectionality as the confluence of oppressions within society. Often these expressed oppressions center on race, class, and gender. Intersectionality focuses on how these oppressions are shaped by one another, and thus, how the sum is greater than its parts. For example, the experience of a Black woman cannot be simply captured by independently examining the experience of being Black or a woman, but needs to be seen in the context of being a Black woman in the specific historical and social context of today's society.

Crenshaw (1991) is credited with the phrase "intersectionality" as a way of capturing how race, gender, and employment "interact to shape the multiple dimensions of Black women's employment experiences" (p. 1244). The notion of intersectionality came into play by Black women, who found that White women's feminism was tied to equality with White men and the Black movement was sexist in the sense that it prioritized Black men's pursuit of equality with White men (Gopaldas, 2013). There was not a space that captured the experience of being both a woman and being Black, although it is impossible to separate one's identities into discrete entities.

Understanding intersectionality involves exploring the concept at both macro and micro levels. The macro level explores the multiple identities of women (e.g., Latinx, woman, bisexual) within the context of race, class, and gender. The micro level examines individual identity positions within society in reference to privilege and disadvantage (Gopaldas, 2013). As a health provider, understanding the complexity of how various factors intersect to create a specific experience of wellness and illness is vital to excellent care and helping patients achieve optimal health.

USING THEORY TO GUIDE PRACTICE

Theory and practice are inextricably linked, each simultaneously creating and reinforcing the other. Theory is used to create practice, and practices change because of emerging theories. Feminist theory is a new application for nursing research and care, which has largely focused on physiologic and symptoms research (which reinforced nursing's search for credibility and authority within the medicine-dominated world of health research). With all new applications, one first must learn the tenets of the theory, begin to identify and uncover situations where the theory is applicable, and ultimately, use the theory to create practice. Feminist theory has spent many years at the margins of theory in nursing, slowly moving toward central positions in research and practice. Nurse researchers and practitioners primarily use feminist theory as a framework to conceptualize issues or as a form of feminist critique of research and practice (Anderson, 2004; Anderson & McCann, 2002; Bunting, 1997; Im et al., 2000; Im & Meleis, 2001; Johnson et al., 2004; Maxwell-Young et al., 1998; Richman et al., 2000; Schroeder & Ward, 1998).

Understanding the theoretical background of the struggles around women's and minoritized gender persons' rights and recognition of the multiple concerns included in these struggles allows providers to better serve this clientele. In using feminist theory to guide practice, the provider can place current struggles in women's and minoritized gender persons' health into context, particularly when considering determinants of health and the economic, political, and social situations that can contribute to poor health outcomes. As with moving away from identifying race as a risk factor, and instead naming the structural power of racism as the relevant risk factor, we must also move away from looking at gender as a risk factor, and instead interrogate minoritizing and examine sexism, misogyny, and trans- and homophobia influences on health. Since women are more likely than men to be disabled during our lives, we must also examine ableism. Women are more likely to live in poverty than are men, so classism and economic justice are relevant. Lorde noted that "There is no such thing as a single-issue struggle, because we do not live single-issue lives" (Lorde, 1984b, p. 2). As nurses, we provide holistic care, and that requires that we see our patients as whole, in all the complexity that entails. We cannot care effectively for a Black woman, for example, without recognizing how the systems of power affect her as a Black person, as a woman, and as a Black woman person, and how these identities interact (Collins, 2000). We cannot care effectively for a genderqueer patient without knowing how sexism and transphobia interact in their life experience. We cannot care for a disabled low-income woman without hearing how sexism, classism, and ableism are experienced by this particular patient. Our patients arrive as whole human beings, and our responsibility as nurses is to see and care for them in that wholeness.

Aside from physiologic and psychological needs, providers need to be involved in issues around safety, esteem, and self-actualization as they pertain to the lives of their patients. There are many problems affecting the health of these populations that may be viewed and better understood as a result of using feminist theory and gaining knowledge around the historical complexities of populations. Some of these problems include (1) violence against women and other minoritized gender persons; (2) social and economic inequities and the effect of these on health; (3) the ways that women's and minoritized genders' healthcare needs are represented to and by large institutions (e.g., state and federal agencies, insurance plans, the media) as priorities for funding and research; and (4) how the intermediate disparities of health (e.g., access to primary care, jobs that pay a living wage) contribute to poor health outcomes.

A related issue in feminist practice is the social construction of women and minoritized genders within the healthcare system. Although a nonhierarchical relationship would be ideal, it is impossible to completely equalize social, political, and historical experiences between providers and their patients. Historically, most providers see themselves as custodians of knowledge versus seeing this relationship as a shared partnership. At the same time, patients enter the healthcare interaction as experts of their own bodies and lives, and desire recognition of this expertise by providers. Disrupting the hierarchical power structure requires that we recognize both its existence within ourselves and how it affects our therapeutic relationships with our patients.

Validation of the nonrational is another dimension of feminist practice. This orientation allows for multiple competing definitions of problems and many "truths." It emphasizes women's and minoritized genders' ability to reconstruct their own experiences and to find meaning in events that they alone can determine. For example, a woman may perceive that her mastectomy is not a sexual phenomenon, but it may raise existential issues for her. Conversely, a patient may regard menopause not as a crisis of identity but as a health condition that impacts her sexuality, comfort, and sense of

wellness. Both of these perspectives, and many others, are valid. In feminist approaches to healthcare, the process of problem definition is recognized as subjective. Nonlinear, multidimensional thinking is encouraged (Bricker-Jenkins & Hooyman, 1986; Weedon, 1997). Beyond feminist theory, this decentering of "objective" knowledge is well established in nursing, in Carper's Ways of Knowing model (Carper, 1975). Practicing from a feminist perspective means being mindful of the ways power relations function and are managed in the healthcare setting, as well as the existence and importance of varied perspectives and meanings to health and health events. The analysis and interpretation of subjective and objective data and treatment plans need to be discussed openly and agreed on by both the provider and the patient. This model of healthcare is often called "shared decision-making," but the provider must also be mindful that despite the power accorded them by hierarchical healthcare systems, the patient is the final decision-maker. The decision-making process may be shared, but the decision is, in the end, that of the patient.

Understanding gender as a social versus biological construction is an important distinction in feminist and nonfeminist perspectives (Allen et al., 1991; Campbell & Bunting, 1991). In addition, providers working within a feminist framework are concerned with ways to transform the social and health-related conditions that effect their patient's health. It is not enough to describe oppression, it is also important to change the conditions that create and sustain it. This concern gives legitimacy to consciousness-raising, advocacy and praxis.

Praxis references the component of feminist consciousness that leads to social transformation: an awareness of the reality that shapes women's and minoritized gender persons' lives becomes infused into public values and actions. Reality is renamed according to their experiences. Recognition of the small group as a unit of social change is explicit. Self-help is one means of change, yet does not substitute for the provision of adequate services from the state. Struggles to implement values such as egalitarianism, consensus democracy, nonexploitation, cooperation, collectivism, diversity, and nonjudgmental spirituality are central to feminist practice (Andrist, 1988; Bricker-Jenkins & Hooyman, 1986; Sampselle, 1990, Seng, 1998).

However, consciousness-raising is an ongoing process, often undertaken at some risk to many of these groups, such as exposing previously unstated vulnerabilities. Facilitating consciousness-raising with women and gender minorities cannot be abandoned midprocess, as this risks leaving them more vulnerable than before the process began. Providing consciousness-raising follow-up support is essential as it allows the woman who has now recognized her vulnerabilities with the additional support required to change them (Wolf, 1996). At the same time, it is essential for White healthcare providers to avoid the tendency to saviorism, or the belief that marginalized persons and groups are somehow less capable of finding solutions and need the intervention of (White, straight, cisgender, affluent) others. Instead, the role of healthcare providers is to support and strengthen existing efforts by individuals and communities, and to direct their research and practice based on the expressed needs of those individuals and communities, not the preferences or beliefs of the healthcare provider.

Chopoorian (1986) urges us to consider multiple dimensions of environments for human health, a perspective consistent with many feminist theories that link health to social, political, and economic structures as context. Moreover, the emphasis on social relationships, including domination, power, and authority within organizations and families, leads one to examine exploitation of and violence toward women and minoritized gender persons and the relationships to their health. Finally, an emphasis on understanding everyday life and its meaning for these populations is consistent with feminist conceptions of the importance of a patient's experience.

An ethical feminist practice in nursing understands the category of "woman," "lesbian," "bisexual," "queer," "nonbinary," "transgender," and others as multiple, shifting, and constantly changing. It is also essential to understand that identity, orientation, and behaviors are possibly overlapping or congruent, or may apparently conflict (people who identify as lesbian may have a male sexual partner, for example, or sex workers may participate in sexual acts with gender[s] other than those of their preferred partners). Nursing practice that understands the complexities of women and minoritized gender persons, the contexts of their lives, and the multiple and shifting landscape of their health is desirable and attainable. Educating nurses about how these populations' health needs vary and how knowledge of the context of their lives is essential to their developing an ethical feminist practice, although it is also critical to acknowledge that different identities and populations may experience those needs in very different ways. Nurses' knowledge about women's and minoritized gender persons' health problems and the differences in how their health is experienced should be offered through work sites, academic settings, and continuing education offerings that are timely and economically accessible to a wide variety of nursing professionals. It is also essential that they be incorporated effectively into prelicensure programs as they currently are not (Orgel, 2017). Encouraging nurses to further their education in master's and doctoral programs translates into improved opportunities for the development of an ethical nursing practice using feminist theory as a central feature of this education. An ethical practice demands attention to intersectionality, reflexive thinking, and self-reflection, while avoiding a narcissistic perseveration and self-awareness, and values local action to influence women's and gender minorities' health on a global level.

COMPETENCIES FOR ADVANCED PRACTICE NURSING

While many competencies expected of APRNs are relevant to a discussion of feminism in women's healthcare, there are several that are key to effective and ethical practice. Because the competencies for women's health nurse practitioners (WHNPs) differ from those for certified nurse midwives (CNMs), and both may differ somewhat from the general APRN competencies espoused by the American Association of Colleges of Nursing (AACN), these are considered separately here, but there is considerable overlap among them.

American Association of Colleges of Nursing APRN Competencies

DOMAIN 1: PATIENT CARE

As noted in the competencies (AACN, 2017), patient care at the advanced practice level requires (a) "a comprehensive evidence-based assessment" and (b) "develop[ing] a patient-centered, evidence-based plan of care." As noted earlier, a comprehensive assessment of the patient and their needs does not include only the immediate physical indicators present at the time of the visit; rather, it must incorporate an understanding of the historical and current systems that affect the health and lives of that patient. This understanding is also crucial to developing an effective and individualized plan of care. Feminist theory brings this structural knowledge into the exam room and enables the APRN to evaluate both the patient and the context in which they live and have lived.

DOMAIN 5: PROFESSIONALISM

Per AACN, "professionalism" at the APRN level requires the nurse to advocate for patients and populations "considering social justice and equity" (AACN, 2017). The knowledge of how lines of power and privilege are arranged by gender and gender expectations, as well as the fallout from those structural arrangements, is essential to effective advocacy for women and gender minorities.

American College of Nurse-Midwives Core Competencies for Basic Midwifery Practice

SECTION I: HALLMARKS OF MIDWIFERY

This section is primarily concerned with the inclusivity and support of patients seeking midwifery care within their individual contexts, including social determinants of health and use of shared decision-making. Without feminist theoretical analysis, it can be difficult to fully understand both the basis for this model of care (centering and empowering the midwifery patient in their care) and the challenges that patients often face in sexual and reproductive healthcare (SRH), as well as in daily life. The history of midwifery in the United States is problematic in many ways, including the erasure of Black midwifery history and the continued disproportionately White midwifery workforce (American College of Nurse-Midwives [ACNM], 2021). An intersectional interpretation of feminism requires the acknowledgment and recognition of racism as well as sexism and/or homophobia, transphobia, and ableism that patients experience in their lives and in healthcare. The work of the Black feminists discussed earlier, among many others, is essential to meeting this competency.

National Certification Corporation Women's Health Nurse Practitioner

Apply ethical, legal, and professional issues inherent in providing care as a Women's Health Nurse Practitioner (WHNP). Ethical norms of nursing require the nurse to act using the basic principles of autonomy, beneficence, nonmaleficence, and justice, among other guidance (American Nurses Association [ANA], 2015). Acting in the interests of justice and patient autonomy, in particular, requires the APRN to be familiar with the fundamental injustices that patients face based on gender, sexual orientation, race, and disability, among other characteristics, and how those injustices fit into the larger systems of healthcare and daily life in the United States. While this competency does not, in contrast to the ACNM core competencies, specifically require advocacy for social justice, ethical practice in nursing does require attention to how injustice appears, and mitigation of that injustice where it is possible. Feminist theory provides a framework for the WHNP to address these ethical obligations in daily practice.

FUTURE DIRECTIONS

As of this writing, we are in a peculiarly critical crossroads for the intersections of feminism and women's health, as well as the health of minoritized genders more broadly. When considering the future directions of feminism and women's health, we must both reflect on the successes and missteps of the past, and the future directions signaled by the diverse grassroots efforts toward justice that are centered in both the American South and in the global South. While second wave activists may have envisioned a 21st century in which economic and legal equity would drive full social equity for women (other minoritized genders were not considered by most of the leaders of this movement), a powerful backlash against the apparent gains of the previous century has changed the anticipated landscape of healthcare for women and other minoritized genders.

Starting with the immediate post-*Roe* era in the mid-1970s and fueled by the Republican Party's anti-civil rights "Southern strategy" to capture power (McKeegan, 1993), abortion opposition was a powerful force motivating conservative voters and inspiring violence against women and others seen to be disrupting gender norms (Williams, 2011). With the 2022 *Dobbs v. Jackson Women's Health Organization* decision, which overturned abortion protections at the federal level and has implications for pregnancy care more broadly, the assumptions of two generations about reproductive health access have been profoundly altered. Without the guarantee of abortion access, and in the context of the highest maternal mortality rates of any wealthy nation—both of which disproportionately impact the Black and Indigenous population, as well as other people of color—there is by necessity a pivot to ensuring the most basic levels of Maslow's hierarchy (physiologic safety) that will move resources away from other issues of justice. When body autonomy is at risk, after all, everything is up for debate.

The potential impact of *Dobbs* goes well beyond abortion legality, which reproductive justice advocates have accurately noted is inadequate to ensure body and social autonomy (SisterSong, n.d.). In his concurring opinion on *Dobbs*, Justice Clarence Thomas took aim at the constitutional basis for other privacy-based rights, including marriage equality and contraception access (Thomas, 2022), and signaled the willingness of the Court to overturn other rights long taken for granted that disproportionately impact women and other minoritized genders. These have significant implications not only for the ability of people to access contraception, for example, but for the interpretations of civil rights law protecting LGBTQ+ people in the workplace, as well as their rights to relationships, to cover their partners under their health insurance, to parental rights for their children, and other protections that are basic to human rights. While LGBTQ+ people may be more vulnerable immediately, the precedent *Dobbs* set for the removal of an affirmative right grounded in the Constitution places cisgender heterosexual women at risk as well.

In this profoundly disrupted legal environment, we must look to the work of reproductive justice activists in the American South, who have worked for justice within restrictive legal environments for decades. Groups like Black Mamas Matter Alliance and SisterSong have long track records of making progress at a grassroots and national level toward comprehensive reproductive justice goals, including reducing Black maternal mortality rates, and can serve as models and leaders for feminist healthcare going forward. Leaders like Stacey Abrams and Rep. Lauren Underwood, as well as Reps. Ilhan Omar, Rashida Tlaib, Alexandria Ocasio-Cortez, Ayanna Pressley, Cori Bush, and Jamaal Bowman, have worked for change in the context of being minoritized both racially and (except for Rep. Bowman) by gender, and are examples of changing leadership within existing systems of power.

Times of disruption are opportunities for change, both positively and negatively, and the shift away from centering legal actions (which have proved to be less resilient than previously believed) and traditional lines of power that have occurred in third- and fourth-wave feminist movements suggests where we can move in the future. Healthcare providers for women and other minoritized genders can look critically at the systems in which they exist and work for change at the individual, clinic, and local levels, as well as in the larger legal and social systems. Understanding the implications of public health action on SRH, for example, has new meaning in a world grappling with the continued fallout from the COVID-19 pandemic and the emergence of other infections, including monkeypox and returning vaccine-preventable diseases such as measles and polio. Rather than reliance on the U.S. Supreme Court to interpret laws favorably for SRH, there is a critical need for nurses at every level to incorporate the work of improving outcomes and access, as well as the larger economic and justice systems that affect people regardless of their need for abortion or contraception. If there is a future direction for feminist healthcare, it must be to bend the arc of history further toward justice.

SUMMARY

Emancipatory feminist paradigms orient practice to praxis and facilitate active engagement and participation in the larger society. Being actively engaged and participating in the larger society unites our individual concerns with the concerns for all populations. The goals of feminist practice thus transcend the boundaries of traditional practice in which the patient is an individual.

Feminism is an integrative process that helps women and gender minorities expand our consciousness about health and identity. In this model, promotion of health is a function of transforming one's life through the expansion of one's consciousness rather than merely engaging in periodic medical checkups (VanderPlaat, 1999). Subjectivity and agency are prominent within a feminist practice. Women and minoritized gender persons have awareness of themselves and others and the ability to appreciate the complexity of many diverse situations while acting in their own best interest (Beasley, 1999).

In a feminist model, caring occurs in the context of an open and collaborative relationship. Mutual recognition of one another's expertise, sharing of information, and defining goals in collaboration are the central elements of the process.

Information is shared freely between nurses and patients. The clinician as a consultant provides information about the full range of alternatives for health. The patients make prescriptions for their own health based on information about self-care options. They are part of a relationship in which they define and strive for optimal health.

REFERENCES

References for this chapter are online and available at https://connect.springerpub.com/content/book/978-0-8261-6722-4/part/part01/chapter/ch06

PART II

Health Promotion and Prevention

CHAPTER 7

Women's Bodies, Women's Health*

IVY M. ALEXANDER, ANNETTE JAKUBISIN-KONICKI, LAUREN EDDY, JENNY YUNG, AND CAROLYN LEVY

Providing women's healthcare affords APRNs a special opportunity to educate women and minoritized gender persons about their bodies and the intricacies of their physical and physiologic form and functions. Established as the major consumers of healthcare and the primary gatekeepers of their family's health, women and other minoritized gender persons are usually eager to learn about how their bodies work and how to keep them healthy (Daniel et al., 2018). When given the chance, they often express curiosity about specific aspects of their anatomy or physiology. Although a frequently neglected topic in routine healthcare, women also wonder about their sexuality and their body's ability to experience pleasure.

Discovering that there are unique biological aspects of having a female body beyond solely the reproductive system interests many women as well. Over the past few decades, the advanced scientific study of cellular and molecular mechanisms of human biology have uncovered new, significant sex-based differences in physiologic functions (Galea et al., 2020). Being familiar with these discoveries in biological sex differences is important to anyone involved in healthcare to promote a better understanding of the implications for disease prevention and health maintenance of women and minoritized gender persons.

To complicate consideration of women's bodies, it is important to recognize that they have been a contested territory for centuries. Demystifying women's bodies was a core element of the popular women's health movement of the 1970s and the feminist movement. Perspectives on embodiment thus inform women's healthcare.

The purpose of this chapter is to briefly highlight perspectives on women's bodies, as well as frameworks for understanding women's relationships to their bodies, focusing on embodiment. In addition, the key aspects of female anatomy and physiology are reviewed so that this information can be shared with women who seek nursing services, consultation, or education about their bodies. The chapter begins with a review of perspectives about women's bodies, followed by consideration of the structural and functional aspects of a woman's unique anatomy. The procreative and recreative functions of women's bodies are considered in the context of women's health. Next, a brief discussion of the reproductive endocrine system and, specifically, the hormonal influences on women's bodies sets the stage for understanding the complexities of women's cyclic rhythms. Descriptions of initial sexual differentiation and development, pubertal development, and changes occurring during menarche and menopause are presented. Two important cyclic phenomena are women's menstrual cycles and sexual response cycles; how women's bodies participate in these cycles is described. Finally, this chapter includes some recently established biological sex differences in the brain, relating them to the body, behavior, and environment to appreciate how they affect women's health and longevity.

WOMEN'S BODIES

Controversies over women's bodies have characterized much of contemporary women's history. The early efforts of the feminist women's health movements in the United States focused on demystifying women's bodies to reduce the alienation women experienced from their bodies as well as the power differential between women and healthcare providers. Understanding the conditions of embodiment for women provides healthcare providers with insight through which the integration of women's everyday life experiences and contexts with their health could be appreciated.

---

*This chapter is a revision of the chapter that appeared in the second edition of this textbook, coauthored with Nancy Fugate Woods and Lucinda Canty, and we thank them for their original contribution.

Embodiment

Embodiment refers to the relationship between subjective experiences one has of one's own body as well as the corporeal experience and identity associated with living in one's body. In nursing science, the notion of embodiment often refers to the intertwining of body and mind, enabling reciprocity between the person and the external world. The body has long been understood to both constitute a material self and simultaneously the self is not viewed as separate from the materiality of the body (Einstein & Shildrick, 2009). In the context of nursing science and practice, the body is viewed in an ecological framework in which the experiences of embodiment are in mutual interaction with the societies, cultures, and physical environments in which women spend their everyday lives. Bodies are viewed as active and engaged entities and in the case of public health, embodiment refers to how bodies incorporate the world in which we live, the ecological circumstances of our lives (Krieger, 2005). Indeed, Krieger points out that embodiment warrants consideration of more than phenotypes and genotypes and an implicitly external environment. Instead, she advocates that we are jointly biological organisms and social beings; we are "multilevel phenomena, integrating soma, psyche, and society within historical and ecological context" (Krieger, 2005, p. 351). Embodiment of social conditions allows the material and social worlds in which we live to become incorporated in our bodies: Thus, life experiences and our histories become part of us, providing biological evidence of life experiences such as adverse childhood experiences and poverty. Old understandings of embodiment emphasized the biological nature of women as separate from the rational mind, with various conceptions of the body as accounting for women's lives and life possibilities, the body as a commodity and an object to be maintained for others' pleasure, and the body as a source of vulnerability as well as needing to be controlled. Contemporary feminist theorists of embodiment have invited consideration of the deterministic link among corporeal experience, mental functions, and social roles, challenging the naturalizing accounts of embodiment. Movement from considering the body as a source of vulnerability to celebration of the body as a source of sensual pleasure and unique capabilities has punctuated the history of women's embodiment and contributed to the philosophical theory that is required to make sense of the embodied self (Lennon, 2014). Piren et al. (2020) relate experiences on five continuous dimensions to the overall experience of embodiment: body connection and comfort, agency and functionality, experience and expression of desire, engagement in attuned self-care practices, and resistance to self-objectification.

Influences on Women's Perceptions of Body Ideal and Body Image

Women's perceptions of their bodies are influenced through many factors. Beginning around adolescence, females become more aware of their bodies and how people view them based on their weight and body shape (Guan et al., 2012). Cultural meanings affect what is considered an ideal body size and shape. Cultural meanings also influence women's perceptions of body image, weight, and what is considered healthy.

The U.S. society frequently uses body mass index (BMI) to define whether an individual is underweight, healthy, overweight, or obese. However, within different cultures, these categories are often defined differently (Andrews et al., 2017). Women may underestimate or overestimate their body size category because of influential cultural norms and ideals (Schuler et al., 2008). Women may also consider a body size to be normal and healthy as perceived through their cultural lens when the BMI rating classification defines that same size as overweight or obese (Schuler et al., 2008).

Women's perceptions of an ideal body size differ with their cultural/ethnic backgrounds. U.S. societal standards impose a more restrictive "acceptable" body size on women (Olson et al., 2020). However, Black and Hispanic women have reported more flexible ideal body shapes and overall accept larger body sizes (Bakhshi, 2011; Olson et al., 2020). Black women perceived heavier body types as ideal compared to White and Hispanic women. White women perceived the thinnest body as ideal. Hispanic women perceived a body type as ideal that was thinner than what was selected by Black women, but thicker than that selected by White women. Black women also identified the larger body sizes as more favorable compared to White and Hispanic women. Body ideal often relates to the culture with which the women most closely associate and the external cultural cues they experience. Asian American women who associate more with Asian versus American culture identify a thinner or smaller body as ideal. In contrast, Black American women who associated more closely with Black versus mainstream American culture identify a thicker or larger body as ideal. Conversely, Asian American women who experienced more American cultural cues identified a thinner or smaller body as ideal than those who experienced more Asian cultural cues. Black American women who experienced more American cultural cues identified a thicker or larger body as ideal than those who experienced more Black cultural cues. Interestingly, bicultural women tended to identify with the body ideal that was prototypically opposite of the dominant cultural cues they experienced.

Positive or negative body images can also be influenced by cultural identity (Tylka & Wood-Barcalow, 2015). Although women of different cultural backgrounds have unique experiences in relation to body image, positive experiences can translate to a positive personal perception of one's own body (Bakhshi, 2011; Tylka & Wood-Barcalow, 2015). White women have been found to express concerns about their weight and body shape, despite most of them having a normal weight (Bakhshi, 2011; Bardone-Cone et al., 2011). Conversely, Black women were less concerned about their weight although most were classified as overweight (Bakhshi, 2011; Bardone-Cone et al., 2011; Olson, et al., 2020).

Receiving conflicting information about what is considered an ideal body type and what body type is considered healthy is common for women regardless of their cultural identity (Capodilupo & Kim, 2014; Franko et al., 2012). Black and Latina women reported receiving messages about thinness being perceived as ideal, while thickness, or having curves, was identified in their culture as being ideal (Franko et al., 2012; Gordon et al., 2010). For example, in the Black culture, if someone loses a significant amount of weight, it may be perceived that they are suffering from a serious illness rather than an effort to improve health purposefully (Capodilupo &

Kim, 2014). Family also had an influence on women's feelings and perceptions of their weight and body shape (Capodilupo & Kim, 2014; Franko et al., 2012).

With the popularity of social media in the U.S. culture among young women, there is increased exposure to idealized body images on Instagram and other social media sites. Often these images depict unrealistic proportions, flawless skin, thin waists, and long thin legs. Research has shown that women who are exposed to idealized bodies internalize this unrealistic standard of beauty. This can result in increased negative mood and increased body dissatisfaction (McComb & Mills, 2021).

Understanding how women from diverse backgrounds and cultural/ethnic groups perceive their bodies can provide healthcare professionals with guidance on how to educate women and nurture positive and healthy body images (Andrews et al., 2017). When approaching a woman, it is important to ask about and understand her perception of her own body, body size, and what she perceives as ideal. This information is important in fostering a successful partnership with a woman and effective education and management plans.

WOMEN'S ANATOMY

Anatomic and Physiologic Dimensions

BREASTS

Although some Western societies socialize women to regard their breasts as symbols of their feminine attractiveness and nurturance while socializing men to regard women's breasts as sexual objects, women's breasts serve to provide both procreative powers and recreative pleasures. Lactation, including the synthesis, secretion, and ejection of milk, is the primary function of a woman's breasts. Indeed, the mammary gland is the distinguishing feature of an entire zoological class—mammals. Naturally round, protuberant breasts are exclusive to the human female and vary in their appearance more than most other parts of the female anatomy. These structures have a unique and complex anatomy (Figure 7.1). Under the influence of ovarian estrogen, maturation of the female breast occurs at puberty. Proliferation and branching of ducts and full development of the nipples and acini are influenced by both estradiol and progesterone. Breast health is discussed in greater detail in Chapter 24, Breast Health Considerations.

Location

Considered organs of the integumentary system, breasts are highly specialized variants of sweat (or apocrine) glands, located between the second and sixth or seventh ribs with an axillary tail projecting laterally and superiorly along the axillary and serratus anterior fascia (Suneja et al., 2020). About two thirds of the breast lies superficial to the pectoralis major, the remainder superior to the serratus anterior, and the lower part of the breast lies over the rectus sheath.

Appearance

The breasts of healthy women are generally symmetrical in shape and amplitude, although they are often not equal in size. Breasts are typically measured by both chest circumference and their fullness. What are commonly defined as plural

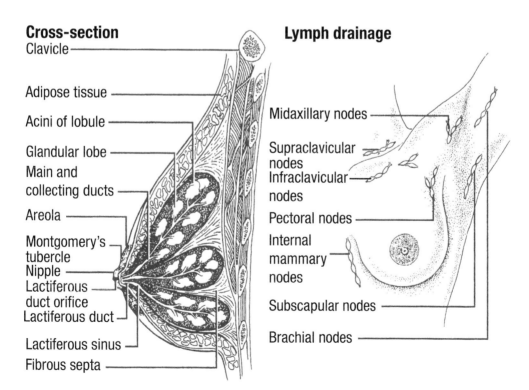

Cross-section

Clavicle
Adipose tissue
Acini of lobule
Glandular lobe
Main and collecting ducts
Areola
Montgomery's tubercle
Nipple
Lactiferous duct orifice
Lactiferous duct
Lactiferous sinus
Fibrous septa

Lymph drainage

Midaxillary nodes
Supraclavicular nodes
Infraclavicular nodes
Pectoral nodes
Internal mammary nodes
Subscapular nodes
Brachial nodes

FIGURE 7.1 Components of breast tissue and lymph drainage. Breast tissue is composed of glandular, fibrous, and fatty tissue. Lymph from the skin of the breast flows to the axillary nodes and lymph from the medial cutaneous area of the breast flows to the opposite breast. Lymph from the areolae and the nipples flows into the mammary nodes.

glands are two parts of a single, contiguous anatomic breast with a proliferation of a shared nerve, vascular, and lymphatic supply (Porth, 2007). The skin covering the breasts is like that of the abdomen. Hair follicles sometimes are noted around the darker pigmented area surrounding the nipple, called the areola. Often, women with fair complexions can note a vascular pattern in a horizontal or vertical dimension under the superficial skin of the breast tissue. When present, this pattern is usually symmetrical (Pandya & Moore, 2011).

The areolar pigment varies in color from pink to brown, in position on the breast, and in size from woman to woman depending on the individual's complexity and parity. The areola surrounds the nipple that is located at the tip of each breast. Several sebaceous glands can be seen on the areola as small elevations that are called Montgomery's tubercles to keep the nipple area soft and stretchy. The nipples are more darkly pigmented and usually protuberant because of erectile muscles. Nipple size and shape are highly variable from woman to woman, and the same woman may notice a great deal of variation in the size and shape of her nipples depending on the extent to which they are contracted. The erectile tissue of the nipple is responsive to emotional and tactile stimulation, thus promoting the recreative function of the breasts. Some women have inverted nipples, a condition in which the nipple is dimpled or its central portion flattened or depressed. A normal nipple that suddenly becomes inverted may indicate the presence of breast cancer.

Some women have supernumerary nipples and breasts, or breast tissue. This supernumerary tissue develops along the longitudinal ridges extending from the axilla to the groin, which existed during early embryonic development.

Visible changes in a woman's breasts occur in conjunction with her development. Before the age of 10 years, there is little visible distinction between boys' and girls' breasts. Between the ages of 10 to 12 years, the mammary buds appear in girls' breasts. The subareolar mammary tissue is not prominent at this point. The adult breast develops under the influence of estrogen and progesterone. During the transition to adulthood, the prominent subareolar tissue of adolescence recedes into the contour of the remainder of the breast and the nipple protrudes. (See the later section Puberty for a more complete description of breast changes that occur during puberty.)

Breast shape and texture are influenced by nutritional factors, heredity, endocrine factors, and hormonal sensitivity in addition to age, muscle tone, and pregnancy. Nodularity, tenderness, and size of the breasts may fluctuate with the menstrual cycle. Usually, women's breasts are smallest during days 4 to 7 of the menstrual cycle, shortly after menstruation. An increase in breast volume, tenderness, heaviness, fullness, and general or nipple tenderness may be experienced just before menstruation.

Short-lived changes of appearance are observed in many women during sexual response, including protuberance of the nipple, increase in breast size, and so forth. The breasts are highly erogenous organs for many women. They do not merely vary in shape and size with sexual excitement, but there is also a great deal of variation from woman to woman in those parts of the breasts that women perceive as erotic. For example, some women perceive erotic sensations in the areolae, others in the nipples, and still others in the breast tissue near the axilla.

A woman's breasts may also double or triple in size during pregnancy when the maximum branching capability of the breast is attained as well as the full extent of glandular differentiation (Harigopal & Singh, 2021). Striae, engorgement of veins, and increased prominence and pigmentation of nipples and areolae are common during pregnancy. The glandular tissue of the breast gradually involutes, with a marked decrease in the number of lobules after menopause and fat is deposited in the breasts. The breasts of postmenopausal women as they age, therefore, take on a more flattened contour and appear less firm than they were before menopause.

A convention useful in describing the appearance of women's breasts during physical examination is a division into four quadrants by vertical and horizontal lines crossing at the nipple (e.g., upper, outer quadrant of left breast). Another landmark, the axillary tail (also called the tail of Spence), is a portion of breast tissue that extends into the axilla. A more precise description of breast landmarks is one that incorporates an analogy to the face of a clock: A lump could be described at 2 o'clock and include the appropriate number of centimeters from the nipple.

Although women are encouraged to wear brassieres to prevent a drooping of Cooper's ligaments, which makes breasts appear pendulous, there is no compelling evidence for the efficacy of the practice. Aside from fatigue or pain that some women with large breasts experience, there are no health consequences associated with not wearing a brassiere.

Components of Breast Tissue

There are three main components of tissue in women's breasts: glandular, fibrous, and fatty tissue. Most of the breast is composed of subcutaneous and retromammary (behind the breast) fat. Breast tissue is supported by fibrous tissue, including suspensory ligaments (Cooper's ligaments), extending from the subcutaneous connective tissue to the muscle fascia (see Figure 7.1).

An important functional component of the breast is the glandular tissue, which consists of 12 to 25 lobes, arranged radially, that terminate in ducts that open on the surface of the nipple. The lobes are separated from one another by various amounts of fat. Each lobe is composed of 20 to 40 lobules, each of which contains 10 to 100 alveoli (sometimes called acini).

The alveolus is the basic component of the breast lobule. The hollow alveolus is lined by a single layer of milk-secreting columnar epithelial cells, which are derived prenatally from an ingrowth of epidermis into the mesenchyme between 10 and 12 weeks of gestation. These cells enlarge greatly and discharge their contents during lactation. The individual alveolus is encased in a network of myoepithelial strands and is surrounded by a rich capillary network. The lumen of the alveolus opens into a collecting intralobar (within the lobe) duct through a thin, nonmuscular duct. The intralobar ducts eventually end in the openings in the nipple and are surrounded by muscle cells.

Supporting Structures

The third and fourth branches of the cervical plexus provide the cutaneous nerve supply to the upper breast and the thoracic intercostal nerves to the lower breast. The perforating branches of the internal mammary artery constitute the chief external blood supply, although additional arterial blood supply emanates from the lateral thoracic arteries (Harigopal & Singh, 2021). Superficial veins of the breast drain into the internal mammary veins and the superficial veins of the lower portion of the neck and from the latter into the jugular vein. Veins emptying into the internal mammary, axillary, and intercostal veins serve deep breast tissue.

The lymphatic drainage of the breast is of special interest and importance to women because of its role in dissemination of tumor cells as well as its ability to respond to infection. The lymphatic system of the breast is both abundant and complex. In general, the lymphatics drain both the axillary and internal mammary areas. Lymph from the skin of the breast, except for areolar and nipple areas, flows into the axillary nodes on the same side of the body, whereas the lymph from the medial cutaneous breast area may flow into the opposite breast. The lymph from the areolar and nipple areas flows into the anterior axillary (mammary) nodes.

Lymph from deep within the mammary tissues flows into the anterior axillary nodes but may also flow into the apical, subclavian, infraclavicular, and supraclavicular nodes. Lymph from areas behind the areolae and the medial and lower glandular areas of breast tissue communicates with the lymphatic systems draining into the thorax and abdomen (see Figure 7.1).

PERINEUM AND PELVIC ORGANS

The perineum is a diamond-shaped structure that is bounded by the symphysis pubis ventrally, the coccyx dorsally, and the pelvic diaphragm. Several structures are visualized on the external perineum during a clinical examination. Starting from the symphysis pubis, the mons pubis is seen, followed by the clitoral hood, clitoris, labia majora and minora, urethra, vestibule, vaginal introitus, perineal body, and then the anus (see Figure 7.2). Chapter 27, Vulvar and Vaginal Health, includes a full discussion of their musculature, bony structures, innervation, and vascular supply.

As with breasts, many of a woman's pelvic structures serve both reproductive functions and recreative (or sexual) pleasures. Despite the unique functions served by their pelvic structures, women may be unaware of their appearance because they are located deep within the pelvic cavity or because women have not had an opportunity to visualize their external genitalia, or they have been discouraged from examining or touching themselves.

Many of a woman's genital structures can be visualized easily with a mirror (see Figure 7.2). The configuration of the genitals is strikingly unique to each woman and highly variable from woman to woman. For example, many paired structures, such as the labia, are not perfectly symmetrical. Indeed, evidence suggests that the anatomic diversity of women's external genitalia is not associated with sexual activity or aspects of sexual response (Krissi et al., 2016).

VULVA

The external female genitalia are commonly referred to as the vulva. An older term for the vulva, the pudendum, derives from the Latin word meaning to be ashamed. For this reason, the term *vulva* is preferable.

The most obvious feature of an adult woman's external genitalia is her pubic hair, which is usually coarse, curly, and darker than the hair on her head. Pubic hair not only covers parts of the vulvar area (mons pubis, labia majora) but may extend upward toward the abdomen and outward onto the inner thighs. The flattened area of pubic hair over the lower abdomen forms the base of an inverted triangle. The triangle is sometimes referred to as the *female escutcheon*. Although this is a somewhat typical pattern, it is not

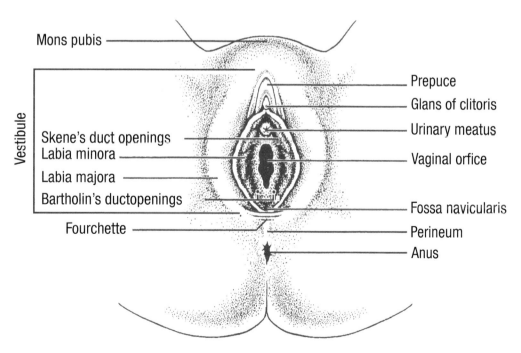

FIGURE 7.2 External genitalia. Note the mons pubis, labia majora, labia minora, clitoris, urinary meatus, vaginal orifice, and anus.

uncommon for healthy women to exhibit variation in this pattern; hair growth may extend up toward the umbilicus in a narrow diamond pattern or back toward the anus. Some women have little pubic hair or a well-delineated triangular area while others have a prolific hair pattern. Pubic hair eventually turns gray and thins with aging.

The mons veneris or mons pubis is composed of soft, fatty tissue and lies over the symphysis pubis. The labia majora consist of two larger, raised folds of adipose tissue. The inner surface of the labia majora consists of apocrine (scent), eccrine (sweat), and sebaceous (oil) glands that serve to lubricate as well as stimulate by releasing a classic, female musk scent during sexual arousal. The labia majora are heavily pigmented, and in postpubertal women, their outer surfaces are covered with hair, whereas the inner surfaces are smooth and hairless. In postmenopausal women, the hair on the labia becomes thinner and the labia and mons appear less full because of the loss of fatty tissue.

The labia minora are two very thin folds of inner skin heavily endowed with blood vessels that lie within the labia majora and extend from the clitoris to the fourchette (vaginal outlet). Each of the labia minora divides into medial and lateral parts. The medial parts join anteriorly to the clitoris to form the clitoral hood (also called prepuce), and the lateral parts join posterior to the clitoris. There are more nerve endings in the labia minora than in the outer labia majora. There are also more sebaceous glands to lubricate the opening into the vagina (the vestibule), and to provide waterproof protection against urine, menstrual bleeding, and bacteria. In some women, the labia minora are completely hidden from view by the labia majora, but in other women the labia minora protrude out from between the labia majora. Frequently, the labia minora are asymmetrical.

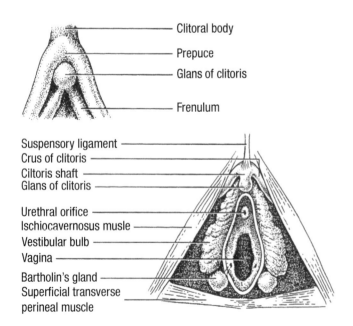

FIGURE 7.3 The clitoris. The sole purpose of the clitoris is reception and transformation of sexual stimuli. Three sections of the clitoris are the glans, the body or corpus, and the crus/crura or root. The crura and the shaft lie below the labia minora, with only the glans of the clitoris directly visible.

The color and texture of the labia minora are highly individual, varying from pink to brown. The clitoral hood covers the clitoris and is believed to protect this extremely sensitive organ from irritation. In some women, the clitoral hood will adhere to the clitoris so that the hood cannot be pulled back very far to reveal the clitoris (see Figure 7.3).

The area between the labia minora, called the vestibule, contains both the urethral and vaginal orifices. The hymen, a membranous covering at the vaginal opening, may be intact, but more frequently is seen as a ring of small, rounded skin fragments attached to the margins of the vaginal opening. This fluted or ruffled appearance is attributed to the natural erosion of the hymen from regular childhood activities such as running, jumping, and riding a bicycle. Some women have a more thick and rigid membrane that remains intact even after penile penetration. Approximately 0.05% to 0.1% of women have an imperforate hymen that requires surgical intervention (Lee et al., 2019).

Skene's glands are tiny, clustered paraurethral organs, the ducts of which open laterally and posteriorly to the urethral orifice. Bartholin's glands, located laterally and slightly posterior to the vaginal introitus, open into the groove between the labia minora and the hymen at the 5 and 7 o'clock positions in relation to the vaginal orifice. Both Skene's and Bartholin's glands are usually not visible, although they are located in tissues that can be visualized, and their openings on the vulva can be seen in some women. These racemose (in the shape of a cluster) glands serve a lubricating function by secreting mucus. The perineum consists of the tissues between the vaginal orifice and the anus. Beneath the vestibule are two bundles of vascular tissue referred to as the bulbs of the vestibule or the perineal sponge. These tissues become congested during sexual response.

Equally important as understanding the anatomic characteristics of a woman's vagina is the new understanding of the vaginal microbiome as it relates to behavior, sexual health, and sexually transmitted infections (Lewis et al., 2017). Recent contributions to molecular techniques and informatics have allowed researchers to assess the composition of microbial communities in the human body. The vaginal microbiome refers to the microbiota, complex microbial communities, and the microbiome to the genetic material, found to differ across anatomic sites, for example, vagina, gut, and across individuals. Study of the vaginal ecosystem, involving the relationship among the bacterial communities, person or host, and the environment, has begun to illuminate understanding of a variety of health outcomes, such as vaginal infection. Some of the most recent understandings about vaginal ecology indicate that vaginal bacterial communities tend to cluster into types of organisms and are also dynamic. Lactobacilli are dominant in most communities, but some types of communities include obligate anaerobic bacteria, such as *Atopobium, Gardnerella,* and *Prevotella* spp., and others. Accumulating evidence suggests that a microbiome with *Lactobacillus* species other than *Lactobacillus iners* is optimal for vaginal health. Production of lactic acid across vaginal microbial communities appears to confer health benefits to women by keeping the pH of the vagina low and inhibiting growth of organisms such as *Candida albicans*, an important cause of vaginitis (Levinson et al., 2022). This new area of investigation has begun to expand our understanding of the relationships of the vaginal microbiome to a variety of health states, including infectious diseases, relationships among bacterial vaginosis and herpes simplex virus, human papillomavirus, HIV, bacterial sexually transmitted infections, trichomonas, pelvic inflammatory disease, and preterm birth (Lewis et al., 2017). Sex hormones and hormonal contraception, sexual behavior, intravaginal practices such as douching, smoking, diet, and environmental factors such as environment, poverty, and characteristics of sexual partners are being investigated for their associations with the vaginal microbiome.

CLITORIS

A woman's clitoris is an erectile organ unique to all human anatomy. Its sole purpose is to serve as a receptor and transformer of sensual stimuli. This unique structure exists to initiate or elevate levels of sexual tension for women (Masters & Johnson, 1966). The various structural components of the clitoris are homologous to similar structures of the male penis (Federation of Feminist Women's Health Centers, 1981). The clitoris, from the Greek word meaning "key," has a similar number of nerve endings at its tip as the glans of the penis, making it extremely sensitive to tactile stimulation.

The clitoris consists of three erectile sections: the glans, the body (corpus), and the crura or root. The clitoris is highly innervated, providing a mechanism uniquely devoted to women's sexual pleasure. The glans and the body of the clitoris sit inside the prepuce or clitoral hood, formed by the lateral parts of the labia minora. It is usually less than 0.5 cm in diameter and is covered by stratified squamous epithelium (Cunningham et al., 2018). The two corpora cavernosa (cavernous bodies) of the clitoris are enclosed in a dense fibrous membrane that is made up of elastic fibers and lies beneath smooth muscle bundles (ischiocavernosus muscles) located beneath the frenulum of the labia minora. Each corpus is connected to the pubic ramus and the ischium. The clitoris is held in place by a suspensory ligament and two small ischiocavernosus muscles that insert into the crura of the clitoris (Cunningham et al., 2018).

Blood supply to the clitoris emanates from the deep and dorsal clitoral arteries that branch from the internal pudendal artery. The vasculature supporting the clitoris plays an important role in increasing its size during sexual response.

The length of the clitoral body (consisting of glans and shaft) varies markedly. The size of the clitoral glans may vary from 2 mm to 1 cm in healthy women and is usually estimated at 4 to 5 mm in both the transverse and longitudinal planes. There is also variation in the position of the clitoris, a function of variation in the points of origin of the suspensory and crural ligaments. The glans is capable of increasing in size with sexual stimulation, and marked vasocongestive increases in the diameter of the clitoral shaft have also been noted (Shindel & Rowan, 2020).

The dorsal nerve of the clitoris is the deepest division of the pudendal nerve, and it terminates in the nerve endings of the glans and corpora cavernosa. Pacinian corpuscles, which respond to deep pressure, are distributed in both the glans and the corpora but have greater concentration in the glans. Their distribution is highly variable from woman to woman, which probably accounts for the rich variation in women's self-pleasuring techniques. For example, some women prefer very light touch whereas others prefer deep pressure. In some women, the anatomic arrangement of the labia minora that forms the clitoral hood makes it possible for mechanical traction on the labia to stimulate the clitoris indirectly. The clitoris is endowed with sensory nerve endings that respond to tactile stimuli as well as pressure. Although afferent stimuli can be received through afferent nerve endings in the clitoral glans and shaft, it is also possible that the clitoris serves as the subjective endpoint or transformer for efferent stimuli from higher neurogenic pathways (Cunningham et al., 2018).

VAGINA

Although the vagina can be considered an internal structure, it can be visualized easily with the assistance of a speculum, a light source, and a mirror. The vagina is a musculomembranous canal connecting the vulva with the uterus. It is lined with a reddish pink mucous membrane that is transversely rugated. Under the stratified squamous epithelial lining (much like the skin on the palm of the hand) is a muscular coat that has an inner circular layer and an outer fibrous layer (see Figure 7.4).

The vagina is typically a potential rather than a real space as it is ordinarily an empty, collapsed tube. Although highly distensible, its unstimulated length is approximately 6 to 7 cm anteriorly and about 9 cm posteriorly. The vaginal canal inclines posteriorly at about a 45-degree angle. The cervix is the neck of the uterus and is encased in the vagina anteriorly and superiorly. There is a recessed portion of the vagina adjacent to the cervix, which, together with the cervix, is called the *vaginal fornix*. The fornix has anterior, posterior, and lateral portions.

Unlike the clitoris, the vagina has procreative as well as recreative functions. One of the important physiologic functions of the vagina during sexual response is its ability to produce lubrication by means of vasodilation lending to liquid transudate through aquaporins located within the vaginal mucosa cells; there are no glandular elements to the vagina (Shindel & Rowen, 2020). In addition, vaginal lubrication occurs in a rhythmic 90-minute cycle throughout the day and night. The

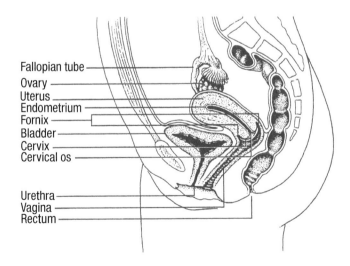

Fallopian tube
Ovary
Uterus
Endometrium
Fornix
Bladder
Cervix
Cervical os

Urethra
Vagina
Rectum

FIGURE 7.4 The internal genitalia. The vaginal canal is a potential rather than a real space and inclines posteriorly at a 45-degree angle. The cervix pierces the anterior superior wall of the vagina.

circulatory venous plexus (including the bulbus vestibuli, plexus pudendalis, plexus uterovaginalis, and possibly the plexus vesicalis and plexus rectalis) encircling the vaginal barrel probably provides the circulatory support for vaginal lubrication and a constant natural sloughing of dead epithelial cells. This vaginal discharge is normal and is called leukorrhea.

In addition to producing lubrication, the vagina demonstrates a remarkable distensive ability during both sexual response and childbirth. Both a lengthening of the vagina and a ballooning out of its inner portions are observed during sexual response. The vascular changes occurring in conjunction with sexual response are profound. The reddish pink hue of the premenopausal woman's vagina changes to a darker purplish vasocongested appearance. In postmenopausal women, the color changes in the vagina and its expansion during sexual response are less pronounced. As the vagina distends, the rugae become flattened as a result of the thinning or stretching of the vaginal mucosa. The vagina, unlike the clitoris, is not well endowed with nerve endings; although there are deep pressure receptors in the innermost portion of the vagina, it is primarily in the outer third of the vagina where women report pleasurable sexual sensations (Masters & Johnson, 1966).

CERVIX

Although the cervix might be regarded as an internal structure because it is a part of the uterus, it can be visualized for a clinician's examination with the aid of a speculum and a light source. The cervix extends from the isthmus of the uterus into the vagina, and it is through the small cervical opening (os) that the uterus and vagina communicate. The cervical os appears as a small, regular, oval opening in nulliparous women and converts to a transverse slit in parous women that can appear irregular, nodular, or stellate (Cunningham et al., 2018). The cervix appears as an oval structure and is usually shiny and pale pink. In postmenopausal women, the cervix may be smaller and less pigmented than that in premenopausal women. The stroma (connective tissue forming the supportive framework) of the cervix consists of connective tissue with unstriated muscle fibers as well as elastic tissue.

The stratified squamous epithelium of the outer cervix (the portio) is made up of several layers. The basal layer is a single row of cells resting on a thin basement membrane and is the layer where active mitosis (cell division) is seen. The parabasal and intermediate layers appear next. In the intermediate layer, vacuoles containing glycogen are seen. The superficial, keratinized layer varies in thickness in response to estrogen stimulation. The desquamation of this surface layer occurs constantly. The superficial layer contains a large amount of glycogen, as does the intermediate layer. It appears that glycogen plays an important role in maintaining the acid pH of the vagina. Glycogen released by cytolysis of the desquamated cells is acted on by the glycolytic bacterial flora in the vagina, forming lactic acid. In a healthy vaginal ecosystem with a basic pH, the vagina will typically smell salty and slightly musky. Each woman has a unique, characteristic odor that is more noticeable during the hormonal influences associated with ovulation, menstruation, and sexual stimulation.

Just as the endometrium is influenced by the hormonal fluctuations of the menstrual cycle, so is the mucus produced by the secretory cells of the glands in the endocervix (interior cervical canal). This is especially noticeable in premenopausal women. The fluctuations in cervical mucus during the course of the menstrual cycle are discussed later in this chapter.

There is an abrupt transition from the stratified squamous epithelium covering the vagina and the outer surface of the cervix to the tall, glandular columnar cells rich in mucin (proteinaceous mucoid substance) located within the internal cervical canal. This junction between ectocervical cells and endocervical cells is designated as the transformation zone. This ever-changing squamocolumnar junction is actually a cellular dividing line where newly forming columnar epithelium in the cervix merge with the encroaching stratified epithelium lining. It is an area of increased susceptibility to infection and carcinogens. During a cervical cytology test for cervical cancer, desquamated (exfoliated) cells from the cervix are examined through cytology for cellular abnormalities. For an adequate test, endocervical cells at the squamocolumnar transformation zone, as well as ectocervical squamous cells, must be included. The transformation zone is sometimes visualized at the cervical os or may be higher up in the endocervical canal.

UTERUS

The uterus is a hollow, pear-shaped organ that is 5.5 to 9 cm long, 3.5 to 6 cm wide, and 2 to 4 cm thick in nulliparous women. The uterus of a parous woman may be 2 to 3 cm larger in any of these three dimensions and typically weighs more than the nulliparous uterus. The uterus is usually inclined forward at a 45-degree angle from the longitudinal plane of the body and is anteverted or slightly anteflexed in position. However, it also may be retroflexed, retroverted, or in a midposition.

The portion of the uterus above the cervix is termed the corpus (body) and is constructed of a thick-walled musculature. It is covered with peritoneum on the exterior and lined interiorly with a mucoid surface called the endometrium. The body of the uterus is divided into three portions: the fundus, the corpus, and the isthmus. The fundus is the prominence above the insertion of the fallopian tubes, the corpus is the main portion, and the isthmus is the narrow lower portion of the uterus adjacent to the cervix. The uterus is not a fixed organ but can be moved about; for example, during the sexual response cycle, the entire uterus elevates from the true pelvis into the false pelvis.

FALLOPIAN TUBES

Two fallopian tubes are laterally located at either horn of the uterine fundus; run laterally toward the ovaries; and are the site for ovum and sperm transport, sperm capacitation, ovum retrieval, fertilization, and embryo transport. Each tube is approximately 8 to 14 cm long. The distal portion of the tube (oviduct) is fimbriated; both the middle portion (the ampulla) and the portion of the tube closest to its insertion in the uterus (the isthmus) are extremely narrow at 5 to 8 mm and 2 to 3 mm, respectively. The wider funnel-shaped end of the tubes is surrounded by irregular, fingerlike extensions called *fimbriae*. Although not actually attached to the ovary, the fimbriae come into contact with the ovary and are lined with ciliated epithelium that sweeps uniformly toward the uterus, acting as a vacuum for any newly released ovum. The outer, serous coat of the oviduct covers a muscular portion consisting of an inner circular layer and a thin, outer longitudinal layer. The mucosal layer, composed of a number of rugae that become more numerous approaching the fimbriated portion, lines the tubes.

OVARIES

The ovaries are paired, almond-shaped, female gonads approximately 3 to 4 cm long, 2 cm wide, and 1 to 2 cm thick. They are located near the pelvic wall at the level of the anterior superior iliac spine. The external ovarian surface has a dull, whitish, opaque appearance. The ovary is composed of three major portions. The first portion is an outer cortex lined by a single layer of cuboidal (cube-shaped) epithelium. Through this layer, blood vessels and nerves enter and leave the ovary. Follicles are embedded in the connective tissue of the outer cortex and are either growing or inactive. The second portion is the central medulla of the ovary, which is composed of loose connective tissue (stroma), lymphatics, and blood vessels. The ovarian stroma comprises contractile cells, connective tissue cells that provide structural support to the ovary, and interstitial cells that secrete sex steroid hormones (primarily androgens). In addition, the stroma contains the primordial follicles yet to be recruited. Not only do the ovaries release gametes, but they also produce sex steroid hormones—including estrogen, progesterone, and androgens—as well as a number of nonsteroidal factors that regulate endocrine regulation of ovarian function. The ovary has a rich lymphatic drainage, and an abundant supply of unmyelinated nerve fibers also enters the medulla through the rete ovarii (the hilum). The hilum is the point of ovarian attachment to the mesovarium, a peritoneal fold on the posterior surface of the broad ligament.

At birth, the ovary contains approximately 1 to 2 million germ cells after reaching the acme of follicular formation at 16 to 20 weeks' gestation (6–7 million oocytes). Research has demonstrated that by the onset of puberty, the total content of germ cell mass is ultimately reduced through the process of atresia to 300,000 follicles, and only 400 oogonia will achieve ovulation during a woman's reproductive life. However, during the past decade, scientists have discovered evidence supporting the capacity for postnatal oogenesis and follicle renewal in mammals, including humans (Truman et al., 2017). These new findings of oogonial stem cells (OSCs) challenge the notion of a fixed ovarian reserve of oocytes that gets depleted over the course of reproductive aging, supporting the fact that generation of new oocytes and follicles occurs. Although prior evidence from follicle counts would suggest that follicles become atretic and their number is reduced by the time of puberty, it remains uncertain how the production of new oocytes and follicles affects follicle counts using current clinical methods.

The follicle is the functional unit of the ovary, the source of both the gametes and the ovarian hormones. Each follicle is surrounded by a circular cellular wall called the *theca folliculi*. The theca contains an inner rim of secretory cells (the theca interna) and an outer rim of connective tissue (the theca externa). Within the theca—but separated from it by a layer of thin basement membrane—are the granulosa cells, which, in turn, surround the ovum. An acellular layer of protein and polysaccharide, the zona pellucida, separates the ovum from the granulosa cells. The theca interna is richly vascularized, although neither the ovum nor the granulosa

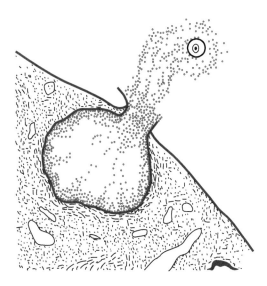

FIGURE 7.5 Ovulation. At ovulation, the ovum, surrounded by the corona radiata and floating in the follicular fluid, ruptures into the peritoneal cavity.

cells are in contact with any capillaries. The theca and granulosa cells are the primary sex steroid–secreting elements. These cells have receptors for gonadotropins and respond to those released by the anterior pituitary: follicle-stimulating hormone (FSH) and luteinizing hormone (LH).

Development and maturation of the follicle are stimulated by FSH and it stimulates proliferation of the granulosa cells and the gradual elaboration of fluid within the follicle. Accumulation of the fluid increases rapidly with follicular maturation and causes the follicle, known as the graafian follicle, to bulge into the peritoneal cavity. As the follicle swells, the ovum remains embedded in granulosa cells (cumulus oophorus), which remain in contact with the theca. As fluid accumulates, the cumulus thins until only a narrow thread of cells connects the ovum with the rim of the follicle. At ovulation, the ovum, surrounded by the corona of granulosa cells (sometimes called the corona radiata) while floating in the follicular fluid, ruptures. The ovum and its corona extrude into the peritoneal cavity in a bolus of the follicular fluid. This sometimes is perceived as a crampy sensation, referred to as mittelschmerz. After ovulation, ingrowth and differentiation of the remaining granulosa cells fill the collapsed follicle to form a new endocrine structure called the *corpus luteum*. The corpus luteum continues to develop when a pregnancy occurs. When the ovum is not fertilized and dies, the corpus luteum no longer develops and leaves a remnant on the surface of the ovary called a corpus albicans (see Figure 7.5).

Pelvic Supporting Structures

The pelvic floor is a complex of interrelated structures that support the pelvic organs. Bones, muscles, ligaments, blood vessels, and nerves form supporting structures of the pelvic organs and are described in the following section.

BONY PELVIS

The pelvis is composed of two innominate bones: the sacrum and coccyx. The innominate bones, in turn, are the ilium, ischium, and pubis. These constitute the hip bones. The pubic bones meet anteriorly at the symphysis pubis, a fibrocartilaginous symphyseal joint. The pubic arch is formed by the inferior borders of the pubic bones and symphysis. The ilium joins with the sacrum posteriorly to form the sacroiliac joint, which is a synovial joint. A woman's pelvis is typically wider and hollower than a man's because of the flaring of the woman's iliac bones and a curved sacrum (see Figure 7.6).

MUSCLES

Several sets of pelvic muscles attach to the bony pelvis and can be divided into two main groups: the urogenital triangle and the pelvic floor. These muscle groups both actively and passively support the pelvis and are involved in the voluntary contraction of the vagina and the anus. The layer of muscles that is closest to the skin is called the urogenital triangle. Two pairs of long, slender muscles (the ischiocavernosus) run alongside the pelvic outlet and form the two sides of the triangle, with

the clitoris at its apex. It then sends fibers to the upper and middle thirds of the urethra, forming the greater part of this organ's voluntary sphincter (Owen & Heitmann, 2019). The superficial transverse perineal muscle extends laterally and forms the base of this triangle. The bulbocavernosus muscles extend from the glans of the clitoris downward under the labia majora, connecting at the perineum, and are shaped like a pair of parentheses. The deep transverse perineal muscle forms a solid triangular base of muscle immediately behind the open urogenital triangle and is bisected by the vagina and urethra. During orgasm, all these muscles contract simultaneously, compressing the engorged clitoral tissue between them, creating muscle tension and sexual pleasure. Behind the urogenital triangle is the pelvic floor, which is made up of the levator ani muscle. The pubococcygeus muscle, part of the levator ani group, has particular significance in women because it is important in sexual sensory function, bladder control, and childbirth—by controlling relaxation and extension of the perineum and expulsion of the infant (see Figure 7.7).

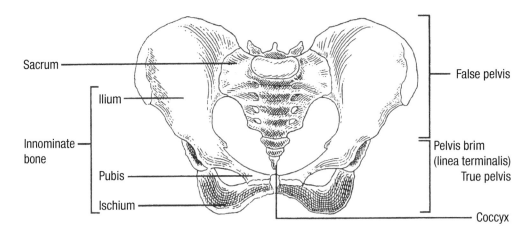

FIGURE 7.6 The bony pelvis. The pelvic spine consists of the sacrum and the coccyx. The innominate bones are the ilium, the ischium, and the pubis, which make up the pelvic girdle.

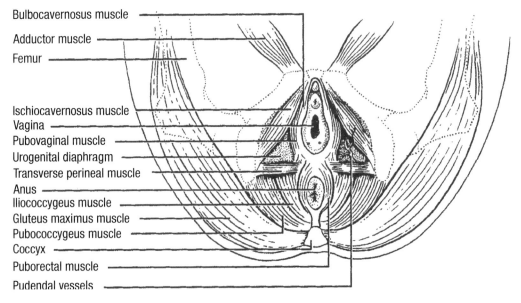

FIGURE 7.7 Pelvic muscles. Several sets of muscles support the pelvic floor. The bulbocavernosus and the pubococcygeus muscles have special significance for sexual function.

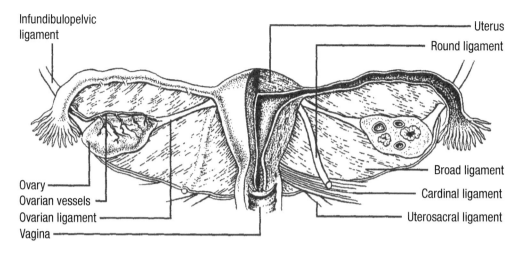

FIGURE 7.8 **Ligaments. Four pairs of ligaments support the uterus, fallopian tubes, and ovaries. These are the cardinal, uterosacral, round, and broad ligaments.**

LIGAMENTS

Four pairs of ligaments—the cardinal, uterosacral, round, and broad ligaments—provide primary support for the uterus, and the ovarian ligaments and infundibulopelvic ligaments provide ancillary support (see Figure 7.8). Overstretching the ligaments is sometimes associated with minor discomfort during strenuous exercise or during pregnancy.

VASCULATURE

The ovarian arteries arise from the abdominal aorta, supply the fallopian tube and ovary, and ultimately anastomose with the uterine artery. The uterine artery arises from the anterior branch of the hypogastric artery and supplies the cervix and uterus. The vaginal artery arises similarly from the anterior branch of the hypogastric artery. The uterine veins run along the same channels as the uterine artery. The ovarian veins from the vena cava pass through the broad ligament en route to the ovarian hilus (neck of the ovary). On the right, the ovarian vein empties into the inferior vena cava; on the left, it empties into the renal vein.

INNERVATION

The internal genitalia are supplied by autonomic as well as spinal nerve pathways. The main autonomic supply to the uterus appears to consist of both sympathetic and parasympathetic fibers of the superior hypogastric plexus, which stems from the second to fourth sacral nerve roots and the sacral sympathetic trunk (Hoffman et al., 2020). The pudendal nerve is the main spinal nerve, providing the source of motor and sensory activation of the lower genital tract.

ENDOCRINE PHYSIOLOGY

Many of the unique functions of the female body are regulated by hormonal influences resulting from the communication between the endocrine system and the central nervous system (CNS). Grasping the basic relationship among the hypothalamus, pituitary, and ovaries is important for understanding sexual differentiation, pubertal development, rhythms of the menstrual cycle, the menopausal transition and postmenopause, and specific biological differences created by classic female steroid hormones, estradiol, and progesterone, as well as oxytocin.

The endocrine system includes all the glands that secrete hormones (considered chemical messengers) that are carried by the blood bound to a plasma protein from the glands to target cells elsewhere in the body to elicit systemic biological responses. In addition to discrete organs such as the adrenal or thyroid glands, the definition of endocrine systems has been expanded recently to include single cells or clusters of cells that are not anatomically definable as a gland but that can also secrete or produce hormones. The effects of hormones can be either rapid or delayed, short or long term, depending on their structure and synthesis. A complex feedback system allows for the intricate balance between the hormones secreted and the responses elicited at the level of the target cells throughout the body.

On the target cell (the cell that responds to the presence of the hormone), receptors on the surface or within the cytoplasm or nuclei are the immediate recipients of the chemical messages or information units of hormones. These receptors are structurally organized so that they can specifically recognize and interact with their own cognate hormone, either inside the cell or, more frequently, on the plasma membrane of the cell. All receptors have two essential components: a ligand-binding region that binds the exact hormone for that receptor and an effector region that recognizes the presence of the hormone bound to the ligand region and then initiates the generation of the biological response. Fat-soluble hormones, such as the steroid hormones estrogen and testosterone, pass through the cell membrane and bind to intracellular receptors, whereas water-soluble hormones (peptides such as FSH) bind to a cellular membrane receptor and subsequently trigger a second messenger that engages protein kinases in producing a cellular response. The steroid and thyroid hormones can produce rapid nongenomic action as well as a less

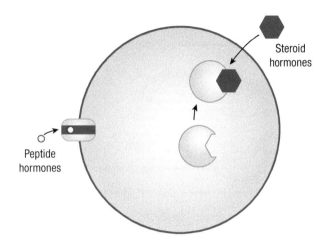

FIGURE 7.9 Hormonal effects within cells: Steroid hormones bind to intracellular receptors and peptide hormones bind to cellular membrane receptors.

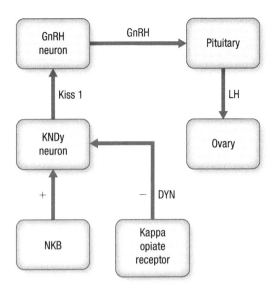

FIGURE 7.10 Regulation of GnRH by the KNDy neurons, modulated by NKB and DYN.
DYN, dynorphin; GnRH, gonadotropin-releasing hormone; LH, luteinizing hormone; NKB, neurokinin B.

rapid response in which they bind to nuclear receptors that alter genome transcription. As a consequence of the specific receptor–hormone interaction (much like a specific lock and key), a cascade of events, or signal transduction pathways, occurs, and a specific biological response is generated in and, in some instances, around the target cell (Figure 7.9).

To maintain system precision, receptors have internal physiologic regulators to maintain a balance between the extracellular hormone messengers and the number of target cell receptor sites that elicit specific cellular responses. One of these mechanisms is called downregulation and has the effect of reducing the number of receptor sites (within target cells) in response to long periods of frequent or intense hormonal bombardment. The other mechanism, upregulation, increases the number of receptor sites on the target cell to increase the cell's response to prolonged periods of low concentrations of particular hormones. In other words, if a gland over- or undermanufactures a particular hormone, the controlling gland in the brain or hypothalamus senses the amount of circulating hormone and responds by modulating hormone secretion (Hsiao & Gardner, 2017).

As key elements of the CNS, the hypothalamus and pituitary glands are located in the middle of the forebrain on its undersurface, inferior to the third ventricle. While these structures occupy a very small portion of the brain and account for less than 1% of the brain's weight, the hypothalamus and pituitary function as the control center for the coordination of both neural and endocrine systems (Javorsky et al., 2017).

The hypothalamus plays a significant role by integrating centrally the neurologic and endocrine systems. In addition to production of releasing and inhibitory hormones and tropic hormones, the hypothalamus regulates homeostasis of the interior climate of the body such as temperature regulation, water balance, and emotional behaviors as well as behaviors related to preservation of the species—hunger, thirst, and reproduction. Recent discoveries indicate that the hypothalamus orchestrates the pituitary and ovarian secretion of hormones by means of neurons that are estrogen-sensitive and synthesize kisspeptin, neurokinin B (NKB), and dynorphin. The neurons involved in this process are referred to as KNDy

neurons and regulate pulsatile secretion of gonadotropin-releasing hormone (GnRH) and LH. Dynorphin can inhibit this system by binding kappa opioid receptors in the area of the KNDy neurons. It is of interest to note that these neurons are adjacent to the thermoregulatory center of the hypothalamus. In brief, the pulsatile activity of KNDy neurons is regulated by NKB and dynorphin acting in a reciprocal fashion (Hoffman et al., 2020; Oakley et al., 2009). NKB stimulates and dynorphin suppresses the pulsatile secretion of GnRH and LH (current investigations are focused on the relationship of the KNDy neurons and hot flashes; Oakley et al., 2015; Figure 7.10).

The pituitary gland sits in a hollow area of the sphenoid bone, called the sella turcica, just below the hypothalamus. This endocrine gland is attached to the hypothalamus by a stalk that contains nerve filaments and small blood vessels. In adults, the pituitary is composed of two lobes—the anterior and posterior—each of which functions essentially as a distinct gland. The anterior pituitary releases hormones responsible for a wide variety of critical functions, including growth, metabolism, steroid release, breast growth, and milk synthesis as well as gamete production and sex hormone secretions. These essential bodily capacities are produced by the release of growth hormone (GH), thyroid-stimulating hormone (TSH), ACTH, prolactin, and two gonadotropic hormones—FSH and LH. The posterior pituitary controls milk let-down and uterine contractility as well as water secretion by the kidneys and blood pressure through release of oxytocin and vasopressin.

The posterior pituitary is an extension of the hypothalamus and communicates through neural connections and electrical messages to release hormones. The anterior pituitary has a unique, localized circulatory connection to the hypothalamus that allows blood to transport special hormones secreted directly from the hypothalamus to the anterior pituitary (hypophysiotropic hormones) to stimulate the release of other, specific anterior pituitary hormones.

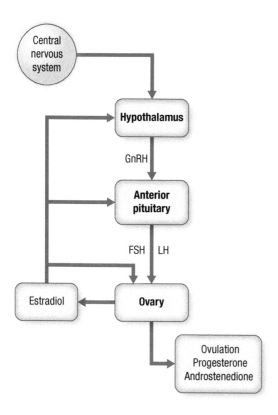

FIGURE 7.11 Hypothalamic–pituitary–ovarian axis.
FSH, follicle-stimulating hormone; GnRH, gonadotropin-releasing hormone; LH, luteinizing hormone.

Of particular importance to the female body is the regulation of the menstrual cycle and the ovaries' ability to produce gametes. This signal transduction pathway is initially stimulated by GnRH secreted by the hypothalamus, which then stimulates the release of FSH as well as LH from the anterior pituitary. FSH and LH are called gonadotropins because they stimulate the target cells—ovaries (gonads)—to release steroid hormones estradiol, progesterone, and androgens while a mature egg follicle develops and is subsequently released. The ovarian hormones feed back to the hypothalamus and pituitary, regulating the secretion of gonadotropins during the phases of the menstrual cycle. The careful monthly orchestration of these various hormonal pathways in the interrelated CNS and endocrine communication system is referred to as the *hypothalamic–pituitary–ovarian (HPO) axis* (Figure 7.11).

Although the dominant ovarian hormones in women are estrogen and progesterone, testosterone and other androgens are produced by the ovary as well as the adrenal gland. These are significant as they serve as precursors to other steroid hormones. Steroidogenesis involves the synthesis from conversion of cholesterol to pregnenolone (McCance & Huether, 2014).

Estrogens

Three estrogens are among the ovarian steroid hormones: estradiol, estrone, and estriol. Estrogens are synthesized by aromatization (CYP19 enzymes) from androstenedione and testosterone; estradiol is synthesized from testosterone and estrone from androstenedione (Barrett et al., 2019; see Figure 7.12). Estrone

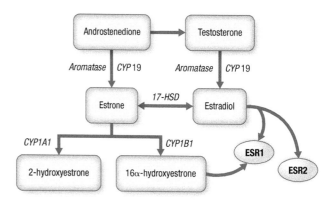

FIGURE 7.12 Sex steroid pathways: synthesis, metabolism, and receptors for estrogens.
Estrogen and estradiol synthesis: CYP19—aromatase, regulated by 17-hydroxysteroid dehydrogenases (17-HSD); estrogen metabolizing: CYP1A1 and CYP1B1; estrogen receptors: ESR1 and ESR2.

and estradiol synthesis is also regulated by 17-hydroxysteroid dehydrogenase (17-HSD) enzymes. Other important aspects of estradiol metabolism include metabolism to 2-hydroxyestrone and 6α-hydroxyestrone by CYP1A1 and CYP1B1 enzymes. Estrogen receptors (e.g., alpha and beta types) provide the means by which circulating estrogens influence biological outcomes in cells and tissues throughout the body.

Although the majority of estradiol is produced by the ovaries (an estimated 95%), adrenal cortical production of estradiol also occurs. Two peaks of secretion occur: one just prior to ovulation and the other during the midluteal phase. Synthesized from testosterone under the influence of the aromatase, estradiol is the most biologically potent of the estrogens. Estrone is the second most potent estrogen, synthesized from androstenedione under the influence of aromatase in adipose tissue and to some extent in the ovaries and adrenals from androgen precursors.

With the transition to menopause, women's metabolism changes from an estradiol-dominant milieu to an estrone-dominant milieu. Estriol, a weak metabolite of estradiol and estrone, is predominantly influential during pregnancy and produced by aromatization of fetal androgen in the placenta.

Estrogens play a significant role in the development of the reproductive organs; secondary sex characteristics; and other organs including bone, liver, blood vessels, brain, kidney, and skin. Adaptations of pregnancy are influenced by estrogens, such as those involved in breast development to support lactation.

Progesterone

Progesterone is released from the corpus luteum during the luteal phase of the menstrual cycle. Released under stimulation of the ovary by LH, which promotes the luteinization of the granulosa in the dominant follicle, progesterone is secreted increasingly after ovulation occurs. In addition, a small portion of progesterone is secreted by the adrenals. During the follicular phase of the menstrual cycle, progesterone is produced in nearly equal amounts by the ovary and the adrenals. Progesterone plays a significant role in the production of androgens. Large doses of progesterone inhibit LH secretion and potentiate the inhibitory effects of estrogen, preventing ovulation.

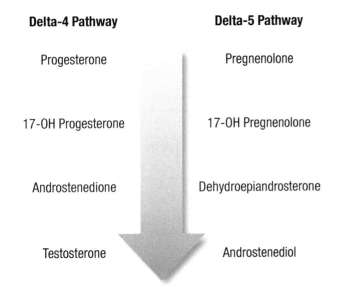

Delta-4 Pathway	Delta-5 Pathway
Progesterone	Pregnenolone
17-OH Progesterone	17-OH Pregnenolone
Androstenedione	Dehydroepiandrosterone
Testosterone	Androstenediol

FIGURE 7.13 Primary steroidogenic pathways. Steroidogenesis involves the synthesis from conversion of cholesterol to progesterone and pregnenolone via two pathways: delta-4 and delta-5 pathways.
Source: Adapted from Lasley, B. L., Crawford, S., & McConnell, D. S. (2011). Adrenal androgens and the menopausal transition. Obstetrics and Gynecology Clinics of North America, 38, 467–475. *https://doi.org/10.1016/j.ogc.2011.06.001*

Androgens

Androgens are produced by the adrenals, ovaries, and peripheral conversion of androstenedione and dehydroepiandrosterone (DHEA) to testosterone. Adrenarche, preceding the onset of puberty, is stimulated by increased production of adrenal androgen. The rapid increase in androstenediol stimulates both adrenal and ovarian production, resulting in long bone growth, pubic and axillary hair, increased sebaceous gland function, and libido.

As seen in Figure 7.13, androgens are synthesized from two primary pathways. The delta-4 pathway supports synthesis of androstenedione and testosterone, which can be aromatized to estrone and estradiol in peripheral tissues, as well as the mineralocorticoids and glucocorticoids. The delta-5 pathway supports synthesis of DHEA and dehydroepiandrosterone sulfate (DHEAS), prohormones for the peripheral conversion to more bioactive steroids. With recent findings that androstenediol is produced in relatively high concentrations, it is considered important during the menopausal transition as a source of estrogen synthesis (Manson & Bassuk, 2018).

Nonsteroidal Ovarian Hormones

In addition to the steroid hormones estrogens and progesterone, the ovaries also produce inhibin, activin, follistatin, and oocyte maturation inhibitor (OMI), peptides that modulate ovarian follicular development and steroid hormone synthesis. FSH stimulates inhibin secretion from the granulosa cells and suppresses FSH synthesis. Inhibin B is secreted in the follicular phase, but spikes at ovulation, whereas inhibin A is secreted in the luteal phase. Activin stimulates secretion

of FSH and increases pituitary response to GnRH. Further activin increases FSH binding in granulosa cells in the dominant follicle. Follistatin, produced by the pituitary, suppresses FSH activity by binding to activin. Inhibin and activin also play a role in regulating LH stimulation of androgen synthesis in theca cells. A follicular factor, OMI, prevents resumption of meiosis by ova of antral follicles before the gonadotropin and LH surge before ovulation. Insulin-like growth factor (IGF) is also produced in the ovary.

In addition, several ovarian hormones serve as markers of follicle counts in women. Anti-Müllerian hormone (AMH) is produced by granulosa cells in the primary follicles produced by a primordial follicle. AMH is regarded as an indicator of the number of antral follicles in the ovary and is being investigated as an indicator of approaching menopause (Grossman et al., 2017).

Oxytocin

Produced by the posterior pituitary, oxytocin stimulates contraction of the uterus and milk ejection in lactating women. Stimulated by suckling and distention of the reproductive tract, release of oxytocin is responsible for the milk let-down reflex. Binding to receptors on myoepithelial cells of mammary tissues, oxytocin causes contraction of cells to increase the intramammary pressure necessary for milk expression. Oxytocin stimulates uterine contraction, enhances the effectiveness of labor contractions, promotes delivery of the placenta, and prevents excessive postpartum bleeding. Recent research suggests that oxytocin modulates responses to stress, especially during pregnancy and the postpartum period. Indeed, some investigators suggest that oxytocin promotes women approaching stressful situations by tending and befriending instead of fight or flight (McCance & Huether, 2014).

Prolactin

Produced by the anterior pituitary, prolactin induces milk production during pregnancy and lactation. The drop in progesterone at the end of pregnancy is the final signal for the beginning of milk production. Suckling by the child stimulates the hypothalamus to continue to promote pituitary gland secretion of prolactin. It has been implicated in immune function and ovulation (Bubier, 2018).

Hormone-Binding Proteins

Hormone-binding proteins play a critical role in regulating the amount of free hormones circulating to cells throughout the body. Sex hormone–binding globulin (SHBG) binds to steroid hormones, for example, testosterone, thus preventing it from binding to cellular receptors and initiating a biological effect.

SEXUAL DIFFERENTIATION AND DEVELOPMENT

Sexual differentiation and development involve a complex series of events that ultimately transform an undifferentiated embryo into a human with a specific sexual determination of female or male designated sex. Early research formulated a model that identified that chromosomal sex would determine gonadal sex and gonadal sex will determine phenotypic sex. As a result of the complexity of sexual differentiation, one can be born with genotypic sex that is inconsistent with one's phenotypic sex. Phenotypic sex can be understood as the total perceptible characteristics displayed by an individual under specific environmental circumstances, regardless of the person's genotype. The developmental process of sexual differentiation begins at fertilization with establishment of genetic sex. *Genetic sex* refers to the chromosomal combination from the ovum and sperm, resulting in XX (female), XY (male), or other combinations. *Gonadal sex* refers to the structure and function of the gonads, whereas *somatic sex* involves the genital organs other than the gonads. *Neuroendocrine sex* refers to the cyclic or continuous production of GnRH. Although gonadal, somatic, and neuroendocrine sexual differentiation begins before birth, sexual differentiation continues after birth. Development of social, psychological, and cultural dimensions of sexuality as well as secondary sex characteristics occurs after birth.

Genetic Sex

Genetic sex is determined at the time of fertilization and is defined by the contribution of an X or Y chromosome from the father. It is of interest that, despite the genotype, sexual differentiation produces a basic female phenotype unless testosterone is present and can be used by the cells of the developing human.

Gonadal Sex

At about 4 to 6 weeks of gestation, germ cells migrate to the site of the fetal gonad. At the sixth week, the gonads are sexually indistinguishable, containing a cortex and medulla layer. Several genes have been identified as important to gonad development, but it is the *sex-determining region of the Y (SRY)* gene that provides the testis-determining factor and it is in the presence of this gene that gonads develop as testes (Hoffman et al., 2020). Up until approximately 7 weeks of embryonic development the male and female sex is indistinguishable from each other. If the chromosomal sex is XX, the cortex will differentiate into the ovaries, and the medulla will regress; if the chromosomal sex is XY, the medulla will differentiate into a testis and the cortex will regress.

Differentiation of the gonad occurs slightly earlier in male than in female fetuses. At 7 weeks, testicular differentiation begins under the influence of testosterone, which is stimulated by human chorionic gonadotropin (hCG). The ovary differentiates about 2 weeks after testicular differentiation and is identifiable by 10 weeks. By 16 weeks, the oogonia become surrounded by follicular cells, composing the primordial follicle. At 20 weeks' gestation, the fetal ovary contains mature stroma organization and compartmentalization with primordial follicles and oocytes, with approximately 5 to 7 million germ cells present. Follicular maturation and atresia are already progressing. Approximately 1 million germ cells remain in the ovary at birth. The oocytes are surrounded by primordial follicles and are arrested in the prophase of the first meiotic (cellular division in which the diploid number of chromosomes is reduced to the haploid) division until the follicle is reactivated at the time of puberty.

No single gene has yet been identified for ovarian determination, though genetic research over the past 2 decades now shows multiple genes that have a synergistic effect to ensure ovarian development (Eggers et al., 2014). Ovarian development has long been thought to result from a default pathway. Research in animal models and gene transcription evaluation in those with ovarian pathologies have identified three genes having some role essential for ovarian determination, differentiation, and/or maintenance: *FOXL2, RSPO1,* and *WNT4* (Elzaiat et al., 2017). The genes influencing testes development are better defined. The sex-determining region on the Y chromosome encodes the *SRY* gene, triggering a genetic cascade. Activation of the *SRY*'s direct target gene *SOX9* (Uhlenhaut et al., 2009) supports differentiation of the testes and inhibits the default ovarian differentiation pathway (Biason-Lauber, 2010). Only one X chromosome is needed for primary ovarian differentiation, explaining why female differentiation may occur in fetuses with XY chromosomes who lack testosterone elaboration at a critical point in development or are unable to use testosterone.

Somatic Sex

The mesonephric (wolffian duct) and the paramesonephric (Müllerian duct) ducts coexist in all embryos regardless of chromosomal sex. During the third fetal month, one persists and the other disappears. The intrinsic tendency toward feminization produces differentiation of the paramesonephric (müllerian) system. In the absence of Müllerian inhibiting factor, *anti-Müllerian hormone (AMH),* which inhibits the further development of the Müllerian ducts in male embryos, the paramesonephric system differentiates into the uterine tubes, uterus, and upper vagina.

At the eighth week of gestation, the embryo is bipotential—that is, it can differentiate into either a female or a male. Between 9 and 12 weeks of gestation, differentiation of external genitalia becomes evident. The urogenital sinus, labioscrotal swellings, and genital tubercle will differentiate into a female pattern in the absence of androgen stimulation and without a Y chromosome. In females, the urogenital folds remain open, developing into the labia minora. The labioscrotal folds differentiate into the labia majora, and the genital tubercle differentiates into the clitoris. The urogenital sinus becomes the vagina and the urethra. The lower vagina is formed as part of the external genitalia. The differentiation of these structures is illustrated in Figures 7.14 and 7.15.

Fetal endocrine glands are supported by the placenta as well as the fetal gonads. By the 10th week of gestation, most of the pituitary hormones are apparent, rising during the first 20 weeks of pregnancy, and then limited by negative feedback mechanisms. LH and FSH are apparent at 9 to 10 weeks and peak at about 20 to 22 weeks' gestation. FSH stimulates follicular development in females; LH stimulates steroid synthesis in the ovary and will later induce ovulation in FSH-primed follicles. Hypothalamic-releasing hormones stimulate ACTH production by about 8 weeks' gestation.

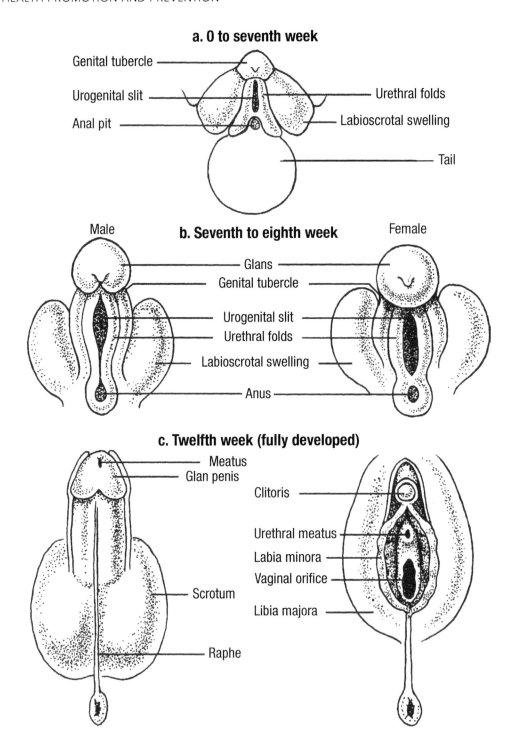

a. 0 to seventh week

Genital tubercle

Urogenital slit

Anal pit

Urethral folds

Labioscrotal swelling

Tail

Male

b. Seventh to eighth week

Female

Glans

Genital tubercle

Urogenital slit

Urethral folds

Labioscrotal swelling

Anus

c. Twelfth week (fully developed)

Meatus
Glan penis

Scrotum

Raphe

Clitoris

Urethral meatus

Labia minora

Vaginal orifice

Libia majora

FIGURE 7.14 Sexual differentiation of the external genitalia. As early as weeks 7 and 8 of fetal life, gender differentiation begins. Before week 6, the embryo appears undifferentiated. By week 12, the external genitalia assume the differentiated appearance.

PUBERTY

Puberty refers to the period of becoming capable of reproducing sexually and is indicated by the maturation of the genital organs, the development of secondary sex characteristics, and the first occurrence of menstruation in young women. Puberty and the menopausal transition share the characteristic of a transitional period during which a biological series of events culminating in a change in fertility occurs. During puberty, menarche occurs in girls; during the menopausal transition, the final menstrual period occurs in women.

A time interval of a decade or more separates birth and puberty. Puberty occurs during the later phases of human growth, long after the initial sexual differentiation. Both growth and differentiation continue during puberty, making it a distinctive part of the life span and requiring complex physiologic mechanisms to initiate its occurrence.

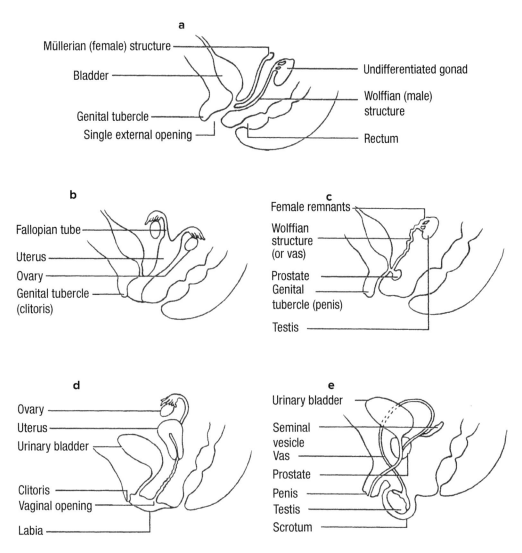

FIGURE 7.15 Sexual differentiation of the internal genitalia. (a) undifferentiated structures, (b) female structure at the third month, (c) male structure at the third month, (d) female mature form, and (e) male mature form.

Initiation of Puberty

The initiation of puberty remains poorly understood, although it is recognized that a highly complex neuroendocrine process is responsible for the onset of puberty and is influenced by both environmental signals and genetic factors (Biro & Chan, 2020). The genes *NKB* and the neuropeptide kisspeptin appear to play a critical role in a control system that modulates the release of GnRH at initiation of puberty (Herbison, 2016). It also appears that the HPO axis in girls develops in two definitive stages during puberty. First, early in puberty, gradually increasing gonadotropin secretion takes place because of a decrease in sensitivity of the hypothalamic centers to the negative inhibitory effects of low levels of circulating sex steroids. This can be viewed as a slowly rising set point of decreased sensitivity, resulting in increasing GnRH pulsatile secretions. This, in turn, leads to increasing gonadotropin production and ovarian stimulation. Second, later in puberty, there is a maturation of the positive feedback response from ovarian estrogen to the anterior pituitary, which stimulates the

midcycle surge of LH with subsequent ovulation (Breehl & Caban, 2022). This explains why the first few menstrual cycles are anovulatory (for as long as 18 months), although there are frequent exceptions (Taylor et al., 2019).

Current data suggest that the CNS inhibits the onset of puberty until the appropriate time. Thus, the neuroendocrine control of puberty is mediated by GnRH-secreting neurons in the hypothalamus that act as an internal pulse generator. At puberty, the GnRH pulse generator is reactivated or disinhibited, leading to increasing amplitude, frequency, and regularity of GnRH pulses, especially at night (Taylor et al., 2019; Welt, 2021). Consequently, the hormonal cascade of reproductive processes is triggered—hypothalamic GnRH pulsations stimulate the release of FSH and LH from the anterior pituitary, which then stimulates ovarian steroidal secretions. Just what causes the disinhibition of GnRH is still unknown. It is important to understand that puberty is not merely turned on like a light switch but rather a functional convergence of all factors. It is more of a concept than an actual focal point of action (Taylor et al., 2019).

Physiologic Development and Puberty

Shortly after birth, neonatal FSH and LH levels are still elevated because of negative feedback provided by the maternal ovarian hormones during pregnancy. The gonadotropins remain high for approximately 3 months with resulting transient elevations of estradiol; FSH and LH then gradually decrease to reach a nadir at 1 to 2 years of age in females. Then, gonadotropin levels begin to rise slightly between 4 and 10 years. Low levels of gonadotropins in the pituitary and circulation during childhood yield little response of the pituitary to GnRH and maximal hypothalamic suppression. LH pulses appear during infancy although they are quite irregular. Thus, it appears that immaturity of the endocrine systems is not the factor that tempers the onset of puberty. Indeed, all components of the HPO axis below the level of the hypothalamus can respond to GnRH from birth.

Prepubertal Phases

In girls, the first steroids to increase in the circulation from the adrenal cortex are androgens—DHEA, DHEAS, and androstenedione—which occurs from about 6 to 8 years of age, shortly before FSH begins to rise. Estrogen as well as LH levels do not begin to increase until 10 to 12 years of age.

During the prepubertal years, three phases are evident: adrenarche, decreasing the suppression of the gonadostat, and amplification of interactions leading to gonadarche. The physiologic event of adrenarche refers to the development of pubic and axillary hair. An increase in the size of the inner zone of the adrenal cortex precedes a classic linear growth spurt by about 2 years. In addition, adrenarche precedes elevation of estrogens and gonadotropins seen during early puberty and menarche in midpuberty. However, adrenarche is independent of puberty. The mechanisms governing adrenarche are not the same as those influencing GnRH–pituitary–ovarian axis maturation and gonadarche (Auchus, 2011). Adrenarche is not a signaled "abrupt" process but a result of a continuous process from birth, though the actual purpose of adrenarche remains unclear (Auchus, 2011). Early adrenarche, occurring before 8 years, is not associated with early gonadarche.

Decreasing repression of the gonadostat refers to the increased responsiveness of the anterior pituitary to GnRH and follicular activity to FSH and LH. Factors that are responsible for de-repressing the gonadostat, allowing the hypothalamus and pituitary to become less sensitive to the negative feedback of low levels of estrogens and permitting gonadotropin concentrations to rise, remain uncertain. Sustained elevation of GH levels may play a role as the factor responsible for de-repressing the gonadostat.

Endogenous GnRH is important in establishing and maintaining puberty. An increasing amplitude and frequency of pulsatile GnRH probably enhances the responses of FSH and LH secretion. GnRH appears to induce cell surface receptors specific for itself and necessary for its action on the surface of gonadotrope cells of the anterior pituitary. Sleep-related pulsations of LH are seen during early puberty. By midpuberty, estrogen enhances LH secretory responses to GnRH (creating positive feedback) and maintains its negative feedback of FSH responses.

Puberty

A cascade of endocrine events initiated by the release of pulsatile GnRH results in elevated gonadotropin levels and gonadal steroids, with subsequent appearance of secondary sexual characteristics and, later, menarche and ovulation. Between the ages of 10 and 16 years, the usual sequence includes the appearance of a pulsatile pattern of LH during sleep, followed by pulses of lesser amplitude throughout the day. Increasing levels of estradiol result in menarche, and by the latter part of puberty, the positive feedback relationship exists between estradiol and LH that is necessary to stimulate ovulation.

Progression of puberty through a sequence of increased rate of linear growth, breast development, pubarche (onset of pubic hair growth), and menarche occurs over a period of approximately 4.5 years. Usually, the first sign of puberty is acceleration of growth, which is followed by breast budding (thelarche; Eckert-Lind et al., 2020). The growth peak (about 2 to 4 inches within 1 year) usually occurs about 2 years after breast budding. Pubarche usually appears following the appearance of breast budding; axillary hair growth occurs approximately 2 years later. In some girls, pubic hair growth is the first sign of puberty. The growth peak in height occurs about 1 year before menarche. Menarche occurs late in this sequence with a median age of about 12.8 years, after the growth peak has occurred. GH and gonadal estrogen are important factors in the increased growth velocity. In addition, increasing estrogen levels produce breast development, female fat distribution, vaginal and uterine growth, and skeletal growth.

Menarche

Menarche is a function of genetic and environmental influences and occurs between 9.1 and 17.7 years of age, with a mean age of 12.8 years. Improvements in the standard of living and nutrition have produced children who mature earlier than in the past. In cultures that are affluent, menarcheal age has become lower. After menarche, growth slows, with approximately 2.5 inches in height gained after menarche. Age of menarche is correlated for mothers and daughters and between sisters.

Although there has been controversial discussion of a critical weight for menarche to occur (47.8 kg), it is likely that the shift in body composition from 16% to 23.5% fat is a more important factor. Adipose tissue secretes the peptide hormone leptin. The concentrations of leptin hormone are directly related to percentage of fat mass. This hormone acts on the CNS to regulate eating behaviors and thermoregulation, and recent research supports leptin's role in pubertal development (Chen et al., 2021). Leptin levels increase during childhood until the onset of puberty. Presumably, the increased concentration of leptin serves as an indicator to the CNS that the body's energy stores are adequate to support the pubertal developmental process. Earlier ages of menarche are associated with higher levels of leptin. What is also clear is that estrogen secretion, which produces endometrial proliferation, is essential for menarche to occur (Taylor et al., 2019).

Fertility

Development of positive feedback effects of estrogen on the pituitary and hypothalamus that stimulates the midcycle LH surge necessary for ovulation is a late event in puberty. For this reason, menstrual cycles are often anovulatory for about 12 to 18 months after menarche. The frequency of ovulation becomes more regular with each menstruation and as girls progress through pubertal changes.

Development During Puberty

The five Tanner (1981) stages are a commonly used indicator of the stage of pubertal development. On the basis of assessment of breast and pubic hair growth, it is possible to assess progression through puberty (see Figure 7.16).

In stage 1, a prepubertal stage, there is elevation of the papilla of the breast only. Although the feminine pelvic contour is evident, the breasts are flat. The labia majora are smooth, and the labia minora are poorly developed. The hymenal opening is small, the mucous membranes are dry and red, and the vaginal cells lack glycogen.

In stage 2, there is elevation of the nipple, with a small mound beneath the areola, which is enlarging and beginning to become pigmented. The labia majora become thickened, more prominent, and wrinkled. The labia minora are easily identified because of their increased size along with the enlarging clitoris. The urethral opening is more prominent,

mucous membranes are moist and pink, and some glycogen is present in vaginal cells. Pubic hair first appears on the mons and then on the labia about the time of menarche. The pubic hair is scanty, soft, and straight. There is increased activity of the sebaceous and merocrine sweat glands and the initial functions of the apocrine glands in the axilla and vulva.

In stage 3, the rapid growth peak has occurred; menarche occurs most frequently during this stage following the acceleration of the growth peak. The areolae and nipples enlarge, and pigmentation is more evident along with increased glandular size. The labia minora are well developed, and the vaginal cells have increased glycogen content. The mucous membranes are increasingly paler. The pubic hair is thicker, coarser, and often curlier at this time. There is increased activity of the sebaceous and sweat glands, with the beginning of acne in some girls along with adult body odor.

In stage 4, the areolae project above the plane of the breast, and the areolar glands are apparent. Glandular tissue is easily palpable. Both the labia majora and minora assume the adult structure, and the glycogen content of the vaginal cells begins its cyclic pattern. Pubic hair is more abundant, and axillary hair is present.

In stage 5, the breasts are more mature, with the nipples enlarged and protuberant and the areolar glands well developed. Pubic hair is more abundant and spreads to thighs in some women or may extend to the umbilicus. Facial hair may increase. Increased sebaceous gland activity of the skin and increased severity of acne may appear.

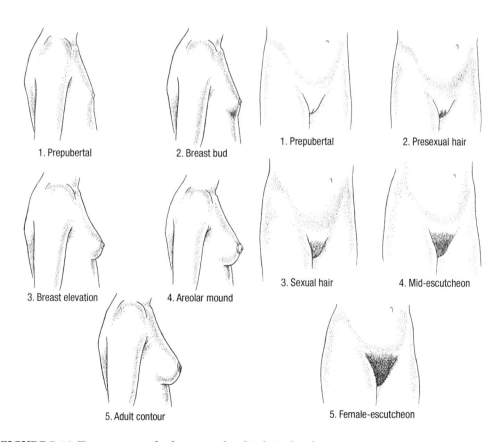

FIGURE 7.16 **Tanner stages for breast and pubic hair development.**

WOMEN'S UNIQUE CYCLES: THE MENSTRUAL CYCLE

Coordination of the Menstrual Cycle

The menstrual cycle requires a complex sequence of physiologic events coordinated by the hypothalamus in conjunction with the pituitary, ovary, and uterus, and that adapts to environmental phenomena. Major components of the system coordinating the menstrual cycle include the GnRH pulse generator, GnRH released by the hypothalamus, the gonadotropins (FSH and LH) secreted by the pituitary, and estrogen and progesterone produced by the ovary and corpus luteum, respectively. GnRH is released from the hypothalamus in a pulsatile fashion into the pituitary portal circulation. The pituitary gonadotropins respond to the stimulus from GnRH with pulses of LH and FSH released into the peripheral circulation. In response to GnRH and the gonadotropic hormones, the follicles produce estradiol, and the corpus luteum produces progesterone in response to elevated LH.

This coordinating system can be modulated by many inputs from higher neural centers and peripheral factors influencing the GnRH pulse generator as well as other hormones. Norepinephrine seems to amplify GnRH secretion, whereas dopamine dampens GnRH secretion. Increased endorphin release inhibits gonadotropin secretion through suppression of the release of GnRH (Taylor et al., 2019).

Ovarian Cycle: The Follicular Phase

The menstrual cycle consists of an ovarian and an endometrial component. The ovarian component is customarily divided into three phases to facilitate discussion: the follicular, ovulatory, and luteal (see Figure 7.17). The follicular phase consists of 10 to 14 days of hormonal influence that supports the growth of the primordial follicle through the preantral, antral, and preovulatory phases. The primordial follicle consists of the oocyte arrested in the diploid stage of development in which it still has 46 chromosomes. The initiation of follicular growth does not appear to be dependent on gonadotropins or estrogen. In fact, follicular growth may have begun during the days of the previous luteal

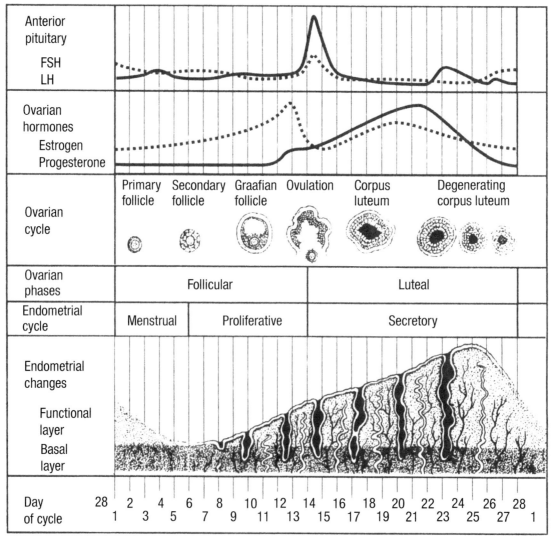

FIGURE 7.17 Coordination of the menstrual cycle.
FSH, follicle-stimulating hormone; LH, luteinizing hormone.

phase, when the regressing corpus luteum secretes decreasing amounts of steroids. Indeed, follicles grow continuously, even during pregnancy, ovulation, and anovulation.

During the first few days of the cycle, the follicle that will ovulate is selected and recruited. The mechanism for determining which follicles or how many will grow appears to be the result of two estrogenic actions: a local interaction between estrogen and FSH with the follicle and the effect of estrogen on pituitary secretion of FSH (Taylor et al., 2019).

Preantral Follicle

A rise in FSH stimulates a group of follicles to grow to the preantral phase (the phase before the antrum is identifiable). During this phase, the zona pellucida appears around the ovum and the thecal layer begins to organize. The granulosa cells synthesize steroids, producing more estradiol than progestins or androgens. The follicle also can convert androgens to estrogens. Activated by FSH, the preantral follicle can generate its own estrogenic microenvironment. FSH can increase the concentration of its own receptors on the granulosa cells, thus inducing the production of estradiol. Moreover, at low concentrations, androgen enhances its transformation to estradiol. At higher levels, androgens cause the follicle to produce a more androgenic environment, leading to atresia of the follicle. The follicle's development depends on its ability to convert androgen to estrogen.

Antral Follicle

Accumulation of follicular fluid in the antral follicle provides nurturance in an endocrine microenvironment. Influenced by FSH, estradiol becomes the dominant substance in the follicular fluid. During the follicular phase, estrogen production occurs by a two-cell, two-gonadotropin mechanism. LH stimulates the theca cells to liberate androgens that are converted to estrogen, and FSH stimulates the granulosa cells to produce estradiol. Sensitivity to FSH determines the capacity for conversion of an androgenic environment to an estrogenic one in the follicle.

Selection of the follicle that will ovulate (often called dominant follicle) occurs during cycle days 5 through 7 and requires estrogenic action. By day 7, peripheral estradiol levels begin to rise significantly. Estradiol produces negative feedback that decreases gonadotropin support to other follicles. To survive, the selected follicle must increase its own FSH production. Because the dominant follicle has FSH receptors in the granulosa cells, it can enhance FSH action. These actions effectively allow the selected follicle to increase its own estradiol levels and suppress FSH release to other follicles. The theca doubles in vascularity by day 9, producing a siphon for gonadotropins for the selected follicle.

Although the midfollicular increase in estradiol levels produces negative feedback to suppress FSH, it exerts a positive feedback on LH. When estradiol levels reach a concentration necessary for positive feedback (more than 200 pg/mL sustained for at least 50 hours), the LH surge occurs (Taylor et al., 2019).

Feedback systems involving the pituitary and hypothalamus also enable the selected follicle to control its own development. Estradiol exerts negative feedback effects on the hypothalamus and anterior pituitary. Progesterone exerts inhibitory feedback at the level of the hypothalamus and

positive feedback at the level of the pituitary. FSH is particularly sensitive to estradiol, whereas LH is sensitive to negative feedback of estradiol at low levels and to positive feedback by estradiol at higher levels. Progesterone slows LH pulses.

GnRH is secreted in the hypothalamus in a pulsatile fashion that changes in amplitude and duration across the menstrual cycle. During the early follicular phase, GnRH is secreted at approximately 94-minute intervals; in the late luteal phase, it is secreted at 216-minute intervals with a decreased amplitude. In turn, the pituitary releases gonadotropic hormones in a pulsatile fashion.

Preovulatory Follicles

Initiated by the LH surge, the oocyte resumes meiosis, approaching completion of reduction division. Estradiol concentrations rise to maintain the peripheral threshold necessary for ovulation to occur. LH initiates luteinization of the granulosa cells and the production of progesterone in the granulosa. The preovulatory increase in progesterone facilitates positive feedback of estradiol and may be necessary for induction of the midcycle FSH peak. The midcycle increase in local and peripheral androgens deriving from the theca of the nonselected follicles may account for the increased libido some women report at midcycle.

Ovulation

Ovulation occurs about 10 to 12 hours after the LH peak and 24 to 36 hours after the estradiol peak. The onset of the LH surge is estimated to occur approximately 34 to 46 hours before the follicle ruptures. LH stimulates the completion of the reduction division in the oocyte (to 23 chromosomes), luteinization of granulosa cells, and synthesis of progesterone and prostaglandins. The continuing rise in progesterone in the follicle up to the time of ovulation may act to end the LH surge. Progesterone also enhances proteolytic enzymes and prostaglandins needed for digestion and rupture of the follicle. Progesterone influences the midcycle rise in FSH, which in turn frees the oocyte from the follicular attachments, converts plasminogen to plasmin (a proteolytic enzyme involved in follicular rupture), and ensures sufficient LH receptors for a normal luteal phase.

Ovarian Cycle: Luteal Phase

The luteal phase is named after the process of luteinization, which occurs following rupture of the follicle and release of the ovum. The granulosa cells increase in size and take on a yellowish pigment, lutein, from which they were named the corpus luteum, or yellow body. Luteinization involves synthesis of androgens, estrogens, and progesterone. The process of luteinization requires the accumulation of LH receptors during the follicular phase of the cycle and continuing levels of LH secretion. Progesterone acts during this phase to suppress new follicular growth, rising sharply after ovulation with a peak at about 8 days after the LH surge. The length of the luteal phase tends to be more constant than that of the follicular phase and is consistently close to 14 days from LH midcycle surge to menses. Luteal phases ranging from 11 to 17 days are within normal limits. The corpus luteum begins a rapid cessation of activity at about 9 to 11 days after ovulation, and the mechanism triggering this remains unknown. Some speculate that estrogen production and alteration in prostaglandin concentrations within the ovary are responsible. When pregnancy occurs, the corpus luteum continues to function with the stimulus of hCG, which appears at the peak of corpus luteum function, 9 to 13 days after ovulation. hCG maintains corpus luteum function until approximately the 9th or 10th week of gestation.

The Endometrial Cycle

The first portion of the menstrual cycle is dominated by follicular development and follicular secretion and causes proliferation of the endometrium. The first portion of the menstrual cycle is named the *follicular phase* with respect to the ovary and the *proliferative phase* with respect to the endometrium. The second portion of the cycle is influenced by the corpus luteum, and the increasing levels of progesterone evoke secretory changes in the endometrium. The second portion of the menstrual cycle is named the *luteal phase* with respect to the ovary and the *secretory phase* with respect to the endometrium.

Immediately after menstruation, the endometrium is thin, only about 1 to 2 mm thick. Its surface endometrium is composed of low cuboidal cells, the stroma is dense and compact, and the glands appear straight and tubular.

Proliferative Phase

Under the influence of estrogen, the endometrium proliferates and thickens. The endometrium becomes somewhat taller, and the surface epithelium becomes columnar. The epithelial lining becomes continuous with the stromal component containing spiral vessels immediately below the epithelial-binding membrane that form a loose capillary network. Although the stroma is still quite compact, the endometrial glands have become more tortuous. Mitotic activity is evident in both the surface epithelium and the basal nuclei of the epithelial cells lining the endometrial glands. Estrogenic effects are also seen in the secretions of the cervical glands and in the vaginal lining. The variability in the length of this phase of the menstrual cycle is greater than that for the luteal phase. Indeed, the varying number of proliferative or follicular phase days accounts for the variation in the total cycle length.

Secretory Phase

As a result of the developing corpus luteum, progesterone evokes and increases the secretory changes in the endometrium. The surface epithelium is now tall and columnar; the stroma is less compact than earlier in the cycle and somewhat edematous and vascular. The endometrial glands become increasingly tortuous and convoluted. In addition, by 7 days after ovulation, the spiral vessels are densely coiled. The confinement of the growing endometrium to a fixed structure produces the tortuosity of the glands and spiral vessels.

Implantation usually occurs within 7 to 13 days after ovulation. At this point, the midportion of the endometrium appears lacelike, a stratum spongiosum. The stratum compactum overlies the inner layers of the endometrium and is a sturdy structure.

Premenstrually, the surface epithelium is quite tall, about 8 to 9 mm. The stroma consists of large polyhedral cells. The endometrial glands are very convoluted and serrated, resembling a corkscrew. The lining epithelium of endometrial glands is less well demarcated and smaller because of loss of glycogen into the gland lumen. A large number of lymphocytes and leukocytes are seen, probably as a result of the beginning necrosis of the endometrium.

Menstruation

In the absence of fertilization, implantation, and sustaining hCG, estradiol and progesterone levels wane as the corpus luteum ceases to function.

Endometrial growth regresses a few days before the onset of menstruation; at the same time, there is stasis of blood flow to the coiled arteries, with intermittent vasoconstriction. Between 4 and 24 hours before the onset of menstrual bleeding, intense vasoconstriction occurs. The menstrual blood flows from coiled arteries that have been constricted for several hours. Prostaglandins, synthesized in the endometrium as result of progesterone stimulation, are released and produce more intense vasoconstriction. Dissolving of the endometrium liberates acid hydrolases from the cell lysosomes. The acid hydrolases further disrupt the endometrial cell membranes, completing the process of menstruation. White blood cells migrate through capillary walls, and red blood cells escape into the interstitial space along with thrombin-platelet plugs that appear in the superficial vessels. Leakage and interstitial hemorrhage occur. With increased ischemia, the continuous-binding membrane becomes fragmented and intercellular blood is extruded into the endometrial cavity. The loose, vascular stroma of the spongiosum desquamates. Menstrual flow stops because of prolonged vasoconstriction, desquamation of the spongy layer of the endometrium, vascular stasis, and estrogen-induced rebuilding. The lower layer of the endometrium (basalis) is retained, and the stumps of the basal glands and stroma for the ensuing cycle continue to grow from them. The surface epithelium regenerates rapidly and may begin even while other areas are being desquamated.

With menstruation, as much as two thirds of the endometrium is lost. The menstrual flow may last from 2 to 8 days. Menstruation fluid consists of cervical and vaginal mucus as well as degenerated endometrial particles and blood. Sometimes clots may appear in the menstrual fluid. Usually, 2 to 3 ounces of fluid is lost with menses, but the amount of flow is highly variable. Women with more rapid loss experience a shorter duration of flow. Heavier flow and greater blood loss may indicate delayed or incomplete shedding of the endometrium.

Cyclic Changes in Other Organs

In addition to the uterus and ovary, other organs experience cyclic changes. The cervical canal contains about 100 crypts referred to as columnar glands; the secretory cells of these crypts secrete mucus into the endocervical canal. The mucus undergoes qualitative and quantitative changes during the menstrual cycle depending on the hormonal environment. Immediately after menstruation, the mucus is sparse, viscid, and sticky. When examined under a microscope, an abundance of vaginal and cervical cells and lymphocytes can be seen. From about the eighth day of the cycle until ovulation, the quantity and viscosity of the mucus increase. Sometimes an obvious plug of yellow, white, or cloudy mucus of a tacky consistency is present. At midcycle, the mucus is a thin hydrogel containing 2% solids and 98% water. The mucus resembles raw egg white, being clear, stretchy, and slippery. It will stretch without breaking or spin a thread (and is called *spinnbarkheit*). The ability of the mucus to stretch at least 5 to 6 cm has been established as a guideline for determining adequacy of the cervical mucus to support sperm transport. When the midcycle mucus is allowed to dry on a slide, it gives a fern or palm-leaf pattern. This pattern is absent after ovulation, during pregnancy, and after menopause. After ovulation, the mucus may again become cloudy, white, or yellow and tacky, and may disappear altogether. Women can use the changes in cervical mucus as an indirect index of ovulation.

The cervix itself changes with the menstrual cycle. During the proliferative phase, the os progressively widens, reaching its maximum width just before or at ovulation. At the point of maximal widening, mucus can be seen extruding from the external os. After ovulation, the os returns to a smaller diameter, with the profuse and watery mucus becoming scanty and viscid. These changes are believed to be estrogen induced and are not seen in prepubertal or postmenopausal women nor in those whose ovaries have been removed.

The motility of the uterine tubes is greatest during the estrogen-dominant portion of the menstrual cycle. They demonstrate a decreased motility during the progesterone-dominant phase.

Estrogen stimulation leads to cornification of the vagina. Following progesterone stimulation, the vaginal epithelium shows an increase in the number of precornified cells, mucus shreds, and aggregates of cells.

WOMEN'S CYCLES: HUMAN SEXUAL RESPONSE CYCLE

Masters and Johnson (1966) characterized physical phenomena that occur as humans respond to sexual stimulation as well as the psychosocial factors that influence how people responded. Their observations during sexual response in 382 women and 312 men ranging from 18 to 89 years of age and representing a wide range of educational levels and ethnic groups contributed significantly to understanding sexual physiology.

Two principal physiologic changes are responsible for events during the human sexual response cycle: vasocongestion and myotonia. Vasocongestion is congestion of blood vessels, usually venous vessels, and is the primary physiologic response to sexual stimulation. Myotonia, increased muscular tension, is a secondary physiologic response to sexual stimulation. These two changes are responsible for the phenomena observed during the sexual response cycle. Human sexual response is a total body response, not merely a pelvic phenomenon. Changes in cardiovascular and respiratory function as well as reactions involving skin, muscle, breasts, and the rectal sphincter occur during sexual response. The sexual response cycle originally included four phases: excitement, plateau, orgasm, and resolution (Masters & Johnson, 1966).

Research on sexual desire by Kaplan (1974) suggested that desire is another essential component of human sexual response. Desire initially supplies the catalyst or motivation for sexual receptivity. As with other aspects of sexuality, desire is influenced by health, physiology, past experiences, and cultural and environmental factors (MacLaren, 1995). Additional discussion of women's sexual response and desire is found in Chapter 19, Women's Sexual Health, and sexual problems are discussed in Chapter 26, Sexual Health Problems and Dysfunctions.

Excitement Phase

Excitement develops from any source of bodily or psychic stimuli, and, if adequate stimulation occurs, the intensity of excitement increases rapidly. This phase may be interrupted, prolonged, or ended by other competing stimuli. During the excitement phase, the clitoral glans becomes tumescent or enlarged, and the clitoral shaft increases in diameter and length. The appearance of vaginal lubrication, caused by vasocongestion and transudation of fluid across the vaginal membrane, occurs within 10 to 30 seconds after initiation of sexual stimulation. The vaginal barrel expands about 4 cm in transcervical width and lengthens 2.5 to 3.5 cm. In addition, the vaginal wall develops a purplish hue because of vasocongestion. Partial elevation of the uterus may occur if it lies in the anterior position.

In nulliparous women, flattening and separating of the labia majora occur. In multiparous women, the labia majora move slightly away from the introitus because of a vasocongestive increase in their diameter. The vaginal barrel is lengthened approximately 1 cm as a result of the thickening of the labia minora.

During the excitement phase, changes also occur in women's extragenital organs. Nipples may protrude, breast size increases, the areolae become engorged, and the venous pattern on the breast becomes more obvious. The sex flush, a maculopapular rash, may appear over the epigastric area, spreading quickly over the breasts. Some involuntary muscle tensing may be evident, as in the tensing of intercostal and abdominal muscles. The heart rate and blood pressure also increase as sexual tension increases (see Figure 7.18A).

Plateau Phase

When stimulation is maintained, sexual tension becomes intensified to the level at which a person may experience orgasm. Like excitement, this phase also may be affected by competing stimuli. During the plateau phase, the clitoris retracts against the anterior body of the symphysis pubis, underneath the clitoral hood. Vasocongestion of the tissues of the outer third of the vagina and the labia minora causes an increase in size of this highly sensitive tissue, referred to as the orgasmic platform. Further increase in the depth and width of the vaginal barrel occurs. The uterus becomes fully elevated, and as the cervix rises, it produces a tenting effect in the inner part of the vagina. Irritability of the corpus uteri continues to intensify.

In both nulliparous and multiparous women, the labia majora continue to become engorged, with the phenomenon being more pronounced in nulliparous women. The labia minora undergo a vivid color change from bright red to a deep wine-colored hue, considered a sign of impending orgasm. During the plateau phase, a drop or two of mucoid material is secreted from Bartholin's glands; this secretion probably assists slightly in vaginal lubrication.

Several extragenital responses occur in women during the plateau phase. Nipple stiffness continues to develop along with an increase in breast size and marked engorgement of the areolae. The sex flush, which began during excitement, may spread over the body. Facial, abdominal, and intercostal muscles contract; muscle tension is increased both voluntarily and involuntarily. Some women use voluntary rectal contractions to enhance stimulation during this phase. Hyperventilation occurs along with a heart rate of 120 to 175 beats per minute, elevation of the systolic blood pressure of 20 to 60 mmHg, and diastolic elevation of 10 to 20 mmHg (see Figure 7.18B).

Orgasmic Phase

Orgasm, the involuntary climax of sexual tension increment, involves only a few seconds of the cycle during which vasocongestion and muscle tension are released. During the orgasmic phase, the primary response occurs in women's orgasmic platform, as illustrated in Figure 7.18C. Approximately five to 12 contractions occur in the orgasmic platform at 0.8-second intervals. After the first three to six contractions, the interval between contractions increases and the intensity diminishes. The pelvic floor muscles that surround the lower third of the vagina contract against the engorged vessels, thus forcing out the blood trapped in them. Contractions of the uterus begin at the fundus and progress to the lower segment of the uterus. The contractile excursion of the uterus parallels women's ratings of the intensity of the orgasmic experience.

Extragenital responses involve several organ systems during orgasm. The sex flush parallels the intensity of orgasmic experience and is present in about 75% of women. Involuntary contraction and spasm of muscle groups may be experienced, including contractions of the rectal sphincter, which occur at the same intervals as those of the orgasmic platform. Respiratory rates as high as 40 breaths per minute have been recorded, along with pulse rates from 110 to 180 beats per minute. Fluctuations in the pulse and respiratory rate tend to parallel the level of sexual tension. The systolic blood pressure may be elevated 30 to 80 mmHg and the diastolic pressure 20 to 40 mmHg.

Resolution Phase

During the resolution phase, involutional changes restore the preexcitement state. With adequate stimulation, women may begin another sexual response cycle immediately before sexual excitement totally resolves. Usually, the length of the resolution period parallels the length of the excitement phase. During the resolution phase, the clitoris returns to its usual position within 5 to 10 seconds after the contractions of the orgasmic platform cease. Vasocongestion or tumescence of the clitoris dissipates more slowly. There is rapid detumescence (loss of vasocongestion) of the orgasmic platform and relaxation of the walls of the vagina. The vaginal wall returns to its normal coloring in about 10 to 15 minutes. Gaping of the cervical os continues for 20 to 30 minutes. The uterus returns to its unstimulated position in the true pelvis, and the cervix descends into the dorsal area of the vagina. The nulliparous labia majora return to their preexcitement position, while in multiparas the labial vasocongestion dissipates more slowly. The labia minora changes from deep red to light pink, and they decrease in size as vasocongestion recedes.

Involution of nipple stiffness, a slow decrease in breast size, and rapid reversal of the sex flush are seen. Some myotonia may still be seen during resolution. The respiratory rate, pulse rate, and blood pressure return to usual levels. An involuntary widespread film of perspiration may appear (Figure 7.18D).

Although these physiologic changes are common in women's sexual response, not every woman experiences each response. Indeed, the same woman may experience different aspects from cycle to cycle. Regardless of the difference in stimuli, some women will experience the same sexual responses whether the stimulus is self-pleasuring, pleasuring from another person, or intercourse (Sherfey, 1972). Women also tend to be more whole-body oriented (vs. genitally oriented) and thus more receptive to sexual touching and experiencing pleasurable, exciting sensations from their skin. Women tend to report a high degree of sensitivity from either mouth or finger contact (Masters & Johnson, 1966).

MENOPAUSE

Between 38 and 42 years of age, ovulation becomes less frequent. Residual follicles decrease in number from about 300,000 at puberty to a few thousand, are less sensitive to gonadotropin stimulation than they were earlier in life, are less likely to mature, and produce less estradiol. Menopause occurs when estradiol is insufficient to stimulate endometrial growth so that a woman no longer menstruates (Crandall, 2019; Taylor et al., 2019).

Menopause is said to have occurred when a woman has not menstruated for a period of 1 full year. Before menopause, women notice changes in their menstrual cycles, most likely because of a shortening of the follicular phase as a result of lower estradiol secretion. As a woman's cycles become more irregular, vaginal bleeding may occur at the end of a short luteal phase or after an estradiol peak without ovulation or corpus luteum formation.

Elevated FSH levels reflect an attempt to stimulate a follicle to produce estradiol. FSH levels of more than 30 to 40 IU/L are used as an indicator that menopause is approaching, although women may still be bleeding. Elevated FSH levels probably reflect the decreased regulation by the negative feedback of inhibin produced by the granulosa cells. Recent studies have revealed that FSH is an unreliable predictor of the final menstrual period: Thus, a single FSH level is not

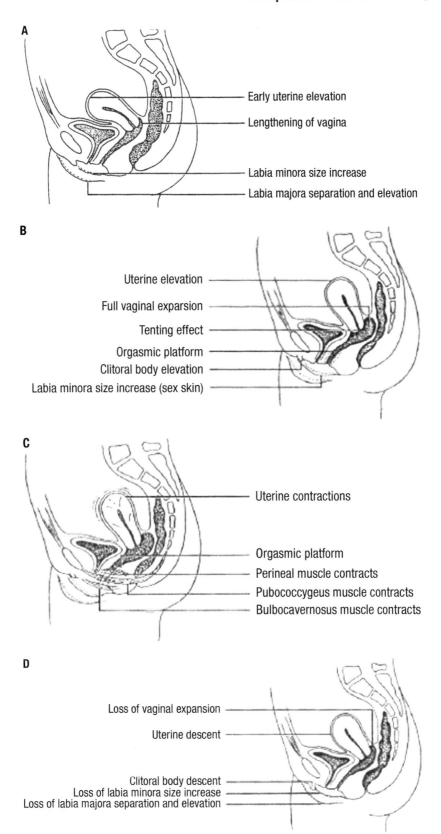

FIGURE 7.18 (A) Excitement phase of sexual response; (B) plateau phase; (C) orgasmic phase; and (D) resolution phase.

a useful clinical tool for predicting menopause (Crandall, 2019). Although FSH rises to 10 to 20 times its premenopausal level and LH rises to three times its premenopausal level within 1 to 3 years after menopause, there is a subsequent decrease in both gonadotropins to a new steady state. In postmenopausal women, the ovary continues to secrete testosterone from the stromal tissue. Indeed, recent studies indicate that dramatic changes in androgen metabolism follow menopause, providing for continued production of estrogen in the form of estrone.

Testosterone and androstenedione both rise in parallel to DHEAS. During the same period, DHEA and androstenediol both increase markedly (up to seven to eight times) during the perimenopause. Given the androgenic and estrogenic biological activity of androstenediol, it makes an important contribution to androgen–estrogen balance during the postmenopause. Conversion of androstenediol is the source of most endogenous estrogen after menopasue (Crandall, 2019). These new findings underscore the transition women experience from an ovarian-driven to an adrenal-driven estrogen metabolism during the postmenopause.

Circulating estradiol levels after menopause range from approximately 10 to 20 pg/mL. Most of this is derived from the conversion of estrone to estradiol in adipose tissue. Circulating levels of estrone are higher than those of estradiol with the mean levels of approximately 30 to 70 pg/mL. Also, an increase in substrate for estrogen production, as occurs in stressful situations that increase adrenal output, may induce a menstrual flow in a woman who is postmenopausal.

Occasionally, ovulation occurs after months of amenorrhea and may result in an unplanned pregnancy during the menopausal transition. Elevation of both FSH and LH is thought to indicate that pregnancy cannot occur. Nonetheless, to prevent unwanted conception, women who are experiencing the menopausal transition need to be aware of their fertility status and use reliable contraceptive methods. Progression through the stages of reproductive aging from the late reproductive stages to the menopausal transition and postmenopause is discussed further in Chapter 9, Midlife Women's Health.

BEYOND REPRODUCTION: SEX-BASED BIOLOGICAL DIFFERENCES

It is evident through recent scientific exploration that there are broader influences beyond the genetic assignment of two X chromosomes on a woman's health. The interplay between genes, prenatal hormone exposure, natural hormone exposure throughout adulthood, female physiologic and biochemical responses, as well as behavioral and socioenvironmental factors and effects of epigenetic changes all contribute to the way a woman's body responds to disease and illness as well as modifiers of health, disease, and healthcare (Institute of Medicine Committee on Understanding the Biology of Sex and Gender Differences et al., 2001; Institute of Medicine Committee on Women's Health Research 2010; Mauvais-Jarvis et al., 2020).

In 1999, the Institute of Medicine organized a large, interdisciplinary committee to evaluate and consider the current scientific evidence related to the determinants of sex differences at a biological level (Institute of Medicine Committee on Understanding the Biology of Sex and Gender Differences et al., 2001). Over the intervening years, there have been many discoveries of sex differences that involve the entire body. Indeed, a recent review of sex differences in the brain revealed that the entire body is sexually differentiated and that sex differences in the nervous system cannot be separated from differences in the remainder of the body (de Vries & Forger, 2015).

Sex Chromosome

A special protective mechanism called X-chromosome inactivation allows females to possess a unique, mixed population of inherited X chromosomes—some from the mother and some from the father. Early in the embryonic development, most female cells randomly inactivate one set of X chromosomes (within their normal XX chromosome genotypic assignment). This ability allows inactivation of potential X chromosome gene mutations that would cause disease or death. This ability is not seen in males (XY), who only have one X chromosome assigned and thus only one copy of the X chromosome gene that is thus vulnerable to any deleterious X chromosome gene mutation inherited from only one parent. Thus, if a male inherits a mutated X chromosome that is incompatible with life, death occurs. If a female inherits a mutated X chromosome, and random X chromosome inactivation occurs to this mutated chromosome, the other X chromosome is able to replace it and sustain life.

Sex Differences in the Brain and Contexts of the Body and Environments

There is extensive evidence that male and female brains differ. De Vries and Forger (2015) point out that the number of motor neurons controlling striated perineal muscles mirrors the size of the perineal muscles in male and female bodies. In addition, some sex differences seem designed to compensate for physiologic differences that may be maladaptive, and these may be evident in the face of perturbation of the system. An example of compensation relates to the inactivation of the one X chromosome in every cell in a female body, noted earlier.

De Vries and Forger also note that sex differences in peripheral systems provide different contexts in which female and male brains operate. The liver and kidneys modulate the environments in which sex hormones function: The liver metabolizes hormones and the kidneys excrete them in ways that modulate their effects in the entire body. De Vries and Forger further explore the causes of sex differences in the brain, providing evidence that hormones may influence differentiation of tissues by acting on steroid receptors in peripheral tissues or the brain and hormone actions affecting peripheral structures may influence the nervous system. In addition, they propose a whole-body perspective of sexual differentiation of the brain that involves the pelvic viscera, adipose tissue, liver, peripheral immune system, gut, kidney, and sensory systems. They support the idea of a sexome, defined by Arnold and Lusis (2012) as the sum of all sex-specific and sex-biased modulatory interactions operating within the intricate network of interactions

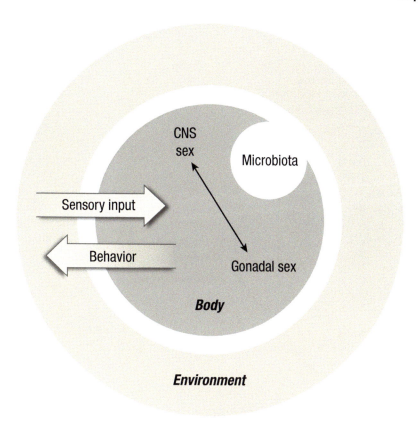

FIGURE 7.19 Sexorganome as suggested by de Vries and Forger (2015). CNS sex and gonadal sex interrelate with muscle, liver, fat, pelvic viscera, kidney, immune cells, and placenta, modulating sensory input and behavioral outputs.
CNS, central nervous system.

among all the different molecules constituting a cell, as foundational to a systems ecological approach to understanding biology of sex differences in interaction with environments. De Vries and Forger build a case for the interaction of the whole body (including organ systems) with its external environments, behavior, and the microbiome, in which the influence of sexual differentiation modulates and is modulated in the "sexorganome" (Figure 7.19).

As more women participate in ongoing research to determine sex-based differences in morbidity and mortality, it will be important to take into account *all* the factors—biological, social, ethnic/cultural, and personal—that contribute to these health differences. Gender differences in social opportunities shape women's choices and expectations regarding role-related activities. This, in turn, can affect women's exposures to various risks (including stress, role overload, and occupational health problems such as carpal tunnel syndrome and exposure to toxic chemicals) and access to appropriate health resources (health insurance, income, and social support; Bird & Rieker, 1999).

Sexualities

Sexuality is a complex personal experience, which is influenced by an individual's sexual and gender identity and expression of each. Asking a woman to define their identity may be difficult, especially for sexual minorities who may defy previously defined categories such as gay, straight, or bisexual (Salomaa & Matsick, 2019). Sexuality may transcend somatic sex when gender identity is considered. For

instance, if Alex was born with male sex organs but identifies as female in gender and she is sexually attracted to males, Alex may identify as a straight transgender woman when questioned about her sexuality for her health history. This can lead to confusion if the provider does not take the time to understand Alex's gender identity, sexual identity, and sexual expression regardless of her history of gender-confirming surgery or hormonal therapies. This is one example of why defining and understanding sexuality is so important in women's healthcare. Mitchell et al. (2021) helped to highlight the importance of sexuality in adults through the creation of a construct that intends to better inform public health. In the Pillars of Sexuality framework, sexuality is approached within four pillars: sexual health, sexual justice, sexual pleasure, and sexual well-being (Figure 7.20). Sexual identity and attraction are discussed more fully in Chapter 20, Primary Care of Lesbian, Gay, and Bisexual Individuals.

CONSIDERATIONS FOR SPECIAL AND MINORITIZED POPULATIONS

Women's and minoritized gender person's bodies are complex and diverse with a variety of procreative and recreative functions. Cultural perspectives and societal beliefs influence women's and other minoritized gender person's relationships with their bodies, as well as their relationship with their health providers. A woman or minoritized gender person may choose to delay care if they believe that their provider

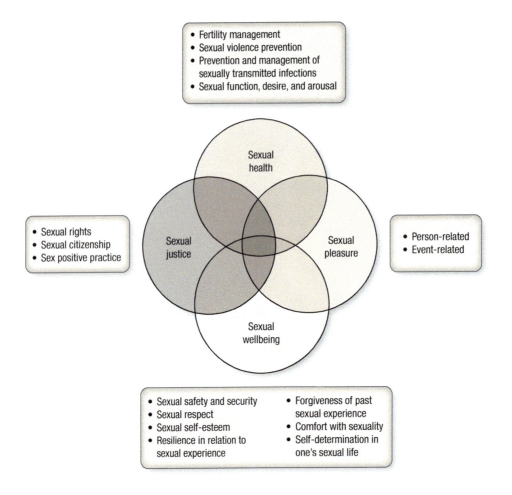

FIGURE 7.20 Four pillars of sexuality.
Source: Adapted from Mitchell, K. R., Lewis, R., O'Sullivan, L. F., & Fortenberry, J. D. (2021). What is sexual well-being and why does it matter for public health? Lancet Public Health, 6(8), e608–e613. *https://doi.org/10.1016/S2468-2667(21)00099-2*

is not accepting of their beliefs or lacks a basic understanding of their care needs in the context of their culture, life, gender, sexuality, or other aspects. Many populations have historically been underrepresented regarding women's and sexual health such as women, minoritized gender persons, and women with disabilities.

Cultural Considerations in Care

The APRN should exercise cultural awareness and respect in all care interactions. Especially in the context of women's reproductive health, these conversations can be particularly intimate with social, cultural, sexual, and gender norms playing a large role in reproductive decisions such as the use of contraceptives, timing of childbearing, or abortion (Rich et al., 2021). For example, Asian Indian immigrant women may face societal pressures from family and the community regarding their decision to have a child. Haredi Jewish women may incorporate faith into family planning decisions by consulting with their rabbi or religious leaders in decisions regarding pregnancy, reproductive technologies, and prenatal testing (Rich et al., 2021). Understanding cultural variations as well as personal preferences in care can help providers

build rapport with their patients and assist in developing a plan of care aligned with the patient's beliefs and priorities, especially in the unfolding and often changing post-*Roe* era.

As previously discussed, women's perceptions of their bodies are influenced by cultural meanings of what is ideal in terms of form (size and shape) and function (procreative and recreative). The Western ideals of body image encourage women to maintain slim and slender physiques, which is linked to attributes such as fitness and self-control (Bakhshi, 2011). For women who identify with another cultural group, these ideals may not be congruent. Larger body sizes were associated with attributes such as health, fertility, affluence, and longevity in various non-Western cultures such as in Indian, Chinese, and Arabic cultures (Bakhshi, 2011). Black and Hispanic women reported variable ideals in body shapes and sizes (Olson et al., 2020).

The understanding of these ideals is essential when discussing healthcare needs assessing for at-risk behaviors with women and minoritized gender persons of various cultures. The perception of their own bodies as seen through their cultural lens influences their health concerns. For instance, it has been documented in a previous study that young African Caribbean and Asian women showed more body satisfaction and fewer weight concerns, whereas White women engaged in unhealthy weight management practices to alter their body image (Bakhshi, 2011). Another study found that low-income Black women were less likely to diet and purge compared to White and Latina women of similar socioeconomic standing (Breitkopf & Berenson, 2004).

The need for care within the context of culture and personal beliefs and choice cannot be overemphasized. While it is necessary to understand cultural variations and beliefs, the practitioner must also understand the limitations of such an approach. APRNs must remain cognizant of the fact that one cannot ever be fully "competent" in another's culture and should not misinterpret cultural beliefs for individual preferences. By practicing self-reflection, maintaining open communication, and respectfully asking for clarification when appropriate, we can learn to provide more effective and more patient-centered care.

Minoritized Sexual and Gender Populations

Sexual minoritized women (SMW) include women who identify as lesbian, bisexual, transgender, queer, or other. Transgender women are individuals who identify as female but were assigned a male sex at birth. Transgender men are individuals who identify as male but were assigned a female sex at birth. Nonbinary persons are those who may have been assigned male or female sex at birth but do not identify with a specific gender. The term minoritized sexual and gender (MSG) persons is the umbrella term that encompasses these groups. The research base regarding MSG women is limited; however, the evidence currently points to worse case outcomes when compared to their heterosexual counterparts (Pharr et al., 2019). Factors that negatively influence health outcomes include social exclusion, social stigma, and institutional heterosexism at the structural level, and microaggressions, discrimination, victimization, and abuse at the individual level (Pharr et al., 2019).

Gender dysphoria or gender incongruence refers to the distress and suffering caused by discordance between one's gender and assigned sex at birth. Previous studies have emphasized that these views can lead to maladaptive behaviors in transgender individuals such as self-harm and disordered eating behaviors as a method to alter their bodies (Mirabella et al., 2020). In a qualitative study of 36 young transgender adults, researchers found that discomfort was an experience mentioned in every interview, with all participants describing feelings of shame and even repulsion about their body and physical appearance. The onset of puberty and bodily changes increased these feelings and led to the development of behaviors such as self-harm, disordered eating, and suicide attempts in an effort to gain a degree of relief from these feelings (Mirabella et al., 2020).

Healthcare providers can mitigate some of these challenges by increasing their own knowledge of MSG experiences and validating MSG women's concerns. Unfortunately, MSG populations do report a high degree of discrimination in healthcare settings. About half of transgender individuals reported that care providers were not knowledgeable about transgender care; about one in four individuals reported verbal harassment in a medical setting, and 19% reported being refused care altogether based on gender identity and expression (Hoy-Ellis et al., 2022). These biases translate into decreased or loss of access to care and/or subpar care. For example, studies have demonstrated that transgender individuals receive preventive services at lower rates than cisgendered individuals (Hoy-Ellis et al., 2022). Lesbian and bisexual women were less likely to have a Pap smear compared to heterosexual women. Bisexual women aged 40 and older were less likely to have a mammogram when compared to straight and lesbian women (Pharr et al., 2019). Rates of unintended pregnancy are higher among SMW than among their heterosexual peers (Stoffel et al., 2017).

By understanding the unique needs of MSG populations, healthcare providers can reverse biases and close the gap in care for these underserved individuals. Further discussion regarding care of lesbian, gay, bisexual, and transgender individuals can be found in both Chapter 20, Primary Care of Lesbian, Gay, and Bisexual Individuals, and Chapter 25, Caring for the Transgender and Gender Binary Patient.

Women With Disabilities

People with disabilities have historically struggled with personal and environmental barriers to their health and sexual lives. Although there has been a global move toward embodiment and sexual awareness, women with disabilities continue to be a group continually affected by lack of access to sexual health resources, women's healthcare, and sexual experiences (Matin et al., 2021). Studies have documented that healthcare professionals may have preconceived assumptions about women with disabilities—about their ability to tolerate screenings, both physically and emotionally, and their level of sexual activity (Conder et al., 2019).

In a systematic review of qualitative articles on sexuality in women with intellectual disabilities (IDs), common themes were lack of education, lack of knowledge, lack of autonomy, and vulnerability to sexual coercion and abuse (Matin et al., 2021). Women with ID reported being excluded from the classroom during school-based sexual education, and stigma associated with wanting to learn more about sex, which resulted in subsequent knowledge deficits about physical intimacy. The combination of limited knowledge and lack of skills needed for healthy sexual interactions make women with ID vulnerable targets of unwanted sexual contact and abuse (Matin et al., 2021).

Additionally, women with disabilities have lower rates of preventive services and screenings. Data from the 2002 to 2008 annual Medical Expenditure Panel Surveys (MEPS) conducted by the Agency for Healthcare Research and Quality (AHRQ) demonstrated that women with disabilities were less likely than women without disabilities to meet U.S. Preventive Services Task Force recommendations for breast and cervical cancer screenings, and the disparity was greater for women with complex limitations (Horner-Johnson et al., 2014).

Healthcare clinicians are in a unique position to support women with disabilities to reclaim their sexual and reproductive rights. The option to discuss sensitive topics should be available to all women; not acknowledging women with disabilities' sexual and women's health needs undermines their autonomy. Health information should be available in plain language to those with ID, and barriers such as knowledge deficits on proper positioning for pelvic exams or screenings in those with physical disabilities should be addressed through training and education.

FUTURE DIRECTIONS

From this discussion, it is evident that certain structures and functions are unique to a woman's body. These are involved in the menstrual cycle and women's sexual response cycles. Several of the structures of a woman's body serve both her reproductive powers as well as her recreative pleasures—with the exception of the clitoris, an organ whose sole raison d'être is to receive and transduce sexual pleasure. Women's bodies develop uniquely from the time of conception and early differentiation through pubertal and menopausal transitions and are affected by multiple stimuli, such as personal perspective, culture/ethnicity, family influences, and more. APRNs must attend to the complex needs of women and minoritized gender persons to assure these patients receive care that aligns with the patients' cultural, sexual, and personal preferences. Navigating these preferences and providing access to care are likely to become more complex in the post-*Roe* era.

WEB/SMART PHONE/CLINICAL GUIDELINES/BOOK RESOURCES FOR PROFESSIONALS

U.S. Preventive Service Task Force (https://www.uspreventiveservicestaskforce.org/uspstf)

Planned Parenthood Organization, Female Sexual Anatomy (https://www.plannedparenthood.org/learn/health-and-wellness/sexual-and-reproductive-anatomy/what-are-parts-female-sexual-anatomy)

Medical News Today, Guide to Female Anatomy (https://www.medicalnewstoday.com/articles/326898)

Western Australia Department of Health, Get the Facts, Female Anatomy (https://www.getthefacts.health.wa.gov.au/our-bodies/female-anatomy)

REFERENCES

References for this chapter are online and available at https://connect.springerpub.com/content/book/978-0-8261-6722-4/part/part02/chapter/ch07

CHAPTER 8

Young Women's Health

CATHERINE TAKACS WITKOP,* DANIELLE WRIGHT,* KRISTI NORCROSS, AND KIM SHAUGHNESSY-GRANGER[†]

Adolescence is a time of significant physical, emotional, social, and cognitive development, and behaviors and habits developed during this time can have a lasting impact in adulthood. The state of a young woman's health and the decisions she makes during the second and into the third decade of her life can jeopardize her short-term health and long-term well-being. On a more positive note, it is precisely during such a formative time that healthcare providers can influence and support development of health-seeking behaviors and the foundation of a healthy lifestyle. Providing impactful preventive guidance and services in a safe and supportive environment can bolster healthy behaviors and establish the young woman on a trajectory toward health.

This chapter contains an overview of young women's health, beginning with considerations of the demographic characteristics of adolescents in the U.S. population. For the purposes of this chapter, adolescents include those between 10 and 19 years of age. However, where appropriate, issues and services pertaining to young women up to age 25 years are addressed. Adolescent development occurs in stages and can be affected by numerous factors such as disabilities, race/ethnicity, and the home environment. Furthermore, several external influences, including family, peers, school, community, and the internet can have an impact on health and development. Health services that adolescents need are driven by challenges in their development and the context in which they live, and healthcare providers can contribute to the accessibility and quality of care. Finally, the chapter concludes with an outline of the female adolescent visit and consideration of specific conditions and challenges.

AN OVERVIEW OF ADOLESCENCE IN THE UNITED STATES

Demographic Characteristics

Adolescents are a large and diverse part of U.S. society. Children and teens ages 10 to 19 make up approximately 13% of the U.S. population, while adolescent females account for approximately 6% of the total population (U.S. Census Bureau, 2020). Geographically, adolescents are concentrated in urban and suburban communities, but their percentage of the overall population of the community is greatest in rural areas. The increasing diversity in the population will be most visible among children, with the percentage of those children who are two or more races anticipated to double from 5.8% in 2020 to 11.3% in 2060, Hispanic children to increase from 25.5% to 31.9%, and children who belong to all ethnic/racial minority groups increasing from 52.4% to 69% of the total youth population (Vespa et al., 2020).

There are several sources for reliable and comprehensive youth data that are referenced throughout this chapter. Each year, the Annie E. Casey Foundation publishes the *Kids Count Data Book*, intended to highlight key indicators of youth health and assess trends at the state and national level. Sixteen key indicators are measured, and four of these specifically target adolescent health: teen birth rate, high school students not graduating on time, eighth graders not proficient in math, and the percentage of teens not attending school and not working (Annie E. Casey Foundation, 2021). The trend for this decade on all four key indicators focused on adolescent

---

*The opinions and assertions expressed herein are those of the author(s) and do not necessarily reflect the official policy or position of the Uniformed Services University or the Department of Defense.
†The views expressed are those of the author and do not reflect the official policy or position of the Department of the Navy, Department of Defense, or the U.S. government.

well-being has been positive. In particular, the teen birth rate has gone from 34 per 1,000 in 2010 to 17 per 1,000 in 2019; however, after a steady decline since 2010, the teen birth rate remained the same from 2018 to 2019 (Annie E. Casey Foundation, 2021). The report also highlights ethnic/racial and regional differences in the data. For example, the teen birth rate for Hispanic or Latina girls is the highest among the major racial/ethnic groups, and regionally, the teen birth rate ranged from 7 per 1,000 adolescents (ages 15 to 19 years) in both Massachusetts and New Hampshire compared with 30 per 1,000 in Arkansas (Annie E. Casey Foundation, 2021). While the *Data Book* report itself is focused on the 16 key indicators, the Kids Count Data Center website (datacenter. kidscount.org) includes data sets that can be manipulated for any number of topics, indicators, demographics, and geography including state, territory, and city. This resource is worthwhile for understanding the needs of a provider's adolescent subpopulation.

Another rich source of adolescent health data is collected to support *Healthy People 2030* (Office of Disease Prevention and Health Promotion [ODPHP], 2022). This program, launched in 1979 by Surgeon General Julius Richmond with the landmark report "Healthy People: the Surgeon General's Report on Health Promotion and Disease Prevention," included quantifiable objectives to achieve health promotion and disease prevention goals for the United States within 10 years (by 1990). *Healthy People 2030* is the fifth iteration of this effort under the Department of Health and Human Services (following *Healthy People 2000, Healthy People 2010,* and *Healthy People 2020)*, and has the updated overarching goals of (a) attaining healthy, thriving lives and well-being, free of preventable disease, disability, injury, and premature death; (b) eliminating health disparities, achieving health equity, and attaining health literacy to improve the health and well-being of all; (c) creating social, physical, and economic environments that promote attaining full potential for health and well-being for all; (d) promoting healthy development, healthy behaviors, and well-being across all life stages; and (e) engaging leadership, key constituents, and the public across multiple sectors to take action and design polices that improve the health and well-being of all (ODPHP, 2022). *Healthy People 2030* has reduced the number of objectives from over 1,200 to 358 core objectives, in order to reduce overlap, and to prioritize the most pressing public health issues. In addition to the 355 core objectives, which all have reliable baseline data from no earlier than 2015, there are a set of 115 developmental objectives and a set of 40 research objectives. The developmental objectives represent high-priority public health issues that do not currently have reliable baseline data but are associated with evidence-based interventions; the research objectives represent issues that may have a high health or economic burden, or have significant disparities between groups, but do not currently have associated evidence-based interventions (ODPHP, 2022). These objectives are organized into five major categories: health conditions, health behaviors, populations, systems and settings, and social determinants of health. There are 10 core and 14 developmental and research objectives specific to adolescent health (see Box 8.1), and an additional 66 objectives that directly or indirectly pertain to

Box 8.1 Objectives Directly Related to Adolescent Health From *Healthy People 2030*

AH-01 Increase the proportion of adolescents who had a preventive healthcare visit in the past year

AH-02 Increase the proportion of adolescents who speak privately with a provider at a preventive medical visit

AH-03 Increase the proportion of adolescents who have an adult they can talk to about serious problems

AH-04 Increase the proportion of students participating in the School Breakfast Program

AH-05 Increase the proportion of fourth graders with reading skills at or above the proficient level

AH-06 Increase the proportion of fourth graders with math skills at or above the proficient level

AH-07 Reduce chronic school absence among early adolescents

AH-08 Increase the proportion of high school students who graduate in 4 years

AH-09 Reduce the proportion of adolescents and young adults who aren't in school or working

AH-10 Reduce the rate of minors and young adults committing violent crimes

AH-D01 Increase the proportion of trauma-informed early child care settings and elementary and secondary schools

AH-D02 Increase the proportion of children and adolescents with symptoms of trauma who get treatment

AH-D03 Reduce the proportion of public schools with a serious violent incident

AH-R01 Increase the proportion of adolescents who get support for their transition to adult healthcare

AH-R02 Increase the proportion of adolescents in foster care who show signs of being ready for adulthood

AH-R03 Increase the proportion of eligible students participating in the Summer Food Service Program

AH-R04 Increase the proportion of eighth graders with reading skills at or above the proficient level

AH-R05 Increase the proportion of eighth graders with math skills at or above the proficient level

AH-R06 Increase the proportion of schools requiring students to take at least two health education courses from grades 6 to 12

AH-R07 Increase the proportion of secondary schools with a start time of 8:30 a.m. or later

AH-R08 Increase the proportion of secondary schools with a full-time RN

(continued)

Box 8.1 Objectives Directly Related to Adolescent Health From *Healthy People 2030* **(***continued***)**

AH-R09 Increase the proportion of public schools with a counselor, social worker, and psychologist

AH-R10 Increase the proportion of students served under the Individuals With Disabilities Education Act who earn a high school diploma

AH-R11 Reduce the rate of adolescent and young adult victimization from violent crimes

Other Relevant Objectives

FP-03 Reduce pregnancies in adolescents

FP-04 Increase the proportion of adolescents who have never had sex

FP-05 Increase the proportion of adolescent females who used effective birth control the last time they had sex

FP-06 Increase the proportion of adolescent males who used a condom the last time they had sex

FP-07 Increase the proportion of adolescents who use birth control the first time they have sex

FP-08 Increase the proportion of adolescents who get formal sex education before age 18 years

FP-11 Increase the proportion of adolescent females at risk for unintended pregnancy who use effective birth control

NWS-04 Reduce the proportion of children and adolescents with obesity

Source: Office of Disease Prevention and Health Promotion. (2022). Healthy people 2030. *U.S. Department of Health and Human Services. http://www.health .gov/healthypeople.gov*

the health and well-being of adolescents (ODPHP, 2022). The need for these objectives will become clear throughout this chapter as they encourage public health interventions and health services initiatives targeted on the most important current health issues for adolescents. Although many of these evidence-based public health objectives fall outside the scope of influence of the health system, healthcare providers should be aware of the objectives and attempt to implement them as appropriate. Healthcare providers who care for adolescents should become familiar with the website in which *Healthy People 2030* progress is continually updated (www.healthypeople.gov).

RISK FACTORS

Risk and Protective Factors

In addition to information on health and well-being, various organizations collect comprehensive data on risk factors that impact the health of adolescents. For example, the Centers for Disease Control and Prevention (CDC), in cooperation with state and local health departments, surveys ninth-through 12th-grade youth in public and private schools with the Youth Risk Behavior Surveillance System (YRBSS). The goals of the survey are to identify health problems in youth and trends in risk-taking behaviors along with focusing the country on adolescent health issues. The YRBSS measures activities that contribute to unintended injuries and violence, tobacco use, alcohol and other drug use, sexual behaviors that contribute to unintended pregnancy and sexually transmitted infections (STIs), unhealthy eating patterns, and physical inactivity (Underwood et al., 2020). In addition to monitoring these risk behaviors, the surveys measure asthma and obesity rates and other health-related behaviors, as well as sexual identity and sex of sexual contacts.

The Youth Risk Behavior Survey Data Summary & Trends Report: 2009–2019 focuses on four priority areas associated with STIs and unintended teen pregnancy: sexual behavior, high-risk substance use, experiencing violence, and mental health and suicide (CDC, 2020). It is developed by the CDC Division of Adolescent and School Health, whose mission is to prevent HIV infection, STIs, and unintended pregnancy by strengthening schools, families, and communities. The most recent report showed trends improving related to sexual behavior and high-risk substance use, including declines in the percentage of students who ever had sex, had four or more sex partners, are currently sexually active, and ever used drugs (CDC, 2020). Bullying and forced sex remained high, but trends remained flat in these areas. Unfortunately, other trends are moving in the wrong direction. Condom use has declined over the past decade, while there has been an increase in STIs including HIV infection, chlamydia infection, gonorrhea, and syphilis, leaving many adolescents vulnerable, particularly young women. Reports of negative mental health and safety issues increased, including the percentage of youth who reported not going to school because of safety concerns, who felt sad or hopeless for at least 2 weeks, and who seriously considered suicide or made a suicide plan. There were stark disparities found in all high-risk behaviors, with sexual minority students more at risk than their heterosexual peers.

The resiliency model recognizes the ability of youth to buffer themselves from harm and remain healthy even when faced with multiple risk factors. Risk and protective factors are inversely related to each other as they affect health outcomes, and these factors can be identified in the individual, peers, family, school, and community. Youth with multiple risk factors and few protective factors have poorer health outcomes than youth with few risk factors and multiple protective factors. Examples of risk factors are an individual's lack of school commitment, friends who engage in drug use, family conflict, violence in the school, and community disorganization. Examples of protective factors include an individual's positive social orientation, bonds with friends and within the family, a school's high expectation of youth, and opportunities for youth participation in the community (Hawkins et al., 2002).

Hall et al. (2021) examined the association of adverse childhood experiences (ACEs) with poor health outcomes including obesity, hypertension, and depression in adolescents in a high-risk urban area, and the impact of resiliency in mitigating those poor health outcomes. Their findings demonstrated that higher ACE scores were associated with a higher risk of negative health outcomes in adolescents, that higher resiliency scores were associated with a lower risk of negative health outcomes, that ACE scores and resiliency are inversely related, and that the relationship with a caregiver was a primary protective factor increasing resilience in this adolescent population. Adelmann (2005) has linked protective factors with positive health behaviors in sixth-grade students: seat belt use, participation in exercise and recreation, quality nutrition intake, and academic achievement. Conversely, his findings reveal that individuals with multiple risk factors had significantly higher negative health behaviors. Barrow et al. (2007) examined the resiliency of African American adolescents and identified specific protective factors to be fostered: self-efficacy, positive racial/ethnic identity, and commitment to the family and community. In African American youth, the development of ethnic pride was linked with parental influence, self-esteem, and self-control and therefore had a protective impact on risk-taking behaviors (Wills et al., 2007).

School environments and academic connectedness combine to create a strong protective factor for youth. Using social and school connectedness as predictors of future health outcomes, Bond et al. (2007) found that positive social and/or school connectedness in eighth-grade students was associated with positive outcomes (school achievement, mental health, and substance abuse) in the 10th and 12th grades. In addition, they found that having both social and school connectedness was associated with the best outcomes. Youngblade et al. (2007) studied a sample of more than 42,000 adolescents ages 11 to 17 years, from the 2003 National Survey of Children's Health. They concluded that multiple family, school, and community protective factors had a positive influence on youth health behaviors. No single influence in an adolescent's life provides protection from violence, substance abuse, or poor health outcomes, but the individual, family, school, and community all contribute to a strong foundation for positive youth development.

ADOLESCENT DEVELOPMENT

Adolescent Stages of Development

During adolescence, development occurs in physical, social, spiritual, and emotional spheres as well as in cognitive and moral spheres. Many theories have been developed to enhance understanding of developmental stages. There are multiple ways to define the boundaries of adolescent development, and there is no consensus between and among researchers, clinicians, parents, and youth themselves. For girls, thelarche marks the first physical sign of pubertal change and is often accompanied by some of the emotional changes of adolescence; this may occur in girls as young as 7 or 8 years old. Considerations for extending adolescence up to 24 or 25 years of age reflect the emerging science on brain development and the tasks of emancipation that extend well into the 20s for some youth (Casey et al., 2008; Galvan et al., 2007; Romer et al., 2017). Others consider adolescence to run through age 19 years and "young adult" up to age 25 years. In a 2009 National Research Council Report on adolescent health services, the committee divided the available evidence into subsets of early adolescence (approximately 10 to 13 years), middle adolescence (approximately 14 to 17 years), late adolescence (approximately 17 to 21 years), and young adulthood (approximately 18 to 25 years; Lawrence et al., 2009). Because there are no exact demarcations among stages, this chapter generally refers to early, middle, and late adolescence, as well as young adulthood, without any discrete ages defining the stages.

Each phase of a young woman's development contributes to the foundation for successful emergence from adolescence and the transition to womanhood. Throughout adolescence, women are seeking independence, identity development, social skills and connections with peers, and body awareness. According to Erickson (1963, 1968), adolescents and young adults must develop their identity to avoid role confusion. In Piaget's (1973) cognitive theory, the adolescent proceeds from concrete operational thinking to formal operational thoughts characterized by abstract thinking. An extension of Piaget's work, Kohlberg's (1981) moral development theory discusses movement from conventional moral reasoning—making judgments based on what is right because of society's regulation—to postconventional morality—making judgments based on universal principles of justice. Carol Gilligan's work developed as a result of her affiliation with Kohlberg and examination of how gender variables challenged the moral development theory. Through further investigation, Gilligan (1982) identified how girls construct moral dilemmas in terms of caring, responsibility, and relationship and not in terms of right, wrong, and rulemaking. Rew (2005) pointed out that adolescent girls recognize a disparity between care and power and that many choose to abandon the concern for attaining and maintaining power and adopt the concern for caring.

Early Adolescence

The developing characteristics of early adolescence often parallel the rapid physical changes of puberty in most girls. These girls become less interested in family activities and may begin to critique parental influences. The struggle for independence while still being dependent frequently creates family discord and is accompanied by wide mood swings in the young adolescent. A young woman often makes strong attachments to a peer group and experiences the ups and downs of that intensity. She becomes increasingly aware and yet insecure about her body, frequently comparing herself with others. A young woman may be confused about her physical body's impact on others in her social network and in the community. She begins to have sexual feelings and begins to privately question her thoughts and emotions. At this stage in a young woman's development, she is expanding her knowledge, beginning to abstractly process information, fantasize about the future, and daydream about idealistic goals. There is an intense focus on the self, accompanied by an overwhelming self-consciousness that Elkind and Bowen (1979) termed the "imaginary audience."

Middle Adolescence

Middle adolescence is marked by continued withdrawal from the family and increasing conflict at home. Young women also have a heightened interest in peer connections and adopt peer-group norms, which may lead to school and community conflicts as well. Middle adolescence sees involvement in more delinquency, gangs, sports, and clubs as a young woman tries to identify and connect with a peer group. The middle adolescent begins to accept the physical changes of puberty and focuses on developing a personal identity within the peer-group norms in terms of clothing, makeup, and hairstyle. This creative self-expression enhances identity development and body image. During middle adolescence, the invincibility felt by a young woman, and her impression that "it can't happen to me," may lead to poor decision-making and risky behaviors.

Late Adolescence

Late adolescence is a time for the young woman to begin the transition to adulthood. If her earlier experiences with independence, peer-group support, and identity development have been empowering, the young woman is well equipped to trust this next phase of her life. If, on the other hand, her early and middle stages of adolescence were complicated by mental illness, an eating disorder, or other chronic problems, the young woman may not be optimally prepared to face the responsibilities and challenges of adult life. The tasks during this phase are to have body acceptance, a clear self-identity, and the ability to critically appraise parents and peers in order to make independent choices.

Physical Development

Before menarche, young women experience dramatic changes in their bodies during a relatively short period, including a deposition of adipose tissue (up to 11 kg of body fat) as well as an increase in height (up to 25 cm), called the *growth spurt* (Tanner, 1962). In addition, premenarcheal girls experience adrenarche (growth of pubic hair, stimulated by androgens), thelarche (breast development stimulated by estradiol), and late in puberty, menarche. Nearly two thirds of girls experience menarche during Tanner's (1981) stage 4 (Brooks-Gunn & Warren, 1985; Brooks-Gunn et al., 1987; Tanner, 1962). Menarche occurs 2 to 2.5 years after breast buds emerge, after the peak height velocity is completed, and at a sexual maturity rating of 3 or 4. The physiologic basis of puberty and menarche is discussed more fully in Chapter 7, Women's Bodies, Women's Health.

In addition to sexual maturation, bone mass or bone mineral density increases. Physical activity level, heredity, nutrition, endocrine function, and medications can positively or negatively affect bone mass in adolescents. Peak bone mass is acquired by early adulthood, so adolescence is a critical time in acquiring bone density necessary for lifelong bone health. Of all the physical changes associated with puberty, among the most dramatic, unexpected, and misunderstood is the change in adipose mass. On average, girls who mature earlier tend to have higher body mass index (BMI), and slightly shorter girls who mature later tend to be lighter, leaner, and slightly taller when puberty is complete.

In recent years, there has been increasing focus on the developing adolescent brain and its role in social, behavioral, and psychiatric disorders. This work has found that social skills, decision-making, and impulsivity are significantly linked to measurable physiologic changes in the brain. Nelson et al. (2005) described the brain's social information processing network and identified three nodes based on function and developmental timing: detection node, affective node, and cognitive-regulatory node. The associations of the adolescent brain's maturation, social inhibition, and risk-taking impulsivity are individualized and remain an area of emerging science (Casey et al., 2008; Galvan et al., 2007; Romer et al., 2017).

PRECOCIOUS PUBERTY

A growing body of literature (Haudek et al., 1999; Hayward et al., 1997, 1999; Mrug et al., 2014; Siegel et al., 1999) indicates that early puberty can be challenging. The girls entering puberty before their peers may not be as well prepared for the physical, psychological, and social changes that occur in puberty (Brooks-Gunn et al., 1985). Early pubertal status has been found to be a predictor of frequent problems seen among adolescent girls, including depression, anxiety, disordered eating, delinquency, substance use, and school failure or dropout (Angold et al., 1998; Hayward et al., 1999; Mendle, 2014).

Some have investigated the implications of pubertal timing for adult functioning. Serepca (1996) examined whether women's objective pubertal timing (their menarcheal age) and subjective timing (perceived timing relative to peers of menarche and breast development) influenced their adult body image and self-esteem. Objective pubertal timing did not differ on any of the body image or self-esteem variables. However, adult women who perceived themselves as early in breast development, compared with their peers, described themselves as heavier and were more preoccupied with being or becoming overweight. They were also less satisfied with their physical appearance than late-maturing women. Late maturers, on both subjective timing measures, reported more positive body-image attitudes than on-time and early maturers. Mendle et al. (2018) investigated the associations of age at menarche with mental health problems in adulthood. They found that earlier age at menarche is associated with higher rates of depressive symptoms and antisocial behavior in early and middle adulthood, demonstrating that emotional effects of puberty extend further than previously identified, and indicating that an elevated mental health risk exists in this population and should be considered by care providers. These suggest that perception of relative pubertal development and overall timing of puberty may have lasting implications for women.

MENARCHE

McDowell et al. (2007) analyzed the change in menarche timing over the past century. Data from the 1999 to 2004 National Health and Nutrition Examination Survey (NHANES) on 6,788 women revealed a 0.9-year decline in self-reported age at menarche in all racial/ethnic groups. For women born before 1920, the mean age of menarche was 13.6 years. For women born in 1980 to 1984, the mean age was 12.5 years. Martinez (2020) recently reviewed trends in menarche in the United States from 1995 to 2013 to 2017. She found that the median age at menarche decreased from

12.1 in 1995 to 11.9 in 2013 to 2017, and that an earlier age at menarche was associated with a higher probability of earlier age at first sexual intercourse. To account for this decrease, researchers have suggested multiple related variables, including nutrition status, obesity, race, socioeconomic class, genetic predisposition, and environmental and societal influences (Cesario & Hughes, 2007; Lee et al., 2007; Martinez, 2020).

FACTORS INFLUENCING ADOLESCENT DEVELOPMENT

Being Different

Feeling "different" during adolescence can have an impact on the transition from adolescence to adulthood, affecting identity formation, engagement with peers, and self-confidence. All youth experience the feelings of not fitting in or questioning, "Am I normal?" However, these feelings may be intensified in adolescents living outside the dominant norms of society. This section of the chapter examines the impact of disability, chronic illness, racial disparities/ethnicity, immigration and refugee status, socioeconomic and family status, sexual orientation, and gender identity on adolescents. It is important to create a safe space for all adolescents, including both the environment and during the medical interview. See recommendations about preparing a safe clinical environment and potential tools for conducting the medical interview later in this chapter.

Intellectual and Physical Disability

Because there is variability in the impact that one or more disabling mental and physical health conditions have on an individual, it is difficult to generalize the effect disability has on the development of an adolescent. Intellectual disabilities (IDs) impact the social skills, reading, writing, learning, and practical day-to-day independent living skills specifically to meet the criteria for the diagnosis before the age of 18.

These physical disabilities also carry with them increased risk for several chronic conditions that are more prevalent in adolescents including obesity, congenital heart defects, constipation, dental caries, endocrine abnormalities, gastroesophageal reflux disease (GERD), hearing loss, seizures, sleep disorders, visual impairment, lead poisoning, cerebral palsy, and other motor impairments (Houdek & Gibson, 2017).

Adolescents with special healthcare needs often require coordinated care by an experienced healthcare team. This type of "medical home" provides services with a focus on transition to adulthood (for more information, consult the American Academy of Pediatrics [AAP] page found at www.MedicalHomeInfo.org). In addition to participating in the multidisciplinary team taking care of the client and being cognizant of the other challenges facing the client, the healthcare provider can assist in facilitating the transition to adulthood by treating the young woman with respect, speaking directly to her during the visit (instead of to the caregiver), and if possible, conducting part of the visit, including the examination,

without the caregiver present (American College of Obstetricians and Gynecologists [ACOG], 2020c). A chaperone should be in the room during the examination, but a positive, dignified experience in which the young adult is treated as such may facilitate her comfort in returning for future visits.

There are additional considerations for the reproductive health visit in adolescent women with disabilities. The rate of sexual abuse among persons with disabilities is three times higher than for their fully bodied counterparts (Iyengar, 2015). This group is less likely to receive adequate sex education and guidance on healthy sexual behavior and is often thought of as asexual (Houdek & Gibson, 2017). It is important therefore for the women's healthcare provider to be aware of this risk and look for possible signs or symptoms of abuse, including significant changes in behavior; depression; sleep disturbances; avoidance or fear of individuals, genders, or situations; refusal to be touched; hints about change in sexual activity; and/or a new understanding of sexual behavior. Physical signs could be bleeding, bruising, or infection of the genitals, rectum, mouth, or breasts; pain with walking or sitting; and nonspecific, unexplained medical problems such as pelvic pain or headaches.

It is important to note that all licensed providers in every jurisdiction in the United States must report suspected sexual or physical abuse of a minor to child protective services. In most jurisdictions, this also applies to young adults with disabilities. If possible, the licensed provider should tell the young woman that reporting will take place, but this needs to be done confidentially and with sensitivity to the client's circumstances.

Adolescents with disabilities may have menstrual issues that are more complex than the common anovulatory cycles experienced by most young women after menarche. These menstrual cycle abnormalities may result from obesity, thyroid disease (particularly in clients with trisomy 21), medications (antiepileptic and psychiatric medications causing hyperprolactinemia and amenorrhea), or polycystic ovary syndrome (PCOS; more common in teenagers with seizure disorders), among others (ACOG, 2016). Cyclic behavior changes, such as changes in mood around the times of her period, may also be more common in women with disabilities, although making the diagnosis of premenstrual dysphoric disorder (PMDD) can be a challenge, especially with cognitive delays. Seizure disorders are more common in adolescents with disabilities, as are catamenial seizures. Using puberty blockers prior to menarche is not recommended. Menstruation confirms a patent genital tract, allows the growth of full adult stature, and gives the young woman an opportunity to achieve maturity (ACOG, 2016). Young women with disabilities can successfully manage menstrual bleeding if desired and capable; however, it may be their desire to utilize available resources for suppression and pregnancy prevention.

Because of complications with menstrual cycles, menstrual manipulation/suppression is frequently considered in women with disabilities, often at the request of her caregiver (ACOG, 2016). Most contraceptive options are also appropriate for women with disabilities, but unique issues, such as difficulty with inserting a contraceptive ring for adolescents with physical disability or weight gain with medroxyprogesterone acetate (Depo-Provera) in an already obese client, should be considered before medications are prescribed (ACOG, 2016). Contraceptives should be discussed not only in the context of menstrual suppression, but also in the context of protection against pregnancy. Adolescents with disabilities should not be assumed to be asexual. It is important to know that permanent sterilization in this population is rarely appropriate and introduces significant ethical issues that must be comprehensively addressed (Li et al., 2018). If the client is deemed competent and she requests sterilization, she may meet the criteria for informed consent. The hospital ethics committee and legal counsel may need to become involved in cases in which sterilization is requested.

Determining the capacity of an adolescent with developmental disabilities to participate in decision-making or an informed consent process can be complex. *Incompetency* is a legal determination and must be assessed at a given time and situation before a client is deemed incompetent. If a legal guardian has been appointed, it is important to understand who can make certain decisions in the adolescent's life. Information on guardianship and consent can be obtained through the National Disability Rights Network (www.ndrn.org).

Chronic Conditions

Although most adolescents are physically healthy when compared with the general population, the rate of adolescents with multimorbidity continues to rise, especially in the United States. Multimorbidity, the concurrence of multiple mental and/or physical chronic health problems, has a staggering effect on our healthcare system (Romano et al., 2018). The CDC (n.d.) reported that two in five adolescents age 6 to 17 have a chronic health condition such as asthma, diabetes, or epilepsy. In addition, 21.2% of age 12 to 19 youth are obese, and 23.6% of these students use at least one tobacco product.

Transitioning from pediatric to adult healthcare adds additional pressure on young women with chronic medical conditions (Butler, 2021). The increased rates of concurrent mental health conditions and unplanned frequent hospitalizations make navigating this time frame more challenging. Often leaving their parents medical insurance policies can have a negative impact on medication compliance and seeking and/or completing recommended preventive services. Attending an educational program or joining the work force can be daunting, as these processes are designed for independent young adults without the complexities of chronic medical condition care. The healthcare system and payers often prevent parental assistance during this transition because of mandated privacy restrictions based on their age.

Racial Disparities and Ethnicity

Adolescents and youth from nondominant racial-ethnic (NDRE) groups experience inequities in health status and outcomes related to structural or institutional racism, personal mediated racism, and internalized racism. Healthcare providers serving this population need to be aware of their own unconscious, and conscious, bias and potential privilege. Providers, like their clients, can experience the chronic minority stress and vicarious trauma effects themselves in working with this population (Society for Adolescent Health and Medicine, 2018). Health disparities between Black, American Indian/Alaska Native, and White women are evident when comparing reproductive health outcomes (infant and maternal mortality, unintended pregnancy, and access to preventive healthcare). According to the Pregnancy Mortality Surveillance System (PMSS) 2011 to 2015, Black and American Indian/Alaska Native women are two to three times more likely to die from pregnancy-related causes than White women. Approximately 60% of these deaths regardless of race were determined to be preventable (Petersen et al., 2019). After age 18 years, many young adults have barriers to health insurance and experience low rates of coverage, but Black and Hispanic young adults are most likely to be uninsured. National, state, and community interventions to address racial/ethnic health disparities among youth must focus on improvements in access and the quality of available care.

Immigration and Refugee Status

The United Nations has called for action against racism, xenophobia, ethnocentrism, and intolerance (Barkley, 2018). In 2017, 27% of children 17 years of age or younger were first- or second-generation immigrants, with the largest numbers of immigrants coming from Mexico (42%), El Salvador (5%), India (5%), and the Philippines (3%; Murphey et al., 2018). In a study using data from the 2017 Current Population Survey, 24% of first-generation immigrant children live below poverty, as compared to 17% of U.S.-native families. At the same time, more of the immigrant youth live in two-parent homes (72%) while more U.S.-native families live in single-parent homes (29%). Many of these families and youth have been exposed to violence and may have experienced or witnessed torture. Studies have identified gender differences among the youth; girls were more likely to report feelings of aloneness, even though they were more likely to be partnered, married, or with their mothers. Yet those same youths often have protective factors that aid in their adjustment to a new country: two-parent and multigenerational households and strong commitment to the family unit (Child Trends, 2018).

Young women as an immigrant population tend to be invisible to policy makers and planners in humanitarian evacuations. In 2021, over 124,000 Afghan civilians were evacuated by a coalition of military forces. Those Afghan civilians included over 2,000 pregnant women processing through Germany, and 200 pregnant women housed on the base (Liebermann & Kaufman, 2021). The women's healthcare needs of this unique group of practicing Muslim young women were initially overlooked until the healthcare mission was extended beyond the initial rescue. Protecting religious-driven modesty while providing sensitive OB/GYN healthcare proved to be daunting. The women travelers only consented to female providers and with translation all through an interpreter in Pashto, Dari, Arabic, and other languages. Term or preterm births occurred frequently and unexpectedly outside of hospital settings. The first birth occurred before the C-17 aircraft landed in Germany, with 800 passengers observing, and subsequent births continued (Kindelan, 2021). Out-of-hospital births were recorded at the traveler camps on the military flight line, in the housing pods and military tents and German ambulances during transport. Because of political agreements and limitations between countries, nongovernment organizations (NGOs) were unable to assist with rescue efforts. Of all the lessons learned, the need to anticipate and prepare for the healthcare needs of large numbers of women and children is essential. Successful planning for future humanitarian missions requires procuring specialized OB/GYN and pediatric equipment in addition to emergency, surgical, medical, and pharmaceutical supplies. This should include, but not be limited to, the following: (1) When initially registering the arrival of individuals, identify all the pregnant women; (2) keep records of approximate due dates and utilize female interpreters to obtain medical and pregnancy history to create an abbreviated health record or pregnancy passport for the client to carry; (3) for success, seek out trained healthcare professionals from within the displaced population to consult on women's healthcare specific to their culture.

Sexual Orientation

Adolescence is a time for sexual identity development, including sexual orientation. There has been an increasing number of studies of lesbian, gay, bisexual, transgender, queer, intersex, asexual, and other (LGBTQIA+) youth to better understand this community, their sexual identity development, and health risks. In a 2021 Gallop poll, 21% of participants from Generation Z (those surveyed who were born 1997–2003) self-identified as LGBT, most identifying as bisexual (J. M. Jones, 2022). In the 2019 CDC YRBSS survey, 47% of youth identifying in this group had considered suicide (CDC, 2020). As a group, LGBTQ youth experience higher rates of family violence, homelessness, substance abuse, depression, and suicidality than their heterosexual peers (CDC, 2020).

The Trevor Project found that at least 1.2 million LGBTQ youth ages 13 to 18 in the United States seriously consider suicide each year (Green, 2019). In examining suicidal ideation and suicide attempts among nearly 22,000 adolescents with same-sex experience in the 2022 Minnesota Student Survey, Eisenberg and Resnick (2006) found that lack of supporting and caring environments (including family connectedness, teacher caring, other adult caring, and school safety) was associated with suicidality and that same-sex experience alone was not a predictive variable. Clinicians can enhance their communication skills, confront personal bias, and develop cultural competency by using available resources such as the following websites: www.pflag.org and genderdysphoria.fyi/en.

Gender Identity

All clients identify somewhere on the continuum of the individual characteristics of sexual orientation and gender identity (see Figure 8.1). For many young adults, these descriptions are more fluid, dynamic, and nonbinary than the terms boy, girl, and cisgender. Providers are essential in locating resources and appropriate healthcare specialists, related to who they identify as, in relation to gender identity and gender expression. Athan (2020) suggests things to consider for putting a young adult client identifying as transgender at ease and establishing a respectful relationship:

- Identify their desired pronouns, (he/him, she/her, they/them).
- Assist with accurate education and support for the client and family (resources).
- Refer to appropriate adolescent specialists (a team that includes mental health professionals for adolescents trained and knowledgeable about diagnostic criteria for gender-affirming treatments, with experience in

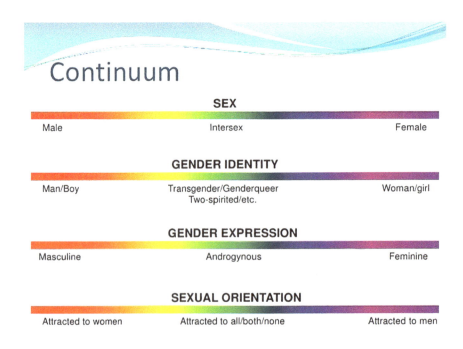

FIGURE 8.1 The gender spectrum: A look into the gender spectrum, which shows the distinction between physical sex and gender identity.
Source: Boyle, J. (2016). The gender spectrum. In The hope for a monstrous world without gender. https://scalar.usc.edu/works/index-2/the-hope-for-a-monstrous-world-without-gender

assessing psychopathology, and, if indicated, who are willing to participate in endocrine transition).

- Provide situationally sensitive care (trauma triggers—physical exams, skin exposure, touch).
- Encourage the young adult to consider and share their reproductive identity. (Athan, 2020)

Reproductive identity is the desire to be a parent or not, and the desire for children to be genetically related to them or not. For those young adults who are contemplating transitioning, fertility preservation can be discussed before hormonal treatments or surgical interventions. Depending on state or national laws, age restrictions vary for gender transition treatments. In the United States, puberty blockers can be used until age 16 to pause the physical attributes of maturity. Hormonal therapy can be offered after informed consent after the age of 16, and the age for surgical intervention consent is after age 18. Young adults with breasts desiring a less feminine appearance often bind their breasts to adapt to their desired image. Young transgender male-to-female clients may desire a more feminine look through estrogen/progesterone therapy and schedule an appointment in a women's health clinic. Despite gender expression or repression by young adults, gender dysphoria has serious consequences if left untreated or unsupported. Rates of suicide attempts, hospitalizations, and self-inflicted injury are statistically higher in studies in the transgender population as compared with their cisgender peers (Thoma et al., 2019). The gender dysphoria diagnosis can be described as a discord between the young adult's gender assigned at birth, usually by external genitalia, and the individual's gender identity. This gender dysphoria is marked by forms of distress or impairment and often presents during puberty but may also occur later in life (Turban, 2020). Not all transgender individuals experience gender dysphoria. In a cross-sectional study involving 27,715 questionnaires from all 50 states and including U.S. territories, along with military bases stationed overseas, transgender respondents recalled exposure to gender identity conversion efforts (GICE). Only 19,741 (71.3%) had spoken to a professional about their gender identity, and of those, 3,896 (19.6%) reported exposure to GICE in their lifetime. Compared to non-GICE therapy participants, the respondents who experienced GICE were 1.56 times more likely to experience severe psychological distress, 2.27 times more likely to attempt suicide in their lifetime, and 4.15 times more likely to attempt suicide if the exposure to GICE was before age 10. No statistical significance was found between secular professionals or religious advisors (Turban et al., 2020).

Assessing the adolescent woman's sexual and gender orientation during a brief exam can overwhelm both the provider and client, but tools exist to help with this segment of the medical history (ACOG, 2020c).

Out-of-Home Youth

Out-of-home youth are those adolescents not living in the home of their immediate family or guardian. These can include youth experiencing homelessness with their family or those living with relatives or friends, in foster care, or in detention facilities, as well as runaway youth or unaccompanied minors. Youth leave home for a variety of reasons, but neglect and sexual abuse are often triggers and consequently put youth at extreme risk for additional victimization (Meinbresse et al., 2014).

Youth living in foster care may have multiple health and educational needs lacking during adolescence that contribute as barriers for successful life outcomes. Teenage pregnancy rates are exceptionally higher for this population. By age 21, over 49% of the females in foster care experienced at least one pregnancy (Combs et al., 2018).

Runaway youth are a transient and ever-changing population. It is estimated that 6% to 7% of youth run away from home; however, half reported they were forced to leave because of family dynamics, all types of abuse, or economic issues (National Clearinghouse on Homeless Youth & Families, 2019). In 2015, the National Center for Missing and Exploited Children reports one in five runaways are forced into sexual trafficking (National Center for Missing and Exploited Children, n.d.). From 2014 to 2015, the number of requests for asylum under the Trafficking Victims Protection Reauthorization Act saw a fourfold increase. Youth seeking healthcare present occasionally with signs of a current or past sexual or labor trafficking history; however, little time is allocated for evaluating these possible victims for indicators. The National Human Trafficking Resource Center (NHTRC) hotline prepares healthcare workers to assist potential victims. The information can be found at humantrafficking-hotline.org. A few of the red flags for trafficking victims include evidence of a controlling relationship in which clients are unable to report their address, the current time, the date, or their location. Be cautious if you note tattoos such as "Daddy," "Property of, …" "For Sale," or sexually promiscuous clients reporting a high number of partners, pregnancies, or STIs. Professional interpreters or services are essential for communicating directly with potential victims and gaining trust. Identify your requirements for reporting suspected and reported trafficking. Providers should gain consent for further actions while safely respecting client confidentiality and decision-making.

Social Contexts for Adolescent Development

PARENTS AND SCHOOLS

Parental influence is linked to multiple health outcomes in adolescents. Positive parental involvement (time together, monitoring whereabouts) influenced an adolescent's health and behavior and was linked with stronger school performance, abstinence from sex and tobacco, and lower rates of delinquency. Adults who experienced strong connections as adolescents reportedly were 48% to 66% less likely to experience negative life outcomes, such as mental health issues, substance use, risky behavior, or violence (Steiner et al., 2019). In 2019, the Minnesota Student Survey (MSS) assessed ACEs in eighth, ninth, and 11th grade students (Minnesota Department of Human Services, 2020). The experiences assessed included living with someone with mental illness, being in jail, using illegal drugs, drinking too much alcohol, and being a victim or witnessing all types of abuse. The higher the ACE score, the more times likely the students were to report experiencing suicidal ideations and attempts, illegal substance use, and violence. Protective factors in this study were simply feeling people in the community, school, family, and friends care about them. Parents providing open communication frequently build those necessary strong connections over time.

School environments have an impact on the development of risk and protective factors in adolescents, and positive interventions are linked with positive outcomes into adulthood (CDC, 2022). Early school connectedness and positive social relationships with peers are predictive of future academic achievement, reduced substance abuse, and improved mental health later in high school. In the presence of peers, adolescents are more likely to partake in risky behaviors such as driving recklessly, smoking, and gambling (van Hoorn et al., 2018). School dropout has been linked with multiple risks to health and overall well-being during adolescence and extending into adulthood. High school graduation leads to lower rates of health problems, reduced risk for incarceration, and improved financial stability as an adult (van Hoorn et al., 2018).

Schools also provide an opportunity for girls to be physically active and to receive health and sex health education. Evidence shows that comprehensive sex education programs that provide information about both abstinence and contraception can help delay the onset of sexual activity among teens, reduce their number of sexual partners, and increase contraceptive use when they become sexually active (Child Trends, 2018). In its School Health Profiles, the CDC provides ongoing evaluation of health education, physical education, health services, food services, school policy and environment, and family and community involvement in schools. The CDC also provides useful tools for parents, teachers, and communities to increase physical activity for adolescents, such as those found at www.cdc.gov/healthyyouth/physicalactivity/toolkit/userguide_pa.pdf (CDC, 2015). For adolescent health education, these programs, generated under the Department of Health and Human Services, are available for promoting positive behaviors and outcomes in the form of the think, act, grow (TAG) call to action found at opa.hhs.gov/adolescent-health?tag/index.html (Office of Population Affairs, n.d.). TAG supports five behaviors that support adolescent health: positive connections with supportive people; safe and secure places to live, learn, and play; access to high-quality, teen-friendly healthcare; opportunities to engage as learners, leaders, team members, and workers; and coordinated adolescent-and-family-centered services, as needed.

COMMUNITIES

Adolescents respond to positive and negative pressure from peers, neighborhoods, families, and schools every day. In addition, young people are continually filtering the powerful media messages that surround them. Youth today have grown up with 24/7 access to the social media, devices, and instantaneous access to information. There is no passive down time in their world, resulting in overstimulated youth. In the new millennium, the influence of media on adolescent health requires additional examination. Adolescents need to be aware of social media safety precautions and responsibilities. The CDC has provided a comprehensive overview of technology and its impacts on teens' sexual health, including recommendations for providers to use technology for health promotion and prevention of STIs or other risky sexual behaviors. Communities working with healthcare providers can build posi-

tive youth development activities including school clubs and community-based activities providing students a network of supportive adults. More information can be found about the CDC recommended positive youth promotion strategies at www.cdc.gov/healthyyouth/protective/youth-connectedness-important-protective-factor-for-health-well-being.htm.

HEALTH SERVICES FOR ADOLESCENTS

Utilization of Health Services

Historically, adolescents and young adults have had the lowest rates of utilization of primary or preventive health services among all age groups and those with behavioral health diagnoses are particularly lacking in accessing care (AAP Committee on Adolescence, 2016) One obstacle has been coverage; when the Patient Protection and Affordable Care Act (ACA) of 2010 was implemented, only 89.3% of adolescents (ages 10 to 17) and 66.7% of young adults (ages 18 to 25) had continuous coverage for at least a year (English & Park, 2012). While the ACA did have several provisions to improve coverage of adolescents and young adults and there were significant gains in coverage between 2010 and 2016, adolescents and young adults saw the least incremental improvement in coverage and access (Spencer et al., 2018).

In 2016, 5.3% of adolescents ages 10 to 14 and 7.6% of those between 15 and 18 were uninsured (Spencer et al., 2018). Further, the overall proportion of adolescents (10 to 17 years of age) who have had a preventive healthcare visit in the past 12 months (a *Healthy People 2030* objective) was 78.7% in 2016–2017, below the target of 82.6% (ODPHP, 2022), and significant disparities exist, ranging from 58.2% of American Indian or Alaskan Native only to 80.3% of White only and 80.6% of Black only (ODPHP, 2022).

Equally or more concerning is the lower quality care available for many adolescents. One potential reason is the lack of a solid model of healthcare between childhood and adulthood. Because healthcare providers specializing in pediatrics often are not trained in the rapidly changing needs of adolescents and adult healthcare providers often do not encourage adolescent clients in their practices, adolescents often do not have a true "medical home." Healthcare providers who see the entire spectrum of clients may close this gap somewhat but often do not have comprehensive training in dealing with the complexity of adolescent clients. It was only during the past several decades that the subspecialty of adolescent medicine appeared, likely in response to increases in morbidity and mortality rates in this age group and greater understanding of the complex changes in development that occur during this time (Alderman et al., 2003). A significant challenge is the adolescent's concern about confidentiality. Some of the concerns are not founded in reality, and healthcare providers should ensure that they educate their adolescent clients about confidentiality. However, given the current structure of our healthcare system and wide variation in public (both federal and state) and private policies and procedures, a young client's concerns about confidentiality may be appropriate and must be handled with respect and honesty to ensure the maintenance of trust of the adolescent client (ACOG, 2020a; English & Park, 2012; Maslyanskaya & Alderman, 2019; Pathak & Chou, 2019).

Consent and Confidentiality

In the United States, rules and regulations regarding adolescent rights to consent for healthcare vary by state. *Consent* defines the legal ability to obtain health services, and *confidentiality* is the ability to choose when to disclose the content of that care. Individual states govern the minor's rights to obtain reproductive healthcare, mental health services, and substance abuse assessment and treatment. Reproductive healthcare can include contraception, sexually transmitted disease and STI assessment and treatment, pregnancy services, and termination of pregnancy care. A helpful review of state laws and policies provides context for this issue (English et al., 2012), but defining current individual minor's rights in each state is outside the scope of this text. Updated information for each state and the District of Columbia can be found through the Center for Adolescent Health & the Law (www.cahl.org) and the Guttmacher Institute (www.guttmacher.org). Rights to confidentiality and the ability to consent change frequently, and each year there are new attempts by state legislatures to limit or expand the rights of parents/guardians and adolescents. A young woman must understand that there are legal and ethical situations when confidentiality will be broken. If she discloses intent to harm herself or someone else, it is the professional responsibility of the healthcare provider to break confidentiality and obtain all necessary services to maintain safety for all involved. In addition, if the young woman is a minor and has been assaulted or abused, she is subject to state laws governing child protection (www.childwelfare.gov). It is the healthcare provider's responsibility to understand and follow the rules in the state where they practice. It is important to note that protecting confidentiality in some cases can be a challenge, especially for minors with private insurance, if a medical bill for a procedure or consultation lists the reason for the bill.

Multiple organizations have provided tools for clinicians and health systems to improve the quality of care for adolescents. The World Health Organization (WHO) created a framework for adolescent-friendly health services (AFHS). The main goals are to support adolescent healthcare that is accessible, acceptable, appropriate, effective, and equitable (Tylee et al., 2007). Preventive healthcare guidelines for adolescent girls have been developed by national health organizations: *Bright Futures: Guidelines for Health Supervision of Infants, Children, and Adolescents,* sponsored by a collaborative based in the Department of Health and Human Services and the AAP (Hagen et al., 2017); *Guidelines for Adolescent Preventive Services,* developed by the American Medical Association (AMA; Elster & Kuznets, 1994); and *Primary and Preventive Health Care for Female Adolescents,* published by the ACOG (2010). National guidelines are utilized to improve the quality of care and to emphasize comprehensive health services, including anticipatory guidance, targeted health screening, immunizations, and physical exam components. *Bright Futures: Guidelines for Health Supervision of Infants, Children, and Adolescents* recommends annual visits for health screening and anticipatory guidance (Hagen et al., 2017). *Bright Futures* incorporates a focus on the major causes of morbidity and death of adolescence and therefore emphasizes the importance of risk reduction, injury prevention, pregnancy and STI prevention, physical growth and development, social and school connectedness, and mental health. National guidelines are reviewed and updated regularly to reflect trends in health indicators and evidence-based research. The recommendations from *Bright Futures* have been translated into a comprehensive toolkit to assist providers in conducting the adolescent healthcare visit, based on phase of adolescence (11 to 14 years of age, 15 through 17 years of age, and 18 through 21 years of age; Shaw et al., 2018).

ACOG also provides guidelines for adolescent care and recommends that the first visit for screening and provision of reproductive preventive health services occur between 13 and 15 years of age, although the guidance is applicable at other ages (ACOG, 2020c). This visit can be done as part of the primary care visit, and if training or experience does not allow or the client prefers to be seen outside the primary care setting, referral is appropriate for any component of the reproductive health visit that is not covered by the primary healthcare provider. ACOG has provided useful recommendations for practices and staff that can help create an office environment that is more comfortable and appealing to adolescents (ACOG, 2020c).

The National Adolescent and Young Adult Health Information Center provides updates and summaries of policies and clinical guidelines; for example, the Summary of Clinical Preventive Services Guidelines for Adolescents Up to Age 18 (CPSG-ADOL Summary) is updated regularly and can be used as a point-of-care tool for clinicians (National Adolescent and Young Adult Health Information Center [NAHIC], 2020).

A model that was developed in response to adolescents' low utilization of traditional health services and high rates of preventable adverse outcomes is that of school-based health centers (SBHCs; AAP Committee on Adolescence, 2016). They have created links from community and education systems to health systems and may serve as a point of entry to primary care for those who would otherwise not have access. Although about half of SBHCs are in urban areas, most new SBHCs since 2010 have arisen in rural areas, addressing the needs of many underserved adolescents (AAP Committee on Adolescence, 2016). An excellent resource is the website for the School-Based Health Alliance available at www.sbh4all.org. Arenson et al. (2019) reviewed outcomes of SBHCs and found that over 83% of SBHCs provide management of chronic health conditions, a challenge for many adolescents, and they have demonstrated success in treating asthma, obesity, substance abuse, and those children with special healthcare needs. The review also reported that nearly 70% of SBHCs offered mental healthcare services, utilizing licensed clinical social workers, psychologists, and substance abuse counselors, and that services have been shown to reduce depressive episodes and suicide risk among adolescents (Arenson et al., 2019). Although these outcomes are promising and SBHCs are viewed as having a critical role in improving screening, the best models for mental healthcare for SBHCs continues to be an area for research, given the complexity of mental health issues for the adolescent population (Arenson et al., 2019).

ASSESSMENT

Healthcare Visits for Adolescent Women

With this background, it is easier to comprehend why providing care to an adolescent can be both challenging and incredibly rewarding. Understanding the rapid development during the adolescent years and the factors and contexts that can significantly affect that development allows the healthcare provider to skillfully approach the encounter with the adolescent client and hopefully provide the quality care that will improve the client's health and well-being.

The clinician begins with an introduction, and clarifying the goals of the visit. For the first time, this client may present for healthcare without their parents or guardian. If an adult is present, it is important for a portion of the visit to be conducted with the client alone. This can be accomplished by stating, for example: "I am glad you are here for this visit together. Now that [name] is getting older, it is important for [appropriate pronoun] to have part of this visit in private. After we have talked together, I will ask you to leave, so [name] and I have a chance to talk in private." This is also the optimal time to help the young client and their parent understand rights to confidentiality and consent. The parent or guardian may also have concerns to address without the adolescent present, and these can be addressed when the parent is out of the exam room. This should be done, however, before the confidential interview with the client to dispel the perception that confidential information that the client provides will be shared with the parent.

The first step in establishing care with adolescents is to create the foundation for a trusting relationship. Making connections is time well spent and requires skill and patience. With an understanding of adolescent development, health status, and health concerns, the healthcare provider may consider a different approach for the teen client (e.g., by incorporating motivational interviewing [MI] into the visit). MI is a directive, client-centered counseling style with the goal of eliciting and strengthening motivation for change and evoking plans for changing behavior (Rollnick & Miller, 1995). The purpose of MI is the establishment of a goal-oriented partnership that empowers the client to initiate and actively take responsibility for change. MI does not utilize direct persuasion by a healthcare provider to resolve conflicts or ambivalence; instead, the healthcare provider quietly and actively listens. MI recognizes that change is not absolute but fluctuates over time.

MI has been adapted to multiple settings other than the field of addiction and substance abuse treatment, where much of the research has been conducted (Resnicow et al., 2006). MI is well suited for clients who may be more difficult to engage in treatment (e.g., adolescents, substance users, those with high-risk lifestyles) and, indeed, results of studies of MI for substance use among adolescents have demonstrated significant and lasting effects (Jensen et al., 2011). Adolescents' developmental goals are to individuate, experiment, and begin to trust their ability to make health decisions independently. Utilization of MI aids the healthcare provider in respectful care of the young woman, recognizing

her current stage of development and working with her to move toward responsible healthcare decisions.

Gold and Kokotailo (2007) developed practical guidance on how to implement MI for adolescents, including the use of Importance and Confidence Rulers, which help make these abstract concepts more concrete, and creating a SMART (Specific, Measurable, Achievable, Realistic, Time-framed) plan.

It is helpful to look to other theories on adolescent development to guide communication techniques in the clinical setting. Based on the imaginary audience theory of Elkind and Bowen (1979), adolescents are naturally self-conscious about personal discussions. It is useful to preface the discussion with something like: "I talk with all the young clients I see about _____." The natural egocentrism of adolescents and the stages of psychosocial development necessitate careful use of feedback. Feedback that is direct, sincere, and

TABLE 8.1 The SSHADESS Dimensions: Protective Factors and Personal Strengths in Young Persons' Lives

SSHADESS DIMENSIONS	SAMPLE QUESTIONS/COMMENTS
Strengths	Tell me some of the things you like best about yourself. Tell me what your friends would say are the best things about you.
School	How is it going for you in school? What are the best and hardest things about school?
Home	How is it going for you at home? What responsibilities or chores do you have in your home?
Activities	What do you like to do with your friends? If you had half a day and could do whatever you wanted, what would you do?
Drugs and substance abuse	At some point in growing up, everyone faces decisions about tobacco, alcohol, and drugs. Do you have friends that smoke or drink?
Emotions and depression	Being healthy is more than being able to run around the track or not having broken bones, but has a lot to do with how we feel about ourselves, how connected we are at home, school, and with our friends. How have you felt over the last couple of months? Do ever think about hurting yourself or dying?
Sexuality	What questions do you have about your body and how it works? If you were with someone you really liked and they wanted to have sex but you did not, what would you do?
Safety	When you are out with your friends, do you feel safe? Do you know how to swim? What would you do if your ride home was drunk or high?

Source: Ginsburg, K. R. (2007). Viewing our adolescent patients through a positive lens. Contemporary Pediatrics, 24(1), 65–76.

hopeful and that builds on the young woman's protective factors and strengths should be provided. Barriers to effective communication with young women include generalizations and labeling, accusations, blaming, and threats. Ginsburg (2007) proposed an acronym that includes protective factors in a young person's life and a review of the person's strengths: SSHADESS (Table 8.1). This tool may also serve as a guide for the healthcare provider interviewing an adolescent.

A questionnaire called the PRAPARE (The Protocol for Responding to and Assessing Patients' Assets, Risks, and Experiences) screening tool was developed as a patient-centered social determinant of health assessment tool by a partnership between the National Association of Community Health Centers, Inc., the Association of Asian Pacific Community Health Organizations, and the Oregon Primary Care Association (2019). The tool is available in over 25 languages to effectively organize the social portion of the healthcare visit and can be found at prapare.org/the-prapare-screening-tool.

General Medical History

Although most teens are healthy without chronic medical conditions, the client's current and past medical history should be reviewed, including any conditions, medications, and allergies. Family history should be documented or updated in the client's medical record; in particular, a history of venous thromboembolism; breast, ovarian, colon, or uterine cancer; and other familial gynecologic issues should be noted. Vaccination history also should be reviewed and any missing or indicated vaccinations discussed with the client (details are given in the following section).

Reproductive Health History

Providing a reproductive health history will likely be a new experience for the client and parent. During the initial discussion with the client and guardian, the provider should explain the difference between a pelvic examination and a Pap test and that the initial visit will not usually require either. Letting the client know that an internal examination is required only if there are particular concerns will alleviate anxiety coming into the visit. The healthcare provider should explain that the first Pap test should be done at age 21. However, at the initial visit, the healthcare provider should discuss normal pubertal development, appropriate menstrual flow and patterns, and menstrual hygiene. An assessment for menstrual issues such as anovulatory cycles, PCOS, menorrhagia, and dysmenorrhea should be conducted and details on these specific conditions are covered in the following discussions.

The first day of the last menstrual cycle should be considered a *vital sign* in each health assessment for young women. ACOG and AAP developed a document to assist healthcare providers in the evaluation of the abnormal vital sign (ACOG, 2015). The normal cycle is between 21 and 45 days; menstruation lasts 7 days or less, and is not excessively heavy (Adams Hillard, 2006).

Amenorrhea

Primary amenorrhea is defined as failure to menstruate by age 15 in the presence of normal secondary sexual characteristics

or no menses by age 13 and the absence of secondary sexual characteristics (Halverson, 2020). *Secondary amenorrhea* occurs after menarche when a young woman fails to menstruate for 3 months or the adolescent has fewer than nine cycles a year. Primary amenorrhea requires an evaluation for potential congenital, neurologic, hormonal, and genetic etiologies while secondary amenorrhea also requires an evaluation for pregnancy, PCOS, psychosocial stressors, extreme weight changes, and causes of premature ovarian insufficiency. It is important to complete the evaluation while attending to the emotional and psychological needs of the adolescent. By conducting a careful history, physical assessment, and standard laboratory tests, the etiology of amenorrhea can be determined. It is essential to rule out pregnancy as the first step in any evaluation.

Abnormal Uterine Bleeding

In adolescent girls, the menstrual cycle ranges from 21 to 45 days and menstruation typically lasts less than 7 days with blood loss of less than 80 mL per cycle (or three to six pads or tampons per day; ACOG, 2015). Any bleeding pattern that varies from this definition can be classified as abnormal uterine bleeding and a menstrual calendar is useful for aiding the adolescent in understanding their menstrual cycle and the healthcare provider in making a diagnosis.

Etiologies for abnormal uterine bleeding in the adolescent population include pregnancy, PCOS, pelvic infection, hormonal contraception, endocrine disorders, and malignancy (Hernandez & Dietrich, 2020). After the onset of menses, cycles can be irregular due to an immature hypothalamic–pituitary–ovarian axis; it can take up to 36 months for cycles to regulate, lasting between 31 and 34 days (WHO Task Force on Adolescent Reproductive Health, 1986). Adolescents who require hospitalization and/or transfusion have a 20% to 30% risk of having a coagulopathy such as von Willebrand disease, and this fact needs to be considered when completing the laboratory assessment. Depending on the severity and suspicion for certain etiologies, laboratory assessment may include: complete blood count and differential, platelet count and aggregation studies, human chorionic gonadotropin, thyroid studies, prolactin, fibrinogen, prothrombin time, partial thromboplastin time, and a von Willebrand's panel (Sanfilippo & Lara-Torre, 2009). If the client is found to have mild (hemoglobin greater than 11 g/dL) or moderate (hemoglobin 9 to 11 g/dL) anemia, iron supplementation should be provided in addition to a hormonal contraceptive (combined hormonal contraceptives, depo medroxyprogesterone, or a levonorgestrel-releasing intrauterine device) if pregnancy prevention is desired. If severe anemia is found along with ongoing bleeding this can be addressed with a contraceptive taper or the client can be referred to a gynecologist for evaluation and either outpatient or inpatient treatment depending on their hemodynamic status (Sanfilippo & Lara-Torre, 2009).

Polycystic Ovary Syndrome

PCOS is a common endocrine disorder with a prevalence of about 4% to 6% of the female population and which results in excessive androgens produced by the ovary and possibly the adrenal gland. It results in a constellation of signs and symptoms, including hirsutism, irregular menstrual cycles, obesity, and acne. Because of the similarity of many of these symptoms with normal puberty, PCOS may be overdiagnosed during adolescence. It is diagnosed using the Rotterdam criteria whereby an affected adolescent has two out of three following symptoms: (a) oligomenorrhea or amenorrhea, (b) clinical or biochemical evidence of hyperandrogenism, and (c) polycystic ovaries on sonography (ACOG, 2018c). Clients with PCOS are more at risk of developing metabolic syndrome, which includes (a) increased abdominal fat mass (waist circumference more than 35 inches), (b) increased triglycerides (150 mg/dL or more), (c) decreased high-density lipoproteins (50 mg/dL or less), (d) increased blood pressure (130/85 mmHg or higher), and (e) increased plasma glucose (100 mg/dL or higher; Sanfilippo & Lara-Torre, 2009). Clients with PCOS also have a 2.7-fold increased risk for developing endometrial cancer due to prolonged exposure of the endometrium to unopposed estrogen that results from anovulation (Dumesic & Lobo, 2013). Because PCOS has future consequences on an adolescent's overall health, early intervention can prevent long-term sequelae such as infertility, insulin resistance, cardiovascular disease, and endometrial cancer. Weight loss of about 10% can help restore regular ovulatory cycles in many women, but this may be difficult to accomplish in adolescent women. Combined oral contraceptive pills may help reduce circulating androgens and improve hirsutism while promoting a regular withdrawal bleeding and decreasing risk of endometrial hyperplasia. Metformin has been used to address the insulin resistance in PCOS, but its use in adolescence is controversial. Shared decision-making is useful in treating adolescents with PCOS, as its treatment relies on both lifestyle changes and possible pharmacologic therapy. Education and discussion of the impact of the symptoms on the client's life are critical. Helpful resources for young women with PCOS can be found at the website of the Center for Young Women's Health at Children's Hospital in Boston (www.youngwomenshealth.org/index.html). Identification of PCOS, treatment goals, and psychological supports must be developed in a partnership with the adolescent and parents, recognizing the complex emotional and identity development of adolescence.

Dysmenorrhea

Most adolescents experience *primary dysmenorrhea*, defined as painful menstruation in the absence of pelvic pathology, which typically begins within 6 to 12 months of menarche (Gantt & McDonough, 1981). *Secondary dysmenorrhea* describes painful menses due to a known pathology with the most common being endometriosis (Laufer et al., 1997). Other causes of secondary dysmenorrhea include leiomyoma, adnexal masses, adenomyosis, infection, and obstructive reproductive tract anomalies. Associated symptoms of dysmenorrhea can include nausea, vomiting, diarrhea, headaches, muscle cramps, poor sleep quality, and recurring absence from school (Woosley & Lichstein, 2014). The initial evaluation includes a detailed history compiling information about the client's medical, surgical,

psychosocial, and family history. A pelvic exam is not necessary when primary dysmenorrhea is suspected. When the history suggests primary dysmenorrhea a 3- to 6-month trial of nonsteroidal anti-inflammatory agents with or without a hormonal agent (combined oral contraceptives, depo medroxyprogesterone, or the levonorgestrel-releasing intrauterine devices) should be considered. If pain has not improved after this time point, and compliance is not an issue, an additional 3 months can be initiated on a different hormonal method (ACOG, 2018b). If the client's pain does not improve after an additional 3 months of therapy a pelvic exam and sonography should be considered (ACOG, 2018b). If endometriosis is suspected, the adolescent has the option to proceed with diagnostic laparoscopy for a definitive diagnosis versus a trial on a gonadotropin-releasing hormone analogue; referral to a gynecologist can be considered in this circumstance.

History of Sexual Activity

During the confidential visit, the healthcare provider should assess the client's history of sexual activity and discuss contraception and STIs. A discussion of sexual and reproductive health is included in the care of all young women regardless of sexual behavior. As seen in the YRBSS from 2019, 27.4% of all high school students reported being sexually active and 26.9% had four or more sexual partners up to that point. Among high school students surveyed, 54.3% reported using a condom during the last act of intercourse; however, condom use was lower for those with other sexually risky behaviors (Szucs et al., 2020). Each year, the Guttmacher Institute publishes *Fact Sheet: American Teens' Sexual and Reproductive Health* (Guttmacher Institute, 2014). This compilation of research on adolescent sexual behavior provides an overview of sexual activity, contraceptive use, access to contraceptive services, and rates of STIs, pregnancy, childbearing, and abortion. Similar to YRBSS, this report states that nearly half of all 15- to 19-year-olds in the United States have had sex at least once. At age 15 years, approximately 16% of youth have had sex, and by age 19 years 71% of teens have engaged in sexual intercourse. Most teens (78% of girls and 85% of boys) report using some form of contraception during their first sexual experience (Guttmacher Institute, 2014). The most common method used by teens is condoms, and most teenage women (96%) report using them at least once. Teens are at risk of STIs; they represent one quarter of the sexually active population yet account for nearly half of all new STIs. In addition to asking about voluntary sexual activity, providers should inquire about intimate partner and dating violence, including unwanted or involuntary sexual activity. In 2019, 8.2% of respondents to the YRBSS reported physical or sexual dating violence (CDC, 2020). The prevalence of having been forced to do sexual acts (kissing, touching, or being forced to have sexual intercourse) while dating was 8.1% among White, 6.2% among Black, and 8.7% among Hispanic females, highlighting that this issue can be present across all demographics (Basile et al., 2020).

Teen Pregnancy

The Guttmacher Institute reported that each year, nearly 615,000 women ages 15 to 19 years become pregnant and that in 2010 there were 57 pregnancies per 1,000 young women ages 15 to 19 years. This represents a significant decline from its peak in 1990, thought to be secondary to delays in sexual activity and more consistent use of contraception in those who are sexually active. Pregnancy rates declined for all racial groups from 1990 to 2010, with the sharpest declines among Black teens (56%). However, Black women continue to have the highest teen pregnancy rate (100 per 1,000 women ages 15 to 19 years), followed by Hispanic (84 per 1,000) and non-Hispanic Whites (38 per 1,000). Teen pregnancies are largely unplanned (82%). Two thirds of teen pregnancies occur in older adolescents ages 18 to 19 years. The birth rate for teens age 15 to 19 years dropped 50% from 1991 (62 births per 1,000) to 2011 (31 births per 1,000). Babies born to teens are at greater risk for health complications including low birth weight. Teen mothers are also less likely to receive prenatal care or to engage in prenatal care late in their pregnancy. In 2010, 26% of 15- to 19-year-olds ended their pregnancies with abortion, and the primary reasons teens gave for having an abortion included concerns about how a baby would affect their lives, an inability to afford a child, and a feeling of being insufficiently prepared to raise a child at that time in their lives. As of May 2014, 38 states required by law that parents of a minor seeking an abortion be involved in the decision (Guttmacher Institute, 2014).

Contraception

When counseling a client on contraception, it is critical to help the client understand their risk of pregnancy with and without various forms of contraception. If a client is having sexual intercourse or planning to in the near future, asking them directly "Do you want to get pregnant?" often is the best way to undermine the invincibility many young clients feel regarding sexual behavior. Using visual aids, videos, or other tools to clearly illustrate the risk of getting pregnant will likely be more effective than listing types of birth control methods and numbers. A useful handout from the CDC can be accessed at www.cdc.gov/reproductivehealth/unintendedpregnancy/pdf/contraceptive_methods_508.pdf. Furthermore, discussing the client's preferences and values regarding contraception is critical to ensuring appropriate compliance. Counseling should not be coercive and using a counseling style that walks the client through her decision-making may be helpful. Shared decision-making is ideal for preference-sensitive decisions such as contraceptive method. Decision aids are tools (e.g., written, videos, or digital) that have been shown to facilitate shared decision-making and are often easily accessible for clients (Witkop et al., 2021).

Long-acting reversible contraception (LARC) should be first-line methods of birth control for sexually active adolescents, whether nulliparous or parous (Adams Hillard, 2013). This includes both intrauterine devices (IUDs) and implants. When appropriately counseled, young women will choose LARC methods over short-acting contraception, as demonstrated in the prospective CHOICE study in which 62% of adolescents chose LARC methods (63% of the 14- to 17-year-olds chose the implant and 71% of the 18- to 20-year-olds chose an IUD; Mestad et al., 2011). Healthcare providers who do not insert IUDs and/or implants should ensure that information is readily available regarding referral to another provider who does. For healthcare providers who insert IUDs but are less experienced with providing this service to nulliparous clients, especially adolescents, tips regarding counseling, preprocedure preparation, and insertion are available (ACOG, 2018a; Adams Hillard, 2013). All five IUDs currently available on the market (Paragard, Mirena, Liletta, Kyleena, and Skyla) can be inserted without concern into a nulliparous uterus. Which option is best for an individual client requires shared decision-making, so the client's concerns and preferences play a role. If LARCs are not desired by the client, combined oral contraceptive pills, the weekly patch, or the vaginal contraceptive ring (placed every 3 weeks) are all effective options for the adolescent, and the type depends on client preference for dosing.

It is important for adolescents to understand that (excluding the copper IUD) contraception is not immediately effective and a backup form of birth control (e.g., condoms) must be used for the 7 days following the initiation of any method. Adolescents should be informed on the availability of emergency contraception (e.g., levonorgestrel pill, ulipristal acetate, and the copper IUD) and their administration restrictions. Adolescents must also understand that contraception does not protect them against the acquisition of STIs and the clinician should encourage them to use condoms for any new partners or partners who partake in risky sexual behaviors. Barrier methods should be highly encouraged for STI prevention.

Adolescent decision-making regarding sexual behavior, contraceptive use, acquisition of STIs, and pregnancy have lifelong impacts on young women's health, as well as that of their families and communities. Ginsburg (2007) emphasized that providers of adolescent healthcare services must balance the identification of risky behaviors with the promotion of the independence that teens crave. Both motivational interviewing and shared decision-making are approaches that might resonate with an adolescent struggling with decisions that affect reproductive health. Healthcare providers can support risk reduction if there is an integration of health promotion, resiliency, and positive youth development during the adolescent health visit.

GUIDELINES FOR HEALTH PROMOTION

Other topics of particular concern in young women's health are nutrition, dieting behaviors, eating disorders, mental health, and substance abuse.

Nutrition

Adolescence places new demands on the nutritional status and emerging body image of developing young women. The body has increased demand for calories, protein, calcium, iron, zinc, vitamin C, and folic acid. Normal adolescent eating patterns are a challenge to evaluate, and in contrast to childhood, teens have more meals independent of the family, often skip breakfast, eat frequent snacks, and increase their consumption of convenience foods.

Eating habits established during the new independence of adolescence are linked with lifelong eating behaviors and may contribute to future health status (Jenkins & Horner, 2005). Food availability and security, family socioeconomic status, and media advertising also play roles in determining food preferences and healthy eating (Taylor et al., 2005). A prospective study of 4,746 adolescents revealed socioeconomic status, family meal frequency, home availability of healthy food, and maternal, paternal, and peer support for healthy eating were positively associated with vegetable and fruit food patterns, and inversely associated with a fast food pattern of eating (Cutler et al., 2011).

Young women are at particular risk for establishing distorted eating patterns during periods of marked change, especially during the transitions of late adolescence. Eating disorders are included in the *Diagnostic and Statistical Manual of Mental Disorders* (5th ed.; *DSM-5*) and include anorexia nervosa, bulimia nervosa, and binge eating disorder (American Psychiatric Association [APA], 2013). The care of young women with disordered eating requires a team of professionals working in collaboration to support the adolescent, her family, and the complex demands of her physical and emotional health.

Overweight and obesity are common issues for young women, have serious implications for long-term health, and have multifactorial etiologies. The CDC (2015) recommends that all children and adolescents participate in physical activity for at least 60 minutes per day. However, as adolescent girls grow older, they are less likely to participate in vigorous physical activity or participate in school-based physical education. In a North Carolina study of eighth grade girls, evaluated again in the ninth and 12th grades, a drop from 45% to 34% participation in vigorous exercise over the 4 years was identified. The results also note that eighth grade participation in exercise was predictive of 12th grade exercise patterns (Pate et al., 2007). Childhood and early adolescence must be the target of efforts to increase physical activity throughout adolescence and extending into adulthood.

Substance Use and Abuse

This chapter addresses alcohol and substance abuse in the context of peer, family, and community influences on adolescents. Individual substance use is best understood as a continuum: abstinence, experimental use, regular use, problem use, substance abuse, substance dependency, and secondary abstinence as part of recovery (Knight et al., 1999). Alcohol use among teenage girls is problematic, and prevalence is significantly higher than their male counterparts. The 2019 YRBSS survey revealed that 31.9% of high school females reported current alcohol consumption and 14.6% reported binge drinking (four or more drinks in a row) on at least 1 day in the 30 days before the survey (C. M. Jones et al.,

2020). In addition to the increased risk of addiction, when alcohol is consumed during the adolescent years, it has been shown that teens who use tobacco, alcohol, marijuana, or other drugs are more likely to engage in risky sexual behavior and to have unwanted consequences of sex, such as STIs and unintended pregnancy, than teens who do not use those substances (Garofoli, 2020). Another study showed that women who engage in preconception binge drinking are more likely to have an unplanned pregnancy and to use alcohol and tobacco during pregnancy (Naimi et al., 2003).

In terms of drug use, 20.8% of female teens reported current marijuana use in the most recent YRBSS survey (one or more times in the 30 days before the survey; C. M. Jones et al., 2020). The prevalence of other substance use indicated that asking adolescent clients about substance use during the confidential portion of the health visit is an important part of the health history.

The CRAFFT screening tool developed by Knight et al. (1999) was designed specifically for adolescents and has been validated repeatedly in many different contexts (Connery et al., 2014; see Box 8.2). Other advantages of the CRAFFT tool are its free public access; brevity (2 to 3 minutes to complete); availability in many languages; good positive and negative predictive probability for alcohol and drug use, abuse, and dependence; and 74% sensitivity and 96% specificity. A computerized version is validated and can simplify administration (Connery et al., 2014; Knight et al., 2007). CRAFFT questions are intended for use in developing a partnership with the adolescent and in forming an alliance for future health promotion. Two or more positive answers suggest a significant problem with alcohol or other drugs and necessitate further evaluation. For example, one study has demonstrated its effectiveness in detecting preconception substance use in pregnant young women 17 to 25 years of age (Chang et al., 2011).

Box 8.2 CRAFFT Questions

C Have you ever ridden in a **c**ar driven by someone (including yourself) who was high or had been using alcohol or drugs?

R Do you ever use alcohol or drugs to **r**elax, feel better about yourself, or fit in?

A Do you ever use alcohol or drugs while you are by yourself, **a**lone?

F Do you ever **f**orget things you did while using alcohol or drugs?

F Do your family or **f**riends ever tell you that you should cut down on your drinking or drug use?

T Have you ever gotten into **t**rouble while you were using alcohol or drugs?

Source: Knight, J. R., Shrier, L. A., Bravender, T. D., Farrell, M., Vander Bilt, J., & Shaffer, H. J. (1999). A new brief screen for adolescent substance abuse. Archives of Pediatrics & Adolescent Medicine, 153(6), 591–596. *https://doi .org/10.1001/archpedi.153.6.591*

TOBACCO USE

One disadvantage of the CRAFFT tool is that it does not screen for use of tobacco products. Tobacco use by teens in all age groups had been declining since its peak in the late 1990s and current use of cigarettes (4.9%), cigars (3.8%), and smokeless tobacco (1.6%) among females is at the lowest levels since the YRBSS began (Creamer et al., 2020). This may be the result of legislation to reduce access to tobacco and restrict smoking in public places, of relatively high taxation of tobacco products, and of social marketing campaigns aimed at youth (Evans et al., 2004). However, newer forms of tobacco delivery are becoming more prevalent among teens with the 2019 YRBSS demonstrating that 40% had ever tried smoking and 33.5% of high school females were considered current users of electronic vapor products (used on at least 1 day during the 30 days before the survey; Creamer et al., 2020). An appropriate screening technique is to ask if the adolescent ever used cigarettes, other tobacco products, e-cigarettes, and other vaping methods (e.g., hookah), followed by an attempt at quantification (Connery et al., 2014).

Prevention of initiation is the ideal, and the U.S. Preventive Services Task Force (USPSTF) recommended in 2020 that healthcare providers provide interventions, including education or brief counseling, to prevent initiation of tobacco use among school-age children and adolescents (USPSTF, 2020b).

Mental Health

Mental health screening and treatment are integral components in the care of adolescent girls. Women are more likely to experience depression across the life span and, during adolescence, are particularly vulnerable (Garber, 2006). In an examination of gender differences in coping styles by Tamres et al. (2022) depressed young women were more likely to utilize ruminating and emotion-focused coping versus problem-focused and distractive coping skills. Studies have estimated anywhere from one tenth to one half of young adults have been diagnosed with a mental health condition (Lawrence et al., 2009). The most common diagnoses in the female adolescent population are anxiety and depression. There continue to be health disparities in access to quality mental health services based on race/ethnicity, geography, socioeconomic status, and insurance coverage (Children's Defense Fund, 2003).

Suicide is the third leading cause of death nationally, and in many states, it is the second cause of death among adolescents. Suicide screening and prevention are recommended as part of healthcare for all adolescents. Suicidality is multifaceted and continues to be investigated to provide insights into adolescent mental health and suffering. It is difficult to estimate the prevalence of current clinical diagnoses of mental disorders in adolescents and the impairment of those diagnosed. However, suicidal behavior among adolescents is a significant public health problem and is more prevalent among female teenagers than males (Ivey-Stephenson et al., 2020). Young men typically choose more lethal methods in suicide, such as firearms, hanging, and motor vehicles, resulting in more deaths. Young women tend to choose medication or overdosing; these methods are usually not immediate and allow for help to arrive or be sought. During the 12 months before the 2019 YRBSS, 24.1% of females reported seriously considering attempting suicide, and 11.0% reported having attempted to commit suicide in the 12 months before the survey (Ivey-Stephenson et al., 2020). Of females who identify as LGB, 49% reported seriously considering suicide and 23.6% reported having attempted suicide (Johns et al., 2020). Although rates of seriously considering suicide are similar among all race/ethnicities (22.7% of Hispanic girls, 23.7% of Black non-Hispanic girls, and 24.3% of White non-Hispanic girls), Black non-Hispanic girls have attempted suicide at higher rates (15.2%) than Hispanic (11.9%) and White (9.4%) women (Ivey-Stephenson et al., 2020). Furthermore, there are disparities in receipt of counseling that may be related to access and cultural differences that may prevent even those who have access to mental healthcare from receiving effective, culturally competent care without language barriers (Center for Health and Health Care in Schools, 2023). Healthcare providers can work within their system and with the community to help facilitate "meaningful access" for immigrants and other adolescents.

Finally, bullying is a growing issue for adolescents. In particular, female adolescents are more likely to be victims of cyberbullying than their male counterparts. In 2019, 30.2% of females reported having been bullied in the 12 months before the survey, higher among White than Black non-Hispanic or Hispanic females and higher among those who identify as LGB than those who identify as heterosexual (Basile et al., 2020). Being a victim of bullying puts adolescents at increased risk of depression, anxiety, and suicide. Asking the client about any experiences with bullying, whether physical, verbal, or electronic, is an important part of the adolescent history.

THE PHYSICAL EXAMINATION AND LABORATORY SCREENING

The physical examination is a small, but often important, component of the overall assessment of the adolescent client. *Bright Futures* recommendations (Hagen et al., 2017) include a physical examination for each health supervision visit. The physical examination includes weight, height, BMI, blood pressure, a complete physical examination including dental screening, sexual maturity rating/Tanner staging, and other components to investigate concerning symptoms such as evidence of hirsutism. Vision and hearing screening questions should be completed during each preventive care visit. Vision testing is recommended during each phase of adolescence: early, middle, and late (Hagen et al., 2017). Audiometry is performed based on risk assessment.

Pelvic Exam

The pelvic exam is no longer an essential part of every young woman's annual examination. With the advent of urine-based sexually transmitted disease and STI screening and the consensus on national cervical screening guidelines, adolescents obtain pelvic examinations based only on risk factors. An internal pelvic examination is generally unnecessary during the first reproductive health visit, but when indicated, the first pelvic examination is an excellent opportunity for health promotion and education about the female body. Providing a clear explanation about the equipment and the procedure, allowing time for the young client to ask questions, and allowing a friend or family member to be present if desired will reduce anxiety and increase cooperation. The client's developmental status, hymenal opening, and sexual experience should guide the selection of speculum, but generally a Pederson speculum (⅞ inch wide by 4 inches long) or Huffman speculum (½ inch wide by 4¼ inch long) is appropriate (ACOG, 2020c). Application of pressure with a single finger to the perineal area may lessen the sensation of the speculum being inserted and may be especially useful for the client who is not yet sexually active (Sanfilippo & Lara-Torre, 2009). Asking the client if has used tampons can assist the provider in determining how comfortable she is with the exam and an estimation of the hymenal opening. Occasionally, during the first pelvic exam, the provider may come across a client with an imperforate hymen, which will need to be addressed. Creating a positive experience for the adolescent's first pelvic exam provides the foundation for future preventive gynecologic care. It is also an investment in developing a respectful partnership with the young client.

Screening for Sexually Transmitted Infections

All young clients who are sexually active (with males, females, or both) must be screened for STIs. Most major organizations recommend screening sexually active young clients age 24 years or younger annually for chlamydia infection and gonorrhea (ACOG, 2020c; USPSTF, 2021). This test can be completed with a vaginal swab (by client or by provider), cervical swab, or urine testing using the nucleic acid amplification technique, which may be the most acceptable option to the client. In September 2006, the CDC released recommendations for HIV testing of adults, adolescents, and pregnant women, advising routine HIV screening of all adolescents in healthcare settings in the United States (Branson et al., 2006). In 2019, the USPSTF released its updated recommendations on screening for HIV, recommending that all adolescents age 15 years and older (and younger adolescents who are at increased risk) be screened for HIV and that all pregnant clients, including those who present in labor or at delivery whose HIV status is unknown, be screened (USPSTF, 2019). A one-time screening is recommended, followed by repeated screening for those at increased risk, those engaged in risky behaviors, or those who live in a high-prevalence setting. Syphilis screening is recommended for pregnant adolescents and high-risk youth, including those who have multiple partners; do not use a condom or barrier method; exchange sex for drugs, money, or services; have spent time in jail or detention; are homeless; use intravenous drugs; or have been diagnosed with another STI (CDC, 2015). Finally, nonjudgmental, risk-reduction counseling appropriate to the individual's developmental age should be provided. This should include counseling about risky behaviors that increase the acquisition of STIs and evidence-based prevention strategies (including abstinence, reduction in numbers of partners, correct condom use; CDC, 2015). The USPSTF also recommends high-intensity behavioral counseling for all sexually active adolescents to prevent STIs (USPSTF, 2020a). Often videos, MI, or other information involving multimedia or social marketing may be more effective.

Immunizations

Immunizations are an essential and changing part of adolescent preventive healthcare services. The CDC Advisory Committee on Immunization Practices (ACIP) currently recommends several vaccines for young adolescents age 11 to 12 years:

- Tetanus-diphtheria-acellular pertussis (Tdap) vaccine
- Meningococcal conjugate vaccine
- Human papillomavirus (HPV) vaccine

See Chapter 32, Human Papillomavirus, for further discussion regarding HPV vaccines. The HPV vaccine, bivalent, quadrivalent, or 9-valent, is recommended routinely for females age 13 to 26 years who have not yet received all doses or completed the vaccination series. Concerns about change in sexual behavior after receiving HPV vaccine have not been substantiated in the literature (CDC, 2015).

It is recommended that all adolescents, if not previously immunized, receive the following vaccinations (CDC, 2023):

- Hepatitis B series
- Hepatitis A series
- HPV
- Polio series
- Measles–mumps–rubella series
- Meningococcal conjugate (MenACWY), with booster at age 16
- Serogroup B meningococcal (MenB) vaccine at age 16–18
- Tdap
- Varicella (chickenpox) series (A second catch-up shot is recommended for adolescents who have previously received only one dose and have no history of chickenpox infection.)

Influenza vaccine is recommended annually, and pneumococcal polysaccharide vaccine is also recommended for certain adolescents with special health conditions.

Two doses of COVID-19 vaccines are recommended for all adolescents, with more doses recommended for some clients based on medical conditions, and boosters available to most clients. ACIP immunization recommendations are reviewed annually because vaccine-preventable diseases or conditions are identified and vaccine schedules change. The CDC maintains up-to-date immunization schedules at www.cdc.gov/vaccines/schedules/index.html.

COVID-19

To control the spread of COVID-19, governments around the world implemented social distancing, mask mandates, and school closures, all of which have impacted the mental health of the U.S. adolescent population. Magson et al. (2021) evaluated the impact of the pandemic on the adolescent population and found that those surveyed had increased depression, anxiety, and decreased quality of life scores. In addition, some children may express more social anxiety as they navigate the process of being reintroduced into social settings in and outside of school (Morrissette, 2021). To help adolescents manage their stress, providers can encourage clients to (1) continue behaviors that help prevent the spread of coronavirus (wash hands, wear a mask, social distance), (2) get vaccinated, (3) complete activities that encourage relaxation (e.g. exercise, meditation, reading), (4) avoid alcohol and drugs, and (5) seek counselling if necessary (Organisation for Economic Co-operation and Development, 2021).

Final Discussion With the Client

Having another discussion with the client and her parent (after any confidential issues were discussed in the exam room or when with the client and/or parent alone) will allow the healthcare provider to discuss the findings of the examination, develop a plan, and answer any additional questions.

The healthcare provider should fully understand and respect any information confidentially shared by the client as well as any that she would like to share with her parent. Acting as a liaison between the adolescent and the parent can sometimes be helpful if the client has provided permission to do so with confidential issues. Clearly, adolescence is a time of great transition for the young woman seeking care. The visit may be more challenging than providing healthcare for women at other times in their life, yet the healthcare provider also has a tremendous opportunity to help set the young woman on a trajectory for healthy behaviors and well-being for the rest of her life.

REFERENCES

References for this chapter are online and available at https://connect.springerpub.com/content/book/978-0-8261-6722-4/part/part02/chapter/ch08

CHAPTER 9

Midlife Women's Health*

IVY M. ALEXANDER, ANNETTE JAKUBISIN-KONICKI, JESSICA L. PALOZIE, AMANDA M. SWAN, CHRISTINE ALEXANDRA BOTTONE, AND RUBBY KOOMSON

MIDLIFE: DEFINITIONS, PERCEPTIONS, AND TRANSITIONS

Midlife women account for a growing proportion of the U.S. population. Only recently have researchers and clinicians devoted attention to midlife women's health concerns. There is a dearth of data available regarding care for other minoritized gender persons at midlife—including transgender men and women, nonbinary persons, and the greater LGBQ community. During the past several decades, there has been increasing interest in the transition to postmenopause (TPM) as a central feature in the lives of those who identify as women. Although the TPM had been a neglected topic, the changing focus of research about midlife has provided important new evidence about the transitions in women's bodies that are intertwined with the transitions in their lives. The purposes of this chapter are to (a) define and summarize evidence about women's experiences and perceptions of midlife and those of other minoritized gender persons when available; (b) review current understanding of the biological changes associated with midlife, with a special emphasis on the TPM; (c) characterize symptoms experienced (hot flashes, sleep disruption, mood changes, cognitive changes, pain, and sexual desire changes) and their correlates during the TPM and postmenopause (PM); (d) explore the relationship of the TPM to healthy aging; and (e) propose a program of health promotion and prevention for midlife women.

In this chapter, the terms woman and women are used when describing biological changes to include both cisgender females and those born with female sex organs even if they do not identify as female. Limitations in language are acknowledged. Given the limited data available that address midlife experiences among other minoritized gender persons, the terms woman and women are used to describe research that has provided guidance to caring for women at midlife.

Midlife can be defined in a variety of ways, often by using age boundaries, such as 35 to 65 years, to differentiate midlife from younger and older adulthood. Alternatively, definitions can be based on reproductive aging stages using indicators of menstrual cycle changes or hormonal changes. Women's changing role patterns, using indicators such as a child leaving home or a woman's return to the workplace to designate the beginning of midlife, provides another option, and using women's own perceptions about whether they are in the middle of their lives provides yet another option. Brooks-Gunn and Kirsh (1984) stressed the multidimensional and multidirectional nature of change in midlife, describing the boundaries as fluid and constructed by the society and the individual rather than being determined by chronological age. This has not changed.

Whatever the markers for midlife might be, understanding the context in which women experience midlife is extremely important. Anticipation of midlife by each woman's age cohort (women born at the same time), as well as socialization by other women about what to expect during midlife, contribute to the framework with which women and others view and interpret the events of midlife. Both anticipated and actual midlife experiences can influence a person's notions of health.

Meanings of Midlife

Midlife women from different birth cohorts, those born during different eras, have lived in different worlds (Bernard, 1981); thus, it is important to locate women's midlife experiences within the sociopolitical and historical context in which they occur. Contemporary midlife women were born in the late 1950s to 1980s, which represents at least three birth cohorts, who have had very different lives. The cohorts represent a generational divide as well; midlife people today include members of the later part of the baby boomer generation in addition to Generation X and the millennial generation. Persons experiencing midlife today

---

*This chapter is a revision of the chapter that appeared in the second edition of this textbook, coauthored by Nancy Fugate Woods, Judith Berg, and Ellen Sullivan Mitchell, and we thank them for their original contribution.

should be considered in the context of their own sociopolitical and historical experiences, which varies by experienced social events, history, political milieu, and personal experience of these.

The perceptions and experiences of baby boomer women during their middle years are likely to reflect dramatic changes in their life course. Gilligan (1982a) proposed restoring the missing text of women's development for this cohort rather than simply replacing it with work about men's development. She saw women's middle years as a risky time because of women's embeddedness in relationships, their orientation to interdependence, their ability to subordinate achievement to care, and their conflicts over competitive success. If midlife brings an end to relationships and, with them, a sense of connection for women, then midlife may be a time of despair. Gilligan stressed that the meaning of midlife events for women is contextual, arising from the interaction between the structures of women's thought and the realities of their lives. Women approach midlife with a different history than do men, and they face a different social reality with different possibilities for love and work (Gilligan, 1982a, 1982b).

Gilligan's perspective that midlife may be a time of despair explains, in part, increases in substance use for some individuals as they attempt to cope with the transition in relation to society's trends and demands. Aging women face both an increase and a change in challenges, which reflects today's more complex society. These challenges are clear in midlife, and the attempt to cope with the transitional despair of the aging process itself, in hopes of discerning a sense of individual meaning and purpose, is reflected in increased rates of substance misuse by today's midlife women (Sarabia & Martin, 2016). Baby boomers are also more vulnerable to resuming prior substance use and even increasing their substance use in the midlife stage (Duncan et al., 2010). Resumed and increased use is thought to relate to the higher rate of substance use among baby boomers in their formative years, when compared to prior generations (Duncan et al., 2010; Patterson & Jeste, 1999). However, this increase can also be explained by current trends and an emerging cultural shift in this group's attitude toward substance use. Policy changes increasing legalization of marijuana have made marijuana more accessible and affordable and have mitigated some stigma midlife women may face surrounding use.

Prescription drug misuse is also a rising concern among midlife women. Healthcare providers are more likely to prescribe mood-altering substances to aging women than any other gender or age group (Blow & Barry, 2012). Since 1992, prescription drug overdoses have tripled (Centers for Disease Control and Prevention [CDC], 2011). This is of vital concern. Societal issues faced by contemporary midlife women are novel. A cultural shift in attitudes, coupled with society's ever-increasing complexity, further complicates the aging process.

Taking this into account, the context in which the midlife woman perceives herself as an individual, in relation to her changing role and to society, deeply affects her meaning of health and well-being and the midlife transition. In this notion, a study of nearly 500 midlife women (35–60 years old in 1986) by the Society for Research on Women in New Zealand (1988) indicated that 80% to 90% had positive attitudes

about life, more than 80% had positive attitudes toward their physical appearance and health, and 80% were positive about their futures. Only 14% were unhappy with their daily lives. One third of women reported some stress in their relationships with husbands or partners, such as unemployment, illness, work demands, or finances. Women's experiences with their children were a function of their ages: Of the 35- to 40-year-olds, two thirds found their children stressful, and of the 50- to 60-year-olds, two thirds rated their children not at all stressful.

While women are experiencing the social transitions associated with parenting responsibilities, they are also experiencing the aging of their bodies. In a series of interviews with a convenience sample of midlife women, Coney (1994) found that signs of aging, such as wrinkles and weight gain, produced grief in some women and no concern in others. Reflections of others' perceptions of aging that included sexist and ageist stereotypes about women, frequently reinforced by mass media, caused some women to be worried about their physical aging. Others were more worried about loss of physical abilities, such as hearing, eyesight, and mobility, and loss of mental powers. Still others felt panicky and negative because they sensed that time was running out for them. The "empty nest" had both positive and negative associations for many of the women Coney studied. Despite negative attitudes toward menopause and aging, and despite inequities in employment and financial security, midlife women had surprisingly high perceptions of well-being. They expressed having had achievements and gaining maturity, experience, and confidence that younger women do not have, as well as knowing what they can do. Having attained some seniority in employment and having launched their children, many women felt freer to concentrate on themselves and decide what they want for the next third of their lives. More secure in their own opinions and beliefs and less afraid of expressing them, the midlife women Coney studied emphasized increasing freedom.

Participants in the Seattle Midlife Women's Health Study (SMWHS)—begun in 1990, when the women were 35 to 55 years of age—responded to these questions: What does "midlife" mean? What events of midlife do women believe are important? Distressing? Satisfying? A particular emphasis of this investigation was to determine whether menopause figured prominently in women's experiences of this part of the life span. Participants' most common image of midlife was getting older (Woods & Mitchell, 1997b). Their emphasis on defining midlife as an age and aging process is consistent with findings from older cohorts of women (Rossi, 1985; Rubin, 1979) and is not surprising, given the youthful value orientation of U.S. society. These women also associated changes of every kind with midlife. They alluded to transitions with respect to their physical bodies, emotions, feelings about being older, outlook on life, relationships, and "change of life." A few referred to their changing health and vulnerability. Given the prevalence of life changes among this cohort of midlife women, their emphasis on transitions is not surprising. The centrality of personal achievements and employment in the Seattle women's lives stands in striking contrast to data from older birth cohorts of midlife women. The distinction between images of midlife described by older women and those of the women in this study reflect the dramatic changes in lifelong employment patterns women have experienced since the 1970s. The baby boomers did describe trying to figure out what to do with the rest of their lives. They were still juggling the demands of integrating work and family responsibilities. Although emphasis on work-related events and personal goal attainment among this cohort resembled that in studies of men's development (Neugarten, 1968), emphasis on family and health-related events were among those considered most important. Children, spouses, and parents were mentioned frequently as women described the important events of midlife.

Participants in the SMWHS (N = 508), with a median age of 41 years at the beginning of the study, reported a variety of stressful or distressing events, which included health problems, deaths, family problems, work-related problems, frustrated goal attainment, and financial problems (Woods & Mitchell, 1997b). Women reported distressing health problems, including their own and those of their parents, with similar frequency. Deaths were also commonly cited as the most distressing event and included the deaths of parents, in-laws, and husbands. Family problems also involved adolescent children, domestic violence, divorce or separation from a spouse, and the ending of relationships. Work problems, including inability to find work, workplace conflicts, and downsizing of workplaces, were also mentioned frequently. Frustrated goal attainment included events such as being unable to finish an academic program on time or having personal time while working on an academic program. Women's financial events included problems such as inability to pay college tuition for a child or afford essentials. When asked to look back over the past 15 years of their study participation and describe the most challenging aspects of their lives, midlife women indicated that most of these events were salient, but only one woman identified menopause as most challenging.

Not surprisingly, the Seattle women's images of midlife and the events they found most important and most stressful reflected their engagement in a broader, more complex world than that of their mothers. No longer focusing only on their roles as mothers and homemakers, contemporary midlife women are attempting to balance the demands of workplace and home, and this is reflected in how they characterized the best and worst of midlife. This sample of midlife women talked freely of their multidimensional selves and the social circumstances that necessitated their viewing themselves differently from their mothers' generation.

A new emphasis on women's preparation for their own aging is evident in both professional and public literature. Sarah Lawrence-Lightfoot (2009) uses the term *third chapter* to designate those years when one is neither old nor young, emphasizing the possibility that these years can be the most transformative time in life. Having courage to challenge ageist stereotypes and creativity to resist old cultural norms (about aging and gender) in combination with curiosity to learn and a spirit of adventure to pursue new passions and experiences are core elements of how one creates the third chapter. In her case studies, Lawrence-Lightfoot explores the themes of engagement over retreat, labor over leisure, and reinvention over retirement, emphasizing the elements of active engagement, purposefulness, and new learning as themes in the life stories that people write about the third chapter of their lives. Indeed, she emphasizes the power of our stories—new narratives or several narratives—to serve as our maps through this third chapter. Often this period becomes a time of public service and growing toward a new direction. In many ways Lawrence-Lightfoot finds this third chapter as a prime time in life.

In *Composing a Further Life*, Mary Catherine Bateson (2010) introduces a modification to Erik Erickson's model of human development by splitting adulthood into two phases: Adulthood 1 includes the challenge of generation versus stagnation, resulting in the strength of care, and Adulthood 2 addresses engagement versus withdrawal, resulting in active wisdom. Bateson's discussion of lifelong learning as part of the developmental processes includes the achievement of receptive wisdom and humility as one resolves the challenges of old age.

Both Lawrence-Lightfoot and Bateson invite us to consider midlife as a period in which we can actively compose a life story or a set of possible stories into which we can live as we age. This theme of creation of our own maps for aging suggests that some of the developmental tasks included in earlier theories need to be revised to accommodate the lengthening life span and women's aspirations for that additional time in one's life.

Contemporary midlife women described midlife similarly to women from earlier birth cohorts with important exceptions, one being the centrality of work and personal achievement in their lives. As women's roles have changed, so have the experiences that women count as important. Personal achievement and work-related events have assumed a central place, along with family events, in how women describe their lives. Another exception unique to contemporary midlife is the increased awareness of inequalities in the structure of today's society. Midlife women are more conscious of inequalities seen in today's social hierarchies as well as other axes of inequalities (e.g., gender, class, race) compared to their predecessors, and are aware of how such inequalities influence health and longevity (Homan, 2019).

Although women have seen significant improvement over the last century in terms of new growth and opportunities for women, gender inequality remains. As an example, the U.S. Department of Labor's research on current trends shows that not only does a gender-wage-gap continue to exist today, this gender-wage gap increases as women age (U.S. Department of Labor, 2017).

Most recently, the unforeseen and ongoing COVID-19 pandemic, first appearing in 2020, has further widened gender gaps in various ways (Al-Rawi et al., 2021; Wenham et al., 2020). For one, community- and state-wide closures resulted in increased caregiving responsibilities for working parents and diminished employment opportunities, even more so for women who were "nonessential" workers (Collins et al., 2020; Wenham et al., 2020). Women also were more highly represented in sectors that laid off employees. The pandemic, as a global health emergency, caused contemporary midlife women to see a limit and disruption to sexual and reproductive health services (Wenham et al., 2020).

The COVID-19 pandemic widened the gender equality gap. Working mothers reduced work hours four to five times more than working fathers from February 2020 to April 2020. The gender gap in working hours has continued to grow an estimated 20% to 50% (Collins et al., 2020). Such negative consequences highlight challenges already seen among contemporary midlife women; the COVID-19 pandemic continues to only amplify challenges women face today (Collins et al., 2020).

With a life course that is made more complex than their mothers' by lifelong employment, contemporary midlife women are not wondering what to do with the rest of their lives as much as they are wondering how to juggle the demands of family- and work-related responsibilities. Meaning in midlife within this age group has also been redefined, separate from prior generations, to consider new conditions and challenges seen following the onset of the COVID-19 pandemic. In addition, many midlife women are anticipating the next stage of their lives and creating the narratives for their own "third chapter."

Midlife as a Transitional Period

Midlife has earned recognition as a period of developmental transition worthy of study. Indeed, an important area of scholarship related to midlife focuses on multiple types of transitions. Transitions have been identified as periods during which change occurs. One can envision midlife as a transitional period between part of the life span during which reproduction and parenting typically occur, occupying a large component of women's lives (see Chapter 8, Young Women's Health), and older adulthood, a period focused on adaptation to aging-related changes and ultimately dying (see Chapter 10, Older Women's Health). During midlife, women experience many types of transitions, including developmental, situational, and health–illness transitions. Although the TPM, the period between the late reproductive years when women have regular menstrual periods and the final menstrual period (FMP), is one that has gained the attention of health professionals, other transitions include changes in marital status and parental roles, which may be more salient to some women than menopause, as well as health–illness transitions to experiencing chronic illness. Transitional periods in life create opportunity for adaptation, and these in turn may lead to either positive or negative changes in health status and well-being. Despite emphasis on the negative outcomes of transitions, midlife women experienced well-being during this period (Smith-DiJulio et al., 2008). Moreover, women's estimates of their own mastery and satisfaction with social support during this period were important predictors of their well-being. As anticipated, women who experienced negative life events during this period also experienced lower well-being. Experiencing the TPM had relatively small effects on well-being.

THE TRANSITION TO POSTMENOPAUSE

During the 20th century, the term *menopause* was used to refer to the period around the time of the FMP. Women were described as premenopausal, menopausal, or postmenopausal, without specific reference to the time period denoted. In the health sciences, the term *menopause* is used to refer to the point in time 1 year following the FMP (North American Menopause Society [NAMS], 2019).

The years during which women make the transition to postmenopause and the first few years after the FMP (early PM) hold great fascination and sometimes frustration for the women experiencing them as well as their healthcare providers. When midlife women were asked about what they anticipated menopause would be like, the most prevalent theme was uncertainty and mixed feelings (Woods & Mitchell, 1999). As women anticipate midlife, menopause is one focus of their concerns. Participants in the SMWHS voiced uncertainty about what to expect menopause would be like, and many had no expectations about the experience, revealing a need for education about the TPM and changing biology (Woods & Mitchell, 1999). Indeed, women defined *menopause* as the cessation of menstrual periods, the end of reproductive capacity, a time of hormonal changes, a new or different life stage, a time of symptoms, a time of changing emotions and changing bodies, and part of the aging process. Of interest is that few defined this period of life as a time of disease risk or one necessitating medical care.

Significant progress has been made in understanding the TPM as part of reproductive aging and as it influences women's health during the transition and ultimately their health as they age. Around the globe there have been several longitudinal studies of midlife and the menopausal transition (MT): the Massachusetts Women's Health Study (MWHS; McKinlay et al., 1992), the Study of Women's Health Across the Nation (SWAN; Sowers et al., 2000), the Melbourne Midlife Women's Health Project (Dennerstein et al., 2000), the Penn Ovarian Aging Study (Freeman et al., 2001), and the SMWHS (Woods & Mitchell, 1997a). Taken together, the results of these studies have contributed to understanding the biological changes that occur during the MT and PM, symptoms women experience, and the influence of the TPM on healthy aging.

How various U.S. ethnic groups of women define menopause (as used in the popular culture to mean the experiences around the time of the FMP) was unknown until the efforts of investigators for SWAN (Sowers et al., 2000). Results from the multisite study of multiple U.S. ethnic groups indicate widespread differences in women's expectations and experiences as well as areas of similarity across groups. Urban Latina women stressed the primacy of health and the importance of harmony and balance in their lives. They described menopause as *el cambio de vida*—a change of life you have to go through. They also stressed that "this time is for me," referring to reorienting and restructuring their lives (Villarruel et al., 2002). Conceptions among Japanese American and European American women differed. Change in self-focus, self-satisfaction, and ability to reprioritize values accompanied the transition to menopause. Japanese American women described a metamorphosis from motherhood to nurturing, becoming a more complete human being (Kagawa-Singer et al., 2002). Black American women's conceptions of menopause emphasized midlife as a period of developmental changes. They recognized their personal mortality, changing family relationships, and increasing authenticity, reevaluating life experiences, setting new goals for personal growth, and experiencing greater self-esteem. They emphasized increased self-acceptance and productivity (Sampselle et al., 2002). Chinese American and Chinese women's conceptions of menopause were inextricably bound with meanings of midlife. For this group, the borders and timing of the TPM are ambiguous. The TPM represents a natural progression through the life cycle.

Interestingly, expectations of women who have not yet experienced their FMP did not match the experiences of women who had. The TPM was viewed as a marker for aging. Women believe that it is important to prepare for and manage the MT (Adler et al., 2000), but this belief exists in the context of a lack of access to information and uncertainty about the process.

CHANGING BIOLOGY: THE TRANSITION TO POSTMENOPAUSE AND BEYOND

During the first 2 decades of the 21st century, efforts to predict the events of the TPM culminated in the creation of a model for staging reproductive aging. As part of this effort, researchers and clinicians proposed and continue to test criteria that women and clinicians can use to anticipate the onset of the TPM and PM. Figure 9.1 presents a model focusing on late reproductive aging through early PM adapted from the Staging Reproductive Aging Workshop + 10 (STRAW+10) held in 2012. The first STRAW workshop was held 10 years earlier (Soules et al., 2001). The STRAW+10 model is oriented around the FMP (represented as time point 0), with the period immediately preceding the FMP labeled the TPM and the period immediately following the FMP labeled the PM. The period that precedes the TPM is referred to as the reproductive stage and begins with menarche. Criteria used to denote the stages in the STRAW+10 model have been validated using data from several longitudinal studies.

STRAW+10 participants divided the reproductive stage into three parts—early, peak, and late—corresponding to women's experience of fertility. The late reproductive stage (stage −3a, just before the TPM), is characterized by rising follicle-stimulating hormone (FSH) levels and regular menstrual cycle length but may include some subtle changes in flow and length of bleeding. Figures 9.2 to 9.4 illustrate the late reproductive and early and late TPM stages as indicated by women's menstrual calendars completed by participants in the SMWHS.

STRAW criteria for staging the TPM were validated by the RESTAGE collaboration that compared results from several longitudinal studies of women's menstrual cycles as they approached the FMP (Harlow et al., 2006). The TPM is divided into two stages: early (−2) and late (−1). The beginning of the early TPM is the beginning irregularity of menstrual cycles, with the length of one cycle varying by 7 or more days from the preceding or following cycle. To define the onset of the early TPM stage, irregularity was observed to repeat itself at least once during the next 10 bleeding segments (Harlow et al., 2008).

The onset of the late TPM is denoted by amenorrhea of 60 or more days (Harlow et al., 2007). One such episode is sufficient to define late TPM for women age 45 years and older. For women younger than 45 years, amenorrhea needs to repeat itself at least once during the next 10 bleeding segments (Taffe et al., 2010).

STRAW+10 participants divided PM into early and late stages, with the early stage spanning the first 6 years after the FMP based on trajectories of FSH and estradiol. Specific attention focused on the year after the FMP (+1a) and the year after that (+1b), when endocrine changes stabilized. During the last 3 to 6 years of early PM (stage +1c), FSH and estradiol continue to stabilize. Late PM (+2) represents the period during which processes of somatic aging become paramount. STRAW+10 participants recommended application of these stages regardless of women's age, ethnicity, body mass index, or lifestyle characteristics.

Women's own definitions of the TPM, based on their observations of their own experiences, differ from the detailed staging of reproductive aging presented earlier. Women not only observe vaginal bleeding, as recorded on menstrual calendars, but also frequently report other types of vaginal blood loss such as spotting (bloody discharge that does not require the use of a sanitary product) and longer, heavier episodes of bleeding (menorrhagia or flooding). Such bleeding may occur before, after, and in between episodes of menstrual bleeding and may cause them to worry and seek healthcare. They may define themselves as "in menopause" or "menopausal" based on their bleeding changes, but their definitions may not be consistent with those in the STRAW+10 staging model. *Menopause* is defined as the final day of the FMP. The

STAGE	−3a	−2	−1	+1a	+1b	+1c
Terminology	Late reproductive	Early menopausal transition	Late menopausal transition	Early postmenopause	Early postmenopause	Early postmenopause
Duration	Variable	Variable	1–3 years	1 year	1 year	3–6 years
Menstrual cycle	Subtle changes in amount of flow and length of bleeding	Variable length with persistent difference in consecutive cycles of ≥7 days	Amenorrhea ≥60 days	Amenorrhea	Amenorrhea	Amenorrhea
				Final menstrual period (FMP)		

FIGURE 9.1 Stages of reproductive aging from late reproductive through early postmenopause.
Source: Adapted from STRAW+10.

Seattle Midlife Women's Health Study
University of Washington
School of Nursing

Late reproductive stage = All segment lengths less than 7 days apart
Bleed-free days after spotting are part of bleeding episode

Year __XXXX___   ID NO___XX____

Day	1	2	3	4	5	6	7	8	9	10	11	12	13	14	15	16	17	18	19	20	21	22	23	24	25	26	27	28	29	30	31
JAN								S	S	B	B	B	B	S	S																
FEB			S	S	B	B	B	S																					■	■	■
MAR	S	S	B	B	B	S	S																				S	S	B	B	B
APR	S																							S	S	B	B				■
MAY																			S		S		B	B	B	S					
JUN																		S	B	B	B	S									■
JUL															B	B	B	B	S												
AUG							S		S	B	B	S																			
SEP			S	B	B	B	S	S																							■
OCT		B	B	B	S																					S		B	B	B	B
NOV	S	S	S																					B	B	B	S	S	S		■
DEC																		S	B	B	B	S	S								

For every day you spot or bleed enter an S or B in the appropriate square. Record a 1, 2, 3 or 4 next to every B day.
(1: light flow, 2: moderate, 3: heavy, 4: very heavy/flooding)
For any month no bleeding or spotting occurs write in NO BLEEDING.
If you forget to record for a month write in FORGOT TO RECORD.

FIGURE 9.2 Menstrual calendar for late reproductive stage.
Source: Adapted from Seattle Midlife Women's Health Study data.

end of menstruation is marked by the last menstrual period, said to have occurred after women have not menstruated for 1 calendar year (NAMS, 2019; Soules et al., 2001).

Staging reproductive aging provides a useful framework for women to use in anticipating their progress through the TPM. It is also useful to clinicians in organizing their understanding of the changing biology around the time of menopause (Santoro et al., 2007). Educating women about standardized stages of reproductive aging can help patients and providers to communicate more clearly so that appropriate guidance and interventions can be provided. This first requires that healthcare providers familiarize themselves with models such as STRAW+10.

Reproductive Aging: The Transition to Postmenopause

In the United States, most women experience their FMP during their late 40s or early 50s, with the median age being 51 to 52 years (NAMS, 2019). Although the FMP occurs only once in a woman's lifetime, the natural TPM is a biological process that usually occupies several years of a woman's life, as opposed to being a single occasion (see Table 9.1 for information on ages at and duration of TPM stages based on findings from

the SMWHS). The early stage of the TPM estimated from U.S. women's menstrual bleeding patterns recorded daily on menstrual calendars started during the mid-40s at a median age of 45.5 years for a population of Midwestern White women (Treloar, 1981), at 47.5 years as reported in telephone interviews by participants in the MWHS (McKinlay et al., 1992), and 46.6 years based on menstrual calendars obtained from participants in the SMWHS (Mitchell & Woods, 2007; Mitchell et al., 2000). The beginning of the late stage of TPM occurred at 49.2 years in the SMWHS. The duration of TPM averages 4 to 5 years across the studies but varies widely, with a range of 2 to 7 years and a median of 4.5 years in the Minnesota and 3.5 years in the MWHS samples. The median duration of the early stage was 2.8 years and, for the late stage, 2.3 years in the SMWHS sample (Cray et al. 2012; Mitchell & Woods, 2007).

Researchers are yet to elucidate the reasons for such variation in length of the TPM among women. However, data analyses from the multiethnic SWAN suggests that the duration of TPM may be influenced by the age of onset of TPM; women in SWAN who began their TPM at younger ages had a longer transition (Paramsothy et al., 2017). The same analysis found smoking to be associated with an earlier onset of TPM, but also a shorter overall transition, likely due to the cytotoxic effect of smoking on the ovaries leading to accelerated ovarian aging. Black women had a longer TPM duration

Seattle Midlife Women's Health Study
University of Washington
School of Nursing

Onset Early Menopausal Transition Stage, July 5
Onset = segment lengths 7 or more days apart, repeated within 10 segments
Bleed-free days between bleeding and spotting are part of bleeding episode
No bleeding in November

Year __ XXXX___   ID NO___ XX ____

Day	1	2	3	4	5	6	7	8	9	10	11	12	13	14	15	16	17	18	19	20	21	22	23	24	25	26	27	28	29	30	31
JAN									B	B	B	B																			
FEB			B	B	B	B																							■	■	■
MAR	B	B	B	B																		B	B	B	B						
APR														B	B	B	B			S	S										■
MAY														S	S	B	B	B													
JUN												B	B	B	B	S															■
JUL					S		B	B	B	B																					
AUG						S	B		B	S																					
SEP			B	B	B		B	S																							■
OCT					B	B	B	B	S																				B	B	B
NOV																															■
DEC	B	B	B																										B	B	B

For every day you spot or bleed enter an S or B in the appropriate square. Record a 1, 2, 3 or 4 next to every B day.
(1: light flow, 2: moderate, 3: heavy, 4: very heavy/flooding)
For any month no bleeding or spotting occurs write in NO BLEEDING.
If you forget to record for a month write in FORGOT TO RECORD.

FIGURE 9.3 Menstrual calendar illustrating early menopausal transition stage.
Source: Adapted from Seattle Midlife Women's Health Study data.

than White women. In contrast to earlier studies, the SWAN analysis found that women with higher body mass index (BMI) experienced a later TPM; however, BMI did not significantly influence duration of TPM.

Endocrine Changes During the Transition to Postmenopause and Early Postmenopause

Irregularity of menstrual periods has been used as an indicator of progression through the TPM and is associated with a logarithmic decrease in the number of ovarian follicles as women age. Comparing women aged 45 to 55 years who were menstruating regularly to women having irregular cycles and women who had stopped menstruating, Richardson (1993) found that follicle counts had decreased dramatically among women having irregular cycles and were nearly absent in the postmenopausal group. Although counts of antral follicles are important indicators of ovarian aging, they are not typically used in primary care. Instead, providers often rely on changes in bleeding patterns and cycle regularity as a basis for helping women estimate whether they may be in the TPM and at what stage. This, understandably, poses a problem for those who are

not menstruating due to hysterectomy, ablation, or underlying medical issues that impact menstrual regularity (polycystic ovary syndrome [PCOS], hypothyroidism, hypothalamic amenorrhea, etc.) and in these instances, other symptoms can help to estimate the stage of reproductive aging.

STRAW+10 workshop participants reviewed potential indicators of the TPM and FMP and recommended further research to identify indicators with greatest predictive power and clinical utility (Harlow et al., 2012). The STRAW framework is anchored by changes in menstrual cycle regularity and is useful as a reference point for examining the changes in ovarian (estrogens, progesterone, testosterone, antimüllerian hormone [AMH], and inhibins A and B) and pituitary (FSH and luteinizing hormone [LH]) hormones. Women nearing and those who have experienced their FMP have complex changes in endocrine levels, which are not simply declining or increasing over time. Some women experience very high estrogen levels in response to increases in FSH before their FMP (Santoro et al., 1996). Similarly, accelerated follicular development has been associated with a monotropic rise in FSH in women between 40 and 45 years who were still cycling (Klein et al., 1996). As women neared the end of regular ovulation, their estradiol levels during the early follicular phases were higher and rose earlier in the follicular phase

Seattle Midlife Women's Health Study
University of Washington
School of Nursing

Onset Late Menopausal Transition Stage, September 14 (Age 50)
Onset = Bleed-free days between segment lengths 60 or more days; repeated within 10 segments if younger than 46
Bleed-free days between bleeding and spotting are part of bleeding episode
SS in February = Intermenstrual spotting, not a bleeding episode

Year __ XXXX___   ID NO___ XX ____

Day	1	2	3	4	5	6	7	8	9	10	11	12	13	14	15	16	17	18	19	20	21	22	23	24	25	26	27	28	29	30	31
JAN								B	B	B	B	B		S																	
FEB				B	B	B	S									S	S												■	■	■
MAR																		B	B	B	B	B	S			S					
APR																			S	S	B	S	B		S						■
MAY																		B	B	B	B	B	B	S	S	S	S				
JUN										B	B	B	B	S																	■
JUL																														S	B
AUG	B	B																		S	B	B	B	B	S						
SEP													B	B	B	B	B	S	S			B								■	
OCT																															
NOV																														■	
DEC	B	B	B	B	B	S	S				S																		S	B	B

For every day you spot or bleed enter an S or B in the appropriate square. Record a 1, 2, 3 or 4 next to every B day.
(1: light flow, 2: moderate, 3: heavy, 4: very heavy/flooding)
For any month no bleeding or spotting occurs write in NO BLEEDING.
If you forget to record for a month write in FORGOT TO RECORD.

FIGURE 9.4 Menstrual calendar illustrating late menopausal transition stage.
Source: Adapted from Seattle Midlife Women's Health Study data.

TABLE 9.1 Duration and Age of Onset of Menopausal Transition Stages

	EARLY STAGE				LATE STAGE				POSTMENOPAUSE			
	N	Mean	SD	Range	*N*	Mean	SD	Range	*N*	Mean	SD	Range
Age of onset	121	46.4	3.4	36.6–53.2	130	49.4	2.7	43.1–55.0	114	52.1	2.9	43.7–58.3
Duration (years)	82	2.8	1.5	0.2–6.5	84	2.5	2.7	0.41–7.0	NA	NA	NA	NA

NA, not applicable; SD, standard deviation.
Source: Adapted from unpublished data from Seattle Midlife Women's Health Study data.

than in younger women. As reproductive age advanced, their progesterone levels diminished.

The SWAN, an ongoing multisite longitudinal study of a multiethnic population of U.S. women extending across the TPM, was designed to characterize the physical and psychosocial changes that occur during the time of the TPM and PM and to observe their effects on later risk factors for age-related diseases and health. SWAN investigators collected data from more than 16,000 women between the ages of 40 and 55 years who were screened from 1995 to 1997. Of these women, 3,302 of them who were between 42 and 52 years of age were enrolled in a longitudinal cohort studied by annual visits and other data-collection efforts for up to 25 years of follow-up, and 900 of these women participated in a daily hormone study (DHS). The data being collected in SWAN include ovarian markers, lifestyle and behavior indicators, and markers of cardiovascular and bone health. The results of the SWAN study will continue to make a significant contribution to the understanding of the natural history of the TPM (Sowers et al., 2000). The multiethnic SWAN cohort has allowed investigators to explore the variability of endocrine levels with racial/ethnic groups as well as the stage of the TPM. A complete list of publications that have come from the SWAN cohort can be found at www.swanstudy.org/publications.

SWAN investigators found a period of about 4 years when maximal changes occurred in FSH and estradiol; changes in FSH levels preceded those in estradiol. After this period of maximal changes, both FSH and estradiol levels stabilized (Randolph et al., 2003, 2011). The rise in FSH accelerated 2 years before the FMP, and deceleration began immediately before the FMP and stabilized 2 years after the FMP (Randolph et al., 2011), consistent with the findings of Sowers, Zheng, et al. (2008) and the prior findings of Burger et al. from the Melbourne Midlife Women's Health Project (Burger et al., 1999, 2000, 2002). Estradiol levels did not change until about 2 years before the FMP, when they began decreasing and then dropping maximally at the time of the FMP and decelerating to stability about 2 years after the FMP. In obese persons, the initial acceleration of FSH occurred slightly later (approximately 5.5 years before the FMP) and was limited compared with the levels for those who were not obese (Randolph et al., 2011). A unique component of the SWAN study was the DHS in which Santoro and colleagues found that cycles became anovulatory before the FMP, with declining progesterone levels as ovulation occurred more irregularly or stopped (Santoro et al., 2007). A more recent analysis of SWAN DHS data found that mean menstrual cycle length was preserved at 26 to 27 days in cycles that were estimated to have luteal activity (meaning they were likely to be ovulatory cycles), regardless of the stage of TPM (Santoro et al., 2017). A high percentage of cycles were estimated to have luteal activity up until 5 years before the FMP. Only 22.8% of cycles within 1 year of FMP were estimated to have luteal activity; however, these cycles exhibited hormone excretion patterns that were remarkably similar to those associated with peak fertility. This suggests that risk of unintended pregnancy remains a concern up until the FMP and clinicians should educate patients about this potential and provide options for pregnancy prevention if pregnancy is not desired.

The precise cause of cessation of menses is unknown; many complex hormonal factors contribute and continue to be studied. Estradiol levels drop as ovulation occurs less frequently and FSH rises in response to ovarian signals from inhibins and AMH (Burger et al., 2007; Randolph et al., 2011; Sowers, Zheng, et al., 2008). AMH, produced in growing ovarian follicles, is a direct indicator of ovarian reserve and as such decreases as women approach their FMP. AMH and AMH rate of change have been associated with time to menopause (Freeman et al., 2012; Kim et al., 2017). Finkelstein and colleagues (2020) suggested that an ultrasensitive AMH assay may be a more accurate predictor of time to menopause than FSH; further investigation is needed before wide use in the clinical setting. Inhibin B, produced by small antral follicles, serves to restrain follicular growth, and serum levels can indicate growth of the antral follicle cohort. In the reproductive years, inhibin B helps to maintain a reserve of antral follicles so that large numbers of follicles do not ovulate at once. Inhibin B suppresses FSH secretion by the pituitary and becomes undetectable 4 to 5 years before the FMP (Sowers, Eyvazzadeh, et al., 2008). Dramatic increases in FSH may be responsible for elevated levels of estrogens during the later phase of the TPM, producing hyperestrogenism in some women. Dominant follicles continue to produce estradiol and inhibin A, probably because of the fall in inhibin B, which allows FSH to rise and stimulate the ovary. As ovulation ceases, the levels of inhibin A fall, reflecting the inability of a dominant follicle to develop (Burger et al., 1999, 2000, 2002).

Current evidence indicates that increasing FSH levels are a useful indicator that the FMP is approaching; however, they are not sufficiently specific to diagnose a TPM stage and there is no clear cut point distinguishing women in the TPM within a specified time period compared with those not yet in the TPM.

In addition to reproductive aging, antral follicle counts (AFCs) may be influenced throughout the life span by exposure to environmental adversity. AFCs are considered a marker of total ovarian reserve. Physiologic stressors of poor sleep quality, excessive exercise, and alcohol intake were associated with lower AFC in infertile women ages 31 to 36 (Dong et al., 2017). In contrast, greater levels of perceived stress during the reproductive years (25–35 years) were associated with higher AFCs while greater perceived stress in midlife (40–45 years) were associated with lower AFCs (Bleil et al., 2012). Greater stress may enhance reproductive readiness in younger women at the cost of accelerating reproductive aging later in the life span. Environmental adversity was hypothesized as promoting the allocation of resources toward greater reproductive readiness by increasing the volume of growing follicles at the cost of depleting more rapidly the ovarian reserve as women aged (Bleil et al., 2012). Further research is needed to determine whether the effects of stress on ovarian aging would differ under conditions of more extreme stressors or whether the difference between perceived stress and physiologic stress is relevant to follicle reserve.

Androgens

Women produce androgens in both the ovary and adrenal cortex, and current data indicate no difference in metabolic clearance of androgens for midlife women regardless of whether they had their FMP. Although the conversion of estrone to estradiol decreased in middle-aged women who continued to menstruate, peripheral aromatization of androstenedione to estrone increased in all women with age regardless of their menopausal status (menstruating to menopausal, and menopausal at both occasions). Women begin producing increasing levels of estrone before FMP (Longcope & Johnston, 1990), presumably to account for decreasing estradiol levels.

The adrenal gland secretes androgen precursors, including dehydroepiandrosterone sulfate (DHEAS), dehydroepiandrosterone (DHEA), androstenedione, and testosterone. Data from the Melbourne Midlife Women's Health Project, a longitudinal study of Australian women during the TPM and PM, revealed that testosterone levels remained unchanged during the TPM (from 4 years before FMP to 2 years after). DHEAS levels decreased as a function of age, not of the TPM (Burger et al., 2000). In addition, sex hormone–binding globulin (SHBG) decreased by 43% from 4 years before to 2 years after FMP, with the greatest drop 2 years before FMP. SHBG levels were associated with a drop in estradiol levels over the same period. Free androgen index (FAI), calculated as the ratio of testosterone to SHBG, rose by 80% during the same period, with the maximal change occurring 2 years before the FMP (Burger et al., 2000).

Androgens have also been studied in the SWAN population. Although DHEAS has been found to decline as a function of age, there was a transient rise in DHEAS noted in some SWAN participants during the transition to late perimenopause (the late stage of the TPM using the STRAW+10 terminology), followed by a decline during the early PM (Crawford et al., 2009; Lasley et al., 2002). Approximately 85% of women experienced increase in DHEAS between the pre/early TPM to the late TPM/early PM stages (Crawford et al., 2009). The transient increase in androgens has also been observed in women who have undergone bilateral salpingo-oophorectomy (BSO), which supports an adrenal source of this change (Lasley, Crawford, Laughlin, et al., 2011) DHEAS provides an important source of estrogen for women during PM because it is converted to estrone. Testosterone levels were stable during the TPM in both the Melbourne Midlife Women's Health and SWAN cohorts (Burger et al., 2000; Lasley et al., 2002).

Lasley, Crawford, and McConnell (2011) found that DHEAS, DHEA, and androstenediol increased at their greatest rate and were at peak variability during the years immediately before the FMP when estradiol levels were low. Androstenediol, a prohormone for peripheral conversion to bioactive steroids, acts as a signal transducer in estrogen and androgen receptors. It is considered a weak estrogen with a potency of 0.01% to 0.1% that of estradiol (Lasley et al., 2012). Androstenediol levels increased fivefold during the time that estradiol levels were decreasing. This negative correlation between androstenediol and estradiol in the late TPM and early PM was also found in Japenese women (Kawakita et al., 2021). Lasley et al. (2012) proposed that disappearance of inhibin B and rising FSH levels triggered an increase in androstenediol production, producing a transition from estrogenic to androgenic metabolism. SWAN participants produced high levels of androstenediol that were 100 times greater than the levels of estradiol. Lasley, Crawford, and McConnell (2011, 2013) proposed that the much higher levels of androstenediol, which has lower bioactivity than estradiol, were needed to compensate for lower estradiol levels. Although the clinical significance of increasing androstenediol is unknown, the greater concentration of androstenediol coupled with lower estradiol levels during the TPM may contribute to the circulating estrogen pool. These insights may prove valuable in better understanding endocrine changes during the TPM, including the ratio of estrogens to androgens.

Cortisol rose between the early and late TPM stages in the SMWHS, in which assays were obtained multiple times per year (Woods, Carr, et al., 2006). No cortisol rise was evident in the annual measures obtained from the SWAN population (Lasley et al., 2002).

Lasley et al. (2013) proposed that the wide range of delta-5 steroid production, especially DHEA and androstenediol, may account for the diversity in phenotypes (symptoms and health conditions) observed in women during the TPM. The adrenal response to LH may be mediated by LH receptors in the adrenal cortex that may shunt metabolism of pregnenolone to the delta-5 pathway. Whereas older theories attribute the transition to an androgenic from estrogenic transition in metabolism to the disappearance of inhibin B and rising FSH triggering increases in delta-5 (androstenediol) production, current theory suggests that LH stimulates receptors on the adrenal cortex to transition to androgenic metabolism (Lasley et al., 2013). The significance for this metabolic shift for women's experiences of symptoms and health conditions during the TPM remains to be investigated.

Data from the multiethnic SWAN study indicate that serum FSH, SHBG, estradiol, testosterone, and DHEAS all are correlated with body mass. Estradiol levels adjusted for body mass do not differ across ethnic groups. Adjusted FSH levels were higher and adjusted testosterone levels were lower in African American and Hispanic women. Thus, while serum sex steroids, FSH, and SHBG levels vary by ethnicity, this relationship is highly confounded by ethnic differences in body mass (Randolph et al., 2003).

The Transition to Postmenopause as a Time of Reregulation

Although some emphasize the physiologic dysregulation of the hypothalamic–pituitary–ovarian (HPO) axis functions during the TPM, this period in a woman's life may instead represent a time of reregulation of endocrine function. The ovary produces lower levels of estradiol as the ovarian follicles decrease in number, but the transition is punctuated by higher levels of estradiol in response to increasing levels of FSH. Ovulation ceases and progesterone levels become extremely low or unmeasurable. During the TPM, a compensatory response with an increase in peripheral aromatization of the androgen androstenedione to estrone and a time-limited increase in DHEAS occur during the late transition stage. These events may signal a transition from ovarian to ovarian-adrenal metabolism of estrogens, thus supporting reregulation of the HPO axis to a new pattern not dependent on the ovarian production of higher levels of estrogen.

The widespread physiologic effects of estrogens, progesterone, and androgens would warrant compensatory changes in response to their production to reregulate the HPO axis, and these alter physiologic functioning. The physiologic effects of estrogen and progesterone seen in menstruating women change over the course of the TPM as estradiol production becomes more variable and eventually diminishes; progesterone production linked to ovulation ceases; testosterone, DHEA, and DHEAS levels remain stable or fluctuate slightly; and androstenediol levels increase dramatically, producing an increasing ratio of estrone to estradiol.

Symptoms During the Transition to Postmenopause

During midlife, women experience a variety of symptoms, some of which are related to the TPM and related endocrine changes and some to aging, as well as a variety of factors influencing symptom experiences across the life span. Hot flashes, night sweats, depressed mood, sleep disturbances, sexual concerns or problems, memory symptoms, vaginal dryness, urinary incontinence (UI), and somatic or bodily pain symptoms are among those reported most frequently.

VASOMOTOR SYMPTOMS

Vasomotor symptoms (VMS), including hot flashes and night sweats, are the most commonly reported symptoms in the

TPM. Hot flashes are sudden sensations of heat that usually arise on the chest and spread to the neck and face and sometimes to the arms. They may be accompanied by sweating and flushing in some women (Voda, 1981), and sometimes anxiety and palpitations. Hot flashes that occur during sleep are referred to as night sweats.

Hot flashes occur in an effort by the body to dissipate heat by means of vascular dilation. Voda (1981) characterized the menopause-related hot flash from women's own experiences, exploring the question, "Who is the woman who has hot flashes and what are the characteristics of the hot flashes?" Using data from their daily self-reports, she sought to describe the frequency, duration, trigger, origin, spread, intensity, and method of coping with hot flashes. Voda found that no single pattern characterized women's experiences. Although most hot flashes began on the upper body (e.g., the chest or face), some women noted their hot flashes started in other parts of their body. Hot flashes tended to spread to other areas on the upper body, but for some women spread to the legs and arms or back. On average, a hot flash lasted about 3 minutes. Women distinguished between mild, moderate, and severe hot flashes. They coped with hot flashes in relation to their duration and severity. Internal strategies included ingesting a cold beverage. External strategies involved fanning oneself, showering, or opening a window. Some hot flash triggers included sleep, work activities, recreation and relaxation, and housework. Voda's study emphasized the variability in women's hot flash experiences and how they managed them. In collaboration with Kay and others, Voda extended this work to characterize the experiences of both Mexican American and Anglo women (Kay et al., 1982). They found that although Anglo women experienced hot flashes negatively, Mexican American women viewed them as positive, a natural part of life, indicating they could no longer have children and meaning they could be confident they would not become pregnant again. SWAN data have provided a cross-cultural assessment of VMS and found that Black women reported VMS most frequently (46%), followed by Hispanic (35%), White (31%), Chinese (21%), and Japanese women (18%; Gold et al., 2000). The reasons behind such differences are unclear. In the SWAN data, racial/ethnic differences persisted even after controlling for covariates (Thurston & Joffe, 2011).

Hot flashes and sweats increase in prevalence as women approach and pass the FMP, with an estimated 20% to 40% of women experiencing them in the TPM and 60% to 80% of women reporting VMS after the FMP (Freeman & Sherif, 2007; Mishra & Dobson, 2012; Politi et al., 2008). Hot flashes have been associated with various physiologic processes including LH pulses (Casper et al., 1979; Freedman, 2005a), low estradiol (Guthrie et al., 1996, 2004, 2005; Woods et al., 2007), rate of estrogen change (Dennerstein et al., 2007), low inhibin levels (Guthrie et al., 2005), and high FSH levels (Freeman et al., 2001; Randolph et al., 2005; Woods et al., 2007). SHBG and free estradiol levels were also associated with a lower prevalence of hot flashes (Randolph et al., 2005), and in one study (Øverlie et al., 2002), androgen levels were associated with a decreased frequency of PM vasomotor symptoms.

In acute studies in which laboratory stimuli were used to provoke hot flashes, elevations in LH, ACTH, and cortisol were closely associated in time with the experience of the hot flash, but no changes were reported in estradiol and FSH levels (Meldrum et al., 1980; Tataryn et al., 1979). In the laboratory, hot flashes were associated with a rise in skin temperature and skin conductance levels, elevated heart and respiratory rates, and reduced blood pH. Lab studies also indicated autonomic nervous system activation, like a stress response, in mediating the vasodilation and elaboration of norepinephrine after the hot flash (Freedman, 2005a, 2005b; Freedman & Subramanian, 2005). Potent vasodilators, including calcitonin gene-related peptide, are released during hot flashes but not during exercise or sweating (Thurston, Sutton-Tyrrell, et al., 2008). Although the etiology of hot flashes and the mechanisms stimulating vasodilation remain unclear, some investigators implicate estrogen withdrawal or changing estrogen levels.

Other theories propose a narrowed thermoneutral zone in perimenopausal women by which small changes in temperature trigger a heat dissipation event (Freedman, 2014). This is believed to have a hypothalamic origin and is related to the relationship between estrogen and the neuropeptides involved in thermoregulation, namely kisspeptin and neurokinin B (Skorupskaite et al., 2014). Serotonin may also play a role in VMS as evidenced by the utility of selective serotonin reuptake inhibitors (SSRIs) for managing VMS. The precise mechanism by which serotonin impacts the thermoregulatory system is not yet known.

SWAN investigators are beginning to characterize the effects of changing estrogen levels on blood vessel structure and function by focusing on the relationship of the TPM and associated physiologic changes to heart disease risk. Thurston, Sutton-Tyrrell, et al. (2008) found that women who had hot flashes experience lower heart rate variability during hot flashes, suggesting that the parasympathetic nervous system, which helps influence the return to normal heart rate after a stressful experience, may function differently in women with hot flashes than in women who do not have hot flashes. SMWHS participants who experienced a cluster of symptoms including severe hot flashes had higher norepinephrine levels than those experiencing low severity symptoms (Woods et al., 2014). Thurston, Sutton-Tyrrell, et al. (2008) also found that women who had VMS had less expansion of their arteries when blood flow was increased than did women without hot flashes, indicating poorer endothelial function. Others have linked hot flashes to calcification of the aorta as seen in heart disease (Thurston, Christie, et al., 2010; Thurston, Kuller et al., 2010) and increased carotid intima media thickness among midlife women (Thurston, Sutton-Tyrrell, et al., 2011). Other evidence indicates that women who experienced hot flashes have higher levels of tissue plasminogen activator (tPA) and factor VII than those without hot flashes (Thurston, Khoudary, et al., 2011). Taken together, these findings suggest that the role of hot flashes as a marker for subclinical heart disease is worthy of further investigation.

Hot flashes have been linked to both increased FSH and lower estrogen levels and to increased bone turnover during the TPM. During the early and late stages of the TPM, women with the most frequent hot flashes tended to have higher N-telopeptide levels, a marker of bone loss (Crandall et al., 2011). However, a population-based longitudinal study from the Canadian Multicentre Osteoporosis Study did not find a significant association between bone mineral density or hip fracture in women who reported VMS (Wong et al., 2018). Limitations of this study include a narrow definition of VMS (night sweats only) and a 2-year time frame. Lower estrogen levels as well as higher FSH levels have been associated with higher levels of interleukins (e.g., interleukin 1 beta [IL-1β]), linking both gonadotropins and estrogen to immune response as well as to hot flashes (Corwin & Cannon, 1999).

As Voda (1981) found, hot flashes may range from barely noticeable to severe, resulting in a high degree of variability of the experience among women (Smith-DiJulio et al., 2007). Thurston, Bromberger, et al. (2008) found that women who were most bothered by hot flashes were those with more negative affect, greater symptom sensitivity, sleep problems, poorer health, longer duration of hot flashes, and younger age and of Black race. Bother related to night sweats was associated with sleep problems and night sweats duration. Hot flashes are sufficiently bothersome to lead many women to seek healthcare during the TPM (Williams et al., 2007, 2008).

Among participants in the SMWHS, hot flash severity increased for women in the late TPM stage or early PM. Those who used hormone therapy had a longer duration of the early TPM stage, were older at the time of their FMP, had higher levels of FSH, and had more severe hot flashes. Anxiety was also associated with hot flash severity. Older age at entry into the early TPM stage and higher urinary estrogen (estrone) levels were associated with decreased hot flash severity. Psychosocial/mood (stress and depressed mood) and lifestyle variables (BMI, activity level, sleep amount, and alcohol use) were not associated with hot flash severity in this study (Smith-DiJulio et al., 2007). In contrast, in daily diary studies, women reported negative affect on the same day and the day after they reported hot flashes, suggesting that negative cognitive appraisal of hot flashes and perhaps other associated symptoms are linked to subsequent experiences of negative affect (Gibson et al., 2011). A study of women from the SMWHS examined the association between self-awareness and hot flash severity and found that women with greater self-awareness reported more severe hot flashes, contrary to the authors' hypothesis (Taylor-Swanson et al., 2019). The authors conclude that women with higher self-awareness may perceive their hot flashes as more severe due to an enhanced ability to evaluate their symptom experience. Further studies evaluating self-awareness and attitudes about menopause may help to guide symptom management.

BMI (Gold et al., 2004), anxiety (Freeman et al., 2005, 2007), and lifestyle behaviors also have been associated with hot flash severity. As one example, women who smoked reported more severe hot flashes (Gold et al., 2004).

It remains unclear how long hot flashes persist (Woods & Mitchell, 2005). Barnabei et al. (2005) found that between 23% and 37% of participants in the Women's Health Initiative Study who were in their 60s and 11% to 20% in their 70s reported hot flashes. Some Melbourne Midlife Women's Health Project participants reported hot flashes for as long as 10 years after the FMP, although the average duration was 5 years (Col et al., 2009). Freeman et al. (2014) assessed hot flashes annually in 255 women who were followed for 16 years. They found the prevalence increased in each year before the FMP, reaching 46% in the first 2 years after FMP. Hot flashes decreased gradually during the PM and did not return to levels like those before the TPM until after 9 years after the FMP. One third experienced moderate to severe hot flashes at 10 years or more during the PM. Black women and obese White women experienced a greater risk of hot flashes. Increasing FSH levels before the FMP, decreasing estradiol, and increasing anxiety increased the risk of hot flashes, and higher education levels reduced the risk (Freeman et al., 2014). Avis et al. (2015) reported that SWAN participants experienced a median duration of hot flashes (on more than 6 days in the previous 2 weeks) of 7.4 years. Based on nearly 900 women who experienced a FMP, the median post-FMP persistence was 4.5 years. Women who experienced hot flashes before the TPM or in early perimenopause had the longest duration (median: more than 11.8 years), and post-FMP persistence was 9.4 years. Those who were postmenopausal when they first experienced hot flashes had the shortest duration (median: 3.4 years). Black women reported the longest duration of hot flashes compared with other racial/ethnic groups. Factors influencing duration of vasomotor symptoms were younger age, less formal education, greater perceived stress, higher symptom sensitivity, and higher depressive and anxiety symptoms when hot flashes were first reported.

Analysis of the severity of hot flashes in the SMWHS population indicated an increase in women's age across the spectrum, from age 35 to 60 years. In addition, hot flash severity was associated with lower estrone and higher FSH levels and the late TPM stage or early PM. Hot flash severity increased most from 2 years before to 1 year after FMP, declining 3 years after, and was highest during the late stage and all life years before FMP (Mitchell & Woods, 2015), consistent with the findings of the SWAN (Randolph et al., 2005) and Penn Ovarian Aging Study (Freeman et al., 2011, 2014). They are also consistent with the relationship between TPM stages and PM as described by Freeman et al. (2011). Of interest is the declining severity of hot flashes seen in the SMWHS cohort after 2 years following the FMP. This finding suggests that as the PM progresses, the severity of hot flashes diminishes.

SLEEP SYMPTOMS

An estimated 30% to 45% of women experience disrupted sleep during the TPM, with the prevalence of symptoms becoming higher during the late MT stage and early PM (Dennerstein, Lehert, Burger, & Guthrie, 2005). Women believe that awakening during the night is caused by hormonal changes and hot flashes (Woods & Mitchell, 1999) and that hot flashes are correlated with sleep disruption and estrogen levels (Woods et al., 2007), but evidence from a recent study indicates that often women awaken, then have a hot flash (Freedman & Roehrs, 2004).

In this specific population, primary sleep disorders are also very common; thus, not all sleep disturbances can be entirely attributed to the TPM. However, the transition itself can aggravate or bring about a primary sleep disorder, particularly for those at increased risk. Taking this into account, a report of 102 women ages 44 to 56 years who had sleep disturbances indicated that 54 (53%) had sleep apnea, restless legs syndrome, or both (Freedman & Roehrs, 2007). Additionally, depression and anxiety play a significant role in sleep disturbances in this population (Freedman & Roehrs, 2007). Shaver was the first to study sleep during the perimenopause using polysomnographic methods in a sleep laboratory, discovering the relationship between sleep problems and ongoing stressful life events and anxiety (Shaver et al., 1988, 1991, 2001). Polysomnographic studies of sleep among women during the TPM and PM demonstrated that there was an increase in sleep disruption as women progressed to the PM, as well as psychological distress associated with subjectively experienced symptoms (Shaver et al., 1988; Shaver & Paulsen, 1993). Sleep symptoms have been associated with higher FSH levels during the late reproductive stage and with lower estradiol levels in women who were still cycling (Hollander et al., 2001), but findings are not consistent across all studies (Woods et al., 2007). When women without hot flashes were monitored overnight, arousals that occurred were associated with sleep-disordered breathing and age (Lukacs et al., 2004).

Findings from a study of relationships between TPM-related symptoms and EEG sleep measures indicate that hot flashes were associated with a longer sleep time. Women with higher anxiety symptoms had a longer sleep latency (took more time getting to sleep) and lower sleep efficiency only if they also had hot flashes. Hot flashes and mood symptoms were unrelated to either delta sleep ratio or rapid eye movement (REM) latency (Kravitz et al., 2011). In this same study, elevated beta EEG power in the non-REM (NREM) and REM sleep in women during late perimenopause (late TPM) and early PM exceeded levels in premenopause (late reproductive stage) and early perimenopause (early TPM). Elevated beta EEG power indicated increased arousal and disturbed sleep quality during the late perimenopause (late TPM) and early PM (Campbell et al., 2011). These study results suggest that sleep symptoms during the TPM may be amenable to symptom management strategies that take into account women's experiences of arousal and their ability to regulate arousal as well as efforts to promote women's general health rather than focusing only on the TPM as a causative factor.

Studies of self-reported hot flashes and sleep symptoms indicate that menopause-related factors may have effects on some, but not all, sleep symptoms. SMWHS participants who experienced more severe difficulty going to sleep had several other symptoms such as anxiety, hot flashes, depressed mood, and joint and back pain; reported more stress; were more likely to be in early PM; had a history of sexual abuse; rated their own health more poorly; had lower cortisol levels; and had greater caffeine and less alcohol intake than women who did not have this problem. Age, exercise, estrogen, and FSH were not related to difficulty getting to sleep. On the other hand, women who had more severe awakening during the night were older, more likely to be in the late TPM stage or early PM, had higher FSH and lower estrogen (estrone) levels, and reported more severe hot flashes, depressed mood, anxiety, joint pain, backache, perceived stress, poorer overall health, less alcohol use, and history of sexual abuse. Women who had more severe problems with awakening early (and not getting back to sleep) were older; reported more severe hot flashes, depressed mood, anxiety, joint pain, backache, and perceived stress; rated their health more poorly; and had higher epinephrine and lower urinary estrogen levels. Exercise, MT stage, and alcohol use were not related to waking up early (Woods et al., 2010). These findings are consistent with those of other studies (Ensrud et al., 2008; Kravitz et al., 2008; Pien et al., 2008).

Freeman et al. (2014) studied the sleep of participants in the Penn Ovarian Aging Study, who were followed for 16 years. They found that women's sleep before the MT predicted sleep around the time of the FMP: Those who had poor sleep before the TPM were at 3.5 times the risk of having poor sleep around the time of the FMP, whereas those who had mild sleep problems were at 1.5 times the risk. There was no relationship between poor sleep and time relative to the FMP among those without poor sleep before the TPM. Hot flashes contributed to poor sleep regardless of the sleep status before the TPM.

Joffe, Crawford, et al. (2013) and Joffe, White, et al. (2013) induced hot flashes measured by skin conductance with a gonadotropin-releasing hormone (GnRH) agonist to determine whether hot flashes induced awakenings measured by polysomnography. The reported frequency of nighttime hot flashes was associated with recorded sleep disturbances, including increasing wake after sleep onset (WASO), awakenings, and early-stage sleep. Nighttime hot flashes were also associated with perceptions of increased WASO, awakenings, and scores on the Insomnia Severity Index and Pittsburgh Sleep Quality Index, and decreased perceived sleep efficiency. In addition, recorded hot flashes were associated with polysomnography-measured WASO. These findings suggest that hot flashes interrupt sleep during the conditions of the TPM.

Clearly, sleep disturbances are commonly experienced during the TPM and PM. The Midlife Women's Health Study sought to describe specific dynamics surrounding poor sleep quality in the TPM using annual response surveys to further identify individual risk factors. Interestingly, for all sleep outcomes studied, a high frequency of depression was highly correlated with a high frequency of poor sleep. Vasomotor symptoms were also significantly related and demonstrated a higher frequency of all poor sleep outcomes in the surveyed group (Smith et al., 2018).

Recent data on chronic stress and sleep among SWAN participants indicate that women experiencing chronic stress over a period of up to 9 years reported lower subjective sleep quality and insomnia and exhibited increased WASO measured by polysomnography compared with women with low to moderate chronic stress profiles (Hall et al., 2015). These findings, taken together with the relationship between EEG measures of arousal and sleep disruption, suggest an important pathway linking cumulative stress experience and poor sleep during midlife.

DEPRESSED MOOD

Depressed mood symptoms are prevalent among midlife women. This phenomenon has been explored in the SWAN, Penn Ovarian Aging Study, and SMWHS longitudinal studies, which collectively suggest a progressive increased risk of depression as women advance through the TPM. The early TPM is associated with a 1.5-fold increased risk of depression while the late TPM is associated with a 1.8- to 2.8-fold increased risk. In some studies, higher FSH and LH levels and increased variability of estradiol, FSH, and LH (within women) were associated with depressed mood symptoms (Freeman et al., 2004, 2006), as were lower levels of estradiol (Avis, Crawford, et al., 2001; Freeman et al., 2006), and DHEAS (Morrison et al., 2001; Schmidt et al., 2002). Other studies show no relationship of depressed mood to endocrine levels (Woods et al., 2008).

Although some would suggest that the TPM may be a period of vulnerability to depression, even for women who have no history of it earlier in life (Bromberger et al., 2001, 2003, 2004, 2007; Freeman et al., 2006; Woods et al., 2008), others argue that menopause is overpathologized by suggesting that menopause-related depression is a model of biologically induced depression (Judd et al., 2012). The literature about depressed mood in midlife women is complex, and studies use both indicators of depressed mood symptoms, such as the Center for Epidemiologic Studies Depression Scale (CESD) and measures of major depressive disorder, such as the Structured Clinical Interview for *DSM-5* Disorders (SCID-5). For this reason, it is important to distinguish the results of studies of depressed mood symptoms from those of major depressive disorder.

Studies of depressive symptoms indicate an increase in severity during the TPM. Freeman et al. (2006) found that during the early TPM stage, women were 1.5 times more likely to have high CESD scores and those in late transition stage were three times more likely to have high CESD scores than women who had not yet begun the TPM. In addition, women with a history of depression were at twice the risk of reporting depressed mood during the TPM, as were women who had severe premenstrual symptoms, poor sleep, and lack of employment. Those with a rapidly increasing FSH level were less likely to develop depressed mood. Participants in the SMWHS completed the CESD scale annually as a measure of depressed mood symptoms. While age was associated with slightly lower depressed mood (CESD) scores, being in the late TPM stage was associated with more severe depressed mood, although there was no effect of being in the early TPM stage or early PM. Hot flash severity, life stress, family history of depression, history of postpartum blues, sexual abuse history, BMI, and use of antidepressants were also individually related to depressed mood. Neither FSH nor estrogen levels were related to depressed mood in this cohort (Woods et al., 2008; Woods, Mariella, et al., 2006; Woods & Mitchell, 1997a).

Several investigators have suggested that the TPM may be a period of vulnerability to the first onset of depressed mood (Bromberger et al., 2007, 2010; Cohen et al., 2006; Freeman et al., 2006). Results of studies of depressed mood symptoms suggest that variability of hormonal levels (estrogen, FSH) and rate of change in FSH are related to depressed mood, although there is no evidence that estrogen levels themselves are related (Avis, Crawford, et al., 2001; Avis et al., 1994; Avis, Stellato, et al., 2001; Freeman et al., 2006). Although women in the late TPM stage are vulnerable to depressed mood, factors that account for depressed mood earlier in the life span continue to have an important influence and should be considered in studies of etiology and therapeutics. Of interest is the potential relationship of androgens to depressed mood: Testosterone rise was associated with depressed mood in a subset of the SWAN study participants (Bromberger et al., 2010), and DHEAS was associated with depressed mood symptoms but not major depression in the Penn Ovarian Aging Study participants (Morrison et al., 2011).

Bromberger et al. (2009, 2011) made an important distinction between studies of major depressive disorder and depressed mood symptoms, as well as between repeat versus first-onset depressive disorder, during the TPM and early PM. Among SWAN participants who responded to a Structured Clinical Interview for *DSM-IV* Axis Disorders (SCID-IV), those in the TPM stages (perimenopause) compared with those who had not yet begun the TPM or were in the early PM were two to four times more likely to experience a major depressive episode, even when prior depression history, upsetting life events, psychotropic medication use, hot flashes, and serum levels or changes in reproductive hormone levels were taken into account. It is of interest that many of the same predictors of depressive disorder at other parts of the life span were important. Indeed, using the Patient Health Questionnaire (PHQ) to measure depression or the Primary Care Evaluation of Mental Disorders (PRIME-MD), Freeman et al. (2006) found that 11% of the Penn Ovarian Aging Study cohort developed major depression over the 8 years of follow-up. Women in the TPM were twice as likely to experience depression as those who had not yet begun the transition and greater variability of estradiol levels was a risk factor for new onset of diagnosed depressive disorder.

In contrast, when Bromberger et al. (2009) considered 266 SWAN participants who had *no* lifetime history of depression and assessed a new onset of depression based on SCID interviews, she found that 42 (16%) met criteria for new-onset major depression. There was no association between becoming depressed and the TPM stages based on either bleeding patterns or reproductive hormones. Instead, women experiencing low role functioning caused by physical health, low social functioning, and anxiety disorder were more likely to experience a first depressive episode during the TPM.

Judd et al. (2012) conducted a systematic review of studies of depressed mood and depressive disorder to determine whether depression at the time of menopause might constitute a reproductive-related depressive disorder, the result of a biological response to hormonal change. She concluded there was not sufficient evidence to support depression during the TPM as part of a distinctive diagnostic group of reproductive-related depressive disorders and cautioned instead that a more plausible explanation is a biopsychosociocultural model of the processes that may lead to a depressive disorder in midlife. Given the prevalence of depression, clinicians should be alert to the possibility of depression in all clinical encounters.

COGNITIVE SYMPTOMS

Women often notice cognitive symptoms such as forgetfulness or difficulty learning and concentrating during midlife, but few rate them as serious, and most attribute these symptoms to changing hormones as well as general aging and life stress (Mitchell & Woods, 2001; Woods et al., 2000). The SWAN reported stage-specific prevalence of forgetfulness ranging from 31% during the late reproductive stage to 42% in PM (Gold et al., 2000). Cross-sectional studies have suggested that memory and other cognitive factors are worse after the TPM than before (Rentz et al, 2017; Weber et al., 2014). Other studies have shown that the minor slowing of learning during the late TPM stage seems to disappear during the early PM (Greendale, 2009; Greendale et al., 2010; Luetters et al., 2007).

SMWHS participants who experienced more severe difficulty concentrating were slightly older; reported more anxiety, depressed mood, night-time awakening, perceived stress, and poorer perceived health; and were employed. The best predictors of forgetfulness included slightly older age, hot flashes, anxiety, depressed mood, awakening during the night, perceived stress, poorer perceived health, and history of sexual abuse, suggesting a multifactorial process of cognitive changes. This is contrasted by the SWAN findings of Greendale et al. (2010) who reported that age, depression, anxiety, sleep disturbance, and VMS did not account for a transient decrease in cognitive function reported by women in late perimenopause. Considering women's ages and the context in which they experience the TPM may be helpful in understanding experiences of cognitive symptoms (Mitchell & Woods, 2011).

PAIN SYMPTOMS

Musculoskeletal and joint aches and pains are a commonly experienced symptom in midlife women and have been reported to be the most troublesome symptom of midlife in around 20% of women in one study (Obermeyer et al., 2005). Fifty-seven percent of participants in the Melbourne study experienced musculoskeletal pain during the late TPM and early PM (Dennerstein et al., 2000). In a follow-up study of Melbourne participants, postmenopausal women were twice as likely to report joint pain and stiffness (Szoeke et al., 2008). Some evidence suggests that pain symptoms may be influenced by estrogen (Popescu, 2010). In the SMWHS, women experienced a significant increase in back pain during the early and late TPM stages and early PM; estrogen, FSH, and testosterone levels were unrelated to back pain (Mitchell & Woods, 2010). Perceived stress and lower overnight urinary cortisol levels were associated with more severe back pain; a history of sexual abuse and catecholamines did not have a significant effect. Those most troubled by symptoms of hot flashes, depressed mood, anxiety, nighttime awakening, and difficulty concentrating reported significantly greater back pain. Of the health-related factors, having worse perceived health, exercising more, using analgesics, and having a higher BMI were associated with more back pain; alcohol use and smoking did not have significant effects. Having more formal education was associated with less back pain; parenting, having a partner, and employment were unrelated. Age was associated with increased severity of joint pain, but TPM-related factors, such as stage or hormone levels, were unrelated, as was anxiety. Symptoms of hot flashes, nighttime awakening, depressed mood, and difficulty concentrating were each significantly associated with joint pain, as was poorer perceived health, more exercise, higher BMI, and greater analgesic use. History of sexual abuse was the only stress-related factor significantly related to joint pain severity. Based on these findings (Mitchell & Woods, 2010), which are consistent with those of others (Dugan et al., 2006, 2009; Szoeke et al., 2008), clinicians working with women traversing the TPM should be aware that managing back and joint pain symptoms requires consideration of their changing biology as well as their ongoing life challenges and health-related behaviors. Moreover, the relationship between pain and sleep symptoms, including sleep hygiene interventions, should be considered (Mitchell & Woods, 2010).

SEXUAL SYMPTOMS

Changes in sexual functioning are troublesome to some women, and these changes become more pronounced in the late TPM stage (Avis et al., 2000; Dennerstein et al., 2002; Dennerstein & Lehert, 2004). Such changes may relate to sexual desire, sexual arousal, ability to achieve orgasm, and discomfort with sexual activity. The Fourth Edition of the *Diagnostic and Statistical Manual of Mental Disorders* (*DSM-IV; American Psychiatric Association [APA]*, 2000) included two diagnoses of female sexual disorders: hypoactive sexual desire disorder (HSDD) and female sexual arousal disorder (FSAD). The Fifth Edition (*DSM-5*; APA, 2013) combines HSDD and FSAD into one disorder, female sexual interest/arousal disorder, but sexual medicine experts have emphasized the importance of keeping HSDD and FSAD unique entities because of their differing clinical manifestations and treatments (McCabe et al., 2016).

Unsurprisingly, hormonal changes have been implicated in changes in sexual function of women in the TPM. Decreased sexual desire was negatively correlated with estradiol levels in one study (Woods et al., 2007), and lower sexual functioning scores in the Melbourne Midlife Women's Health Project were associated with higher FSH levels and lower estradiol levels (Dennerstein et al., 2002). Although there was no relationship with testosterone in the Melbourne study, participants in the Penn Ovarian Aging Study who experienced fluctuations in testosterone levels experienced more problems with sexual desire (Gracia et al., 2004). Several studies have found correlations between androgen levels and sexual interest and arousal in women during the TPM (Davis et al., 2005; Randolph et al., 2015; Wåhlin-Jacobsen et al., 2015).

Dyspareunia can contribute to decreased sexual interest and has been associated with low estradiol levels (Avis et al., 2000). Vaginal dryness, a key player in the dyspareunia of the TPM, has been associated with higher FSH levels and lower testosterone levels (Woods et al., 2007). Vaginal dryness increases in frequency as women progress from the TPM to PM; 21% of participants in the Melbourne study reported vaginal dryness during the late TPM stage and 47% during early PM (Dennerstein et al., 2000).

SMWHS participants experienced a significant decrease in sexual desire during the late TPM stage and early PM (Woods et al., 2010). Those with higher urinary estrone (E1) and testosterone (T) reported significantly higher levels of sexual desire, whereas those with higher FSH levels reported significantly lower sexual desire. Women using hormone therapy also reported higher sexual desire. Those reporting higher perceived stress reported lower sexual desire, but history of sexual abuse did not have a significant effect. Those most troubled by symptoms of hot flashes, fatigue, depressed mood, anxiety, difficulty getting to sleep, early morning awakening, and awakening during the night also reported significantly lower sexual desire; there was no effect of vaginal dryness, perhaps because of low prevalence in this cohort. Women with better perceived health reported higher sexual desire, and those reporting more exercise and more alcohol intake also reported greater sexual desire. Having a partner was associated with lower sexual desire. Women's sexual desire during the TPM and early PM is related to both biology and the social situation in which she finds herself (Avis, Zhao, et al., 2005; Dennerstein, Lehert, & Burger, 2005; Gracia et al., 2004; Woods et al., 2010).

Longitudinal data about sexual functioning as women experience the TPM indicate that the odds of vaginal or pelvic pain increased and sexual desire decreased by late perimenopause (approximation of late MT; Avis et al., 2009). Women used masturbation more frequently during early perimenopause (approximation of early TPM) but less during PM. Health, psychological functioning, and the importance of sex were related to each of the sexual function outcomes (self-reports of importance of sex, frequency of sexual desire, arousal, masturbation, sexual intercourse, pain during intercourse, degree of emotional satisfaction, and physical pleasure). Age, race/ethnicity, marital status, change in relationship, and vaginal dryness were associated with sexual functioning. When other factors were considered, the TPM was not associated with reported importance of sex, sexual arousal, frequency of sexual intercourse, emotional satisfaction with partner, or physical pleasure.

URINARY INCONTINENCE SYMPTOMS

Urinary incontinence (UI) symptoms are prevalent among women and appear to increase with age as well as during and after the TPM. Approximately 47% of the Melbourne study participants reported being bothered by urinary leakage during the late TPM and 53% during early PM (Dennerstein et al., 2000). U.S. data from the National Health and Nutrition Examination Survey (NHANES) indicated that the prevalence of stress urinary incontinence (SUI) peaks in the 50- to 59-year age group, urge urinary incontinence (UUI) peaks in women 80 years and older, and that mixed incontinence is associated with increasing age (Dooley et al., 2008).

Data from the SWAN revealed that nearly 47% of participants reported at least monthly UI at baseline when the cohort was an average age of 45.8 years and an average increase in incidence of 11% per year. The most prevalent type of UI was SUI: 7.6% of women experienced SUI at baseline, and this increased to 15.9% over the course of the study (Waetjen et al., 2007). Black and Hispanic women had the lowest incidence and White women had the highest. Although progression to early and late perimenopause (estimates of STRAW early and late TPM stages) from premenopause (STRAW late reproductive stage) was associated with an increase in the incidence of any UI, the transition from the TPM stages to PM resulted in a reduced incidence of newly reported UI (approximately half that observed in the late TPM stage; Waetjen et al., 2009) UI became more prevalent as women progressed to the late TPM (Waetjen et al., 2008). Of interest is that estradiol, FSH, testosterone, and DHEA were unrelated to any type of incontinence in the SWAN participants (Waetjen et al., 2011).

Participants in the SMWHS who experienced SUI were more likely to perceive their health as poor, have a history of more than three live births, and were likely to be White. Those experiencing urge incontinence were older, perceived their health as worse, and had a BMI of 30 or higher (Mitchell & Woods, 2013). Women who experienced incontinence reported lower levels of self-esteem and mastery but did not report effects on mood, attitudes toward aging, and menopause on perceived health. TPM stage, exercise, estrone, and FSH were not associated with either SUI or UUI (Woods & Mitchell, 2013). Clinicians working with midlife women who experience UI can be alert to the stigmatizing nature of this set of symptoms and to the erosion of self-esteem and sense of control associated with the symptoms.

VULVOVAGINAL SYMPTOMS

Many women experience bothersome vulvovaginal changes as they progress through the TPM. These may include vaginal dryness, vaginal irritation and burning, and vulvar pain as well as urinary symptoms. In 2014, the NAMS and the Inter-

national Society for the Study of Women's Sexual Health (ISSWSH) terminology consensus conference proposed using the term *genitourinary syndrome of menopause* (GSM) to describe such changes, as it is a more accurate, all-encompassing, and publicly acceptable term than vulvovaginal atrophy, which was previously used. GSM is defined as a collection of symptoms and signs associated with a decrease in estrogen and other sex steroids and involving changes to the labia majora and minora, clitoris, vestibule and introitus, vagina, urethra, and bladder. The syndrome may include, but is not limited to, genital symptoms of dryness, burning, and irritation; sexual symptoms of lack of lubrication, discomfort or pain, and impaired function; and urinary symptoms of urgency, dysuria, and recurrent urinary tract infections. Women may present with some or all the signs and symptoms, which must be bothersome and should not be better accounted for by another diagnosis (Portman et al., 2014). Research to establish the syndrome versus clusters of symptoms is needed to guide treatment.

Symptoms of GSM often progress as a woman transitions through the various stages of midlife. Melbourne Midlife Women's Health Project participants reported a progressively increasing prevalence of bothersome vaginal dryness: 3% of women in the reproductive age, 4% in the early TPM, 21% in the late TPM stage, and 47% who were 3 years PM. Findings from the SWAN cohort were consistent with the Melbourne findings and indicated that women experienced vaginal dryness more frequently as they aged (Gold et al., 2000). Vaginal dryness has been associated with lower estrogen levels in the SMWHS cohort (unpublished data). Current research on vulvovaginal symptoms is focusing on understanding GSM, and some investigators are beginning to study groups of symptoms related to GSM, reflecting their effects on quality of life, including sexual function and interpersonal relationships.

Interference With Daily Living and Symptoms

Women indicate that symptoms they experience during the TPM and early PM interfere with many aspects of their daily lives (e.g., work, relationships with family and friends; Carpenter, 2001). SMWHS participants rated each day how their symptoms interfered with their ability to work and their relationships. Hot flashes, depressed mood, anxiety, sleep problems, cognitive and pain symptoms, and perceived health were related individually to work interference; the most influential factors interfering with work were perceived health, stress levels, depressed mood, and difficulty concentrating. Age was not related to work interference. The most influential factors interfering with relationships were younger age, stress, depressed mood, and difficulty concentrating. TPM stage did not affect either type of interference (Woods & Mitchell, 2011).

A Menopausal Syndrome?

Although many assume that there is a "menopausal syndrome" that affects women universally, Avis, Stellato, et al. (2001) found there was no evidence to support this assertion. Findings from the SWAN study revealed that there is no universal menopausal syndrome consisting of a variety of vasomotor and psychological symptoms. Instead, during the

TPM, women who used hormones and women who had surgical menopause reported more vasomotor symptoms but no more psychological symptoms than did their counterparts. White women reported more psychosomatic symptoms than other ethnic groups, and African American women reported more VMS than other ethnic groups in the SWAN study (Avis, Brockwell, et al., 2005).

The relationships among symptoms any individual woman experiences are important for clinicians to consider. Mitchell and Woods (1996) found that the trajectory of groups of symptoms (e.g., VMS, dysphoric mood, sleep symptoms, and others) changed differently during the TPM. The VMS were least reliable across multiple occasions, indicating they were most likely to change across the TPM. Avis, Crawford, et al. (2001) and Avis, Stellato, et al. (2001) found that participants in the MWHS experienced multiple types of symptoms: Those who had hot flashes, night sweats, and trouble sleeping also had more depressed mood. Thus, Avis proposed a "domino" hypothesis: Depressed mood occurs among women who have VMS and sleep problems related to their changing hormone levels. When the VMS and sleep symptoms are considered, Avis, Stellato, et al. found that estradiol had no effect on depressed mood.

Despite lack of evidence for a menopausal syndrome, it has become evident that women experience multiple symptoms, with some experiencing multiple severe symptoms. Moreover, researchers studying symptoms have identified the importance of studying co-occurring symptoms, or symptom clusters, as a basis for identifying mechanisms that may be common to several symptoms or explain relationships among symptoms. As an example, Joffe and colleagues have found that induced, objectively recorded hot flashes influenced sleep efficiency, creating fragmentation, and that perceived hot flashes were associated with perceived poor sleep quality (Joffe, Crawford, et al., 2013; Joffe, White, et al., 2013). In addition, investigators studying symptom clusters are concerned about identifying therapeutics that will maximize effects of an intervention on all or most symptoms and minimize the likelihood that a therapy will have positive effects on one symptom, but exacerbate others (Woods & Cray, 2013).

Cray et al. (2012) identified three clusters of symptoms that women in the SMWHS experienced during the TPM and early PM. Among these were clusters of (a) low-severity symptoms of all types (hot flashes, mood, sleep disruption, cognitive, pain, and tension symptoms), (b) moderately severe hot flashes with moderate levels of other symptoms, and (c) low-severity hot flashes with moderate levels of all other symptoms (Figure 9.5). The high hot flash cluster versus the low symptom severity cluster was associated with being in the late TPM stage as well as with higher levels of FSH, lower levels of estrogen, and higher norepinephrine and lower epinephrine levels. The moderate severity symptom cluster versus the low severity cluster was associated only with having lower epinephrine levels (Woods et al., 2014). A similar set of symptom clusters has been reported in the Menopause Strategies: Finding Lasting Answers for Symptoms and Health (MsFLASH) trial participants, who were selected for their experience of bothersome hot flashes (Woods et al., 2016).

In contrast to a symptom cluster, a syndrome is a pattern of symptoms that is presumably disease specific and results from

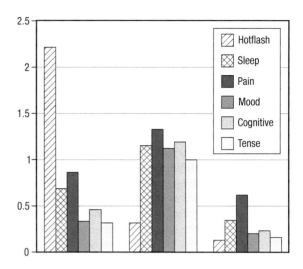

FIGURE 9.5 Symptom clusters during the transition to and early postmenopause.
Source: Adapted from Cray, L. A., Woods, N. F., Herting, J. R., & Mitchell, E. S. (2012). Symptom clusters during the menopausal transition and early postmenopause: Observations from the Seattle Midlife Women's Health Study. Menopause, 19(8), 864–869. https:// doi.org/10.1097/gme.0b013e31824790a6

a common underlying mechanism. It is likely that symptom clusters may be a more useful concept for clinicians caring for midlife women than a menopausal syndrome, which implies a disease. A careful history could elicit from women the symptoms they are experiencing and their impressions of which are related. Knowing the complement of symptoms may help clinicians suggest a tailored therapy regimen (e.g., one that is effective for both hot flashes and sleep disruption).

Symptoms and Culture

There is some evidence that symptoms women report during the TPM and PM are a culture-bound phenomenon because women from cultures not influenced by Western medicine reported few symptoms or different symptoms than did Western women. For example, Lock et al.'s (1988) work with Japanese women revealed that their most frequently reported symptom was shoulder pain, not hot flashes. Whether infrequent reporting of hot flashes by Japanese women may be attributable to the high phytoestrogen content in their diets or other features by which culture influences biology remains to be seen.

When considering the relationship of symptoms to the TPM, it is important to consider the context in which they occur. Many women juggle multiple obligations for their families, such as parenting adolescent or young adult children, providing caregiving services for their older family members, being grandparents, and dealing with employment or the challenges of relationship stress. The participants in the SWAN study who have trouble paying for basics are at greater risk for nearly every kind of symptom (Gold et al., 2000). Viewing symptoms in the broader context of women's lives may help tailor therapies likely to be most effective.

Given the global nature of healthcare, it is important to focus on women's experiences of menopause in many parts of the world. Although a detailed review of the symptoms women experience around the globe is beyond the scope of this chapter, Sievert (2006) has led research identifying ways in which diverse populations of women experience menopause. Her work includes a biocultural model in which environment, culture, and biology intersect to influence the expression of symptoms such as hot flashes. Sievert notes that environment prompts consideration of the climate and altitude in which women live their lives and that culture warrants consideration of practices related to marriage, religion, attitudes, medicalization, hysterectomy, smoking, reproductive patterns, and diet. Finally, because different populations of the world have different genetic characteristics, they also may have differing hormone levels and sweating patterns. Thus, variation across populations and the variation within populations of women are complex and together influence women's individual experiences. Indeed, Sievert points out that cross-country comparative studies illustrate the differences between cultures, whereas cross-cultural studies of menopause can facilitate understanding of women's place in society and the influence of social context on symptom experience (Sievert, 2013). In a comparison of symptom experiences across countries, women from different countries report some similar symptoms but may cluster their symptoms differently. For example, expression of somatic with emotional complaints varies across populations, possibly reflecting comfort with expression of emotional symptoms (Sievert & Obermeyer, 2012). These influences can be considered when caring for the U.S. population given the diversity across the nation with regard to culture, diet, activity, and other norms in various areas.

Symptoms and Gender Identity

Transgender and gender-nonbinary individuals represent an important and growing segment of the population, yet there are large gaps in research and clinical guidelines when it comes to their care. Transgender women and individuals who identify as gender-nonbinary are often overlooked in conversations about the TPM. Transgender women may have undergone gender affirming surgery and/or may be taking gender-affirming hormone therapy (GAHT), and little is known about how they feel about approaching the age where cisgender women experience the TPM. Nonbinary individuals may have conflicting feelings about experiencing the symptoms of a process that is strongly associated with femininity. Mohamed and Hunter (2019) conducted a mixed-methods cross-sectional study to investigate menopausal beliefs, expectations, and experiences among transgender women. The study also examined beliefs about long-term GAHT use in this population. The authors found a general dismissal of the relevance of menopause, and most participants expressed a desire to continue GAHT indefinitely, rather than decrease GAHT doses to mimic the TPM. Some transgender women in the study expected that their medical providers would make decisions for them about hormone therapy doses when they reached "menopausal age." Overall, there was uncertainty about how the TPM would be approached, suggesting that better communication between transgender women and their practitioners is crucial, and more research is needed in this arena. Studies are lacking that investigate the TPM for nonbinary individuals and how the psychological and physical changes of the TPM might impact

their experiences of self. Healthcare providers should openly communicate with transgender women and nonbinary individuals at the time of the TPM to discuss anticipated changes and explore how the individual might feel about such changes so that the appropriate support and care can be provided.

Stress and the Menopausal Transition

Given the nature of symptoms that women experience during the TPM, one might ask whether the TPM itself is stressful. We found that there was little change in perceived stress as women transitioned from the late reproductive stage to the early and late TPM stages and PM. Instead, women who were employed and had a history of sexual abuse and depressed mood experienced greater stress. Those who experienced an improvement in the burdens associated with their roles, more social support, and more adequate incomes reported less stress. Those who appraised aging changes in their bodies as negative and perceived their health as poorer reported higher stress levels (Woods et al., 2009).

A recent report of chronic stress and sleep in midlife women from the SWAN cohort indicated that upsetting life events assessed annually for up to 9 years were related to women's sleep. Using the Psychiatric Epidemiology Research Interview (PERI) Life Events Scale to assess life events across eight domains (school, work, romantic relationships, children, family, criminal and legal matters, finances, and health), investigators found that relative to women with low or moderate levels of chronic stress, those with high chronic stress had lower sleep quality (Pittsburgh Sleep Quality Index) and were more likely to report insomnia (Insomnia Symptom Questionnaire). They also exhibited increased WASO measured by polysomnography in the home. These results underscore the importance of the cumulation of stress across the life span (Hall et al., 2015).

Exposure to chronic stress appears to relate to symptom experience during this part of the life span. Clinicians working with women traversing the TPM should remain vigilant to the social circumstances of women's lives, focusing on the social as well as endocrine features of this transition. Of interest is that when women who had participated in the SMWHS for 15 years were asked about the most challenging aspect of their lives during this period, only one said that it was the TPM (Woods & Mitchell, unpublished).

Well-Being and the Transition to Postmenopause

Despite the symptoms and experiences of stress during this period, midlife women report high levels of well-being. Although estrone, FSH levels, and hot flash severity had no effect on well-being in the early transition stage, in the late TPM stage, they predicted a decrease in well-being, but this decrease did not persist into early PM. The significant variability in women's well-being was affected more by life events and the personal resources available to meet transition demands, such as satisfaction with social support and feelings of mastery, than by the TPM (Smith-DiJulio et al., 2008).

THE TRANSITION TO POSTMENOPAUSE AND HEALTHY AGING

Metabolic Changes

Over the past several decades, research about menopause and midlife health has focused on the relationship of the TPM to healthy aging, including studies linking dimensions of the TPM to health outcomes through metabolic changes affecting bone, muscle, and fat. During the TPM and early PM, women experience changes in body composition affecting both lean body mass (bone density and muscle mass) and fat deposition (subcutaneous and intra-abdominal).

Changing Bone

Bone loss accelerates in the late TPM and continues in the early PM in both the spine and hip areas. For some women, the decrease in bone mass may progress to osteoporosis. The acceleration of bone mineral density (BMD) occurs 1 year prior to the FMP and decelerates 2 years following the FMP (El Khoudary et al., 2019; Greendale et al., 2012). The pulse of these changes is influenced by hormonal and metabolic changes (Karlamanga et al., 2018). The physiologic cascade of bone demineralization occurs when N-telopeptide, a by-product of collagen breakdown, increases in the urine as estradiol levels decrease. Once estradiol nadir levels are reached, there is stabilization of the N-telopeptide, decelerating bone resorption (El Khoudary et al., 2019). Estrogen is necessary for closure of the epiphyseal plates at puberty; during the TPM, there is a disruption at the estrogen alpha sites (receptive to skeletal muscle) and beta sites (receptive to osteoblastic activity). The decrease in estrogen creates an opposition at these two receptor sites, resulting in bone degradation (Raisz, 2005).

After follow-up of SWAN participants that included 5 years before and 5 years after the FMP, Greendale et al. (2012) described the time of onset and offset of BMD loss in relation to the timing of the FMP, age at FMP, BMI, and race/ethnicity in the multiethnic SWAN cohort. Bone loss began 1 year before and slowed 2 years after the FMP in the lumbar spine and femoral neck sites. Bone loss rates occurring between 2 and 5 years PM were lower than those observed from 1 year before to 2 years after the FMP. The cumulative 10-year bone loss was 10.6%; however, the majority (7.4%) occurred during the period between 1 year before and 2 years after the FMP (Greendale et al., 2012).

For ethnic/racial groups, SWAN found Japanese and Chinese women have lower BMD compared to White women, but fewer fracture rates and stronger strength indices (El Khoudary et al., 2019). These findings provide important confirmation of a period of acute bone loss near the time of the FMP, as reported in earlier studies of smaller and less heterogeneous populations of women. It remains uncertain whether changes in the microarchitecture of bone during this period permanently damages bone (Greendale et al., 2012).

A recent analysis of SWAN data using estimates of bone strength instead of BMD calculated the compression, bending, and impact strength of bone. These, as well as C-reactive protein (CRP), a measure of inflammation, were associated with fracture risk (Ishii et al., 2013).

Muscle

Estrogen beta receptor sites are sensitive to skeletal muscle function, and muscular satellite cells depend on adequate circulating estradiol. The degeneration of muscle quality and function during the TPM, known as sarcopenia, results from a release of inflammatory cytokines. Insufficient estradiol leads to abnormal cell proliferation, creating muscular functional changes (Geraci et al., 2021). These physiologic changes lead to decreased lean body mass, lean body mass index, right leg mass, and absolute and relative muscle cross-sectional area (Juppi et al., 2020). Participants in the SWAN study had a 0.2% decrease in lean body mass and 0.6% decrease per year (Greendale et al., 2012).

Although most studies of body composition and physical function have involved older PM women, research examining the contributions of body composition, physical activity, muscle capacity, and muscle quality to physical function performance in midlife women revealed relationships between optimal body composition (lower adiposity and higher lean body mass) and function. Nyberg et al., (2017) observed that PM women had significantly reduced exercise endurance with leg blood flow, oxygen delivery and oxygen uptake, lactate release, and blood pressure/heartrate workloads compared to women in the TPM. However, with regular aerobic exercise, there was improvement in muscular mitochondrial activity in the TPM and PM group. Degree of sedentary lifestyle and limited physical activity can pronounce the muscular dysfunction confronted during the TPM.

Overall, the TPM-induced weaker muscle mass lends to overall decline in functionality. Ward-Ritacco et al. (2014) assessed body composition using dual-energy x-ray absorptiometry, physical activity indicated by accelerometer (steps/day), and physical function using the Timed Up and Go test, 30-second chair stand test, and 6-minute walk test. Leg strength was measured by isokinetic dynamometry and leg power with the Nottingham Leg Extensor power rig. Women who had greater fat mass performed more poorly on the gait measure, although effects were not noted on the measures of endurance or speed and agility in the midlife women. Muscle quality was influential in tests of endurance, gait, and speed and agility. Bondarey et al. (2018) had similar findings; while PM women had the significantly weakest handgrip, TPM women had significantly reduced jumping height in comparison to premenopausal women. These findings support clinicians' attention to both muscle and fat mass in midlife women, given their potential functional consequences in midlife and old age.

The consequences of loss of skeletal muscle mass may include health outcomes during the postmenopausal period, such as development of sarcopenia, one component of frailty in older adults (Finkelstein et al., 2002; Sowers et al., 2003, 2006). Loss of muscle mass may lead to changes in physical functioning in PM women, as reflected by the measures of hand grip, ability to move from a sitting to a standing position, velocity of walking, and perceived physical functioning. Juppi et al. (2020) discovered in muscle biopsies of women experiencing the TPM that type 2 muscle fibers (fast twitch) were smaller than type 1 muscle fibers (slow twitch). The role of muscle in glucose metabolism and physical functioning has not yet been characterized fully in longitudinal studies of the TPM. To date, evidence about the influence of changing levels of endogenous estrogen and androgens on muscle function in women during the TPM and early PM has not been available from human studies. Studies of frailty in older women in whom multiple low anabolic hormone levels (insulin-like growth factor [IGF-1], free testosterone, DHEAS) and higher levels of IL-6, IL-18, and tumor necrosis factor-alpha (TNF-α) have been found, suggesting generalized endocrine dysfunction, emphasize the value of understanding the role of endocrine changes of the TPM in the development of sarcopenia and frailty in old age (Li et al., 2019). Physical inactivity, protein intake, and oxidative stress have also been linked to PM sarcopenia and are modifiable factors that clinicians can consider in promoting the health of midlife women (Maltais et al., 2009).

McClure et al. (2014) examined the influence of inflammatory and hemostatic markers (CRP, plasminogen activator inhibitor type 1 [PAI-1], tPA, fibrinogen, and factor VIIc) on physical functioning. They found that higher CRP and tPA were associated with greater limitations in physical functioning. African American women's higher fibrinogen levels were associated with greater physical functioning limitations. The relationship between hemostatic factors and cytokine levels may help account for inflammatory effects on muscle mass and strength.

In addition, El Khoudary et al. (2014) found that reduced estradiol or testosterone was associated with greater physical functioning decline. This is important given that changes in physical function may be a pathway to disability. Moreover, by age 56 to 66 years, nearly 50% of SWAN participants reported limitations in physical functioning, but these levels of function fluctuated, suggesting that interventions may be able to alter functioning levels. Ylitalo et al. (2013) found that higher BMI and arthritis were both associated with the prevalence and onset of limitations in physical functioning.

Fat

With the increasing prevalence of obesity in the United States, understanding changes in fat metabolism during midlife has become increasingly important. The SWAN study discovered fat mass and proportion of fat mass increased by 1% and 0.4%, respectively. Each year, there is a 1.7% increase of fat mass and 1% increase in proportion of fat mass (El Khoudary et al., 2019). Research conducted by Greendale et al. (2021) revealed similar findings during the TPM; truncal adiposity, or android fat, increased by 5.54% per year, along with visceral and gynoid fat. Waist girth grew by 0.94% per year during the TPM (Greendale et al., 2021). Changes in HPO hormones were related to changing fat metabolism. Increases in FSH have been associated with changes in levels of substances that regulate appetite, fat deposition, and inflammation. Increases of FSH were positively associated with leptin and adiponectin and negatively associated with ghrelin (Sowers, Wildman, et al., 2008).

SWAN data indicate that changes in sex hormones followed changes in waist circumference over a 9-year period when women were experiencing the TPM. Increased waist circumference was associated with subsequent lower SHBG levels, increased testosterone, and lower FSH. Estradiol levels were negatively associated with waist circumference in the early TPM and positively associated with waist circumference during the late transition stage. Women in late TPM or PM had a higher BMI and were more likely to be African American. Moreover, estradiol and waist circumference exhibited reciprocal effects. Waist circumference as a marker of weight predicted lower SHBG levels, possibly operating through adiposity-induced hyperglycemia, which may suppress SHBG. Hyperinsulinemia, hyperglycemia, and fatty liver are higher in the presence of greater abdominal fat, thus making it plausible that weight gain lowers SHBG by increasing insulin and glucose and/or by promoting hepatic fat accumulation. Taken together, these findings suggest that weight gain may set in motion endocrine changes during the TPM and bear observation for the health promotion of midlife women (Wildman et al., 2012).

Metabolic Syndrome

As changes in both intra-abdominal and subcutaneous fat mass occur, women experience changes in lipid patterns, glucose levels and insulin resistance, and thrombotic and inflammatory responses. Collectively, these have been characterized as the metabolic syndrome. As seen in Box 9.1, metabolic syndrome includes several risk factors for cardiovascular disease (CVD). Many of these risk factors become more prevalent as women complete the TPM. Changes in lipid patterns, glucose and insulin, thrombotic and inflammatory processes that compose the metabolic syndrome become more prevalent as women reach the late TPM stage and PM.

There is mounting evidence linking endocrine changes during the TPM to risk factors for heart disease, including the metabolic syndrome. Higher free androgen and lower SHBG levels are associated with cardiovascular risk factors for women during the TPM. Recent evidence suggests that an increasing ratio of testosterone to estrogen is implicated in developing metabolic syndrome. Women with low SHBG and FAI and high total testosterone at baseline experienced increased risk of metabolic syndrome over 5 years of follow-up. Both the baseline total testosterone:estradiol ratio and its rate of change were associated with the increased incident metabolic syndrome (Torréns et al., 2009; see Chapter 43, Cardiovascular Disease in Women, and Chapter 44, Endocrine-Related Problems).

Box 9.1 Indicators of Metabolic Syndrome

Abdominal obesity (waist >35 inches)
Atherogenic dyslipidemia, with triglycerides >150 mg/dL, HDL <50 mg/dL, and elevated LDL and small, dense LDL
Hypertension (blood pressure >130/85 mmHg)
Fasting blood glucose >110 mg/dL
Insulin resistance and glucose intolerance
Prothrombotic state
Proinflammatory state

HDL, high-density lipoprotein; LDL, low-density lipoprotein.

Lipid Patterns

The SWAN study cohort experienced changing levels of lipids during the late stage of the TPM and early PM consistent with cross-sectional findings from an earlier study (Carr et al., 2000). Total cholesterol, low-density lipoprotein (LDL) cholesterol, triglycerides, and lipoprotein (a) levels peaked during the late TPM and early PM. High-density lipoprotein (HDL) cholesterol also peaked during this period (Derby et al., 2009). Greater increases in ghrelin levels (important in appetite regulation) over the TPM were associated with increases in LDL cholesterol (Wildman et al., 2011).

Multiple hormonal changes during the TPM and early PM have been implicated in changes in fat deposition and lipid metabolism. In SWAN participants, FSH was associated with increased total cholesterol and LDL cholesterol. Estradiol was associated with increased triglycerides, lower LDL, and higher HDL. Higher testosterone was associated with greater BMI and higher triglyceride levels. SHBG was associated with lower waist circumference, BMI, total cholesterol, LDL, and HDL levels. FAI (a measure of bioavailable androgen) was associated with greater waist circumference, BMI, total cholesterol, and triglycerides (Sutton-Tyrrell et al., 2005).

SWAN data also revealed that lower levels of estradiol and SHBG and higher levels of FAI were associated with a higher atherogenic profile of lipoproteins. El Khoudary et al. (2015) found that lower levels of estradiol and SHBG and higher levels of FAI were associated with multiple indicators of a more atherogenic profile of lipoprotein subclasses. Estradiol was negatively related to medium–small LDL particle concentration and positively to HDL particle sizes. SHBG was related negatively to small LDL particle concentration and positively to LDL and HDL particle sizes. FAI was associated negatively with large HDL particle concentration and HDL and LDL particle sizes. These results underscore the important relationship of endocrine metabolism and heart disease risk factors during the TPM and PM.

Total cholesterol, LDL cholesterol, and apolipoprotein B (ApoB) increased 1 year before and 1 year following the FMP. Data demonstrate an increased prevalence of carotid plaque formation with these metabolic changes in cholesterol. Findings revealed the lipid patterns in women in TPM had a significant increase in the first 3 years following the FMP. Women who had an FMP at an older age fared better with greatest decline in total cholesterol, LDL cholesterol, and triglycerides (Matthews et al., 2021).

Glucose and Insulin

In another longitudinal study of midlife women, increases in leptin over the TPM were associated with greater glucose and insulin, insulin resistance, and greater diastolic blood pressure. Larger decreases in adiponectin over the TPM were associated with greater increases in insulin and insulin resistance as well as increases in systolic blood pressure and greater decreases in HDL cholesterol (Khan et al., 2014). FSH levels were associated with increased insulin resistance and lower insulin levels. Testosterone was associated with higher glucose levels. SHBG was associated with lower insulin, glucose, and homeostatic measurement of insulin resistance (HOMA-IR)

measures. Free androgen was associated with greater insulin, glucose, and HOMA-IR levels (Sutton-Tyrrell et al., 2005).

A report of data from the SWAN cohort indicates that bioavailable testosterone was associated with visceral fat, was a stronger predictor than estradiol, and was similar in effect to SHBG (Janssen et al., 2011). In addition, recent SWAN data implicate the effects of liver fat and insulin resistance in midlife women, indicating that the association between SHBG and insulin were greater among women who had fattier livers (Kavanagh et al., 2013). Moreover, as women progressed in the TPM, they had significantly higher prevalence and incidence of nonalcoholic fatty liver disease (Ryu et al., 2015). These data suggest that liver fat and SHBG both have important roles in metabolic risk among midlife women.

In addition, cardiovascular fat has been examined in relation to TPM status and endogenous sex hormones in the SWAN population. Women in the late TPM had approximately 10% more epicardial adipose tissue, 21% more pericardial adipose tissue, and 12% more total heart adipose tissue than those in the late reproductive stage or early TPM stages. Aortic perivascular adipose tissue was not associated with the TPM stages. Lower estradiol levels were associated with greater pericardial adipose tissue and total heart adipose tissue, and women with the greatest reduction in estradiol had greater volumes of pericardial fat (El Khoudary et al., 2015). Increases in pericardial heart fat deposits positively correlate with coronary artery calcifications (El Khoudary et al., 2017). The relationship between TPM changes with adiposity and insulin resistance leading to fulminant diabetes mellitus remains unknown.

Thrombotic Changes

Studies of hemostatic factors and hormone levels during the TPM revealed that both testosterone and estrogen play important roles. Androgens (testosterone and FAI) were positively associated with PAI-1 and tPA. FAI was positively associated with high-sensitivity C-reactive protein (hs-CRP). Lower SHBG levels, which were associated with greater levels of bioavailable testosterone, were also associated with higher levels of PAI-1, hs-CRP, and factor VIIc (Sowers et al., 2005). Compliment protein C3 was positively correlated with menopausal stage, significantly in women with obesity. Moreover, C3 levels were independently associated with higher levels of PAI-1, tPA-ag, factor VIIc, and fibrinogen (El Khoudary et al., 2013).

Estrogen was significantly related to some hemostatic factors in the SWAN cohort. Lower estradiol was associated with higher PAI-1 and tPA, but not with fibrinogen, factor VIIc or hs-CRP. Elevated FSH was related to higher levels of PAI-1 and factor VII and to lower fibrinogen and hs-CRP. The TPM was not associated with different levels of hemostatic factors. It is possible that endogenous estrogens may be associated with lower CVD risk via fibrinolytic but not coagulation or inflammatory mechanisms (Wildman et al., 2008).

Inflammatory Responses

Changes in intra-abdominal fat metabolism during midlife have been associated with inflammatory markers and adipokines. An increase in intra-abdominal fat from premenopause to PM was correlated positively with the change in serum alpha-amylase (SAA), CRP, tPA, and leptin and negatively correlated with the change in adiponectin (Lee et al., 2009). These are each involved in regulation of fat metabolism, inflammation, and appetite. During the TPM, women also experience changing levels of inflammatory markers, including IL-6.

A recent report indicates that there are between-group differences among women who have not yet begun the TPM, women in the TPM, and women in early and late PM. IL-4 was higher in late PM women, and IL-2 was higher in women in early PM, as was granulocyte-macrophage colony-stimulating factor (GM-CSF). Age was negatively related to IL-6, but the TPM and PM were unrelated. Estradiol was negatively related to IL-6 levels and weakly negatively related to IL-2, IL-8, and GM-CSF (Yasui et al., 2007). IL-6 levels were higher in women who were in late TPM compared to premenopausal women. Menopause stage and confrontation of stressors that promote inflammation was positively correlated with IL-6, IL-1β, and TNF-α (Metcalf et al., 2021). Healthcare providers must be aware that while the TPM extends fluctuating adjustments in inflammatory markers, inflammatory activity is further pronounced during encounters of situational stress.

The consequences of changes in inflammatory markers for physical functioning are of interest, given the risk of disability in older women. McClure et al. (2014) reported that higher levels of tPA-antigen and hs-CRP were associated with subsequent reports of greater limitation in physical functioning in SWAN participants. These findings prompt further consideration of longitudinal changes in inflammatory and hemostatic markers that may help understand and prevent the development of mobility limitations and other types of disability in later life.

Blood Pressure

Healthcare providers must consider the effects of TPM on a woman's hemodynamics. Changes in blood pressure are of concern because of their relationship to stroke and coronary artery disease. A systematic review revealed that women who became PM early (before age 45) had a higher incidence of arterial hypertension in comparison to women who became PM at a normal age (>45 years of age). It is presumed women with shorter durations of endogenous estrogen are more likely to develop arterial hypertension (Anagnostis et al., 2020). The prevalence of hypertension among the SWAN cohort varies significantly by racial/ethnic group, with White, Black, Hispanic, Chinese, and Japanese women having respective prevalences of hypertension of 14.5%, 381.%, 27.6%, 12.8%, and 11.0% (Lloyd-Jones et al., 2005). Current research focuses on controlling incidence of hypertension in perimenopausal and PM women. However, a gap remains to elaborate how TPM affects blood pressure, eliminating influence from comorbidities such as metabolic syndrome, obesity, dyslipidemia, and diabetes mellitus and social practices of smoking and alcohol intake.

Adaptation to Stress

A final set of changes observed in relation to the TPM is adaptation to stress. Studies of autonomic nervous system responses across the TPM stages and PM have revealed differences in stress response when comparing premenopausal and PM women. PM women exhibited greater increases in heart rate during all laboratory stressors compared with premenopausal women, with a pronounced increase during a speech task stressor deemed to be socially relevant to middle-aged women. PM women exhibited greater increases in systolic blood pressure and epinephrine during the speech task, but not in response to other stressors (Saab et al., 1989). Subsequent experiments confirmed this effect and demonstrated that women receiving estrogen therapy had an attenuated stress response (Lindheim et al., 1992), but a more recent study with transdermal estrogen in PM women 52 to 56 years of age revealed that acute transdermal estrogen administration did not attenuate norepinphrine spillover or sympathetically mediated hemodynamic responses (Sofowora et al., 2005). Recent findings relating chronic stress to sleep disruption in midlife women from the SWAN cohort suggest that increased physiologic arousal as indicated by beta EEG power may be involved (Campbell et al., 2011; Hall et al., 2015). Further research is needed to clarify the relationship of the TPM to this marker of arousal and related health effects.

Data from the SWAN study have illuminated characteristics of women's lives that have multisystem, cumulative, burdensome effects on physiologic dysregulation, termed *allostatic load* (AL). Investigators modeled effects of race/ethnicity, discrimination, hostility, socioeconomic status (SES), and perceived stress on AL. They found racial and SES differentials in AL in which African American women and women of lower SES had the highest AL. In addition, among African American women, the indirect effects of increased discrimination and hostility were predictive of a higher AL. For lower income women, the indirect effects of discrimination and hostility were predictive of greater AL, and greater perceived stress was predictive of more rapid increases in AL. For women with lower education, indirect effects through hostility were predictive of a greater AL. Chyu & Upchurch (2018) hypothesized that AL would increase 2%, but it actually increased 4% for each additional year from baseline. These results illuminate complex ways in which race, SES, and psychosocial factors influence AL, suggesting longer term health effects (Upchurch et al., 2015).

HEALTH PROMOTION FOR MIDLIFE WOMEN

Health promotion in midlife women includes promoting healthy behaviors to avoid disease plus early detection through regular screening for diseases, with early intervention as a goal. Healthy behaviors include the lifestyle elements of eating healthy foods, engaging in physical activity, and avoiding tobacco use and alcohol or if used at all, using them in moderation. Adopting healthy lifestyle behaviors can achieve the goal of preventing heart disease, cancer, diabetes, and other chronic diseases (Colditz et al., 2016). The focus of this discussion is on general health-promoting behaviors and age-appropriate screening practices. Discussion of health promotion and symptom management related to the TPM can be found in Chapter 34, Menopause.

Health-Promoting Behaviors

Health-promoting behaviors can reduce risk factors that play a significant role in disease development for midlife women. These health-promoting behaviors, considered primary prevention, target modifiable risk factors such as overweight and obesity, tobacco use, alcohol overuse, suboptimal nutrition, and sedentary lifestyle or physical inactivity (Stampfer et al., 2000). *Primordial prevention* is defined as healthy lifestyle behaviors that do not permit the appearance of risk factors. Most urgent among primordial prevention lifestyle habits is lowering the prevalence of obesity, as it affects blood pressure, lipid profiles, glucose metabolism, inflammation, and atherothrombotic disease progression. Advocating for universal healthy eating and physical activity are primordial prevention approaches to obesity. Routine physical activity also has overwhelming evidence for primary and secondary prevention for at least 25 chronic diseases and in reducing the risk for premature death (Warburton & Bredin, 2017). Of 84,129 midlife women participating in the Nurses' Health Study who had no diagnosis of CVD, cancer, or diabetes at baseline, those who scored in the low-risk range had fewer coronary events. A low-risk profile included women who did not smoke cigarettes, were within the normal weight range (BMI <25), maintained a healthy diet (low in transfat and glycemic load; high in cereal fiber, marine omega-3 fatty acids, and folate, with a high ratio of polyunsaturated to saturated fats), exercised moderately or vigorously for half an hour a day, and consumed alcohol moderately. Women with this low-risk profile had an incidence of coronary events that was more than 80% lower than that in the rest of the population across the 14 years of follow-up (Stampfer et al., 2000).

Elements of a healthy lifestyle, as defined by the U.S. National Library of Medicine, National Institutes of Health (2022), include the following:

- Do not smoke or use tobacco
- Get plenty of exercise
  1. Women who need to lose or keep weight off need at least 60 to 90 minutes of moderate-intensity exercise on most days
  2. For health maintenance, women need at least 30 minutes of exercise a day, 5 days a week
- Maintain a healthy weight; BMI between 18.5 and 24.9; waist less than 35 inches
- Get screened and treated for depression if present
- Women with high cholesterol or triglyceride levels may benefit from omega-3 fatty acid supplements
- Limit alcohol consumption to no more than one drink per day

Coronary Heart Disease

Heart disease is the leading cause of death among U.S. women (CDC & National Center for Health Statistics, 2020). In recent years a decline in the actual number of women dying from heart disease has been noted and is attributed to the reduction in risk factors and advancements in treatment of heart disease (Benjamin et al., 2019; Office of Women's Health, 2019). The American Heart Association (AHA) identified seven cardiovascular health (CVH) metrics consisting of four health behaviors and three health risk factors for the Life's Simple 7 tool (Lloyd-Jones et al., 2010) Long-term observational studies have noted that an overall healthy lifestyle (prudent diet, not smoking, healthy weight, and physical activity) in midlife may prevent the development of CVD risk factors and CVD events (Chiuve et al., 2014). Healthy lifestyle recommendations have remained consistent and are included in various guidelines to aid in reducing risk of CVD (Stewart et al., 2017). Health promotion related to reducing modifiable CHD risk factors includes reducing overweight and obesity, eliminating or controlling hypertension, reducing or eliminating dyslipidemia, reducing type 2 diabetes, avoiding tobacco use, and preventing stroke.

OVERWEIGHT AND OBESITY

Disease burden associated with obesity has grown in proportion to the increasing weight of the U.S. population (CDC, n.d.-b). Women are advised to maintain their BMI under 25 kg/m² (Mosca et al., 2011). The prevalence of obesity in the United States was 42.4% in 2018, an increase from 30.5% in 2006, with severe obesity rates increasing to 9.2% from 4.7% (Hales et al., 2020). Research findings consistently identify that a healthy diet is higher in vegetables, fruits, whole grains, low-fat or nonfat dairy, seafood, legumes, and nuts; moderate in alcohol; lower in red and processed meat; and low in sugar-sweetened foods and drinks and refined grains (Cespedes & Hu, 2015; U.S. Department of Agriculture [USDA], 2015). Eating a healthy diet is an important aspect of health promotion related to reducing or eliminating overweight and obesity, which can reduce the incidence of CHD and its risk factors as well as type 2 diabetes.

Physical activity has a positive effect on overweight and obesity, producing caloric consumption and regulation of adipose and pancreatic function. Additionally, exercise or physical work improves the capillary system and oxygen supply to the brain, thus enhancing metabolic activity, neuron oxygenation, and neurotropin levels and resistance to stress (Chedraui & Perez-Lopez, 2013; Kaliman et al., 2011). Any health promotion related to reducing overweight and obesity risk factors must include a component of physical activity. The AHA (2014a) recommends:

- At least 30 minutes of moderate-intensity aerobic activity at least 5 days per week for a total of 150 minutes
- *Or* at least 25 minutes of vigorous aerobic activity at least 3 days per week for a total of 75 minutes; or a combination of moderate- and vigorous-intensity aerobic activity
- *And* moderate- to high-intensity muscle-strengthening activity at least 2 days per week for additional health benefits (AHA, 2014a, 2014b)

HYPERTENSION

Health promotion related to reducing hypertension, according to the CDC (n.d.-c), includes (a) following a healthcare provider's prescription for medication use; (b) eating a healthy diet low in salt, total and saturated fat, and cholesterol but high in fresh fruits and vegetables; (c) taking a brisk 30-minute walk at least 5 days per week; (d) eliminating smoking, and if smoking, quitting as soon as possible; (e) limiting alcoholic drinks to one per day for women; and (f) getting between 7 and 8 hours of sleep each day. The optimum blood pressure is less than 120/80 mmHg, and guidelines recommend pharmacologic treatment of blood pressure of 140/90 mmHg or higher in adults younger than 60 years (Whelton et al., 2018). Guidelines for blood pressure management in individuals over 60 years of age are based on the clinical judgment of life expectancy and presence of comorbid conditions; the threshold for treatment may be an aggressive targeted blood pressure of 130/80 mmHg or raised to 150/80 mmHg (Kulkarni et al., 2020). Selecting a diet consistent with current dietary guidelines lowers blood pressure and lipids, which is expected to reduce the risk of CVD in healthy middle-aged and older persons by one third (Reidlinger et al., 2015).

DYSLIPIDEMIA

Higher-than-normal cholesterol levels can lead to CVD. Lowering cholesterol can reduce women's risk of heart disease and stroke. Health promotion related to lowering cholesterol includes encouraging patients to take responsibility for their diets. Eating foods low in saturated fats, trans fats, and cholesterol plus eating foods high in fiber, monounsaturated fats, and polyunsaturated fats can prevent high levels of LDL cholesterol and triglycerides while increasing HDL cholesterol levels. Specific recommendations are:

- Eat less saturated fats from animal products (cheese, fatty meats, and dairy desserts) and tropical oils (such as palm oil)
- Avoid trans fats, which are often found in baked goods (cookies, cakes), snack foods (such as microwave popcorn), fried foods, and margarines
- Limit foods high in cholesterol, including fatty meats and organ meat (liver, kidney)
- Choose low-fat or fat-free milk, cheese, and yogurt
- Eat more foods high in fiber, such as oatmeal, oat bran, beans, and lentils
- Eat a heart-healthy diet that includes more fruits and vegetables and foods low in salt and sugar

Additional health promotion related to lowering cholesterol levels is to exercise at a moderate intensity for at least 2.5 hours each week with activities such as bicycling or brisk walking. This can lower LDL and raise HDL. Furthermore, those prescribed cholesterol-lowering medication should take it as prescribed (CDC, n.d.-e).

TYPE 2 DIABETES

Type 2 diabetes results from the body's ineffective use of insulin; more than 95% of people with diabetes worldwide have this form of the disease (World Health Organization [WHO], 2021). Diabetes can damage the heart, blood vessels, eyes, kidneys, and nerves, resulting in (a) an increased risk of heart disease and stroke; (b) combined with reduced blood flow, increased nerve damage (neuropathy) in the feet and increased risk of foot ulcers, infection, and possible eventual limb amputation; (c) increased diabetic retinopathy, an important cause of blindness as a result of long-term damage to the small blood vessels in the retina; (d) kidney failure; and (e) doubled overall risk of dying compared with peers without diabetes (Sarwar et al., 2010; WHO, 2016).

The prevention of type 2 diabetes involves simple lifestyle measures (WHO, 2016):

- Achieve and maintain a healthy body weight.
- Avoid physical inactivity—get at least 30 minutes of regular, moderate-intensity activity on most days. More physical activity is required for weight control.
- Eat a healthy diet of between three and five servings of fruits and vegetables each day and reduce sugar and saturated fat intake.
- Avoid tobacco use—smoking increases the risk of CVD.

Observational studies found that a healthy lifestyle (regular physical activity, moderate alcohol consumption, not smoking, healthy diet, and normal weight range) greatly reduced the risk of developing type 2 diabetes (Galaviz et al., 2015). According to the U.S. Diabetes Prevention Program, the strongest predictor of type 2 diabetes prevention was weight loss. The risk of diabetes was 16% lower for every kilogram of weight lost (Knowler et al., 2009).

TOBACCO AVOIDANCE

Smoking is a major cause of CHD, with the risk associated with number of cigarettes smoked and the duration of smoking. A decline in smoking rates occurred from 20.9% in 2005 to 14% in 2019, with approximately 13% of women being smokers (CDC, n.d.-a). Through complex and interconnected mechanisms, cigarette smoking promotes atherogenesis and consequently atherosclerosis, endothelial dysfunction, altered lipid stimulation, and prothrombotic and proinflammatory states, all of which contribute to CVD pathology (Roy et al., 2017).

The major health promotion element for reducing risks associated with smoking is to stop smoking. Many venues, including in-person or telephone counseling, nicotine replacement, and pharmacologic therapies, are available to help women stop smoking (U.S. Department of Health and Human Services [DHHS], 2014).

STROKE PREVENTION

Stroke is the second leading cause of death worldwide and was responsible for 8.9 million deaths worldwide in 2019 (WHO, 2020). Accumulating risk factors and the aging population have contributed to the global lifetime risk of stroke increasing from approximately 23% in 1990 to 25% in 2016 (Virani et al., 2020). Direct and indirect costs of stroke in the United States in 2019 were estimated at $45.5 billion (AHA, 2019. Stroke is preventable by engaging in healthy lifestyle behaviors (CDC, n.d.-d; Meschia et al., 2014).

STRESS REDUCTION

A common definition of *stress* is when the demands of the stressor threaten to exceed the resources of the individual (Lazarus & Folkman, 1984). Stress has been identified as a major influence upon mood, well-being, behavior, and health. Long-term unremitting stressors can damage health. The relationship between psychosocial stressors and disease is affected by the nature, number, and persistence of stressors as well as by the individual's biological vulnerability (genetics, other constitutional factors), psychosocial resources, and learned patterns of coping (Schneiderman et al., 2005). Studies have demonstrated consistent associations between stress and level of health, particularly in CVD risk (Gallo et al., 2014).

Ten healthy habits that can protect from the harmful effects of stress have been recommended by the AHA (2014b). These recommendations include talk with family and friends, engage in daily physical activity, embrace the things you are able to change, remember to laugh, give up bad habits (drink alcohol in moderation, do not smoke), slow down, get enough sleep, get organized, practice giving back, and try not to worry. Incorporating these recommendations and adopting a healthy lifestyle, especially physical activity, can assist individuals in managing stress more effectively.

Osteoporosis

Osteoporosis is characterized by low bone mass and deterioration of structural bone tissue in aging adults resulting in increased risk of fractures. Women are four times more likely to develop osteoporosis and two times more likely to have osteopenia than men (Alswat, 2017). The WHO first convened a group of experts in 1994 to assess fracture risk and its application to screening for PM osteoporosis. It was this group that first defined the diagnostic thresholds for low bone mass and osteoporosis using a standardized score, known as a *T-score*, that compared BMD to average values for healthy young persons. Thresholds for diagnosis of osteoporosis based on T-scores are normal (T-score: −1.0 and greater); low bone mass or *osteopenia* (T-score: between −1.0 and −2.5); osteoporosis (T-score: −2.5 and below); and severe osteoporosis (T-score: −2.5 and below with a history of fracture; 4Bone-Health, 2015). Revised recommendations in 2004 included BMD plus selected risk factors for fracture along with height and weight. A Fracture Risk Assessment Score (FRAX) is calculated to determine a 10-year probability of fracture and is given in two scores: probability of hip fracture and probability for a major osteoporotic fracture, defined as wrist, shoulder, hip, or painful spine fractures (4BoneHealth, 2015).

Of the estimated 10.2 million Americans with osteoporosis 80% are women (Sarafrazi et al., 2021). One in two women older than 50 years will break a bone because of osteoporosis. This is attributed to the facts that women tend to have smaller, thinner bones than men and that estrogen decreases sharply in early PM, which can cause bone loss. Approximately 20% of White and Asian American women age 50 years and older, 10% of Latinas, and 5% of Black women older than 50 years have osteoporosis.

Osteoporosis is largely preventable by achieving maximal BMD (Nguyen, 2017) and yet is the most common bone disease in humans (Cosman et al., 2014). The main controllable determinants of bone health are nutrition with adequate calcium and vitamin D intake, physical activity, healthy weight, smoking cessation, avoidance of heavy alcohol ingestion, and fall prevention (Yedavally-Yellayi et al., 2019). The 2004 Surgeon General's Report on Bone Health and Osteoporosis proposed the following seven lifestyle approaches to bone health:

- Eat a well-balanced diet containing the following each day: 6 to 11 servings of grains; three to five servings of vegetables; two to four servings of fruits; two to three servings of dairy or other calcium-rich foods; and two to three servings of meat or beans.

- Get adequate calcium intake.
- Get recommended intake of vitamin D. Most individuals need 200 IU/day; individuals age 50 to 70 years need 400 IU/day; and individuals older than 70 years need 600 IU/day. Sunlight and dietary sources of vitamin D are recommended.
- Get at least 30 minutes of weight-bearing exercise every day (high impact: stair-climbing, hiking, dancing, jogging, downhill and cross-country skiing, aerobic dancing, volleyball, basketball, gymnastics, weight lifting or resistance training; low-impact weight bearing: walking, treadmill walking, cross-country ski machines, stair-step machines, rowing machines, water aerobics, deep-water walking, low-impact aerobics; non-weight-bearing: lap swimming, indoor cycling, stretching or flexibility exercises, yoga, Pilates).
- Maintain a healthy body weight.
- Avoid smoking.
- Drink alcohol in moderation (for women, one drink per day).

It is also important that midlife women prevent falls. Recommended actions for avoiding falls include (a) exercising regularly; (b) making the home safer (remove things that may cause tripping, remove small rugs or use tape to keep them from slipping, keep frequently used items in easy-to-reach cabinets, put grab bars next to toilets and in bathtubs/showers, use nonslip mats in bathtub/shower floors, improve lighting, have handrails and lights put in all staircases, wear shoes that give good support and avoid wearing slippers or athletic shoes with deep treads); (c) renewing prescriptions and taking medications; and (d) having vision checked. Measures that reduce fall risk provide secondary prevention of fractures (Santy-Tomlinson et al., 2018).

Cancer

Cancer cannot be prevented completely, but there are ways to reduce risk. Modifiable risk reduction for breast, cervical, ovarian, and lung cancer has many elements in common. Commonalities include limiting alcohol, being physically active, maintaining a healthy body weight, never smoking or stopping smoking, following recommended dietary guidelines for healthy living, and obtaining recommended screening (Gapstur et al., 2018). Breast and ovarian cancers have additional health-promotion options for women who carry one of the *BRCA* gene mutations: chemoprevention in the form of selective estrogen-receptor modulators (SERMs) or prophylactic surgery (bilateral mastectomy, bilateral oophorectomy). Prophylactic mastectomy results in a 90% decrease in breast cancer risk in these high-risk women (De Felice et al., 2015), and prophylactic oophorectomy can decrease the risk of breast cancer as well as the risk of ovarian cancer (Marchetti et al., 2014). Risk reduction and health promotion for midlife women related to cervical cancer is to follow guidelines for cervical cancer screening and to adopt lifestyle changes, such as using safer sex practices, stopping smoking, and getting vaccinated when appropriate (American Cancer Society, 2020). Lung cancer risk can be reduced by not smoking or quitting smoking, avoiding secondhand smoke, testing the home for radon (and reducing/eradicating as needed), avoiding carcinogens at work (exposure to toxic chemicals, use of a face mask for protection if toxins do exist), eating a diet full of fruits and vegetables, and exercising most days of the week (American Cancer Society, 2019).

Depression and Anxiety

The cause of depression and anxiety disorders is not completely clear, but it is known that both are more common in women (National Institute of Mental Health [NIMH], 2021a). Both disorders are thought to be triggered by stressful life events and/or ongoing stressful social conditions. However, there may also be biological, genetic, and psychosocial factors such as hormonal imbalance, brain chemistry changes, socioeconomic issues, lack of support network, diet, premorbid medical conditions, cognition, personality, and gender (DHHS, 1999). Major depressive disorder is one of the most common mental disorders in the United States, and women are 70% more likely than men to be diagnosed with depression in their lifetime. Major depression is growing in overall disease burden around the world; it is predicted to be the leading cause of disease burden by 2030 (Albert, 2015). Depression and anxiety are leading and increasing causes of disability worldwide, especially for women (Griffiths et al., 2014). Signs and symptoms of anxiety and depression are common during midlife and may occur concurrently with menopause-related symptoms. Some of these symptoms may mirror those of anxiety and depression and can be difficult to distinguish (Hickey et al., 2012).

Major risk factors for depression in midlife women include family or personal history of depression, history of postpartum depression, history of or current anxiety disorder, and alcohol and other substance abuse or dependence. Depression may occur concomitantly or because of other serious medical illnesses such as heart disease, stroke, cancer, HIV/AIDS, diabetes, or Parkinson disease (NIMH, 2021b). Many of the risk factors are not modifiable unless associated with lifestyle, such as physical inactivity and obesity, smoking, and intimate partner violence. Savoy and Penckofer (2015) noted that depressive symptoms are an independent risk factor of CVD and may also negatively affect health-promoting lifestyle behaviors and quality of life in women. Therefore, early detection and treatment are key. Signs and symptoms of depression include persistent sad, anxious, or "empty" feelings; feelings of hopelessness or pessimism; feelings of guilt, worthlessness, or helplessness; irritability, restlessness; loss of interest in activities once found pleasurable; fatigue and decreased energy; difficulty concentrating; insomnia, early-morning wakefulness, or excessive sleeping; overeating or appetite loss; thoughts of suicide or suicide attempts; and aches or pains, headaches, cramps, or digestive problems that do not decrease even with treatment (NIMH, 2021b).

Anxiety is often a normal reaction to stress and can be beneficial. When it becomes excessive, the individual may find that the anxiety is not controllable and that it may have negative effects on daily living (NIMH, 2022). Anxiety disorders and all other mental illnesses are complex and are likely a result of genetic, environmental, psychological, and developmental factors (NIMH, 2022). Women are 60% more likely

to experience an anxiety disorder in their lifetime compared with men. Little is known about the risk of anxiety in women during midlife and TPM. The SWAN study examined the association between TPM/PM stage and high anxiety during a 10-year follow-up of 2,956 women of multiple races and ethnicities. The study concluded that those with high anxiety during premenopause may be chronically anxious and not at increased risk of high anxiety at specific stages of TPM. In contrast, women with low anxiety during premenopause may be more susceptible to high anxiety during and after the TPM than before. Those with high anxiety were more likely to have a high school education or less, have difficulty paying for basics, be early in the TPM, and report frequent vasomotor symptoms, worse health characteristics, and at least one very upsetting event in the previous year (Riley et al., 2013). Anxiety disorders commonly occur with other mental or physical illness, including alcohol or substance abuse, which may mask anxiety symptoms and sometimes heighten them (NIMH, 2022). There is no specific risk reduction applicable; however, like depression, early diagnosis and treatment are key. General lifestyle health promotion, such as optimal diet and nutrition and physical activity, may positively affect anxiety disorders.

Purpose in life has been linked with better mental and physical health. As previously discussed, midlife holds different meanings for different women. Women who identify a renewed interest in health can be encouraged to draw on this newfound meaning to establish a new purpose in life. For example, in a nationally representative study of U.S. adults older than 50 years, a higher purpose in life was associated with a higher likelihood of use of preventive healthcare services (Kim et al., 2014). Several promising interventions have demonstrated that purpose, along with facets of psychological well-being, can be improved (Davidson & McEwen, 2012; Ryff, 2014). Ryff (2014) reviewed a dozen psychiatric intervention studies using cognitive behavioral therapy, meditation, or emotional disclosure and found these all enhance facets of well-being. As people with a higher purpose in life use more preventive health services, it is likely that they will have less of a negative effect on the cost of healthcare. It would seem prudent to add improving purpose in life to health promotion related to both depression and anxiety disorders.

In a sample of 48,273 Finnish women with a mean age of 45.6 years, physical activity provided a protective effect for later mental health in women. The study suggests that increasing physical activity levels may be beneficial in terms of mental health among midlife and older women (Griffiths et al., 2014). There are many commonalities in health promotion for disease prevention. Most commonly, experts recommend a healthy lifestyle, as well as primary prevention for diseases that have modifiable risk factors, as primordial. It would be prudent for clinicians to recommend all elements of a healthy lifestyle to their clients and particularly to midlife women who are more vulnerable to the onset of chronic disease than younger women. In this way, morbidity may be averted or ameliorated.

Health Screening

Health screening is defined as the use of a test or series of tests to detect health risks or preclinical disease in healthy individuals. The purpose is to permit prevention and early intervention (Dans et al., 2011). Health screening is not limited to conducting screening tests, such as cervical cancer testing. Instead, screening must include obtaining personal and family data to establish baseline and determine risk factors, performing a physical examination, and finally conducting screening tests. It should be noted that screening tests do not determine disease presence, and a single test is rarely sufficient to establish a diagnosis (Dans et al., 2011). Often at least two tests in sequence (screening followed by a confirmatory test) are necessary to determine a diagnosis. This approach is practical and generally more economical than using confirmatory tests for screening purposes, as confirmatory tests are usually more accurate but also more expensive. Screening coupled with personal and family history and physical examination data can uncover unrecognized health risks, such as preclinical diabetes and other diseases in an asymptomatic stage, such as breast cancer (Dans et al., 2011). The patient history should include screening for tobacco use, alcohol misuse, intimate partner violence, anxiety, and depression (Riley et al., 2013; USPSTF, 2016, 2022).

Health screening has been a widely accepted practice in healthcare, and proponents of screening programs emphasize the potential for early disease detection or assistance in changing unhealthy lifestyles (Hackl et al., 2015). However, screening is known to increase healthcare costs, which may underlie policy decisions to reduce health screening or eliminate it altogether. Recent debate has underscored the potential physical and psychological harm to healthy individuals from health screening and confirmatory testing (Ilic et al., 2013; Sabbath & Indik, 2006). An example of physical harm is pain or bruising related to a blood draw. Psychological harm usually occurs when an individual tests positive for the condition being screened for, such as a positive finding on mammogram, when being screened for breast cancer (Brewer et al., 2007). Confirmatory testing can also cause physical or psychological harm. Therefore, it is prudent to weigh the risks and benefits of health screening. Dans et al. (2011) developed the following criteria for evaluating screening strategies: (a) The burden of illness must be high, (b) the tests must be accurate, (c) early treatment should be more effective than late treatment, (d) tests and early treatment must be safe, and (e) the cost of the screening strategy must be justified by the potential benefit. Using evidence-based practice and updated recommendation guidelines, healthcare providers should discuss these issues with their patients and come to a mutual decision about recommended screening tests acknowledging patient values and goals of care.

Despite issues related to healthcare costs and potential physical or emotional harm, health screening is still considered a valued aspect of health promotion and maintenance. To that end, a number of organizations have made recommendations related to health screening for midlife women (American Academy of Family Physicians: www.aafp.org; USPSTF: www.uspreventiveservicestaskforce.org; DHHS: www.hhs.gov; American College of Obstetricians and Gynecologists: www.acog.org; and CDC: www.cdc.gov). Listed in Table 9.2 are recommendations for screening midlife women by these organizations on overweight, obesity, diet and nutrition, physical activity, tobacco and alcohol use, depression, intimate partner violence, diabetes, sexually transmitted infections (including HIV), CHD (hypertension, dyslipidemia), osteoporosis, and cancer (breast, ovarian, cervical, colorectal, and lung). Blank

cells in the table occur where organizations have made no specific screening recommendation.

CONSIDERATIONS FOR SPECIAL AND MINORITIZED POPULATIONS

Biologically, the physiology of menopause is similar at the core for most women. However, the TPM is arguably confounded by differences in culture, race/ethnicities, demographics, socioeconomic status, access, level of education/health literacy, and other social determinates that affect perceptions of the transition. Understanding cultural contextual factors that may influence the TPM symptom experience is essential. Special and minoritized populations perceptions, reflections, and experiences with the TPM must be considered.

There is currently limited research on perceptions and experience of TPM in specialized and minoritized populations. SWAN explored how ethnic background influences the perception of a woman's symptoms. The study concluded that ethnicity should be a vital component considered when interpreting menopause-related symptom presentation (El Khoudary et al., 2019).

Understanding the historical backdrop of these minoritized groups provides a better understanding of how various populations of women relate to the TPM as well as the challenges and barriers that influence their health outcomes. In U.S. society, women fall into a minoritized group when considering gender. Within that is another subgroup of individuals categorized as sexual and gender minority. Although the push for gender equality has afforded women some advances in society, women continue to face inequalities and health disparities in the form of access to and affordability of care. Being a woman from a minoritized racial/ethnic group exacerbates such inequalities even further and increases the risk of developing depressive and anxiety symptoms during the midlife transition (Im et al., 2009). The history of Black women in the United States positioned them to suffer from disproportionate adverse health outcomes stemming from a history of enslavement and systematic oppression compared to U.S. women of other ethnicities (Jones et al., 2016). According to the DHHS Office of Minority Health (OMH), U.S. Hispanic women have the highest uninsured rates of any racial/ethnic group. They have higher rates of obesity, with Mexican Americans suffering disproportionately from diabetes (2021), both conditions exacerbated by TPM. Asian Americans are most at risk for cancer, heart disease, stroke, unintentional injuries (accidents), and diabetes. They also tend to have infrequent medical visits because of language and cultural barriers (DHHS & OMH, 2021). Native Americans suffer from adverse health outcomes and have a high prevalence and risk factors for mental health and suicide, substance use, and obesity with 42.1% of them relying on Medicaid or other public health insurance coverage. It is worth mentioning that this ethnic group also frequently contends with issues that prevent them from receiving quality medical care such as cultural barriers, geographic isolation, inadequate sewage disposal, and low income (DHHS & OMH, 2021).

Other minoritized groups include transgender women; lesbian, gay, and bisexual persons; nonbinary persons; incarcerated women; and women living with disabilities. The plights of the transgender woman have only recently gained attention, and despite this increasing awareness, a paucity of research

TABLE 9.2 Health Screening Recommendations for Women by the AAFP, USPSTF, DHHS, ACOG, and CDC

SCREENING TARGET	AAFP	USPSTF	DHHS	ACOG	CDC
Overweight, obesity, and diet/nutrition	Annually; CAV	Screen all adults, NRSI	Same as USPSTF	BMI each visit	NRSI
Physical activity	CAV	CAV	CAV	CAV	CAV
Tobacco and alcohol use	CAV	CAV	CAV	CAV	CAV
Depression	CAV	CAV	CAV		
Intimate partner violence	CAV	CAV	CAV	CAV	CAV
Diabetes	Same as USPSTF plus recommendations from American Diabetes Association: all adults 45+ years; all adults with BMI ≥25 kg/m² and one of following additional risk factors: physical inactivity; first-degree relative with diabetes, high-risk race or ethnicity (Black, Hispanic, Native American, Asian American, Pacific Islander); delivered baby >9 lb or history of gestational diabetes, high-density lipoprotein cholesterol <35 mg/dL or triglyceride level >150 mg/dL, polycystic ovary syndrome, hemoglobin A1c level >5.7%, impaired glucose tolerance or fasting glucose previously, conditions associated with insulin resistance (obesity, acanthosis nigricans), or history of cardiovascular disease. If results normal, repeat screening in 3 years. Repeat yearly screening if prediabetes, and consider more frequent screening, depending on risk status.	Asymptomatic adults with sustained blood pressure (treated or untreated) >135/80 mmHg; insufficient evidence to recommend for or against screening adults with blood pressure ≤135/80 mmHg. Optimal screening interval is unknown.	Screening recommended for patients who have high blood pressure or take medication for high blood pressure.		
Sexually transmitted infections	Same as USPSTF plus all adults 65 and younger should be screened for HIV. High-risk women should be screened for gonorrhea, syphilis, and chlamydia infection.	The USPSTF recommends behavioral counseling for all sexually active adolescents and adults who are at increased risk for sexually transmitted infections.			
CHD: hypertension	Yearly in those with normal blood pressure CAV	CAV	CAV At least q 2 years	CAV	CAV

Topic				
CHD: dyslipidemia	Same as USPSTF	Screen women 45+ years if at increased risk of CHD; NRSI but reasonable option is q 5 years with longer or shorter intervals based on risk factors and lipid levels.	Recommend regular screening if patient uses tobacco, is overweight/obese, has personal history of heart disease and male relative had heart attack before 50 or female relative before age 60.		Screening at least q 5 years
Osteoporosis	Same as USPSTF	Women age 65+ years: DEXA screening NRSI. Women younger than 65 years: Use WHO Fracture Risk Assessment Tool to risk-stratify.	Age 65+ years get DEXA; age 50–65 years ask clinician if bone density test is needed.	Age 65+ DEXA screening interval no less than q 2 years in the absence of new risk factors. Postmenopausal women with fracture are screened to confirm diagnosis of osteoporosis and assess severity. Screen women <65 years with one or more risk factors for osteoporosis.	Same as ACOG
Cancer: breast	Same as USPSTF	Women age 40–49 years: provider/patient decision; biennial mammography screening beginning at 50 years with insufficient evidence to determine risk/benefit after age 75 years. Advise against teaching breast self-examination; insufficient evidence to assess additional benefits/harms of clinical breast examinations in women 40 years and older	Same as USPSTF	Begin annual mammography at age 40 years; clinical breast examinations annually at age 40 years and older	Same as USPSTF
Cancer: ovarian	Routine screening not recommended	Against routine screening			No screening recommendations; discuss symptoms with clinician

(continued)

TABLE 9.2 Health Screening Recommendations for Women by the AAFP, USPSTF, DHHS, ACOG, and CDC *(continued)*

SCREENING TARGET	AAFP	USPSTF	DHHS	ACOG	CDC
Cancer: cervical	Same as USPSTF	Screen women age 21–65 years with Pap smear q 3 years or, for women 30–65 years who want to lengthen screening interval, screen with combination of Pap smear and human papillomavirus testing q 5 years; recommends against screening in women older than 65 years who have adequate prior screening and are not at high risk; recommends against screening women who have had total hysterectomy with removal of cervix and who have no history of a high-grade precancerous lesion. In 30- to 65-year-old women, if Pap and human papillomavirus are negative, wait at least 5 years to rescreen.	Pap smear q 3 years or a combination Pap smear and human papilloma virus (HPV) test q 5 years until age 65	Same as USPSTF	Same as USPSTF
Cancer: colorectal	Same as USPSTF	Screen adults 50–75 years: annual fecal occult blood test; sigmoidoscopy q 5 years plus fecal occult blood q 3 years; colonoscopy q 10 years—all acceptable. Discontinue screening at age 75 (however, certain persons 76 to 85 years of age may warrant screening). No screening after 85 years of age. Insufficient evidence to recommend for or against CT colonography or fecal DNA testing.	75 or younger, get a screening test for colorectal cancer; NRSI		Same as USPSTF
Cancer: lung		Age 50–80 years with history of smoking: annual screening with LDCT with 30 pack-year smoking history and currently smoke or have quit within past 15 years; Discontinue when person has not smoked for 15 years or develops health problem that limits life expectancy or ability/ willingness to have curative lung surgery.	Screen if patient is between the ages of 55 and 80, have a 30 pack-year smoking history, and smoke now or have quit within the past 15 years.		Same as USPSTF

AAFP, American Academy of Family Physicians; ACOG, American College of Obstetricians and Gynecologists; BMI, body mass index; CAV, by convention, screen at all visits; CDC, Centers for Disease Control and Prevention; CHD, coronary heart disease; DEXA, dual-energy x-ray absorptiometry; DHHS, U.S. Department of Health and Human Services; LDCT, low-dose computed tomography; q, every; NRSI, no recommendation for screening interval; USPSTF, U.S. Preventive Services Task Force.

Sources: American College of Obstetricians and Gynecologists. (2013). Well-woman health care. http://www.acog.org/topics/well-woman-health-care; American Diabetes Association. (2012). Standards of medical care in diabetes—2012. Diabetes Care, 35(Suppl. 1), S11–S63. https://doi.org/10.2337/dc12-s011; Centers for Disease Control and Prevention. (n.d.). What screening tests are there? http://www.cdc.gov/cancer/dcpc/prevention/screening.htm; Centers for Disease Control and Prevention, Division of Cancer Prevention and Control. (n.d.). What should I know about screening? http://www.cdc.gov/cancer/dcpc/prevention/screening.htm; http://healthfinder.gov/HealthTopics/Category/doctor-visits/screening-tests/get-your-blood-pressure-checked; http://healthfinder.gov/HealthTopics/Category/health-conditions-and-diseases/heart-health/drink-alcohol-only-in-moderation; http://rethinkingdrinking.niaaa.nih.gov/IsYourDrinkingPatternRisky/WhatsYourPattern.asp; http://www.healthfinder.gov/HealthTopics/Category/nutrition-and-physical-activity; http://www.smokefree.gov; Moyer, V. A. (2012). Screening for and management of obesity in adults: U.S. Preventive Services Task Force Recommendation Statement. Annals of Internal Medicine, 157(5), 373–379. https://doi.org/10.7326/0003-4819-157-5-201209040-00475; Riley, M., Dobson, M., Jones, E., & Kirst, N. (2013). Health maintenance in women. American Family Physician, 87(1), 30–38; U.S. Department of Health and Human Services. myhealthfinder.gov; U.S. Preventive Services Task Force. (2003). Screening for obesity in adults: Recommendations and rationale. Annals of Internal Medicine, 139(11), 930–932. https://doi.org/10.7326/0003-4819-139-11-200312020-00012; U.S. Preventive Services Task Force. (2021). Lung cancer: Screening. http://www.uspreventiveservicestaskforce.org/Page/Document/UpdateSummaryFinal/lung-cancer-screening; U.S. Preventive Services Task Force. (2016). Breast cancer: Screening. http://www.uspreventiveservicestaskforce.org/Page/Document/UpdateSummaryfinal/breast-cancer-screening; U.S. Preventive Services Task Force. (2021). Colorectal cancer: Screening. http://uspreventiveservicestaskforce.org/Page/Document/UpdateSummaryfinal/colorectal-cancer-screening

data and clinical protocols of care continue to exist (Francis et al., 2018). Clinicians should be on the forefront of promoting strategies that forge a meaningful and collaborative relationship for sexual and reproductive healthcare needs with both transgender women and transgender men (female to male) as they experience the TPM (Francis et al., 2018). For transgender men in midlife who have a uterus, contraceptive concerns may be an important part of their annual wellness visit, and asking about what is needed and including appropriate care are important (Francis et al., 2018). Similarly, adherence to recommended mammogram screenings are important for transgender women on hormone therapy, those who have had breast augmentation, and transgender men who have not had top surgery (Francis et al., 2018). Patient education is key for all patients; in these subgroups where health literacy and access are limited, education is paramount in empowering them to take ownership of their health and seek healthcare or resources for health promotion and disease and symptom management (Jaffe et al., 2021). It is vital to teach these women about important screening and tests relevant to this phase of life, including what is normal and expected as well as symptoms that warrant seeking medical advice.

There are critical gaps in access to menopause-related resources and medical care for incarcerated women. Lifestyle changes and medical interventions to mitigate menopause-related symptoms in prison are largely inaccessible; untreated symptoms contribute to significant distress (Jaffe et al., 2021). Incarcerated women report feeling as though medical staff did not believe their concerns and were dismissive of their complaints. In some cases, menopause-related symptoms and symptom management exacerbated the ways in which institutional barriers reproduce criminalization within the carceral system (Jaffe et al., 2021).

The reality of the woman with disability living through TPM also cannot be overlooked. This minoritized group of women already face an ongoing struggle to promote their health and prevent secondary disabling conditions, which may be exacerbated by menopause. Thus, issues of midlife onset, progression of disability, and racial/ethnic disparities in disability prevalence and trajectories are particularly concerning given the effects that the burgeoning issue of midlife disability has on productivity, healthcare costs, and risk for future adverse health events (Karvonen-Gutierrez & Strotmeyer, 2020). The healthcare provider should be aware of these challenges and account for appropriate screening and testing needed when counseling and creating a plan of care.

From the SWAN study, Hispanic and Black women were more likely to report depressive symptoms, while Chinese and Japanese women were the least likely to report depressive symptoms (El Khoudary et al., 2019). Despite the adversities and challenges of midlife faced by minoritized women, they continue to show resiliency and positivity throughout this phase of life. Hispanic women viewed menopause as "just a change of life" (*cambio de vida*) from one stage to another stage, which is accompanied with physical changes moving

them from their ability to conceive to loss of that ability. Many of the women perceived these physical changes as positive, liberating them from a monthly menstrual period. They typically treated menopause with lowest priority due to their perception that it is a normal life stage (Im et al., 2009). For the urban Latina, the TPM signified a time for reorientation and restructuring for rediscovery and redefinition as opposed to being defined by physical symptoms (Villarruel et al., 2002). Based on the SWAN study, Black women were significantly more positive in their attitude toward menopause, agreeing that menopause signaled freedom and independence. The least positive groups were the less acculturated Chinese American and Japanese American women, which was attributed to cultural upbringing (El Khoudary et al., 2019). Native Americans view the TPM as a neutral or positive experience and PM women are considered "women of wisdom" within their communities (Jones et al., 2012).

Healthcare providers treating these groups of patients should educate themselves on the barriers and challenges that these groups face and provide patients with tools to combat some of these challenges. In the minoritized sexual and gender populations, identifying patients by their preferred pronoun is an important way to make them feel welcomed and open to further discussion about themselves. Acknowledgment and validation of a woman's experience as an intervention in itself can help to build a strong provider–patient relationship. Open provider–patient communication can allow for recognition of problem stressors and can facilitate effective interventions (Jones et al., 2016). It is our duty to continue to advocate and provide adequate equitable culturally appropriate care to all patients, especially those belonging to minoritized populations.

FUTURE DIRECTIONS

Research in the past several decades has provided a lens to better understand women's perspectives and experiences in the TPM. Providers can use this information to inform preventive and health-promoting care for midlife women. Much more research is needed to similarly inform care for other minoritized gender persons. In the interim, providers are urged to ask patients about their individual perceptions about, needs, and hopes for care at midlife.

REFERENCES

References for this chapter are online and available at https://connect.springerpub.com/content/book/978-0-8261-6722-4/part/part02/chapter/ch09

CHAPTER 10

Older Women's Health*

CHRISTINE ALEXANDRA BOTTONE

Our beliefs and assumptions about older women—their capabilities, interests, and goals—influence how we behave toward them. Likewise, our behavior and the care we provide to older women affect their images of themselves. Just as sexism and racism are associated with stereotyping and discrimination simply because of one's gender or skin color, ageism can lead to systematic stereotyping of and discrimination against people because they are aging (Burnes et al., 2019; Ochida & Lachs, 2015). Growing older is an inevitable and universal process, but personal fears and denial about our own aging can negatively influence our attitudes toward older women

The World Health Organization (WHO) defines ageism as any form of prejudice, discrimination, or stereotyping toward people on the basis of age (WHO, 2018). Additionally, ageism has been linked to negative physical and mental health outcomes in older women (Vahia et al., 2020). The added challenges wrought by the COVID-19 pandemic have further propagated long-standing notions of ageism within our society (Fraser et al., 2020). Self-isolation disproportionally affects older adults, placing them at increased risk for seclusion and isolation (Armitage & Nellums, 2020). This is significant, as most of this group's socialization occurs outside the home—in community centers, day care venues, and places of worship (Armitage & Nellums, 2020). To add, the media and public discourse during the COVID-19 crisis have created misrepresentation of the virus as "an older adult problem"—linking older age to comorbidities and frailty—further exacerbating ageism on a global level (Fraser et al., 2020). Older adults also may have fewer resources to cope with social isolation during the pandemic than younger individuals, as technology use in the older adult population is less frequent and was a key means of maintaining social connections (Vahia et al., 2020). Changing social behaviors and attitudes toward older age and the aging process itself is both possible and essential to promote health and longevity across populations (Officer & de la Fuente-Nunez, 2018). However, this is difficult—and intergenerational solidarity is important to maximize support of older adults (Fraser et

al., 2020). While societal attitudes are not easily changed, an understanding of aging and older adults' strengths and challenges can increase the effectiveness of the care we provide to this population—"for a society is measured by how it cares for its elderly citizens" (WHO, 2019).

The goal of this chapter is to increase understanding of the multifaceted nature of being an older woman in America today and to serve as a knowledge base for providing appropriate healthcare. The population of older adults in America is composed mostly of women, many of whom are poor, living alone, and dealing with chronic illness. Therefore, most issues of aging and older adults' health can be thought of as women's issues. Although many of the challenges facing older women today are gender based, the context within which these issues arise can be more broadly described as a sociocultural phenomenon in which youth is valued over age and independence is valued over interdependence, regardless of gender.

The term *women* is used in this chapter versus the more inclusive terms of *individuals* or *people* because most of the research cited in this chapter specifically involved cisgender women as subjects. It is not known if the research findings apply as stated to transgender or nonbinary women and individuals as gender is a social construct and a social identity. The term *older women*, as used in this chapter, refers to women age 65 years and older. Women's health issues have often focused on reproductive health and the changes associated with menopause, but until recently, women's postmenopausal years have been largely neglected. The lives of older women may span three or four decades (e.g., young old, middle old, oldest old, centenarians), such that this age group encompasses three or more birth cohorts of women who have led diverse lives and experienced a wide variety of challenges and opportunities. As young girls, some of these women experienced the Great Depression, whereas others were born just before Pearl Harbor was attacked. The sociocultural contexts of these older women's lives have been influenced by history and personal experience, changing norms and expectations, and visions and possibilities for the future. These powerful

---

*This chapter is a revision of the chapter that appeared in the second edition of this textbook, coauthored with Barbara B. Cochrane and Heather M. Young, and we thank them for their original contribution.

contextual factors shape individual and collective views of what it means to age well. Topics included in this chapter, therefore, encompass the demographic patterns and social forces that shape older women's lives, age-related changes, key health concerns experienced by older women, and considerations for healthy aging and health promotion.

Over the past 2 decades, there has been a dramatic increase in evidence related to older women's health and factors that influence health and quality of life. Much of what we know about older women's health comes from long-term, observational studies of men and women, such as the Baltimore Longitudinal Study of Aging, the Framingham Heart Study, the Rancho Bernardo Study, the Seattle Longitudinal Study, and the Health and Retirement Study. Longitudinal studies of women's health have included the Nurses' Health Study and the Women's Health Initiative. All of these studies have followed participants for 2 or more decades. Some of these studies included only older adults; others enrolled young or midlife adults (and, in some, their children) and followed them through their older adult years. Most of these studies, and many others, are still ongoing. Analyses of their data will contribute to our understanding of older women's health for many years to come.

DEMOGRAPHIC AND ECONOMIC CONSIDERATIONS

Population Trends

The older population in the United States, those 65 years and older, has grown rapidly throughout the 20th century. For example, the group grew over 10-fold at the start of the century, from 3.1 million in 1900, to 35 million in 2000, 40.3 million in 2010, and 52 million in 2018, now representing almost 17% of the nation's population (Administration on Aging, 2021; Roberts et al., 2018b; U.S. Census Bureau, 2021). Per U.S. Census Bureau projections, by the year 2034, older adults are projected to outnumber children under 18 for the first time in U.S. history. In some states, this demographic change has already occurred (U.S. Census Bureau, 2021).

Why this rapid increase? It is a combination of improvements in infant mortality, treatment of infectious diseases, and maturation of a large cohort, the baby boomer generation. This large segment of the U.S. population was born between 1946 and 1964 and started turning 65 years beginning in 2011, and the older population will continue to expand in the next decades (Roberts et al., 2018b). While the most recent census year was in 2020, only partial census data has been made available.

In the United States, as in most countries of the world, adult women outnumber adult men (Statista, 2020). Although male births outnumber female births, men generally have higher mortality rates at every age (National Center for Health Statistics, 2019), so the higher percentage of women compared with men is most pronounced at older ages, reflecting their increased life expectancy. Based on 2016 estimates, women composed approximately 53% of the 28.7 million

individuals between the ages 65 to 74 years in the nation (Roberts et al., 2018b). However, women outnumber men 2:1 in the 85 years and older age group—with an estimated 4.1 million and 2.2 million, females and males, respectively, based on 2016 data (Roberts et al., 2018b). In the 2010 census data, women accounted for 57% of adults 65 years and older and 67% ages 85 years and older (Federal Interagency Forum on Aging-Related Statistics, 2020).

Economics

The economic status of older women is an important factor in their health status and is influenced not just by current income and poverty rates, but by their Social Security and retirement benefits such as pensions, relative healthcare costs, and healthcare insurance coverage. Although economic trends for older women are rapidly changing as the U.S. economy has changed—and particularly, as more women enter and remain in the workforce full time—women still experience profound economic disadvantages compared with men, in part because of historical differences in life trajectories. For example, men and women in younger cohorts are earning college degrees at about the same rate, but the economic status of the current cohort of older women has been influenced by previous gender gaps in educational opportunity. In 2016 it was estimated that 22% of women and 32% of men aged 65 and older held at least a bachelor's degree (Roberts et al., 2018b). For the older adult age group, those 85 years and up, about 15% of women versus about 28% of men hold a bachelor's or higher degree for education (Roberts el al., 2018b).

INCOME AND POVERTY

In each age group of working adults, women earn approximately 82% of what men earn for comparable work and this gap increases with age (U.S. Bureau of Labor Statistics, 2021). For the older adult population participating in the labor force, 22% are men and 14% are female (Roberts et al., 2018b). However, it was true of every age group that men outnumbered women in the workforce (Roberts et al., 2018b). Occupational differences also exist with all ages of women, with women more likely to have an office or sales occupation (Roberts et al., 2018b). More older women than older men will live lives of poverty, regardless of race/ethnicity, geographic residence, age, or labor force participation (Bond et al., 2020). The poverty threshold was $12,261 in 2019 for individuals age 65 and older and living alone (Administration on Aging, 2021). Although poverty rates of older adults in the United States have decreased over the last half century (from 35% in 1959 to 9% in 2010 to 8.9% in 2019), age and sex disparities still exist (Administration on Aging, 2021).

Women who earn less than men for comparable work have lower total lifetime earnings (U.S. Bureau of Labor Statistics, 2021). This disparity is even more pronounced for racial/ethnic minority women, with these women in the workforce more commonly receiving lower wages and fewer benefits (American Association of University Women [AAUW], 2019). In the United States, the financial gender gap in wage earnings is so pronounced that it is predicted to not close until 2093 (AAUW, 2019). Hispanic and Black women are paid an estimated 54 cents and 62 cents on each dollar earned by men, respectively (AAUW , 2019). More recently, this disparity has increased. In the year 2019, the highest poverty rates in the nation were among Hispanic and Black women who lived alone (32.1% and 31.7%, respectively; Administration on Aging, 2021). Being older, female, a member of a minority group, and living alone constitute the greatest risk for poverty. Compared to the poverty rate for females within the total population, the rate for those 65 years and older was significantly lower—with 11% of women and 7% of men in the older adult age group living in poverty (Roberts et al., 2018b). Yet, in 2019, one in 10 individuals in the United States 65 years and older lived below poverty level (Administration on Aging, 2021).

Unfortunately, the COVID-19 pandemic has affected the number of older adults in the labor force. For example, per recent data about 18% or 9.8 million older Americans were either currently working or actively seeking work, versus 20.2% or 10.7 million older adults seeking work or in the work force the year before in 2019 (Administration on Aging, 2021).

SOCIAL SECURITY AND RETIREMENT BENEFITS

Initially planned in 1935, Social Security benefits were designed for dependents after the wage earner's retirement, disability, or death. Under the current regulations, Social Security is biased against some older adults and nearly all older women because benefits are still calculated based on pre-1950s family and work structures and more continuous career trajectories. Many older women have functioned in the dual role of homemaker and head of household while employed in low- or minimum-wage jobs with much lower lifetime earnings than men. In addition, women live longer than men and thus are more likely to outlive their savings and be more dependent on Social Security benefits. Women are penalized because they have a career trajectory that has been interrupted by childbearing, child rearing, and care of other family members, including elder care toward the end of their careers. Family caregiving does not generally provide a pension or individual retirement account (IRA) contributions. Due to complex Social Security calculations, single heads of families or spouses earning equal amounts of pay find such calculations benefit married couples with a primary wage earner (Hanna & Goldman, 2017). The disparity in benefits is further widened by women's lower wages for work comparable with their male counterparts', with 80% of female Social Security beneficiaries in 2018 age 62 and older receiving earned worker benefits (Federal Interagency Forum on Aging-Related Statistics, 2020). Of interest is that the percentage of females receiving earned worker Social Security benefits increased from 43% in 1960 to 80% in 2018 (Federal Interagency Forum on Aging-Related Statistics, 2020). However, it is noted that Social Security does constitute the most common form of income for older adults in general—regardless of gender (Roberts et al., 2018b).

HEALTHCARE COSTS

Older adults use more healthcare services than any other age group and make up a significant percentage of the acute care population- and most older adults have one or more chronic conditions (Administration on Aging, 2021). These trends are only expected to increase as the baby boomers age. Although there has been a decline in long-term care or nursing home use by older adults, a greater percentage of long-term care residents are women, and more women than men will live their final days in long-term care, which also represents the longer life expectancy of women (Federal Interagency Forum on Aging-Related Statistics, 2020). Additionally, in the nursing home setting, women represented 60.3% and 67.9% of short- and long-term residents, respectively (National Center for Health Statistics, 2019). There are various national and state health programs to which older women may turn, but significant barriers still exist to good healthcare. In many situations the criteria for employer and supplemental medical insurance coverage are more easily met by men than by women, and women are likely to have greater out-of-pocket expenses for healthcare over their older adult years, in part because of their increased longevity (Weller & Karakilic, 2020).

The two major sources of reimbursement for healthcare used by older women are Medicare and Medicaid. Interestingly, nearly all (94%) of those 65 years and older were covered under Medicare, with 99% having some type of health insurance coverage, and over half (52%) having some form of private insurance (Administration on Aging, 2021). Although most older women have health insurance through Medicare, they still spend the same proportion of out-of-pocket income (15% or more) on healthcare as they did before the passage of Medicare in 1965, despite recent changes brought on by the Patient Protection and Affordable Care Act (Kaiser Family Foundation, 2022). Out-of-pocket healthcare expenditures have only increased—with the average American age 65 and older with $6,833 out-of-pocket healthcare expenditures in 2019, which represents a 41% increase from 2009 when average out-of-pocket expenditures were $4,846 for the older adult age group (Administration on Aging, 2021). While one in 10 beneficiaries spent at least 52% of their income on healthcare in 2018, healthcare expenses pose a significant financial burden for women, with half of those with traditional Medicare spending at least 16% of their income on healthcare (Noel-Miller, 2021). In 2016, the percentage of income spent on out-of-pocket health expenses for Medicare beneficiaries was 13% for women versus 11% for men (Cubanski et al., 2019). Furthermore, healthcare costs are projected to equate to half of the average Social Security income by 2030 (Kaiser Family Foundation, 2022).

Although some preventive and behavioral counseling services are now covered by Medicare, only about 48% of older adults' healthcare costs overall are covered (Noel-Miller, 2021). These costs are disproportionately borne by women, who have a higher burden of chronic illness but are less likely than men to have Medicare Advantage or supplemental insurance and available family caregivers. The current reimbursement system discriminates against women because of its heavy emphasis on high-technology medical care and acute illness, whereas women are more likely to be diagnosed with chronic diseases and autoimmune conditions when compared to men (Daniel et al., 2018). Increased out-of-pocket costs for healthcare therefore become a considerable worry for many older women and may, in fact, limit or prevent their access to care.

Out-of-pocket expenses will continue to increase with females 85 years and older spending 83% of individual per capita income on out-of-pocket healthcare expenses in 2013 and this percentage predicted to increase to 98% by the year 2030 (Cubanski et al., 2018). This expense is significantly more than what males spent in the same age group, which was 58% of individual per capita income on out-of-pocket healthcare expenses in 2013 and predicted to increase to 68% by the year 2030 (Cubanski et al., 2018). There is a clear gender gap. Recent federal legislation has capped annual Medicare pharmaceutical expenses to $2,000 annually. The drug cap aspect of the Inflation Reduction Act is expected to be fully implemented by 2025 and will change the percentage of out-of-pocket expenses under Medicare.

Each of the potentially reimbursable services has exceptions, copayments, deductibles, and other requirements that place considerable limitations on the coverage overall and cause considerable confusion for older adults. In addition to these restrictions, Medicare does not cover, or covers in extremely limited ways, many important healthcare services, such as extended long-term care in nursing homes, hearing aids, eyeglasses, and dentures. In turn, individuals have extensive out-of-pocket expenses for medical devices and services not covered by traditional Medicare (Noel-Miller, 2021). The U.S. Congress has attempted to pass legislation to cover hearing aids, eyeglasses, and dental coverage for Medicare enrollees, but all attempts have failed to date.

Medicare Part D was instituted in 2006 to provide Medicare recipients with coverage for prescription drugs, regardless of income, health status, or prescription drugs used. Although many issues and concerns associated with the implementation of this coverage have been addressed, including a low-income subsidy, there remains a great deal of confusion and concern about appropriate coverage, enrollment periods, and the wide variety of plans and associated formularies and costs. The Centers for Medicare & Medicaid Services (CMS; www.medicare.gov), AARP (www.aarp.org/health/medicare-insurance), and other groups offer helpful online information about coverage, as well as searchable databases to identify plans from which to choose, given an individual's current prescription drug needs.

The feminization of poverty among older women, particularly women who live alone and women of color, makes out-of-pocket costs a critical issue that can become untenable for some. Exemplifying this notion is that out-of-pocket spending by women in traditional Medicare was higher than out-of-pocket spending by men ($5,748 versus $5,104 in the year 2016; Koma et al., 2021). Moreover, the share of Medicare beneficiaries' average out-of-pocket spending per capita Social Security income drastically increases with age and is higher for women than men, particularly for those age 85 and over and for those who identify as Black or Hispanic (Kaiser Family Foundation, 2022; Noel-Miller, 2021). Total spending for healthcare services and premiums increases with age but is also higher for women in general, and for those with higher incomes as well as for White people (Noel-Miller, 2021). Research has shown that a primary reason why women pay more out of pocket than men overall is because they use more healthcare (Daniel et al., 2018).

Additionally, the financial burden of healthcare as a share of income impacts lower-income Medicare beneficiaries disproportionately when compared to beneficiaries with higher incomes (Koma et al., 2021). In 2016, half of Medicare beneficiaries with incomes under $10,000 spent at least 18% of per capita income on healthcare costs when compared to only 7% for beneficiaries with incomes of at least $40,000 (Koma et al., 2021). Moreover, healthcare costs are borne disproportionately by women not only because of their higher burden of chronic illness and need for long-term services and supports, but also because they are less likely to have private insurance and available family caregivers. Out-of-pocket expenses also greatly differ for race and ethnicity with 12%, 11%, and 7% of individual per capita income being spent for individuals identifying as White, Black, or Hispanic, respectively (Koma et al., 2021).

As the primary source of healthcare coverage for the poor in America, Medicaid becomes an important healthcare support for older women, particularly women age 85 years and older. Older women are more likely than men to be poor, so Medicaid coverage is both a class and a gender issue, with women representing 59% of those individuals "dually eligible" for both Medicare and Medicaid in 2019 (Medicare Payment Advisory Commission & Medicaid and CHIP Payment and Access Commission, 2022).

CONTEXTS OF OLDER WOMEN'S LIVES

Relationships With Family and Friends and Caregiving

Demographic trends for older adults help explain why older women are much less likely to be married than older men; 46% of women 65 years and older are married compared with 71% of men of the same age range (Federal Interagency Forum on Aging-Related Statistics, 2020). Predictably, widowhood is more common than widowerhood, with 11% of men 85 years and older being widowed compared with 32% of women in the same age group, making older women about three times more likely to be widowed than older males (Federal Interagency Forum on Aging-Related Statistics, 2020). Research has shown that older individuals who value friendships have a more successful strategy for coping with the challenges of older age (Lu et al., 2021). However, women, individuals with a higher level of education, and individuals residing in countries low in inequality place a higher value on friendship in terms of its relative importance in an individual's life (Lu et al., 2021). With the higher likelihood of being unpartnered with age, close and intimate relationships for older women, many of which are long-term friendships, take on even more importance.

Older women enact many roles in the lives of their families. One of the most important roles is that of a caregiver. Individuals 65 years and older represent about 18.8% of total caregivers in the United States (National Association of Chronic Disease Directors, 2018). However, approximately, 75% of all caregivers are women, and they spend as much as 50% more time providing care compared to men (Daniel et al., 2018). Astoundingly, the economic value of the informal care that caregivers provide to adults with Alzheimer disease or dementia (not all chronic disease) is estimated to be $470 billion (Alzheimer's Association, 2022). Women as caregivers also partake in the responsibility of decision-making for others; in this sense, women reported making 20% of decisions affecting their spouse or partner and 27% of decisions affecting their children (Daniel et al., 2018). Women caregivers of a close relative are also at a higher risk for poor health outcomes due to the emotional and physical stress associated with the caregiver role (Daniel et al., 2018). More than half of caregivers (53%) experience a decline in individual health, thus compromising their ability to continue to provide care (Centers for Disease Control and Prevention [CDC], n.d.-a).

Additionally, in 2019, 1.1 million grandparents were responsible for the basic needs of at least one of their grandchildren under age 18 living with them, and 60% of these grandparents are women (Administration on Aging, 2021). In terms of caregivers assisting community-living older adults with activity limitations, approximately 64% of such caregivers are women, with the average age being 59.4 years for this particular group (Wolff et al., 2020). Caregiving prevalence at the household level varies among ethnic groups, with estimates of family caregiving occurring in 10.2% of Asians and Pacific Islanders, 17.9% of Hispanics, 24.3% of African Americans/Black Americans, and 23.1% of White households (National Association of Chronic Disease Directors, 2018). Racial disparities also vary on the premise of specific caregiving tasks, with Black and Hispanic caregivers completing more health-related tasks than White caregivers (Leggett et al., 2022). Hispanic caregivers were more likely to use their own money to pay for the care recipient's medications and medical care (25.9%) when compared to non-Hispanic Black (25.7%) and White caregivers (14.2%; Leggett et al., 2022). Additionally, the cultural and generational context of the individual caregiver shapes both expectations about caregiving and the experience of caregiving, including role and identity, rewards and challenges, and resources and supports (Apesoa-Varano et al., 2015–2016). Race, ethnicity, and gender disparities result in barriers to education and to a lower lifetime income which may be associated with more disability and health care needs in aging. Informal supports systems maybe be insufficient to meet caretaking needs (Spillman et al., 2020).

Midlife and older women are the most frequent caregivers of aging parents and spouses, with about 25% spending 5 years or more providing care and higher hour caregivers (who spend more than 20 hours a week providing care) spending 10 years or more providing care. This fact is quite extraordinary when one considers the 17 years spent, on average, caring for their own dependent children and the fact that some older women are the primary caregivers for their grandchildren. Although midlife women are sometimes described as being in the "sandwich" generation (caring for both their children and their parents), some older adult women may also be providing care for three generations of family members or more. During the COVID-19 pandemic, caregivers faced additional burdens as the need to shelter in place for an extensive period of time aggravated their existing scenarios Caregivers during the pandemic were more likely to be women, slightly older, married or partnered, unemployed/retired, live alone, and have a health condition or disability in comparison to noncaregiver counterparts (Gallagher & Wetherell, 2020).

Although, the rate of depression increased for both caregivers and noncaregivers during the COVID-19 pandemic, caregivers were more likely to report new depressive symptoms (21.6%) when compared to noncaregivers (17.9%; Gallagher & Wetherell, 2020). An estimated 45% of women provided child care during the pandemic compared to only 14% of men (Zamarro & Prados, 2021). Moreover, women generally have incurred a greater burden than men in the COVID-19 crisis, in terms of the need to provide child care even when continuing to work. This workload was associated with the reduction of employment hours and the increased likelihood for women to transition out of employment as an undue consequence (Zamarro & Prados, 2021). Caregivers play a vital role, and the lack of individual caregivers is a public health priority. In 2019, it was estimated that seven potential family caregivers exist per adult; however, by 2030, there will be only four potential family caregivers for every adult (CDC, n.d.-a).

An extensive literature on caregiving has established both the rewards and strains of this experience, including a sense of meaning, meeting of interpersonal obligations, pleasure in providing care to a loved one, and satisfaction, as well as feelings of burden and emotional stress. The impact of caregiving on the older women is a function of many factors, including vulnerability and strengths, the demands of the care situation, social support, characteristics of the care recipient, the type and quality of the dyad's relationship, and health (AARP & National Alliance for Caregiving [NAC], 2020). The physical and emotional demands over a long period can result in negative health outcomes, including increased morbidity and mortality risks for caregivers (Gallagher & Wetherell, 2020; National Association of Chronic Disease Directors, 2018).

Many older women will be the primary providers of end-of-life care for their spouses, and their release from caregiving responsibilities comes with the death of the spouse. However, the death of a spouse, particularly after long-term caregiving, is one of the most significant losses for older women, often requiring great changes in lifestyle. Spousal bereavement and widowhood have become almost normative for aging women. However, many aging women demonstrate an extraordinary degree of resiliency, resourcefulness, and adaptability after the death of a spouse (King et al., 2019).

Living Arrangements

Older women in every racial/ethnic group, as well as in each age group, because of their increased longevity and fewer available potential partners, are more likely than men to live alone. However, non-Hispanic White women and Black women are more likely to live alone than Hispanic and Asian women, who are more likely to live with relatives (Federal Interagency Forum on Aging-Related Statistics, 2020). Marital history and number of children may influence these findings, as may cultural variations in beliefs about the care of older relatives or more available extended family members and thus more resources for care. Older women were more likely than men to live in multigenerational households (15% vs. 7%; Federal Interagency Forum on Aging-Related Statistics, 2020). Most older women live in independent housing with only 3% living in group care facilities (Federal Interagency Forum on Aging-Related Statistics, 2020). Rates of nursing home residence have declined overall in recent years, reflecting both shorter stays in these settings for acute rehabilitation and wider variety of long-term care living arrangements available for older adults.

Aging in place, or aging at home, has been considered both a goal and a desirable response to the needs of aging individuals (Ahn et al., 2020). Health disparities exist and reflect inequalities associated with aging itself but also reflect the accumulation of disparities faced throughout the individual's lifetime (MacGuire, 2020). Evidence has shown that in order to reduce health inequalities at older ages, interventions must address the social determinants of health in early life and continue through the life course (Macquire, 2020). While disparities indicate that women may be more reliant on family care, there is often a lack of family caregivers to meet the needs of the aging individual (Wang et al., 2020). With older age, the individual's social network tends to shrink and family support, as a critical component of social support, has been shown to have greater significance than nonfamily support for older adults (Wang et al., 2020).

Rural and Urban Contexts

The percentage of all older adults in rural areas is slightly higher than in urban areas (17.8% compared with 15.5%; Tuttle et al., 2020). Interestingly, the population of rural communities has a higher percentage of older adults (age 65 and over) while urban communities have a higher percentage of the oldest adults (age 85 and over; Tuttle et al., 2020). Rural communities are not keeping pace with urban communities on life expectancy, mortality rate, and other major health indicators (Health Resources and Services Administration, Office of Health Equity, 2018).

Economic security and access to healthcare are significant problems for many older adults; however, rural residents have lower average incomes and higher poverty rates than urban residents. Urban older adults possess nearly twice as much total household wealth and assets ($471,290) compared to older adults residing in rural communities ($264,573; Tuttle et al., 2020). Individuals in rural communities are more geographically isolated, have fewer financial resources, have higher rates of chronic disease with fewer community-based resources for managing chronic illness, and thus experience poorer health outcomes than their urban counterparts (Tuttle et al., 2020). The trend in closure of rural hospitals has reduced access to care. Facilities that closed both inpatient and outpatient services more likely served a higher proportion of people of color (Office of Health Equity, 2020). In rural areas where healthcare access is not a barrier, health outcomes may still remain poor. Many of these communities are dealing with the impact of multigeneration poverty with limited economic and educational opportunities, complicated even more by the ever-growing drug abuse problem (Office of Health Equity, 2020).

Retirement

Women are less prepared and less likely to retire when they reach retirement age, in large part because of the economic disadvantages related to their work and work-related benefits (Dowell, 2022). However, participation in the labor force is changing, and the gap between men's and women's participation is narrowing considerably. These trends mandate a closer examination of women's adjustment to retirement and the changes in social and personal resources as well as psychological and physical well-being after retirement. Women's adjustment to retirement is reflective in part to the age that a woman retires, and recent data has shown a gap in monthly wages of almost $4,000 for women who hold a bachelor's or advanced degree compared to men with such degrees (Dowell, 2022).

The COVID-19 pandemic has impacted older women's ability to retire and their adjustment to retirement (American Society of Pension Professionals and Actuaries, 2022). Men were shown to be more likely to increase their retirement savings in response to the pandemic when compared to women. Reports show that in response to the pandemic 41% of women are saving more for retirement when compared to 59% of their male counterparts (American Society of Pension Professionals and Actuaries, 2022).

Most studies of women and retirement focus on the timing of retirement and retirement planning. Reviews of retirement research on women have indicated that because of different life paths and career trajectories, women do not prepare for retirement in the same way that men do, in terms of their decision-making or their consideration of risk (Wanka, 2019). For women, their choices about retirement may be based on being able to contribute to social life more than their productivity. Women report less subjective well-being and satisfaction during retirement than men (Calasanti et al., 2021), although this difference is small. Compared to men, women derive less overall life satisfaction associated with entering retirement and this disparity is representative of women's lower satisfaction with their savings and overall finances (Calasanti et al., 2021). Factors that contribute to women's perceptions of a good retirement include good health, fewer years spent in part-time employment as they lack the financial means to stop working, an early retirement, a good postretirement income, volunteer work, as well as more frequent and a greater variety of social activities. As a culture, we lack the societal map for ongoing engagement and meaning after retirement, and this is further aggravated by the complex patterns of social inequalities associated with the transition to retirement unchanged in decades (Wanka, 2019). Retirement is associated with an increased risk of cognitive decline and this in part reflects the issue of finding meaning and further social engagement without employment (Hamm et al., 2020). One of the developmental challenges of late life, as described by Erik Erickson, is determining how one remains involved in connections and activities that are meaningful, despite changes in social networks (Erikson et al., 1986).

Racial/Ethnic Contexts

Population projections suggest that by 2030, the older adult population in the United States will be much more diverse. This represents the demographic changes in the overall U.S. population during past several decades (Federal Interagency Forum on Aging-Related Statistics, 2020). Taking this into account, in 2018, 77% of the population was composed of non-Hispanic White individuals, 9% non-Hispanic Black individuals, 5% non-Hispanic Asian individuals, and 8% Hispanic individuals (of any race; Federal Interagency Forum on Aging-Related Statistics, 2020). However, by 2060, it is projected that non-Hispanic White individuals will represent 55% and Hispanic individuals 21%, compared to 13% non-Hispanic Black individuals and 8% non-Hispanic Asian individuals (Federal Interagency Forum on Aging-Related Statistics, 2020). The population of individuals of Hispanic ethnicity is predicted to grow the fastest (Federal Interagency Forum on Aging-Related Statistics, 2020). There is also expected to be increasing numbers of immigrant women and older women classified as "other" because they are of two or more races. Older Hispanic and Asian people have more likely immigrated while most older White and Black Americans were born in the United States (Roberts et al., 2018a). Immigrant older adults represent considerable diversity in their countries of origin, with wide-ranging languages and cultural traditions. Women from underrepresented racial/ ethnic groups will face the greatest challenges with poverty and illness, and it is this segment of the population that is growing the fastest.

Any consideration of the status of older women of color must be tempered by the fact that accurate information on the demographics of this population has been lacking until recent times, and moreover, the current information that is available regarding this population does not include their perspectives nor the issues that reflect their specific aging community (Newcomb, 2021). Newcomb (2021) notes that the undercounting of African American and Hispanic populations in the 1970 census led to a political advocacy movement by these groups to obtain more accurate national data. Accurate documentation of the increasing diversity of older adults now challenges the healthcare system to incorporate greater inclusiveness in its programs and services to meet the varying needs of the changing population.

Lesbian Older Women

With the aging of the population, there are a growing number of older LGBTQ adults. Although older women with female partners may not have revealed their sexual identity publicly during the earlier years of their lives, they have unique health concerns and often remain relatively invisible and underserved within the healthcare system and by healthcare researchers (Laramie, 2021). The majority of available research on aging ignores women's sexual orientation; however, sexual orientation–related discrimination that older women have faced across the life course may influence a corresponding increased risk for poorer health (Jabson Tree et al., 2021). Even less research has focused on the transgender older adult.

In the context of societal intolerance for same-sex relationships, older lesbians can face particular challenges in advocating for and participating in decision-making for their partners during acute and chronic illness episodes, as well as accessing partner health benefits for their own healthcare. LGBTQ older women have identified several areas for improvement in health and social services to address needs for LGBTQ-oriented/friendly legal advice, social events, grief and loss counseling, social workers, and assisted living (Jabson Tree et al., 2021; Valenti et al., 2021). An increasingly

salient issue is effective end-of-life planning, including ensuring legal rights and designated decision-makers such as durable powers of attorney, areas where both older LGBTQ adults and healthcare providers lack adequate preparation (see Chapter 20). End-of-life planning and grief support are also lacking for this specific group of older women. However, of note, interactions with healthcare professionals during the end of life and bereavement process are improving (Valenti et al., 2021).

AGE-RELATED PHYSICAL CHANGES

Is the end of life built into its beginning? Several theories of aging focus on aging at a cellular level. For example, the free radical theory of aging suggests that aging is due in part to by-products of oxidative metabolism that attack cellular DNA and result in mutations (Martin, 1992); the thesis of genetic instability refers to faulty copying in dividing cells or the accumulation of errors in information-containing molecules (Kane et al., 2003). In general, the literature shows that psychological stress has been related to biological stress (Chang et al., 2018). More recently, the study of telomeres—DNA caps on the end of chromosomes, which protect the genetic material and shorten with each replication to a critical point signaling the end of the cell's replicative life—has contributed to our understanding of biological aging and age-related diseases by exhibiting the aging process and age-related disease in terms of telomere dysfunction (Rossiello et al., 2022). For example, osteoporosis, commonly seen in older women, is associated with changes in aging bone and is related to the shortening of telomere length (Pignolo et al., 2021; Rossiello et al., 2022). Recent research is exploring the longer telomere length in women compared with men as a possible linkage to women's greater longevity (Sutphin & Korstanje, 2016). The faster shortening of the telomere lengths in men has been explained as the major reason for shorter life expectancy (Öngel et al., 2021).

Additionally, recent research has studied how physical activity and cognition affect the telomere length of older women—with studies demonstrating that participation in a physical exercise program for at least 6 months can lead to an improvement in both cognitive functions and telomere length (Sánchez-González et al., 2021). Interestingly, caregiver stress and depressive symptoms also have been shown to affect telomere length in older women. In this respect, the chronicity of the caregiver role (measured in years) was significantly associated with a shorter telomere length in older women when compared to older women who were not in the caregiver role (Chang et al., 2018). However, there is very little existing literature regarding the intensity of the caregiver role and telomere length when compared to literature regarding depression and telomeres (Chang et al., 2018). Lastly, recent studies have explored diet as a regulator of telomere length through its impact on entropy and the overall aging process (Öngel et al., 2021). For example, when using telomere length as a basis for predicting life expectancy, it is estimated that the lowest length and highest life expectancy for women are associated with vegetarian and Mediterranean diets (Öngel et al., 2021).

The sentinel Baltimore Longitudinal Study of Aging study (Shock et al., 1984) identified six patterns of physical changes that can be viewed as age related: (a) the stability or the absence of significant change with age (e.g., personality); (b) declination with age resulting from age-related illnesses (e.g., arthritis); (c) steady declines in physical function even in the context of general good health (e.g., muscle strength); (d) more precipitous change in function, often associated with disease (e.g., dementia); (e) compensatory change to maintain function (e.g., aerobic capacity); and (f) changes over time that are unrelated to aging but instead reflect more secular trends (e.g., changes in diet resulting from increased processing of foods). Most physical changes of aging are not gender specific, but age-related changes do occur at different rates among individuals, and systems age at different rates within an individual, resulting in the great heterogeneity of aging processes among older adults (Kaeberlein & Martin, 2016).

Cardiovascular

Age-related structural and functional changes within the heart are similar for both older men and women and include increased vascular thickening and resultant stiffness, which correlates with the onset of hypertension in advancing age. Although not strictly a normal change of aging, the effects of lifestyle and heredity on atherosclerotic changes begin fairly early in life and accumulate over time such that most older women and men have some degree of subclinical or clinical coronary vascular disease (CVD). Women have some protective effects with estrogen and as levels decline after menopause, the rates of heart disease increase (see Chapter 43, Cardiovascular Disease in Women, for a discussion on the effect of menopause on heart health).

Women in midlife experience a change in body fat distribution from a premenopausal gynoid pattern (more hips and thighs weight distribution) to a preferential android pattern (more abdominal/visceral weight distribution). Abdominal fat is an endocrine organ producing adipokines and inflammatory factors that impact hepatic metabolism altering the level of triglycerides and increasing insulin resistance and thus a risk factor for cardiovascular disease. Such changes may lead to the development of metabolic syndrome, type 2 diabetes, and cardiovascular disease. Neither aging nor menopause is thought to cause weight gain per se; more likely the weight gain is from a decline in physical activity and lower quality of dietary intake.

Immune Function

Age-related changes in both cell-mediated and humoral immune systems, sometimes described as biological immunosenescence, are often accompanied by an increased incidence of malignancy, autoimmune diseases, inflammation, and infections in older adults. Cellular senescence is thought to contribute to aging through two pathways: (1) senescence of stem cells leads to dysfunctional stem cells, which in turn, decrease tissue regeneration, and (2) cells secrete proinflammatory, tissue destructive accumulations in various tissues with aging and at sites of pathogenesis in many chronic conditions

(Kang, 2019; Kirkland & Tchkonia, 2017). Prior to the development of COVID-19 vaccines, older adults were at higher risk of COVID-19–related illness and complications, hospitalization, and death than younger people through the age-related decline in immune function. Another example of the decline of immune function is the reactivation of the herpes zoster virus to cause shingles in older adults. Age-related immune function decline is a risk factor for many of the cancers that affect older women, such as breast, colorectal, and ovarian cancer.

Cognition

Cognition refers to the various mental functions—such as thinking, decision-making, memory, attention, and problem-solving—that are important for gaining, storing, using, and expressing knowledge as well as engaging in daily functional activities. Cognitive aging involves a gradual and dynamic process of changes in cognitive function that occur as a person gets older; these changes involve varying capacities, such as motivation, short- and long-term memory, intelligence, learning and retention of tasks, and other factors that facilitate or impede these capacities. Common age-related cognitive changes are manifested as slow retrieval of names, feeling the word is at "the tip of the tongue" or misplacing objects around the house. There is significant interindividual and intraindividual variation in cognitive aging with the differences due to health status, lifestyle, education, mental health, and other life experiences. Some abilities decline, whereas others, such as wisdom, remain stable, and yet others, such as knowledge, can improve with age. Some memory impairment may occur as women get older, but dementia, even mild cognitive impairment (MCI), is not considered a part of typical cognitive aging. Currently, there is not an effective, safe, economical pharmacologic treatment for cognitive decline and neurodegeneration. Modifying risk factors over a lifetime, however, could delay or prevent 40% of dementia cases (Livingston et al., 2020). The modifiable risk factors include reducing: smoking, exposure to air pollution and second-hand tobacco smoke, hearing loss by protecting ears from high noise levels, obesity, alcohol intake, head injury, hypertension, and diabetes. Positive activities include providing primary and secondary education to all, promoting an active lifestyle, and providing hearing aids to anyone in need (Livingston et al., 2020).

Sensory

Presbyopia, a gradual loss of the eyes' focusing ability because of lens changes, results in slightly increased far-sightedness (i.e., decrease in ability to see up close) and some difficulty with accommodation and is a typical change of aging. Other typical changes associated with the aging process include needing longer to adjust to changes in levels of light and difficulty in distinguishing certain similar color variation such as blue from black (National Institute on Aging, n.d.-a). Other vision changes, such as glaucoma, cataracts, and age-related macular degeneration are more age-related conditions; they occur more commonly in older adults but not in all (National Institute on Aging, n.d.-a). Certain age-related vision changes however are further aggravated or triggered by prolonged, uncontrolled hypertension or hyperglycemia, which exemplifies microvascular changes occurring with chronic conditions, such as diabetes and hypertension through resulting diabetic and hypertensive retinopathies and vision loss (National Institute on Aging, n.d.-a). For example, elevated systolic blood pressure increases individual risk for glaucoma (Hua et al., 2021).

Similarly, presbycusis, like presbyopia, results from sensory changes in the aging process. Presbycusis, a gradual and very slight impairment in hearing primarily for higher pitched tones, is considered a normal change of aging. In fact, age has been shown to be the strongest predictor for presbycusis, yet there has not been an intervention identified that can prevent age-associated hearing loss (National Institute on Deafness and Other Communication Disorders, 2021).

Visual and/or hearing impairments have been reported by approximately 15% and 31% of women aged 65 years and older, respectively (Federal Interagency Forum on Aging-Related Statistics, 2020). Data also show that in recent years there has been an overall increase in adults age 65 years and older reporting functional limitations in association with vision and hearing changes—with 3.1% and 5.2%, in 2018, reporting vision and hearing loss, respectively, compared to 2011 when these changes were reported by 2.8% and 5%, respectively (Federal Interagency Forum on Aging-Related Statistics, 2020).

An estimated 28.8 million U.S. adults could benefit from using hearing aids; however, only about 16% of people in the younger age group of 20 to 69 years who could be helped by hearing aids have ever used them (National Institute on Deafness and Other Communication Disorders, 2021). Sadly, for those ages 70 and older who would benefit from hearing aids, it is estimated that only 30% have ever used them (National Institute on Deafness and Other Communication Disorders, 2021).

Unfortunately, the purchase of appropriate corrective devices, such as eyeglasses and hearing aids, for these sensory impairments is a challenge for many older women, who may have insufficient supplemental insurance and income to cover out-of-pocket expenses that are not covered by Medicare. Hearing loss is considered a modifiable risk factor for dementia (Livingston et al., 2020). The recent approval of over-the-counter hearing aids should increase access and spur innovation for new, and hopefully more affordable, devices.

SELECTED HEALTH ISSUES FOR OLDER WOMEN

Given the diversity of older women's experiences and daily lives, their health issues vary widely. Older women report higher levels of hypertension, asthma, chronic bronchitis, and arthritis than men, and their lives are affected by a high risk of heart disease, cancer, and diabetes (Federal Interagency Forum on Aging-Related Statistics, 2020). These chronic illnesses cause much of the morbidity that older women experience, and women's increasing longevity places them at high

TABLE 10.1 Screening for Geriatric Health Issues: The 4M Framework

4M FRAMEWORK CORE ISSUES	APPLICATION
Matters Most	Understand each individual's health outcome goals and care preferences.
Mind	Screen for depression, dementia, and delirium.
Mobility	Assess gait, balance, and fall injury prevention.
Medication	Consider polypharmacy, optimal prescribing, deprescribing, adverse medication effects, medication burden.

Source: Adapted from Institute for Healthcare Improvement. *(2021, December 7). Using the age-friendly 4Ms to better advocate for older adults (and geriatric care). https://www.ihi.org/communities/blogs/using-the-age-friendly-4ms-to-better-advocate-for-older-adults-and-geriatric-care*

risk for multiple, concurrent chronic conditions. One way to approach the care of the older adult is to conceptualize a clinical encounter in terms of the "4Ms" conceptualized by the Institute for Healthcare Improvement (2021; see Table 10.1).

Cardiovascular Disease

Clinical manifestations of cardiovascular disease, including hypertension, coronary heart disease (CHD), and stroke, are known to develop at a later age in women than in men (Mozaffarian et al., 2016). Unlike men, women are also more likely to be diagnosed with CVD based on clinical signs and symptoms of angina, rather than myocardial infarction. In addition, women more frequently experience atypical myocardial infarction symptoms (e.g., jaw aching, profound fatigue, arm pain without chest discomfort), rather than the more typical substernal chest pain, and may have no symptoms at all (van der Ende et al., 2020). In fact, women are twice as likely to have unrecognized myocardial infarctions, and it has been described that unrecognized myocardial infarctions in women compared to men are more strongly associated with lower pain sensitivity (Ohrn et al., 2016; van der Ende et al., 2020). These atypical or even absent symptoms lead to missed opportunities to implement preventive therapies and unrecognized myocardial infarctions (van der Ende et al., 2020). Strategies for preventing cardiovascular disease focus on the control of risk factors, including controlling smoking, hypertension, high cholesterol, obesity, and diabetes and increasing physical activity.

Additionally, women have a higher prevalence and lifetime risk of stroke than men, primarily because of greater longevity (Mozaffarian et al., 2016). Hypertension is an important risk factor for CHD and stroke, and increases in prevalence among older women, disproportionately affecting African American women. Stroke risk for African Americans is estimated to be two to three times higher than that of non-Hispanic Whites (Der Ananian et al., 2018). Atrial fibrillation increases the risk of stroke more in women than men despite atrial fibrillation being more prevalent in men (Corbière & Tettenborn, 2021). Other cardiometabolic risk factors include diabetes mellitus and smoking, which also demonstrate gender differences in age-adjusted stroke incidence and prevalence (Madsen et al., 2018, 2019). Ironically, women are less likely to call an ambulance for themselves yet are more likely to know symptoms of a stroke compared to their male counterparts (Corbière & Tettenborn, 2021).

Cancer

More than 80% of all cancers are diagnosed at age 55 years or older (American Cancer Society, 2022). Although breast cancer is diagnosed more frequently in women than any other cancer, lung cancer is the leading cause of cancer death. Early detection through regular screening (e.g., mammography, colonoscopy) is critical for minimizing morbidity and mortality. Many older women survive cancer and live with it as a chronic disease. Treatment goals in this phase emphasize symptom management, ongoing monitoring, and optimization of function. Strategies for preventing cancer, similar to preventing cardiovascular disease, focus primarily on lifestyle modification, including healthy eating, weight control, increasing physical activity, limiting sedentary time, abstinence from smoking and alcohol, avoiding sun damage, and vaccinations as appropriate (human papillomavirus [HPV], hepatitis B; American Cancer Society, 2022; Rock et al., 2020).

Diabetes

Type 2 diabetes mellitus, characterized by an increased resistance and decreased sensitivity to insulin, confers a greater risk for CHD in women than in men (Bertoluci & Rocha, 2017). Additionally, new research has been done regarding adult-onset autoimmune diabetes, which presents as classic type 1 diabetes with insulin requirement at diagnosis, and latent autoimmune diabetes in adults (LADA; Fadiga et al., 2020). Women are more likely to be diagnosed later in life with LADA with one study demonstrating the median age of diagnosis to be 42 years (Fadiga et al., 2020). Overall, obese and overweight older women are at a greater risk for developing diabetes. Adults ages 65 years and older have the greatest percentage of those diagnosed with diabetes at about 29%, with the prevalence of diagnosed diabetes being the highest among Alaska Natives and American Indians (CDC, n.d.-c). Currently, prevention and management of diabetes are key areas of research and clinical interventions to decrease morbidity and mortality and enhance quality of life (Stetson et al., 2017).

Arthritis

Arthritis is one of the leading chronic conditions and affects approximately one in two individuals 65 years and older (Administration on Aging, 2021). Approximately, 54% of older women report arthritic conditions when compared to 46% of older men (Federal Interagency Forum on Aging-Related Statistics, 2020), which may be classified as degenerative or osteoarthritis, with changes in the cartilage of the joint and associated pain, and inflammatory or rheumatoid arthritis,

with joint inflammation and stiffness. Medications or surgery can address some of the functional difficulties and pain associated with arthritis, but weight loss and judicious physical activity remain important interventions for arthritis-associated symptoms.

Osteoporosis and Fractures

Hip fractures, usually related to low bone density or osteoporosis, are not only a major cause of morbidity and death in older women, but are considered the most deadly of fractures, with one in three requiring long term care and one in five dying within a year of injury (Bone Health and Osteoporosis Foundation, 2022). Vertebral fractures may be even more common than hip fractures and can have a marked impact on women's functional health, particularly activities that involve bending and reaching, because of debilitating back pain, loss of height, and kyphosis. See Chapter 34, Menopause, and Chapter 35, Osteoporosis, for a discussion of the effects of menopause on bone health. Vertebral column fractures, when left untreated, lead to changes that eventually cause a variety of pulmonary, cardiovascular, digestive, and neurologic disorders in addition to chronic pain—and weak back muscles lead to hyperkyphosis, which is linked to higher morbidity and mortality in older women (Bone Health and Osteoporosis Foundation, 2022). Prevention strategies include adequate dietary calcium and exercise. Vitamin D has been considered an important supplement for bone health, although vitamin D supplementation may not offer the benefits once thought (LeBoff et al., 2022).

Cognitive Impairment, Alzheimer Disease, and Related Dementias

MCI, a syndrome distinct from cognitive aging and associated with an increased risk of dementia, is characterized by a measurable change in at least one domain of cognition (learning and memory, language, executive function, complex attention, perceptual-motor, social cognition) without an impact on daily activities (Guagler et al., 2022). MCI is an intermediate state between normal cognition and dementia. However, MCI is reversible if it is a transient state due to illness, medications or depression, or it may not progress (American Psychiatric Association, 2013).

The most common form of dementia in older adults (60% to 80%) is Alzheimer disease (AD). AD and related dementias are brain disorders characterized by impairments in two or more mental functions, such as memory, language, visual perception, attention, and the ability to reason and solve problems. Forgetfulness is the most common complaint. Manifestations of dementia can include confusion, behavior and personality changes, and other progressive declines such that a person cannot carry out normal activities of daily living. Being that advancing age is the single greatest risk factor for AD and that the population of those 65 years and older is growing rapidly, AD and other dementias will continue to increase in prevalence (Alzheimer's Association, 2019). In 2019, it was estimated that 5.8 million Americans were living with Alzheimer dementia, and of these individuals, 85% were age 75 or older. Alzheimer dementia affects one in 10 individuals age 65 and older, and nearly one in three individuals 85 years and older (Alzheimer's Association, 2019). It is also estimated that by the year 2060, the population of those with AD will triple to 14 million Americans (CDC, n.d.-b; Matthews et al., 2019).

For Americans 71 years and older, more women (16%) than men (11%) have dementia (Alzheimer's Association, 2019). There are some indications that the prevalence of MCI is higher in men than in women; but because of women's increased longevity, the majority of individuals with prevalent dementia are older women (Alzheimer's Association, 2019; CDC, n.d.-b). Women have twice the lifetime risk for Alzheimer dementia, and worldwide, women with dementia outnumber men by two to one (Kiely, 2018). While women's longevity is a factor to consider, dementia is caused by diseases, not aging. Brain scans have shown that the rate of brain cell death is faster for women compared to men (Kiely, 2018). Additionally, research has demonstrated an association with the hormone changes during and after menopause as a risk factor (Kim et al., 2021). However, the risk for Alzheimer and other dementias is greater in minority groups, with Hispanic (sevenfold) and African Americans (fourfold) expected to see the largest overall increases from 2015 to 2060 (CDC, n.d.-b; Matthews et al., 2019).

AD is irreversible, but medical treatment options have been developed that slow its progression, enhance memory, improve functioning, and minimize problem behaviors, such as agitation, sleep disturbances, and wandering. While extensive research continues to be done on disease-modifying treatment, medications approved to treat AD generally act by inhibiting cholinesterase or lowering glutamate levels in the brain and therefore improving certain cognitive skills and behavioral symptoms (Yiannopoulou & Papageorgiou, 2020). Currently, donepezil, rivastigmine, and galantamine are acetylcholinesterase inhibitors approved for treatment, while memantine is an N-methyl-D-aspartate (NMDA) receptor antagonist approved for moderate to severe AD (Cummings et al., 2019). An amyloid beta–directed antibody medication approved for the treatment of AD has had mixed results and has been mired with controversary about the Food and Drug Administration (FDA) approval process. Studies of nonpharmaceutical approaches, such as exercise, are encouraging. The EXERT study suggests that vigorous exercise or simple exercises such as stretching, balance, and range of motion simple exercise may slow the progression of MCI (Baker et al., 2022).

Depression

Depression is an important mental health indicator that may represent a recurrent, chronic condition in older adults, and its rate is steadily increasing (Reinert et al., 2021; Yelton et al., 2022). Clinically relevant depression affects a higher percentage of older women than men, but it often goes underdiagnosed or undertreated. Women with depressive symptoms often experience high rates of physical illness, functional disability, and greater use of health services. Research on depression in older women has identified important racial/ethnic considerations, including the finding that African American women have higher levels of depression throughout later life, a difference

attributable, in part, to both physical health and socioeconomic status (Amutah-Onukagha et al., 2017). Current research has also found significantly higher depression severity among Black, Hispanic, and multiracial older adult females when compared to their non-Hispanic White counterparts (Vyas et al., 2020). Additionally, poverty and smoking showed a significant association with increased rates of major depressive disorder among Black women, and depression has also been shown to be linked to increased intimate partner violence in Black transgender women (Amutah-Onukagha et al., 2017; Bukowski et al., 2019). Medication, counseling, and physical activity, ideally in combination, have been effective in treating depression in older adults (Hidalgo et al., 2021), but access, insurance coverage, and other barriers can exist. Similarly, there are gender and racial/ethnic disparities with treatment, as evidence strongly shows disparities in counseling and antidepressant treatment among depressed older adults—which particularly affects older Black women (Vyas et al., 2020).

Urinary Incontinence

Although not a disease, urinary incontinence (UI) has been described as a geriatric syndrome because of its impact on daily life and its prevalence in older adults, which is estimated to be 37% in older women (Batmani et al., 2021). UI increases with age and is higher in frail nursing home residents, with one study demonstrating that it affects one in four nursing home residents (Tai et al., 2021). UI is twice as likely in women as men with stress incontinence the most common type for females (Ching Lim, 2017). Many studies show prolonged sedentary behavior and low levels of physical activity to be common risk factors (Farrés-Godayol et al., 2022; Jerez-Roig et al., 2020; Rodolfo et al., 2021). Types of UI include stress (leakage brought on by coughing, sneezing, laughing, or straining), urge (associated with overactive bladder syndrome or inability to get to the toilet in time), nocturnal, or a combination of types (Ching Lim, 2017). Effects of UI include decreased quality of life, depression, social isolation, and restricted sexual activity, along with increased risk for pressure ulcers and urinary tract infections. Financial concerns as well as falls and fractures, are frequent consequences of UI (Ching Lim, 2017). Transient UI may be an outcome of urinary tract infections, which are frequent among older women, as well as with commonly prescribed medications such as antihypertensives and antidepressants (Anderson et al., 2015).

Functional Changes and Frailty

Functional ability is a major determinant of a living situation and the need for supportive services. Acute or chronic illness, injury, or mental health problems can all have an impact on the ability of an older woman to manage instrumental activities of daily living (e.g., doing light housework, doing laundry, preparing meals, grocery shopping, getting around outside, managing money, taking medications), as well as basic activities of daily living (e.g., bathing, dressing, getting in or out of bed, getting around inside, toileting, and eating). Although disability and functional limitations among older populations are declining, older women residing in lower-income communities continue to bear the greatest burden of disability due to impaired physical functioning with disability prevalence higher in Alaskan Natives and American Indians (Okoro et al., 2018; Orellano-Colón et al., 2021). Older women, in general, have a higher estimated prevalence of self-care disability (53.6%) and functional mobility disability (60.4%) when compared to men (Orellano-Colón et al., 2021).

When considering six disability types (mobility, self-care, independent living, cognition, hearing, vision), recent reports indicate impaired mobility (26.9%) as the most common type among those 65 years and older (Okoro et al., 2018). Additionally, the prevalence of any of these disability types, apart from self-care and hearing, were shown to be highest among females (Okoro et al., 2018).

Older women with severe functional limitations, disability, or multiple comorbid conditions may be described as frail, but specific research definitions of frailty have evolved over time. *Frailty* has been described variously as a reaction of older adults to adverse events (Sobhani et al., 2021) and more recently frailty has been characterized by the individual's response to exogenous and endogenous stressors—ultimately leading to their excessive vulnerability (Proietti & Cesari, 2020). Research on frailty, including its measurement, neurocognitive indicators, other risk factors, and biomarkers, as well as trajectories, interventions, and outcomes, is expanding rapidly and more recently has been including gender differences (Gordon & Hubbard, 2020). Unfortunately, to date, the effectiveness of interventions addressing frailty has not been sufficiently addressed in the research literature (Gordon & Hubbard, 2020). Thus, our understanding of this phenomenon may one day help prevent its development and minimize its effects on older women's lives.

Elder Mistreatment

Elder mistreatment is a growing, but often hidden, problem in the United States. The current prevalence is underestimated, as incidences of elder abuse remain drastically underreported—with an estimated 24 cases going undetected for every case reported (National Center on Elder Abuse, 2022; Pillemer et al., 2016). Elder abuse includes physical, sexual, emotional, or psychological abuse, and financial or exploitative acts, as well as neglect (CDC, n.d.-d). These acts may be intentional or unintentional, may occur in the community or institutions, and occur across socioeconomic groups. Risk factors for elder mistreatment include dependency/vulnerability of the elder (e.g., functional impairment), female sex, social isolation, abuser psychosocial problems (e.g., alcohol/substance abuse, mental health issues), and shared living arrangements.

Although there has been an increased awareness of elder mistreatment, research and advocacy have focused on intimate partner violence of women, so the special problems of older women are sometimes ignored, particularly regarding long-standing unreported wife abuse, abuse by caregivers, and exploitation and neglect of older women (Yon et al., 2019). It is estimated that among older women, one in seven have been affected by abuse within the past year, and yet this has not received the same level of public health attention as other forms of violence (National Center on Elder Abuse, 2022; Yon et al., 2019). Elder mistreatment is sometimes

difficult to identify with certainty, but clinicians have a responsibility to ensure that it does not go unrecognized, unreported, or untreated. Identification and management of this complex phenomenon, which are best accomplished through interprofessional collaboration, can be challenging.

COVID-19: Health Consequences of the Pandemic

While the COVID-19 pandemic has served to further propagate ageism within our society, the disproportionate effect of the virus on the older adult population also cannot be denied. One study showed that severity and mortality were higher in middle-aged and older women with COVID-19 than in younger females (Balcázar-Hernández et al., 2021). Data collected by the CDC concluded nationwide vaccination rates among older adults were higher among person 65 to 74 than among adults aged 75 and older and higher in older men compared to older women (Whiteman et al., 2021). Recent studies have suggested a connection between estrogen and the hormone's ability to serve as a protective mechanism against COVID-19 infection in females (Sund et al., 2022). If true, given the decline in estrogen after menopause, this provides additional information as to a greater risk in older women (Sund et al., 2022). Additionally, initial COVID-19 vaccination rates in the United States further exemplified existing gender and age disparities.

HEALTHY AGING/HEALTH PROMOTION

Healthy aging for older women can involve negotiating a wide variety of challenges and transitions, as well as recognizing and building on various opportunities for growth. It does not necessarily represent a life that is free of chronic illness or functional impairment (Grami et al., 2022). Although some older women without chronic conditions live for several decades with excellent health and high function, others with chronic conditions still view themselves as healthy and functional. This latter view is inconsistent with earlier research studies that define *successful aging* as the absence of disability or disease, high cognitive and physical function, and active engagement in life (Rowe & Kahn, 1998). A phenotype of positive aging and health promotion focused on physical, social, and emotional functioning has been found to predict health outcomes, such as decreased mortality, risk of major health conditions or hospitalizations, and risk of dependent living (Grami et al., 2022). Therefore, engaging in health promotion and maintenance of function are key goals for many older women, regardless of their current health condition. Lifestyle modifications, including engaging in physical activity, eating a good diet, enhancing safety (e.g., fall prevention), minimizing risk (e.g., vaccinations), taking an active role in one's healthcare management, and engaging socially are important components for healthy aging in older women.

Self-Management of Health

To promote personal growth and optimal aging, women need adequate information about their bodies as well as behavioral strategies that ensure a healthy lifestyle. Meeting these goals requires skills in information processing, decision-making, integration of change into one's daily life, and action. Older women have been described as health conscious and resilient and are more likely than older men to have a regular clinician, to have seen their clinician in the past year, and to seek immediate care if symptomatic. With adequate information and skills, and an environment that promotes physical, mental, economic, and social health, older women are well positioned to maintain independence and achieve late-life health goals. Chronic conditions pose the greatest threat to health, quality of life, and functional ability and, at the same time, are the most amenable to improvement with behavioral health changes, such as healthy eating, activity, reduction of alcohol intake, and smoking cessation. Novel strategies to support chronic disease management have accelerated in recent years. Wearable medical tracking devices monitor blood pressure, temperature, respiratory rate, heart rate, and oxygen saturation and send EKG information to clinicians, and fall detection devices will automatically call 911 if they detect that the wearer is not moving. The full potential of such devices has not yet been realized.

The use of telehealth increased during the COVID-19 pandemic. Some recent studies demonstrate that older adults of color with chronic conditions, requiring a high level of self-management, tend to be less satisfied with telehealth, due to concerns regarding the clinician's understanding of their chief complaint (Ladin et al., 2021). Despite this and barriers unique to the older adult population when adopting telehealth (e.g., design challenges, access, cost, privacy concerns), telehealth has been shown to be beneficial during the pandemic for older Americans (Goldberg et al., 2021; Roberts & Mehrotra, 2020).

RECOMMENDED SCREENING

Guidelines for screening for older women are a function of age, risk factors, and multiple comorbidities. Evidence is evolving regarding recommendations. The American Geriatrics Society (2022) synthesizes current recommendations and hosts both general and condition-specific current guidelines for care of older adults. Federal websites provide detailed information about coverage under Medicare and eligibility for preventive services (www.medicare.gov and www.healthcare.gov). Table 10.2 summarizes current preventive services available through Medicare for older women.

Physical Activity

There is growing evidence that, with appropriate cautions, the benefits of physical activity in older adults, particularly weight-bearing aerobic exercise such as walking and exercises to improve balance, far outweigh possible risks. Physical activity has also been shown to decrease risk of frailty while improving overall functional, physical, and cognitive status (Gammack, 2017). Americans of all ages are advised to do a minimum of 150 to 300 minutes a week of moderate exercise or 75 to 150 minutes a week of vigorous exercise, or an equivalent combination of both, although even small amounts of physical activity are beneficial (U.S. Department of Health and Human Services, 2018). Older adults are advised to add balance training and aerobic and muscle-strengthening activities. Physical activity not only helps to prevent chronic disease but helps to manage chronic disease as well (U.S. Department of Health and Human Services, 2018).

Despite these benefits and increased participation in physical activity in the last 20 years among older adults, participation among older women compared with older men remains low; 12% of older women versus 16% of older men met federal guidelines for regular physical activity (Federal Interagency Forum on Aging-Related Statistics, 2020). Racial differences were noted with non-Hispanic Whites over age 65 reporting higher levels of physical activity than their non-Hispanic Black counterparts (15% compared to 9%). Barriers to exercise for many Black populations include lack of access to safe neighborhoods, lack of sidewalks, high heat temperature islands in inner city neighborhoods, and concern of racial profiling while exercising outdoors (U.S. Environmental Protection Agency, 2022; Hornbuckle, 2021). With physical activity rates low, it is essential for clinicians to promote a physically active lifestyle to improve both the current and future level of health and state of well-being among the older adult population (Rivera-Torres et al., 2019) and to advocate for safe neighborhoods in which to exercise.

Healthy Eating

Healthy eating can play an important role in preventing or delaying the onset or morbidity associated with many chronic diseases, such as CVD, cancer, stroke, and diabetes (Federal Interagency Forum on Aging-Related Statistics, 2020). In addition, adhering to recommended dietary guidelines can reduce controllable risk factors for chronic diseases, such as obesity, hypertension, and hypercholesterolemia (Federal Interagency Forum on Aging-Related Statistics, 2020). For older women, many of whom tend to gain weight as they age, healthy eating can also be synonymous with weight control along with reduced risk of frailty (Struijk et al., 2020). Diet changes are important as elderly adults are less responsive to the anabolic stimulus of low doses of essential amino acid intake compared to younger individuals. Since protein is a key nutrient for muscle health and prevention of sarcopenia., higher levels of dietary protein are needed. This lack of responsiveness in older adults can be overcome with higher levels of protein (or essential amino acid) consumption. The current research is unclear as to the necessary total amount of protein or the distribution, quality (eating more fish and legumes vs. red meat), or timing of protein intake related to exercise (Kiesswetter et al., 2020). Vitamin B_{12} is of concern for some older adults as the ability to absorb this vitamin decreases with age and adsorption can be affected by certain medications. Although there are many guidelines for calcium and vitamin D supplementation in older, community-dwelling women, the U.S. Preventive Services Task Force (USPSTF) has not found sufficient evidence for supplementation recommendations (USPSTF, 2018a).

TABLE 10.2 Screening and Preventive Services for Older Women Under Medicare Coverage

PREVENTIVE SERVICE	WHAT IS COVERED	WHO MEDICARE COVERS
Alcohol misuse counseling	Annual screening and up to four face-to-face counseling sessions/year if misusing alcohol	All
Breast cancer	Screening mammograms annually Diagnostic mammograms more frequently than once a year, if medically necessary	Older than 40 years Recommendations vary and are ever changing; most do not have an upper age limit to screening but rather base screening on each woman's health status (CDC, 2020).
Cardiovascular screening	Cholesterol, lipid, triglyceride Recommended every 5 years and more often in those with a diagnosis of coronary artery disease, diabetes, peripheral arterial disease, or prior stroke (Reuben et al., 2022)	All
Cervical and vaginal cancer	Pelvic examinations and breast exams every 2 years HPV tests (as part of a Pap test) every 5 years in asymptomatic women age 30–65 years	Screening not needed after age 65 if no history of cervical intraepithelial neoplasia grade 2 or more severe disease within the past 25 years, and who have documented adequate negative prior screening in the prior 10 years (American Cancer Society, 2022; USPSTF, 2018)
Colorectal cancer	Fecal occult blood test, flexible sigmoidoscopy, screening colonoscopy	Yearly for FOBT and FIT, 1–3 years for FIT-DNA screening, every 5 years for sigmoidoscopy and CT colonography, and every 10 years for colonoscopy for average risk
Depression screening	One per year	All
Diabetes screening	Fasting blood glucose test	At risk: may be eligible for up to two screenings each year depending on risk factors
HIV screening Hep B and Hep C screenings	HIV test Lab work	Covers annual screening for ages 15–65, or if >65 and at risk Covers if at risk for Hep B Covers if at risk for Hep C from IV drug use (annually), had a blood transfusion prior to 1992 (annually), or born between 1945 and 1965 (if not at other risk, covers only once)
Obesity screening/ counseling	Screening and face-to-face counseling	BMI >30 kg/m²
Osteoporosis	Bone density test/BMD every 2 years if criteria met.	Risk criteria: • Estrogen-deficient and at risk for osteoporosis, based on medical history and/or other findings • X-rays show possible osteoporosis, osteopenia, or vertebral fractures • On prednisone or steroid-type drugs • Primary hyperparathyroidism • For monitoring response to drug therapy
Tobacco use cessation	Up to eight face-to-face counseling sessions per year	However, recommend smoking cessation at every office visit for primary prevention
Vaccinations	Flu/pneumoccal/hepatitis B	All flu, COVID-19 vaccinations and boosters If at risk for Hep B 65 years and older adults receive PCV13 followed by PPSV23 6 months to 1 year later; for adults age 65 years and older who have already received PPSV23 but not PCV13, they can receive one dose of PCV13 at least 1 year after PPSV23 vaccination

BMD, bone mineral density; BMI, body mass index; FIT, fecal immunochemical test; FOBT, fecal occult blood test; Hep, hepatitis; HPV, human papillomavirus; IV, intravenous; PCV, pneumococcal conjugate vaccine; PPSV, pneumococcal polysaccharide vaccine; USPSTF, U.S. Preventive Services Task Force.

Sources: Adapted from American Cancer Society. (2022). Cancer facts & figures 2022. https://www.cancer.org/content/dam/cancer-org/research/cancer-facts-and-statistics /annual-cancer-facts-and-figures/2022/2022-cancer-facts-and-figures.pdf; Centers for Disease Control and Prevention. (2020). Breast cancer: Things you should know. https://www.cdc.gov/cancer/breast/pdf/breast-cancer-fact-sheet-508.pdf; Centers for Medicare & Medicaid Services. (2022). Preventive & screening services: Part B. https://www.medicare.gov/coverage/preventive-screening-services; Reuben, D., Herr, K., Pacala, J., Pollock, B., Potter, J., & Semla, T. (2022). Geriatrics at your fingertips. American Geriatrics Society; U.S. Preventive Services Task Force. (2018b). Cervical cancer: Screening. https://www.uspreventiveservicestaskforce.org/uspstf/recommendation /cervical-cancer-screening

Weight Control

Obesity, described as an epidemic in the United States today, has increased among older women in recent decades, yet it is a key modifiable risk factor for disease, morbidity from chronic disease, and death. The prevalence of severe obesity is lowest in the over-60 age category, although the prevalence is affected by gender, race, and ethnicity. Severe obesity is highest in non-Hispanic Black women and lowest among non-Hispanic Asian women (Stierman et al., 2021). Obesity is associated with an increased risk of CHD, hypertension, diabetes, some cancers, osteoarthritis, and disability, among other chronic conditions. Obese older women can derive multiple health benefits from weight loss; however, careful ongoing health assessments are warranted during weight loss to evaluate the impact on lean muscle mass, fracture risk, and other health parameters. It is important in the older adult to avoid losing muscle mass with weight loss. There appears to be a consensus that a moderate weight loss of 5% to 10% results in significant health benefits, and that to counteract muscle loss due to aging, the American College of Sport Medicine guidelines recommend resistance training with muscle-strengthening exercise twice a week (Fiataraone Singh et al., 2019). The Women's Preventive Services Initiative (WPSI) has recommended counseling midlife women age 40 to 60 years with normal or overweight body mass index (BMI) to maintain or limit weight gain through healthy eating and physical activity to prevent obesity as women age (Health Resources and Services Administration [HRSA], 2022). HRSA has approved this recommendation, and insurance plans must cover weight counseling in this age group beginning in 2023.

Sleep

Older adults do not always report problems with sleep to their healthcare providers because the common wisdom has held that sleep disturbances are to be expected as one grows older. Sleep architecture changes—decreased rapid eye movement and slow wave sleep, increased awakenings at night, and a "phase advance" in circadian rhythms (becoming sleepy earlier)—are seen with aging and contribute to sleep changes. More prominent in sleep disturbances are comorbidities such as depression, anxiety, chronic respiratory illnesses, CVD, gastroesophageal reflux disease (GERD), chronic pain, neurodegenerative disorders, and movement disorders (e.g., restless legs syndrome), which affect sleep quality. Medication side effects and interactions and primary sleep disorders, lifestyle patterns, psychosocial factors, and late life stressors also affect sleep quality. Geriatric pharmacotherapy guidelines can aid the clinician in cautious prescribing: to avoid prescribing certain medications or to prescribe only under specific conditions (American Geriatrics Society Beers Criteria Update Expert Panel, 2019). Self-managed approaches to better sleep hygiene include consistent bedtime and awaking, 7 to 9 hours of sleep each night, exercise prior to 3 hours before bedtime, avoidance of large meals close to bedtime, and reducing screen time prior to sleep (National Institute on Aging, n.d.-b).

Prevention of Falls

Because fall-related fractures increase the risk for further decline, the prevention of falls is a top priority. Hip fractures and most other nonvertebral fractures in older women occur because of a fall (North American Menopause Society, 2021), making fall prevention a key safety concern for older women. Falls can have a major impact on women's morbidity and mortality (Burns & Kakara, 2018; Florence et al., 2018). The most recent Cochrane Review of fall-prevention interventions showed that programs likely to be beneficial included multidisciplinary and multifactorial programs with both health and environmental risk factor screening and modification in the community and residential facilities; home hazard assessment and modification; muscle strengthening and balance retraining programs; and withdrawal of psychotropic medications (Gillespie et al., 2012).

Vaccinations

Because of immune system changes with aging (e.g., immunosenescence) and an increased prevalence of multiple chronic illnesses, older adults can be particularly vulnerable to infectious conditions, associated profound morbidity with complications, and increased risk of mortality. Therefore, older adults will particularly benefit from vaccinations. Annual influenza, two-dose pneumococcal (after age 65 years), and two-dose herpes zoster (after age 50 years) vaccinations are recommended for older adults (CDC, n.d.-d). It is imperative for clinicians to discuss the benefits of vaccinations with their clients. Vaccination against COVID-19 may become part of the routine vaccination schedule as recent data have shown that the highest impact of vaccination against infection and death includes booster doses among the older adult population (Johnson et al., 2022).

Medication Management

Prescription drug use has increased dramatically over the years as more and more new medications are introduced. Polypharmacy, can be defined as taking five or more medications while hyperpolypharmacy, also becoming more common, is defined as 10 or more medications (Masnoon et al., 2017). Polypharmacy increases with age, and remains a significant safety issue for older adults, particularly older women who consume the majority of prescription medications. In fact, a recent large study involving nearly 2 million older adults showed the prevalence of polypharmacy among this population to be approximately 44% (Khezrian et al., 2020; Sheikh-Taha & Asmar, 2021). With the higher number of chronic illnesses with age, the drug burden, along with the potential for drug interactions, increases. Optimal medication management occurs with appropriate prescription given the goals of the older woman, coupled with evidence-based guidelines that take comorbid conditions into account. Adherence can be improved by addressing both health literacy and financial considerations, as well as the deployment of enabling technology for reminding and tracking medications.

Social Relationships

Connection with others is core to healthy aging. Women often survive spouses and friends, resulting in changes in their social network, with losses and opportunities to develop new relationships. Women more readily form and nurture relationships and commonly possess skills and abilities to sustain and develop meaningful connections across the life span. Compared with most men, women play a key role in ensuring family connectivity, sustaining friendships over longer periods of time and actively engaging in friendships throughout life. Women without social connections will benefit from suggestions and referrals to community social activities.

Sexuality

Older women are sexual beings who are capable of meaningful sexual relationships. Normal changes with age do not need to affect women's sexual desires and the ability to experience an orgasm; however, about 50% to 70% of postmenopausal women do experience symptoms of genitourinary syndrome of menopause (GSM; Angelou et al., 2020). Physiologic changes associated with lowered estrogen and other sex steroid hormones affecting vaginal blood flow can make sexual activity uncomfortable. The estrogen changes lead to thinning of vulvar tissue; narrowing, shortening, and loss of elasticity of the vaginal walls; and a reduction of glandular secretions with an increase in vaginal pH. A number of additional factors influence sexual function for older women: established behavioral patterns and preferences, illness, certain medications such as SSRIs (selective serotonin reuptake inhibitors), relationship quality, self-esteem, life stressors, and societal values. Vaginal dryness is the most bothersome GSM symptom, affecting up to 93% of older women with irritation, burning, and itching of vulva/vagina experienced by 63% whether sexually active or not (Moral et al., 2018). Loss of a partner has been reported to be the main reason older women are no longer sexually active, with older women identifying emotional intimacy as an important reason for sexual activity (Granville & Pregler, 2018). The prevalence of sexual activity declines as widowhood increases with age. More than 60% of older women between ages 57 and 64 years are sexually active, 40% among those between 65 and 74 years are active, and less than 20% of women between 75 and 85 years remain active. Among those who are sexually active, approximately half report issues that are bothersome to them, most commonly low desire (43%), difficulty with vaginal lubrication (39%), and inability to have an orgasm (34%). These concerns are more likely among women with chronic health conditions (Merghati-Khoei et al., 2016).

Discussion of sexual concerns remains limited, with only 22% of women older than 50 years having conversations about their sexuality with healthcare providers, and usually it is the patient who will initiate the discussion rather than the clinician (Granville & Pregler, 2018). The low rate of sexual health discussions highlights the need for clinicians to initiate such dialogue. A thorough sexual history will guide possible treatments, such as lubricants, vaginal moisturizers, or estrogen creams to reduce physical discomfort or counseling for issues of relationship quality. If a healthy older woman has remained sexually active, is not inhibited by societal stereotypes and myths against sex with advanced age, and has a partner who has maintained sexual interest and ability to engage in sexual activity, it is likely that she will have continued satisfactory sexual relationships (see Chapter 19, Women's Sexual Health, for a comprehensive life span discussion of sexuality).

SUMMARY

This chapter focuses on older women and their experiences of aging, shaped by the sociopolitical context of women's lives and the disparities in access to healthcare and services that are related to gender, race, and class. The economic lives of older women are improving, but their economic disadvantages compared with older men are expected to continue; this is particularly true for women of color who experience the triple effects of gender, age, and ethnicity. Transgender people continue to face discrimination as they age. The diversity of the older population is growing, and the coming wave of baby boomers represents a challenge for policy makers, private enterprises, families, and healthcare providers (Thorpe & Whitfield, 2017). As baby boomers attain their eighth decade of life in large numbers, it is highly likely that aging in our culture will be redefined and new solutions and innovations will proliferate in the coming decades.

A woman's experience of aging depends on her personal characteristics and history, access to resources that promote health, and ability to develop strategies for coping with loss and change. Coping with the changes that accompany aging involves some losses that may not be anticipated, but many of the normal psychological and physiologic changes that affect older women may be predicted. Improving outcomes for older women starts with primary prevention to improve general health, delay the onset of disability, and increase productivity and well-being; it continues with health promotion to minimize the effects of chronic conditions and optimize quality of life and functional capacity. If women are educated about age-related changes and given time to assimilate and plan for the process of transition from one phase of life to the next, the potential for optimal aging will be enhanced. Sensitivity to the needs and issues of older women and advocacy for appropriate access and service are essential for promoting the health and well-being of this significant population.

REFERENCES

References for this chapter are online and available at https://connect.springerpub.com/content/book/978-0-8261-6722-4/part/part02/chapter/ch10

CHAPTER 11

Well Women's Health*

ELDORA LAZAROFF, LYNN M. GADDIS, AND VERSIE JOHNSON-MALLARD

The practice of well women's health is not of a reactive health-care system that responds to acute and urgent needs, but rather one that nurtures health, well-being, and minimized health risk (American College of Obstetricians and Gynecologists [ACOG], 2018; National Women's Law Center [NWLC], 2022). The modern approach to addressing the physical and mental healthcare needs of women from adolescence to older age is a team approach. Providers of sexual and reproductive health (SRH) services to women range from gynecologic care to geriatric services. Healthcare professionals nurture the optimal health and well-being of women at significant stages of their lives. This chapter offers suggestions and new evidence-based research, clinical updates, drug information, clinical guidelines, information related to COVID-19, racism and health disparities, emerging topics in women's health, and expanded information on the care of transgender individuals as well as enhanced information on pregnancy and related issues as these clients are increasingly treated in primary care settings.

Healthcare providers educated in primary care specialties, such as family, adult/gerontology, and pediatrics, are knowledgeable to provide SRH care services to women. The Agency for Healthcare Research and Quality (AHRQ) supports the National Academy of Medicine (NAM) assessment of possible gaps in evidence expressed by the U.S. Preventive Services Taskforce (USPSTF; Institute of Medicine [IOM], 2011). The Mary Horrigan Connors Center for Women's Health and Gender Biology at Brigham and Women's Hospital developed resources for consumers, healthcare providers, and policy makers to help women navigate the SRH preventive services available to them under the Patient Protection and Affordable Care Act (ACA; IOM, 2011; NWLC, 2022). Clients come from varied cultural and socioeconomic backgrounds with a host of personal beliefs regarding their health. The NAM provides resources on transgender and gender diverse inclusivity, sex as a biological variable, and sex-specific illnesses and vulnerabilities (IOM, 2011) Furthermore, clients are surfing the web, reading medical literature, and becoming self-educated in mainstream medicine along with alternative and complementary medicine. Women entering the clinician's office often have thought-out questions and suggestions for their plans of care.

COMPONENTS OF A WELL-WOMAN VISIT

The yearly well-woman visit is an opportunity to promote health by addressing health concerns and educating women about health risks and disease prevention across a lifespan.

A woman's health history should be collected while she is clothed. The healthcare provider should sit at eye level and face the woman. If language is a barrier for the client, a qualified, professional translator may be necessary to collect health information correctly. Begin the history with social conversation. Asking sensitive questions in front of family or friends may result in incomplete answers and missed information. Interview your client alone, if possible. If unable to interview the woman alone, attempt to contact her later to fill in any important missing information. The well-woman visit, at minimum, should include:

- Review of health history
- Assessment of physical and psychosocial well-being
- Primary and secondary screening
- Review of prescription and over-the-counter medications, vitamins, and supplements
- Counseling/education
- Preconception, prenatal, and interconception care
- Updates on risk factors and immunizations (Women's Preventive Services Initiative [WPSI], 2022)

Health History

The health history is a fundamental part of the annual visit and may vary depending on age, risk factors, and the woman's and/or her healthcare provider's preferences (ACOG, 2018; WPSI, 2022). The best time to begin establishing a relationship with a woman is during your interview to collect her and her family's health history.

An annual visit for an established female client may consist of:

- Counseling about health maintenance
- Risk assessment

---

*This chapter is a revision of the chapter that appeared in the second edition of this textbook, coauthored with Barbara B. Cochrane and Heather M. Young, and we thank them for their original contribution.

- Body mass index (BMI) assessment
- Screening
- Immunizations

An established client will require a thorough review and update of her past medical history and social history, as well as a three-generation family history (if known, see Table 11.1). Updating a woman's health history is the opportune time to, together, determine what healthcare needs may be indicated and how the woman views her personal health. The health history is an investigation of current health, real and potential risks, and discovery of knowledge gaps and is a time to gather information to support any indicated referrals.

Developing a rapport with the woman may decrease any discomfort that might occur when asking personal and often difficult questions such as drug use, sexual history, and abuse. Asking the question does not imply judgment when asked in a respectful manner and without criticism. Active

listening skills, such as leaning forward, nodding, and encouraging further description while saying *tell me more* or *go on* all indicate interest and serve to instill a sense of trust in the client–healthcare provider professional relationship.

It is critical to listen to the woman's response while paying attention to the language and words she uses, as well as her facial expressions and body language. Furthermore, it is important to do everything possible to avoid interruptions while the woman is explaining her concerns and reasons for her health visit. It is very important that the healthcare provider maintain good eye contact with the woman (not the computer screen) while addressing her. If necessary, the typing of information into the electronic medical chart should be kept to a minimum.

Routine Health Screening

LIPID PROFILE ASSESSMENT

A lipid profile provides healthcare providers with a risk assessment for morbidity related to coronary heart disease (CHD; Table 11.2). CHD is the most common cause of death in adults in the United States (Bays et al., 2014). Women considered to be at high risk are those with a family history of premature cardiovascular disease, previous personal history of CHD, a BMI greater than 30, a personal and/or family history of peripheral vascular disease, and diabetes mellitus (Bays et al.,2014; USPSTF, 2014). The recommended timing for dyslipidemia screening in women ages 20 to 45 years with increased risk for CHD is every 5 years (Fitzgerald et al., 2015; USPSTF, 2014).

ENDOCRINE SCREENING

The endocrine system is a complex system using hormones that target organs throughout the body. Hormones affect the development of sexual characteristics, fertility, fluid balance, and maintenance of blood pressure (BP). Disorders of the endocrine system are categorized as:

TABLE 11.1 Components of Client History

PAST MEDICAL HISTORY	SOCIAL HISTORY
• Medical • Medications • Allergies • Surgery • Immunizations	• Occupation • Diet • Exercise • Tobacco • Alcohol • Illicit drugs • Sexual history • Last menstrual period • Last Pap smear
FAMILY HISTORY	
• Mother—e.g., HTN, alive • Father—e.g., healthy, alive • Siblings	**OBSTETRIC HISTORY**

HTN, hypertension (high blood pressure).

TABLE 11.2 Lipid Profile Components and Levels

LIPID PROFILE	COMPONENTS	LEVELS
Total cholesterol	Measures all of the cholesterol	*Desirable:* <200 mg/dL (5.18 mmol/L) *Borderline high:* 200–239 mg/dL (5.18–6.18 mmol/L) *High:* 240 mg/dL (6.22 mmol/L) or higher
High-density lipoprotein (HDL) cholesterol	"Good cholesterol"; removes excess cholesterol	*Low level, increased risk:* <50 mg/dL (1.3 mmol/L) for women *Average level, average risk:* 50–59 mg/dL (1.3–1.5 mmol/L) for women *High level, less than average risk:* 60 mg/dL (1.55 mmol/L) or higher
Low-density lipoprotein (LDL) cholesterol	"Bad cholesterol"; deposits excess cholesterol	*Optimal:* <100 mg/dL (2.59 mmol/L); for those with known disease (ASCVD or diabetes), <70 mg/dL (1.81 mmol/L) is optimal *Near/above optimal:* 100–129 mg/dL (2.59–3.34 mmol/L) *Borderline high:* 130–159 mg/dL (3.37–4.12 mmol/L) *High:* 160–189 mg/dL (4.15–4.90 mmol/L) *Very high:* > 190 mg/dL (4.90 mmol/L)
Fasting triglycerides	Measures all the triglycerides in all the lipoprotein particles	*Desirable:* 500 mg/dL (5.6 mmol/L) *High:* 200–499 mg/dL (2.3–5.6 mmol/L) *Very high:* >500 mg/dL (5.6 mmol/L)

ASCVD, atherosclerotic cardiovascular disease.
Source: Adapted from National Lipid Association. (2017). NLA recommendations for patient-centered management of dyslipidemia. https://www.lipid.org/recommendations

- **Primary disorders**: those affecting target organs (e.g., the thyroid or adrenal glands)
- **Secondary disorders**: those that affect regulation of target organs (e.g., the pituitary gland)
- **Tertiary disorders**: those that arise from the hypothalamus

Diabetes is the most common endocrine disorder in the United States. Adults with surveilled BP readings ≥135/80 mmHg should be screened for diabetes.

Ambulatory BP monitoring is the best method for confirming elevated BP. *Ambulatory monitoring* is defined as measuring BP every 30 minutes over the course of 24 to 48 hours of normal activity. Ambulatory BP monitoring is recommended at intervals of every year for high-risk adults and every 3 to 5 years for those who are at low risk.

Women with a history of gestational diabetes mellitus (GDM) should have lifelong screening for the development of diabetes or prediabetes at least every 3 years. A fasting plasma glucose, 2-hour postload plasma, and hemoglobin A1c (HgA1c) tests are approved for diabetes screening at 3-year intervals. Regardless of the woman's age, glycemic target goals are a fasting plasma glucose ≤126 mg/dL (7 mmol/L, a HgA1c <6.4% or a 2-hour plasma glucose <200 mg/dL (11.1 mmol/L; American Diabetes Association [ADA], 2021).

COLORECTAL SCREENING

The goal of colorectal screening in women is to reduce mortality from gastrointestinal system cancer. Colorectal cancer is the third leading cause of cancer death in women. The lifetime risk of developing colorectal cancer for women is one in 26, or about 4% (American Cancer Society [ACS], 2023). The ACOG (2014) endorses the USPSTF recommendation to begin screening with colonoscopy at age 50 through age 75 (Davidson et al., 2021). Because of the high mortality risk, all African American women should begin screening at age 45 years (Davidson et al., 2021). The most effective screening interval for colonoscopy is every 10 years.

Sigmoidoscopy is recommended every 5 years. It is recommended that high sensitive guaiac and fecal immunochemical testing (noninvasive methods used to detect occult blood in the stool) accompany sigmoidoscopy. The guaiac test requires two samples from each of three consecutive bowel movements at home. It is important to note that a single stool sample collected from a healthcare provider's rectal examination is not adequate for the detection of colorectal cancer (Davidson et al., 2021).

SCREENING MAMMOGRAPHY

Breast cancer is the second leading cause of death from cancer in American women and the most commonly diagnosed cancer in women (ACOG, 2017). The ACS estimates that in 2023, there will be 297,790 newly diagnosed cases of invasive breast cancer and 55,720 case of ductal carcinoma in situ in women. Of those newly diagnosed cases, it is estimated that 43,700 American women will die from the disease (ACS, 2021). It is important to note that although breast cancer is typically associated with women, approximately 1% of all cases are diagnosed in men.

Historically, breast cancer screening has included three aspects: (1) breast imaging (e.g., mammography), (2) the clinical breast examination (CBE), and (3) the woman's self-breast screening (monthly breast self-examination [BSE]). The significance and impact that each of these aspects has on the early diagnosis, detection, and prognosis, as well as the appropriate age to initiate and discontinue and the frequency of screening, remain controversial. ACOG (2017) endorses the inclusion of all three aspects in breast cancer screening (Table 11.3). Breast

TABLE 11.3 Breast Cancer Screening Recommendations

PROFESSIONAL ORGANIZATION	MAMMOGRAPHY	CLINICAL BREAST EXAM (CBE)	BREAST SELF-EXAM (BSE)	BSE AWARENESS
American College of Obstetricians and Gynecologists	Annually or biennial in women ≥40 years of age	Every 1–3 years in women age 20–39 years Annually in women ≥40 years of age	Consideration when caring for high-risk women	Recommended
American Cancer Society	Annually in women 40–50, recommended at age 45; biennial with the option to continue annual screening for women ≥55 years of age	Does not recommend	Optional for women ≥20 years of age	Recommended
National Comprehensive Cancer Network	Annually in women ≥40 years of age	Every 1–3 years in women age 25–39 years Annually in women ≥40 years of age	Recommended	Recommended
National Cancer Institute	Every 1–2 years in women ≥40 years of age	Recommended	Not recommended	
U.S. Preventive Services Task Force	Age 40–49 years should be individualized; age 50–74 years biennially	Insufficient evidence	Not recommended	

Source: American College of Obstetricians and Gynecologists. (2017). Practice bulletin number 179: Breast cancer risk assessment and screening in average-risk women. Obstetrics and Gynecology, 130(1), e1–e16. https://doi.org/10.1097/AOG.0000000000002158

cancer morbidity and mortality can be effectively reduced through screening mammography.

Screening mammography is recommended for women who are not at an increased risk by known genetic workup or personal or family history. Increasing age is the most important risk factor. Known risks include:

- Early menarche
- Nulliparity
- Not breastfeeding
- Higher BMI
- Dense breast on mammogram
- Prior exposure to high-dose therapeutic chest irradiation in young women (10 to 30 years old)
- Breast cancer diagnosis before age 50 years
- Personal and/or family history of bilateral breast cancer
- Family history of breast and ovarian cancer
- Presence of breast cancer in at least one female family member
- Multiple cases of breast cancer in the family
- One or more family member with two primary types of *BRCA*-related cancer
- Ashkenazi Jewish ethnicity
- History of positive *BRCA* mutations (ACOG, 2017; USPSTF, 2014)

Genetic risk assessment for breast cancer (*BRCA*) mutation testing is a multistep process that includes genetic counseling by trained providers. Interventions in women who are *BRCA* mutation carriers should have early, more frequent, and intensive cancer screening. High-risk women with known *BRCA* mutations should be evaluated for treatment with interventions such as risk-reducing medications (e.g., tamoxifen or raloxifene), and risk-reducing surgery (e.g., mastectomy or salpingo-oophorectomy; ACOG, 2017; USPSTF, 2014).

Breast cancer risk assessment tools, such as Breast Cancer Risk Assessment Tool, Gail Model Assessment Tool, and Tyrer-Cuzick Model, are available to use for women with known risk factors for breast cancer. Women who score 20% to 25% or higher using these models are considered high risk for breast cancer and should get breast MRI and a mammogram every year, typically starting at 30 years of age. Specific risk factors include a known *BRCA1* and *BRCA2* gene mutation, a first-degree relative (parent, brother, sister, or child) with a *BRCA1* or *BRCA2* gene mutation and have not had genetic testing themselves, radiation therapy to young women, and Li-Fraumeni syndrome, Cowden syndrome, or Bannayan-Riley-Ruvalcaba syndrome or first-degree relatives with one of these syndromes (ACS, 2022).

Women who have never performed BSE or those with questions about BSE technique should be educated and encouraged to palpate breast tissue and structures monthly so that they become familiar with their breast tissue. Increasing one's awareness as to what her *normal* breast tissue feels like may lead a woman to seek her healthcare provider when aberrancies occur.

CERVICAL CANCER SCREENING: PAP TEST

Screening has been successful in lowering morbidity and mortality from cervical cancer and is defined as an internal examination using cytology (Pap test). Cervical cancer screening is age specific and should begin at age 21 years. A Pap test is not recommended on an annual basis for any woman at any age. Cytology alone every 3 years is the recommended screening method for women age 21 to 29 years (ACOG, 2021a). For women 30 to 65 years of age, any one of the following screening methods can be utilized; cytology alone every 3 years, Food and Drug Administration (FDA)–approved primary high-risk human papillomavirus (hrHPV) testing alone every 5 years, or cotesting hrHPV and cytology every 5 years (ACOG, 2021a). Women with screening results indicating HPV infection/underlying CIN 3 (cervical intraepithelial neoplasia grade 3) should be followed with repeat HPV testing or cotesting at 1 year. (See Chapter 32, Human Papillomavirus, for detailed information on the association between HPV and cervical cancer.)

For women older than 65 years, no screening is recommended with adequate negative prior screening and no history of moderate or severe CIN grade 2 or 3 within the past 20 years (ACOG, 2021b). Cervical screening should not be resumed in this age group for any reason (including the introduction of a new sex partner). Furthermore, women with a history of hysterectomy for benign disease do not require cervical screening. However, women older than 65 years of age with a history of CIN 2 or 3 should continue to undergo screening (ACOG, 2021b). Any woman with a cervix and a positive history for CIN 2 or 3 or adenocarcinoma in situ should continue to be screened (ACOG, 2021b). Cervical screening practices after HPV vaccination are recommended and should not change.

Sexual and Reproductive Health Examination

CLINICAL BREAST EXAMINATION

CBE was designed to monitor breast size, symmetry, contour, skin color, texture, venous patterns, and lesions (Table 11.4). The healthcare provider should begin by inspecting a woman's breasts while noting any dimpling, venous patterns, and symmetry. It is not uncommon for one breast to be slightly larger or smaller. During the CBE and while sitting up, the woman should place her hands on her hips while flexing her pectoral muscles. The healthcare provider should note any breast changes (e.g., nipple retraction, puckering, and/or changes in vascular patterns). With the woman in the supine position, the healthcare provider can place a small towel or pillow behind the woman's scapula on the side to be examined. The breast tissue should be distributed by asking the woman to raise her arm above her head.

The keys to an effective CBE are examination, palpation, and inspection of the entire breast—from the woman's midchest to the clavicle to the midaxillary areas, as well as the tail of Spence (ACOG, 2017). It is critical that the healthcare provider document all findings from the CBE into the electronic medical record. Many electronic medical records also provide the ability to draw or mark areas of concern noted on the CBE onto an electronic diagram. This diagram can then be accessed any time follow-up is indicated.

TABLE 11.4 Clinical Breast and Axillae Examination

EXAMINATION	RECORD ABNORMALITY
Examine breasts for size, symmetry, contour, skin color and texture, venous patterns, and lesions. Use several positions for inspection: • Seated, arms hanging loosely at sides • Seated, arms extended over head or flexed behind neck • Seated, hands pressed against hips with shoulders rolled forward (or seated, hands pressed together) • Seated or standing, and leaning forward from waist	• Use nipple as center of clock face. • Draw or mark diagram to depict size and location of abnormalities. • Describe lesion by the following: • Clock position • Distance from nipple • Relative depth from skin • Described contour (linear, round, or lobulated) • Texture (fluctuant, soft, firm, rock hard) • Mobility (fixed, mobile) • Note inflammation, if present (warm, red, tender). • Note associated skin changes (peau d'orange or ulceration).
Nipples Examine nipples for symmetry, direction, contour, color, and texture.	
Breast and Axillae Perform bimanual digital palpation, compressing tissue between fingers and flat of hand.	
Use palmar finger surface to palpate into axillary hollow for lymph nodes: • Palpate medially, anteriorly, and posteriorly.	
Palpate infraclavicular and supraclavicular nodes.	
Continue palpation with woman in supine position. Have her raise one arm behind her head and place small folded towel under shoulder. Use finger pads and push toward chest in systematic pattern. • Use light, medium, and deep pressure without lifting fingers. • Include tail of Spence.	

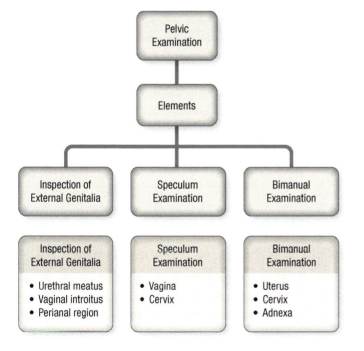

FIGURE 11.1 Components of the pelvic examination.

PELVIC EXAMINATION

The components of a pelvic examination may vary depending on a woman's age, risks, and assessment findings (Figure 11.1). The ACOG (2021a) recommends that a pelvic examination be performed on all women beginning at age 21 years. The decision to collect cervical and/or vaginal specimens while performing a pelvic examination for the asymptomatic woman is a shared decision between a woman and her healthcare provider. Together, they will use sound clinical judgment as a guide to any decision-making.

Examination of the external and internal sexual organs is an appropriate component of a comprehensive evaluation of any woman reporting genital symptoms. Women with menstrual disorders, vaginal discharge, infertility, or pelvic pain should undergo a pelvic and bimanual examination. Women presenting with complaints of abnormal uterine bleeding, a change in bowel or bladder function, and/or vaginal discomfort should undergo a pelvic examination (Fitzgerald et al., 2015).

The initial pelvic examination for an adolescent is usually a source of fear. Furthermore, a pelvic examination in a postmenopausal woman experiencing atrophic vaginitis and/or vaginal or cervical stenosis can be challenging for the novice healthcare provider. A woman's hesitancy, concern, and fears may be alleviated by first demonstrating how the speculum works, offering a mirror to reflect the external and internal genitalia, and defining and explaining commonly used medical terminology.

Gloves are worn throughout the pelvic examination, which should begin with the inspection of the soft tissues of the lower and then upper genital tract. With the woman supine, in a lithotomy position and draped, the healthcare provider should visually inspect the mons and vulva for symmetry and hair quality and growth distribution. It is important to note and later document any piercings, bruising, discharge, rashes, lacerations, and/or tattoos. Next, the healthcare provider should palpate. To avoid startling the woman and before beginning palpation, the healthcare provider should inform the woman of the intention to touch her. This is effectively done by first touching the woman's inner thigh and moving up to the labia, then perineum. The healthcare provider should palpate for lumps and tumors as well as note any elicited pain. Bartholin glands are then palpated to look for a cyst or mass. Bartholin glands are located at approximately the 5 and 7 o'clock positions, in the most distal part of the vagina. The healthcare provider should note and document any lesions, discharge, erythema, and/or edema.

If indicated, the healthcare provider should perform a speculum examination and collect specimens for cytology. Using a gentle touch, the healthcare provider should separate the labia, placing light pressure on the bulbocavernosus muscles, and then insert the speculum (while in the mind's eye, drawing an imaginary line to the woman's rectum) toward the woman's rectum. The selected size of the speculum is based on the size of a woman's vaginal opening. In an adolescent, the Pederson speculum may be appropriate. A Graves speculum is commonly selected for a parous and sexually active woman with a normal BMI. Using a good light source, the healthcare provider should inspect the walls of the vagina for discharge, erythema, and lesions. The cervix should then be examined for color, shape, discharge, lacerations, polyps, and lesions. A normal cervix is moist, pink, and rounded. Nulliparous women tend to have a closed cervical os. In parous women, the cervix usually appears to have a slit-shaped os. The healthcare provider should note common cervical variations, which may indicate all of the following: paleness (a possible sign of anemia or menopausal state), bluish (pregnant), or protrusions (polyps). A woman's vaginal discharge should be assessed—noted for odor, color, and consistency. If appropriate, the healthcare provider should use the appropriate supplies to collect cervical and vaginal specimens. The healthcare provider should warn the woman that she may feel pressure or fullness during specimen collection and during any manipulation of the cervix. It is not a normal finding for a woman to experience any pain upon cervical and vaginal specimen collection. Healthcare providers should be careful to follow manufacturers' directions when collecting specimens. Finally, the healthcare provider withdraws the speculum from the cervix by gently closing the blades before removal from a woman's vagina.

BIMANUAL EXAMINATION

The bimanual examination is performed to determine the size, shape, lie, and location of a woman's uterus and her ovaries. With the woman lying in a lithotomy position and the healthcare provider standing, the clinician, with gentle pressure, inserts the index and middle fingers into the woman's vaginal canal (taking care that the thumb does not brush or compress the clitoris or urethra; Figure 11.2). The healthcare provider's internal finger is then used to palpate the cervix for tenderness/pain, masses, and/or any irregularities. The bimanual examination should not be painful. Cervical motion tenderness (CMT) is an abnormal finding and may indicate ectopic pregnancy, pelvic inflammatory disease, or infections of the cervix. Assessment of the ovaries is accomplished by shifting the internal fingers first to the right ovary and then to the left ovary.

The external hand presses downward toward the internal finger to capture the ovary and uterus (Figure 11.3). With the tips of the fingers and with gentle pressure, start at the umbilicus and work down to the symphysis. In obese, prepubescent, and postmenopausal women, the ovaries may not be palpable. When

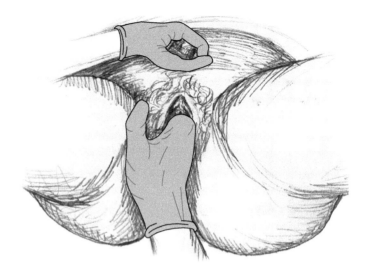

FIGURE 11.2 Bimanual examination, frontal view.

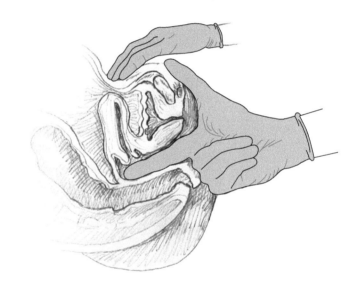

FIGURE 11.3 Bimanual pelvic examination, lateral view.

palpable, the ovaries should normally be about 5 cm in diameter, firm, oval, and nontender, depending on phase of a woman's menstrual cycle. The fallopian tubes are not palpable. The ability to palpate the fallopian tubes is an abnormal finding and may indicate, for example, the presence of an ectopic pregnancy.

The healthcare provider should also assess the uterus for mobility and tenderness. The uterus should be firm, smooth, and nontender. The normal uterus is anterior, pear-shaped, and the size of an average women's fist. An enlarged uterus may indicate a pregnancy, fibroid tumors, endometriosis, or carcinoma. The healthcare provider should estimate the size of a woman's enlarged uterus by weeks of gestation. For example, if the uterus is midpoint between the umbilicus and symphysis pubis, the estimated size of the uterus would be 12 weeks. A uterus that is found to be immobile is an abnormal finding. An immobile uterus may indicate uterine infection, carcinoma, or adhesions.

A cervix positioned toward the anterior canal indicates a retroflexed uterus. A retroverted uterus is not an abnormal finding and does not usually cause health issues for a woman. However, if a woman with a retroverted uterus presents with complaints of pelvic pain, for example, the healthcare provider should add endometriosis, adhesions, and fibroids to the differential list and rule out pathology (Figure 11.4).

If on evaluation, a woman's uterus and cervix are shifted left or right, this may be an indication of a pelvic mass. Further evaluation with diagnostic imaging (an ultrasound exam) would be necessary. Palpation of the anterior vaginal fornix (above the cervix) can be used to determine the degree of an anteflexed uterus (Figure 11.5). Palpating the fundus of a woman's uterus down to the posterior fornix supports the finding that a woman's uterus may be retroverted. It is important that the healthcare provider note if a woman exhibits guarding during the bimanual examination. Guarding is an abnormal finding and is indicative of pain.

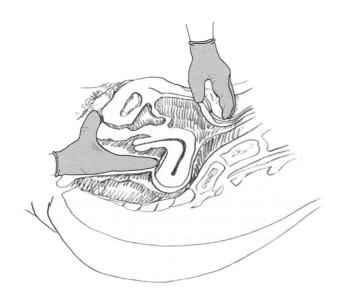

FIGURE 11.4 Retroflexed uterus.

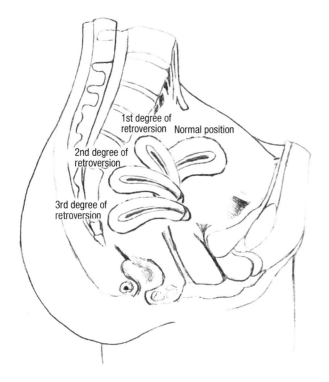

1st degree of retroversion   Normal position

2nd degree of retroversion

3rd degree of retroversion

FIGURE 11.5 Degrees of retroversion of the uterus.

RECTOVAGINAL EXAMINATION

A retroverted uterus and adnexal masses can be palpated on rectovaginal examination. The healthcare provider should first visually examine a woman's external anal area for hemorrhoids, lesions, and/or masses and then ask the woman to bear down. While the woman is bearing down, the healthcare provider should slowly and carefully, place a gloved and lubricated finger, into the woman's anus, noting the presence of polyps and/or hemorrhoids, as well as the tone of the anal sphincter. It is very important that the healthcare provider change gloves after performing pelvic and bimanual examinations and before performing a rectovaginal examination. This will avoid cross-contamination (ACOG, 2018).

SPECIAL CONSIDERATIONS

The Adolescent Well-Woman Exam

Expanding access to primary screening and family planning methods to adolescents improves health outcomes. For the first time in history, the United States is experiencing 4 decades of low adolescent pregnancy rates (Pascale et al., 2016; Sawaya, 2016). Medicaid and the 2010 ACA are posited as part of the reason for these unprecedented low rates. These provisions have allowed significantly improved adolescent access to highly effective methods of birth control (e.g., long-acting reversible contraceptive methods [intrauterine devices and systems and implants]; IOM, 2011). Long-acting reversible contraceptive methods have been proved to be both safe and highly effective in reducing the rates of unintended pregnancy (Richards, 2016).

The initial reproductive health visit can be scheduled as early as 13 years old. This visit should be handled with confidentiality, one on one between client and clinician. Confidentiality laws very state by state. Talk the adolescents through access of patient portal within the electronic health record system. Respect, trust, and comfort are important for the provider and office staff to establish with adolescents. Suggestions include offering afterschool appointments and offering cultural and age-appropriate literature in the reception and examinations room. Give attention to how the adolescent self identifies gender, name they prefer, and preferred contact information such as cell phone number. During the visit address immunization history including COVID vaccine, mental health, and sexuality. Follow-up visits should be individualized based on each client encounter (ACOG, 2020).

Adolescents younger than 21 years should not be screened with a cytology test/Pap test regardless of age at sexual initiation, sexually transmitted infection (STI) history, parity, or other risk factors (ACOG, 2021a). Testing and screening adolescents for HPV infection leads to unnecessary evaluation and overtreatment, which can increase the risk of reproductive problems such as incompetent cervix, stenosis, and/or scarring (ACOG, 2021a). Adolescents who underwent cervical cancer screening (e.g., cervical cytology) and had one or more Pap tests with normal results before the screening guidelines changed should *not* be screened again until they reach age 21 years. Adolescents with a previous abnormal Pap test, followed by two normal tests, should wait until age 21 years to be rescreened (ACOG, 2021a).

Cervical cancer screening every 3 years is recommended for women 21 to 29 years of age. Recent evidence supports addressing any of these reproductive health issues regardless of a woman's cervical cancer screening status (ACOG, 2021a). It is not necessary to perform cervical cancer screening in order to provide most contraceptive services (e.g., oral, implants, injections, patches), initiate hormone management of dysmenorrhea or menstrual health, or provide STI screening. Vaginal swabs or urine tests are appropriate, effective alternatives for STI screening.

Reproductive Age

For women in their childbearing years, an annual well-woman visit is the perfect opportunity to provide SRH education, immunizations, health screening, and family planning services. Pelvic and bimanual examinations are indicated before procedures such as the insertion of an intrauterine device or system, the fitting of a diaphragm or pessary, and an endometrial biopsy.

One innovative, reproductive health needs measure that came from the Oregon Foundation for Reproductive Health is the One Key Question' Initiative (OKQ, 2012). The OKQ concept was designed to encourage primary care providers to query women about their reproductive health needs. By asking women one question, "Would you like to become pregnant in the next year?" healthcare providers can support women's preventive reproductive health needs (e.g., pregnancy prevention, preparation for a healthy pregnancy; OKQ, 2012).

Mature Women

The mature women, defined as 46 to 64 years of age, has special health concerns. The North American Menopause Society (NAMS), estimate that 2 million women reach menopause in the United States each year and there is an estimated 45 million women older than the median age of menopause, which is 51 years of age (NAMS, 2018). Our new generation of healthcare provider graduates often lack the training and core competencies needed to manage a woman experiencing menopausal symptoms, as well as the necessary knowledge needed to prescribe hormonal treatment (see Chapter 34 for management/treatment guidelines). Inconsistent practice protocols exist based on personal interpretation of the Women's Health Initiative (WHI) study findings and given the many hormonal, bioidentical, *natural,* and complementary and alternative therapies touted as safe and effective.

An annual flu shot, a tetanus booster every 10 years, pneumococcal vaccine PPSV23, and screening for hepatitis C are recommended for women older than 65 years. The zoster recombinant or shingles vaccine is recommended for all women at age 50 (Center for Disease Control and Prevention [CDC], 2023) Screening for osteoporosis is recommended for women starting at age 65 years (ACOG, 2021b). See Figures 11.6 and 11.7 for additional recommended immunizations.

Mature women have sexual concerns and sometimes want their healthcare provider to first address the subject—thereby opening the door to an open and trusting conversation. Age should *not* be a barrier to sexual health topics. Women experience aging differently and should be managed based on a woman's and her healthcare provider's joint decision-making.

SUMMARY

Well women's healthcare provisions have improved preventive healthcare service for women across their lifetime by promoting a paradigm shift from reactive healthcare to encouraging health and well-being (Figure 11.8). An annual, well-woman visit is a covered benefit under the ACA and by most private insurance and Medicaid plans. With no out-of-pocket cost requirements, private insurance plans, Medicaid, and Title X allow greater access for women to include low-income women who continue to be disproportionately affected by limited information and limited access to preventive care. In 2016, more than 55 million women have access to their choice of safe and efficacious birth control methods approved by the FDA. Well-woman visits are a vital element and entry to preventive care as well as a new paradigm for healthcare practices. Reproductive healthcare needs, from adolescence through the reproductive years and into maturity, continue to be managed by healthcare providers—including specialty and primary care healthcare providers across a variety of healthcare disciplines. Nurse practitioners, nurse midwives, physicians, and physician assistants are trained to translate evidence into practice at the point of care, thereby improving the quality of healthcare delivery and access to comprehensive preventive care.

FUTURE DIRECTIONS

Future directions include client-centered medical homes led by nurse practitioners and other healthcare professionals. This new wave in healthcare emphasizes coordination, communication, and the practice of putting women *front and center* as active participants in their healthcare decision-making (Sawaya, 2016). Shared informed decision-making has been challenging to implement because of clinic time constraints and patient loads that are needed to meet the economic requirements of healthcare organizations. This model of healthcare delivery demands a *huge* paradigm shift, not only in moving to a focus in prevention, but also in the manner in which third-party payers will reimburse healthcare providers and hospitals, where quality and health outcomes are used to determine reward and monetary compensation. A change of such magnitude will necessitate guidance for healthcare providers and women as this new model of healthcare is incorporated into healthcare delivery. This is an exciting time to be a healthcare provider and a woman—the opportunities to help shape these changes are appreciated daily in healthcare delivery settings. The well-woman visit is an opportunity to provide care that is evidence based, has high value, and is woman centered (Sawaya, 2016).

REFERENCES

References for this chapter are online and available at https://connect.springerpub.com/content/book/978-0-8261-6722-4/part/part02/chapter/ch11

Vaccine	19–26 years	27–49 years	50–64 years	≥65 years
COVID-19	2- or 3- dose primary series and booster (See Notes)			
Influenza inactivated (IIV4) or Influenza recombinant (RIV4) **or**	1 dose annually			
Influenza live, attenuated (LAIV4)	1 dose annually			
Tetanus, diphtheria, pertussis (Tdap or Td)	1 dose Tdap each pregnancy; 1 dose Td/Tdap for wound management (see notes) — 1 dose Tdap, then Td or Tdap booster every 10 years			
Measles, mumps, rubella (MMR)	1 or 2 doses depending on indication (if born in 1957 or later)			For healthcare personnel, see notes
Varicella (VAR)	2 doses (if born in 1980 or later)	2 doses		
Zoster recombinant (RZV)	2 doses for immunocompromising conditions (see notes)		2 doses	
Human papillomavirus (HPV)	2 or 3 doses depending on age at initial vaccination or condition	27 through 45 years		
Pneumococcal (PCV15, PCV20, PPSV23)	1 dose PCV15 followed by PPSV23 OR 1 dose PCV20 (see notes)		See Notes / See Notes	
Hepatitis A (HepA)	2, 3, or 4 doses depending on vaccine			
Hepatitis B (HepB)	2, 3, or 4 doses depending on vaccine or condition			
Meningococcal A, C, W, Y (MenACWY)	1 or 2 doses depending on indication, see notes for booster recommendations			
Meningococcal B (MenB)	19 through 23 years	2 or 3 doses depending on vaccine and indication, see notes for booster recommendations		
Haemophilus influenzae type b (Hib)	1 or 3 doses depending on indication			

Recommended vaccination for adults who meet age requirement, lack documentation of vaccination, or lack evidence of past infection

Recommended vaccination for adults with an additional risk factor or another indication

Recommended vaccination based on shared clinical decision-making

No recommendation/ Not applicable

FIGURE 11.6 Recommended immunization schedule for adults aged 19 years or older, United States.
These schedules indicate the age groups and medical indications for which the administration of currently licensed vaccines is commonly recommended for adults age 19 years or older, as of January 2023. For all vaccines being recommended on the Adult Immunization Schedule, a vaccine series does not need to be restarted, regardless of the time that has elapsed between doses. Licensed combination vaccines may be used whenever any components of the combination are indicated and when the vaccine's other components are not contraindicated. For detailed recommendations on all vaccines, including those used primarily for travelers or that are issued during the year, consult the manufacturer's package inserts and the complete statements from the Advisory Committee on Immunization Practices (www.cdc .gov/vaccines/schedules/hcp/imz/adult.html). Use of trade names and commercial sources is for identification only and does not imply endorsement by the U.S. Department of Health and Human Services. Covered by the National Vaccine Injury Compensation Program.
Recipients of a hematopoietic stem cell transplant (HSCT) should be vaccinated with a three-dose regimen 6 to 12 months after a successful transplant, regardless of vaccination history; at least 4 weeks should separate doses.
Source: Reproduced from Center for Disease Control and Prevention. (2023). Recommended adult immunization schedule. U.S. Department of Health and Human Services. https://www.cdc.gov/vaccines/schedules/downloads/adult /adult-combined-schedule.pdf

Vaccine schedule — indications by condition

Vaccine	Pregnancy	Immuno-compromised (excluding HIV infection)	HIV infection CD4 percentage and count <15% or <200 mm³	HIV infection CD4 percentage and count ≥15% and ≥200 mm³	Asplenia, complement deficiencies	End-stage renal disease, or on hemodialysis	Heart or lung disease; alcoholism[a]	Chronic liver disease	Diabetes	Health care personnel[b]	Men who have sex with men
COVID-19			See Notes								
IIV4 or RIV4 **OR** LAIV4			1 dose annually							1 dose annually	
			Contraindicated (LAIV4)				Precaution				
Tdap or Td	1 dose Tdap each pregnancy	1 dose Tdap, then Td or Tdap booster every 10 years									
MMR	Contraindicated*	Contraindicated	Contraindicated	1 or 2 doses depending on indication							
VAR	Contraindicated*	Contraindicated	Contraindicated	2 doses							
RZV		2 doses at age ≥19 years					2 doses at age ≥50 years				
HPV	Not Recommended*	3 doses through age 26 years		2 or 3 doses through age 26 years depending on age at initial vaccination or condition							
Pneumococcal (PCV15, PCV20, PPSV23)					1 dose PCV15 followed by PPSV23 OR 1 dose PCV20 (see notes)						
HepA							2, 3, or 4 doses depending on vaccine				
HepB	3 doses (see notes)				2, 3, or 4 doses depending on vaccine or condition						
MenACWY		1 or 2 doses depending on indication, see notes for booster recommendations									
MenB	Precaution	2 or 3 doses depending on vaccine and indication, see notes for booster recommendations									
Hib		3 doses HSCT[c] recipients only			1 dose						

Legend:
- Recommended vaccination for adults who meet age requirement, lack documentation of vaccination, or lack evidence of past infection
- Recommended vaccination for adults with an additional risk factor or another indication
- Recommended vaccination based on shared clinical decision-making
- Precaution–vaccination might be indicated if benefit of protection outweighs risk of adverse reaction
- Contraindicated or not recommended–vaccine should not be administered. *Vaccinate after pregnancy.
- No recommendation/Not applicable

a. Precaution for LAIV4 does not apply to alcoholism. **b.** See notes for influenza; hepatitis B; measles, mumps, and rubella; and varicella vaccinations. **c.** Hematopoietic stem cell transplant.

FIGURE 11.7 Vaccines that might be indicated for adults age 19 years or older based on medical and other indications.

Source: Reproduced from Center for Disease Control and Prevention. (2023). Recommended adult immunization schedule. U.S. Department of Health and Human Services. https://www.cdc.gov/vaccines/schedules/downloads/adult/adult-combined-schedule.pdf

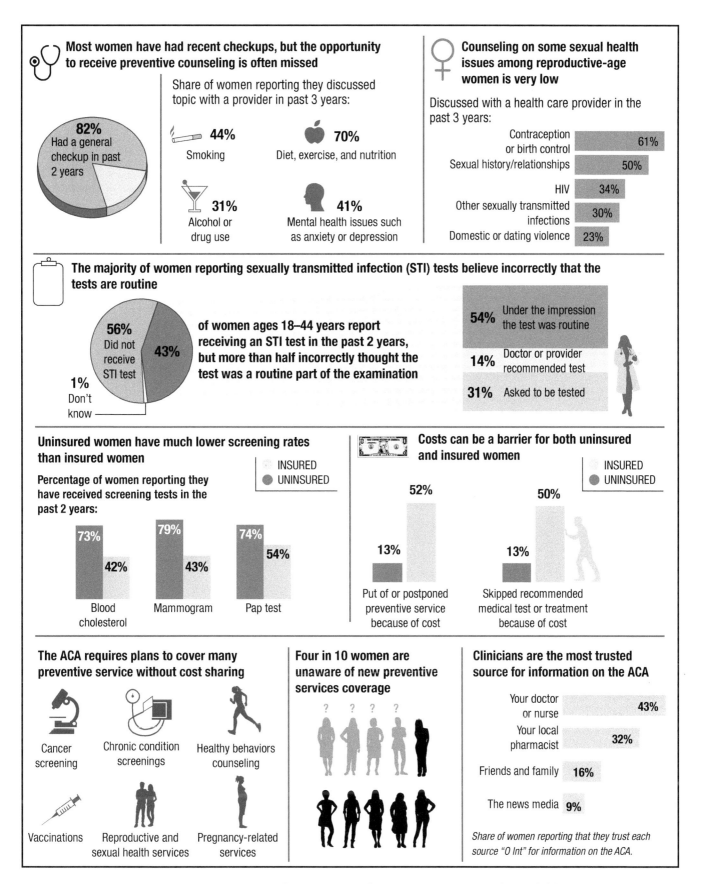

Most women have had recent checkups, but the opportunity to receive preventive counseling is often missed

82% Had a general checkup in past 2 years

Share of women reporting they discussed topic with a provider in past 3 years:

44% Smoking

70% Diet, exercise, and nutrition

31% Alcohol or drug use

41% Mental health issues such as anxiety or depression

Counseling on some sexual health issues among reproductive-age women is very low

Discussed with a health care provider in the past 3 years:

Contraception or birth control	61%
Sexual history/relationships	50%
HIV	34%
Other sexually transmitted infections	30%
Domestic or dating violence	23%

The majority of women reporting sexually transmitted infection (STI) tests believe incorrectly that the tests are routine

56% Did not receive STI test

43%

1% Don't know

43% of women ages 18–44 years report receiving an STI test in the past 2 years, but more than half incorrectly thought the test was a routine part of the examination

54% Under the impression the test was routine

14% Doctor or provider recommended test

31% Asked to be tested

Uninsured women have much lower screening rates than insured women

☐ INSURED
● UNINSURED

Percentage of women reporting they have received screening tests in the past 2 years:

Blood cholesterol **73%** / **42%**
Mammogram **79%** / **43%**
Pap test **74%** / **54%**

Costs can be a barrier for both uninsured and insured women

☐ INSURED
● UNINSURED

Put of or postponed preventive service because of cost **13%** / **52%**

Skipped recommended medical test or treatment because of cost **13%** / **50%**

The ACA requires plans to cover many preventive service without cost sharing

Cancer screening

Chronic condition screenings

Healthy behaviors counseling

Vaccinations

Reproductive and sexual health services

Pregnancy-related services

Four in 10 women are unaware of new preventive services coverage

? ? ? ?

Clinicians are the most trusted source for information on the ACA

Your doctor or nurse	43%
Your local pharmacist	32%
Friends and family	16%
The news media	9%

Share of women reporting that they trust each source "O Int" for information on the ACA.

FIGURE 11.8 Preventive services for women and the Patient Protection and Affordable Care Act (ACA).

Source: Salganicoff, A., Ranji, U., Beamesderfer, A., & Kurani, N. (2014). Women and health care in the early years of the ACA: Key findings from the 2013 Kaiser Women's Health Survey. Kaiser Family Foundation. http://kff.org/womens-health-policy/report/women-and-health-care-in-the -early-years-of-the-aca-key-findings-from-the-2013-kaiser-womens-health-survey. Reprinted by per-mission of the Henry J. Kaiser Family Foundation. All rights reserved.

CHAPTER 12

Mental Health*

SANDRA J. JANASHAK CADENA

There is no health without mental health.

—World Health Organization (2004)

INTRODUCTION

This chapter reviews the evolving world view of mental health and mental illness, the unique incidence and prevalence of mental disorders in women, and women's vulnerabilities to specific mental illnesses based on the stages of her reproductive life cycle. Women's struggles with mental health often go undetected and untreated (Izutsu et al., 2015; World Health Organization [WHO], 2004). These mental disorders can impact a woman's life, fluctuating throughout her lifetime. A depressive disorder, for example, may begin with the start of one's menstrual cycle, increase during young adulthood that precipitates alcohol abuse, then evolve into a bipolar disorder with mania during pregnancy and in the postpartum phase, become less dominant until reappearing at perimenopause, and finally contribute to cognitive disorders and dementia during postmenopause.

The biopsychosocial model is used in this chapter to explain the etiology of mental illness in women, with an overview of identifying risk and protective factors when evaluating a woman and her mental health. Common mental disorders (CMDs), including mood and anxiety disorders, as well as other diagnoses such as psychosis and eating, sleep, and cognitive disorders, that may dominate a specific point in a woman's reproductive cycle are reviewed. Issues that contribute to women's poor mental health are also addressed, including intimate partner violence (IPV), suicide, alcohol and substance use, nonsuicidal self-injuries, and trauma. Considerations for special and minoritized groups include racism and mental health disparities, transgender and gender nonconforming (TGNC) persons, and the impact of the COVID-19 phenomenon on women's mental health. Finally, the chapter considers the future of mental health and mental illness identification and consequences for girls and women in need of such care.

Integrated in conjunction with mental health challenges of women in this chapter is use of standardized and international screening instruments. Screening is the health practitioner's first step in evaluating the need to delve further into the presence or absence of a mental disorder. This determination may signal a crisis and the need for immediate intervention or suggest when to refer the woman to a mental health professional. Employing these screening instruments are strategies paramount in reducing risk and enhancing opportunities for the woman to understand and self-manage her stresses and build upon her own protective factors to increase resiliency.

DEFINITIONS OF MENTAL HEALTH AND MENTAL ILLNESS

For many years, mental health was viewed primarily as the absence of mental illness. In 2004, WHO defined mental health as "a state of well-being in which the individual realizes his or her own abilities, can cope with the normal stresses of life, can work productively and fruitfully, and is able to make a contribution to his or her community" (WHO, 2004, p. 69). This state of well-being includes psychological, social, and emotional well-being. But differences in approaches and definitions cloud what multidimensional aspects should be include in the definitions of mental health. The Committee on Ethical Issues of the European Psychiatric Association (Galderisi et al., 2015) attempted to be more comprehensive, culturally and globally flexible, and inclusive in their definition:

Mental health is a dynamic state of internal equilibrium which enables individuals to use their abilities in harmony with universal values of society. Basic cognitive and social skills; ability to recognize, express and modulate one's own emotions, as well as empathize with others; flexibility and ability to cope with adverse life events and function in social roles; and harmonious relationship between body and mind represent important components of mental

---

*This chapter is a revision of the chapter that appeared in the second edition of this textbook, authored by Gail M. Houck, and we thank her for her original contribution.

health which contribute, to varying degrees, to the state of internal equilibrium. (pp. 231–232)

The Canadian Public Health Association (2021) historically utilized a more socially integrated definition that went beyond the biological model. It has since updated the embracing of this more encompassing model:

Mental health is the capacity of the individual, the group and the environment to interact with one another in ways that promote subjective well-being, the optimal development and use of mental abilities (cognitive, affective and relational), the achievement of individual and collective goals consistent with justice and the attainment and preservation of conditions of fundamental equality. (p. 6)

Not until recent years has there been an embracing of this definition that contributes to a more holistic understanding of women's mental health. Bhagawati (2020) states that using this multidimensional definition for women and girls

- emphasizes the intricacies of mutuality and interrelations among a host of variables that determine mental health and that the determinants of health function at multiple stages;
- looks and reaches beyond the "biological" and "individual" and concedes the significance of the society and the "social";
- acknowledges the primal importance of values and principles of justice and equality in configuring mental and emotional well-being. (pp. 772–773)

Global Perspectives

Global interest in women's health has grown over the past 3 decades and now takes a seat at the forefront of the world, facilitated by the United Nations (2018) and the 17 Sustainable Development Goals (SDGs). SDG 3 of the 2030 Agenda for Sustainable Development *"ensures healthy lives and promoting well-being for all at all ages."* Associated targets specific to mental health include the goal to "reduce mortality from non-communicable diseases and strengthen the prevention and treatment of substance abuse." Target indicators' accomplishments for 2030 include:

3.4 Reduce by one third premature mortality from non-communicable diseases through prevention and treatment and promote mental health and well-being (including mental illness),
3.5 Strengthen the prevention and treatment of substance abuse, including narcotic drug abuse and harmful use of alcohol. (United Nations, 2018)

Goal 5 of the SDGs also focuses on concerns of women: to *"achieve gender equality and empower all women and girls."* This goal's indicators and 2030 target accomplishments include:

5.1 End all forms of discrimination against all women and girls everywhere,
5.2 Eliminate all forms of violence (physical, sexual, or psychological) against all women and girls in the public

and private spheres, including trafficking and sexual and other types of exploitation,
5.3 Eliminate all harmful practices, such as child, early and forced marriage and female genital mutilation,
5.6 Ensure universal access to sexual and reproductive health and reproductive rights. (United Nations, 2018)

Such lofty goals with the emphasis on "elimination" of inequality throughout the world underscore the long path that individuals, institutions, governments, and national policies have yet to travel. North America, including the United States, continues attempts at advancing women's health initiatives and efforts at the Office of Research on Women's Health at the National Institutes of Health (NIH), the Office of Women's Health in the U.S. Department of Health and Human Services (DHHS), and through the U.S. Food and Drug Administration (FDA) guidelines and policies. The U.S. Preventive Services Task Force (USPSTF) clinical guidelines and recommendations often focus on needs of women across a variety of medical diagnoses, symptom presentations, interventions, and health promotion and illness prevention strategies (Feltner et al., 2022).

These institutional and federal guidelines emphasize the value of mental health and well-being for women and girls. It is an integral part of their capacity to lead a fulfilling life, including the ability to form relationships, study, work, or pursue leisure interests, as well as to make day-to-day decisions and choices. Women's mental health, therefore, impacts a full range of health and illnesses and is often seen as worthy of more attention than many other illnesses (Feltner et al., 2022).

The National Institute of Mental Health (NIMH; 2023) reports that one in five U.S. adults, approximately 52.9 million people, live with a mental illness. Mental illnesses include many different conditions that vary in degree of severity and affect men and women differently (NIMH, 2023). For example, depressive disorders are about twice as common in women than men (Brody et al., 2018). Women also are also more likely to experience the full range of anxiety disorders, including panic, generalized anxiety disorder (GAD), and posttraumatic stress disorder (PTSD; Jalnapurkar et al., 2018). Over 90% of all persons identified with an eating disorder are women (Smink et al., 2012). Although alcoholism is much more prevalent in men, Males accounted for the majority (76%) of alcohol-related deaths. However, a steeper increase was observed for females between 1999 and 2017 (White, 2020).

Reproductive life cycle events are often critical points in a woman's mental health. Mental disorders in girls and women are most often diagnosed coinciding with the beginning of one's menstrual cycle (11 to 15 years of age) and during childbearing (11 to 40 years old; Altemus et al., 2014). Pregnancy, nonviable births, and terminated pregnancies can act as triggers for the initial onset or exacerbations of disabling symptoms (O'Hara, 2009). Women living through perimenopause and postmenopause can experience a wide range of disabling mental health symptoms. The stage in a woman's reproductive life cycle may influence how illnesses present, complicate responses to treatment, and contribute to shortening her life.

ETIOLOGY OF MENTAL ILLNESS

What components contribute to mental health and mental illness, particularly in women? One paradigm looks at current biological, psychological, and social aspects, the biopsychosocial model of mental health and illness. This model is embraced by the American Psychiatric Nurses Association (APNA), American Psychiatric Association, American Psychological Association, World Psychiatry Association (WPA), and an array of additional mental health professional groups (Tripathi et al., 2019). It is helpful to understand and integrate these concepts specific to women's mental health.

Biological perspectives of mental health include one's genetic predisposition and vulnerabilities. With the advancements of science utilizing MRI, both static and functional technologies, neuroscientists can (1) predict and identify many mental illnesses, (2) develop and test pharmacologic interventions, (3) evaluate the efficacy and effectiveness of alternative strategies, and (4) reinforce resiliency approaches and mental well-being, all based on structural and functional components of the central and peripheral nervous systems (Falkai et al., 2018). Laboratory studies, including genetic studies, have continued to evolve in the identification and treatment options available to persons with mental health disorders. Testing can now be utilized, for example, to select the most efficacious antidepressant for a person with a major depressive disorder (MDD) at the initial point of treatment (Baldessarini et al., 2019). No longer do prescribers need to depend solely upon patient's report of symptoms as the only guideline when selecting from the myriad of available pharmacologic and psychological treatment options.

Psychological causes of mental health and illness continue to evolve as classic theories and models are refined, building upon psychodynamic, familial, and trauma-based ramifications of experiences throughout the lifespan. Frequently encountered women with histories of childhood sexual trauma such as incest, for example, present with a myriad of physical problems and concerns that often mask a cascade of emotional, self-esteem, and psychological struggles (Tripathi et al., 2019).

Social determinants of mental health have taken the forefront implicating causes of mental illnesses (Jeste et al., 2022). Poverty, pollution, and inadequate means to meet basic needs of food, water, shelter, and safety contribute to the vulnerabilities of persons with these unfortunate barriers in life. WHO (2012) encourages policy makers and clinicians to integrate diagnostic approaches and interventions addressing these complex aspects of the patient who seeks mental healthcare. It is truly an approach that allows the practitioner to "*meet the patient where they are*" in a comprehensive etiologic perspective. Understanding the complexity and fluidity of possible causes for mental health and illness is critical when evaluating and treating a patient. Identifying risk factors and protective factors of mental health is paramount in understanding and providing comprehensive care (Prince et al., 2007).

RISK AND PROTECTIVE FACTORS

Risks and Vulnerabilities

Mental health and well-being are influenced not only by individual attributes but also by the social circumstances in which persons find themselves and the environment in which they live; these determinants interact with each other dynamically and may threaten or protect an individual's state of mental health.

Risks to mental health manifest themselves at all stages in life and risk exposures specifically in the formative, reproductive stages of life—insecure attachment in infancy, family violence in childhood, and substance use in pregnancy—can affect mental well-being or predispose toward mental disorders many years later (Carter & Kostaras, 2005). Certain groups and subgroups in society may be particularly susceptible to experiencing mental health problems from the biopsychosocial paradigm (Box 12.1).

Being diagnosed with a chronic mental disorder has its own additional set of vulnerabilities and risks such as an increased likelihood of experiencing disability and premature death, stigma and discrimination, social exclusion, and impoverishment (Centers for Disease Control and Prevention [CDC], 2016). As many persons with a mental illness will tell you, they are "*more than their illness.*" This mantra, supported by NAMI, emphasizes a focus on strengths, resiliency, and identification of protective factors throughout many of one's formative life stages.

Protective Factors

Just as we assess the mental health risk factors of our clients, it warrants the practitioner to also identify and emphasize protective factors for the client. Enhancing their awareness of risks for mental health problems empowers the client to also evaluate factors to incorporate in protection of one's mental health.

WHO (2012) delineates fundamental factors throughout life that may enhance effective coping skills that can be learned as well as built upon when facing past problems or in anticipation of coping with many of life's difficulties (Box 12.2).

Establishing a positive relationship begins with an understanding of both risk and protective factors when taking

---

Box 12.1 Risk Factors and Vulnerability for Mental Illness

- Living in poverty
- Chronic health conditions
- Racial minority groups
- Ethnic minority groups
- Sexual minority groups
- Exposure to war or conflict
- Displaced by war or conflict

Source: Adapted from World Health Organization. (2012, October 16). Risks to mental health: An overview of vulnerabilities and risk factors. Author. https://www.who.int/publications/m/item/risks-to-mental-health

Box 12.2 Protective Factors for Mental Illness

- Flexibility and coping
- Problem-solving skills
- Development and maintenance of connections to friends, family, and community support
- Minimal use of mind-altering substances, including alcohol, tobacco, and psychoactive substances
- Awareness of both positive and negative self-talk
- Cultural and religious beliefs that support resilience
- Supportive relationships with care providers
- Availability of physical and mental healthcare

Source: Adapted from the World Health Organization. (2012, October 16). Risks to mental health: An overview of vulnerabilities and risk factors. Author. https://www.who.int/publications/m/item/risks-to-mental-health

the initial history and completing a physical examination. Women struggling with mental health concerns may be cautious in sharing details of their emotional, situational, social, or cognitive concerns. Whether the practitioner suspects a patient may be experiencing a mental health problem for the first time or knows this patient lives with a chronic mental disorder such as schizophrenia for over 30 years, for example, a practitioner gains knowledge of the client by always asking about these critical factors. Identifying when the patient is experiencing a range of signs and symptoms indicative of distress, mental health concerns, or a mental health disorder warrants deeper exploration and evaluation.

Comprehensive biopsychosocial assessment incorporates selected assessment and screening instruments, based on the information the patient has shared. The practitioner also brings a range of knowledge, education, and experiences that guide one to selecting the most useful assessment and screening tools.

Mental Health and Mental Illness: Two Continuums

Mental health and illness have traditionally been viewed on one continuum (Luijten et al., 2019). Keyes and colleagues, however, spearheaded international research of mental health (often called well-being) and mental illness as a dual-continuum model (Keyes, 2005; Keyes & Haidt, 2003; Keyes & Westerhof, 2012). Individuals with a mental illness, for example, can still experience high levels of well-being, whereas individuals without a mental illness can also experience low levels of well-being.

Mental illness symptoms, such as intense sadness and lack of motivation, cluster around the concept of *languishing* (Keyes, 2005). According to Keyes, mental health includes happiness and positive functioning, labeled *flourishing*. There are 13 symptoms that meet this criterion, including a designated length of time, very much like the presence of a mental illness symptom. When asking a client about her happiness in life, are they (1) regularly cheerful, in good spirits, happy, calm and peaceful, satisfied, and full of life for the past 30 days, and (2) feel happy or satisfied with life overall or domains of life (relationships, employment, etc.)? Experiencing high levels of

positive functioning include domains of (1) self-acceptance, personal growth, purpose, autonomy; (2) social acceptance, actualization, coherence, contribution, integration; (3) environmental mastery; and (4) positive relations with others (Keyes, 2005; Ryff & Singer, 2003).

Understanding these aspects of well-being/mental health assists practitioners to observe and assess a client's perception of function, resilience, available resources, and adaptability in times of stress as well as personal satisfaction with life. Questions with purpose, such as asking about the client's own views of their life, function, positive support of friends, family, or community can gauge the level and intensity of a need to delve deeper in uncovering potential problems in function and mental health.

Screenings Instruments

Nursing and medicine have a long history of viewing health as the absence of illness (Compton & Shim, 2015). Hence, there are several screening instruments that have been deemed valid and reliable when initially attempting to identify a mental illness. Providing a mental disorder diagnosis requires multiple steps in obtaining a history and physical evaluation, conducting diagnostic tests, and collecting additional information. Consistently including screening instruments, many of them self-administered, can assist the practitioner to identify signs and symptoms of specific mental disorders. Mental illness, distress, and problems can be categorized based on severity utilizing such tools. This dual approach of (1) assessing mental health, including resiliency, function, and resource availability, and (2) evaluating mental illness with an emphasis on psychopathology, improves diagnostic accuracy and treatment. It also provides guidance to the practitioner when to (1) use active listening skills, (2) select the correct screening tool when mental health problems are of concern, (3) focus on positive, resilient aspects of the patient, and (4) determine need (acute or chronic) for referrals to mental health professionals (Feltner et al., 2018).

REPRODUCTIVE LIFE CYCLE

As women's health practitioners, it is helpful to categorize specific mental health vulnerabilities based on age, life experiences and reproductive category when women may be most susceptible. This section divides the reproductive life of women into four stages: (1) preadolescence and adolescence, (2) early and later adulthood, (3) pregnancy and the postpartum period, and (4) perimenopause and postmenopause. Women's life experiences, of course, may overlap and repeat. And mental health problems may begin prior to the onset of menarche and fluctuate throughout the woman's entire life. We know, however, that there are points in time in relation to a woman's reproductive life cycle that an increased occurrence of mental health problems and diagnoses occur (Rahman et al., 2013). Understanding these stages allows the practitioner opportunities to focus on specific mental illnesses that can occur during specific points in a woman's life. Identifying these potential mental health flashpoints can best be integrated into a plan of treatment and care by selecting the appropriate screening instruments

Preadolescence and Adolescent Mental Health Risk Assessment

According to WHO, one in six people in the world are age 10 to 19 years. Globally, it is estimated that one in seven (14%) of 10- to 19-year-olds experience mental health conditions, yet remain unrecognized and untreated (WHO, 2021). Preadolescents and adolescents are at high risk for developing mental problems and disorders.

Adolescence is a developmental stage during which dependent children grow into independent adults. This period usually begins at about the age of 10 years and lasts until the late teens or early 20s. During adolescence, children undergo powerful physical, intellectual, and emotional growth. Adolescent girls are faced with increased peer pressure, perceived stress, and fluctuating abilities to accept or reject all the alterations they experience. Besides the perception of high demands, girls and young women struggle with low levels of global self-esteem, sleep disturbances, and poor social support. These aspects play a crucial role in the prediction of stress-related symptoms (Wiklund et al., 2010). Girls as young as 10 years of age are at risk of experiencing increasing and ongoing psychological distress, develop inadequate coping styles, struggle with poor self-esteem, and often have unhealthy social relations. Preadolescents, adolescents, and young adults experience many risk factors of the social determinants of mental health, including exposure to poverty, abuse, and violence, contributing to adolescents' vulnerability to mental health problems. Matud et al. (2020) report that young women, ages 19 to 29 years, scored higher than men of the same ages in psychological distress, chronic stress, and minor daily hassles. Adolescents with mental health conditions are even more susceptible to a range of stress-producing experiences, as presented in Box 12.3.

Protecting individuals from adversity, promoting socioemotional learning and psychological well-being, and ensuring access to mental healthcare are critical for their health and well-being during adolescence and adulthood. When these protective factors are not sufficiently present, women's health practitioners are often faced with girls and young women, ranging from age 12 to their early 20s, who struggle with a myriad of emotional and psychological concerns that may or may not meet criteria for a referral to a mental health professional. These patients may never be evaluated or treated for a diagnosable condition. Using a self-report screening tool of 20 questions with yes or no responses can capture if there is a need for further evaluation for mental health concerns (Patel, 2003).

CMDs impact on the mood or feelings of affected persons; symptoms range in terms of their severity (from mild to severe) and duration (from months to years). These disorders are diagnosable health conditions, and are distinct from feelings of sadness, stress, or fear that anyone can experience from time to time in their lives. Anxiety disorders involve a general mood condition involving feelings of uneasiness, being fearful or feeling nervous, whereas depressive disorders have emotions that involve feeling low, sad, fed up, or miserable (Patel, 2003).

SELF-REPORTED QUESTIONNAIRE

The Self-Reported Questionnaire (SRQ-20) was initially developed by WHO, Buesenberg, and Orley in 1994 to screen for CMDs, referring to two main diagnostic categories: depressive disorders and anxiety disorders. It has been validated over the past four decades in multiple countries throughout the world and is often utilized in primary care settings, particularly where there is a lack of mental health professionals or access is limited for psychiatric care (Buesenberg et al., 1994; Scholte et al., 2011; van der Westhuizen et al., 2016).

The SRQ-20 (Box 12.4) is a screening tool, or a case-finding instrument, that the patient answers if they have experienced feelings, vague physical symptoms, or certain thoughts within the past 30 days. It is a good introductory tool when the practitioner is concerned about a patient's mental health

---

Box 12.3 Stress-Producing Experiences for Those With a Mental Health Disorder

- Social exclusion
- Discrimination
- Stigma (affecting readiness to seek help)
- Educational difficulties
- Risk-taking behaviors
- Physical ill health
- Human rights violations

Source: Adapted from the World Health Organization. (2012). Risks to mental health: An overview of vulnerabilities and risk factors. Author. https://www.who.int/publications/m/item/risks-to-mental-health.

Box 12.4 Relevant Mental Health Assessment Tools

- The Alcohol Use Disorders Identification Test (AUDIT)
- The Brief Non-Suicidal Self-Injury Assessment Tool (BNSSI-AT)
- Columbia-Suicide Severity Rating Scale (C-SSRS)
- Edinburgh Postnatal Depression Scale (EPDS)
- Generalized Anxiety Disorder-7 (GAD7)
- Humiliation, Afraid, Rape, Kick Questionnaire (HARK)
- Mini-Mental Status Exam (MMSE)
- Mood Disorder Questionnaire (MDQ)
- Patient Health Questionnaire (PHQ-9).
- Pittsburgh Sleep Quality Index (PSQI)
- Prodromal Questionnaire-Brief Version (PQ-B)
- Self-Report Questionnaire-20 (SRQ20)
- Short Post-Traumatic Stress Disorder Rating Interview (SPRINT)
- Stanford-Washington University Eating Disorder screen (SWED)
- The Transgender Congruence Scale (TCS)

but is uncertain about their presentation of symptoms. The SRQ-20 is used throughout the world, has been translated into numerous languages, and has been culturally adapted to identify CMDs of anxiety, depression, and somatoform disorders (Buesenberg et al., 1994). Questions that are answered "yes" indicate the immediate need to ask additional questions about safety, availability of support, and previous experiences.

EATING DISORDERS

Adolescent girls and women in the early adulthood stage of life are most vulnerable for the development of eating disorders (Feltner et al., 2022). The etiology and history of eating disorders is not well understood. Underlying causes of eating disorders are categorized into predisposing (background vulnerabilities), precipitating (environmental context at onset), and perpetuating factors (secondary aspects of the illness that cause it to be valued and maintained). Predisposing risk factors for eating disorders can be biological, psychological, or socioenvironmental (Graham et al., 2019).

Eating disorders are associated with significant short-term and long-term adverse health outcomes, including physical, psychological, and social problems. Eating disorders can lead to physical complications affecting all organs and systems. Specific complications vary by diagnosis and frequency of certain behaviors (Treasure et al., 2020). For example, purging behaviors (e.g., self-induced vomiting, laxative abuse, and diuretic abuse) are associated with morbidity affecting the teeth, esophagus, gastrointestinal system, kidneys, skin, cardiovascular system (e.g., arrhythmias, cardiac failure), electrolyte disturbances, and musculoskeletal system and as low bone density and increased fracture prevalence. Chronicity of illness increases the risk of complications. Binge eating disorder, if untreated, can contribute to obesity (30% to 45%) and related metabolic disorders. Evidence also suggests that individuals with eating disorders have higher mortality rates than the general population. Anorexia nervosa is associated with physical complications directly attributed to weight loss and malnutrition (National Collaborating Centre for Mental Health, 2004).

Eating disorders consist of three most prevalent types: (1) anorexia nervosa (AN), (2) bulimia nervosa (BN), and (3) binge eating disorder (BED; American Psychiatric Association, 2013). Adolescent girls and young women are three times more likely compared to older women to develop an eating disorder. Often, however, girls and women struggle with eating problems that can go undetected. College age women, for example, are most vulnerable to having an eating disorder that was occurring for several years before the symptoms and physical changes became evident to others. It behooves the practitioner to understand the importance of identification and screening of patients who may be seeking treatment for other health concerns. Eating disorders have a significant component of shame and denial, adding to problems with identification. Descriptions and prevalence of the three eating disorder types (American Psychiatric Association, 2013) are as follows:

1. Anorexia nervosa (AN): An eating disorder that entails excessive restrictions of foods, excessive exercises, purging behaviors (self-induced vomiting or use of laxatives), and a distorted body image. Many of these girls and young women report having been influenced by social media that glorifies women who are very thin, such as models and athletes. AN is more common among girls and younger women than older women. On average, girls develop AN at age 16 or 17. Teen girls between 13 and 19 and young women in their early 20s are most at risk (Smink et al., 2012). AN can evolve into a lifelong illness with medical comorbidities and potential impairment or death. The mortality rate of women ages 20 to 40 with this illness is 5% of the population (Feltner et al., 2022).

2. Bulimia nervosa (BN): Women with BN eat a lot of food in a short amount of time and feel a lack of control over eating during this time (binging). They then try to prevent weight gain by getting rid of the food (purging). Purging may be done by making oneself vomit and/or taking laxatives. Women with BN may also try to prevent weight gain after binging by exercising more than normal, eating very little or not at all (fasting), or taking pills to urinate often. Women with BN usually have self-esteem that is closely linked to their poor body image. Their weight may not significantly fluctuate over time, making them difficult to identify.

3. Binge eating disorder (BED) affects more than 3% of women in the United States. More than half of people with BED are women. BED affects women of all races and ethnicities. It is the most common eating disorder among Hispanic, Asian American, and Black women. Some women may be more at risk for BED. Women and girls who diet often are 12 times more likely to binge eat than women and girls who do not diet. BED affects more young and middle-aged women than older women. On average, women develop BED in their early to mid-20s.

   It can be difficult to tell whether a patient has BED. Many women with BED hide their behavior due to shame or embarrassment. To arrive at a diagnosis, for at least once a week over the past 3 months, the patient will have at least three of the following symptoms:

   - Eating faster than normal
   - Eating until uncomfortably full
   - Eating large amounts of food when not hungry
   - Eating alone because of embarrassment
   - Feeling disgusted, depressed, or guilty afterward

   People with a BED may also have other mental health problems, such as depression, anxiety, or substance abuse. It is imperative for the practitioner to identify and use a screening tool with all girls and women, even though there may not be a clear indication of medical, psychological, or emotional complications (Smink et al., 2012).

The USPSTF published a review and recommendations in the use of screening tools with persons with eating disorders (Feltner et al., 2022). Most studies utilize girls and young women and a variety of screening tools, reviewing the validity and reliability of identifying those at risk of an eating disorder. The *Stanford-Washington University Eating Disorder* (SWED) screen is one example of a valid and reliable screening tool for women of all ages (Graham et al., 2019). It is an 11-item self-report measure derived from existing questionnaires assessing eating disorder behaviors (e.g., dietary restriction, self-induced vomiting) and weight concerns (Box 12.4).

Treatment

Adolescent girls and young women are most at risk of developing an eating disorder that may progress to a lifetime of dysfunction and evolving comorbidities. According to recommendations by the National Eating Disorders Association (2022) and supported by Zerwas and Claydon (2014), development of treatment plans may include one or more of the following:

- **Nutrition therapy:** To maintain a healthy weight. This may involve hospitalization, residential treatment centers and ongoing outpatient monitoring.
- **Psychotherapy:** To facilitate the exploration and enhance coping skills for detrimental emotions and behaviors.
- **Support groups:** Meetings of girls or women with similar eating disorders to share their struggles and success with eating problems. Groups may include family.
- **Medications:** Psychopharmacology is often utilized to treat the concomitant depressive symptoms or anxiety disorders often evident in a female with an eating disorder.

NONSUICIDAL SELF-INJURY

Defined as behaviors in which an individual intentionally harms the body without overt suicidal intent and for reasons that are not socially sanctioned, nonsuicidal self-injury (NSSI) typically includes behaviors such as cutting, burning, scratching, and self-battery. It often begins in early adolescence and can continue through young adulthood. NSSI is considered a deliberate act that reflects the adolescent's inability to express themself and a lack of impulse control behavior (Williams et al., 2018). Owens and colleagues (2002) conducted a systematic review and postulate that the link between self-harm and suicide is a strong one; subsequent suicide occurs in somewhere between one in 200 and one in 40 self-harm patients in the first year and approximately one in 15 people after 9 or more years Nonfatal repetition is common also after the initial self-harm behavior; about one in six patients repeats over the next year and one in four after 4 years (Owens et al., 2002).

Adolescent girls are a high-risk group for self-injury (Williams et al., 2018). They may not have current clinical diagnoses of substance use or depressive or anxiety disorders. However, these comorbid conditions can evolve if girls are untreated or self-harm goes undetected (Muehlenkamp et al., 2010; Verroken et al., 2018).

Whitlock and colleagues (2011, 2013) developed the Brief Non-suicidal Self-Injury Assessment Tool (BNSSI-AT), a valid and reliable screening instrument. It consists of 12 questions that address primary and secondary functions of self-harm: why an adolescent would harm themselves (Likert-type responses), how recent and frequent the person does self-injury behaviors and when (if) they ceased those behaviors, how old they were when they started, how often and what body parts were affected by types of self-harm, how many times they have self-harmed, and what are their motivations for intentionally hurting themselves (Whitlock et al., 2011, 2013; Box 12.4).

Treatment

Results of a screening instrument such as the BNSSI-AT can guide the practitioner on what areas of concern can be discovered with a girl or young woman who is suspected of self-harm behaviors. Once the practitioner establishes a trusting relationship, referral to a mental health provider, specifically one knowledgeable with these behaviors, is paramount. Psychotropic medications can be utilized in the treatment of co-occurring disorders such as depressive or anxiety disorders. The prevention of further self-injury is paramount, as many young people commit suicide in later years.

Ougrin and colleagues conducted a review of 19 randomized clinical trials (RCTs) including the analysis of 2,176 adolescents. Treatment interventions included psychological and social interventions. The proportion of the adolescents who self-harmed over the follow-up period was lower in the intervention groups (28%) than in control groups (33%). Dialectical behavior therapy (DBT), cognitive behavioral therapy (CBT), and mentalization-based therapy (MBT) were approaches specifically utilized in the clinical trials with positive effects (Ougrin et al., 2015).

Eating disorders and nonsuicidal self-harm behaviors start in early adolescents and may continue into adulthood. Young women may continue to struggle with these problems into the next reproductive life stage, emerging adulthood.

Emerging Adulthood

In the past decade the existence of a new life stage at ages 18 to 29 years, known as emerging adulthood, has been proposed (Arnett et al., 2014). It is a distinct period from adolescence and young adulthood that has its own demographic and identity-related characteristics. This is considered a critical period of life and is the most unstable period of the life span (Arnett et al., 2014). This period often entails many life transitions in living arrangements, relationships, education, and employment (Bonnie et al., 2015). It is a time of heightened instability in which young people can experience a series of loving relationships and frequent job changes before making lasting decisions. The important changes of this period can generate instability, uncertainty, and a significant mental health risk. One of these risks is for depression.

DEPRESSIVE DISORDERS

Depressive disorders are prevalent in all countries and cultures throughout the world (Evans-Lacko et al., 2018; GBD 2019 Mental Disorders Collaborators, 2022; Woody et al., 2017). Over 280 million people, 5% of the global population, suffer from depression. It is estimated that over 130 million women ages 15 through 29 years experience a diagnosable depressive disorder (Institute of Health Metrics and Evaluation, 2021). One in eight women in the United States experience depressive symptoms during her lifetime, two to three times more than men (Substance Abuse and Mental Health Services Administration [SAMHSA], 2020).

specific phobia (SP), and social anxiety disorder were also greater in women (Baxter et al., 2013).

The emergence of anxiety disorders is typically during childhood, adolescence, or early adulthood, with a peak occurring in middle age and a subsequent decline in older individuals (Jalnapurkar et al., 2018). Anxiety disorders can lead to the development of several adverse consequences including reduced educational and occupational opportunities, greater functional impairment, and overall increase in morbidity and mortality rates as compared to those without an anxiety disorder (McLean et al., 2011). Persons with anxiety disorders utilize emergency medical and mental health services and have been linked to elevated rates of teenage pregnancy and parenthood (Altemus et al., 2014). Suffering with an anxiety disorder can also result in having several comorbid psychiatric diagnoses, especially mood disorders like MDD (Box 12.4).

Women with symptoms of anxiety tend to develop additional anxious features, somaticize often, and become more limited in their overall ability to function (McLean et al., 2011). Identification of women with an anxiety disorder as soon as possible enhances their willingness and responsiveness to treatment (Jalnapurkar et al., 2018). Practitioners can utilize a screening instrument with patients who have physical complaints that appear unfounded to establish the possibility of anxiety symptoms and potentially a treatable disorder. The most used instrument is the Generalized Anxiety Disorder-7 (GAD-7; Spitzer et al., 2006).

The GAD-7 is a seven-item self-report questionnaire that asks the patient to identify how often they are bothered by seven problems and whether it is not at all, several days, most days, or every day in the past 2 weeks. When screening for anxiety disorders with the GAD-7, a score of 8 or greater represents a reasonable cut-point for identifying probable cases of GAD; further diagnostic assessment is warranted to determine the presence, type, and intensity of an anxiety disorder. The following score ranges correlate with the severity of the level of anxiety:

- Score 0–4: Minimal anxiety
- Score 5–9: Mild anxiety
- Score 10–14: Moderate anxiety
- Score greater than 15: Severe anxiety

Although the GAD-7 was initially developed for identification of GAD, it also has validity in accurately screening for three other common anxiety disorders—PD, social anxiety disorder, and PTSD (Kroenke et al., 2001; Box 12.4).

Treatment

Despite the availability of efficacious treatments, research suggests that most patients with a GAD remain untreated (Crits-Christoph et al., 2011). In a survey conducted with 127 patients meeting criteria for GAD, the average interval between the onset of GAD and the initiation of the first adequate medication trial was 81.6 months (Jalnapurkar et al., 2018). Antidepressants in the class of selective serotonin reuptake inhibitors (SSRIs such as paroxetine, citalopram, sertraline, fluoxetine, and escitalopram) are first line in the treatment of GAD. Norepinephrine and serotonin reuptake inhibitor (NSRI) antidepressants (duloxetine and

venlafaxine) are also considered to be highly effective pharmacotherapy for GAD. If effective, antidepressant treatment for GAD should be continued for at least 12 months (Jalnapurkar et al., 2018).

Psychotherapy, specifically CBT, has demonstrated significant value and similar treatment effect as those associated with effective pharmacotherapeutic agents (SSRIs and NSRIs) in GAD (Linden et al., 2005). Treatment response rates in GAD range between 47% and 75% for CBT, whereas response rates with pharmacotherapy range between 44% and 81% (Bandelow et al., 2013). Alternatives to SSRI and SNRI antidepressants for treatment-resistant or treatment-intolerant GAD patients include tricyclic antidepressants, buspirone, second-generation antipsychotics (quetiapine), and valproate (Abejuela & Osser, 2016).

SCHIZOPHRENIA SPECTRUM AND OTHER PSYCHOTIC DISORDERS

According to the *DSM-5* (American Psychiatric Association, 2013), persons with a psychosis may have temporary or chronic symptoms of psychosis with the following four hallmarks:

- Delusions (false beliefs)
- Hallucinations (hearing, seeing, touching, or smelling what other people do not)
- Disorganized speech (incoherent, rambling)
- Grossly disorganized behavior (behaviors without goal-directed purpose)

Although these symptoms are present at times in persons with schizophrenia, they may also occur in persons who have a bipolar disorder experiencing acute mania, substance-induced psychosis, psychosis related to severe depressive disorder, or postpartum depression with psychosis (American Psychiatric Association, 2013). Women are less frequently diagnosed with schizophrenia than men (Nagle-Yang et al., 2022). Psychosis, however, can become evident in women suffering from the other disorders throughout the reproductive life cycle. Identification of psychotic symptoms in women may indicate an urgent situation. A woman experiencing postpartum psychosis, for example, may have delusions that her infant is "evil" and she should destroy it. It is imperative to evaluate the severity of the psychotic thinking and intervene in an urgent fashion (Nagle-Yang et al., 2022).

A screening instrument, the Prodromal Questionnaire-Brief Version (PQ-B) can be used by practitioners who may be suspicious of patients who demonstrate "odd" thinking or behaviors or have stated thinking or beliefs that seem implausible or not believable. This 16-item questionnaire evolved from a more comprehensive instrument used in prodromal psychosis research clinics that includes in-depth interviews. As a screening tool, however, Loewy and colleagues determined that an abbreviated instrument could identify individuals with a risk of developing psychosis as well as delineating those currently with psychotic symptoms. The PQ-B asks the patient to respond "true" or "false," and if they respond positively they are then asked to identify the severity of any distress experienced (Loewy et al., 2011; Box 12.4).

Treatment

Persons with a psychotic disorder such as schizophrenia should be evaluated by a mental health professional who can prescribe and monitor psychotropic medications. This chronic, debilitating illness challenges the person through fluctuating episodes of acute illness, often requiring hospitalization and periods of partial remission. Selection and adherence to antipsychotic medications is most effective with attention to the impact of the community and support for the patient. Women with a psychotic disorder respond best to a multidisciplinary approach to both physical and mental health strategies (Fear et al., 2009).

Pregnancy

Pregnancy brings with it a range of potential stresses resulting in vulnerability for a variety of mental health problems. Reports of mood and anxiety disorders may increase as the pregnant woman experiences a multitude of physical, emotional, social, and relational changes.

Depression in pregnancy is relatively common with at least 15% of postpartum episodes occurring during pregnancy. Gavin and colleagues reported that the incidence of new-onset depression in pregnancy (14.5%) was the same as the incidence in the first 3 months after delivery (Gavin et al., 2005).

Childbirth and reproductive events can be significant and stressful for women, often triggering mood disorders, such as depression with psychotic episodes and mania affiliated with bipolar disorders (Sharma & Pope, 2012). Identifying and screening newly pregnant women becomes critical in anticipation of the physiologic and hormonal fluctuations attributable to pregnancy. Discontinuation of psychiatric medications the woman may have been taking to treat these disorders must be discussed and incrementally introduced, since abrupt discontinuation may precipitate a relapse, increasing stress and risk to the pregnant woman and fetus. A history of depression, poorer overall health, greater alcohol use, smoking, being unmarried, unemployment, and lower educational attainment were significantly associated with symptoms of depression during pregnancy (Nau & Peterson, 2014; Sharma & Pope, 2012).

Marcus and colleagues' study of pregnant women identified that over 20% had significant symptoms of depression. Most of these women had no prior diagnosis of depression nor had they been in treatment. Elevations in depressive symptomatology have been associated with adverse maternal and infant outcomes, and they strongly urged practitioners to utilize screening tools on an ongoing basis during pregnancy and the postpartum period (Marcus et al., 2003).

INTIMATE PARTNER VIOLENCE

It is well established that women are vulnerable to mental health problems and crises during this reproductive stage of life. What is profound is that the frequency of domestic violence, whether it is an intimate or nonintimate perpetrator, significantly increases during pregnancy and the postpartum period in most countries throughout the world (USPSTF, 2018; WHO, 2010). The USPSTF concludes that "screening for IPV in women of reproductive age and providing or referring women who screen positive to ongoing support services has a moderate net benefit" (2018). When the practitioner uses a screening instrument for IPV, women do self-identify (Cadena, 2012). Evidence finds that providing information about referrals alone is not very effective. There also needs to be ongoing supportive intervention components (Taft et al., 2013).

IPV including physical, sexual, and emotional abuse is a major public health problem. Prevalence rates from the Centers for Disease Control and Prevention (CDC, 2020; National Center for Injury Prevention and Control, 2016) continue to be high for women, estimated at more than 4.2 million intimate-partner-related physical assaults, rapes, and stalking perpetrated against women annually.

Research suggests that women who experience violence during pregnancy may be more likely than those who do not experience violence while pregnant to be victims of severe violence (Campbell et al., 2007). In a classic study, Stewart and Cecutti (1993) reported that 66.7% of women abused during pregnancy sought medical treatment for the abuse. Pregnant women have also been found to be more likely to experience attempted and completed femicide (Campbell et al., 2007; Decker et al., 2004; McFarlane et al., 2002). Women who are victims of IPV when they are pregnant are three times more likely to die at the hands of their perpetrators than women who are victims of IPV when they are not pregnant (McFarlane et al., 2002). Past research also reported that pregnant women who are most at risk for homicide may be more likely to leave their partners during their pregnancy (Decker et al., 2004).

Potentially life-threatening situations for the pregnant woman, therefore, warrant initial and ongoing screening for IPV during as well as at the postpartum stage. There are several screening instruments available (Feltner et al., 2018) and the following tool can be integrated into the practitioner's toolbox.

The HARK screening instrument (Humiliation, Afraid, Rape, Kick) is a four-question self-response survey that evolved from the Abuse Assessment Screen (AAS; Soeken et al., 1998). The most effective way to use the HARK is if a woman answers "yes" to any one of the four questions, there is an 83% chance that she has been abused within the past year (Sohal et al., 2007). If she answers "yes" to three of the four questions, there is 100% accuracy that she has been abused. Hence this simple and quick screening tool is helpful for the practitioner to incorporate in the evaluation with pregnant as well as nonpregnant women (Box 12.4).

Treatment

A vital role for healthcare practitioners is to assess the safety of the woman who may be suspected of being a victim of violence. Women in the United States may leave their perpetrator five times or more before they are able to establish a plan for safety, self-sufficiency, and adequate support. Ongoing use of a screening tool such as the HARK assists the practitioner to provide ongoing assessment. This approach allows the woman repeated opportunities to share her concerns with a nonjudgmental and compassionate listener (Warshaw et al., 2013).

Referral to a mental health professional is also helpful in this disengaging process. Multiple therapy approaches have been utilized with success, decreasing the increasing threats of physical, sexual, and psychological violence. Psychotropic medications to assist with symptoms of PTSD, anxiety, and depressive disorders are also indicated.

PERIPARTUM AND POSTPARTUM STAGE

Women's vulnerability to mental health problems and disorders becomes enhanced not only during pregnancy but in the postpartum or peripartum stage of the reproductive life cycle. This category includes not only viable births but nonviable births, miscarriages, and abortions. Peripartum depression is the most common complication of childbearing, affecting one in seven women (Wisner et al., 2002). Due to the severity of fluctuations in physiologic, social, economic, and relationship status following birth or termination of a pregnancy, women often experience the "baby blues." This is a transitory change, usually lasting a few weeks. Postpartum depression usually starts during pregnancy. Peripartum depression, however, can extend to months after birth, jeopardizing the mental health and well-being of the mother, child, and family (American Psychiatric Association, 2013). In addition to symptoms indicative of an MDD, postpartum depression may also display the following symptoms (Sharma & Pope, 2012):

- Increase in purposeless physical activity (e.g., inability to sit still, pacing, handwringing) or slowed movements or speech (these actions must be severe enough to be observable by others)
- Feeling worthless or guilty
- Difficulty thinking, concentrating, or making decisions
- Thoughts of death or suicide
- Crying for "no reason"
- Lack of interest in the baby, not feeling bonded to the baby, or feeling very anxious about/around the baby
- Feelings of being a bad mother
- Fear of harming the baby or oneself

Cox et al. (1987) and Glaze and Cox (1991) sought to identify the increasing presence and intensity of depressive symptoms in women following birth by developing the Edinburgh Postnatal Depression Scale (EPDS), a 10-item scale that has been used and validated in multiple countries over the past three decades. The gold standard screening instrument, the EPDS is also valid when screening women during pregnancy as well as months into the postpartum stage (Wisner et al., 2002). The EPDS is a valuable and efficient way of identifying patients at risk for "perinatal" depression. The 10-question, Likert scale tool is easy to administer and interpret. With a maximum score of 30, a score of 10 indicates depressive symptoms that should trigger further evaluation and referral to a mental health professional (Box 12.4).

Pregnant women also suffer anxiety symptoms sometimes more than postpartum depression during and after pregnancy (Fairbrother et al., 2016). Utilization of a screening instrument such as the GAD-7 can identify women with anxiety disorders prior, during, and after pregnancy (Spitzer et al., 2006).

Treatment

Peripartum and postpartum women with mood and anxiety disorders must be monitored for their responses throughout pregnancy and for several months after birth (Nau & Peterson, 2014). Standard treatment approaches for these disorders should be followed. It is not advisable to initiate psychotropic medications if the woman is breastfeeding, unless the risks of suicide or infanticide exist (Sharma & Pope, 2012). Infamous cases exist when the postpartum woman suffers a severe depressive disorder with a psychotic episode, resulting in the killing of her child and herself. Ongoing assessment and urgent referral are paramount if the practitioner suspects increasing symptoms of mental disorders in a vulnerable woman.

PERIMENOPAUSE AND POSTMENOPAUSE

Menopause is a 4- to 10-year multidimensional process experienced by women in the midlife reproductive stage. It is associated with many factors that can trigger or enhance a woman's sleep disturbance, including hormonal alterations that can increase vasomotor symptoms, such as hot flashes and night sweats and increases of symptoms of depression, anxiety, and stress (Sowers et al., 2008). These alterations also result in physical and emotional changes ranging from uncomfortable to severe. Women who also undergo surgery such as hysterectomies will experience similar hormonal and physical changes if not prescribed hormone replacement therapy. An increase in mood and anxiety disorders can occur during this reproductive life stage. Women also have a five to six times greater chance of developing a sleep disorder, increasing intake of alcohol, and over the passage of time, developing cognitive impairment (Sowers et al., 2008).

SLEEP DISORDERS

Sleep disorders occur in 40% to 70% of all women 60 years of age and older (Luyster et al., 2015). A sleep disorder is defined as a predominant complaint of dissatisfaction with sleep quality and quantity (American Psychiatric Association, 2013). It can result in a decrease of function and daily activities, impaired problem-solving skills, compromised driving capability, and poor concentration. Sleep deprivation, particularly in the older woman, can contribute to feelings of agitation, depression, and lethargy. Age-related changes in sleep combined with medical and psychiatric conditions that accompany older age, lead to many older adults having sleep complaints, with approximately 50% reporting difficulty sleeping (Beaudreau et al., 2012).

A screening instrument is helpful in identifying a sleep disorder to differentiate from other medical or psychiatric disorders. The Pittsburgh Sleep Quality Index (PSQI) was initially developed in 1989 by Buysse and colleagues. The PSQI is a self-rated questionnaire that assesses sleep quality and disturbances over a 1-month time interval. Nineteen items generate seven "component" scores: subjective sleep quality, latency, duration, efficiency, disturbances, use of sleeping medication, and daytime dysfunction. The sum of scores for these seven components yields one global score (Buysse et al., 1989). Since that time, multiple studies have supported the validity and reliability of this instrument in persons 60 years and older and among diverse populations of urban and rural, Black, White, and Asian populations (Luyster et al., 2015; Sowers et al., 2008; Box 12.4).

Treatment

Nonpharmacologic first-line interventions are strongly recommended to assist a woman in managing her sleep disorder. Caution must be exercised when considering benzodiazepines and should only be prescribed for a limited time. In addition to over-the-counter products, complementary and alternative medicines (CAM) are frequently used for the treatment of sleep disorders. There is a growing body of studies using CAM that have shown the following: (1) melatonin is an effective agent for the treatment of circadian phase disorders that affect sleep, but the role of melatonin in the treatment of primary or secondary insomnia is less well established, (2) valerian has shown a benefit in some, but not all, clinical trials, and (3) several other modalities, such as tai chi, acupuncture, acupressure, yoga, and meditation have improved sleep parameters in a limited number of trials (Gooneratne, 2008; Pearson et al., 2006). Sleep problems become increasingly present as a woman ages. Her cognitive capabilities that can impact functioning may also decline as she ages.

NEUROCOGNITIVE DISORDERS AND IMPAIRMENT

In 2019, the number of people age 60 years and older was 1 billion and increasing. WHO predicts that by 2030 this number will increase to 1.4 billion and 2.1 billion by 2050. This unprecedented pace is expected to accelerate in coming decades, particularly in developing countries (WHO, 2019). Women are currently 49.6% of the total world population; 10.35% of these women are 76 and older (World Bank, 2022). In the United States, 50.5% (166,449,500) of the total population are women. Those who are 65 years of age and older make up 18.1% of this population, compared to 15.1% men (World Bank, 2022). WHO reports that currently there are over 55 million people with dementia (WHO, 2020). Those who are 75 or older have increased risks of developing one of the several types of dementia. This spectrum of diseases affects older women who, on average, have a longer life expectancy (WHO, 2020). These vulnerable women may not always initially have cognitive difficulties. They deny any functional limitations, are anxious about being restricted, and threatened with losing their ability to drive, live independently and make their own decisions (Beaudreau et al., 2012).

When there is a decline in one's previous level of performance and function, early assessment for possible cognitive impairment allows for early intervention that may correct the underlying causes or slow the progression of untreatable etiologies (Levine et al., 2021). Cognitive impairment categories are mild, moderate, severe, and profound cognitive impairment (American Psychiatric Association, 2013). Although cognitive impairment is attributable to neurologic disorders of any age, cognitive disorders in older women and the impact on the last reproductive stage in life is this focus.

Neurocognitive impairment is defined as a decrease in thinking capabilities such as problem-solving and executive functioning (decision-making). Often the person themselves raises concerns about memory, language, or daily functioning. Other times a knowledgeable informant (e.g., relative, neighbor, spouse) identifies changes in function and decision-making. Getting lost in a familiar community, being unable to pay bills, and poor everyday memory are benchmarks to seek an evaluation.

Levine and associates (2021) conducted several pooled analyses of individual participant data from over 34,000 people in five cohort studies from 1971 to 2017. Results provide some evidence suggesting that women had higher baseline performance than men in global cognition, executive function, and memory. Women experienced significantly faster declines in global cognition and executive function but not memory. These sex differences persisted after accounting for the influence of age, race, and education (Levine et al., 2021).

Screening for cognitive impairments should be routine for the health professional evaluating the perimenopausal and menopausal woman. One standard cognitive screening instrument is the Mini-Mental Status Exam (MMSE). This widely used tool is a 30-item questionnaire that measures cognitive function among older adults; it includes tests of orientation, attention, memory, language, and visual-spatial skills. It is not usually self-administered but is used as a screening instrument for the practitioner to have a global assessment of the older person's capacities (Box 12.4).

Treatment

Identification of any cognitive impairment indicates a complete physical examination, laboratory testing, and detailed history to differentiate medical conditions that can be addressed. Involving family members can also be helpful to obtain a complete picture of the woman's daily functioning and decision-making. Referral to a neurologist or psychiatrist, as well as connecting with a multidisciplinary team, is recommended to obtain an accurate diagnosis and develop treatment plans for the trajectory of the woman's life (Rocca et al., 2014).

Although age is the strongest known risk factor for dementia, it is not an inevitable consequence of aging. Reducing risks for cognitive decline and dementia is emphasized in healthcare of the older woman. Research evidence indicates that people can reduce their risk of cognitive decline and dementia by being physically active, not smoking, avoiding harmful use of alcohol, controlling their weight, eating a healthy diet, and maintaining healthy blood pressure, cholesterol, and blood sugar levels (WHO, 2020).

CONSIDERATIONS OF SPECIFIC MENTAL HEALTH CONCERNS AND MARGINALIZED POPULATIONS

Suicide

According to the CDC (n.d.) suicide is "death caused by injuring oneself with the intent to die" (para. 1) A suicide attempt is when someone harms themselves with any intent to end their life, but they do not die because of their actions (Crosby, Ortega, et al., 2011).

Suicide is the 10th leading cause of death in the United States. Suicide attempts continue to be an increasing public health problem with suicide rates increasing 33% between 1999 and 2019. It was responsible for more than 47,500 deaths in 2019, which is about one death every 11 minutes. In 2020, there was a reported 5% decrease to 44,834 deaths in the United States The number of people who think about or attempt suicide is likely to be even higher. In 2019, 12 million

American adults seriously thought about suicide, 3.5 million planned a suicide attempt, and 1.4 million attempted suicides (CDC, 2020).

There are specific factors that increase the risk for suicide or protect against it. Suicide is often connected to other forms of injury and violence. People who have experienced physical violence, including child abuse or sexual violence, for example, have a higher overall suicide risk. Suicide affects all ages. It is the second leading cause of death for people ages 10 to 34, the fourth leading cause among people ages 35 to 44, and the fifth leading cause among people ages 45 to 54 (Chapman & Dixon-Gordon, 2007).

Suicide statistics reveal that women are three times more likely to attempt suicide, though men are two to four times more likely to die by suicide (Vijayakumar, 2015). Compared to men, women show higher rates of suicidal thinking, nonfatal suicidal behavior, and suicide attempts (Crosby, Han, et al., 2011).

The differences in attempts and completed suicides in women have erroneously led many people to believe that suicide attempts in women are often a method of "getting attention" rather than a serious risk. This is far from true. It is important to note that among women, an attempted (but failed) suicide attempt is the greatest risk factor for suicide in the future, and all suicide attempts, whether in men or in women, need to be taken very seriously (Callanan & Davis, 2012).

Some groups have higher suicide rates than others. Suicide rates vary by race/ethnicity, age, and other factors. The highest rates are among American Indian/Alaska Native and non-Hispanic White populations. Other Americans with higher-than-average rates of suicide are veterans, people who live in rural areas, and workers in certain industries and occupations, such as mining and construction (Stone et al., 2017).

Women of all ages are at risk of suicide. As practitioners, it is helpful to know the risk factors for suicide (see Box 12.5). Assessing for risk of suicide and preventing an attempt often depends on the practitioner to quantify the immediacy and severity of the risk. Three behaviors may indicate that a person

Box 12.5 Risk Factors for Suicide

- Prior suicide attempt(s)
- Misuse and abuse of alcohol or other drugs
- Mental disorders, particularly depression and other mood disorders
- Access to lethal means
- Knowing someone who died by suicide, particularly a family member
- Social isolation
- Chronic disease and disability
- Lack of access to behavioral healthcare

Source: Adapted from Stone, D., Holland, K., Bartholow, B., Crosby, A., Davis, S., & Wilkins, N. (2017). Preventing suicide: A technical package of policies, programs, and practices. Centers for Disease Control and Prevention, National Center for Injury Prevention and Control. https://doi.org/10.15620/cdc.44275

Box 12.6 Serious Risk Behaviors for Suicide

- Talking about feeling trapped or in unbearable pain
- Talking about being a burden to others
- Increasing the use of alcohol or drugs
- Acting anxious or agitated, behaving recklessly
- Sleeping too little or too much

Source: Adapted from Stone, D., Holland, K., Bartholow, B., Crosby, A., Davis, S., & Wilkins, N. (2017). Preventing suicide: A technical package of policies, programs, and practices. Centers for Disease Control and Prevention, National Center for Injury Prevention and Control. https://doi.org/10.15620/cdc.44275

Box 12.7 National Suicide Prevention Hotline

U.S. National Suicide Prevention Lifeline

Phone: Dial 988

The Lifeline is a 24-hour toll-free phone line for people in suicidal crisis or emotional distress.

Online: 988lifeline.org

is at immediate risk for suicide and are warning signs that require a rapid response of the practitioner:

- Talking about wanting to die or to kill oneself
- Looking for a way to kill oneself, such as obtaining a gun, hoarding medications, finalizing plans
- Talking about feeling hopeless or having no reason to live

Other behaviors may indicate a serious risk—especially if the behavior is new, has increased, and/or seems related to a painful event, loss, or change. Box 12.6 lists serious risk behaviors for suicide, and Box 12.7 provides the Suicide Prevention Hotline contact information.

A multiorganizational, international standard for screening and assessing for suicide is the Columbia-Suicide Severity Rating Scale (C-SSRS). The complete C-SSRS was designed to explore definitions of suicidal ideation (thinking) and behaviors and to quantify the severity over time (Posner et al., 2011).

The abbreviated, consolidated version, known as the Columbia Protocol, is a six-item screening tool designed using simple, plain-language questions that help to identify whether someone is at risk for suicide, assess the severity and immediacy of that risk, and gauge the level of support that the person needs. Practitioners ask the patient:

- Whether and when they have thought about suicide (ideation)
- What actions they have taken—and when—to prepare for suicide
- Whether and when they attempted suicide or began a suicide attempt that was either interrupted by another person or stopped of their own volition

Substance Abuse

Substance-related and addictive disorders, according to the *DSM-5* (APA, 2013), include 10 separate classes of psychoactive substances that have addictive qualities (Box 12.8). Categories of drug use are further divided into two groups: substance use disorders and substance-induced disorders. Substances can precipitate a psychiatric disorder—at intoxication or withdrawal—and trigger disorders such as psychotic, bipolar, depressive, anxiety, sleep, delirium, and neurocognitive (American Psychiatric Association, 2013). This section focuses on alcohol use and abuse among all women throughout the reproductive life cycle. It is the most prevalent reported "drug of choice" for women of all ages in the United States (WHO, 2006).

According to WHO (2019), men consume more alcohol and account for more alcohol-related harms to self and others than women do across countries. In 2016, for example, 54% of males (1.46 billion) and 32% of females (0.88 billion) age 15 and older worldwide consumed alcohol. Alcohol caused roughly 3 million deaths (5% of all deaths) that year, including 2.3 million deaths for men (8% of deaths) and 0.7 million deaths for women (3% of deaths; WHO, 2019). There are significant variations across countries. In Norway, for example, males consume alcohol 32 times more often than women. In the United States the traditional gap is dramatically decreasing.

Over the past 3 decades, there have been considerable changes in alcohol consumption and the physical and psychological consequences of alcohol use and abuse. According to White and colleagues (2015), among adolescents and emerging adults, gaps in drinking have narrowed primarily because alcohol use among males has declined more than alcohol use among females. Alcohol use is increasing among adults for women but not for men. Rates of alcohol-related ED visits, hospitalizations, and deaths all have increased among adults during the past two decades (White et al., 2015). Consistent with the changing patterns of alcohol use, increases in these outcomes have been larger for women. Recent studies also suggest that females are more susceptible than males to alcohol-induced liver inflammation, cardiovascular disease, memory blackouts, hangovers, and certain cancers (White, 2020).

Grucza and colleagues conducted an analysis of six different U.S. national surveys between 2000 and 2016, suggesting that the number of women age 18 and older who drink increased every year by 6% but decreased by 0.2% for men, and the number of women who binge drink increased by 14% but by only 0.5% for men (Grucza et al., 2018).

When considering women throughout the reproductive life cycle, a troubling trend becomes apparent in the United States. Adolescents in the 12th grade, for example, self-reported in 2018 that their past-month alcohol use was equally prevalent among males (30%) and females (30%). Gender differences in self-reported past-month drunkenness among 12th graders also narrowed between 1991 (37% males, 25% females) and 2018 (19% males, 16% females; Johnston et al., 2018).

Emerging and young adult alcohol consumption has been decreasing for the past 2 decades. The frequency of drinking and reported drunkenness have decreased more in men but increased in women (White, 2020). There was little difference when comparing those men and women who were attending college and those who were not. Another troubling trend for young women is the tendency to drink alone and to experience drunkenness more often (Grucza et al., 2018). These women in their childbearing years are high risk for multiple physical and psychological complications as they navigate pregnancy and motherhood.

Alcohol consumption and binge drinking seems to increase in all adults, but particularly for women over the age of 30 and significantly higher in those over 50 years of age (Johnston et al., 2018). Continuation of pregnancies, postpartum and peripartum mental health disorders, and perimenopause and menopause increase the burden on women's mental health when complicated by alcohol use and abuse (White, 2020). Despite reports of declines in drinking during pregnancy, one in 10 pregnant women still drink each month in the United States (Charness et al., 2016).

Sexual orientation also has a significant influence on alcohol consumption and binge drinking. Lesbian, bisexual, and transgender women, for example, report consuming 12 drinks in a 2-hour period, which is the definition of binge drinking. The legal 0.8% blood alcohol level for men and women is five drinks in a 2-hour period (White et al., 2015). This population is at a significantly higher risk of mental disorders due to alcohol abuse and chronic medical consequences.

It is imperative to detect excessive and potentially harmful drinking behaviors, particularly in women of any age. The Alcohol Use Disorders Identification Test (AUDIT) is a screening instrument developed by WHO (2019) to be used by health professionals in the primary care arena. It is a 10-item questionnaire for all ages of adolescents and adults. It can be completed as a self-report or used in an interview by the practitioner. The 10 items address three domains of drinking behavior: hazardous alcohol use, dependence symptoms, and harmful alcohol use. A score of 8 or more may indicate hazardous use or dependency (Babor et al., 2001; Box 12.4).

Box 12.8 Classes of Psychoactive Substances

- Alcohol
- Caffeine
- Cannabis
- Hallucinogens
- Inhalants
- Opioids
- Sedatives, hypnotics, and anxiolytics
- Stimulants
- Tobacco
- Other (unknown) substances

Transgender and Gender Nonconforming Individuals

Research has found that suicidal thoughts and rates are much higher among those who are lesbian, gay, bisexual, transgender, and nonbinary individuals (Meyer, 2015). Johns et al.,

(2019) reports that lesbian, gay, and bisexual youth are three times more likely to think about suicide and seven times more likely to attempt suicide than heterosexual youth.

The report of the 2015 U.S. Transgender Survey found:

- 40% of transgender adults have attempted suicide.
- 50% of trans males reported a suicide attempt in the past year.
- 42% of nonbinary teens reported some type of self-harm in the previous year.
- Less than 10% of cisgender males and 17% of cisgender females (those whose gender identity matches the gender that is most often correlated with their biological sex) reported suicidal behaviors. (James et al., 2016)

Rejection and bullying have both been implicated in the increased suicide rates among the transgender and gender nonconforming (TGNC) community. Young people who are rejected by their families due to their identity or sexual orientation are 8.4 times more likely to attempt suicide than those who have more family support and acceptance. A study published in the *American Journal of Public Health* found that every incident of TGNC harassment or abuse, both verbal and physical, more than doubles the risk of self-harming behaviors (Mustanski et al., 2010).

TGNC individuals are at significant risk for anxiety, substance abuse, and depressive disorders (Meyer, 2015). There is a growing understanding that individuals of a sexual minority are often subject to significant stress due to discrimination and stigma. Identifying these individuals at critical reproductive stages in life can impact the quality of life and decrease potential suicide (Meyer, 2015).

Shulman and colleagues (2017) discuss the psychological aspects of minority stress and stigma that strongly impact many TGNC individuals. These aspects have significant ramifications in the development of mental health disorders present in the TGNC population. Identification of such stressors as well as the acceptance or nonacceptance (gender dysphoria) of one's gender identity is critical when evaluating persons from a women's health perspective (Ryan et al., 2009). There are several instruments that have been developed, such as the Gender Minority Stress and Resilience Scale (GMRS). Testa et al. (2015) developed the 58-item GMRS to measure the difficulties associated with identifying as a gender minority and protective factors for psychological well-being.

The Transgender Congruence Scale (TCS; Box 12.4) was developed by Kozee et al. (2012) to measure congruence between desired gender and the current expression of gender. The TCS has 12 items related to quality-of-life variables consistent with contemporary understandings of gender dysphoria. Two factors of the TCS were identified: appearance congruence and gender identity acceptance. Appearance congruence measures whether the individual's physical appearance matches their desired ideal gender expression. Gender identity acceptance measures the individual's pride of their gender expression and identity. If gender identity is of concern to patients, it can be helpful to focus more on acceptance of appearance and gender identity than on any transitions that may occur or be contemplated (Kozee et al., 2012).

Research suggests that taking steps to facilitate friendships between TGNC and heterosexual students may help reduce these rates. A study conducted by researchers from the University of British Columbia found that simply having a gay-straight alliance (GSA) at school reduced suicidal thoughts and attempts among all students, regardless of their sexual orientation (Shulman et al., 2017). The researchers suggest having a long-standing GSA reduces homophobic bullying and improves student mental health no matter their sexual orientation.

Trauma and Trauma-Informed Care

There is no universal definition of trauma. The SAMHSA describes trauma as resulting from "an event, series of events, or set of circumstances experienced by an individual as physically or emotionally harmful or life-threatening with lasting adverse effects on the individual's functioning and mental, physical, social, emotional or spiritual well-being" (SAMHSA, 2014).

Trauma-informed care (TIC) is an approach in healthcare delivery that assumes that an individual is more likely than not to have a history of trauma. TIC recognizes the presence of trauma symptoms and acknowledges the role trauma may play in an individual's life, including service staff. TIC requires an organization as well as practitioners to make a paradigm shift from asking, "What is wrong with this person?" to "What has happened to this person?" (SAMHSA, 2016). Trauma results from exposure to an incident or series of events that is emotionally disturbing or life-threatening. Examples of events that may be traumatic include:

- Physical, sexual, and emotional abuse;
- Childhood neglect;
- Having a family member with a mental health or substance use disorder;
- Violence in the community;
- Natural or human-made disasters and forced displacement;
- Sudden, unexplained separation from a loved one;
- Poverty and discrimination (SAMHSA, 2016).

Symptoms of trauma can be present following an acute event and may evolve to a more chronic experience over the years. According to the American Psychiatric Association (2013), the hallmarks of PTSD are that the person has recurrent, intrusive, and distressing memories and/or dreams of the traumatic event. There often is a persistent avoidance of any reminders (people, places, activities, objects, situations) that "trigger" distressing feelings and thoughts. Intrusive memories can result in "flashbacks" by the person thinking and feeling that they are reliving the traumatic event. Over time, the person can experience negative changes in cognition and mood with alterations in arousal and reactivity. There can be angry outbursts, reckless or self-destructive behavior, hypervigilance, and problems with concentration and sleep (American Psychiatric Association, 2013).

Studies reveal that being female or an ethnic minority increases the risk of experiencing trauma and poor outcomes (Briere, 2004). Girls are vulnerable to high-impact trauma like rape, sexual and physical abuse, and dating violence. Women are twice as likely to receive a PTSD diagnosis. Girlhood trauma leads to higher risk of revictimization and psychological and physical health problems (Johnson, 2014).

Girls who experience adverse childhood events (ACEs) may develop resiliency in living with PTSD, particularly if they have social supports (Cheong et al., 2017). In contrast, however, others evolve coping activities that enhance self-destructive behaviors such as prostitution, engaging in abusive relationships, and alcohol and substance abuse (Johnson, 2014). It is imperative for practitioners to identify trauma-induced symptoms in women who seek care as soon as possible after the traumatic event.

One such screening instrument is the Short Post-Traumatic Stress Disorder Rating Interview (SPRINT) developed by Connor and Davidson (2001). It is an eight-item self-report measure that assesses the core symptoms of PTSD (intrusion, avoidance, numbing, arousal), somatic malaise, stress vulnerability, and role and social functional impairment. Symptoms are rated on five-point scales from 0 (not at all) to 4 (very much). The authors suggest a cutoff score of 14 for this screen. Those screening positive should then be referred for further assessment by mental health professionals (Connor & Davidson, 2001; Box 12.4).

Referrals to Mental Health Professionals

Evaluating women utilizing one or more of the screening instruments that has been discussed, always concludes that if the girl or woman meets a cutoff point in the scoring, they should be referred to a mental health professional. Some general guidelines, supported by the NAMI and the National Association of Social Workers (NASW) can be helpful (see Box 12.9).

There are several different types of mental health professionals who specialize in different treatment modalities.

Box 12.9 When to Make a Mental Health Referral: Signs and Symptoms

- Showing depressive symptoms, especially a decline in the ability to experience pleasure, or prolonged sadness
- Any suicidal or homicidal gestures (immediate referral)
- Any dangerous behaviors such as self-harming behavior (cutting)
- Excessive anxiety (panic attacks, irrational fears, phobias)
- Intrusive, uncontrolled thoughts
- Periods of euphoria associated with a reduced need for sleep or impulsive or risk-taking behavior (an increase in promiscuous sex, excessive drug or alcohol use, or spending sprees)
- Severe irritability or outbursts of anger (argumentative, easily annoyed, easily upset)
- Psychosis (hallucinations, delusions, paranoia)
- Addictive behaviors (drug use, excessive alcohol use, excessive overeating)
- Signs and symptoms of abuse (physical, emotional, or sexual)

Source: Adapted from Gruttadaro, D., & Markey, D. (2011). The family experience with primary care physicians and staff: A report by the National Alliance on Mental Illness. *National Alliance on Mental Illness.*

Depending upon the state in the United States, there are differing educational requirements and certified and/or licensed titles. In general, psychiatrists (MD and DO) and psychiatric APRNs can diagnose, treat with a variety of psychotherapeutic interventions, and prescribe psychotropic medications. Psychologists diagnose and treat patients with an emphasis on utilizing psychological testing and types of CBT. Counselors, therapists, and mental health counselors vary with their license and degree requirements. They often are case managers for those with chronic mental illness (NAMI, 2022). Licensed clinical social workers can specialize in psychotherapy and family therapy modalities. Patients who may benefit from psychotherapy and counseling include those with:

- Noncompliance with medical treatment
- Unresolved grief
- Parenting or family issues
- Struggles with adjustment to major life changes (e.g., death, move, divorce)
- Anger issues or poor impulse control
- Significant relationship problems (e.g., dependency, manipulation, infidelity)
- Identity confusion (e.g., gender, race, sexual orientation; NAMI, 2022)

MENTAL HEALTH DISPARITIES

In 2003, the Institute of Medicine (IOM) in the United States published *Unequal Treatment*, which served to elevate racial-ethnic healthcare disparities to the forefront of clinical and policy attention. The IOM defines disparities as differences between racial-ethnic minority groups and Whites that are attributable to socioeconomic factors and insurance but not to clinical need and treatment preferences (IOM, 2003).

The American Psychological Association (2022) recently published recommendations for mental health reform for the United States. They and other professional organizations concur that "mental and behavioral health is a critical and frequently unaddressed matter in racial and ethnic minority communities" (p. 1). Ethnic and racial groups, including Blacks, Latinxs, American Indians/ Alaska Natives, and Asian Americans are overrepresented in populations that are particularly at risk for mental health disorders. Additionally, minority individuals may experience symptoms that are undiagnosed, underdiagnosed, or misdiagnosed for cultural, linguistic, or historical reasons (Cook et al., 2017).

Multiple studies have contributed to expanding evidence that Blacks and Latinxs are less likely than Whites to receive mental health or substance abuse services and are more likely than Whites to delay seeking care. Even when Blacks and Latinxs do receive mental health/substance abuse services, they are more likely than Whites to obtain inappropriate diagnoses, terminate treatment early, report less satisfaction with treatment, and receive inadequate or substandard care (Cook et al., 2014, 2017; SAMHSA, 2015).

Khan and colleagues' study focused on discrimination, particularly as it applies to persons of color who also may be a sexual minority, and suggest that among minority populations, discrimination during healthcare is significantly associated with delayed care and stopped treatment. Disengagement with the healthcare system due to negative patient–provider interactions resulting from discrimination may partially explain poor health outcomes across marginalized communities. Given that discrimination affects disease outcomes through its effect on healthcare access, the "institutionalizing" of discrimination contributes to a revolving cycle of inadequate social determinants of health, translated into stigma and followed by the behaviors of discrimination (Khan et al., 2017). Discrimination can also be reinforced by social inequities, including economic, education, environment, and access (Cadena & Arguello Durante, 2019).

Aneshensel (2009) emphasized "how social inequities become mental health disparities," addressing the mental health social determinants of health. These main mental health "core" social determinants, according to Compton and Shim (2015) include:

- Racial discrimination and social exclusion
- Adverse early life experiences
- Poor education
- Unemployment, underemployment, and job insecurity
- Poverty, income inequality, and neighborhood deprivation
- Poor access to sufficient healthy food
- Poor housing quality and housing instability
- Adverse features of the built environment
- Poor access to healthcare.

Mental healthcare requires practitioners to embrace both clinical and public policy responsibilities. To promote mental health at the population level and to reduce the risk of mental illnesses and substance use disorders, health professionals have a role in altering clinical interventions, implementing and evaluating programs, and advocating for policy change. Only in this fashion can there be an impact to reduce vulnerabilities, facilitate adequate care, and move forward to face the "unequal distribution of opportunity" (Compton & Shim, 2015).

COVID-19 PHENOMENON

Starting in late 2019 during the global COVID-19 pandemic, the overall suicide rate in the United States decreased by 5% (CDC, n.d.). But studies looked closer and found that the decrease was in White, non-Hispanic communities. In some disenfranchised communities of color, there was a sixfold increase in suicides in 2019 and 2020 (Thibaut & van Wijngaarden-Cremers, 2020).

Mental distress during the pandemic is occurring against a backdrop of high rates of mental illness and substance use that existed prior to the current crisis. The pandemic's mental health impact has been pronounced among the communities of color also experiencing disproportionately high rates of COVID-19 cases and deaths. Black and Hispanic adults have been more likely than White adults to report symptoms of anxiety and/or depressive disorder during the pandemic. This disparate mental health impact comes in addition to Black and Hispanic communities experiencing disproportionately high rates of coronavirus cases and deaths (Roesch et al., 2020).

According to Thibaut and van Wijngaarden-Cremers, the COVID-19 pandemic has affected women more profoundly than men in several areas, both in the workplace (especially health and social sectors) and at home with an increased workload due to "lockdown" and quarantine measures (2020). Worldwide, 70% of the health workforce is made up of women who are often frontline health workers (nurses, midwives, and community health workers). Most of health facility service staff (cleaners, laundry, catering) is also made up of women (WHO, 2019). In the United States, women hold 78% of all hospital jobs, 70% of pharmacy jobs, and 51% of grocery store positions. Consequently, women are more likely to be exposed to the virus (Thibaut & van Wijngaarden-Cremers, 2020). Guo and colleagues reported that COVID-19 positive patients in China and healthcare professionals had higher levels of depression, anxiety, and PTSD symptoms as compared with normal control subjects. Women reported significantly more "perceived helplessness" as compared to men and control subjects. There were reports of increased fear about the stigma of being COVID-19 positive and anxiousness about the uncertainty of the disease's progression (Guo et al., 2020).

There are reports of increased violence against women worldwide, with increases of 25% to 30% during the pandemic in countries that collect data (Roesch et al., 2020). These figures may reflect only the worst cases. More complex forms of violence may also develop when perpetrators further restrict access to services and psychosocial support. Lockdowns at home when home is not a safe place result in staggering increases of IPV (Capaldi et al., 2012; United Nations Women, 2020). Women in their reproductive stage of pregnancy and the peripartum stage are at particular risk for initial or worsening of mental health disorders, primarily anxiety and depressive symptoms (Berthelot et al., 2020).

The world's workforce for healthcare and auxiliary healthcare is over 50% women (Sampaio et al., 2020). WHO postulated that many nurses and physicians could develop PTSD, depression, anxiety, and burnout during and after the pandemic peak, particularly those who struggled with insufficient PPE (personal protective equipment; WHO, 2021). History has shown that disasters go beyond the physical impact, suggesting today's elevated mental health needs will continue well beyond the coronavirus outbreak itself. For example, the psychological toll on healthcare providers during outbreaks found that psychological distress can last up to 3 years afterward (Savage, 2020). Due to the financial crisis accompanying the pandemic, there are also significant implications for the mortality rate due to "deaths of despair." Based on the economic downturn and social isolation, additional deaths due to suicide and alcohol or drug misuse may occur until 2029 (Sampaio et al., 2020).

FUTURE DIRECTIONS FOR MENTAL HEALTH

"There is no health without mental health," a statement by WHO, should also expand to "and there is mental health when there are equitable opportunities" (Compton & Shim, 2015; WHO, 2004). The social determinants of mental health and negative lifelong impacts of poverty, pollution, climate change, and violence have once again become the focus on changing the future of mental health through the prevention of illness, promotion of health, and social responsibility to address policy and discrimination (Compton & Shim, 2015). Mental health is a growing public health problem reflected in national and global studies. We are challenged to look toward other options in seeking more equitable opportunities for the lives of the patients we touch.

One expanding opportunity is the future of mental health and technology that is rapidly changing, in part due to the COVID-19 pandemic and the need for easy and remote access for mental healthcare. Not imagined even 10 years ago, the drive for research exploring the use of mental healthcare, held in the hands of the mental health consumer, continues to revolutionize accessibility, improve access,, and reduce discrimination across the globe. Leaders, such as Australia's Black Dog Institute, drive evidence-based cognitive and behavioral therapies that can be delivered safely online (Black Dog Institute, 2022). Digital technologies, and the world's population with cellular phone access, can increase options by putting their mental health access and management into their own hands.

WHO, along with the Pan American Health Organization (PAHO) spearheaded the integration of mental healthcare into primary care projects such as the Mental Health Gap Action Programme (MH-GAP; WHO, 2008). Research has uncovered both opportunities and challenges in the integration of quality services, and efforts continue to expand adequate referral systems providing ongoing evaluation and support (WHO, 2012). Adequate management of the three most common mental illnesses in the world—depressive and anxiety disorders and PTSD—benefits most from a multidisciplinary team approach that requires the integration of primary care practitioners (Bandelow et al., 2013).

The inequities of mental health professional distribution continue to challenge the world. Whether low-, middle-, or high-income countries, the lack of access to mental health professionals deters patients from receiving specialized care. Expanding the use of trained community mental health workers is one expanding strategy, particularly in countries with a dearth of mental health professionals. The Friendship Bench organization, for example, has an established project of evidence-supported interventions, reaching thousands of persons with CMDs in countries with little or no access (Abasa et al., 2020; Chibanda et al., 2016).

Stigma and discrimination also impact a person's willingness to acknowledge their need for mental health assessment and care. Byrne (2000) defines stigma "as a sign of disgrace or discredit, which sets a person apart from others" (p. 65).

The stigma of mental illness, although more often related to context than to a person's appearance, remains a powerful negative attribute in all social relations. Stigma is the community's fear, attitudes, and beliefs about a person with a mental health problem. Discrimination is the unfair or prejudicial behaviors of people and groups based on characteristics such as race, gender, age, or sexual orientation. The future of mental health in the United States and the world depends upon practitioners understanding their role and responsibilities in mitigating negative effects of discrimination and policies and that support continuation of inequities.

Finally, mental health's future is brighter when there is a focus on building resiliency. Health professionals have a long history of learning about illness and pathology. They are now learning how to integrate aspects of resiliency using today's advancing technology, address social determinants of mental health in daily practice, and view opportunities as well as challenges of primary care for mental health delivery. The complexities of women's reproductive life cycle, ranging from the first stage of menarche through postmenopause, can emphasize the vulnerabilities and fragility of many women. Shifting our focus to encompass resiliency, including the knowledge, identification and implementation of resiliency-based screening, along with treatment and support will make mental healthcare more accessible and meaningful for all women.

RESOURCES

COVID-19 PHENOMENON

https://www.kff.org/coronavirus-covid-19/issue-brief/the-implications-of-covid-19-for-mental-health-and-substance-use

DEPRESSIVE DISORDERS

https://www.mayoclinic.org/diseases-conditions/depression/in-depth/depression/art-20047725
https://adaa.org/find-help-for/women/depression#Trending%20Articles
https://www.nimh.nih.gov/health/statistics/major-depression
https://www.samhsa.gov/data/release/2020-national-survey-drug-use-and-health-nsduh-releases
https://www.psychiatry.org/patients-families/postpartum-depression/what-is-postpartum-depression

EATING DISORDERS

https://pubmed.ncbi.nlm.nih.gov/29979922
https://www.womenshealth.gov/mental-health/mental-health-conditions/eating-disorders/bulimia-nervosa
https://www.womenshealth.gov/mental-health/mental-health-conditions/eating-disorders/anorexia-nervosa

INTIMATE PARTNER VIOLENCE

https://www.ncbi.nlm.nih.gov/labs/pmc/articles/PMC2034562/table/T1
https://www.ahrq.gov/ncepcr/tools/healthier-pregnancy/fact-sheets/partner-violence.html

MENSTRUAL CYCLE: ADOLESCENTS

https://www.msdmanuals.com/professional/pediatrics
/growth-and-development/adolescent-development
#v7821280

NATIONAL ALLIANCE ON MENTAL ILLNESS

https://www.nami.org/Home

PSYCHOSIS

https://www.ementalhealth.ca/index.php?ID=6&m=survey

SUICIDE

https://www.verywellmind.com/gender-differences-in-suicide
-methods-1067508

SUICIDE PREVENTION RESOURCE CENTER

https://www.sprc.org/about-suicide/warning-signs
https://www.cdc.gov/suicide/facts/index.html

TRANSGENDER AND GENDER NON-CONFORMING INDIVIDUALS

https://transcare.ucsf.edu/guidelines/mental-health

TRAUMA

https://www.acesaware.org/ace-fundamentals/principles
-of-trauma-informed-care

WORLD HEALTH

https://sdgs.un.org/topics/health-and-population

REFERENCES

References for this chapter are online and available at https://
connect.springerpub.com/content/book/978-0-8261-6722
-4/part/part02/chapter/ch12

CHAPTER **13**

Nutrition for Women

HEATHER HUTCHINS-WIESE

Until recently, women's health and subsequent nutrition implications revolved around the reproductive system. Now more research and clinical efforts address a broad spectrum of women's health concerns, especially those unique to or more prevalent in women. With increased life expectancy, many women in the United States live 35 to 40 years after childbearing years cease. Those later years can be productive, healthy, and mobile if acute or chronic diseases are prevented or well managed. Lifestyle choices can have a significant role in controlling or modifying the course of diseases, even for those with a genetic predisposition. Of the 10 leading causes of death in females (Table 13.1), nutrition is involved in the etiology or treatment of five of them—heart disease, cancer, stroke, diabetes, and kidney disease (Centers for Disease Control and Prevention [CDC] Office of Women's Health, n.d.-a). This chapter focuses on the contributions of nutrition and dietary behaviors for

women throughout the life cycle as well as the prevention and management of selected diseases and conditions that place women at increased risk of death and morbidity.

THE NUTRIENTS—A BRIEF REVIEW

Food provides the energy needed for biological processes and materials to build and maintain all body cells. These materials are referred to as *nutrients*; each plays a role in ensuring that the biochemical machinery of the human body runs smoothly.

Nutrients are classified into six categories: carbohydrates, lipids, proteins, vitamins, minerals, and water (Table 13.2). Carbohydrates, lipids, and protein are sources of energy and are called macronutrients; vitamins and minerals are micronutrients. Energy released from the macronutrients can be measured in calories—tiny units of energy so small that the typical measure is in kilocalories (kcal) or 1,000 calorie metric units. The basic features of nutrients are as follows:

- Carbohydrates contain carbon, hydrogen, and oxygen combined in small molecules called *sugars* and large molecules represented mainly by starch. Carbohydrates provide 4 kcal/g.
- Lipids (fats and oils) contain carbon, hydrogen, and oxygen (like carbohydrates), but the amount of oxygen is much less. Triglyceride is the main form of fat in food. Fats provide 9 kcal/g.
- Proteins contain carbon, hydrogen, nitrogen, oxygen, and sometimes sulfur atoms, arranged in small compounds called *amino acids*. Chains of amino acids make up dietary proteins. Protein provides 4 kcal/g.
- Vitamins are organic compounds that serve to catalyze or support a number of biochemical reactions in the body.
- Minerals are inorganic compounds (do not contain carbon atoms) that play important roles in metabolic reactions and serve as structural compounds of body tissue, such as bone.
- Water is vital to the body as a solvent and lubricant and as a medium for transporting nutrients and waste. Water is also an inorganic compound, as it does not contain carbon.

TABLE 13.1 Leading Causes of Death in Females in the United States, 2017

RANK	CAUSE OF DEATH
1	Heart disease[a]
2	Cancer[a]
3	Chronic lower respiratory diseases
4	Stroke[a]
5	Alzheimer disease
6	Unintentional injuries
7	Diabetes[a]
8	Influenza and pneumonia
9	Kidney disease[a]
10	Septicemia

[a]Causes of death with nutritional implications.
Source: Centers for Disease Control and Prevention Office of Women's Health. (2021). Leading causes of death in females, United States, 2017. https://www.cdc.gov/women/lcod/2017/all-races-origins/index.htm

247

TABLE 13.2 Essential Nutrients

CARBOHYDRATE	FAT (LIPIDS)	PROTEIN (AMINO ACIDS)	VITAMINS	MINERALS (MAJOR)	MINERALS (TRACE)	WATER
Glucose (or a larger carbohydrate containing glucose)	Linoleic acid (omega-6), alpha-linolenic acid (omega-3)	Histidine, isoleucine, leucine, lysine, methionine, phenylalanine, threonine, tryptophan, valine	Thiamin, riboflavin, niacin, pantothenic acid, biotin, folate, vitamin B_6, vitamin B_{12}, vitamin C, vitamin A, vitamin D, vitamin E, vitamin K	Sodium, chloride, potassium, calcium, phosphorus, magnesium, sulfate	Iron, zinc, iodine, selenium, copper, manganese, fluoride, chromium, molybdenum	Water

Some nutrients the body can make, but others cannot be made in the body or the amount the body can make is insufficient to meet our needs. Therefore, it is essential to obtain some nutrients from the foods we eat. Table 13.2 lists essential nutrients that must be consumed from food to meet the body's needs.

As knowledge of nutrition and health continues to expand, the Food and Nutrition Board of the Institute of Medicine (IOM, now the National Academies of Sciences, Engineering, and Medicine [NASEM]) updates dietary intake recommendations regularly. The recommendations for individuals are *recommended dietary allowances* (RDAs) and are scientifically calculated recommendations based on current research to meet the needs of 98% of healthy individuals in a group. When not enough research is available to make a calculated recommendation, an adequate intake (AI) is designated to cover the needs of all healthy individuals in age/gender groupings. The tolerable upper intake level (UL) is the highest level of daily nutrient intake that is likely to pose no risk of adverse health effects to almost all individuals in the general population (IOM, 2005). The RDA, AI, and UL recommendations are for macronutrients, water, vitamins, and elements. A range of macronutrient intake can also be used for recommendations and is called the acceptable macronutrient distribution ranges (AMDRs) and includes the essential fats, linoleic acid (LA), and alpha-linolenic acid (ALA), as well as dietary cholesterol, trans fatty acids, saturated fatty acids, and added sugars. The AMDR recommendations do not, however, differentiate between genders. A new category for dietary intake recommendation was recently added, called the *chronic disease risk reduction* (CDRR) recommended intake; this was first used for sodium and potassium recommendations. The CDRR recommendations are nutrient intakes that are expected to reduce the risk of disease development (Stallings et al., 2019). The CDRR differs from the RDA or AI; for instance, the sodium AI for those age 14 through older adults is 1,500 mg per day and the CDRR is a recommendation to reduce sodium intake if it is above 2,300 mg per day (Stallings et al., 2019). This means that 1,500 mg per day of sodium is what is needed for the body but if there are intakes above 2,300 mg per day, this should be reduced for disease risk reduction. All recommendations—the RDA, AI, UL, AMDR, and CDRR—are part of what is called the *dietary reference intakes* (DRIs); see Table 13.3 for RDA and

AI vitamin and mineral requirements for females and Table 13.4 for the vitamin and mineral UL).

Supplements

Women report greater dietary supplement use compared to men (Mishra et al., 2021). Supplement use increases with age, with women over age 60 reporting the highest dietary supplement use in the United States (Mishra et al., 2021). The most commonly reported dietary supplements are multivitamin-mineral supplements followed by vitamin D and omega-3 fatty acids (Mishra et al., 2021). Healthcare professionals, including nurses, should screen for use *and* dose of dietary supplements as well as other complementary and alternative therapies with appropriate counseling (or appropriate referrals) on safe and effective use as needed. Screening for supplement use is important because combining supplements and dietary sources of nutrients can provide levels that exceed the UL and pose risk of negative consequences. Additionally, there can be negative interactions between supplements and some medications. The National Institutes of Health Office of Dietary Supplements provides resources for professionals and consumers (ods.od.nih.gov).

REVIEW OF NUTRITIONAL NEEDS THROUGHOUT THE LIFE CYCLE

Infancy and Childhood

The quality and quantity of children's diets are the most constant environmental factors affecting growth and development. Food, feeding, and the satiation of hunger are also important contributors to parent–infant bonding, parent–child interactions, and the child's ability to attend to the environment and learn. Feeding progresses from the newborn's total dependence on breast milk or formula to the preschool girl, who can feed herself, use utensils, make food choices, and communicate clearly regarding hunger and satiety. Food habits developed in childhood can have far-reaching effects on adult nutritional status and eating patterns. Excess weight gain in childhood or adolescence can increase the risk of adult

TABLE 13.3 DRIs: Vitamin and Mineral RDAs and AIs for Healthy, Nonpregnant, Nonlactating Females

	AGE					
	9–13 YEARS	**14–18 YEARS**	**19–30 YEARS**	**31–50 YEARS**	**51–69 YEARS**	**70 YEARS AND OLDER**
Vitamin A (mcg)	600	700	700	700	700	700
Vitamin D (mcg)[a]	11	15	15	15	15	20
Vitamin E (mg)	11	15	15	15	15	15
Vitamin K (mcg)	60	75	90	90	90	90
Vitamin C (mg)	45	65	75	75	75	75
Thiamin (mg)	0.9	1	1.1	1.1	1.1	1.1
Riboflavin (mg)	0.9	1	1.1	1.1	1.1	1.1
Niacin (mg)	12	14	14	14	14	14
Vitamin B$_6$ (mg)	1	1.2	1.3	1.3	1.5	1.5
Folate (mcg)	300	400	400	400	400	400
Vitamin B$_{12}$ (mcg)	1.8	2.4	2.4	2.4	2.4	2.4
Biotin (mcg)	20	25	30	30	30	30
Pantothenic acid (mg)	4	5	5	5	5	5
Choline (mg)	375	400	425	425	425	425
Calcium (mg)	1,300	1,300	1,000	1,000	1,200	1,200
Chromium (mcg)	21	24	25	25	20	20
Copper (mcg)	700	890	900	900	900	900
Fluoride (mg)	2	3	3	3	3	3
Iodine (mcg)	120	150	150	150	150	150
Iron (mg)	8	15	18	18	8	8
Magnesium (mg)	240	360	310	320	320	320
Manganese (mg)	1.6	1.6	1.8	1.8	1.8	1.8
Molybdenum (mcg)	34	43	45	45	45	45
Phosphorus (mg)	1,250	1,250	700	700	700	700
Potassium (mg)	2,300	2,300	2,600	2,600	2,600	2,600
Selenium (mcg)	40	55	55	55	55	55
Sodium (mg)	1,200	1,500	1,500	1,500	1,500	1,500
Zinc (mg)	8	9	8	8	8	8

Note: RDAs are indicated by boldface type; AIs are in lightface type.
[a]As cholecalciferol. 1 mcg cholecalciferol = 40 IU vitamin D.
AI, adequate intake; DRIs, dietary reference intakes; RDAs, recommended dietary allowances.
Source: Stallings, V. A., Harrison, M., & Oria, M. (Eds.). (2019). Dietary reference intakes for sodium and potassium. *National Academies Press. https://doi.org/10.17226/25353*

TABLE 13.4 DRIs: Vitamin and Mineral UL Intakes for All Females

VITAMIN/ MINERAL	AGE					
	9–13 YEARS	14–18 YEARS	19–30 YEARS	31–50 YEARS	51–69 YEARS	70 YEARS AND OLDER
Vitamin A (mcg)	1,700	2,800	3,000	3,000	3,000	3,000
Vitamin D (mcg)	100	100	100	100	100	100
Vitamin E (mg)	600	800	1,000	1,000	1,000	1,000
Vitamin K (mcg)	ND	ND	ND	ND	ND	ND
Vitamin C (mg)	1,200	1,800	2,000	2,000	2,000	2,000
Thiamin (mg)	ND	ND	ND	ND	ND	ND
Riboflavin (mg)	ND	ND	ND	ND	ND	ND
Niacin (mg)	20	30	35	35	35	35
Vitamin B_6 (mg)	60	80	100	100	100	100
Folate (mcg)	600	800	1,000	1,000	1,000	1,000
Vitamin B_{12} (mcg)	ND	ND	ND	ND	ND	ND
Biotin (mcg)	ND	ND	ND	ND	ND	ND
Pantothenic acid (mg)	ND	ND	ND	ND	ND	ND
Choline (mg)	2	3	3.5	3.5	3.5	3.5
Calcium (mg)	3,000	3,000	2,500	2,500	2,500	2,500
Chromium (mcg)	ND	ND	ND	ND	ND	ND
Copper (mcg)	5,000	8,000	10,000	10,000	10,000	10,000
Fluoride (mg)	10	10	10	10	10	10
Iodine (mcg)	600	900	1,100	1,100	1,100	1,100
Iron (mg)	40	45	45	45	45	45
Magnesium (mg)[a]	350	350	350	350	350	350
Manganese (mg)	6	9	11	11	11	11
Molybdenum (mcg)	1,100	1,700	2,000	2,000	2,000	2,000
Phosphorus (mg)	4,000	4,000	4,000	4,000	4,000	4,000
Potassium (mg)	ND	ND	ND	ND	ND	ND
Selenium (mcg)	280	400	400	400	400	400
Sodium (mg)	ND	ND	ND	ND	ND	ND
Zinc (mg)	23	34	40	40	40	40

[a]UL for magnesium represents pharmacologic intake only and does not include intake from food and water.
DRIs, dietary reference intakes; ND, not determined; UL, upper limit.
Source: Stallings, V. A., Harrison, M., & Oria, M. (Eds.). (2019). Dietary reference intakes for sodium and potassium. *National Academies Press. https://doi.org/10.17226/25353*

obesity and its related diseases. Inadequate calcium intake in the growing years is an environmental factor that can lead to a reduced bone density in adulthood and elevated risk for osteoporosis later in life. Maternal body size and food intake patterns may even have an impact on an infant and child's health. At the opposite end of the spectrum, malnutrition in the prenatal period or in the early years can have a negative effect on developmental and reproductive abilities later, even in subsequent generations. Although small body composition differences are seen in boys and girls from about age 6, the nutritional needs do not differ by gender until puberty. The DRIs are delineated by gender from 9 years of age.

Dietary eating patterns of children can affect future health and are influenced by family and caregivers. The role of family eating patterns should be addressed in childhood and into the teen years to establish healthy eating patterns at an early age.

Adolescence

Adolescence is a dynamic period in human development, with pubertal changes beginning between ages 9 and 11 years in girls. Factors such as body fat percentage and racial/ethnic differences can affect the onset and completion of puberty. Rapid physical growth and the development of secondary sexual characteristics increase the demand for energy and other nutrients. At the same time, tremendous social, cognitive, and emotional growth occurs. There is increased nutritional vulnerability in the teenage years because of the high nutrient demand, which is affected by lifestyle and food habits, possible use of alcohol and drugs, and special situations such as pregnancy, sports, and excessive dieting or eating disorders (EDs).

Changes in body composition are likely triggers for the initiation of puberty and menarche. Data from the National Health and Nutrition Examination Survey (NHANES) 1999 to 2004 showed that girls, typically prepuberty at age 8 years, have an average body fat percentage of 31%, whereas 19-year-old adolescents have an average body fat percentage of 37% (Ogden et al., 2011). Because changes in physical growth can occur at different ages in girls, using age as an indicator of nutrient needs is limiting. The use of sexual maturity ratings (or Tanner stages), body composition, and level of physical activity should all be included in the consideration of energy and nutrient needs for the adolescent.

Developing an adult body image is an emotional and cognitive task for adolescent girls that has nutritional implications. The maturing female body, with increased body fat, is in direct contrast to the American culture "ideal" of excessive thinness, reinforced by popular media, social media, fashion, and emphasis on dieting. Thus, teenage girls can be dissatisfied with their bodies, frequently attempt weight-loss diets, and are vulnerable to developing EDs (Rohde et al., 2015; Stice et al., 2011). Disordered eating behaviors in transgender and gender diverse (TGGD) adolescents and young adults are reported more often compared to cisgender youth and young adults and have a consistent theme: to prevent or delay onset of the pubertal progression (Coelho et al., 2019). Those who rely on unhealthy eating behaviors to lose weight are more likely to have poorer nutrient intake than those who

do not (Larson, Neumark-Sztainer, & Story, 2009). Furthermore, unhealthy and disordered eating behaviors tend to remain prevalent as the adolescent becomes a young adult (Neumark-Sztainer et al., 2011).

The other end of the dietary spectrum is childhood and adolescent obesity. Children and adolescents who are overweight are more likely to become obese adults and carry increased risk for chronic health conditions such as diabetes, stroke, heart disease, and certain cancers (Singh et al., 2008; Whitlock et al., 2005). Furthermore, prediabetes in adolescence is more likely to occur in conjunction with obesity as well as other unfavorable cardiometabolic risk factors (Andes et al., 2020). The rise in prediabetes seen in children and adolescents with obesity warrants screening and intervention for this vulnerable population. In 2017/2018 in the United States, 19.2% of girls age 6 to 11 years and 19.9% of girls age 12 to 19 years were obese; rates differed by race and Hispanic origin (Fryar et al., 2021). Non-Hispanic Black (29.1%), Mexican American (24.9%), and Hispanic (23.0%) girls age 2 to 19 had the highest prevalence of obesity (Fryar et al., 2021). Unfortunately, data from early in the COVID-19 pandemic, when many American children and adolescents experienced a change in their usual school day routines, corresponded with an increase in obesity prevalence for all children age 2 to 19; the greatest rate increase was experienced in 6- to 11-year-olds (Lange, Kompaniyets et al., 2021). The high prevalence of obesity highlights the need for dietary monitoring and guidance at a young age (Federal Interagency Forum on Child and Family Statistics, 2022).

NUTRITIONAL NEEDS

Energy needs in adolescent girls are determined by rate of growth, stage of maturation, and physical activity. This individual variability is shown in the DRIs for energy for healthy, active girls compared with sedentary girls: 2,071 versus 1,538 kcal/day (11 years old); 2,368 versus 1,731 kcal/day (15 years old), and 2,403 versus 1,690 kcal/day (18 years old), respectively (IOM, 2005). Protein needs parallel the growth rate; the typical diet in the United States provides adequate protein and sometimes more than needed. Protein intake becomes a concern when the energy intake is so low that dietary protein is used for energy needs rather than synthesis of new tissue and tissue repair.

Micronutrients and their dietary sources are often lacking in the diets of teenage girls. Fruits and vegetables are excellent sources of many vitamins and minerals; additionally, consumption is linked to a reduced risk of cancers and other chronic diseases. The *Dietary Guidelines for Americans, 2020–2025* (U.S. Department of Agriculture [USDA] & U.S. Department of Health and Human Services [DHHS], 2020) recommend 1.5 cups of fruit and 2.5 cups of vegetables for females age 14 to 18 years to promote health and for disease prevention; few teens, however, meet these recommendations (Lange, Moore et al., 2021).

Calcium needs are high during puberty and adolescence, with approximately 45% of the adult skeletal mass added between the ages of 9 and 17 years (Weaver & Heaney, 2014). Because the greatest retention of calcium as bone mass occurs in early to middle adolescence, the recommended AI is 1,300 mg for all adolescents age 9 to 18 years. By comparison, less than 20% of adolescent girls consume that amount, and intake decreases as the adolescent approaches young adulthood (Larson, Neumark-Sztainer, Harnack et al., 2009). Beverage choice is important as it can be a source of needed nutrients (e.g., milk) or a source of empty calories (e.g., soda). The Youth Risk Factor Surveillance System (YRFSS) monitors health behaviors of high school students in the United States. Beverage intake data from YRFSS demonstrated a significant decrease (13%) in daily soda consumption from 2007 to 2015. Milk consumption was stagnant between 2007 and 2011, with a smaller but still significant (6.9%) decline in intake between 2011 and 2015 (Miller et al., 2017). While the decline in soda intake is encouraging, the concurrent decline, albeit to a lesser degree, for milk intake is equally important to consider. Soda is only one of the sources of sugar-sweetened beverages—there are many other beverage choices, such as energy drinks or sports drinks, that contribute to added sugar intake. Milk is one of the best sources of dietary calcium as it also contains vitamins and minerals that promote absorption; however, it is often not the adolescent's beverage of choice. Therefore, conversations with teenagers should include alternative sources of dietary calcium such as yogurt, cheese, and nondairy sources, such as nondairy milk substitutes and calcium-fortified orange juice, which provide calcium amounts that are nearly equal to a serving of milk. Other nondairy food sources of calcium with slightly lesser absorption due to the coingestion of fiber include almonds, chia seeds, tofu, white beans, dried figs, and some vegetables such as leafy greens (kale, mustard and collard greens), broccoli rabe, broccoli, and sweet potatoes. Of note, cola drinks in particular have a high phosphorus content; a low calcium-to-phosphorus ratio may be an added negative impact on bone (Calvo & Tucker, 2013). Calcium intake can set the stage early in life for bone health and lower risk for osteoporosis in later years.

Iron requirements are high in adolescent girls because of the increased muscle mass and blood volume, as well as the iron loss that occurs with menses. The RDAs for iron increase from 8 mg/day in 9- to 13-year-old girls to 15 mg/day in 14- to 18-year-old girls and then increase again as girls enter young adulthood (18 mg/day for 19- to 30-year-old women). National studies have noted that iron consumption is often less than the RDAs in this population (Lytle et al., 2002). Although the incidence of iron deficiency anemia is low, the problem of low iron stores is common.

The need for vitamins and other minerals increases in adolescence but can be met by a well-chosen diet. The risk for marginal or inadequate intakes increases with the omission of fruits and vegetables, food insecurity, skipping meals, eating food prepared away from home, cigarette use, EDs, chronic diseases, and fad diets. A recent assessment of food security in children and adolescents from a U.S. national survey, NHANES 2011–2016, showed that food insecurity was associated with lower micronutrient intake; this association was most pronounced for adolescent girls and demonstrates the importance of food security assessment and resources in clinical and community settings (Jun et al., 2021).

Nutritional needs are determined by gender- and age-specific cut points and ranges of intake recommendations. This presents a unique situation for practitioners working with TGGD individuals. Work in this area is evolving; at this time there are some clinical practice guidelines and standards of care for transgender populations, but they are not specific to nutritional care. Therefore, recommendations for the nutritional assessment and care of TGGD patients are devised from clinical reasoning and the broader medical community (Linsenmeyer et al., 2022; Rozga et al., 2020). Three recommendations for application to nutritional assessment are based upon medical transition status, individualization, and using reference values in a range (Linsenmeyer et al., 2022). Specifically, for adolescents on pubertal suppression therapy or adolescents/adults who have not medically transitioned using hormone therapy, sex-specific nutritional recommendations are consistent with the sex assigned at birth. Individuality is needed for those undergoing hormone therapy as changes occur at differing times and scales. Lastly, for total energy and macronutrient intake recommendations a range using both female and male reference values can be used as a range of parameters are used in clinical practice (Linsenmeyer et al., 2022). Ranges of intake recommendations may be best applied to those early in the hormone therapy process or at low-moderate regimens (Linsenmeyer et al., 2022).

Young Adulthood

Young adulthood, or the childbearing years, is a time when women may attend college and university or join the workforce, create and establish careers, have babies and nurture families, actively participate in their communities, and attempt to balance it all. Nutrient needs are less than in the growing years, yet a variety of scenarios make achievement of optimal nutrition a challenge for many. These possible scenarios can include stressful work and family schedules; a single lifestyle with little desire to cook for one; single motherhood (which constitutes the majority of women who have limited food resources); and/or a lack of basic food and cooking knowledge, skills, and/or desire among some young women that can lead to little time or energy for meal planning or food preparation, frequent reliance on meals prepared away from the home, and irregular intakes resulting in poor diet quality.

A common complaint of young women is mood changes that accompany the premenstrual period. Numerous diet and lifestyle theories and interventions are proposed to aid in the relief of symptoms of premenstrual syndrome (PMS) and premenstrual dysphoric disorder (PMDD); however, study quality, outcomes, and findings vary. Although evidence is still limited for PMDD, as well as PMS, calcium and vitamin B_6 have the most consistent findings (Arab et al., 2020; Kashanian et al., 2007). A small randomized controlled trial found that the combination of calcium with vitamin B_6 provided greater benefit in PMS symptoms than either supplement alone (Masoumi et al., 2016). One should include supplemental and dietary sources of intake when determining total calcium intake for women. A number of herbal supplements have been proposed to support relief of PMS and/or PMDD symptoms. There is not enough evidence, however, to support use of herbal supplements such as chasteberry, gingko, evening primrose oil, or valerian for the management of PMS and/or PMDD (National Center for Complementary and Integrative Health, 2023).

Routine vitamin and mineral supplementation is not generally indicated for healthy young adult women with a well-balanced diet; the exception is folic acid supplementation. Folic acid is the form of folate that is found in fortified foods and supplements. Randomized trials have demonstrated the role of folic acid in the prevention of neural tube defects (NTDs), such as spina bifida and anencephaly. Studies have shown that the optimal red blood cell folate levels for preventing NTDs (906 mmol/L) are achieved from folic acid supplementation, not from diet alone (Shabert, 2004). Because the neural tube closes by day 28 of gestation (before most women realize they are pregnant), folic acid is needed before conception. Therefore, the CDC (1992) recommends that all women of childbearing years increase their intake of folic acid. One public health measure to address this was the implementation, in 1998, of the addition of folic acid to enriched flour or grain products, such as bread, rice, and pasta. In 2016, the U.S. Food and Drug Administration (FDA) approved the voluntary supplementation of folic acid to corn masa flour; because of the voluntary nature of the corn flour approval, it is important to advise those who use these products frequently to check product labels. In combination with good dietary sources of folate (dark green leafy vegetables, legumes, enriched cereals and grains, orange juice, soy, wheat germ, and almonds and peanuts), women of childbearing age and especially those who are planning a pregnancy should supplement their diets with 400 mcg/day of folic acid (CDC, n.d.-b).

Perimenopause/Postmenopause

Decreased estrogen production during the transition to postmenopause leads to physiologic changes that affect nutritional needs. The loss of estrogen affects the cycle of bone turnover necessary for the maintenance of bone mass in that bone resorption is greater than re-formation, resulting in loss of bone mass by the end of the early postmenopausal period and placing women at increased risk of osteoporosis. However, optimal prevention in the early decades (adequate calcium intake and weight-bearing activity) promotes optimal bone density at menopause. Reduced estrogen levels can also have an effect on blood lipids—higher total cholesterol and low-density lipoprotein (LDL) cholesterol levels along with lower high-density lipoprotein (HDL) levels—all negatively affect cardiovascular health.

The use of natural hormone replacement, namely, soy isoflavones, has grown in popularity, especially in light of potential adverse effects of hormone replacement therapy (HRT; Mangano et al., 2013). Isoflavones are a class of phytoestrogens under the larger umbrella of phytochemicals. Genistein and daidzein are the two most common isoflavones found in soy products. These phytochemicals have weak, nonsteroidal estrogen effects when bound to estrogen receptors and have been studied for effects on menopause-related symptoms and related morbidities. Isoflavones in soy may decrease the frequency of hot flashes in midlife women. A review and meta-analysis of randomized, controlled studies, however, showed that they had a modest or inconsistent effect on hot flashes (Nelson et al., 2006). A benefit of HRT was prolonged cardiovascular and bone health. When soy proteins were tested in randomized, controlled trials, there was little to no effect on serum lipids (Campbell et al., 2010; Mangano et al., 2013; Wofford et al., 2012). Related to bone health, a 1-year, randomized, controlled trial failed to find a benefit for soy protein or isoflavones (together or alone) on bone turnover or bone density (Kenny et al., 2009). Although other studies have evaluated different outcomes with varied dosages and sources of soy in different study populations, the evidence as a whole points to a lack of effect of soy, isoflavones, and phytoestrogens for the prevention of bone loss.

Post- and perimenopausal women may seek out other alternative nutritional therapies for symptom relief. However, there is no clear evidence for the effectiveness of phytoestrogens, herbs, or other dietary supplements for menopause-related symptom relief. Likewise, dietary pattern and diet quality research findings are inconsistent and inconclusive as there are only a small number of studies in this area (Noll et al., 2021). A healthy diet that focuses on intake of fruits, vegetables, and whole grains and limits refined carbohydrates and sugars may help to promote healthy sleep patterns in menopause (Laudisio et al., 2021).

Postmenopausal Years and the Aging Woman

As the number of people age 65 years and older continues to increase, there is more interest in the health and nutritional needs of this population. With the natural aging process, many physiologic, metabolic, and psychosocial changes can alter appetite, digestion, absorption, nutrient requirements, and functional skills needed for food acquisition and preparation (Table 13.5). As women get older, there is increased prevalence of chronic diseases such as heart disease, hypertension, diabetes, and cancer. These conditions may require a modified diet or changes in eating patterns that can be particularly challenging to this population.

There is growing evidence for the intersection of nutrients and dietary patterns with mental well-being. Insomnia and depression are common complaints for the postmenopausal women. Data from the Women's Health Initiative prospective cohort study show that diets with a higher glycemic index (a measure of how much a specific food raises blood glucose compared to a standard food, which can be either white bread or sugar) have more added sugars, starch, and refined grains and are associated with higher levels of insomnia and depression. More favorable dietary qualities, such as higher intakes of dietary fiber, whole grains, whole fruit, and vegetables, were inversely associated with insomnia and depression in postmenopausal women (Gangwisch et al., 2015, 2020).

The nutritional status of otherwise healthy older adults can deteriorate without much notice; screening tools are commonly used to help practitioners determine if an older adult is at risk. The American Dietetic Association, the American Academy of Family Physicians, and the National Council on Aging developed the Nutrition Screening Initiative for older adults who live independently (Nutrition Screening Initiative, 1991). The simple screening tool evaluates risk factors such as body weight, living environment, eating habits, and functional status (Box 13.1). Based on the National Screening Initiative results, a more thorough nutritional assessment can be completed and followed by appropriate intervention. This kind of early detection and prevention can be used to promote healthy behaviors and catch early warning signs to reduce hospitalizations and disease.

NUTRITIONAL NEEDS

Energy requirements decrease with age, and although the etiology is multifactorial, this decrease is largely a result of reduced basal metabolic rate and physical activity. Weight gain and an increase in body fat can occur despite decreasing dietary intake. Although energy requirements and intake often decrease with age, the requirements for protein, vitamins, and minerals do not decline, and some increase. Therefore, it is essential for the older female to choose nutrient-dense foods.

TABLE 13.5 Factors With Potential to Affect Nutritional Status in Older Women

FACTOR	NUTRITIONAL IMPACT
Decreased lean body mass and strength	Possible increase in protein requirement
Loss of independence and mobility	Limited food access and ability to prepare meals
Decreased energy expenditure, physical activity	Decreased energy requirement, increased need for nutrient-dense diet
Xerostomia (dry mouth)	Chewing and/or swallowing problems, food avoidance
Dysgeusia/hyposmia	Reduced sensory stimulation and appetite changes
Decreased immune function	Possible increased requirement for iron, zinc, and other nutrients
Atrophic gastritis	Increased requirement for folate, calcium, vitamin K, vitamin B_{12}, and iron
Increased blood pressure	Reduced sodium requirement and unprocessed food sources
Menopause	Decreased iron requirement
Reduced skin production and reduced metabolism of vitamin D to physiologically active form	Increased requirement for vitamin D and calcium
Increased retention of vitamin A	Reduced requirement for vitamin A
Constipation	Possible increase in fluid and fiber requirements
Depression, social isolation	Poor appetite and limited food intake
Changes in financial status	Possible reduced food access and choices, limited food variety and intake

Box 13.1 Checklist to Determine Your Nutritional Health

The warning signs of poor nutritional health are often overlooked. To see whether you (or people you know) are at nutritional risk, take this simple quiz. Read the statement below and circle the number in the Yes column for those that apply. To find your total nutritional score, add up all the numbers you circled.

	Yes
I have an illness or condition that made me change the kind and/or amount of food I eat.	2
I eat fewer than two meals per day.	3
I eat few fruits, vegetables, or milk products.	2
I have three or more drinks of beer, liquor, or wine almost every day.	2
I have tooth or mouth problems that make it hard for me to eat.	2
I do not always have enough money to buy the food I need.	4
I eat alone most of the time.	1
I take three or more different prescribed or over-the-counter drugs a day.	1
Without wanting to, I have lost or gained 10 lb in the past 6 months.	2
I am not always physically able to shop, cook, and/or feed myself.	2
Total nutritional score:	

If your total nutritional score is

0 to 2: Good! Recheck your nutritional score in 6 months.

3 to 5: You are at moderate nutritional risk. See what can be done to improve your eating habits and lifestyle. A local office on aging, senior nutrition program, senior citizens center, or health department can help. Recheck your nutritional score in 3 months.

6 or more: You are at high nutritional risk. Bring this checklist next time you see your doctor, dietitian, or other qualified health or social service professional. Talk with them about any problems you have experienced. Ask for nutritional counseling.

Source: Reprinted from Nutrition Screening Initiative. (1991). Report of nutrition screening I: Toward a common view: Executive summary: A consensus conference, Washington, D.C., April 8–10, 1991. *The Nutrition Screening Initiative is a project of the American Academy of Family Physicians, the American Dietetic Association, and the National Council on the Aging, and is funded in part by a grant from Ross Products Division, Abbott Laboratories.*

Dietary protein needs may increase in the older female as a result of diminished protein stores in the declining muscle mass, as well as altered gastrointestinal (GI) function and the presence of acute and chronic diseases. Although the RDA for protein for all adults is 0.8 g/kg/day, evidence indicates that 1.0 to 1.5 g/kg/day may better maintain positive nitrogen balance in older adults (Paddon-Jones et al., 2015). Furthermore, some experts recommend consumption of protein (25 to 30 g) at each meal from a variety of high-quality protein sources along with regular physical activity before or after the protein-rich meal to prevent the onset or slow the progression of sarcopenia (Paddon-Jones et al., 2015).

The nutritional status of older adults is varied. Age, geographic location, culture, and disease conditions are contributing factors to the heterogeneity of older adult nutrition status. National surveys of food consumption and nutritional status indicate that older adults in the United States are at nutritional risk. With decreased mean energy intakes, nutrients at greatest risk for deficiency are calcium, riboflavin, folate, vitamin B_{12}, vitamin B_6, iron, and zinc (Jain, 2015). Older women have increased needs for vitamins C, D, and the B vitamins as well as calcium, magnesium, and zinc. One nutrient that is often chronically low in older adults is vitamin D, which is necessary for absorption of calcium and phosphorus. In addition to possible limited dietary intake, skin efficiency in converting vitamin D from sunlight cannot be counted on due to multiple variables that affect how much vitamin D is converted (such as skin color, location, weather, and liver and kidney function). Sun exposure for the purpose of converting vitamin D is also discouraged because of the documented increased risk for skin cancers from sun exposure. Supplementation of vitamin D should be considered for those who do not obtain enough vitamin D through enriched dietary sources. In addition to providing calcium and vitamin D supplements to achieve RDIs and promote bone health, other nutrients important for bone health also need to be provided including protein; vitamins A, C, and K; magnesium; and possibly omega-3 fatty acids.

PREGNANCY

Nutritional and lifestyle choices of pregnant women are key contributors to the progression and health of a pregnancy. A pregnancy is considered healthy when the mother is without physiologic or psychological pathology and it results in a healthy baby (Kaiser et al., 2014). One area with health disparities is maternal deaths; this is a significant public health concern and was identified in *Healthy People 2030* as a leading health indicator (LHI). *Healthy People* (originally published in 1979) is updated each decade with specific health objectives based on priority areas. LHIs are a group of topics determined to be high-priority health issues. Black and American Indian/Alaskan Native women have significantly higher pregnancy-related deaths compared to White, Asian/Pacific Islander, and Hispanic women (Petersen et al., 2019). A reduction in maternal mortality is the focus for this LHI.

Points in history have demonstrated the impact of food deprivation and malnutrition on reproduction. Studies from Russia and the Netherlands during World War II demonstrated a decrease in fertility and an increase in stillbirths, neonatal deaths, and infants with low birth weight (LBW; Shabert, 2004). LBW remains a public health concern; 8.31% of U.S. newborns are of LBW (less than 2,500 g; Martin et al., 2021). Birth defects and LBW are the number 1 and 2 causes, respectively, of death in U.S. infants (Murphy et al., 2021).

The timing and duration of nutritional restriction are significant. During the embryonic stage of fetal development, cells differentiate into three germinal layers. Growth during this time occurs only by an increase in the number of cells. The fetal stage is the time of most rapid growth. During this time, growth is almost continuous and is accompanied by increases in cell size. Most organ cells continue to proliferate after birth. It is thought that growth in cell size begins at around 7 months' gestation and can continue for 3 years after birth. Given this sequence of growth, it is possible to suggest the effects malnutrition might have at different stages of gestation. During the embryonic phase, a severe limitation in nutrients could have teratogenic effects, causing malformation or death. Although malnutrition occurring after the third month of gestation would not generally have teratogenic effects, it could cause fetal growth restriction. During the last trimester, nutritional needs are at a peak as cells increase in both size and number. Poor nutrition in the latter stages of pregnancy affects fetal growth, whereas malnutrition in the early months affects embryonic development and survival.

Maternal size at conception and nutritional history also influence pregnancy outcomes. Prepregnancy body mass index (BMI) is an independent predictor of adverse outcomes of pregnancy. The prevalence of overweight and obesity in women of childbearing years has increased; nearly half of all pregnant women are either overweight (24%) or obese (24%) prepregnancy. There are racial and ethnic differences in prepregnancy weight. Alaskan Native/American Indian (36.4%), Black (34.7%), and Hispanic (27.3%) women have higher rates of prepregnancy obesity compared to White (23.7%) and Asian women (7.5%; U.S. Preventive Services Task Force [USPSTF], 2021a). Maternal size is believed to be a controlling factor on the ultimate size of the placenta, which in turn determines the amount of nutrition available to the fetus. Women who have lower prepregnant weights tend to have lighter placentas than women with higher prepregnant weights (Shabert, 2004). Short- and long-term effects of overweight and overconsumption on maternal health risk include obesity, diabetes, dyslipidemia, and cardiovascular disease (Procter & Campbell, 2014). Preconception healthcare providers should assess weight status of women who eventually plan to get pregnant and provide support (or possibly consultation with a registered dietitian) for healthy eating and weight loss efforts, prepregnancy, to promote optimal health of the mother and child. Weight loss or weight maintenance during pregnancy, however, is not recommended as inadequate gestational weight gain during pregnancy is associated with increased risk of adverse events and infant mortality (Wang et al., 2021).

Weight Gain During Pregnancy

Gestational weight gain (GWG) follows a typical pattern of little gain in the first trimester, a rapid increase in the second, and a slightly slower rate of gain in the third. Most of the weight gain associated with the products of conception (placenta, fetus, and amniotic fluid) takes place in the second half of pregnancy, whereas maternal stores are laid down very rapidly before midpregnancy and then slow down and appear to stop before term. By the time of delivery, the weight gain can be accounted for in the fetus, placenta, amniotic fluid, maternal blood, maternal extracellular fluid, maternal breast and uterus, and maternal fat (Pitkin, 1976). The amount of fat stores gained parallels GWG.

Monitoring weight gain during pregnancy serves to estimate the adequacy of pregnancy progression, including dietary sufficiency. Historically, weight gain in pregnancy was restricted even through the 1960s. The current recommendation for women of normal body weight for height (BMI 18.5–24.9) is to gain a total of 25 to 35 lb, at a rate of about 1 lb per week. The IOM, in 2009, updated guidelines for pregnancy weight gain for subgroups of American women (Rasmussen & Yaktine, 2009). The weight gain goals are based on prepregnancy BMI, which is weight (in kilograms) divided by height (in meters squared). Women who are underweight (BMI <18.5) are recommended to gain 28 to 40 lb at a rate of about 1 to 1.3 lb per week. Those who are overweight (BMI 25.0 to 29.9) or obese (BMI ≥30) are recommended to gain only 15 to 25 lb and 11 to 20 lb, respectively. Their weekly rates of weight gain are about 0.6 lb for overweight women and 0.5 lb for those who are obese (Rasmussen & Yaktine, 2009).

Both insufficient and excessive weight gain during pregnancy can affect fetal and maternal outcomes. Poor weight gain is associated with poor fetal growth, LBW, and risk for a preterm delivery (Rasmussen & Yaktine, 2009). Excessive weight gain affects infant growth, increases chances for large-for-gestational-age birth weight and cesarean delivery, and is associated with the longer-term outcome of higher body fatness in childhood (Turner, 2014).

To help patients meet healthy weight gain recommendations in pregnancy, the USPSTF recommends that clinicians offer pregnant women effective behavioral counseling interventions (USPSTF, 2021a). Implementing this recommendation is dependent on the care setting and patient needs. The most used, successful interventions include activity/supervised exercise, counseling about diet and physical activity, and/or lifestyle and behavioral change counseling from clinicians, registered dietitians, qualified fitness specialists, physiotherapists, and/or health coaches across a variety of settings such as group or individual counseling delivered in person, virtually, or by telephone (USPSTF, 2021a). Behavioral counseling interventions to promote healthy weight gain can improve maternal and infant outcomes such as a decreased risk of gestational diabetes mellitus, emergency cesarean delivery, infant macrosomia, and large-for-gestational-age infants (USPSTF, 2021a). The number of contacts with patients also matters. Interventions with 12 or more contacts were more effective at reducing excess GWG and infant macrosomia compared to interventions with fewer contacts

TABLE 13.6 DRIs: Vitamin and Mineral RDAs[a] and AIs for Pregnant and Lactating Females

VITAMIN/MINERAL	PREGNANCY	LACTATION
Vitamin A (mcg)	**14–18 years: 750**	**14–18 years: 1,200**
	770	1,300
Vitamin D (mcg)	**15**	**15**
Vitamin E (mg)	**15**	**19**
Vitamin K (mcg)	14–18 years: 75	14–18 years: 75
	90	90
Vitamin C (mg)	**14–18 years: 80**	**14–18 years: 115**
	85	120
Thiamin (mg)	**1.4**	**1.4**
Riboflavin (mg)	**1.4**	**1.6**
Niacin (mg)	**18**	**17**
Vitamin B$_6$ (mg)	**1.9**	**20**
Folate (mcg)	**600**	**500**
Vitamin B$_{12}$ (mcg)	**2.6**	**2.8**
Biotin (mcg)	30	35
Pantothenic acid (mg)	6	7
Choline (mg)	450	550
Calcium (mg)	**14–18 years: 1,300**	**14–18 years: 1,300**
	1,000	1,000
Chromium (mcg)	14–18 years: 29	14–18 years: 44
	30	45
Copper (mcg)	**1,000**	**1,300**
Fluoride (mg)	3	3
Iodine (mcg)	**220**	**290**
Iron (mg)	**27**	**14–18 years: 10**
		9
Magnesium (mg)	**14–18 years: 400**	**14–18 years: 360**
	19–30 years: 350	**19–30 years: 310**
	31–50 years: 360	**31–50 years: 320**
Manganese (mg)	2	2.6
Molybdenum (mcg)	**50**	**50**
Phosphorus (mg)	**14–18 years: 1,250**	**14–18 years: 1,250**
	700	700
Selenium (mcg)	**60**	**70**
Zinc (mg)	**14–18 years: 12**	**14–18 years: 13**
	11	12

[a]DRIs presented for ages 19–30 years and 31–50 years. Unless otherwise indicated, RDAs are noted in bold, AIs in ordinary type.
AIs, adequate intakes; DRIs, dietary reference intakes; RDAs, recommended dietary allowances.
Source: Otten, J. J., Hellwig, J. P., & Meyers, L. D. (Eds.). (2006). DRI, dietary reference intakes: The essential guide to nutrient requirements. National Academies Press.

(USPSTF, 2021a). The lifestyle skills gained from behavioral health interventions during pregnancy may also be applied to healthy living postpregnancy.

Energy and Macronutrient Needs

ENERGY

As growth requires energy, additional energy above that required for maintenance is needed for pregnancy. RDAs for energy aim to provide optimal weight gain at various stages; meet growth needs of the fetus, placenta, and other maternal tissues; and account for the increased maternal basal metabolism. The RDA for pregnancy includes an additional 340 kcal/day for the second trimester and an additional 452 kcal/day for the third trimester; this varies with the woman's level of physical activity during her pregnancy. If the rate and amount of weight gain are within acceptable limits, the range of energy intake can be quite variable. More energy expenditure for movement is required with increasing body weight; however, most pregnant women slow or decrease their activity as pregnancy progresses. Enough energy is needed to protect protein to be used for growth rather than energy expenditure. Caloric restrictions in animals and humans have demonstrated profound negative effects on maternal physiologic adjustments and fetal growth and development.

PROTEIN

Dietary protein needs increase during pregnancy to support increases in whole body protein turnover and accumulation of protein for growth of the fetus, uterus, blood volume, placenta, amniotic fluid, and maternal skeletal muscle (IOM, 2005). The RDA for protein during pregnancy is 71 g/day, which is 25 g more than the RDA for nonpregnant women.

CARBOHYDRATE

Glucose is the fetus's primary energy source, with an estimated transfer from mother at a rate of 17 to 26 g/day. All glucose transferred to the fetus is used by the growing brain by the end of pregnancy (IOM, 2005). The RDA increases to 175 g/day of dietary carbohydrate for pregnant women.

FAT

Fat is an energy source and is essential for fat-soluble vitamin and carotenoid absorption (Turner, 2014). Intake recommendations for essential omega-3 and omega-6 fatty acids were determined based on median intakes among pregnant women in the United States, the AI method for estimating nutrient needs. The AI for linoleic acid (LA), the essential omega-6 fatty acid, is 13 g/day. The AI for ALA, the essential omega-3 fatty acid, is 1.3 g/day (IOM, 2005). The longer chain omega-3 fatty acid, docosahexaenoic acid (DHA), accumulates in large amounts in the prenatal and postnatal brain. DHA can be formed from ALA in fetal tissues; therefore, ALA intake at recommended levels can meet essential DHA needs. Direct DHA intake occurs via seafood intake, particularly oily fish. Improved infant and childhood outcomes are associated with maternal seafood consumption (Heppe et al., 2011; Noakes et al., 2012). Balancing seafood intake recommendations for a healthy pregnancy while avoiding high methylmercury

content can be achieved. A good rule is to consider the size of the fish; larger fish have higher methyl-mercury content. The top sources of high-mercury fish in the United States should be avoided and include tilefish from the Gulf of Mexico, shark, swordfish, king mackerel, marlin, orange roughy, and bigeye tuna (FDA, 2021). Fatty fish such as salmon, sardines, anchovies, and light canned tuna are low in methylmercury and good sources of omega-3 fatty acids. White albacore tuna should be limited to 4 oz (or approximately the size of the palm of a hand) per week for pregnant women and is also a good source of omega-3 fatty acids. Two to three 4-oz servings of low methylmercury-containing fish per week is recommended for pregnant women (FDA, 2021).

Micronutrient Needs

The need for most vitamins and many minerals increases during pregnancy. Many of the water-soluble vitamins are used as cofactors in metabolic exchanges and processes essential for growth; therefore, needs increase for thiamin, riboflavin, niacin, vitamin B_6, folate, vitamin B_{12}, pantothenic acid, choline, and vitamin C (Suitor & Meyers, 2007). The requirements for fat-soluble vitamins A and D are also increased during pregnancy (Table 13.6). Element needs that increase are iron, magnesium, chromium, copper, iodine, manganese, molybdenum, selenium, zinc, and chloride. Some highlights of vitamins and minerals are given in the following sections, along with their importance during pregnancy.

VITAMIN NEEDS
Vitamin A

The RDA for vitamin A for pregnant women, 770 retinol activity equivalents (RAE), is slightly more than the nonpregnant level. The concern is that excessive intake of vitamin A can be teratogenic. Cases of adverse pregnancy outcomes, such as malformations, have been associated with a daily ingestion of 25,000 IU (7,500 RAE) or more of vitamin A (Rosa et al., 1986). In addition, epidemiologic evidence indicates that the drug isotretinoin (or Absorica, a vitamin A analog used to treat cystic acne) causes major malformations involving craniofacial, central nervous system, cardiac, and thymic changes (Lammer et al., 1985). Use of this drug is contraindicated in pregnancy. Some findings indicate that pregnant women who take vitamin A supplements at levels as low as 2.5 times the RDA increase the risk of delivering a baby with a cranial neural crest defect (Rothman et al., 1995). The Teratology Society (1987) urges that women in their reproductive years be informed that the excessive use of vitamin A shortly before and during pregnancy could be harmful to their babies. It also suggests that manufacturers of vitamin A–containing supplements should lower the maximum amount of vitamin A per unit dosage to 5,000 to 8,000 IU and identify the source of vitamin A. Beta-carotene, a precursor of vitamin A, is not associated with these pregnancy risks.

Vitamin D

The IOM recommendation for vitamin D intake in pregnancy does not differ from that for nonpregnant women: RDA of 600 IU (15 mcg) and UL of 4,000 IU/day (Ross et al., 2011). Vitamin D is necessary for fetal growth and development, particularly of the skeleton and tooth enamel. Vitamin D can be produced in the body from UV sunlight exposure and is found in some foods such as fatty fish, egg yolks, liver, and fortified milks and orange juice. Sunlight exposure for converting vitamin D is not recommended; rather, dietary sources and supplements are recommended. Serum levels of vitamin D are measured as 25-hydroxyvitamin D [25(OH)D]; low levels are common in the United States. The American College of Obstetricians and Gynecologists (ACOG), however, does not recommend vitamin D assessment for all pregnant women to detect vitamin D deficiency (ACOG, 2011). Additionally, the most recent World Health Organization (WHO) updated nutrition recommendation for antenatal care of pregnant women does not recommend vitamin D supplementation for all pregnant women to improve maternal and perinatal outcomes (WHO, 2020). Rather, women are recommended to focus on dietary sources and sunlight exposure. Women at higher risk for vitamin D deficiency or for conditions associated with reduced risk from vitamin D supplementation may benefit from a more thorough assessment. Supplementation of vitamin D, alone, compared to placebo or no vitamin D intervention had low to moderate evidence for risk reduction of preeclampsia and gestational diabetes but does increase infant serum 25(OH)D levels for approximately 8 weeks postpartum (March et al., 2015; Palacios et al., 2019; WHO, 2020). Examination of longer-term outcomes of prenatal vitamin D supplementation found that high-dose supplementation (2,800 IU/day) resulted in greater bone mineral density of children, at age 6 years, who were vitamin D sufficient from mothers who received the high-dose supplementation during pregnancy (Brustad et al., 2022). These findings highlight the need for more research on immediate maternal and infant outcomes, as well as long-term outcomes of prenatal vitamin D supplementation.

Folic Acid

Folic acid requirements increase during pregnancy because of augmented maternal erythropoiesis and fetal and placental growth. It is also an essential coenzyme in metabolism and in DNA synthesis. Folic acid deficiency results in megaloblastic anemia. Although it is not as common as iron deficiency anemia, megaloblastic anemia can occur in high-risk women, such as those of low socioeconomic status and those with a multiple pregnancy or chronic hemolytic anemia. Diagnosis may not occur until the third trimester, but biochemical and morphologic signs may be seen earlier. Maternal folic acid deficiency in animals is associated with congenital malformations; some evidence in humans suggests an association with pregnancy complications, but high-quality studies have not been conducted (Tamura & Picciano, 2006).

The current RDA for folate is 600 mcg for pregnancy, 200 mcg more than the recommendation for nonpregnant women. Synthetic folic acid as a fortified or supplemental source (400–800 mcg/day), in addition to food forms of folate from a variable diet for women who are capable of becoming pregnant, is recommended (USPSTF, 2017). It is important to note, however, that the tolerable UL of 800 to 1,000 mcg/day from fortified foods and supplements is only double the recommended dose.

The most significant influence of folic acid in pregnancy is its role in preventing NTDs. Randomized clinical trials of several thousand women in Europe in the late 1980s and early 1990s resulted in unequivocal results (Tamura & Picciano, 2006). Good dietary sources of folate and folic acid supplements are needed before and between conceptions; in fact, the public health recommendations are that "all women who are planning or capable of pregnancy take a daily supplement containing 400 to 800 mcg of folic acid" (USPSTF, 2017).

Vitamin B$_{12}$

Vitamin B$_{12}$ accumulates in the placenta and fetus and is essential for normal blood formation and neurologic function. At birth, fetal vitamin B$_{12}$ levels are twice that of the mother. Only new vitamin B$_{12}$ is transferred to the placenta, so supplementation is required for those who limit the intake of meats and meat products. Vegans in particular need supplemental sources of vitamin B$_{12}$. Deficiency during pregnancy can increase the risk for maternal and fetal megaloblastic anemia, fetal demyelination, and NTDs (Turner, 2014).

Choline

Large amounts of choline are transferred to the fetus from maternal stores. Therefore, the AI for choline increases to 450 mg/day for pregnant women. Maternal deficiency can negatively affect fetal brain development (Caudill, 2010). Choline intakes may be lower than the recommended intake for many pregnant women. Suggestions for increased dietary intake are needed, as choline is often not included in prenatal vitamin and mineral supplements. Good dietary sources include eggs (best source), meat, salmon, kidney or navy beans, and low-fat milk (Kaiser et al., 2014).

MINERAL NEEDS
Iron

Pregnancy imposes a severe burden on the maternal hematopoietic system. With the natural increase in maternal blood supply in pregnancy, total erythrocyte volume increases by 20% to 30%. Normal hematopoiesis requires a nutritionally adequate diet. To produce hemoglobin, there must be protein to provide essential amino acids and sufficient additional iron. Other vitamins and minerals, such as copper, zinc, folic acid, and vitamin B$_{12}$, are needed to serve as cofactors in the synthesis of heme and globin. The limiting factor in this synthesis is usually the availability of iron. Heme iron, found in animal products, is more easily absorbed than nonheme iron found in beans, peas, lentils, and dark green vegetables. Absorption can be enhanced by the addition of vitamin C rich foods such as citrus and peppers. Women following vegan, vegetarian, or "plant-based" diets prior to or during pregnancy, minority populations, or low-income women may be at increased risk for iron deficiency during pregnancy.

Iron deficiency prevalence in the United States increases by trimester and is higher in Mexican American and non-Hispanic Black pregnant women as well as women with parity greater than two (Mei et al., 2011). Recommendations for iron deficiency anemia screening and supplementation vary by expert group. The most conservative recommendation comes from the USPSTF, which found limited evidence for the screening of all pregnant women for anemia and supplementation and identified a number of research gaps (Siu & USPSTF, 2015). ACOG recommends low-dose iron supplementation to decrease maternal anemia at delivery based on good and consistent evidence (ACOG Committee on Practice Bulletins, 2021). Most prenatal vitamins contain a low-dose iron source to meet this recommendation. Based on limited or inconsistent evidence, ACOG recommends treatment of iron deficiency anemia during pregnancy at levels above prenatal vitamin iron content. Additionally, parenteral iron may be considered for those who do not respond to oral iron supplementation or for women with severe iron deficiency in late pregnancy. Lastly, based on consensus and expert opinion, all women should be screened for anemia with a complete blood count in the first trimester and again between weeks 24 and 28 (ACOG Committee on Practice Bulletins, 2021).

Calcium

Calcium deposition in fetal bones and teeth occurs primarily in the third trimester; by the time of a full-term birth, the newborn has accumulated approximately 25 to 30 g of calcium. The current RDA for calcium during pregnancy (1,000 mg/day for adults and 1,300 mg/day for those younger than 19 years) is not an increase over the nonpregnant state because of the increased efficiency of intestinal calcium absorption.

Although available data are insufficient to support routine calcium supplementation for the prevention of osteoporosis in younger women, prenatal nutrition counseling should address dietary strategies to meet calcium needs. In situations in which dairy products are omitted or restricted in the diet (allergy, lactose intolerance, and veganism) or in which calcium intake is chronically low, calcium supplementation should be considered. The goal is for dietary intake plus supplementation to meet the RDA for calcium; care should be taken so the RDA is not exceeded.

Sodium

Sodium restriction in the diet of pregnant women was standard practice for decades. It is now recognized, however, that healthy pregnant women retain salt normally, and moderate edema appears to be a normal consequence of pregnancy. Fluid retention increases the body's need for sodium.

A positive sodium balance occurs in normal pregnancy, resulting from significant changes in renal and hormonal function. The glomerular filtration rate increases by 50% in early pregnancy and remains elevated until late in the third trimester, filtering sodium into the renal tubules. Simultaneously, progesterone produces a salt-losing action in the kidneys, slowing absorption of filtered sodium through the tubules.

To prevent an electrolyte imbalance, the renin–angiotensin–aldosterone system acts as a compensatory mechanism in normal pregnancy. This counterbalances the salt-losing tendencies of progesterone and decreases urinary sodium excretion. The result is that sodium is conserved to meet the needs of the expanded tissue and fluid. Severe sodium restriction can stress the physiologic mechanism of sodium conservation, resulting in hyponatremia. Moderation in sodium intake is appropriate for everyone; pregnancy recommendations mirror those for the nonpregnant population.

Zinc

Zinc has wide-ranging enzymatic, structural, and regulatory functions. Zinc deficiency in pregnancy can cause intrauterine growth retardation, teratogenesis, and embryonic or fetal death (King, 2000). The RDA for zinc during pregnancy is 11 mg/day (12 mg/day for those younger than 18 years), 3 mg/day more than the RDA for the nonpregnant female population. Because iron inhibits zinc absorption, high levels of prenatal iron supplementation may have a negative impact on maternal zinc status. For women taking more than 30 mg/day of iron, supplements of 15 mg/day of zinc and 2 mg/day of copper are recommended (Procter & Campbell, 2014); these are mineral amounts typical in prenatal vitamins that contain iron. Good sources of dietary zinc include meat, fish, poultry, dairy products, nuts, whole grains, and legumes. The bioavailability of zinc can be inhibited in vegetarian diets because of phytates, fiber, and/or calcium that may inhibit absorption (Kaiser et al., 2014). Therefore, the needs of pregnant vegetarians may be higher than those of nonvegetarians.

Alcohol, Artificial Sweeteners, and Caffeine

The teratogenic effects of excessive alcohol consumption are well accepted. In addition to the outcomes of fetal alcohol syndrome and fetal alcohol effects, alcohol use in pregnancy is associated with spontaneous abortion, LBW, and abruptio placentae. As no safe level of alcohol intake in pregnancy can be guaranteed, promoting abstinence before and during pregnancy is recommended. Inquiring about alcohol intake can sometimes be less threatening when done within the context of a dietary history and usual patterns of food and beverage intake.

Artificial sweeteners used in the U.S. food supply include saccharin (e.g., Sweet 'n Low), aspartame (e.g., Equal), sucralose (e.g., Splenda), acesulfame K (e.g., Sweet One), and steviosides (e.g., Truvia, or Stevia in the raw). Saccharin has been shown to be a weak carcinogen in animals but is not teratogenic. Acesulfame K is considered safe, but is relatively new in food use, so no long-term studies during pregnancy have been conducted. A product of aspartame metabolism is the amino acid phenylalanine, which can cause brain damage in persons with phenylketonuria. Moderate intake of aspartame in women without phenylketonuria, however, does not increase serum phenylalanine levels high enough to affect the fetal brain. There are few human studies on the effects of artificial sweeteners during pregnancy; findings in animal studies indicate a need for more research in humans (Palatnik et al., 2020). Dietary assessment of pregnant women should include the use of artificial sweeteners, found primarily in soft drinks but also in flavored yogurt, in baked goods, and as a substitute for added sugar. Counseling should encourage moderation in artificial sweetener intake for the pregnant woman and encourage nutrient-containing milk and 100% juice or water instead of soft drinks.

Extensive research has been conducted on caffeine's effect on pregnancy outcome, with mixed results depending on study design and population. A large prospective study out of the United Kingdom found that caffeine intake is associated with fetal growth restriction (CARE Study Group, 2008); other studies have had mixed results. Although there is controversy surrounding the recommendation to eliminate or restrict caffeine intake, women should limit their intake to no more than 200 mg/day (ACOG, 2010). In addition to coffee and tea, soft drinks are a major source of caffeine in the United States. The average caffeine content of common beverages is 137 mg in an 8-oz cup of regular coffee, 40 mg in a 1-oz espresso, 48 mg in an 8-oz cup of tea, and 37 mg in 12 oz of cola. Dark chocolate also provides 30 mg caffeine in a 1.45-oz serving (ACOG, 2010).

Diet-Related Problems in Pregnancy

COMMON GASTROINTESTINAL COMPLAINTS

Nausea and vomiting, commonly called *morning sickness*, are reported in 70% to 85% of pregnant women. Standard dietary recommendations for mild nausea include eating frequent, small meals; avoiding offensive odors and spicy or greasy foods; drinking adequate fluids; and getting fresh air (Kaiser et al., 2014). There is limited support for the use of complementary therapies or supplements (typical practices include acupuncture, vitamin B_6, or ginger products) to help alleviate GI symptoms. Rather than a specific diet for managing nausea, pregnant women should be encouraged to eat whatever they tolerate and avoid odors that result in nausea. For some women, nausea is caused by getting overly hungry and may be prevented by ingesting small, frequent snacks.

For a small percentage of pregnant women, the vomiting can be frequent and severe enough (hyperemesis gravidarum) to affect their nutritional status, resulting in weight loss, decreased nutrient intake, and electrolyte imbalance. These women need medical management and frequently require hospitalization for fluid and electrolyte replacement and possibly nutrition support in severe cases.

Acid reflux, or heartburn, is reported in approximately two thirds of pregnant women (Turner, 2014). Calcium-based antacids have been tested in randomized, controlled trials and are effective for rapid relief of symptoms. Additional, but not empirically tested, common recommendations for heartburn relief include avoiding the supine position for 3 hours after eating; sleeping with an elevated head; eating small, frequent meals; and avoiding greasy and/or spicy foods, as well as tomatoes, highly acidic citrus, carbonated beverages, and caffeine-containing beverages (Kaiser et al., 2014).

Constipation occurs among 11% to 38% of pregnant women and is attributed to the slowed digestive changes of pregnancy and/or a side effect of iron supplementation (Vazquez, 2010). Adequate fluid and fiber intake recommendations (28 g/day for pregnant women) and regular physical activity can help alleviate constipation.

PREGNANCY-INDUCED HYPERTENSION

The cardinal symptoms of pregnancy-induced hypertension (PIH) are hypertension, proteinuria, and edema, usually occurring after the 20th week of gestation. This condition is unique to pregnancy and resolves only by the termination of the pregnancy. PIH is sometimes referred to as *preeclampsia* and *eclampsia*; the latter is an extension of preeclampsia, with more severity (i.e., seizures and high risk of maternal and infant death). PIH, a more appropriate description of this disorder, is most often seen in first pregnancies, obesity, history of preeclampsia, chronic hypertension, older age, and African American race. Criteria for diagnosing PIH include:

- **Hypertension:** Blood pressure of 140/90 mmHg or an increase of 20 to 30 mmHg systolic or 10 to 15 mmHg diastolic above the woman's usual baseline; at least two observations at 6 or more hours apart
- **Proteinuria:** 500 mg or more in a 24-hour urine collection or random 2+ protein; develops late in PIH
- **Edema:** Significant; usually in hands and face; if left unattended, seizures may occur; can be fatal to either mother or infant

The etiology of PIH is unknown. Nutritional deficiency is suspected; however, because of the socioeconomic and other confounding factors (age, preconception weight, health status, and prenatal care) the etiology remains undetermined. Protein, total energy intake, macronutrient imbalances, omega-3 fatty acids, calcium, sodium, zinc, iron, magnesium, and folate have been studied as potential nutritional triggers; however, definitive findings remain elusive. A basic, healthy diet—including good potassium sources (fruits and vegetables), low-fat dairy products, and high fiber—is associated with a reduced risk of preeclampsia (Frederick et al., 2005). Women at risk for PIH should receive early prenatal care and guidance on following a balanced diet that provides adequate energy and protein.

DIABETES

With the prevalence of overweight and type 2 diabetes mellitus (DM) on the rise in the general population, more women are entering pregnancy with DM, insulin resistance, or high risk for the development of gestational diabetes. This increases the risk for pregnancy complications and poor birth outcomes.

Pregnancy is a diabetogenic event in which energy needs and fuel requirements are increased. Glucose is the primary fuel, particularly for the growing fetus, who has an uptake rate of glucose at least twice that of an adult. To meet fetal needs, glucose is transferred rapidly from mother to fetus through simple diffusion and active transport. Although glucose crosses the placental barrier, insulin does not, so the fetus is dependent on its own supply for development. Maternal fasting blood glucose levels drop because of rapid fetal uptake, which decreases maternal fasting insulin levels. Even brief fasting can result in the production of ketones, which is an alternative fuel source, but carries the risk of fetal brain damage.

The normal energy metabolism of pregnancy and the maternal–fetal relationship have implications for women with insulin-dependent DM. During the first half of pregnancy, the increased transfer of maternal glucose to the fetus, along with the potential lower food intake because of nausea, may result in reduced insulin requirements. In the second half of pregnancy, the diabetogenic effects of the placental hormones override the continuous fetal drain of glucose, so insulin requirements are increased by as much as 70% to 100% over prepregnant requirements. The risk of ketoacidosis is also increased; pregnant women with DM need frequent monitoring. Because of frequent changes in diet and insulin, these women are best served by a team of professionals, including a registered dietitian experienced in DM management.

Diet is critical in the management of pregnant women with DM. Increased energy intake is dependent on prepregnancy weight, physical activity level, and adequacy of weight gain. It is important to maintain regular meals and snacks, including a bedtime snack to avoid overnight ketonemia. More structured eating schedules and balanced distribution of food in the pregnant state are usually needed to achieve a normoglycemic state. More frequent follow-up visits are needed for women with DM so that the team can monitor weight gain, blood glucose control, and energy and nutrient intake and adjust meal and snack plans or insulin doses as needed.

GESTATIONAL DIABETES

Pregnant women without known prior diabetes should be screened for gestational diabetes between the 24th and 28th weeks of gestation (USPSTF, 2021b). A two-step approach for gestational diabetes is more commonly used in the United States (ACOG, 2017). The two-step approach employs a 50-g oral glucose tolerance test (OGTT) between 24 and 28 weeks of gestation. If the screening threshold is exceeded, the OGTT is repeated and a diagnosis is made after two or more glucose values are at or above the specified glucose thresholds (ACOG, 2017).

The nutritional recommendations for gestational diabetes are like those for preexisting DM, with more frequent prenatal evaluations. Management goals include providing adequate energy and nutrients to support optimum weight gain without episodes of hyperglycemia or ketonemia. Intensive and frequent self-monitoring and healthcare team evaluations of blood glucose, weight gain, dietary intake and meal and snack timing, and urinary ketones are essential, followed by appropriate adjustments in food intake and meal plans (American Diabetes Association, 2023).

Women with gestational diabetes are at increased risk for postpartum type 2 DM and should be tested for persistent diabetes or prediabetes at 4 to 12 weeks postpartum with a 75-g OGTT using nonpregnancy criteria (American Diabetes Association, 2023).

PICA

Pica is the behavior of eating nonfood substances. Although occurring in the broad population, it is most common in pregnant women. Usual substances consumed are clay, starch (laundry starch and chalk), and ice. Pica is associated with a higher incidence of malnutrition because it displaces foods providing needed nutrients. There is a strong link between pica and iron deficiency; it is thought that some of those substances may bind to iron, preventing absorption (Rainville, 1998). Other negative consequences from pica can include intestinal obstruction and toxic levels of heavy metals such as lead.

The reasons for pica are not clearly identified. Culture and tradition passed from generation to generation are important factors. Some reports indicate that women believe these substances relieve nausea, prevent vomiting, relieve dizziness, cure swelling, and stop headaches. Pica behavior is not easy to discourage, but the potentially dangerous consequences should be avoided.

For the practitioner, the immediate need is to identify the pica behavior, which is rarely revealed spontaneously. A dietary intake assessment can address this by asking about cravings or eating unusual substances while obtaining an overall diet pattern. If pica behavior is acknowledged, the practitioner should identify the extent of the amount and frequency, followed by a more thorough dietary and biochemical assessment. The client then can be offered nutrition education regarding the potential harm of the pica behavior, as well as nutritional guidance for strategies to improve their diet for pregnancy.

FOOD SAFETY

Pregnant women should take caution to avoid food-borne illnesses. Bacteria of greatest concern for this special population are *Listeria monocytogenes, Toxoplasma gondii, Brucella* species, *Salmonella* species, and *Campylobacter jejuni*. Listeriosis, caused by *L. monocytogenes*, can cause premature delivery, stillbirth, or newborn infection. During pregnancy, women should avoid unpasteurized (raw) juices; raw sprouts; and unpasteurized (raw) dairy products, including soft or homemade cheese; and raw or undercooked meat, fish, eggs, and poultry (USDA & DHHS, 2020). Luncheon meat and hot dogs, if consumed, should be heated to steaming hot (165°F) to kill the *Listeria* organisms (Kaiser et al., 2014).

The FDA also recommends that pregnant women avoid eating large fish that accumulate high levels of methylmercury (see discussion of Fat, under Energy and Macronutrient Needs). Women are also advised to contact their state or local health departments regarding methylmercury or other contaminants in local fish and seafood, as noted (FDA, 2021).

FOOD TABOOS

Superstitions and taboos about food are as old as human life. Pregnancy seems to be a time of great concern about food taboos, with strong connotation as to what is beneficial or harmful. When these taboos are grounded in ignorance, they can have a deleterious effect on the pregnant woman's diet. Many superstitions have been associated with protein and protein-rich foods, which can be particularly harmful if the taboo leads to restricted consumption and the pregnant women not meeting needs. Alternatively, if the taboo leads to consumption over the tolerable upper limit, this too may be problematic. Some food beliefs in pregnancy center on limiting weight gain to have a smaller baby who is easier to deliver. Many food avoidances are rooted in religious or cultural practices that are believed to impart positive qualities in the offspring.

Healthcare practitioners should remember that a belief does not necessarily imply practice. In our rapidly changing multicultural society, assumptions cannot be made about dietary beliefs and practices based on ethnicity or culture alone. In working with pregnant women who have unhealthy dietary practices based on beliefs or taboos, it is essential to understand and listen to the woman's view, provide explanation and information, and then negotiate.

ADOLESCENT PREGNANCY

Pregnancy in adolescence poses potential physical and psychological risks because adolescence is a period of rapid growth and development with increased nutrient

production, regular suckling is required, which triggers the hormonal response of prolactin secretion. The hormone oxytocin is also triggered by suckling for milk ejection and letdown (O'Connor & Picciano, 2014).

Time and maternal diet are significant factors in the determination of milk composition, as early milk has a higher composition of nitrogen and total protein, fat-soluble vitamins, phosphorus, sodium, potassium, chloride, and micronutrient minerals but less lactose, total lipids, and water-soluble vitamins; other constituents are similar between early and mature milk (Picciano, 2001). Maternal intake of fatty acids, vitamin B_{12}, thiamin, riboflavin, vitamin B_6, vitamin A, selenium, and iodine, as well as alcohol and caffeine, are reflective from mother's diet to milk. Independent of maternal intake, milk can maintain adequate levels of nutrients when maternal intake is suboptimal by drawing upon maternal stores. However, if a deficiency persists, milk concentrations of the deficient nutrient can also become inadequate. Lipids are the most variable constituents of human milk, which is a rich source of the essential fatty acids LA and ALA, as well as their long-chain polyunsaturated fatty acid (LCPUFA) derivatives, arachidonic acid (AA) and DHA. AA and DHA can be found in some infant formula, as they are major components of the brain, retina, and nervous tissue lipids early in life. Studies have inconclusive evidence for the supplementation of the mother or formula with LCPUFA to enhance infant and child visual acuity or neurodevelopment (Delgado-Noguera et al., 2015). One of the benefits of breastfeeding is that the infant receives more than nutrients alone from human milk. Some additional components include anti-inflammatory agents, immunoglobulins, antimicrobials, antioxidants, oligosaccharides, cytokines, hormones, and growth factors (Chirico et al., 2008).

The recommended energy increase for a breastfeeding mother reflects the production of approximately 750 mL of milk per day but varies with each woman. This assumes exclusive breastfeeding; mothers of infants who receive supplemental infant formula will produce less milk and require less energy. Energy needs are higher if the postpartum woman is also very active or nursing more than one infant. The amount of milk produced usually decreases after 6 months of age as solids are added to the infant's diet. Women who are obese before pregnancy or gain excessive weight during pregnancy may not need much more energy intake. The maternal fat stores accumulated during pregnancy are expected to provide some of the energy for breast milk production in the early months of breastfeeding.

The postpartum pattern of weight loss during lactation varies greatly from woman to woman. Many will gradually lose 1 to 2 lb per week while nursing, whereas others do not. Continued breastfeeding, moderate to high levels of physical activity, and less than 20 lb GWG are factors that promote postpartum weight loss in women with prepregnancy obesity (Dalrymple et al., 2021).

Early in lactation, primary issues include sore nipples, engorgement, infection, and leaking. Clinicians who counsel lactating women should reinforce a varied and healthy diet, urge avoidance of restrictive dieting attempts, and recommend 3,800 mL/day of total liquid for adequate milk production. As women may not automatically feel thirsty to consume that amount, practitioners suggest that the nursing mother drink something each time they sit down to nurse. Consuming 16 oz

(1-pint glass or approximately 475 mL) at each of six feedings in a 24-hour period results in an intake of 2,850 mL and requires only an additional 1,000 mL at other times during the day to meet the recommended fluid intake for lactating women.

Breastfed infants as a group tend to grow somewhat slower than do bottle-fed infants. On occasion, a nursing infant may fail to thrive while appearing to nurse adequately. Rather than providing a supplemental bottle right away, possible contributing factors should be thoroughly explored. These include maternal factors (stress, fatigue, use of oral contraceptives or other drugs, smoking, illness, poor diet, and excessive caffeine) and infant factors (poor suck, infrequent feeding, increased energy needs, infection, malabsorption, reflux, vomiting, and diarrhea). The healthcare practitioner can be critical in identifying the contributing factors and working with the mother and infant to find the best strategies to solve the problem.

Nursing mothers are likely to voice other concerns about diet and breastfeeding issues such as:

1. **Vitamin and mineral supplementation for the infant:** Vitamin D (400 IU) is recommended.
2. **Allergic reaction of the baby to a compound in the breast milk:** Most babies tolerate breast milk very well. A minority, however, may demonstrate an adverse reaction to a diet-derived component in breast milk. This is more often seen in highly allergenic families. Cow's milk protein is reported to be the major culprit. If this occurs, lactating women should be advised to avoid the potentially problematic food and assess the infant's behavior in the next few days. If the dietary change is beneficial for the baby, the mother should make sure her own diet is adequate.
3. **Contaminants in breast milk:** Lactating women are often exposed to a variety of non-nutritional substances that may be transferred to their milk. These substances include drugs, environmental pollutants, viruses, caffeine, and alcohol. Although moderate amounts of many of these agents are believed to pose no risk to nursing infants, some substances provoke concern because of known or suspected adverse reactions (Lawrence & Lawrence, 2005).
4. **HIV/AIDS and breast milk:** Evidence suggests that HIV can be transmitted through breast milk. In developed countries, it is recommended that HIV-positive mothers do not breastfeed their infants (Committee on Pediatric AIDS, 2013).
5. **COVID-19 and breast milk:** There is growing evidence concerning the safety of breast milk from SARS-CoV-2 positive mothers (Kalampokas et al., 2021). For example, one study tested multiple samples of milk and breast skin swabs from SARS-CoV-2 positive lactating mothers; SARS-CoV-2 was not detected in any milk sample; rather it is likely a contributor to passive immunity through the identification of anti-SARS-CoV-2 immunoglobulin A in the extracted breast milk (Pace et al., 2021). Further, 71% of the breast skin swabs were negative for SARS-CoV-2 and after washing the breast skin, 93% (27/29) of skin swab samples tested negative for SARS-CoV-2 (Pace et al., 2021). This data demonstrate that lactating women with COVID-19 illness can continue to breastfeed and that simple precautions

such as masking, handwashing, and breast washing prior to feeding reduce airborne or household COVID-19 transmission to the breastfeeding infant. COVID-19 vaccination can affect lactation and milk content. Lactating women who obtained the messenger RNA COVID-19 vaccine have reported a reduction in milk supply, which rebounded to normal within 72 hours of the vaccine without any intervention (Bertrand et al., 2021). After vaccination a sample of pregnant and lactating women's breast milk and infant cord blood contained SARS-CoV-2 specific antibodies, which suggests transfer of immunity for neonates and newborns (Collier et al., 2021).

Promotion of Breastfeeding

The decision to breastfeed or not to breastfeed is usually made during pregnancy. Therefore, information and counseling about nursing should be provided to the mother and her partner during prenatal visits, in childbirth classes, and through community programs. Nurses working in a variety of settings can play an important role in providing this education and counseling. Additional knowledge (the specific how-to) and supportive counseling are key to later successful and sustained breastfeeding. The hospital nurse or lactation specialist can provide practical tips and demonstration before the mother and baby go home. Hospitals that adopt the guidelines of the Baby-Friendly Hospital Initiative provide trained staff that support initiating breastfeeding in the first half hour of life, offer 24-hour rooming-in, do not give bottles or pacifiers, and provide discharge support or referral for breastfeeding assistance (Baby-Friendly USA, 2018).

The La Leche League International, an educational and support group founded by nursing mothers, is found in most communities. Hospitals with a large obstetrics department often have lactation specialists or other trained nurses available for phone consultation to new mothers. Those with the credentials, such as international board-certified lactation consultants (IBCLCs), have completed the International Board of Lactation Consultant Examiners certification process. The national Healthy Mothers, Healthy Babies programs include breastfeeding promotion, as does the Special Supplemental Nutrition Program for Women, Infants, and Children program. Trained peer counselors are available in some community programs; they frequently work with groups who have low rates of breastfeeding, such as low-income women, teens, and minority women.

NUTRITION–RELATED CONCERNS OF WOMEN

Obesity and Weight Management

OBESITY PREVALENCE

Obesity is a serious public health concern in the United States and all North America. Data from 2017/2018 show that 42.4% of adults in the United States are obese with a BMI of 30 kg/m^2 or more (Hales et al., 2020). There were no gender differences in the prevalence of obesity as a whole; however, the prevalence of obesity was highest in non-Hispanic Black adult women compared to all other race/ethnic groups and compared to non-Hispanic Black men (Hales et al., 2020).

DEFINITION OF OVERWEIGHT AND OBESITY

BMI is calculated by dividing a person's weight in kilograms by height in meters squared. For instance, a woman who is 64 inches (1.63 m) tall and weighs 130 lb (59 kg) has a BMI of 22.3. The use of BMI eliminates the dependence on body frame size. A limitation of BMI is the use in populations with greater muscle tone, as some would be categorized as overweight or obese because of a muscular build. Health risks from excess weight begin when BMI exceeds 25, called *overweight*. *Obesity* is defined by a BMI of 30 or greater (Table 13.9). Obesity can be further categorized as grade 1 (BMI 30–34.9), grade 2 (BMI 35–39.9), and grade 3/severe obesity (BMI ≥40). Severe obesity is more prevalent in women compared to men (11.5 vs. 6.9%, respectively) and most prevalent in non-Hispanic Black adults (13.8%) compared to all other groups (Hales et al., 2020).

Abdominal obesity may be a better predictor than overall obesity for disease risks and causes of death. Waist circumference (WC) is the most common, noninvasive measure of abdominal obesity and can replace use of the waist-to-hip ratio as a routine clinical assessment measure (Ross et al., 2020). When used with BMI, the combination is a predictor for increased risk of type 2 DM, hypertension, and CVD; see Table 13.9 for risk assessments. Trends over time have shown increases in BMI and WC, with differences by gender and race or ethnicity. Using age-adjusted BMI and age-adjusted WC data from NHANES 2011–2012 to 2017–2018, significant increases in BMI were observed in non-Hispanic Asian women and women categorized as "other race." A nonsignificant increase was seen in Hispanic, non-Hispanic White, and non-Hispanic Black women (Liu et al., 2021). Likewise, overall increases in WC were observed for all racial and ethnic groups; however, the increases could be attributed to increases in male WC as there were no significant changes observed for women, except for women categorized as "other race" (Liu et al., 2021). It is important to note that the prevalence of obesity in these studies, measured by BMI, was higher than *Healthy People 2030* targets for all race and ethnic groups and for both genders. So while it seems that obesity rates may be plateauing, the prevalence remains an issue.

CONSEQUENCES OF OBESITY

Adults with obesity are at increased mortality risk and the risk grows with each obesity category (Flegal et al., 2013). It is well known that obesity increases the risk of many chronic diseases such as hypertension, coronary heart disease, DM, stroke, gallbladder disease, osteoarthritis, asthma, sleep apnea, and certain cancers (e.g., ovarian, breast, endometrial, colon). More recently, obesity was recognized as a risk factor for severe COVID-19 infection and is associated with greater risk for hospitalization, greater hospital care needs, and death in a dose response relationship with increasing BMI (Kompaniyets et al., 2021). Women with obesity are

TABLE 13.9 BMI Categories and WC Measurements With Associated Disease Risk

CATEGORY	BMI (KG/M²)	OBESITY CATEGORY	DISEASE RISK[a] RELATIVE TO NORMAL WEIGHT AND WC	
			WOMEN ≤88 CM (35 INCHES)	WOMEN >88 CM (35 INCHES)
Underweight	<18.5			
Normal	18.5–24.9			
Overweight	25.0–29.9		Increased	High
Obesity	30.0–34.9	I	High	Very high
	35.0–39.9	II	Very high	Very high
Severe obesity	≥40.0	III	Extremely high	Extremely high

[a]Disease risk for type 2 diabetes, hypertension, and cardiovascular disease.
BMI, body mass index; WC, waist circumference.
Source: *National Heart, Lung, and Blood Institute. (n.d.).* Classification of overweight and obesity by BMI, waist circumference and associated disease risks. *https://www.nhlbi .nih.gov/health/educational/lose_wt/BMI/bmi_dis.htm*

more likely to present with reproductive dysfunctions resulting from alterations in the hypothalamic–pituitary–ovarian axis, oocyte quality, and endometrial receptivity (Klenov & Jungheim, 2014). More difficult to measure is the stigma that is often experienced by women with obesity. Weight stigma and weight bias are common for healthcare professionals, including nurses, to express when working with clients with obesity. A first step in exploring personal attitudes is self-assessment. Box 13.2 contains questions that you can ask yourself and strategies to consider to reduce bias. Weight bias in healthcare can have negative effects on the client's mental and physical health and need to be minimized whenever possible.

Box 13.2 Questions for Identifying Personal Attitudes About Body Weight

- What assumptions do I make based only on weight regarding a person's character, intelligence, professional success, health status, or lifestyle behaviors?
- Could my assumptions be impacting my ability to help my patients?
- How comfortable am I working with patients of different sizes?
- What kind of feedback do I give to obese patients?
- Do I give appropriate feedback to encourage healthful behavior change?
- Am I sensitive to the needs and concerns of obese individuals?
- Do I consider all of the patient's presenting problems, in addition to weight?
- What are my views about the cause of obesity? How does this impact my attitudes about obese persons?
- Do I treat the individual or only the condition?
- What are common stereotypes about obese persons? Do I believe these to be true or false? What are my reasons for this?

Strategies for Providers to Reduce Bias

- Recognize the complex etiology of obesity and its multiple contributors, including genetics, biology, sociocultural influences, the environment, and individual behavior.
- Recognize that many obese patients have tried to lose weight repeatedly.
- Consider that patients may have had negative experiences with health professionals, and approach patients with sensitivity and empathy.
- Explore all causes of presenting problems, in addition to body weight.
- Emphasize the importance of behavior change rather than just weight.
- Acknowledge the difficulty of achieving sustainable and significant weight loss.
- Recognize that small weight losses can result in meaningful health gains.

Source: UConn RUDD Center for Food Policy and Health. (n.d.). Weight bias and stigma: Healthcare providers. *https://uconnruddcenter.org/research /weight-bias-stigma/healthcare-providers*

ETIOLOGY OF OBESITY

The etiology of obesity is multifactorial with varying degrees of contribution from genetics, obesogenic environments, and sociobehavioral factors. The dramatic increase in obesity in the past few decades can be attributed to interactions between genes and environmental and lifestyle/behavioral choices. The obesogenic environment, where high-fat, energy-dense foods and large portion sizes are palatable, have a low cost, and are easily available in combination with less work-related physical activity and more sedentary behavior in general, has resulted in an imbalance in which there is greater energy in and less energy out, tipping the scale toward a higher body fat mass (Hill et al., 2000).

The study of hormonal control of food intake and related obesity is an exciting area with new developments on a regular basis. The discovery of leptin fueled research on the genetic basis of obesity. Further, research on the adipokine leptin became more complex with each discovery. We now know that individuals with obesity have high circulating leptin levels; however, the issue presents at the receptor level, where individuals with obesity are more likely than lean individuals to be leptin resistant. Leptin receptors are located at the arculate nucleus of the hypothalamus, and stimulation of these receptors promotes satiety; however, with leptin resistance the signal for satiety is diminished. Gut-derived hormonal signals are also of interest when examining the etiology of obesity. The hormones cholecystokinin, peptide YY, glucagon-like peptide-1 (GLP-1), oxyntomodulin, and glucose-dependent insulinotropic peptide (GIP) are gut-derived hormonal signals that promote satiety. Ghrelin is the only gut-derived signal to stimulate appetite. These hormones are reactive to food intake and some, GLP-1 in particular, are also being used and studied as therapeutic treatment options for obesity and type 2 DM management (Khoo & Tan, 2020).

WEIGHT MANAGEMENT

Americans spend billions of dollars each year on a multitude of weight-loss efforts, including diet books, commercial weight-loss programs (some providing food), weight-loss and healthy lifestyles classes, exercise programs and equipment, liquid and powdered meal replacements, drugs, herbal products and supplements, acupuncture, hypnosis, and surgery. Despite the high level of resources spent on various weight-loss efforts, the percentage of Americans who are overweight or obese has plateaued at approximately two thirds of the population. Many of the aforementioned weight-loss efforts are not successful over time because they have a single narrow treatment focus, appeal to individuals as a new diet but are too restrictive, do not address needed changes in eating and activity behaviors, and/or do not provide information and support. A focus on lifestyle behavior change and a sustainable lifestyle behavior rather than a "diet" is an important distinction to make with clients. A "diet" is often considered a temporary or "quick fix" for weight loss that often results in weight regain when the client returns to their prior habitual intake. A lifestyle change, however, can help the client develop a mindset that focuses on eating behaviors for the long term. Furthermore, the individual-focused approach to weight management disregards the obesogenic culture we live in. To fully address the obesity epidemic, the physical and social environment must be adjusted to promote a culture change to one that reflects health and wellness. Efforts to reduce obesity on a public health scale that are directed toward larger, societal issues have the largest impact.

As healthcare professionals, obesity and weight-management must be understood within the context of the physical and social environment, striving to understand individual, interpersonal, and societal obesogenic environmental challenges to support change. Most long-term successful weight-management efforts for the individual are neither fast nor flashy. They work over time because they include modifications in food choices, activity, and lifestyle and often also include social support. Dieting alone rarely addresses the weight problem on a permanent basis; behavioral techniques incorporated with weight-loss counseling, are a recommended approach at the individual level to promote sustained weight loss (Seagle et al., 2009). Many women trying to lose weight set ideal goals for themselves that are hard to achieve, thus resulting in disappointment and a sense of failure, which colors future attempts. Weight cycling (losing and gaining weight several times over years) is particularly common in overweight women. Many health professionals recommend a gradual reduction in weight with a focus on healthy lifestyle choices, to a level of better overall health if not slimness (Seagle et al., 2009). A 5% to 10% weight loss for those with excess body weight can improve cardiometabolic risk factors. What is important to emphasize is weight management and strategies to maintain weight loss once it occurs. After the weight is lost, energy requirements, for most people, are permanently lower (Polsky et al., 2014). A return to dietary behaviors before weight loss results in rapid weight regain. What needs to occur after weight loss is consumption of fewer calories or an increase in physical activity compared with before weight loss (Polsky et al., 2014). The need for less energy after weight loss has been qualified. To maintain a 10% weight loss in an adult with a starting weight of 100 kg would require a permanent caloric deficit of 170 to 250 kcal/day. To maintain a 20% weight loss in the same individual would require a 325- to 480-kcal/day deficit (Hill, 2009). These quantifications are estimates and individual needs must be considered. A dedicated and significant behavior change must be maintained to achieve consistent, permanent caloric deficits. Determinants of weight loss maintenance include dietary behaviors such as removing unhealthy foods, decreased sugar-sweetened beverage consumption, portion control, and increased fruit and vegetable intake to replace added sugar consumption. To elicit these food behaviors, monitoring behaviors are also determinants of long-term weight loss maintenance as well as increased physical activity. Self-efficacy (the notion that one can complete the desired activity) for exercise and weight management and a high physical self-worth are strong predictors of long-term weight loss maintenance. Programs that promote these behavioral factors are more likely to promote long-term weight loss maintenance (Varkevisser et al., 2019). Overall, a well-rounded weight loss strategy should:

- Meet nutritional needs—except for energy
- Allow adaptation to individual habits and tastes (emphasize slow and steady weight loss)
- Minimize hunger and fatigue
- Contain common, readily available, culturally acceptable foods
- Be socially acceptable and incorporated into family meals
- Help promote regular and healthy eating habits (provide enough energy for regular physical activity)
- Promote self-efficacy for weight loss, physical activity/exercise, and weight loss maintenance

Exercise is an important aspect of weight loss programs and maintenance. A combination of aerobic and resistance training is optimal. The aerobic exercise helps use fat stores for fuel and has positive cardiovascular effects. Strength training increases resting metabolic rate and lean body mass, as well as improves bone density. Exercise alone, without changing diet, can result in slow weight loss. Other benefits of physical activity include stress reduction, a sense of accomplishment, relief of boredom, increased self-control, and improved sense of well-being. Consistency with the exercise program is important in weight management; the activity should be convenient, affordable, pleasant, and relatively easy to do. Many women find classes and group activities to be supportive and reinforcing, but any activity that a woman enjoys should be encouraged (e.g., walking the dog or gardening).

Lifestyle modification in successful weight-management efforts includes analyzing and modifying behaviors relating to weight gain. The use of self-monitoring, problem-solving, stimulus control, and cognitive restructuring help implement these changes (Gee et al., 2008).

Examples include:

- Self-monitoring—Recording the what, where, and when of food intake, as well as feelings and actions affecting eating, helps identify the settings where eating occurs and the antecedents.
- Problem-solving—Defining the eating or weight problem, considering possible solutions, choosing one to implement, evaluating the outcome, reimplementing that one or trying another, and reevaluating.
- Stimulus control—Altering the environment to minimize the stimuli for eating (e.g., storing food out of sight in the kitchen, slowing the pace of eating by putting down the utensils between bites, avoiding the purchase of "problem" foods).
- Cognitive restructuring—Helping identify and correct the negative thoughts that undermine weight-management efforts. For example, instead of overeating when angry, call a friend or go for a walk; rather than considering a dietary lapse as "blowing my diet," use positive self-talk to continue healthy eating.

Many Americans use commercial weight-loss programs, including internet-based programs. Some include meal replacement formulas instead of, or with, food. The diets used are generally well balanced, but each program has different components, such as behavior modification and group sessions. In addition, there are always new popular diets in the media—the dietary approach may vary from appropriate to unhealthy. Diets promising fast results with little effort are appealing to those who are overweight but usually have unrealistic expectations and result in feelings of failure. Consumers should be helped to evaluate these popular diets (Gee et al., 2008).

Heart Disease

Heart disease, a catch-all phrase for conditions of the heart and its functions, is the leading cause of death for women in the United States, accounting for approximately one in every five female deaths in 2019 (Heron, 2021). Cardiovascular disease (CVD) encapsulates heart disease and diseases of the vascular system, such as a stroke. Disparities are present in this national data. Heart disease was the leading cause of death for Black and White women in 2019; however, heart disease was a close second to cancer as a leading cause of death for American Indian and Alaska Native, Native Hawaiian or

other Pacific Islander, Asian, and Hispanic women in 2019 (Heron, 2021). Heart disease is historically thought of as a "man's disease," although nearly the same number of men and women die each year of heart disease in the United States. Much advocacy is placed on heart disease education and prevention for women; however, only 56% of women recognize that heart disease is their number 1 killer (CDC, n.d.-a). For more information on heart disease in women, please see Chapter 43, Cardiovascular Disease in Women.

Diet and a healthy weight are two items of the American Heart Association's (AHA) Life's Simple 7, which notes seven core behaviors and health factors that affect cardiovascular health (Tsao et al., 2022). Nutrition-related findings for cardiovascular health have shown that consuming the recommended five servings of fruits and vegetables a day is associated with 12% lower CVD mortality. For several years, a low-fat diet was recommended for weight control and cardiovascular health; however, the type of fat is more important than total fat within caloric recommendations. Polyunsaturated and monounsaturated fatty acids are associated with lower total mortality. The evidence for saturated fatty acid intake and total or CVD mortality remains controversial (Tsao et al., 2022). These dietary factors support the AHA dietary recommendations, which recommend the consumption of:

- A variety of fruits and vegetables*#
- Whole grains*#
- Healthy sources of protein such as legumes and nuts, fish and seafood, low-fat or nonfat dairy, and lean and/ or unprocessed meats and poultry (if chosen)*#
- Liquid, nontropical vegetable oils (olive oil for Mediterranean diet*)
- Minimally processed foods*
- Minimized intake of added sugars*# (and/or limited desserts*)
- Foods prepared with little or no salt#
- Limited or no alcohol intake (AHA, n.d.)

Recommendations that align with a Mediterranean diet are noted with an asterisk (*) in the list above. Recommendations of the Dietary Approaches to Stop Hypertension (DASH) diet are noted with a hashtag (#) sign in the list above. The DASH diet overlaps in many attributes to the Mediterranean diet but typically includes more nonfat/low-fat dairy and lean meat products while limiting total and saturated fats. The Mediterranean diet is higher in total fat, primarily from the specific use of olive oil, which is high in monounsaturated fat. Both dietary plans are heart healthy and have demonstrated benefits for cognitive and metabolic health. The Mediterranean diet is explained in more detail in the Nutrition and Health Promotion section of this chapter and in Figure 13.1. What is most important when considering the usefulness of dietary recommendations is helping individuals to find a well-balanced and healthy dietary and lifestyle pattern, with attributes to the diets discussed here, that they can follow long term.

Cancer

Cancer is the second leading cause of death for all women, and the leading cause of death for American Indian and Alaska Native, Native Hawaiian or other Pacific Islander, Asian, and

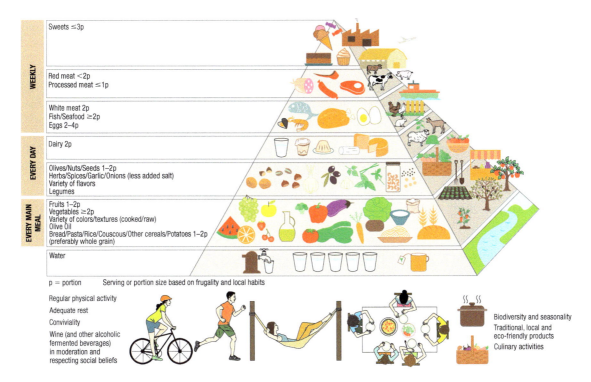

Figure 13.1 New pyramid for a sustainable mediterranean diet.
Source: Serra-Majem, L., Tomaino, L., Dernini, S., Berry, E. M., Lairon, D., Ngo de la Cruz, J., Bach-Faig, A., Donini, L. M., Medina, F. X., Belahsen, R., Piscopo, S., Capone, R., Aranceta-Bartrina, J., La Vecchia, C., & Trichopoulou, A. (2020). Updating the Mediterranean diet pyramid towards sustainability: Focus on environmental concerns. International Journal of Environmental Research and Public Health, 17, 8758–8778. https://doi.org/10.3390/ijerph17238758

Hispanic women (Heron, 2021). Breast cancer accounts for nearly 33% of all female cancer diagnoses and 15% of estimated deaths (Siegel et al., 2022). Lung, breast, and colorectal cancers account for 51% of all new cancer diagnoses and 44% of estimated deaths (Siegel et al., 2022). Death rate disparities are quite large; for instance, Black women have a 4% lower incidence rate of breast cancer yet have a 41% higher mortality rate compared to White women (Siegel et al., 2022). Both incidence and mortality remain higher for men compared to women.

Dietary choices, alcohol intake, and body weight are related to cancer incidence, treatment, and survival. The American Cancer Society recommendations include:

- A healthy body weight throughout life and avoidance of weight gain in adult life
- Following a healthy dietary pattern including nutrient-dense foods, variety of fruits and vegetables, and whole grains while limiting red and processed meats, sugar-sweetened beverages, and highly processed foods and refined grain products
- Physical activity following the DHHS Physical Activity Guidelines for Americans to "move more and sit less"
- Avoidance of alcoholic beverages; if one chooses to consume, women should limit intake to one drink per day (Rock et al., 2020)

Greater adherence to a Mediterranean diet, DASH diet, Healthy Eating Index (HEI) and Alternative HEI (measures of compliance to *Dietary Guidelines for Americans*) dietary patterns are associated with 8% to 17% lower risk of cancer deaths for women (Rock et al., 2020). Similarities among these and other healthy dietary patterns are the emphasis on vegetables, fruits, whole grains, legumes, nuts/seeds, fish, and unsaturated fats, with limited processed and red meats, added sugar, saturated and/or trans fats, and overall excess caloric intake.

Osteoporosis

Osteoporosis is a bone disease characterized by low bone strength, predisposing a person to increased risk of fracture. Bone strength reflects the combination of bone density and bone quality. Women are more likely than men to develop the condition, but the prevalence of men with osteoporosis is rising as the male life expectancy increases. For more information, please see Chapter 35, Osteoporosis.

Dietary measures to promote bone health are lifelong, although most women experience the effects of low bone quality later in life. High diet quality, specifically meeting calcium and vitamin D intake requirements, promotes bone growth to reach peak bone mass in young adulthood and to maintain bone quality throughout adulthood and into older age. Maximizing peak bone mass early in life and establishing positive dietary and exercise habits can sustain the natural bone changes of menopause and aging. Positive dietary habits for bone health include a high-quality diet with adequate protein (at least the RDA of 0.8 g/kg/day, up to 1.2 g/kg/day) coupled with adequate calcium and vitamin D (Anam & Insogna, 2021). Other specific nutrients are associated with bone health and include magnesium, potassium, vitamin K, and vitamin C (Munoz-Garach et al., 2020). Nutrients that may be protective for bone health include folate, vitamin B_{12}, and omega-3 fatty acids (Munoz-Garach et al., 2020).

To help slow the progression of osteoporosis, specific nutrient recommendations include 1,200 mg calcium with 800 IU of vitamin D as well as weight-bearing exercise (Roberts et al., 2021). The DRI for calcium increases from 1,000 to 1,200 mg/day for those older than 50 years (Table 13.3). For many women, this level of calcium intake cannot be achieved with diet alone, so supplements are needed. Although calcium supplementation does not have much effect on bone mineral density (BMD) in the first few years of postmenopause, it does slow bone loss in the late postmenopausal period (Heaney & Weaver, 2005). Food sources to emphasize include low-fat dairy products, small or canned fish with edible bones, calcium-set tofu, and fortified nondairy milk or juice products. Vitamin D supplementation in combination with calcium (dietary sources first, supplementation when needed) is considered the favored dietary treatment for preventing BMD loss and reducing risk of fracture in older adults (Anam & Insogna, 2021).

Adequate vitamin D is required for normal bone metabolism because it is integral to calcium absorption. Older persons are more at risk for vitamin D deficiency because their skin is less able to convert sunshine exposure to vitamin D and because they may have less sun exposure overall, even though sun exposure is not a recommended source for vitamin D conversion. Most studies show positive benefits from vitamin D intake (dietary and supplement combined to meet age-appropriate RDAs). The recommended amounts of this nutrient are increased for older women (see Table 13.3). Epidemiologic trials found that a vitamin D intake of 700 to 800 IU can promote a 26% risk reduction in hip fracture and a 23% risk reduction of nonvertebral fractures in adults over age 60 (Bischoff-Ferrari et al., 2005).

In more recent years, there has been a shift from looking at specific nutrients to understanding how dietary patterns can benefit health. A higher adherence to the Mediterranean diet is associated with lower risk of hip fracture and higher bone density in postmenopausal women (Munoz-Garach et al., 2020). In a study of postmenopausal Puerto Rican women living in Boston, MA, the DASH diet, Mediterranean diet, and AHEI positively associated with bone health, the DASH diet being slightly more protective (Noel et al., 2020). There are few studies on vegetarian or vegan diets; however, those who follow a vegan dietary pattern should aim to obtain calcium from nondairy sources such as tofu or fortified products.

Eating Disorders

EDs, which include anorexia nervosa (AN), bulimia nervosa (BN), binge-eating disorder (BED), other specified feeding disorders or EDs, and other unspecified feeding disorders or EDs, are psychiatric and medical conditions described in the *Diagnostic and Statistical Manual of Mental Disorders* (5th ed.; *DSM-5*; American Psychiatric Association [APA], 2013). These conditions are characterized by eating- and feeding-related behavior that results in altered consumption or absorption of food with significant physical and psychosocial consequences (APA, 2013). Prevalence of EDs is far more common in females than males with approximately a

10:1 female/male ratio (APA, 2013). EDs are more often diagnosed during adolescence or young adulthood; however, EDs can present across age groups with women over 45 years of age accounting for approximately 25% of hospital admissions due to ED (Zhao & Encinosa, 2011). Unfortunately, midlife and older women's ED symptoms are more likely to be overlooked and take longer to diagnose (Samuels et al., 2019). Weight preoccupation, food control, and psychological vulnerability are hallmarks of EDs. Although AN and BN have been identified and treated for many decades, the range of EDs to include recurrent binge eating indicates a wider spectrum. See Box 13.3 for diagnostic criteria for EDs.

An ED may be undiagnosed for some time because of the secretive behaviors and sensitive nature of the diseases. The onset of AN is typically during adolescence, but there is an emergence of late-onset AN in midlife women (Malatesta, 2007). BN can be first observed in adolescence and can continue into adulthood (Ozier et al., 2011). The lifetime prevalence of AN, as characterized in the *DSM-5*, is estimated at up to 4% in females and 0.2% in males (Gorrell & Murray, 2019). The prevalence of BN and BED is estimated at approximately 2% for women and 0.4% for men (Field et al., 2014; Smink et al., 2013).

ETIOLOGY AND MEDICAL COMPLICATIONS

The etiology of EDs is thought to cover three domains: genetic/biological, psychological, and socioenvironmental; those with a biological predisposition are often triggered by an environmental factor (Bakalar et al., 2015).

ANOREXIA NERVOSA

A genetic component for AN is indicated by the observation that the disorder is much more common in pairs of identical twins than in pairs of fraternal twins. It is well documented that there is a disturbance in the hypothalamic–anterior pituitary–gonadal axis, which is likely secondary to malnutrition. The chronic dieting appears to trigger a continuous weight loss and hypometabolic adaptation in vulnerable individuals, leading to a vicious cycle that becomes self-perpetuating.

The medical complications relate primarily to the progressive starvation. These include protein-energy malnutrition, hypoproteinemia, hypokalemia, decreased gastric motility, hypotension, arrested growth, and prolonged reduction of estrogen, which leads to low bone mass and osteoporosis (Ozier et al., 2011). In children and adolescents, normal growth and development may be compromised by pubertal delay, reduction in peak bone mass, and brain abnormalities (Ozier et al., 2011). Serious electrolyte imbalances can occur when vomiting, laxative abuse, or diuretic abuse is present. Muscular weakness, cardiac arrhythmias, and renal impairment may occur. These complications can lead to cardiac and renal damage or to sudden death.

BULIMIA NERVOSA

The etiology theories for BN include addiction, family dysfunction, and cognitive behavioral, sociocultural, and psychodynamic factors (Schebendach, 2008). Depending on the model, different treatment strategies are emphasized. The onset of this disorder is most often seen in the late teens or early 20s, when young women leave home to attend college

Box 13.3 Diagnostic Criteria for Feeding and Eating Disorders

Anorexia Nervosa (AN)

A. Restriction of energy intake relative to requirements, leading to a significantly low body weight in the context of age, sex, developmental trajectory, and physical health. *Significantly low weight* is defined as a weight that is less than minimally normal or, for children and adolescents, less than that minimally expected.

B. Intense fear of gaining weight or of becoming fat, or persistent behavior that interferes with weight gain, even though at a significantly low weight.

C. Disturbance in the way in which one's body weight or shape is experienced, undue influence of body weight or shape on self-evaluation, or persistent lack of recognition of the seriousness of the current low body weight.

Specify whether:

Restricting type: During the past 3 months, the individual has not engaged in recurrent episodes of binge eating or purging behavior (i.e., self-induced vomiting or the misuse of laxatives, diuretics, or enemas). This subtype describes presentations in which weight loss is accomplished primarily through dieting, fasting, and/or excessive exercise.

Binge-eating/purging type: During the past 3 months, the individual has engaged in recurrent episodes of binge eating or purging behavior (i.e., self-induced vomiting or the misuse of laxatives, diuretics, or enemas).

Specify if:

In partial remission: After full criteria for anorexia nervosa were previously met, Criterion A (low body weight) has not been met for a sustained period, but either Criterion B (intense fear of gaining weight or becoming fat or behavior that interferes with weight gain) or Criterion C (disturbances in self-perception of weight and shape) is still met.

In full remission: After full criteria for anorexia nervosa were previously met, none of the criteria have been met for a sustained period of time.

Specify current severity:

The minimum level of severity is based, for adults, on current body mass index (BMI) (see below) or, for children and adolescents, on BMI percentile. The ranges below are derived from World Health Organization categories for thinness in adults; for children and adolescents, corresponding BMI percentiles should be used. The level of severity may be increased to reflect clinical symptoms, the degree of functional disability, and the need for supervision.

Mild: BMI $\geq$ 17 kg/m^2
Moderate: BMI 16–16.99 kg/m^2
Severe: BMI 15–15.99 kg/m^2
Extreme: BMI < 15 kg/m^2
Bulimia Nervosa (BN)

A. Recurrent episodes of binge eating. An episode of binge eating is characterized by both of the following:

  1. Eating, in a discrete period of time (e.g., within any 2-hour period), an amount of food that is definitely larger than what most individuals would eat in a similar period of time under similar circumstances.

  2. A sense of lack of control over eating during the episode (e.g., a feeling that one cannot stop eating or control what or how much one is eating).

B. Recurrent inappropriate compensatory behaviors in order to prevent weight gain, such as self-induced vomiting; misuse of laxatives, diuretics, or other medications; fasting; or excessive exercise.

C. The binge eating and inappropriate compensatory behaviors both occur, on average, at least once a week for 3 months.

D. Self-evaluation is unduly influenced by body shape and weight.

E. The disturbance does not occur exclusively during episodes of anorexia nervosa.

Specify if:

In partial remission: After full criteria for bulimia nervosa were previously met, some, but not all, of the criteria have been met for a sustained period of time.

(continued)

Box 13.3 Diagnostic Criteria for Feeding and Eating Disorders *(continued)*

In full remission: After full criteria for bulimia nervosa were previously met, none of the criteria have been met for a sustained period of time.

Specify current severity:

The minimum level of severity is based on the frequency of inappropriate compensatory behaviors (see below). The level of severity may be increased to reflect other symptoms and the degree of functional disability.

Mild: An average of 1–3 episodes of inappropriate compensatory behaviors per week
Moderate: An average of 4–7 episodes of inappropriate compensatory behaviors per week
Severe: An average of 8–13 episodes of inappropriate compensatory behaviors per week
Extreme: An average of 14 or more episodes of inappropriate compensatory behaviors per week

Binge-Eating Disorder

A. Recurrent episodes of binge eating. An episode of binge eating is characterized by both of the following:

1. Eating, in a discrete period of time (e.g., within any 2-hour period), an amount of food that is definitely larger than what most people would eat in a similar period of time under similar circumstances.
2. A sense of lack of control over eating during the episode (e.g., a feeling that one cannot stop eating or control what or how much one is eating).

B. The binge-eating episodes are associated with three (or more) of the following:

1. Eating much more rapidly than normal.
2. Eating until feeling uncomfortably full.
3. Eating large amounts of food when not feeling physically hungry.
4. Eating alone because of feeling embarrassed by how much one is eating.
5. Feeling disgusted with oneself, depressed, or very guilty afterward.

C. Marked distress regarding binge eating is present.
D. The binge eating occurs, on average, at least once a week for 3 months.
E. The binge eating is not associated with the recurrent use of inappropriate compensatory behavior as in bulimia nervosa and does not occur exclusively during the course of bulimia nervosa or anorexia nervosa.

Specify if:

In partial remission: After full criteria for binge-eating disorder were previously met, binge eating occurs at an average frequency of less than one episode per week for a sustained period of time.

In full remission: After full criteria for binge-eating disorder were previously met, none of the criteria have been met for a sustained period of time.

Specify current severity:

The minimum level of severity is based on the frequency of episodes of binge eating (see below). The level of severity may be increased to reflect other symptoms and the degree of functional disability.

Mild: 1–3 binge-eating episodes per week
Moderate: 4–7 binge-eating episodes per week
Severe: 8–13 binge-eating episodes per week
Extreme: 14 or more binge-eating episodes per week

Avoidant/Restrictive Food Intake Disorder

A. An eating or feeding disturbance (e.g., apparent lack of interest in eating or food; avoidance based on the sensory characteristics of food; concern about adverse consequences of eating) as manifested by persistent failure to meet appropriate nutritional and/or energy needs associated with one (or more) of the following:

1. Significant weight loss (or failure to achieve expected weight gain or faltering growth in children).
2. Significant nutritional deficiency.
3. Dependence on enteral feeding or oral nutritional supplements.
4. Marked interference with psychosocial functioning.

B. The disturbance is not better explained by lack of available food or by an associated culturally sanctioned practice.
C. The eating disturbance does not occur exclusively during the course of anorexia nervosa or bulimia nervosa, and there is no evidence of a disturbance in the way in which one's body weight or shape is experienced.
D. The eating disturbance is not attributable to a concurrent medical condition or not better explained by another mental disorder, the severity of the eating disturbance exceeds that routinely associated with the condition or disorder and warrants additional clinical attention.

Specify if:

In remission: After full criteria for avoidant/restrictive food intake disorder were previously met, the criteria have not been met for a sustained period of time.

Rumination Disorder

A. Repeated regurgitation of food over a period of at least 1 month. Regurgitated food may be re-chewed, re-swallowed, or spit out.
B. The repeated regurgitation is not attributable to an associated gastrointestinal or other medical condition (e.g., gastroesophageal reflux, pyloric stenosis).
C. The eating disturbance does not occur exclusively during the course of anorexia nervosa, bulimia nervosa, binge-eating disorder, or avoidant/ restrictive food intake disorder.
D. If the symptoms occur in the context of another mental disorder (e.g., intellectual disability or another neurodevelopmental disorder), they are sufficiently severe to warrant additional clinical attention.

Specify if:

In remission: After full criteria for rumination disorder were previously met, the criteria have not been met for a sustained period of time.

Other Specified Feeding or Eating Disorder

This category applies to presentations in which symptoms characteristic of a feeding and eating disorder that cause clinically significant distress or impairment in social, occupational, or other important areas of functioning predominate but do not meet the full criteria for any of the disorders in the feeding and eating disorders diagnostic class. The other specified feeding or eating disorder category is used in situations in which the clinician chooses to communicate the specific reason that the presentation does not meet the criteria for any specific feeding and eating disorder. This is done by recording "other specified feeding or eating disorder" followed by the specific reason (e.g., "bulimia nervosa of low frequency").

Examples of presentations that can be specified using the "other specified" designation include the following:

1. Atypical anorexia nervosa: All of the criteria for anorexia nervosa are met, except that despite significant weight loss, the individual's weight is within or above the normal range.
2. Bulimia nervosa (of low frequency and/or limited duration): All of the criteria for bulimia nervosa are met, except that the binge eating and inappropriate compensatory behaviors occur, on average, less than once a week and/or for less than 3 months.
3. Binge-eating disorder (of low frequency and/or limited duration): All of the criteria for binge-eating disorder are met, except that the binge eating occurs, on average, less than once a week and/or for less than 3 months.
4. Purging disorder: Recurrent purging behavior to influence weight or shape (e.g., self-induced vomiting; misuse of laxatives, diuretics, or other medications) in the absence of binge eating.
5. Night eating syndrome: Recurrent episodes of night eating, as manifested by eating after awakening from sleep or by excessive food consumption after the evening meal. There is awareness and recall of the eating. The night eating is not better explained by external influences such as changes in the individual's sleep-wake cycle or by local social norms. The night eating causes significant distress and/or impairment in functioning. The disordered pattern of eating is not better explained by binge-eating disorder or another mental disorder, including substance use, and is not attributable to another medical disorder or to an effect of medication.

(continued)

Box 13.3 Diagnostic Criteria for Feeding and Eating Disorders *(continued)*

Unspecified Feeding or Eating Disorder

This category applies to presentations in which symptoms characteristic of a feeding and eating disorder that cause clinically significant distress or impairment in social, occupational, or other important areas of functioning predominate but do not meet the full criteria for any of the disorders in the feeding and eating disorders diagnostic class. The unspecified feeding and eating disorder category is used in situations in which the clinician chooses *not* to specify the reason that the criteria are not met for a specific feeding and eating disorder, and includes presentations in which there is insufficient information to make a more specific diagnosis (e.g., in emergency room settings).

Source: American Psychiatric Association. (2013). Diagnostic and statistical manual of mental disorders *(5th ed.). https://doi.org/10.1176/appi.books.9780890425596*

or to join the workforce. This transitional time in life appears to be a high-risk period for developing problematic eating behaviors. Since persons with BN are usually in a normal weight range and they are also very secretive, symptoms are more difficult to detect. Most of the medical complications are a result of the inappropriate compensatory behaviors used to counter the binge eating—self-induced vomiting and excessive use of laxatives, diuretics, and enemas.

INTERVENTION FOR EDS

Persons with EDs are best served by interdisciplinary teams, which include primary care providers, nutritionists, and psychotherapists. These teams should be trained and experienced in working with this population. Settings may include outpatient, day treatment, or psychiatric units; for some patients with AN, a crisis medical state may warrant hospitalization and nutritional rehabilitation, including tube feeding.

NUTRITION ASSESSMENT AND INTERVENTION

In addition to the standard diet history, anthropometric (height, weight, and BMI) indices, biochemical data, and a comprehensive nutrition assessment (by a specially trained dietitian) should be obtained. The nutrition assessment should include eating, weight, and body shape attitudes and behaviors, as well as an assessment of behavioral–environmental symptoms such as food restriction, binging, preoccupation, rituals, secretive eating, affect and impulse control, vomiting, other purging, and/or excessive exercise (Ozier et al., 2011). Reported energy intakes may be less than 1,000 kcal/day in young women with AN; caloric intake of those with BN is quite varied. Because of the often limited quantity and variety of food consumed, attention must be given to nutrient adequacy (macronutrients and micronutrients) and fluid and electrolyte balance. Taking the time to determine attitudes, beliefs, and behaviors regarding food and eating is essential to developing appropriate nutrition education and therapy objectives. Some red flags to look for include:

- Avoidance of certain foods or food groups (e.g., animal foods, all fats, sweets)
- Preoccupation with food and calorie content
- Strictly grouping foods as "good" or "bad"
- Ritualistic eating schedules, preparation, and timing and misconceptions regarding usual portion sizes
- Certain foods that can trigger a binge episode

Nutrition therapy for AN initially focuses on refeeding to promote a positive energy balance and eventual weight gain. Increments of the caloric prescription are increased slowly, and weight gain goals may be as modest as 1 to 2 lb/week, with emphasis placed on mutual goal setting between patient and practitioner. The dietary plan should address diet quality, variety of foods consumed, perceptions of hunger and satiety, and potential need for dietary supplements. Psychosocial support and positive reinforcement from caregivers are also essential components of the care plan for individuals with EDs.

For patients with BN, nutrition therapy depends on current weight status. For someone trying to lose weight, a diet plan that does not promote weight gain yet stimulates increased metabolic rate is appropriate. A balanced diet providing DRI of vitamins and minerals eaten at regular meals and snacks will begin to address the cycling periods of restrained eating and binging. The use of self-monitoring techniques, such as keeping a food diary, can sometimes provide a sense of control about eating and help avoid binging. As with other ED patients, mutual goal setting, psychosocial support, and positive reinforcement are important components of the care plan. From the counseling theory standpoint, an approach incorporating cognitive behavioral therapy, interpersonal psychotherapy, or dialectical behavior therapy can be helpful in challenging the erroneous beliefs and thought processes of the person with EDs (Ozier et al., 2011).

Nutrition education, combined with psychotherapy, is key in addressing the long-term outcomes of EDs. The specific nutrition therapy will work best when there is a collaborative relationship between the patient and the nutritionist. Helping the patient separate the food and weight issues from the psychological issues will help ensure more cooperation and progress. Although many of these patients appear to be knowledgeable about nutrition, they have many misconceptions. Nutrition education sessions can include metabolism, energy expenditure, nutrient and energy values of foods, and other topics, while using abstract thinking and a problem-solving process approach.

MONITORING AND OUTCOME

Regular and ongoing monitoring by appropriate team members is important in the care of ED patients, as these disorders tend to be chronic conditions. Outcome criteria include appropriate weight for height; adequate and balanced food intake; regular menses; realistic understanding of food, weight, and shape; and improved psychological adjustment. Therapy can last for years. Follow-up studies indicate that one third of persons with AN recover fully and the remaining demonstrate lifelong problems with disordered eating (APA, 2006). Although early identification and treatment have significantly reduced mortality from EDs, this population is vulnerable to relapse.

EATING DISORDERS IN PREGNANCY

If a woman with a past or lifelong ED becomes pregnant, the healthcare team needs to screen for signs of active behaviors or depression throughout the pregnancy and postpartum period. Postnatal depression is high in women with a history of or a lifelong ED, averaging over 30% (Micali, 2010). Conception and a healthy pregnancy are often a challenge for those with a history of an ED, particularly AN when amenorrhea was long standing. For active BN patients, conception carries an increased risk of miscarriage by two thirds (Micali, 2010). Women with BED who become pregnant are also at higher risk for large-for-gestational-age babies and cesarean section births (University of Arkansas for Medical Sciences [UAMS], 2021). If a woman can conceive, the pregnancy is considered high risk because of the psychiatric history. Screening for past or present EDs should occur at the initial prenatal visit including a thorough medical and nutrition history and the five-question, validated SCOFF questionnaire (https://www.psychtools.info/scoff; Morgan et al., 1999). Assessment should include questions related to body weight, eating behaviors, and weight-control behaviors on a regular basis, especially early in pregnancy (Micali, 2010). Much emphasis must be placed on appropriate food choices to promote healthy weight gain during pregnancy and a return to a healthy weight after birth while paying sensitive attention to body image issues. It is advised for the patient to have regular care visits with a nutritionist specializing in EDs. An interdisciplinary healthcare team of nurses, obstetricians, and registered dietitians is essential in promoting a healthy pregnancy. Additional prenatal visits are also warranted to closely monitor the growth of the fetus, especially in women with an active or a significant history of AN. Babies of women with active or lifelong AN are more likely to have lower birth weight (Micali et al., 2007). Postpartum follow-up is also particularly important, as women with active or lifetime EDs often can see an improvement of symptoms during pregnancy and can have severe reemergence of symptoms postpartum (UAMS, 2021).

NUTRITION AND HEALTH PROMOTION

Nutrition and dietary factors are associated with the major causes of morbidity and death in U.S. women; hence, it makes sense that nutrition is a key component of health promotion and disease-prevention efforts. The role of nutrition and diet in promoting health and reducing chronic diseases is documented for many chronic conditions, including DM, CVDs, cognition and mood disorders, and some cancers. *Healthy People 2030* includes Nutrition and Healthy Eating with 27 nutrition-related objectives that support the goal to improve health by promoting healthy eating and making nutritious foods available (ODPHP, n.d.-b). See Box 13.5 for a list of the *Healthy People 2030* Nutrition and Healthy Eating and Related Objectives.

Box 13.5 *Healthy People 2030* Nutrition and Healthy Eating and Related Objectives

Nutrition and Healthy Eating – General (baseline only, unless otherwise noted)

NWS-01	Reduce household food insecurity and hunger
NWS-02	Eliminate very low food security in children
NWS-06	Increase fruit consumption by people age 2 years and over
NWS-07	Increase vegetable consumption by people age 2 years and older
NWS-08	Increase consumption of dark green vegetables, red and orange vegetables, and beans and peas by people age 2 years and over
NWS-09	Increase whole grain consumption by people age 2 years and over
NWS-10	Reduce consumption of added sugars by people age 2 years and over
NWS-11	Reduce consumption of saturated fat by people age 2 years and over
NWS-12	Reduce consumption of sodium by people age 2 years and over
NWS-13	Increase calcium consumption by people age 2 years and over
NWS-14	Increase potassium consumption by people age 2 years and over
NWS-15	Increase vitamin D consumption by people age 2 years and over
NWS-16	Reduce iron deficiency in children age 1 to 2 years
ECBP-D02	(Developmental) Increase the proportion of schools that don't sell less healthy foods and drinks

(continued)

Box 13.5 *Healthy People 2030* Nutrition and Healthy Eating and Related Objectives (*continued*)

| AH-04 | Increase the proportion of students participating in the School Breakfast Programs |
| AH-R03 | (Research) Increase the proportion of eligible students participating in the Summer Food Service program |

Cancer

| C-R01 | (Research) Increase quality of life for cancer survivors |

Diabetes

| D-D01 | (Developmental) Increase the proportion of eligible people completing CDC-recognized type 2 diabetes prevention programs |

Heart Disease and Stroke

| HDS-04 | Reduce the proportion of adults with high blood pressure |
| HDS-06 | Reduce cholesterol in adults |

Infants

| MICH-15 | Increase the proportion of infants who are breastfed exclusively through age 6 months |
| MICH-16 | Increase the proportion of infants who are breastfed at 1 year |

Overweight and Obesity

| NWS-03 | Reduce the proportion of adults with obesity |
| NWS-05 | Increase the proportion of healthcare visits by adults with obesity that include counseling on weight loss, nutrition, or physical activity |

Women

| MICH-12 | Increase the proportion of women of childbearing age who get enough folic acid |
| NWS-17 | Reduce iron deficiency in females age 12 to 49 years |

Workplace

| ECBP-D05 | (Developmental) Increase the proportion of worksites that offer an employee nutrition program |

CDC, Centers for Disease Control and Prevention.
Source: Adapted from Office of Disease Prevention and Health Promotion. (n.d.). Healthy People 2030: Nutrition and healthy eating. *https://health.gov/healthypeople/objectives-and-data/browse-objectives/nutrition-and-healthy-eating*

Nutrition can be applied to the three levels of disease prevention: primary prevention (aimed at disease risk factors), secondary prevention (screening to detect risk followed by early intervention), and tertiary prevention (treatment and rehabilitation for identified health conditions). An example of primary nutrition prevention is the 5 A Day Program, an education program to encourage people to eat a minimum of five servings of fruits and vegetables a day. Blood pressure screenings and the DASH diet nutrition education program are examples of secondary prevention programs for individuals at risk for hypertension. The DASH diet is high in fruits and vegetables and low in saturated and total fat, with moderate intakes of low-fat dairy. The DASH diet can also be considered a primary prevention for the broad population as well as part of a medical management program for those with identified hypertension. Studies have also identified the DASH diet as one that may delay cognitive decline in older adults (Tangney et al., 2014). Tertiary prevention is the management of chronic conditions through diet, such as application of Medical Nutrition Therapy with a registered dietitian.

The *Dietary Guidelines for Americans* are the current national recommendations for dietary guidance upon which nutritional health promotion programs are based. The DHHS and USDA have jointly published the *Dietary Guidelines* every 5 years since 1990 under the National Nutrition Monitoring and Related Research Act (1990). The *Dietary Guidelines* are based on current scientific and medical knowledge. Current knowledge shows the importance of healthy eating patterns and regular physical activity for good health and for chronic disease risk reduction. The *Dietary Guidelines* are designed for health promotion and disease prevention and is especially focused on CVD, type 2 DM, and obesity, which have a high prevalence in the United States and a strong direct link to nutrition. These guidelines are not, however, designed for disease treatment (USDA & DHHS, 2020). The 2020–2025 *Dietary Guidelines* provide four overarching guidelines for healthy eating at every life stage. (See Box 13.6 for the guidelines.) The 2020–2025 *Dietary Guidelines* emphasize dietary patterns rather than specific nutrients, as well as nutrient-dense foods and beverages to promote a healthy weight (USDA & DHHS, 2020).

A dietary pattern represents the totality of what individuals habitually consume; the parts of the pattern act synergistically to affect health (USDA & DHHS, 2020). Elements central to a healthy dietary pattern include a variety of vegetable types such as dark green, red, and orange vegetables; beans, peas, and lentils; starchy and other vegetables; fruit, especially whole fruit; grains, with at least half as whole grains; diary, including fat-free or low-fat yogurt and cheese, or other nondairy alternatives; protein sources such as lean meats, poultry, eggs, seafoods, beans, peas, lentils, nuts and seeds, and soy products; and oils such as vegetable oils and oils in foods such as fatty fish and nuts (USDA & DHHS, 2020). These core foods can be found in several healthy dietary patterns such as the DASH diet, Mediterranean diet, and with the omission of animal proteins, a vegetarian diet pattern. As stated in Guideline 4 (see Box 13.6), some food qualities should be limited for a healthy dietary pattern. The recommended limits are as follows: less than 10% of calories per day from added sugars starting at age 2; less than 10% of calories per day from saturated fat; less than 2,300 mg per day of sodium and even less for those younger than 14 years of

age; and limit alcoholic beverage consumption to one drink or less for women of legal drinking age, and women who are pregnant should avoid alcoholic beverages (USDA & DHHS, 2020). Nutrient density is a way to evaluate food and dietary quality considering the nutrients the food provides in a standardized (usually 100 kcal) serving and the contribution that food provides to meeting food group recommendations (Drewnowski et al., 2019). Foods and dietary patterns with more of the core elements and less of the food qualities to avoid have greater nutrient density. Unfortunately, the typical dietary pattern for Americans does not align with the *Dietary Guidelines* as it contains too many foods with components to avoid (sugar, sodium, saturated fat) and not enough of the core element foods.

Along with the general guidance that the 2020–2025 *Dietary Guidelines* provide, nutritional goals are summarized into actionable dietary pattern plans. Three healthy dietary pattern plans are provided in the *Dietary Guidelines*: a healthy U.S. dietary pattern, a vegetarian dietary pattern, and a Mediterranean diet pattern. The diet pattern plans can be found for toddlers through older adults by activity and caloric level needs on the *Dietary Guidelines* website (www. dietaryguidelines.gov). Table 13.10 includes food intake recommendations at the 1,600 calorie and 2,000 calorie goals for adult women who are sedentary or more active. These dietary patterns provide recommendations at the daily and weekly level. To further support translation of the *Dietary Guidelines* into action for consumers is the USDA MyPlate campaign (USDA, 2020). The MyPlate icon and message replaced the Food Guide Pyramid, which was active for nearly 20 years from 1992 to 2011. The MyPlate system emphasizes dietary variety from all food groups and portion control using a plate icon to serve as a reminder of healthy eating, but not intended to provide specific messages (Center for Nutrition Policy and Promotion, 2011). See Figure 13.2 for a visual representation of the MyPlate icon. In general, half of a plate should be filled with vegetables and fruits, with grains and protein sources on the remaining half, and diary is included as a glass beverage at the side of the plate. What the MyPlate message does not convey is the heavy reliance that Americans have on processed foods that are high in added sugars, sodium, and saturated fats.

The two additional dietary pattern plans included in the *Dietary Guidelines for Americans* have robust research to support their use to promote health. A vegetarian dietary pattern can promote health when the basics of good nutrition are followed with emphasis on consumption of fruits and vegetables, whole grains, and nonanimal protein sources and with less intake of high sugar, salt, and saturated fat products. The Mediterranean diet has received much attention in recent years for quality of the diet and ease of adoption. This dietary pattern emphasizes fruits, vegetables, whole grains, and olive oil as the main source of fat as well as fish consumption to offset the recommendation for limited red and processed meats. Sweets and desserts are also limited. The Mediterranean diet pyramid (Figure 13.1) is a visual representation of these food-based recommendations with emphasis on the promotion of global health as well as human health promotion. This dietary pattern can also be considered a lifestyle, which is demonstrated by physical activity and culinary activities

Box 13.6 Dietary Guidelines for Americans, 2020–2025: Four Guidelines

Guideline 1: Follow a healthy dietary pattern at every life stage.

Guideline 2: Customize and enjoy nutrient-dense food and beverage choices to reflect personal preferences, cultural traditions, and budgetary considerations.

Guideline 3: Focus on meeting food group needs with nutrient-dense food and beverages, stay within calorie limits.

Guideline 4: Limit foods and beverages higher in added sugars, saturated fat, and sodium, and limit alcoholic beverages.

Source: Adapted from U.S. Department of Agriculture, & U.S. Department of Health and Human Services. (2020). Dietary guidelines for Americans, 2020–2025 (9th ed.). https://www.dietaryguidelines.gov/resources/2020-2025 -dietary-guidelines-online-materials

TABLE 13.10 HEALTHY U.S. STYLE DIETARY PATTERN[a,b]

FOOD GROUP OR SUBGROUP	DAILY OR WEEKLY AMOUNT		EQUIVALENT (EQ) SERVING SIZES
	1,600 KCAL[c]	2,000 KCAL[d]	
Vegetables (cup eq/d)	2	2½	1 cup eq = 1 cup raw or cooked vegetable, 1 cup vegetable juice, 2 cups leafy salad greens, ½ cup dried vegetable
Dark green vegetables (cup eq/wk)	1½	1½	All fresh, frozen, and canned dark-green leafy vegetables and broccoli, cooked or raw
Red and orange vegetables (cup eq/wk)	4	5½	All fresh, frozen, and canned red or orange vegetables or juice, cooked or raw
Beans, peas, lentils (cup eq/wk)	1	1½	All cooked from dry or canned beans, peas, chickpeas, and lentils
Starchy vegetables (cup eq/wk)	4	5	All fresh, frozen, and canned starchy vegetables
Other vegetables (cup eq/wk)	3½	4	All other fresh, frozen, or canned vegetables
Fruits (cup eq/d)	1½	2	1 cup eq = 1 cup raw or cooked fruit, 1 cup fruit juice, ½ cup dried fruit
Grains (ounce eq/d)	5	6	1 ounce eq = 1 cup cooked rice, pasta, or cereal; 1 oz dry pasta or rice, 1 medium (1 ounce) slice of bread, tortilla, or flatbread; 1 ounce ready-to-eat cereal (about 1 cup of flaked cereal)
Whole grains (ounce eq/d)	3	3	All whole-grain products and whole grains used as ingredients
Refined grains (ounce eq/d)	2	3	All refined-grain products and refined grains used as ingredients
Dairy (cup eq/d)	3	3	1 cup eq = 1 cup milk, yogurt, or fortified nondairy milk; 1½ ounces natural cheese
Protein foods (ounce eq/d)	5	5½	1 ounce eq = 1 ounce lean meats, poultry, or seafood, 1 egg, ¼ cup cooked beans or tofu, 1 tablespoon nut or seed butter, ½ ounce nuts or seeds
Meats, poultry, eggs (ounce eq/wk)	23	26	Meats and poultry should be lean cuts
Seafood (ounce eq/wk)	8	8	Includes low mercury fish and shellfish
Nuts, seeds, beans, soy products (ounce eq/wk)	4	5	Beans, peas, lentils can be considered as part of protein or vegetable groups, but should only be counted in one group.
Oils (g/d)	22	27	
Limit on calories for other uses (kcal/d)	100	240	
Limit on calories for other uses (%/d)	6%	12%	

[a]The vegetarian dietary pattern recommends slightly more grains (+0.5 ounce eq/d), and less protein foods total, with a removal of meats, poultry, and seafood. The protein food recommendations for 1,600/2,000 kcal become: eggs (3/3 ounce eq/wk); beans, peas, lentils (4/6 ounce eq/wk); soy products (6/8 ounce eq/wk), and nuts and seeds (5/7 ounce eq/wk). There are more calories available for other uses as well.

[b]The Mediterranean dietary pattern also differs slightly from the healthy U.S. style dietary pattern in that fruit (+ 0.5 ounce eq/d) and total protein food recommendations are increased, the specific increase for seafood is 11 ounce eq/wk for the 1,600 kcal pattern, and 15 ounce eq/wk for the 2,000 kcal pattern. The Mediterranean dietary pattern also has more calories available for other uses.

[c]1,600 kcal are recommended for sedentary women over age 50. Sedentary is a lifestyle that includes only physical activity of independent living.

[d]2,000 kcal are recommended for sedentary women between 19 and 25 years old, moderately active women 26–50 years old, and active women over age 60. Moderately active is characterized as a lifestyle that includes physical activity equivalent to walking about 1.5 to 3 miles per day at 3 to 4 miles per hour, in addition to the activities of independent living. Active refers to a lifestyle that includes physical activity equivalent to walking more than 3 miles per day at 3 to 4 miles per hour, in addition to the activities of independent living.

Source: U.S. Department of Agriculture, & U.S. Department of Health and Human Services. (2020). *Dietary guidelines for Americans, 2020–2025 (9th ed.).* https://www.dietaryguidelines.gov/resources/2020-2025-dietary-guidelines-online-materials

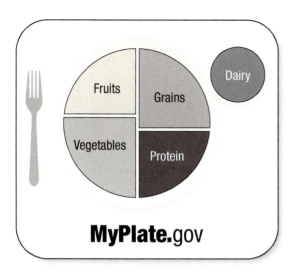

Figure 13.2 MyPlate icon.
Source: U. S. Department of Agriculture. (2020). MyPlate style guide and conditions of use for the icon. *https://www.myplate.gov /resources/graphics/myplate-graphics#*

with others to promote conviviality. As shown throughout this chapter, there are many potential health benefits from following a Mediterranean dietary pattern such as metabolic, endocrine, oncologic, and cognitive health promotion and disease prevention.

The differing approaches to meet guidelines set forth by the DHHS and USDA in the *Dietary Guidelines* demonstrates the importance of individualized nutrition assessment and plans based on cultural practices and personal preference. Registered dietitians (RDs) as part of a healthcare team are best suited for developing specific plans with patients and clients to meet health and medical needs. Interprofessional collaborations and communication among RDs, nurses, physicians, and other healthcare professionals (speech language pathologists, physical therapists, athletic trainers, and/ or occupational therapists) are key to promote health and well-being for patients.

The *Dietary Guidelines* serve as a reference for policy makers and for federal and local health and nutrition programs. Several federal food and nutrition programs from the USDA and the DHHS use these guidelines to serve the most vulnerable— infants and children, pregnant women, and those with low income. These nutrition programs include the National School Lunch and Breakfast Program (all school-age children can obtain school meals; low-income children receive free or reduced-price meals); Summer Food Service Program (free meals for low-income children at day camps and summer programs); Special Supplemental Nutrition Program for Women, Infants, and Children (low-income pregnant women and children up to 5 years of age who have nutritional risk are provided with nutritious foods, information on healthy eating, and referrals to healthcare); Head Start and Early Head

Start (child-focused child-development program for low-income children from birth to 5 years, pregnant women, and their families); the Older Americans Act Nutrition Program (congregate and home-delivered meals for seniors); Supplemental Nutrition Assistance Program– Education program (SNAP-Ed); and direct payments in the form of electronic benefits transfer (EBT) to low-income households.

Many national health organizations also provide community-based nutrition prevention programs, such as the AHA, American Cancer Society, March of Dimes, and American Diabetes Association. Nutrition efforts in health promotion and disease prevention for women are most likely to succeed if they address lifestyle factors, environment, economics (personal and public), and the social and political climates that affect individuals and communities. Partnerships and coalitions among a variety of agencies and organizations can utilize limited resources, even though they take time and energy to develop. Possible partners for promoting good nutrition include public health agencies, primary care providers, schools (early childhood through college), supermarkets, the food industry, agricultural growers and farmers' markets, and print and electronic media.

Nurses working in a variety of settings, including public health, primary care, ambulatory care, school health, and teaching, can have a positive effect on preventive nutrition in the female populations they serve. They are also key team members for initiating nutrition awareness, supporting healthy eating and lifestyle practices, and providing consultation to dietitian and nutritionists when nutrition intervention and counseling are required or requested.

FUTURE DIRECTIONS

Nutrition is an evolving science, with new discoveries and a deeper understanding of mechanisms of action occurring on a regular basis. Minimal nutritional needs to prevent deficiency have been well studied; however, the fundamental shift to understanding nutritional needs or excesses and dietary patterns as they relate to chronic disease and health promotion are more complex. Health disparities and individual genetic underpinnings also add to this complexity. An initiative supported by the National Institutes of Health (NIH) is the concept of Precision Nutrition. This area with ongoing research will enhance our understanding of nutrition for women throughout the life cycle, at important life transitions, and for overall health promotion.

REFERENCES

References for this chapter are online and available at https:// connect.springerpub.com/content/book/978-0-8261-6722 -4/part/part02/chapter/ch13

CHAPTER 14

Healthy Practices: Physical Activity

JiWon Choi

Regular physical activity is an essential component of health practices for optimal health. The accumulating evidence shows that physical activity is linked with numerous health benefits including fostering normal functions and reducing the risk of many chronic diseases (Centers for Disease Control and Prevention [CDC], n.d.; Perez-Lasierra et al., 2022). In 2008, the U.S. Department of Health and Human Services (DHHS) released the first edition of the physical activity guidelines for Americans, which was updated in 2018 (DHHS, 2008, 2018). The key points of the 2018 physical activity guidelines for Americans are listed in Table 14.1. Both the initial and updated 2018 guidelines recommended that adults engage in aerobic exercise at least 150 minutes per week at a moderate intensity or 75 minutes per week at a vigorous intensity. The guidelines also recommended at least 2 days a week of muscle-strengthening activities that involve all the major muscle groups such as legs, hips, back, chest, abdomen, shoulders, and arms. However, only 19% of women report performing sufficient activity to meet the relevant aerobic and muscle-strengthening guidelines compared to 26% of men in 2016 according to National Health Interview Survey (NHIS; DHHS, 2018). The barriers to involvement in physical activity, including, sports are numerous and complex. Sociocultural norms and women's time constraints may deeply relate to the gender inequality in leisure time (Lancet Public Health, 2019).

Because women often put their own health needs after those of their family, a focus on the importance of regular physical activity is especially important for women. As beneficial effects of moderate-intensity physical activity are confirmed, active lifestyle during leisure time as well as nonleisure time should be encouraged. Women need to be counseled about how important it is for them to keep their health maximized so they can effectively care for their families.

PHYSICAL ACTIVITY, EXERCISE, AND FITNESS

The terms *physical activity, exercise,* and *fitness* are often interchanged, yet they are not the same. The definitions that Caspersen and his colleagues proposed to distinguish them have been widely used since the 1980s. *Physical activity* is defined as "any bodily movement produced by skeletal muscle that results in energy expenditure" (Caspersen et al., 1985, p. 126). It includes occupational work, household chores, yard work, transportation-related activity such as walking and biking, leisure-time activity, playing sports, and exercising. Exercise is a subset of physical activity, which is planned, structured, and repetitive and has the purpose of improving or maintaining physical fitness, physical skills, or health (Caspersen et al., 1985). *Physical fitness* is defined as "a set of attributes that people have or achieve that relates to the ability to perform physical activity" (DHHS, 1996, p. 21). The attributes can be categorized into health- or performance-related components of physical fitness, depending on their relevance to health or athletic performance. Health-related fitness components are later discussed in detail in this chapter in the section discussing the assessment of physical fitness.

RISK FACTORS AND HEALTH CONSIDERATIONS RELATED TO EXERCISE

Physical Activity and Cardiovascular Disease

High levels of physical activity lower the risk of cardiovascular disease (CVD) mortality in adults, even after statistically

TABLE 14.1 Key Points of the 2018 Physical Activity Guidelines for Americans	
POPULATION GROUP AND RECOMMENDED ACTIVITIES	
Preschool-age children	Preschool children (ages 3–5 years) should be physically active throughout the day.
Children and adolescents	Children and adolescents (ages 6–17 years) should do at least 60 minutes of moderate-to-vigorous physical activity daily. The activity should include aerobic, muscle-strengthening, and bone-strengthening activities.
Adults	Adults should do at least 150 minutes to 300 minutes a week of moderate-intensity exercise or 75 minutes to 150 minutes a week of vigorous-intensity aerobic activity. Preferably, aerobic activity should be spread throughout the week. Adults should also do muscle-strengthening activities that involve all major muscle groups on at least 2 days a week.
Older adults	Older adults should do multicomponent physical activity that includes aerobic, muscle-strengthening, and balance training exercise. They should be as physically active as their abilities and conditions allow.
Women during pregnancy and the postpartum period	Pregnant and postpartum women should do at least 150 minutes of moderate-intensity aerobic activity a week during pregnancy and the postpartum period.
Adults with chronic health conditions or disabilities	Adults with chronic conditions or disabilities, who are able, should do at least 150 minutes to 300 minutes a week of moderate-intensity, or 75 minutes to 150 minutes a week of vigorous-intensity, aerobic activity. Adults with chronic conditions or disabilities, who are able, should also do muscle-strengthening activities that involve all major muscle groups on at least 2 days a week. Older adults should determine their level of effort for physical activity relative to their level of fitness.

Source: Adapted from U.S. Department of Health and Human Services. (2018). Physical activity guidelines for Americans (2nd ed.). Author. https://health.gov/sites/default/files/2019-09/Physical_Activity_Guidelines_2nd_edition.pdf.

controlling for the modifiable risk factors (Kraus et al., 2019). Studies have shown that aerobic exercise produces favorable anatomic and physiologic changes, including increased heart size, increased size of coronary vessels, and increased cardiac work capacity. In addition, physical activity influences cardiovascular risk factors, including blood pressure, lipid metabolism, glucose metabolism, and body composition. The role of physical activity on these modifiable risk factors and health outcomes are discussed in the following section.

National surveys have shown that majority of U.S. adults do not meet the physical activity guideline recommendations. According to the U.S. 2015 Behavioral Risk Factor Surveillance System, the proportion of those who met both aerobic physical activity and muscle-strengthening guidelines was higher among men than women (22.9% vs. 18%; Bennie et al., 2019). Physical activity declines with age and is lower in non-White women than in White women (Nagata et al., 2021). Women are reported to participate in leisure-time physical activity, such as sports and recreational activities, less often than their male counterparts (Saint-Maurice et al., 2021). Since people can achieve the recommended amount of physical activity by engaging in physical activity during leisure time, at work, doing household chores, or for transportation to/from places, healthcare providers should encourage people to accumulate physical activity across various life domains.

CVD is the leading cause of death, responsible for about one of every three deaths in the United States (Mozaffarian et al., 2015). Among postmenopausal women, CVD is the number 1 cause of death, affecting approximately one of every two individuals. CVD is a disorder affecting the heart or blood vessels and includes coronary heart disease (CHD), stroke, hypertension, heart failure, and other diseases. The risk factors for CVD can be classified as ones that cannot be controlled and ones that can be controlled. Age and family history of early onset of CVD are risk factors that cannot be

controlled. Age older than 55 years for females is considered a risk factor. Having a parent or sibling with premature (younger than 55 years of age if male; younger than 65 years of age if female) CVD or death from CVD also increases the risk. The modifiable risk factors include elevated blood pressure, elevated serum total cholesterol (TC) and low-density lipoprotein cholesterol (LDL-C), low serum high-density lipoprotein cholesterol (HDL-C), diabetes mellitus (DM), physical inactivity, and obesity.

Women are also at increased risk for disorders of glucose metabolism and DM as they age. Other important health issues that are potentially modified or prevented by exercise include osteoporosis, depression and mood/affective disorders, and menstrual cycle changes and dysfunction. Exercise is also an important factor in pregnancy.

DIAGNOSTIC CRITERIA

People who plan to initiate a physical activity program should be screened for the presence of risk factors for various cardiovascular, respiratory, and metabolic diseases, as well as other conditions (e.g., pregnancy, orthopedic injury) that require special attention when developing the exercise prescription. Although exercise testing before initiating a physical activity program is not routinely recommended except for those at high risk, the information obtained from an exercise test is helpful for the development of a safe and effective exercise prescription. Before the exercise testing, an informed consent form should be obtained from the participant. Exercise testing of individuals at high risk should be supervised by a clinician in a setting where emergent care is readily available. Testing of healthy individuals for research purposes may not require clinician supervision. However, all research procedures must be approved by institutional review boards, and a plan for managing emergency events should be in place.

EKG, heart rate, and blood pressure readings are obtained before, during, and after exercise testing. The EKG is monitored to detect any abnormalities in heart rhythm and electrical conductivity. Blood pressure is monitored to determine if any abnormal changes in systolic and diastolic blood pressure occurs as the rate of work progresses from low intensity to maximal or submaximal levels. It is also important to check with the client, asking about perceived exertion and observing signs and symptoms during the exercise test, such as chest pain or pressure, unusual shortness of breath, and lightheadedness or dizziness.

ASSESSMENT

Physical Activity

Because physical activity is a complex set of behaviors, a good measure of it is required to provide reliable and valid information on its specific components, including type, intensity, duration, and frequency. Several methods are available for physical activity assessment, including self-report instruments, physiologic markers, and motion sensors.

Self-reported information, including diaries, logs, or recall surveys, is often converted to estimate energy expenditure (i.e., kilocalories [kcal] or kilojoules [kJ]). A total of 1 kcal is the amount of heat required to increase the temperature of 1 kg of water 1°C, and 1 kcal = 4.2 kJ. Because the goal of most self-report instruments is to estimate the energy expenditure attributable to participation in specific types of physical activity, a variety of physiologic and mechanical methods can be used to validate the self-reported information by assessing energy expenditure.

Physiologic methods include direct calorimetry (requiring the participant to remain in a sealed, insulated metabolic chamber) and indirect calorimetry (requiring the participant to wear a mask and to carry portable equipment for analyzing expired air). Another method of physiologically monitoring energy expenditure is doubly labeled water (requiring the participant to drink a measured amount of water that has been labeled with stable isotopes of hydrogen and oxygen and collect urine over a 7- to 14-day period). Although the use of doubly labeled water is considered the most accurate measure of daily energy expenditure, the lack of information on specific components of physical activity and high cost for the procedure and equipment for analysis for the urine sample make this method infeasible in large-scale studies. A heart rate monitor is a useful tool for helping the participant maintain the optimal heart rate target zone and assess the intensity of physical activity. However, it still lacks other components of physical activity, such as type.

Pedometers are designed to count steps and can measure the distance walked when stride length is programmed into the device. Some pedometers even provide caloric expenditure. They are relatively inexpensive and easy to use. However, they lack information about the intensity of walking. Thus, pedometers are accurate for measuring steps but are less accurate for measuring distance and energy expenditure. Accelerometers are also motion sensors that measure movements in terms of acceleration. They operate by detecting accelerations along a given axis, and a single monitor can capture a movement in multiple axes, converting the movement into electrical signals (counts). These counts are used to estimate energy expenditure. Compared with pedometers, accelerometers are considered to provide more accurate and detailed information about the frequency, duration, and intensity of physical activity. However, accelerometers are relatively expensive and do not accurately capture certain types of activities (e.g., stationary biking).

Physical Fitness

The health-related components of physical fitness are cardiorespiratory endurance, body composition, muscular strength, muscular endurance, and flexibility (Caspersen et al., 1985; DHHS, 1996). The performance-related components of physical fitness are agility, balance, coordination, power, speed, and reaction time (Caspersen et al., 1985). Cardiorespiratory endurance refers to the ability of the circulatory and respiratory systems to supply oxygen to working muscles for an extended time. The best criterion of an individual's cardiorespiratory endurance is the direct measurement of Vo_2 max, which is the rate of oxygen uptake during maximal exercise (i.e., collection and analysis of expired gas samples). It is expressed in milliliters of oxygen used per kilogram of body weight per minute (mL/kg/min), allowing for meaningful comparisons among individuals with differing body weight. However, the measurement procedure requires expensive equipment, qualified personnel, and a considerable time to administer; thus, its use is limited in large epidemiologic studies and usual primary care practices.

Alternatively, a number of maximal and submaximal exercise test protocols using the treadmill, cycle ergometer, and bench stepping have been validated to estimate Vo_2 max without measuring respiratory gases. In addition, performance tests such as distance runs (e.g., 1-mile walk test, 1-mile run test, and 12-minute run test) are devised to predict Vo_2 max. The individual with a higher degree of fitness is expected to walk or run a greater distance in a given period of time or a given distance in less time. Although performance tests may not provide an accurate index of Vo_2 max, they may be useful for clinicians and researchers to establish a baseline of performance and evaluate interventions. Through regular aerobic exercise, people can increase their Vo_2 max.

Body composition is a component of an individual's physical fitness and refers to the relative amount of body fat and lean body mass. Hydrostatic (underwater) weighing is a method used to measure body volume and density from the water displacement. Although it is used as the criterion for assessing percentage of body fat, this method requires time, expense, technical expertise, and the participant's discomfort with being underwater during the procedure. Another method for determining the percentage of body fat is air displacement plethysmography. In this method, body volume is estimated while the client is sitting in a sealed chamber. Compared with hydrostatic weighing, it is quick to administer and requires less client compliance and less technical expertise. However, the equipment is expensive.

Dual-energy x-ray absorptiometry (DEXA) is gaining wide acceptance as a reference method for measuring body composition. This method provides estimates of bone mineral, fat, and lean soft tissue as the x-rays pass through the client. The radiation exposure is minimal, and the method requires minimal client cooperation and minimal technical skill. The major disadvantages of this method are cost and less-than-easy access to the equipment.

Widely used methods for assessing body composition include the body mass index (BMI), waist circumference, and skinfold measurement. BMI is calculated by dividing the weight in kilograms by the height in meters squared. It is a quick and easy method but can be problematic because it does not differentiate between fat and fat-free weight. Waist circumference can alone provide valuable information about disease risk as a measure of regional adiposity (i.e., abdominal obesity; Ross et al., 2020). Skinfold measurement is the quick, noninvasive, inexpensive method for estimating the percentage of body fat. Commonly used skinfold sites include the abdomen, triceps, chest, midaxillary area, subscapular area, suprailiac area, and thigh.

Muscular strength is the ability of a muscle or a muscle group to generate force, and muscular endurance is the ability of the muscle to continue to perform without fatigue. Tests of muscular strength and endurance include sit-ups, push-ups, bent-arm hangs, and pull-ups. *Flexibility* refers to the range of motion (ROM) available at a joint. As flexibility is specific to each joint of the body, there is no general indicator of flexibility. The criterion method of measuring flexibility is goniometry, which is used to measure the angle of the joint at both extremes in the ROM. Sit-and-reach tests are used to evaluate the flexibility of the hamstring muscles, and the back scratch test is used to assess upper body (shoulder joint) flexibility.

GUIDELINES FOR PROMOTING EXERCISE PRESCRIPTIONS

The basic elements of the exercise prescription include frequency (how often), intensity (how hard), time (how long), and type (mode), with the addition of total volume (amount) and progression (advancement), or the FITT-VP principle. The exercise prescription should be made based on the client's characteristics, including age, capabilities, preferences, fitness level, and goals. For details of exercise prescription for healthy populations as well as clinical populations, refer to *ACSM's Guidelines for Exercise Testing and Prescription* by the American College of Sports Medicine (ACSM, 2021).

INTERVENTIONS/STRATEGIES FOR RISK REDUCTION AND MANAGEMENT

Physical Activity and Blood Pressure

Several mechanisms are proposed to explain the blood pressure–lowering effects of physical activity. First of all, a bout of physical activity has the immediate and temporary effect of lowering blood pressure through dilation of the peripheral blood vessels. Repeated and regular exercise training induces remodeling of the vasculature of the heart and other blood vessels. Existing arterial vessels are enlarged, and new capillaries developed in large muscles. Furthermore, regular exercise training has the ongoing effect of lowering blood pressure by attenuating sympathetic nervous system activity (Hegde & Solomon, 2015).

The American Heart Association and the American College of Cardiology recommend physical activity for the prevention and treatment of elevated blood pressure (Gibbs et al., 2021). Research demonstrates the role of physical activity in the prevention as well as the treatment of hypertension. Longitudinal studies show that high levels of physical fitness are associated with decreased risk of developing hypertension. In a study involving 91,728 Swedish adults, those whose cardiorespiratory fitness decreased over time (1982–2019) had an increased risk in developing hypertension compared to those whose fitness increased (Holmlund et al., 2021). An increasing pattern of cardiorespiratory fitness observed in a longitudinal study over time with at least four time points for calculating cardiorespiratory fitness change also showed the lowest risk of hypertension in the middle-aged adults (Sui et al., 2017). When acute effects of different types of exercise on blood pressure among 30 hypertensive older women were examined in a randomized controlled trial, a decrease in systolic blood pressure occurred only after aerobic exercise. However, aerobic exercise in the interval mode and resistance exercise were more effective in reducing blood pressure over a period of 24 hours (de Oliveira Campos et al., 2021).

According to meta-analyses including normotensive and hypertensive populations, engaging in aerobic, resistance, or combined exercise training has significant effects on blood pressure (Cornelissen & Smart, 2013; Corso et al., 2016). However, in a recent systematic review and meta-analysis of 15 randomized controlled trials, aerobic exercise was effective in reducing ambulatory blood pressure whereas resistance and combined training showed no benefits among individuals with hypertension (Saco-Ledo et al., 2020). Due to the small number of studies on resistance training exclusively in people with hypertension, further research is needed to confirm the comparative health effects of aerobic vs. resistance training among patients with hypertension. Since the benefits of regular physical activity outweigh the risks, physical activity should be recommended for the majority of people with hypertension.

Physical Activity and Blood Lipids

Because lipids or fats are water-insoluble substances, they need to bind with some other substance to be transported in the blood. Lipoproteins are a group of proteins to which a lipid molecule can attach. Classifications for lipoproteins are based on their size and makeup. The major forms of lipoproteins are LDL-C and HDL-C. The TC content of plasma is a measure of LDL-C, HDL-C, and other lipid components. LDL-C is composed of protein, a small portion of triglyceride (TG), and a large portion of cholesterol. It transports cholesterol and TG in the body to all cells except liver cells and is involved in the development of atherosclerotic plaque in the arteries. On the other hand, the HDL-C is a lipoprotein composed primarily of protein and a minimum of cholesterol or TG. It transports cholesterol from the cells and returns it to the liver to be metabolized. Increased levels of HDL-C help prevent the atherosclerotic process.

Physical activity positively affects lipid metabolism and lipid profiles. The studies have shown that HDL-C levels are more sensitive to aerobic exercise than LDL-C and TG (Wang & Xu, 2017). TG and LDL-C reductions occur when dietary fat intake is reduced and body weight loss is associated with physical activity (Clifton, 2019). Although the biological mechanism is not fully understood, physical activity seems to promote the effect of regulatory lipoprotein enzymes on the increased use of TGs as energy. Lifestyle (e.g., diet with reduced fat intake, weight loss) or pharmacologic interventions, in addition to physical activity, may be required to maintain normal ranges of lipid and lipoprotein profiles for those with dyslipidemia (Mannu et al., 2013).

A systematic review with a meta-analysis of 69 clinical trials in which resistance training was used as the primary intervention among adults found that resistance exercise caused significant decreases in TC, LDL-C, and TG, with an increase in HDL-C (Costa et al., 2019). These data overall suggest that the greatest benefits on lipids and lipoproteins may be derived from participating in both aerobic and resistance activities.

Physical Activity and Glucose Metabolism

During physical activity, energy demands for muscular contraction require that more glucose be made available to the muscles. Because glucose is stored in the body as glycogen, primarily in the muscles and the liver, glucose must be freed from its storage and then enters the blood (glycogenolysis). Plasma glucose concentration also can be increased through gluconeogenesis, which uses noncarbohydrate sources such as pyruvate, lactate, and some amino acids to produce glycogen, which is then converted to glucose. Once glucose is delivered to the muscle, insulin facilitates its transport into cells.

Aerobic exercise has been shown to increase glucose uptake by skeletal muscles, but plasma levels of insulin tend to decline. In addition, the ability of insulin to bind to its receptors on muscle cells increases during exercise, thereby reducing the need for high concentrations of plasma insulin to transport glucose into the cell. However, for the diabetic, special consideration should be given to maintain appropriate blood glucose levels during exercise.

DM is a disease characterized by an elevated blood glucose concentration as a result of defects in insulin secretion and/or an inability to use insulin. Type 1 DM results from severe insulin deficiency, whereas type 2 is caused by insulin-resistant skeletal muscle, adipose tissue, and liver combined with defects in insulin secretion. The management of DM is glycemic control using diet, exercise, and in many cases, medications such as insulin or oral hypoglycemic agents. The beneficial effect of exercise on glucose metabolism is increased insulin receptor activity. Meta-analyses confirmed that regular exercise causes meaningful improvements in glycemic control among people with type 2 DM (Umpierre et al., 2011).

The Diabetes Prevention Program (DPP), a randomized, controlled trial of 3,234 overweight prediabetic adults, found that lifestyle modification aimed at reducing weight by 7% through a low-fat diet and exercise (150 minutes per week) was effective in preventing type 2 DM (Knowler et al., 2002). After 3 years of the intervention, 14% of the group using lifestyle modifications developed diabetes, whereas 29% of the placebo group and 22% of the metformin group (oral hypoglycemic drug) developed diabetes. The lifestyle modification was effective in both men and women across all ethnic groups. These data suggest that interventions aimed at lifestyle modifications can prevent or delay type 2 DM. However, most persons in each treatment group had developed diabetes after 15 years after enrollment, indicating that we still need more effective interventions for diabetes prevention (Diabetes Prevention Program Research Group, 2015).

Physical Activity and Bone Health

The type of exercise or activity performed greatly influences skeletal adaptations. Weight-bearing exercise is activity in which the body weight is supported by muscles and bones, thereby working against gravity (e.g., walking, running, resistance training). Nonweight-bearing exercise, in contrast, refers to activity in which the body weight is artificially supported (e.g., stationary cycling, swimming). Weight-bearing activities are more likely to stimulate increased bone mass than nonweight-bearing activities.

Overall, studies suggest that weight-bearing and resistance exercise improve bone mass during childhood and adolescence, increasing or maintaining bone mass through adulthood (Beck et al., 2017; Weaver et al., 2016). However, cessation of endurance and muscle-strengthening training results in a loss of the positive adaptation obtained by training; the increased bone mineral resulting from exercise is lost if exercise is discontinued (Iwamoto et al., 2001).

Loss of bone mineral (osteoporosis) is a serious health problem affecting millions of Americans. Clinical problems associated with osteoporosis include greater incidence of fractures and considerable pain from the fractures and curvature of the spine. It is believed that the rapid loss of bone mineral density after menopause is associated with the decrease in estrogen levels. However, postmenopausal women are not the only people at risk for developing osteoporosis and subsequent bone fractures. Young female athletes who experience training-related amenorrhea or menstrual irregularity are at risk for bone loss. Individuals with chronic conditions, such as organ transplantation, autoimmune disease, and seizure disorders, are also at increased risk of osteoporosis as a result of either physical inactivity or drug therapies (e.g., glucocorticoids, antiepileptics). In addition to its positive effect on bone mineral density, exercise may help reduce the risk of fractures by increasing muscular strength and balance, thereby decreasing the risk of falling (Cadore et al., 2013).

Physical Activity and Mood and Affect

The therapeutic benefits of physical activity for reducing depression and anxiety were found among people with or without diagnosed depression or anxiety in meta-analyses (Ensari et al., 2015; Rebar et al., 2015). It has been established since the 1980s and 1990s that exercise induces changes in neurobiological mechanisms involving elevations in endogenous opioids and neurotransmitters in the brain, which may be associated with elevating mood and reducing pain (Ransford, 1982; Thorén et al., 1990). Current evidence, however, is limited to provide a biologically plausible explanation for the role of physical activity on mental disorders.

Recently, affect or mood has received more attention as an important determinant of future physical activity. A 2015 review shows that positive changes in the affective response during moderate-intensity exercise was associated with future physical activity behavior in the small–large effect size range (Rhodes & Kates, 2015). However, the relationship of affective response to exercise with key potential mediators of behavior, such as intention and self-efficacy, were inconclusive. More research is needed to understand the process by which affect may influence behavior. Although exercise is considered to produce the positive changes in affect, overtraining athletes are known to experience mood disturbances in addition to physical symptoms, such as bradycardia, tachycardia, muscle soreness, and sleep disturbances (Kreher, 2016). The optimal exercise program for improving or maintaining mental health has yet to be determined.

Physical Activity and the Menstrual Cycle

Female athletes who perform vigorous exercise training can be placed at high risk for menstrual dysfunction. Low energy availability resulting from exercise and/or dietary restriction is hypothesized to cause disruption to the hypothalamic–pituitary–ovarian (HPO) axis (Sokoloff et al., 2016). Decreased gonadotropin-releasing hormone (GnRH) release from the hypothalamus results in the suppression of the release of pituitary follicle-stimulating hormone (FSH) and luteinizing hormone (LH), which in turn causes attenuated estrogen (estradiol) and progesterone concentration. It has been also proposed that the physical and psychological stress from exercise elevates cortisol levels, resulting in the suppression of the GnRH release and disruption of the normal menstrual cycle.

Menstrual dysfunction can include delayed menarche, shortened luteal phase, anovulation, oligomenorrhea (irregular or inconsistent menstrual cycles), and amenorrhea (complete cessation of menstrual cycle). One of the major concerns with absence of the menstrual cycle is the low levels of circulating estrogen (hypoestrogenia) that may negatively affect bone mass. Almost half of bone mass is attained during adolescence and young adulthood. However, late maturing adolescents may be at increased risk of failure to reach potential peak bone mass. There is an increased risk of premature bone loss in women with amenorrhea (Holtzman & Ackerman, 2021).

Physical Activity During Pregnancy and Postpartum

Pregnancy places enormous changes on a body and requires special consideration regarding the amount and type of exercise for the safety of the fetus and the mother. Overall, substantial evidence indicates that exercise is safe and beneficial for healthy pregnant women (Berghella & Saccone, 2017).

The benefits include reduced risk of excessive gestational weight gain, gestational diabetes, gestational hypertensive disorders, and symptoms of postpartum depression (Dipietro et al., 2019). The American College of Obstetricians and Gynecologists (ACOG, 2020) recommends that women with uncomplicated pregnancies should engage in aerobic and strength exercises before, during, and after pregnancy, following the 2018 Physical Activity Guidelines for Americans, which is an accumulation of 30 minutes or more of moderate exercise a day on most days of the week during pregnancy and the postpartum period. ACOG also suggests that activity restriction such as bed rest during pregnancy should not be routinely recommended for the prevention of preterm labor and preeclampsia since there is no evidence documenting an improvement in outcomes and there are multiple studies documenting negative effects of routine activity restriction on the mother.

Pregnant women with cardiovascular, pulmonary, or metabolic disease, as well as those who were physically inactive before pregnancy or who are severely underweight or obese, should seek a healthcare provider's guidance concerning exercise. In addition, the Physical Activity Readiness Medical Examination (PARmed-X) for pregnancy is a useful tool for screening for potential medical problems and assists with exercise prescription for pregnant clients (ywcavan.org/sites/default/files/assets/media/file/2021-01%20/parmed-xpreg.pdf). Maximum exercise testing should be avoided during pregnancy. If a submaximal exercise test is needed, it needs to be done under the supervision of a physician (ACSM, 2021).

Because of the demands of pregnancy, certain types of activities are not safe. After the first trimester, pregnant women are advised to avoid supine positions during exercise because the enlarged uterus can apply pressure to the surrounding blood vessels and obstruct venous return leading to decreased cardiac output and orthostatic hypotension. In addition, pregnant women should not participate in activities with a high potential for contact, falling, and trauma. Exercise involving extremes in air pressure such as scuba diving and exercise at altitudes more than 6,000 feet (1,829 m) could be potentially dangerous.

During the postpartum period, the return to prepregnancy activity should be gradual and based on individual response. There is no evidence to suggest that exercise negatively affects lactation. Findings of studies with lactating mothers suggest that exercise does not affect breast milk composition and volume or infant growth (Be'er et al., 2020; Daley et al., 2012). In addition, the potential beneficial effects of resistance training on bone mineral density were reported in lactating people (Colleran et al., 2019).

THE IMPACT OF THE COVID-19 PANDEMIC ON PHYSICAL ACTIVITY

The coronavirus disease 2019 (COVID-19) pandemic has resulted in a tremendous impact on people's lives worldwide. After the initial outbreak, state governments in the United States issued "shelter-in-place" orders. Federal, state, and local public parks, trails, and beaches were closed, and nonessential services including gyms and fitness facilities were suspended. Overall, physical activity levels declined during the early COVID 19 period when "shelter-in-place" orders were in force (Dunton et al., 2020; Meyer et al., 2020). In addition, individuals from lower-income households showed larger decrease in walking during this period and were less likely to report engaging in physical activity on the sidewalks and roads in their neighborhood (Dunton et al., 2020). They may have poor conditions of sidewalks or crime in their neighborhood, which can deter them from walking. COVID-19-related restrictions and social distancing measures seem to bring more challenges to people from underserved communities who lack resources for active communities.

SOCIAL DETERMINANTS OF HEALTH AND PHYSICAL ACTIVITY

The World Health Organization (n.d.) defines *social determinants of health* as the conditions in which people are born, grow, live, work, and age that influence health outcomes. The social determinants of health include factors associated with physical activity such as walkable neighborhoods, safety, and income that contribute to health disparities and inequities. Compared with White populations, some barriers to physical activity participation are reported more often among Black and Hispanic populations. According to the 2015 NHIS, Black and Hispanic respondents reported crime and animals as barriers to walking more frequently than White respondents (Whitfield et al., 2018). Black and Hispanic adults were also less likely to engage in any leisure-time aerobic activity and meet the aerobic physical activity guideline across all income levels compared with White counterparts (Watson et al., 2021). However, research on broader structural and contextual factors for the promotion of physical activity among diverse population groups is still lacking (Ball et al., 2015).

According to the data from the National Health and Nutrition Examination Survey from 2007 through 2016, significant disparities by sex, race/ethnicity, and income were reported in the proportions of individuals who were meeting the national physical activity guidelines (Armstrong et al., 2018). In the study, female adolescents and young adults reported less physical activity than did their male counterparts in all age and race/ethnicity categories. Also, minority race/ethnic (Black and Hispanic) and low income were associated with lower likelihood of any moderate or vigorous physical activity among females of all ages. Cultural and social contextual factors may need to be explored to address the disparities among Black and Hispanic female adolescents and young adults.

A large number of racial/ethnic minority women are not reported as engaging in regular physical activity. For example, Becerra et al. (2015) reported that among Japanese and Korean Americans in California, being middle aged, currently married, feeling unsafe in ones neighborhood, and being female were significantly associated with lower odds of meeting physical activity recommendations in the 2007 California Health Interview Survey, a population-based survey with six Asian American subgroups (Chinese, Filipino, South Asian, Japanese, Vietnamese, and Korean).

In a systematic review on physical activity interventions conducted among African American women, a few studies reported barriers to physical activity (e.g., family and work responsibilities, unsafe neighborhood) although seven out of the 13 interventions showed significant changes in physical activity (Bland & Sharma, 2017). These findings show that future research is needed to target multilevel components by incorporating individual-level behavioral components as well as interpersonal-level and physical and social environments for interventions for racial/ethnic minority women.

THE CONTROVERSY OF TRANSGENDER ATHLETES IN COMPETITION

Since 2019, state lawmakers have enacted legislation to ban or limit transgender youth from participating in school sports that differ from their sex at birth, mostly often in K-12 schools but sometimes including college (Chen, 2021). The supporters of the legislation claim that transgender athletes who have transitioned from male at birth to female have an unfair advantage to cisgender girls (those who identify with the sex assigned to them at birth) due to inherent differences between men and women. Opponents, however, view the legislation a way to discriminate against transgender athletes and that the reason to block their participation in women's sports is lacking in scientific evidence.

There are no uniform guidelines to determine the eligibility of transgender women and girls in participating in sports. There is also little research regarding the performance of elite transgender athletes (e.g., how much testosterone-suppression regimens reduce physiologic advantages that male athletes generally gain at puberty). The International Olympic Committee (IOC) currently allows transitioned male to female athletes to compete in the games if they reduce their serum testosterone levels below 10 nmol/L for at least 12 months prior to and during competition. However, a recent review shows that the effects of testosterone suppression on muscle mass and strength in transgender women are very modest, indicating that current policies regarding participation of transgender women in the female sport should be reassessed (Hilton & Lundberg, 2020).

FUTURE DIRECTIONS

Women are at increased risk of several conditions that can be effectively modified or prevented with exercise. Partnering with clients to identify clear exercise prescriptions that are feasible in their individual lives is critical. More research is needed that focuses on how exercise can further modify or prevent health risks and how exercise can be effectively integrated into daily life patterns. As technology continues to advance, research examining the efficacy of technology-based physical activity interventions have increased in recent years. Although technology-based interventions using mobile phones, apps, wearable devices, or online social networking are efficacious for increasing physical activity, there is still a need for large-scale randomized controlled trials (Lewis et al., 2017). Additional research is needed to understand how technology can be used to promote physical activity by integrating theory-based behavior strategies into technology-based interventions. Furthermore, it is important to explore multilevel factors associated with physical activity in diverse sociodemographic groups for appropriate adjustments.

REFERENCES

References for this chapter are online and available at https://connect.springerpub.com/content/book/978-0-8261-6722-4/part/part02/chapter/ch14

CHAPTER 15

Healthy Practices: Sleep*

JULIE L. OTTE AND SHALINI MANCHANDA

Sleep is essential for life, health, and well-being. The American Academy of Sleep Medicine (AASM) in collaboration with the Sleep Research Society (SRS) published a consensus statement with a recommendation that adults 18 to 60 years of age should obtain *at least* 7 hours of sleep per night (Watson et al., 2015). In a similar fashion, the American Thoracic Society (ATS) published a policy statement on the importance of obtaining adequate and good-quality sleep (Mukherjee et al., 2015). They also recommend that adults obtain between 7 and 9 hours of nightly sleep. The Centers for Disease Control and Prevention (CDC) awarded the AASM a cooperative agreement project called the National Healthy Sleep Awareness Project (2013–2018; CDC, 2014). The project goals were focused on generating awareness of the growing epidemic of insufficient sleep and subsequent health consequences among children, youth, and adults in the United States. The outcomes from the funding produced numerous public sleep campaigns that promote healthy sleep and supported the current revision of the sleep-specific objectives of *Healthy People 2030* (Office of Disease Prevention and Health Promotion, n.d.; Box 15.1). For the purposes of this chapter, the terms *woman* and *women* refer to those born with a uterus. It is unclear based on a lack of comparative research if sleep needs, insomnia, and sleep disruptions are the same across cisgender, transgender, and other minoritized gender persons. Therefore, that is an area for future direction and need of better research studies.

The continued emphasis on advocating and promoting adequate sleep can be noted in several national surveys that included questions on insufficient sleep. The national Behavioral Risk Factor Surveillance System Survey of adults in the United States and National Sleep Foundation (NSF) Survey are two national telephone surveys that provide global metrics of sleep health (NSF, 2021). The data from these surveys reveal that one in three adults reported sleeping less than 7 hours per night. The problem of daily insufficient sleep increases with each adult age group but is noted to decrease in the ≥65 age group. The 45 to 54 age group has the highest percentage of

people (39%) with short sleep durations (below 7 hours) compared to all other adult age groups. Men had slightly higher reporting of short sleep duration (35.5%) compared to women (34.8%) in the same poll (CDC, 2020), although recent data show women report greater daily impact of sleep insufficiency (NSF, 2021). There are noted racial differences in the percentage of adults with insufficient sleep duration. Native Hawaiian/Pacific Islanders (46.3%) tend to report shorter sleep durations compared to all other racial groups (CDC, 2020). In the United States and other developed countries, many adults and teenagers obtain fewer hours of sleep than the recommended amount per night. It has been estimated that adults in modern society sleep more than 2 hours less compared with 100 years ago before the widespread use of electric lighting extended daily activities into the nighttime. Several studies show that access to electric lights affects sleep duration in studies of indigenous groups in South America (Casiraghi et al., 2020). When participants with access to electricity were compared with those without access, the latter slept about an hour longer, mostly explained by going to bed earlier. Most adults believe that insufficient sleep leads to poor job performance, a higher risk for injury, and health problems, yet 62% of adults normalize daytime sleepiness and often "shake off" sleepiness (the top-rated coping mechanism; NSF, 2020). The prevalence of insufficient sleep coincides with rising rates of obesity, diabetes, and developing other chronic conditions (Mukherjee et al., 2015). Insufficient sleep has been documented to contribute to developing these conditions, and its etiologic role is an active area of investigation (see section on Sleep Health Promotion).

Obtaining adequate quality sleep is a struggle for many women of all ages. Across the adult life span, women complain about poor sleep to a greater extent compared with men and are at higher risk of developing insomnia (Pengo et al., 2018). However, investigators from several studies reported that while women have higher sleep duration than men on objective sleep measures, women have more nighttime awakenings (e.g., determined with wearables, polysomnography

---

*This chapter is a revision of the chapter that appeared in the second edition of this textbook, authored by Carol A. Landis, and we thank her for her original contribution.

Box 15.1 Sleep General Objectives of *Healthy People 2030*

- Increase the proportion of adults with sleep apnea symptoms who get evaluated by a healthcare provider.
- Increase the proportion of adults who get enough sleep.
- Reduce the rate of motor vehicle crashes due to drowsy driving.
- Increase the proportion of high school students who get enough sleep.

Source: Office of Disease Prevention and Health Promotion. (n.d.). Healthy people 2030: Sleep. *U.S. Department of Health and Human Services. https://health .gov/healthypeople/objectives-and-data/browse-objectives/sleep*

[PSG]; Jonasdottir et al., 2021). In one population-based study of 609 men (age 49.1 ± 13.8 years) and 715 women (age 47.0 ± 13.3 years), women showed a higher amount of total sleep time (TST), less stage 1 (of light sleep) and more slow-wave sleep (deep sleep; Bixler et al., 2009). This paradox could be explained on the basis of a higher prevalence of anxiety and depression in women compared with men because insomnia often occurs in these disorders, yet this does not explain observations of better objectively measured sleep in healthy women. An alternative explanation could be stress exposure, which has been shown to be a significant predictor of insomnia onset in good sleepers; women also show a significantly higher risk for developing insomnia. However, these explanations fail to take into consideration the gendered nature of women's lives.

Women's social roles, economic status, and responsibilities, as they endeavor to balance work and family demands, may be an important influence on the assessment of sleep health and sleep problems. An analysis of survey data obtained in 2000 from 8,578 British men and women ages 16 to 74 years revealed that women self-reported significantly more trouble sleeping on at least 4 nights per week compared with men (odds ratio [OR] = 1.49). The odds of poor sleep were reduced by half (OR = 1.27) in models adjusted for age, marital status, socioeconomic factors, worries about life, health status, and mood (anxiety and depression; Arber et al., 2009). In this analysis, four measures of socioeconomic status (not working for pay, income, educational attainment, and living in rented housing) each showed an independent, statistically significant association with sleep problems. The results from this survey raise doubts about the "primacy" of a biological explanation for poor self-reported sleep among women compared with men. A comprehensive understanding of the gender differences in the prevalence of and risk for sleep problems between women and men will require multidisciplinary and social science studies that take into account the gendered nature of women's multiple roles and responsibilities and how these affect time available for sleep. Although men are taking a greater role in family caregiving (Sharma et al., 2016), women are still generally primary caregivers and managers of family activities and health practices; thus, a careful evaluation of women's sleep, risks for poor sleep quality, and the health consequences of inadequate or insufficient sleep is needed.

WHAT IS SLEEP?

Sleep can be defined in multiple ways: a behavioral state, a complex physiologic process uniquely distinct from resting, and as a temporary, reversible suspension of consciousness or conscious awareness. Based on PSG data (see Box 15.2 for common sleep terminology), sleep is divided into two main behavioral states: nonrapid eye movement (NREM) and rapid eye movement (REM). NREM sleep is subdivided into three stages based primarily on different frequency and amplitude of electroencephalographic (EEG) and electromyographic (EMG) waveforms, which are called *N1, N2,* and *N3.* The criteria for visual scoring of sleep stages were revised in 2007 resulting in NREM stages 3 and 4 being combined into one stage, N3, which represents slow-wave sleep (SWS; Carskadon & Dement, 2022).

Figure 15.1 is a hypnogram of a night of sleep consistent with that of a young adult. It shows five complete sleep cycles with only two very brief periods of waking during the night. At sleep onset, after a brief waking period, the first sleep cycle begins with a short amount of time spent in N1 and N2 stages,

Box 15.2 Sleep Terminology and Common Abbreviations

AASM: American Academy of Sleep Medicine

ACT: actigraphy

AHI: apnea–hypopnea index

CBT-I: cognitive behavioral therapy-insomnia

EDS: excessive daytime sleepiness

ISI: Insomnia Severity Index

MSLT: multiple sleep latency test

NREM: nonrapid eye movement

NSF: National Sleep Foundation

OSA: obstructive sleep apnea

PSG: polysomnography

PSQI: Pittsburgh Sleep Quality Index

REM: rapid eye movement

RLS: restless legs syndrome

SDB: sleep-disordered breathing

SE: sleep efficiency (TST/TIB × 100)

SEM: standard error of the mean

SOL: sleep onset latency

TIB: time in bed

TST: total sleep time

WASO: wake after sleep onset

WHIRS: Women's Health Initiative Insomnia Scale

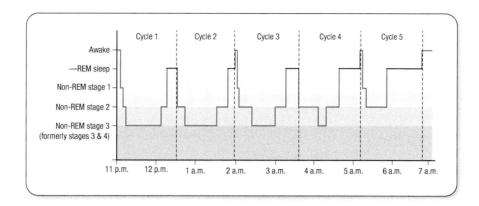

FIGURE 15.1 A typical hypnogram showing sleep stages and cycles in adult sleep.
REM, rapid eye movement.
Source: Mastin, L. (2022). Types and stages of sleep. *http://www.howsleepworks.com/types_cycles.html*

followed by a longer interval of N3 and a short bout of REM sleep. This first cycle is followed by repeating cycles during which the amount of N3 gradually declines, N2 increases, and the bouts of REM are longer, with the longest bout in the early morning before awakening. As one grows older, N3 still predominately occurs during the first half of a night of sleep, but the amount of N3 declines substantially by the fourth and fifth decades, whereas N2 and more frequent brief awakenings increase, and bouts of REM become shorter.

Sleep and Wake Regulation

Sleep and wake are highly regulated processes controlled by brain networks. Humans ordinarily are day active, night sleepers. Sleep and wake are under both homeostatic and circadian (*circa dies*, about a day) control (Carskadon & Dement, 2022). The homeostatic component regulates sleep intensity and duration such that longer intervals of waking are followed by more intense sleep episodes usually of longer duration. Simply put, the longer people are awake, the sleepier they become. The homeostatic drive for sleep rises during the day and dissipates after one falls asleep and throughout a night of sleep. From PSG recordings of sleep-deprived subjects, we know that amounts of both SWS and REM sleep stages increase after a period of sleep deprivation. The intensity of SWS can be measured by the number of delta waves (frequency from 0.5 to 4 Hz), which is increased substantially in the first NREM period after even one night without sleep.

The timing of sleep and wake is controlled by a circadian clock mechanism located in the suprachiasmatic nucleus (SCN) in the hypothalamus. This clock mechanism and genes control the sleep–wake cycle (Hastings et al., 2019). The hypothalamus is considered the master clock or pacemaker for the body, but all cells contain clock genes and show circadian rhythmicity. Clock genes control the timing and distribution of sleep and wake in the daily cycle, and select SCN neurons are thought to operate as an internal alarm clock to actively promote wakefulness (Ma & Morrison, 2021). Circadian rhythms (CRs) persist when people are placed in isolated environments free from external time cues. Light is the main input for synchronizing the SCN to the environment

through specific light detectors in the retina (Saeed et al., 2019). Physical activity and melatonin, a hormone secreted from the pineal gland, also aid the entrainment of the endogenous clock to the environment. This entrainment is important for both optimal functioning and health. CRs are quite stable in an individual, but variations exist among people, called chronotypes. Some people are morning types, called *larks*, who get up early and function best in morning hours; others are evening types, called *night owls*, who stay up late and function best in evening hours. Some data show that the 24-hour endogenous CR is slightly shorter in women (circa 10 minutes) compared with men, which may contribute to the observation that more women self-report being morning types compared with men (Potter et al., 2016).

Sleep Patterns Across the Human Life Span

SLEEP CYCLE DEVELOPMENT

Sleep cycle development from infancy to old age is shown in Figure 15.2. Infants have an ultradian sleep–wake rhythm, sleeping in short intervals of time and waking primarily for periodic feeding. By the time children are 4 years of age, they usually have only one nap in the afternoon and by age 10 years, the monophasic pattern of one long sleep episode at night is fully developed. Whether daytime napping continues into adolescence and adulthood is influenced more by volitional choice, individual sleep hygiene behaviors, and culture than by physiology.

NORMATIVE SLEEP VALUES IN ADULTS

Large studies that provide normative sleep values based on PSG are limited because it is expensive to gather such data from a large number of healthy adults and because most data are limited to White participants. A meta-analysis of PSG sleep parameters from 169 studies using data from 5,273 participants ages 18 to ≥80 years revealed that total sleep time (TST) and sleep efficiency (SE) declined while wake after sleep onset (WASO) increased with aging (Boulos et al., 2019). Mean TST ranged from more than 394 minutes (approximately 6.6 hours) in adults age 18 to 34 years to less than 198 minutes (less than 4 hours) in adults older than 80

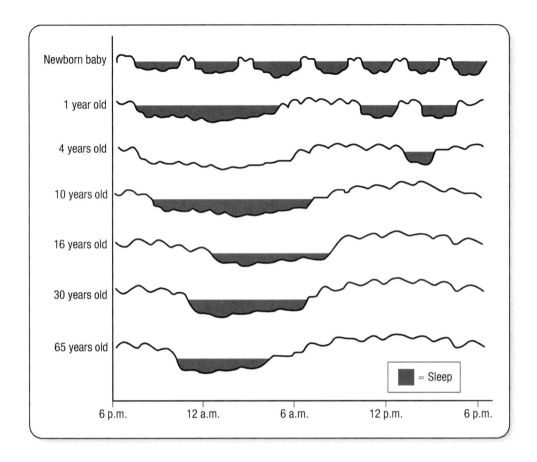

FIGURE 15.2 Sleep cycle development throughout the life span.
Source: Mastin, L. (2022). Sleep cycle development. *http://www.howsleepworks.com/need_age.html*

years; mean WASO ranged from 48.2 minutes in 18 to 34 year age group to more than 77 minutes in adults age 65 years and older. The amount of stage N3 sleep or SWS declined after early adulthood, and was reduced considerably, whereas N2 stage was consistent among the young adults to middle-age groups but decreased in those age 80 years and older. The amount of REM sleep as a percentage of recording time was also consistent during early adulthood to middle age (19.0% to 17.7%) but declined significantly in those over 80 years old (9.9%). Few differences were found between the sleep of women and men; however, the magnitude of age effects was attenuated as participants were not screened for mental disorders, use of alcohol and other drugs, or sleep disorders such as obstructive sleep apnea (OSA) in all the studies. Of note, no data on race/ethnicity were reported from these data.

RACIAL DIFFERENCES IN NORMATIVE SLEEP

Research on normative values for PSG sleep among different racial/ethnic groups is emerging. One historical narrative review (Durrence & Lichstein, 2006) of four PSG studies comparing sleep in healthy White and Black adults revealed Black participants showed more N1 and N2 stages of sleep and less SWS. One of the studies controlled for sleep disorders and compared laboratory with home sleep and found that although Black adults had lower SWS compared with Whites in both settings, they had more SWS at home compared with sleep in the laboratory. Data from the Study of

Women's Health Across the Nation (SWAN) PSG home sleep study showed that among a racially diverse group of 368 predominantly premenopausal women, Black women showed on average significantly reduced TST (363.3 minutes [approximately 6 hours]) relative to White women (393.9 minutes [approximately 6.5 hours]) and Chinese women (390.4 [6.5 hours]; Hall et al., 2009). Black women also took longer to fall asleep (sleep onset latency [SOL] in Black women, 24.5 minutes; White women, 4.4 minutes; Chinese women, 3.2 minutes); had more WASO (Black, 62.5 minutes; White, 47.7 minutes; Chinese, 43.4 minutes); and lower percentage of SWS (Black, 2.5%; White, 4.4%; Chinese, 3.2%). Both Black and Chinese women had SEs of less than 85% and Pittsburgh Sleep Quality Index (PSQI) scores higher than five, indicating poorer sleep when compared with White women. Racial differences persisted after adjustment for socioeconomic status. Another study, based on AASM scoring criteria (Mitterling et al., 2015) in 100 carefully screened White adults 19 to 77 years of age revealed findings similar to those of the meta-analysis: decreased SE, TST, and SWS, although the percentage of WASO increased with a young group (30 years or younger) compared with a group of older adults (60 years or older). No data on gender differences were reported in this study.

Data on self-reported sleep duration yield additional information about differences in sleep among racial/ethnic groups of adults in the United States. The 2007 to 2008 National

Health and Nutrition Examination Survey (NHANES) data demonstrate that Black adults have greater odds of reporting sleep duration of both less than 5 hours (OR = 2.34, p <.002) and less than 6 hours (OR = 1.85, p <.001) compared with white adults (Whinnery et al., 2014). Hispanics/Latinxs and Asians also had higher odds of reporting very short sleep duration (Hispanics/Latinxs, OR = 2.69, p <.025; Asian, OR = 3.99, p <.002). Those with lower incomes and educational attainment were also more likely to report shorter sleep duration, and these associations remained after controlling for health status. In other studies, Black adults have been more likely to report both short (less than 6 hours) and long (less than 9 hours) hours of sleep (Basner et al., 2014; Knutson, 2013). Among short sleepers, regardless of sociodemographic characteristics (except those who were unemployed or retired), adults spend time working rather than sleeping; adults working more than one job had the highest odds of sleeping less than 6 hours on weekdays (Basner et al., 2014).

Whether race or ethnicity is a defining feature of greater risk for sleep-related morbidity and mortality compared with socioeconomic status, living in impoverished neighborhoods, or educational attainment awaits results from future research.

ETIOLOGY AND RISK FACTORS OF SLEEP DISRUPTIONS

Sleep Habits Among U.S. Women

The NSF Sleep in America Poll is a telephone survey with a specific sleep-focused topic conducted annually (NSF, 2021). In an historically relevant 2007 survey, the focused topic was women's perspectives of sleep habits and problems. The survey included 1,003 women 18 to 64 years of age who were primarily White (77%). The major findings from the survey revealed that poor sleep affected all aspects of the women's lives. Many women were struggling to "do it all" and as a result sacrificed time for sleep as well as healthy practices, such as exercise. Biological as well as many lifestyle factors had an impact on their sleep quality. Sixty percent of the women reported obtaining a good night's sleep only a few times per week. Two thirds of the women reported sleep problems a few nights per week, and 46% reported sleep problems every single night. Working mothers (72%) and single working women (68%) were more likely to experience sleep problems and insomnia symptoms. Other factors associated with nighttime awakenings included noise (39%), child care (20%), and pets (17%). Nearly 50% of women reported that they were the only care providers for children at night. Women also reported excessive daytime sleepiness (EDS) accompanied by (a) experiencing high stress, anxiety, and worries (80%); (b) feeling unhappy or sad (55%); spending less time with friends (39%); (c) being too tired for sex (33%); (d) driving drowsy at least once a month; and (e) being late for work (20%). Some of the women in this survey routinely used prescription antidepressants (12%) or hypnotics (8%), or over-the-counter sleep aids (15%). Compared with women who reported excellent to very good health, women who reported

fair to poor health or had a body mass index (BMI) of 30 or above were more likely to experience symptoms of a sleep disorder or had been given a diagnosis of a sleep disorder, missed work because of sleepiness, and use a sleep aid a few nights per week. The findings in this survey are remarkable in that 80% of the women considered daytime sleepiness as something to accept and to keep going through (NSF, 2007). The 2020 poll reaffirms that women on average feel sleepy 3.4 days per week with 44% noting occasional interference with activities of daily living. This is higher compared to men who feel sleepy 2.7 days with 36% reporting occasional effects of sleepiness. To cope with daytime sleepiness, 30% to 33% of women often consume caffeinated beverages (e.g., coffee, soda) to deal with sleepiness (NSF, 2020). Caffeine is an antagonist for adenosine receptors in the brain, and adenosine is thought to be an endogenous substance underlying the sleep drive that rises during the day (Porkka-Heiskanen et al., 2013). Caffeine has at least a 6-hour half-life, probably longer in older adults, such that caffeinated beverages consumed in the afternoon or early evening may lead to difficulty falling and staying asleep. Thus, consuming caffeine, although an effective countermeasure for daytime sleepiness, eventually may contribute to a vicious cycle of poor sleep, daytime sleepiness, more caffeine consumption, and poor sleep (Clark & Landolt, 2017).

SLEEP IN A SOCIAL CONTEXT

Women are vulnerable to limiting sleep time because of work schedules, family routines, and especially caring for children. Data from a report from an analysis of the 2011 to 2013 American Time Use Survey (ATUS) provided insights into who provides the majority of "informal" or "nonpaid" care to others, mostly in the form of family obligations to care for children and/or elders living in the same household (Dukhovnov & Zagheni, 2015). The sample of approximately 12,000 persons was designed to be representative of the U.S. population. These analyses revealed that nearly one third of adults in the United States provide informal care to others, and among these, women between the ages of 30 and 50 years made up the highest proportion. Women in the so-called sandwich generation spend more time per day in providing care compared with the general population and the highest proportion of time was spent in parenting, caring for one's children rather than elders (Evans et al., 2017). It is important to note that during the stage of life when sleep patterns change the most, women experience high demands on their time in caring for others. This pattern has been highlighted during the COVID-19 pandemic with women taking on additional responsibilities with at-home learning with children and/or additional elder care. Thus, it comes as no surprise that women sacrifice sleep time to meet work and family responsibilities.

In U.S. families with at least one school-age child, parents (n = 1,103) reported that frequent evening activities and the use of technological devices in the bedroom were associated with fewer hours of sleep, reduced sleep quality, and more complaints of disturbed sleep (Buxton et al., 2015). In this study, more than 90% of parents reported sleep was "very to extremely important," yet 90% of all children did not obtain recommended amounts of sleep. The best predictors for children obtaining recommended amounts of good quality sleep included enforcing rules about limited caffeine intake, not using technological devices in the bedroom, and going to bed at a regular time. Perhaps, not surprising, if parents used technological devices in the bedroom, their children were more likely to use devices in the bedroom.

Women's Sleep During Life Stages

Before mandates from National Institutes of Health (NIH) that required the inclusion of women in federally funded research studies, many laboratory sleep studies included only men. Although current studies include men and women participants, the sample size often lacks sufficient power to analyze results based on gender, leaving many unanswered questions regarding sex differences and sleep. Nevertheless, beginning with the onset of menarche and continuing throughout life's transitions, women experience changes in reproductive hormones that affect sleep quality and quantity. Gender differences in sleep emerge with the onset of puberty; girls are at higher risk of developing insomnia and report more insomnia symptoms after puberty (Pengo et al., 2018). Whether the increased risk can be explained primarily on the basis of hormonal changes with puberty is an open question. Sleep complaints are frequently reported during menses, pregnancy, and the transition to postmenopause (TPM).

MENSTRUAL CYCLE

Scheduling sleep study research in women needs to include documentation of, and preferably control for, where they are in their menstrual cycle. Overall, women are more likely to self-report sleep complaints in the late luteal phase and during menstruation (Pengo et al., 2018). They complain of trouble falling asleep or long SOL, increased number of awakenings and increased WASO, leading to reduced SE, and in some studies, increased EDS. The odds of reporting trouble sleeping were 29% higher in perimenopause compared with premenopause among women from the initial SWAN report; both groups of women reported more trouble sleeping at the beginning and end of a menstrual cycle. Most women (74.5%) reported trouble sleeping for at least 1 night and 19.2% met criteria for chronic insomnia (Kravitz et al., 2005). Subsequent ancillary studies of the SWAN data continue to show similar patterns of trouble sleeping among women with greater impact on cognitive functioning and mood, and effects on diverse populations of women (Bowman et al., 2021; Matthews et al., 2019; Solomon et al., 2020).

There are data that suggest that subjective sleep reports in middle-aged to older adults do not correlate with objective sleep measures such as PSG (Kaplan et al., 2017). However, objective measures of sleep often can be used to explain the physiologic impact of hormone change and the impact on sleep. One PSG study of a small sample of 11 women with insomnia compared with nine control subjects revealed that both groups showed more awakenings ($p = .003$) and arousals ($p = .025$) per hour of sleep and less percentage of SWS ($p = .024$) during the luteal phase compared with the follicular phase (de Zambotti et al., 2015). Women with insomnia had shorter sleep duration ($p = .012$), more WASO ($p = .031$), and a lower SE ($p = .034$) than women without insomnia, regardless of menstrual cycle phase. In

another PSG study of 33 perimenopausal women ages 43 to 52 years (16 with a clinical diagnosis of insomnia) and 11 premenopausal women without sleep complaints (ages 18 to 27 years), follicle-stimulating hormone (FSH) levels were positively associated with WASO, number of awakenings, and arousals in perimenopausal women ($p < .05$) without sleep complaints independent of age, BMI, and hot flashes (de Zambotti et al., 2015). Similarly, FSH correlated with wakefulness after sleep onset and a light N1 sleep stage in premenopausal women ($p < .05$). In perimenopausal women with insomnia, there was no correlation with FSH, yet there was with anxiety and depression ($p < .05$). Estradiol did not correlate with sleep in perimenopausal groups; it did correlate negatively with arousals in premenopausal women ($p < .01$). In summary, sleep is more disrupted in the luteal phase compared with the follicular phase in midlife women. Women with insomnia are more vulnerable to experience and self-report poor sleep that may be related to factors intrinsic to insomnia, such as mood disturbances and night-to-night variability, rather than to changing levels of reproductive hormones.

PREGNANCY AND POSTPARTUM

There is ample evidence that pregnant women experience sleep disturbances, both from self-report and from objective sleep measures. Throughout pregnancy there are many changes in physiology associated with hormones, increased body temperature, increased respiratory rate, decreased functional residual capacity, frequent urination, increased abdominal mass, and vascular load that could contribute to changes in sleep. From a recent meta-analysis of 24 studies that included 11,002 women, 45% reported poor sleep quality during pregnancy. Poor sleep quality ratings on the PSQI were noted overall during pregnancy ($M = 6.07$) and worsened significantly from the second ($M = 5.31$) to third trimester ($M = 7.03$; Sedov et al., 2018).

Data from an internet survey of 2,427 women showed that across all months of pregnancy, 76% reported poor sleep quality, 38% reported insufficient sleep, 49% reported EDS, and 78% took daytime naps (Mindell et al., 2015). Based on the Insomnia Severity Index (ISI), 57% reported insomnia symptoms with no differences across months of pregnancy. Frequent urination and inability to find a comfortable sleeping position were also common complaints. Most women fail to sleep through the night by the third trimester of pregnancy and napping during the day becomes more frequent, often to make up for shorter sleep duration, which has been verified with actigraphy (Tsai et al., 2013). Lower socioeconomic status is associated with self-reported poor sleep quality and more fragmented sleep documented with actigraphy during the first trimester (Okun et al., 2014).

Changes in PSG-recorded sleep during pregnancy vary, and most studies conducted in the past decade have measured indices of sleep-disordered breathing (SDB) with other comorbidities (e.g., diabetes, hypertension) in high-risk women. One PSG study of secondary data of a prospective study compared 127 early pregnancy with 97 receiving a repeated PSG in late pregnancy (Izci-Balserak et al., 2018). Investigators reported that during late pregnancy women had shorter sleep duration, worse sleep efficiency, increased awakenings and N2 sleep, decreased SWS and REM, increased AHI, and more periodic limb movements compared to the early pregnancy stage (Izci-Balserak et al., 2018).

Pregnant women are at risk for developing sleep disorders besides insomnia. Signs and symptoms of SDB or restless legs syndrome (RLS) may manifest for the first time during pregnancy, so screening is recommended. In an online survey, symptoms of SDB and RLS were reported by 19% (Berlin Questionnaire) and 24%, respectively (Mindell et al., 2015). The risk of SDB occurs because of changes in physiology, including weight gain, larger neck circumference, nasal congestion, reduced functional residual capacity from diaphragmatic elevation, and reduced oxygen saturation in the supine position from increased ventilation/perfusion mismatch, particularly in the third trimester. The onset of snoring during pregnancy is common and is associated with a higher risk (OR = 2.34) of gestational hypertension and preeclampsia (Dunietz et al., 2014; Pamidi et al., 2014) and for gestational diabetes (OR = 1.86; Pamidi et al., 2014). Women who are overweight and obese are at even higher risk of pregnancy-associated SDB. Hypertension during pregnancy is associated with the development of cardiovascular disease (CVD) in later life. Since SDB contributes to the development of CVD (hypertension, myocardial infarction, and stroke) in nonpregnant individuals, SDB during pregnancy may well contribute to cardiovascular morbidity and mortality in older women (Dunietz et al., 2014). Proposed mechanisms for the higher risk of CVD in association with SDB include heightened sympathetic activity, oxidative stress, inflammatory reactions from repeated apneic episodes, and metabolic syndrome. Efforts have been made to predict the presence of SDB in pregnancy with the Berlin Questionnaire and the Multivariable Apnea Risk Index in association with a respiratory disturbance index obtained from PSG. A BMI of at least 32 kg/m^2 and tiredness on awakening were the strongest, independent SDB predictors during pregnancy (Wilson et al., 2013). Findings from the Nulliparous Pregnancy Outcomes Study Monitoring Mothers-to-be (nuMoM2b) showed self-reported late sleep midpoint had a higher risk of gestational diabetes mellites (OR = 1.67) and no associations with pregnancy hypertension (Facco et al., 2018).

Using that same dataset, investigators determined that around 4% of early-pregnancy women have SDB and that rate increases to around 6% in midpregnancy. However, fetal birth weights were not affected when controlling for BMI of the mother (Hawkins et al. 2021).

RLS is a common sensorimotor neurologic disorder with a prevalence influenced by ethnicity, age, and gender. RLS is associated with unusual "creepy-crawly" sensations in the legs, which are relieved by moving them. Symptoms of RLS can occur at any time of day or night but most often occur when lying quietly after going to bed. In pregnancy, RLS most often is related to iron or folate deficiency, and symptoms often subside with adequate supplementation and/or after birth. There is evidence that a family history of RLS can contribute to development and progression of RLS independent of pregnancy. In a study of 1,563 pregnant women in the third trimester, 36% had symptoms of RLS with moderate to severe symptom profiles that contributed to increased poor sleep quality (OR = 2.2) and poor daytime functioning (OR = 1.9) with no significant relationship to delivery outcomes (Dunietz et al, 2017). Iron is a cofactor in the synthesis of dopamine, and iron deficiency in the central nervous system is known to lead to RLS. It is quite challenging to treat RLS during pregnancy, as most central nervous system–acting dopaminergic medications routinely used have not been studied in pregnant women, so risks to the fetus are unknown.

Sleep problems have been associated with potential effects on delivery and adverse pregnancy outcomes. As an example, a recent meta-analysis of 120 studies (n = 58,123,250) of pregnant women found sleep disturbances (e.g., poor sleep quality, changes in sleep duration, insomnia symptoms, RLS, SDB) were associated with higher risks of preeclampsia (OR = 2.80), gestational hypertension (OR = 1.74), gestational diabetes (OR = 1.59), cesarean birth (OR = 1.47), and stillbirth (OR = 1.25). The study also presented higher morbidity rates in women over 30 years old and those with higher prebirth BMI (Lu et al., 2021). Additionally, persistent sleep problems (e.g., poor sleep quality, short sleep duration, sleep disorders) throughout pregnancy have been associated with various adverse pregnancy outcomes (e.g., prenatal depression, gestational diabetes, hypertension, preeclampsia, duration and type of delivery, preterm birth, and low birth weight) across multiple studies (Palagini et al., 2014). Shift work, with disturbed sleep and circadian misalignment, is associated with the development of CVD morbidity and early death (Gu et al., 2015) and could be an occupational hazard for women working during pregnancy.

Most women are sleep deprived during the first postpartum month, and persistent short sleep duration increases the risks for mental and physical morbidity. In the 2007 NSF poll, 42% of women reported that they rarely or never got a good night's sleep and 19% of these women experienced postpartum "blues." Poor sleep quality can predict time to recurrence of postpartum major depression (PPMD), such that over a 17-week interval after delivery for every 1-point elevation in the PSQI global score, the risk of depression recurrence increased 25% among women with a history of major depression or PPMD (Okun et al., 2011). Weight gain is normal during pregnancy, and failure to return to prepregnancy weight at 1-year postpartum places women at greater risk of midlife obesity compared with women who return to prepregnancy weight (Xiao et al., 2014). Because obtaining less than 5 or 6 hours of sleep per night has been associated with weight gain and obesity in nonpregnant women, postpartum women may be at an even greater risk. In fact, one recent review found that women who continued to self-report sleep an average of at least 5 hours per day at 6 months postpartum had 3.13 greater odds (adjusted) of a weight retention of 5 kg or more at 1 year (Bazzazian et al., 2021; Gunderson et al., 2008). Other studies have shown similar associations at reduced levels of risk (Xiao et al., 2014). Finding ways for women to increase the amount of sleep they obtain every 24 hours has the potential to enhance women returning to prepregnancy weight.

MIDLIFE, TRANSITION TO POSTMENOPAUSE, AND EARLY POSTMENOPAUSE

Sleep changes are often experienced most notably after age 30 years and before the seventh decade of life (Pengo et al., 2018). Sleep problems in midlife women are common and cause significant daytime sleepiness and functional impairments (Viola-Saltzman & Attarian, 2020). A number of studies have reported greater amounts of sleep-related daytime sleepiness and fatigue in women compared with men, both in clinic-based and population-based studies; the reasons for these differences, especially the effects of different gender role and societal expectations, continue to be investigated (Landis & Lentz, 2006). In general, women report more symptoms than men, are more likely to seek healthcare, and are overrepresented in general clinic populations such that the prevalence of disorders based exclusively on symptom criteria is much greater in women compared with men. Insomnia is a disorder of symptoms related to initiating and maintaining sleep, as well as waking early in the morning and being unable to fall back to sleep; thus, it is not surprising that the prevalence of insomnia is twofold higher in women compared with men (Baker et al., 2018).

The Transition to Postmenopause

As women approach menopause, it has been reported that 26% experience severe symptoms of poor sleep (Baker et al., 2018). As women transition to postmenopause, they often complain of insomnia symptoms that are related to hot flashes; these symptoms are also associated with mood disturbances (anxiety and depression) and perceived stress, and the prevalence of sleep complaints varies widely. The overall effects on daytime functioning typically lend to a diagnosis of a sleep disorder, typically insomnia (Baker et al., 2018). One of the central questions in studying sleep during the TPM is whether complaints of sleep disturbance are specifically related to menopause per se rather than to the effects of aging, changes in mental health status, or increased perceived stress associated with other life changes commonly experienced during midlife. The overall odds of reporting poor sleep among 67,542 women in a 24-study meta-analysis were significantly higher in all the stages of menopause (perimenopause, postmenopause, and surgical menopause) compared with premenopause (all OR >1.39, p <.01), with the highest odds after surgical menopause (OR = 2.17, p <.001), despite a large variability of poor sleep symptoms across all the studies (Xu & Lang, 2014). The OR for postmenopause compared with perimenopause was lower and very small (OR = 1.09). Asian and White women experienced the most disturbed sleep, whereas Hispanic women experienced no sleep changes during the transition. Measures for identifying sleep disturbance varied widely across studies. Based on data from validated questionnaires used in a trial focused on treatments for hot flashes, baseline PSQI (mean = 8.23) and ISI (11.6) scores were elevated among healthy women selected for hot flashes, not for sleep disturbance (Ensrud et al., 2012). According to categories of the ISI, 37.6% of the women had mild (8–14), 26.8% had moderate (15–21), and 5.9% had severe (22–28) insomnia. Of note, to be included in this trial, women had to meet the Stages of Reproductive Aging Workshop (STRAW) criteria for the late and early postmenopause stages (Harlow et al., 2012). One limitation of this trial is the failure to screen women for SDB or other sleep disorders using PSG. There is evidence that SDB is largely underdiagnosed or often co-occurring with other sleep disorders, which often go undiagnosed in women due to lower referral rates for evaluation (Viola-Saltzman & Attarian, 2020).

Data from at least two longitudinal studies show distinct differences from cross-sectional analyses with respect to sleep disturbance being related specifically to menopause stages. Based on 14-year follow-up data from a retrospective questionnaire completed annually, the prevalence of moderate to severe poor sleep ranged from 28% to 35% with no relation to the final menstrual period (Freeman et al., 2015; Shaver & Woods, 2015). However, women who experienced moderate to severe poor sleep premenopause had greater odds (OR = 3.8) of poor sleep during the transition, whereas women who reported mild sleep disturbance before menopause were 1.5 times more likely to have moderate to severe sleep during menopause. In this analysis, the adjusted odds of experiencing poor sleep if a woman reported hot flashes were increased significantly (OR = 1.79) independent of baseline sleep reports. Insomnia symptom severity (e.g., difficulty getting to and especially staying asleep and early morning awakening) was greatest during the late and early postmenopause stages of the transition. Poor sleep also was significantly related to many symptoms (e.g., perceived stress, history of sexual abuse, perceived health, alcohol use, depressed mood, anxiety, and pain). In a review of sleep and menopause, Shaver and Woods (2015) point out that comparing studies of sleep during the TPM is quite challenging because of the heterogeneity of samples, inconsistency in screening and evaluation for sleep disorders, failure to verify menopausal stage, variety of self-report measures used to assess sleep and sleep disturbances, and still relatively few studies of sleep physiology and sex differences.

The SWAN Sleep Study

An important contribution to understanding the nature and extent of sleep problems during the TPM is derived from the SWAN study of midlife women and the ancillary study of sleep conducted at four of the seven original sites in the United States (Kravitz & Joffee, 2011). This historically important set of studies provided data to better understand how the TPM affects sleep.

The first SWAN sleep study, in which 67% of the 370 women were in the premenopausal or early perimenopausal stage, assessed self-report, behavioral (actigraphy), and PSG measures of sleep. The protocol involved three nights of PSG, followed by approximately a month of diary and actigraphic data. The second sleep study involves two nights of PSG along with 14 days of diary and actigraphy. Data from this study should permit longitudinal analyses of changes in sleep according to both self-report and physiology as women move through the TPM stages (Kravitz & Joffe, 2011). The self-report measure of sleep from the initial SWAN study asked women about problems sleeping (Yes, No) in the previous 2 weeks. Thirty-seven percent of 12,603 women reported sleep problems; this estimate excludes women on hormones or surgical menopause (Kravitz & Joffe, 2011). The prevalence of sleep problems increased from premenopause to the late phase and early postmenopause in cross-sectional analysis and controlling for age. Among ethnic groups represented,

Japanese women reported the lowest (28.2%), and White women reported the highest (40.3%) prevalence; Chinese (31.6%), Hispanic (38%), and Black (35.5%) fell in between the two extremes. In multivariate analysis, vasomotor symptoms (VMSs), psychological symptoms (depression and anxiety), perceived health, pain (arthritis), quality of life, lower income, and marital happiness were associated with sleep problems. In a longitudinal follow-up analysis, three types of insomnia symptoms (trouble falling and staying asleep, early morning awakening) were analyzed if symptoms were present at least three nights each week in the previous 2 weeks. Of the women who transitioned to postmenopause, difficulty staying asleep (analogous to increased WASO) increased the most, from slightly more than 20% before menopause to nearly 50% after menopause. From this longitudinal analysis of data representing a few years, the odds of developing trouble falling asleep or staying asleep on six or more nights of 2 weeks increased dramatically (OR ~>2.5; Kravitz & Joffe, 2011). These data, albeit representing only a few women in the late TPM stage or postmenopause, are consistent with subsequent research (Gracia & Freeman, 2018).

A distinct advantage of the data derived from the SWAN sleep study was the use of self-report sleep, actigraphy, and at-home PSG measures. Nearly two thirds of the women in this study reported poor sleep quality, with PSQI scores exceeding the cutoff point of greater than 5 (6.6 ± 2.4; Kravitz & Joffe, 2011). PSG measures of clinical sleep problems showed that 20% of the sample had an apnea–hypopnea index (AHI) of greater than 15 per hour of sleep, which is much higher than the 4% reported from a cohort of women of similar age from the initial report of SDB prevalence from the older Wisconsin study (Young et al., 1993). An AHI of greater than 15 per hour of sleep is used as the clinical cutoff point for the diagnosis and treatment of OSA, because it is used by Medicare for reimbursement. The overall SWAN AHI mean was 10.4 per hour of sleep, indicating a mild form of SDB. In addition, 8% of the women had periodic leg movements associated with EEG arousals of greater than 10 per hour of sleep, which is indicative of the periodic limb movement disorder (PLMD) often manifested with complaints of poor sleep or insomnia symptoms.

PSG data can be analyzed to yield estimates of slow versus fast EEG frequencies. Slow or delta frequency is indicative of SWS and is used as a measure of sleep intensity, whereas fast frequency or beta activity is indicative of the waking state and has been identified as a feature of primary insomnia (Buysse et al., 2011). Higher beta EEG activity could provide an explanation for the increased complaints of poor sleep quality as women experience TPM. Quantitative analysis of the EEG from night 2 in the first SWAN sleep study showed that beta frequency power was higher both in NREM and in REM sleep in late and early postmenopausal stages relative to premenopausal and perimenopausal stages, despite no differences in sleep stage amounts (Campbell et al., 2011). However, there were significant covariates, including hot flash frequency, overall health status, and antidepressant drug use that attenuated the association of EEG power with menopausal stage. In another report, cross-sectional analysis revealed higher risk for metabolic syndrome in association with SE and NREM

beta power (both OR = 2.1) and AHI (OR = 1.9); all remained significant after adjustment for covariates (Hall et al., 2012). In a subsequent follow-up analysis of 310 women, although the average AHI was similar (8.1/hour), BMI was slightly increased and each hour of less sleep time recorded by actigraphy was inversely related to BMI. However, there was no longitudinal association between sleep duration and BMI change for more than 4.6 years (Appelhans et al., 2013).

In general, it is thought that PSG used at home will be more ecologically valid than the same data obtained in a laboratory setting. In laboratory studies, we usually use the first night as an adaptation night because of the well-known "first night" effect (Byun et al., 2019). Despite the use of in-home PSG, a first-night effect was observed in the SWAN sleep study with increased TST on nights 2 and 3 and reduced sleep fragmentation compared with night 1 (Zheng et al., 2012). Additional sources of higher night-to-night variability included obesity, smoking, and financial strain. PSG recordings, regardless of setting, may be a source of sleep disruption and overweight; smoking women with financial concerns may be at even higher risk of a "first night" effect.

Data from the SWAN sleep study from a community sample yield interesting results. An analysis of 314 women showed higher pain reports (bodily pain score from the short-form health survey) in association with actigraphically recorded longer sleep duration but with lower SE and self-reported less restful sleep (Kravitz et al., 2015). Women with any pain (*n* = 211), compared with those without pain (*n* = 103), were slightly heavier, and were more likely to report taking sleep, antidepressant, and pain medication at some time during the month-long study. Regardless of pain, hot flashes occurring at night were associated with higher odds for restlessness, lower SE, and lower odds of feeling rested in the morning.

Menopausal Strategies: Finding Lasting Answers to Symptoms and Health

In 2008, the MsFLASH network was funded by the NIH and conducted a set of clinical trials to investigate new ways to alleviate menopause-related symptoms in peri- to postmenopausal women (Reed et al., 2020). In one study examining symptom clusters during the TPM and early postmenopause, women with hot flashes showed multiple co-occurring symptoms that grouped or clustered into five classifications or classes (Woods et al., 2016). Women in class 1 (10.5%) experienced severe hot flash interference, severe sleep symptoms, and moderate levels of pain. Class 2 (14.1%) contained severe hot flash interference, severe sleep symptoms, moderate-severe depression, and anxiety. Class 3 (39.6%, the largest group) included moderate hot flash interference, moderate-severe sleep symptoms but lower on mood and pain. These findings emphasize that symptoms can vary by severity and type during the TPM (Woods et al., 2016).

POSTMENOPAUSE AND OLDER WOMEN

Sleep complaints are quite common after menopause and among older women. In the 2007 NSF survey, 61% of postmenopausal women reported insomnia symptoms at least a few nights each week, with 41% reporting the use of some type of sleep aid. This group of women had the highest BMIs, with 36% reporting being overweight and 30% obese. In the self-reported data from the Women's Health Initiative (WHI; $N = 98,705$), the frequency of sleep-related symptoms occurring at least 3 days per week included daytime sleepiness (26%), napping during the day (12%), trouble falling asleep (10%), waking up frequently (40%) with trouble getting back to sleep (15%), early morning waking (18%), and reports of snoring (34%; Kripke et al., 2001). Minority women (Black, Hispanic, other) reported more trouble falling asleep, more daytime sleepiness, and more naps and snoring compared with White women; they also reported less nocturnal waking and use of sleep aids. Women who were obese or had a history of depression reported the highest frequency of both short (no more than 5 hours) and long sleep duration (at least 10 hours) in an ancillary study using wrist actigraphy. While Black women showed the lowest sleep duration (315 minutes, 5.3 hours) compared with the other racial/ethnic groups, all groups obtained less than 7 hours of sleep (Kripke et al., 2004). An analysis of survival data up to 2009 from 444 women from the original sample of 459 showed that after controlling for chronic conditions such as hypertension, diabetes, myocardial infarction, cancer, and major depression, those who slept less than 300 minutes (5 hours) had a 61% mean survival rate, those who slept more than 390 minutes (6.5 hours) had a 78% mean survival rate, while those with a 90% survival rate had actigraphic sleep durations between 300 and 390 minutes (Kripke et al., 2011). Many more women slept more than 390 minutes compared to those who slept less than 300 minutes; these women who slept less than 300 minutes represented 50 of the 86 deaths that could be verified.

In an examination of the findings from the Midlife Women's Health Study, the aim was to determine risk factors of poor sleep from the TPM to postmenopause from 776 women in various stages (R. L. Smith et al., 2018). The results indicate that symptoms experienced during each transitional phase did not predict the symptom experience for each subsequent phase, suggesting poor sleep in premenopause to perimenopause was not predictive of poor sleep during perimenopause to postmenopause. The one exception was women with severe insomnia symptom experiences during perimenopause (five nights per week or more), which were more likely to carry over into postmenopause.

The optimum nighttime sleep duration for older adults is dependent on various factors and tends to stabilize after 60 years of age (Li et al., 2018). The recommendations for at least 7 hours of sleep for adults (Watson et al., 2015) did not include adults older than 60 years. The meta-analysis of PSG sleep from control participants in laboratory studies showed that for those over the age of 60 years, the number of studies in which sleep duration was less than 400 minutes far exceeded those reporting more than 400 minutes, or 6.6 hours (Ohayon et al., 2004). An elegant laboratory study of sleep propensity comparing healthy young adults (mean age of 21.9 ± 3.3 years) to a group of healthy older adults (mean age of 67.8 ± 4.3 years) revealed a reduced capacity for the older adults to sleep during daytime naps as well as at night (Klerman & Dijk, 2008). Sleep duration on average was 1.5 hours shorter in older adults (7.4 ± 0.4, SEM) compared with young adults (8.9 ± 0.4). This study revealed that older adults were less sleepy

in the daytime and objective sleep is not always a predictor of feeling tired during the day (Chen et al., 2014).

Why healthy older adults report lower amounts of daytime sleepiness compared with young adults runs counter to common beliefs and observations of older adults frequently reporting napping or falling asleep while engaged in quiet activities such as watching television (TV) or attending evening concerts or shows. However, many older adults have sleep disorders, such as SDB or PLMD and multiple chronic conditions with comorbid insomnia, which could account for differences unobserved from their healthy counterparts (Li et al., 2018). An observational study of actigraphically derived sleep duration in midlife and older adults showed that more frequent napping was associated with shorter subsequent nighttime sleep duration; more daytime sleepiness, pain, and fatigue; and increased cardiovascular risk factors of a higher BMI and a bigger waist circumference (Valiensi et al., 2019). However, the research studies on napping are not consistent and often not in the natural setting suggesting short naps are not consistently found to impact nighttime sleep (Irish et al., 2015). The prevalence of SDB is known to be much higher in postmenopausal women compared with those who are premenopausal or in the early stages of the TPM. The proportion of older women with SDB is nearly equal to that of men. Higher BMIs and neck circumference relative to younger women place postmenopausal women at greater risk for SDB (Orbea et al., 2020). Observations from the Study of Osteoporotic Fractures in community-dwelling women older than 65 years have provided evidence of significant increased risk of morbidity among those with poor sleep quality or indications of sleep disorders. Among all participants in this study, after 5 years ($N = 817$, mean age = 87.3 ± 3.3), average actigraphically derived sleep duration was 409.2 ± 66.0 minutes (approximately 6.8 hours), WASO was 65.9 ± 40.4 minutes, and SE was 79.9 ± 9.9% (Spira et al., 2012). In this analysis, 41% developed at least one functional impairment, and those with the shortest TST had an increased risk (OR = 1.93). A subsequent analysis of PSG data from a subset of the participants ($n = 302$) from two study sites showed that after adjustment for comorbidities and baseline daily function scores, an AHI of greater than 15 increased the risk of functional difficulties (OR = 2.2) compared with women with an AHI of less than 5 (Spira et al., 2014). Data from this study also revealed that older women with short sleep duration or greater WASO are at greater risk for falls (Stone et al., 2008) or depression (Maglione et al., 2014), respectively. However, women in this study who habitually sleep more than 9 hours in 24 hours are at higher risk for dying from CVD compared with women who sleep 8 hours (Stone et al., 2009). Thus, older women are at increased risk for poor sleep quality and sleep disorders. Helping women during midlife to develop healthy sleep habits, along with sufficient exercise and weight control, has the potential to assist them to lead healthy lives beyond menopause.

Sleep Deficiency

The most common type of sleep deficiency, a concept introduced in the 2011 NIH Sleep Disorders Research Plan (Box 15.3), is voluntary sleep restriction consistent with reports of sleep duration of less than 6 hours nightly sleep. Individuals

Box 15.3 Sleep Deficiency

Sleep deprivation is a condition that occurs if you don't get enough sleep. Sleep deficiency is a broader concept. It occurs if you have one or more of the following:

- You don't get enough sleep (sleep deprivation).
- You sleep at the wrong time of day (i.e., you are out of sync with your body's natural clock).
- You don't sleep well or get all of the different types of sleep that your body needs.
- You have a sleep disorder that prevents you from getting enough sleep or causes poor quality sleep.

Source: National Heart, Lung, and Blood Institute. (n.d.). What are sleep deprivation and deficience? Retrieved February 2022, from https://www.nhlbi.nih.gov /health/sleep-deprivation

simply do not set sleep as a priority and sacrifice time for sleep to other activities. Evidence continues to accumulate that an increasing number of adults in the United States report short sleep duration. Although the average sleep duration reported in a 1985 survey was 7.4 hours compared with 7.18 hours in 2012, the proportion of adults older than 18 years and under 75 years of age reporting no more than 6 hours of nightly sleep increased from 22.3% in 1985 to 29.2% in 2012 (Ford et al., 2015). These proportions are estimated to represent 38.6 and 70.1 million adults, respectively.

HEALTH CONSEQUENCES OF SLEEP DEFICIENCY

There are wide variations in responses to acute sleep deprivation because some individuals appear more sensitive or vulnerable to the effects of sleep loss and others appear resistant. Common responses include increased sleepiness, irritability, lower pain thresholds, difficulty concentrating and other cognitive impairments, poor mood and judgment, attention deficits, dietary changes, and reduced energy and motivation to engage in activities. Maximal physiologic sleepiness accumulates quickly after 24 or 48 hours of acute sleep loss. Microsleeps, very short periods of sleep, commonly occur. Performance tasks that depend on frontal/parietal lobe function, such as logical reasoning or complex mathematical tasks, seem particularly affected by acute sleep deprivation (Goel et al, 2013; Troynikov et al., 2018). However, a reliable test of sleepiness from sleep loss is a simple psychomotor vigilance test (PVT). This is a valid and reliable test of sustained attention and reaction time to a visual stimulus over a 5- to 10-minute period. Performance on this test deteriorates the longer one stays awake.

Chronic sleep deficiency has been shown to impair immune responses to vaccination, reduce antibody production to the cold virus, produce hyperalgesia, raise circulating levels of proinflammatory cytokines, and increase sympathetic activity (e.g., blood pressure and heart rate; Mullington et al., 2009). Knutson (2013) reviewed the consequences of chronic sleep deficiency with cardiometabolic disease risk, especially diabetes and CVD. Experimental studies have revealed that sleep restriction of 4 to 5 hours compared with 7 or more hours of time in bed (TIB) over a varying number of consecutive days leads to reduced glucose tolerance and insulin sensitivity, as well as increased caloric intake associated with, and changes in appetite regulation that favors, increased "hunger" (ghrelin) and reduced "satiety" (leptin) hormones. Epidemiologic observational studies have shown an increased risk for weight gain and obesity with self-reported short sleep duration. From a meta-analysis of 19 cross-sectional studies in children and 26 cross-sectional studies in adults, the odds of developing obesity (higher BMI) were greater for children ($n = 30,002$, OR = 1.89) than adults ($n = 604,509$, OR = 1.55; Cappuccio et al., 2008). Another meta-analysis of 12 studies representing 18,720 cases and 70,833 control subjects revealed increased odds (OR = 1.27) of developing metabolic syndrome with short sleep duration (Xi et al., 2014). Knutson (2013) summarized potential determinants of sleep deficiency as older age, female sex, depression, stress, loneliness, and Black race (compared with White). Allostatic load is a concept representing the accumulation of biological disease risk from prolonged or poorly regulated responses to stressors and has been linked to sleep apnea, insomnia, and short sleep duration (Chen et al., 2014). The prevalence of allostatic load was higher among Blacks (26.3%) and Hispanics (20.3%) compared with Whites (17.7%). After adjustment for sociodemographic and lifestyle variables, allostatic load was associated with sleep apnea (OR = 1.92), snoring (OR = 2.2), and short sleep duration of less than 6 hours (OR = 1.35). Finally, among adults more than 45 years of age, 31% reported sleeping no more than 6 hours and only 4.1% reported sleeping at least 10 hours; when compared with the majority who reported sleeping 7 to 9 hours, both short and long sleep durations were associated with obesity, poor mental health, CVD, stroke, and diabetes (Liu et al., 2013). One of the challenges with interpreting these types of data is that it is unknown if the presence of a chronic condition leads to or is the consequence of short or long sleep durations.

The impact of the global SARS-CoV-2 (COVID-19) pandemic on sleep patterns, sleep quality, and treatment of sleep disorders is associated with stress, fear, anxiety, and viral infections associated with the virus (Jahrami et al., 2021). The impact of the various social and physical effects on sleep continues to evolve. In one review of 45 articles, 74.8% of COVID-positive patients had sleep problems compared to 35.7% of the overall population of 54,231 participants. A recent study found OSA patients were eight times more likely to be hospitalized with COVID-19 (OR = 1.65) and experience respiratory failure (OR = 1.98; Maas et al., 2021). Obesity has been associated with worse outcomes from COVID-19 (Soeroto et al., 2020). There are still several unanswered questions related to immune interruptions related to long-term sleep problems and how that predicts overall outcomes of the infection with the virus.

Although associations between sleep duration and morbidity are robust, the association between sleep duration and mortality is less clear. Several recent studies focus on individual sleep disorders as they relate to morbidity and mortality (e.g., OSA) or focus on the effects of a specific comorbid condition with a type of poor sleep (e.g., short sleep duration). In historically relevant data from a survey of more than 1 million adults, both short and long sleep durations were associated with early death (Kripke et al., 1979, Kurina et al., 2013). Other studies have shown a similar U-shaped curve, with a sleep duration of no more than

6 hours and at least 9 hours associated with increased mortality risk. In a critical review of these studies, Kurina et al. (2013) found that two studies supported the association of only short sleep duration and increased mortality risk, 16 supported an association with only long sleep duration, 14 supported a U-shaped effect (both short and long sleep duration), and 23 found no association at all. Furthermore, the way the survey question was worded is important. An association with mortality was more likely to be present if participants were asked to respond to a question about the number of hours they usually sleep versus if they reported their usual bedtime and rise times. There was no association with the latter method of reporting, which required investigators to calculate sleep duration. Self-reported estimates of sleep duration tend to be longer than that measured via actigraphy or PSG. This observation suggests that if people overestimate the amount of sleep they obtain versus what is recorded with actigraphy or PSG, then the proportion of individuals with short duration of less than 6 hours may be higher than current surveys have reported.

Although sleep is variable from night to night and no two nights of sleep are exactly the same, high intraindividual night-to-night variability in sleep duration is associated with poor sleep quality and is a common feature of chronic insomnia.

DIAGNOSTIC CRITERIA AND RISK FACTORS

Sleep Measures

Sleep indicators fall into three main categories: self-report, behavioral assessments, and sleep physiology (PSG). Self-report measures include daily logs or diaries, sleep quality and hygiene assessments, insomnia, and sleepiness scales, among others (Chen et al., 2018). Variability in measurements exists between self-report, actigraphy, and PSG. Each category of sleep measure provides a distinctly different dimension of the sleep experience. Self-report is an important indication of one's perception of sleep. Behavioral assessments provide a portrait of rest/activity patterns, especially over time. Finally, PSG enables detection of multiple physiologic parameters during sleep that are not subject to recall bias or distortion.

SELF-REPORT MEASURES

Sleep diaries are used routinely in insomnia research and clinical practice (Figure 15.3). An example of a 2-week sleep diary is available to download from the AASM Sleep Education website (AASM, 2023).

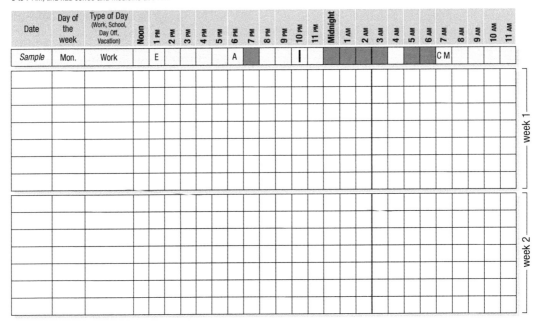

FIGURE 15.3 Self-report 2-week sleep diary.
Source: American Academy of Sleep Medicine. (2023). Sleep education: Sleep diary. *https://sleepeducation .org/resources/sleep-diary. Used with permission.*

This type of diary, when completed, provides a visual representation of one's sleep pattern and daily variation in sleep onset, offset, and duration over a 2-week period. Although considered the least accurate measure of sleep compared with actigraphy and PSG, sleep logs and diaries are a necessary and an important component both in research and in clinical sleep medicine. Diaries provide prospective recordings of self-reported daily sleep patterns, habits, lifestyle factors, and symptoms affecting sleep quantity and quality. Diaries usually include quantitative assessments of SOL, number of nighttime awakenings, minutes of WASO, TST, bedtime, and rise time, from which TIB can be determined and SE calculated (SE = TST/TIB × 100). To provide easier comparison across future research studies, sleep investigators have developed a standard sleep dairy for use in research on insomnia (Carney et al., 2012). Diary applications for use on smartphones are available for research and being used in clinical practice. The Veterans Administration has developed a cognitive behavioral therapy (CBT) phone app for insomnia, called the *CBT-I coach app*, which includes a sleep diary and is designed for use by patients with posttraumatic stress disorder (PTSD) undergoing therapy to help them sleep better (mobile.va.gov/app/cbt-i-coach).

Various other types of sleep questionnaires and instruments have been used to measure sleep quality and insomnia symptoms in women (Table 15.1). Because the instruments in Table 15.1 are not capable of establishing a case definition of insomnia consistent with diagnostic criteria, the Insomnia Symptom Questionnaire was developed to measure chronic insomnia in participants in the SWAN sleep study (Okun et al., 2009). The initial evaluation of this retrospective questionnaire had high reliability and specificity and excellent face validity; however, concurrent validity with sleep measures from a prospective diary or PSG (e.g., SOL, WASO, or SE) could not be established. Nevertheless, the questionnaire identified 9.8% of the sample screened for sleep apnea with PSG as meeting criteria for chronic insomnia. This proportion is consistent with epidemiologic estimates of chronic insomnia and continues to increase (Dopheide, 2020). A 2017 NSF panel provided evidence-based recommendations for indicators of good sleep quality reaffirming that measures that capture sleep latency, number of awakenings, WASO, and SE are good indicators of sleep quality across the lifespan (Ohayon et al., 2017). Several other self-report instruments that assist with assessing aspects of sleep are also available (Tables 15.2 and 15.3).

BEHAVIORAL ASSESSMENTS

Behavioral assessments are based on visual observation of sleeping behavior via video recordings or in real-time by personal observations. Monitoring body movements with wrist actigraphy provides an objective measure of sleep and wake behavior. Both types of measures are used in clinical sleep medicine. Sleep has certain behavioral characteristics across species: little movement, specific posture, lack of awareness of surrounding environment, and for most, closed eyes.

Although it is easy to observe a person asleep—video recordings are a routine aspect of a clinical sleep study—it is possible for an individual to "play possum," acting as if they are asleep. Using personal real-time observational methods to measure sleep is labor intensive and not likely to be of much use except in hospitals or other institutional care settings.

Actigraphy is based on recordings of body movements with accelerometers placed in small devices, about the size of a typical watch and usually worn on the wrist. Sleep is associated with little movement such that periods of wrist/arm immobility are indicative of sleep, whereas periods with wrist/arm movements are indicative of wake. Sleep and wake episodes

TABLE 15.1 Sleep Quality and Insomnia Scales for Use With Women

SCALE	USE	DESCRIPTION	NOTES	SOURCES
PSQI (Pittsburgh Sleep Quality Index)	Sleep quality	19-item, validated questionnaire with seven subscales	Originally developed as a screening tool for sleep problems in psychiatric disorders	Buysse et al. (1989)
PSQI	Sleep quality	19 item, validated questionnaire with seven subscales	Summary global score of either ≥5 or ≥8 can be used as a valid measure of poor sleep quality both in research and in clinic populations	Buysse et al. (1989) Smith & Wegener (2003) Carpenter & Andrykowski (1998)
ISI (Insomnia Severity Index)	Insomnia symptom severity: can use to identify insomnia and treatment response	Seven-item validated questionnaire Score 0–7 = absence of insomnia Score 8–14 = mild insomnia Score 15–21 = moderate clinical insomnia Score 22–28 = severe insomnia	• Difficulty falling asleep • Difficulty staying asleep • Early wakening • Sleep satisfaction • Interference with daily functioning • Noticeability of improvement • Degree of distress attributable to sleep problem	Bastien et al., (2001) Morin et al. (2011)
Insomnia scale used in Women's Health Initiative	Insomnia	Five-item insomnia rating scale: reliability and validity assessed in a very large group of older women representing multiple racial and ethnic groups	Detected sleep disturbances between women taking hormone therapy from placebo and those with mild vs. moderate-to-severe hot flashes	Levine et al. (2003, 2005)

TABLE 15.2 Self-Report Scales for Sleep Hygiene and Sleep Disturbances

SCALE	USE	DESCRIPTION	NOTES	SOURCES
Berlin Questionnaire	Sleep apnea	10-item instrument	Notes snoring, restfulness, and patient hypertension	Kang et al. (2013)
STOP-Bang Questionnaire	Sleep apnea	Eight-item instrument	Identifies presences of risk factors and symptoms for sleep apnea	Orbea et al. (2020)
Sleep Hygiene Awareness and Practice Scale	Sleep hygiene	Multiple questions that identify common hygiene practices	Identifies awareness of hygiene and hygiene practices	Glovinsky and Spielman (2006, 2018)
General Sleep Disturbance Scale	Sleep disturbances	21-item instrument scored 1–7	Identifies common sleep concerns	Lee (1992)
PROMIS (Patient Reported Outcomes Measurement Information System)	Sleep disturbance and wake impairment	Preliminary validity established for both short forms (27 items for sleep disturbance and 16 items for sleep-related impairment) in the PROMIS databank of items	The PROMIS short forms for sleep disturbance and for sleep-related impairment have been found to correlate well with the Pittsburgh Sleep Quality Index (PSQI) and Epworth Sleepiness Scale (ESS) scores	Amedt (2011) Yu et al. (2011)

TABLE 15.3 Self-Report Instruments for Measuring Sleepiness

SCALE	USE	DESCRIPTION	NOTES	SOURCES
Epworth Sleepiness Scale (ESS)	Likelihood to doze or fall asleep during typical daily activities (e.g., quietly reading, watching TV, riding in a car, or sitting in traffic waiting for a light to change)	Eight-item scale	Used most extensively in clinical sleep medicine	Johns (1991, 1992)
Stanford Sleepiness Scale	Level of sleepiness at a given point of time	Eight levels of rating from awake to asleep	Can use at multiple times in a given day	Hoddes et al. (1973)
Karolinska Sleepiness Scale	Level of drowsiness at a given point of time	Nine-point Likert scale	Can use at multiple times in a given day	Akerstedt and Gillberg (1990)

are scored with the use of specialized algorithms in commercially available software specific to each type of actigraphic device. Figure 15.4 is a sample of an actigram (Actiware, 5.0, Philips/Respironics, Inc.) with data obtained over a period of 2.5 weeks from an older woman (Taibi et al., 2009).

As can be seen from this sample, an actigraph can be worn continuously more than 24 hours for several weeks at a time. These devices are water resistant (not waterproof) and are removed for bathing or swimming. The validity of actigraph-derived sleep variables has been established and are most reliable for data obtained from healthy individuals. However, although sensitivity is high for measuring sleep in older women with insomnia, the specificity of measuring WASO with actigraphy is poor relative to PSG (Taibi et al., 2013). Actigraphy will overestimate sleep and underestimate wake behavior in individuals lying quietly in bed while awake, which may be one reason that actigraphy is less accurate in measuring SOL (Smith et al., 2018b) and WASO in insomnia (Taibi et al., 2013). Nevertheless, in conjunction with sleep diaries, increasingly, actigrapy is used in sleep medicine practice as an objective measure of sleep disturbance (Smith et al., 2018b), and updated practice parameters for actigraphy have been published (Smith et al., 2018a).

SLEEP PHYSIOLOGY ASSESSMENTS

PSG is the most accurate, valid sleep measure and remains the gold standard against which other measures of sleep and wake are compared. PSG measures brain waves, muscle tone, eye movements, recordings of heart rate, respiratory rate, airflow, chest and abdominal muscle movements, leg movements, oxygen saturation, and exhaled carbon dioxide. PSG is usually conducted in a laboratory setting; however, portable equipment can be used in homes or in institutional settings. PSG recordings are the only accurate way to measure sleep stages and cycles. PSG is more expensive; while consecutive recordings are often limited to two or three nights in case control studies, a clinical sleep study usually involves only one recording night. PSG is also used to measure daytime physiologic sleepiness in a series of naps, called *multiple sleep latency tests (MSLTs)*. Participants are placed in a quiet bedroom for 20 minutes at 2-hour intervals throughout the day and EEG is recorded. The time from lights out to the first few epochs of sleep is used as a measure of physiologic sleepiness. Individuals who are sleep deprived will often fall asleep within less than 5 minutes. In adults, a cutoff of 10 minutes is used to indicate EDS.

Home-based screening for OSA is a common practice with the use of devices such as the WatchPAT 200 (Itamar Medical,

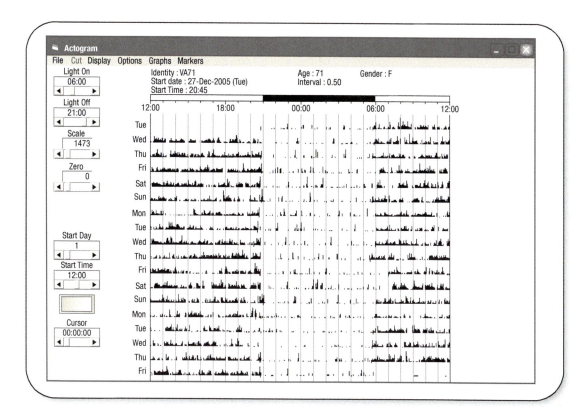

FIGURE 15.4 Actigraphy recording from an older woman whose sleep was recorded for 2.5 weeks. The recording begins just before sleep onset on Tuesday evening and continues until the actigraph was removed in the morning on the final day of the recording.
Source: University of Washington, Sleep Research Laboratory.

Caesarea, Israel), which measures peripheral arterial tone (PAT), pulse oximetry, and heart rate in combination with actigraphy (Yuceege et al., 2013). Although this type of device does not measure EEG, changes in arterial tone, heart rate, and oxygen desaturation are used as indirect indicators of episodes of apnea (pauses in breathing). The WatchPAT 200 and PSG measures of respiratory events (apnea and hypopneas) have shown reasonably good agreement, especially in adults older than 45 years (Yuceege et al., 2013). OSA occurs because of repeated pauses (apneas) or reductions in airflow (hypopneas) that occur frequently during sleep in association with complete or partial airway obstruction. OSA is a common sleep disorder in U.S. adults, with a prevalence of 6% in women and 13% in men, and is associated with significant cardiovascular morbidity (Mukherjee et al., 2015). A clinic sleep study is still required to make a definitive diagnosis of OSA.

GUIDELINES FOR HEALTH PROMOTION AND INTERVENTIONS/STRATEGIES FOR RISK REDUCTION AND MANAGEMENT

Modern sleep research has grown substantially since the discovery of REM sleep in the early 1950s. Much of basic sleep research has been oriented toward understanding neurobiological mechanisms and networks that control sleep and wake, describing the consequences of sleep deprivation with the goal of answering questions about the function sleep serves, or more recently, discovering the genetic basis of CRs or sleep phenotypes (duration, continuity, disorders). Current clinical sleep research focuses on describing the extent of deficient sleep and its consequences and primary and comorbid sleep disorders in diverse populations, as well as testing appropriate treatments. Research studies have emerged that focus on understanding sleep health. The statements from professional societies (Mukherjee et al., 2015; Watson et al., 2015) recognize the importance of sleep health, and reviews highlight the perils of inadequate sleep (Albakri et al., 2021; Grandner, 2017).

Buysse (2014) introduced a definition of sleep health (Box 15.4). Inherent in this definition are the dimensions suggested as appropriate for measuring sleep health: satisfaction,

Box 15.4 Sleep Health

Sleep health is a multidimensional pattern of sleep–wakefulness, adapted to individual, social, and environmental demands, which promotes physical and mental well-being. Good sleep health is characterized by subjective satisfaction, appropriate timing, adequate duration, high efficiency, and sustained alertness during waking hours.

Source: Buysse, D. J. (2014). Sleep health: Can we define it? Does it matter? Sleep, 37(1), 9–17. https://doi.org/10.5665/sleep.3298

alertness, timing, efficiency, and duration. Buysse (2014) developed a scale, SATED, to measure sleep health and recently added a dimension, regularity. This scale with six items rated "rarely/never = 0," "sometimes = 1," and "usually/always = 2" will yield a total score of "12 = good sleep health." It is designed for screening purposes and could easily be used in a clinical setting. A recent psychometric evaluation study validated this instrument with a noted Cronbach's alpha (α = .64) in 3,401 adults (47.8% female; Ravyts et al., 2021).

Sleep Health Promotion

SLEEP HYGIENE PRACTICES

Messages about good sleep practices are well known and easy to find with a simple internet search (sleep hygiene practices). Box 15.5 contains tips for better sleep. Sleep hygiene includes practices such as presleep routines (getting ready for bed) using goals for timing (bedtime), turning lights off in the house to allow the brain to have less stimulation (including electronics), relaxation techniques to remove cognitive stimulus, and avoiding food and drinks that interfere with sleep. Using the same cues on a regular basis alerts the reticular activating system (RAS, the system that control the brain during sleep) that it is time to take over.

Although these practices are well known to sleep scientists and clinicians, and many parents employ them to assist their children with sleep, many adults do not employ them for themselves and are unaware of their own habits and practices that are not conducive to good sleep. The empirical basis for sleep hygiene recommendations is largely based on findings from laboratory studies (e.g., caffeine, nicotine, and alcohol). Whether other individual components of sleep hygiene recommendations, such as reducing noise, keeping the bedroom dark and cool, and managing stress, improve sleep has not been well tested (Irish et al., 2015). In their review, Irish et al. summarize practice points for sleep hygiene, as follows:

> Although each recommendation is theoretically sound and plausible, a review of individual sleep hygiene recommendations regarding caffeine use, smoking, alcohol use, exercise, stress, noise, sleep timing, and napping revealed that empirical support for these recommendations in the general population is lacking. (Irish et al., 2015, p. 33)

As noted previously, caffeine is an effective countermeasure for daytime sleepiness. However, from laboratory studies, caffeine consumed before bedtime disrupts sleep in a dose-dependent manner, with the doses of more than 250 mg associated both with self-reported and with actigraphic disrupted sleep, and tolerance may develop quickly (Irish et al., 2015). Fewer studies have examined effects of either reducing caffeine intake or limiting use to morning hours only, as sleep hygiene recommendations suggest. The amounts of caffeine available in some commercial products are large, as shown in Box 15.6. For individuals who are particularly sensitive to the alerting effects of caffeine, a short nap of 15 to 20 minutes midafternoon could be a better option than consuming a latte or a cappuccino. Irish et al. (2015) found that short napping (less than 30 minutes) could be beneficial to those suffering from daytime

Box 15.5 Tips for Better Sleep

Create a Conducive Environment

Turn down the lights in the house as bedtime approaches.

Keep your bedroom quiet, dark, and cool.

Go to bed only when sleepy.

Turn off electronic devices such as laptops and phones.

Avoid Certain Behaviors

Avoid heavy meals before bed.

Avoid strenuous exercise close to sleep (within 2–3 hours).

Avoid tobacco, alcohol, and caffeine.

Avoid napping during the day.

Establish a Bedtime Routine

Assume a comfortable posture.

Clear the mind and tune out distractions.

Use muscle relaxation, pleasant visual images, and relaxing bodily sensations.

A light snack (starch, protein) can be relaxing.

Be Consistent

Use the bedroom only for sleep (and sex).

Go to bed at the same time every night to obtain sufficient sleep.

Get up at same time every morning, even on weekends, to set up a regular sleep pattern.

Be physically active; regular daily exercise may help sleep.

If not asleep in 20 minutes, get up and do something relaxing; go back to bed when tired.

sleepiness and, in some studies, had minimal adverse effects on nighttime sleep.

For individuals who suffer from chronic insomnia, sleep hygiene instructions alone have not been very effective, however, when coupled with CBT they are considered quite effective for improving sleep in adults (Chung et al., 2018). Telephone delivery of CBT-I is quite effective for improving sleep and reducing insomnia symptoms in women in the late stage of TPM and early postmenopause (McCurry et al., 2016). Results of a clinical trial of older adults with osteoarthritis recruited from a primary care setting showed that those who improved their sleep with the initial treatment of combined CBT-I and CBT for pain intervention showed sustained significant improvements in reduced insomnia symptoms (ISI), improved sleep quality, and pain severity at 18-month follow-up (Vitiello et al., 2014). A self-help–oriented 6-week intervention program was effective in improving

Box 15.6 Examples of Caffeine Content in Commercial Products

Coffee

Starbucks Coffee, Pike Place (venti, 20 fl oz) 410 mg

Starbucks Coffee Blond Roast (grande, 16 fl oz): 330 mg

Starbucks Coffee Dark Roast (grande, 16 fl oz): 260 mg

Starbucks Caffe Latté, Cappuccino, Caramel Macchiato (grande 16 fl oz): 260 mg

Dunkin' Donuts Coffee (large, 20 fl oz): 270 mg

Dunkin' Donuts Coffee (medium, 14 fl oz): 210 mg

Starbucks Decaf Coffee, Pike Place (grande, 16 fl oz): 25 mg

Bottle Coffee Drink

High Brew Nitro Black Cold Brew (10 fl oz): 200 mg

Starbucks Vanilla Latte Chilled Espresso (12 fl oz): 125 mg

Starbucks Mocha Frappuccino (13.7 fl oz): 110 mg

Tea

Starbucks Tazo Awake (grande, 16 fl oz): 135 mg

Black tea, brewed for 3 minutes (8 fl oz): 30–80 mg

Soft Drinks (All 12 fl oz)

Pepsi Zero Sugar: 69 mg

Mountain Dew: 54 mg

Diet Coke: 46 mg

Seven-Up, Fanta, Fresca, ginger ale, or Sprite: 0 mg

Energy Drinks

5-hour Energy Extra Strength (1.9 fl oz): 230 mg

Monster Energy (16 fl oz): 160 mg

Red Bull (8.4 fl oz): 80 mg

Chocolate Candy and Drinks

Hershey's Special Dark (1 bar, 1.5 oz): 20 mg

Hershey's Milk Chocolate (1 bar, 1.6 oz): 9 mg

Dannon Lowfat Coffee Yogurt (5.3 oz): 40 mg

Source: Center for Science in the Public Interest. (2022). Caffeine chart. https://www.cspinet.org/caffeine-chart

sleep quality (PSQI) and insomnia symptoms (ISI) compared with standard sleep hygiene among older adults with comorbid medical conditions (Morgan et al., 2012). Glovinsky and Spielman's text, *The Insomnia Answer* (2006) and follow-up book, *You Are Getting Sleepy: Lifestyle-Based Solutions for Insomnia* (2018), provide a personalized program for identifying and managing sleep onset, maintenance, and early morning insomnia symptoms. Glovinsky and Spielman

advocate assessing sleep hygiene practice to assist individuals to identify habits and behaviors that may be disturbing sleep, and attending to them, rather than ignoring them, will aid in sleeping better.

EXERCISE EFFECTS ON SLEEP

Among the components of good sleep hygiene practices, evidence for the beneficial effects of regular exercise on sleep seems the most robust. Both regular and, especially, acute bouts of exercise have been shown to improve sleep quality and duration, both by self-report and by PSG measures (Irish et al., 2015). However, data from exercise training of at least 4 weeks' duration have shown mainly improvement in self-reported sleep quality, with limited data available on objective sleep measures. A 12-week intervention trial of yoga (Buchanan et al., 2017; Newton et al., 2014) and aerobic exercise (Sternfeld et al., 2014) yielded small, significant improvements in ISI compared with usual activity in women with hot flashes; aerobic exercise also was associated with improved sleep quality. Exercise may be quite beneficial for improving sleep quality (Irish et al., 2015). However, exercise is complex, and at present, there are few clear guidelines as to the type, duration, intensity, and timing associated with improving sleep (Irish et al., 2015).

Over the past few years, many technological devices for personal monitoring of physical activity have become commercially available, and some also monitor sleep. These devices may work well for counting steps, providing estimates of energy expenditure and heart rate, or assisting individuals to reach performance goals, but the ability to monitor sleep quality accurately is questionable because they reply on time of inactivity, which may or may not represent actual sleep as described above. Additionally, these devices may have not undergone reliability or validity testing with PSG or been compared with actigraphs that have been validated for sleep.

SLEEP MEDICATION

The use of medications to treat sleep disorders has increased with the evolution of prescription and over-the-counter sleep aids. The AASM has published several clinical guidelines for treatment of several sleep disorders and these should be the gold standard when considering oral medications for treatment. Oral sleep medications can be categorized into prescription and over the counter (e.g., herbal and nonherbal). The majority of sleep medications focus on sleep-enhancing agents that promote sleep. However, sleep disorders include other conditions such as RLS and narcolepsy, which require different classifications of prescription and nonprescription medication intervention. The following will provide brief information according to the type of sleep disorder.

Since insomnia is the most common sleep disorder, this section focuses on drug classifications called benzodiazepines and nonbenzodiazepines. Benzodiazepines are the traditional agents used for short-term treatment of sleep–wake disturbances (Holbrook, 2004). Benzodiazepine compounds are agonists that mimic the action of the neurotransmitter gamma-aminobutyric acid (GABA). Nonbenzodiazepines are considered the newer generation of sedative-hypnotics (Holbrook, 2004). The mechanism of action for nonbenzodiazepines is similar to benzodiazepines but binding is selective to certain receptor sites and thus are more selective in their action. Both types of drugs remain the most prescribed hypnotics for the treatment of sleep–wake disturbances. The current practice recommendations divide medication recommendations for insomnia as treatment of sleep initiation (ability to fall asleep) and sleep maintenance (staying asleep; Sateia et al., 2017). Current recommendations include Food and Drug Administration (FDA) recommended medications for the short-term use for treatment of insomnia such as eszopiclone, doxepin, and zolpidem. Currently, the recommendations do not support use of nonprescription sleep medications purchased over the counter and include sleep aids such as melatonin, CBD oil, and diphenhydramine derivative agents for the treatment of insomnia (Sateia et al., 2017).

Other practice guidelines can be found for treatment of RLS (Allen et al., 2018) and hypersomnolence disorders (Maski et al., 2021), These both note the recommendations for various populations such as pregnancy. See Appendix 15A at the end of this chapter for additional details on medications used to treat sleep disorders and medications that can exacerbate or cause sleep disorders.

CONSUMER TECHNOLOGIES FOR SLEEP PROMOTION

Along with technologies for monitoring physical activity, many types of commercial devices have become available to measure sleep with a primary goal of improving it. Consumer sleep technology (CST), also known as *wearables*, are accessible in the form of downloaded apps to smart phones or wearable wrist devices (e.g., Fitbit or Apple Watch). These devices may aid in sleep or wake induction, provide self-guided sleep assessment, entertainment, information sharing, and education about sleep cycle quality or quantity.

The AASM issued a position statement in 2018 to provide guidance for healthcare providers to educating patients regarding the use and accuracy of these products (Khosla et al., 2018). Most wearable products are not approved by the FDA, diminishing the utility to help clinicians with usable data and should not be used as substitutes for medical evaluation (Khosla et al., 2018). The technology of wearables is improving. Although most of these products have not undergone reliability or validity testing to verify the acceptable use in practice, a group of investigators recently evaluated the validity of two wearables developed for measuring sleep on an iPhone and Oura Ring compared with laboratory-based PSG and wrist actigraph (Respironics Aciwatch Spectrum Plus; Roberts et al., 2020). They found strong correlations between the two devices compared to comparable research devices of actigraphy and PSG and the application for SE, sleep stages, or SOL. Furthermore, an epoch-by-epoch comparison showed moderate accuracy through sensitivity between 0.88 and 0.98 and specificity between 0.41 and 0.82 in detecting sleep using machine learning methods suggesting wearable multisensory data could be used in research studies.

In a review and commentary on some of the most popular devices (Ko et al., 2015), the app "Go! to Sleep" created by the Cleveland Clinic Sleep Disorders Center, a lifestyle and sleep habit questionnaire is used to create a sleep score, track the score over time, and provide daily sleep advice to improve

one's score (my.clevelandclinic.org/mobile-apps/go-to-sleep-app). Consumer sleep technologies have the potential to raise awareness of and promote education about sleep health, but they may have an unintended consequence of providing inaccurate information about one's actual sleep. The number of devices oriented to monitoring sleep, along with physical activity and nutritional intake, is likely to increase with people relying more on technology and the focus of healthcare becoming more oriented toward healthy lifestyles. Understandably, wearables are popular and can be used to encourage consumers to seek guidance when sleep becomes problematic and further engage in an appropriate evaluation by a provider.

FUTURE DIRECTIONS

Investigators continue to study the empirical basis for sleep hygiene practices. More research is needed in naturalistic settings as opposed to the laboratory (Irish et al., 2015). Important questions remain unanswered. At present, unlike physical activity and nutrition, there are no validated, broadly disseminated global or U.S.-based public health programs for sleep. Does following sleep hygiene recommendations (such as keeping a regular sleep and wake pattern; keeping the bedroom quiet, dark, and cool; or avoiding caffeine after lunch) really improve sleep quality and duration? What is an optimal dose of caffeine or alcohol that is associated with good sleep? Do rituals and relaxation exercises before bedtime improve sleep quality and duration? Does reducing caffeine lead to more napping behavior with unintended consequences such as feeling too tired to exercise? How do racial differences in poor sleep impact pregnancy and postpartum outcomes? How does hormone therapy for transgender persons affect sleep? What might be the best combination of sleep hygiene practices for various diverse populations? Just as important as studies about the effectiveness of sleep hygiene practices are questions about extending sleep time. Does making more time for sleep lead to longer sleep duration and better health outcomes? Do intervention programs fail to assist people to lose weight or sustain weight loss because they are not getting enough sleep? Do community-based walking programs fail to engage and sustain large numbers of participants because people are just too tired to attend? Are the recommended sleep health programs delivered in a culturally sensitive manner? What are the sleep issues and needs for the LGBTQ+ population? Among older adults, about 50% complain of sleep problems, but 50% do not. Why not? What motivates individuals to obtain adequate sleep? The overall average of sleep duration from a survey in 1985 fell only by approximately 13 minutes, yet the number of individuals reporting less than or at least 6 hours' sleep increased 7%, estimated to represent approximately 31 million in the United States (Ford et al., 2015). Why are more people sleeping fewer hours? What interventions will work to assist individuals and families to prioritize sleep? How does the long-term impact of the COVID-19 pandemic affect our understanding of the illness trajectory and sleep health?

In the United States and especially in advanced practice nursing, a paradigm shift continues in healthcare, from an emphasis on treating medical disorders to preventing them. Simultaneously, in the field of sleep medicine, a paradigm shift continues from an emphasis on studies and treatments for sleep disorders to a focus on sleep health and ways to assist people to obtain good, adequate sleep. The evolution of the NSF's quality indicators provides evidence-based recommendations to the public and needs wider dissemination through public health campaigns across the life span. Perhaps a good starting place is in the home, with families of all backgrounds addressing typical household routines to tailor culturally and individually sensitive information. Findings from a clinical trial focused on family routines known to influence the growing epidemic of obesity in preschool children yielded positive benefits for sleep duration, although BMI was the primary target (Haines et al., 2013). After a 6-month trial, families ($n = 62$) who received the intervention program (promoting family meals, adequate sleep, limited TV time, and removal of technologies from the child's bedroom through motivational interviewing) reported that their children slept 0.56 hour more per day compared with control subjects ($n = 59$), who slept 0.19 hour per day less. There were no group differences in number of family meals or TVs removed from the child's bedroom; TV viewing was reduced by 1.06 hours in the intervention group. Children in the intervention group had lower BMIs after the intervention, whereas BMI in control children increased. Families in the study were predominately Black and Hispanic with annual incomes of $20,000 or less. The findings from this study are important, and the authors noted that of the 500 families contacted, only 24% enrolled, and thus the findings are not generalizable. However, bundled lifestyle interventions such as the Healthy Habits, Happy Homes trial hold promise for future prevention studies. Obtaining efficient, restful, satisfying sleep of adequate duration synchronized with one's internal "clock" is key to staying alert throughout the day.

As the NSF Women and Sleep poll found, and continues to be a repeated finding in research, far too many women are trying to do it all, perhaps burning the candle at both ends, placing themselves and their families at risk for sleep problems and sleep-related morbidity. APRNs, especially in women's health, family, and primary care settings, are at the forefront to understand changes in sleep as women age and the hazards of inadequate sleep and are poised to help improve the sleep of their patients.

RESOURCES

1. Weblink or app resource for insomnia: https://support.myshuti.com/hc/en-us/articles/115004286247-What-is-SHUTi-
2. Clinical practice guidelines for sleep disorders: American Academy of Sleep Medicine: https://aasm.org
3. National Foundation of Sleep: https://www.thensf.org
4. *Sleep Disorders in Women* textbook (Viola-Saltzman & Attarian, 2020)

APPENDIX 15A. MEDICATIONS USED IN SLEEP DISORDERS

Appendix 15A is online and available at https://connect.springerpub.com.

REFERENCES

References for this chapter are online and available at https://connect.springerpub.com/content/book/978-0-8261-6722-4/part/part02/chapter/ch15

CHAPTER 16

Genetics and Women's Health*

SARAH E. MARTIN AND ELIZABETH A. KOSTAS-POLSTON

OVERVIEW OF THE REACH OF GENETICS AND CLINICAL CARE

Rapid scientific advances and the emergence of direct-to-consumer (DTC) genetic testing are pushing clinicians in all practice communities to become more knowledgeable about genetics. Although the basic tenets of inheritance have been known (and manipulated) since antiquity, the biological mechanisms responsible for an individual's unique characteristics remained shrouded in mystery until very recently. The molecule that forms the foundation for DNA (nucleic acid) was described in 1869 (Dahm, 2008), but nearly a century passed before DNA's precise molecular structure was determined (Pray, 2008), and another 50 years ticked by before the first draft of the human genome was completed in 2003 (Collins et al., 2003). Over the past decade, the pace of scientific and technological advances has continued to accelerate, with sequencing speed doubling every 4 months and costs plummeting from hundreds of millions of dollars to just a few thousand dollars during that time (National Human Genome Research Institute [NHGRI], 2013). Researchers are now conducting highly complex genome-wide association studies (GWASs), combining phenotype, family health history (FHH), and genomics to better explain the development of complex health conditions such as hypertension and diabetes.

Educational leaders across all healthcare professions are looking for ways to infuse this important (and rapidly evolving) information into curricula effectively, but nursing has the additional challenge of meeting the needs of a professional community that is evolving rapidly as well. This chapter provides an overview of some of the important genomic concepts that all clinicians should know but places particular emphasis on the intersection between genomics and women's health.

GENETIC AND GENOMIC COMPETENCIES FOR NURSES

Virtually every disease has a genetic or genomic component and treatment options increasingly involve genetics in disease prevention, screening, diagnosis, prognosis, and monitoring. In 2005, committed to addressing the practice and knowledge gap in the nursing profession, a panel of nursing leaders, cosponsored by the American Nurses Association (ANA), NHGRI, National Cancer Institute (NCI), and Office of Rare Diseases (ORD), gathered to identify essential genetic and genomic competencies that all registered nurses should have. The following year *The Essential Nursing Competencies and Curricula Guidelines for Genetics and Genomics* was published. In 2009, an updated version added curricular guidelines for nursing educators to use when creating nursing curricula (Jenkins, 2011). Three years later, an expanded set of genetic/genomic competencies guiding the education of nurses at the graduate level was published. These competencies, the *Essential Genetic/Genomic Competencies for Nurses With Graduate Degrees*, were developed specifically for nurses with advanced degrees, including, but not limited to, advanced practice registered nurses (APRNs), clinical nurse leaders, nurse educators, nurse administrators, and nurse scientists (Greco et al., 2011). None of these documents replaces or recreates existing standards of practice, but rather they incorporate genetic and genomic perspectives into nursing education and practice. It is important to note that all three documents were created by consensus, informed by public opinion, and endorsed by more than 30 nursing organizations.

---

*This chapter is a revision of the chapter that appeared in the second edition of this textbook, coauthored with Diane C. Seibert, and we thank her for her original contribution.

SEX, GENDER, AND GENETICS

Genetics plays a role in the majority of the leading causes of death in the United States (Centers for Disease Control and Prevention [CDC], 2015a). Diseases such as cancer, diabetes, and cardiovascular disease are related to epigenetic influences—the complex interactions among shared genes, behaviors, cultures, and environments that influence health and risk (CDC, 2015; Scheuner et al., 2004).

Biological differences between women and men result from sex determination and differentiation. The sex determination process determines if the female or male sexual differentiation pathway will be followed. Sex differentiation, the development of a given sex, involves many genetically regulated and developmental steps. For example, the Y chromosome produces testicular differentiation of the embryonic gonad. Gender, usually described as masculinity and femininity, is a social construct and varies across cultures and time. Biological differences between women and men manifest differently when considering health risk. Table 16.1 describes sex and gender influences on health across the life span.

An FHH is an important tool used to identify and prevent or reduce risk. If used properly, it allows the healthcare provider to take steps toward the early diagnosis and management of disease as well as make appropriate referrals.

GENETICS AND TRANSGENDER CONSIDERATIONS

With the paradigm shift in societal and cultural norms, there is a growing population of individuals who identify as transgender or nonbinary in healthcare settings. Therefore, healthcare professionals should have the cultural competencies and medical knowledge needed to provide appropriate genetic counseling, testing, and referrals (von Vaupel-Klein & Walsh, 2021). For example, a transgender client who is biologically female (XX) but identifies as male or nonbinary (not specific to either gender) will still need to be counseled on the importance of cervical cancer screening (Pap smears) unless they undergo hysterectomy to remove the uterus and cervix. In addition, *BRCA1/BRCA2* genetic mutation screening may still be warranted based on cascade testing and FHH. As healthcare professionals and nurses, it is important to recognize your personal beliefs and cultural barriers so that optimal health screening and genetic services can be provided to all clients and referrals can be made when appropriate.

WOMEN AS GATEKEEPERS OF FAMILY HEALTH HISTORY AND HEALTH

The collection of an accurate FHH is an essential element of client assessment, but although most clinicians appreciate how important the FHH is, this important information is rarely collected, updated, or recorded systematically (Welch

TABLE 16.1 Sex and Gender Influences on Health

FEMALES	MALES
Mental Health	
• Twice as likely to experience depression • More likely to develop eating disorder, panic disorder, and PTSD • Depressed middle-aged women have almost double risk of having a stroke • Experience mood symptoms related to hormone changes during puberty, pregnancy, and perimenopause	• More likely to show aggressive, impulsive, coercive, and noncompliant behaviors
Cardiovascular Disease	
• Low-dose aspirin reduces risk of ischemic stroke. • Blood vessels of a woman's heart are smaller in diameter and much more intricately branched. • Cholesterol plaque may not build up into major artery blockages. Instead, they spread evenly over the entire wall of the artery. This makes diagnosis of artery blockages more difficult. • Onset of cardiovascular disease occurs later in women.	• Low-dose aspirin reduces risk of heart attack.
Osteoporosis	
• More common because of less bone tissue • Experience a rapid phase of bone loss because of hormonal changes at menopause	• Worse health outcomes post fracture
Osteoarthritis	
• More common ≥45 years of age • Severity significantly worse because of knee and hip anatomy, imbalanced leg muscle strength, and loose tendons and ligaments • Black women at greater risk for osteoarthritis complications	• More common ≤45 years of age
Autoimmune Disorders	
• 80% affected • Pain mechanisms in female brain not found in men; pain associated with irritable bowel syndrome greater in women • In animal models, female chromosome set (XX) stimulates development of lupus	• Type 1 diabetes and ankylosing spondylitis more common
Cancer	
• Lung cancer leading cause of death • For any given number of cigarettes smoked (when compared with men), appear to be at higher risk of developing lung cancer • Breast cancer more common • Greater incidence across the life span, and risk increases in seventh decade and beyond	• Male teens and young men 55% more likely to die of melanoma • Prostate cancer is the leading cause of death • More prone to liver cancer

PTSD, posttraumatic stress disorder.
Source: Adapted from Canadian Institutes of Health Research, Institute of Medicine (IOM), National Institute of Arthritis and Musculoskeletal and Skin Diseases (NIAMSD), National Institutes of Health (NIH), National Institute on Drug Abuse (NIDA), NIH Osteoporosis and Related Bone Diseases, National Resource Center (NIH ORBD NRC), and World Health Organization (WHO).

et al., 2015). Gathering an accurate and complete FHH involves both trust and collaboration; clients have to believe that if they disclose sensitive information, it will be used appropriately, and providers need to ask the right questions at the right time and verify the accuracy of the information they gather. In some families "kinkeepers" play an important role in facilitating family communication (Giordimaina et al., 2015) because they maintain and disseminate family health information; although they are not formally recognized, they are often the ones other family members consult when family medical information is needed. It is interesting to note that kinkeepers are often middle-aged women and are more often identified in White families than in African American or Hispanic American families for reasons that have yet to be completely elucidated (Giordimaina et al., 2015; Thompson et al., 2015).

Disparities in genetic counseling and screening have been identified within medically underserved and minority populations (Hinchcliff et al., 2019). Lack of trust, poor communications, and financial constraints may all contribute as barriers to genetic counseling and missing opportunities for cancer prevention. More research needs to be done to identify the key socioeconomic barriers to genetic counseling services so that the healthcare community can develop mitigation strategies and ensure all women have equitable access for disease prevention and identification. Detailed knowledge of the FHH may be known to these women, not because they are simply curious and ask health-related questions but because women are often responsible for managing the family's health needs.

FAMILY HISTORY AS A MEANS OF EVALUATING RISK

Family Health History

Inquiring about the health history of one's immediate family is a critical part of collecting an individual's medical history. FHH is the most consistent tool for determining risk factors for human disease across the life span; it reveals diseases (e.g., heart disease, diabetes, cancer, osteoporosis, asthma, hypertension, hypercholesterolemia) that carry significant public health concern (Khoury & Mensah, 2005; Yoon et al., 2003). It brings to light the complex interactions among shared genes, behaviors, cultures, and environments that influence families' health and disease risk. In fact, the FHH is so important that it has been referred to as the best genetic test available (Genetic Alliance, n.d., 2009; MedlinePlus, 2021; Scheuner et al., 2004). Although one's FHH cannot be changed, an increased awareness provides healthcare providers with the opportunity to, for example, personalize and target disease prevention, treatment, and management (Khoury, 2003; U.S. Department of Health and Human Services [USDHHS], n.d.). One such method of identifying specific genetic mutations through FHH and genetic counseling is called *cascade testing*. A thorough FHH can help identify relatives with hereditary cancer syndromes and determine if specific genetic testing is

recommended. In women's health, for example, mutations with *BRCA1* and *BRCA2* genes are commonly associated with hereditary breast and ovarian cancer (HBOC). Genetic mutations have also been identified in Lynch syndrome, an autosomal dominant condition causing an increased risk of endometrial, ovarian, and colon cancer. In addition, cascade testing is considered more cost effective because it targets specific genetic mutations instead of the more expensive whole-gene sequencing (Committee on Gynecologic Practice, 2018).

Healthcare providers are armed with a variety of tools for evaluating health risk. The FHH is one such important screening tool. It brings to light epigenetic influences, characterizes trends and patterns of disease that may lead to prevention and treatment, and increases knowledge about health and genetics for individuals and their family members (Genetic Alliance, 2009). As a diagnostic tool, the FHH is used to guide medical decisions about genetic testing and disease risk.

Precision Medicine Initiative

In 2015, the brightest leaders in the United States in science (National Institutes of Health [NIH], 2015) rolled out the Precision Medicine Initiative. This initiative came about as a result of the sequencing of the human genome, improved technologies for biomedical analyses, and new tools for the use of large data sets. The hope is that new scientific evidence will be generated to inform clinical practice. In fact, the overall aim is to integrate this genomic approach for disease prevention and treatment, necessitating a marked paradigmatic shift in the manner in which healthcare providers currently deliver healthcare. Overcoming drug resistance, adopting advanced pharmacogenomics (the right drug for the right patient at the right dose), using new targets for prevention and treatment, and using mobile devices to encourage healthy lifestyle behaviors are but a few of the projected goals. Central to the Precision Medicine Initiative is the FHH.

Contemporary Clinical Practice

In contemporary healthcare education and training programs, graduate students are taught how to take a thorough family medical history using questions and pedigree collection. It is unfortunate that in clinical practice, time constraints necessitate, at best, an abbreviated collection of family medical history, often focusing only on diseases with high prevalence (e.g., heart disease, cancer, hypertension, diabetes; Yoon et al., 2003). The result is an incomplete FHH that is missing critical health information. What is more, the incomplete FHH limits the healthcare provider's ability to accurately determine health risk as well as to identify potential preventive and treatment measures.

Family Health History Tools

Because time constraints are a reality, FHH tools have been developed so that clients may complete them before clinic visits.

An FHH should reflect the gold standard, a three-generation pedigree (if possible and at minimum) of biological relatives as well as age at diagnosis and age and cause of death of family members. There are many tools available. One such tool, My Family Health Portrait (USDHHS, n.d.), is a computerized tool that runs on any web-connected computer or laptop. There is no cost, and once an individual has created a family health portrait, they can download the file to their personal computer and even share it with other family members. This way, family members can share their accurate FHH with their healthcare providers. This particular tool is part of the U.S. Surgeon General's Family History Initiative (USDHHS, n.d.) that encourages family gatherings to incorporate time to talk about and document health problems that run in families. It is important that the information gathered be reliable, which may require family members checking old health records of loved ones as well as death certificates. Other tools are also available at no cost.

The emergence and popularity of DTC genetic testing has shifted the platform of genetics from the healthcare sector into the private sector. The low costs and convenience of obtaining genetic testing has enabled the population at large to identify one's pedigree and medical risk factors. In 2017, 23andMe Personal Genome Service became the first DTC test for genetic health risk (GHR) to be approved by the Food and Drug Administration (FDA; Allyse et al., 2018). Many other DTC genetic testing companies are also seeking FDA approval, such as Color Genomics, Good Start Genetics and Counsyl, and Ancestory.com. DTC genetic testing has many pros and cons for consideration by the healthcare community and we must stay informed of the latest developments in "infotainment" so we can adapt accordingly to our patient needs.

Genetics, Genomics, and Advanced Practice Nursing

Today, tumultuous changes resulting from advances in biomedical technology are evidenced in all healthcare disciplines and settings. These advances are redefining the understanding of health and illness and are necessitating changes in education, training, and clinical practice. APRNs are positioned to contribute significantly to the genetic and genomic transformation of healthcare for the purpose of improving clinical outcomes.

For the purpose of defining genomic competencies in advanced nursing practice, the *Essential Genetic and Genomic Competencies for Nurses With Graduate Degrees* (Greco et al., 2012) were developed in 2006 (revised in 2009). These competencies of professional advanced practice nursing are organized under seven topics: (a) risk assessment and interpretation; (b) genetic education; counseling, testing, and results interpretation; (c) clinical management; (d) ethical, legal, and social implications (ELSIs); (e) professional role; (f) leadership; and (g) research (Greco et al., 2012). The FHH serves as the clinical starting point (risk assessment and interpretation). Evaluation of the FHH brings to light genetic red flags (reported family health issues, which become suspect for possible increased health risk; Seibert, 2014). Genetic red flags serve to shape the professional conversation between the healthcare provider and client. Genetic and

genomic competencies provide a framework to be used in advanced practice nursing.

Pedigrees

FHH data can be captured in several ways: provided in oral communication, written in a narrative, or displayed graphically in a drawing, called a *pedigree*. Pedigrees are particularly useful because they reveal the influence of both heredity and environment on an individual and within a particular family. The pedigree can trace how traits are passed along within a family, and the incidence of a particular characteristic in a family can actually be counted. Standardized symbols (Figure 16.1) can be used to document and communicate the FHH. Because the FHH constantly evolves, clients should be encouraged to ask about changes in the FHH from their family members, and pedigrees should be reviewed and updated regularly by providers.

The complete pedigree contains information about three generations of family members including first-degree (parents, siblings, and children), second-degree (half-siblings, grandparents, aunts, uncles, and grandchildren), and third-degree (cousins) relatives. Whenever possible, data should be recorded electronically to facilitate retrieval, review, and updating.

As time consuming and challenging as collecting an accurate and complete FHH might be, accurately assessing risk to an individual is more difficult because information from disparate (and often multiple) sources must be appraised and synthesized. Several mnemonics have been developed to help clinicians assess genomic risk (Table 16.2). The first, SCREEN, is used to elicit concerns and/or risk factors regarding a client's family history; the second, F-GENES, helps stratify clinical features into red-flag categories; and the words *too* and *two* are often used to describe individuals or families with genetic conditions because a particular condition occurs too

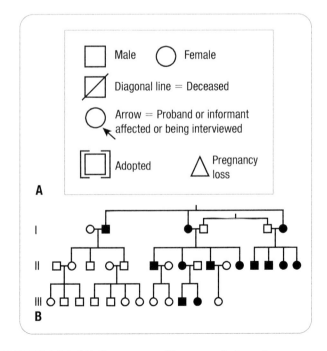

FIGURE 16.1 (A) Common pedigree symbols and **(B)** a three-generation pedigree.

TABLE 16.2 Three Mnemonics for Gathering and Interpreting the Family Health History

MNEMONIC	DEFINITION/INTERPRETATION
SCREEN	Some concern: Do you have any (some) concerns about diseases or conditions that seem to run in your family?
	Reproduction: Have there been any problems with pregnancy, infertility, or birth defects in your family?
	Early disease/death/disability: Have any members of your family been diagnosed with a chronic disease at an early age, or have members of your family died at an early age?
	Ethnicity: How would you describe your ethnicity? What country did your ancestors come from?
	Nongenetic or not necessarily genetic: Are you aware of any nonmedical conditions or risk factors, such as smoking or problem drinking, that are present in your family?
F-GENES	Family history: Multiple affected siblings or individuals in multiple generations
	Groups of congenital anomalies
	Extreme or exceptional presentation of common conditions (e.g., early age of onset, condition manifesting in a less-often-affected sex)
	Neurodevelopmental delay or degeneration
	Extreme or exceptional pathology
	Surprising laboratory values
Rule of Too/Two	Too something (tall, short, early, young, many, different)
	Two of something (tumors, generations, in the family, congenital defects)

Source: Adapted from The Jackson Library. (n.d.). Core principles in family history: Interpretation. Retrieved October 14, 2022, from https://www.jax.org/education -and-learning/clinical-and-continuing-education/clinical-topics/core-principles -in-family-history/interpretation#:~:text=In%20general%2C%20identifying%20 %E2%80%9CGenetic%20Red,genetic%20disorder%20in%20family%20members

often, affects too many individuals, or appears in two locations (two primary cancers) or in two generations of family members, and so forth.

Other genetic red flags include disease in the absence of known risk factors, ethnic predisposition to certain genetic disorders, and close biological relationship between parents, such as consanguinity, all of which, if present, raise the index of suspicion that an individual might be at increased risk for developing a particular condition (Arnold & Self, 2012; Borgmeyer, 2005). Referring back to the competencies in the *Essential Genetic and Genomic Competencies for Nurses With Graduate Degrees* (Greco et al., 2012), other questions that might be asked include:

- Is other information (assessment, history, diagnostics) needed to assess their risk?
- Do other family members need to be tested?
- Should a genetic test be offered? If so, which one?
- Is a genetics referral indicated?
- Who will offer posttest counseling and education?

- Assuming a genetic mutation is found, how will clinical care be affected?
- What ELSI issues should be discussed before or after testing?
- Does this case raise any nursing "professional responsibility" concerns?

SCENARIOS

This final section contains three examples that provide a brief case narrative, a pedigree, and a glimpse into a healthcare provider's thoughts as they integrate and synthesize the individual and family health histories with physical examination findings and other clinical data (e.g., laboratory and/or diagnostic testing results) to assess an individual's risk for having (or developing) a particular condition and select an appropriate management strategy.

Scenario 1

JC, a 32-year-old Black female, presents for a routine well-woman examination. Her past medical history is significant for three uncomplicated vaginal deliveries and hypothyroidism, which is well managed. She reports no surgeries except for wisdom tooth extraction at age 19. She has no allergies, takes no over-the-counter medications, and regularly takes Synthroid 75 mcg and NuvaRing (contraception). JC is a good historian, providing a thorough FHH (see Figure 16.2).

As you evaluate JC's FHH (Figure 16.2) you immediately notice that she and several other family members have different autoimmune disorders and you suspect that other family members may be at an increased risk for developing autoimmune diseases as well. You also wonder if a gene is involved, whether it may have been inherited from her 72-year-old father, because he, too, has an autoimmune condition. Her mother died relatively young from a stroke, at age 62 years, so family members may share genes that put them at an increased risk for cardiovascular disease, but because the genetics of many complex conditions like autoimmune and cardiovascular disease are unknown, you really cannot evaluate the risk in an empiric way. The NIH estimates that 5% to 8% of Americans have an autoimmune disorder, and alterations in immune response are involved in more than 80 human diseases (National Institute of Allergy and Infectious Disease, 2016). Related individuals may not always develop the same autoimmune disease, and the risk may be greater or smaller depending on the specific disease, but in general, close relatives are more likely to develop related autoimmune disorders. Many genes have been implicated in causing autoimmune disease, primarily genes related to the human major histocompatibility complex (human leukocyte antigen [HLA]), the most gene-dense region in the human genome, containing around 250 genes, nearly 100 of which are thought to regulate immune function (Goris & Liston, 2012). However, genes associated with the development of autoimmune disease do not usually act in isolation. Environmental exposures and viral infections are common triggers in the development of autoimmune disease. The FHH can be useful in

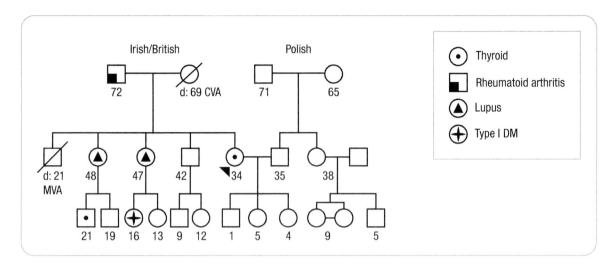

FIGURE 16.2 JC's family health history.
CVA, cerebrovascular accident; DM, diabetes mellitus; MVA, motor vehicle accident.

highlighting shared environmental exposures, but in most cases, clear evidence of a specific environmental trigger causing autoimmune disease is absent (Ray et al., 2012).

Because those conditions seen in JC's family are so complex, no specific genetic tests are currently available, and no referrals or other diagnostic testing is currently needed. JC should be told that she might be at an increased risk for developing other autoimmune conditions and should be alert to the appearance of unusual symptoms (joint pain, polyuria, polydipsia) and clinicians should carefully assess for early manifestations of other autoimmune conditions.

Scenario 2

DG, a 32-year-old White female, presents requesting a genetic test for breast cancer stating she has a "strong family history of breast cancer" (Figure 16.3).

To determine whether she is, in fact, at an increased risk for developing breast cancer compared to other White women, the FHH is scrutinized for red flags that might

indicate that she is at an increased risk for inherited breast disease (see Figure 16.3):

- Ashkenazi Jewish ancestry (UNKNOWN)
- FHH of breast, ovarian, or pancreatic cancer (YES)
- Ovarian cancer at any age (NO)
- FHH of breast *and* ovarian or breast *and* pancreatic cancer (NO)
- More than two family members with breast cancer, one at a young age (NO)
- More than three family members with breast cancer at any age (NO)
- Breast cancer in a male relative (NO)
- Breast cancer diagnosed before menopause (≤50 years) (NO)
- One or more primary breast cancers in one individual or on the same side of the family (NO)
- Triple negative breast cancer (UNKNOWN)

DG might be at an increased risk for developing breast cancer because she does have two second-degree relatives who

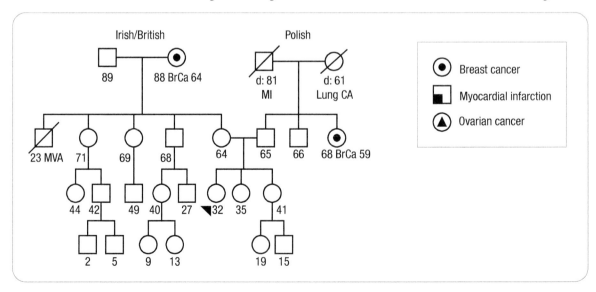

FIGURE 16.3 DG's family health history.
BrCa, breast cancer; CA, cancer; MI, myocardial infarction; MVA, motor vehicle accident.

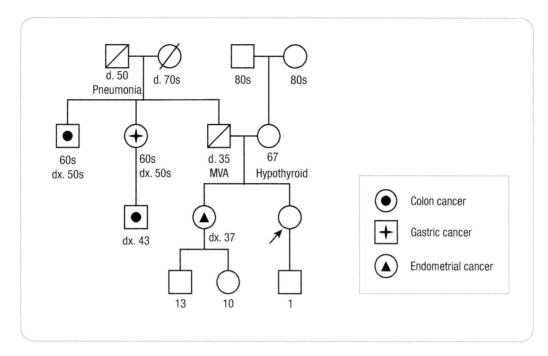

FIGURE 16.4 MB's family health history.
dx, diagnosis; MVA, motor vehicle accident.

have had breast cancer, but she is much more likely to be at "population" (or average) risk because the two affected women are on opposite sides of the family, and both developed postmenopausal breast cancer (ages 64 and 59 years). She does not know whether either woman had any genetic testing nor whether either of the tumors were tested for hormone receptor status. She does not think that she has any relatives who were Ashkenazi Jewish, although it is possible as her grandfather was from Poland. Although pieces of information are unknown, DG's FHH is not provocative for inherited breast disease and no further genetic testing for HBOC genes is indicated at this time.

DG should be reminded, however, that one in every eight women (12.4%) born in the United States will develop breast cancer at some time during their lifetime. Although current screening recommendations for women at population risk are inconsistent, you should have a conversation with her about when and how often to screen given her FHH, her personal risks (age of menarche and menopause, pregnancy and breastfeeding history, radiation exposure, etc.), and her anxiety about developing breast cancer.

Scenario 3

MB, a 34-year-old White female, is concerned about developing uterine cancer because her older sister was just diagnosed with it and was told by *her* doctor that MB should see a genetics specialist. You have known MB for several years and believe you have a good relationship with her. You last saw her 2 months ago when you started her on oral contraceptive pills after she stopped breastfeeding her son. MB has mild anxiety that is somewhat worse now that she is nearly as old as her father was when he died in a car accident, but she is otherwise healthy, has never had any surgery, and takes only combined hormonal birth control pills and multivitamins. Although

you have known MB for several years, you have never gathered a detailed, three-generation FHH on her before, and you are surprised at what you learn (see Figure 16.4).

Although you do not know much about hereditary colorectal cancer (CRC) syndromes, you recognize that there are some significant red flags in her FHH.

- Three or more family members have been diagnosed with a CRC-associated cancer (YES)
- One affected family member must have been diagnosed before age 50 (YES)
- One affected family member must be a first-degree relative to the other two (YES)
- At least two consecutive generations must be affected (YES)

Several family members on MB's paternal side have developed a CRC-syndrome cancer: one first-degree relative (her sister), two second-degree relatives (paternal aunt and paternal uncle), and one third-degree relative (paternal cousin).

SHOULD MB BE OFFERED A GENETIC TEST? IF SO, WHICH ONE?

Genetic testing is appropriate in this case, but the biggest question is what test to order and who to test. The first question to ask is whether any of MB's affected relatives had been tested for a CRC-syndrome mutation; if the family gene is known, MB can be screened for just the familial mutation. If no one in the family has been tested, however, the best person to test is someone with the disease, such as MB's uncle, sister, or cousin, because they are still alive. Genetic testing is expensive when the familial mutation is unknown because several genes have to be tested and additional confirmatory tests may also be necessary. Because MB's sister developed a CRC-associated cancer, MB's father likely had the mutation as well, but because he died at a young age, he never manifested the disease.

TABLE 16.3 Phenotype Variations in Lynch Syndrome

ASSOCIATED CONDITION	LIFETIME RISK OF CONDITION	NOTES
Colon cancer	*MLH1, MSH2* (43%–82%) *MSH6* (20%–44%) *PMS2* (15%–20%) *EPCAM* (75%)	For *MLH1, MSH2,* and *MSH6,* risks are lower in women
Endometrial cancer	*MLH1, MSH2,* and *MSH6* (44%) *PMS2* and *EPCAM:* unknown	In 50% of Lynch syndrome women, this is the initial presentation
Gastric cancer	*MLH1* and *MSH2* (6%–13%)	Highest in males with *MSH2* mutation; *Helicobacter pylori* coinfection may raise risk
Ovarian cancer	*MLH1* (4%–6%) *MSH2* (8%–11%)	30% diagnosed before age 35 years
Bladder cancer	*MSH2 > MLH1* Males > Females	Interaction of risks can give dramatic findings, but they are just estimates; women with *MLH1* mutation have 1% risk; men with *MSH2* mutation have 27% risk

IS A GENETICS REFERRAL INDICATED?

The importance of counseling prior to genetic testing cannot be overstated. Genetic screening tests are being developed very rapidly. Because most are covered by insurance, testing has become standard in many women's health and obstetric offices. However, this is one of the situations in which it is more appropriate to refer to a genetic professional. Genetic testing can be straightforward and relatively inexpensive when the family mutation is known, but when the mutation is unknown, things become complicated very quickly. This FHH is very likely Lynch syndrome, a hereditary CRC syndrome, in which mutations in any of five different "mismatch repair" genes have been associated with the development of different cancers (Lindor et al., 2006).

Later, you learn that MB's cousin had genetic tumor testing, which was initially inconclusive but later found to contain a mutation associated with Lynch syndrome, and therefore, the family cancer gene was confirmed. Referral to a genetic professional is most appropriate because MB and her family will be offered the time and expertise they need to get their questions and concerns addressed.

DO OTHER FAMILY MEMBERS NEED TO BE TESTED?

There are no other family members on the paternal side who are alive or unaffected except MB's son and typically children are not offered genetic testing for adult-onset disorders unless a treatment is available that prevents or delays development of disease (Caga-anan et al., 2012).

IF MB HAS A DELETERIOUS MUTATION, WILL HER CLINICAL MANAGEMENT BE ALTERED?

First, clinicians should be prepared to communicate the increase in risk in a way that MB can understand it. MB may be able to understand statistical risks if they are presented mathematically but may grasp the concepts better when a more simplistic approach is used to explain risk (e.g., coloring in stick figures). Before risk is discussed, however, a careful review of the literature

(or current resources) should be conducted to ensure that the risk numbers being provided are accurate. As knowledge advances, these numbers adjust over time (see Table 16.3).

If MB is found to carry a deleterious familial mutation and has received appropriate genetic counseling, the focus can then shift to reducing risk and identifying clinical manifestations as early as possible. This can be challenging even for oncologists who work with these patients on a daily basis, so the best course of action would be to refer MB and her family to a center specializing in managing people with Lynch syndrome, which can develop a comprehensive management plan that can then be communicated back to the family's primary care providers.

ARE THERE ANY ENHANCED SURVEILLANCE AND/OR RISK REDUCTION OPTIONS FOR MB?

Several screening options are recommended for individuals with Lynch syndrome mutations: annual colonoscopy starting at age 20; upper endoscopy (esophagogastroduodenoscopy [EGD]) annually starting at age 40; annual urinalysis starting at age 30; and endometrial and ovarian cancer symptom education and discussion of prophylactic hysterectomy and oophorectomy by age 40, or when childbearing is complete (Lindor et al., 2006).

WHAT ARE THE REPRODUCTIVE IMPLICATIONS?

Because Lynch syndrome is inherited in an autosomal dominant manner, MB should be informed that with each pregnancy the risk for passing the mutation to each child is 50%. Because the familial mutation in MB's family is known, pregestational diagnostic (PGD) testing and prenatal screening would be available to her, but additional counseling from a reproductive geneticist is highly recommended.

WHAT ETHICAL, LEGAL, AND SOCIAL IMPLICATIONS SHOULD BE DISCUSSED BEFORE OR AFTER TESTING?

There are several ELSIs in this scenario. Beneficence is applied when MB's increased risk for developing a

Lynch-syndrome cancer is identified before the onset of disease. This early recognition of risk offers her the opportunity to discuss options, such as enhanced screening, chemoprevention, or surgery before she develops cancer, improving her longevity as well as the quality of her life. Justice is applied when MB's family members are offered the same counseling and screening services she is. Autonomy is applied when adult family members are offered genetic counseling, testing, and treatment options, but each person has the right to refuse any or all of these interventions. Two ethical constructs, nonmaleficence and privacy, are competing priorities and, depending on the preferences of individual family members, are potentially the most difficult ethical principles to apply evenly. If everyone in MB's family considered to be at increased risk is interested in being counseled and tested, and genetic information is shared freely among family members, then these ethical principles are satisfied; no one is harmed by the information, and the concept of privacy, as it relates to carrier status, has been addressed. When *some* but *not all* family members want to know their mutation status, maintaining privacy and minimizing harm become more difficult. Finally, Genetic Information Nondiscrimination Act (GINA) insurance and employment protections may apply to some, but not all, family members. MB is protected because she has not been diagnosed with breast or ovarian cancer, but several of her family members (including her sister) have been diagnosed with cancer, so GINA protections do not apply.

SUMMARY

Assessing genetic risk can be complicated and collecting an FHH can be challenging. The genomic landscape is evolving rapidly, and specialized knowledge is often needed to interpret and translate this information for colleagues, clients, families, and communities. The potential power of genomics to improve health and healthcare is truly stunning. Very basic information, such as an accurate FHH, can open the door to critical conversations about individual and familial risk, offering the opportunity to make presymptomatic or early diagnoses, choosing the most effective interventions (e.g., pharmacogenomics), increasing communication among family members, and informing reproductive decisions. Everyone on the healthcare team needs to be fully engaged in working in a community in which genomics features prominently, and partnership with other healthcare team members (e.g., genetic counselors, medical geneticists, maternal–fetal medicine specialists, oncologists, social workers, dietitians, dentists) will be the way healthcare is delivered in the future.

REFERENCES

References for this chapter are online and available at https://connect.springerpub.com/content/book/978-0-8261-6722-4/part/part02/chapter/ch16

CHAPTER 17

Women and the Workplace*

KIM SHAUGHNESSY-GRANGER,† CYNTHIA A. KUEHNER,† LANA J. BERNAT,†
TIMOTHY G. WHITING,† AND BROOKES WILLIAMS

Work provides a foundation of personal dignity and a source of stability for individuals and their families; good paying, intellectually rewarding jobs are instrumental in building societal strength and personal resilience, particularly for women. Work is often connected with identity, meaning, and social connection as well as access to medical insurance and retirement benefits. Alternatively, the lack of work, unemployment, or underemployment has been associated with higher rates of illness and low self-esteem (Linn et al., 1985). Work itself may also have deleterious consequences, particularly when that work involves exposure to hazards or injury risks.

Healthcare professionals must understand work from two perspectives. During individual client encounters, professionals need to gather an adequate occupational history in order to understand the impact to the holistic health of the individual and family unit. With this information, caregivers can anticipate and capitalize on opportunities to protect their patients from adverse health outcomes associated with their occupations. A global perspective is also necessary to understand the impact of policy on communities and societies. Action-oriented, visionary nurse leaders empower individual women and explore ways to influence the local, national, and global community in order to advance policy in support of women in the workplace.

America has an increasing number of women in the workplace and an increasing number of women serving in leadership roles. According to the U.S. Bureau of Labor Statistics (2021), 57% of all women participated in the workforce in comparison to 69% of all men. In comparison to past decades, women are more likely to seek higher education. Since 1970, women in the 25- to 64-year age group are four times as likely to have a college degree. The percentage of women with children who participate in the labor force ranges from 63.8% to 72.4%, depending on the age of their children. Despite the increased number of women in the workforce, disparities remain, and women still face challenges that affect their health.

The major factors influencing a woman's experience in the workplace fall into two broad categories: systemic influences and environmental influences. Systemic influences include overarching factors that affect the larger workforce such as racial disparities or gender inequalities or factors that affect special populations such as women with children, aging women, or military veterans. Environmental influences are more specific to a particular organization or profession and encompass many different types of workplace hazards. This chapter will explore how these systemic and environmental influences affect women in the workplace and will help prepare APRNs to address workplace challenges when caring for working women.

Women have always worked, but in the United States they have increasingly participated in compensated employment. In an agrarian society, most workers were self-employed or worked for family members. The work, while often accompanied by long hours and risky activities, was small scale (one man and one animal, and one woman and one loom). Opportunities for injury and death related to work certainly existed, but most people in agrarian societies died of infectious diseases, poor nutrition, poor sanitation, or war. The Industrial Revolution, starting in the mid-1700s, brought with it an increase in work-related accidents and illnesses. Mechanization and mass production were accelerated by the advent of the steam engine, and people were drawn or enticed off the farms to the new production facilities in small towns or villages, increasing the concentration of workers near these facilities. Machines were built for production and not with the safety of workers in mind. During this time women were increasingly working outside their homes. In fact, women and children

---

*This chapter is a revision of the chapter that appeared in the second edition of this textbook, authored by Janice Camp, and we thank her for her original contribution.
†The views expressed are those of the authors and do not reflect the official policy or position of the Department of the Navy, Department of the Defense, or the U.S. government.

were highly desirable, cheap sources of labor and often exploited labor as was the case in the early textile mills.

Work-related injuries reached an all-time high in the late 1800s and early 1900s, which led to investigation into the challenges faced by employed women (Centers for Disease Control and Prevention [CDC], 1999). This ultimately resulted in some protective legislation, restricting women from some forms of work. However, women continued to enter the workforce, and with the production needs associated with World Wars I and II, women were increasingly engaged in hazardous work. The U.S. Army sponsored a comprehensive investigation of the occupational health problems of women, "Women in Industry" (Baetjer, 1946). Dr. Anna Baetjer warned of the reproductive effects for pregnant women of benzene, carbon monoxide, carbon disulfide, lead, mercury, and radiation. After World War II, many women experienced social pressure to leave the workforce; however, by 2015 about 57% of American women were reported to be in the workforce (www.dol.gov/wb/stats/stats-data.htm). Employment is no longer restricted by gender; women find themselves in all workplaces, and many of them are doing hazardous work.

Occupational or workplace health and safety fit well within a public health framework. Care providers often find the assessment and treatment of work-related injuries similar to the care and treatment of non-work-related illnesses and injuries. Care of a severed finger or broken arm is the same regardless of the precipitating event. However, understanding the population-based model of occupational health as it fits into an overall context of health can assist the care provider in anticipating and preventing similar injuries or illnesses in other members of the community, understanding the interaction between workplace exposures and health in general, and helping return the patient to an optimal state of wellness. An ecological or population health model takes a broader perspective and examines the relationship between the biological characteristics of individuals and their interactions with their peer groups, families, communities, schools, and workplaces, as well as the broad economic, cultural, social, and physical environmental conditions at all levels. An ecological model emphasizes the importance of the social and physical environments that strongly shape patterns of disease and injury, as well as the responses to them over the entire life cycle, providing a broader conceptualization of well-being and not merely the absence of disease (Fielding et al., 2010).

Within the public health framework are the concepts of primary, secondary, and tertiary prevention. Primary prevention seeks to reduce the incidence of disease by altering risk factors or improving resistance through efforts to alter individual or collective behaviors or eliminating or mitigating exposures. Some examples are smoking-cessation programs, drinking-water treatment, and installation of machine guards on saws or punch presses. Secondary prevention includes procedures for the early detection of diseases or early treatment of preclinical forms of diseases to reduce or control disease progression. Examples include mammograms to detect early-stage breast cancer, blood lead testing, and surveillance of battery reclamation workers to prevent lead-related disease and symptoms. Tertiary prevention seeks to reduce the impact of diseases or injuries on patient function and well-being; examples here might include quality disability management and return-to-work programs. Providing healthcare to people who work (about 60% of the American population participate in the labor force) requires incorporating these principles into care strategies and integrating them into workplace health and safety programs.

SYSTEMIC INFLUENCES

The *workplace* is a broad term that can include the home office, corporate office, a factory, a vehicle, and nearly any place in between. Data have shown since the inception of tracking labor statistics there has been significant gender disparity in the U.S. labor force. According to a U.S. Bureau of Labor Statistics report released in 2021, women's participation in the labor force peaked at 60% in 1999. Figure 17.1 illustrates the ratio of women to men in the U.S. labor force from 1948 through 2019.

Males have disproportionately dominated the labor force as well as the institutions responsible for setting policies and regulations that affect the workplace. As such, it can be reasonably inferred those policies and regulations have been shaped by masculine defaults and have been void of considerations that may afford women equality in the workplace. Masculine defaults exist when characteristics and behaviors typically associated with men are rewarded and considered standard practice. They make it more challenging for many women to enter and succeed in organizations (Cheryan & Markus, 2020). An ugly by-product that can in part be attributed to a historically male dominated labor force are the systemic inequities and subsequent inequalities that have manifested. To understand how systemic factors play a role in the health of women within the workplace the APRN should understand the terms *inequity* and *inequality*.

Inequality, Inequity, and Intersectionality

According to the *Oxford English Dictionary* (n.d.-b), *equity* is defined as the quality of being fair and impartial. The World Health Organization (WHO) defines *equity* as the absence of unfair, avoidable, or remediable differences among groups of people. The definitions highlight in different manners that equity is ultimately about fairness and ensuring access to the same opportunities. WHO further elaborates to say health equity is achieved when everyone can attain their full potential for health and well-being (WHO, n.d.-b). Significant literature and research findings articulate that women have been disadvantaged in the workplace for decades and that systemic inequities are a plausible factor resulting in women not being afforded the opportunity to attain their full potential for health and well-being.

According to the *Oxford English Dictionary* (n.d.-a), *equality* is the state of being equal, especially in status, rights, and opportunities. *Gender equality*, as defined by the United Nations, is the equal valuing by society of the similarities and the differences of men and women, and the roles they play (UNICEF, 2017). These definitions highlight that equality

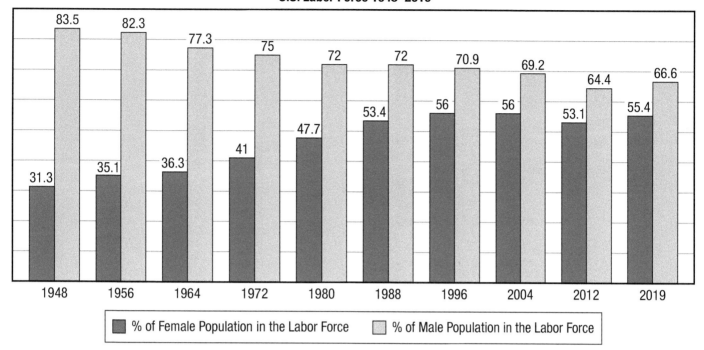

U.S. Labor Force 1948–2019

Legend: ■ % of Female Population in the Labor Force ☐ % of Male Population in the Labor Force

FIGURE 17.1 Ratio of women to men in the U.S. labor force.
Source: U.S Bureau of Labor Statistics. https://www.bls.gov/opub/reports/womens-databook/2020/home.htm

is present when everyone is provided the same opportunity. Gender inequality within the workplace has been studied in depth by scholars and government bodies. Well-studied issues that contribute to gender inequality in the workpace include unequal pay, sexual harassment, and merit-based promotion, just to list a few. As the impact of inequality on women's health in the workplace is discussed in this section it is important to also understand intersectionality. *Intersectionality* is an analytical framework designed to promote understanding about how social identities, such as gender, socioeconomic class, and race, can lead to advantage and disadvantage or marginalization of individuals.

An example of intersectionality is illustrated in a report by McKinsey & Company titled, "Women in the Workplace 2021" (Burns et al., 2021; Figure 17.2). In this report, the percentage of White women represented in the corporate setting lagged behind White men across six corporate level roles, from entry level to C suite, by an average of 25.8%. The disparity across levels ranged from 5% at the entry level to 42% at the C-suite. By comparison women of color lagged behind White women in the same corporate roles by an average of 16%. However, women of color lagged behind White men across the same six corporate roles by an average of 42% and ranged from 18% at entry level positions to 58% in the C-suite (Fuller & Raman, 2022). The intersectionality of being a woman of color exacerbates the systemic inequalities experienced. This is an important concept for the healthcare provider to understand as it may potentially provide a greater holistic understanding of factors that are impacting the health of a woman in the workplace. It is important for the APRN to understand and appreciate how systemic inequity and inequality contribute to the health of women in the workplace. Where inequality exists inequities must be explored.

FACTORS CONTRIBUTING TO SYSTEMIC INEQUALITY

Systemic inequity is not necessarily deliberate. A look back through time will illustrate that the vast majority of countries and cultures have been dominated by male figures throughout history. As a result, societal rules were largely developed by males. When males dominate the policy making, elements that impact women are generally not considered. This phenomenon can more technically be defined as *androcentrism.* Androcentrism refers to a societal system organized around men and evident in both individual biases and institutional policies (Bailey et al., 2018). It is important to understand that androcentrism is not a term for male superiority or female inferiority. An argument can be made that androcentrism has culturally shaped the world as we know it and as such has perpetuated the masculine default. Masculine defaults include ideas, values, policies, practices, interaction styles, norms, artifacts, and beliefs that often do not appear to discriminate by gender but result in disadvantaging more women than men (Cheryan & Markus, 2020). As society has evolved, advancements have been made and efforts continue to increase female representation, but there is still much more that needs to be done to achieve equality. Nevertheless, let's explore where gender disparities that are influenced by systemic factors impact the health of women in the workplace.

As previously stated, *workplace* is a broad term, but potentially one that has not had broad representation in shaping its design. An example of this may be the standard office temperature. The formula for setting the standard office temperature was developed in the 1960s and was based around the metabolic resting rate of the average 40-year-old man (at that time) weighing 70 kg (Kingma & van Marken Lichtenbelt, 2015). This bias persists, as current offices are as much as 5 degrees too cold for women. It is unlikely that a standard

At every step up the corporate ladder, women of color lose ground to White women and men of color.

Representation by corporate role, by gender and race, 2021, % of employees

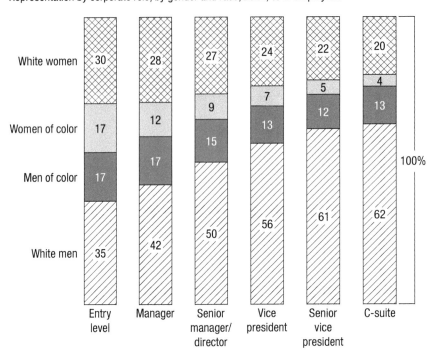

FIGURE 17.2 Intersectionality by corporate role.
Source: Burns, T., Huang, J., Krivkovich, A., Yee, L., Rambachan, I., & Trkulja, T. (2021). Women in the workplace 2021. McKinsey & Company. https://www.mckinsey.com/featured-insights/diversity-and -inclusion/women-in-the-workplace. Copyright © 2022 McKinsey & Company. All rights reserved. Reprinted by permission.

developed and intended for the use in design, operation, and commissioning of buildings was deliberately established with the intent of making females in the workplace uncomfortable, yet it is precisely the type of standard regulation that manifests into inequalities that affect females to a greater degree than males in the workplace. There are common conditions that may exclusively be experienced by females and which the typical workplace environment may not have been designed to accommodate. A common shortcoming for a typical workplace setting is the absence of maternity-related accommodations. Females can experience adverse health outcomes for themselves or their newborn as a result of insufficient building accommodations such as available parking near an entrance or appropriate spaces for breastfeeding and pumping. Outside of maternity-related issues, work environments could benefit from more favorable accommodations related to menstrual health. While many women have a regular menstrual cycle, it is normal for the cycle to vary by a few days from month to month. Readily available feminine hygiene products in workplace restrooms would alleviate a significant source of stress for women, and although sanitary bins have been readily available for decades, it is not uncommon for them to be absent in the workplace. More significantly, between 10% and 30% of premenopausal women experience abnormal uterine bleeding (Wouk & Helton, 2019); these challenges can keep women from the workplace altogether.

Beyond the design of the built environment, organizations must also scrutinize the safety of women in the workplace by ensuring appropriate fitting personal protective equipment (PPE). Studies in both the United States and United Kingdom have found that women often do not have access to correctly fitting PPE. Research has also shown that ill-fitting PPE can hinder rather than protect (Ghani, 2017). Women are not scaled down versions of men. It cannot be assumed that small sized PPE fit for a male will be an appropriate fit for a woman. A well-documented example of ill-fitting PPE was demonstrated by NASA in 2019 when the agency had to scrap the first all-female spacewalk from the International Space Station due to not having enough space suits to fit two women scheduled for the spacewalk (Koren, 2019). NASA is arguably considered the world's premier space agency so it should be reasonable to think that the appropriate gear would be available for all personnel aboard the International Space Station. It may be reasonably inferred that if NASA is not prepared with the appropriate PPE for astronauts, other organizations may be missing the mark as well. The prevalence of the examples used in this section should be considered endemic across the world. APRNs should understand these systems-level influences that confer risk specifically to women in the workplace.

It is well established in literature and research that health is an important determinant of labor force participation. Furthermore, there are social and cultural determinants of health that may be systemic in nature, but not deliberate, impacting women's health in the workplace. One such well-documented factor is unequal division of labor related to responsibilities at home. According to observed data and prevailing social and cultural norms, women have been bearing the primary burdens of housework, child care, and other family responsibilities even as they participate in the paid labor force (Mussida & Patimo, 2021). A scholarly search on disparities in family care responsibilities returns a multitude of literature globally that provides empirical studies on the topic. All workers experience time conflicts, but working mothers are disproportionately impacted because in addition to paid employment they often come home to a second shift of unpaid work that includes household labor and child care (Glynn, 2018). The greater number of hours of unpaid work by women makes them more susceptible to stress. This is substantiated in epidemiologic and psychological literature, which has shown that caregivers suffer from high stress that can often lead to deteriorating health (Mussida & Patimo, 2021). Understanding workplace policies such as paid leave, workplace flexibility, scheduling predictability, and affordable child care may assist the healthcare provider as women, low-wage workers, and people of color are less likely to have access to the policies that would help them address their family caregiving responsibilities (Glynn, 2018). In addition to addressing the symptoms and manifestations that may be related to increased stress, healthcare providers should be prepared to provide family resource options.

Another systemic issue that impacts women's health in the workplace is sexual harassment. *Sexual harassment* is defined as unwelcome sexual advances, requests for sexual favors, and other verbal or physical harassment of a sexual nature (U.S. Equal Employment Opportunity Commission [EEOC], n.d.-c). A 2018 survey reported that 38% of women have experienced sexual harassment in the workplace. Those most vulnerable to sexual harassment are female, younger, in low or subordinate positions, and migrant or temporary workers (Raj et al., 2020). Although many women have experienced sexual harassment in the workplace, many events have gone unreported. Explanations for the lack of reporting relate to threats to self-esteem and risk of secondary victimization. Women fear facing doubts, scrutiny, and blame for the harassment they experience. The impacts can be devastating to the health of the victim and can manifest in various ways that may include physical health concerns, substance abuse, depression, and other forms of psychological distress. The effects of harassment can be seen for nearly a decade following the harassing event (Keplinger et al., 2019). A significant number of studies have been published since 2018 evaluating multiple components of two key social movements, the #MeToo movement and the subsequent #TimesUp movement. The #MeToo movement became the largest social movement related to sexual harassment in history (Raj et al., 2020). Studies suggest these movements may have led to a decrease in sexual harassment in the workplace. A key tenet following the #MeToo movement was victims feeling empowered to speak up. Understanding the resources available to victims of sexual assault that may have occurred in the workplace will be a key component to caring for this population.

Solutions for systemic inequities need to be rooted in data. The importance of data in eliminating systemic factors cannot be understated as data and information must be available for policy makers to assess and develop appropriate, evidence-based responses and policies. However, data alone is not enough. The diversity of research teams and of research participants is a key element to ensuring policies enacted as a result of data analysis do not contribute further to systemic inequities. Representation of women conducting research varies by country, but it has been well established that women are underrepresented in all regions. Only four nations within the 38-nation Organisation for Economic Co-operation and Development (OECD) show a percentage of women researchers greater than 40% (Abramo & D'Angelo, 2015). It is a well-established fact that women are underrepresented in science, technology, engineering, and math (STEM). The lack of diversity in conducting research may perpetuate systemic factors that contribute to inequality by creating a void in perspective.

In addition to gender diversity in conducting research, it is also of significant importance that studies have parity in the gender representation of participants. The CDC plays an important role in the collection of public health data through a multitude of surveillance networks. An analysis of the CDC's public health data collection systems shows that 94% of the systems collect data on sex (Kress et al., 2021). This would establish the United States as a global leader when it comes to collecting sex as a data point in the surveillance of health data. However, there is a significant gap between sex being reported as a data point and the representation of women in studies that may result from the collection of sex disaggregated data. An analysis conducted in 2021 reviewed 20,020 studies registered in the ClinicalTrials.gov database with over 5 million participants enrolled. The analysis found that female participants were underrepresented in oncology, neurology, immunology, urology, cardiology, and hematology relative to the burden of disease women experience in these areas. There are many concerns that can be expressed but most notable is the underrepresentation in cardiology and oncology, as diseases in these fields are the leading cause of death among females in the United States (Steinberg et al., 2021).

To ensure a workplace free of policies that are rooted in systemic inequity, healthcare providers must be prepared to advocate for their patients and confront systems and policies that result in adverse health outcomes due to workplace inequality. Understanding systemic factors that impact the workplace provides a greater opportunity for healthcare providers to identify when the physical and psychological manifestations are the result of factors systemic in nature. Gender statistics that adequately reflect the lived realities of women are indispensable tools for developing evidence-based policies and solutions that can help eliminate systemic inequities. Such statistics, which include but are not limited to sex-disaggregated data and sex as a biological variable in research, shed light on areas where progress is made, provide evidence of what works, and reveal gaps where further efforts are needed (U.N. Women, n.d.). It is important that all healthcare providers are familiar with systemic inequities and the impacts they have on the workplace, and subsequently women's health, as well as the gender data gaps that result.

Working Mothers

Women represent nearly half of the American workforce, and more than one-third of working women are mothers with children under the age of 18 (U.S. Department of Labor, 2016). Pregnancy, childbirth or adoption, and work reintegration all represent major life transitions for working women. Women have concerns about work safety during pregnancy. Pregnancy discrimination, lack of parental leave benefits, inability to access quality and affordable child care services, and inadequate lactation support are among the challenges that working mothers face. Healthcare professionals have an opportunity to help shape workplace environments in support of women during these life transitions through healthcare policy work, involvement in local organizations, and patient education. This effort begins by gaining an understanding of these challenges working women face, reviewing current policies, and exploring resources to advocate for women both in patient encounters and through strategic healthcare work.

PREGNANCY AND WORK

Pregnancy is a transition of life and working throughout the pregnancy is largely safe for women with uncomplicated pregnancies. Work accommodations are often sufficient to support women who have pregnancy complications or who work in high-risk occupations. However, long work hours and night shift work have been associated with increased risk of adverse pregnancy outcomes including miscarriage, preterm labor, hypertensive disorders of pregnancy, vacuum/forceps delivery, and small-for-gestational-age babies (Begtrup et al., 2019; Quenby et al., 2021; Suzumori et al., 2020). Unfortunately, these associations are not well understood, and there is often limited ability to reduce work hours and shift work for most women.

Physical discomforts are common in pregnancy, and many can be addressed with simple adjustments or accommodations. Low back pain is one of the most common complaints in pregnancy, and physically demanding tasks can exacerbate low back pain. Simple accommodations such as floor mats, ergonomic workstations, support belts, compression stockings, and comfortable shoes can ease these discomforts. In addition, the change in center of gravity and ligament laxity can predispose pregnant women to falls (American College of Obstetricians and Gynecologists, 2018). In order to mitigate these risks, the National Institute of Occupational Safety and Health lifting guidelines for the general population were adapted for application to pregnant workers (MacDonald et al., 2013).

Many women report feeling stressed during pregnancy. Low-level stress is usually manageable; however, chronic high levels of stress or stress from a catastrophic event during pregnancy is associated with increased complications of pregnancy such as high blood pressure, preterm birth, and low birth weight babies (March of Dimes, n.d.). The impact of pregnancy discrimination includes economic and psychological stressors that can contribute to these complications of pregnancy.

PREGNANCY DISCRIMINATION

The Pregnancy Discrimination Act (PDA) is an amendment to the Civil Rights Act of 1964 that was passed in 1978 and applies to employers who have 15 or more employees. The PDA protects a pregnant woman from unfavorable treatment as an applicant or employee due to pregnancy, childbirth, or a pregnancy-related medical condition. Sometimes pregnant women experience a complication that falls within a definition of disability. In this case, the PDA also requires employers to extend disability benefits and workplace accommodations to women who require a change in duties in accordance with the Americans With Disabilities Act (Box 17.1). Examples of workplace accommodations include ergonomic office equipment, lifting restrictions, or altered work schedules or work breaks (EEOC, 2016).

Pregnant women still experience formal and informal discrimination in the workplace despite laws to prohibit discrimination. The EEOC (n.d.-b) reported a 65% increase in pregnancy-related discrimination charges in 2007 as compared to 1992. As a result of this increase, National Partnership, a national nonprofit organization, researched to understand the reasons for the increasing trend. The research identified no single cause; however, the analysis revealed an intersection with race and ethnicity, because claims filed by women of color accounted for a significant portion of the increased charges. The research also found that having large numbers of women in a particular organization did not protect against discrimination, because more than half of the claims stemmed from industries with the highest percentages of women workers (National Partnership for Women & Families, 2008). This research demonstrates that discrimination is a common experience for women, particularly through the lens of intersection from race and gender, despite having a large circle of women in the workplace and despite laws to prevent discrimination. Pregnancy adds another layer to this intersection.

PARENTAL LEAVE

Parental leave provides benefits beyond physical recovery of the birthing parent. A number of studies over the past 2 decades highlight several benefits of parental leave: fewer low birthweight births, decreased infant mortality, increased breastfeeding rates, improved compliance with childhood immunizations, and better mental health (Burtle & Bezruchka, 2016). Not all working women have access to parental leave benefits. Under the Family Medical Leave Act (FMLA) established in 1993, federal policy provides for 12 weeks of unpaid employment leave, which includes childbirth. Many

---

Box 17.1 EEOC and ACOG Pregnancy Discrimination Act Information

The Equal Employment Opportunity Commission (EEOC) website www.eeoc.gov offers information to help providers understand how to assist patients who have pregnancy-related limitations that affect their work.

The American College of Obstetricians and Gynecologists (ACOG) publishes a committee opinion available at www.acog.org that includes guidance on how to write a work accommodation note.

women do not have access to this FMLA benefit, however, because eligibility is based on a 12-month work history with an employer. Women may also work for employers who are not required by law to extend the benefit because they have fewer than 50 employees (U.S. Department of Labor, 2023). Access to the parental leave benefit through FMLA remains a limited benefit policy that disparately affects lower-income families who cannot afford unpaid absences.

More than 80% of employees in the United States do not have access to paid parental leave (Miller, 2020). Among 41 other developed countries, the United States is the only country that does not mandate paid maternity leave, despite many attempts toward its legislation (OECD, 2021). While employers may be concerned about the cost, studies have shown women with paid parental leave are more likely to return to work following childbirth, especially low-income women (Council of Economic Advisors, 2014). Access to parental leave policies affect women's decision about when to return to the workforce. According to research conducted by Paid Leave for the United States (n.d.), 25% of working mothers return to work just 10 days following birth due to the lack of access to a paid parental leave plan.

RETURN TO WORK AFTER CHILDBIRTH

The percentage of women returning to the workforce following childbirth varies based on parity and level of education. Following the birth of the first child, the rate of working women decreases by 18%, and fewer working mothers participate in the workforce with subsequent births. Over 80% of women with professional degrees returned to work in comparison to about half of women who had a high school degree or less (Sandler & Szembrot, 2020). About 64% of mothers with children under the age of 3 and 60% of mothers with children under the age of 1 participate in the labor force (U.S. Bureau of Labor Statistics, 2021). Despite the advances in women's workforce participation in the United States, working mothers face problems when reintegrating to the workforce following childbirth.

Access to quality and affordable child care is a significant issue for working women, especially for mother-only families, who represent 25% of U.S. households with families (U.S. Department of Labor, 2016). The COVID-19 pandemic resulted in a significant decline of working mothers due to drastic decreases in child care availability and shifts in education modalities due to public health concerns. Women of color and low-income women were disproportionately affected by unemployment related to the pandemic (Ranji et al., 2021).

LACTATION IN THE WORKPLACE

Lactation is beneficial for women, reducing the risk of breast and ovarian cancer, type 2 diabetes, cardiovascular disease, and postpartum depression. Human milk benefits infants and children, who are less likely to develop acute infections such as upper respiratory illnesses and ear infections as well as chronic medical problems such as asthma. In the long-term, infants fed with human milk are less likely to develop obesity in their lifetime (United States Breastfeeding Committee, 2010). As a result, the American Academy of Pediatrics (2021) recommends exclusive breastfeeding for the

first 6 months and continuing breastfeeding up to 2 years of life while introducing other foods.

Despite the numerous advantages and benefits of lactation, women who intend to work full time are less likely to initiate breastfeeding (Attanasio et al., 2013). Full-time mothers are 19% less likely to breastfeed for more than 6 months (Ogbuanu et al., 2011). Barriers to workplace lactation include lack of schedule flexibility, lack of space to pump or store milk, perceived lack of support from employers or colleagues, and concerns about low milk supply (Lauer et al., 2019). These barriers illustrate the need to continue developing national policy and education based on the benefits of lactation.

Research shows that lactation programs increased breastfeeding duration among middle- and high-income workers who had an intent to breastfeed; however, more research is needed to understand how lactation programs benefit low-income workers (Kim et al., 2019). Businesses can benefit from supporting lactation in the workplace, because babies fed with human milk are not as likely to become sick, translating to fewer missed workdays for the mother (American Academy of Pediatrics, 2021). According to a publication by the U.S. Department of Health and Human Services, Office on Women's Health (2023), companies both large and small experience significant returns from investing in lactation support programs. In the United States, one 2-year study of 343 employees who participated in a lactation support program found the program resulted in an annual savings of $240,000 in healthcare expenses, 62% fewer prescriptions, and $60,000 savings in reduced absenteeism rates. Globally, according to the World Bank, investment in breastfeeding promotion and protection has the potential to yield a return of about $35 to $1 invested over the 10 years (Dixon, 2018). As of 2021, 30 states (60%) have laws supporting workplace lactation (National Conference of State Legislatures, 2021). This is a 14% increase over the past decade, when just 23 (46%) states had adopted laws in support of workplace lactation (Murtagh & Moulton, 2011).

A major advance occurred in 2010 through an amendment to Section 7 of the Fair Labor Standards Act of 1938. This amendment requires employers to support nursing mothers in the workplace by providing reasonable time to express milk for the first year following birth. Employers must also provide a private space other than a restroom for an employee to express milk. This law does not require an employer to compensate the employee for time spent expressing milk, though the lactating employee could choose to express milk during usual break times, which would require usual compensation. Certain exceptions apply to this labor law (e.g., if an employer has fewer than 50 employees and it would cause undue hardship to the employer, then the employer is not required to adhere to the law). Employers must also adhere to any state laws related to lactation in the workplace (U.S. Department of Health & Human Services, Office on Women's Health, 2023). With the exception of grandfathered plans, U.S. insurance plans must provide support, counseling, and equipment for breastfeeding (U.S. Centers for Medicare & Medicaid Services, n.d.). Insurance covers the cost of a breast pump, decreasing cost for the lactating employee.

Women are an important segment of the American workforce, and women face many challenges in the workplace, particularly in the childbearing years. Advocacy is part of the professional responsibility of the nursing profession. APRNs have an essential role in educating and assisting women with navigating these challenges in the workplace. As credible servants to the public, APRNs have the opportunity to shape local and national policy through conversations and work, leveraging evidence and social justice concepts that support improvements for women in the workplace (Box 17.2).

Veteran and Military Service Women

To care for him who shall have borne the battle, and for his widow and his orphan.

—Abraham Lincoln, March 4, 1865

The direct quote from President Lincoln's second inaugural address, delivered at the conclusion of the Civil War, just weeks before Lincoln's assassination, has served as the basis for the U.S. Government's commitment to caring for our nation's veterans and stands as the motto of the U.S. Department of Veterans Affairs (VA). Lincoln's words have come under modern-day criticism, described by some as *sexist* and *exclusionary*. Legislation has been introduced in both the House and the Senate to update the wording of the motto, replacing *him* and *his* with the gender-neutral pronouns *they* and *their*. While much has changed in the gender demographics of uniformed service members since Lincoln's remarks, the nation's commitment to caring for its service members, veterans, and their families remains steadfast. As a well-established subset of military and veteran service, women who serve or have served require specific consideration with regard to prevalent and unique military service and veteran health issues and concerns.

APRNs and professional nursing organizations are proactively establishing initiatives, contributing to the science, and committing resources toward military and veteran women's healthcare needs in the context of individual and community health policies and practice. The American Academy of Nursing, in collaboration with state VA directors, launched the "Have you ever served in the military?" campaign in 2013. This campaign was in cooperation with the White House's *Joining Forces* military family and veteran support

initiative and by 2015 the campaign had rolled out in all 50 states (Collins et al., 2013). The purpose of the campaign is to identify all military and veteran service members during clinical settings intake assessments. By asking the simple question, "Have you ever served in the military?" APRNs will specifically identify veteran and military women service members, better target their assessments and treatment plans in specific consideration of uniformed service, and identify additional resources as part of clinical care. A pocket guide for clinicians, including intake questions, is available online at haveyoueverserved.com.

National defense and the roles of military service members continue to evolve. Women are now able to serve in every military specialty, providing they meet all required standards. The traditional domains of military service —air, land, and sea—have expanded, and now include cyber and space, as well as defense and deterrence, enhanced by diplomacy and allied partnerships. The opportunities for women to serve in exciting, evolving, and diverse career fields continue to expand, and as they do, the number of women actively serving and the veteran populations will continue to grow.

As data science improves, and military and veteran women's needs are better understood, it is critical that APRNs and healthcare teams identify uniformed and veteran service women in their clinical practice and incorporate military and service-unique employment considerations. Individual, family, and population health outcomes, specific to uniformed service and veteran status, are enhanced through the use of evidenced-based practice when available, but gaps in research are prevalent. Women service members' needs may be generally similar to all women's health needs; however, the context of military service, including employment and deployment settings, military organizational structure, workplace hazards, and prevalence of military-unique stressors add dimension and special considerations in caring for women whose employment or careers commit them to public service in defense of the nation.

It is helpful to understand women service members in the context of military service composition, and the evolution of demographic changes over time. The U.S. Government Accountability Office (GAO) Report to Congressional Committees (2020) describes gender demographics in military service between 2004 and 2018. Women in uniformed service remain a minority of the total military force. In 2004, 15.1% of the military was female; by 2018, the percentage had increased only minimally, to 16.5%, in spite of previous policies on role restrictions (e.g., serving in combat specialties) being eliminated in 2013. Female attrition rates continue to exceed male attrition for both commissioned officers and enlisted personnel, with women separating from service 28% faster than males.

Women are underrepresented in top tier military leadership ranks; female admirals and generals make up only 7% of the highest pay grades (GAO, 2020), while women make up more than double that percentage of the military's total force. It is recognized that women leaders in military service are optimally suited to lead critical defense initiatives, through global conflict prevention, mitigation, and resolution, in addition to more traditional military assignments. Public law prescribes specific Department of Defense (DoD) actions

Box 17.2 Helpful Websites for Workplace Pregnancy and Breastfeeding Advocacy

www.abetterbalance.org/know-your-rights

https://pregnantatwork.org

www.usbreastfeeding.org

www.cdc.gov/breastfeeding/pdf/bf_guide_2.pdf

https://web.uri.edu/worklife/files/BF_entire_toolkit_FINAL.pdf

including training relevant military personnel, as codified in the landmark legislation, the Women, Peace, and Security Act of 2017, which asserts that meaningful participation by women results in greater efficacy and durability of global peace initiatives. In recent conflicts (e.g., Operation Iraqi Freedom, Operation Enduring Freedom) military women-specific roles have expanded, to include specific operations as leaders and members of female engagement teams (FETs), cultural support teams (CSTs), and provincial reconstruction teams (PRTs). Women in uniform have historically responded to military operations other than war, including humanitarian assistance and disaster relief, both domestically and globally, frequently alongside other government or nongovernment agencies and departments (e.g., the Department of State and U.S. Agency for International Development).

While the literature identifies multiple variables that affect the status and health of women in the services, gaps persist. The GAO report (2020) identifies key areas that affect women's experience and decisions to stay in or leave military service. These six broad areas include organizational culture, work schedules, family planning, sexual assault, dependent care, and deployments. This is not an exhaustive list; however, these factors and others, in the context of military service, may have significant bearing and influence on the physical and mental health of veteran and military service women. APRNs will be better positioned to care for this population by pursuing further baseline knowledge and specific study with regard to military occupations (e.g., aviation, submarines, surface combatant ships, infantry, intelligence, cybersecurity), exposures to known and potential hazards, workplace physical demands, rules for compliance with military and fitness standards, environmental risks and occupational safety, relationship issues (both personal and professional), and unique stressors affected by arduous demands of military service.

Readiness is a central tenet of military service eligibility and incorporates both physical and mental fitness (capacity and qualification) for military service. The Department of Defense Instruction (DoDI) 1332.45 (DoD, 2018), updated in 2021, establishes policy for determining whether nondeployable service members may be retained in military service. This policy prescribes that "to maximize the lethality and readiness of the joint force, all service members are expected to be deployable" (p. 4), and a nondeployable status for more than 12 months must be evaluated for military retention. APRNs must focus on the occupation-specific requirements of women in military service, in order to promote an optimized state of physical and mental well-being and a continuous state of military readiness. In the case of injury or illness, service members are expected to expeditiously pursue appropriate care that enables rapid recovery or rehabilitation and return to full duty when possible. Military members with chronic or disqualifying illness or disability, and who are unable to maintain standards for physical and mental fitness (and worldwide assignment or deployment) may be released from active service. Each of the service branches' medical departments have additional policies and procedures for determining qualification for initial and ongoing service eligibility.

Civilian health records may be utilized in evaluating service members' medical conditions and military service qualification. It is important that military service members' complete health records be available to military medical authorities in order to make reliable determinations. Many military women seek or obtain care in civilian facilities (e.g., urgent or emergent care, obstetric services, or for mental health services). Some medications may be contraindicated for some occupations (e.g., flying or diving), and prescriptions for any controlled substances must be carefully documented in the health record, as all military members are subject to mandatory and random urinalysis testing. A discrepancy (lack of corresponding medical record documentation) may result in removal of a security clearance, or separation of the service member for violation of DoD substance abuse policies.

The organizational structure of the military relies upon a unique hierarchy known as the chain of command. Military personnel have supervisory-subordinate relationships that are governed by the Uniformed Code of Military Justice, in order to provide for good order and discipline in the context of military mission accomplishment. These concepts and the provisions inherent to them may be foreign to civilian personnel, but they have their basis in military policy and precedent and allow for regulation of unique military circumstances. Some provisions apply in the context of healthcare delivery and govern some exceptions to privacy protection normally afforded within a confidential provider-patient relationship.

The Health Insurance Portability and Accountability Act (HIPAA) allows for (and even obligates) protected health information (PHI) of service members to be disclosed to military command authorities under specific circumstances. The Military Health System (2022) Privacy and Civil Liberties internet page provides guidance and descriptions of the provisions commonly known as the *Military Command Exception*. Healthcare providers who manage military patients for conditions that may affect their ability to perform military duties may have an obligation to report pertinent PHI to military command authorities. Examples would include a patient who had entered an inpatient treatment facility for a substance misuse disorder, or a patient admitted for suicidal behavior. Pregnant female service members are required to notify their commanding officer of pregnancy confirmation, in accordance with service-specific regulations or policies, as some assignments may not be available to pregnant service members (e.g., shipboard duty after 20 weeks' gestation in naval service).

Veteran and military service women are affected by federal laws and regulations that may impact their ability to access specific care or health services. For example, Tricare (2022), the health benefit plan for active-duty service women, advises on their website the limitations for covered abortion services, which include only two circumstances; the pregnancy must be determined (and documented by a physician in the health record) to be the product of rape or incest, or the life of the mother is threatened if the pregnancy is carried to term. The basis for this provision is commonly referred to as the Shaheen Amendment, introduced during the 112th Congress of the United States, and in 2013 was added to Title X of U.S. Code (Performance of Abortions: Restrictions, 1985 & rev. 2013). In the context of military service, restrictive provisions like this may have significant impacts to women serving abroad, or while on deployment. A study by Fix et al. (2020) highlights military women's concerns surrounding access to abortion services, specific to military assignment, including access to care in remote or austere service settings, inability to maintain workplace privacy and confidentiality, legality of abortion services while overseas, deployment suspension, career disruptions, and even punitive or adverse employment actions, among other considerations. While abortion services represent a single example, healthcare providers must be aware of laws and regulations that specifically impact federally insured service women and veterans, specific to healthcare eligibility and benefits coverage.

It is useful during clinical intake and health history to identify the nature of any military work, past or present, that may influence health status. Knowledge and exploration of duty assignments, environmental exposures, workplace hazards, safety and risk conditions, injury prevention, PPE availability and use, and any other imposed conditions will lead the clinician to additional screenings, specialty referrals, and comprehensive care. Collaboration with occupational medicine specialists should be considered in order to ensure military women's occupational safety, risk reduction, and safeguarding of health.

Military work settings and employment conditions for uniformed service women may impose physical and mental demands and occupational hazards that may not be familiar to civilian healthcare providers. For example, women identified as radiation workers or who work aboard nuclear-powered aircraft carriers or submarines may have occupational screening and surveillance requirements, in order to detect and prevent exposure to ionizing radiation. Healthcare professionals who provide care to military women should be cognizant of publications that govern occupational risks and management of military personnel, such as the Navy's Bureau of Medicine and Surgery's *Radiation Health Protection Manual* (2011) and the DoD Instruction 6055.08 (DoD, 2021), both of which address surveillance, and quantify radiation exposure limits and provision for safety to pregnant service women.

Deployment and service-related exposures may present acute and long-term risks to service members, including females. While research gaps exist, and some areas of study are inconclusive, the VA continues to monitor for disease and chronic illness that may have been precipitated by hazardous exposures. Veterans are eligible for disability compensation and provision of medical care for service-related injury and illnesses. The VA Public Health website (ww.publichealth.va.gov/exposures/categories/index.asp) makes available information and links to resources for possible military service hazardous exposures by different types. Current categories include chemicals (e.g., Agent Orange, pesticides, water contaminants), radiation, occupational hazards (e.g., asbestos, lead, vibration, noise), air pollutants (dust, smoke, burn pits, oil well fires, etc.), and warfare agents (e.g., chemical, biological, and nerve agents). Depending on service occupation, geographical location, and deployment time frames and locations, service women and veterans may have been exposed to multiple hazards and be susceptible to higher disease burden (e.g., respiratory illness, cancers) as a result.

Some exposures may also have teratogenic effects and elevate risks to offspring. A thorough history of military service and specific questions regarding air quality, proximity to burn pits, mandatory vaccine and medication prophylaxis (e.g., malaria), and chemical and other hazards or exposures will help clinicians to determine the need for additional screening and diagnostic examinations, referral, and follow-up.

Fortunately, interest in female military health continues to increase, and specific conditions that are prevalent among veteran and military service women continue to be identified, studied, and reported. A very large-scale scoping review and gap analysis evaluated all peer-reviewed literature published between 2000 and 2015 to determine the content and quality of research specific to women in the military, and to identify research gaps (Yablonsky et al., 2017). Of 14,999 articles identified, 979 met inclusion criteria, and were categorized into eight broad topic areas, with 73 subtopic areas. Seven of the eight broad categories demonstrated research gaps, with obstetrics and gynecology and psychological health leading as the two categories with the greatest gaps in research. Perhaps surprisingly, obstetric and gynecologic health of female service members was determined to be the major category with the highest number of research gaps, including many relevant subcategories such as menstrual suppression; fertility; unplanned pregnancy; antepartum, intrapartum, and postpartum periods; breastfeeding; and contraception (Englert & Yablonsky, 2019). Injury was the only category for which no research gaps were identified specific to military women. Many additional subtopic areas demonstrated gaps in the literature and a need for expanded and high-quality research in areas such as sleep, sexual and physical assault, gynecologic care during deployment, and sexually transmitted infections, to name a few.

Topics of congressional interest and growing research focus include women's health conditions impacted by military service and veteran status. Legislative attention, and increasing elected representation by veterans of military service, prompt deliberate attention and policy actions that continue to address the interests of veteran and military service women. Military-specific women's health research and interest groups continue to expand and commit resources toward the improved understanding of women in military service and veteran women's health. The TriService Nursing Research Program and Military Women's Health Research Interest Group, currently nested under the Uniformed Services University of the Health Sciences, continue to build a repository of collaborative and interdisciplinary nurse-led research, focused on these dynamic interest areas.

A journal supplement from *Women's Health Issues* (Trego, 2021; Trego & Wilson, 2021) describes a framework for understanding and ultimately promoting military health policy development through a social ecological model for military women's health (SEM-MWH). This framework identifies ecosystems of military service that surround military women and impact health. The framework described acknowledges layers of complexity that surround the features of military service, specific to women and their health, inclusive of the individual (roles, personal values and beliefs); the microsystem (physical, social, and work environments of military service); the mesosystem (how the military woman interfaces with a larger military community, including medical treatment facilities, and virtual community, such as social media groups); and the exosystem (influence on an individual woman from larger systems such as a service branch or the DoD). This model is a useful foundation for understanding the many areas of health influence that are within or beyond an individual veteran or military service woman's control. These concepts emerge throughout the literature, specific to military women's health.

The focus on women's military service, as the context and construct for workplace and employment considerations, provides a backdrop and reference for clinicians' understanding of available and future research into veteran and military service women's health. By way of example, a growing body of evidence and published research recruit all layers of the SEM-MWH model in describing prevalence of gender-specific distinctions among veteran and military service women, while addressing gaps in current research and novel or emerging areas for exploration.

Cazares et al. (2021) examines recent research in women's mental health, reviewing topics of perinatal mental health, posttraumatic stress disorder (PTSD), depression, and a newer area of research focus, gender isolation specific to military service women. The summary identifies a lack of focused research on perinatal mental health among active-duty women and acknowledges previously identified and recurrent incidence of higher odds ratios for depression and PTSD among active duty and veteran service women, compared to male service members. Watrous et al. (2021) highlights similar findings with regard to PTSD and depression among women injured in military service and offers insights into correlational issues among female veteran health, such as indications to screen for substance abuse, sleep disturbance, and physical sequelae related to military service and injury history.

A study by Sienkiewicz et al. (2020) revealed that trauma exposure (commonplace in military service) among military women also contributes to occupational outcomes in the women veteran population. Worse occupational functioning is associated with a history of military trauma, including military sexual trauma (MST), military sexual assault/harassment, and nonmilitary trauma, suggesting a need for trauma history screening, and evaluation of mental health and employment needs specific to women veterans. Adverse childhood experiences (ACEs) are also identified in the literature as being more prevalent among women veterans (Gaska & Kimerling, 2018), and there is some suggestion that additional military-service imposed trauma may be additive and cumulative for women veterans with military exposures (e.g., military combat or MST). Research on cumulative adversity and trauma-informed care is growing, and the authors suggest that universal screening among female veterans, as well as DoD initiatives to eliminate preventable trauma and harm to female service members, should continue in the active-duty population.

Veteran and military service women present unique opportunities for APRNs and healthcare team members to identify women who are serving and have previously served in the military. This population has unique health and healthcare needs in the context of military employment and will best be served by clinicians who are educated and sensitized to features of military service, unique risks and hazards, health policies, and common conditions that warrant initial screening and follow-through. Veteran and military service women represent a small segment of the population. Clinicians who ask, "Have you ever served in the military?" will quickly identify and be better positioned to care for their women clients who answer, "Yes."

Aging Women in the Workforce

Women represent almost half of the nation's workforce. Projections estimate that women over 55 will account for more than half of all working women by 2024. As the baby boom generation ages, the U.S. Bureau of Labor Statistics (Toossi & Torpey, 2017) expects the fastest growth in labor participation rates for people over the age of 55, and especially for people over the age of 65. This projected increase is due to improved health and life expectancy as well as the need to save more for retirement. Despite the increase in women in the workforce, age discrimination and menopause are among the unique challenges that women face in the workplace.

AGE DISCRIMINATION

The rates of age discrimination are on the rise, and 64% of women report age discrimination as compared to 59% of men. Furthermore, race and ethnicity intersect with gender and age discrimination. Age discrimination is experienced by 40% Asian women, 34% Hispanic women, 31% Black women, and 29% White women (AARP, 2021). The Age Discrimination in Employment Act (ADEA) protects workers who are over age 40. Workers have 180 days to file a charge for age discrimination to the EEOC (n.d.-a), and federal employees have a 45-day deadline to initiate an informal complaint to an Equal Employment Opportunity specialist.

MENOPAUSE AND WORKING WOMEN

Menopause is a transition of life that occurs naturally around 51 years for most women and typically lasts for 4 years, but can take many more years for some women. Women may experience menopause earlier as a consequence of medical diseases or surgical procedures. Common menopausal symptoms include hot flashes, night sweats, and sleep disruption. Sleep disruption can contribute to further symptoms such as fatigue, irritability, musculoskeletal discomforts, and difficulties with memory and concentration (U.S. Department of Health and Human Services, 2019).

As a result of the increased rates of women and aging women in the workforce, menopause is a relevant gender- and age-specific issue. Research indicates that many women consider their menopausal symptoms to have a negative impact on their work. About 80% of menopausal women in a 2014 study reported vasomotor symptoms, and most of these women categorized the symptoms as moderate to severe (Avis et al., 2014). Severe menopausal symptoms put women at risk for increased stress, burnout, and work absences. Decreased cognition as a result of sleep deprivation can also contribute to errors that can lead to disciplinary action. Despite the fact that the menopausal transition affects many women in the workplace, menopause is typically considered a "taboo" subject, which further contributes to women's sense of burden (Rees et al., 2021).

The timing of menopause also intersects with critical career advance, as age 45 to 55 is the most common age bracket for women to move into leadership positions. Considering the increased numbers of women in the workplace and the length of time for menopausal transition, women advancing into top leadership positions are simultaneously experiencing menopausal symptoms. Addressing these women's health issues is important to retaining aging women in the workforce and supporting women in leadership roles (Patterson, 2020).

Healthcare professionals should have an understanding of the effect of menopause on working women. Conversations during well-women encounters should include information about evidence-based recommendations for managing menopausal symptoms. Employers can support women through this transition by promoting education about menopause and considering practices such as allowing flexible dress codes or thermoregulated fabrics, improving ventilation or temperature control, improving access to cold drinking water, and supporting breaks to manage severe vasomotor symptoms (Rees et al., 2021).

ENVIRONMENTAL INFLUENCES

Environmental influences are those factors specific to organizations or a particular profession, encompassing many types of workplace hazards. Healthcare occupations are often heavily populated with women and are notable for the particular hazards associated with this work. Preventing workplace injuries and illness requires anticipation of the possible hazards present, recognition and evaluation of exposures and risks identified, and development of ways to correct or control identified hazards. Anticipation and recognition of hazards is a disciplined analysis of the production facility and activities that includes understanding the production processes, raw materials used, and possible by-products produced. Many workplace hazards affect employees the same, indiscriminate of gender. One factor altering the severity of a workplace hazard is the size of an individual. In the United States, the average woman is 5 feet 4 inches tall and weighs approximately 171 pounds, while the average man is 5 feet 9 inches weighing roughly 200 pounds (CDC, n.d.-a). The Occupational Safety and Health Administration (OSHA) offers a variety of resources on their website (OSHA, n.d.-b) for clinicians. This section reviews chemical, physical, biological, musculoskeletal, psychosocial, sleep, and reproductive hazards of the workplace and aims to provide a heightened awareness for concerns specifically related to women.

Chemical Hazards

The use of both natural and synthetic chemicals is pervasive in current manufacturing and commerce. Most workers are highly likely to be exposed to some chemical compounds in the course of their employment. The American Chemical Society has more than 194 million organic and inorganic substances registered in the Chemical Abstracts Service (CAS) Registry (American Chemical Society, 2022), of which 40,000 are in commercial use (GAO, 2019). The Environmental Protection Agency (EPA) is responsible for enforcing regulations for chemical development under the Toxic Substances Control Act (2016) and for protecting the environment and the public from untoward chemical exposures. The U.S. Department of Labor, via OSHA, has established permissible exposure limits (PELs) for 400 chemicals in the workplace (OSHA, n.d.-d).

Chemicals in the workplace may be found in a variety of forms: dust (formed from mechanical action), smoke (formed from combustion), fumes (formed from volatilizing metal), mists (water droplets), vapors (evaporate of liquid), gases (particles without defined shape or volume), aerosols (atomized particulate), and liquids. Adverse health effects can occur with acute or chronic exposures to chemicals and can affect any or all body systems (dermal, cardiovascular, neurologic, and bone) depending on the composition and molecular makeup of the chemical. The APRN should be aware of occupational worksites where chemicals are present, such as shipyards, beauty spas/cosmetology, textile factories, medical/dental/veterinary facilities, laboratories, laundry services, housekeeping, electronics factories, fire departments, agricultural and animal farming, pest control/pesticides, plastic factories, and weapons ranges. This is not a comprehensive list; clinicians should consider a patient's occupation while examining patients and establishing differential diagnoses. For example, healthcare workers mix, administer, and dispose of hazardous drugs, such as antineoplastic cytotoxic medications, anesthetics, antiviral drugs, and hormones. Chemotherapeutic drugs in particular have been linked to cancers and other health outcomes in the workers mixing and administering these agents. Because of the complexity of chemical effects on women's health and reproductive repercussions, clinicians should maintain close collaborative relationships with occupational medicine teams and should refer patients early and often when a potential or known exposure exists.

Adverse health effects in response to chemical exposures depends on an interaction between the intrinsic toxicity of the chemical, the amount of substance actually delivered (the dose), the exposure conditions, and the physiologic response of the recipient. The concept of dose is particularly useful when considering the interaction between exposure and the worker. For example, a small person has a higher respiratory rate than a larger person; consequently, they will receive a greater dose with the same exposure. The route of exposure, whether by inhalation, ingestion, or skin contact, will also influence the potential for adverse effects. Some chemicals may be more, or less, biologically available depending on the route of exposure (e.g., asbestos inhaled vs. applied to the skin).

In the workplace, attention is primarily paid to the acute effects of exposure to a single chemical, such as headache, respiratory irritation, or skin rashes, or to the effects of very high concentrations leading to loss of consciousness or loss of life. Less attention is paid to health effects related to low-level exposures, exposures to mixtures, or subacute or chronic effects on neurologic or reproductive systems. Cancer has been a concern for long-term outcomes in that a growing number of chemicals have been identified as carcinogenic. The WHO International Agency for Research on Cancer (IARC) lists 121 agents known to be carcinogenic to humans and another 412 compounds that are probably or possibly carcinogenic to humans (WHO, n.d.-a). Of additional concern are chemicals that are cocarcinogenic in that the risk of cancer is increased by the interaction between two chemicals, one or both of which may be found in the workplace. An example of this is the greatly increased risk of lung cancer in asbestos-exposed workers who also smoke cigarettes as opposed to asbestos workers who do not smoke. Diet, medications, air pollution, and non-work-related chemicals or activities may also substantially affect the risk of cancer or other adverse health outcomes produced by chemicals found in the workplace.

One example of the interactive effect of workplace and nonworkplace exposures is seen with lead exposures, which occur in occupations such as construction, battery reclamation, and recycling, but also in hobbies such as stain glass construction and shooting activities at firing ranges. Although OSHA workplace allowable limit is of 50 mcg/m³ 8-hour time-weighted average (TWA; OSHA, n.d.-c), there are no regulatory guidelines for limiting exposures for non-work activities. Women may be uniquely at risk for the effects of lead exposures. The allowable workplace exposure limit does not take into account small-stature workers, pertinent to some women; consequently, these workers may be subjected to a higher dose relative to the same exposure. Furthermore, lead substitutes for calcium in the body and thus accumulates in the bone. The lead can mobilize out of the bone during pregnancy, potentially affecting the developing fetus. In addition, lead can be tracked home from the workplace if workers do not leave contaminated clothes at work, thus contaminating the home and potentially exposing others in the household. Children are particularly vulnerable to lead exposure in that they can absorb up to 50% of ingested lead, whereas adults absorb less. Workplaces using lead should ensure that they are compliant with OSHA lead standard (OSHA, n.d.-c).

Physical Hazards

Physical hazards are factors that may cause harm without direct contact with the worker. The most common physical hazards found in the workplace include noise, temperature extremes, ionizing and nonionizing radiation, and vibration.

NOISE

Noise is unwanted sound. Exposure to high sound levels can be stressful and contributes to noise-induced hearing loss. Noise triggers physiologic changes in the endocrine, cardiovascular, and auditory systems and interferes with a worker's ability to concentrate and adequately communicate with coworkers. (Münzel et al., 2018).

The pituitary–adrenal axis has a very low threshold for stimulation by noise, estimated to be as low as 68 dB. Activation of the pituitary–adrenal axis leads to increased secretion of ACTH and subsequent increase in adrenocortical activity. Thus, noise can be considered a nonspecific stimulus capable of inducing ACTH release.

Noise also appears to stimulate the adrenal medulla, resulting in increased urinary excretion of epinephrine and norepinephrine. The cardiovascular response to noise includes peripheral vasoconstriction. It is believed that vasoconstriction in the spiral vessels supplying the organ of Corti is the change probably responsible for noise-induced hearing loss in humans. Noise exposure in the presence of some chemicals and metals may increase the potential for hearing loss.

The OSHA Technical Manual (Driscoll, 2022) states noise is measured in decibels (dB) and is typically reported as dBA. OSHA regulates noise levels in the workplace and requires regular measurements of noise levels using specially calibrated instruments. According to OSHA requirements, workers may be exposed to average noise levels of up to 90 dBA for no more than 8 hours; however, workers must be enrolled in a hearing conservation program when their 8-hour average noise exposure is at or above 85 dBA. On the decibel scale, pain occurs at 140 dB, jet taking off 200 feet away is 130 dB, a construction site is 100 dB, boiler room is 90 dB, and a conversation 3 feet away is 60 dB (Driscoll, 2022).

WHO identified occupational noise exposure as the second highest workplace risk factor with noise exposure contributing to 22% of work-related health issues (WHO, 2018). An initial assessment for noise-induced hearing loss includes an occupational history of exposure to high sound levels, symptom reporting (inability to hear normal conversation at about 3 feet, tinnitus after leaving a noisy environment), and the use of a screening audiogram. Work-related hearing loss may be temporary, resulting in a "temporary threshold shift" with workers recovering their hearing perception after a period of time away from noisy environments, or it may be permanent, resulting in a "permanent threshold shift." Permanent hearing loss resulting from documented workplace exposures may be compensated through state workers' compensation programs.

HEAT

Exposure to hot environments reduces work efficiency and productivity and can be life threatening. With increasing ambient temperatures related to climate change, heat exposure is of particular concern for women living or working in buildings without climate control or who are working outdoors (e.g., agricultural workers). High humidity slows the evaporation process, increasing the potential stress on the body. In addition to agricultural workers, other occupations at risk for heat exposure include laundry and construction workers, fire fighters, hazardous waste workers, and highway flaggers.

Physical exertion decreases the tolerance for heat and interferes with the body's ability to dissipate heat, particularly if evaporation is impeded or slowed. Workers not accustomed to heat exposure may experience compensatory vasoconstriction to the kidney, liver, and digestive organs as the cutaneous vessels dilate. Persons not acclimatized to heat may not perspire efficiently, thus limiting the amount of effective heat dissipation. Underlying chronic health conditions, such as diabetes or cardiovascular disease, and advanced age reduce the body's ability to compensate for exposure to hot environments.

Workers exposed to elevated temperatures in the workplace acclimate over a period of a few weeks. Over time, the cutaneous blood vessels are better able to dilate and dissipate body heat; however, unusual and acute spikes in ambient temperature may cause heat stress in even the most acclimated worker. During the acclimatization period, workers should avoid continuous and strenuous work, take frequent rest breaks in a shady area, and stay hydrated (cool drink every 15–20 minutes). Salt supplements are not usually recommended or needed. Acclimatization periods vary dependent on protective clothing and job specific requirements (CDC, n.d.-b). OSHA published an Advance Notice of Proposed Rulemaking for Heat Injury and Illness Prevention in Outdoor and Indoor Work Settings in October 2021 as a first step for establishing workplace policy and standards for heat injury and illness prevention (OSHA, 2022).

IONIZING RADIATION

The principal hazard from ionizing radiation (UV light, x-rays, gamma rays, or alpha or beta particles) is its ability to pass through biological tissue and excite atoms, changing them to electrically charged ions and damaging DNA. The health effect varies with the type of radiation and the dose received and may range from no noticeable change in organ function to genetic damage or cancer. The health effects associated with radiation exposure have been modeled primarily on a 70-kg male. Exposures to and protection of women should take into account the unique vulnerability of their reproductive role.

Women can be exposed to ionizing radiation in occupations such as dentistry, x-ray technology, radiology, nuclear medicine, quality control in metal industries, nuclear power, or some laboratory or research work. A common form of environmental exposure to radiation is radon gas, found in a variety of geographical areas of the United States and elsewhere. Radon comes from the breakdown of naturally occurring uranium in rocks and soil and can become airborne. Radon has been linked to high rates of lung cancer (EPA, 2021).

Symptoms of acute high-dose exposure to ionizing radiation range from burns to "radiation sickness," which is characterized by loss of hair, sore throat, diarrhea, rash, and damage to rapidly proliferating tissues, such as bone marrow. Such an exposure would be expected only in the event of an accidental exposure or ingestion of isotopes of high specific radioactivity. Radiation exposure effects are cumulative with regard to changes in biological tissues, and risk of adverse outcomes increases with continued exposure.

A more insidious form of occupational radiation poisoning comes from long-term exposure to low-level radiation sources or to exposures when proper protective measures are not used. Animal studies suggest that exposure for long periods may produce subcellular tissue damage that can lead to a variety of adverse health outcomes, including cataracts and cancer.

The OSHA's Ionizing Radiation Standard (2016) establishes the maximum allowable radiation exposure levels at which no further exposure is permitted until a designated time has elapsed. Protection from the adverse health effects of ionizing radiation includes the use of proper shielding (lead for x-ray or gamma radiation and protective clothing for other forms of radiation such as alpha particles). Persons working in areas where there is a source of radiation should wear personal radiation-monitoring devices for cumulative exposure assessment, and all radioactive chemicals should be appropriately labeled and properly stored and disposed of.

NONIONIZING RADIATION

Nonionizing radiation (also known as *electromagnetic frequency [EMF] radiation*) refers to radiation with enough energy to cause molecules to vibrate but not enough to remove electrons or ionize biological tissue. Electrical fields are characterized by an electrical charge and are easily shielded, whereas moving electrical charges create magnetic fields and are difficult to shield. Common forms of nonionizing radiation include lasers (light amplification by stimulated emission of radiation), UV light, radio frequency or microwaves, infrared light, and visible light. Common sources of UV light, the type of nonionizing radiation that presents the greatest health concern, include sunlight, welding, mercury vapor lamps, tanning booths, and black lights. UV light does not penetrate deeply, so the eyes and skin are the primary organs of concern related to exposure. Chronic overexposure may lead to cataract and skin cancer. UV light is listed as a group 1 human carcinogen by the IARC. Some nonspecific, vague, and poorly documented symptoms may be related to nonionizing radiation exposure and include increased fatigue, dizziness, headaches, and changes in sensitivity to light and sound.

Occupations or work activities with possible exposure to nonionizing radiation include welders, telecommunication, electricians, glass and steel making, surgical and other lasers, heat lamps, high-voltage power lines, and a wide range of electrical equipment. Exposures can be prevented or mitigated by increasing the distance from the source, as well as using protective glasses, face shields, or goggles and protective clothing. The American Conference of Governmental Industrial Hygienists (ACGIH) has published a consensus standard providing exposure limit guidance to reduce adverse health effects. OSHA and other regulatory agencies have also published PELs and other guidance for nonionizing radiation and lasers in particular.

Biological Hazards

Work with and around microorganisms, mold allergens, fungi, viruses, or plant and animal poisons places workers at risk of exposure to potentially harmful infectious agents and associated diseases. Healthcare and laboratory workers are the primary at-risk professionals and are at risk for exposures to diseases from needlesticks and general exposure to bodily fluids. Since 1991, OSHA has enforced the Bloodborne Pathogens Standard(2019), which focuses on hepatitis B and C, HIV, and other potentially infectious materials. Workers in child care, laboratories, public utilities, heating and air conditioning ventilation systems, tattoo parlors, swimming pools, and lifeguards at public beaches may be at risk as well (OSHA, n.d.-a).

Musculoskeletal Hazards

Musculoskeletal injuries may occur due to tool design, work-station design, prolonged sitting or standing, lifting, pushing or pulling heavy loads, performing highly repetitive movements, or being in awkward postures. Carpal tunnel syndrome is a common musculoskeletal condition frequently reported by working women. Low back injury and pain is a leading cause of disability and is particularly prevalent among healthcare workers due to patient handling including inconsistent use of assistive devices (Andersen et al., 2019). Work-related musculoskeletal injuries result in high costs related to absenteeism, decreased productivity, healthcare expenses, and Workers' Compensation claims (CDC, n.d.-e). Ergonomic (fitting the work to the worker) programs and interventions such as sit–stand workstations, adjustable table heights, lifting aids, and redesigned production methods and tools can reduce or eliminate musculoskeletal injuries.

Psychosocial Hazards

Workplace stress is probably the major psychosocial hazard faced by American workers. *Work-related stress* can be defined as harmful physical or emotional responses that occur when the requirements of the job do not match the capabilities or resources of the worker. Stress is not altogether undesirable; in fact, some stress helps motivate and focus the learning necessary to master new skills and to be productive. Individual coping skills may moderate or accentuate the effects of stressful situations. Some working conditions are considered stressful for nearly all personality types and coping skills. These include heavy workloads with infrequent breaks, long hours, and irregular shift work; organizational challenges such as poor communication of organizational culture or goals, poor relationship with supervisor or coworkers, lack of support from coworkers, tight production schedules, inadequate resources, and lack of opportunity for growth or advancement; unreasonable job expectations including too many responsibilities with too little control, role ambiguity, and insufficient training; and physical conditions such as dangerous or hazardous conditions without control strategies, excessive noise, poor housekeeping, and lack of adequate ventilation or light.

Most workers can adapt to short-term stresses but may have difficulty compensating for chronic or unresolved stress. Stressful conditions that continue unabated can increase physiologic and psychological wear on biological systems and lead to disturbances in sleep patterns, headaches, difficulty in problem-solving and maintenance of relationships, and increased risk of injury or illness. There is some suggestion that stressful working conditions interfere with safe work practices and may contribute to absenteeism, tardiness, and staff turnover.

Violence in healthcare settings is surprisingly high and disconcerting because of the vulnerability of the patients and the caregiver's commitment to patient safety and well-being. Workplace bullying is the behavior of individuals or groups that includes repeated aggressive acts against a coworker or subordinate. Workplace bullying can also involve an abuse or misuse of power; it creates feelings of defenselessness and undermines an individual's right to dignity at work. Bullying has also been linked to adverse health outcomes.

Sexual harassment as a form of workplace violence is an unfortunate and all too frequent reality in many workplaces and can be stressful and affect mental and physical health. Although women are often the victim of sexual harassment, men are not immune. Sexual harassment can come in the form of implying job security or benefits in return for sexual favors or in the form of a hostile work environment where unwelcome sexual verbal comments, visual images, or psychological harassment is tolerated. Sexual harassment is a violation of the 1964 Civil Rights Act, which was expanded in 1991 to include gender bias and harassment against both men and women and includes same-sex harassment.

Addressing workplace stress and violence requires organizational change, education, resiliency, and stress management. This might include working with management to adjust workloads, review or modify job expectations, provide adequate training, and improve environmental conditions. Stress-management programs might include education on multiple sources of stress, time-management skills, relaxation exercises, or other personal skills to reduce stress.

Shift Work and Extended Shifts

Shift work and extended work hours (beyond 8 hours per day) is an integral and accepted practice in healthcare and other industries. Up to 30% of healthcare workers are engaged in some degree of night shift work. Not only is the healthcare industry dependent on workers willing to work nonstandard shifts, but globalization has pushed numerous other industries to a 24-hour work cycle, with more employees working nights and rotating shifts.

Shift work and extended hours have been related to increased injury and illness rates, weight gain, fatigue, lower cognitive function, and increased fatality rates (Leso et al., 2021). Shift work, particularly night shift, can lead to excessive sleepiness, insomnia, disrupted sleep schedules, depression, irritability, and poor performance. Night shift work may also be related to cancer outcomes (Kolstad, 2008). Not surprisingly, shift work can contribute to challenging personal relationships and difficulty meeting family responsibilities. Strategies for addressing some of the effects of shift work include staying active and consuming caffeinated beverages during waking hours but avoiding them just before sleeping. Sleeping in a dark and quiet environment is advised, as is considering using eye shades and ear plugs.

Reproductive Hazards

In general, healthy women with a normal pregnancy and fetus can work throughout their pregnancy. The fetus is highly vulnerable to exposures in the mother's workplace, particularly during the first trimester (CDC, n.d.-c). All parents should be equally watchful for exposures to compounds that can be carried home on clothing or skin, thereby exposing other family members, particularly children, and the home environment. In addition, women should be aware that some compounds, such as lead and some pesticides, can bioaccumulate before pregnancy and affect the developing fetus during gestation. Work-related pesticide exposures can precipitate adverse reproductive outcomes in both men and women. Companies are prohibited from excluding women from hazardous exposure jobs under Title VII of the 1964 Civil Rights Act. With regard to mitigating exposures to reproductive hazards, the focus should be on making jobs safe for all workers, including women of reproductive age, and on increasing awareness among women and their employers regarding exposures that may affect reproduction and offspring.

Materials that can affect reproduction have several mechanisms of action, including mutagenesis, teratogenesis, and epigenetic transmission. Each is discussed in the following sections.

MUTAGENESIS

Mutagenesis is the process that occurs when chemicals, radiation, or biological agents interact with living cells to cause a change in the genetic material of that cell. The genetic change is called *mutation,* and the substance producing the change, a *mutagen.* Most mutations are harmful and often result in the death of the individual cell. However, mutations may also cause abnormal cell division, which can result in cancer or altered cell function. If a mutation occurs in a germ cell (sperm or egg) before conception, it may be incompatible with life, resulting in infertility of the parent or death of the fetus. Alternatively, mutations in the offspring may also occur, manifesting as congenital defects. It is not known to what extent the rate of mutations is in human cells and to what degree those mutations are increased or influenced by occupational or environmental exposures.

TERATOGENESIS

Teratogenesis is the process that occurs when exposures alter fetal development during gestation to cause fetal death or abnormalities such as cleft lip. Exposures to the fetus generally occur from the mother's blood by way of the placenta, although direct exposures, such as radiation, may also occur. The developing fetus is uniquely sensitive to some chemicals that may not be harmful to the mother. The first trimester (up to 60 days after conception) is thought to be the period of greatest susceptibility to teratogenic insult, although teratogens may affect the fetus to various degrees throughout gestation. There is growing concern that even low-level exposures to the mother can result in fetal anomalies. For example, phthalate exposure may result in male offspring with undescended testicles or hypospadias. Subtle or dramatic damage to the fetus can also occur with prenatal exposure to a variety of compounds such as thalidomide, some antibiotics, alcohol, lead, and mercury.

EPIGENESIS

Epigenetics is the process by which environmental or external factors regulate the timing, duration, and/or intensity of gene expression. In turn, gene expression may cause variations in phenotypic traits. Some epigenetic changes can be inherited across generations without changing the underlying DNA. External factors are naturally occurring, whereas other factors may be related to lifestyle or various diseases. Recent research suggests that there may be a relationship between epigenetic changes and various health outcomes, such as cancers, immune disorders, and neuropsychiatric disorders. For example, prenatal and early postnatal environmental factors influence the adult risk of developing various chronic diseases and behavioral disorders (Gartstein & Skinner, 2017).

ADDRESSING WORK–RELATED ADVERSE HEALTH OUTCOMES

Occupational Health History

An occupational health history is an invaluable tool for understanding workers' symptoms and designing effective treatment plans. An occupational health history is a chronological list of all the worker's employment with more detail collected to identify occupational exposure to potentially hazardous agents and related health effects. Because work-related illness can present with common symptoms, an occupational health history can help determine whether or not work is a cause or aggravation of adverse health conditions. It helps link health problems to specific workplace exposures or hazards. Also, it can help determine whether or not the patient has the capacity to work and whether or not short- or long-term restrictions are necessary when returning to job tasks.

Assessment forms can be developed for workers/patients to list current and previous jobs or work activities, but more specific information regarding exposures may need to be elicited by interviewing the worker/patient. Questions should explore all current and previous jobs, (including part time or temporary jobs). In addition, the interview should include questions about hobbies, military service exposures, and work overseas.

Interpreting the information gleaned from an occupational health history interview should be conducted in consultation with occupational health professionals who can assist with follow-up questions to better understand workplace processes and materials and possible links between exposures and health outcomes. Screening or ongoing surveillance may be required for some exposures covered by OSHA regulations and standards, such as for working with lead or cadmium. Workers with work-related injuries are entitled to Workers' Compensation benefits for medical care, possibly time-loss payments, and/or a disability pension. Application for Workers' Compensation benefits often requires the healthcare provider to complete necessary forms and refer the patient to the relevant state agency or insurance carrier.

Workers' Compensation

Caring for working populations, particularly injured workers, necessitates a basic understanding of Workers' Compensation programs in the United States. Workers' Compensation is a form of insurance that provides medical benefits, time-loss wage replacement, and disability pension to employees injured in the course of employment. In the event of a fatality, Workers' Compensation programs pay benefits to the immediate family. Workers' Compensation is administered on a state-by-state basis, with a governing board overseeing varying public–private combinations of compensation systems. The benefit award amounts vary widely across the states. Every state except Texas requires employers to carry some form of Workers' Compensation insurance. The Workers' Compensation insurance scheme was the result of the "grand bargain" negotiated between workers and employers over several decades in the United States. In exchange for medical care and time-loss wage replacement in the event of an injury, workers are required to relinquish their right to sue their employer for negligence or for general damages of pain and suffering.

Employers, with a few exceptions, completely fund the programs by purchasing commercial insurance, setting up a "self-insured" account, or paying into state-managed programs. The goals of the insurance programs are to provide "sure and certain relief" by paying for the financial consequences of treated work-related injuries, compensating the injured for time loss, and paying any temporary or permanent disability benefit that is incurred. Some states allow employers to optionally carry insurance; however, the majority of American businesses carry some form of Workers' Compensation insurance. Notably, some groups (e.g., agriculture, some domestic workers, longshore workers, and railroad workers) are not covered by state Workers' Compensation programs. Some are not covered at all, and others are covered under separate and specific federal compensation programs (Federal Employers Liability Act of 1908; Longshore and Harbor Workers' Compensation Act of 1927).

The definition of *work-related injury* or *illness*, the extent of compensation, the benefit rates, administrative rules and practices, the terms for disability pensions, and caregiver reimbursement schedules are highly variable across the United States and often the source of continued political tension between business and labor groups. Some states permit workers to select their own caregivers, whereas others allow employers to manage care either through third-party administrators (TPAs) or through employer-selected caregivers. In addition, the difference between *impairment* (the degree of loss of anatomy or function of a body part or system) and *disability* (degree of impaired ability to perform required work) can be contentious and confusing. The interaction between state Workers' Compensation systems and the Americans With Disabilities Act (1990) and Patient Protection and Affordable Care Act (2010) relative to comprehensive care for injured workers is still evolving. One of the early hopes of the Workers' Compensation scheme was that it would incentivize employers to work to prevent workplace injuries; however, this goal was imperfectly achieved. It was not until the passage of OSHA in 1970 that meaningful prevention efforts in American workplaces were undertaken.

Guidance for the Care Provider

Care of injured workers triggers interactions with insurance carriers, TPAs, claims adjudicators, case managers, employers, and other healthcare disciplines. In addition to immediate care of the injury or illness, it is important to try to return the injured worker to work as soon as possible and to avoid long-term disability for the benefit of both the worker and the employer. Interacting with a Workers' Compensation system is as legal as it is clinical; clinicians should consult with occupational and environmental healthcare specialists to navigate the system for the benefit of the patient and best clinical outcomes. In addition, the relevant state agency that manages Workers' Compensation can provide state-specific program information.

Disability Prevention

The goal of tertiary prevention is to prevent disability progression and to reduce residual deficits and dysfunction in workers with established disability. Unfortunately, injured workers with compensation claims are at risk of slipping into long-term disability. Some injuries are so catastrophic that full recovery is unlikely. Efforts to improve the integration of care with strong communication between the injured worker, healthcare provider, the workplace, and the Workers' Compensation agency have been suggested to reduce the risk of long-term disability. Others have worked to understand the early issue or conditions that might predict which injured worker might slide into chronic disability. Careful management of chronic pain is an important aspect of care of the injured worker, particularly since opioid use within 90 days from injury has been shown to significantly increase the incidence of long-term and permanent disability (Haight et al., 2020).

Caring for injured workers can be complicated, time consuming, and at times frustrating. It requires an in-depth understanding of state-specific Workers' Compensation laws and regulations, as well as clinical best practices and workplace issues, in order to return the injured worker to optimal health and to prevent permanent disability. Clinicians are encouraged to collaborate with occupational and environmental healthcare specialists when providing care to patients with work-related injuries or illnesses.

Controlling Workplace Hazards

Although treating work-related injuries and illness is the most common opportunity practitioners have to deal with occupational health issues, preventing adverse health outcomes related to exposures at work should be the primary strategy. Primary prevention requires the recognition of workplace hazards with a keen understanding of specific production processes, raw materials used, by-products of the production process, available engineering controls, use of PPE, and relevant regulatory guidelines. The standard strategy for controlling workplace exposures is termed the *hierarchy of controls,* a ranking of interventions by first eliminating hazardous materials or operations, substituting for hazardous materials with less hazardous ones, instituting engineering controls such as ventilation systems or machine guarding, and exploring administrative controls such as worker rotation through less hazardous jobs. The last control strategy to consider within the hierarchy of controls paradigm is the use of PPE. A significant consideration is the likelihood of a worker removing PPE if the fit is poor or the effectiveness is altered if someone wears additional layers under PPE in an attempt to make equipment fit.

The Role of Government in Controlling Workplace Hazards

Historically, the costs of caring for injured workers and even for preventing injuries and illnesses were largely externalized by business and industry. The resulting social costs, as well as pressure from injured workers and their families, motivated government involvement. Most industrialized countries recognized that eliminating and reducing the adverse health effects associated with the production of goods and services require some form of government intervention. Even the most well-meaning company may not have the information or the political will to fully anticipate, evaluate, and control workplace hazards. A high workplace fatality rate in the late 1800s and early 1900s incentivized some states to start state-level safety programs and to initiate Workers' Compensation programs.

After the death of 68 miners in a mine explosion in West Virginia in 1968, occupational health and safety legislation was a priority. Occupational Safety and Health Act was signed into law in 1970 and went into effect the following April establishing the Occupational Safety and Health Administration within the Department of Labor. The law made provisions for each state to develop its own OSHA program, and 22 states (OSHA, 2020) have done so. State OSHA plans must have regulations that are at least as effective as the federal OSHA regulations. States that did not develop their own "state plan" are covered by the federal OSHA regulations.

OSHA regulations are wide ranging and include guidance and enforceable standards for both safety and health. In addition to the basic OSHA regulations, other regulations are relevant for occupational health, such as the Workplace Right to Know, which requires labeling of chemicals in the workplace and training on their use and directs that chemical manufacturers must supply safety data sheets with each shipment of chemicals. Community right to know made information available to emergency responders and others on chemicals in use in manufacturing firms in their area.

OSHA works to update its regulatory standards, though political pressure has often delayed the setting of new standards. Among the OSHA regulations that are frequently referred to are the Permissible Exposure Limits (PELs), which is a listing of several hundred chemicals with their allowable or legal level for exposure on a daily basis over the course of a working lifetime. PELs are usually designated as 8-hour TWA, short-term exposure limits (usually 15 to 30 minutes), or ceiling limits and are reported as parts per million or milligrams per cubic centimeter. If workers are exposed to regulated compounds for more than 8 hours, a reassessment of the allowable limits is required. Some state programs may regulate exposures to compounds not regulated by OSHA.

The PELs have been criticized for being set by what industry found to be achievable levels rather than levels related to health outcomes. In addition, political pressure has limited OSHA's ability to update the PEL with new scientific findings; consequently, many of the PELs reflect science and industry control abilities present in the 1960s or 1970s. The OSHA PELs are therefore considered by many occupational health and safety practitioners to be minimal standards.

OSHA met with considerable pressure from business interests, and Congress has not funded the agency to the level necessary to fully implement its mandate. There are not enough inspectors to review company compliance with state and federal regulations, resulting in some companies never being inspected. To effectively use limited resources, the federal agency and state counterparts often prioritize inspections according to high-risk industries or complaints. Consequently, strategies for preventing workplace injuries and illness rely on the companies themselves and on local occupational safety and health professionals. OSHA also posts directives, fact sheets, and other information to assist employers in complying with regulations.

Other federal agencies such as the EPA are responsible for implementing other laws with relevance for workplaces and communities, such as the Toxic Substances Control Act (sets expectations for testing and labeling chemical substances), the Clean Air Act (addresses air pollution), the Clean Water Act (addresses allowable pollution of waterways), the Resource Conservation and Recovery Act (addresses hazardous waste), and the Federal Insecticide, Fungicide, and Rodenticide Act (addresses pesticide use), among others. The regulations associated with these laws are often administered by state as well as the federal agency. Knowledge of the provisions of these regulations is critical in helping clients understand to what protections they are entitled.

In addition to establishing the parameters of OSHA, the Occupational Safety and Health Act outlined the requirement for a federal agency to conduct research and professional training in the area of occupational health. The National Institute for Occupational Health and Safety (NIOSH) implemented these requirements, publishing numerous research findings, reports, criteria documents, guidance documents, and fact sheets on the practice of occupational health and helped establish guidance for state and federal rule making as well as corporate policies to protect worker health (www.cdc.gov/niosh).

International Standards

The United States lags behind many industrialized democracies in the type and level of protection they provide for working people. For example, the European Commission has established a policy on the Registration, Evaluation, Authorisation, and Restriction of Chemicals (REACH; European Commission, 2015). Since 2007, the regulations have required manufacturers and importers of chemicals to compile and distribute information on the properties and safe use of their chemicals. Chemicals that cannot be used safely may have restrictions on their use or must be phased out. These regulations place more responsibility than is currently required under U.S. regulations. U.S.-based companies wishing to do business in the European Union are required to comply with REACH, and some want to see these regulatory requirements to ultimately be the standard in the United States. Practitioners interested in the understanding of safe chemical compositions and their use may find more current information through the REACH regulations than the U.S. chemical regulations under the Toxic Substances Control

Act. OSHA works to maintain some consistency with newer international regulatory developments. Of particular interest for practitioners is the Globally Harmonized System (GHS) of Classification and Labeling of Chemicals to improve the consistency internationally of labeling and training on the use of chemicals.

Professional Collaborators

NIOSH established a strategic plan for fiscal years 2019 to 2026 (CDC, 2022). Strategically, NIOSH is focused on addressing health and safety in the U.S. workforce to reduce occupationally related chronic diseases and cancer, hearing loss, integumentary diseases, musculoskeletal disorders, respiratory diseases, and safety and traumatic injuries, and to promote healthy work design and well-being.

Despite efforts to mitigate and prevent occupational injuries and illness, occupational medicine remains an invaluable component in healthcare delivery. Caring for injured workers and preventing future injuries requires a strong collaboration with occupational and environmental physicians, nurses, industrial hygienists, safety professionals, toxicologists, health physicists, case managers, and vocational rehabilitation counselors. These professionals have the expertise and knowledge of best practices to address workplace exposure and healthcare management, and as stated previously, APRNs should refer early and often for support in caring for women with workplace-related health and wellness concerns.

Unions

No discussion of occupational safety and health is complete without the inclusion of organized labor. Unions were not always supportive of federal legislative effort to protect workers or provide injured workers compensation for injuries, as some union leadership felt it was the union's role to provide health and safety support to its members. Over the years, however, organized labor became a strong advocate for workplace health and safety protections and partnered with many occupational health and safety professionals to oversee implementation of hazard controls. Labor representatives have the right to accompany OSHA inspectors on a site visit and often provide helpful information on work processes and exposures. If an injured worker is a member of a union, it will be useful for the caregiver to reach out to union representatives for assistance in return-to-work efforts and help in understanding work requirements.

Integrating the Workplace and General Health

Increasingly it has been acknowledged that the work is not, and should not be, isolated from the rest of a worker's life and that the health and safety of people who work should be dealt with holistically. Workplace exposures and stressors have a great influence on the health of the individual and general health. Alternatively, living conditions and the environment contribute to worker health and workplace productivity. To be fully effective in building health and well-being, efforts to prevent workplace injuries and illnesses inside the factory walls must be integrated with promotion of health. Early activities in this arena included vendor-supplied health promotion, smoking cessation, exercise, or weight-loss programs offered at the workplace. Others pushed their corporate sustainability commitments beyond being environmentally "green" to incorporating worker health, safety, and well-being into their corporate efforts. NIOSH responded to this goal by developing their Total Worker Health program (CDC, n.d.-d) with guidance on integrating workplace illness prevention with health promotion. Evaluation of the effectiveness of these various approaches in improving worker health, safety, well-being, job satisfaction, work–life balance, and productivity is ongoing.

Women are an indispensable part of the American workforce, where many find themselves exposed to hazardous compounds and risky situations. Healthcare providers have an opportunity to anticipate, evaluate, and control hazards while caring for workplace injuries or illnesses. Clinicians play a vital role in supporting working women by providing individualized care and advocating for policy modification and addressing the differences between genders.

REFERENCES

References for this chapter are online and available at https://connect.springerpub.com/content/book/978-0-8261-6722-4/part/part02/chapter/ch17

CHAPTER 18

Health Considerations for Women Caregivers*

CHRISTINE DILEONE

WOMEN AS CAREGIVERS

The lion's share of caregiving work continues to fall to women, who are more likely than men to find themselves providing care for ill and disabled children, parents, and spouses; roughly 60% of caregivers in the United States are women (Family Caregiver Alliance, 2016). Current estimates from the American Time Use Survey (ATUS) indicate that nearly one third of the population composes informal caregivers, contributing 1.2 billion hours of unpaid work annually. Women's involvement in caregiving to children is prominent when women are in their 30s, coinciding with their working years, and also during their 50s and beyond, during years of grandparenting. In addition, women in their 70s and 80s make noteworthy contributions to spousal care (Dukhovnov & Zagheni, 2015). In the United States, estimates indicate that a majority of caregivers are women, some of whom simultaneously care for aging parents, spouses, children, and more recently, grandchildren. Indeed, the term *sandwich generation* has been used to describe women's position in the middle of aging parents and children needing care. Informal caregiving was valued at $691 billion in 2012, constituting 4.3% of the gross domestic product (GDP) and is predicted to reach $838 billion by 2050 owing to the aging of the population. Nonetheless, informal caregivers usually are not compensated for their services.

How did this arrangement evolve? Sociological studies reveal that caregiving is a product of gender-role socialization, with women being allocated the relational work of families and men the instrumental, external work to generate resources to support the family. That women are "ordered to care" by social convention has been examined by Susan Reverby, who studied the social arrangements that affect women in general and nurses in particular (Reverby, 1987). Indeed, gender-role socialization expectations are that women will assume responsibility for elder caregiving as well as that for their children. In some societies, the care for family members extends to members of the husband's family, increasing the expectations that women will be constantly available as wives, mothers, daughters, and caregivers. Socially constructed arrangements dividing labor in families also extend to women's voluntary contributions of many hours to support community agencies, often viewed as an extension of their family's contributions. In addition, women who do not provide caregiver service to their families may be made to feel guilty about their decisions.

Of consequence for women is that their informal caregiving is contributed as voluntary and without pay. Often women's caregiving work remains hidden and is taken for granted, resulting in the failure of social and health policy makers to consider their contributions to the economy. Many Western countries' healthcare systems, including home care, rely on women's unpaid work but do not account for their contribution to the GDP. The estimated economic value of this unpaid labor in the United States is significant (Dukhovnov & Zagheni, 2015). Moreover, unpaid caregiving often interferes with women accruing retirement benefits such as Social Security, healthcare benefits such as insurance, or other employee benefits, and their absence from the labor force results in their lagging behind men in promotions, salary increases, and the development of skill sets that command higher salaries. Because women are overrepresented in lower paying, lower status occupations, their incomes are often assumed to be discretionary or expendable; thus their willingness to provide caregiving services is assumed to be a "natural" arrangement in families. In turn, the gender disparities in occupational strata are reinforced and are evident even in healthcare (see Chapter 2, Women and Healthcare Workforce: Caregivers and Consumers).

Lost opportunity costs for women who may need to modify employment commitments or leave their paid work to

---

*This chapter is a revision of the chapter that appeared in the second edition of this textbook, authored by Judith Berg and Nancy Fugate Wood, and we thank them for their original contribution.

provide care for their families do not appear in the calculation of the GDP, nor do they afford tax breaks or benefits for women's families. The loss of accrued salary plus Social Security benefits for women's own retirement and employee benefits packages that include health insurance coverage together are missing from our national calculation. When women are able to reenter the workforce after providing caregiving, their past absences from work places them in jeopardy because of lost opportunities for training in new skills, reduction of their seniority, or even loss of their jobs, despite the provisions of the Family and Medical Leave Act. The loss of networking opportunities also removes them from sources of social support, friendship, and professional and occupational information flows and may constrain their friendship networks.

For women who are mothers as well as caregivers, becoming a caregiver increases the demands on relationships, sometimes requiring women to balance the needs of their developing children against the needs of family members, including their spouses or their own parents. An estimated 67% of U.S. women with preschool children are employed, and the absence or low availability of workplace-based child care or leave policies such as in Scandinavian countries complicates the demands they face in providing informal caregiving services (U.S. Bureau of Labor Statistics, 2022).

Caregiving experiences punctuate women's lifespans. In addition to the assumptions about being the constantly available mother to infants and young children, women are also assumed to be willing and available to provide grandparenting, spousal care, and parent care. Some may provide care to all of these family members over the course of a lifetime and sometimes simultaneously.

The demand for informal caregivers has increased for a variety of reasons. Among the most pressing is the aging of the population. An estimated 65% of older adults rely on family caregivers, with 30% of these also using formal caregivers (Family Caregiver Alliance, 2015). In addition, the shortening

of hospital stays has resulted in a transfer of healthcare responsibilities to families earlier in the course of an illness. The use of increased home care technology, such as monitoring devices and even ventilators that can be used in home settings, has shifted many procedures from the healthcare system to informal caregivers.

In addition to social and economic consequences, recent research findings indicate that caregiving may affect women's health–related behaviors and their health. In this chapter we examine (a) a framework for considering the factors affecting caregivers' health and health promotion practices, (b) assessment and interventions for caregivers: a review of evidence, and (c) clinical applications of what we know about promoting caregivers' health.

FACTORS AFFECTING CAREGIVERS' HEALTH AND HEALTH PROMOTION: A FRAMEWORK

Figure 18.1 provides a framework depicting possible relationships among personal characteristics of the caregiver, caregiver resources, life demands and their relationships to caregiving processes, meaning of caregiving, and health outcomes of caregiving. Each of these components is discussed in this chapter.

Personal Characteristics

Personal characteristics describe people who are the caregivers and include their age, education, personal development, life opportunities, health status, and health-promoting practices as they begin caregiving work (Leveille et al., 2000). The ages of caregivers in the United States cross the life span. Young adults to the oldest old provide caregiving services.

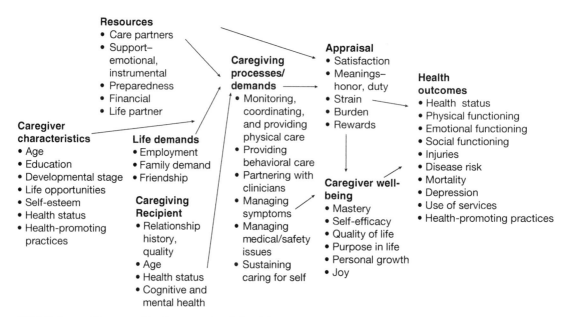

FIGURE 18.1 Factors affecting caregiver's health
Caregiver characteristics, resources, life demands, caregiving recipient, caregiving processes/demands, appraisal, and caregiver well-being influence health outcomes.

In some circumstances, children and adolescents assume some caregiving responsibilities for family members, sometimes for siblings and parents or grandparents. Middle-aged and older women, including those who are remaining in the workforce, provide the majority of the care to U.S. family members. Indeed a recent Behavioral Risk Factor Surveillance System survey indicated that the largest proportion of family caregivers was 50 to 64 years of age, female, Black/non-Hispanic, and married and had some college education (Anderson et al., 2013).

A caregiver's education may provide access to information that may be useful in providing caregiver services and obtaining information about the health problem of the person who is the care recipient. The developmental history of the caregiver influences the ability of caregivers to find meaning in the work of caregiving and possible outcomes of caregiving. For example, an adolescent daughter who is caring for a parent might narrow her range of friendships and opt out of continuing school beyond high school and experience the lower income associated with lower educational preparation that persists across her remaining life span. In contrast, an older woman who provides care for a husband may view herself as doing what is consistent with her life stage and personal history.

As women develop health-promoting practices, they may accrue health benefits that sustain their health across their life span. The type of health-promoting practices in which women engage (e.g., physical activity such as walking and eating fresh fruits and vegetables) may become difficult to continue in the face of caregiving demands. Women who are in good health enter caregiving relationships with health advantages, but maintaining their health in the face of caregiving demands may present challenges. Those who assume caregiving in poor health begin this part of their lives having attenuated possibilities for health promotion and illness management, although evidence suggests the possibility for their experiencing well-being despite their health problems.

Women's Roles and Relationships in Caregiving

As women enter caregiving arrangements, they bring with them the complement of roles and responsibilities that characterize their lives. Many perform roles of wife, mother, employee, volunteer, grandparent, or even great-grandparent. The demands of these roles influence not only women's energy levels, but also financial obligations that may be delicately balanced with their incomes and financial reserves. Consequently, the commitment to be a caregiver brings with it financial as well as energy commitments.

Caregiving implies creating or maintaining a relationship with the care recipient. Often the relationship to the person for whom one provides care has been established before the commitment to caregiving is made (Pinquart & Sorenson, 2011). Some women may find themselves caring for family members with whom the relationship does not have a long history, such as in the case of caring for an orphaned young grandchild or a more distant relative with whom there is little opportunity to have developed a relationship. When caregiving results from a family crisis, the demands of new roles may be immediate, as in assuming the care of a young grandchild,

and may allow limited time to adapt to new demands (Moore & Rosenthal, 2014; Musil et al., 2010, 2013). Also, caregiver strain arises from conflicting demands with other roles, including parenting, employment, friendships, and other volunteer efforts, each of which may have special meanings for the caregiver.

When there is a history of a relationship with the care recipient, the caregiver may be challenged by its nature. Caring for a family member with whom the relationship has been abusive or distant may pose some risk for caregivers. Hodgins et al. (2011) found that health outcomes and health promotion for women caregivers were affected by their becoming caregivers because of a sense of duty or obligation and by the quality of their past relationship with the caregiving recipient. Women who had better past relationships were less likely to assume caregiving because of duty or obligation. Indeed, having an abusive parent or partner increased the sense of obligation to provide care for them. Obligation, in turn, influenced caregivers' health such that women who provided care out of a sense of duty had poorer health, including physical, emotional, and relational health and material well-being indicators.

Caregiving During a Pandemic

Beach et al. (2021) found "the coronavirus disease 2019 (COVID-19) pandemic has negatively affected persons with existing chronic health conditions [and has] the potential to exacerbate the stresses of family caregiving" ("Abstract"). The authors compared family caregivers with noncaregivers on physical, psychosocial, and financial well-being outcomes during the pandemic and determined that family caregivers were more at risk for adverse outcomes. Family caregivers reported higher anxiety, depression, fatigue, sleep disturbance, lower social participation, lower financial well-being, increased food insecurity (all $p < .01$), and increased financial worries ($p = .01$). Caregivers who reported more COVID-19–related caregiver stressors and disruptions reported more adverse outcomes (all $p < .01$). In addition, caregivers who were female, younger, lower income, providing both personal/medical care, and providing care for cognitive/behavioral/emotional problems reported more adverse outcomes. The challenges of caregiving are exacerbated by the COVID-19 pandemic. Family caregivers reported increased duties, burdens, and resulting adverse health, psychosocial, and financial outcomes. Results were generally consistent with caregiver stress–health process models. Family caregivers should receive increased support during this serious public health crisis.

Caregiving Resources

One's ability to provide care for a family member or friend may be enhanced by having access to resources that support the caregiver and their efforts. Among these resources are access to help, including care partners who share the responsibility, provide substitution to afford the caregiver respite and opportunity to engage in valued activities or rest, and instrumental assistance, such as access to information about options in caring for someone who is bedridden or incontinent, as well as providing physical assistance. Access to emotional support, such as provided by a life partner or a close friend, can sustain women in their caregiving efforts. Emotional support in the form of encouraging the caregiver, affirming and valuing the commitment to caregiving, and listening to the expression of feelings can help sustain the emotional energy needed for caregiving as well as support emotional regulation of the caregiver.

Financial resources that support access to respite and instrumental assistance, such as by purchasing home care services, enable caregivers to balance their own personal needs with the care recipient's needs. Long-term care insurance that pays for home care services, as well as other types of health insurance, may contribute to the success of caregiving relationships, but access to these types of insurance benefits are limited. Moreover, these benefits often are associated with one's employment, thus making them inaccessible when a caregiver must resign from employment in order to assume caregiving responsibilities.

Caregiving Processes

At the center of this framework are caregiving processes. What do caregivers do? Despite the impressive contributions of caregivers, there is often limited understanding of the activities in which they engage. Caregiving processes can be described by focusing on meeting the needs of the care recipient for assistance in activities of daily living (ADLs), such as bathing, dressing, grooming, moving from one place to another, toileting, feeding, and continence care. In addition, caregivers often provide assistance with instrumental ADLs (IADLs), including conducting financial transactions, such as paying bills; shopping for food and preparing meals; doing housework and laundry; managing transportation; conducting phone conversations; and coordinating and performing medical regimens. What is not included in a simple enumeration of these tasks is the coordination of elements of care; these may include managing multiple caregivers (informal and formal) who may contribute a variety of services; monitoring the care recipient to promote safety and prevent injury, such as falls; anticipating and planning for the needs of the care recipient over a period of time; and maintaining an interpersonal relationship with the care recipient that is appropriate to one's family role, such as wife or mother. Caring for a person with dementia provides some unique challenges, as discussed later in this chapter.

In addition to the informal caregiving activities enumerated earlier, caregivers provide essential health-related services that may include the management of a variety of medications (some with serious side effects), administration of treatments such as the application of dressings or external medications, and performance of prescribed physical activity routines such as those prescribed by a physical therapist. Often the informal caregiver assumes responsibility for identifying health issues, contacting the healthcare provider about health issues, and communicating about health issues, as well as coordinating healthcare services for the care recipient (Sadak, Souza et al., 2015).

Many caregivers may assume these responsibilities gradually, providing time to learn best practices. Some, however, assume extensive responsibility for caregiving abruptly, such as at the time of hospital discharge of a family member, and may have little time to prepare for these responsibilities.

CAREGIVER BURDEN

Caregiver burden has been described in multiple ways, but common to most definitions is the realization that burden is multidimensional. Some differentiate objective indicators of burden, such as the hours devoted to caregiving or the tasks performed, from subjective experiences of burden, such as the impact caregiving has on one's quality of life. Others focus on the perception of burden or strain. Emotional distress may serve as an important indicator of strain or burden, revealing the meaning of the experience to the caregiver. Strain is often expressed as a conflict between two sets of role obligations, such as caregiver–employee, caregiver–parent, caregiver–spouse, and caregiver–friend conflicts. Interventions can be directed at reducing the level of strain or burden as well as reducing the impact of strain or burden on health outcomes (Schumacher et al., 2007).

More dementia caregivers were classified as having a high level of burden than caregivers of people without dementia (46% vs. 38%) based on the AARP Public Policy Institute & the NAC (2015) survey's Burden of Care Index, and 59% of family caregivers of people with Alzheimer disease (AD) or other dementias rated the emotional stress of caregiving as high or very high. Approximately 30% to 40% of family caregivers of people with dementia suffer from depression, compared with 5% to 17% of noncaregivers of similar ages (Alzheimer's Association, 2020).

As it relates to caregiving in the community, with and without dementia, Kasper et al. (2015) found caregiving is most intense for older adults with dementia in community settings and from caregivers who are spouses or daughters or who live with the care recipient. This intensity of caring that daughters experience as they care for their parent in the home has long-term effects on them. Figure 18.2 depicts these effects as found by DiLeone (2021).

HEALTH EFFECTS OF CAREGIVING

Caregiving for family members with dementia and other health problems has been associated with caregivers' chronic physical and mental health problems in some studies, particularly when the caregiving is perceived as stressful (Buyck et al., 2011; Fredman et al., 2010; Goode et al., 1998; Gouin et al., 2012; Lovell & Wetherell, 2011; Pearlin et al., 1990; Pinquart & Sorensen, 2003; Roth et al., 2009; Schulz et al., 1997; Vitaliano et al., 2003). Based on these findings, one might anticipate that caregiving would be associated with poor health of caregivers (Ho et al., 2009). In contrast, some studies have revealed the benefits of caregiving for physical health, cognition, and mortality (Bertrand et al., 2012; Brown et al., 2009; Fredman et al., 2008, 2009; O'Reilly et al., 2008; Roth et al., 2013). Caregivers may be more physically robust as a prerequisite for becoming caregivers, especially if they

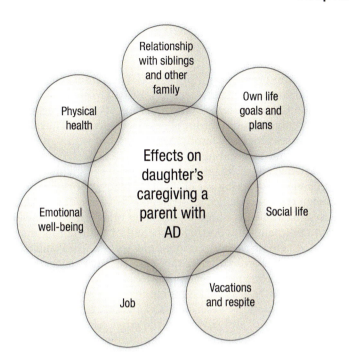

FIGURE 18.2 The combined effects on daughter's caregiving a parent with Alzheimer disease.
Source: Adapted from DiLeone, C. (2021). Experiences of daughters caring for a parent with Alzheimer's disease living at home. Research in Gerontological Nursing, *14(4), 191–199. https://doi .org/10.3928/19404921-20210428-02*

must spend many hours giving care. In addition, the effects of caregiving-related physical activities may build capacity for physical function (Chappell & Reid, 2002; Fredman et al., 2006; Rosso et al., 2015) and mental health (Gruenewald et al., 2007; Kim et al., 2007). Conversely, those whose health worsens may end their caregiving commitments (McCann et al., 2004). The "healthy caregiver hypothesis" asserts that not only would healthier adults be more likely to take on caregiving and to remain in that role, but also that the activities of caregiving would promote their health (Fredman et al., 2015).

A recently reported set of analyses from the longitudinal Women's Health Initiative study of 5,600 women age 65 years and older revealed that there was no difference in the changes observed in grip strength, walking speed, or number of chair stands among older women who were caregivers compared with noncaregivers over a 6-year period but that women who engaged in low-level caregiving, compared with those who did not, had greater grip strength at the first observation (Rosso et al., 2015). Sorting out the effects of caregiving on health versus the influence of the burden of existing chronic disease at the time that older women become caregivers is complex, but the propensity for high-frequency caregivers to have more chronic disease burden at the outset of caregiving, instead of the caregiving demands, may be responsible for higher disease rates observed among these caregivers (Pinquart & Sorensen, 2003). Also, in some studies, women who elected to provide high-frequency caregiving were healthier than those who were noncaregivers or low-frequency caregivers, and this bias toward caregivers being healthier at the

outset may be responsible for their continued health during the time they are caregivers. In addition, study results related to the type of caregiving demands will be important in future research. Based on research that investigated caregiver stress, caregivers with greater burden experienced worse physical and mental health and quality of life (Dias, et al., 2015). Understanding caregiver strain or stress and its effects on health may require more careful analysis of the nature of the caregiving activities, such as caregiving for someone with dementia versus someone without dementia. Likewise, understanding the influence of the frequency of caregiving or hours spent in caregiving versus the actual demands of the caregiving situation will be important for future research. Based on findings from the Women's Health Initiative study, Rosso et al. (2015) concluded that caregiving may not have universally negative consequences for caregivers. Indeed, Roth et al. (2015) reexamined the impact of caregiving on mortality risk, confirming that caregivers experience significantly reduced mortality rates compared with noncaregiving counterparts.

Fredman et al. (2015) investigated the relationship between caregiving and mortality, considering the transitions that caregivers make in and out of their roles as well as caregiving intensity. Caregivers were older women with an average age of 81 years who provided care for a spouse or another care recipient who required care because of dementia, frailty or health decline, stroke, or other health problems or who was recovering from fracture or surgery. Caregivers provided assistance with an average of 1.5 ADL and 3.9 IADL tasks, and 38% had been in the role for more than 5 years. Compared with noncaregivers, caregivers experienced a more pronounced reduction in mortality rate that diminished over time. Caregiving stopped because of the death of the care recipient, transfer of the care recipient to a long-term care facility, move of the care recipient to live with other caregivers, improvement of care recipient's health, or a decline in the caregiver's health. In this same population, an investigation of the effects of caregiving intensity on perceived stress revealed that high-intensity caregivers (those who provided more assistance with ADLs and IADLs) reported the highest levels of stress. Women who assumed caregiving responsibility over the course of the study and those whose levels of caregiving intensity increased both had increasing stress levels (Lyons, Cauley et al., 2015).

Factors that influence the intensity and stress of caregiving may include challenges related to the types of assistance provided, as well as the types of health problems experienced by the care recipients. These may differ when caring for persons with dementia, life-threatening and chronic health problems, end-of-life (EOL) care needs, and care according to the age of the care recipient (e.g., caregiving for one's child vs. one's parent).

Positive Consequences of Caregiving

Among the benefits of caregiving was a sense of meaning attributable to caregivers' relationships with the caregiving recipient and their contributions as caregivers to a sense of purpose in life. Opportunities for generativity are linked to theories about aging and human development (e.g., Erickson's description of generativity as central to late-life development). In addition, there may be personal growth related to learning new information and ways of functioning in response to caregiving challenges.

Well-being refers to people's experience of feeling well or positive, as assessed with measures of positive mood, and their evaluations of their lives, as estimated by ratings of the quality of their lives. In addition, eudemonic well-being, as reflected in purpose in life and personal growth, is a commonly used indicator of well-being. Chappell and Reid (2002) assessed the effects of the care recipient's cognitive status, needs for assistance with ADLs, and behavioral problems as they affected caregivers' well-being and estimates of burden. A majority of caregivers and caregiving recipients were women: The average age of caregivers was 51 years (range, 21–85 years), and for caregiving recipients, the average age was 80 years (range, 65–99 years). Caregivers' well-being was positively related to perceived social support and self-esteem but negatively related to the burden of caregiving and informal hours of care. In contrast to well-being, burden was positively related to the provision of more informal hours of care, lower frequency of getting a break, caregiving recipient behavioral problems, and lower self-esteem (Chappell & Reid, 2002). The care recipient's cognitive status and ADL needs were both related to the use of formal services, although neither of these factors directly affected caregiver burden or well-being.

Habermann et al.'s (2013) qualitative descriptive approach was used to analyze semistructured interviews conducted with 34 adult children providing care for a parent with either Parkinson disease (PD) or AD. As part of a larger randomized clinical trial, the authors explored only the positive effects of caregiving. Eighty-two percent of participants were adult daughters. Themes such as spending and enjoying time together, appreciating each other and becoming closer, and giving back care were found. These themes illustrate the various ways (e.g., time, appreciation, and giving back) through which relationships between adult children and their parents are strengthened during the caregiving process and the benefits that adult children derive from providing care to their parents during their illness. In addition, these themes underscore the underlying quality and nature of the relationship between the adult child and the parent with AD or PD, and they suggest the history of the relationship between the adult child and their parent prior to their impairment may partially determine the quality of the current caregiving experiences. A small number of caregivers (*n* = 6) could not identify positive experiences and described their situations as "doing what needs to be done" (Habermann et al., 2013, p. 186). They were often motivated to continue as a caregiver to avoid nursing home placement of their parent. Their narratives centered heavily on the difficulties, often identifying multiple difficulties. They found the caregiving to be "every minute of the day" (Habermann et al., 2013, p. 186) and often spoke of feeling all alone. These caregivers, despite interviewers' probing, could not express satisfying experiences or any joy in caregiving. Narrative regarding the parent and adult child's relationship was lacking. Caregivers who had positive experiences in caregiving expressed fewer feelings of being overwhelmed or distressed by their situation.

Risk for Health Problems Among Caregivers

Those who provide both professional and informal caregiving warrant special consideration. Ward-Griffin et al. (2015) studied Canadian nurses who were negotiating professional family care boundaries (double-duty caregivers). They found that nurses providing family care were faced with striving for balance and responding to familial care expectations. They experienced both "reaping the benefits of caregiving" as well as caregiving "taking a toll." Nurses who were double-duty caregivers used multiple strategies to strive for balance: assessing the care situation, advising others about illnesses and treatments, advocating on behalf of their family member, collaborating and cooperating with unpaid and paid caregivers, coordinating family care through delegation to others, and consulting when they needed further knowledge or expertise. Nurses who were family caregivers experienced different situations described as "making it work," "working to manage," and "living on the edge" as they negotiated professional and familial care boundaries. The investigators recommend that the health of nurses and other health professionals who are caregivers for relatives may be at risk if the blurring of professional and family boundaries is not acknowledged. Furthermore, failure to provide adequate resources supporting double-duty caregivers may result in fewer human resources in healthcare, as some nurses may be lost to practice. Recommendations for policy can be found in Supporting Double-Duty Caregivers: A Policy Brief (www .uwo.ca/nursing/cwg/docs/PolicyBrieffinal.pdf).

ASSESSMENT AND INTERVENTIONS FOR CAREGIVERS: CONTEMPORARY EVIDENCE

Assessment of Caregivers' Health and Fitness with Caregiving Demands

Clinicians can provide useful information, emotional support, and coaching to women who are considering assuming the role of a caregiver. An assessment of the caregiver's general health includes an age-appropriate history and physical examination of general health. In addition, advanced practice clinicians can use these tools to appraise the potential demands of caregiving and the caregiver's health status as a basis for planning interventions.

The Caregiver Mastery Scale asks caregivers to rate overload, relational deprivation, economic strains, role captivity, loss of self, caregiving competence, and expressive support. Higher caregiver mastery was associated with a lower number of patient problem behaviors and lower caregiver depression. Gitlin and Rose (2014) assessed caregiver readiness to care for a person with dementia by using a single item that reflects caregiver understanding of behaviors as dementia related and willingness to try strategies to manage behaviors. High caregiver readiness was associated with lower caregiver depression and financial strain despite greater patient cognitive and behavioral burden.

According to DiLeone (2021) there are numerous instruments used to assess the impact of informal caregiving on the informal caregiver's life. Several studies (Gaugler et al., 2016, 2019; Koo & Vizer, 2019) aimed at supporting the caregiver. Mosquera et al. (2016) conducted a systematic review of 93 instruments that measured caregiver burden, quality of life and well-being, management and coping, emotional and mental health, psychosocial impact, and physical health and healthy habits. The authors confirmed the complexity and multidimensionality of the effects of elderly caregiving on the informal caregiver's life and explained the difficulties to assess these effects in practice. Additionally, they found caregiver burden and emotional and mental health were the most evaluated dimensions.

Sadak, Karpa et al. (2015) recently reviewed several measures assessing dementia caregiver readiness or activation. Missing from these measures was an assessment of caregiver activation focused on healthcare for the person living with dementia (Hibbard et al., 2004). They have recently developed and tested a measure for caregiver activation for healthcare, the Partnering for Better Health–Living With Chronic Illness: Dementia. This 32-item measure reflects seven domains, covering the ability to (a) recognize and anticipate the day-to-day symptoms and challenges with multiple dimensions of patient health; (b) manage sudden changes in the dimensions of the patient's health, engage health services, and practice self-care; (c) manage the patient's medications; (d) manage day-to-day symptoms and challenges with the patient's health; (e) understand basic aspects of the patient's dementia; (f) recognize sudden/worrisome changes in the dimensions of the patient's health, and (g) advocate for the patient in healthcare situations. Scores on this scale were related to the caregiver's quality-of-life ratings as well as other measures of caregiving readiness and stress.

Assessing the caregiving demands and capacity of the potential caregiver is an important basis for determining the caregiver's fit with the demands of the care process. When there is discretion in choosing to be a caregiver (often there is not), an enumeration of the kinds of activities that are required of caregivers can be a useful guide for women. Types of caregiving activities may range from providing assistance with ADLs, IADLs, and health and healthcare.

The nature of the caregiving tasks may have different effects on caregivers, and recently developed assessment tools reflect these differences. For example, the Caregiver Demands Scale for use with caregivers of people with cancer (Stetz, 1987) focuses on burden related to meals, intimate care, movement and comfort, medications and treatments, supervision, rest, and acquisition of new skills. Some have employed the Zarit Burden Interview (first designed in 1980 and modified in 2001; Bédard et al., 2001), an instrument that assesses burden related to health, psychological well-being, finances, social life, and relationship with the patient (Zarit & Zarit, 1990). Others have focused on burden related to self-esteem; lack of family supports; and impact on finances, schedule, and health (Given et al., 1992). Still others have related burden to the frequency, severity, and distress of patient symptoms. A review of caregiver measurement instruments focusing on providing care to patients with cancer illustrates the importance of using a multidimensional, valid, reliable, and clinically relevant tool for this type of assessment (Honea et al., 2008). Specific assessment approaches have been developed for caregivers of people with dementia, such as those described earlier. Most of the assessment tools have been developed for research purposes, but some authors advise that use of a brief screening tool or selected subscales of a long instrument may improve clinical applicability (Honea et al., 2008).

Evaluating who is prepared be an informal caregiver can include an assessment of the fit between the demands of caregiving and the potential caregiver's' skills, knowledge, and well-being, as well as their physical and emotional capacity. Several of the assessment tools mentioned earlier provide important dimensions to assess and have been tailored to the age and caregiving needs of care recipients. Translating these research instruments to formats useful in practice warrants the attention of researchers.

Interventions for Caregivers

Given the prevalence of informal caregiving, many interventions to support caregivers are being developed and tested. The high prevalence of dementia and its consequences for caregivers have stimulated numerous trials of interventions supporting dementia caregivers. As the population ages and the prevalence of chronic illnesses increases, the need for caregiving for older adults with multiple chronic illnesses, such as cancer and heart failure and their associated disabilities, is escalating. In addition, family members provide care for children with chronic illnesses and often provide care for family members at the EOL. Increasingly, grandparents have assumed the role of caregivers to their grandchildren. Research on how to support these diverse populations of caregivers and their unique needs for support will be critical to ensuring the well-being of caregivers and care recipients alike (McGuire et al., 2007).

According to Wennberg et al. (2015), evidence has suggested that for an intervention to be effective, it must (a) consist of multiple components, (b) be individualized and person centered (e.g., possibly by using a care service "menu" of options for each dyad or family based on their desires and needs), and (c) involve both the caregiver and care recipient, while maintaining patient dignity. In this way, caregivers would participate in therapies that are most effective for their situation, without feeling overwhelmed by a myriad of additional strategies. Table 18.1 displays common caregiver interventions according to the Alzheimer's Association (2020) and displays interventions such as counseling, respite, and support groups.

INTERVENTIONS FOR CAREGIVERS OF PEOPLE WITH DEMENTIA

Currently, more than 16 million Americans provide unpaid care for people diagnosed with AD and other dementias, and the number of people diagnosed with the disease is predicted to rise to 14 million by 2050. Although the person with the disease is the most affected, the emotional, psychological, and physical effects of caregiving are overwhelming. As estimated by the Alzheimer's Association (2020), approximately two thirds of caregivers are women; more specifically, over one third are daughters. Daughters may also be in what is

TABLE 18.1 Type and Focus of Caregiver Interventions	
TYPE	**FOCUS**
Case management	Provides assessment, information, planning, referral, care coordination, and/or advocacy for family caregivers
Psychoeducational approaches	Include a structured program that provides information about the disease, resources and services, and about how to expand skills to effectively respond to symptoms of the disease (i.e., cognitive impairment, behavioral symptoms, and care-related needs). Include lectures, discussions, and written materials and are led by professionals with specialized training.
Counseling	Aims to resolve preexisting personal problems that complicate caregiving to reduce conflicts between caregivers and care recipients and/or improve family functioning
Support groups	Are less structured than psychoeducational or psychotherapeutic interventions. Support groups provide caregivers the opportunity to share personal feelings and concerns to overcome feelings of social isolation.
Respite	Provides planned, temporary relief for the caregiver through the provision of substitute care; examples include adult day services and in-home or institutional respite for a certain number of weekly hours.
Psychotherapeutic approaches	Involve the establishment of a therapeutic relationship between the caregiver and a professional therapist (e.g., cognitive behavioral therapy for caregivers to focus on identifying and modifying beliefs related to emotional distress, developing new behaviors to deal with caregiving demands, and fostering activities that can promote caregiver well-being)
Multicomponent approaches	Are characterized by intensive support strategies that combine multiple forms of interventions, such as education, support, and respite, into a single long-term service (often provided for 12 months or more)

Source: Adapted from Alzheimer's Association. (2020). Facts and figures. https://www.alz.org/alzheimers-dementia/facts-figures

called the sandwich generation—still caring for children under age 18 while caring for their parent (Alzheimer's Association, 2020). Caring for family members with dementia produces many stressors for caregivers, beyond the care recipient's memory and behavior problems, communication challenges, interpersonal conflicts, and role strain; these can precipitate caregiver health problems, compromise well-being, and disrupt social relationships (Black et al., 2010). A recently reported analysis of the National Study of Caregiving indicated that baby boomers who were caregivers for a family member with dementia, when compared with those who were caregivers for family members with other health problems, experienced similar rates of health problems, including high blood pressure and arthritis, and did not differ in how they rated their own health. Significant differences were observed among caregivers for relatives with dementia who provided more help with daily activities, experienced a higher level of caregiving and social activity conflict and more interrupted sleep, and were more likely to feel depressed than caregivers for someone without dementia. Also, dementia caregivers were more likely than caregivers providing care for someone without dementia to have engaged paid help, experienced higher caregiving–work conflict, and higher caregiving–other family care (e.g., children) conflict. Outcomes of caregiving included depressed mood, which was increased by caregiving/social activity conflict but lessened by having a higher level of informal support. Caregiving–other family care conflicts were negatively related to how dementia caregivers rated their own health. Being married offset the effects of dementia caregiving on general health. Caregivers for family members without dementia who reported greater levels of interrupted sleep, caregiving–family activity conflict, caregiving–social activity conflict, and less informal support were

likely to perceive their own health as poor. Those with more formal education reported lower levels of depressed mood and better perceived health (Moon & Dilworth-Anderson, 2015).

A variety of interventions for informal caregivers has been evaluated, with several Cochrane Reviews available summarizing evidence for their effectiveness. Among these are educational interventions, functional analysis-based interventions for challenging behaviors, cognitive reframing for caregivers, and respite care, among others. Educational interventions for caregivers of people with dementia living in the community include teaching skills for dementia caregiving, such as communication skills, coping and management strategies, information about dementia, and availability of support services. A review of seven trials revealed that educational interventions moderately reduced caregiver burden (Jensen et al., 2015), but in a smaller number of studies, there was a small effect on depression but no effect on the number of transitions of care recipients with dementia to long-term care was observed. Effects of educational interventions on quality of life of the caregiver could not be estimated from the existing studies (Jensen et al., 2015).

Psychosocial interventions for caregivers of people with dementia often are multicomponent, are tailored to the caregivers and persons with dementia, and have multiple mechanisms of action. Cognitive reframing is an important element of cognitive behavioral therapy (CBT) interventions, often used to reduce stress, depression, and anxiety. In dementia care, cognitive reframing interventions may focus on changing caregivers' beliefs about their care recipient's behaviors and their own performance as caregivers that are maladaptive, self-defeating, or distressing. A Cochrane Review of effects of cognitive reframing interventions for family caregivers of people with dementia examined effects on caregiver stress and mental health (Vermooji-Dassen et al., 2011). Results indicated a beneficial effect of these interventions on caregiver anxiety, depression, and subjective stress, but no effects were seen on caregiver coping, appraisal of the burden of caregiving, reactions to the behaviors of the person with dementia, or institutionalization of the person with dementia (Vermooji-Dassen et al., 2011).

Often, interventions focused on helping caregivers manage the challenging behaviors of the person with dementia promote caregiver well-being. A study examined the effects of behavioral activation for dementia caregivers that involved scheduling pleasant events and enhancing communications. Behavioral activation and psychoeducational interventions provided more than eight biweekly sessions that led to increased relationship satisfaction and decreased depressed mood for dementia caregivers when compared with the effects of the psychoeducational intervention (Au et al., 2015).

A Cochrane Review of studies of functional analysis-based interventions for challenging behavior in dementia examined the effects of approaches that explore the meaning or purpose of an individual's behavior, extending the activator–behavior–consequences (ABC) approach of behavioral analysis to allow for more than a single explanatory hypothesis for the person's behavior (Moniz et al., 2012). Often, these interventions are taught to caregivers to manage agitation and aggression. Typically, a therapist develops and evaluates strategies that aid family and staff caregivers to reduce a person's distress and associated challenging behaviors. Analysis of trials that were conducted predominantly in family care settings revealed that functional analysis was one of many components of the care program. Overall, these types of interventions tended to reduce the frequency of challenging behaviors and improve the caregiver reaction, but not their experience of burden or depression. The effects were short lived in these studies (Moniz et al., 2012).

A well-established program of research incorporating functional analysis approaches is the STAR-C program, which has been translated recently for use in community-based settings. Teri et al. (2012) used the ABC approach to behavioral analysis, engaging caregivers in identifying the ABC relationships as a basis for generating problem-solving strategies. The STAR-C program exposes family members to dementia education, effective communication, and implementation of pleasant activities to reduce mood and behavioral disturbances. Strategies to improve their own well-being and reduce adverse reactions to challenging behaviors also are provided in eight weekly sessions in the care recipient's home with four monthly phone calls. In translating the program to a community-based setting, Teri et al. (2012) reduced the intervention to eight weekly sessions. Outcomes included reduction in caregiver depression, burden, and reactivity to care recipients' behavior problems, the latter of which was maintained across 6 months. Reductions in depression and better quality of life were important outcomes for care recipients. Caregivers expressed high satisfaction with STAR-C.

Interventions specifically focused on the caregiver often include stress management strategies. Lewis et al. (2009) developed and trialed a stress-busting program (SBP) for caregivers who were providing care for a family member with dementia. The SBP included education, stress management, problem-solving, and support delivered in a group setting over 9 weeks. Caregivers experienced improvements in general health, vitality, social function, and mental health and decreases in anxiety, anger/hostility, depression, perceived stress, and caregiver burden. Investigators concluded that when weighed with the potential cost of increased use of acute care and institutionalization of the care recipient, the program was a cost-effective health-promotion strategy for caregivers who manage substantial ongoing stress (Lewis et al., 2009).

Interventions to promote self-care among caregivers have focused on promoting caregiver physical activity and sleep. McCurry et al. (2009) found that caregivers for persons with dementia who reported sleep problems at the beginning of a longitudinal study had worse scores on caregiver burden, memory, and measures of quality of life. In addition, sleep quality was reduced by caregiver depression as well as care recipient characteristics, such as amount of assistance needed with ADLs. McCurry et al. (2009) studied the effects of standard sleep hygiene, stimulus control, and sleep-compression (limiting time in bed for sleep) strategies, plus education about community resources, stress management, and ABC training to reduce disruptive behaviors. Caregivers' sleep improved immediately after treatment and at 3 months after treatment. King et al. (2002) also studied ways to promote caregiver sleep, comparing a moderate-intensity exercise intervention with a nutrition education attention control condition. Caregivers exercised (walking) for four 30- to 40-minute periods weekly for 1 year. Those who exercised experienced improved sleep and lower systolic blood pressure at the end of the year.

Another important option for some caregivers is the use of respite care, an intervention designed to provide relief to caregivers. A Cochrane Review of intervention studies indicated that there was no difference between the use and the nonuse of respite care in several outcomes, including rates of institutionalization of the person with dementia and caregiver burden. There were few studies available to evaluate, so further evidence is needed about the effects of respite care on caregivers and care recipients, including consideration of the type, duration, and nature of respite services (Maayan et al., 2014).

As indicated earlier, many intervention programs for caregivers of people with dementia incorporate multiple components that reflect the multiple complex needs of both persons in the dyad. Education, emotional support, social network enhancement, and interventions to change the care recipient's behaviors are commonly directed at enhancing caregiver coping efforts and well-being. In some approaches, they are combined with more complex behavioral strategies, such as incorporated in functional analysis approaches of the care recipient's behavior.

Multicomponent interventions present challenges for translation beyond research projects to practice arenas, such as clinical and social service agencies. Gitlin et al. (2015) estimate that more than 200 caregiver interventions have been reviewed from 1966 to 2013, but few have been translated into practice. Some of the treatment modalities in the programs that have been evaluated include professional and informal support, psychoeducational interventions, behavior management/skills training, counseling/psychotherapy, self-care/relaxation techniques, and environmental redesign. In addition, care management, specific disease education, skills to manage dependencies in functional ADLs, strategies specific to managing behavioral symptoms, and activities to effectively engage patients have been evaluated. Gitlin et al. (2010, 2015) assert that meaningful benefits to caregivers are often unclear in these studies and that long-term effectiveness, cost-effectiveness, and populations for whom the interventions are most effective remain undefined. Moreover, development and testing of the interventions most often occurs outside the traditional care systems used for people with dementia. Thus, translation of research is of high priority to make programs accessible. Programs that have been evaluated in translational studies include the Skills Care Intervention (Gitlin, Jacobs, & Earland, 2010) that led to the improvement in caregiver knowledge and skills, including their ability to understand memory loss and ways to engage the care recipient; confidence managing behaviors of the care recipient; and self-care. The Resources for Enhancing Alzheimer's Caregiver Health (REACH) program (Nichols et al., 2011) and a version translated by the Veterans Affairs (REACH-VA; Easom et al., 2013) improved caregiver burden, depression, impact of depression in everyday life, and frustration, health, and confidence in caregiving skills. The Reducing Disability in AD (RDAD; Menne et al., 2014; Teri et al., 2012) and STAR-C (McCurry et al., 2017) programs led to improvements in caregiver strains and reduction of unmet caregiver needs.

Considering all the interventions that have been translated for care systems or communities, Gitlin et al. (2015) concluded that most have improved caregiver outcomes. Among these outcomes are caregivers' competence, confidence, knowledge, skills, social support, tangible assistance, reaction to care recipient behaviors, caregiver strain, improvement of care recipient activity, positive aspects of caregiving, depression, and self-care. The availability of interventions such as these through community organizations, such as the Alzheimer's Association, Area Agencies on Aging, and others can be a significant resource for caregivers.

Caregiver interventions have been delivered using a variety of media, with many intensive interventions delivered by a professional in the home. Given the difficulty some caregivers experience in arranging respite care for the care recipient, use of approaches that do not require caregivers to leave the home is potentially valuable. An increasing interest in the use of internet-based interventions for caregivers of people with dementia is evident. The internet intervention Mastery Over Dementia (MOD; Blom et al., 2015) was evaluated recently in comparison with minimal intervention consisting of e-bulletins. MOD is an innovative guided self-help internet course designed to reduce caregivers' symptoms of depression and anxiety. MOD was developed using findings from reviews that identified effective face-to-face interventions to diminish caregivers' mental health symptoms, including psychoeducation and active participation of the caregiver, management of behavioral problems, coping strategies, cognitive behavior therapy that included cognitive reframing, and an increase in social support. MOD involved caregivers

in eight lessons and a booster session with guidance from a coach, who monitored progress and evaluated homework. The course topics included coping with behavioral problems by solving problems, relaxing, arranging help from others, changing nonhelping thoughts (cognitive restructuring), and communicating with others (assertiveness training). The e-bulletins were provided to the comparison group over a 6-month period. Topics included driving, holiday breaks, medication, legal affairs, activities throughout the day, help with daily routines, safety measures in the home, and possibilities for peer support, but there was no contact with a coach. Effects on depression and anxiety were significantly greater for the internet course than for the e-bulletins alone.

INTERVENTIONS FOR CAREGIVERS OF PEOPLE WITH CANCER

The caregiving trajectory in the cancer population tends to be nonlinear. It is often characterized by the rapidity with which caregivers have to take on the role as treatment decisions are made and treatment begins. As the cancer experience unfolds, caregiving transitions may occur in rapid succession, each having its own learning curve in movement from one treatment modality to the next (e.g., from postoperative recovery at home to beginning radiation or chemotherapy). Transitions among care settings also occur unpredictably. For example, transitions from home to ED to hospital are unpredictable but not uncommon. Moreover, the functional abilities of older adults with cancer may fluctuate rapidly, resulting in intense but short periods of caregiving. Rapid transitions in the caregiving role may occur in the context of advanced cancer as well, as the care recipient moves from management of advanced cancer symptoms (e.g., pain, sleep disturbance, and lack of appetite) through a succession of changes in functional status and self-care ability, leading ultimately to EOL care and bereavement. The rapid succession of caregiving transitions, some of which may occur with little warning, challenge caregivers' ability to provide care, as ability during one phase of the caregiving trajectory may or may not be sufficient to meet the demands of the next phase (Schulz et al., 2016).

Psychoeducational interventions include structured programs of information for caregivers that include teaching about the person's disease process, symptom management, psychosocial issues, caregiving resources, coordination of services, and caregiver self-care. These interventions are offered in group formats and may include lectures by people trained to deliver the intervention, opportunity for discussion with other caregivers, and often, written materials for reference. Support may also be part of these interventions.

Supportive interventions focus on building rapport with caregivers and creating opportunities for discussing difficult caregiving issues, successes, and feelings regarding caregiving. Mutual support, among caregivers includes not only emotional support, but also instrumental support such as strategies for caregiving and problem-solving opportunities.

Psychotherapy is another option for caregivers and typically involves individual counseling with a professional related to strategies for managing distress. This service may be particularly valuable for caregivers who have a past conflicted relationship with the care recipient, such as a history of abuse. Cognitive behavioral strategies engage caregivers in learning self-monitoring, addressing negative thoughts and assumptions, promoting problem-solving, and encouraging engagement in pleasant experiences.

Caregiving work often includes physical work, and some therapies focus on the caregiver's body. Therapeutic massage uses manipulation of soft tissues to induce relaxation. Healing touch involves noninvasive approaches that use hands to balance human energy fields. Respite care provides services inside or outside the home and may include assistance with ADLs or skilled care with the aim of giving the caregiver time away from caregiving.

An Oncology Nursing Society Putting Evidence Into Practice (PEP) project team concluded that no single intervention could be recommended for nursing practice for caregiver strain or burden based on studies published before their review (up to 2006). Interventions likely to be effective included psychoeducational, psychotherapy, and supportive programs (Honea et al., 2008).

According to Northouse et al. (2010), types of interventions for family caregivers of people with cancer indicated that several have efficacy on different caregiver outcomes. Types of interventions included psychoeducational support, skills training, and therapeutic counseling, with some including multiple components. In addition, some trials included content for caregivers that addressed the caregivers' own needs for self-care as well as those of the care recipient. Caregiver outcomes examined included three domains: illness appraisal, coping resources, and quality of life. Interventions in the illness appraisal domain addressed appraisal of caregiving burden, caregiving benefit, and information needs. Small effects of interventions on caregiving burden and caregiving benefit were noted, but large and significant effects of interventions on caregivers' appraisal of their information needs were evident. Interventions in the coping resources domain addressed enhancing active coping strategies, such as problem-solving and/or reducing ineffective coping. Persistent moderate effects were evident. In addition, interventions in the coping resources domain focused on increasing self-efficacy, including ability to manage symptoms and provide care, and had small but persistent effects. Interventions in the quality-of-life domain focused on enhancing physical functioning by promoting performance of caregivers' self-care behaviors, such as increasing exercise and improving sleep. These had small but persistent effects. Other quality-of-life interventions that focused on reducing distress and anxiety had small but persistent effects beyond 6 months after intervention. In contrast, interventions did not reduce caregivers' depression. Interventions focused on promoting marital or sexual satisfaction, family support, and couple communication had small, immediate effects, but these did not persist beyond the first few months after intervention. Interventions that focused on social functioning of caregivers led to delayed effects with family members, friends, and peers that did not occur until after 6 months after the intervention (Northouse et al., 2010).

Most of the interventions reviewed by Northouse et al. (2010) were delivered jointly or separately to patients and family. Taken together, the results of the studies indicated that multiple outcomes were affected by the interventions, most of which were multidimensional. The timing of different effects varied, likely influenced by the time necessary for caregivers to make changes in order to achieve caregiver benefits, such as those focused on improvement in physical or social function. Sustained effects for some interventions included changes in coping strategies, sense of self-efficacy, and distress/anxiety outcomes. Large effects were observed for increases in knowledge. Limited translation of these interventions to practice settings was noted (Northouse et al., 2010).

Since the *Oncology Nursing Society Review* was published in 2008, an array of new interventions has been studied for caregivers. Modes of delivery of interventions for caregivers are variable and include in-person individual and group formats, telephonic intervention, online interventions, and interactive health communication technologies (IHCTs) that make use of internet 2.0/social media types of applications. The emerging use of technology in providing support to caregivers is providing access to an array of new interventions.

IHCTs are being used to deliver psychosocial interventions to couples and families. Badr et al. (2015) found evidence from a systematic review that incorporating IHCTs in psychosocial interventions with cancer patients and their caregivers was feasible and, in some, effective. Of note is the Comprehensive Health Enhancement Support System (CHESS), an extensively studied IHCT with information, support, and coaching components that together facilitate decision-making and communication with caregivers (Gustafson et al., 2013). Of the multiple features to provide tailored cancer information are "Ask an Expert," recent news, and resource guide. Support is provided through facilitated bulletin boards, written and video accounts of how other patients and families cope, and interactive tools, including decision-making support, action planning, skills building for easing distress, and journaling. Clinicians are able to receive a report of the patient's health status and questions for the next visit from either the patient or the caregiver. The version of CHESS for lung cancer (CHESS-LC) patients and their caregivers was successful in reducing caregiver burden and negative mood after 6 months use when compared with internet-only interventions (DuBenske et al., 2014).

CHESS exemplifies an IHCT in a comprehensive interactive system. In addition IHCTs are being developed and tested to facilitate treatment decision-making, enhance patient–caregiver communication, and promote lifestyle behavior change (Badr et al., 2015). Nonetheless, of all the caregiver interventions reviewed for cancer care, the multicomponent interventions were rated as most likely to be effective because they use a variety of techniques to reduce burden and thus are able to address a variety of needs (Honea et al., 2008).

INTERVENTIONS FOR CAREGIVERS OF PEOPLE WITH CHRONIC ILLNESSES

Caregiver interventions for those providing care for people who have experienced a chronic illness with consequent disability, such as stroke or congestive heart failure, have also been developed and tested. With the aging of the population and anticipated increased prevalence of complex chronic illnesses requiring caregiver support, these programs will increase in importance.

For stroke caregivers, the trajectory may begin with sudden intensity, gradually decrease as the older adult regains function, and then remain relatively stable over a long period of time (perhaps punctuated by short-term acute illnesses or setbacks). Alternatively, caregiving may gradually increase with stroke complications, recurrence, or new comorbid conditions. Transitions in the caregiving trajectory may be planned, as in the transitions from hospital to skilled rehabilitation facility to home, or they may be unplanned, as in an ED visit and rehospitalization (McLennon et al., 2014). Stroke often leads to severe and long-term disability for survivors and presents family caregivers with significant challenges. Family caregivers often experience stress, challenges related to rehabilitation, and health concerns for themselves, as well as depression. Recognizing the risk of depression for stroke caregivers as well as stroke survivors, McLennon et al. (2014) investigated perceived task difficulty and life changes among stroke caregivers who experienced mild to moderate depressive symptoms shortly after discharge of the care recipient who had survived stroke. Caregivers with more depressive symptoms reported more difficulty performing tasks and worse life changes. In addition, the gender of the caregivers (female) and their number of chronic illnesses, as well as the effects of survivor mobility and thinking, were associated with depressive symptoms. Among the most difficult tasks were arranging care while away, providing personal care and emotional support, watching and monitoring the stroke survivor, talking with healthcare providers, assisting with walking, coordinating care, and providing transportation (McLennon et al., 2014).

Despite challenges associated with providing care to stroke survivors, stroke caregivers reported positive aspects of their roles, as revealed by a 2012 systematic review; Mackenzie and Greenwood (2012) found that perceptions of improvements in the survivor's physical condition, including being able to prevent deterioration and seeing the care recipient being well cared for, were sources of positive experiences. In addition, progress or recovery indicators were sources of pride and satisfaction. Strengthened relationships, feelings of love, and other positive emotions were seen as positive dimensions of caregiving, as was feeling appreciated by the care recipient and the community. These experiences were described as giving meaning to life and reciprocation for past caring. Identifying what was important in life as well as learning new skills and ways of managing difficulties were associated with caregivers' self-esteem and perceptions of strength and mastery. Seeing more positive aspects of caregiving increased over time as caregivers gained more experience (Mackenzie & Greenwood, 2012).

Cheng et al. (2014) conducted a meta-analysis of psychosocial interventions for stroke family and examined effects of psychoeducation and social support groups on caregiver burden, caregiving competency, depression, anxiety, social support, family functioning, physical health, quality of life, satisfaction with the intervention, and use of health services. Limited numbers of studies precluded clear conclusions, but the effects of psychoeducation that focused on improving caregivers' family functioning were small. Training in problem-solving and stress coping when offered by telephone may reduce depression and enhance sense of competency of caregivers, but evidence was not sufficient to recommend this approach. Nonetheless, equipping caregivers with caregiving skills was associated with the reduced use of healthcare resources for stroke survivors (Cheng et al., 2014).

A statement by the American Heart Association and American Stroke Association examined evidence for stroke family caregiver and dyad interventions (Bakas et al., 2014). Reviewing 17 caregiver intervention studies and 15 caregiver–survivor dyad interventions, investigators focused on determining whether family caregivers and dyad interventions improved stroke survivor and caregiver outcomes and the types of interventions that were most effective. Caregiver outcomes included:

- Preparedness—confidence, self-efficacy, competence, quality of care
- Burden, stress, and strain—task difficulty of care, threat appraisal, and mood
- Anxiety and depression
- Quality of life, including life changes
- Social function—social activity, family functioning
- Coping—confronting, social support, problem-solving, optimism
- Service use—healthcare visits
- Knowledge and satisfaction

Kim et al. (2020) employed the meta-ethnography methodology approach to the experiences of caregivers caring for a family member with heart failure. Living with heart failure, a debilitating disease with an unpredictable course, requires ongoing adaptation and management not only from patients but also from their families. Family caregivers have been known to be key facilitators of self-management of heart failure. The authors identified three themes: "shouldering the entire burden," "starting a new life," and "balancing caregiving and everyday life." These three themes illustrate how family caregivers fulfilled caregiving roles, what helped them juggle their multiple responsibilities, and how they struck a balance between life as caregivers and individuals in their own right.

The nature of interventions for caregivers included three main categories: skill building, psychoeducation, and support. Skill-building interventions involved processes to facilitate problem-solving, goal setting, and communication with healthcare providers; stress management; hands-on training, such as lifting and assisting with ADLs; and communication tailored to the stroke survivor's needs. Psychoeducational interventions focused on providing information such as warning signs of impending stroke, lifestyle changes, and resources, as well as managing survivor emotions, medications and personal care, finances and transportation, and the emotions and healthcare needs of the stroke survivor. Support interventions included interactions with peers for emotional support and advice, offered through support groups or online discussion forums. A combination of skill building and psychoeducational interventions resulted in positive caregiver outcomes. Psychoeducational interventions alone increased caregiver knowledge, but did not offer improvement in caregiver depression or quality of life. As with interventions for dementia and cancer caregivers, multicomponent approaches appear to be most effective. In addition, offering interventions, both in person as well as via telephone, was associated with more positive effects than either alone, but further investigation is needed of the mode by which the intervention is offered, including the use of internet-based approaches for this population. Information alone cannot address the complex needs of caregivers (Rodriguez-Gonzalo et al., 2015).

Recommendations with the strongest level of evidence based on this review include interventions with these elements:

- Combining skill building (e.g., problem-solving, stress management) with psychoeducational strategies versus interventions with only psychoeducational strategies
- Tailoring or individualizing to the needs of stroke caregivers versus using nontailored approaches
- Delivering information face to face and/or by telephone (Forster et al., 2012)
- Consisting of five to nine sessions

With the growing prevalence of heart failure among older adults, there is an increasing emphasis on interventions for caregivers who are assuming responsibility for their care (Stamp et al., 2015). Investigators have studied the experiences of spouses or partners of people living with advanced heart failure, learning that spouses with higher levels of perceived control had greater levels of well-being and that older spouses enjoyed greater levels of well-being than younger ones. Dracup et al. (2004) recommended that interventions, including information and counseling directed toward enhancing the spouse caregiver's level of control, would be advantageous.

Sullivan et al. (2015) identified three areas of needs among family caregivers of people with heart failure: competence, compassion, and care of the self. Competence concerns included those related to the ability to perform caregiving tasks safely. Caregivers expressed worry about doing things right, making a serious mistake, and being uncertain about their ability to be a family caregiver. Their descriptions of their concerns included worry about harming the person with heart failure (e.g., giving the wrong medications). They also described vigilance behaviors, such as monitoring activity and dietary restriction, regulating patients' activities, preventing activities, and engaging in anticipatory helping behaviors. In addition, caregivers were concerned about their ability to maintain compassion and provide emotional support to the person with heart failure. A final theme, care of the self, related to caregivers' abilities to juggle multiple responsibilities, obtain personal care for themselves, and have some modicum of escape in which to maintain fitness and well-being (Sullivan et al., 2015). Confidence was an overarching consideration of caregivers in another study and was associated with quality of life in patients and social support of caregivers (Lyons, Vellone et al., 2015).

Caregiver intervention trials for heart failure are limited but have included several dimensions. A trial of integrated dyad care compared usual care with a psychoeducational intervention delivered in three modules over a 12-week period through nurse-led, face-to-face counseling, computer-based education, and other written teaching materials (Ågren et al., 2012). The modules included cognitive, sup-

port, and behavioral components, as well as teaching materials over the three sessions. These addressed topics such as the definition of heart failure, medications, symptom management, and lifestyle modification, as well as direction of care, relationships, and sexual activities. In addition, support components included patients' and partners' need for support and caregiver burden. Behavioral components included intentions, abilities, and self-efficacy related to self-care, barriers to lifestyle modification, and strategies to improve or maintain self-care behavior. There were no significant effects of the interventions on the partners of heart failure patients, but the skill-building and problem-solving education and psychosocial support was effective in enhancing patients' level of perceived control. Additional trials are needed to evaluate the impact of being a family caregiver for heart failure patients.

INTERVENTIONS FOR CAREGIVERS OF CHILDREN WITH CHRONIC ILLNESSES

Parent caregivers of children with chronic and acute illness experience unique sets of challenges as they integrate the roles of parent and caregiver. A review of studies on caregivers of children with chronic illness indicated that they report significantly greater parenting stress than do caregivers of healthy children (Cousino & Hazen, 2013). Greater general parenting stress was related to greater parental responsibility for treatment management but was not related to illness duration and severity across illness populations (Cousino & Hazen, 2013).

In an integrative review of nursing research about parenting children with complex chronic conditions (CCCs) spanning 2002 to 2012, Rehm (2013) identified a wide array of impacts of providing care for children with CCCs in the home. Among these were emotional impacts (stress, worry, fear, anxiety, and feelings of being overwhelmed, including depression symptoms) and positive impacts (rewards of parenting a child with a CCC, commitment to the child and role in providing care, pride, empowerment, and personal growth in achievements as caregivers, increased empathy for others, and increased closeness to family members). In addition, Rehm identified parental role challenges that included facing conflict between the role as a parent and as a caregiver, difficulty in switching from the affectionate parent to the technical/procedural caregiver, legal barriers to decision-making for foster parents, and inadequate preparation for care provision. Family members also reported challenges related to working with healthcare providers that for some, included changes in their home life when professional providers were always present; constrained communication, affection, privacy, and discipline in the presence of the professional caregivers; negotiations to clarify parental roles versus nursing roles; and lack of clarity of roles for parents and nurses when the child was hospitalized. Another set of themes in this literature was efforts at normalizing family life that were parental efforts to emphasize the normal aspects of life when complete normalization was not possible because of ongoing demands, the intrusiveness of equipment, and stigma. The impact on social relationships and activities families reported included isolation when parents were unable to leave home because of care demands, difficulty arranging child care or respite care because of the child's complex care needs, stigmatizing aspects of the child's condition, constrained interactions with family and friends, and excursions from home requiring extensive planning and needs for equipment for providing ongoing care. This body of literature also revealed moral implications associated with parenting children with CCCs. Rehm identified parents' concerns about the unfairness of their situations, lack of viable alternatives to home care for children with CCCs, parents' unwillingness to live without their child, and shifts of responsibility and expenses to families from the healthcare system and society. This extensive review underscores the challenges that face parents who are simultaneously caregivers for children with CCCs.

Kieckhefer et al. (2014) developed and evaluated the Building Family Strengths Program, an educational program provided in the context of a social and supportive environment of parents and facilitators, for parents of children with a variety of chronic health conditions whose children ranged in age from 2 to 11 years. Parents were exposed to seven sessions of a curriculum derived from the Chronic Disease Self-Management Program produced by the Stanford Patient Education Research Center that included an array of topics: impact of living with a childhood chronic illness; emotional dimensions of parenting a child with chronic illness; impact of chronic illness on the child; impact on relationships and family communication; impact on parenting; work with large systems and discovery of resources; skills for effective partnering and shared decision-making within the family; and transitions, finding meaning and approaching the future with confidence. These topics were explored using a variety of facilitation techniques, among these brief presentations by cofacilitators related to knowledge, topically structured parent discussions, facilitated peer exchange information and insights, modeling by the cofacilitators providing examples of newly learned skills, and parent development of weekly individualized action plans promoting their practice of the new skills. The intent of these approaches was to honor and encourage the unique support that parents could offer to one another within the context of the curriculum. The processes encouraged parents to practice positive, practical coping strategies and supported them in determining how they could involve their child in developmentally appropriate ways in shared management tasks.

At baseline 56% of parents had high depressive symptoms, which improved significantly when measured 6 months after treatment. In addition, parents experienced improved self-efficacy to manage their child's condition, coping, and family quality of life. Parent–child shared management also increased, but the change was not statistically significant. Most parents completed all or all but one class (86%; Kieckhefer et al., 2014).

A Cochrane Review of psychological interventions for parents of children and adolescents with chronic illnesses, including painful conditions, cancer, diabetes mellitus, asthma, traumatic brain injury, and skin disorders, revealed a limited number of studies. The average age of children in these studies was 14.6 years. Results were analyzed according to disease and by treatment classes that included CBT, family therapy (FT), problem-solving therapy (PST), and

multisystemic therapy (MST). Parent behavior and parent mental health outcomes were assessed in relation to the types of therapies. Across all conditions PST led to improved adaptive parenting in families with children with cancer after treatment and improved parent mental health. There were no effects of CBT and limited or no data on FT or MST (Eccleston et al., 2015).

INTERVENTIONS FOR CAREGIVERS PROVIDING END-OF-LIFE CARE

The aging of populations across the globe has prompted societies to rethink EOL care, with shifting emphasis from cure to palliative care and from institution-based care to care at home, with most approaches dependent on caregiving provided by family members. Palliative care practice has stimulated research about pain and symptom management as well as support for dying individuals and families (see Grady & Gough, 2015; McGuire et al., 2012). Promoting death with dignity has guided the development of new models of care, most of which include family members, in particular, family caregivers.

Caregiver well-being is key to providing palliative/EOL (P/EOL) care at home. Williams et al. (2011) noted that efforts to promote caregiver well-being have included grief counseling, educational workshops, and group interventions to provide peer support. Individual countries have created fiscal policy to support P/EOL caregivers, including paid employment leave to care for family members in Canada (Compassionate Care Benefits [CCBs]) and provisions for unpaid leave for some employees in the United States (Family and Medical Leave Act). Caregivers providing P/EOL care face many of the same challenges as those who care for chronically ill family members, including providing for physical care needs; managing complex symptoms; organizing and coordinating care from health professionals and others; acting as a spokesperson, advocate, or proxy; and providing spiritual, emotional, and psychological support. Like other caregivers, P/EOL caregivers experience positive outcomes, as well as burden, strain, and health effects associated with caregiving. Women caregivers tend to experience more demands owing to their multiple roles and strain among them linked to caregiving demands. In addition to stressful roles and role strain, caregivers also experience financial stress, challenges related to lack of family or friendly work environments that allow flexibility and absences to provide care, and lack of available health and social services. Michaels et al. (2021) aimed to describe and explain the process of EOL caregiving as experienced by family caregivers of older adults residing in the home setting. They found family caregivers engaged in the process of "navigating a caregiving abyss" when providing and managing EOL care for older adults at home. The "caregiving abyss" consisted of four phases: (1) managing multiple roles, (2) encountering challenges, (3) mobilizing resources, and (4) acknowledging death is near. During the process family caregivers strived to "live day by day" and "maintain normalcy" to achieve the goals of honoring life's final wishes and provide home death.

Although the population receiving P/EOL care is growing, little is known about the effects of caregiving on caregiver outcomes. Hoefman et al. (2015) evaluated caregiver outcomes in palliative care, identifying both caregiver experiences of care and caregiver quality of life as important features. Caregiver experiences incorporated into a Carer Experience Scale included caregiver appraisals of the impact of P/EOL care on activities outside of caring, such as socializing, physical activity, and hobbies; support from family and friends, such as personal help in caring or emotional support; assistance from organizations and government, such as help from voluntary groups with respite and practical information; fulfillment from caregiving, such as positive feelings; control over caregiving; and a successful relationship with the care recipient, such as being able to talk and discuss issues without arguing. In addition, the investigators assessed caregiver quality of life by asking caregivers to appraise the extent to which they experienced fulfillment from carrying out care tasks, relational problems with care recipient, problems with their own mental health, problems combining care tasks with their own daily activities, financial problems related to care tasks, support with carrying out care tasks when needed, and problems with their own physical health. Higher negative effects of caregiving experiences were associated with higher negative effects on caregiver quality of life. Lower scores on both were associated with less strain from caregiving, more positive care experiences, and less process utility (reflected in ratings of happiness if all of the caregiving tasks were taken over by another person who would provide all care free of charge at his or her own house).

Of note is a research program conducted by Hudson and Aranda (2014), the Melbourne Family Support Program. Hudson and Aranda (2014) tested a program of psychoeducational interventions using four psychoeducational interventions, incorporating one-to-one and group format delivery in home and inpatient hospital/hospice settings. Outcomes included family caregivers' preparedness, competence, positive emotions, psychological well-being, and reduction in unmet needs.

Interventions to provide P/EOL caregiver peer support, individual and group counseling, psychoeducation, respite care, and home care are being studied in relation to outcomes, such as caregiver knowledge, personal renewal, community support, and health promotion and prevention of health problems of caregivers. Reduced burden in this population may be associated with efforts to provide caregivers encouragement, assistance, and emotional support, and personal health practices and coping strategies have been enhanced by teaching caregivers coping strategies and health-enhancing behaviors (Williams et al., 2011). Although limited information is available specific to caregivers of children with acute and chronic illness or EOL care, those areas of science are growing. Future research in these areas would be extremely helpful for caregivers whose focus is on children or EOL care, as targeted interventions might provide resources for information, respite care, or additional helpful ways to manage this care.

Health Policy and Caregiving

Policies supportive of family caregivers have been developed. Canada's CCBs offer full-time workers meeting criteria the option to contribute to family caregiving by providing 6 weeks of income support with a 2-week unpaid waiting period before payments begin, with payments of up to 55% of regular earnings, up to a maximum of $457 (Canadian dollars) per week. Job security is ensured for 8 weeks. These benefits can be shared between family members and the benefit can be taken consecutively or broken into shorter periods within a 26-week period. Nonetheless, an interview study of caregivers revealed that the CCB is not sustaining all informal P/EOL caregivers: Gender, income and social status, working conditions, health and social services, social support networks and personal practices, and coping strategies all influenced caregiver burden (Williams et al., 2011). In the United States, the Family and Medical Leave Act provides support for caregivers that may include their ability to return to their employment when their caregiving is completed, although it does not provide for compensation of employees during the caregiving leave. The Patient Protection and Affordable Care Act made it now possible for caregivers to receive up to 12 weeks leave through their employer. More information can be found at www.aarp.org.

Next Steps

Despite many studies of interventions developed for caregivers, the majority have addressed caregiver capacity to provide care (Table 18.2). Fewer efforts have focused on promoting caregiver well-being and health and preventing disease or injury. Missing from most intervention research are studies of the effects of financial strain and the physical challenges of caregiving for caregivers. Given the large number of older caregivers, managing symptoms and comorbidities of both the care recipient and the caregiver warrant increased attention by both researchers and policy makers.

In addition, a new area of investigation in caregiving will focus on multicultural caregiving and interventions that have been culturally tailored to specific populations of caregivers (Apesoa-Varano et al., 2015). This effort will provide important perspectives to inform support for caregivers from the diverse cultural backgrounds of North America.

CAREGIVER HEALTH

Assessment of Women Caregivers' Health

Central to clinical assessment of a caregiver's health is the consideration of the woman's age and personal and family history. In addition, prevailing literature concludes that caregivers are more likely to experience depressive symptoms and have poorer physical health outcomes compared with noncaregivers (Pinquart & Sorensen, 2003; Schulz & Sherwood, 2008; Vitaliano et al., 2003). In most studies reporting increased risk to health, the poorer health outcomes are linked to stress. However, in an analysis of health consequences of caregiving, Roth et al. (2015) noted that caregivers experience symptoms

TABLE 18.2 Summary of Interventions for Caregivers and Care Recipients

INTERVENTIONS FOCUSED ON ENHANCING CAREGIVER CAPACITY TO PROVIDE CARE	INTERVENTIONS FOCUSED ON CAREGIVER WELL-BEING AND HEALTH
• Education: increase knowledge about disease • Caregiving skills • Functional analysis of challenging behaviors (e.g., ABC) • Care coordination	• Stress management • Cognitive strategies (e.g., reframing) • Support (e.g., emotional) • Counseling, psychotherapy • Respite care • Massage
INTERVENTIONS DIRECTED AT BOTH CAREGIVER AND CARE RECIPIENT	
• Problem-solving related to needs of care recipient • Interventions promoting pleasant events • Interventions promoting physical activity • Interventions promoting sleep and regulating activity • Environmental redesign for care recipient (e.g., safety)	• Problem-solving related to caregiver challenges • Interventions promoting pleasant events • Interventions promoting physical activity • Interventions promoting caregiver sleep • Environmental redesign (e.g., ergonomics of caregiver)

ABC, activator–behavior–consequences.

of emotional distress possibly more related to watching a family member struggle with a medical condition and not to the stress of caregiving per se. Also, there is no clear evidence that caregiving presents increased risk for mortality (Roth et al., 2015), but clinicians must consider caregiver age and health status independent of caregiving tasks. Analysis of data from a national epidemiologic study that matched caregivers with noncaregivers on multiple confounders that could bias caregiving–mortality association found that caregivers had an 18% survival advantage over a 6-year period compared with the matched noncaregivers (Roth et al., 2013). Certainly there is a prevailing view, despite these more recent findings across larger population-based analyses, that informal caregiving is a stressful obligation that is hazardous to caregivers' health (Carroll, 2013).

Of note, however, spouses who provided care but reported no caregiving strain had mortality rates similar to those for spouses of nondisabled partners (Roth et al., 2015). In a large population-based study, it was found that 44% of spouse caregivers reported no strain (Schulz & Beach, 1999), and in another study, 17% of caregivers reported a lot of strain, and 33% reported no strain (Roth et al., 2009). When *stress* is defined as a relationship between the person and environment that is interpreted by the person as taxing or exceeding personal resources and endangering well-being (Lazarus & Folkman, 1984), it is understandable that caregivers who are confident that they have sufficient resources to manage caregiving situations do not feel stressed (Roth et al., 2015). Alternatively, caregivers might report high levels of stress if they have less-than-adequate information, skills, coping behaviors, help from other family members, or formal care resources.

ASSESSMENT OF PHYSICAL AND EMOTIONAL HEALTH

Because there are conflicting viewpoints on the risks associated with caregiving, clinicians must assess all aspects of a caregiving woman's physical and mental health based on age and individual circumstances. Special attention should be paid to her personal and family health history, relationship to the person receiving care, and the hours per day engaged

in caregiving. Screening must encompass cardiovascular disease and pertinent risk factors (hypertension, hypercholesterolemia, smoking, physical inactivity, overweight and obesity, diabetes), osteoporosis, cancer (breast, cervical, and colon), depression and anxiety, menopause transition and/or menstrual issues, and physical abuse by the person receiving care (Berg et al., 2015). Attention to all of these factors accommodates potential risks that may or may not be associated with informal caregiving. Moreover, an essential assessment step is to ask the caregiver if she has stress associated with caregiving as well to ask about the rewards she attributes to these activities. See Assessment and Screening of Caregivers' Health in Box 18.1.

There are a number of instruments to measure caregiver burden (Herbert et al., 2000), perceived benefits (Beach et al., 2000), caregiving self-efficacy (Steffen et al., 2002), and perceived social support (Krause, 1995; Krause & Borawski-Clark, 1995). The choice of instrument to use should be determined by the clinical setting and caregiver situation, use, and number of items because some are quite brief and others take more patient time. The assessment scale developed by Picot and Youngblut (1997) to assess external and internal rewards experienced by caregivers may be a useful tool for additional clinical assessment. On this scale, caregivers who scored high on rewards of caregiving scored lower on depression and caregiver burden. This 16-item revised scale is unidimensional and measures the positive consequences of caregiving with acceptable internal reliability consistency (0.8–0.83). Whichever instrument is selected should be intended to determine the caregiver's level of stress and coping, health-promotion practices, and resources, such as social support networks, economic resources, and care respite resources.

Health Promotion

Health promotion for women caregivers is multifaceted and ranges from living a healthy lifestyle, screening for common health conditions encountered as women age, employment, sexuality, accessing economic and respite resources,

Box 18.1 Assessment and Screening of Caregivers' Health

Physical Health

- Cardiovascular disease
  - Hypertension
  - Hypercholesterolemia
  - Smoking
  - Physical inactivity
  - Overweight and obesity
  - Diabetes
- Osteoporosis
- Cancer
  - Breast
  - Cervical
  - Colon
- Menopause transition or menstrual issues
- Physical abuse

Emotional Health

- Depression
- Anxiety
- Caregiver stress
- Caregiver rewards

Box 18.2 Elements of Caregiver Health Promotion

Healthy lifestyle

Screening for age-appropriate common physical and emotional health conditions

Employment satisfaction

Sexuality

Accessibility of economic and respite resources

Accessibility to innovative support services

Promotion of positive body image

Promotion of health self-esteem

Promotion of emotional health and well-being

Cultivation of healthy relationships

- For women with high cholesterol or triglyceride levels, take omega-3 fatty acid supplements.
- Drink alcohol in moderation; limit intake to no more than one drink per day.

Healthy lifestyle recommendations related to nutrition (Berg et al., 2015) include a diet rich in fruits, vegetables, and whole grains:

- Choose lean proteins (chicken, fish, beans, legumes).
- Eat low-fat dairy products.
- Avoid sodium (salt) and fats found in fried foods, processed foods, and baked goods.
- Eat fewer animal products that contain cheese, cream, or eggs.
- Read labels and avoid saturated fats, partially hydrogenated fats, and hydrogenated fats.

Culture influences healthy lifestyle choices. In some cultures, engaging in physical activity is not promoted, and it is therefore difficult to motivate caregivers to adopt routine physical activity in these groups of women (Im et al., 2011). Mexican American women place their own health below that of family, so engaging in positive health behaviors take the second place or even the last place (Berg et al., 2002). Hoffman et al. (2012) found that caregiving is associated with poor health behaviors that put baby boomer caregivers' health at risk in the long term. This may be attributed to caregivers' lack of social support (Ostwald, 2009), or it may be a result of caregiver burden that prevents engagement in health-promotion behaviors (Sisk, 2000).

Discussed previously, screening for physical and emotional health conditions is an important aspect of health promotion. Clinical guidelines related to cardiovascular disease and screening for risk factors (hypertension, hypercholesterolemia, smoking, physical inactivity), osteoporosis, common cancers in women (breast, cervical, colon, and lung), depression and anxiety, and menopause transition and menstrual issues are readily available. Less is understood about health promotion related to employment,

innovative support services, and promoting positive body image and healthy self-esteem. Furthermore, mental health promotion and cultivation of healthy relationships are important aspects of health promotion in women caregivers (Berg et al., 2015; see Box 18.2).

LIVING A HEALTHY LIFESTYLE

Poor lifestyle behaviors include suboptimal diet, physical inactivity, and tobacco use (Mozaffarian et al., 2012). Challenges for women caregivers' healthy lifestyle activities relate to work-related roles, economic stability, health status, and caregiving activities (Moen, 1996; Moen et al., 1992). Multiple role challenges may affect a caregiver's engagement in physical activity and dietary behaviors, which are likely to have a significant effect on their overall healthy lifestyle choices (Berg et al., 2015). Caregivers may neither consider their own health compared with that of the person they take care of nor be encouraged to maintain their own health (Beach & White, 2015). Although there are multiple definitions of maintaining a healthy lifestyle, commonalities include preventing heart disease, cancer, diabetes, and a number of chronic diseases (Berg et al., 2015). The National Library of Medicine (2015) define behaviors of a healthy lifestyle as:

- Do not smoke.
- Exercise. To lose or keep off weight, get moderate exercise for at least 60 to 90 minutes on most days; to maintain health, get at least 30 minutes of exercise per day for at least 5 days per week.
- Maintain a healthy weight, which for women is between 18.5 and 24.9 body mass index (BMI).
- Get checked for depression and treated if necessary.

sexuality, positive body image and healthy self-esteem, and healthy relationships.

EMPLOYMENT

Evidence suggests that paid employment improves the health of women who have positive attitudes toward employment (Repetti et al., 1989). This may result from social support afforded in a work setting. However, for some women, paid employment may be related to overload or multiple role strain (Repetti et al., 1989) or resultant stress. Also, there is some evidence that employment can lead to negative health behaviors, such as smoking, increased alcohol use, and more sedentary behavior (Hazuda et al., 1988). Informal caregivers often leave paid work for periods of time, work part time, or take low-paying jobs (Repetti et al., 1989), contributing to lost income, retirement, or health insurance benefits (Berg & Woods, 2009). Therefore employment-related health promotion must weigh the benefits of employment versus role burden and stress. Already working women should be asked about job satisfaction and the number of roles they simultaneously occupy. Women whose employment is stressful might benefit from employment-related counseling and/or conflict resolution training, and clinicians need to have resources available to suggest to these women as a way to reduce situational stress (Berg et al., 2015).

SEXUALITY

Participation in partnered sexually intimate activities has been linked to increased social support and improvement in well-being (Praire et al., 2011). An important aspect of health promotion related to sexuality is to ask women about their sexuality satisfaction and sexual partner. Caregiving women may be caring for their spouses, which may negatively affect engagement in sexual activity and their overall satisfaction with the sexual aspect of her health. This warrants open conversation with the clinician, who must have counseling resources to offer. Women in troubled relationships need encouragement to seek counseling related to improving their relationship and self-esteem. It is important that clinicians make sexual assessments part of their routine examinations and be able to discuss sexual matters with their patients in an open and nonjudgmental manner (Berg et al., 2015).

HEALTH PROMOTION RELATED TO EMOTIONAL HEALTH

Caregivers are likely to have higher levels of stress, depression, and psychological distress than noncaregivers (Pinquart & Sorensen, 2003; Roth et al., 2009, Schulz & Sherwood, 2008). Therefore, it is important to assess depression and anxiety in those who report a new onset of symptoms and provide appropriate interventions. The first step in promoting emotional health is to assess for depression and anxiety and, if not present, reassure the caregiver that she does not have these clinical conditions. However, women with depressed mood or who report undue stress from their caregiving activities should be offered resources that may be helpful in alleviating these conditions. Overall, health promotion of emotional health involves all aspects of health promotion already

suggested, particularly making healthy lifestyle choices related to nutrition and physical activity (Berg et al., 2015).

HEALTH PROMOTION RELATED TO CULTIVATING HEALING RELATIONSHIPS

Relationships are key contributors to health. Zender and Olshansky (2015) note that women's relationships with spouses, parents, work colleagues, and friends actually interact with their own personalities and psychological makeup, genetic predispositions, history of relationships, and even physiology to affect health and well-being. It is known that women grow toward relationships throughout life, and healthy development hinges on healthy interpersonal relationships (Jordan et al., 1991). The ways in which relationships affect health are complex and include behavioral, psychosocial, and physiologic/biological aspects (Zender & Olshansky, 2015). A greater degree of high-quality social interactions extends the life span; reduces morbidity from cardiovascular disease, depression, recovery from cancer, wound healing, autoimmune diseases, and inflammation-related diseases such as arthritis or kidney disease; improves quality of life; and promotes greater meaning of life for women (Cohen et al., 2007; Fagundes et al., 2013; Strating et al., 2006; Uchino, 2006).

Health promotion related to relational health includes interventions to improve social engagement, relational capacity, or natural social networks (Cohen & Janicki-Deverts, 2009). One major aspect is to reduce social isolation and loneliness through group or one-on-one interventions. Many of these interventions provide activities and instrumental support by engaging women through active participation (Dickens et al., 2011). For women caregivers, these interventions are more likely to be obtained through referrals to counseling or by linking caregivers with support groups that hold regular meetings and activities. That in itself affords the caregiving woman with activities that engage her with others.

It is known that relationships are often marred by disconnections and misunderstandings that breed conflict (Zender & Olshansky, 2015). Caregiving situations may involve conflicted relationships with the caregiver and the person or persons being cared for, other relatives and friends who have emotional investment, or healthcare providers or individuals who represent potential physical or economic resources for the caregiver. Each situation may require a different intervention to promote resolution; thus, healthcare providers assess carefully and then prescribe referral resources that can improve relationship health. These resources may include counseling referrals, support group information, potential economic resources, and respite services.

Caring for Yourself While Caring for Others

Healthcare providers may overlook the importance of the caregiving woman's need to care for herself and avoid *burnout, which is* defined as subjective burden related to caregiving. Tips for caring for yourself from Ask Medicare (www.medicare.gov/files/ask-medicare-caregiver-support.pdf), include

(a) identifying local support services, (b) making connections with others, (c) asking for help, and (d) taking care of personal health through nutrition, regular exercise, and enjoyable activities.

Maslach and Jackson (1982) identified three aspects of burnout among workers in health settings: (a) emotional exhaustion, or loss of emotional resources and a lack of energy to invest in human relationships; (b) depersonalization of the individuals for whom one cares, which refers to a negative and indifferent attitude toward patients; and (c) personal accomplishments, which refer to feelings of self-efficacy and satisfaction in caring for patients. In burnout, a lack of personal accomplishments is the third aspect and may result from emotional exhaustion and depersonalization of patients (Maslach & Jackson, 1982, 1986).

SUPPORT SERVICES AND RELATED ISSUES

Support Services

Support services for caregivers do not always fall into the usual categories of physical, emotional, or financial support. Sometimes these services involve "how to" or other means for assisting in caregiving activities or to prevent caregiving burnout. Often the activities of caregiving require education or enlightenment as to how to do something. Support services might be related to demonstrating particular procedures or planning for issues that might come along. Financial issues resources might be related to how to manage money or plan for billing or managing another person's money.

Related Issues

Resources for caregivers are abundantly available and range from educational to special resources for respite care, financial and legal issues, and skill building. These resources are ever changing, and it is important for clinicians to update their referral and resource lists quite regularly for the benefit of their caregiving patients. Overall, the literature related to caregiving and caregiving resources is growing, probably relative to the increased need for informal caregiving and recognition of caregivers' special needs. However, there are still many unmet needs for informal caregivers, and future research must target those gaps in knowledge, resources, and special assistance to relieve caregiving burden. At the same time, it is important to recognize that some caregivers report their caregiving role provides meaning and gives satisfaction in their lives. From these caregivers, clinicians can learn ways to enhance these benefits in caregivers who report increased burden leading to physical and emotional health issues.

REFERENCES

References for this chapter are online and available at https://connect.springerpub.com/content/book/978-0-8261-6722-4/part/part02/chapter/ch18

CHAPTER 19

Women's Sexual Health*

SUSAN M. SEIBOLD-SIMPSON AND JUSTIN M. WARYOLD

All human beings have the "right to bodily integrity, sexual safety, sexual privacy, sexual pleasure, and sexual healthcare; the right to make free and informed sexual and reproductive choices; and the right to have access to sexual information based on sound scientific evidence (Sexuality Information and Education Council of the United States [SIECUS], 2018, para. 4). Due to a variety of societal pressures and cultural norms, as well as the reproductive outcome of pregnancy, women have unique needs related to sexuality and sexual health. Addressing healthy sexuality and sexual health, particularly around sexual pleasure, is not always included in nurse practitioner education and training programs (Cappiello & Boardman, 2022; Cappiello et al., 2017). A recent study by Simmonds et al. (2019) found that while *either* sexual health promotion or assessment clinical or didactic training were often (91.7%) offered in transition to practice training programs for primary care nurse practitioners in the United States, *both* were infrequently being required (18.8%). Accurate, honest information needs to be provided to APRN students in order to deliver optimal care to their clients. When women express concerns regarding sexuality, sexual health, and sexual activity, they have the right to expect that APRNs will provide accurate sexual assessment and interventions, including information, counseling, or therapy. The goal of this chapter is to provide a knowledge base from which nurse practitioners can assess women's concerns about sexual health, provide comprehensive and complete sexual healthcare, and make appropriate referrals for their sexual problems. This chapter includes a focus on healthy, positive sexuality and sexual health, moving beyond reproductive health, with an updated look at dimensions of women's sexuality and sociocultural influences on sexuality and sexual health as well as the sexual assessment of women and individuals across a variety of perspectives.

While the focus on this chapter is on women's sexuality, we recognize that not all individuals who identify as female are assigned female at birth (AFAB). Though gender has traditionally been considered dichotomous, it is more commonly being seen as a spectrum, with female being on one end, male being on the opposing end, and a wide variety of identities contained within (DuBois & Shattuck-Heidorn, 2021). Consequently, women's sexual health includes women who were AFAB and are cisgendered, transwomen, transmen who continue to have female reproductive organs, individuals who are two-spirit, and individuals who are genderqueer/gender diverse/nonbinary. Correspondingly, pronouns for this chapter may include they/them or be absent entirely. Given that sexuality moves beyond reproduction, it is essential to acknowledge when anatomy and biology are necessary for inclusion in sexual health and when it is necessary to be more expansive of gender identity and sexual orientation. To do less would be a disservice to women everywhere. As appropriate, references will be made to other chapters in this text that provide greater detail than in this chapter.

SEXUALITY AND SEXUAL HEALTH

It is helpful to consider sexuality and sexual health in women from a sex positive and intersectionality frame. Sex positive is important to assist with viewing sexual health as an expectation for all women, regardless of age, culture, or religion. Addressing intersectionality is critical: it requires examining where personal identities overlap, identities that include race, ethnicity, sexual orientation, gender identity, disability, class, and other markers of discrimination. It is specifically related to addressing inequities and is especially relevant to women's sexuality.

According to the World Health Organization (WHO, 2017, p. 3):

Sexuality [italics added for emphasis] is a central aspect of being human throughout life and encompasses sex, gender identities and roles, sexual orientation, eroticism, pleasure, intimacy and reproduction. Sexuality is experienced and expressed in thoughts, fantasies, desires, beliefs, attitudes, values, behaviours, practices, roles and relationships. While sexuality can include all of these dimensions,

---

*This chapter is a revision of the chapter that appeared in the second edition of this textbook, authored by Elizabeth Kusturiss and Susan Kellogg Spadt, and we thank them for their original contribution.

not all of them are always experienced or expressed. Sexuality is influenced by the interaction of biological, psychological, social, economic, political, cultural, ethical, legal, historical, religious and spiritual factors.

WHO (2017) goes on to state:

Sexual health [italics added for emphasis] is a state of physical, emotional, mental and social well-being in relation to sexuality; it is not merely the absence of disease, dysfunction or infirmity. Sexual health requires a positive and respectful approach to sexuality and sexual relationships, as well as the possibility of having pleasurable and safe sexual experiences, free of coercion, discrimination and violence. (p. 3)

Sexuality is present throughout the life span, although the various influences and expressions affecting sexuality may differ over time. One's sexuality is circumscribed by cultural, socioeconomic, geopolitical, and legal contexts (WHO, 2017, p. 9).

Sex Positivity and Pleasure

The World Association for Sexual Health defines *sexual pleasure* as:

Sexual pleasure is the physical and/or psychological satisfaction and enjoyment derived from shared or solitary erotic experiences, including thoughts, fantasies, dreams, emotions, and feelings. Self-determination, consent, safety, privacy, confidence and the ability to communicate and negotiate sexual relations are key enabling factors for pleasure to contribute to sexual health and well-being. Sexual pleasure should be exercised within the context of sexual rights, particularly the rights to equality and nondiscrimination, autonomy and bodily integrity, the right to the highest attainable standard of health and freedom of expression. The experiences of human sexual pleasure are diverse and sexual rights ensure that pleasure is a positive experience for all concerned and not obtained by violating other people's human rights and well-being. (Ford et al., 2022)

Women's sexual pleasure and desire have been presented as both positive and negative in our society (Chmielewski et al., 2020; Dobson, 2019; Fava & Fortenberry, 2021; Laan et al., 2021). A growing body of work shows that sexual pleasure is integral to broader health, mental health, sexual health, and well-being (Coleman et al., 2021; Fava & Fortenberry, 2021; Ford et al., 2022; Kashdan et al., 2018; Lorenz, 2019). Acknowledgment of sexual pleasure is a key aspect of sexual positivity (Fava & Fortenberry, 2021). Burnes and colleagues (2017) noted,

As many White, Western, paradigms have understood sexuality using evolutionary theory, cisgender, heterosexual couples that engage in procreative sex are often seen as [the] standard, and other individuals are shamed, silenced, hypersexualized, or asexualized. However, sex positivity helps to expand the notion that sexual diversity does not only include sexual orientation identities. Rather, sex positivity represents physical wellness and the presence of safe (noncoercive), pleasurable sexual experiences and relationships. (p. 474)

Gendered sexual scripts, where the man is expected to be sexually dominant and the woman to be sexually passive, can have a negative impact on a women's sexual desire (Rubin et al., 2019; Schneider, 2022). Rubin et al. (2019) noted that, "research highlights the pursuit of pleasure as an important force in women's sexual desire—in other words, for some women to desire sex, it must be pleasurable sex worth desiring" (p. 7). While the reasons for pursuing sex are many, having fun and receiving pleasure are an important aspect of sexual behavior.

Little has been written in the nursing literature regarding sex positivity. Much in healthcare has focused on the *disease model* or *sex negativity* perception of sexuality, with sexually transmitted infections (STIs), HIV, and unwanted pregnancy being in the forefront (Fava & Fortenberry, 2021; Ford et al., 2022). However, it is appropriate and necessary to embrace sex positivity when working with individuals throughout their lifespan. Incorporating intersectionality adds additional depth to understanding women's sexuality. For example, Hargons et al. (2021), when examining sex positivity in Black women's sexuality research, found that, out of 265 articles, only 6.5% utilized a sex-positive perspective. As women's sexuality is presented, it is necessary to consider varying intersectionalities and resist viewing only from the prevailing majority perspective. The impact of culture on sexuality cannot be stressed enough.

Culture, including religion, can play a key role in how sexuality is expressed (Agocha et al., 2014). Not that long ago, virginity in women until marriage was the norm, and sex outside marriage was considered immoral. Although conservative religious groups and older Americans may still view all nonmarital sex as sinful, values are shifting, and nonmarital sex among women in a relational context is the norm (National Center for Health Statistics, n.d.-a) and sexual hookups are common in young adults (Hollis et al., 2022). Contraception, legal abortion, and changing gender roles legitimizing female sexuality have helped to lead to the shift away from *sin* to acceptance. Although some women report having sex purely for physical release, many women view sex from within a love and commitment perspective (Meston et al., 2020). Although nonmarital sex in women has become the norm, the attitude that *slutty* women are passionate, experienced, autonomous, and independent has not entirely changed. Despite changing gender norms, society continues to be hesitant to fully embrace women who are sexually outspoken and experienced (Dobson, 2019). APRNs can assist women in having positive self-esteem regarding their sexual persona and enjoying their sexual being.

Sexual and Intimate Relationships

Multiple factors are associated with sexual pleasure and satisfaction. *Sexual satisfaction* is a term that refers to "an effective response arising from one's subjective evaluation of the positive and negative dimensions associated with one's sexual relationship" (Lawrance & Byers, 1995, p. 268). Relationships, and correspondingly, the quality of relationships, are one factor that contributes to sexual pleasure and satisfaction and can vary across lifecycle and other demographics. Communication, intimacy, and commitment in a relationship have been associated with greater sexual satisfaction, but women in casual sexual relationships may also have strong sexual satisfaction, particularly when the casual sex is in the context of a greater predisposition to engage in uncommitted sex (Wongsomboon et al., 2020). Women's choices of relationships are individual and unique; the role of the APRN is to provide corresponding assessment, education, counseling, and treatment that supports the woman's choices.

Celibacy is a lifestyle in which a woman makes a conscious choice to abstain from sexual activity. It is different from asexuality, not being sexually attracted toward individuals of any gender (discussed later in this chapter). Relationships can be committed or casual and can be monogamous or nonmonogamous. Consensual nonmonogamy includes swinging, open, and polyamorous relationships (Moors et al., 2021). In polyamorous relationships, individuals are committed to being open about each of the relationships in their lives, and this should not be synonymous with infidelity. Moors et al. (2021) note that "polyamorous relationships typically encourage romantic love and sexual activity with multiple concurrent partners." They go on to identify different types of polyamory including with three, four, or five partners, or when one partner is monogamous and the other partner is polyamorous. Moors et al. (2021) found that in their study, "Approximately 1 out 6 people desire to engage in polyamory and 1 out of 9 people have engaged in polyamory at some point during their life" and this was associated with "people who identified as lesbian, gay, or bisexual (compared to people who identified as heterosexual) and men (compared to women) were more likely to report desire to engage in polyamory and previous engagement in polyamory."

Sexuality and Masturbation

Masturbation is manual stimulation of the clitoris with or without a partner. It can include the use of mechanical instruments such as vibrators, and despite a perceived stigma (Meiller & Hargons, 2019), it is a healthy part of women's sexuality. Regrettably, research about masturbation in women is lacking (Fischer et al., 2022; Rowland et al., 2020). Reasons for masturbation in women include sexual pleasure and satisfaction as well as helping to relieve stress (Rowland et al., 2020).

Dimensions of Women's Sexuality

Sexuality is multidimensional and includes sexual orientation, gender identity and expression, and sexual behaviors. These factors, along with the addition of biological sex and social sex-role, make up an individual's sexual identity (Edwards & Brooks, 1999; Larson, 1981; Shively & De Cecco, 1977). Sexual identity is how we perceive ourselves as sexual beings (Dailey, 1981).

SEXUAL ORIENTATION

Sexual desire, sexual attraction, and sexual pleasure are integral to sexual orientation. Multiple theories exist to explain sexual desire and attraction and include biological, psychological, cultural, and social components (Atallah et al., 2016; Brotto et al., 2016; Toates, 2009). *Sexual desire* is defined as, "the presence of sexual thoughts, fantasies, urges, and motivations to engage in sexual behavior in response to relevant internal and external cues" (Cherkasskaya & Rosario, 2019, p. 1661). Sexual desire is a highly subjective experience, and it is critical to consider women within their cultural contexts when addressing sexuality. It is also critical to note that many internal and external factors can negatively impact sexual well-being, such as body image (Avery et al., 2021; Gillen & Markey, 2019). While much of the healthcare literature focuses on sexual dysfunction and absence of sexual desire, or libido, it is important to begin with a clear understanding of what is considered to be healthy and functional. Libido is considered to be a basic human need, along with eating and sleeping. Yet, as noted by Brotto and Graham (2022), "no one model captures all women's experiences of sexual desire and arousal" (p. 13).

Sexual orientation includes multiple dimensions: sexual attraction, fantasy, emotional attraction, and sexual behavior (Massey et al., 2021; Salomaa & Matsick, 2019). Sexual orientation is not static and can change over time (Salomaa & Matsick, 2019). Sexual orientation is a spectrum of sexual attraction from asexual to pansexual, with terminology rapidly changing (Garrett-Walker & Montagno, 2021; Salomaa & Matsick, 2019). It can be necessary to use reliable websites, frequently associated with colleges and universities, to remain current with nomenclature.

It is helpful to begin with definitions of common terms used when discussing sexual orientation. *Asexuality* refers to not being sexually attracted toward individuals of any gender (Brotto & Milani, 2022). The term *heterosexual* refers to a woman whose sexual orientation is toward members of the opposite gender. The term *lesbian* is generally used for women whose sexual orientation is toward members of her own gender. Within the lesbian community, often there are women who identify as more feminine (femme) and women who identify as more masculine (butch) or women who identify as androgynous (Luoto et al., 2019; Rothblum et al., 2018). *Pansexual* or *omnisexual* refers to individuals who are attracted to all genders and sexes. The term *queer* is often used as an umbrella term for LGBTQ and can refer to sexual orientation or gender identity.

It is important to note that sexual attraction exists on a continuum, with exclusive sexual attraction to the same sex and sexual attraction to the opposite sex on either end of the scale (Copen et al., 2016; Lorenz, 2019). The most recent National Survey on Family Growth (NSFG) from 2015 to 2019 found that 89.6% of women identified with a heterosexual sexual orientation, 2.7% with a gay sexual orientation, and 7.7% with a bisexual orientation. Seventy-seven percent indicated being attracted only to the opposite sex with 14.2% being attracted mostly to the opposite sex, 4.8% attracted equally to both sexes, 1.4% being mostly attracted to the same sex, 1.5% being only attracted to the same sex, and 1.3% answering "not sure" (National Center for Health Statistics, n.d.-b). A previous analysis of the NSFG data found that sexual behavior, sexual attraction, and sexual orientation vary by age, marital or cohabiting status, education, and race/Hispanic origin (Copen et al., 2016). See Chapter 20, Primary Care of Lesbian, Gay, and Bisexual Individuals, and Chapter 25, Caring for the Transgender and Gender Nonbinary Patient, for a more in-depth discussion of healthcare issues of lesbian, gay, bisexual, and transgender health.

GENDER IDENTITY AND GENDER EXPRESSION

Sexual orientation is frequently discussed with gender identity/expression, resulting in an international term known as SOGI, to be more inclusive and representative (Phillips et al., 2021). Gender identity refers to a person's internal sense of gender, which may or may not align with their biological sex assigned at birth, while gender expression refers to how people express their gender, usually through characteristics such as dress or speech or behaviors (Phillips et al., 2021, p. 226). As with sexual orientation, gender exists on a continuum with some individuals identifying solely as male or female, some as two-spirit, and others identifying as gender diverse/nonbinary/genderqueer or genderfluid (DuBois & Shattuck-Heidorn, 2021; Garrett-Walker & Montagno, 2021). Women's healthcare subsequently includes not only women who were AFAB and identify as female (also known as *cisgender*) but also women whose gender identity is male but have female reproductive organs. *Transgender* refers to people whose gender identity does not align with their sex assigned at birth, and *gender diverse/nonbinary/genderqueer* refers to identities that are somewhere between or outside the gender binary regardless of sex assigned at birth (DuBois & Shattuck-Heidorn, 2021, p. 4). See Chapter 25, Caring for the Transgender and Gender Nonbinary Patient, for more about transgender health. An additional category for inclusion in gender identity and expression is *intersex*, which is an "umbrella term for unique variations in reproductive or sex anatomy, compared to the two usual paths of human sex development" (InterACT, 2021). APRNs need to inquire of individuals as to their preferred gender pronouns to know what their preferred gender identity is and not rely on presentation or assumptions.

WOMEN'S SEXUAL RESPONSE

Sexual arousal includes both physiologic and psychological experiences. Physiologic changes include genital vasocongestion as a result of increased heart rate and blood pressure and increases in pelvic muscle tone. This results in "vulvar, clitoral, and vaginal vasoengorgement, genital lubrication, and increased tactile sensitivity" (Chivers & Brotto, 2017, p. 6). A woman's sexual response is a complex interplay of psychological, physiologic, and interpersonal components (Cherkasskaya & Rosario, 2019). Major differences exist in terms of expectations and perceptions of normal sexual response in women and can vary from one culture to another (Agocha et al., 2014). Additionally, within cultural groups it is essential to consider levels of acculturation, social structure, and socioeconomic status (Agocha et al., 2014). However, research suggests that women who identify as heterosexual, lesbian, bisexual, queer, or questioning tend to experience comparable levels of sexual desire and identify similar motivating factors (e.g., physical pleasure, emotional connection) regardless of the sex of the partner (Cherkasskaya & Rosario, 2019). Although physiologic aspects of the sexual response, such as orgasmic contractions or vasocongestion of the genitals, can be universal in women without

sexual dysfunction, the subjective and emotional aspects of sexual response are highly individual and subject to learning and cultural factors

Various models have been proposed to describe the human sexual response and more continue to be developed. Masters and Johnson, in the 1960s, described the cycle for both men and women as consisting of four stages, which progressed in a *linear* fashion beginning with excitement, which leads to plateau, orgasm, and finally resolution (Masters & Johnson, 1966). According to this response cycle, each stage had genital and extragenital responses and involved a gradual buildup of sexual tension, which culminated in the release of orgasm. Masters and Johnson were the first researchers to describe the possibility of multiple orgasms in the female response cycle (Rosen & Barsky, 2006). Their model was later modified by Kaplan (1974) in the 1970s, and was represented in a triphasic model, which emphasized desire as the initial and critical phase, which then led to excitement, followed by orgasm. The introduction to Kaplan's model brought libido into the picture, as it has been viewed until recently as a necessary precursor to the development of adequate excitement and orgasm.

Earlier models of the female sexual response focused on a linear biological progression, lacked a focus on psychological or interpersonal issues, and were not always reflective of women's actual experiences of sexual response. A different model, proposed by Basson in 2000, was based on a female-focused *circular* model, which redefined the phases of the female sexual response and their relationship to one another (Cherkasskaya & Rosario, 2019; Hayes, 2011; Rosen & Barsky, 2006). The Basson model includes a complex interplay of sexual stimuli, emotional intimacy, psychological factors, and relationship satisfaction and refuted the notion that all sexual activities are prompted by a woman's own innate and spontaneous desire or libido (Cherkasskaya & Rosario, 2019; Hayes, 2011; Kingsberg & Rezaee, 2013). Basson (2008) noted that women can enter a sexual scenario from a position of sexual neutrality and commence sexual activity for reasons other than innate desire. Reasons for engaging in sex play can include emotional reasons (e.g., love and commitment), physical reasons (e.g., stress reduction and pleasure), goal-attainment reasons (e.g., revenge and social status), and insecurity reasons (e.g., mate guarding, a sense of duty, or low self-esteem). Although noting that spontaneous sexual desire in women is more typical in the early phase of a relationship and less common for sexually content women in long-term relationships, Basson described "responsive" female desire as an event that is triggered or reactive to incoming sexual stimuli and/or physiologic arousal (Basson, 2008; Hayes, 2011). "Responsive sexual desire," Basson posited, could feed back into the cycle, leading to increased arousal. In this model, sexual satisfaction with sexual activity (in which orgasm and resolution are not essential) is suggested to be more representative of a woman's experience. Positive sexual experiences provide further motivation to engage in sexual activity and contribute toward a woman's reasons for allowing sexual stimuli and moving from a sexual-neutral state to a sexual-aroused state (Basson, 2008).

Another essential element in the female sexual response is the disconnect that often exists between a woman's subjective feelings of sexual arousal and the actual physiologic changes, such as genital vasocongestion, that have more typically represented sexual arousal. In her research, Basson (2000) discovered that subjective arousal does not always correlate with physiologic measures of genital congestion, and emotions or thoughts have a greater influence on the subjective experience of sexual excitement. Typical women have the ability to experience vaginal lubrication or genital engorgement without the subjective perception of sexual excitement and vice versa (Rosen & Barsky, 2006).

Work on women's sexual response continues to evolve. Cherkasskaya and Rosario (2019) provide a thorough description of sexual response that builds upon the work done by Basson, Kaplan, and Masters and Johnson, and proposed a new theory, the Relational and Bodily Experiences Theory that incorporates the additional concepts of "women's internalized models of self, attachment styles, and sexual body self-representations that incorporates the constructs of self-objectification, sexual subjectivity, and genital self-image" (p. 11). Genital self-image refers to a woman's thoughts and feelings about how her genitalia look, smell, or function (Velotta & Schwartz, 2019). This theory provides a deeper exploration of the psychological aspects of sexual arousal and how they impact sexual functioning. This complexity contributes to the etiology of female sexual interest/arousal disorder.

Sexual Behaviors

Sexual activity is more than vaginal/penile intercourse or masturbation. Healthy sexual behaviors can include kissing, cuddling, breast touching and/or nipple stimulation, hand-penis stimulation ("hand job"), vaginal fingering, anal fingering, receiving oral sex, giving oral sex, rubbing genitals together, vaginal intercourse, receptive anal intercourse, and insertive anal intercourse (Townes et al., 2022). Sexual activity can occur alone, partnered, or with multiple partners. It can include the use of toys and other mechanical tools (e.g., vibrators and dildos). This is only a sampling of the variety of sexual behaviors that can occur.

SEXUALITY ACROSS THE LIFE SPAN

Healthy sexuality evolves and changes across the lifespan beginning in infancy and continuing through old age. It is present in all stages, with variations occurring over time. Challenges may develop based on social, cultural, psychological, and legal impacts. Advance practice nurses can assist in maintaining optimal sexual health. See also Chapter 8, Young Women's Health; Chapter 9, Midlife Women's Health; and Chapter 10, Older Women's Health.

Childhood

Sexuality occurs across the life span and is present during childhood. Children acknowledge gender around age 3 (Kar et al., 2015). Work done by Friedrich et al. (2003) highlighted common sexual actions in children during the ages of 2 to 5 years old, 6 to 9 years old, and 10 to 12 years old. Friedrich found that it is common for young boys and girls to touch their genitals and to try to see adults when they are nude or undressing, and this behavior decreases with increasing age (p. 114). Friedrich cautioned that sexual behaviors vary across "age, gender, family sexuality, life stress, family violence, peer relationships, number of days in daycare, and maternal attitudes toward sexuality" (Friedrich et al., 2003, p. 107).

Adolescence and Emerging Adulthood

Adolescence is the social and psychological state that occurs between the beginning of puberty, when the body becomes capable of reproduction, and acceptance into full adulthood. Experts suggest that there is an additional phase between adolescence and full adulthood known as emerging adulthood (Arnett, 2000). Adolescence is typically divided into three stages: early (10–13 years), middle (14–16 years), and late (17–19 years; Kar et al., 2015), with emerging adulthood focusing on the years between 18 and 25 (Arnett, 2000).

A primary task of adolescence is establishing a sense of self or identity and, through dating and romantic and sexual experiences, constructing themselves as sexual beings. Developing a healthy sense of sexuality is an essential task in adolescence. During this time, adolescent girls make discoveries about their bodies and sex, struggle with self-esteem, develop crushes and begin dating, explore their sexual orientation, and often experience their first heartbreak. It is a time that helps define how a woman views herself and as others as sexual people.

During adolescence, the female body undergoes rapid physical changes triggered by the hypothalamus, development of secondary sexual characteristics, increased growth velocity, changes in body composition, and capability of reproduction. Girls typically begin to experience physical changes at age 7, known as adrenarche, which precedes the development of secondary sex characteristics (Archibald et al., 2003). Gonadarche begins approximately 2 years later with rises in luteinizing hormone and follicle-stimulating hormone (Archibald et al., 2003). Breast buds develop between the ages of 8 and 13, followed by the development of pubic hair and increases in height (Archibald et al., 2003). The median age of menarche is 12.2 years (Biro et al., 2018). The age at menarche varies by race/ethnicity and body weight, with some studies suggesting that overweight girls reach menarche earlier than girls who are not overweight or obese (Biro et al., 2018). Early pubertal debut can be associated with adverse health outcomes, including more depressive symptoms, worse self-reported health, and higher body mass index (BMI); later pubertal debut can be associated with fewer sex partners, less drug use, more physical activity, better self-report health, and lower BMI during adolescence (Hoyt et al., 2020).

Onset of sexual activity begins in adolescence. Current data indicate that by age 15, 21% of young females aged 15 to 24 had ever had sexual intercourse; by age 17, this increased to 53% of young females, and by age 20, 79% of young females had ever had sexual intercourse (Martinez & Abma, 2020). Young women are more likely to use a method of contraception at first intercourse when then are older (≤14 years old—57%; 15 to 17 years old—79%, and 17 to 19 years old—83% (Martinez & Abma, 2020). The most common method of contraception in adolescents remains the condom, followed by withdrawal (65%) and the pill (53%; Martinez & Abma, 2020). Ethier et al. (2018), in their recent analysis of the 2005–2015 National Youth Risk Behavior Survey found that it appears fewer students are having sex during the earlier years of high school and that there were decreases in the prevalence of sexual intercourse among Black and Hispanic students, who had traditionally been reported as having sex at a young age and being at risk for negative outcomes. Early onset of sexual activity has been associated more sexual partners, more STIs, and adolescent pregnancy (Ethier et al., 2018; Sprecher et al., 2019).

Work is being done to examine what healthy adolescent sexuality comprises (Kågesten & van Reeuwijk, 2021; Landers & Kapadia, 2020). Sexual activity should be safe, free from coercion, protected from STIs and HIV/AIDS, and mutually respectful (SIECUS, 2018). Adolescents benefit from comprehensive sexuality education that provides the necessary knowledge along with healthy communication among family and with partners. Adolescents also benefit from developing a positive sense of one's own (sexual) self, identity, and body, which includes the capacity to be aware of one's sexual desires and develop sexual self-esteem (sense of self-worth and attractiveness) and self-efficacy (perceived ability to assert preferences; Kågesten & van Reeuwijk, 2021). Kågesten and van Reeuwijk (2021) have identified "six key domains of competencies in the form of knowledge, skills and attitudes that support adolescent sexual wellbeing: 1) sexual literacy, 2) gender equitable attitudes, 3) respect for human rights and understanding of consent, 4) critical reflection skills, 5) coping skills and stress management, and 6) interpersonal relationship skills." (p. 5)

Sexuality and sexual activity in adolescence and emerging adulthood may include the use of technology, such as sexting or other forms of sextech (discussed later in this chapter). It may also include the use of pornography (Bridges et al., 2016).

Adulthood

In early adulthood, women have a greater understanding of themselves as sexual beings and develop a more mature sexuality. Women establish their sexual orientation, integrate love and sexuality, forge intimate connections, make commitments, make decisions regarding their fertility, and develop a coherent sexual philosophy. The sexual orientation of women is often established by adolescence or early adulthood, including for lesbian, bisexual, or queer women (Bishop et al., 2020). Often early- to mid-adulthood is a time for consideration of developing a long-term, committed relationship and considering childrearing, although rates of intended childlessness are increasing slightly (Hartnett &Gemmill, 2020).

CHILDBEARING

Pregnancy and childbirth represent a unique period in a woman's life, which involves significant physical, psychological, hormonal, social, and cultural changes that may greatly affect sexuality. These factors may include changes in the couple relationship; planned/unplanned and desired/ undesired pregnancy; prior pregnancy, abortion, or miscarriage history; physical and hormonal changes causing poor self-image; mood instability; and difficulty or pain with vaginal intercourse (McBride & Kwee, 2017). Not all couples experience the same level of challenges, however, and sexuality, sexual activity, and sexual desire can change over time (Rosen et al., 2020). See also Chapter 39, Intrapartum and Postpartum Care.

INFERTILITY

Struggles with infertility and repeated attempts to conceive can compromise sexual self-esteem, expression, activity, and desire. A diagnosis of infertility may negatively affect a woman's sense of sexuality and her self-image and have a profound impact on her relationship. Studies have shown that women with infertility have an increased risk of sexual dysfunction, including lower sexual desire, lower sexual satisfaction, and lower orgasm (El Amiri et al., 2021).

Women in treatment for infertility experience sex that is prescribed and planned around ovulation, having little to do with pleasure or sexual desire. Women may experience frustration that their reproductive as well as sexual life is out of their control during infertility treatment. Years of attempting to conceive makes spontaneous sex difficult to maintain and couples often find it difficult to separate spontaneous sex for pleasure from "functional" sex for conception. See also Chapter 37, Infertility.

Midlife

In middle adulthood (approximately 40–60 years of age), work and family often play major roles in women's lives. Personal time is spent primarily on marital and family matters, which can affect sexual expression by its decreasing intensity, frequency, and significance. Sex in the context of committed relationships may change and become less central to relationship satisfaction (Yarber & Sayad, 2022). Overall, sexual frequency is decreasing in the United States and this trend increases with aging (Herbenick et al., 2022; Twenge et al., 2017).

One of the greatest barriers to a woman's sexuality in midlife is ageism. Our cultures' preoccupation with equating sexiness to youth often leaves the vibrant sexuality of women in midlife socially invisible. This is a time when women may feel sexually unappealing and withdrawn because of the physical changes in their body shape. During this time, women's bodies undergo a number of changes associated with menopause and aging; however, many women in their 40s and 50s continue to be sexually robust and develop increased confidence, which gives them the courage to be more passionate in their sexuality and identity.

Menopause and adolescence are the two times in a woman's life in which she undergoes dramatic physiologic changes, which can have a profound effect on her sexuality. Common sexual difficulties experienced by women in midlife include inability to relax, loss of interest in sex, dyspareunia, arousal difficulties, and anorgasmia (Yarber & Sayad, 2022). Perimenopause, or the years leading to menopause, is characterized by fluctuating estrogen levels and irregular menses that result in vasomotor symptoms, anxiety, and sleep disturbances, which can negatively impact a woman's sexual interest and ability to become aroused and/or achieve orgasm (Yarber & Sayad, 2022). In the United States, the average age of menopause is 51 (Yarber & Sayad, 2022). It is marked by the cessation of ovarian estrogen production and a decline in estrogen levels, a dominant factor that can affect sexual function. This decrease in estrogen affects the urogenital tissues, including the pelvic floor musculature, bladder, urethra, and vagina. Reduced vaginal estradiol alters the microbial environment, predisposing postmenopausal women to vaginal infections and/or urinary tract infections. Up to 50% of postmenopausal women experience symptoms of vaginal atrophy from a decreased elasticity of the vulvovaginal tissues, a thinning vaginal wall, and decreased vaginal lubrication, causing dryness, itching, irritation, burning, and dyspareunia (Yarber & Sayad, 2022). See also Chapter 34, Menopause.

Older Adulthood

Aging is a physiologic, psychological, and social transition that often affects a woman's sexuality. Sexuality and sexual activity do not end in older adulthood. As with other aspects of sexuality, there is variation in what occurs in older adults. For example, Kolodziejczak et al. (2019) found that almost one-third of participants between the ages of 60 to 82 years old reported both more sexual activity and sexual thoughts than the average younger adult (p. 396). Although research has shown that women are less likely than men to report being sexually active, this has been attributed primarily to health or lack of a partner (Sinković & Towler, 2019; Yarber & Sayad, 2022). The capacity to enjoy sexual activity is not lost with advancing age. For some women, a new partner following divorce or widowhood can lead to more frequent and higher quality sexual activity (Sinković & Towler, 2019). However, while older adults may perceive a stigma around being sexual, they noted they often feel more comfortable in their own skin (Towler et al., 2021).

Age-related physiologic changes in later adulthood can contribute to painful sexual symptoms, and these, in turn, may be associated with reduced sexual desire and activity. Reduced tissue elasticity and thinning of the vaginal tissues may cause irritation or discomfort with penetration, contributing to a reduced desire for sexual activity (Srinivasan et al., 2019; Yarber & Sayad, 2022). In addition, loss of fatty tissue of the labia and mons may contribute to tenderness, and these tissues may be easily damaged or abraded with sexual stimulation.

Many psychosocial factors affect a woman's sexuality as she ages. As women continue to age, their sexuality becomes less genitally oriented, with a greater focus on the emotional, sensual, and relationship aspects (Srinivasan et al., 2019). Although sexual frequency may decrease, intimacy is especially valued and is an essential element for an older woman's well-being (Yarber & Syad, 2022). Chronic illness, hormonal changes, and vascular changes in a woman or her partner can result in decreased sexual activity. Furthermore, older women may experience difficulty seeing themselves as sexual beings because of culture's association of sexuality, romance, and sexual desires with youth (Towler et al., 2021). Social constructions of desirability influence a woman's view of herself as a sexual being. Cultural and social constructs of sexuality frequently influence a woman's perceptions of the physical

signs of aging and losing attractiveness and femininity. If a woman has this negative association, she will frequently also have a poor body image and a detrimental effect on sexuality. Conversely, a woman who perceives the aging process in a positive manner with confidence may even experience enhancement of her sexual desire and desirability. Age is not a reliable predictor of the quality and type of intimate relationships, and emotional intimacy typically remains an essential need regardless of a woman's age.

SOCIOCULTURAL ASPECTS OF SEXUALITY AND SEXUAL HEALTH

Sexuality, sexual health, and sexual behaviors evolve over time and reflect cultural, environmental, and technological changes. Sociocultural aspects of sexuality vary across age groups, racial/ethnic groups, and SOGI groups. This section addresses some of the current sociocultural aspects of sexuality that are particularly important to be aware of when providing care to women.

Hookups, Dating Apps, and Sextech

Hookup behavior is common among young adults, both in and out of college (Garcia et al., 2015). Hooking up refers to a spontaneous sexual encounter when there is no expectation of an ongoing relationship (Garcia & Reiber, 2008). A great deal of research has been conducted related to hooking up, particularly around psychological factors, within concerns having been identified related to guilt, remorse, or coercion, particularly for women (de Jong et al., 2018; Fielder et al., 2014). Hookups often result from use of online dating apps such as Tinder or Bumble (Petrychyn et al., 2020). There have been concerns related to increased risk of unwanted sexual harassment and rape for women who use online dating apps and hookups. However, many women have identified strategies to ensure their own personal safety and in turn find that using dating apps can result in increased confidence and self-esteem (Petrychyn et al., 2020). Hookups occur in straight and queer women and are often used as an opportunity to find longer-term relationships (Cama et al., 2021; Petrychyn et al., 2020; Weitbrecht & Whitton, 2020). They are also used for experiencing pleasure and intimacy, particularly when individuals are focused on other goals in their life (Anders et al., 2020; Garcia et al., 2018; Jamison & Sanner, 2021). There may be racial/ethnic differences related to hookup behavior and sexual satisfaction, but more work is needed to clarify this (Harris, 2020; Helm et al., 2015).

Another area where technology has influenced sexuality and sexual behaviors is sexting and other types of technology for sexual engagement (Gesselman et al., 2022). Gesselman et al. (2022) in their study of 7,512 American adults ages 18 to 65 years found that "participants indicated their engagement with eight forms of sextech, including six emerging forms of sexual technology (visiting erotic camming sites, participating in camming streams, teledildonic use, accessing virtual reality pornography, playing sexually explicit video games, and sexual messaging with chatbots or artificially intelligent entities) as well as two more common domains (online pornography and sexting)" (p. 1). The COVID-19 pandemic and corresponding social distancing clearly contributed to this use of sextech (Lehmiller et al., 2021). Sexting refers to "sharing of personal, sexually suggestive text messages, or nude or nearly nude photographs or videos via electronic devices" (Mori et al., 2020, p. 1103) and is common among adolescents and young adults (Madigan et al., 2018; Mori et al., 2020; Symons et al., 2018). As with other forms of technology, sexting can have positive and negative outcomes, particularly for females (Madigan et al., 2018; Reed et al., 2020). For example, sexts can be forwarded without an individual's consent, an individual can be coerced to send a sext, or a sext can be unwanted by the recipient (Klettke et al., 2019; Reed et al., 2020). However, sexting can also be a way to increase intimacy and enjoyment (Symons et al., 2018).

Bondage, Discipline, Dominance, Submission, and Sadomasochism and Kink

Bondage, discipline, dominance, submission, and sadomasochism (BDSM) or other forms of kink are not uncommon in men and women. It has been suggested that the BDSM community offers its members "access to a social network, friendship, a sense of community, and acceptance" (Erickson et al., 2022). Formerly considered a mental health disorder, it is common to see studies related to BDSM in the healthcare literature as a healthy activity for experiencing sexual pleasure. BDSM "generally includes sexual behaviors that involve some sort of power exchange between two or more partners and/or the use of pain to elicit sexual pleasure, though sensations other than pain (e.g., pleasure) are also frequently used in play" (Brown et al., 2020, p. 781). This power exchange is based in affirmative consent; all parties involved consent to the behaviors taking place and can withdraw consent at any time (e.g., through the use of a safeword; Brown et al., 2020, p. 781). Studies suggest that BDSM practitioners are often White, well-educated, young, and frequently nonheterosexual (Brown et al., 2020; De Neef et al., 2019). It has been noted that the BDSM community has elements of racial discrimation, however (Erickson et al., 2022).

There remains a perception of stigma associated with being a member of the kink community and participating in BDSM activities (Brown et al., 2021; De Neef et al., 2019). However, estimates of prevalence of BDSM fantasies (69%–76% of the population) and engagement (20%–30% of the population) suggest that it is likely that nurse practitioners will have clients who are involved in BDSM (Brown et al., 2021; De Neef et al., 2019). It is suggested that heterosexual, cisgender women are more likely to identify as being in the submissive category while genderqueer, pansexual participants were more likely to be "switches," that alternate between submissive and dominant (Brown et al., 2021; De Neef et al., 2019).

Sex Work

The exchange of sex for money, goods, and services by consenting adults has been in existence for centuries (Grittner & Walsh, 2020; Sawicki et al., 2019). Sex work "refers to

prostitutes, escorts, strippers, porn actors, sex phone operators; however not all people who participate in these acts identify as sex workers" (Sawicki et al., 2019, p. 355). Issues associated with sex work include violence, housing instability, mental health issues, drug use, and increased risk for HIV/STIs (Platt et al., 2018). The perception of sex work being a choice for employment is controversial (Grittner & Walsh, 2020; Platt et al., 2018; Sawicki et al., 2019). In one study of sex workers in Baltimore City, Maryland, "73% of women entered the sex trade to get drugs, 36% of women entered to get basic necessities such as food or housing, and 17% of women entered to support their children or family" (Footer et al., 2020, p. 406). Footer and colleagues (2020) found that women who entered sex work before the age of 18 were more likely to report "to get food" and "to get a place to stay" as reasons for current sex work. This is also known as "survival sex." Sex work is highly stigmatized, and this negative stigma can correspondingly increase exposure to violence (Grittner & Walsh, 2020).

Intimate Partner Violence and Rape

Intimate partner violence (IPV) includes rape or sexual assault, sexual coercion, and any unwanted sexual contact and can occur between a stranger or a known partner (Tarzia, 2021). IPV can result in injury and death and has social and economic repercussions as well (Palmieri & Valentine, 2021). The Centers for Disease Control and Prevention (CDC; n.d.) note that about one in four women have experienced contact sexual violence, physical violence, and/or stalking by an intimate partner during their lifetime and reported some form of IPV-related impact. Rates are higher in bisexual women than heterosexual women (Chen et al., 2020). Palmieri and Valentine (2021) noted that survivors of IPV are at risk for long-term psychological issues including substance abuse, depression, suicide, and posttraumatic stress disorder. It is essential to normalize screening for women, and to conduct screening and referrals on a regular basis (Curry et al., 2018; Lutgendorf, 2019). See Chapter 42, Gender-Based Violence and Women's Health, for more information related to violence and women's health.

SEXUAL HEALTHCARE

Assessment

With continually increasing public and professional awareness of sexuality and evaluation/management of patients for sexual problems, providers struggle with the complexity of obtaining adequate and meaningful information from the individual. Nevertheless, providers and patients alike struggle to establish a rapport to discuss the patient's sexual identity and relationships.

Although sexual health may include concerns related to sexual intercourse, such as contraception and STIs, these are not the only aspect of one's sexual health. Studies have shown that many adult women continue to go without appropriate guidance and only raise questions when they experience symptoms, such as decreased desire or pleasure (Kingsberg et al., 2019). Many patients have expressed the desire for their healthcare provider to inquire about their sexual history, including having a question on an intake form to address sexual concerns (Ryan et al., 2018).

Establishing rapport and putting patients at ease in a kind and understanding manner are essential when conducting a sexual health history. All are vital components to obtaining an adequate and meaningful history, from minimizing interruptions to providing appropriate eye contact to ensuring that the person is appropriately dressed. Healthcare providers should be comfortable discussing sexual concerns and be aware of their tone and nonverbal expressions during this interaction. Some providers may benefit from practicing using explicit sexual terminology in order to desensitize themselves. One technique that may be helpful is to ask these questions aloud in front of a mirror, observing one's nonverbal presentation. Using appropriate, objective terminology may be challenging, especially when trying not to be offensive. When inquiring about sexual acts, use terminologies based on the anatomy present, such as penis-to-vagina or mouth-to-vagina. This technique will allow a person to describe the act without associating it with their inner sexual identity, which may be fluid (Waryold & Kornahrens, 2020).

Taking a sexual history during a patient visit is an effective way to begin the conversation, as it conveys that discussing sexual concerns and functioning is encouraged and appropriate. A patient's sexual history may also be obtained via a questionnaire that the person completes in the waiting room. This ensures that the provider is aware of any sexual concerns that the patient wishes to discuss. Ideally, a sexual history should be incorporated within the review of systems. This discussion should occur in a private setting, and confidentiality must be ensured. Allowing the person to be clothed helps eliminate the anxiety, vulnerability, and discomfort that are commonly experienced when sitting in an examination gown (Kingsberg, 2006).

Before engaging in a conversation regarding a patient's sexual history or concerns, the provider can ask for permission and assess the situation for opportunities to discuss these concerns. By asking for permission, the provider is able to factually state that although these questions are of a sensitive nature, they are necessary to evaluate the patient's concerns further and promote a healthy sexual outlook. An example of this type of questioning might look like this: "I'm going to ask you a few questions about your sexual health. Since sexual health is essential to overall health, I ask all my patients these questions. If you're uncomfortable answering any of these, just let me know, and we'll move on. To begin, what questions or sexual concerns would you like to discuss today?" (Altarum Institute, 2016). This technique can help establish a rapport and provide comfort for continued discussion of one's sexual history and/or concerns.

Providers can continue approaching the topic by mentioning the importance of assessing sexual function with all patients and starting with the presenting issue or reproductive stage concerning their sexual function, which is helpful. Normalizing or universalizing techniques beginning the question with "many patients…" or "other patients have told me…" can help relieve anxiety. For example, "Many people who are menopausal often notice problems with decreased lubrication or discomfort during vaginal intercourse. Have you noticed this or any changes in your sexual functioning you would like to discuss?" Most patients are eager to tell their story to a compassionate provider and often do so if given the opportunity (Althof et al., 2013). Therefore, it is indispensable to use open-ended questions when conducting the sexual health history. Closed questions generally follow to gather specific information such as medical history, menstrual history, and drug reactions.

A comprehensive sexual history should include medical, reproductive, surgical, psychiatric, social, and sexual information. As sexual functioning is multifactorial, each domain of function must be examined in terms of its individual or combined impact. Relevant medical information pertinent for a thorough sexual assessment includes:

- Past medical history
- Current health status
- Current use of prescription and over-the-counter medications, as they may contribute to or cause sexual dysfunction
- Cardiovascular disease, as it has been linked to difficulties with arousal
- Endocrine conditions such as diabetes, androgen insufficiency, estrogen deficiency, and thyroid conditions
- Reproductive history inclusive of last menstrual period, age at menarche, menstrual history, and obstetric history, including spontaneous or induced abortions, history of infertility, contraception history, STI history, age at menopause if pertinent, gynecologic pain, surgeries, and urologic functioning
- Neurologic diseases, such as multiple sclerosis and injuries to the spinal cord, which may impair arousal and orgasm
- Psychiatric illness

Clarification should be sought when necessary (e.g., to clarify the degree of lubrication present during sexual arousal if pain occurs during vaginal intercourse). The patient should be asked to describe their current relationship briefly and rate their relationship concerning communication, affection, whether sexual needs are met, and sexual contact. Acknowledging that it may be difficult for any person to discuss the intimate details of their sexual life may also help reassure and encourage them to proceed (Althof et al., 2013).

Opportunities for sexual health screenings include visits based on organs present in the person, including gynecologic examinations, menopause-related concerns, antenatal or postpartum appointments, infertility assessment and treatment, and management of chronic illness and depression. Primary screening for sexual functioning may progress into a more detailed evaluation after normalizing the importance of assessing for sexual function. Questioning might begin with, "Are you currently involved in a sexual relationship?" If the patient reports that they are, an example of a follow-up might be, "Are you sexually active with men, women, or both?" or simply, "Tell me about your partners." Asking the question in this fashion allows the patient to express their sexual activity on their own terms, not limited to gender identity, gender expression/presentation, or sex assigned at birth.

Lastly, suppose the answer is "no" in response to being involved in a sexual relationship. In that case, the provider should further inquire with, "Are there any sexual concerns you would like to discuss or that have contributed to a lack of sexual behavior?" Providers mustn't make any assumptions about the person's age, appearance, marital status, or any other factor. Providers cannot know a person's sexual orientation, behaviors, or gender identity unless they inquire (Altarum Institute, 2016). Providers should be aware that one's sexual orientation, behaviors, or gender identity may be fluid, and may change from encounter to encounter.

A physical exam may be completed if the health history indicates the need, if it is the person's reason for seeking care, if it is part of their treatment goal(s) or a need for referral. The examination may include obtaining vital signs and general aspects of a physical exam, particularly abdominal and pelvic. The pelvic examination should include inspecting the external and internal genitalia using specula and bimanual techniques.

TRAUMA-INFORMED CARE

Trauma is experienced throughout the life span, and traumatic experiences may be remote events or current and ongoing. In the United States, about one in five women have experienced childhood sexual abuse and a similar proportion experience rape as adults (Finkelhor et al., 1990). Providers must recognize the prevalence and effect of trauma on patients and the healthcare team and incorporate trauma-informed approaches to the delivery of care. Understanding trauma, its prevalence, and its effect on health is an initial step to improve the patient experience. Still, to fully optimize outcomes for those who have survived trauma, providers should become familiar with the trauma-informed model of care. Implementing this approach is critical in creating an environment that emphasizes physical, psychological, and emotional safety for both practitioners and survivors and creates opportunities for survivors to rebuild a sense of control and empowerment (American College of Obstetricians and Gynecologists' Committee on Health Care for Underserved Women, 2021). Survivors of trauma may be "triggered," consciously or unconsciously, by situations they encounter in the healthcare setting. The need to undress, undergo procedures, wait in a room with a closed door, or see blood are all concrete ways of the patient becoming retraumatized while obtaining medical care. Traumatic memories provoked by healthcare encounters may make medical care intolerable to patients and contribute to worsened health outcomes (Kimberg & Wheeler, 2019). Engaging in patient-centered

communication and care can be accomplished by seeking patient input on how best to make them comfortable and can be particularly valuable for establishing trust and rapport. Maintaining a calm, supportive, nonjudgmental, and resiliency-promoting demeanor that can stabilize and assure patients with a history of trauma can be challenging even for experienced clinicians. It requires a commitment to ongoing self-reflection, practice, and individual and systems transformation. The provider may use the four Cs of trauma-informed care to better support patients and facilitate a meaningful evaluation (Table 19.1; American College of Obstetricians and Gynecologists' Committee on Health Care for Underserved Women, 2021).

Trauma-informed care promotes a safe environment for patients who are trauma survivors and provides considerations for staff and clinicians who may have experienced trauma in their lives. Patients, providers, and staff alike may experience stress reactions and symptoms because of exposure to another individual's traumatic experiences, commonly known as secondary trauma. Utilizing the four Cs of trauma-informed care can limit this distress.

DIFFERENTLY-ABLED

Providers may see a differently-abled person as asexual and ignore their natural urges and desires. This should not be. Recent literature has shown that physical disabilities associated with such conditions as multiple sclerosis, spinal cord injury, cerebral palsy, deafness, blindness, and arthritis lead to reduced sexual activity and satisfaction compared with levels before the disability and among the disability-free population (Mamali et al., 2020). Resources are widely available to individuals who have different physical capabilities. A consultation with a physical and/or occupational therapist may be warranted to examine the person's sexual needs and desires. Providers need to give their patients permission to engage in sexual activities and suggest new activities or techniques for them to have complete and satisfying sex lives (Yarber & Sayad, 2022).

Intellectual disability refers to a significant general impairment in intellectual functioning acquired during childhood, commonly described as scoring more than two standard deviations below the population mean on general intelligence tests (IQ <70). Research has shown that most young people with mild/moderate intellectual disabilities have had sexual intercourse by age 19 and are more likely to have unsafe sex; girls are likely to have been pregnant and become a mother (Baines et al., 2018). Within this population, if a person can provide consent, it is essential to debunk myths of enjoyable

TABLE 19.1 The Four Cs of Trauma-Informed Care

Calm	Pay attention to how you are feeling when you are caring for the patient. Breathe deeply and calm yourself to model and promote calmness for the patient, yourself, and your colleagues.
Contain	Limit trauma history detail to maintain emotional and physical safety. Invite the patient to share what changes would make visits more tolerable and healing. Normalize fear of returning to the healthcare setting if the triggering of a trauma response occurs.
Care	Emphasize self-care, compassion, and equity. The provider should continue to practice cultural humility.
Cope	Emphasize coping skills, positive relationships, and interventions that build resilience.

Source: Adapted from Kimberg, L., & Wheeler, M. (2019). Trauma and trauma-informed care. In M. Gerber (Ed.), Trauma-informed healthcare approaches *(pp. 25–56). Springer. https://doi.org/10.1007/978-3-030-04342-1_2*

sexual encounters and give education about one's body and physical response to sex, protection from STIs, and contraception methods. If the person cannot provide consent, sex education should be delivered in a way that the person can understand. Patients without the capacity to give consent should be referred to a mental health specialist for further evaluation. In cases such as these, abuse is a concern. Research has shown that the people at highest risk of abuse are institutionalized females, with the abuser being a peer with intellectual disability. Particular attention should be paid to early detection and intervention in high-risk situations (Tomsa et al., 2021).

Before performing a sensitive exam, such as examining female genitalia, the person should be asked if she prefers a chaperone. Informed consent and explanation of what is being performed before it is done are essential. Patients should be undressed from the waist down and covered to maintain modesty. The provider will only uncover if it is necessary for the exam. Instruct the patient to lie on their back on the table in the dorsal lithotomy position. The patient's buttocks should be at the edge of the table to better mobility of the speculum and better visualization. When performing an examination, start with examining external features of the anatomy, followed by the internal speculum examination. With every aspect of the physical exam, the provider should obtain consent and observe the patient for verbal and nonverbal communication. If a bimanual exam is warranted, again, obtain permission, describe the procedure, and inform the person of what is to be expected.

Laboratory Studies

Although no studies are specific to sexual assessment, laboratory studies are often indicated when dysfunction is suspected. Screening for STIs should be obtained if there is a risk of contracting an STI of all possible exposed areas (mouth, vagina, and rectum). Suppose the person presents with a history of purulent discharge, postcoital bleeding, or excessive discharge noted at the time of the physical examination. In that case, additional studies can be ordered to determine the etiology of the findings. If a bladder infection is suspected or if a person complains of dyspareunia, a clean-catch urine specimen for culture and sensitivity should be collected. Refer to Chapter 11 (Well Women's Health) for a more comprehensive review.

SEXUAL HEALTHCARE INTERVENTIONS

Framework for Intervention

A simple, but effective, framework for providing sexual healthcare interventions is the Permission, Limited Information, Specific Suggestions, and Intensive Therapy (PLISSIT) model developed by Jack Annon (1976). This approach, which many healthcare professionals use for sexual counseling, comprises four levels of intervention: PLISSIT. As the complexity of intervention levels increases, additional knowledge and skills are needed. All practitioners should be able to provide permission and limited information related to many of the sexual concerns of clients. All providers should be able to intervene at the specific suggestion level. Intensive therapy requires

special training and requires that the patient be referred to a licensed mental health professional who has extensive education and training in sex therapy in addition to mental health.

Permission is the first step when discussing a person's sexual concerns. The simple act of asking permission when talking about sexual functions conveys respect and sensitivity toward the patient. It gives the implicit message that it is permissible to discuss sexuality either now or in the future. This step involves giving the patient permission to express herself sexually and reassurance that her behaviors are "normal" or "okay" (Nusbaum & Hamilton, 2002). Permission is given if the behavior is realistic, is something both partners are comfortable with, involves no danger or coercion, or causes no harm. Permission involves answering questions about sexual fantasies, feelings, and dreams and may include permission for self-pleasuring (masturbation); initiation of sexual encounters; and the use of fantasy, erotica, and sexual aids such as oils, objects, or devices used to enhance one's sexual pleasure. Asking about the effect of developmental changes, illness, or lifestyle alterations on sexuality may be ways of permitting to be a sexual being throughout their life span. Permission giving is particularly helpful for patients who are anxious about their sexual adequacy or have a sexual dysfunction concern related to guilt over the enjoyment of sexual practices. Examples of interventions at this level are permission to be sexually aroused by normal feelings, engage in arousing activities such as masturbation and fantasizing, and have sexual intercourse as often as desired.

Limited Information serves the role of providing education and information about anatomy and physiology, the sexual response cycle, myths about relationships, life-cycle changes, and effects of illness on sexuality (Nusbaum & Hamilton, 2002). The information given at this level includes specific facts directly related to the sexual concern. This level of intervention helps change potentially negative thoughts and attitudes about particular areas of sexuality and refute sexual myths. Any information offered should be immediately relevant and limited in scope. To provide this level of sexual healthcare, providers need to be familiar with various sexual behaviors, norms, and forms of expression. This level is beneficial when women have a sexual knowledge deficit or anxiety associated with sexual misinformation.

The provider can offer *Specific Suggestions* if the patient responds positively. Specific suggestions provide additional information that the patient may or may not choose to use, although they do not "prescribe" sexual practices but offer suggestions that might improve one's sexual concern (Nusbaum & Hamilton, 2002). The recommendations do not need to be exotic, complex, or imaginative; usually, they are suggested based on the situation. Specific suggestions entail giving direct behavioral suggestions to relieve a sexual problem that is limited in scope or of brief duration. The provider and client agree on specific goals, and the clinician offers specific behavioral suggestions that are assessed at a follow-up visit.

Numerous suggestions can be made to clients, but they are always tailored to individual needs and situations. For example, the provider may suggest that many people find the side-lying position to be a pleasurable sexual position for the person who may have pain with deep penetration or for those who desire clitoral stimulation during coitus. Additional examples of specific suggestions are the use of a water-soluble lubricant or moisturizer to relieve vaginal dryness and prevent dyspareunia in postmenopausal persons, sensate focus exercises (mutual erotic stimulation excluding the genitals) to increase arousal, medication to treat vaginal infection, and alternative ways of sexual pleasure (e.g., oral–genital contact, mutual masturbation, cuddling, holding, massage) when traditional intercourse is not possible or undesired.

Providers should refer for *Intensive Therapy* if the sexual concerns are not fully addressed after offering limited information and specific suggestions and when the problem interferes with sexual expression. This level of intervention is the most complex and should be provided only by professionals with advanced training in sexual counseling and therapy. Referral to a sex therapist for further assistance is often the appropriate intervention.

To understand your patient's sexual health, determine the frequency of STI/HIV screenings, vaccinations, and/or medications; and guidance counseling, questions from the CDC's five Ps of sexual history taking (Partners, Practices, Past history of STI[s], Protection, and Pregnancy Prevention/Reproductive Life Plan) has been expanded to include a sixth P (Plus), as well as Pleasure, Problems, and Pride, developed by National Coalition for Sexual Health's Health Care (NCSH; Reno et al., n. d.). The addition of the sixth P allowed an opportunity to explore sexual satisfaction, functioning, concerns, and support for one's gender identity and sexual orientation. The National Coalition for Sexual Health has a variety of free, user-friendly resources for providers to decrease barriers to competent, appropriate sexual care (nationalcoalitionforsexualhealth.org/tools/for-healthcare-providers).

SEXUAL HEALTH CHALLENGES

Many health-related factors can affect sexual health. Experiencing illness and/or living with specific pathologies, prior surgery, challenges in performing activities of daily living, and using medications (prescription, nonprescription, and herbal supplements) can impact sexual health. Many medications can alter sexual functioning and cause sexual dysfunctions, including decreased sexual desire, lack of sexual arousal, inadequate lubrication, and delayed or absent orgasm. Depending on the dosage and the individual's mental and physical state, some medications known to inhibit sexual function may also enhance it. Sexual dysfunction can occur with the use of substances such as alcohol, amphetamines, cocaine, opioids, sedatives, and tranquilizers (Teets, 1990). Substance use and abuse can have an adverse effect on sexual functioning and sexuality. Advertisements and social media images continue to present provocatively clothed women drinking, leading to the belief that alcohol and sex usually go together. The belief that alcohol is a sexual enhancement product is also a popular myth. Alcohol leads to disinhibition, causes decreased lubrication, dulls stimulation, and contributes to sexual risk-taking. Like alcohol use, most recreational drugs interfere with libido and sexual functioning, making it difficult to achieve an orgasm. Drug use has been linked to a greater risk of acquiring STIs, including HIV. Addiction to various drugs, such as cocaine, increases the risk of bartering sex for drugs (Yarber & Sayad, 2022).

The CDC (2021) estimates approximately 26 million new STI infections each year, with the cost estimated to be as much as $16 billion annually. Risk factors for STIs include not using condoms, using drugs or alcohol before intercourse, having multiple sex partners, and having concurrent partners. It is essential to recognize that STIs are prevalent in persons AFAB regardless of their sexual orientation (Lindley et al., 2013). Research has shown that STIs (especially genital herpes and human papillomavirus [HPV]) often have a negative impact on a person's sexuality. An STI diagnosis has been shown to strongly influence feelings of sexuality and desirability (Newton & McCabe, 2008). AFAB people with genital herpes and HPV are more sexually anxious, more afraid of sex, more concerned about the impression created by their sexuality, and more sexually depressed than those without an STI. Individuals may decide to be celibate to avoid risk, choose to decrease the number of their partners or avoid certain partners, and change or avoid specific sexual activities that increase risk. Additionally, these individuals are less sexually satisfied, have lower self-esteem, and have a negative sexual self-concept. For a more comprehensive review of the adoption of safer sex practices, refer to Chapter 30, Sexually Transmitted Infections.

Relationship Issues

Research has shown that love in conjunction with social rewards, intimacy, commitment, and equity is an important determinant of sexual satisfaction. Communication is the thread that ties sexuality and intimacy. The quality of the communication affects the quality of the relationship, which affects the quality of sex. Sex often serves as the barometer of the relationship: Good relationships consist of satisfying sex, whereas bad relationships tend to consist of unsatisfying sex (Yarber & Sayad, 2022). Sexual communication difficulties can be exacerbated by distrust, feelings of betrayal, and fear of disease when sex has occurred outside a committed relationship. Sexual dysfunction in one partner may precipitate dysfunction in the other partner; for example, erectile difficulty is sometimes accompanied by lack of vaginal lubrication, orgasmic difficulties, and impaired desire disorders in a partner.

Loss of a Partner

Loss of a partner can adversely affect opportunities for intimacy and sexual expression. Some people define their identity through their relationships; thus, losing a partner can create a loss of the sense of self. Furthermore, the typical image of a widow is that of a person who is grieving, implying that their sexual life has ended. Factors related to one's sexuality after the loss of a partner are extramarital sexual experiences, age, and sexual satisfaction in the marriage (Bernhard, 1995). Remarriage is correlated with age. As a person ages, it becomes less likely they will remarry.

SEXUAL DYSFUNCTIONS

Female sexual dysfunction (FDS) describes various sexual problems associated with decreased arousal or desire, difficulty with orgasm, and dyspareunia or sexual pain (Shifren et al., 2008). Sexual dysfunction in women dramatically impacts the quality of life, self-esteem, body image, and interpersonal relationships. Sexual dysfunction is mainly underdiagnosed and undertreated. Practitioners are frequently limited in the time available to assess sexual problems and understand the multifactorial nature of sexuality and appropriate treatment options for dysfunction. Although many are reluctant to discuss sexual issues, as awareness increases in society, people become more comfortable opening up about their sexual difficulties and seeking treatment. The ability of clinicians to have a comprehensive understanding of the evaluation and current diagnostic classification of FSD is essential to the comprehensive care of women (Latif & Diamond, 2013).

Research on FSD documents that sexual dysfunction is a common condition and concern among women in the United States. In a national probability survey of 1,749 women, the U.S. National Health and Social Life Survey estimated that 43% of women reported sexual dysfunction (Laumann et al., 1999; Waite et al., 2009). This survey noted a strong association between sexual problems and decreased emotional satisfaction, physical satisfaction, and overall life satisfaction. More recent data from a large cross-sectional population-based study of 31,581 female adults age 18 years and older in the United States, the Prevalence of Female Sexual Problems Associated with Distress and Determinants of Treatment Seeking (PRESIDE) study, evaluated the self-reported sexual problems of desire, arousal, and orgasm. Data from this study support earlier research that sexual problems are common among women, with the prevalence of reported sexual problems at 44.2% (Shifren et al., 2008). The most common sexual problem was low desire, with a prevalence of 38.7%, followed by low arousal at 26.1% and difficulty with orgasm at 20.5%. The majority of sexual problems increased with age, with 27.2% of women ages 18 to 44 years compared with 44.6% of middle-aged women and 80.1% of older women reporting any sexual dysfunction. It should be noted that these statistics may be misleading, as the criteria used to assess these data are not those currently used to diagnose sexual dysfunction (Latif & Diamond, 2013).

There is considerable variation in how women rate the importance of sex, their optimal sexual frequencies, preferred sexual practices, and the amount of stimulation they require for arousal and satisfaction. It is important to note that although many women report sexual dysfunction, this problem causes actual distress in only a small percentage. The PRESIDE study also evaluated the prevalence of personal distress associated with sexual problems. Although more recent studies have reported increased levels of sexually related personal distress, PRESIDE noted it in just 12% of women. Distress was lowest in women age 65 years and older (8.9%), intermediate in those age 18 to 44 years (10.8%), and highest in those age 45 to 64 years (14.8%). It is crucial to correlate distressing sexual problems with factors such as age, current partner/marital status, poor self-assessed health, current anxiety or depression, menopause (natural and surgical) status, and a history of urinary incontinence or other issues (Shifren et al., 2008).

Dyspareunia

Dyspareunia is recurrent or persistent and distressing genital pain with sexual intercourse. Dyspareunia may be superficial, causing pain with attempted vaginal insertion or deep vaginal insertion. Women with dyspareunia are at increased risk of sexual dysfunction, relationship problems, diminished quality of life, anxiety, and depression. It has been reported that women who suffer from deep dyspareunia are less fulfilled and relaxed after sex, have a limited number of intercourse episodes per week, have fewer satisfying orgasms, and often avoid sexual contact and refuse sexual advances in an attempt to avoid or reduce pain (Ferraro et al., 2008; Hill & Taylor, 2021; Sadownik, 2014). Women with vestibulodynia—chronic discomfort that occurs in the area around the opening of the vagina, inside the inner lips of the vulva—also report decreased sexual interest, arousal, satisfaction, and self-esteem. Women with this type of sexual dysfunction can be less relaxed as well as less fulfilled after sex, have a limited number of intercourse episodes per week, have fewer satisfying orgasms, and often avoid sexual contact and refuse a partner's sexual advances in an attempt to avoid or reduce pain (Ferraro et al., 2008; Sadownik, 2014).

Partners of those experiencing dyspareunia often feel that physical intimacy becomes an unwelcome physical and emotional challenge (van Lankveld et al., 2010). This often leads to them feeling helpless, angry, and depressed. They believe their partner avoids sex for reasons beyond pain and feel rejected (Goldstein et al., 2011). Therefore, such couples must discover other ways to be intimate. They must learn that sex involves more than just intercourse and that communicating is a necessary part of a sexual relationship, especially when pain is involved (Goldstein et al., 2011).

Dyspareunia also exhibits a profound impact on one's psychological status. Unfortunately, even when dyspareunia is resolved, the psychological dysfunction often persists (Goldstein & Burrows, 2008). Although sexual pain is one of the most common complaints in the gynecologic setting, it is never normal. Dyspareunia is often a symptom of a complex multitude of disease states that are poorly understood. In addition, women complaining of sexual pain often have multiple related conditions, further exacerbating their pain and complicating the diagnosis (Steege & Zolnoun, 2009). Providers must assess for dyspareunia in their practice in that many of these conditions are progressive and detrimental to one's life.

Assessing for sexual dysfunction or sexual pain should include a thorough evaluation of the pain (in terms of its quality, quantity, location, duration, and aggravating and relieving factors). A complete medical, surgical, obstetric, gynecologic, and contraceptive history should be collected and include questions about previous vaginal or pelvic surgeries and pelvic trauma such as rape and sexual abuse. The patient should always be questioned about the use of medications, douching, and perineal products such as sprays, deodorants, and sanitary pads. Furthermore, various validated questionnaires have been developed to assess sexual dysfunction and assist the clinician in establishing a diagnosis. The Brief Sexual Symptoms Checklist for Women (Figure 19.1; Hatzichristou et al., 2010) is a valuable self-report tool in the primary care setting. It consists of four basic questions regarding the patient's satisfaction with their sexual function, details about specific sexual problems, and willingness to discuss them with a provider.

Please answer the following questions about your overall sexual function:

1. Are you satisfied with your sexual function? ❏ Yes ❏ No

If no, please continue.

2. How long have you been dissatisfied with your sexual function? _____

3. Mark which of the following problems you are having, and circle the one that is most bothersome:
   - ❏ Little or no interest in sex
   - ❏ Decreased genital sensation (feeling)
   - ❏ Decreased vaginal lubrication (dryness)
   - ❏ Problem reaching orgasm
   - ❏ Pain during sex
   - ❏ Other: _____

4. Would you like to talk about it with your clinician? ❏ Yes ❏ No

FIGURE 19.1 Brief sexual symptoms checklist.
Source: Adapted from Hatzichristou, D., Rosen, R. C., Derogatis, L. R., Low, W. Y., Meuleman, E. J., Sadovsky, R., & Symonds, T. (2010). Recommendations for the clinical evaluation of men and women with sexual dysfunction. Journal of Sexual Medicine, 7(1 Pt. 2), 337–348. https:// doi.org/10.1111/j.1743-6109.2009.01619.x

Genitourinary Syndrome of Menopause/Vulvovaginal Atrophy

Vulvovaginal atrophy (VVA) in menopause related to declining estrogen levels is common and is a frequent cause of sexual dysfunction and pain in this population. Loss of estrogen results in thinning of the vaginal epithelium, loss of collagen, and decreased blood flow in the tissue, leading to reduced lubrication, shortening and narrowing of the vaginal wall, and pale, dry mucosa. Because of the decreased genital perfusion, estrogen deficiency prolongs the time to vaginal vasocongestion, thus contributing to reduced intensity of orgasm (Palacios et al., 2018). VVA is also termed *genitourinary symptom of menopause* (GSM) because estrogen deficiency can affect both the genital system and the lower urinary tract. The initial symptom is often a lack of lubrication during intercourse. Eventually, persistent vaginal dryness may occur. Thinning of the epithelial lining may also cause pruritus, soreness, and stinging pain in the vaginal and vulvar area, which, in turn, may further contribute to dyspareunia. Vaginal spotting, due to small tears in the vaginal epithelium, may also occur. VVA often reports urgency, frequency, nocturia, and urge incontinence symptoms. Urinalysis may show microscopic hematuria. Recurrent urinary tract infections can also result (Mac Bride et al., 2010).

Approximately half of postmenopausal women in the United States report symptoms of VVA, which causes a significant negative effect on the quality of life. Menopausal symptoms, such as hot flashes, typically resolve over time, whereas the symptoms of VVA usually persist or increase without treatment (Portman et al., 2014). Although atrophy-related symptoms are common, only approximately half seek medical care or are offered help by their healthcare provider (Rahn et al., 2014).

Treatment of VVA seeks to restore the vagina and genital tissue to a healthier state and aims to alleviate symptoms associated with estrogen deficiency. Nonhormonal treatments that are available over the counter include vaginal moisturizers, which are water based, are available as liquids, gels, or ovules inserted every few days. Vaginal moisturizers can be safely used long term, but they need to be used regularly for optimal effect. Hormonal treatments such as low-dose vaginal estrogen are available (Mac Bride et al., 2010). Although systemic estrogen effectively treats vasomotor symptoms, studies have shown it to provide adequate relief of vaginal dryness in only 40% of women (Portman et al., 2014). Local vaginal estrogen is available in a vaginal cream, ring, or tablet; the vaginal estrogen cream Premarin is also indicated to treat moderate to severe dyspareunia. Local vaginal estrogen cream has been shown to decrease vaginal pH, increase vaginal blood flow and lubrication; improve arousal, orgasm, and sexual satisfaction; and reduce vaginal dryness, pain, and dyspareunia (Simon, 2011). Ospemifene (Osphena) is the first nonhormonal oral alternative to estrogen to treat VVA and dyspareunia. It is a selective estrogen receptor modulator (SERM) that exerts agonist effects on the vulvovaginal tissue and has been shown to significantly reduce vaginal dryness and dyspareunia symptoms. Osphemifene is a safe and effective option for the treatment of postmenopausal VVA to treat moderate to severe dyspareunia (Portman et al., 2014).

FUTURE DIRECTIONS

When patients express concerns regarding sexuality and sexual activity, they have the right to expect that APRNs will provide accurate sexual information, counseling, and/or appropriate therapy. This chapter provides an overview of sexual health and sexual dysfunction and a basis for nurse practitioners to assess concerns about sexual health, provide sexual healthcare, and make appropriate referrals for their care. Future directions should allow providers to reframe and expand one's clinical thinking regarding women's health from a binary term to a nonbinary standpoint. When providers hyperfocus on the term *women's health*, opportunities may be missed to appropriately screen and manage people who may or may not have typical female anatomy. With the increase of people discovering their gender fluidity, providers must establish a safe and welcoming environment to express one's sexual identity, expression, and anatomy present for the appropriate evaluation. Providing this inclusivity promotes individualized evaluation required to have the person live their best life.

REFERENCES

References for this chapter are online and available at https://connect.springerpub.com/content/book/978-0-8261-6722-4/part/part02/chapter/ch19

CHAPTER 20

Primary Care of Lesbian, Gay, and Bisexual Individuals*

KATHRYN S. TIERNEY

There is an ongoing effort to better understand the specific healthcare needs of lesbian, gay, and bisexual (LGB) people. LGB people experience health disparities at a higher rate than the general population (Lunn et al., 2017). These disparities exist, not because of inherent differences in people who identify as LGB, but because of external factors such as minority stress and stigmatization, and lack of healthcare provider (HCP) knowledge. Insufficient education in nursing and medical schools, inadequate data collection and research, and lack of understanding of the specific healthcare needs of LGB people continue to be barriers to care in this group. *Healthy People 2030*, which outlines areas of focus to reduce healthcare disparities in the United States, as well as ongoing academic research, aims to improve the health and well-being of LGB people (Office of Disease Prevention and Health Promotion [ODPHP], n.d.). This chapter focuses on what is known about the health of LGB persons and suggests strategies for providing evidence-based care to this population. For information on how to care for transgender and nonbinary people, please see Chapter 25, Caring for the Transgender and Gender Nonbinary Patient.

REVIEW OF TOPIC

LGB persons live in almost every, if not every, county in the United States and represent people from all ethnic backgrounds, socioeconomic statuses, and ages. The most recent estimates suggest that there are at least 646,000 same-sex U.S. households (U.S. Census Bureau, 2011) and that approximately 3.5% (Gates, 2011) of the U.S. population identifies as LGB. It is believed that a higher percentage of people have attraction to or engage in same-gender sexual behaviors but do not identify as gay, lesbian, or bisexual, and thus may not be counted in official demographic reports (Gates, 2011). Table 20.1 lists various ways to categorize sexual orientation. This is not an exhaustive list and nurse practitioners (NPs) should ask patients to self-describe their sexual orientation and should use the wording provided by the patient. The use of *LGB* in this chapter is meant to encompass anyone who does not identify as heterosexual. It is important to note that sexual orientation is a label or identity based on the genders of the people involved, and that one cannot assume the genitalia of the patient based on sexual orientation or romantic interest.

NPs need to be proactive about asking patients about their sexual orientation and sexual relationships in order to tailor healthcare based on personal risk factors. Open-ended questions regarding sexual orientation and relationships allow the NP to address specific risk factors as well as incorporate what is known about population level health disparities to provide appropriate care.

ETIOLOGY

There is no known genetic, social, or hormonal etiology for determining an individual's sexual orientation. As with many human traits, development of sexual orientation is likely influenced both by biological factors and environmental circumstances. Identifying as LGB is not a medical disorder, and as such, the etiology or reason for identifying as LGB is important only as it relates to determining specific risk factors and supporting patients.

RISK FACTORS

Identifying as LGB or having same-gender romantic or sexual attraction is not a risk factor for any health issue. NPs need to be cognizant of population-level health issues that

---

*This chapter is a revision of the chapter that appeared in the second edition of this textbook, coauthored with Caroline Dorsen, whom we thank for her original contribution.

TABLE 20.1 Sexual Orientation Vocabulary

TERM	DEFINITION
Gay (sometimes called homosexual)	Relationship between people of the same gender or sex
Lesbian	Relationship between people who identify as female
Bisexual	Romantic or sexual interest in both male- and female-identified people regardless of the person's own gender identity
Straight or heterosexual	Relationship between two people of the opposite sex or gender
Asexual	A person with reduced or lack of sexual interest or desire
Aromantic	A person who has no interest in or desire for romantic relationships
Polyamorous	A person with interest in romantic or sexual relationships with more than one person concurrently

disproportionately affect LGB persons, as well as individual risk factors that may place patients at greater risk than their heterosexual counterparts. LGB health can be considered from the development/population perspective (i.e., what are the pressing issues for LGB youth or elders) or health risk perspective (i.e., what health risks are important to identify for this person related to behavior, socioeconomical status, and family history). An understanding of these perspectives allows NPs to explore the complexities of LGB health and translate this knowledge to direct patient care. A more detailed look at the health risks particular to each age group is outlined and suggestions for reducing those risks are reviewed later in this chapter.

Fear of negative interactions with healthcare providers (HCPs) or frank discrimination may decrease access to and use of healthcare services, including preventive care services and chronic disease management. Similarly, lack of provider knowledge about LGB health disparities and how being part of the LGB community may affect health can translate to a lack of individualized and culturally competent care. HCPs, including clinicians and NPs, often receive little or no training regarding LGB healthcare (Lim et al., 2015). NPs are encouraged to read evidence-based literature and seek out continuing education opportunities to support ongoing knowledge building on how to best care for people in this population.

DIAGNOSTIC CRITERIA

Homosexuality was considered pathologic and was included in the first edition of the *Diagnostic and Statistical Manual of Mental Disorders* (*DSM-I*, 1952) of the American Psychiatric Association until 1973. Many older LGB people may remember a time when their sexual orientation was considered pathologic. While advances have been made in addressing inequalities in healthcare for LGB people, many still experience discrimination, both at the personal and population levels, because of their sexual orientation (Casey et al., 2019).

Major health organizations and LGB advocacy groups, such as the Fenway Institute, recommend that HCPs ask all patients basic questions about their sexual orientation during routine assessments (Box 20.1). Knowing this information

Box 20.1 Sample Conversation to Assess Sexual Orientation and Sexual Activity

Are you sexually active? Do you have a regular partner? *Sexual health screening is a key assessment for all individuals.*

How do you identify sexually? What is your sexual orientation? *If the person does not understand, provide options such as, "Do you identify as straight, gay, lesbian, bisexual, or something else?"*

In order to know which screenings would benefit you, can you tell me with whom you have sex? What parts of your body do you use when having sex? How do your partners identify their gender and sexual orientation? *If the person does not understand, provide options such as, "Do you have sex with women, men, both? Are your partners cisgender? Do you participate in oral sex (receptive/insertive), oral–vaginal contact, oral–anal contact, anal sex (receptive/insertive), vaginal sex (receptive/insertive)? Do you use shared sex toys or have any type of genital-to-genital contact?" Note: For individuals who identify as transgender, it may be important to first ask about "triggering" labels for body parts; for example, an individual who identifies as transgender male may prefer to use the term* frontal canal *instead of vagina and may find that the term* vagina *triggers feelings of gender dysphoria. Reflecting preferred labels or terms within sexual health history questions is most appropriate.*

Are you in a relationship? *Not all people who are sexually active, even with regular partners, are in a relationship, and a relationship is not always exclusively between two people.*

Is your relationship open or closed? *Some relationships have consensual agreements that partners have other sexual partners outside the relationship. Some relationships are between multiple people, rather than two.*

Are you satisfied with your sexual function? *Key assessment for all individuals.*

How do you protect yourself from sexually transmitted infections (STIs)? *If using barrier protection such as condoms ask, "Do you wear protection 100% of the time? Are barriers used for oral–genital contact?"*

When was the last time you had STI screening? *Key assessment related to sexual health for all individuals.*

Do you use drugs or alcohol when having sex? Do you exchange sex for money, drugs, or a place to stay? *These questions are intended to identify behaviors and situations that increase risks to health and well-being.*

Do you desire to have biological children? Do you desire pregnancy? *For transgender patients, also ask if they desire to have preserved fertility, such as cryopreservation of sperm and eggs, prior to starting hormonal or surgical transition. This issue is especially complicated in individuals on puberty blockers as they are never exposed to natal hormones necessary for gamete development.*

Have you felt isolated, trapped, or like you are walking on eggshells in an intimate relationship? Has someone pressured or forced you to do something sexual that you didn't want to do? Has someone hit, kicked, punched, or otherwise hurt you? *Screen for intimate partner violence, as well as past and/or current history of physical, sexual, emotional, economic, or verbal abuse.*

about every patient allows HCPs to tailor episodic and ongoing medical care according to the specific risks and needs of the patient, as well as open a dialogue about whether previous negative interactions with HCPs have influenced the patient's access to, and receipt of, medical care. This also helps to build trust with patient populations who have experienced discrimination and stigma in medical settings, which will allow for a more open, comfortable, and affirming patient/HCP relationship. NPs should respect patient choices and assess patients based on risk behaviors and risk factors, rather than on identity labels.

ASSESSMENT

LGB Youth

Although some LGB adolescents live in supportive environments and experience the normal challenges of the teen years, research suggests that LGB teens may experience increased rates of bullying and violence; substance abuse; depression, anxiety, and suicidality; higher risk sexual behavior; and homelessness compared with the general adolescent population

(Hafeez et al., 2017). NPs should be aware that some of these risk factors are ameliorated by the support of parents and/or other influential adults, including teachers and HCPs (Kaczkowski et al., 2022). Asking youth about issues related to their sexual orientation, and providing them with a safe space to discuss their concerns, is an essential role for NPs.

LGB in Midlife

During midlife, issues related to accessing preventive care and chronic disease management, having relationships (including marriage equality), and becoming and being parents figure prominently for some LGB persons. NPs can support midlife LGB patients by asking them about their family structure, recognizing that the definition of family for many LGB persons may be based on biology or on "family of choice" in whatever constellation they identify. NPs must be sensitive to the possibility of previous stigma and discrimination and the way that this history might affect accessing and receiving healthcare services.

LGB Older Adults

Many of the same concerns of older age that affect LGB persons also affect the general population; these include financial issues, long-term care decisions, and end-of-life issues. However, many concerns may be amplified in LGB populations, including issues related to social isolation caused by rejection by, or disengagement with, families of origin. There are also some institutional concerns unique to this population. Acute care institutions, such as hospitals, have historically limited LGB people from visiting and making healthcare decisions for their loved ones. Since 2011, all hospitals receiving federal funds must allow the patient to designate their visitors without restriction. There are currently no antidiscrimination requirements for outpatient centers. Some older LGB persons may still be hesitant to identify as LGB while hospitalized or in long-term care environments because of fear of discrimination. The Supreme Court decision legalizing same-sex marriage in the United States inherently provides same-gender spouses certain rights and improves some aspects of health, including the ability to direct medical decision-making and access to healthcare.

GUIDELINES FOR HEALTH PROMOTION

Sexually Transmitted Infections and Sexual Behavior

Risk for sexually transmitted infections (STIs) depends not on a patient's self-identified sexual orientation, but rather on individual patient behaviors. Using open-ended questions and allowing patients to self-describe their sexual activity will help the NP provide appropriate screening and education and avoid unnecessary testing. Particular attention should be paid to finding out from the patient what words they use to describe their body parts and how they use them for intimacy, as well as safer sex practices. See Chapter 30, Sexually Transmitted Infections, and Chapter 32, Human Papillomavirus.

Depression, Anxiety, and Suicidality

LGB persons across the life span often have increased rates of depression, anxiety, and suicidality than their heterosexual counterparts (Gmelin et al., 2022). NPs should be aware of increased risk of mental health concerns and use validated tools, such as the PHQ-2, PHQ-9, or Geriatric Depression Scale, to screen all clients, keeping in mind that these scales were not developed for or validated in the LGB population specifically. Prompt referral to LGB-affirming mental health-care is of absolute importance. Lists of LGB and LGB ally providers are available online, such as the database provided by the Gay and Lesbian Medical Association (www.GLMA.org). Educating HCPs, including mental health specialists; creating awareness in school systems and communities; and using available online tools to reach isolated persons are all ways to increase access to care and decrease stigma (Committee on Lesbian, Gay, Bisexual and Transgender Health Issues and Research Gaps and Opportunitieset al., 2011). NPs can help reach clients who are battling depression and anxiety by creating a safe space in their offices with signs to alert LGB clients they are LGB allies, educating staff, asking open-ended questions regarding feelings of depression and anxiety, and providing appropriate referrals to mental health specialists. See Chapter 40, Mental Health Challenges.

Cancer and Cardiovascular Disease

Identifying as LGB does not inherently increase risk for cancer or cardiovascular disease (CVD). It is essential to recognize that some of the risk factors for CVD and cancer, such as tobacco use, alcohol use, and decreased access to care, may be higher for LGB individuals than the general population. LGB persons may have lower rates of early detection via screening and diagnostic tests and may not receive care until late in the course of the disease (Fredriksen-Goldsen et al., 2013). NPs should follow the same national guidelines for CVD and cancer screening for LGB patients as in all other individuals. See Chapter 43, Cardiovascular Disease in Women.

Overweight and Obesity

Lesbians and bisexual cisgender women are more likely to be overweight or obese compared to their heterosexual counterparts (Azagba et al., 2019). Weight and weight management in the United States is a complicated topic that, when addressed in the healthcare space, needs to take into account risk for food insecurity and lack of affirming or affordable exercise options. See Chapter 13, Nutrition for Women.

Substance Abuse, Including Alcohol, Tobacco, and Drugs

Rates of tobacco, alcohol, and substance abuse appear to be higher in the LGB population compared with the heterosexual population (Felner et al., 2021). As with all patients, LGB persons should be screened for substance abuse and culturally competent care and resources for treatment should be offered. See Chapter 41, Substance Abuse and Women.

Trauma and Violence

LGB persons are at an increased risk for hate crimes and violence compared with the general population. The risk can be as much as two to nine times higher than for their heterosexual counterparts (Bender & Lauritsen, 2021). Questions regarding safety at home and school or the workplace should be part of routine primary care screening at all ages and for all patients, LGB and non-LGB patients alike. See Chapter 42, Gender-Based Violence and Women's Health.

INTERVENTIONS AND STRATEGIES FOR RISK REDUCTION

NPs must use existing health-promotion guidelines established for all adolescents and adults and tailor them to individual clients, with a clear understanding of individual risk-taking behaviors, along with an understanding of population-level health inequities. For example, a nuanced understanding of some of the causes of decreased utilization of preventive care services by LGB persons can aid NPs in communicating with clients about why preventive services are important to use and troubleshoot how to access them in a way that is comfortable and safe for the individual. Likewise, an understanding of structural issues that create barriers to care, such as decreased rates of health insurance among LGB persons, can inform NPs' work with clients and other providers, such as social workers, to facilitate access to, and use of, health services.

FUTURE DIRECTIONS

As cultural acceptance progresses and more HCPs are educated in the particular needs of the LGB population, the health of the community will improve. NPs can help improve the health of LGB persons by providing a safe space in which they can explore health promotion and educating their peers about current resources. Simply having pamphlets or posters in the waiting room that picture LGB individuals and asking clients about their sexual identities in a nonjudgmental way will indicate to LGB patients that they are welcome in a practice. In addition to this, it is essential to follow evidence-based practices of and continually seek out education on clinical care specific to this population.

REFERENCES

References for this chapter are online and available at https://connect.springerpub.com/content/book/978-0-8261-6722-4/part/part02/chapter/ch20

CHAPTER 21

Fertility Self-Management and Shared Management

RICHARD M. PRIOR, HEATHER C. KATZ, AND LESLIE L. BALCAZAR DE MARTINEZ*

The journey that led to the development of highly effective, safe, reliable, affordable, and well-tolerated contraceptive options for women has been long and challenging, and is ongoing. The result, however, has been nothing short of a renaissance. By allowing women to control their sexuality and decisions to procreate, they have enjoyed greater freedom to pursue family, economic, and personal goals. An astute provider must gain an understanding of the variables that influence a woman's contraception decisions, her past medical history, and her personal risk factors in order to appropriately filter through the available contraceptive options and provide her the best possible contraceptive solutions. In this chapter, we discuss the variables that contribute to individual choice and the natural, hormonal, barrier, and sterilization contraceptive methods that are widely available in the United States.

HISTORICAL AND SOCIAL CONTEXT

No scientific breakthrough has altered as many women's lives so momentously as the development of safe, effective methods for fertility control. Before these methods were available, women suffered chronic illness, fatigue, and even death from unpreventable pregnancy (Cooke & Dworkin, 1979). Multiple pregnancies and unspaced births not only affect women's physical health negatively, but also reduce their economic productivity, leading to increased dependence on others and unfulfilled human potential.

Today, a sexually active woman can affect her physical, educational, socioeconomic destiny—and that of her family and significant others and partners—by choosing to use or not to use contraception. By using a highly effective contraceptive method, she reduces the risk of unplanned pregnancy, which enables her to plan her family along with other aspects of her life. When a woman is able to control her fertility, she gains the opportunity to plan and limit family size or to remain childless.

The ability to prevent or defer childbearing allows a woman to pursue educational opportunities and participate in the labor force. A woman's knowledge that she can, if she wishes, control her childbearing, and society's understanding that women can do so, may broaden her outlook when she considers other life opportunities. Because a planned birth can be integrated into a woman's career or job more readily than an unplanned birth, a planned birth has fewer negative effects on her employment or education. Some women use contraceptive methods successfully to take advantage of educational and employment opportunities. Others are not as successful. Instead, they learn by experience that few events change a woman's life as much as the fear of conception or the reality of an unintended pregnancy.

Margaret Sanger and the Birth Control Movement

In the latter years of the Victorian age, an individual was born who would create a new episode in the contraception drama for U.S. women. Margaret Louise Higgins Sanger, born in Corning, New York, in 1879, dedicated herself to this work after seeing her mother die from tuberculosis and the burden of bearing 11 children and after observing women in New York's Lower East Side die from childbirth or illegal abortions. In 1902, she completed nursing school at White Plains Hospital in New York. Inspired by Emma Goldman, the first nurse to lecture on birth control in the United States, in 1912, Sanger began to publish information about women's

The opinions and assertions expressed herein are those of the author(s) and do not necessarily reflect the official policy or position of the U.S. Air Force, Department of Defense, or the U.S government.

reproductive concerns. Her first efforts were a series of articles describing puberty and the functions of a woman's body for the *Call,* a socialist newspaper (Gordon, 1990). These articles were the basis for *What Every Girl Should Know,* a pamphlet published in 1915 and later published as a book (Sanger, 1920a). The first issue of *The Woman Rebel* was published in March 1914. In the same year, Sanger prepared the pamphlet *Family Limitation* and organized a committee called the *National Birth Control League.* She fled to England in October 1914 to avoid prosecution for violating the Comstock Law; federal legislation prohibiting the mailing of obscene material, which included birth control information and devices (Tannahill, 1980). In England, Sanger met C. V. Drysdale, head of the international birth control movement, and Havelock Ellis, author of *Studies in the Psychology of Sex.* An unfortunate consequence of these meetings was Sanger's introduction to the eugenics movement. That association was to affect views of Sanger's work throughout her life. From England, Sanger went to Holland, where she learned how to fit "pessaries," now known as contraceptive diaphragms, and studied that country's birth control clinic system.

On October 16, 1916, Sanger and her sister Ethel opened the Brownsville Clinic in Brooklyn, New York—America's first birth control clinic. The clinic provided birth control information and education, although both were illegal at the time. From 1916 to 1934, Sanger established birth control clinics, published birth control articles and pamphlets in defiance of the Comstock Law, worked to change birth control laws, organized the American Birth Control League (1921), attended national and international conferences on birth control, lectured around the world, and was jailed more than once for her activities. In 1922, she engaged Dorothy Bocker to run the Clinical Research Bureau. The next year, she hired James F. Cooper to lecture to physicians across the United States about birth control. She smuggled pessaries into the United States through her husband's factory in Canada until 1925, when she convinced two of her supporters to establish the Holland Rantos Company and begin U.S. production. In 1926, she traveled to London, Paris, and Geneva to prepare for a 1927 international meeting, which led to the formation of the International Union for the Scientific Investigation of Population Problems (Himes, 1936). In 1928, she resigned as president of the American Birth Control League but continued to edit the *Birth Control Review* until 1929, when she withdrew from the league and the paper. In April that year, police raided the Clinical Research Bureau, because this research was also considered in violation of the Comstock Law, but Sanger did not give up.

The 1930s brought some victories for the birth control movement. In the summer of 1930, the Seventh International Birth Control Conference was held under Sanger's leadership. In 1934, Sanger went to Russia to gather data about the birth control movement there. The next year, she attended the All India Women's Conference, met Mohandas Karamchand (Mahatma) Gandhi, and gave 64 lectures across India. The U.S. Congress finally revised the Comstock Act in 1936, redefining obscenity to exclude birth control information and devices; 1 year later, the American Medical Association resolved that contraception was a legitimate medical service. By 1938, more than 300 clinics were in operation in the United States. In 1939, the American Birth Control League and

the Voluntary Parenthood League merged and named Sanger honorary president of what is now Planned Parenthood.

Throughout the 1930s, Sanger continued to promote birth control. In 1952, she persuaded Katherine McCormick, widow of the founder of International Harvester, to fund the research that produced the oral contraceptive (OC). She also traveled to India to help organize the International Planned Parenthood Federation; the next year in Stockholm, Sanger was elected president of this organization. In 1959, the 80-year-old Sanger attended the International Conference on Population in New Delhi, where she met Prime Minister Nehru. She died in 1966, in Tucson, Arizona (Douglas, 1970; Gordon, 1990; Gray, 1979; Lader, 1955; Marlow, 1979; Sanger, 1920b, 1931, 1938; Sicherman et al., 1980).

The New Feminism

Although Sanger was establishing birth control clinics, other U.S. women were working to obtain the right to vote, which they finally gained with the passage of the 19th Amendment in 1920 (Kerber & De Hart, 1995). The suffrage movement reflected women's growing opportunities for paid employment in nursing, teaching, offices, factories, and other fields.

During this period, some advocates saw birth control as a tool, not only for limiting pregnancies, but also promoting social revolution. They believed the solution for many social ills lay in population control (Gordon, 1990). Thus, most birth control advocates were social radicals; some were also socialists or political radicals. After World War I, women returned to work in the home and the birth control movement changed considerably. As healthcare professionals made birth control an integral part of their practices, they moved it into the mainstream of society. Birth control, which had begun as a radical social movement, shifted decisively into the medical arena, ensuring medical control of contraception (Gordon, 1990).

Recent efforts of feminists to wrest control of reproduction from the hands of medicine have their roots in the birth control movement of the 1920s and 1930s. In 2015, in the United States, the most effective means of contraception—intrauterine devices (IUDs), OCs, hormonal implants, rings, patches, and injectables—remain under physician control. As clinical nurse specialists, nurse practitioners, nurse-midwives, and physician assistants gained prescriptive authority, control of these methods passed to healthcare professionals other than physicians and into the hands of more women.

Sexual Beliefs and Practices

From the time when the *Kinsey Report* (Kinsey et al., 1953) revealed that some women masturbated, had premarital sexual experiences, and were orgasmic, the U.S. public has lived through: (a) the baby boom of the 1950s when many middle-class women returned to or stayed home to raise families; (b) the new wave of feminism of the 1960s beginning with Betty Friedan's *Feminine Mystique* (Friedan, 1963); and (c) the sexual revolution of the 1970s.

Although the feminist movement of the 1960s was gaining momentum, scientists were developing OCs promising freedom from unwanted pregnancy in a pill—a contraceptive method totally disassociated from intercourse. However, physicians controlled this method, as well as abortions (legalized in 1973 with *Roe v. Wade,* a decision overturned by the U.S. Supreme Court in *Dobbs v. Jackson Women's Health Organization,* 2022). To counter medical control of women's bodies, the Boston Women's Health Book Collective published the first edition of *Our Bodies, Ourselves* in 1970, which was a motivation for the rise of women's self-help groups. At the same time, many authors addressed the new sexuality of women, allegedly discovered during the sexual revolution. Thus, although women worked for liberation from feminine stereotypes, they experienced a bombardment of expectations about their sexuality. The role of superwoman took on new qualities; not only were U.S. women expected to be faultless wives, mothers, and career women, but they were also supposed to be able to fulfill all their partners' sexual fantasies. However, the sexual revolution did not relieve women of the burden of contraception. Even today, most sexually active fertile women make most decisions about contraception.

Patterns of Contraceptive Use

During the period of 2006 to 2010, 86.6% of women ages 15 to 44 years reported that they had been sexually active during their lifetimes. Of this group of sexually active women, 99.1% reported that they had experienced some form of contraception. The most commonly used forms reported were the male condom (93.4%) and OCs (81.9%). It is noteworthy that 59.6% had reported using withdrawal, the third most commonly reported method. The average woman uses 3.1 methods of contraception throughout her lifetime (Daniels et al., 2013).

At any given moment, approximately 65% of women in the United States use contraception. The most commonly used methods are female sterilization (18.1%), OCs (14%), long-acting reversible contraceptives, and the male condom (8.4%). White women are most likely to be currently using contraception (69.2%), followed by Black women (61.4%) and Hispanic women (60.5%; Daniels & Abma, 2020).

Contraceptive Decision-Making

From menarche to menopause, women must make decisions about their fertility, including if, how, and when they will regulate it. Women may choose to abstain from heterosexual vaginal intercourse, engage in such intercourse and risk pregnancy, or engage in intercourse and prevent pregnancy by using contraception. Making a decision about contraception is more than selecting among attractive alternatives. It requires strategies and compromises that satisfy personal, social, cultural, and interpersonal needs influenced by constraints, opportunities, values, and norms. When made in cooperation with a healthcare provider, these characteristics are filtered through the additional variables of medical history and possible contraindications, future healthcare, personal goals (such as timing of future pregnancies), and cost.

Deciding to Use Contraception

Decision models assume that individuals' choices are determined by beliefs about their consequences and perceptions of their advantages and disadvantages. Although individuals try to make the best possible choices, they can be hampered by the complexity of a situation, conflicting beliefs and motives, misinformation, social constraints, and intrapsychic conflicts (Adler, 1979). When making a decision, an individual's values and perceptions of probable outcomes and values are valid, even if they are not objective or consistent with cultural values. Some investigators believe that the decision not to use contraception can be sensible even when pregnancy is not intended. In fact, it may be based on a decision model in which a woman decides that benefits associated with not using a contraceptive outweigh the risks associated with pregnancy (Luker, 1978). Each decision has antecedents and consequences. Antecedents initiate the decision-making process. These are events or incidents that cause doubt, wavering, debate, or controversy. In turn, these lead to a search for options, followed by a gathering of information about these options. Before making a decision, the individual examines and evaluates the feasibility of each option and considers the possible risks and consequences. Consequences are the events or incidents that result from the decision.

When the individual makes a decision, stabilization occurs because the decision ends the doubt, wavering, debate, or controversy. Then the individual may affirm the decision by implementing it, affirm it but postpone implementation, reverse it, or reconsider it and make new decisions as circumstances and desires change. For example, a woman is considering switching from OCs to a barrier device. She may have used other contraceptive methods in the past and probably will consider those along with the numerous choices for barrier contraception. Then she compares the advantages and disadvantages of the various barrier methods with those of other options. After considering the consequences of using a barrier method (such as its use must be linked to intercourse), the necessity of inserting the device in her body, and the need to remove the device in a prescribed time frame, the woman decides to use this contraceptive method. After choosing the particular barrier method, the woman might then consider the consequences of that decision on her relationship with her partner, the need to learn insertion and removal techniques, and other factors unique to her lifestyle and roles.

Before deciding to contracept, a woman must perceive herself as sexually active and at risk for becoming pregnant. A sexual self-concept is strongly correlated with contraceptive use (Winter, 1988). The decision to use contraception is influenced by many factors, such as age, family patterns of healthcare, advice from a healthcare provider, the influence of culture (Lethbridge, 1997), socioeconomic status, locus of control, knowledge of pregnancy risks, availability of contraception, approach to risk taking, and relationship with partner (Lethbridge & Hanna, 1997; Mills & Barclay, 2006).

A woman's opinions about contraceptive methods may change with her age, relationships, number of children, plans for future children, and experiences with methods (Grady et al., 2002; Huber et al., 2006; Mathias et al., 2006; Mills & Barclay, 2006). A woman's choice on the type of contraception may be influenced by her partner's preference. Women entering new relationships may desire the flexibility for future pregnancies. Women's choices may be influenced by health concerns related to side effects or safety. Some women's primary concern may revolve around the ability to control when the contraceptive method is used and when it is not. (Alspaugh et al., 2020)

Some women manage their fertility regulation without the assistance of a healthcare provider. These women do not feel a need for educational services or prescription methods. Favorable attitudes toward methods are a prerequisite for contraceptive use and for seeking assistance from a healthcare provider when a woman believes she needs help choosing a method or accessing a prescription method. The attitudes of healthcare providers affect women's perceptions of methods, especially when a prescription is required (or other assistance) to procure a birth control method (Bird & Bogart, 2005; Mills & Barclay, 2006; Wysocki, 2006). Sometimes women see a healthcare provider, obtain a contraceptive method, and then never return. If the prescription expires or the method needs replacement, the woman may discontinue it rather than return to see the healthcare provider. Still other women switch from one healthcare provider to another for various reasons. The quality of the interaction between healthcare providers and their clients can also positively or negatively affect a woman's level of contraceptive use over time (Bird & Bogart, 2005; Mills & Barclay, 2006).

Transgender and Gender Nonbinary Individuals

It is important for healthcare providers to pay careful attention to patient populations that are LGBTQIA. These patients have historically suffered marginalization with surveys showing as little as 29% of healthcare providers feeling comfortable with caring for these individuals (Schwartz et al., 2019). The discomfort and lack of training of healthcare providers to care for this population has led to less than half of persons identifying as transgender presenting for healthcare. However, it is vital that these individuals receive care and are offered the same contraception options as the cisgendered population. It is reported that the rates of unintended pregnancy for these individuals are similar to that of the cisgendered population (Reynolds & Charlton, 2021). A person's sexual activities cannot and should not be assumed based on a person's sexual identification or presenting gender. Providers also cannot make assumptions about future pregnancy desires or plans for patients in this population (Britton et al., 2020). Testosterone therapy is not a guaranteed form of contraception and persons using this method of hormone therapy should be counseled as such. Many of these individuals desire control over their fertility options. Often same-sex couples or transgendered men will present with a request for contraception with the intention of conception later in their relationships.

Family Planning Service Settings

Agencies offering family planning services should provide patients free access to current developments through the use of state-of-the-art media. Clinics should be open at convenient hours for all patients. They should welcome a woman and, with her permission, her partner's participation in method selection and educational sessions. The setting should be conducive to teaching and learning. Waiting and counseling rooms should be large enough to permit various seating arrangements for several persons. To promote teaching and learning, these areas should have adequate lighting and ventilation. Because individuals have different learning styles and educational backgrounds, healthcare providers should use various teaching methods, such as one-to-one discussions and group sessions. Women should have access to appropriate and up-to-date educational materials, including those available in print and in the social media, to include "apps" for smartphones and other devices, hands-on displays, and online access (Bird & Bogart, 2005; Tabeek, 2000).

Changing from a technically oriented family planning care delivery system to an educational delivery system with product and nonproduct methods requires fertility awareness education—a basis for all contraception. Increased involvement and control over method selection may increase a woman's use of the method she chooses. The current delivery system of family planning services does not meet the needs of all patients. Drastic change in the system is unlikely, however, unless patients demand more from the system. Patient education may help solve this problem. However, changing the knowledge, attitudes, and behaviors of some family planning healthcare providers presents a greater challenge. Addressing the role of healthcare providers in the provision of care will also help to individualize care. Fortunately, most healthcare providers are enthusiastic about the future of family planning and are eager to participate in new care delivery systems and to integrate new methods of contraceptive teaching and counseling into their practices (Herrman, 2006; Mills & Barclay, 2006; Tabeek, 2000).

Several types of healthcare providers offer a range of family planning services, such as counseling; prescribing OCs, the ring, or the patch; fitting diaphragms; inserting contraceptive implants or IUDs; administering injectables; and providing family planning education. Healthcare providers offer these services in private practices; community health centers; hospital-based, public health, and freestanding clinics; and family planning agencies (Herrman, 2006).

Healthcare providers' roles range from assisting women with decision-making to direct hands-on care. Social workers, counselors with various educational backgrounds, health educators, and lay volunteers also participate in family planning programs. All healthcare providers bring their personal agendas, biases, values, and cultures to the family planning setting, affecting care delivery and interactions with patients. The style of healthcare delivery ranges from giving a method to a woman and assuming she will use it to being a partner in the decision-making process.

Healthcare providers use a variety of interaction styles when caring for women who are making choices about their reproductive health. Healthcare providers with a paternalistic style assume they know what is best and make decisions for their patients. They commonly use statements beginning with, "I will . . . " and "You will. . . ." Those with a maternalistic style attempt to influence the woman's choices and gain her acquiescence by stating consequences of an action rather than the alternatives to it. This approach puts the focus on potential outcomes and the effects of the woman's choice on herself or others. Providers using this approach commonly use statements that begin with, "If you don't . . . then. . . ." Providers using either style of interaction focus on outcomes and attempt to gain adherence with their own predetermined goals.

Healthcare providers using a participatory style demonstrate respect for a woman's autonomy and ability to make decisions. They focus on the process she uses to reach a decision, presenting alternatives and encouraging her to participate in the decision-making. They use statements that begin with "What do you think about . . . ?" or "We can talk about. . . ." The woman's needs and concerns are more likely to emerge in participatory interactions than in maternalistic or paternalistic ones (Scott & Glasier, 2006; Wysocki, 2006). As Orne and Hawkins (1985) pointed out, "Providers must avoid the temptation to prescribe 'for clients.' Clients must make their own informed choice in collaboration with providers; they should feel supported in their right to choose" (p. 33).

CONTRACEPTIVE METHODS

For most women in the United States, fertility regulation is a major concern. Ideally, young women should be taught about their bodies before menarche (the onset of menses) and learn about the developmental changes of puberty and the signs and symptoms of fertility. After menarche, they may begin the journey along the sometimes-tortuous path of contraception decision-making. During the fertile years, women may decide the number and timing of any pregnancies they choose to have.

Before deciding to use a particular contraceptive method, a woman should weigh the effectiveness against risks (if any), advantages, disadvantages, and adverse effects. She should also consider any contraindications that relate to her health history. The effectiveness among contraceptive methods varies considerably. Each method has a theoretical effectiveness (effectiveness under ideal laboratory conditions, which depends solely on the method and not the human user) and use effectiveness (effectiveness under real-life or human conditions, which allows for the user's carelessness or error as well as method failure). Healthcare providers often use this information when counseling a woman about contraceptive choices and risks. When a woman seeks assistance with family planning, care would ideally include a detailed personal and family health history (focusing on hypertension, strokes, thromboembolism, smoking status, migraines, current medications, and allergies). Although important, perceptions have changed over time, deemphasizing the need for a physical exam or a Pap smear to start contraception. Telemedicine visits provide a unique opportunity to avoid office visits for those for whom an office visit is a barrier (Lesnewski, 2021). The cost of contraception is a significant consideration. For example, some long-acting reversible contraceptive (LARC) methods may be more expensive up front, yet more cost-effective in the long term. A 2015 in-depth analysis calculated costs based on the purchase price of the method, the administration and clinical costs, and costs of failure. This analysis found that IUDs (both copper and progesterone) were the least expensive at around $300 per patient per year. Injections ($432) and patches ($730) were the more expensive per patient/per year options (Trussell et al., 2015). In 2015, some large retailers offer generic combined OCs (COCs) and progesterone-only OCs for $4 per month. The 2010 Patient Protection and Affordable Care Act mandates that employers provide contraceptive coverage as a part of their employee insurance plans.

Natural Family Planning Methods

Fertility regulation and awareness is the cornerstone and basis for understanding all contraceptive methods; especially the fertility awareness (natural family planning [NFP]) methods. This information assists the woman in knowing when or if she ovulates. Therefore, the healthcare provider should explore a woman's awareness of her fertility patterns and provide additional information, if needed, before assisting her with the selection of a contraceptive method (Hawkins et al., 2008; Tabeek, 2000). Additionally, some healthcare providers have taught aspects of fertility awareness to couples who wish to conceive, but are having difficulty (Thijssen et al., 2014).

Fertility awareness education refers to imparting information about male and female reproductive anatomy and physiology, primary and secondary signs of fertility, and cyclical changes in these signs. All fertility awareness methods use this information, as well as knowledge of female fertile and infertile phases and their relationship to male fertility and require abstinence from vaginal–penile intercourse during the fertile phase to prevent conception. Because NFP methods are unmodified by chemical, mechanical, or other artificial means, they represent a natural way to regulate fertility (World Health Organization [WHO], 2011).

Evidence from ancient times suggests rudimentary knowledge of periods of relative infertility during the menstrual cycle, as well as at other times in a woman's life. For example, East African women believed that avoiding intercourse for a few days after menstruation would prevent pregnancy (Gordon, 1990). Breastfeeding was recognized as a means to prevent pregnancy and was used by Alaska Natives, Native Americans, and ancient Egyptians (Gordon, 1990). This latter method gained popularity in the 1990s under the title of lactation amenorrhea method (LAM), and is still practiced today (Díaz, 1989; France, 1996; WHO, 2018).

NFP includes cervical mucus, basal body temperature (BBT), and symptothermal methods and LAM. Except for LAM, these methods use normal signs and symptoms of ovulation and the menstrual cycle to prevent or achieve pregnancy (Finnigan, 2008). The woman is taught the methods and then asked to observe several cycles to best understand and recognize her fertile and infertile phases.

CERVICAL MUCUS METHOD

The cervical mucus method is based on detecting signs and symptoms of ovulation through consistent observation of the cervical mucus, which is produced by cells in the cervix. Throughout the menstrual cycle cervical mucus changes. Immediately after the menstrual period, cervical mucus is scant and the woman should notice vaginal dryness for a few days. Then mucus is present for a few days, in which the woman should feel vaginal wetness. After this, the mucus becomes clear (as differentiated from milky white, translucent, or creamy color) and slippery or stretchy, similar to raw egg white. The woman should notice increased wetness or a slippery sensation. The peak day of wetness signals ovulation.

During ovulation, cervical mucus nourishes sperm, facilitates their passage into the intrauterine cavity, and probably helps select sperm of the highest quality. However, the peak day is only obvious the day after it occurs, when the mucus becomes less slippery and stretchy. After this day, the mucus starts to lose its slippery, stretchy, wet quality, and becomes cloudy and sticky until menses begins (Simmons & Jennings, 2020). The Billings Ovulation Method is one of the more common cervical mucus methods and is 97% effective with perfect use and 77% effective with typical use. More information to include tracking applications can be found at billings.life/en.

To use the cervical mucus method, the woman should check her cervical mucus daily, beginning when menstrual bleeding ends or becomes light enough to allow assessment of the mucus. The woman can check her mucus in several ways, depending on her level of comfort with her body. She can wipe a folded piece of toilet tissue across her vaginal opening, and then feel whether the tissue slides across easily or drags, pulls, or sticks. If mucus is present, she can place it between two fingers and check its wetness and stretchiness. These characteristics are referred to as *spinnbarkheit*. As an alternative, she can check for these characteristics by holding the toilet tissue with both hands and pulling it apart (Finnigan, 2008; Tabeek, 2000).

BASAL BODY TEMPERATURE METHOD

The BBT method is based on the temperature change triggered by the progesterone rise that occurs when the ovum leaves the ovary. To use this method, the woman takes her temperature at the same time every day and immediately upon waking, using a digital basal thermometer, before she eats, drinks, smokes, and/or participates in any physical activity. Then she documents her daily temperature on a chart, noting any variations. During ovulation, the temperature typically rises up to 1° above the preovulatory BBT. To prevent conception, the woman should abstain from intercourse until after 3 days of temperature rise. Infections, illnesses, and other conditions such as fatigue, anxiety, sleeplessness, some medications, use of an electric blanket, and/or a heated waterbed can also increase the body temperature. Therefore, applying the rules for taking and interpreting the BBT are crucial to the effectiveness of this method.

The natural cycles method incorporates BBT into a smart phone–based application. Women enter their BBT into the application or use a Bluetooth-enabled thermometer that automatically uploads their temperature for her. The application assesses that day as being either red (fertile) or green (infertile). The natural cycles method is estimated as being 99% effective with perfect use and 92% effective with typical use (Simmons & Jennings, 2020). More information can be found at www.naturalcycles.com.

SYMPTOTHERMAL METHOD

The symptothermal method uses a combination of BBT and cervical mucus monitoring to avoid fertile periods. Users of this method track both BBT and cervical mucus on a daily basis. Some symptothermal methods use cervix position as an additional indicator of fertility. A safe time to engage in intercourse is determined by 3 days of higher BBT and a change in cervical mucus. Charts are available for this method as well

as smart phone applications. There are formal symptothermal programs that are provided by individuals trained in the method. With perfect use, the symptothermal method is estimated to be 99.4% effective, and it is 98% effective with typical use (Simmons & Jennings, 2020).

LACTATIONAL AMENORRHEA METHOD

The lactational amenorrhea method is predicated upon the fact that a new mother who is exclusively or nearly exclusively breastfeeding their infant ovulate while experiencing amenorrhea. In order for this method to be used, three conditions must all be met:

1. The patient must be not be menstruating.
2. The infant must nearly fully breastfeed. Occasional liquids are acceptable, but the mother must be regularly and frequently nursing, at a minimum of eight to 10 times per day.
3. The infant must be less than 6 months old.

With perfect use, the lactational amenorrhea method is 99% effective. With typical use, it is 98% effective (WHO, 2018).

ELECTRONIC HORMONAL FERTILITY MONITORING

Electronic hormonal fertility monitors were developed and marketed for the purpose of helping women determine when they are ovulating so they could optimally time intercourse and maximize the opportunity to conceive. The monitors work by detecting the level of luteinizing hormone (LH) and estrogen in urine, identifying peak fertility days.

Recently, however, fertility monitors have begun to be used also as a method of avoiding intercourse during fertile periods. The Marquette Model uses electronic fertility monitors to identify elevations of LH and progesterone in combination with cervical mucus monitoring. Women interested in the Marquette Method can be trained by certified instructors. More information can be found at www.marquette.edu/nursing/natural-family-planning-model.php. More research is needed on the feasibility of using electronic fertility monitoring as a standalone strategy for NFP. In time, it may prove to be useful for women who are very comfortable with technology, are uncomfortable with using traditional NFP methods, and/or are looking for confirmation of existing solutions.

PRESCRIPTION HORMONAL AND OVER-THE-COUNTER METHODS

Planning when and when not to conceive is an important part of being in a responsible, healthy, and sexually active relationship. Women and men use birth control methods to prevent pregnancy, plan the interval of time between pregnancies, prevent the spread of sexually transmitted infections, and regulate menstrual cycles (Shields, 2020). There are a multitude of hormonal prescription and over-the-counter methods available to assist couples in preventing pregnancy. Understanding the advantages, disadvantages, cost, and health risks is critical in helping advise a couple on a birth control method that fits their needs and wants for whatever stage of life they are in.

Combined Oral Contraceptives

In 1960, the Food and Drug Administration (FDA) ushered in the era of COCs with the approval of the drug Envoid (Christin-Maitre, 2013). Initial research was conducted in the 1950s by Gregory Pincus and was financed by Sanger's colleague Katharine McCormick, who spent $2 million of her own money on the project. Even with advancements in other methods of contraception, COCs remain the most commonly used reversible contraceptive method in the United States. In the most recent National Survey for Family Growth, 82% of U.S. women reported using COCs at some point in their lives (Hatcher, 2022). The modern COC has two components. The first component, estrogen, provides some contraceptive effect by suppressing the release of follicle-stimulating hormone (FSH) but more importantly stabilizes the endometrium in order to maintain bleeding regularity (Frye, 2006). In the United States, ethinyl estradiol and less commonly mestranol are the synthetic estrogens used in COCs. In the 1960s, Envoid used 150 mg of ethinyl estradiol, which caused a wide variety of unpleasant side effects that included thromboembolic events. Since then, the amount of estrogen contained in COCs has been decreased to less than 35 mg, thereby significantly improving both safety and tolerability (Christin-Maitre, 2013).

The other component of COCs is a synthetic progesterone, which is classified by "generation." Progesterone provides the vast majority of the contraceptive effect by suppressing both FSH and LH. The result of these altered hormonal conditions is suppression of ovulation, thickening of cervical mucus, and the creation of hormonal conditions within the uterus that are unfavorable for implantation (Frye, 2006). A side effect of the progestin component is androgenization, which can cause acne, hirsutism, and weight gain. Third- and fourth-generation progestins were developed to be less androgenic and minimize these unpleasant symptoms (Sitruk-Ware & Nath, 2010).

COC packs contain both active pills and inert pills. The purpose of the inert pills is to withdraw hormones in order to promote bleeding, as the initial developers believed that women would be reassured by the monthly demonstration of the fact that they are not pregnant. Most monophasic preparations contain a pill that is taken for 21 days followed by 7 days of inert pills that exist only as a daily placeholder until the next round of active pills begins. Multiphasic COCs were developed in the 1980s to lessen side effects by varying the amount of hormones over the course of the first 3 weeks. Multiphasic COCs exist in biphasic, triphasic, and newer quadriphasic regimens.

COC HEALTH ADVANTAGES

There are significant advantages to COCs that make them a strong birth control option for many women. When taken perfectly, COCs are 99.7% effective at preventing an unintended pregnancy in a year of use (Hatcher, 2022). They offer a quick return to fertility, as women often ovulate within a few cycles of ceasing use. Furthermore, COCs are easy to take, are well tolerated, maintain efficacy when an occasional dose is forgotten. However, it is important to remind patients that COCs provide no protection from sexually transmitted infections (STIs) to include HIV, and for that reason, many women require the addition of a barrier method (e.g., condoms).

The use of COCs provides many health benefits that extend beyond contraception. Because OCs tend to stabilize the endometrium, women often experience a lighter menses that benefits women with anemias and heavy or frequent menses. A lighter menses can also reduce painful cramps and pelvic pain related to endometriosis. Some women use the pills to alter the timing of their periods or prevent periods altogether by taking the pills continuously. Many women who take COCs (particularly triphasic preparations) experience a significant improvement in acne. COCs have demonstrated effectiveness in decreasing the severity of premenstrual mood symptoms (headaches, irritability, and depression). There is also a decreased incidence of ovarian cancer in women who take COCs, particularly for longer than 10 years of use. Additionally, COC users demonstrate a decrease in the incidence of fibrocystic breasts and endometrial cancers (Shields, 2020).

CONTRAINDICATIONS

Although COCs are very safe, some women are not ideal candidates for their use. It is imperative that healthcare providers take a detailed medical history before discussing contraceptive options in order to identify conditions that make some women poor candidates or optimal candidates for contraceptive methods. Fortunately, many of the contraindications to COCs do not apply to progesterone-only methods, IUDs, or barrier methods, ensuring that there is a safe and effective option for almost any woman.

WHO has produced helpful guidelines that identify conditions and states that are contraindications to COCs. These guidelines are available and may be accessed online at no cost (www.who.int/reproductivehealth/publications/family_planning/Ex-Summ-MEC-5/en). Absolute contraindications to COCs include (a) women who are breastfeeding and less than 6 weeks postpartum; (b) those who are older than 35 years and smoke greater 15 or more cigarettes per day; (c) women with a systolic blood pressure greater than or equal to 160 mmHg; (d) those with vascular disease; (e) those with known heart disease, valvular disease, or stroke; (f) those with current breast cancer; (g) those with a history of diabetes with target end-organ damage; and (h) those with active viral hepatitis, cirrhosis, or liver cancer (WHO, 2015), and (i) those who experience migraines with auras (WHO, 2015; Shields, 2020).

Blood pressure must be monitored with each visit, as COCs may raise both the systolic and diastolic blood pressure in some women; although the effect is not usually clinically significant. Negative changes in blood pressure will normalize after cessation of COCs (Chrousos, 2021). Generally, it is considered safe to prescribe COCs to women with normal blood pressures (less than 140/90 mmHg; American College of Obstetricians and Gynecologists [ACOG], 2019). Women who have well-controlled hypertension, are younger than 35 years, and do not smoke are reasonable candidates for COCs. Women with poorly controlled hypertension and those who are smokers are better candidates for progesterone-only methods, IUDs, or barrier contraception.

On occasion, COCs have been known to cause thromboembolic events, such as deep vein thrombosis (DVT) and thromboembolic stroke. Although venous thromboembolism is estimated to occur at a three times higher rate for COC users, the risk is still low (Peragallo Urrutia et al., 2013). COCs should be avoided in women with a history of DVT or pulmonary embolus (PE), those who have prolonged immobilization due to surgery or other conditions, and those with a history of heart disease or stroke (WHO, 2015). Progesterone-only methods are generally safe for use in women with these conditions and are a viable alternative.

Women who have a history of migraines with auras are thought to have a significant risk of ischemic stroke (ACOG, 2019). Like many other serious COC adverse effects, this risk appears to increase with higher doses of ethinyl estradiol and in women who smoke. Although the risks are low, because of the morbidity associated with ischemic stroke current recommendations are that women who have a history of migraines with auras are prescribed an alternative form of contraception. Women who have a history of migraines without aura, however, are generally considered to be safe to take COCs.

There continues to be a concern over the role of COCs in the development or acceleration of breast cancer. Many studies have found that COCs are not associated with an increased risk of breast cancer, while others have found a statistically significant but low increase in risk. For some women the benefits of a reduction in risk of ovarian cancer may outweigh a potential slight risk in the development of breast cancer (Del Pup et al., 2019). Both the CDC's U.S. medical eligibility criteria for contraceptive use (Curtis, Tepper et al., 2016) and WHO's medical eligibility criteria for contraceptive use (2015) recommend no restrictions for women with a family history of breast cancer, recommend against prescription for women with current breast cancer, and believe that the risks outweigh the benefits for a woman with a past history of breast cancer. One approach to counseling a woman who is concerned about breast cancer risk but wishes to be prescribed COCs could include focusing on lifestyle changes that reduce risk of breast cancer to include weight loss and exposure to sunlight/vitamin D (Del Pup et al., 2019).

HEALTH BENEFITS

The use of OCs provides many health benefits that extend beyond contraception. Because OCs tend to stabilize the endometrium, women often experience a lighter menses that benefits women with anemias and heavy or frequent menses. Many women who take COCs (particularly triphasic preparations) experience a significant improvement in acne. COCs have demonstrated effectiveness in decreasing the severity of premenstrual mood symptoms. There is also a decreased incidence of ovarian cancer in women who take COCs, particularly for longer than 10 years of use. Additionally, COC users demonstrate a decrease in the incidence of fibrocystic breasts and endometrial cancers (Schindler, 2013).

ASSISTING PATIENTS WITH THE SELECTION OF COMBINED ORAL CONTRACEPTIVE

Obtaining and understanding a woman's health history and reproductive health goals is the key to selecting a COC. While the patient may be due for a breast and pelvic exam, neither is required to initiate COC use in an asymptomatic, healthy patient. Patients who desire a short-acting reversible method or desire the noncontraceptive benefits of COCs should be provided the opportunity to express what type of pill regimen might work best for them. While most COCs provide the traditional 21/7 preparations, there are several others to choose from. For example, women who dislike the inconvenience or symptoms associated with menses may prefer preparations that contain 84 active pills and 7 inactive pills, resulting in a period only once every 3 months. Regardless of the desired regimen, timely access to pills is critical. Requiring patients to return each month or every 90 days for refills constitutes a major barrier to successful COC use. Healthcare providers should consider dispensing a 1-year supply in order to reduce barriers to continuous use.

Traditionally, women have been instructed to begin taking COCs on either the first day of menses or the first Sunday after menses begins, known as the *conventional start method*. The advantages of this method are that the days of the week are aligned with those on the pack and establish that the woman is unlikely to be pregnant. Another approach, known as the *quick start method*, has the patient take the medication on the day they are prescribed as long as the healthcare provider and patient are reasonably sure that the patient is not pregnant. Although studies have shown little difference in the incidence of unintended pregnancies with the quick start method, it provides yet another opportunity for patient choice (Lopez et al., 2012). Patients should be encouraged to associate taking their COCs with another daily activity (such as brushing their teeth) in order to develop habit-forming behavior. Those who forget to take one pill should take two the next day. Several smartphone applications exist to help women remember to take their medication and anticipate their periods. Patients who miss two or more pills should continue with the aligned days of the pack and use barrier contraception for the remainder of the cycle. Women who miss pills frequently should explore other types of contraception that do not require daily intervention. Women who miss more than 1 day of triphasic or quadriphasic preparations may benefit from checking manufacturer instructions on product websites.

MANAGING SIDE EFFECTS

Thirty percent of women who have used COCs have discontinued use due to side effects (Daniels et al., 2013). Therefore, it is important for the healthcare provider to set expectations and assess and manage side effects with each patient visit to ensure continued use or to partner with the patient to make a change. The most common side effects of COCs include breakthrough bleeding (BTB), nausea, and mild headaches. Most patients simply require reassurance that the side effects will improve after two to four cycles. BTB is a frequent occurrence and is often due to missed pills. With extended regimens, stopping the pills for 4 days and causing a short withdrawal bleed may prove helpful. Some women will eventually require a formulation with higher doses of estrogen, or, conversely, lower doses of the progestin (Lohr & Creinin, 2006). Headaches are common with all formulations, and may improve with extended regimens (Barr, 2010). Some women may experience melasma (patches of pigmented skin discoloration), which usually dissipates slowly when the medication is stopped.

As a part of patient education, it is important to counsel the patient on the signs and symptoms of serious side effects. The mnemonic ACHES was developed to help women remember these potential serious adverse effects. Any woman who experiences ACHES should immediately stop taking her COCs and notify her provider. ACHES represents

- Abdominal pain (severe)
- Chest pain (severe), cough, or shortness of breath
- Headaches (severe), dizziness, weakness, or numbness
- Eye problems (vision loss or blurring) or speech problems
- Severe leg pain (calf or thigh)

Contraceptive Patch

The contraceptive patch and the contraceptive ring are estrogen/progesterone combination products that have the same mechanism of action as COCs. The patch and the ring are particularly advantageous to women who find the ritual of remembering a daily medication burdensome. They share the same side effects, risks, contraindications, and noncontraceptive benefits as combined oral products. Both products have a quick return to fertility, as ovulation usually occurs within a few cycles of cessation.

The contraceptive patch was introduced in the United States in 2002, providing a unique alternative to daily dosed COCs. The oldest patch consists of a 14 cm² square adhesive patch combining .75 mg of ethinyl estradiol with 6 mg of norelgestromin (sold under the brand names Ortho Evra and Evra; Figure 21.1). A newer patch (sold under the brand name Twirla) was approved in 2020 and is a 15 cm² adhesive patch combining 2.3 mg of ethinyl estradiol with 2.6 mg of levonorgestrel (LNG). With perfect use, the patch is 99.7% effective in preventing pregnancy. With typical use, efficacy falls to 93% (Gatcher, 2022).

USAGE

Applied on the first Sunday after menses, the patch is worn for a week and then replaced for three consecutive weeks. A quick start method similar to COCs is considered an acceptable alternative. On the fourth week, no patch is worn, creating a withdrawal bleed. The cycle is then repeated. If a woman desires to control or skip her period, they can use the patch continuously. Menses will resume a few days after the patch is removed (Shields, 2020). The patch is placed on clean skin on any of the following areas: lower abdomen, upper arms, buttocks, and upper torso. The breasts are to be avoided. A patch that partially detaches or becomes completely removed can be reapplied or taped on as long as it has been off for less than 24 hours. A common additional side effect to the patch is skin irritation (WHO, 2018).

Contraceptive patches should not be prescribed to women with a body mass index ≥30 kg/m². The FDA has issued a black box warning for this population due to concerns over reduced effectiveness and a higher risk of venous thromboembolic events.

Contraceptive Ring

The original vaginal contraceptive ring (sold under the brand name Nuvaring) was approved for use by the FDA in 2001. It is a soft and flexible 54-mm diameter ring (Figure 21.2) that releases 120 mcg/day of etonorgestrel and 15 mcg/day of ethinyl estradiol and must be replaced every 21 days. A newer product (sold under the brand name Annovera) releases 150 mcg/day of segesterone acetate and 13 mcg/day of ethinyl estradiol in a 56-mm ring and lasts for 1 year. It is 93% effective in preventing pregnancy with typical use and 99.7% effective with perfect use (Hatcher, 2022).

USAGE

The contraceptive ring is used very similarly to the contraceptive patch. On the first Sunday after menses, the patient compresses the opposite sides of the ring and inserts it into her vagina. Although the ring can be anywhere in the vagina to be effective, it tends to be less apparent to the patient and their partner in the deeper, posterior portion of the vagina. The patient starts the vaginal ring on the Sunday following menses and replaces it once a week for a total of 3 weeks. A ring-free fourth week creates a withdrawal bleed (WHO, 2018). The etonorgestrel/ethinyl estradiol ring is designed to be discarded after each cycle, whereas the segesterone acetate/ethinyl estradiol ring lasts for 13 cycles.

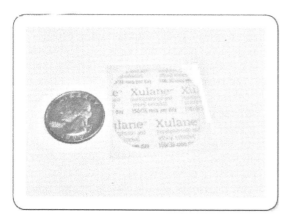

FIGURE 21.1 Contraceptive patch.

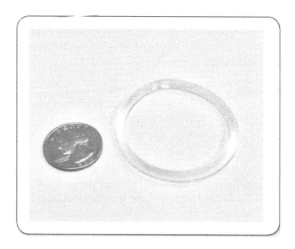

FIGURE 21.2 Contraceptive ring.

The segesterone acetate/ethinyl estradiol should be washed with mild soap and water and placed its case for each of the ring-free weeks.

The etonorgestrel/ethinyl estradiol ring should remain in place at all times throughout the week, to include intercourse. If it falls out, the patient should rinse it with water and put it back in place. If the ring is out of the vagina for less than 48 hours, it should be put back as soon as possible with no further concern. If the ring is out of the vagina for more than 48 hours during the first 2 weeks, it should be reinserted and a barrier method should be used for 7 days. If the ring is out of place for more than 3 hours during the third week then a new ring should be inserted and a barrier method should be used for 7 days (WHO, 2018).

The segesterone acetate/ethinyl estradiol ring loses efficacy quickly when outside the vagina. A backup method of contraception should be used if the ring has been out of the vagina for more than 2 cumulative hours during the 21 days of continuous use or for more than 7 days during the ring-free interval (TherapeuticsMD, 2022).

Progesterone-Only Pills

Progesterone-only pills (POPs; also known as "mini-pops") provide an alternative to traditional COCs for women who are not candidates for the estrogen component. POPs' contraceptive efficacy is thought to approximate that of COCs at 93% effective with typical use and 99.7% effective with perfect use (Hatcher, 2022). POPs are most commonly used by lactating mothers who are in the immediate postpartum period and do not wish a long-term progesterone-only solution, such as injectable medroxyprogesterone acetate. Efficacy rates may be lower for women who are not lactating. As there is no estrogen component, breakthrough vaginal bleeding is a common side effect.

USAGE

Progesterone-only pills can be started without a backup method any time after birth as long as menses has not returned. A woman who starts within 5 days of menses does not require a backup method. A woman who starts more than 5 days after the start of menses requires a backup method for the first 2 days of taking pills. POPs lose effectiveness if not taken at the same time every day. A woman who is more than 3 hours late taking her medication should use a barrier method for any intercourse in the following 48-hour period (WHO, 2018).

Emergency Contraception

Since the 1970s, both COCs and POPs have been used as emergency contraception (EC). Common reasons for prescribing EC include unprotected intercourse, a mistake in or failure of a contraceptive, or sexual assault. EC is not an abortifacient and does not harm an existing pregnancy.

Dr. Albert Yuzpe pioneered the practice of using two doses of a COC within 72 hours of unprotected sexual intercourse or barrier contraception failure to prevent pregnancy. The *Yuzpe method* used large doses of ethinyl estradiol that often caused unpleasant adverse effects (Li et al., 2014). Current methods achieve the same results but with more tolerable, lower amounts of hormone. It is believed that the mechanism of action is to prevent or delay ovulation and to thicken cervical mucus.

OPTIONS AND USAGE

Any COC could feasibly be used as EC. The *World Health Organization Family Planning Global Handbook* (available free online at www.who.int/reproductivehealth/publications/fp-global-handbook/en) provides charts with detailed instructions for using almost any existing COC or POP as EC (WHO, 2018). However, if financial resources and availability allow, two FDA-approved commercial products may offer more convenient and potentially efficacious choices.

LEVONORGESTREL

The common, over-the-counter option for EC is levonorgestrel, a progesterone-only product sold in the United States and licensed under the brand Plan B One-Step. This regimen calls for one 1.5-mg tablet to be taken within 72 hours of unprotected intercourse. LNG should not be taken if the patient believes she is pregnant; yet it will not harm an already existing pregnancy. LNG is most effective if taken within 48 hours of unprotected intercourse; efficacy decreases at 48 to 72 hours post intercourse (Hang-Wun et al., 2014; Li et al., 2014). Package inserts estimate the product to be around 85% effective in preventing a pregnancy, which otherwise would have occurred. Common side effects include spotting, mild abdominal pain, fatigue, headache, dizziness, and breast tenderness.

ULIPRISTAL

An alternative and arguably more effective prescription-only solution for EC is the progesterone uliprital acetate (UPA), sold in the United States under the trade name Ella. UPA is to be taken as a single 30-mg dose after unprotected intercourse. The advantage of UPA over LNG is that it can be taken up to 120 hours after unprotected intercourse. One study demonstrated a failure rate of only 2.1% from 48 to 120 hours after intercourse. The disadvantage of UPA is that it is not available over the counter (Hang-Wun et al., 2014; Li et al., 2014).

Intrauterine Device

The IUD, discussed in more detail in a separate section later in this chapter, is also a very effective choice for EC. It is 99% effective as an EC and can be placed up to 5 days after the unprotected sexual intercourse event. Traditionally, copper IUDs were the treatment of choice for a woman who wished for an EC solution that could also serve as a long-acting reversible contraceptive. A recent randomized control trial comparing the effectiveness of a 52-mg LNG IUD with the copper IUD found that both options had comparable, near zero rates of pregnancy when placed within 5 days (Turok et al., 2021).

Healthcare providers should carefully and nonjudgmentally explore the reason(s) that EC was required. This information is *key* to determining if the current contraceptive option is failing for reasons that require a change, or if the situation requires a discussion about a reliable, long-term contraceptive option. The discussion may also provide insight as to whether or not a woman is at risk for pregnancy due to sexual assault. Additionally, a discussion on EC might prompt discussions about risk for STIs.

Barrier Methods

Barrier contraception remains a popular and effective birth control choice. Barrier contraception includes male and female condoms, the diaphragm, and the cervical sponge. Barrier contraception is unique in that it provides (particularly with male and female condoms) protection against STIs. An additional benefit is that many barrier methods (with the exception of diaphragms) are available over the counter at low cost.

MALE CONDOM

The male condom is the oldest, most widely known and most commonly available form of barrier contraception. It is 98% effective at preventing pregnancy when used perfectly and is 87% effective if used typically (Hatcher, 2022). Condoms are arguably the only form of contraception that is primarily managed by the male partner. It is around 90% effective at preventing HIV transmission. The male condom is potentially a good choice for a woman and her partner who cannot or do not wish to engage in hormonal birth control methods.

The correct use of a condom is imperative in order to ensure maximum efficacy. The condom should have at least half an inch of space at the tip of the penis to serve as a reservoir for ejaculation. Immediately upon ejaculating, the male should withdraw from intercourse and the condom should be carefully removed and disposed of. A new condom should be used for any subsequent sexual activity. Condoms can be used with either a water- or silicon-based lubricant—never with an oil-based lubricant as it places the integrity of the condom at risk. Condoms can be used with spermicidal applications. If a condom breaks or spills during sexual activity, healthcare providers should advise patients to consider EC.

FEMALE CONDOM

Female condoms provide an alternative to male condoms and are almost as effective at preventing pregnancy. With perfect use, female condoms are 95% effective and with typical use they are 79% effective in preventing pregnancy (Hatcher, 2022). They are made of a soft plastic film and are lubricated on both the inside and outside. They are made of two rings, one at the closed end to assist with insertion and one at the open end to keep the condom open (Figure 21.3). They are effective at preventing sexually transmitted disease and are available over the counter. They are, however, a bit more difficult to properly place than a male condom.

Female condoms are prelubricated. However, they can be used with any type of additional lubricant to include those that are oil based. After intercourse, the female condom is removed by twisting the outer ring in order to form a seal, and then gently pulling it out of the vagina. As with the male condom, any contraceptive failures that include breaking or the spilling of semen into the vagina can be mitigated with EC (WHO, 2018).

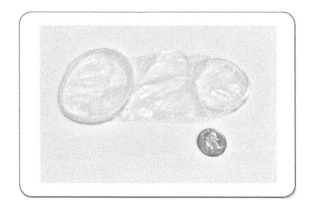

FIGURE 21.3 Female condom.

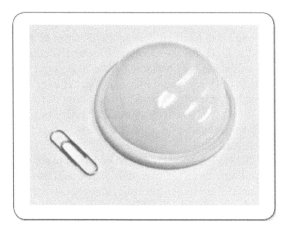

FIGURE 21.4 Diaphragm.

DIAPHRAGM

The diaphragm is an older form of barrier contraception that has lost popularity due to newer, well-tolerated, long-acting hormonal contraceptives. It consists of a soft plastic or silicone cap that is placed in the vagina before intercourse in order to cover the cervix (Figure 21.4). It is used with a spermicidal agent to increase efficacy. With perfect use, the diaphragm is 84% effective in preventing pregnancy and with typical use, efficacy declines to 83% (Hatcher, 2022). It requires some dexterity to correctly place the diaphragm before intercourse, which may prove to be a disadvantage to some women.

A visit with a provider who is skilled and experienced in fitting diaphragms is necessary, as there are multiple available sizes. The diaphragm should fit against the vaginal walls but should not be so tight that it causes discomfort or loose enough to easily dislodge. Women who have a prolapsed uterus are poor candidates due to inadequate diaphragm fitting. A diaphragm must remain in place for at least 6 hours after intercourse, and for no more than 24 hours. Many healthcare providers suggest that women try a diaphragm while they continue their current method of contraception (WHO, 2018).

CONTRACEPTIVE SPONGE

Another older form of barrier contraception is the contraceptive sponge. It is a one-size, absorptive polyurethane device that is impregnated with spermicide (Figure 21.5). The Today

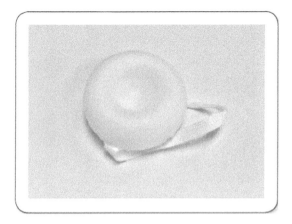

FIGURE 21.5 Contraceptive sponge.

brand sponge has been sold over the counter in the United States and is marketed as an alternative to the condom. The device is moistened with water before placement. The concave portion of the device is placed against the cervix and the opposite side has a loop to use for removing the device after use. The sponge is significantly more effective in nulliparous women than parous women (91% vs. 80%, respectively, with perfect use and 86% vs. 73%, respectively, with typical use; Hatcher, 2022). The sponge should be left in place for at least 6 hours and may be left in place for 24 hours. It does not need to be replaced if there are multiple intercourse sessions within the 24-hour period (Yranski & Gamache, 2008). At the time of this writing, although approved for use in the United States, the contraceptive sponge is largely unavailable due to manufacturer production issues.

INJECTABLE CONTRACEPTION

The only injectable form of contraception available in the United States is depot medroxyprogesterone acetate (DMPA), marketed as Depo-Provera. DMPA is available in two formulations: DMPA-IM, given as a deep intramuscular injection, or DMPA-SC, given subcutaneously. These progestin-only contraceptive injectables are highly effective, safe, convenient, long acting, and reversible, and can be used by most women in most circumstances (Raine-Bennett et al., 2019). Since FDA approval for contraceptive use in 1992, DMPA has been used by millions of women. Although women using this progestin-only contraceptive injectable often initially experience irregular bleeding and spotting, long-term DMPA use typically results in amenorrhea. Currently available by prescription only, DMPA can range from $0 to $250 with initial clinic visit and $0 to $150 thereafter (Planned Parenthood, 2021). DMPA is safe for most women and most medical conditions and is safe for women of any age and parity and for women living with HIV. DMPA can be used postabortion or in postpartum breastfeeding mothers.

Because DMPA does not contain any estrogen, it represents a good contraceptive choice for postpartum and lactating women, as well as women who cannot or do not want to take estrogen. DMPA prevents pregnancy primarily through suppression of ovulation. A possible secondary mechanism of action includes thickening of cervical mucus, which decreases sperm penetration, and endometrial atrophy, which prevents implantation (Curtis, Jatlaoui et al., 2016).

Both DMPA-IM and DMPA-SC are highly effective. Data from the United States suggest that 0.2% of women with perfect use and 6% of women with typical use of DMPA will experience an unintended pregnancy within the first year of use (Curtis, Jatlaoui et al., 2016). It is important to note progestin-only contraceptive injectables are not expected to have lower efficacy in overweight or obese women. Additionally, because DMPA avoids first-pass metabolism, its efficacy is unaffected by a women's use of other medications (Wu & Bartz, 2018).

DMPA is available in two formulations: (a) DMPA-IM, 150 mg given as a deep intramuscular injection every 12 weeks; and (b) DMPA-SC, 104 mg given subcutaneously every 12 weeks. The CDC in 2021 evaluated the recommendation from WHO for self-administration of DMPA-SC (Curtis et al., 2021). The adoption of the recommendation is a result of evidence supporting higher continuation rates and higher patient satisfaction (Curtis et al., 2021). This decision could decrease disparities for access to contraception for women who cannot take off work to go the clinic for an injection or do not have reliable transportation.

Usage

DMPA can be started at any time during a woman's menstrual cycle, as long as the healthcare provider is reasonably sure that the patient is not pregnant (Curtis, Jatlaoui et al., 2016). Requiring that a woman needs to be menstruating in order to receive DMPA is an unjustified barrier to care. DMPA can be initiated without a pelvic examination, blood or other lab tests, cervical cancer screening, and/or breast examination (Curtis, Jatlaoui et al., 2016).

DMPA-IM is injected into the upper arm or buttock. DMPA-SC can be injected into the upper thigh, upper arm, or abdomen (Curtis, Jatlaoui et al., 2016). DMPA has a 14-week duration of action and is recommended to be administered every 12 weeks, thereby providing a 2-week "grace" period for the patient. The possibility of pregnancy should be ruled out in the case of any woman who is more than 2 weeks late for her DMPA injection.

Side Effects

Thorough counseling, patient education, and anticipatory guidance regarding side effects of DMPA are critical. Side effects of DMPA include menstrual disturbances, weight gain, depression, decrease in bone density, allergic reactions, metabolic effects, headaches, nervousness, decreased libido, and breast tenderness (Hadji et al., 2019; Raine-Bennett et al., 2019).

There is a black box warning for DMPA indicating use of this product beyond 2 years is not recommended due to potential bone loss that is potentially irreversible. Studies indicate that it may be the decrease in estradiol to levels between 20 and 30 pg occurring secondary to the use of DMPA that is responsible for the bone density loss, leading to a slight risk increase of fracture. However, this risk was not observed after discontinuation (Hadji et al., 2019).

Menstrual changes occur in almost all women who use DMPA and are the most common cause for dissatisfaction and discontinued use. Bleeding patterns are initially unpredictable, with approximately 70% of women experiencing infrequent but prolonged episodes of bleeding or spotting. Irregular bleeding typically decreases with each reinjection. After the first year of use, close to 50% of women will experience amenorrhea (Sims et al., 2020).

Weight gain is commonly reported as a side effect of DMPA and can lead to method discontinuation or reluctance to initiate the method (Wu & Bartz, 2018). Although weight gain is not consistent for all women, recent studies have shown an overall 2.40-kg (5-lb) weight gain with younger age of initiation being a contributing factor (Sims et al., 2020).

Some women may experience an increase in depression when they use DMPA. However, data are limited and conflicting, and a history of depression is not a contraindication to DMPA use (Singata-Madliki et al., 2020). Long-term DMPA users may develop a decrease in bone mineral density, but this side effect is temporary and reversible on discontinuation of DMPA. Although rare, allergic reactions to DMPA may occur. Some healthcare providers encourage women to remain in the clinic for 20 minutes after an injection. In addition, women should be asked if they have ever experienced severe itching or redness at the site of a previous DMPA injection site. If so, another DMPA dose should not be repeated.

Because DMPA is an injection, it is not possible to immediately discontinue. Menstrual irregularities, weight gain, depression, allergic reactions, breast tenderness, and headaches may continue until DMPA is cleared from the woman's body, anywhere from 6 to 8 months after her last injection.

Health Benefits

DMPA is associated with certain noncontraceptive benefits, such as a reduction in or elimination of premenstrual symptoms, absence of menstrual bleeding, a reduced risk of pelvic inflammatory disease (PID), a reduced risk of ectopic pregnancy, decreased risk of endometrial cancer, improvement in grand mal seizure control, and hematologic improvement in women with sickle cell disease. DMPA-induced amenorrhea may make it a good contraceptive choice for women with menorrhagia, dysmenorrhea, fibroids, and iron deficiency anemia.

Contraindications

There are some conditions for which risks may outweigh the benefits. These conditions include cardiovascular disease, liver disease, a history of breast cancer, and unexplained vaginal bleeding before a thorough evaluation. Providing DMPA in these circumstances requires careful clinical consideration (Ju et al., 2018). When counseling women who have conditions such as diabetes mellitus (DM) it is important to discuss risk of a negative effect on lipid metabolism as a result of hypoestrogenic effects. If a women experiences complications from DM the risk may begin to outweigh the benefit (Robinson et al., 2016). A current diagnosis of breast cancer is the only absolute contraindication to DMPA use.

Women need to be informed of the likely delay in fertility after DMPA use. Return to fertility after a DMPA-IM injection averages between 9 and 10 months, with some studies showing that fertility may not be restored for as long as 22 months (Ju et al., 2018). DMPA is not the best choice for women who wish to become pregnant within the next 1 to 2 years and these women should be counseled about alternative contraceptive options.

Serious health issues are rare with DMPA use. However, a woman should immediately contact her healthcare provider for any of the following warning signs:

- If you think you might be pregnant
- Repeated, very painful headaches
- Depression
- Severe, lower abdominal pain
- Pus, prolonged pain, redness, itching, or bleeding at the injection site
- Any other concerning symptoms

CONTRACEPTIVE IMPLANTS

In 1990, the contraceptive LNG (Norplant) ushered in the era of implantable progestin rods. Norplant consisted of six LNG-containing rods that were inserted into the subdermal layer of the upper, inner arm. It lost popularity when reports about the difficulty in removal of the implant arose (Pushba et al., 2011). Although Norplant is no longer being manufactured, there is currently one contraceptive implant available in the United States. It was originally marketed under the brand name Implanon but has been subsequently marketed as Nexplanon.

Nexplanon

Nexplanon is a hormone-releasing birth control implant for use by women to prevent pregnancy for up to 3 years. Nexplanon is a thin, silicon-free flexible plastic rod, about the size of a matchstick, containing 68 mg of the progestin etonogestrel. The rod slowly delivers an average of 40 mg of etonogestrel every day for at least 3 years, inhibiting ovulation and thickening cervical mucus. The etonogestrel implant is not biodegradable and requires removal either when the patient desires or when the device expires. Nexplanon is reported to be 99.9% effective at preventing pregnancy (Britton et al., 2020).

MECHANISM OF ACTION

The contraceptive effects of Nexplanon are similar to that of other progestin-containing contraceptives. The progestin etonogestrel, used in Nexplanon, thickens cervical mucus, making it difficult for sperm to penetrate, and it also inhibits ovulation. In addition, this progestin thins the uterine or endometrial lining, which makes it unreceptive to implantation.

Implants are in the top-tier effectiveness category of contraceptives and, like IUDs, offer women a private, low-maintenance, long-acting, and rapidly reversible method of contraception with relatively few side effects. In addition, implants do not interfere with the spontaneity of sex, and can be used by women who want or need to avoid estrogen

TABLE 21.1 Nexplanon Use	
IMPLANT ADVANTAGES	**IMPLANT DISADVANTAGES**
High effectiveness	Menstrual disturbances
Ease of use	Rare insertion and removal
Discreetness	complications
No adverse effect on acne	Possible weight gain and other
Relief of dysmenorrhea	hormone-related adverse
Relief of pelvic pain related to	symptoms
endometriosis	Ovarian cysts
Few clinically significant	Clinician dependency
metabolic effects	No protection against STIs
Reduced risk of ectopic	Drug interactions
pregnancy	Possible decrease in bone
No estrogen	density
Reversibility	Possible increased risk of
High acceptability and	thromboembolic conditions
continuation rates	
Cost effective	

STIs, sexually transmitted infections.
Source: Adapted from Nelson, A. L., Crabtree Sokol, D., & Grentzer, J. (2018). Contraceptive implant. In R. A. Hatcher, A. L. Nelson, J. Trussel, C. Cwiak, P. Cason, M. S. Policar, A. R. A. Aiken, A. Edelman, & J. M. Marrazzo (Eds.), Contraceptive technology *(pp. 129–155). Ayer Company Publishers.*

(Moray et al., 2021). From a clinical standpoint, their efficacy is indistinguishable from that of sterilization and IUDs (Moray et al., 2021). In addition, a woman's body weight does not appear to play a role in effectiveness (Table 21.1). Based on current data, an approximate failure rate of Nexplanon is 0.2 per 100 user-years with a Pearl Index of 0.38% (Nelson et al., 2018).

ELIGIBILITY CRITERIA

The vast majority of women are good candidates for Nexplanon. Implants are particularly suitable for women who desire safe, effective, long-term, maintenance-free, reversible contraception. Nexplanon offers women reproductive control, allowing them to postpone a first pregnancy, space pregnancies, or to provide long-term contraception once the desired family size is reached. Like other progestin-only contraceptives, implants may be of interest to women who cannot or do not wish to use a contraceptive that contains estrogen.

Nexplanon can be used by teens, nulliparous women, women with multiple sex partners, and women with HIV. However, women who fall into the aforementioned categories should be counseled on the use of barrier methods as Nexplanon does not protect against STIs.

Nexplanon should not be used in women who have:

- Known or suspected pregnancy
- Current or past history of thrombosis or thromboembolic disorders
- Benign, malignant, or active liver disease or liver tumors
- Undiagnosed abnormal genital bleeding
- Breast cancer, history of breast cancer, or other progestin-sensitive cancer
- Women who are taking antiretroviral agents, antiepileptics, and rifampicin. *Pregnancies have been reported in women taking these medications.*
- Allergic reaction to any of the components of Nexplanon

INSERTION

A healthcare provider trained in Nexplanon insertion can perform this minor surgical procedure in the office. One Nexplanon package consists of a single implant that is 4 cm in length and 2 mm in diameter, which is preloaded into a disposable needle applicator. The rod is typically inserted into the inside portion of arm 8 to 10 cm from the epicondyle inferior to the groove between the biceps and triceps muscles in order to avoid the brachial artery and vein that travel in that sulcus. Local anesthetic can be administered to ease any discomfort with insertion (Nelson et al., 2018). The rod is then inserted into the subdermal tissue. Insertion deeper than recommended can risks migration causing a more complicated surgical removal (Nelson et al., 2018). Complications of rod insertion are very rare. Infection, bruising, skin irritation, or pain may occur immediately after insertion.

Timing of insertion depends on the woman's recent contraceptive history. If the woman has not used any hormonal contraception in the past month, Nexplanon should be inserted between day 1 and day 5 of the menstrual cycle. If the rod is inserted within 5 days of the start of menses, a backup form of contraception is not needed during the remainder of the cycle. However, if insertion occurs outside the recommended window, the woman should either abstain from intercourse or use a backup method for the first 7 days after insertion (Nelson et al., 2018).

ADVERSE EFFECTS/SYMPTOM CONTROL

Similar to all progesterone-releasing contraceptive methods, Nexplanon causes changes in vaginal bleeding patterns in a large majority of women. These changes vary from amenorrhea, infrequent bleeding, irregular bleeding, or prolonged or frequent bleeding. Although these changes are rarely clinically significant, and many women consider amenorrhea or infrequent bleeding to be a benefit, changes in vaginal bleeding patterns are the most common reason for discontinuation of implant use (Moray et al., 2021).

The most common complaints associated with progesterone-releasing implants are related to the hormonal side effects. These side effects include weight gain, headache, changes in mood, breast pain, abdominal pain, nausea, loss of libido, ovarian cysts, and vaginal dryness.

MONITORING

Women considering implants should be advised on the advantages, disadvantages, and insertion and removal procedures before use. A user card is included in the Nexplanon packaging. This card should be filled out and given to the patient after insertion so that she will have a record of the location of the implant in the upper arm and when it should be removed.

Pregnancy is extremely rare with the use of Nexplanon. In general, hormonal contraceptives are not dangerous for either the pregnant woman or a developing fetus (Raymond, 2011). If a woman using Nexplanon is found to be pregnant and wishes to continue the pregnancy, the implant should be removed, and no other evaluation or care is needed.

REMOVAL

Before initiating removal of the implant, positive identification of the location of the rod is required. Once the location has been verified, local anesthetic can be injected under the distal end of the rod. The clinician will then push down on the proximal end of the implant to stabilize it, in turn forming a bulge indicating the distal end of the implant. Then, a 2-mm incision can be made from which to remove the rod. The clinician will gently push the implant toward the incision until the tip is visible. Lastly, the clinician will grab the implant with forceps and gently remove it (Nelson et al., 2018).

RETURN TO FERTILITY

Nexplanon prevents pregnancy for up to 3 years and does not interfere with fertility once the rod is removed. In clinical trials, pregnancies occurred as early as 7 to 14 days after the rod was removed. Upon removal, if continued contraception is desired, another form of birth control should be initiated immediately.

INTRAUTERINE DEVICES

IUDs or intrauterine systems (IUSs) are small, T-shaped devices made of flexible plastic. In this chapter, the term IUD is used generically in reference to all types of intrauterine contraception unless otherwise noted. An IUD/IUS is inserted into a woman's uterus only by trained healthcare providers, in this case, for pregnancy prevention. There are five IUD/IUS brands available in the United States: the copper ParaGard and the hormonal Mirena, Liletta, Kyleena, and Skyla. They are among the most cost-effective contraceptive options available, costing from $0 to $1,300 depending on IUD/IUS type and the patient's insurance (Planned Parenthood, 2021). Although the cost of an IUD might seem high for some, one office visit for an IUD placement can provide anywhere from 3 to 10 years of reliable contraception.

IUDs are one of the most safe, reliable, and cost-effective contraception options available today (Bellows et al., 2018). Modern IUDs have an impressive safety record and are safe for most women, including teens, nulliparous women, and HIV-positive women. There are few contraindications to its use (Hou & Roncari, 2018). They are highly effective and comparable to surgical sterilization and implants (Curtis, Jatlaoui et al., 2016). IUDs also offer women a private, low-maintenance, long-acting, and rapidly reversible method of contraception with relatively few side effects (Hou & Roncari, 2018). In addition, IUDs do not interfere with the spontaneity of sex, offer several noncontraceptive health benefits, have high continuation rates, and can be used by women who want or need to avoid estrogen (Phillips et al., 2017). There is no delay in return to fertility with either the copper IUD or the LNG IUSs.

There are some lingering negative perceptions relating to the IUD that still persist based on first-generation models. In 1970, the Dalkon Shield, a smaller IUD marketed for nulliparous women, was introduced. However, there were multiple reports of serious side effects including infection, septic abortion, perforation of the uterus, heavy bleeding, cramping, ectopic pregnancy, infertility, and death (Britton et al., 2020). Lawsuits as well as the FDA's mandate against the manufacturer of the Dalkon Shield resulted in its removal from the market in the early 1970s. The failure of this IUD was caused in part by a design flaw. The increased risk of pelvic infection appeared to be related to the IUD's multifilament strings, which acted like a wick drawing bacteria from the lower genital tract up into the uterus (Britton et al., 2020). Although these complications were not experienced by users of other IUDs, they caused fear and confusion for both patients and healthcare providers, essentially leading to the demise of IUD use in the United States.

The current generation of IUDs is much safer and has been engineered to mitigate these and other adverse effects that plagued their first-generation predecessors. Rebranding combined with a push to educate providers and patients has made the IUD/IUS a first-line choice for long-term contraception and cycle control in the United States.

The vast majority of women are good candidates for an IUD. IUDs can be used by teens, nulliparous women, women with multiple sex partners, and women who have had ectopic pregnancies (Hou & Roncari, 2018). However, IUDs should not be prescribed for women with known pregnancy, with an active STI or active PID, in the period immediately after a septic abortion, presenting with unexplained vaginal bleeding, or with anatomic abnormalities of the uterus (such as fibroids that disrupt the uterine cavity, a bicornuate uterus, or cervical stenosis; Curtis, Jatlaoui et al., 2016).

IUDs appear safe and effective for women who are immunocompromised due to organ transplantation, autoimmune disease, or HIV (Hou & Roncari, 2018). They can be used safely in women with cardiac disease and structural heart abnormalities, diabetes, venous thromboembolism, and a history of cesarean section and other cervical surgery (Hou & Roncari, 2018). The IUD should not be newly inserted in a woman with cervical cancer, but the method can be continued if the woman desires. IUDs can be used safely in women with a history of breast cancer (Hou & Roncari, 2018). New studies indicate that the LNG releasing device may be beneficial in treating low-risk endometrial cancer (Pal et al., 2018).

Women who are at risk of acquiring STIs should be advised to use condoms and are generally still good candidates for an IUD (Hou & Roncari, 2018). If a woman does acquire an infection with chlamydia or gonorrhea, the IUD does not need to be removed. Standard treatment for the woman and her partner is sufficient.

Copper Intrauterine Devices

The copper T 380 (ParaGard) was developed in the 1970s and approved by the FDA for use in the United States in 1984 and became available for use 1988. It is a T-shaped device with a polyethylene stem and cross arms partly covered by copper wire (see Figure 21.6). It is approved for 10 years of use, although studies indicate effectiveness for up to 12 years (Phillips et al., 2017). The pregnancy rate in women who use the copper IUD is less than 1% in the first year of use (Sundaram et al., 2017).

The copper IUD prevents fertilization primarily by creating a spermicidal environment. It causes the uterine endometrium to initiate a foreign body reaction, which results in sterile inflammation and inhibits sperm from reaching the fallopian tube. Additionally, the copper ions permeate the cervical mucus and decrease sperm motility (Hou & Roncari, 2018).

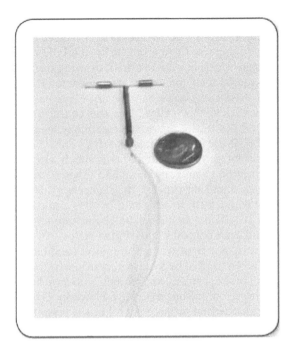

FIGURE 21.6 Copper intrauterine device.

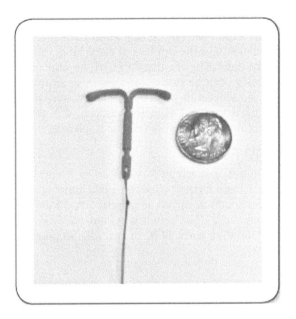

FIGURE 21.7 Levonorgestrel intrauterine system.

Some women who use a copper IUD complain of heavier, longer, and more uncomfortable menstrual periods. Average monthly menstrual blood loss may be increased by up to 55%. For some, these side effects may decrease over time.

Levonorgestrel IUSs

The hormonal IUSs exist in the United States under the brand names Mirena, Liletta, Kyleena, and Skyla. All the IUD/IUSs are made of soft, flexible plastic in a T shape and contain a hormone-releasing reservoir impregnated with LNG (see Figure 21.7). Mirena was originally approved for 5-year use. The FDA approved Mirena for 7-year use in 2021 with the same formulation of 52 mg of LNG releasing an average 20 mcg of LNG per day (Hou & Roncari, 2018). Liletta was released to offer a more economically friendly IUS with the same 52 mg formulation of LNG. Prior to Mirena's approval for 7 years a new 5-year IUS brand name Kyleena with 19.5 mg LNG debuted and was marketed as a smaller option similar to the Skyla with a lower daily release of LNG at an average daily release of 9.8 mcg per day. Skyla at 13.5 mg LNG releases 8 mcg of LNG per day and is approved for 3 years. LNG works by thickening cervical mucus (making it difficult for sperm to penetrate) and by inhibiting ovulation in some patients (Hou & Roncari, 2018).

Intrauterine Device Insertion Procedure

When inserting an IUD, the provider should confirm to the best of their ability that the patient is not pregnant (Curtis, Jatlaoui et al., 2016). The provider will also review the risk and benefits of the particular IUD being inserted. An informed consent must be signed by both the provider and the patient prior the procedure. An IUD can only be inserted by a healthcare provider who has received special training.

Insertion of an IUD may take place at any time during the menstrual cycle, provided the woman is not pregnant. Current preprocedure counseling recommendations for an IUD include warning women of the very low risk of PID in the 20-day postinsertion period. Only women who are symptomatic or those who are at risk for having an STI should be tested before insertion. Women who develop PID can be treated with antibiotics while the IUD is in place. The IUD should be removed only if the patient fails to improve within 72 hours of initiation of antibiotic therapy (Curtis, Jatlaoui et al., 2016).

Before insertion, a bimanual examination is done to determine the uterine position. The procedure to place the IUD begins similar to a Pap smear, with the insertion of a speculum into the patient's vagina. If clinically indicated, a test for chlamydia and gonorrhea can be performed. The cervix is then thoroughly cleansed and sounding of the uterus, with appropriate instrumentation, takes place. The IUD is then inserted through the cervix, into the uterus per manufacturer guidelines, using sterile technique. The IUD threads are made of a monofilament-type string and should be cut at a length to allow the thread to wrap up and around the cervix, approximately 3 cm. The length of the strings should also be noted in the patient's record for future reference. If the threads are cut too short, the woman's partner may complain of discomfort or a poking sensation with intercourse and/or the IUD may be more difficult to reach when removing.

As part of patient education (before discharge), it is important to remind the patient to manually feel for her strings after each menstrual period in order to verify placement of the IUD. If the patient is unable to locate the IUD strings, she should follow up with her healthcare provider.

The IUD/IUSs can be placed immediately postpartum (Curtis, Jatlaoui et al., 2016). Appropriate counseling is important prior to delivery and immediate postpartum insertion of the LGN IUD/IUS. Studies indicate the expulsion rate of the LGN system is statistically significant higher than the copper IUD (Jatlaoui et al., 2018). Studies are mixed on the effect immediate placement of hormonal IUD/IUSs have on breastfeeding. Essentially it is important to have an open discussion with the patient to collaboratively determine if the benefit is greater than the risks (Hou & Roncari, 2018; Turok et al, 2017).

Adverse Effects

Although adverse effects have significantly decreased since the first-generation models were released, they do still exist. The most common side effect related to IUD use includes change in menstrual patterns. Although not medically harmful, menstrual pattern changes may prove uncomfortable or even unbearable to the patient. Irregular bleeding is common in the first few months of use and is a common reason for discontinuation.

For women using progesterone-releasing IUSs, light bleeding or irregular spotting is to be expected in the early months of use. Once endometrial suppression has been achieved, Most women will experience decreased menstrual bleeding while 20% experience amenorrhea or no menstrual bleeding (Sergison et al., 2019).

The most common complaints related to progesterone-releasing IUSs are related to the hormonal side effects. These side effects can include hirsutism, acne, weight changes, nausea, headache, mood changes, and breast tenderness. These symptoms can lead to an elective removal of IUSs (Hou & Roncari, 2018).

Within the first year of IUD use, 2% to 10% of users spontaneously expel the device. Nulliparity, age less than 20 years, menorrhagia, severe dysmenorrhea, and placement immediately postpartum or post second trimester abortion increase the chance of expulsion (Hou & Roncari, 2018). Although expulsion is not a medical emergency, patients should use a backup method of birth control until they can see their healthcare provider.

Pregnancy is extremely rare with an IUD in place. However, when a patient does become pregnant, she may be at an increased risk of having an ectopic pregnancy (Hou & Roncari, 2018). In the rare event of a confirmed pregnancy, the healthcare provider must make a determination about whether or not the pregnancy is ectopic. If the pregnancy is ectopic, this complication must be managed using best practice standards. If the pregnancy is intrauterine and the device is confirmed to be in the uterus, removal is most often recommended due to increased risk for sepsis, spontaneous abortion, and preterm birth (Hou & Roncari, 2018).

Patient education should include information about checking monthly for the IUD strings as well as signs and symptoms of possible complications, including pain, bleeding, odorous discharge, fever, chills, and missed menses.

Anticipatory counseling about expected menstrual changes is critical. Women who choose a copper IUD need to be counseled that they may experience heavier, longer, and more painful menstrual periods. The use of nonsteroidal anti-inflammatory drugs (NSAIDs) may help with bleeding and pain. Conversely, women using progesterone-releasing IUSs may completely stop having menstrual periods. This is not harmful and does not require any treatment. Women should understand that menstrual periods will return once an IUD/IUS is removed.

Intrauterine Device Removal

There are numerous reasons and various times when an IUD can or should be removed (Hou & Roncari, 2018):

- The patient requests removal.
- The device reaches its expiration date.
- The patient develops a contraindication.
- If adverse effects do not resolve.

The IUD is removed by securely grasping the threads at the external cervical OS with ring forceps and gently and evenly pulling the IUD out. Asking the patient to bear down and cough three times can be a useful distraction technique during removal. If significant resistance is met, all removal attempts should cease until it is determined why the IUD is not moving. Once the IUD is removed, it is prudent to show the device to the patient so they are confident that the device has been removed.

STERILIZATION

At one time two methods of female sterilization were available in the United States: transcervical sterilization and tubal ligation. As of 2018, only tubal ligation remains. For men and couples who make sterilization decisions together, vasectomy remains an attractive alternative to female methods. Advantages of sterilization include its permanence, high rate of efficacy, cost effectiveness, lack of significant long-term side effects, and lack of need for partner adherence (Hou & Roncari, 2018).

Permanence may also be viewed as a disadvantage of sterilization. Most women who choose sterilization as their contraceptive method never regret their decision. However, due to relationship changes and other life events, regret is always possible. Women who undergo sterilization at a young age, who have a low parity, or who may be in unstable relationships tend to have a greater risk of regret (Edelman et al., 2019). The CREST study found the overall regret rate to be 12.7% with patients under 30 years old having a 20.3% rate of regret (Hou & Roncari, 2018). Although sterilization may be reversed with varying degrees of success, it is difficult and expensive.

Transcervical Sterilization

Essure was the only FDA-approved transcervical sterilization method that was available in the United States. However, it was voluntarily removed from the market in December 2018 due to declining sales that resulted from FDA actions addressing increasing claims of adverse reactions (Edelman et al., 2019). Studies are ongoing to gather more data about the risks and benefits.

Surgical Sterilization

Tubal ligation sterilization is performed using a laparoscopic approach under general anesthesia. Surgical sterilization for women prevents fertilization by cutting, tying, or clipping the fallopian tubes. Tubal ligation can be done as a planned, laparoscopic procedure in the operating room or as part of a planned cesarean delivery. Surgical tubal sterilization is highly effective with only a 0.5% failure rate (Hou & Roncari, 2018).

Major complications from female tubal sterilizations are uncommon. As with any surgery, there is a risk of hemorrhage, infection, and death from anesthesia-related complications. If the procedure fails and the patient becomes pregnant, the chance that it will be ectopic is considerable (Roncari & Jou, 2011). According to data from the CREST study, 30% of pregnancies achieved after tubal surgery were ectopic (Hou & Roncari, 2018). This varied greatly with the method of tubal surgery.

Male sterilization, or vasectomy, blocks fertilization by cutting or occluding both vas deferens so that sperm can no longer pass out of the body in the ejaculate (Hou & Roncari, 2018). Male sterilization is not recommended for anyone who is not sure of his desire to end future fertility. Success of a vasectomy must be confirmed through a semen analysis with only azoospermia or rare nonmotile sperm (RNMS) left.

Vasectomies are highly effective with only a 0.15% failure rate. A vasectomy is a minor surgical procedure. Fewer than 3% of cases require any follow-up medical attention (Hou & Roncari, 2018). Postoperative complications, such as bleeding or infection as well as failure can occur. The most common complaints after the procedure are swelling of the scrotum, bruising, and minor discomfort. Pain medication and local application of ice are helpful in the immediate post-procedure period.

SUMMARY

Modern contraception began with Margaret Sanger's vision to develop long-lasting, effective, safe, highly reliable, and reversible contraception. Current forms of contraception are ever evolving and improving. Today's healthcare providers must understand the factors that influence a woman's life and contraceptive choices, her medical history, and her personal goals in order to partner with her in selecting contraception that meets both her short-term needs and long-term goals.

REFERENCES

References for this chapter are online and available at https://connect.springerpub.com/content/book/978-0-8261-6722-4/part/part02/chapter/ch21

CHAPTER 22

Preconception Counseling*

KRISTI RAE NORCROSS, JACQLYN C. SANCHEZ, AND ELIZABETH A. KOSTAS-POLSTON

PRECONCEPTION CARE

Preconception care should be a part of preventive health care for all women of reproductive age (including all sexual orientations and gender identities), including and for those planning to initiate a pregnancy (American College of Obstetricians and Gynecologists [ACOG], 2019). This care should be delivered in a culturally competent manner beginning with the simple question, "Are you planning a pregnancy in the next year?" Reproductive health planning and preconception care are not a specific entity but have evolved into a health promotion expectation for every clinician caring for women of childbearing age and capacity. According to the ACOG, the challenge of preconception care lies not only in addressing pregnancy planning for women who seek medical care and consultation specifically in anticipation of a planned pregnancy, but also in educating and screening all reproductively capable women on an ongoing basis to identify potential maternal and fetal risks and hazards to pregnancy before and between pregnanciesy (ACOG, 2019). Reproductive health planning and pre-pregnancy and preconception care, then, are considered critical to improving the health of women.

UNINTENDED PREGNANCY

Pregnancy Intention Status

An unintended pregnancy is defined as a pregnancy that is either mistimed or unwanted at the time of conception (Guttmacher Institute, 2019). Providers can further delineate pregnancy intention by asking the following questions, which are framed either at the onset of a pregnancy or retrospectively.

- At the time of conception, was the client wanting to get pregnant? (*planned pregnancy*)

- At the time of conception, was the client wanting to get pregnant, but not at this time? (*mistimed pregnancy*)
- At the time of conception, was the client not wanting to become pregnant at all, ever? (*unwanted pregnancy*)

Between 2015 and 2019, 40% of pregnancies in the United States (U.S.) were unintended (CDC, 2022f; Martinez & Abma, 2020). Births resulting from unintended pregnancy are at much greater risk for poor pregnancy outcomes, including birth defects, preterm labor, small for gestational age, maternal death-mortality, and neonatal death (CDC, 2023d). What is more, U.S. women at-risk for unintended pregnancy have been reported to be more likely to consume alcohol (10%), use tobacco (10%), be exposed to teratogenic medications that may cause birth defects (3%–6%), have chronic diseases such as diabetes (up to 9%), or be classified as overweight or obese (50%; Guttmacher Institute, 2019). These exposures further contribute to poor pregnancy outcomes and developmental disabilities. Despite many 20th century medical advances, poor pregnancy outcomes remain a problem in the United States, partly due to the lack of pre-pregnancy, preconception planning and preconception care. Each year in the United States, 10.2% of babies are born premature. Exposure to infectious diseases, such as chlamydia infection, or inadequate immunization to preventable diseases, such as rubella and hepatitis B, are also more likely when a pregnancy is unintended. There is a greater risk of nutritional deficiencies such as inadequate folic acid, nutritional excesses such as foods high in mercury, and excess caloric intake leading to obesity (Guttmacher Institute, 2019).

In addition to the preconception risks associated with lack of pregnancy planning that result in teratogen exposures and chronic medical conditions, there are social and genetic factors to consider. For example, a pregnant woman has a greater risk of being a victim of violence than a nonpregnant woman (Gelles, 1988). The risk of intimate partner violence (IPV) increases when the pregnancy is not planned. Women experiencing an unintended pregnancy often seek prenatal care later than those experiencing an intended pregnancy.

---

*This chapter is a revision of the chapter that appeared in the second edition of this textbook, coauthored with Debbie Postlethwaite, and we thank her for her original contribution.

Seeking late prenatal care precludes genetic screening and diagnostic testing, which are often performed earlier in the pregnancy. Hence, genetic diseases often go undetected (Guttmacher Institute, 2019).

Prevalence of Unintended Pregnancy

Pregnancy intention is assessed periodically in U.S. reproductive-age women. This assessment is performed by the National Center for Health Statistics through the use of the NSFG. This survey asks women and men about topics related to childbearing, family planning, and maternal and child health. Additionally, the survey asks about pregnancy intention retrospectively for the past pregnancy and for pregnanciesthose experienced in the past 5 years. Women surveyed in the most recent NSFG survey (2017–2019) reported that 15.7% of their pregnancies were unwanted ever, that 22.2% were mistimed, and that 62% were intended. Although the overall rate of unintended pregnancies in the United States is decreasing, there remain disparities among race/ethnicity, education, income, and other social determinants of health. In the United States, the proportion of unintended pregnancies that ended in an elective abortion increased among women aged 20 years and older but decreased among teenagers who were now more likely than older women to continue their unplanned pregnancies (Guttmacher Institute, 2014). The unintended pregnancy rate was highest among women who were agesd 18 to 24 years, unmarried, low income, or Black or Hispanic. The Healthy People 2030 objectives call for an overall reduction in unintended pregnancies in the United States from 43% to 36.5% (Office of Disease Prevention and Health Promotion, n.d.).

Risk Factors for Unplanned Pregnancy

Almost all women of reproductive age are at risk of an unintended pregnancy and would benefit from preconception health strategies. Let us look more closely at specific subgroups of women at risk. Women exposed to teratogens (substances that may cause birth defects) may be at highest risk of an unintended pregnancy that could result in a poor pregnancy outcome. A teratogen is a substance, organism, or physical agent capable of causing abnormal development and can cause abnormalities of structure or function, growth retardation, or death of the organism (Dutta, 2015). Teratogens may be prescribed or purchased in the form of over-the-counter medications; environmental reproductive toxicants (hyperthermia, lead, mercury, ionizing radiation) or infectious diseases may act as teratogens.

PLANNED PREGNANCY AND RISK SCREENING PRECONCEPTION HEALTH

The target population for preconception counseling consists ofare women presenting for premarital counseling, for vaginitis or sexually transmitted infection (STI) screening, after a negative pregnancy test, and during every postpartum visit (ACOG, 2019). In addition to these reproductive

health planning educational opportunities, preconception counseling given to women with chronic medical conditions, those with certain lifestyle choices, women in work environments involving teratogens, sexual minority women (SMW), and women of color can promote planned pregnancies and therefore prevention of increasing numbers of birth defects (Higgins et al., 2019). With limited time allotted for education during healthcare visits, it is essential to stress preventive information likely to be adopted by women. In a retrospective study with a sample population of 10,267 participants, among those who received education and recommendations from their clinician on prenatal vitamin use, weight loss, exercise, and smoking and alcohol use, statistically significant changes in behavior were noted only with vitamin use and smoking. The group of women who reported receiving education regarding daily intake of a prenatal vitaminPNV with folic acid reported taking the vitamins more often than the group who didn't receive education (77% vs. 40%; $p <.01$; adjusted odds ratio [AOR] 2.99; 95% CI 2.24–4.00). The opposite effect was reported by women who received smoking cessation education, as these participants smoked more during the 3 months prior to the pregnancy (47% vs. 27%; $p < .01$; AOR 2.22; 95% CI, 1.21–4.09) (Oza-Frank et al., 2015). Health care providers tailoring their education to a woman's needs are more likely to see changes in behaviors. Barriers to providing preconception counseling by clinicians were identified by Mazza and colleagues (2013). They reported a lack of scheduled time, competing priorities with prevention, and a lack of preconception guidelines/checklists, brochures, or waiting room posters.

Special Populations of Women Needing Preconception Care Assessment

Women with chronic medical conditions are less likely to plan pregnancies. Chronic conditions that may adversely affect pregnancy include pre-existing diabetes mellitus, thyroid disease, seizure disorders, hypertension, psychiatric illness, and cardiac disease (ACOG, 2019). In women with Human Immunodeficiency Virus (HIV) infection, there is an increased risk of several major complications, including perinatal morbidity and infection. The most important benefit of pregnancy planning for an HIV-infected mother is the ability to provide medical intervention to minimize the risk of vertical transmission to the neonate (CDC, 2023c). Another example of a chronic medical condition requiring preconceptual attention is thyroid disease. Untreated or inadequately treated thyroid disease may lead to maternal anemia, low birth weight, and impaired brain development of the fetus. High circulating human chorionic gonadotropin (hCG) in the first trimester may result in lowering thyroid-stimulating hormone (TSH) levels, resulting in inadequate levels of circulating thyroid hormones triiodothyronine and thyroxine (T3 and T4; American Thyroid Association, n.d.).

Another important subgroup of women at risk of unintended pregnancy is adolescents. Approximately 47% of all high school students report ever having had sexual intercourse (Henry J. Kaiser Family Foundation, 2014). The NSFG (2015–2019) reported the average age of first heterosexual vaginal intercourse to be 17.6 years for women and 17.2 years for men. Teens also report that the most commonly used method of contraception is condoms. However, when asked if they used a condom at last intercourse, only 59% of sexually active adolescents reported that they had actually used a condom (Child Trends Data Bank, 2014). About one third of all U.S. girls become pregnant before the age of 20 years. Of those pregnancies resulting in birth, greater than 80% are unintended (CDC, 2021). U.S. adolescent pregnancy rates are higher than those in almost every other country in the developed world including Canada, Great Britain, Japan, and Sweden. Teen mothers are more likely to drop out of school and remain single parents, which may contribute to the cycle of poverty as well as contribute to poor birth outcomes (CDC, 2021; Office of the Assistant Secretary for Health, n.d.).

Women with a previous unintended pregnancy constitute another important subgroup. It is estimated that 43% of all U.S. women will have has an abortion by 45 years of age (Guttmacher Institute, 2019). More than half of U.S. women (51%) obtaining an abortion report that they were using a method of contraception the month they became pregnant (Guttmacher Institute, 2019). Births resulting from subsequent unintended pregnancies pose the same or even greater risks for poor pregnancy outcomes resulting from exposure to teratogens, fetotoxins, or adverse social situations such as IPV, child abuse, and neglect (Dutta, 2015; Gelles, 1988).

Women of reproductive age are at risk of unintended pregnancy unless they are using long-acting, highly effective, reversible methods of contraception (intrauterine contraception or subdermal implants) or permanent sterilization (www.cdc.gov/reproductivehealth/unintendedpregnancy/contraception.htm). Contraception is a very important component of preconception healthcare because it promotes planned pregnancies. The more effective and less user-dependent the contraceptive method is, the more reliable the method is at reducing the risk of an unintended pregnancy and protecting preconception health. The 2017–2019 NSFG survey participants reported their use of any method of contraception ever as 99.2%; however, that percentage dropped to 65.3% of current contraceptive users. The report further demonstrated that 33% of respondents cited the reason for cessation of their contraceptive method was side effects. Clinicians lack adequate time to assess and prescribe contraception for complex patients. In 2016, to standardize knowledge, the CDC updated a summary chart for medical eligibility criteria for contraception prescriptions. This chart can be found at: www.cdc.gov/reproductivehealth/contraception/pdf/summary-chart-us-medical-eligibility-criteria.

SEXUAL MINORITY WOMEN AND LGBTQIA IDENTIFYING PERSONS

SMW experience an even higher risk for unintended pregnancy than their cisgender peers (Higgins et al., 2019). Almost 20% of U.S. youth identify as SMW, making up as many as 1 in 3.5 contraceptive seeking clients. In those who reported penile–vaginal intercourse (PVI) engagement in the last year, barriers and facilitators were identified for contraceptive use (Table 22.1).

Racism and Health Disparities

The March of Dimes (2022) annual review of 13.5 million birth records pointed to large disparities in the risk of preterm birth (PTB) and birth defects among racial and ethnic groups of women. In 2019, the March of Dimes reported that 14% of Black infants were born before 37 weeks' gestation, as compared to the 10.2% combined PTB rate. Native American and Alaskan Native babies have a higher rate of cleft lip with or without cleft palate, and Hispanic women gave birth to more babies with spina bifida when compared to non-Hispanic

---

TABLE 22.1 Contraceptive Barriers and Facilitators as Described by Sexual Minority Women[a]

CONTRACEPTIVE BARRIERS[b]	CONTRACEPTIVE FACILITATORS[c]
1. Excluding queer women from contraceptive messaging leads to likelihood that they will not think of themselves as contraceptive users.	1. Queer women who have "come out" may be sexually empowered, and therefore more likely to seek care to meet their contraceptive needs.
2. In addition to facing the challenges of their queer identity, queer women face challenges navigating contraceptive use.	2. Importantly, the noncontraceptive benefits associated with contraceptive use are underemphasized in queer women.
3. More effective contraceptive methods use by women participating in penile-vaginal intercourse may not be as relevant in queer women.	
4. Contraceptive use may be more challenging due to queer women's experiences with gender-based violence and power differences.	
5. Queer women may be hesitant to seek contraceptive care based on any anticipated or experienced stigma from within the healthcare system.	

[a]From focus groups and interviews conducted from August 2017 to April 2018 with young adult cisgender sexual minority women in three cities: Chicago, IL; Madison, WI; and Salt Lake City, UT.
[b]Conflicts between contraceptive use and queer identity; potential contributors to unintended pregnancy among queer women.
[c]Areas of alignment between queer identity and contraception; potential ways to amplify positive aspects of contraception among queer women.
Source: Adapted from Higgins, J. A., Carpenter, E., Everett, B. G., Greene, M. Z., Haider, S., & Hendrick, C. E. (2019). Sexual minority women and contraceptive use: Complex pathways between sexual orientation and health outcomes. American Journal of Public Health, 109*(12), 1680–1686. https://doi.org/10.2105/AJPH.2019.305211*

White women. The CDC reported that the infant death rate was 34% higher for non-Hispanic Black babies with birth defects, and 26% higher with Hispanic babies than non-Hispanic White babies. Access to prenatal care is not always available for women across the United States, and even when prenatal care is available, the recommended number of prenatal care visits are not attended by 25% of all pregnant women. Racial disparities are further noted as 41% of Native American and Alaska Native women and 32% of Black women are reported to receive inadequate prenatal care; although what is meant by inadequate prenatal care is not clearly defined (Petersen et al., 2019).

BIRTH DEFECTS

Birth defects affect about 1% to 3% (one in every 33) babies born in the United States each year. They are the leading cause of infant death, accounting for more than 20% of all infant deaths and attributing to the likelihood of illness and long-term disability (CDC, 2023b). Although most birth defects result from genetic, environmental, and lifestyle factors, some may be preventable by improving preconceptual and interconceptual advice, education, and care (ACOG, 2019; CDC, 2023b).

Etiology

When a change to the structure of the body occurs during fetal development, the result is defined as a birth defect. Birth defects can alter the shape or function of one or more parts of the body, causing problems to overall health, how the infant's body develops, and/or how the infant's body works.

Embryo Development and Organogenesis

The fetus is most susceptible in the first 4 to 10 weeks' gestation before most prenatal care is initiated (Figure 22.1). The embryonic period (up to 8 weeks of gestation) is the most vulnerable time for the development of major morphologic abnormalities of the heart, central nervous system, and the skull and face (craniofacial abnormalities), as well as limb defects. Nutritional, drug, and environmental exposures and infectious agents interrupting normal cell organization and differentiation can cause birth defects (King et al., 2015). The dark gray in the schematic in Figure 22.1 (primarily in the embryonic period) represents when the major congenital anomalies occur to the most vital organs such as the central nervous system, heart, eyes, limbs, and ears. The period when the major organ systems are forming is referred to as organogenesis, which primarily occurs between 17 and 56 days after conception. When there is exposure of great magnitude in the first 2 weeks, it is most likely to result in an early spontaneous abortion (see first two columns). Exposure(s) to toxic substances in the embryonic period (up to 8 weeks' gestation) have traditionally been considered teratogens, whereas exposures after 8 weeks are usually referred to as fetotoxins (represented by the shaded light green bars). Fetotoxins are substances that cause no structural changes like those that occur in the embryonic stage of development, but are toxic to the fetus and can impair normal growth and function (Dutta, 2015; King et al., 2015). Examples of fetotoxins include:

- Nicotine
- Cocaine (both teratogen and fetotoxin)
- Amphetamines
- Angiotensin-converting enzyme inhibitors (ACE-I; antihypertensive, both teratogenic and fetotoxic; King et al., 2015)

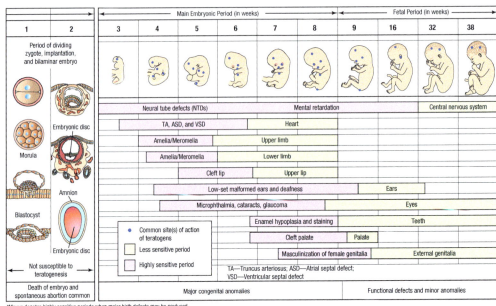

FIGURE 22.1 Embryo development and organogenesis.
Source: Adapted from Moore, K. L., & Persaud, T. V. N. (1998). The developing human: Clinically oriented embryology (6th ed.). W. B. Saunders.

Teratogen and fetotoxins are dependent on the following elements (Dutta, 2015):

- Genotype susceptibility (genetically coded information of the individual)
- Timing of exposure (determines whether teratogen or fetotoxin)
- Specific mechanism (such as gene mutation)
- Manifestation (dependent on stage of development exposure occurs)
- Agent (drug, disease, or environmental agent)
- Dose effect (from no effect to lethal)

Because of greater physiologic vulnerability in the preconception and early gestational periods, many exposures (medications, nutritional deficiencies, other toxic substances) put women at risk of birth defects that are preventable.

Prescription Medications That Increase the Risk of Birth Defects

Because of the number of unplanned pregnancies, development of the fetus can be affected by prescription medications that may be harmful even before the pregnancy is confirmed. In 2014, the U.S. Food and Drug Administration (FDA) Pregnancy Lactation Labeling Rule (PLLR) for all prescribed medications changed to include more information on pregnancy, lactation, and females and males of reproductive potential replacing the Class A, B, C, D, X system used previously. This change does not apply to over-the-counter medications (Food and Drug Administration [FDA], 2021, para. 1). More information can be found at www.fda.gov/drugs/labeling-information-drug -products/pregnancy-and-lactation-labeling-drugs-final-rule.

Interventions and Strategies for Risk Reduction and Management

It is imperative, then, that all clinicians caring for women taking potential teratogenic medications provide reliable and efficacious contraception as well as accurate preconception risk information at the time of prescribing. Because the use of potentially teratogenic medications is at times necessary to maximize the health of women of reproductive age, clinicians must engage women in shared decision- making around the use of contraception when these medications are prescribed, and improved drug-labeling systems should be developed. Given the high rate of unintended pregnancies even with the use of reliable and effective contraception, it is critical that women understand exposure to teratogens and any potential dangers to a pregnancy. One simple step is to promote timely access to emergency contraception when prescribing a potential teratogen to women of reproductive age (ACOG, 2010/2015b).

PREVIOUS PREGNANCY HISTORY

When evaluating pregnancy history, there are high-risk conditions that require further referral beyond the scope of an APRN practitioner. Any condition that may cause death or permanent injury to the mom, fetus, or newborn requires a higher level of consultation with either an obstetrician or a maternal fetal medicine specialist. The goal of multidisciplinary and specialized preconception care is to optimize pregnancy and birth outcomes.

PRECONCEPTION HEALTH AND LIFESTYLE RISK SCREENING

Smoking, Vaping or Electronic Nicotine Delivery Systems, and Cannabis

ETIOLOGY

Tobacco products and smoke contain more than 7,000 chemicals, including formaldehyde, cyanide, and nicotine. Nicotine produces serious side effects and is addictive. Smokers are exposed to carbon monoxide that constricts blood vessels, which in turn decreases oxygen levels in the blood (CDC, 2020). Additional smoking types are becoming more popular, such as hookah, cigars, and the electronic nicotine delivery system (ENDS), also known as e-cigarettes or vaping (ACOG, 2020b). Although there areis insufficient data to evaluate the effects of cannabis use during preconception and pregnancy, it has been shown to impact spermatogenesis and has been linked to impaired sperm function. On the other hand, cannabis use has not been associated with sexual dysfunction in healthy individuals, and delays in conception have not been demonstrated.

PREVALENCE

Actual smoking use rates vary by geography, age, education, and race; however, the overall rates have dropped to 7.2% in the last 10 years (ACOG, 2020b). In the 2015 Pregnancy Risk Assessment Maternal Study (PRAMS), when studying data from only Oklahoma and Texas, 7% used ENDS around pregnancy. When looking at smoking, to include ENDS, 38% reported using either or both during the 3 months prior to a pregnancy. Nearly half of women (45%) cited a belief that ENDS would help stop smoking or that it was safer than cigarettes.

Smoking is fetotoxic as it reduces fetal oxygenation by decreasing placental blood flow. All smoking products expose the consumer to nicotine and unhealthy chemicals with no added benefit. Although there are no safe levels of smoking in pregnancy, the fetotoxic effects are dose related. PTB, premature rupture of membranes, low birth weight, stillbirth, placental abruption, miscarriage, congenital anomalies, and other adverse perinatal outcomes associated with maternal smoking in pregnancy can be prevented if women stop smoking before or during early pregnancy (ACOG, 2020b; CDC, 2020). Cannabis use during pregnancy has been associated with an increased risk for low birth rate, small for gestational age, and NICU admission (Singh et al., 2020). Cannabis use prior to conception is associated with reduced fecundability among women with pregnancy loss despite increased sexual intercourse (Mumford et al., 2021). Disparities in smoking rates have been noted by race/ethnicity and by maternal education.

INTERVENTIONS AND STRATEGIES FOR RISK REDUCTION AND MANAGEMENT

Clinicians should promote smoking cessation before pregnancy even with women with low-level exposures. Because the rate of successful smoking cessation is low, it is recommended that smoking is assessed at every encounter within the healthcare system (ACOG, 2020b). The March of Dimes promotes a 5- to 15-minute, five-step counseling approach called the 5 As (Ask, Advise, Assess, Assist, and Arrange; ACOG, 2020b). The clinician can perform this approach during routine preconception or prenatal visits. Studies suggest that certain factors make it more likely that a woman will be successful in her efforts to quit smoking during pregnancy. These include:

- Attempting to quit in the past
- Having a partner who does not smoke
- Getting support from family or other important people in her life
- Understanding the harmful effects of smoking

Smoking and alcohol cessation interventions have been demonstrated to be effective in certain populations but have been shown to be less effective with persons at highest risk (e.g., injection-drug users and multiple substance users; ACOG, 2020b). More tools for cessation can be found at smokefree.gov.

At-Risk Drinking and Alcohol Dependence

ETIOLOGY

Alcohol is an organic solvent and acts as a neurotoxicant when consumed by crossing the placenta (ACOG, 2021a). Prenatal exposure to alcohol can damage the developing fetus and is the *leading preventable cause* of birth defects and intellectual and neurodevelopmental disabilities (ACOG, 2021a). Besides fetal alcohol syndrome (FAS), alcohol consumed in pregnancy can also lead to low-birth-weight infants, miscarriages, and stillbirths (ACOG, 2014). Fetal alcohol spectrum disorder (FASD) covers a range of impairments from severe, such as Karli's FAS, to mild. Its effects can include impaired growth, intellectual disabilities, and such neurologic, emotional, and behavioral issues as attention deficit hyperactivity disorder (ADHD), vision problems, and speech and language delays. These disabilities last a lifetime—there is no cure, only early intervention treatment, which can improve a child's development. FASD is also sometimes characterized by a cluster of facial features: small eyes, a thin upper lip, and a flat philtrum (the ridge between the nose and upper lip).

PREVALENCE

Although the prevalence of FAS in the United States during the 1980s and 1990s was reported as 0.5 to two2 cases per 1,000 live births, recent studies aggressively diagnosing FASD have reported FAS rates and FASD estimates up to 5%, respectively, while continuing to consider these rates underestimates (ACOG, 2021a). There is *no safe time* during pregnancy to *drink any amount of alcohol* (ACOG, 2021a). Often, irreversible harm occurs before a woman realizes that she is pregnant. The Behavioral Risk Factor Surveillance System (BRFSS) reported that 13.5% of pregnant women used alcohol (Gosdin et al., 2022). Women who binge drink are more likely to have unprotected sex and multiple sex partners, thus increasing the risk of unintended pregnancy and sexually transmitted infections (STIs; CDC, 2022c).

INTERVENTION AND STRATEGIES FOR RISK REDUCTION AND MANAGEMENT

Clinicians should promote cessation or limiting of alcohol use especially in reproductive-age women. FAS and other alcohol-related birth defects can be prevented if women cease intake of alcohol before conception and throughout a pregnancy and while breastfeeding (March of Dimes, 2022). This includes beer, wine, wine coolers, and hard liquors. Provide nonjudgmental support and appropriate chemical dependency referrals to promote alcohol cessation and recovery.

It is important to educate patients so that they understand the implications of drinking during pregnancy:

- Alcohol-related birth defects and developmental disabilities are completely preventable when pregnant women abstain from alcohol use.
- Neurocognitive and behavioral problems resulting from prenatal alcohol exposure are lifelong.
- Early recognition, diagnosis, and therapy for any condition along the FASD continuum can result in improved outcomes for the child.
- During pregnancy:
  - No amount of alcohol intake should be considered safe.
  - There is no safe trimester to drink alcohol.
  - All forms of alcohol, including beer, wine, and liquor, pose similar risk.
  - Binge drinking poses dose-related risk to the developing fetus.

Recreational Drugs

ETIOLOGY

Recreational drugs interrupt the way the brain's cells communicate through neurotransmission. The exact response, whether dampened or stimulated by a drug, varies greatly depending on which neurotransmitters are affected. During the early stages of drug use, the effects wear off with the drug; however, with chronic abusers, long-term changes in cell-to-cell communication result (National Institute on Drug Abuse [NIDA], 2017).

PREVALENCE

According to a 2020 U.S. national survey on drug use, 27.3% of respondents over age 12 reported using drugs in the last year, and twice as many pregnant women tested positive for marijuana use as compared to the number self-identifying. Nearly 5% of pregnant women have been found to use illicit drugs such as cocaine, ecstasy, other amphetamines, and heroin. Despite a large number of pregnant women who stop use, the rates of relapse 3 to 12 months postpartum is very high (U.S. Department of Health and Human Services [DHHS], 2022). It is often difficult to delineate what adverse perinatal outcomes are attributed to specific illicit drugs because of inherent impurities in street drugs, and because of multiple drug, smoking, and alcohol use in some women.

INTERVENTION AND STRATEGIES FOR RISK REDUCTION AND MANAGEMENT

When screening for smoking, or other sensitive subjects, frame the questions for building trust and for the purpose of improving health. The following are some examples to assist the clinician.

Framing Statement:
"Because smoking, alcohol, and recreational drug use have become so mainstream, I have started to ask all my clients routinely about it."

Indirect Question:
"*Have* you and your friends tried any recreational drugs in the past?"

Direct Question:
"In the past 1 to 3 months, have you taken any recreational drugs such as marijuana, speed, cocaine, ecstasy, or heroin?"

Affirmation:
"Thank you for sharing this information with me today. Would you be interested in learning more about the health effects to you should you become pregnant? Are you interested in a drug cessation program?"

Provide nonjudgmental support and provide appropriate referrals for drug use cessation.

Reproductive and Developmental Toxicants at Home and at Work

ETIOLOGY

Reproductive toxicants can affect people's fertility, result in teratogenic effects during pregnancy, increase pregnancy loss (spontaneous abortions and fetal death), and contribute to developmental delays and learning disabilities in children (Kumar et al.IJMR, 2019). Toxic substances that can affect people's fertility and childbearing include: (a) neurotoxicants such as lead, mercury, and organic solvents (degreasers); (b) endocrine disruptors such as polychlorinated biphenyls (PCBs, found in old electrical transformers, hydraulic systems, welding equipment, broken fluorescent light fixtures), polybrominated diphenyl ethers (PCBEs, flame retardants), dioxins (waste incineration, backyard fires), and phthalates (used in plastics, cosmetics, and pesticides); and (c) thyroid toxicants such as perchlorate (dry-cleaning solution). These substances may contribute to neurobehavioral and cognitive disorders, reproductive abnormalities, thyroid dysfunction, and other adverse health effects if exposure occurs during the prenatal period, infancy, childhood, and adolescence. See https://www.ncbi.nlm.nih.gov/pmc/articles/PMC7038808/ for more information (Kumar et al., 2019).

PREVALENCE

About one in six children in the United States now suffer from one or more learning, behavioral, or developmental disabilities (CDC, 2022b). The relationship between exposures to toxic substances and this increase is unknown, but many researchers speculate that these increases in chronic health conditions are associated with exposures to toxicants in the work and home environment. Toxic substances such as lead, mercury, organic solvents, ionizing radiation (x-ray), and chemotherapeutic drugs have been associated with adverse pregnancy outcomes including spontaneous abortion, low birth weight, and birth defects (ACOG, 2019). It is thought that the earlier the exposure after conception and the greater the magnitude of exposure, the greater the risk of a lethal outcome. When toxicant or teratogen exposures occur from conception to day 14 postconception, there is a much higher rate of spontaneous abortion. The magnitude of the exposure depends on several factors: (a) active metabolites within the chemical or substance, (b) duration of exposure, (c) fat solubility of chemical or substance, (d) placental transfer of substance or chemical, (e) maternal disease (e.g., epilepsy or diabetes), and/or (f) genotype of fetus. Some chemicals are commonly thought to be toxic to the fetus without supporting evidence. Although these chemicals are known as respiratory and skin irritants, they have not been associated with harm to the fetus (Box 22.1). Specific teratogens can be found at www.ncbi.nlm.nih.gov/pmc/articles/PMC7038808 (Kumar et al., 2019).

Workplace Toxicant Exposures

ASSESSMENT OF RISK

If a woman reports concerns about possible exposures to potential toxicants at work or symptoms she believes are associated with her work environment such as dizziness or nausea, she should take the following steps (Occupational Safety and Health Administration [OSHA], 2012):

Box 22.1 Common Chemicals Unlikely to Harm a Fetus

Ammonia

Chlorine

Hydrochloric acid

Nitric acid

Sulfuric acid

Sodium hydroxide

Glutaraldehyde (Cidex)

Potassium hydroxide

Sodium hypochlorite (bleach)

Asbestos

Fiberglass

Silica

Source: Adapted from California Department of Health Services, Hazard Evaluation System and Information Service. (2007). If I'm pregnant, can the chemicals I work with harm my baby? https://www.cdph.ca.gov/Programs/CCDPHP/DEODC /OHB/HESIS/CDPH%20Document%20Library/pregnant.pdfAuthor.

1. Request a Material Safety Data Sheet (MSDS) from her employer. The MSDS is a document prepared by the manufacturer that contains information about the hazards of working with a given product or material and how to work safely with that material. All U.S. employers are required by law in most states to make available and to provide training on the health hazards of toxicants used in the workplace and how to protect against harmful exposures, including those that pose a risk to reproduction and pregnancy (Lassi et al., 2014; OSHA, 2012).
2. The employee should report her concern about a possible exposure and resulting injury or illness to her employer.
3. Call the local or regional hazard evaluation service (contact Environmental Protection Agency for more information; OSHA, 2012).
4. If injury or illness has resulted from toxicant exposures in the workplace, consult and refer to an occupational medicine specialist for further evaluation and treatment (Lassi et al., 2014; OSHA, 2012).

INTERVENTION AND STRATEGIES FOR RISK REDUCTION AND MANAGEMENT

- Encourage planned pregnancies to mitigate risks.
- Encourage all reproductive-age people to find out about environmental and workplace hazards *before* pregnancy.
- If employers and employees follow the MSDS recommendations and the workplace is made safe for all employees, then the workplace is safe for pregnancy.
- Remind couples that male exposure also has potential for harm and that harm, caused by reproductive toxicants, can occur through all developmental stages. Whenever possible it is best to prevent or minimize exposure as much as possible.
- Do not eat or drink in the same area when working with toxicants.
- Avoid exposure to toxicants, especially during preconception and pregnancy.
- Provide adequate ventilation and use proper protective equipment (e.g., gloves) when handling toxicants.
- Avoid "take home" exposures by showering/changing to clean clothing before entering the home.
- Use only cold tap water for cooking and drinking. Run the water for at least 30 seconds before use to help reduce lead exposure from old plumbing.

Common Preventable Birth Defects

NEURAL TUBE DEFECTS

Neural tube defects (NTDs) are the most common preventable birth defect and are associated with a nutritional deficiency in folic acid or food folate, a type of B vitamin (CDC, 2023a).

Etiology

The neural tube develops in the first 4 weeks of pregnancy, often before many women even know they are pregnant. Inadequate closure of the neural tube results in an NTD, specifically spina bifida or anencephaly. Babies with anencephaly will result in either a stillborn birth or a neonatal death. Unlike anencephaly, which is 100% fatal, 80% of babies born with spina bifida survive (CDC, 2023a; March of Dimes, 2022). The average lifetime cost for caring for a child with spina bifida ranges from $791,900 to more than $1,350,000 (Mai et al., 2019). These medical costs do not take into account the physical and emotional costs to the family. It is important to note that research has shown that getting enough folic acid before and during pregnancy can prevent most NTDs.

Prevalence

Each year in the United States, there are more than 4,000 pregnancies or 2,500 to 3,000 births (1/1,000 births) affected by NTDs, which include both spina bifida (when the fetal spine column does not close causing paralysis below the affected area), and anencephaly (when most of the brain does not develop; CDC, 2023a).

Assessment of Risk of Neural Tube Defect

Obesity, diabetes, and convulsant disorders as well as certain medications have been shown to increase the risk of NTDs by interfering with folic acid absorption (CDC, 2023a). Obesity has been shown to double the risk of NTDs, despite the use of folic acid, but weight loss before pregnancy may reduce NTD risk.

Health Promotion

Folic acid has been shown to reduce the risk of NTDs by 50% to 70% (CDC, 2023a). In order to reduce the risk of NTDs, the CDC recommends that all women of childbearing age, who are capable of becoming pregnant, take in 400 mcgmicrograms of folic acid each day—even those not trying to get pregnant. The easiest way to obtain adequate folic acid is by consuming a diet filled with folate- rich foods (dark leafy greens, legumes, broccoli, and asparagus), with foods fortified with folic acid (such as cereals, pasta, and bread), and/or by taking a daily multivitamin (ACOG, 2019).

Interventions and Strategies for Risk Reduction and Management

Adequate folic acid has been shown to reduce the risk of NTDs by two thirds (CDC, 2023a). Synthetically produced folic acid has twice the bioavailability as food folate. Consumption of folic acid fortified foods produced in the United States isare estimated to add 100 mcgmicrograms of folic acid per day to the average person's dietary intake of essential nutrients. Almost all multivitamins that contain 100% of the recommended dietary allowances (RDA) will contain at least 400 mcgmicrograms of folic acid (ACOG, 2019).

CHRONIC MEDICAL CONDITIONS AS TERATOGENS

Chronic medical conditions may affect the quality of preconception health (Table 22.2). These include medical conditions such as hypertension, obesity, diabetes, HIV/AIDS,cquired immune deficiency syndrome (AIDS), cardiovascular diseases (CVDs), systemic lupus, seizure disorders, thyroid disease, and chronic depression. Some of these medical conditions may increase the risk of congenital malformations and they

TABLE 22.2 Health Conditions, Related Risks, and Treatment Goals During Pregnancy

HEALTH CONDITION	RELATED RISKS	GOALS
Pregestational diabetes mellitus	Congenital anomalies	Hemoglobin A1c ≤6.5%
Chronic hypertension	Preeclampsia, IUGR	SBP ≤140 mmHg DBP ≤90 mmHg
Untreated/inadequately treated hypothyroidism	Increased risk of spontaneous abortion, placental abnormalities, preeclampsia, preterm birth, fetal death	TSH ≤2.5 mU/L
Bariatric surgery	Prematurity, SGA, IUGR	
Mood disorders	Maternal–infant bonding disorder, postpartum psychiatric illness	• Optimal functioning of mother • Achieving/maintaining euthymia • Relapse prevention • Monitor risk for suicide
HIV	Vertical transmission	• Prenatal care delivered in conjunction with an HIV specialist • Undetectable viral loads • Interventions to prevent/reduce risk of vertical transmission
Thrombophilia (high or low risk)	Pregnancy and/or postpartum DVT and PE	Consider anticoagulation therapy and dosing regimen when appropriate

DBP, diastolic blood pressure; DVT, deep vein thrombosis; IUGR, intrauterine growth restriction; PE, pulmonary embolism; SBP, systolic blood pressure; SGA, small for gestational age; TSH, thyroid-stimulating hormone.
Source: Adapted from American College of Obstetricians and Gynecologists. (2019). Committee Opinion No. 762: Prepregnancy counseling. https://www.acog.org/clinical/clinical -guidance/committee-opinion/articles/2019/01/prepregnancy-counseling

may also require the use of medications that may be teratogenic (e.g., ACE-Is, some anticonvulsants, some antidepressants; American Diabetes Association [ACOG, 2019]).

Diabetes Mellitus

One of the best examples of a medical condition increasing risk is diabetes mellitus. Since the advent of insulin, there has been dramatic improvement in maternal–fetal health outcomes in all areas except for congenital anomalies (ACOG, 2018a).

ETIOLOGY

These malformations occur by the seventh week of gestation and are primarily caused by inadequate glycemic control. Inadequate maternal glycemic control leads to hyperglycemia, hyperketonemia, hypoglycemia, excess somatomedin inhibitor (insulin-like growth factors), deficiency of arachiadonic acid (essential fatty acid), and excess oxygen free radicals. Deficiency in arachiadonic acid and excess free radicals can lead to embryonic malformations (ACOG, 2018a). Despite these known risks, diabetic women are less likely to plan their pregnancies compared with the general population.

PREVALENCE

The rate of congenital anomalies ranges in women with pregestational diabetes is 10% to 12% versus 3% in the nondiabetic population (Riskin et al., 2020). Cardiac malformations linked to pregestational diabetes account for 35% to 45% of these anomalies. Congenital anomaly deaths primarily involve the central nervous system: anencephaly, spina bifida, holoprosencephaly (10-fold increase); cardiac anomalies:

ventricular septal defects, transposition of the great vessels (fivefold increase); and sacral agenesis or caudal dysplasia (200-fold increase; Riskin, 2020).

ASSESSMENT OF RISK

Initial laboratory testing includes assessment of hemoglobin (Hb) A1c and a random albumin-to-creatinine ratio (ACR). If the ACR is elevated, a 24-hour microalbumin level should be collected and evaluated. Increased HbA1c levels that are greater than or equal to 8.0 elevate a woman's risk of congenital malformations to 20% to 25%. Consideration for assessment of blood pressure, retinopathy and kidney function must be included.

HIV/AIDS

ETIOLOGY

HIV attacks the immune system CD4 cells, preventing natural immunity, and resulting in increasing viral load levels from undetectable at 40 to 75 copies per milliliter of blood to millions of copies. Through contact with blood and body fluids, labor, prechewing baby's food, and sharing needles, razors, or drug equipment, HIV is transmitted. When there is a coexisting STI, such as herpes simplex virus (HSV) or hepatitis, HIV is three to five times more likely to spread. With viral loads as low as 3,500 copies, HIV transmission risk exists (CDC, 2023c). AIDS diagnosis is confirmed with viral loads by laboratory testing (CDC, 2023c) or by AIDS-defining conditions found at *Mortality and Morbidity Weekly Report* (MMWR; CDC, 2023c).

PREVALENCE

Since the 1990s, the rates of perinatal transmission have decreased by 95% (CDC, 2023c). Risk of transmission of HIV to infants of infected mothers has been reduced to less than 1% in women taking antiretroviral medication during pregnancy as recommended (CDC, 2023c). HIV is disproportionately greater in Black children in the United States (CDC, 2023c; Henry J. Kaiser Family Foundation, 2020).

ASSESSMENT OF RISK

One of the most important benefits of pregnancy planning for an HIV-infected mother is being able to provide medical intervention to minimize the risk of vertical transmission to her baby. The CDC recommends universal screening of all men and women of reproductive age before pregnancy and at the onset of prenatal care. If an individual is a known HIV/AIDS carrier, then the use of two methods of contraception (barrier protection plus a more effective method) is recommended to prevent an unplanned pregnancy and HIV transmission (CDC, 2023c). When HIV is detected early in pregnancy, the risk of HIV transmission from an HIV-positive mother to the fetus and newborn can be reduced to 1% or less (CDC, 2023c). Risk reduction may be achieved through universal screening, early detection, early treatment, delivery by cesarean section, and avoidance of breastfeeding (CDC, 2023c).

Chronic Hypertension

ETIOLOGY

Hypertensive disorders complicate 5% to 10% of pregnancies (Khedagi & Bello, 2021, para. 1). Hypertensive risks presented in pregnancy are related to treatment (e.g., ACE-Is and beta blockers such as atenolol, which pose teratogenic risks), and adverse sequelae such as maternal and infant morbidity and mortality (e.g., superimposed preeclampsia, eclampsia, acute kidney failure, pulmonary edema, stroke/cardiovascular complications, postpartum hemorrhage, gestational diabetes, premature delivery, low birth weight, NICU admission, placental abruption, congenital malformations, and stillbirth), and a long-term risk of maternal CVD (Khedaji & Bello, 2021).

PREVALENCE

Hypertension is the most common medical disorder of pregnancy, is reported to complicate up to one in 10 gestations, and affects a 5% to 10% of pregnant women in the United States every year (ACOG, 2022). Preeclampsia complicates 2% to 4% of all pregnancies, causing 46,000 maternal deaths and 500,000 fetal deaths worldwide (Magee et al., 2022).

ASSESSMENT OF RISK

In 2022, ACOG released new guidelines for the diagnosis and management of hypertension in relation to pregnancy. Hypertension is classified as chronic (before pregnancy), gestational (after 20 weeks' gestation), preeclampsia (elevated blood pressure with proteinuria or any of listed severe features), and chronic with superimposed preeclampsia. Preconception counseling focuses on lifestyle modifications and management or elimination of comorbidities before conception for decreasing risk. In future pregnancies ensure folic acid supplementation and consider low-dose aspirin for women who experience preeclampsia (Khedaji & Bello, 2021). Dietary modifications

regarding salt, vitamin A, vitamin E, and calcium supplementation demonstrated no effect on risk in the U.S. pregnant population; however, consideration can be offered for women for low-dose aspirin after the first trimester (12 weeks) to decrease risk of adverse perinatal outcomes and preeclampsia (ACOG, 2022). Finally, women who experienced a PTB because of preeclampsia have increased risk of CVD later in life CVD. Annual visits for blood pressure evaluation, cholesterol, fasting glucose, and body mass index (BMI) are recommended by ACOG (2019).

Phenylketonuria

ETIOLOGY

Phenylketonuria (PKU) is another example of a chronic disease that can act as a potent teratogen. PKU is an autosomal recessive disease causing a deficiency in phenylalanine hydroxylase (ACOG, 2020a). This deficiency prevents phenylalanine from being metabolized into tyrosine after the intake of proteins (American Academy of Pediatrics Committee on Genetics, 2001).

PREVALENCE

In the United States, about 1 in 10,000 to 15,000 infants are born with PKU each year (March of Dimes, 2022). If identified and treated, intellectual and developmental disabilities in infants can be prevented. Left untreated, high levels of phenylalanine can lead to microcephaly and developmental delays in 75% to 90% of babies exposed (American Academy of Pediatrics Committee on Genetics, 2001).

ASSESSMENT OF RISK

PKU testing has been standard for many years in all newborns born in the United States, consisting of a simple heel stick blood draw. Females born with PKU must maintain strict dietary control throughout their reproductive years to limit their levels of phenylalanine. ACOG recommends a blood level < 6 mg/dL for 3 months prior to pregnancy and maintaininged 2 to –6 mg/dL to prevent crossing the placenta and causinge embryonic and fetal damage, for example, fetal growth retardation, microcephaly, psychomotor handicaps, and congenital heart defects (ACOG, 2020a).

Pregnancy and Chronic Medical Conditions

Chronic medical conditions can stress and therefore negatively impact a woman's pregnancy. Additionally, a woman's pregnancy may stress a woman's chronic health condition, leading to exacerbation. Chronic medical conditions include heart disease, systemic lupus, rheumatoid arthritis, seizure disorders, thyroid disease, inherited thrombophilia, asthma, and psychiatric conditions (e.g., depression, psychosis). Women with these and other chronic medical conditions should receive expert advice (from a high-risk perinatologist or maternal–fetal medicine specialist) in anticipation or when planning pregnancy.

INTERVENTIONS AND STRATEGIES FOR RISK REDUCTION AND MANAGEMENT

All pregnancies in women with chronic medical conditions should be planned.

Diabetes

- Promote glycemic control and highly effective contraception in all women with preexisting diabetes to reduce the increased risk of birth defects.
- The two- to threefold increase in the prevalence of birth defects among infants of women with type 1 and type 2 diabetes is substantially reduced through proper management of diabetes.
- Screen all women annually for diabetes mellitus with prior gestational diabetes mellitus (GDM).
- Before conception, promote the use of highly effective reversible contraception until glycemic control is achieved.

Hypothyroidism

- The dose of levothyroxine, for treatment of hypothyroidism, will need to be adjusted during early pregnancy. This is necessary to ensure proper neurologic development of the fetus (American Thyroid Association, n.d.).

Heart Disease and Hypertension

- Avoid prescribing ACE-Is, atenolol, and statins in reproductive-age women whenever possible.
- Reevaluate cardiovascular function before a planned pregnancy.
- Promote the use of appropriate contraception to facilitate a planned pregnancy.
- Consider screening all women using the CMQCC algorithm during pregnancy and the postpartum period to stratify risk level (Chambers et al., 2022).
- Help women be realistic about their pregnancy risks and the consequences of aging and heart disease.

Maternal Phenylketonuria

- Adverse outcomes can be prevented when afflicted mothers adhere to a low-phenylalanine diet before conception and continue throughout pregnancy (ACOG, 2020a).
- Check phenylalanine levels frequently during reproductive years.

HIV/AIDS

- Preexposure prophylaxis (PrEP) and postexposure prophylaxis (PEP) medications reduce the risk of high-risk exposure groups.

Infectious Diseases as Teratogens

Infectious diseases may also act as teratogens when exposure occurs in the immediate preconception period and/or during pregnancy. Examples of infectious diseases that may be teratogenic or fetotoxic include toxoplasmosis (caused by *Toxoplasma gondii*), HIV infection, syphilis, rubella, varicella (chickenpox), cytomegalovirus (CMV) infection, parvovirus infection, and herpes. The common acronym that describes the screening test for most of these congenital infections is TORCH, which stands for *Toxoplasma gondii*; *o*ther viruses (syphilis, HIV, measles, and more); *r*ubella (German measles); *c*ytomegalovirus; and *h*erpes simplex.

ETIOLOGY

TORCH and other congenital infections may cause damage to the central nervous system and other organs leading to mental retardation, microcephaly, learning disabilities, eye and hearing defects, cardiac anomalies, gastrointestinal anomalies, and damage to the liver and spleen (ACOG, 2019).

PREVALENCE

TORCH infectious agents affect 1% to 3% of all live births and are among the leading causes of neonatal morbidity and death (Neu et al., 2015).

ASSESSMENT OF RISK

It is recommended that all women of reproductive age know their immune status for rubella and varicella before pregnancy (ACOG, 2019).

Toxoplasmosis

ETIOLOGY

The single-cell protozoan parasite called *Toxoplasma gondii* causes this rare disease. Toxoplasmosis is commonly transmitted in cat feces and through consumption of raw and undercooked meat, and it is rarely congenital or contracted through organ transplant. After eating infected rodents, cats shed the parasite oocytes in their feces (either in the litter box or outside in the soil) for up to 3 weeks (CDC, 2022i). The period of highest risk of acquiring primary toxoplasmosis infection is 10 to 24 weeks of gestation.

PREVALENCE

In the United States, toxoplasmosis is considered to be a leading cause of death attributed to foodborne illness. In fact, one in five adults older than 12 years hasve been infected and carriesy the *Toxoplasma* parasite. Ironically, though, few have symptoms because their immune system is intact, thereby keeping the parasite from causing illness (CDC, 2022i).

ASSESSMENT AND MANAGEMENT

After determining precise exposure date, serological testing for immunoglobulin G (IgG) and immunoglobulin M (IgM) is routinely used; however, parasites directly observed in bodily fluids can be used to make the diagnosis (CDC, 2022i). With congenital transmission, the amniotic fluid can be tested for *Toxoplasma*-infected DNA (CDC, 2022i). Risk reduction for transmission of toxoplasmosis can be achieved through good hand washing; washing of vegetables; proper cleaning (hot soapy water) and handling of cutting boards during food preparation; avoidance of handling cat feces, changing cat litter, and/or avoiding dirty cat litter boxes; and wearing gloves when gardening. High-risk women are screened via laboratory testing (CDC, 2022i).

Varicella

ETIOLOGY

The greatest risk period for malformations caused by varicella (chickenpox) infection is within the first 6 to 18 weeks of gestation (CDC, 2019a). There is also a risk of varicella infection to the newborn if infection occurs in late pregnancy near delivery. Varicella infection is not only dangerous to the growing fetus. Up to 20% of pregnant women who become infected with varicella develop pneumonia. Pneumonia acquired as a result of a varicella infection is associated with a maternal mortality rate as high as 40% (CDC, 2019a).

PREVALENCE

Most women (between 85% and 95%) will be immune to varicella before pregnancy. Approximately 1.5% of infants will acquire congenital varicella syndrome if a nonimmune pregnant woman contracts the virus during the first 28 weeks of pregnancy (CDC, 2019a).

ASSESSMENT AND MANAGEMENT

Verification of varicella immunity is determined by laboratory testing, proof of previous vaccination, or a clinician's confirmation of infection. Women who are rubella nonimmune and not pregnant should receive the varicella vaccine. During routine obstetric care, it is standard of care to screen all pregnant women for immune status. Those who are nonimmune receive the varicella vaccine after delivery.

Parvovirus B19 Infection

ETIOLOGY

Infection with parvovirus B19 (also called fifth disease) is commonly known as erythema infectiosum. The virus is transmitted through sputum, saliva, and nasal secretions. The initial mild symptoms of fever, headache, and runny nose present for 80% of those affected followed with a characteristic rash on the cheeks ("slapped cheek" appearance) from 4 to 14 days following exposure. By the time the rash appears, the virus is no longer infectious (CDC, 2019b).

Parvovirus B19 can infect the fetus before birth. Although no birth defects have been reported as a result of fifth disease, it may cause the death of an unborn fetus (CDC, 2019b). If acquired in the first trimester (rare), parvovirus B19 can contribute to spontaneous abortion. Although rare (less than 5% of pregnant women are infected with parvovirus B19), if exposed during the second trimester, the risks of severe fetal anemia, hydrops fetalis, and stillbirth are significantly increased (CDC, 2019b).

PREVALENCE

In the general population, 35% to 53% of pregnant women have antibodies to parvovirus B19; therefore, preexisting IgG means the mother–baby pair are already protected. The risk of fetal death is 5% to 10% if the mother becomes infected.

ASSESSMENT AND MANAGEMENT

Pregnant women who have not previously had fifth disease should avoid contact with patients who are actively infected. Individuals are contagious during the mild symptoms before the rash or joint pain and not contagious during the rash or

"slapped cheek" appearance (ACOG, 2018b). Circulating IgM antibodies can be detected 10 days after exposure and can be detected for 3 months. The IgG antibody can be detected immediately after the IgM antibodies are detectable and remain present for the rest of the woman's life. Fetal parvovirus infection can be detected in amniotic fluid with a polymerase chain reaction (PCR) test. Pregnant women exposed or with symptoms should have serologic testing for IgG/IgM (Saarainen et al., 1986).

Rubella

ETIOLOGY

Rubella (German or three-day measles) is a viral infection spread through coughing and sneezing of an infected person. In approximately half of those infected, following fever symptoms, a facial rash spreads to the rest of the body lasting 2 to 3 days (CDC, 2022h). Lack of rubella immunity appears to be associated with a generation of young people who were born too late to acquire rubella immunity through natural infection, yet too early to receive vaccine mandated by school entry laws. The lack of immunity has also been associated with foreign-born women of mostly Hispanic descent, especially those with little or no access to immunization programs (CDC, 2022h). Congenital rubella syndrome consists of multiple severe anomalies: eye defects resulting in vision loss or blindness, hearing loss, heart defects, mental retardation, and occasionally movement disorders, all of which frequently result in miscarriage or stillbirth.

PREVALENCE

Rubella exposure within the first 8 weeks of gestation will cause congenital rubella syndrome in ~85% of exposed pregnancies. The highest rates (up to 90%) are associated with infections occurring during the first trimester. Birth defects caused by maternal rubella infection, after 20 weeks' gestation, are rare. Additionally, adolescents and young women aged 12 to 19 years have the lowest immunity (CDC, 2022h).

ASSESSMENT AND MANAGEMENT

Titers for rubella are standard of care with each pregnancy. Laboratory testing is done for the purpose of assessing a pregnant woman's immunity status.

Cytomegalovirus Infection

ETIOLOGY

CMV is prevalent in the excretions of infants and toddlers as well as of adults who are immunosuppressed (e.g., those undergoing organ transplant, HIV positive). Women working in healthcare settings with immunosuppressed patients or those working in child care should be screened before a planned pregnancy as they are at greater risk of contracting CMV infection (ACOG, 2018b). Although the CMV IgG antibody test determines whether a person has been infected, the CMV IgM and IgG avidity tests determine whether the infection is recent or not. It is important to note that these tests are not always commercially available and are not always accurate (ACOG, 2018b; CDC, 2022a).

CMV is a member of the herpesvirus group, which also includes herpes simplex types 1 and 2, varicella-zoster virus (chickenpox), and Epstein–Barr virus (infectious mononucleosis; ACOG, 2018b; CDC, 2022a).

PREVALENCE

CMV is common among adults and infects between 40% and 85% of adults by 40 years of age. Annually, one child in 150 is born and is affected by a CMV infection (ACOG, 2018b).

ASSESSMENT AND MANAGEMENT

Because it is so pervasive, routine screening is not currently recommended. Instead, *meticulous handwashing* should be stressed to prevent transmission of CMV in healthcare and child care settings.

Herpes

ETIOLOGY

There are two types of HSV: type 1 (usually oropharyngeal in origin) and type 2 (usually genital in origin). There is a greater likelihood of subclinical viral shedding with type 2 than with type 1 HSV (Workowski & Bolan, 2015).

PREVALENCE

With most neonatal herpes infections, there is a 30% to 50% transmission rate to the newborn (Workowski & Bolan, 2015). Acquiring a primary herpes outbreak in the genital area late in pregnancy and/or near delivery carries greater risk of fetal diagnosis with congenital herpes.

ASSESSMENT AND MANAGEMENT

Women with a history of genital herpes lesions (type 1 or type 2) should inform their clinician before or at the first prenatal visit. Pregnant women with a history of herpes will be given prophylactic treatment for HSV suppression, beginning at 36 weeks' gestation. Routine serologic testing for HSV remains controversial. We currently have no immunizations for infections with HIV, CMV, *Toxoplasma*, parvovirus, and HSV. Prevention of transmission, appropriate screening, and awareness of the importance of screening high-risk populations are essential.

Zika Virus Infection

ETIOLOGY

Zika virus (ZIKV) is transmitted by infected mosquitos in affected regions of the world. Vertical transmission in pregnancy is associated with birth defects such as microcephaly, ocular abnormalities, and hearing loss.

PREVALENCE

The rate of microcephaly is 1% to 5% with exposure to ZIKV during pregnancy.

ASSESSMENT AND MANAGEMENT

Assess for past travel experiences in areas endemic to ZIKV for both the woman and her partner. Advise women to avoid travel to those areas, avoid sexual partners at risk, and practice mos-

quito protection day and night. Couples planning to conceive who are from high-prevalence areas should discuss all the latest guidance with the clinician and consider delaying conception. Diagnostic assessment in pregnancy is different as the ZIKV RNA remains in the bloodstream three times as long. Symptoms of a ZIKV infection include acute onset of fever, conjunctivitis, arthralgia, and a maculopapular rash (Suy et al., 2016).

Interventions and Strategies for Risk Reduction and Management

Assess immunization status on all women of reproductive age.

- *Rubella seronegativity.* Rubella vaccination provides protective seropositivity and prevents congenital rubella syndrome.
- *Human papillomavirus (HPV)*
  - ○ Assess need for quadrivalent HPV vaccine before pregnancy.
  - ○ Vaccinate all women younger than 26 years old.
- *Hepatitis B virus (HBV).* Screen for exposure and vaccinate to prevent exposure during pregnancy.
- *Varicella immune status*
  - ○ Check for seronegativity and vaccinate in women with no history of chickenpox or if their status is in question.
- *Tetanus, diphtheria, pertussis (T*dap*)*
  - ○ Assess the need for vaccine before pregnancy; recommended every 10 years or after 5 years in the case of a wound or burn.
  - ○ Vaccinate all women early in the third trimester of pregnancy for passive transmission to the fetus for whooping cough protection in the first months of life.
- *COVID-19.* Educate, then offer and recommend the vaccine to all women.
- *Influenza.* Educate, then offer and recommend starting September or October of each year. Routinely offer and encourage effective contraception after administration of vaccines.

Screen for Sexually Transmitted Infection Exposure Before Pregnancy

Early STI screening and treatment may prevent associated adverse outcomes in pregnancy. STIs are strongly associated with ectopic pregnancy, infertility, and chronic pelvic pain, resulting in fetal death or substantial physical and developmental disabilities, including mental retardation and blindness.

- Screen all women younger than 26 years old annually for *Chlamydia trachomatis* and *Neisseria gonorrhoeae* (Workowski & Bolan, 2015).
- Ask about HSV exposure with women and partners and consider serologic screening (controversial) and prophylactic treatment near delivery in women with positive partners.
- Screen for HBV and vaccinate before pregnancy if a woman is negative. Prevention of HBV infection in women of childbearing age prevents transmission of infection to infants. HBV screening and vaccination also eliminate

risk of sequelae, which include possible hepatic failure, liver carcinoma, cirrhosis, and death (Workowski & Bolan, 2015).

- Screen all women for HIV before pregnancy. If HIV infection is identified before pregnancy, women (or couples) should be given additional information and timely antiretroviral treatment can be administered, which is known to prevent mother-to-child transmission (Workowski & Bolan, 2015).
- Encourage safe sex practices for reducing STI risk as part of preconception care. *Safe sex* includes abstinence, mutual masturbation, dry kissing, hugging, body massage, and condom use with intercourse and/or oral sex.

Risk of Preconception Overweight and Obesity

ETIOLOGY

Preconception obesity leads to greater risk of NTDs, gestational diabetes, gestational hypertension, congenital anomalies, and difficult management of labor resulting in operative deliveries (ACOG, 2021b). Postpartum obesity elevates the risks for recurrent medical problems with each subsequent pregnancy.

PREVALENCE

Obesity and diabetes are epidemic in the United States. More than half of U.S. women are overweight and one third of them are considered obese (CDC, 2022g). Diabetes affects 9.1 million or 8.9% of women age 20 years and older and it is estimated that one third of women go undiagnosed (ACOG, 2018a). The prevalence of diabetes is two to four times higher in women who are of Black, Hispanic, Latin American, Native American, or Asian/Pacific Islander descent (ACOG, 2018a). In women of reproductive age, 2% to 5% of them will develop gestational diabetes, which may result in a greater risk of developing type 2 diabetes (ADA, 2013). It is estimated that obesity can also lead to a greater risk of NTDs, despite the recommended 400 mcg daily intake of folic acid likely because of lower circulating blood levels (ACOG, 2018a). Pregnancy complications such as gestational hypertension, gestational diabetes, preeclampsia, PTB, and large-for-gestational-age neonates are amplified or can be attributed to maternal obesity nearly one third of the time.

MANAGEMENT AND HEALTH PROMOTION

Weight loss before pregnancy was also shown to reduce risks of NTDs in overweight women (ACOG, 2019). Women avoiding consumption of carbohydrates for weight loss purposes are at risk of folic acid deficiency; low-carbohydrate diets usually limit folate- fortified carbohydrate-rich foods (e.g., breads, cereals, pasta; ACOG, 2019). Being either overweight or underweight may also contribute to difficulty with conception because of an increased risk of infrequent ovulation or anovulation.

INTERVENTIONS AND STRATEGIES FOR RISK REDUCTION AND MANAGEMENT

Maternal obesity increases the risk of preterm delivery, diabetes, cesarean section, and hypertensive and thromboembolic disease (ACOG, 2021a; CDC, 2023a). Pregnant women

with a BMI > 50 have 2.5 times the risk of poor outcomes for both mom and baby than women with a BMI < 50; poor outcomes includeing severe maternal morbidity and even deathmortality (Platner et al., 2021). This classification has been defined as "super obese" andwhich is associated with a greater risk of renal failure, air and thrombotic embolism, the need for blood transfusion, heart failure, and the need for mechanical ventilation (Platner et al., 2021).

Lead and Mercury

ETIOLOGY

Lead and mercury are widespread in the environment. The most common source of mercury is from the burning of wastes contaminated with inorganic mercury and the burning of fossil fuels, primarily coal. Methyl mercury is formed from inorganic mercury through anaerobic organisms in aquatic environments. The natural food chain in aquatic environments results in higher levels of methyl mercury in larger predator fish, leading to human exposure from consumption of seafood. Lead and mercury are neurotoxicants and may also harm the kidneys of a developing fetus (ACOG, 2019). Exposure to heavy metals, such as lead and mercury, during pregnancy is potentially harmful to a developing fetus.

PREVALENCE

Mercury and lead levels among pregnant women vary by race and ethnicity. Mean lead levels in U.S. pregnant women are generally low (less than 5 mcg/dL; ACOG, 2019). In the United States, there is no standard for blood mercury levels in pregnant women, although blood mercury levels greater than 5.8 mcg/L have raised concerns (ACOG, 2019; U.S. Environmental Protection Agency [USEPA], 2023). There appears to be a negative relationship between prenatal lead and mercury exposure and fetal growth and neurodevelopment (USEPA, 2022).

When testing mercury and lead levels in pregnant women, a single blood lead test may not reflect cumulative lead and/or mercury exposure. Therefore, results from a single blood test may not be sufficient to establish the full nature of the developmental risk to the fetus. Repeat testing may be necessary (EPA, 2023).

ASSESSMENT AND MANAGEMENT

The FDA and the EPA recommend that all pregnant women avoid swordfish, shark, tilefish, and king mackerel, and should limit consumption of other seafood to a maximum of 12 ounces per week (FDA, 2016). Methyl mercury is removed from the body naturally but may take more than a year to return to safe levels once they have become high. Therefore, all women who could become pregnant should also follow the same recommendations (FDA, 2016). To avoid excessive lead exposure from old plumbing, use only bottled or cold tap water for cooking or drinking and let the tap run for at least 30 seconds before using. Lead is also used in paint found on pottery, especially terra cotta. Always recommend lead-free pottery or clear glass for baking and reheating (EPA, 2015).

Testing lead levels is important. The CDC recommends counseling on supplemental calcium, iron, and prenatal vitamins for levels ≥greater than or equal to 5 mg/dL

(CDC, 2022d). A thorough investigation of both occupational and home -risk factors, conducted by the local health department, is indicated for levels ≥greater than or equal to 15 mg/dL. Treatment through chelation for lead levels ≥greater than or equal to 45 mg/dL is also recommended (CDC, 2022d). Mercury levels are tested in the first morning urine preferably; blood levels can be assessed as early as 3 days after exposure (CDC, 2022d).

Listeria

ETIOLOGY

Listeriosis is a foodborne infection caused by the bacterium *Listeria monocytogenes*, which is found in soil and water. Animals carry the bacterium without appearing ill and contaminate foods, such as meat and dairy products, as well as vegetables grown from manure used as fertilizer (CDC, 2022e). Unlike most foodborne bacteria, listeria can grow at refrigerator temperatures. Listeria is most frequently found in nonpasteurized cheeses (e.g., feta, brie, camembert, blue-veined cheeses, some white Mexican cheeses, and panela), hot dogs, lunch meat (unless reheated until steaming hot), refrigerated pates and meat spreads, and refrigerated smoked seafood (e.g., salmon, trout, whitefish, cod, tuna, or mackerel), as well as other unpasteurized milk-containing products (CDC, 2022e).

Symptoms of listeriosis include flu-like symptoms (e.g., stiff neck, fever, muscle aches, nausea, diarrhea), and if infection spreads to the central nervous system, symptoms may include headache, stiff neck, confusion, loss of balance, or convulsions. Infected pregnant women may experience only mild, flu-like symptoms. There is no screening test for listeriosis. In suspected cases, listeriosis is confirmed with blood and cerebrospinal fluid cultures. Once confirmed, prompt intravenous antibiotic treatment is recommended. If diagnosed and treated quickly, the likelihood of transmission to the fetus may be minimized. Even so, prompt treatment is not a guarantee of fetal survival (CDC, 2022e).

PREVALENCE

Listeriosis is recognized as a serious public health problem in the United States because it affects an estimated 2,500 persons each year. Those infected become seriously ill, and approximately 500 die from the infection (CDC, 2022c). Pregnant women are 20 times more likely to contract listeriosis (CDC, 2022e). Approximately one third of all cases of listeriosis occur during pregnancy. Spontaneous abortion, stillbirth, premature delivery, and/or infection of the newborn are negative health outcomes associated with listeriosis during pregnancy (CDC, 2022e).

INTERVENTIONS AND STRATEGIES FOR RISK REDUCTION AND MANAGEMENT

Prevention of exposure to *Listeria* organisms is the best way to prevent infection (CDC, 2022e; FDA, 2016). Prevention of listeriosis can be achieved by:

- Avoiding unpasteurized dairy-containing foods
- Thoroughly cooking all meats before eating
- Washing all vegetables before eating

- Good handwashing and washing all knives and cutting boards after handling uncooked foods
- Storage of uncooked meats separately from all other foods
- Consumption of all ready-to-eat and perishable foods as soon as possible (CDC, 2022e; FDA, 2016)

GENETICS

The Risk of Genetic Anomalies and the Role of the Family History

ETIOLOGY

Mutations in single genes (monogenetic), multiple genes (multifactorial inheritance disorders), and combination genes; environment; and damaged chromosomes can cause genetic anomalies (ACOG, 2017a; National Human Genome Research Institute [NHGRH], 2018). The mother or father may pass on genetic abnormalities to the infant. Genetic abnormalities occur when a gene becomes flawed because of a mutation. In some cases, a gene or part of a gene may be missing. These defects occur at fertilization and are mostly nonpreventable. A particular genetic defect may be present throughout a family history of one or both parents. Before a planned pregnancy, it is optimal to know about family history for inherited diseases and congenital anomalies. In this multicultural world, it is also important to know whether partners planning pregnancies are related by blood (consanguineous), such as first cousins.

PREVALENCE

In the United States, approximately one out of every 33 babies is born with a birth defect, of which many are related to genetics. Across the world, 6% percent of births are affected by a serious genetic or partially genetic defect (ACOG, 2019; March of Dimes, 2022).

INTERVENTIONS AND STRATEGIES FOR RISK REDUCTION AND MANAGEMENT

Cultural sensitivity and a nonjudgmental attitude to consanguineous couples are essential to foster good working relationships between the medical profession and communities, with clinicians offering more targeted or expanded screening based on information desired by the members the individual calls family (ACOG, 2017a).

Assessment of family medical history for three to four generations back is recommended for those individuals with a known history of genetic conditions (ACOG, 2017a). Some genetic conditions are more common in certain ethnic backgrounds. For instance, women of Southeast Asian or Mediterranean background should be tested for Hb E/beta thalassemia. If a woman or her male partner has any Black/African American background, she should be tested for sickle cell disease. Whites (non-Hispanic) should be tested for cystic fibrosis. Couples with an Eastern European Jewish (Ashkenazi) background should be tested for Tay-Sachs disease, Canavan disease, and familial dysautonomia (ACOG, 2017a).

TABLE 22.3 Counseling and Carrier Testing Recommendations for Individuals with a Personal or Family History of Genetic Diseases and Syndromes

GENETIC DISEASE AND/OR SYNDROME	COUNSELING AND RECOMMENDATIONS
Leukodystrophies *Canavan disease*: Gene-linked neurologic disorder in which the white matter in the brain degenerates into spongy tissue with microscopic fluid-filled spaces.	• Counsel and recommend carrier testing if one partner is of Ashkenazi Jewish descent; if carrier status confirmed, offer carrier testing for other partner also.
***CFTR* Mutation** *Cystic fibrosis (CF)*: Caused by a cystic fibrosis transmembrane conductance regulator (*CFTR*) gene that leads to progressive, impaired respiratory function and severe damage of the lungs, digestive system, and other organs.	• If woman or partner is living with CF, counsel and recommend carrier screening to determine chances of *CFTR* penetrance.
Hereditary Sensory and Autonomic Neuropathies (HSANs) *Familial dysautonomia*: Autosomal recessive pattern caused by pathogenic variants in the *ELP1* gene, leading to disturbance in the development and survival of cells in the autonomic and sensory nervous systems. Individuals with an autosomal recessive condition carry one copy of the mutated gene and usually are asymptomatic.	• Counsel and recommend carrier testing if one partner is of Ashkenazi Jewish descent; if carrier status confirmed, offer carrier testing for other partner also.
Mental Retardation and Autism Spectrum Disorders *Fragile X syndrome (FXS)*: Inherited syndrome characterized by changes in the X-linked, fragile X messenger ribonucleoprotein 1 (*FMR1*) gene, leading to a spectrum of mild to severe developmental cognitive delays and learning disabilities.	• Counsel and recommend carrier testing to individuals with symptoms of FXS or those at risk for carrying the *FMR1* mutation.
Hemoglobinopathies Inherited blood disorders passed down through families, causing abnormal production or structure of the hemoglobin molecule (i.e., sickle cell disease [SCD], thalassemia).	• Counsel and recommend prenatal screening to identify offspring at risk of an inherited fetal hemoglobinopathy.
Spinal Muscular Atrophy (SMA) An inherited neuromuscular disease that progressively destroys the motor neurons, brainstem and spinal cord nerve cells that control speaking, walking, breathing, and swallowing.	• All women considering pregnancy should be screened. If the recessive gene is detected, the partner should be tested, as well.
Tay-Sachs Disease A rare, autosomal recessive, inherited, neurodegenerative disease that is passed from parents to their offspring.	• Counsel and recommend carrier testing if one partner is of Ashkenazi Jewish, Pennsylvania Dutch, Southern Louisiana Cajun, or Eastern Quebec French Canadian descent.

Source: Adapted from American College of Obstetricians and Gynecologists. (2007). ACOG Practice Bulletin No. 78: Hemoglobinopathies in pregnancy. Obstetrics & Gynecology, 109(1), 229–237. https://doi.org/10.1097/00006250-200701000-00055; American College of Obstetricians and Gynecologists. (2017). Committee Opinion No. 691: Cancer screening for genetic conditions. Obstetrics & Gynecology, 129(3), e41–e55. https://doi.org/10.1097/AOG.0000000000001952; American College of Obstetricians and Gynecologists. (2019). Committee Opinion No. 762: Prepregnancy counseling. https://www.acog.org/clinical/clinical-guidance/committee-opinion/articles/2019/01/prepregnancy-counseling

Inherited Medical Conditions

If a woman, her partner, or any close family member (children, parents, sisters/brothers, aunts/uncles) has a history of genetic/birth defects or inherited conditions, they should be referred for genetic counseling. Genetic counselors will obtain a family history, screen, and test pregnant women as determined appropriate (Table 22.3). The following medical conditions should be evaluated by a genetic counselor for possible genetic predisposition:

- NTDs (e.g., spina bifida, anencephaly)
- Down syndrome
- Mental retardation
- Bleeding disorder (e.g., hemophilia/thrombophilia)
- Muscular dystrophy, other muscle/nerve disorder
- Cystic fibrosis
- Tay-Sachs disease
- Sickle cell anemia
- Polycystic kidney disease
- Heart defect at birth
- Cleft lip/palate

Genetic Counseling Before Planning a Pregnancy

INTERVENTIONS AND STRATEGIES FOR RISK REDUCTION AND MANAGEMENT

Preconception counseling should include a review of personal, family, and medical health history. The U.S. Surgeon General has developed an internet-based tool, My Family Health Portrait (cbiit.github.io/FHH/html/index.html), in which individuals can create their family health history. This tool can assist families in organizing their family tree while identifying common diseases that may run in their family. It is also an effective way pregnant women can provide their family health history to their clinician who then can identify risk of disease. This tool is available in different languages (National Human Genome Research Institute, 2023).

Pregnant women and their family members should be encouraged to gather and write down familial health problems. To learn about their family history, pregnant women should ask questions, talk about family history at family gatherings, and even review information on death certificates and family medical records. If possible, they should collect information about their grandparents, parents, aunts and uncles, nieces and nephews, siblings, and children. Important information includes (a) major medical conditions (e.g., heart disease, stroke, cancer, diabetes, Alzheimer disease, obesity, blindness, deafness); (b) age of disease onset; (c) age at and cause of death; (d) history of infertility, miscarriages, stillbirths, and/or infant deaths; (e) history of birth defects, learning disabilities, and/or mental retardation; and (f) ethnic background. Pregnant women with a family history of a genetic disorder(s) should be referred for genetic counseling.

ASSESS FAMILY MEDICAL AND GENETIC RISKS BEFORE PREGNANCY

- Provide culturally sensitive family history and genetic screening.
- Refer for genetic counseling with family history of specific medical conditions and thorough ethnicity-based screening.

INTIMATE PARTNER VIOLENCE

ETIOLOGY

IPV is a preventable public health problem that affects millions of women regardless of age, economic status, race, religion, ethnicity, sexual orientation, or educational background. IPV includes overpowering a partner using physical and psychological abuse, sexual violence, and reproductive coercion (ACOG, 20129). Physical abuse can include throwing objects, pushing, kicking, biting, slapping, strangling, hitting, beating, threatening with a weapon, and/or use of a weapon against the victim. Psychological abuse is targeted at decreasing a woman's self-worth and can include harassment, and verbal abuse (e.g., name calling, degradation, blaming, threats, stalking, and isolation). The abuser will oftentimes isolate the woman from her family and friends as well as leave the woman without food, money, and/or transportation. Sexual violence can range from unwanted kissing, touching, and/or fondling to sexual coercion and rape. Reproductive coercion involves the control of a woman's reproductive health. In these situations, the abuser may disrupt a woman's effort at contraception, intentionally expose the abused woman to STIs (including HIV), and/or control the outcome of a pregnancy (for example, force the woman to have an abortion or injure her in a way that leads to or causes a miscarriage;) (ACOG, 20129).

IPV has been linked to early parenthood, miscarriage, severe poverty, overwhelming emotional distress, suicide, acute and chronic physical health problems, and unemployment (Bush & Nash, 2019). The consequences of IPV in pregnancy result in later entry to prenatal care and poor pregnancy outcomes such as preterm labor, low-birth-weight babies, fetal trauma, unhealthy maternal behaviors (e.g., inadequate diet, substance abuse, inadequate exercise), as well as peripartum and postpartum depression, and difficulty breastfeeding (Hrelic, 2019).

Roughly 25 million individuals are transgender worldwide, meaning the gender they identify as is different from their birth gender (Peitzmeier et al., 2020). Transgender

individuals reportedly suffer disproportionate IVP burden when compared to nontransgender individuals (Peitzmeier et al., 2020). In addition to the aforementioned forms of IPV, transgender individuals experience misgendering by using incorrect pronouns, taking advantage of insecurities associated with societal stigma, and/or making threats to reveal their transgender identity in an effort to blackmail (Peitzmeier et al., 2020). Additionally, social isolation (lack of support from family and friends) and economic challenges, such as employment discrimination and being homeless, can foster reliance on a violent partner (Peitzmeier et al., 2020).

PREVALENCE

IPV (also referred to as domestic violence) includes physical, sexual, and/or emotional abuse by a current or ex-intimate partner. Annually, it is estimated that 1.5 million women in the United States are victims of IPV; about 4% to 8% of pregnant women and 54% of transgender people are affected (DynaMed, 2018; Kurdyla et al., 2019; Weil, 2020). Associations between greater risk of unintended pregnancy and IPV due to reproductive coercion have been reported; specifically, women are noted to be at twice the risk for unintended pregnancy (Samankasikorn et al., 2019). Female victims of IPV are also at increased risk of urinary tract infection, gastrointestinal disorders, gynecologic disorders, and musculoskeletal pain (Weil, 2020). Interestingly, an association between IPV and the development of type 2 diabetes and cardiovascular disease has also been identified as a greater risk of all causes of death (Weil, 2020). In comparison with cisgender individuals, transgender individuals experience any form of IPV 1.7 times more often, physical IPV 2.2 times more often, and sexual IPV 2.5 times more often (Peitzmeier et al., 2020).

INTERVENTIONS AND STRATEGIES FOR RISK REDUCTION AND MANAGEMENT
Screening for Intimate Partner Violence

Although women of all ages may be subjected to IPV, it is most prevalent among women of reproductive age. Clinicians are in a unique position to assess and provide support for women subjected to IPV. The U.S. Department of Health and Human Services (DHHS) has recommended that IPV screening and counseling be a part of every woman's preventive health visit,; during new client visits, annual examinations, and at other times when a woman presents for health care (ACOG, 20129). Clinicians must not rule out the possibility of IPV with women who present with injuries, somatic complaints without diagnosis (e.g., chronic pain, fatigue, headache, neurologic symptoms), gastrointestinal pain, pelvic pain, STIs, depression, anxiety, insomnia, and/or multiple or erratic visits with a series of vague complaints. Screening for IPV may be difficult.

IPV screening for the obstetric client should be conducted privately at the first prenatal visit and at least once each trimester (ACOG, 2012). Clinicians should take care to avoid questions that use stigmatizing terms (e.g., abuse, rape, battered, violence; see Box 22.2). Clinicians should:

- Screen women for IPV in a private and safe setting with the woman alone.

Box 22.2 Exemplar Intimate Partner Violence Screening Questions

Introducing or Framing Question

"Unfortunately, violence is a problem for many women. Because it affects health and well-being, I ask all my patients about it."
"Because violence is so common in many women's lives, I have begun asking about this routinely."

Indirect Inquiry

"How are things at home?"

Direct Inquiry

"Do you ever feel physically or emotionally threatened or hurt by your intimate partner?"
"Have you been hit, kicked, punched, or otherwise hurt by someone in the past year? If so, by whom?"
"Do you feel safe in your current relationship?"
"Is there a partner from a previous relationship who is making you feel unsafe?"

After receiving a positive response to questions about intimate partner violence (IPV), the next step is to offer an affirmation to the woman:

"I am so glad you shared this with me."
"This can have a significant effect on your health."
"There are resources available to help you."

If IPV is confirmed, the next step is to assess safety:

"Is it safe for you to go home today?"
"Is there some place you can go that you feel safe?"

Source: Adapted from American College of Obstetricians and Gynecologists. (2012). *Committee Opinion No. 518: Intimate partner violence.* https://www.acog.org/clinical/clinical-guidance/committee-opinion/articles/2012/02/intimate-partner-violence

- When appropriate, use a professional language interpreter only.
- At the beginning of the assessment offer a framing statement to show that screening is done universally, not because IPV is suspected.
- Inform the woman of the confidentiality of the discussion as well as any state law disclosure mandates.
- Incorporate IPV screening into the woman's routine medical history.
- Identify community resources for women affected by IPV.

Screening at periodic intervals, including during well-woman visits and prenatal care visits, can improve the lives of women who experience IPV. Preventing the lifelong consequences associated with IPV can have a huge impact on the reproductive, perinatal, and overall health of women.

PHYSICAL EXAM

A preconception physical examination includes assessment of the heart, breasts, lungs, thyroid, abdomen, mouth, and genital tract, as well as blood pressure and BMI. This exam-ination includes a pragmatic approach to detection of the most common conditions that can affect maternal health and pregnancy outcome.

LABORATORY EXAM

- STIs
- Hepatitis C: History of intravenous (IV) or injected drug use, ever having received maintenance hemodialysis, persistent elevated ALT levels, or transfusion before 1992
- Rubella immunity
- Varicella immunity
- Evaluate for risk and offer the following tests:
  - Genetics (screening and diagnostic testing)
  - Tuberculosis
  - PKU
  - Toxoplasmosis
  - CMV infection

EMERGING TOPICS: CLINICAL GUIDELINES, EVIDENCE-BASED PRACTICE

The concept of reproductive identity is fairly new in the literature. Reproductive identity helps clarify current and future parenting desires, including the desire to parent biological children, nonbiological children, or no desire to be a parent. Intentions of one's reproductive identify impact decisions regarding birth control, cycle control, and if relevant, timing of conception or fertility preservation. Such considerations drive discussions about planned versus unplanned pregnancies, potential or actual teratogenic effects on a fetus, reduced elective terminations, and pregnancy interval timing.

FERTILITY PRESERVATION (LGBTQIA+ INDICATIONS)

Transgender males and females identify on a spectrum of gender (social construct) as opposed to their assigned sex (biological construct) at birth. As part of the preparation for hormonal treatments or gender-aligning surgeries, patients who at some time in the future desire genetically related children can decide if fertility preservation is desired. Options for fertility preservation are constantly evolving; however, currently transmale oocyte retrieval and transfemale sperm extraction with cryotherapy can be reserved for future Reproductive Endocrinology (RE) treatments. Factors such as Tanner's stages of puberty/adulthood, availability of storage facilities, financial concerns present or future, and additional factors are unique. Gender neutrality for all previously female-identified aspects of motherhood should be considered. For instance, breastfeeding or chestfeeding should be discussed in relation to health benefits and the possibility of lactation triggering symptoms of gender dysphoria.

SUMMARY

Promote Planned Pregnancy and Reproductive Identity

All pregnancies should be planned. Contraception is an essential component of preconception health because it facilitates a planned pregnancy. Adequate contraception is especially important in women exposed to teratogens (prescription medications and other reproductive toxicants), women with chronic conditions (e.g., diabetes), women who have had a previous unintended pregnancy (whether they resulted in a birth or abortion), and all sexually active adolescents. Clinicians should refer to and use the U.S. Medical Eligibility Criteria for Contraceptive Use USMEC (Curtis et al., 2016) to determine which contraceptive methods are safe for women with chronic conditions.

To increase the chances of a planned pregnancy:

- Assess type of contraception as a *vital sign* before prescribing all medications and when treating women of reproductive age for medical conditions (ACOG, 2019).
- Assist and promote achieving and maintaining a healthy weight or BMI.

- Counsel and offer emergency contraception (EC) with every prescription to reproductive-aged women who also are using a high-risk or teratogenic medication (ACOG, 2019; see Table 22.1).
- Counsel and offer EC for all women of childbearing age with chronic conditions.
- Promote the use of highly effective methods of contraception such as long-acting reproductive contraception (LARC) when women are exposed to high-risk medications or teratogens that cannot be avoided (e.g., statins, antihypertensives, anticoagulants, antiseizure medications, isotretinoin).
- Whenever possible, prescribe lower risk or nonteratogenic medications to reproductive-age women. Recommend prenatal vitamins with folic acid for all women of childbearing years.

REFERENCES

References for this chapter are online and available at https://connect.springerpub.com/content/book/978-0-8261-6722-4/part/part02/chapter/ch22

CHAPTER 23

Prenatal Care and Anticipating Birth

LISA L. FERGUSON

PRENATAL CARE

The maternal mortality rate in 1920 was 690 per 100,000 births but by 2008 it had dropped to eight per 100,000 births. Cunningham et al. (2018) attribute this decline in maternal mortality to prenatal care. Prenatal care was designed to decrease the morbidity and mortality risks of mothers and infants alike (Cunningham et al., 2018; Lockwood & Magriples, 2021a). This is achieved by early and accurate dating of gestational age, early risk identification, continued monitoring of maternal and fetal well-being, recognition of problems with appropriate interventions, and patient education (Lockwood & Magriples, 2021a). Prenatal care provides opportunities for education to assist the new mother and family in adjusting to the physical changes of pregnancy as well as the psychological adjustments required in an expanding family unit.

This chapter discusses prenatal care of the pregnant person and their fetus. Common discomforts of pregnancy are introduced and described, and the etiology, risk factors, and treatment are discussed. The structure and composition of clinic visits are defined to include screening tests, fetal well-being monitoring strategies, and patient education topics. Finally, medical conditions affecting pregnancy are outlined with strategies to manage them and points at which referral is necessary.

Discomforts of Pregnancy

NAUSEA AND VOMITING

Nausea and vomiting of pregnancy (NVP) are complaints shared by up to 90% of women in the United States (Smith et al., 2021a). Undertreatment of NVP frequently results because of the conviction that nausea and vomiting are an expected course of pregnancy, the fear of medications harming the fetus, or the historical lack of effective pharmacologic management (Niebyl & Briggs, 2014). As a result, pregnant women often experience negative impact on their quality of life (QoL) as well as adding to the economic burden on society in increased healthcare costs and loss of work productivity.

The cause of NVP is unclear; however, multiple theories have been proposed. Rapid rises in hormone concentrations such as estrogen and human chorionic gonadotropin (hCG); delayed or dysrhythmic gastric motility; *Helicobacter pylori* infection; and genetic factors are all thought to contribute to NVP (Smith et al., 2021a; Thomson et al., 2014).

Pregnancy-related risk factors include hydatidiform mole, multiple gestation, and history of previous NVP. Nonpregnancy associated causes encompass a history of nausea and vomiting while taking estrogen-derived medications, the absence of a multivitamin regimen before pregnancy, and a history of gastroesophageal reflux disease (GERD; Smith et al., 2021a; Taylor, 2014; Thomson et al., 2014).

There are no clear diagnostic criteria for NVP; thus, the diagnosis is determined by clinical presentation. Some clinicians have found the Motherisk-PUQE Scoring Index and the Rhodes Index useful in evaluating the severity of a patients' symptoms (Smith et al., 2021a). Average onset of NVP is between 5 and 9 weeks of gestation and usually resolves by 20 weeks (Niebyl & Briggs, 2014; Smith et al., 2021a; Thomson et al., 2014). Although symptoms may only occur in the morning, they frequently take place throughout the day. Symptoms can include "nausea, gagging, retching, dry heaving, vomiting, odor and/or food aversion" (Niebyl & Briggs, 2014, p. S31).

Initial evaluation begins with a review of weight, orthostatic blood pressure measurements, heart rate, serum electrolytes, and a urinalysis for ketones and specific gravity. Comparing the weight from this visit to that of the last visit reveals any weight loss sustained by the patient. Orthostatic blood pressure, heart rate, and specific gravity of the urine can indicate hydration status and need for possible intravenous (IV) fluids. Ketosis confirms lack of adequate food intake and must be addressed if present.

A thorough patient history related to the symptoms is paramount in determining the difference between NVP and non-pregnancy-related causes of nausea and vomiting. Obtain and document from the patient the onset, timing, severity, aggravating and alleviating factors, and appearance of the vomitus (Niebyl & Briggs, 2014). Emesis should not contain bile or blood if pregnancy is the cause. Often, NVP is elicited by motion, heartburn, certain foods, and odors. Ask about fever, abdominal pain, change in bowel habits, headache, neck stiffness, and changes in vision (Niebyl & Briggs, 2014). What has she tried to alleviate the nausea and vomiting herself?

Physical examination encompasses assessing for signs of dehydration, such as skin turgor and mucous membrane quality; evaluation of skin and sclera color for signs of jaundice; auscultation of bowel sounds; palpation of the abdomen for masses (other than a gravid uterus), distention, elicited pain, and hepatosplenomegaly; and evaluating for costovertebral angle tenderness (CVAT).

Simple interventions such as changes in diet, avoidance of triggers, and complementary and alternative therapies should be first-line treatment for NVP (American College of Obstetricians and Gynecologists [ACOG], 2018a; Smith et al., 2021b). If her prenatal vitamin or iron preparation are contributing to nausea and vomiting, reassure her that they may be safely discontinued until her symptoms abate. She may also substitute a children's chewable vitamin that contains folic acid (FA). Encourage the patient to discover what foods she can tolerate and build her menu around these items. Avoiding things such as coffee; spicy, acidic, or high-fat foods; and fried foods may be helpful. Protein-containing foods have been proved to decrease nausea and should be consumed before rising from bed (Jednak et al., 1999; Smith et al., 2021b). Several small meals, every 1 to 2 hours, should be ingested slowly throughout the day. Chilled, transparent, sour, and carbonated beverages are easier to tolerate in small amounts between meals and snacks. With a lack of research into the efficacy of diet changes on NVP, surveys given to affected women who did make dietary adjustments described moderate relief of their symptoms (Ebrahimi et al., 2010).

Many things may act as triggers for nausea and vomiting and should be identified and avoided. Odors such as foods, perfumes, and chemicals; optical or physical motion such as flashing lights and driving; rapid positional changes; and excessive heat can elicit NVP (Smith et al., 2021b). Left side lying can sometimes alleviate NVP, but the efficacy of this simple technique has not been well studied.

Acupressure, a mode of treatment used in Chinese medicine, has demonstrated the ability to decrease the sensation of nausea. Devices using this technique, such as Sea-Bands, are available in most drug stores and are easy to use (Sea-Band Ltd., 2016). Although acupressure has been found to be helpful in decreasing the sensation of nausea, a systematic review of available research suggests that acupressure does not significantly reduce nausea in NVP (Smith et al., 2021b). Sucking on peppermint candy or consuming ginger in the form of supplements, biscuits, tea, or candy can reduce the symptoms of nausea (Smith et al., 2021b; Thomson et al., 2014). Ginger capsules containing 250 mg taken by mouth four times daily are recommended. Ginger is more effective than placebo and as effective as vitamin B_6 in reducing NVP (Ding et al., 2013).

Vitamin B_6 improves mild to moderate nausea when 10 to 25 mg is taken orally every 6 to 8 hours (ACOG, 2018a; Smith et al., 2021b). The combination of vitamin B_6 and the antihistamine doxylamine is modestly effective for symptom relief and is available both over the counter (OTC; in the form of half a tablet of Unisom [25 mg] and the vitamin as recommended previously) and as a prescription medication. This regimen is recommended by the ACOG as first-line pharmacotherapy for NVP (ACOG, 2018a).

Second-line pharmacotherapy can be considered in women with NVP refractory to first-line treatments. This includes the addition of any one of the following to the first-line regimen: dopamine antagonist's promethazine and prochlorperazine and antihistamines dimenhydrinate and diphenhydramine (ACOG, 2018a). OTC antihistamines, such as dimenhydrinate and diphenhydramine, have been shown to be both safe and effective in significantly reducing nausea and vomiting in pregnancy (ACOG, 2018a). Table 23.1 contains dosing recommendations for these medications.

Metoclopramide, ondansetron, and trimethobenzamide are added as third-line therapy, if NVP is resistant to second-line treatment. Metoclopramide, promethazine, prochlorperazine, and ondansetron are equally efficacious in treatment of NVP (Archer et al., 2014; Smith et al., 2021b). Third-line therapy regimens hinge on whether dehydration is present or not. When dehydration is not a factor, an additional medication can be added either orally or intramuscularly. If the patient is dehydrated, IV rehydration is recommended prior to augmenting treatment with additional medication. Patients who have vomited for more than 3 weeks should have 100 mg thiamine added to the rehydration fluid and continue taking 100 mg of thiamine for 2 to 3 days to avoid Wernicke encephalopathy. If symptoms persist after rehydration therapy, additional medications may be added intravenously to the current treatment. See Table 23.2 for recommended dosages for third-line therapy.

Fourth-line therapy in dehydrated patients who do not respond to the addition of third-line treatment after rehydration consists of either chlorpromazine 25 to 50 mg, intravenously or intramuscularly, or 10 to 25 mg orally every 4 to 6 hours; or methylprednisolone 16 mg, orally or intravenously, every 8 hours for 3 days. Methylprednisolone must be tapered over 2 weeks to the lowest effective dose and may be used for up to 6 weeks if beneficial in decreasing nausea and vomiting.

TABLE 23.1 Antihistamine and Dopamine Antagonist Dosing

Dimenhydrinate	25–50 mg by mouth every 4–6 hours (not to exceed 200 mg per day if patient is also taking doxylamine)
Diphenhydramine	25–50 mg by mouth every 4–6 hours
Prochlorperazine	25 mg rectally twice daily
Promethazine	12.5–25 mg by mouth, rectally, or intramuscularly every 4 hours

Source: Adapted from American College of Obstetricians and Gynecologists. (2018). ACOG Practice Bulletin Summary No. 189: Nausea and vomiting of pregnancy. Obstetrics and Gynecology, 131(1), e15–e30. https://doi.org/10.1097/AOG.0000000000002450

TABLE 23.2 Third-Line Therapy Dosing for Nausea and Vomiting of Pregnancy

DEHYDRATION PRESENT		DEHYDRATION NOT PRESENT	
Metoclopramide	5–10 mg by mouth or IM, every 6–8 hours	Dimenhydrinate	50 mg (in 50 mL saline, over 20 min) IV, every 4–6 hours
Ondansetron	4 mg by mouth every 8 hours	Metoclopramide	5–10 mg IV, every 8 hours
Promethazine	12.5–25 mg by mouth, rectally, or IM, every 4–6 hours	Ondansetron	8 mg IV, over 15 minutes, every 12 hours
Trimethobenzamide	200 mg IM every 6–8 hours	Promethazine	12.5–25 mg IV, every 4–6 hours

IM, intramuscularly; IV, intravenously.

Source: Adapted from American College of Obstetricians and Gynecologists. (2018). ACOG Practice Bulletin Summary No. 189: Nausea and vomiting of pregnancy. Obstetrics and Gynecology, 131*(1), e15–e30. https://doi.org/10.1097/AOG.0000000000002450*

One possible risk reduction strategy is to ensure the patient is taking a daily prenatal vitamin before conception. Continuing appropriate management of preexisting GERD may forestall nausea and vomiting in some women with this condition.

HEARTBURN

From 30% to 50% of women describe symptoms of heartburn during pregnancy and up to 80% have symptoms by the third trimester (Thélin & Richter, 2019). These symptoms have adverse effects on a pregnant woman's QoL and capability to work (Law et al., 2010; Naumann et al., 2012).

Heartburn manifests as many symptoms, such as retrosternal pain or burning, indigestion, regurgitation, belching, and the taste of acid in the mouth (Clark et al., 2014; Malfertheiner et al., 2012; Thélin & Richter, 2019). These symptoms are similar to those of myocardial infarction and panic attack and, therefore, must be differentiated from those diagnoses.

Decreased lower esophageal sphincter (LES) pressure is caused by increased progesterone, the growing uterus increasing intra-abdominal pressure, abnormal gastric emptying, and delayed small bowel transit (Phupong & Hanprasertpong, 2014; Théil & Richter, 2019). Estrogen and progesterone decrease the LES tone by 50% (Naumann et al., 2012; Théil & Richter, 2019).

Although most pregnant women experience heartburn, certain risk factors make this discomfort more likely. A prior history of heartburn will almost certainly guarantee its occurrence in pregnancy. Elevated prepregnancy body mass index (BMI), multiparity, advancing gestational age, and Caucasian ethnicity all increase the risk of heartburn in pregnancy (Naumann et al., 2012; Phupong & Hanprasertpong, 2014).

There are no existing diagnostic criteria for heartburn, it is diagnosed based on the clinical picture (Phupong & Hanprasertpong, 2014). Physical exams are typically normal; however, some patients may experience midepigastric pain (MEP) with or without palpation. History can reveal retrosternal pain, often characterized as a burning sensation; frequent burping; regurgitation of acid or stomach contents into the esophagus or mouth; or a "bad" acidic taste in the mouth. Patients may report they have tried OTC antacids such as TUMS or Maalox with or without relief.

Making the same dietary changes as are recommended in NVP can help decrease its occurrence. Lifestyle changes including elevating the head of the bed (helps diminish gastric secretion and reflux), chewing gum (stimulates saliva, helps neutralize acid), and not eating late at night are all ways to help eliminate this pregnancy discomfort (Phupong & Hanprasertpong, 2014).

OTC preparations can be used to enhance the self-management of heartburn in pregnancy. Three classes of medications that are available without a prescription and can be used safely in pregnancy are antacids, histamine-2 antagonists (H2 blockers), and proton pump inhibitors (PPIs). Aluminum-, calcium-, and magnesium-containing antacids neutralize stomach acid. Histamine-2 receptor antagonists work to reduce acid production in the stomach by the parietal cells. PPIs stop the production of acid in the stomach by the proton pumps. One final OTC preparation, Gaviscon, is an alginate-based reflux suppressant and in one study showed an efficacy of 91% (Strugala et al., 2012).

Beginning pregnancy with a healthy BMI is one way to mitigate heartburn. Good medical management of heartburn before pregnancy may reduce its severity during the gestational period.

BACK PAIN

Musculoskeletal discomfort is a common complaint in pregnancy with back pain constituting the majority of those complaints. Low back pain during or after pregnancy contributes to driving up healthcare costs. In Scandinavian countries, one fifth of women who are pregnant take up to 7 weeks of sick time during their pregnancies as a result of back pain. Of women who experience back pain in their first pregnancy, 94% will have back pain in succeeding pregnancies and two thirds of these women become temporarily disabled, placing them on leave from work (George et al., 2013).

In pregnancy, low back pain is caused by the enlarging uterus pulling the abdomen and spine forward, straining the supporting back muscles. It can also occur because the gravid uterus is exerting pressure on the nerve roots, causing sciatica. Professions requiring lifting, pushing, pulling, sitting, and twisting for long periods of time increase the risk of incurring low back pain. Other risk factors include obesity, increasing age, cigarette smoking, depression/anxiety, tall height, and decreased abdominal and spinal muscular strength.

There are no diagnostic criteria for back pain in pregnancy. The diagnosis is based on the symptoms described by the patient. To ensure there are no other physiologic causes of back pain, exploration of symptomatology and a physical exam should be done. Questions should focus on the following: onset of symptoms (abrupt or gradual); prior history of back pain and its course; history of back surgery; history of recent fall, motor vehicle accident, or other trauma; any heavy lifting, to include lifting of children; or recent fever or chills. Characterize the pain using the mnemonic OLDCAART: onset; location; duration; characteristic of pain; aggravating, associated, and relieving factors; and treatments done. Inspect the skin of the back for signs of bruising or trauma. Palpate the area of concern for any masses that may indicate possible muscle spasms.

Stretching exercises can be recommended for low back pain, especially in early pregnancy. Water-based exercise such as water gymnastics has demonstrated a reduction in the intensity of low back pain in pregnancy and a drop in the number of pregnant women out sick for low back pain (Chen et al., 2020). Yoga is safe in pregnancy and can help strengthen back muscles. A maternity belt or band can be used to support the gravid uterus, thus relieving stress on the back muscles. These garments are readily available at department stores, maternity shops, and places such as Target and Walmart. Wearing shoes with low (not flat) heels and good arch support helps ease back pain. Using a board under a too-soft mattress can relieve back pain as can sitting in a chair with good back support or a pillow in the small of the back. Heat, cold, and massage are alternative methods to ease back pain. Tylenol may be recommended in the lowest dose that provides relief, using no more than 4 g in 24 hours. Referral for physical therapy can be given for those whose symptoms interfere with their ability to work and perform activities of daily living (ADLs).

PELVIC PAIN

Pelvic pain is described in one fifth of pregnant women and becomes worse as the pregnancy advances, affecting work, ADLs, and sleep (Pennick & Liddle, 2013). Many times, the etiology is musculoskeletal; however, more serious causes such as ectopic pregnancy, appendicitis, and spontaneous abortion (SAB) need to be ruled out.

In pregnancy, pelvic pain can be attributed to the stretching of any of the supporting structures in the pelvis, including the round ligaments. As the gravid uterus enlarges, it puts additional weight and therefore stress on the supporting apparatus. Ligaments resist stretching and, as a result, cause symptoms of pain such as burning, stabbing, pinching, or soreness. Other structures of the abdomen and pelvis are tested as well as the ligaments. Muscles must stretch to accommodate the growing uterus and occasionally result in a widening of the gap between the abdominal muscles, causing diastasis recti. The symphysis pubis begins to relax because of the effects of the hormone relaxin at about 10 to 12 weeks of gestation. Rearrangement of the pelvic organs can trigger pain and is self-limiting. Other causes of pelvic pain, which require immediate attention, are infection, appendicitis, ectopic pregnancy, ovarian mass, ovarian torsion, and SAB. Nonemergent sources of pelvic pain in pregnancy may also come from the bowels. Gas passing through the intestines can cause significant pain, as well as constipation. Advancing gestational age is the highest risk factor for pelvic pain related to pregnancy.

The clinical picture supplies the diagnosis. A history of bowel movements, recent diet, travel outside of the country, and exposure to illnesses should be elicited. Again, OLDCAART is used to assess the pain. Auscultation for bowel sounds can differentiate between gastrointestinal (GI) and other causes of pelvic pain. Palpation of the abdomen and pelvis can localize the pain and reveal any abnormal masses that may be present. A pelvic exam must be performed to detect any abnormal masses not palpable externally. Note the color and consistency of the cervical discharge and the condition of the cervix itself. Collection of a wet prep and specimen for chlamydia and gonorrhea testing is done at this time. During both external and internal palpation, distract the patient with conversation unrelated to her pain. If she is distractable, the etiology is unlikely to require a surgical response. Severe and exquisite pain requires further evaluation. An emergent US exam can rule out ectopic pregnancy, ovarian masses, and ovarian torsion. It can also inform of the viability of the pregnancy if it is beyond 8 weeks.

Treat any signs of infection. The presence of numerous white blood cells in the wet prep, with or without mucopurulent discharge, warrants treatment for chlamydia and gonorrhea to protect both the mother and the fetus. Treatment of infections is discussed further in this chapter. Tylenol is the only OTC medication that can be prescribed for pain in pregnancy. If pain is severe enough for anything stronger, a referral to an OB/GYN is necessary. Most of the time, education and reassurance is all that is needed to ease the fear of pelvic pain in pregnancy. The pregnant woman should be given anticipatory guidance about how the growing uterus will affect her body. If she is aware there is a normal cause, the pain can be better understood and tolerated.

SLEEP DISTURBANCE

In 2013, Nodine and Matthews, through a literature review, described three sleep disorders in pregnancy: breathing-related sleep disorders, restless legs syndrome (RLS), and insomnia. Interrupted sleep is common in pregnancy, affecting up to 97% of women. This has traditionally been thought of as a common discomfort of pregnancy and not much effort has been put into its treatment. New research has associated sleep disturbance with negative outcomes in pregnancy, thus increasing the need for effective management strategies of these complaints.

Breathing-related sleep disorders include snoring, upper airway resistance syndrome, and obstructive sleep apnea (OSA). Diagnosis of these conditions requires a sleep study done overnight in a sleep lab. Hormonal and physiologic adaptations in pregnancy contribute to these conditions as well. Weight gain and an enlarging gravid uterus cause a rising level of the diaphragm and less space for lung expansion. The swelling of mucous membranes by the action of estrogen can lead to nasal congestion and restricted pharyngeal area. As it has been well established that these disorders are linked to hypertension in adults, increasing evidence supports an association between breathing-related sleep disorders and gestational hypertension and preeclampsia. Management of these disorders is related to the extent of the condition. For simple upper airway resistance, nasal strips have been shown to be efficacious in the nonpregnant population. Other recommendations include regulation of weight gain, elevation of the head, refraining from sleeping in the supine position, and limited ingestion of sedatives and alcohol. Efficacy of these interventions has not been evaluated in pregnancy. Management of OSA relies on continuous positive airway pressure (CPAP), which is well tolerated, safe, and effective in pregnancy.

Approximately 30% of women who are pregnant experience RLS, which contributes to sleep deprivation and fatigue during waking hours (Nodine & Matthews, 2013). Diagnosis of RLS is made through data collected from a sleep history and must include all four of the following *International Classification of Sleep Disorders (ICSD)* criteria: a strong urge to move the legs, usually accompanied by discomfort; the urge to move and discomfort occur during inactivity; movement such as stretching or walking immediately relieves the symptoms, but they recur with subsequent inactivity; and symptoms occur primarily in the evening/night (Nodine & Matthews, 2013). Iron or folate deficiencies are well-known causes of RLS, a condition that is exacerbated during pregnancy. Management strategies include sleep hygiene and lifestyle changes; massage and acupuncture; treatment of folate and iron deficiencies; and medications such as codeine, clonidine, gabapentin, levodopa, pramipexole, pregabalin, ropinirole, tramadol, and zolpidem (Miller et al., 2020). As with any opioid, codeine should be used with caution and as a last resort for severe symptoms.

More than 80% of women suffer from insomnia at some time in their pregnancy, with complaints more prevalent in the third trimester (Nodine & Matthews, 2013). Consequences of insomnia consist of daytime sleepiness, irritability, decreased energy levels, adverse moods, increase in work accidents, car mishaps, and sick leave time. Late pregnancy insomnia has been shown to increase pain perception in labor, increase labor time, and increase rates of operative deliveries. Discomforts of pregnancy, such as back pain, nocturia, active fetal movement, breast tenderness, and leg cramps contribute to insomnia. Increases in estrogen and progesterone decrease the rapid eye movement sleep stage, increase release of cortisol (which increases arousal), and change nocturnal breathing patterns. Diagnosis is made using a sleep history and careful documentation in a sleep diary. Management of insomnia involves sleep hygiene and lifestyle changes; acupuncture; relaxation techniques such as yoga and massage; light therapy; treatment of depression; cognitive behavioral therapy for insomnia; exercise; treatment of physical discomfort; and medications such as zolpidem, trazodone, diphenhydramine, and doxylamine (Miller et al., 2020).

SHORTNESS OF BREATH

Shortness of breath (SOB) is experienced by 60% to 70% of women during pregnancy. For the majority of women, this is a common discomfort. However, a small percentage of pregnancies can be affected by other disorders that manifest as dyspnea and must be evaluated to ensure the health and safety of the mother and fetus (Weinberger, 2021).

The onset of SOB is gradual, begins in the first or second trimester, increases in frequency in the second trimester, and stabilizes in the third trimester. It is not associated with exercise, coughing, wheezing, or pain, and is at its worst with sitting. A careful history and auscultation of the lungs will guide diagnosis. The etiology is not well known but is likely caused by progesterone-mediated hyperventilation. Increased blood volume and cardiac output, physiologic anemia, and changes in respiratory physiology also contribute to dyspnea in pregnancy. Evaluation of dyspnea must be accomplished to differentiate between dyspnea of pregnancy and other underlying conditions such as peripartum cardiomyopathy, asthma, anemia, pulmonary embolism or edema, amniotic embolism, and preeclampsia/eclampsia.

Discussion of normal physiologic changes in pregnancy and reassurance will help the patient understand this process and reduce anxiety related to this normal discomfort of pregnancy. Advice to minimize SOB during pregnancy can include not overeating and taking frequent breaks when exercising.

Clinic Visits

INITIAL VISIT

The initial visit should occur before 10 weeks of gestation to allow for recommended screening to be performed and provide early identification of risk factors that may negatively affect the pregnancy. This is an optimum time to deliver health and safety information, offer anticipatory guidance, and answer patient questions, for both first-time mothers and multiparous women.

A complete history should take place during this visit and include personal, family, and father of the baby (FOB) information. Obtain demographic data such as patient name, birth date, race, address and phone number, emergency contact information, marital status, occupation, education, primary language spoken, and FOB name and phone number. Document prior pregnancies by including gravida, full-term births, premature births, induced abortion, SAB, ectopic pregnancies, multiple births, and living children. Record menstrual history with date of last menstrual period (LMP), whether known, approximate, or unknown. Continue with a description of how many days between cycles, age of onset of menses, whether a birth control method was used at the time of conception, and the date of the first positive pregnancy test. Gather a history of prior pregnancies, noting date of delivery, gestational age, length of labor, birth weight of infant, type of delivery, whether anesthesia was used or not, place of delivery, and whether it was a preterm delivery, and list any complication of the pregnancy and/or deliveries. It is essential to complete a comprehensive medical history of the patient and family. Although not exhaustive, Table 23.3 lists items to be included in this history.

Risk assessment incorporates genetic/hereditary, environmental, occupational, and recreational exposures that may pose a risk to the pregnancy. Genetic and hereditary risk factors are considered within the medical history, but occupational, environmental, and recreational factors are not always explored there. The type of work the patient performs and the work environment can give clues to hazards they may not be aware of. A factory worker may be exposed to elevated noise and vibration levels or be required to do heavy lifting. Healthcare and child care workers risk exposure to infectious

TABLE 23.3 Patient and Family Medical History

Cardiovascular Disease
Hypertension
Arrhythmia
Congenital anomalies
Thromboembolic disease

Endocrine Disorder
Diabetes, including gestational
Thyroid disease

Gastrointestinal Disease
Hepatitis
Gallbladder disease
Inflammatory bowel

Kidney Disease
Pyelonephritis
Urinary tract infections
Congenital anomalies

Neurologic/Muscular Disorders
Seizures
Aneurysm
Arteriovenous malformation
Headaches

Psychiatric Disorders
Eating disorder
Depression, including postpartum
Psychosis

Autoimmune Disorder
Lupus
Rheumatoid arthritis

Pulmonary Disease
Asthma
Tuberculosis

Blood Dyscrasias
Anemia
Thrombophilia

Infectious Diseases
Herpes
Gonorrhea
Chlamydia infection
HIV infection
Syphilis

Gynecologic History
Diethylstilbestrol (DES) exposure
Abnormal Pap history and treatment
Genital tract disease or procedures

Substance Use
Alcohol
Tobacco
Illicit or recreational drugs

Other Indicators
Breast disorders
Cancer
Mental retardation
Birth defects/genetic disorders
Trauma/violence/abuse
Blood transfusion
Surgical procedures
Hospitalizations
Allergies
Medications
Nutrition

diseases. Cosmetologists work with chemicals that may be breathed in or absorbed through the skin. The location and type of housing a person dwells in can also contribute to unforeseen dangers such as airborne toxic chemicals and lead. Some hobbies and recreational activities can be dangerous. Skydiving and underwater diving are contraindicated in pregnancy. Any contact sport should be avoided. Painting, soldering, glass fusing, and welding all produce fumes, which should be well ventilated or avoided altogether. Modifiable risk factors include smoking, drug and alcohol use, and dangerous sports or activities. A discussion about smoking, drug, and alcohol cessation is warranted if these are current risk factors. Make appropriate referrals for assistance in discontinuing these behaviors.

The physical exam performed on the initial visit is similar to a well-woman exam (see Chapter 11, Well Women's Health). Vital signs are examined at every prenatal visit, before the exam, and include height, weight, temperature, respiratory rate, blood pressure, and pulse. Auscultate lung and heart sounds and a heart murmur may be appreciated. A grade II systolic ejection murmur is the physical manifestation of increased plasma volume and cardiac output and is normal in pregnancy. Palpate the thyroid for nodules; a slight increase in size typically occurs. Perform a gentle breast exam as the breasts and nipples can be very tender. Palpate the abdomen for masses; assess for CVAT. Conduct a pelvic

exam, beginning with visual evaluation of the vulva. Examine for lesions, abnormal discharge, and varicosities. Palpate for masses and lymphadenopathy. Insert a speculum, noting the condition of the vaginal walls. Examine the cervix for masses, blood, and discharge. The cervical os should be closed, although in a multiparous woman, it may be gaping. This is the opportunity to take samples for a Pap smear and human papillomavirus (HPV) testing if indicated, wet prep, and testing for chlamydia and gonorrhea. Gently remove the speculum and insert two lubricated fingers into the vagina. Abdominally palpate the gravid uterus and determine its size. Palpate the adnexa for masses and tenderness. It is not necessary to search for fetal heart tones (FHTs). Before 10 to 12 weeks of gestation, heart tones are not audible with a portable Doppler. The timing and elements of subsequent prenatal visits can be done in either individual or group visits and are listed in Table 23.4.

For first-time mothers and women who have had babies alike, as long as the pregnancy is progressing normally without any complications, group prenatal care can provide more patient education and improved outcomes. Centering Healthcare Institute developed CenteringPregnancy as a vehicle to provide prenatal care, highlighting education and support, to help decrease preterm births by 33% (Garretto & Bernstein, 2014). This form of prenatal care affords the clinician the opportunity to provide education while encouraging family

TABLE 23.4 Elements of Prenatal Visits

PRENATAL VISIT	INITIAL VISIT	10 TO 12 WEEKS	16 TO 18 WEEKS	20 TO 24 WEEKS	28 WEEKS	32 WEEKS	36 WEEKS	38 TO 41 WEEKS
HISTORY	COMPLETE	UPDATE	UPDATE	UPDATE	UPDATE	UPDATE	UPDATE	UPDATE
PHYSICAL EXAM								
Complete	*							
BP	*	*	*	*	*	*	*	*
Weight	*	*	*	*	*	*	*	*
Pelvic/cervix exam	*							*
Fundal height	a			*	*	*	*	*
Fetal heart rate/position		*	*	*	*	*	*	*
LAB TESTS								
Hct or Hb	*				*			
ABO/Rh	*							
ABS	*				If indicated			
Pap smear		If indicated						
GTT		If indicated			*			
Fetal aneuploidy screen		b						
CF screen	Offer		Offer					
Urinalysis/culture	*	Offer						
Urine protein	*							
RPR	*				c			
Rubella titer	*							
GC/CT	*				c			
Hep B	*							
HIV	*				d			
Group B strep							*	
PSYCHOSOCIAL								
Barriers to care	*		*			*		
Housing	*		*			*		
Nutrition	*		*			*		
Smoking	*		*			*		
Substance abuse	*		*			*		
Depression	*	*	*	*	*	*	*	*
Safety	*	*	*	*	*	*	*	*

[a]Bimanual exam.
[b]First trimester screen 10 to 14 weeks, or cell-free DNA testing beginning at 9 weeks.
[c]Retest in third trimester if high risk.
[d]Some states require third trimester screen.
ABO/Rh, blood types A, B, AB, and O/rhesus blood type + or −; ABS, amniotic band syndrome; BP, blood pressure; CF, cystic fibrosis; GC/CT, gonorrhea/*Chlamydia trachomatis*; GTT, glucose tolerance test; Hct or Hb, hematocrit or hemoglobin; Hep B, hepatitis B; RPR, rapid plasma reagin; strep, streptococcus.

member participation, support among group members, and self-reliance. Typical total time spent on prenatal care over the course of a pregnancy is roughly 2 hours (Garretto & Bernstein, 2014). With CenteringPregnancy, about 20 hours are devoted to education in health promotion and self-management, performing prenatal examinations, and fostering peer support. This model does not affect clinician productivity and allows for more in-depth discussion of pregnancy-related issues. Supportive Pregnancy Care program, created by the March of Dimes, enhances health literacy and health equity while providing group prenatal care. This program differs from CenteringPregnancy in that it focuses on social determinants of health in addition to medical issues (March of Dimes, n.d.). The Yale School of Public Health, UnitedHealth group, and Vanderbilt University Medical Center clinicians developed Expect With Me group prenatal care. Expect With Me provides an information technology platform that not only helps patients track their weight and vital signs, but also allows them to connect with group members and clinicians and view videos and tip sheets that have been medically reviewed, and provides links to local and nationwide resources.

Laboratory tests usually done in addition to those gathered during the physical exam include urinalysis with culture and sensitivity, urine pregnancy test, serum rubella and varicella titers, complete blood count, ABO/Rh and antibody screen, rapid plasma reagin (RPR), HIV, hepatitis B and C, sickle cell screen, and other lab tests as indicated by the patient's history. A history of a first-degree relative with diabetes, patient BMI in the obese category, or a prior diagnosis of gestational diabetes warrants an early 1-hour glucose tolerance test (GTT). Laboratory tests performed during later visits are listed in Table 23.5.

Continued physical activity or activity begun early in the prenatal course contributes to decreased weight gain and better delivery outcomes. Any physical activity that does not involve contact such as walking, jogging, swimming, and cycling can be a part of an exercise program for the pregnant woman. Care must be taken when engaging in these activities as the center of gravity changes with increased uterine size, and the hormones relaxin and progesterone loosen the body's tendons and ligaments, rendering the patient prone to tripping. The heart rate should be kept below 140 bpm. Safety devices appropriate to the activity, such as eye protection and helmets, should be used. Sexual activity can continue during pregnancy, as long as there is no risk of preterm labor. A well-balanced diet is essential in fueling both the mother and the growing fetus. Avoid shark, swordfish, king mackerel, white or albacore tuna, and tilefish, which contain high levels of mercury. Eat no more than 12 oz of other fish and shellfish weekly. Avoid eating unpasteurized milk and soft cheeses; hot dogs, deli, and luncheon meats (unless cooked to steaming hot); and raw meat and eggs. The craving for unusual substances such as chalk, clay, laundry detergent, laundry starch, and others is called pica. Discourage the ingestion of these substances and ask the patient to inform you if she is having these cravings as they may be manifestations of iron deficiency.

Discuss the care plan with the patient. Visits will be every 4 weeks until 28 weeks. Talk to her about nausea and vomiting, heartburn, and dizziness that she may experience and strategies to treat them. Let her know you will offer her fetal aneuploidy screening at her next two visits, depending on her risk factors. Warning signs that should be discussed are bleeding and abdominal pain. She should not be experiencing any vaginal bleeding and should be evaluated either in the office or the nearest ED if bleeding occurs. Persistent abdominal pain should also be evaluated to rule out appendicitis or an ectopic pregnancy.

Patient vaccination status, ideally, is determined during preconceptual counseling. Often, women do not avail themselves of this service and may not be sufficiently protected from certain diseases. All women should be immunized against influenza during the recommended season and COVID-19 with recommended boosters. The flu is most dangerous to the young, older adults, and pregnant women. COVID-19 is dangerous to pregnant women and those with specific comorbidities. No live vaccines are given during pregnancy because of their teratogenic effects.

Iron and FA supplementation are necessary to both maternal and fetal health. Often, the mother cannot tolerate iron early in pregnancy because of constipation and/or nausea and vomiting. Some clinicians will recommend chewable children's vitamins (containing folic acid) to help decrease these side effects. OTC docusate sodium is helpful in reducing constipation. If iron is not at all tolerated because of nausea and vomiting, taking it can be suspended until NVP subsides.

10 TO 12 WEEKS

At this and each subsequent visit, the following data should be obtained and assessed: patient weight, blood pressure, pulse, and FHTs; signs of depression and domestic violence; and iron and FA intake (American Academy of Pediatrics and American College of Obstetricians and Gynecologists, 2017). After the initial pelvic exam, there is no need to do another one unless there are signs of infection, bleeding, or abdominal pain/contractions. Cell-free DNA testing for fetal aneuploidy can be done at any time after the start of the 9th week of gestation. This test offers the highest detection rate of all fetal screening tests, but still can report false positive and false negative results. If a first trimester fetal aneuploidy screen is desired or necessary by history, blood can be drawn between 10 and 14 weeks (ACOG, 2020b). A US exam is also done during this period and provides two crucial pieces of early data, fetal gestational age and nuchal translucency. An accurate fetal gestational age is vital to offering properly timed obstetric care and establishes a baseline to gauge fetal growth throughout the pregnancy. It is also helpful in scheduling and interpreting

TABLE 23.5 Laboratory Tests Performed During Clinic Visits

VISIT	TEST
Weeks 9–18	Fetal aneuploidy screening (cell-free DNA or first trimester screen)
Week 28	Rh antibody testing and RhoGAM (if not received this pregnancy); 1-hour GTT; chlamydia/gonorrhea testing if high risk
Week 36	GBS
Weeks 28–36	HIV

GBS, group beta streptococcus; GTT, glucose tolerance test.

antepartum tests and allows creating interventions aimed at preventing preterm and postterm births (ACOG, 2017). An early ultrasound is used to measure the fetal nuchal translucency (NT) or the amount of fluid behind the fetal neck, present in all fetuses. An excessive amount of fluid can be an indication of an aneuploidy. The serum analysis and US scan must be evaluated together in order to give a positive screen.

Preterm labor is not a concern at this stage of pregnancy. If an SAB is to occur, there exists neither the means to stop it or the ability to save the fetus. Generally, the age of viability is considered somewhere between 22 and 24 weeks. Discussion about the approximate size of the fetus and how big it will be at the next visit is appropriate. Anticipatory guidance about NVP, if this has not already been discussed, should be given. Open a dialogue on breastfeeding with the patient. The longer she has to learn and think about it, the more prepared and willing she will be to attempt it. Let her know what physiologic changes she will be experiencing, such as skin changes, soft tissue swelling, physiologic anemia, weight gain, increased breast size and sensitivity, alterations in taste, and cravings.

Review lab results from the initial visit with the patient. Anticipatory guidance about the need for RhoGAM and its timing should be done if applicable. If the patient began this pregnancy with an elevated BMI or excessive weight is an issue, ask about current eating habits and review normal weight gain in pregnancy with her. A woman with a healthy BMI will gain between 25 and 35 pounds during pregnancy. Table 23.6 depicts weight gain goals for pregnancy. Emphasize that exercise is important to maternal/fetal health and delivery of the baby. Review any modifiable risk factors identified at the initial visit.

16 TO 18 WEEKS

A second trimester fetal aneuploidy screen, also known as the quad screen, can be done between 15 and 22 weeks of gestation. Maternal blood is drawn and using demographic data such as age, weight, gestational age, and race, serum factors are analyzed, and the risk of aneuploidy calculated and reported. A fetal anatomic survey is performed after 18 weeks of gestation and reports normal versus abnormal fetal anatomy.

A common concern for mothers at this stage of pregnancy is fetal movement. Quickening is the first time a mother can feel her fetus moving. This feeling can be described as bubbles, gas, or flutters. The time when quickening occurs varies with each individual and pregnancy. It can begin as early as 16 weeks to as late as 22 weeks. Reassurance that with good FHTs, the absence of fetal movement is not concerning, is often enough to satisfy an anxious mom. Discuss any lab results from the last visit and follow up on modifiable risk

factors. Ensure the patient is taking prenatal vitamins and FA; review nutrition in pregnancy.

20 TO 24 WEEKS

Beginning with the 20-week visit, measure the fundal height. This is done with a disposable measuring tape, marked in centimeters. The zero point of the tape is placed and held on the upper edge of the symphysis pubis and pulled taut over the abdomen until the fundus is palpated. The measurement recorded is known as the fundal height and is usually within 2 cm of the estimated gestational age (EGA). Three or more centimeters greater or less than the EGA warrants a US scan to observe fetal growth.

Preterm labor education and prevention continue during this visit. Signs of preterm labor, prevention strategies, and when to seek emergency care should be discussed with the patient. Anticipatory guidance about expected body changes and fetal growth is appropriate during this visit as well. Discussion about how this family unit plans to integrate the coming new member should begin. Exploring emotions, changes in couple relationship, daily schedules, parental responsibilities, and expectations has likely already begun. Encourage continued evaluation of these topics to help ease the transition to parenthood and a new family dynamic. Continue to inquire about modifiable risk factors and attempt to mitigate any that exist. Suggest considering and enrolling in breastfeeding and childbirth education classes. Prepare the patient for the hospital stay by discussing items to bring, length of stay, and hospital policies such as number of people allowed in the delivery room, use of recording devices, and presence of children.

28 WEEKS

At this visit, a 1-hour GTT is ordered to screen for gestational diabetes. The only instruction for testing is that the patient needs to be fasting for the first blood draw. Inform the patient that if the test is abnormal, she will be sent for a 3-hour GTT that will diagnose whether she is affected by gestational diabetes. Anti-D immune globulin is given to women who are Rh(D) negative. If needed, Tdap (tetanus, diphtheria, and pertussis) vaccination is ideal for the infant if given between 27 and 36 weeks.

Continue preterm labor education and prevention, physiology of pregnancy, modifiable risk factor, and fetal growth discussions. Hospital preregistration and tour of the labor and delivery (L&D) unit can relieve some of the burden of delivery day. Discuss plans for work, such as plans to stop work before delivery, how long maternity leave will be, and even the possibility of no longer working after delivery. Teach the patient the rationale behind and how to do fetal kick counts. Give guidance on when she should seek emergency care if she is not feeling fetal movement.

32 WEEKS

Warning signs related to preeclampsia and eclampsia are given at this visit. Educate on acceptable travel restrictions for the upcoming weeks. Continue preterm labor education and prevention, physiology of pregnancy, modifiable risk factors, and fetal growth discussions.

Prompt the patient to begin considering what type of contraception she desires after delivery, where she will obtain child

TABLE 23.6 Weight Gain Goals in Pregnancy	
BMI	RECOMMENDED WEIGHT GAIN (LB)
<18.5	28–40
18.5–24.9	25–35
25–29.9	15–25
>30	11–20

BMI, body mass index.

care, and who will be her pediatrician. Introduce the possibility of an episiotomy during delivery and reassure her about her continued ability to participate in and enjoy sex. This is also an opportunity to inform her about changing sexuality for her, her partner, and their relationship. If lab results from the last visit have not been reviewed, it can be done during this visit. Mothers with prior cesarean sections may want to discuss their desire for a vaginal birth for this pregnancy. A referral to an obstetrician will help inform her of this possibility.

36 WEEKS

At this visit, some clinicians will begin cervical examinations to determine the readiness for delivery. Others will not do a sterile vaginal exam unless there is an indication there will be cervical change. The fewer vaginal exams, the less likely it is to introduce infection. Leopold's maneuvers are performed during the examination to confirm fetal position. If there is any doubt of the presenting part of the fetus, a quick look with a US scan can offer confirmation. A culture of the vagina and anus is taken for group beta streptococcus (GBS) screening. In some states a third trimester HIV test is mandatory and can be done at this visit. If the patient is high risk, a repeat gonorrhea/*Chlamydia trachomatis* (GC/CT) and RPR is recommended at this time.

Loss of the mucous plug can occur at any time but is more likely to occur between now and delivery. Discussion that this is not a sign of imminent delivery is appropriate. Continue preterm labor education and prevention, physiology of pregnancy, modifiable risk factors, and fetal growth discussions. Introduce education about routine postpartum care and management of late pregnancy symptoms. Reiterate observing for symptoms of preeclampsia and give L&D warnings. Postpartum depression can occur as early as late third trimester; the patient should be aware of these signs and when she should seek emergency care.

38 TO 41 WEEKS

A sterile vaginal exam for cervical dilatation can be performed at this visit if the patient desires. At term, some clinicians will offer to "strip" or "sweep" the membranes in an attempt to induce labor. Other clinicians will offer advice for natural ways to induce labor. Semen contains prostaglandins, a hormone used to ripen the cervix. Intercourse, if comfortable at this point, can bring about labor. Some recommend rides down bumpy roads, drinking raspberry leaf tea, and eating borscht, based on anecdotal reports. None of these methods have been proved to bring about labor.

Elective induction of labor can be offered at 39 weeks to nulliparous women who are at low-risk. The ARRIVE Trial results, published in 2018, support induction of labor in this group of patients and ACOG recommends that shared decision-making should be based on the values and preferences of each patient, the availability of resources, and the practice setting where induction takes place (ACOG, 2018b).

Discuss postpartum vaccinations for the mother, postterm pregnancy management, and breastfeeding. Preeclampsia warnings should continue to be given along with L&D warnings. Discuss GBS results and, if positive, antibiotic use in labor. Advise patient that this would be an ideal time to learn infant cardiopulmonary resuscitation (CPR) and recommend resources for classes.

POSTPARTUM (4–6 WEEKS)

Vital signs, weight, height, and BMI calculation are recorded. The patient will want a baseline postpregnancy weight to evaluate her weight loss efforts. A depression screening tool such as the Edinburgh Postpartum Depression Screen (EPDS) should be administered to assess the extent, if any, of postpartum depression. A score of 12 or greater warrants referral to a mental health professional. History at this visit should include information about the delivery: infant sex and weight, EGA at time of delivery, hours of labor, type of delivery, whether anesthesia was used, and complications, if any, of the delivery. Document current state of vaginal bleeding (has her bleeding stopped, has her menses returned). A full well-woman exam is done as a postpartum exam with a few additions. The breasts are examined for redness; excessive warmth; hard, painful masses; and cracked nipples. Assess breastfeeding success and refer as needed to a lactation consultant for any breastfeeding problems. During the pelvic exam, assess the perineum for healing of any tears and/or repairs that may have been done and document. Chart any lochia that is present. Evaluate that the uterus has nearly or fully involuted. If the patient had GDM, a 6-week postpartum 2-hour GTT should be ordered to evaluate normalization of glucose tolerance.

As long as any lacerations are healed, it is okay to resume intercourse at this time. Determine the type of contraception desired and educate the patient on its use. Postpartum depression is possible up until 6 months after delivery. The mother should be aware of signs and notify her clinician if any of these are present. Optimally, the infant's pediatrician will be evaluating the mother for postpartum depression at the well-baby visits.

Medical Conditions During Pregnancy

ASTHMA

Asthma is seen often in pregnancy as it is a common disease among younger females, affecting 1% to 13% of all pregnancies (Robijn et al., 2019). Asthma in pregnancy follows the rule of thirds: one third of affected women will get better, one third will remain the same, and one third will get worse. This disease should be carefully monitored in pregnancy, as it increases the chances of perinatal death, preeclampsia, preterm delivery, and low-birth-weight infants (Schatz & Weinburger, 2021).

Asthma is usually a preexisting condition in which the patient is either on medication or has not been affected by the symptoms since childhood. New-onset asthma can be diagnosed with history of sudden onset when exposed to a trigger with wheezing, coughing, and/or dyspnea. Auscultation of the lungs will reveal global, high-pitched expiratory wheezing. In severe attacks, tachypnea, tachycardia, and use of accessory muscles may also be appreciated. Pulmonary function tests are used to evaluate suspected asthma. Spirometry measures forced expiratory volume in 1 second (FEV_1) and forced vital capacity (FVC). A decrease in the FEV_1/FVC ratio below normal demonstrates airflow obstruction. The measured FEV_1 compared with normal predicted value describes the degree of airflow limitation. Bronchodilator response can be assessed with repeat spirometry 10 to 15 minutes after administration of a rapid-acting bronchodilator, two to four puffs. A 12% or

TABLE 23.7 Pharmacologic Management of Asthma in Pregnancy	
SEVERITY	THERAPY
Intermittent	Step 1: Inhaled SABA such as albuterol as needed
Mild persistent	Step 2: Low-dose ICS daily with SABA as needed Or Low-dose ICS plus SABA, concomitantly administered, as needed **Alternative option** Daily LTRA and SABA as needed
Moderate persistent	Step 3: Combination low-dose ICS-formoterol daily and 1 to 2 inhalations as needed up to 12 inhalations/day (preferred) **Alternative options** Medium-dose ICS and SABA as needed OR Low-dose ICS-LABA combination daily or low-dose ICS plus LAMA daily or low-dose ICS plus LRTA daily and SABA as needed OR Low-dose ICS daily plus zileuton and SABA as needed
Severe persistent	Step 4: Combination medium-dose ICS-formoterol daily and 1 to 2 inhalations as needed to 12 inhalations/day (preferred) **Alternative options** Medium-dose ICS-LABA daily or medium-dose ICS plus LAMA daily and SABA as needed OR Medium-dose ICS daily plus LTRA or zileuton and SABA as needed Step 5: Medium- to high-dose ICS-LABA plus LAMA daily and SABA as needed (preferred) **Alternative options** Medium-high dose ICS-LABA daily or high-dose ICS + LTRA daily and SABA as needed Possible addition of asthma biologics Step 6: High-dose ICS-LABA daily; consider LAMA as substitute for LABA or as add-on therapy if not done previously Oral glucocorticoids, titrated to optimize asthma control and minimize adverse effects Possible addition of asthma biologics

ICS, inhaled corticosteroid; LABA, long-acting beta-agonist; LAMA, long-acting muscarinic antagonist; LRTA, leukotriene receptor agonist; SABA, short-acting beta-agonist.
Source: Adapted from Schatz, M., & Weinberger, S. E. (2021). Management of asthma during pregnancy. UpToDate. *https://www.uptodate.com/contents/management-of-asthma-during-pregnancy*

greater increase in FEV_1 with an absolute rise in FEV_1 of a minimum of 200 mL indicates a positive response.

Initial management of asthma consists of identifying and avoiding triggers, monitoring peak expiratory flow rate (PEFR) twice daily, and education about recognizing when to seek emergency care. Pharmacologic therapy may be required in pregnancy and is a stepwise approach as recommended by the National Asthma Education Program (Schatz & Weinburger, 2021). Table 23.7 describes this recommended therapy. Acute exacerbations of asthma not relieved by self-treatment require immediate medical attention.

DIABETES

Diabetes affected 8.6% of females in the United States in 2018 (Centers for Disease Control and Prevention [CDC], n.d.-c). It is thought that the rate of diabetes has increased because of the poor Western diet and lack of exercise in the population. Certain ethnic groups tend to have higher rates, such as Hispanics, non-Hispanic Blacks, and Native Americans (American Diabetes Association, n.d.). Lower socioeconomic status contributes because patients may not be able to afford lean meats, fresh fruits, and vegetables. Women who have preexisting diabetes must be counseled and carefully monitored during pregnancy. Some women may develop diabetes during pregnancy caused by the change in carbohydrate metabolism. Untreated diabetes in pregnancy results in stillbirth, macrosomia, increased cesarean delivery rates,

birth trauma, and infant hypoglycemia, and exposes the child to future risks of childhood obesity, gestational diabetes mellitus (GDM), diabetes mellitus (DM) type 2, and metabolic syndrome (Federico & Pridjian, 2012).

Autoimmune destruction of pancreatic beta cells results in complete insulin deficiency and is known as DM type 1 (DM1). This form of diabetes accounts for about 5% to 10% of all cases of DM (CDC, n.d.-b). Risk factors for DM1 are genetic predisposition and ill-defined environmental factors.

Type 2 DM (DM2) is characterized by insulin resistance and relative insulin deficiency. The etiology of DM2 is unknown, likely multifactorial, and does not involve beta-cell destruction. This form accounts for 90% to 95% of all cases of diabetes. Risk factors include genetic predisposition; history of gestational diabetes; hypertension; low HDL or high triglycerides; obesity; increased age; lack of exercise; Black, Alaska Native, Native American, Asian American, Hispanic/Latinx, Native Hawaiian, or Pacific Islander descent; history of heart disease or stroke, and depression (National Institute of Diabetes and Digestive and Kidney Disorders, n.d.).

Insulin resistance is a normal physiologic occurrence in pregnancy that begins in the second trimester. When the pancreas cannot overcome this resistance, GDM occurs (Durnwald, 2021). The incidence of GDM is between 2% and 10% of all pregnancies (CDC, n.d.-d). Women are at increased risk for GDM if they have a personal history of impaired glucose tolerance or GDM; are of Hispanic, Black, Native American,

South or East Asian, or Pacific Islander descent; have a first-degree relative with diabetes; have a BMI of greater than 30; are older than 40 years; deliver a baby more than 9 lb; or have medical conditions associated with diabetes such as polycystic ovary syndrome (Durnwald, 2021).

Although 90% of women who are pregnant carry at least one risk factor for impaired glucose tolerance, nearly 20% of women diagnosed with GDM have no risk factors (Durnwald, 2021). As a result, screening for gestational diabetes is routinely done between 24 and 28 weeks of gestation in women who are at low or no risk of diabetes. For women who carry GDM risk factors, an early GTT should be performed during the first trimester. Diagnosis of GDM can be made based on serum glucose testing. A 1-hour GTT consists of a 50-g glucose-containing liquid administered orally irrespective of last oral intake. At 1-hour postingestion, serum glucose is measured and patients with results above the cutoff value are scheduled for a 3-hour GTT. Because there is no evidence to support one value over another, the ACOG recommends clinicians select one of three cutoff values (130 mg/dL, 135 mg/dL, or 140 mg/dL) to use consistently in their practice (ACOG, 2018c). In a 3-hour GTT, the patient drinks a 100-g glucose-containing liquid after an initial fasting blood draw. Every hour after ingestion of the glucose, blood is taken, and the serum glucose level evaluated. Table 23.8 describes the diagnostic criteria required to diagnose GDM from a 3-hour GTT. A diagnosis of overt diabetes can be made with results of fasting glucose levels of 126 mg/dL or greater.

Risk reduction for GDM focuses on the overweight or obese patient. Weight loss and increased physical activity, during and before pregnancy, have both been demonstrated to reduce the risk of GDM in several observational studies (Artal, 2015; Durnwald, 2021). A healthy diet can lead to weight loss and, therefore, decrease GDM risk. The efficacy of exercise and healthy diet in reducing GDM risk increases when these two interventions are combined (Artal, 2015).

Women who have DM1 must be counseled before pregnancy and carefully monitored during the gestational period. Tight glucose control is key to a healthy pregnancy with positive outcomes. Establishing normal blood glucose levels before conception is the first step. Diet and exercise can help maintain this normal equilibrium along with correct insulin dosing. These women are typically managed with insulin therapy by an obstetrician or maternal–fetal medicine physician.

Women with DM2 and GDM must also monitor their blood glucose levels. This is done four times daily (fasting and 1–2 hours postprandial), documented, and brought to the clinician for evaluation. Goals for glycemic control should be below 95 mg/dL fasting, less than 140 mg/dL 1-hour postprandial, and 120 mg/dL 2 hours postprandial (ACOG, 2018c). Treatment modalities for GDM are similar to those used for risk reduction. Dietary restriction and moderate-intensity physical activity are recommended, although carbohydrate restricting that results in ketosis starvation is to be avoided (Federico & Pridjian, 2012). For those women who cannot maintain glycemic control with lifestyle interventions, referral to an obstetrician for initiation of oral glyburide, metformin, or insulin therapy is recommended.

Women with preexisting diabetes and those with poorly controlled GDM undergo regular antepartum fetal testing because of the higher risk of fetal death. US evaluation for fetal growth starts at 28 weeks of gestation and is performed every 3 to 4 weeks. Beginning at 32 to 34 weeks of gestation, biweekly to weekly biophysical profile (BPP) and nonstress testing (NST) is performed. The frequency of this testing increases to twice weekly beginning at 36 weeks until delivery.

HYPERTENSION

Hypertensive disorders in pregnancy are a leading cause of maternal death in the world and affect 5% to 10% of pregnancies (ACOG, 2020a; Lahti-Pulkkinen et al., 2020). These diseases are a major factor in the incidence of stillbirths and the morbidity and mortality of the neonate. Hypertension in pregnancy contributes to the occurrence of abruptio placentae, acute renal failure, cerebral hemorrhage, disseminated intravascular coagulation, and hepatic failure. Etiology of hypertensive disorders in pregnancy is not well known and is likely multifactorial. Risk factors for hypertension include obesity, advancing age, race, family history, decreased adult nephron mass, high sodium diet, physical inactivity, and excessive alcohol intake (Basile & Bloch, 2021).

The ACOG (2020a, 2020b) classifies the hypertensive diseases affecting pregnancy as follows: gestational hypertension, preeclampsia with and without severe features, HELLP syndrome, eclampsia, chronic hypertension with superimposed preeclampsia, and chronic hypertension. A short description of each disease is described in the following text.

By definition, gestational hypertension is "systolic blood pressure of 140 mm Hg or more or a diastolic blood pressure of 90 mm Hg or more, or both, on two occasions at least 4 hours apart after 20 weeks of gestation in a woman with a previously normal blood pressure" (ACOG, 2020a, p. e238). If the blood pressure remains elevated after the typical postpartum period, chronic hypertension becomes the diagnosis (ACOG, 2019). Management of gestational hypertension is dictated by severity, gestational age, and whether or not preeclampsia is present. Pharmacologic treatment is begun when systolic blood pressure reaches 160 mmHg or greater or diastolic blood pressure is 110 mmHg or greater, or both. Labetalol and hydralazine intravenously and nifedipine orally are the three most commonly used agents. Diuretics are not used because of the risk of decreased plasma

TABLE 23.8 Diagnostic Criteria: GDM Using the 3–Hour GTT

	PLASMA OR SERUM GLUCOSE LEVEL		PLASMA LEVEL	
	mg/dL	mmol/L	mg/dL	mmol/L
Fasting	95	5.3	105	5.8
One hour	180	10.0	190	10.6
Two hours	155	8.6	165	9.2
Three hours	140	7.8	145	8.0

GDM, gestational diabetes mellitus; GTT, glucose tolerance test.
Source: Adapted from Durnwald, C. (2021). *Gestational diabetes mellitus: Screening, diagnosis, and prevention.* UpToDate. https://www.uptodate.com/contents/gestational -diabetes-mellitus-screening-diagnosis-and-prevention

TABLE 23.9 Hypertensive Treatment in Pregnancy

MEDICATION	DOSE/TIMING	SIDE EFFECTS
Labetalol	10–20 mg IV, then 20–80 mg every 10–30 min to a maximum cumulative dosage of 300 mg; or constant infusion 1–2 mg/min IV	Dizziness, fatigue, nausea
Nifedipine	10–20 mg orally, repeat in 20 minutes if needed; then 10–20 mg every 2–6 hours; maximum daily dose is 180 mg	Nausea, heartburn, headache, dizziness, peripheral edema, reflex tachycardia and headache
Hydralazine	5 mg IV or IM, then 5–10 mg IV every 20–40 min to a maximum cumulative dosage of 20 mg; or constant infusion of 0.5–10 mg/hr	Frequent doses and use of higher doses can result in maternal hypotension, headaches, and abnormal fetal heart tracing

IM, intramuscularly; IV, intravenously.
Source: Adapted from American College of Obstetricians and Gynecologists. (2020). ACOG Practice Bulletin No. 222: Gestational hypertension and preeclampsia. Obstetrics and Gynecology, 135(6), e237–e260. https://doi.org/10.1097/AOG.0000000000003891

volume in the mother. Angiotensin-converting enzyme (ACE) inhibitors, angiotensin II receptor blockers (ARBs), and direct renin inhibitors are absolutely contraindicated in pregnancy. See Table 23.9 for dosing schedules related to these antihypertensive agents in pregnancy.

Preeclampsia affects every organ system with reduced perfusion associated with vasospasm and initiation of the coagulation cascade. It is diagnosed after 20 weeks of gestation when the patient with gestational hypertension also presents with proteinuria (greater than or equal to 0.3 g of protein in a 24-hour urine specimen) or one of the following: thrombocytopenia, renal insufficiency, impaired liver function, pulmonary edema, new-onset headache unresponsive to medication and not caused by alternative diagnosis, or visual changes (ACOG, 2020a). Complaints of visual disturbances and epigastric or right upper quadrant pain in the presence of gestational hypertension without proteinuria should lead the clinician to be highly suspicious of preeclampsia. Gestational hypertension pressures of less than 160 mmHg systolic, 110 mmHg diastolic, or both give the diagnosis of preeclampsia without severe features. When blood pressures reach the severe range (at or greater than the preceding mmHg readings) the diagnosis is preeclampsia with severe features. Laboratory studies such as liver enzymes and platelet count should be monitored with this diagnosis (Table 23.10). Risk factors for preeclampsia include previous history of preeclampsia or chronic hypertension, diabetes, kidney disease, obesity, gestation of multiples, age greater than 35 years, nulliparity, thrombophilia, lupus, antiphospholipid antibody syndrome, assisted reproductive technology, and OSA (ACOG, 2020a). There are no prevention strategies that have proved effective in reducing the incidence of preeclampsia. Eclampsia is diagnosed with the onset of seizures in a preeclamptic patient. Management and treatment of the patient with preeclampsia should be referred to an obstetrician.

Chronic hypertension with superimposed preeclampsia offers a poorer prognosis than either chronic hypertension or preeclampsia alone. This hypertensive disorder can be difficult to recognize, but because of its prognosis, a high degree of suspicion is warranted. The chronic hypertensive pregnant woman garners close monitoring for and early treatment of preeclampsia.

Chronic hypertension is defined as hypertension existing before pregnancy or is diagnosed before 20 weeks of gestation (Cunningham et al., 2018). Women with chronic

TABLE 23.10 Hypertensive Lab Tests in Pregnancy

LABORATORY TEST	COMMENT
Complete blood count with differential	
Blood urea nitrogen	
Urine protein	Spot urine protein/creatinine ratio or 24-hour urine for total protein and creatinine as appropriate
Serum creatinine	
Serum electrolytes	Potassium
Serum aspartate aminotransferase (AST) and alanine aminotransferase (ALT)	

hypertension require prenatal counseling and lifestyle modification in order to prepare for a safe and healthy pregnancy. Patients may remain on prepregnancy pharmacotherapy as long as the medication is not contraindicated for pregnant women. Diastolic blood pressure should be maintained between 80 and 110 mmHg in these patients.

Monitoring for fetal well-being in hypertensive pregnant women is essential in producing positive birth outcomes. Accurate dating must be performed in the event that early delivery is required. A baseline fetal measurement should also be obtained to monitor growth. A US exam done between 18 and 20 weeks of gestation will provide these data and growth can be followed through fundal height assessment. If fetal growth restriction is suspected, NST and BPP should be implemented.

BLEEDING IN PREGNANCY

Although alarming to the mother, bleeding is quite common throughout pregnancy (Norwitz & Park, 2018). Despite its frequent occurrence, bleeding in pregnancy must be evaluated when it occurs.

First trimester vaginal bleeding often does not have a known etiology. Evaluation is directed toward a definitive diagnosis, if there is one, and elimination of serious pathology. A history of the current episode of bleeding is gathered, including the onset, duration, and characteristics of bleeding (pad count, clots, and size of clots); associated symptoms such as lightheadedness, pain, and/or cramping; and passage of tissue. Prior obstetric and medical history should contain past ectopic pregnancies or miscarriages, pelvic inflammatory disease, current use of an intrauterine device (IUD), medication use, and blood dyscrasias. Obtain a serum hCG, Rh(D) typing with antibody screen, and hematocrit or hemoglobin level. Vital signs can often point to the severity of bleeding; evaluate for tachycardia, hypotension, orthostatic hypotension, and dizziness.

Physical evaluation begins with checking FHTs in a gestation of greater than 10 to 12 weeks. Detection of a fetal heartbeat with a portable Doppler is reassuring of fetal well-being. Inability to locate the FHTs at this gestation or greater requires further evaluation with an obstetric US exam. Examine the vulva for presence of blood, clots, and tissue. Insert a speculum to evaluate the vaginal walls and cervix. Look for tears, lesions, warts, abnormal discharge, and polyps. Remove any tissue visible in the vault or extruding from the cervix. All recovered tissues, whether brought in by the patient or removed by the clinician, are sent to pathology for evaluation for products of conception. Take and send specimens for chlamydia/gonorrhea testing and perform a vaginal smear (wet prep). Visible lesions of the cervix warrant a Pap smear. An open cervical os indicates impending abortion. Perform a bimanual exam for estimation of gestational age, presence of uterine and/or adnexal masses, and pain and palpate the internal cervical os to estimate the amount of dilatation, if any.

An obstetric US exam can help direct treatment of the woman with bleeding in pregnancy. If the pregnancy is determined to be nonviable because of lack of cardiac activity, an abortion is likely. Refer to the section on SAB for further information. An ectopic pregnancy may be detected via US; this is discussed in one of the following sections. Evaluation of the wet prep may reveal a large amount of white blood cells, yeast, or trichomonads. Treatment of these findings is outlined in the section on Vaginal Infections and Sexually Transmitted Infections (STIs). If no etiology has been found for bleeding, the patient should be reassured that the cause of bleeding is likely nothing that will jeopardize her or the baby. Regardless of the etiology, all Rh(D) negative women who bleed in pregnancy require anti-D immune globulin for protection against alloimmunization.

ECTOPIC PREGNANCY

Implantation of the blastocyst outside the uterine cavity, known as an ectopic pregnancy, occurs in about 2% of all pregnancies, and results in 4.4% of deaths related to pregnancy (Hoyert & Miniño, 2020). Until definitively excluded, all bleeding and pelvic pain in early pregnancy is thought to be an ectopic pregnancy.

Tubal damage related to sterilization, corrective surgery, or prior ectopic pregnancy gives the highest risk for an ectopic pregnancy. Other risk factors are failed contraceptive method, IUDs, prior genital/pelvic infection, smoking, prior cesarean section, multiple sex partners, history of abortion, infertility, and assistive reproductive technology.

Clinical presentation of ectopic pregnancy is diverse and is contingent on rupture of the gestation. Signs and symptoms include pelvic pain, vaginal bleeding, and abdominal or pelvic tenderness. Severe sharp, stabbing, or tearing lower abdominal/pelvic pain, cervical motion tenderness, bulging of the vaginal cul-de-sac, dizziness, syncope, and neck or shoulder pain indicate a ruptured ectopic pregnancy. Frequently, women will have very elusive or no signs or symptoms of an ectopic pregnancy. Vital signs may be normal, or pulse may be tachycardic and blood pressure may drop.

History concentrates on risk factors and the characteristic of bleeding and pain. A serum beta-hCG, blood typing with antibody screening, and a hematocrit must be drawn. Physical exam includes blood pressure for postural changes, abdominal palpation for tenderness and distention, speculum exam to assess bleeding, bimanual exam of the uterus for size, and careful examination of the adnexa for masses and tenderness and to check for cervical motion tenderness.

Diagnosis is made using a combination of the beta-hCG levels and transvaginal ultrasound (TVUS). The TVUS may reveal a frank ectopic pregnancy, an adnexal mass suggestive of an ectopic pregnancy, an intrauterine pregnancy (IUP), or no sign of pregnancy at all. Management of a frank ectopic or adnexal mass is left to the obstetrician. An IUP with bleeding and/or pain should follow the workup for vaginal bleeding and pelvic pain. If there is no ultrasonographic evidence of a pregnancy with levels of beta-hCG equal to or greater than 2 mIU/mL, the diagnosis of pregnancy of unknown location is made with scheduled serial beta-hCG and TVUS performed under the supervision of an obstetrician. As in all cases of vaginal bleeding in an Rh(D) negative woman, ensure anti-D immune globulin is administered.

SPONTANEOUS ABORTION

Also known in lay terms as a miscarriage, an SAB is the premature delivery of a fetus before the age of viability. SAB incidence is highest in the first trimester with 80% occurring during this time.

Chromosomal anomalies are responsible for 55% of these early pregnancy failures (Cunningham et al., 2018). Other causes include teratogens, uterine anomalies, maternal infections, hypothyroidism, diabetes, radiation, and thrombophilias. Increased risks for SAB are advanced maternal age, a history of SAB, smoking, moderate to high alcohol use, high caffeine intake, and cocaine use.

A woman having an SAB generally presents with either vaginal bleeding and cramping or with absent FHTs, via portable Doppler, in a pregnancy with an established presence of FHTs. The history concentrates on the presenting symptoms and gestational age. Baseline beta-hCG and hematocrit are drawn, along with blood typing and antibody screen. A pelvic exam is performed to assess the amount of bleeding, search for fetal tissue, and assess the condition of the cervical os. Bimanual exam determines the size of the uterus and gentle probing of the internal cervical os reveals whether it is open or not. TVUS is completed in order to detect cardiac activity, first seen at about 5.5 to 6 weeks of gestation. The presence of a gestational sac with its EGA, yolk sac, and fetal pole are also components of the TVUS report.

There are five categories of SAB based on the dilatation of the internal cervical os and the whereabouts of the products of conception. A threatened abortion is one in which there is still fetal cardiac activity, the internal cervical os is closed, but the mother is suffering from vaginal bleeding. This bleeding may or may not be accompanied by pelvic pain or cramping. Watchful waiting is the intervention used in this instance. Most cases of vaginal bleeding in a threatened abortion subside and the pregnancy advances normally. In a missed abortion, there is no cardiac activity, the cervical os is closed, and the products of conception are retained in the uterus. There may or may not be vaginal bleeding and pelvic pain in this type of abortion. Inevitable abortion is characterized by vaginal bleeding, pelvic cramping, and a dilated cervical os. Often, products of conception can be seen or felt in the os. Management of the missed and inevitable abortion can be expectant, medical, or surgical, based on the preference of the mother. In an incomplete abortion, the internal cervical os remains open while some or all products of conception remain in the uterus. Management of this type of SAB tends to be more conservative. An internal os that is open for prolonged time periods can result in uterine infection, and retained products may produce hemorrhage. In a hemodynamically stable woman with a closed os, a period of expectant management of 3 to 4 weeks can be used. If products are not expelled or hemorrhage occurs, the patient should be admitted for observation of blood loss and shock, and if needed, immediate surgical management is performed (Redinger, 2021). In addition to the aforementioned management strategies, if the patient is Rh(D) negative, anti-D immune globulin should be administered.

VAGINAL INFECTIONS AND SEXUALLY TRANSMITTED INFECTIONS

The same vaginal infections and STIs that affect any woman, as discussed in Chapter 29, Urologic and Pelvic Floor Health Problems, can affect a pregnant woman. Etiology, risk factors, diagnostic criteria, assessment, and patient education remain the same. The few medication restrictions in pregnancy for treatment of vaginal infections and STIs are discussed here.

Yeast infections pose no danger to mother or fetus if left untreated but can be quite uncomfortable for mom. Intravaginal imidazoles for 7 days is safe in pregnancy as well as 100,000 units of nystatin intravaginally for 14 days (obtainable from a compounding pharmacy). Terconazole has not been well studied in pregnancy and safety information regarding this treatment in pregnancy is minimal. Fluconazole should be avoided in pregnancy as it has been demonstrated to produce birth defects in women who took high doses of the drug in the first trimester of pregnancy (Sobel, 2021).

Asymptomatic bacterial vaginosis (BV) was once treated to prevent preterm labor in pregnant women; however, the ACOG no longer recommends this as routine practice as it has no effect on decreasing the incidence of preterm labor in infected women (ACOG, 2021). The three treatment options for BV in pregnancy are metronidazole 500 mg orally twice daily for 7 days, metronidazole 250 mg orally three times daily for 7 days, or clindamycin 300 mg orally twice daily for 7 days. The CDC has removed its recommendation for restriction of metronidazole in the first trimester; however, some clinicians still avoid its use in early pregnancy (Sobel, 2021).

Maternal infection with syphilis can cause fetal infection at any stage, although it is uncommon before 20 weeks of gestation (Cunningham et al., 2018). This can lead to preterm labor, fetal demise, and neonatal infection. Treatment for the pregnant woman is the same as benzathine penicillin G treatment for the nonpregnant woman. Infection discovered in the second trimester warrants referral to a maternal–fetal medicine specialist for sonographic evaluation of the placenta and fetus (Workowski et al., 2021). Treatment in the latter half of pregnancy can result in preterm labor and/or fetal distress if treatment triggers a Jarisch–Herxheimer reaction. Patient education should include seeking care for contractions, decreased fetal movement, and fever.

Gonorrhea in pregnancy can result in preterm labor, premature rupture of membranes, chorioamnionitis, and postpartum infection and affects all stages of pregnancy. Treatment for pregnant patients with noncomplicated gonorrhea consists of ceftriaxone 250 mg intramuscularly and azithromycin 1 g orally (Cunningham et al., 2018).

Chlamydial infection in pregnancy does not carry the risk of abortion or preterm delivery, but vertical transmission to the fetus can cause pneumonia and conjunctivitis. Treatment with azithromycin 1 g one time and amoxicillin 500 mg three times a day for 7 days is safe in pregnancy (Cunningham et al., 2018).

Primary herpes simplex virus (HSV) infection in the first half of pregnancy and recurrent infection near delivery offer the least risk for neonatal transmission of the disease. Risk is highest with primary infections close to delivery. That being said, treatment for outbreaks during pregnancy and prophylactic treatment beginning at 36 weeks of gestation for any HSV-infected woman will provide shortened course of disease manifestation and prevent outbreaks near time of delivery. Acyclovir and valacyclovir are the only antivirals safe in pregnancy (Cunningham et al., 2018).

Genital warts, caused by the HPV, tend to grow in number and size during pregnancy and may prevent vaginal delivery by blocking the vaginal outlet. Although rare and benign, vertical transmission of HPV to the neonate can cause juvenile-onset recurrent respiratory papillomatosis. Because transmission risk is so low, the current recommendation is not to deliver infants of affected mothers via cesarean section unless the vaginal outlet is blocked, preventing vaginal delivery. Treatment of genital warts in pregnancy is limited to trichloroacetic acid (TCA) or bichloroacetic acid (BCA) weekly, cryotherapy, laser ablation, or surgical excision (Cunningham et al., 2018).

The care of the woman who has HIV in pregnancy, whether diagnosed previously or during pregnancy, can be complicated and is best done in consultation with a physician who has experience in treating this disease. Treatment is advised for all pregnant women infected with HIV as it decreases the risk of transmission to the fetus. If the patient is already on highly active antiretroviral therapy (HAART), she may remain on it as long as it is successful in suppressing the viral load and the treatment does not contain didanosine, stavudine or full-dose ritonavir (toxic in pregnancy; Cunningham et al., 2018). Newly diagnosed pregnant women will need counseling to decide on the best course of HAART for them.

HYPEREMESIS GRAVIDARUM

Although nausea and vomiting are common discomforts of pregnancy, when they are severe and recalcitrant to antiemetic therapy and dietary modification, they can adversely affect both mother and fetus. Hyperemesis gravidarum is severe prolonged nausea and vomiting resulting in weight loss, dehydration, and ketosis (Miller & Gilmore, 2013). Complications from this illness include rapid, excessive weight loss, esophageal rupture, Mallory–Weiss tears, hypoprothrombinemia, renal failure, and Wernicke encephalopathy (a neurologic condition resulting from thiamin deficiency that requires immediate treatment to prevent death; So, 2020).

Elevated or rapidly increasing levels of hormones in pregnancy seem to be the cause of hyperemesis gravidarum. A woman is at increased risk for this complication with prior history of hyperemesis, a GI illness, hyperthyroidism, prior molar pregnancy, multiple gestation, depression or psychiatric disorder, female fetus, or diabetes (Cunningham et al., 2018; Graham et al., 2014).

Diagnosis is based on clinical picture and laboratory results. Other underlying illnesses should be ruled out using the same workup as recommended in NVP discussed earlier in this chapter. A weight loss of 10% or greater, ketonuria, and a urine specific gravity of greater than 1.030 are laboratory indicators of hyperemesis. Treatment involves hospitalization with IV rehydration, thiamine supplementation, IV antiemetics or corticosteroids, and in some cases, parenteral nutrition therapy (Miller & Gilmore, 2013).

ANEMIA

Anemia is defined as a drop in hemoglobin levels less than 11 g/dL (hematocrit less than 33%) in the first and last trimesters and less than 10.5 g/dL (hematocrit less than 32%) in the second (Bauer, 2020). This blood condition causes fatigue, dizziness, mild dyspnea, and weakness (Friel, 2021). In pregnancy, anemia increases the risk for venous thromboembolism, preterm delivery, and postpartum infections in the mother (Cunningham et al., 2018; Friel, 2021).

Hematologic changes in pregnancy are responsible for creating physiologic anemia of pregnancy (Bauer, 2020). As the plasma volume increases, red blood cell production also increases, but at much smaller volume. This disproportion is at its height during the second trimester. Iron requirement in pregnancy is near 1,000 mg for a singleton gestation. With anemia affecting up to 38% of pregnancies in the United States, most pregnancies begin with lower iron stores than needed for support of both the mother and fetus (Cunningham et al., 2018).

Replacement of iron stores is accomplished with daily oral iron preparations, which contain 200 mg of elemental iron. Iron can cause nausea and constipation, further complicating normal discomforts of pregnancy. Ducusate sodium 100 mg twice daily will avert constipation and iron may be avoided if NVP is an issue but should be reinstated as soon as tolerated by the patient. In a patient with severe iron deficiency anemia who cannot tolerate oral iron, parenteral therapy is given. Blood transfusion for anemia is rarely recommended.

Prepregnancy administration of iron supplements can build iron stores and decrease the incidence of iron deficiency anemia in pregnancy. Supplementation should begin 3 months before conception.

SICKLE CELL TRAIT AND DISEASE

Worldwide, 300 million people have sickle cell trait; it affects people of African, Mediterranean, Middle Eastern, Indian, and Hispanic descent (Vichinsky, 2021). Sickle cell trait does not confer sickle cell disease; however, pregnant women with this carrier condition do require prenatal counseling and increased monitoring during pregnancy. Sickle cell disease, on the other hand, increases the risk of complications for both mother and fetus. Because of the seriousness of these complications, care of the pregnant woman with sickle cell disease is best left to an experienced obstetrician.

Women with sickle cell trait are at a substantially higher risk for asymptomatic bacteriuria and pyelonephritis than nonaffected pregnant women (Cunningham et al., 2018). Urinalysis should be conducted during each trimester and a symptom history obtained at each visit. History, physical exam, and diagnostic criteria are discussed in the next section.

URINARY TRACT INFECTIONS

The most common bacterial infection in pregnancy affects the urinary tract, and if not treated can evolve into a serious medical complication, pyelonephritis. Bacteriuria, if left untreated, can increase the risk of preterm delivery, low-birth-weight infant, anemia, and gestational hypertension (Cunningham et al., 2018; Gupta, 2021). Many pregnant women have bacteriuria and are unaware of its presence. Others will complain of the same symptoms experienced by nonpregnant women.

Etiology of urinary tract infections (UTIs) in pregnancy is the same as in nonpregnant women. The gravid uterus exerting pressure on the bladder and relaxation of smooth muscles leading to dilatation of the ureters may assist in movement of bacteria from the bladder to the kidney, increasing the risk of pyelonephritis. Women with diabetes, sickle cell trait, and sickle cell disease are at increased risk for cystitis (Gupta, 2021).

Often, a woman will have no complaints at the visit, but a dipstick test of her urine will demonstrate the presence of bacteria. This is known as asymptomatic bacteriuria (ASB) and, as 25% of infected women will progress to UTIs, is treated as a UTI (Cunningham et al., 2018). Patients with frank UTIs present with painful urination. Frequency and urgency are normal physiologic changes in pregnancy and, while they may be a presenting symptom, may not be helpful in diagnosis. A history of these symptoms includes timing, characteristics of dysuria, characteristics of the urine, number of times the restroom is used, how many nighttime visits occur, and presence of back or flank pain. The physical exam comprises two elements: suprapubic tenderness and CVAT. Suprapubic tenderness makes the diagnosis of cystitis more likely but should not preclude empiric treatment if absent. The presence of CVAT accompanied by temperature greater than 100.4°F is suspicious for pyelonephritis and requires referral and workup. Diagnosis is made based on symptoms and/or urinalysis with a culture for sensitivity. A urine specimen is obtained for a urine dipstick, and a positive nitrite and/or leukocyte reading is indicative of a UTI. A urinalysis will reveal pyuria and bacteriuria. Most clinicians will treat a pregnant patient with complaints of a UTI, whether or not the urine dipstick test is suspicious for infection.

Most UTI treatments in pregnancy run a 5- to 7-day course; however, trimethoprim-sulfamethoxazole double strength can be used for 3 days and fosfomycin can be given as a one-time dose. See Table 23.11 for other pharmacologic treatment options.

| | | | | TABLE 23.11 Oral Pharmacologic Management of Cystitis in Pregnancy | | | |

ANTIBIOTIC	DOSE	TREATMENT DURATION	NOTES	SUPPRESSIVE THERAPY (CONTINUOUS OR POSTCOITAL)
Amoxicillin	500 mg TID or 875 mg BID	5 to 7 days	Resistant in gram-negative bacteria	
Amoxicillin-clavulanate	500 mg TID or 875 mg BID	5 to 7 days		
Cefpodoxime	100 mg BID	5 to 7 days	Only use when first-line agents can't be used	
Cephalexin	250 to 500 mg QID	5 to 7 days		250 to 500 mg at bedtime or after each episode of intercourse
Nitrofurantoin	100 mg BID	5 to 7 days	Avoid during first trimester and at term if other options available	50 to 100 mg at bedtime or after each episode of intercourse
Trimethoprim-sulfamethoxazole	800/160 mg (one double-strength tablet) BID	3 days	Avoid during first trimester and at term if other options available	
Fosfomycin	3 g single dose	One time		

BID, twice a day; QID, four times a day; TID, three times a day.
Source: Adapted from Gupta, K. (2021). Urinary tract infections and asymptomatic bacteriuria in pregnancy. UpToDate. *https://www.uptodate.com/contents/urinary-tract-infections-and-asymptomatic-bacteriuria-in-pregnancy*

MULTIFETAL GESTATION

With advancements in infertility treatments, multifetal gestations have risen sharply in the United States since the 1980s (Cunningham et al., 2018). This creates an increased burden on the healthcare system and society because of the cost of premature births, long-term disability care, and maternal morbidity (Cunningham et al., 2018). Maternal deaths, preeclampsia, and postpartum hemorrhage risk are doubled, and the risk of fetal malformation rises with multifetal gestation. Because of the increases in both maternal and fetal risks, multifetal pregnancies are considered high risk.

Other than through assisted reproductive therapy (ART), multifetal pregnancies result from either the splitting of one fertilized ovum or the fertilization of multiple separate ova. Risk factors for dizygotic (two fertilized ova) twinning include Black race, maternal history of twins, increased parity, obesity, height 65 inches or greater, increasing maternal age, and good nutrition (Chasen, 2021). The only reliable method to diagnose multifetal pregnancy is with ultrasonography (Chasen, 2021). At any time during the pregnancy, demonstration of size greater than dates, based on initial bimanual exam or fundal height measurement, warrants US examination. Once identified, these high-risk pregnancies should be referred to an obstetrician.

OBESITY

In 2020, Hales et al. reported the 2018 prevalence of obesity in women aged 20 years and greater was 41.9%. Therefore, more than one third of patients who are pregnant may present as obese. According to the CDC, obesity is defined as a BMI of 30 kg/m² or greater (CDC, n.d.-a).

Obesity in pregnancy carries multiple maternal and perinatal risks. Antepartum dangers include gestational diabetes, pregnancy-associated hypertension and/or preeclampsia, post-term pregnancy, multifetal pregnancy, UTIs, OSA, miscarriage, and venous thromboembolism. Problems in labor consist of dysfunctional labor, cesarean section, shoulder dystocia, and both spontaneous and medically indicated preterm delivery. Threats to the fetus and infant are congenital anomalies and death. Postpartum risks involve postpartum infection and postpartum hemorrhage (Cunningham et al., 2018; Ramsey & Schenken, 2021).

Before conception, obese women should lose weight to decrease their BMI below 30 kg/m², thus mitigating some of the risks obesity brings to pregnancy. Losing weight during pregnancy is not recommended. Limiting weight gain in pregnancy is a management strategy that can reduce associated risks. Cunningham et al. (2018) recommend gaining no more than 11 to 20 pounds. Meal planning and exercise work together to control weight gain in pregnancy. An early or first trimester GTT can discover an unknown diabetic condition and give clinicians an opportunity for early intervention. First and second trimester US exams confirm gestational age, number of fetuses, and congenital defects. Routine monitoring of blood pressure will detect the onset of pregnancy-associated hypertension (Ramsey & Schenken, 2021).

Obese women who have had bariatric surgery should wait 12 to 18 months after surgery to become pregnant. If gastric banding was performed, the bariatric clinician should monitor the pregnant woman throughout her pregnancy for the need for band adjustments. Nutritional and vitamin deficiencies can be a problem in a patient who has had bariatric surgery, and monitoring for these conditions in pregnancy is extremely important (Cunningham et al., 2018).

INTRAUTERINE DEVICE IN SITU

Although failure rates in women who use IUDs or intrauterine systems (IUS) range from 0.2% to 0.8%, pregnancy still does occur. An IUD in situ constitutes a threat to the pregnancy and must be removed.

The majority of the time, pregnancy with IUD use occurs because of a malpositioned device or the pregnancy was undetected before insertion. Risk factors include noncompliance with abstinence before insertion and inexperience of the inserting clinician. The risk of SAB is higher with the IUD in place, although removing the device does not guarantee there will not be a subsequent pregnancy loss.

Generally, the patient is aware that she has an IUD in place. A US exam is performed to understand the position of the device in relation to the pregnancy. The patient is counseled on the risks for removal of the IUD with a current pregnancy versus the risks of leaving the IUD in situ. If the strings are visible, the IUD can be removed from the uterus or endocervical canal and disposed of. The patient should be counseled that some bleeding is normal, but she should return if, during a 2-hour period, she soaks two pads each hour (Tulandi & Al-Fozan, 2023).

FUTURE DIRECTIONS

Reducing the Number of Prenatal Visits

Typical prenatal care in the United States provides 16 prenatal appointments for an uncomplicated pregnancy that lasts at least 41 weeks. This is nearly twice as many visits as our international peers whose maternity outcomes have improved, while ours have gotten more deadly (Peahl et al., 2020). In the advent of the COVID-19 pandemic, care delivery had to change to reduce exposure of clinician and patient to this deadly virus. These changes highlighted the damaging consequences of adverse social and structural determinants of health and inferior pregnancy outcomes. The ACOG and the University of Michigan assembled a panel of stakeholders to reformulate prenatal care delivery in the United States. The results of this endeavor produced in the Michigan Plan for Appropriate Tailored Healthcare in pregnancy (MiPATH). This revised schedule of prenatal services for average-risk pregnant women recommends at least four key in-person visits with additional visits completed either in person or remotely. Implementation of this schedule requires early risk assessment of medical and obstetric risk factors and social and structural determinants of health for all patients. MiPATH is the first step in redesigning prenatal care in this country to be effective, efficient, and equitable (Peahl et al., 2021).

Alternative Models of Prenatal Care

As group prenatal models are growing in number and being offered in more practices, researchers continue to explore new models of prenatal care delivery that may provide greater access to those facing barriers to receiving healthcare. Nurse home visits and telemedicine are examples of the types of alternative care models being evaluated by randomized controlled trials for their impact on outcomes as compared to the traditional model. Additionally, research on patient-centered outcomes can inform us which components of prenatal care have evidence to support their continued use (Gourevitch et al., 2020). The Mayo Clinic offers OB Nest, a telemedicine model whereby half of the prenatal care visits are done in the patient's home or "nest." This program seeks to de-medicalize pregnancy, empower women, and offer more home-based care (Mayo Clinic, 2021).

REFERENCES

References for this chapter are online and available at https://connect.springerpub.com/content/book/978-0-8261-6722-4/part/part02/chapter/ch23

Managing Symptoms and Health Considerations

Chapter 24

Breast Health Considerations*

Leslie L. Balcazar de Martinez† and Annesley W. Copeland

Clinical evaluation of the breast, indications for screening and diagnostic imaging, and appropriate follow-up of findings are major issues in women's healthcare for patients and healthcare providers. Meticulous attention to examination techniques, referral for screening and diagnostic testing, and close attention to follow-up of referrals are essential for optimizing breast health through early identification of disease and the minimization of patient nonadherence and provider liability. Early detection and treatment of breast cancer are the ultimate purpose of screening and breast healthcare.

DEFINITION AND SCOPE

Anatomy

The breast is an enlarged and modified sweat gland made up of ducts and lobules. The mature breast borders the second rib or clavicle superiorly, the lateral edge of the sternum medially, the sixth rib inferiorly, and the midaxillary line laterally. Breast tissue extends into the axillary tail of Spence. Blood is supplied from the internal mammary and lateral thoracic arteries and drains into the axillary, internal mammary, and intercostal veins. The breast lymphatics drain centrally to the axillary nodes and less often to the internal mammary or supraclavicular nodes. Muscles that surround and support the breast include the pectoralis major, pectoralis minor, serratus anterior, and latissimus dorsi.

The pigmented nipple, surrounded by the areola at the center of the breast, becomes more prominent at puberty. It enlarges and pigmentation increases during pregnancy due to increased vascularity. Montgomery tubercles, the openings of small pimple-like sebaceous glands called Montgomery glands, are located on the surface of the areola and provide lubrication during lactation. Each nipple has multiple openings for milk ducts. Each duct connects to a lactiferous sinus which then branches into a lobe containing a network of ducts and lobules. There are 12 to 18 lobes arranged around the

nipple like the spokes on a wheel. The lobules end in terminal ductal lobular units (TDLUs) where milk is produced, and most cancers originate. The lobule is the functional unit of the breast and consists of terminal ducts and acini. Each lobe contains an independent ductal system that transfers milk to the nipple. Milk collects in the lactiferous sinuses for breast-feeding. The breast is composed of epithelial and stromal tissue. The epithelial component consists of the ductal and lobular units. The stroma composes most of the tissue in the nonlactating breast and is made up of fibrous connective tissue and fat. Cooper's ligaments are made up of stromal tissue and attach to the skin and the fascia of the pectoralis major muscle suspending and supporting the breast parenchyma.

Breast Development

Breast development starts from the hormonal changes that begin at puberty. Estrogen stimulates the development of ducts and connective tissue. Lobes, which form after ovulation begins, are thought to be a result of progesterone secretion. Breast development stages are known as Tanner phases (1–5). Phase 1 consists of elevation of the nipple with no palpable glandular tissue or pigmentation of the areola. In phase 2, glandular tissue develops under the areola, and the nipple and breast project as a single mound. Phase 3 is marked by palpable glandular tissue and the increase in size and pigmentation of the areola. During phase 4, there is enlargement of the areola that forms a secondary mound above the level of the breast. Phase 5 is the final phase. During this phase, the breast assumes a smooth contour with no projection of the areola and nipple (Osborne & Boolbol, 2014).

Life Cycle Variations

Young women tend to have dense breast tissue due to a larger amount of stroma and parenchyma compared to fat. Estrogen and progesterone stimulation during the

---

*This chapter is a revision of the chapter that appeared in the second edition of this textbook, authored by Deborah G. Feigel and Kathleen Kelleher, and we thank them for their original contribution.

†The opinions and assertions expressed herein are those of the author(s) and do not necessarily reflect the official policy or position of the U.S. Air Force, Department of Defense, or the U.S. government.

menstrual cycle causes enhanced ductal and stromal pro-liferation resulting in fullness, nodularity, and tenderness. With the onset of menses, the decline in hormone levels causes proliferation to regress, improving breast tender-ness and nodularity. Days 3 to 10 in the cycle are optimal for self-breast examination (SBE) and clinical breast exam-ination (CBE) for accuracy and patient comfort. Preg-nancy results in marked ductal and lobular proliferation that increases over the course of the pregnancy, making a CBE at the first prenatal visit an important baseline exam-ination. After the discontinuation of breastfeeding, epithe-lial breast tissue regresses and the ratio of adipose tissue to parenchyma increases. In perimenopause, ductal and lobular elements regress and are replaced by adipose tis-sue, a process known as involution. Some research suggests that incomplete postmenopausal involution in breast tissue may contribute to increased breast cancer risk (Milanese et al., 2006). In the postmenopausal breast, the stromal and epithelial tissue regresses and is replaced with adipose tissue; however, genetic predisposition and exogenous hormone therapy influence this process, resulting in con-siderable variation in postmenopausal breast tissue density and nodularity.

BENIGN BREAST CONDITIONS

Abnormal Breast Development

Breast development before 8 years of age is known as pre-mature thelarche. This usually occurs in the first 2 years of life without other signs of puberty. It is bilateral and usually resolves without treatment in 3 to 5 years. If accompanied by other signs of puberty, before 8 years of age, it is known as precocious puberty. Precocious puberty is usually idio-pathic but a workup by a pediatrician or endocrinologist is recommended.

Abnormal breast growth in adolescents such as amastia (congenital absence of the breast), Poland syndrome (con-genital absence of both the breast and pectoralis muscle), or trauma resulting in damage to the breast bud (e.g., chest tube placement in infancy is a common cause) usually requires mammoplasty after the age of 16 years (when breast devel-opment is usually completed). Juvenile gigantomastia and hormonal or medication-induced macromastia often cause physical and emotional distress and can be treated with elec-tive breast reduction.

Breast growth in adolescents can be uneven, leading to breast asymmetry, which can be distressing. Young women often need reassurance that small differences in size are nor-mal and may resolve with time. Major asymmetry is uncom-mon but may require surgical intervention if emotional distress is severe.

Polythelia, or accessory nipple tissue, is a frequently encountered congenital abnormality and can occur anywhere along the "milk line" from the axilla to the groin. Accessory mammary tissue, or polymastia, is also seen, most frequently in the axilla. This tissue may enlarge or function during preg-nancy and lactation, even producing milk if associated with an accessory nipple.

Elective Breast Surgery

Once breast development is complete, women may elect to undergo elective surgery to change the appearance of their breasts. Women with significant breast asymmetry, very small breasts, or very large breasts may have difficulty find-ing clothes that fit well or may wish to change their appear-ance for a variety of reasons.

Women with very large breasts may suffer from back pain, neck pain, shoulder grooving, and difficulty in exercising. Breast reduction (reduction mammoplasty) is often per-formed to lessen the physical and emotional effects of breast hypertrophy. Women need to be counseled in depth about potential risks and long-term effects. Asymmetry, signifi-cant scarring, fat necrosis, and infection may occur; however, most patients are very relieved and pleased with the results.

Breast enlargement or augmentation mammoplasty is performed by a plastic surgeon. During this procedure, an implant is placed behind the breast tissue or pectoralis mus-cle through a periareolar, inframammary, or transaxillary incision. Risks include contracture, infection, hematoma, and possible mammographic distortion. Implants will likely need replacement every 10 to 15 years. Mammograms in women with implants are more difficult to perform and require addi-tional views to image all breast tissue. MRI can be used to evaluate breast implants for rupture. Decreased sexual plea-sure may occur due to firmness and loss of nipple sensation. To date, there have been no reliable scientific data linking sil-icone implants to connective tissue diseases, and implants do not appear to increase the risk of breast cancer.

Mastopexy is performed to improve ptosis or raise sagging breasts. As a result of this procedure, scarring may be exten-sive, and women should be counseled that ptosis may recur.

Patients undergoing elective breast surgery should follow surgical instructions carefully. A preoperative mammogram and a new baseline mammogram 6 months after surgery are usually recommended for women older than 30 years or for those women who have significant family histories for breast disease. It is important to note that breast surgery alters the mammographic appearance of breast tissue.

Breast Pain

Mastalgia can be cyclical or noncyclical and may present unilaterally or bilaterally (Ader, 2002). Mastalgia that occurs cyclically is usually considered normal and is related to hor-monal stimulation of the breast during the menstrual cycle. Causes of noncyclical breast pain include large cysts, infec-tion, benign and malignant masses, inflammatory breast cancer, hormone therapy, macromastia, ductal ecstasis, and hidradenitis suppurativa. Diet and lifestyle causes of breast pain, such as caffeine, smoking, high fat diets, and iodine deficiency, have also been proposed, but not firmly estab-lished. Breast examination in women with breast pain should include a careful examination while assessing for signs suggestive of malignancy, such as a mass, asymmetry, skin changes, and/or bloody nipple discharge. All areas of the breast including the axilla and supraclavicular and infracla-vicular spaces should be examined in both sitting and supine positions. Palpation of the breast away from the chest wall with the patient sitting or in a side-lying position can help to differentiate parenchymal pain versus a chest wall etiology. Palpation of the ribs and musculature posterior to the breast mound can reproduce the pain. Mammograms and ultrasound (US) for focal pain should be performed. Any breast pain that occurs with redness and inflammation needs immediate evaluation to rule out inflammatory breast cancer. Persistent localized breast pain should also be referred for evaluation to rule out occult malignancy. Once breast disease is eliminated as a cause, reassurance is often the only treatment indicated. Some women anecdotally note slight relief with less caffeine, but this has not been reproduced reliably in clinical trials. Breast and chest wall pain can be treated conservatively with oral and/or topical over-the-counter nonsteroidal anti-inflammatory drugs (NSAIDs), application of ice or heat, and good support or sports bras. For severe pain, a variety of medications are available, including danazol, bromocriptine, low-dose oral contraceptives, and tamoxifen. Except for low-dose oral contraceptives, women with severe breast pain should be treated by breast specialists due to significant risk and side effect profiles associated with these other prescription medications.

Infections

Mastitis is an infection of the breast tissue that usually occurs in lactating women but can occur infrequently in nonlactating women. Treatment with antibiotics and analgesics is indicated. If untreated, an abscess can result that usually requires surgical incision and drainage. Any breast infection not responding rapidly to antibiotic treatment should be referred to a specialist to rule out inflammatory breast cancer. Nonlactational abscesses may be more common in women who smoke, have inverted nipples, or have implanted foreign bodies (such as nipple piercings). Infection of sebaceous glands and cysts may also be encountered.

Mondor's Disease

Superficial thrombophlebitis or Mondor's disease is uncommon. This condition usually results from trauma, surgery, or pregnancy, but can be spontaneous. The palpable thrombosed vein is usually linear and tender. Treatment consists of analgesics and warm compresses and does not require anticoagulation.

Nipple Discharge

Breast discharge is usually benign and may be caused by high prolactin levels, medications, or breast stimulation. History and examination should determine if the discharge is spontaneous or induced, from one duct or multiple ducts, and from one or both breasts. The discharge should be described as serous, serosanguineous, bloody, brown, clear, milky, green, or blue black. Frequency and amount should be documented.

Galactorrhea occurs in nonlactating women and may be caused by medications (commonly estrogens, antihypertensives, antidepressants, and antipsychotics). Galactorrhea usually is spontaneous, ample in amount, from both breasts, and from multiple ducts. Pregnancy testing should be performed if the patient is of childbearing age and prolactin levels should be obtained. Prolactin levels more than 20 ng/mL

are abnormal and may indicate the presence of a pituitary adenoma or prolactinoma. Prolactin should be drawn early in the morning and should precede breast examination or any breast stimulation. An MRI or CT scan of the brain is used to evaluate the pituitary gland if prolactin levels are elevated. Other causes of galactorrhea include hypothyroidism, renal disease (Dietz & Crowe, 2002), and Forbes–Albright syndrome.

Pathologic breast discharge is characterized as spontaneous, is usually unilateral, and comes from a single duct. Persistent discharge and discharge that is serosanguineous, brown, or contains gross blood is worrisome and requires further evaluation to rule out malignancy. Bloody nipple discharge can occur in pregnancy due to increased vascularity. Intraductal papilloma, a benign condition that is rarely palpable, is the most common cause of bloody discharge. Breast discharge can be checked for blood with a Hemoccult card. It is important to note that absence of blood *does not rule out malignancy*. Discharge can be placed on a slide and fixed for cytologic analysis; however, this is not widely recommended as a negative test is usually nondiagnostic, and a result of atypical cells may not necessarily indicate malignancy. Ductography of the breast and/or ductal lavage is sometimes used to evaluate breast discharge; however, evidence of its diagnostic value and clinical application has been mixed. Surgical removal of the duct is the standard treatment for bloody and pathologic discharge.

Masses

PUBERTY/ADOLESCENCE

A normal breast bud, or mammary tissue growth at puberty, may feel like a retroareolar mass. Most breast masses in adolescence are fibroadenomas that feel smooth and rubbery on palpation, or cysts that often feel like marbles. These masses should be imaged with US to rule out suspicious features and should be followed carefully in adolescents and young women. Palpable masses in young women should be referred to a specialist for evaluation unless clearly benign, and biopsy should be considered if there are any suspicious clinical or imaging features. Occasionally, fibroadenomas can become very large and should be referred for surgical excision. Most fibroadenomas are benign, but can uncommonly consist of abnormal stromal hyperplasia, which then is classified as a benign or malignant phyllodes tumor. Phyllodes tumors arise from the stromal or fibrous supportive tissue, are similar in character to sarcomas, and are very rare. Treatment usually consists of wide local excision only.

ADULTS

A breast mass in an adult woman should be considered *cancer until proved benign*. Most masses are found by women or their partners incidentally or on SBE, and are also detected by a clinician on CBE. Common masses include fibroadenomas, cysts, fibrocystic nodules and ridges, lipomas, and carcinomas. If the area in question matches symmetrically in the opposite breast, it is probably an individual finding particular to the patient and should be referred for imaging (usually mammograms and targeted US) as well as to a surgeon breast specialist if not clearly benign. Evaluation of a mass in a menstruating woman should include a thorough examination before and after menses. If the mass persists, a mammogram and targeted US, in all women older than 30 years, should be done. In women younger than 30 years of age, a breast mass can initially be evaluated by US alone. Mammogram and/or breast MRI may also be indicated.

US can help to determine whether a breast mass is a simple cyst, complex cyst, solid, or normal glandular tissue. Simple fluid-filled cysts may be followed without intervention, while complex cysts and solid masses may need further evaluation by aspiration, biopsy, or serial imaging follow-up. Once women have reached menopause, many palpable masses are potentially malignant. Careful evaluation is indicated, including history, date of onset, how it was discovered, practice of SBE, location, size, character, and any recent changes. Mammograms and US should always be performed; MRI may also be indicated.

There are multiple conditions within the breast that are found by women and their clinicians, which may be asymptomatic or result in nodularity, pain, and/or masses. Cystic breast changes are the most common due to parenchymal hormonal stimulation and cyst formation. These changes usually decrease after menopause without exogenous estrogen stimulation. Fibrocystic changes are too common to be called a disease; this common condition ranges from harmless changes in tissue to changes that are associated with an increased risk of cancer. A broad group of tissue changes is known as benign breast disease; these changes generally fall into two categories: proliferative and nonproliferative lesions. Generally, nonproliferative lesions do not increase the risk of breast cancer, while proliferative lesions are associated with varying degrees of increased cancer risk (Table 24.1).

Nonproliferative lesions include cysts, metaplasia, adenosis, papillomas, fibroadenomas, fibrosis, and ductal ectasia. A single papilloma is a benign lesion that often occurs in the subareolar breast tissue but can be present anywhere in the ductal system. It is the most common cause of bloody or serous nipple discharge. Papillomas are usually not palpable and are usually not seen on mammography. Multiple papillomas, or papillomatosis, are considered a proliferative lesion. Fibroadenomas are benign tumors of the stroma, are often palpable, and can be seen on mammograms and US images. Ductal ectasia is a dilated, thickened, and tortuous duct(s). Other benign breast conditions include galactoceles, hematomas, fibroadenolipomas, lipomas, neurofibromas, tubular adenomas, sarcoidosis, diabetic mastopathy (typically seen in women with type 1 diabetes with associated retinopathy and neuropathy), and fat necrosis. Fat necrosis usually results from trauma and may feel like small firm nodules that can be difficult to differentiate from a malignancy. The presence of oil cysts on a mammogram is indicative of this condition.

Proliferative lesions associated with a small increase in risk include ductal hyperplasia without atypia, sclerosing adenosis, papillomatosis, complex fibroadenomas (fibroadenoma-associated proliferative changes, sclerosing adenosis, or papillary apocrine changes), and radial scar. Radial scar is a benign lesion found on mammography that is not related to trauma or previous surgery. The cause is unknown. This finding usually requires a biopsy to differentiate it from carcinoma. Atypical ductal hyperplasia (ADH), atypical lobular hyperplasia (ALH), and lobular carcinoma in situ (LCIS) are proliferative lesions associated with a moderate increased risk of breast cancer. ADH can be associated with malignancy. ALH and LCIS can be associated with neighboring malignancy as well. Complex lesions containing atypia are also seen, such as atypical papilloma, columnar alteration with atypia, or fibroadenoma associated with atypia. Referral to a surgeon for excision is necessary for all atypical lesions to exclude the possibility of breast cancer; however, most lesions will not be associated with malignancy and are considered "markers" for increased risk of cancer in either breast.

Skin Changes

Many benign skin changes can occur on the breast skin, including moles, skin tags, keloids, inclusion cysts, and sebaceous cysts. Any lesions that have changed or have an irregular appearance need prompt referral to a dermatologist for evaluation and possible biopsy. Skin retraction or dimpling is a sign of breast cancer, often advanced, but can also be associated with benign processes such as scar tissue from previous surgery. Redness or inflammation with or without peau d'orange (orange peel skin) may indicate an infection or inflammatory breast cancer.

Nipple Changes

Nipple fissures can occur in lactating women. Cleanliness, the application of lanolin, and air drying are preventive. Nipple shields and/or a referral to a lactation consultant may also be helpful. Any scaling, eczematous changes, redness, erythema, a recurring scab, and/or nonhealing area on the nipple requires prompt referral to rule out Paget disease, a rare form of breast cancer that presents in the nipple.

BREAST ASSESSMENT

Clinical Breast Examination

Average risk women should have a CBE every 3 years in their 20s to 30s, and every year for women age 40 years and older. CBE is an effective diagnostic skill, often related to the experience and training of the examiner. Between 5% and 10% of masses are found during clinical examination. CBE may

TABLE 24.1 Approximate Relative Risk of Breast Cancer Associated With Benign Breast Disease and Atypia

BREAST PATHOLOGY RESULTS	RELATIVE RISK (RR)
Nonproliferative changes	One to two times increase in RR
Proliferative changes	Two times increase in RR
Atypia	Four times increase in RR

detect 3% to 45% of masses that mammography misses. The average amount of time required to perform a good CBE is 6 to 8 minutes. This time is challenged by the discomfort and embarrassment that some patients experience during a breast examination, particularly those who are young or have a history of physical or sexual abuse. A good examination needs to cover all breast tissue including the axilla. Breast awareness should be discussed with the patient with advice to report changes to her healthcare provider. A CBE involves visual inspection of the breasts with the woman sitting with arms at her sides, raised overhead, and with shoulders hunched and her hands at waist height to evaluate any visible dimpling, puckering, or skin changes. Palpation of the entire breast (from the clavicle to the inframammary crease vertically, and the sternum to the midaxillary line horizontally) and axilla is done with the patient sitting and supine. Supraclavicular and axillary nodes are best evaluated in the sitting position. The effectiveness of SBE has been questioned and various health agencies have ambivalent or conflicting recommendations regarding this practice. SBE may result in increased benign biopsies and psychological distress. Although recommendations are mixed, SBE or breast awareness continues to be advocated by most breast cancer organizations and clinicians. The accuracy of the practice varies with the skill of the patient. A study conducted in China found that there was no difference in breast cancer mortality rates between women who did SBE and those who did not (Thomas et al., 2002). Until further data are available, breast awareness continues to play an important role for younger women who are not having other screening tests and it is important for all women to monitor their own health. Women can be advised that performing SBE may result in identification of benign processes but also early detection of a malignancy. Early detection and treatment are associated with increasing survival of patients diagnosed with breast cancer. Any patient presenting with an abnormal finding should have a complete medical and breast history, including documentation of risk factors for breast cancer. A current mammogram is mandatory, and a thorough CBE must be performed. Clinical examination must correlate with diagnostic findings (concordance); mammograms do not have 100% sensitivity and may miss some lesions. A negative mammogram in the presence of a clinical palpable mass *does not rule out breast cancer.*

CBE, breast imaging, and needle biopsy are referred to as *the triple test*. If the triple test indicates a benign process, the likelihood of error is small; however, if there is any clinical concern, even with negative imaging, or if the patient may be nonadherent or have difficulty returning, further evaluation by a specialist should be immediate (Bleicher, 2014).

Liability and Documentation

Breast care is a critical area of patient care and a potential liability. Patient presentation, history, physical examination, all testing, and follow-up plans and visits must be documented in detail (if it is not documented then it did not take place). Meticulous patient education throughout the diagnostic process and follow-up is important to prevent unrealistic patient expectations, facilitate early diagnosis, and help prevent loss to follow-up and liability.

Diagnostic Testing

MAMMOGRAM

Mammography continues to be the gold standard for breast cancer screening but has an overall false-negative rate of 10% to 15%, whichith isa slightly higher rate in younger women. Therefore, mammography cannot exclusively rule out cancer (Bleicher, 2014). Patients should be made aware of the shortcomings of mammography screening so as to eliminate the unrealistic expectation that a normal mammogram means there is no possibility of malignancy. False-positive results may also occur; 5% to 10% of all screening examinations are reported as abnormal, and 80% to 90% of women with abnormal results do not have breast cancer (American Cancer Society [ACS], 2022). All mammography facilities should be accredited by the American College of Radiology. Facility certification can be verified at www.acr.org.

Types of Mammograms

Mammograms are ordered as (a) a screening test, a routine mammogram on a patient without a problem, or as (b) a diagnostic examination in a patient with a breast complaint or abnormal examination. The screening mammogram consists of two standard views of each breast: the medial-lateral-oblique (MLO) and the craniocaudal (CC). Diagnostic mammograms usually include more views than a four-view screening mammogram (90-degree medial-lateral [ML], spot compression, or magnification views). Diagnostic mammograms are indicated when a screening mammogram is abnormal, a patient has a history of breast cancer or a high-risk benign lesion, or there is a new palpable mass. Diagnostic mammography is best performed with a radiologist on site so that additional views can be taken if indicated. A sonogram is usually indicated for any abnormal density or mass seen on the mammogram and for any palpable abnormality. Mammography is digital (similar to a digital camera) or analog (like a regular camera with the image printed on film). Both modalities are certified by the American College of Radiology. Digital mammography is more effective in women with dense breast tissue. Density is determined by the radiologist and is included in the report. Computer-assisted detection (CAD) is a computer program that aids the radiologist when reading digital breast films. CAD may, at best, be equivalent to double read (two radiologists) mammograms, and may lead to increased patient callbacks for additional imaging as well as more benign breast biopsies (false-positives). Findings on mammograms can include nodules, asymmetry, densities, or calcifications. Mammography is the only reliable tool available for the detection of breast microcalcifications that may indicate early, therefore potentially curable, ductal carcinoma in situ (DCIS). Breast calcifications are detected commonly on screening mammograms and are most often benign and classified accordingly without any additional workup. In women with indeterminate (possibly malignant) calcifications on screening studies, additional mammogram views, such as ML and microfocus magnification views, are usually obtained to determine the need for short-term (usually 4–6 months) follow-up or biopsy.

Women may be puzzled and alarmed by calcifications and ask if they should discontinue their calcium supplements or dairy intake and/or request a biopsy. They should be reassured that calcifications are common; most are noncancerous and related to benign tissue changes, and have no relationship to calcium intake. Worrisome calcifications are usually those that are very small (micro) and are new or increased, with a clustered or branching pattern. These patterns of calcification need further exploration to determine if a biopsy is indicated to rule out early malignancy. A breast biopsy using the mammogram to guide the biopsy (an image-guided biopsy) is known as a stereotactic biopsy.

Women should be given yearly prescriptions for mammograms beginning at age 40 years and follow-up should be meticulously tracked. More than seven major health organizations have recommendations on age to start and frequency of mammography. Most suggest starting at age 40 years and then repeating every 1 to 2 years (Mahon, 2007). Women with significant risk factors should have their first baseline mammogram at age 35 years or earlier if there is an abnormal examination finding or very significant family history. Furthermore, they should consider seeing a breast specialist for guidance. Healthcare providers need to review each patient's history individually before deciding on frequency and initiation.

The American College of Radiology Breast Imaging Reporting and Data System (BI-RADS) is a standardized reporting system resulting in an assessment of findings and recommendations. Mammogram reporting is as follows:

- BI-RADS 0: Needs additional imaging evaluation and/or earlier mammograms for comparison
- BI-RADS 1: Negative
- BI-RADS 2: Benign findings
- BI-RADS 3: Probably benign finding; short interval follow-up suggested
- BI-RADS 4: Suspicious abnormality; biopsy should be considered
- BI-RADS 5: Highly suggestive of malignancy; appropriate action should be taken
- BI-RADS 6: Known biopsy-proven malignancy; appropriate action should be taken (D'Orsi, 2005)

ULTRASOUND EXAMINATION

US exam, or sonogram, is an adjunct diagnostic method for a CBE and/or mammogram and can assess the nature of a mammographic nodule, density, or palpable mass. It is also helpful in dense breasts. US imaging should be ordered for further evaluation of mammographic findings and of any palpable mass, even in the setting of a normal mammogram. US is not helpful in diagnosing or clarifying calcifications. It is used as guidance for core breast biopsies, fine needle aspiration (FNA), and cyst aspiration. Its low specificity and high false-positive rate mean the use of US, in the general population, is uncertain. There is no evidence for screening asymptomatic women with this modality (Mahon, 2007).

MAGNETIC RESONANCE IMAGING

Breast MRI is a costly examination that may be very helpful in assessing high-risk patients or those with very dense breast tissue and is an adjunct to standard breast imaging. Breast MRI scans breast tissue using a magnet, not ionizing radiation. A breast MRI can cost much more than $1,200, making it a

substantially more expensive test than mammograms and US exam. The cost of a breast MRI may not be covered by health insurance and usually requires preauthorization. Breast MRI may be indicated in women who are newly diagnosed with breast cancer to rule out occult locally advanced disease, multifocal disease (more than a single tumor), and contralateral disease (cancer in the opposite breast; Mahon, 2007).

MRI may also be helpful in high-risk women. The ACS has published guidelines for MRI screening in high-risk women (ACS, 2022). The ACS recommends MRI screening in women (a) with a documented breast cancer *BRCA1* or *BRCA2* mutation; (b) with an untested blood relative of a *BRCA* mutation carrier; (c) with a 20% to 25% or greater lifetime risk of breast cancer based on accepted risk calculation models; (d) who have received chest radiation (such as for lymphoma) between ages 10 and 30 years; and (e) with several other less common genetic abnormalities involving genetic mutations in gene *TP53* (Li-Fraumeni syndrome) and *PTEN* (Cowden and Bannayan–Riley–Ruvalcaba syndromes) and their first-degree relatives (ACS, 2022). MRI is also indicated when findings are indeterminate after a conventional imaging workup, for evaluation of the effect of neoadjuvant chemotherapy, and when evaluating the local extent of disease in patients with known cancer (Saslow et al., 2007).

BIOPSY

Patients who are found to have a suspicious palpable mass or suspicious density or calcifications on mammogram or US exam need to have breast tissue sampled for an accurate diagnosis. The goal of any method of biopsy is to remove as little tissue as possible, and to make the diagnosis with as little trauma as possible and with as close to 100% accuracy as possible. Biopsies can be performed in multiple ways. The simplest is FNA, which may or may not require local anesthesia. When performing FNA, a small-gauge needle is inserted into the abnormal area and the cells that are sheared off are fixed on a slide and analyzed. If the abnormality is a cyst, the fluid can be sent for cytologic exam. Aspiration should resolve a cyst and it should not recur. If it does not disappear or if it recurs, further assessment is required. FNA does not allow for histologic (tissue) examination; instead, FNA consists only of examination of the cells placed on the slide. FNA performed with image guidance tends to be more accurate than without. A negative FNA does not rule out malignancy.

A core needle biopsy (CNB) can be performed under mammogram (stereotactic), US, or MRI guidance for almost any abnormality, and without imaging guidance for a palpable mass. It is performed with a large-gauge needle to obtain tissue "cores" following injection of a local anesthetic. CNB provides breast tissue for architecture and histology and can usually rule out breast cancer if the histology is concordant (makes sense) with the imaging. Stereotactic CNB is performed using the mammogram as a guide. A three-dimensional mammographic image is obtained with the patient in a prone, sitting, or side-lying position and a computer helps the radiologist or surgeon guide the needle placement. CNB is performed in a radiology department under a radiologist's guidance. If findings from a CNB are inconclusive (not concordant), a surgical biopsy may be required.

An MRI-guided CNB is done when the lesion is best visualized or only seen on an MRI. The same CNB technique is used as described earlier, except that the biopsy must be approached from the lateral breast, making biopsies in the medial breast somewhat more challenging. In most image-guided biopsies a small surgical marker is placed at the site of the biopsy to provide guidance for the surgeon, if surgery is necessary or to provide a reference area for future mammographic evaluation.

SURGICAL BIOPSY

Incisional biopsy removes a piece of the mass and is used for diagnosis alone. Excisional biopsy of a palpable mass (removing the entire lump) is also done for diagnosis, but may also serve as treatment (e.g., removing the lump). Cancer treatment is usually not accomplished with excisional biopsy alone.

If a lesion is nonpalpable (such as with calcifications) and is seen on a mammogram or US, it must be localized for the surgeon before excision. This is accomplished by the radiologist placing a thin surgical wire through or next to the site (wire localization) to guide the surgeon. Placement is confirmed by mammogram and the surgeon removes the tissue around the wire. The specimen removed undergoes x-ray evaluation to confirm that the correct tissue was obtained. For the purposes of diagnosing a breast abnormality, wire localization has largely been replaced in tertiary care and cancer centers where patients have access to CNB. Core biopsy allows diagnosis and cancer surgery planning without a surgical procedure for diagnosis alone. Excisional biopsy is necessary with lesions that cannot be reached with CNB (such as a very far posterior lesion), vague lesions where risk of a false negative is higher, in patients without access to CNB, and for discordant CNB histology (e.g., the mammogram is highly suspicious for cancer, but the biopsy shows completely normal breast tissue).

The majority of CNBs performed are found to be benign. Those that are cancerous will almost always require surgery (the biopsy only samples the area and does not remove it completely). Additional surgery is required to obtain clear margins when excisional biopsy has been performed leaving residual cancer in the breast. Surgical evaluation of the lymph nodes may also be necessary. Bruising and slight tenderness are very common after CNB and surgical biopsy. A good support bra, ice, and over-the-counter analgesics are usually all that are required for pain relief. Small hematomas often occur, but large hematomas are not uncommon. If a patient requires anticoagulation for a medical reason, consultation with the patient's primary physician is indicated regarding the suspension of therapy before biopsy and/or surgery.

BREAST CANCER

Although breast cancer is the most common female malignancy and the second leading cause of cancer death in U.S. women (lung cancer is the first), worldwide, breast cancer has surpassed lung cancer as the leading cause of cancer death among women (ACS, 2022; Sung et al., 2021). One in eight women will develop breast cancer in her lifetime and risk increases with age. It was estimated that 287,850 cases of invasive breast cancer, 51,400 in situ breast cancers, and about 43,250 deaths would occur in the United States in 2022. Furthermore, of all the cases estimated in 2022 for breast cancer, 2,710 were estimated to occur in men (ACS, 2022). The cause of most breast cancer is unknown and is probably multifactorial. Breast tumors are most often sporadic while a small portion is attributed to inherited familial syndromes. Hormone therapy and radiation may also be causative. Dietary fat intake and body weight have been studied but have not been shown to be causative (Willett et al., 2014).

Breast cancer can develop anywhere in the breast, and anywhere there is breast tissue, including the axilla and in the inframammary crease. Breast cancer may be present for 5 years or more before it becomes palpable and begins in the terminal ductal lobular unit. Noninvasive or in situ breast cancer that is contained within the ducts is known as DCIS. DCIS is most often treated by wire-localized lumpectomy followed by radiation; however, debate is ongoing about optimal treatment. Some patients with DCIS will eventually develop invasive carcinomas, but it is impossible to predict which patients will advance or not (ACS, 2022). LCIS is not considered a malignancy or noninvasive cancer but is a marker for increased risk of future breast cancer in either breast.

Invasive cancer breaks through the basement membrane of the duct or lobule, thereby gaining access to blood vessels and the lymphatic system, giving it the ability to spread outside the breast. Biopsy and surgery establish the type and extent of disease.

Risk Factors for Developing Breast Cancer

1. The *number one risk factor* for breast cancer is being female.
2. *Age* is the second most significant risk factor.
3. *Family history of breast cancer*, particularly in first-degree relatives (parent, sibling, and child), increases risk; however, only 5% to 10% of breast cancer is classified as hereditary. Inherited breast cancer involves the *BRCA1* or *BRCA2* tumor suppressor genes. Mutations of these genes result in an increased risk of cancer at an earlier age, cancer in both breasts, and an increased risk of ovarian cancer. Males can carry these genes and may have an increased risk of early prostate and male breast cancer. Many mutations have been identified and are inherited from either the maternal or paternal side in an autosomal dominant manner. Carriers of *BRCA1* have a 65% chance of developing breast cancer by age 70 years, and *BRCA2* carriers have a 45% chance (Antoniou et al., 2003). MRI screening and/or consideration of prophylactic/preventive mastectomy and/or oophorectomy may be recommended. Genetic counseling should be conducted and is often advised before genetic testing due to medical, ethical, psychosocial, legal, and privacy issues. Other genetic disorders that may predispose women to breast cancer include Li-Fraumeni syndrome, Cowden syndrome, Bannayan–Riley–Ruvalcaba syndrome, and Peutz-Jeghers

syndrome (Garber & Offit, 2005). Genetic counselors play an essential role in decision-making related to this type of testing, together with the patient's other healthcare providers who need to assist the patient with decisions as testing has become more available. Probability tools to evaluate the need for genetic testing in women at potential risk are used. Careful selection is important due to cost and ethical issues including possible insurance discrimination, although national legislation has made this practice illegal. The results may often have a strong emotional impact on a patient and family members, who may require supportive intervention.

4. *Reproductive factors* such as age at menarche (less than 12 years), menopause (greater than 55 years) and first birth (later or no children = increased risk), and long-term exogenous hormone exposure are factors in increased breast cancer risk. The Women's Health Initiative reported that women without a uterus, who used exogenous estrogen alone, did not have an increased risk for developing breast cancer at 8 years of follow-up (Ravdin et al., 2007). Findings did support an increase in breast cancer risk in women with a uterus who used exogenous estrogen and progesterone in combination at 4 years of therapy (Rossouw et al., 2002). Oral contraceptives do not seem to increase risk (Willett et al., 2014).

5. *Ethnicity*: Breast cancer incidence is higher in White women but risk of death from breast cancer is higher in minority women (ACS, 2022). Later identification, more aggressive and hormone-negative tumors, and shorter time to recurrence are factors lending to this difference. Racial disparities may exist in treatment and access to screening (Centers for Disease Control and Prevention [CDC], 2012). Incidence for Black women younger than 35 years is twice the rate for young White women and the mortality rate is three times higher ACS, 2022. Black women have fewer mammograms than White women of the same socioeconomic status (ACS, 2022; CDC, 2012). Caregiving responsibilities are often described as impediments to annual screening. Patients might be asked about their ability to follow through on recommended testing by their healthcare provider. Latinas have lower breast cancer rates but tend to be diagnosed later, possibly contributing to more aggressive disease. Asian women have lower risk; however, the risk increases after immigration to the United States (Willett et al., 2014).

6. *Previous breast biopsies and history of ADH, ALH, or LCIS*: Atypical hyperplasia is associated with a fourfold increase in relative risk of breast cancer (Degnim et al., 2007). LCIS is not considered as a noninvasive cancer and is a marker for increased risk of future breast cancer in either breast. DCIS confers a significantly elevated risk of associated and future invasive breast cancer and is usually managed similarly to invasive carcinoma (described later in this chapter).

7. *Exposure to ionizing radiation*: Radiation treatment to the chest, for conditions such as lymphoma and benign thyroid disease, increases risk (Willett et al., 2014).

8. *Alcohol intake*: Women who consume more than one to two alcoholic beverages per day have a higher risk of breast cancer than those who do not. Alcohol may impact endogenous estrogen levels (Willett et al., 2014).

9. *Obesity*: Recent evidence suggests obesity may be a risk factor, particularly in postmenopausal women (Willett et al., 2014). Weight loss has the potential to change breast cancer incidence, morbidity risk, and mortality risk (Gucalp et al., 2014).

10. *Breastfeeding*: Studies show a probable protective benefit of breastfeeding (Willett et al., 2014).

There is no scientific evidence that breast implants, abortions, or deodorants cause or increase the risk of breast cancer (Willett et al., 2014).

Risk Assessment

The known risk factors that place a woman at greater risk of developing breast cancer need to be considered to individualize patient care. Clinical tools, such as the Gail model and Claus model (discussed later in this chapter) are used in assessing breast cancer risk and can assist healthcare providers in their practice. Women who are identified to have increased risk should be closely followed with yearly mammograms (age appropriate), early CBE, and possibly screening breast MRI (as per ACS guidelines), and should be encouraged to perform regular SBE.

Risk Modification

In addition to very close clinical and radiologic monitoring of women who have been determined to be at increased risk, modification and reduction of risk should be considered and discussed. Most risk factors are not modifiable (e.g., age, family history, age at first childbirth), while others are modifiable lifestyle choices, which are not easily or realistically changed (e.g., alcohol consumption). Risk modification should include a discussion about, for example, avoidance or reduction in alcohol intake, and either reduction in dosage or the possibility of eliminating hormone therapy. Publication of findings from the Women's Health Initiative (WHI) in 2002 was likely a contributing factor for the observed national decrease in breast cancer rates in subsequent years (Ravdin et al., 2007; Rossouw et al., 2002). No solid data exist supporting increased physical activity and reduced fat intake as a means for decreasing breast cancer risk; however, there is a trend suggesting that these actions may be helpful. Women who lowered their dietary fat in the WHI had a lower incidence of hormone receptor–positive (HR+) breast cancer (Prentice et al., 2006). Weight gain before and after menopause is associated with increased risk. Encouraging patients to lose excess weight for the purpose of decreasing breast cancer risk may motivate improvement in diet and exercise levels (Eliassen et al., 2006). A healthy diet and exercise are also overwhelmingly beneficial in reducing the risk of heart and vascular disease, both of which contribute to the death of four times more women than breast cancer each year in the United States.

Chemoprevention

A woman's breast cancer risk can be assessed with the use of a breast cancer risk model. Several models are available and easily accessible. The Gail model is available on a disk from the National Cancer Institute (www.cancer.gov) or online at www.cancer.gov/bcrisktool. This model can underestimate risk in women with a possible genetic predisposition to breast cancer because it does not calculate for second-degree affected relatives, early age at diagnosis, and family history of ovarian cancer. The Claus model estimates risk solely based on family history, ages at cancer diagnosis, and patient age. It does not identify individual breast cancer risk but predicts the probability of finding a *BRCA* mutation. BRCAPro (among other models) predicts risk of carrying a *BRCA* mutation based on family history (available at www.southwestern.edu). The IBIS or Tyrer-Cuzick model (www.ems-trials.org/riskevaluator) assesses more family members than only first degree, and also incorporates hormone use, menarche, and family incidence of ovarian cancer. There is no perfect model to assess risk in any one patient, and genetic counselors often use several models to assess risk.

Myriad Genetics also has a tool that predicts for *BRCA* mutations and is available online through Myriad and can be downloaded (www.myriad.com). In women suspected of carrying a mutation, a referral for genetic counseling is highly recommended. Women with a 1.67% or greater 5-year risk of developing breast cancer, based on the Gail model, should consider medication to reduce breast cancer risk (chemoprevention; Vogel, 2006). Tamoxifen, a selective estrogen receptor modulator (SERM) that is also used for treatment of breast cancer, has been shown to reduce the risk of breast cancer by up to 49% over 5 years in this population of women at increased risk for developing breast cancer (Vogel, 2006). The SERM raloxifene has been shown to have a similar preventive effect with fewer risks (Vogel, 2006). Raloxifene has been approved by the Food and Drug Administration (FDA) for breast cancer risk reduction. Breast cancer treatment drugs called aromatase inhibitors (AIs), such as anastrozole, letrozole, and exemestane, by reducing estrogen levels, show promise in reducing breast cancer risk and risk of recurrence by 50%, but may lessen bone density (Rimawi & Osborne, 2014).

Tamoxifen and raloxifene have potentially significant risks and side effects. Some women who would benefit from risk-reduction medication have opted not to, due to fear of complications or underestimation of benefits (Rimawi & Osborne, 2014). Healthcare providers need to be familiar with assessing breast cancer risk and discussing prevention options in high-risk patients; or referring patients to a breast specialist, genetic counselor, or medical oncologist for careful consideration of preventive medications. Careful consideration of risks and benefits is essential as there are risks associated with these medications (Gradishar & Cella, 2006). Women are frequently not made aware of their risk status and therefore not afforded the opportunity to participate in discussions that can lead to informed decisions about preventive treatment options (Salant et al., 2006). High-risk women considering risk-reduction drug therapy are best referred to and monitored by a specialist.

Surgical Prophylaxis

In women who have a very significant lifetime risk of breast cancer (such as *BRCA* mutation carriers), prophylactic mastectomy can be considered. Prophylactic mastectomy is performed by a surgeon and/or plastic surgeon and reduces the woman's lifetime risk of breast cancer by more than 90%. The emotional toll of this type of surgery and the physical changes that will result need to be thoroughly discussed with the patient by her surgeon.

Types of Breast Cancer

Malignant changes usually occur in the ducts or lobules of the breast. Approximately 80% of breast cancers originate in the ducts and most of the remaining 20% in the lobules. Noninvasive breast cancer is classified as DCIS. DCIS is further classified by growth pattern and architecture, which includes comedo, noncomedo, solid, cribriform, micropapillary, and papillary types. DCIS is a breast cancer precursor at its earliest and the most curable stage and consists of a neoplastic lesion confined to the ducts and lobules of the breast. DCIS is often discovered by abnormal calcifications seen on a mammography and now accounts for up to 20% of newly diagnosed breast cancers.

Ideal local therapy (surgery and/or radiation) for treatment of DCIS is currently being debated. The goal of treatment for DCIS involves reducing the risk of a recurrent ipsilateral or contralateral breast cancer. It is generally agreed that DCIS should be treated by wide surgical excision (lumpectomy and related procedures) or by mastectomy if extensive. Radiation to the breast following excision (breast conservation therapy [BCT]) is currently considered standard of care; however, controversy exists in the breast cancer treatment community on how much treatment for DCIS is required. Studies have been done or are underway using tumor characteristics and genetics to determine risk stratification and thus determine which patients may benefit from surgery alone (Hughes et al., 2009). However, risk stratification to determine treatment is not being performed outside the clinical trial setting. Systemic therapy such as tamoxifen does reduce the risk of ipsilateral or contralateral breast cancers in patients treated with BCT and estrogen receptor–positive (ER+) tumors (Wapnir et al., 2011). The 2013 National Comprehensive Cancer Network (NCCN) guidelines recommend women with ER+ tumors consider the addition of tamoxifen after BCT and in women undergoing surgical excision alone. The incidence of DCIS is increasing; this is thought to be due to better mammographic imaging and biopsy techniques and more women having mammograms. Although DCIS is an early and most likely curable breast cancer, it is still a difficult and stressful diagnosis as most women consider DCIS no different from invasive cancers when initially diagnosed. Clinicians can be helpful by supporting and reassuring patients and referring them to support groups and/or reliable resources (Nekhlyudov et al., 2006).

Invasive or infiltrating breast cancer is ductal or lobular in origin. Invasive ductal carcinoma (IDC) is the most common form of breast cancer. It begins in the duct, grows into the surrounding tissue, and has the ability to spread outside the breast by lymphatics or blood vessels. It is the most common type of breast cancer and usually presents as a palpable mass or as an abnormal nodule or density on a mammogram and/or US image. Medullary, tubular, and mucinous carcinomas are less common types of ductal carcinoma. Treatment is initially surgical with wide excision (lumpectomy, partial mastectomy, segmentectomy, quadrantectomy) or mastectomy, with surgical evaluation of the lymph nodes for spread of the cancer. Radiation to the remaining breast tissue, after lumpectomy, is performed to reduce the risk of cancer recurrence in the breast and may be indicated after mastectomy in certain patients deemed at high risk for local cancer recurrence. Antihormonal therapy in hormonally responsive cancers (tamoxifen, aromatase inhibitors) and/or chemotherapy are frequently recommended as additional therapy.

Inflammatory breast cancer is an aggressive form of breast cancer that presents as swelling, redness, warmth, and possibly peau d'orange (orange peel) of the breast skin due to blocked lymph drainage from cancer within the dermal lymphatic system. This can mimic mastitis, but is usually not painful or accompanied by fever or leukocytosis. *Any patient with breast inflammation treated with antibiotics that does not completely resolve should be referred to a breast cancer specialist or surgeon immediately.* Initial treatment is often with chemotherapy and/or radiation followed by surgery.

Paget disease is an uncommon presentation of ductal carcinoma that infiltrates the nipple causing changes that range from a rash, itching, redness, flaking, bleeding, or a recurrent scab or nonhealing sore. Diagnosis is made by breast examination, mammogram, and a nipple biopsy. Mastectomy is the recommended treatment, although less invasive surgery has been explored and used.

Infiltrating or invasive lobular carcinoma (ILC) makes up about 5% to 10% of breast cancers (Li et al., 2003). The cancer cells originate in the lobules, invade the surrounding tissue and can spread via the lymph channels or bloodstream. Lobular carcinoma is more likely to be multicentric or multifocal (two or more separate tumors) and bilateral than IDC. It can also be more difficult to identify on mammography and CBE because it tends to more closely mimic the texture and mammographic appearance of normal breast tissue. As a result, it is often more advanced when detected compared with IDC.

Other cancers are found in the breast including phyllodes tumor, angiosarcoma, and lymphoma, as well as metastatic cancers from other sites in the body that are rare.

Breast Cancer in Pregnancy

Breast cancer that occurs in pregnancy is rare (ACS, 2022). Although rare, when diagnosed, breast cancer is often advanced as the breast undergoes extensive, normal, physiologic changes readying for lactation, making CBE and breast awareness more difficult and less effective. Treatment depends on trimester and stage of malignancy at diagnosis. Patients in their first trimester need to decide on mastectomy or lumpectomy, and radiation therapy is delayed until after delivery leading to an increase in the risk of recurrence. Patients in their second and third trimesters experience less of a delay in time to delivery, so lumpectomy is a better

option. Pregnant women with more advanced disease may be started on chemotherapy in their second or third trimester but there is little data regarding fetal safety or long-term consequences available (Litton & Theriault, 2014). Some patients who are diagnosed with advanced breast cancer may opt for pregnancy termination but this is a very personal decision that must be made by a fully informed patient (Litton & Theriault, 2014). Breast cancer in pregnancy is a crisis for both the pregnant woman and her family, and a supportive oncology team is needed.

Breast Cancer Staging

The stage of breast cancer helps to determine adjuvant or additional treatments. Stages 1 to 4 are a combination of the size of the tumor (T), lymph node involvement (N), and distant metastasis (M; Harris, 2014), spread outside the breast and lymph nodes to other parts of the body, most commonly to the bone, lung, liver, and brain.

Axillary lymph node involvement is the most important prognostic indicator. If malignant cells are found in lymph nodes, there is an increased risk of metastasis. Pathology is described as negative, microscopic (few cells), or gross (visible malignancy in the node), and will describe whether extracapsular extension from the lymph node is present. Traditionally, evaluation of lymph nodes involves axillary lymph node dissection (ALND), which removes most of the affected nodal and fatty tissue in the axilla. This procedure may result in loss of sensation or pain under the arm and, more troubling, lymphedema. Lymphedema occurs in up to 20% of patients who have ALND (DiSipio et al., 2013) and can be chronic and difficult to manage. Axillary sentinel lymph node biopsy (SLNB), a less invasive procedure, is associated with lower rates of lymphedema, 5% to 6% (DiSipio et al., 2013). Blue dye and/or a radioisotope are injected and used to map the lymph node basin drainage of the breast, identifying the first or sentinel node(s) that a cancer would spread to if it is going to spread. The surgeon then removes the node(s) for histologic evaluation and analysis. This procedure is used in invasive breast cancer but not usually in DCIS unless it is high grade or extensive. If positive nodes are found on SLNB, ALND is usually indicated. Tables 24.2 and 24.3 describe tumor staging and nomenclature.

TABLE 24.2 TNM Staging	
Stage 0	Tis, N0, M0
Stage 1	T1, N0, M0
Stage 2	T1, N1, M0 T2, N1 or 2, M0 T3, N0, M0
Stage 3	T1, 2, 3 or 4; N2, M0 T3, N1, M0
Stage 4	Any T, N3, M0 Any T, Any N, M1

is, in situ; TNM, tumor, node, metastasis.

TABLE 24.3 Tumor Staging Nomenclature

T STAGE (SIZE OF TUMOR IN CENTIMETERS)	N: NODAL STATUS	M: PRESENCE OF METASTASIS	STAGE
Tis (DCIS)	N0 = Negative	M0 = Negative	0 = In situ carcinoma
T1 = 2 cm or less	N1 = Positive	M1= Positive	1 = Invasive tumors ≤2 cm in size with negative nodes and no distant metastasis
T2 = 2–1.5 cm	N2/3 = Positive nodes outside axillary nodes (e.g., supra- and/or infraclavicular)		2 = Any tumor with positive lymph nodes is stage 2 or above
T3 >5 cm	N2/3 = Positive nodes outside axillary nodes (e.g., supra- and/or infraclavicular)		3 = Any T4 tumor or tumors >5 cm with positive lymph nodes
T4 = Locally advanced breast cancer			4 = Any size tumor with any lymph node status but with distant metastasis

DCIS, ductal carcinoma in situ; Tis, tumor in situ.

TUMOR GRADE

Tumor grade is not part of the staging system but plays an important part in decision-making about adjuvant treatment. Grade is based on the degree of cell abnormality compared to normal ductal or lobular cells and is classified as grade 1, 2, or 3. Specific cytologic and histologic attributes are associated with each tumor grade. Grade I tumors, which are slower growing than higher grade tumors, are well differentiated, with normal appearing ductal or lobular cells. These cells become more abnormal in appearance in the moderately differentiated grade 2 tumor. They are very abnormal in the poorly differentiated faster growing grade 3 tumors (Harris, 2015).

BIOLOGICAL MARKERS

Tumor markers are used to determine prognosis and treatment. Estrogen and progesterone receptors on cancer cells mediate the cells' response to estrogen and progesterone. About 75% of breast cancers express one or both receptors that indicate a tumor should respond to hormonal therapy (Breastcancer.org, 2023). *HER2* is an oncogene, which is overexpressed in 18% to 20% of invasive cancers, is more aggressive, and indicates a poorer prognosis, especially if lymph nodes are positive (Mahon, 2007). Herceptin is a targeted biological therapy specific for the overexpressed HER2 (human epidermal growth factor receptor 2) protein. Studies have shown great promise in reducing cancer recurrence and possibly mortality in HER2+ cancers (Romond et al., 2005). Genetic evaluation of the tumor is also being used to help predict a tumor's response to endocrine and chemotherapy. The most common profiles used are the 21-gene recurrence score, MammaPrint, and the Risk of Recurrence score.

SURGICAL MARGINS

When breast cancer is removed surgically, a margin of normal tissue around it is removed as well. This margin is important in gauging the risk of leaving tumor behind in the breast and therefore risk of local recurrence. Clear or negative margins

are the gold standard for adequate tumor excision with the amount of gross margin (not microscopic) varying by institutional practice (Moran et al., 2014). When tumor sections are examined microscopically the entire tumor is inked externally for margin reference. "No tumor on ink" is the widely accepted standard for excision (surgonc.org; Moran et al., 2014).

Treatment

Breast cancer is a complex heterogeneous disease and its management is tailored to the individual woman's cancer and to her preferences. Surgical and adjuvant therapy options are based on many factors, including tumor size and characteristics, tumor stage, biological markers, comorbidities in the patient, and genetic profiling of the tumor. The field of breast cancer research is rapidly expanding, leading to frequent changes in standard treatment. Breast cancer treatment is a topic too broad to cover in detail in this chapter. What follows is a comprehensive overview for the nonspecialized healthcare provider.

SURGERY

Surgery continues to be the mainstay of breast cancer treatment. Surgical options are selected based on the extent of the cancer and patient preference. Most women diagnosed with breast cancer are candidates for breast conservation therapy (BCT), which is lumpectomy (surgical resection of the tumor with negative margins) and adjuvant radiation. Re-excision lumpectomy is performed if one or more margins are positive on the initial lumpectomy. The amount of tissue removed varies but can be up to one quarter or more of the breast. Lymph node positivity has no bearing on whether a woman is a candidate for BCT. Radiation to the remaining breast tissue to reduce the risk of recurrence is considered the standard of care in both invasive cancer and DCIS, but this recommendation may be modified based on the tumor type, size, margins, and patient age and comorbidities (Kunkler et al., 2015).

Some patients are not candidates for BCT. When a tumor is large (particularly as compared to breast size), or multicentric with tumors in different quadrants of the same breast, the patient is better served with mastectomy than BCT. Inflammatory breast cancer is a contraindication to BCT. Patients who cannot receive adjuvant radiation therapy are not candidates for BCT; this includes pregnant patients, patients who have previously received therapeutic radiation to the breast or chest, and patients with collagen vascular diseases particularly scleroderma. Patients who are found on genetic testing to have certain germline mutations (*BRCA1* or *BRCA2, ATM,* or *CHEK2*) are also encouraged to undergo mastectomy. Simple or total mastectomy removes the entire breast and may be done in DCIS, invasive cancer, or as a risk-reducing measure for women at high risk. If a patient undergoes mastectomy, she may elect to have breast reconstruction, or to "go flat" which is an increasingly popular choice. For patients who eschew reconstruction, there are specially fitted surgical bras and prostheses that enable the patient to appear entirely normal when clothed. Prostheses have been improved and are lighter and more comfortable than earlier models. The American Cancer Society, the Breast Cancer Network of Strength, Komen for the Cure, and other local societies often provide financial assistance for patients (see www.acs.org, www.y-me.org, and ww5.komen.org/BreastCancer/FinancialResources.html).

For patients who choose breast reconstruction, there are a number of options, including tissue-based and implant-based techniques, which are discussed in the next section.

For all patients with invasive cancer and clinically negative axillary lymph nodes, part of their surgical care will include an SLNB. This is true whether the patient opts for BCT or mastectomy. Patients with DCIS undergoing mastectomy will also have an SLNB performed, in case invasive cancer is found on final pathologic exam. The primary role of SLNB is staging of the breast cancer. ALND, once a common procedure, is now relegated to circumstances in which the axillary lymph nodes are clinically positive, a sentinel node cannot be identified, more than two sentinel nodes are positive for cancer, or the axillary node(s) remain positive following neoadjuvant chemotherapy.

For women who are judged to be good candidates for BCT, the choice of BCT or mastectomy is ultimately up to the patient, with guidance from her surgeon and other members of the multidisciplinary cancer team (Harris & Morrow, 2014). The goals of BCT are to provide the survival equivalent of mastectomy, a cosmetically acceptable breast as the final outcome, and a low rate of recurrence in the treated breast. While historically the risk of local recurrence was higher in patients who underwent BCT, contemporary multimodality treatment significantly reduces the risk of breast cancer recurrence at the original tumor site compared to historical protocols, and in modern series the recurrence rate ranges from 2% to 10%, which is comparable to the rate of local recurrence following mastectomy (Early Breast Cancer Trialists' Collaborative Group [EBCTCG], 2011, 2014). Among women with operable breast cancer, trials dating back to the 1970s have demonstrated at least equivalent disease-free and overall survival rates between mastectomy and BCT. Some more recent observational studies have even shown improved survival in patients with stage 1 or 2 breast cancer undergoing BCT compared with mastectomy (Wrubel et al., 2021).

BREAST RECONSTRUCTION

Breast reconstruction may be done at the time of mastectomy, later, or not at all depending on patient preference. Surgeons make recommendations individually tailored to the patient's needs and desires, keeping in mind that the foremost objectives are oncologic rather than cosmetic. However, quality of life is also an important part of the patient's total care, and many patients experience less emotional distress with immediate reconstruction. Skin-sparing techniques and nipple-sparing surgery are being performed more frequently in certain subsets of women to aid in breast reconstruction and have been shown not to compromise oncologic outcomes (Blanckaert & Vranckx, 2021). Assessment of each individual patient (breast size, lesion size, and so on) helps to determine the use and may result in a better cosmetic outcome (Mehrara & Ho, 2014). Some patients are not good candidates for immediate reconstruction. Postmastectomy chest wall radiation increases the risks for surgical complications due to impaired wound healing, fibrosis, and infection, and is associated with an increased risk of extrusion of the implant in implant-based reconstruction and of poor cosmesis in tissue-based reconstruction options. If the need for radiation cannot be determined before mastectomy, delayed reconstruction may be preferable (Mehrara & Ho, 2014).

Breast reconstruction can be accomplished in many ways, with continued advances in the field. The most common reconstruction technique begins with the insertion of an implant-shaped tissue expander that is placed under the skin (either under or over the pectoral muscle) after the breast is removed, and saline is injected gradually over a few weeks to months to stretch the overlying tissues. When the desired size is achieved, the expander is then surgically exchanged for a permanent saline or silicone implant. Silicone implants provide a more natural-looking result than saline implants. Implant reconstruction requires less extensive surgery and less hospital time than tissue reconstruction, but does involve a second procedure to insert the permanent implant. Patients who do not have nipple-sparing procedures may decide to have the nipple areolar complex reconstructed at a later date; this is typically accomplished as an outpatient procedure and/or a medical tattoo. Implants have a more "youthful" contour with less droop (ptosis) than a natural breast; therefore, some patients will elect to have surgery on the opposite breast to uplift, augment, or reduce the remaining breast for symmetry. Federal law dictates that breast reconstruction surgery as well as contralateral procedures for symmetry be covered by health insurance plans. Implants do carry a risk of capsular contracture in which scar tissue around the implant tightens, resulting in painful hardening and distortion. Radiation to the implant increases the risk of contracture. Like any mechanical device, implants have a finite life expectancy, and should be assessed for replacement beginning at 10 years.

TISSUE RECONSTRUCTION

Autologous tissue reconstruction or "tissue flaps" require more extensive surgery and hospital time but can result in a more anatomic cosmetic appearance. Tissue from the back, abdomen, or other sites can be used to form a tissue mound in place of a breast or to create a pocket for an implant. Not every patient is a candidate for these procedures, as they involve an extended amount of time under anesthesia and require excellent vascularity; comorbidities such as obesity, poorly controlled insulin-dependent diabetes, COPD, and active smoking are generally disqualifiers. A latissimus flap involves moving an oval section of skin, muscle, fat, and blood vessels from the back, below the shoulder blade, through a tunnel made under the skin of the underarm; it can be used with or without an implant. A TRAM (transverse rectus abdominis muscle) flap takes tissue from the transverse rectus abdominis muscle. A section of fat, muscle, and skin is tunneled under the skin up to the breast, or can be attached with microvascular surgery to blood vessels in the chest wall as a free flap. A "tummy tuck"-type closure is performed at the donor site. TRAM flaps have a significant complication rate including partial to complete loss of the flap, fat necrosis, and weakening of the abdominal wall resulting in hernias or back pain. Morbidity can also be significant and donor site asymmetry can be a distressing problem. A variation of the TRAM flap is the DIEP (deep inferior epigastric artery perforator) flap, which has fewer long-term complications such as hernia and muscle weakness, and has gained in popularity in recent years. Variations of these surgical procedures are common and the field is rapidly advancing with newer, less invasive, and innovative techniques.

SURGICAL COMPLICATIONS

The risks of any surgical procedure include risks related to anesthesia, as well as infection, bleeding, scarring, pain, inadvertent injury to normal structures, venous thromboembolism, and other complications. A complication unique to breast surgery that is greatly feared by patients is lymphedema. The risk of lymphedema following ALND is in the range of 20% and is as high as 40% in patients who have had both ALND and regional lymph node radiation. While the risk for patients who have had SLNB alone is smaller, it is in the 5% range. Patients who are obese are at increased risk.

Lymphedema is a very challenging problem to manage. All women who have surgery for breast cancer should be educated about this risk. The onset may be insidious, and symptoms typically include a sensation of tightness, heaviness, or swelling in the ipsilateral limb, usually occurring within 2 years of treatment. Early identification is important because initiation of treatment can slow progression to a higher stage. Bioimpedance spectroscopy (BIS) is currently being used to detect lymphedema early, when treatment is most effective. This technology is used in clinical assessment of symptoms associated with unilateral lymphedema. Specifically, the technology measures resistance to electrical current while comparing fluid compartments between the affected and the nonsurgical side.

In patients who have lymphedema, treatment consists of a multimodality regimen that includes general measures for care, physiotherapy (e.g., simple lymphatic drainage, manual lymphatic drainage, complete decongestive therapy), and compression therapy (compression bandaging, compression garments, intermittent pneumatic compression), the type and the intensity of which depend upon the clinical stage. Women

with lymphedema and those who have undergone ALND are advised to avoid any injuries or infection in the surgical arm. Injections, vaccinations, venipuncture, intravenous (IV) lines, and blood pressure readings are best administered, accessed, and/or obtained from the unaffected arm when possible. There is evidence to support these patients avoiding saunas and steam rooms. Many other recommendations are made to prevent lymphedema, including (a) using electric razors for axillary hair removal; (b) avoiding manicures; (c) wearing gloves during gardening or contact with chemicals; (d) avoidance of constrictive clothing or jewelry; and (e) wearing a compression sleeve on airplanes; while some of these recommendations are "common sense," they may have very little actual scientific evidence to support them.

RADIATION THERAPY

Radiation is almost always advised after lumpectomy for invasive breast cancer to reduce the risk of recurrence in the remaining breast tissue, and it is usually advised after lumpectomy for DCIS (EBCTCG, 2011). Radiation therapy after mastectomy is sometimes indicated to reduce the risk of recurrence in the chest wall or axilla. Postmastectomy radiation therapy to the chest and regional nodes is indicated if the invasive tumor is larger than 5 cm, involves the skin or chest muscle, or involves more than three axillary lymph nodes; if there are positive margins with high-risk features; and in all cases of inflammatory breast cancer.

Whole breast radiation therapy (WBRT) is usually administered as a standard total dose, which is administered on a fractionated or hypofractionated schedule, 5 days a week, for 3 to 5 weeks and which may or may not include a "boost" to the tumor bed. CT planning and small tattoos guide the angle of the beam to help minimize injury to the heart, lungs, and other normal tissues. Fatigue and skin irritation (sometimes severe) are the most troubling side effects during treatment. The breast skin may become hyperpigmented, may thicken or become edematous or fibrous, and may shrink or tighten following completion of therapy. These changes usually become less pronounced with time.

Radiation may also be delivered to the lumpectomy site by a technique known as accelerated partial breast irradiation (APBI). Options for the delivery of APBI include brachytherapy, intraoperative radiation therapy, or external beam radiation. APBI offers a shorter course of treatment than WBRT (e.g., 5 days versus several weeks) and may have similar oncologic outcomes, particularly among those with low-risk disease. Trials have yielded differing results regarding acute and late toxicities for APBI versus WBRT, although cosmesis seems to be more consistently better with WBRT. Vicini et al. (2019) found that APBI did not meet the criteria for equivalence to whole-breast irradiation in controlling ipsilateral breast-tumor recurrence (IBTR) for breast-conserving therapy. For patients with early-stage breast cancer, findings supported whole-breast irradiation following lumpectomy; however, with an absolute difference of less than 1% in the 10-year cumulative incidence of IBTR, APBI might be an acceptable alternative for some women. Therefore, properly selected patients may be potential candidates for APBI; however the results of the NSABP-B39 and RAPID trials will better inform this issue.

CHEMOTHERAPY

The decision to recommend chemotherapy for a given breast cancer patient depends on many factors including the size of the tumor, biological markers, lymph node status, and increasingly, tumor genetics. Chemotherapy is not indicated for DCIS. Patients with invasive cancer determined to be at significant risk for cancer recurrence are usually treated, including all patients with ER$^-$ and HER2$^+$ tumors, and premenopausal patients with node-positive disease. In patients with ER$^+$, HER2$^-$ tumors that are demonstrated to be node-negative, the primary tool to determine whether a patient will benefit from adjuvant chemotherapy is a multigene diagnostic test, such as Oncotype or MammaPrint, which will determine the recurrence risk by examining the genetic profile of the patient's particular tumor (Harris, 2014).

Chemotherapy is prescribed by a medical oncologist. Most cytotoxic chemotherapy agents work by interfering with cells that are rapidly dividing (hair follicles, bone marrow, intestinal tract cells) and can result in hair loss, nausea, mouth sores, changes in taste and/or smell, and gastrointestinal disturbances. Premature menopause can also result. Agents are often used in combination or can be used alone. Herceptin may be administered in combination with chemotherapy for HER2$^+$ disease.

Dosages and regimens of chemotherapy, known as protocols, vary based on tumor profiles, tumor response, and patient comorbidities. There are many chemotherapeutic agents that can be used in early, advanced, recurrent, or metastatic disease. Chemotherapy has historically been most often used in the adjuvant setting, after surgery, but is increasingly being given as neoadjuvant therapy, prior to surgery. Chemotherapy drugs are given intravenously, often via a port device, which is removed when treatment is completed; in some cases, it is given orally.

Chemotherapy is almost always a frightening prospect and a challenging experience for patients. The risk of serious adverse effects is not small, and they include infection, fever, neutropenia, thrombocytopenia, anemia, constitutional symptoms, dehydration, electrolyte disorders, nausea, emesis, diarrhea, deep vein thrombosis (DVT), and pulmonary embolus (PE), as well as toxicities peculiar to the individual agents. Breast cancer is the most common indication for chemotherapy among women in the United States, and chemotherapy accounts for the largest number of serious adverse events among treatment options. Patients will be better prepared to make informed treatment decisions if counseled about the possible risks associated with each type of recommended chemotherapy. The benefits and risks of any therapy should be fully disclosed to all breast cancer patients by a medical oncologist using the best information available to allow informed decision-making.

HORMONAL THERAPY

Hormonal therapy is often recommended alone or in addition to chemotherapy in HR$^+$ invasive breast cancer, and in cases of ER$^+$ DCIS. There are two classes of hormonal therapy: (1) the selected estrogen receptor modulators (SERMs), which include tamoxifen, and (2) the aromatase inhibitors (AIs). Tamoxifen is the most commonly prescribed antihormonal agent and works by binding to breast cell receptors to block the uptake of estrogen. The primary side effects of tamoxifen are hot flashes that mimic menopause; toxicities include an increased risk of venous thromboembolism and an increased risk of endometrial cancer. The AIs include letrozole, exemestane, and anastrozole and work by disrupting the production of aromatase, which is needed to synthesize estrogen in postmenopausal women. Their primary toxicity is accelerated osteoporosis, so bone health must be monitored closely in these patients. Tamoxifen, an AI, or a sequential combination is generally used for treatment for a minimum of 5 years. AIs are not effective in pre- or perimenopausal women whose ovaries still produce estrogen, whereas tamoxifen can be used in both pre- and postmenopausal patients.

BIOLOGICAL THERAPY

Trastuzumab (Herceptin) is a monoclonal antibody that targets the HER2 protein that is overexpressed in HER2$^+$ breast cancer. Nearly all patients with HER2$^+$ tumors will be offered adjuvant (or neoadjuvant) systemic therapy with HER2$^+$-directed therapy in combination with chemotherapy. Patients receiving trastuzumab have an increased risk for cardiac toxicity (congestive heart failure or declines in left ventricle function). All patients receiving adjuvant trastuzumab should undergo routine monitoring of their left ventricular ejection fraction over the course of their treatment. Other newer biological agents are being used and tested in clinical trials: three other HER2-targeted agents have been developed for treatment of HER2-overexpressing breast cancer: (1) lapatinib; (2) ado-trastuzumab emtansine (T-DM1), an antibody-drug conjugate composed of trastuzumab, a thioether linker, and a derivative of the antimitotic agent, maytansine; and (3) pertuzumab.

CLINICAL TRIALS

Many clinical trials are available for patients undergoing breast cancer treatment. The purpose of a clinical trial is to identify a new treatment technique or drug that will be better at treating the cancer than standard therapy. Participants will never receive any treatment in a clinical trial that is less than standard of care. All the recent advances in radiation techniques, biological therapy, chemotherapy, and antihormonal therapy, and in tumor genetic profiling, have come to fruition as a result of patient participation in clinical trials. A comprehensive searchable list of open clinical trials is available at www.cancer.gov/clinicaltrials.

ALTERNATIVE TREATMENTS

Alternative therapies in treating breast cancer have not been well studied. Their effectiveness is unknown and most cancer specialists do not recommend them as a sole treatment option. Complementary and integrative medicine consist of vitamins, herbs, special diets, and spiritual healing. Until further research is available, complementary and integrative therapy should only be recommended in addition to conventional therapy and under the direction of an oncologist.

Breast Cancer Patient Support and Education

Patients going through breast cancer diagnosis and treatment are frequently apprehensive, frightened, and confused. Excellent communication between the patient, oncologist, surgeon, and other members of the multidisciplinary team can be very helpful. There are many excellent breast cancer websites, literature, and peer-to-peer patient support networks available to assist patients in decision-making. Women should be encouraged to access and use these resources for themselves and for family members.

SUPPORT DURING TREATMENT

Women will be counseled to complete any dental work before chemotherapy, as they are more prone to infection during treatment. Nausea is treated preventively with medication. Fatigue is a common problem that may not readily resolve, leading to patient frustration and depression. Vomiting, diarrhea, mouth ulcers, and throat soreness can be troublesome but are usually controllable with medication. Hair loss is very common and can be emotionally and physically painful. Women describe the feeling of hair coming out as uncomfortable and are advised to have it cut short as soon as it starts to fall out to lessen the discomfort. Wigs and specially made head coverings in many styles are available.

During chemotherapy bone marrow suppression occurs and avoidance of infections is extremely important. Women should be counseled to stay out of large crowds, wash their hands often, practice careful oral hygiene, get plenty of rest, and keep any cuts or scratches clean. Exposure to sexually transmitted infections should be minimized. Eating a healthy diet is important to minimize weight gain that often occurs during chemotherapy; however, some dietary restrictions may be advised by the oncologist, such as avoiding soft cheeses, deli meats, and salad bars because these foods and sites may have bacteria that can impact an immunocompromised patient. Chemotherapy patients can gain 5 to 15 lb and possibly more with longer treatment and with prednisone therapy. The reasons for creeping weight gain and stalled weight loss during cancer treatment are unknown, but may be related to the sudden onset of menopause, changes in metabolism, less physical activity during recovery due to fatigue, snacks to lessen nausea, and increased appetite from steroids. Muscle mass can also decrease during chemotherapy, leading to fat increases.

Patients should be encouraged to fend off unwanted pounds with careful diet and exercise including careful weight training with specialized instruction for cancer patients and aerobic exercise as tolerated. Sessions with a registered dietitian and physical trainer can be very helpful.

A premenopausal woman's menstrual periods may stop during chemotherapy and may not restart, leading to premature menopause. However, pregnancy may still occur, even after long periods of amenorrhea, and birth control should be discussed with women during this time. Nonhormonal methods of contraception and control of menopausal symptoms (e.g., vasomotor symptoms) should be offered in this population.

In young women who may want to start or add to their family after treatment, protection of ovarian function with medication or egg harvesting should be discussed prior to initiation of chemotherapy. Referral to a reproductive endocrinologist is important to review all reproductive options. Pregnancy after breast cancer should be a decision made by the patient and her oncologist and obstetrician and should be considered high risk (Ruddy & Ginsburg, 2014).

Follow-Up Care

EMOTIONAL IMPACT

Four times more women die of heart disease than from breast cancer in the United States, but women tend to fear the risk of breast cancer much more. Survivors of breast cancer go on to live healthy and productive lives, but the trauma of the diagnosis and the difficulty of some treatment combinations can result in mild to severe psychological distress and often lasting physical effects. Psychosocial concerns of survivors include fear of recurrence, fatigue, trouble sleeping, pain, body image disruption, sexual dysfunction, intrusive thoughts about illness and persistent anxiety, feelings of vulnerability, and concerns about mortality. The experience of breast cancer has several phases, each with its own issues. Diagnosis, treatment, completing treatment, reentry, survivorship, recurrence, and palliation for advanced cancer all need to be dealt with along with socioeconomic factors, cultural issues, availability of support, access to care, and the presence of other illnesses or life crises (Hewitt et al., 2004).

Patients who have survived cancer have gone through difficult and challenging times and may struggle with depression, physical changes, changes in their sexual relationship, changes in libido, and fear of recurrence, and often require time, empathy, and reassurance. Posttraumatic stress disorder (PTSD)-like syndromes are not unusual. It is important to assess coping mechanisms, psychological adjustment to cancer, and perceived family support, and to refer for psychological assessment and counseling as appropriate. Patient participation in peer support groups is often of benefit. Providers may benefit from reading patient narratives to more fully understand the challenge of cancer (Trillin, 1981).

Breast cancer survivors have a higher risk of developing a second breast cancer, so regular follow-up and annual mammograms are very important. Some survivors experience gaps in care, which may be due to fear of recurrence and dread of repeated treatment (Snyder et al., 2009). Providers caring for breast cancer survivors need to be aware of previous treatments to design posttreatment care plans while coordinating with the multidisciplinary oncology team. Many formal survivorship programs are being designed and implemented to address surveillance and the wide range of needs and issues that survivors face.

Women who have completed treatment for early breast cancer may be discharged from an oncologist's care, but should have continued regular follow-up care at least annually that should include history, physical examination including a CBE, review of systems (recurrence can often show up subtly, such as nagging back or abdominal pain), mammograms, and any other testing based on an oncologist's or survivor clinic's recommendations.

RECURRENT BREAST CANCER

Local recurrence (in the breast or chest wall) or regional recurrence (in the lymphatics) of breast cancer is a distressing event for cancer survivors, but is often salvageable with additional treatment. In both cases, metastatic disease needs to be ruled out as a first step, as synchronous metastases will be found in up to 15% of patients treated with BCT and a third of patients treated with mastectomy. In the case of an in-breast recurrence after BCT, mastectomy is indicated because radiation cannot be performed again. An isolated chest wall recurrence after mastectomy requires wide local excision followed by radiation; because of the high risk of systemic failure, chemotherapy may be advised as well. Isolated axillary lymphatic recurrence is treated with ALND followed by radiation, also typically with adjuvant systemic therapy.

Distant recurrence of breast cancer in the body, metastatic disease, is traumatic and emotionally challenging for all survivors as it is not curable. However, newer therapies have led to better treatment responses and control of disease, and treatment options can have a positive effect on both duration and quality of life for these patients. Many clinical trials are available for women who have progressive disease on standard therapy, using new drugs, drug combinations, and innovative therapies.

SURVIVORSHIP

In the United States in 2021, there were more than 280,000 new cases of invasive breast cancer diagnosed in women, and an additional 49,000 cases of DCIS diagnosed in women. From 2008 to 2017, invasive female breast cancer incidence rates increased by about 0.5% per year. Since its peak in 1989, the female breast cancer death rate had declined by 41% in 2018 because of earlier detection (through screening as well as increased awareness of symptoms) and improved treatment. Although more than 43,000 women in the United States died of breast cancer in 2021, there are more women living with and surviving breast cancer today than ever before. The 5- and 10-year relative survival rates for women with invasive breast cancer are 91% and 85%, respectively. Although survival has improved over time, large inequalities remain, especially for Black women. For example, the survival rate is 9% to 10% lower (in absolute terms) for Black women than for White women overall and for regional- and distant-stage disease (ACS, 2023). As healthcare providers, it is essential to educate women about risks, screening, prevention, and new therapies available to continue to advance survivorship and continue the favorable trends that are being realized in breast cancer care.

REFERENCES

References for this chapter are online and available at https://connect.springerpub.com/content/book/978-0-8261-6722-4/part/part03/chapter/ch24

CHAPTER 25

Caring for the Transgender and Gender Nonbinary Patient*†‡

NATHAN LEVITT

Learning about the care of transgender and gender nonbinary (TGNB) populations is essential to eliminate healthcare disparities, yet there is very limited education and training on the healthcare needs of this population within health professional education. Transgender refers to a person whose internal sense of their gender (gender identity) does not correspond to their sex assigned at birth. Transgender woman refers to someone assigned male at birth who identifies as a woman. Transgender man refers to someone assigned female at birth who identifies as a man. Nonbinary refers to someone whose gender identity falls outside of what is typically labeled woman or man. See Table 25.1 for a glossary of definitions. Providing gender-affirming care to this population falls under the scope of a primary care provider and any practitioner providing sexual and reproductive healthcare (Morenz et al., 2020). In order to provide sensitive and clinically informed care, it is important for healthcare providers to understand the terminology, barriers to care, and factors that affect long-term health maintenance.

BARRIERS TO HEALTHCARE

Social determinants of health are essential to understand and integrate into care of TGNB populations and all communities that healthcare providers work with. Housing, employment, safety, wellness, and access to competent informed care greatly affect the health of TGNB communities (Seelman et al., 2017). In addition to gender-affirming medical transition care, TGNB communities have similar needs to other patients such as access to routine primary care. However, many in the TGNB community are met with discriminatory, insensitive, and uninformed care and may avoid both regular healthcare maintenance screenings and urgent care due to previous negative experiences (James et al., 2016). According to the 2015 U.S. Transgender Survey, a third of respondents who had seen a healthcare provider in the past year reported having at least one negative experience related to their gender identity within a healthcare setting (James et al., 2016). These negative experiences included having to teach the provider about transgender care, being refused treatment, being verbally harassed, or being physically or sexually assaulted (James et al., 2016). The National Transgender Discrimination Survey identified issues with denial of healthcare; provider ignorance of transgender health needs in preventive medicine, routine healthcare, and emergency care; and transgender-related services in 2011 and again in 2016 (Grant et al., 2011; James et al., 2016). There are additional barriers to care for certain segments of the TGNB community such as people of color, disabled people, low-income persons, and immigrant populations (James et al., 2016).

In 2011, the Institute of Medicine (IOM) addressed health needs of transgender persons in their document *The Health of Lesbian, Gay, Bisexual, and Transgender People: Building a Foundation for Better Understanding* describing stigma, discrimination, and lack of provider knowledge and training as barriers to transgender healthcare leading to significant health disparities (IOM, 2011). Although many barriers to care have been identified, transgender healthcare is currently

---

*This chapter is a revision of the chapter that appeared in the second edition of this textbook, authored by Kathryn Tierney and Caroline Dorsen, and we thank them for their original contribution.

†**Note on language:** The author acknowledges the limitations of the language used for this textbook, and the credentialing body, of *women's health nurse practitioner*. The term *women* often implies only cisgender women (people who were assigned female at birth and identify as female) and is not inclusive of vulnerable communities who need these services such as transgender and gender nonbinary (TGNB) people. We recommend using inclusive language that focuses on the care that is provided and the body parts being cared for, rather than gendered language that is not clinically specific or transgender sensitive. To be gender affirming and inclusive of all sexual and reproductive care is to be reflective of the bodies and identities of those who need these medically necessary services and to reduce health disparities.

‡**Note on WPATH:** The World Professional Association for Transgender Health Standards of Care (WPATH SOC) was not yet published at the time this chapter was written. It is now available at: https://www.wpath.org/publications/soc.

TABLE 25.1 Glossary of Terms Relevant to Transgender and Gender Nonbinary Identities

TERM	DEFINITION
Cisgender (adjective)	A person whose gender identity is consistent in a traditional sense with their sex assigned at birth; for example, a cisgender woman is a person assigned female sex at birth whose gender identity is woman/female.
Gender affirmation (noun)	The process of making social, legal, and/or medical changes to recognize, accept, and express one's gender identity. Although this process is sometimes referred to as transition, the term *gender affirmation* is recommended.
Gender dysphoria (noun)	Distress experienced by some people whose gender identity does not correspond with their sex assigned at birth.
Gender expression (noun)	The way a person communicates their gender to the world through mannerisms, clothing, speech, behavior, etc. Gender expression varies depending on culture, context, and historical period.
Gender identity (noun)	A person's inner sense of being a girl/woman/female, boy/man/male, something else, or having no gender.
Gender nonbinary (adjective)	Describes a person whose gender identity falls outside the two-gender binary structure of girl/woman and boy/man.
Intersex (adjective)	Describes a group of congenital conditions in which the reproductive organs, genitals, and/or other sexual anatomy do not develop according to traditional expectations for females or males. The medical community sometimes uses the term "differences (or disorders) of sex development" to describe intersex conditions.
Sex assigned at birth (noun)	The sex (male or female) assigned to an infant, most often based on the infant's anatomic and other biological characteristics.
Sexual orientation (noun)	How a person characterizes their emotional and sexual attraction to others.
Transgender (adjective)	Describes a person whose gender identity and sex assigned at birth do not correspond based on societal expectations.
Trans man/transgender man (noun)	A transgender person whose gender identity is boy/man/male may use these terms to describe themselves. Some will use the term *man*.
Trans woman/transgender woman (noun)	A transgender person whose gender identity is girl/woman/female may use these terms to describe themselves. Some will use the term *woman*.

Source: Adapted from Harris, M. S., Goodrum, B. A., & Krempasky, C. N. (2022). An introduction to gender-affirming hormone therapy for transgender and gender-nonbinary patients. Nurse Practitioner, 47(3), 18–28. https://doi.org/10.1097/01.NPR.0000819612.24729.c7; National LGBTQIA+ Health Education Center. (2020). LGBTQIA+ glossary of terms for health care teams. https://www.lgbtqiahealtheducation.org/publication/lgbtqia-glossary-of-terms-for-health-care-teams

not required in medical provider education (van Heesewijk et al., 2022). Within nurse practitioner (NP) education there is also no curriculum requirement to specifically include transgender health, although, like medical school education, transgender issues are sometimes included under diversity in general (Kellet & Fitton, 2017). Most general nursing education programs have not included transgender health in their curriculum, and some spend an average of 2 hours on the topic (Kellet & Fitton, 2017). Lack of knowledge within healthcare professional schools, especially on populations experiencing health disparities, has been known to produce negative health outcomes (IOM, 2011). Paradiso and Lally (2018) looked at NP knowledge, attitudes, and beliefs when caring for transgender people, and their study revealed NPs' knowledge gaps, lack of education, and lack of availability of resources related to transgender health, and stressed the importance of integrating transgender health into NP curriculum to improve healthcare.

Unger (2014) reported that only 36% of 141 surveyed obstetrics and gynecology providers were comfortable with caring for transgender women clients, and 29% were comfortable with caring for transgender men clients. About 59% did

not know the recommendations regarding cancer screening for this population (Unger, 2014). Overall, 80% of providers sampled had no transgender-specific healthcare training in residency regardless of how long they had been in practice (Unger, 2014). Only 33% of providers reported feeling comfortable with their skills in providing care for transgender men (Unger, 2014); 88% of providers were willing to perform routine Pap screening, felt comfortable performing a gynecologic examination for transgender men, and recognized that these examinations would not differ from those for cisgender women (Unger, 2014).

In March 2021, the American College of Obstetricians and Gynecologists (ACOG) released guidance on healthcare for transgender and gender diverse individuals providing clinical guidance for caring for TGNB patients and information to assist in offering inclusive patient care. In it, they recognized the lack of awareness, knowledge, and sensitivity as well as bias from healthcare professionals, which leads to "inadequate access to, underuse of, and inequities within the health care system for transgender patients (ACOG, 2021, p. e76)" and recommended in order to address the significant health care disparities of transgender individuals and to improve their access to care, obstetrician gynecologists (OB/GYNs) should prepare to provide routine treatment and screening, use inclusive language, and consult with transgender health experts (ACOG, 2021).

Any gendered procedure, screening, or other form of clinical care can be traumatic for a TGNB patient. For example, a prostate or cervical cancer screening or a breast exam, while clinically necessary, can be incredibly distressing for TGNB patients. In addition, the community may face insurance denials for gender-specific care, such as a transgender male who is listed as male on his health insurance receiving a denial for cervical cancer screening due to gender marker "mismatch." Some ways to improve comfort and provide advocacy is to ask all clients what words they use to describe their body parts, using less gendered words (Table 25.2), and collaborating with an insurance navigator or patient advocate. Healthcare provider education can remove barriers for TGNB individuals. Lelutiu-Weinberger et al. (2016) found improvement in licensed and unlicensed medical staffs' knowledge and attitudes and a more welcoming clinic physical environment for transgender persons after training.

GENDER INCONGRUENCE AND GENDER DYSPHORIA

The *Diagnostic and Statistical Manual of Mental Disorders* (5th ed.; *DSM-5*) diagnostic criteria for gender dysphoria (or gender identity disorder, as it appears in *International Statistical Classification of Diseases and Related Health Problems* [10th ed.; *ICD-10; World Health Organization (WHO), 2016]*) are used to assess patients seeking gender-affirming hormone therapy (GAHT) and gender-affirming surgery (American Psychiatric Association [APA], 2013). Gender dysphoria describes the "clinically significant distress or

TABLE 25.2 Less Gendered Language Guide	
USE (LESS GENDERED LANGUAGE)[a]	**INSTEAD OF (GENDERED LANGUAGE)**
People who menstruate, people who are pregnant	Female, women; pregnant women
People who produce sperm	Male, men
Not trans, nontrans, cisgender	Biologically male/female
Assigned male at birth	Biologically male
Assigned female at birth	Biologically female
Sexual or genital (gen) health	Women's/gynecologic healthcare
External genitals, external pelvic area	Vulva, clitoris
Outer parts	Penis, testicles
Genital opening, frontal opening, internal canal	Vagina
Outer folds	Labia, lips
Internal reproductive organs	Female reproductive organs
Internal organs	Uterus, ovaries
Internal gland	Prostate
Chest	Breasts[b]
Chestfeeding or breastfeeding[b]	Breastfeeding
Absorbent product	Pad/tampon
Internal condom	Female condom
Uterine bleeding	Period/menstruation
Parent or gestational parent	Mother
Hypothalamic pituitary gonadal–ovarian axis	Female gonadal steroid axis
Hypothalamic pituitary gonadal–testicular axis	Male gonadal steroid axis

[a]The terms in this column are offered as suggestions, but it is recommended to ask clients which words they use for their own body parts and experiences.
[b]Transfeminine persons may prefer breasts.

impairment that may arise from the incongruence between a person's gender identity and their sex assigned at birth" (APA, 2013). For many in the community, the discomfort or distress associated with the incongruence between gender identity and sex assigned at birth is often attributed to societal discrimination and ignorance that lead to depression and anxiety, rather than a disorder.

As not all TGNB people experience gender dysphoria, diagnostic criteria for "Gender Incongruence of Adolescence and Adulthood" from WHO's *International Statistical Classification of Diseases and Related Health Problems*, version 11 (*ICD-11*)—which is not yet in use in the United States—defines it as "a marked and persistent incongruence" between the patient's gender identity and sex assigned at birth, which may lead the patient to seek medical and/or surgical interventions to better align their body with their gender identity ([WHO, 2019]. In the interim before *ICD-11* is adopted, some providers may continue to use the diagnosis of "gender dysphoria," while others may use "endocrine disorder, unspecified." It is important to discuss coding with patients when appropriate as codes selected may affect insurance coverage.

MEDICAL TRANSITION

There are many ways to transition including changing name, pronoun, and gender expression (clothes, mannerisms, etc.). Healthcare professionals have a responsibility to help all clients live their authentic lives in a safe, affirming way. Not all TGNB people will be able to afford, or will have desire for, medical transition. It is a very personal decision with many factors involved. *Medical transition* is a term used to refer to using hormones and/or surgery to change the physical body to more closely align with gender identity. The terms *gender-affirming hormone therapy* and *gender-affirming surgery* are often used by both medical professionals and those in the TGNB community.

The role of the NP is to determine the healthcare needs regardless of where the person is in their transition process. For TGNB people on the masculine spectrum, for example, depending on whether they have had any gender-affirming surgery or not, this may mean determining the need for pelvic exams and cervical cancer screenings, as well as mammograms. For TGNB people on the feminine spectrum, depending on whether they have had any gender-affirming surgery, this may involve evaluation of the neovagina, as well as screening and treatment of breast tissue. It is also essential that the NP manage the patient's other primary care screenings such as chronic disease and cancer screenings that may or may not be related to the transition process. The World Professional Association for Transgender Health (WPATH) and University of California San Francisco (UCSF) Center of Excellence for Transgender Health (Deutsch, 2016) are two institutions that help to provide the standards of care for this population.

GAHT can involve what is called puberty blockers or gonadotropin releasing hormone (GnRH) agonists for TGNB adolescents and/or exogenous hormones postpuberty to create what is often termed "masculine" and "feminine" secondary characteristics. While this chapter will not go into the specifics of GnRH agonists for TGNB adolescents, there

are many guidelines and resources on the subject (Deutsch, 2016). As with all patients, the goals of medical transition are unique to each person. Some may identify more on the binary (male or female), and some may identify as nonbinary (outside the male and female binary) and have different needs for transition. Prescribing and managing gender-affirming hormones fall within the scope of any primary care provider and there are many opportunities for training, international protocols, guides to starting a transgender health program, and evidence-based practice (Morenz et al., 2020).

The healthcare provider's role is to provide education, assess readiness and expectations, and ensure support, follow-up visits, and medical clearance. What is utilized in healthcare settings is informed consent for all patients over 18 (those under 18 would need parental/guardian consent, which can be challenging when parents/guardians are not accepting). This helps break down historical barriers for the communities and allows for more access to lifesaving medications. As with all patients, the healthcare provider's role is to counsel on risks and benefits and assess for capacity to make informed decisions. For many, finding a TGNB-sensitive medical provider is a huge undertaking and may involve many traumatic, discriminatory experiences. For this reason, it is incredibly important for healthcare providers to educate themselves on sensitive language and informed clinical care.

MASCULINIZING GENDER-AFFIRMING HORMONE THERAPY

Masculinizing GAHT involves the use of testosterone to create masculine secondary sex characteristics in people assigned female at birth. Testosterone can be administered as an intramuscular or subcutaneous injection, topical gel or patch, or implantable pellet. Providers should review specific changes resulting from masculinizing GAHT and the time course of these changes with patients considering this therapy (Table 25.3;) Harris et al., 2022. It is important to counsel patients on what changes are reversible (such as increased muscle mass and cessation of menses) and what changes are permanent (such as deepening of the voice, clitoral enlargement, facial and body hair growth, and scalp hair loss; (Hembree et al., 2017). Most patients achieve amenorrhea on masculinizing hormone therapy within 6 months of testosterone initiation; however, breakthrough bleeding is common. There are several guidelines for evaluation and management of breakthrough bleeding (Grimstad et al., 2021). Hysterectomy and/or oophorectomy is not indicated in the absence of other risk factors, although some patients may desire this surgery for gender affirmation (Harris et al., 2017).

Absolute contraindications to masculinizing GAHT include active hormone-sensitive cancer, pregnancy, and polycythemia with a hematocrit of 54% or higher (Harris et al., 2020). Providers can refer to the UCFS *Guidelines for the Primary and Gender-Affirming Care of Transgender and Gender Nonbinary People* (UCSF *Guidelines*) for masculinizing GAHT dosing recommendations, lab monitoring, and long-term management (Deutsch, 2016).

TABLE 25.3 Expected Changes and Time Course of Masculinizing Gender–Affirming Hormone Therapy[a]

MASCULINIZING EFFECTS IN TRANSGENDER MALES[b]		
EFFECT	ONSET	MAXIMUM
Skin oiliness/acne	1–6 months	1–2 years
Facial/body hair growth	6–12 months	4–5 years
Scalp hair loss	6–12 months	–[c]
Increased muscle mass/strength	6–12 months	2–5 years
Fat redistribution	1–6 months	2–5 years
Cessation of menses	1–6 months	–[d]
Clitoral enlargement	1–6 months	1–2 years
Vaginal atrophy	1–6 months	1–2 years
Deepening of voice	6–12 months	1–2 years

[a]Estimates represent clinical observations: Toorians et al. (2003), Asscheman et al. (1988), Gooren et al. (1985), and Wierckx et al. (2014).
[b]The authors note that not all people using masculinizing gender-affirming hormone therapy will necessarily identify as transgender males.
[c]*Prevention and treatment as recommended for persons assigned male at birth.*
[d]*Menorrhagia requires diagnosis and treatment by a gynecologist.*
Source: *Adapted from Harris, M. S., Goodrum, B. A., & Krempasky, C. N. (2022). An introduction to gender-affirming hormone therapy for transgender and gender-nonbinary patients.* Nurse Practitioner, *47(3), 18–28. https://doi.org/10.1097/01.NPR.0000819612.24729.c7*

FEMINIZING GENDER–AFFIRMING HORMONE THERAPY

Feminizing GAHT consists of the use of any combination of estradiol, antiandrogens, and progesterone to create feminine secondary sex characteristics and to suppress masculine secondary sex characteristics in people assigned male at birth (Harris et al., 2022). Expected changes can include softening of skin, breast growth, and decrease sperm production. Providers should review expected changes resulting from feminizing GAHT and the time course of these changes with patients considering this therapy (Table 25.4).

Estradiol may be administered via oral or sublingual tablets, transdermal patches, and intramuscular injection. Providers can refer to the UCFS *Guidelines* for feminizing GAHT dosing recommendations, lab monitoring, and long-term management (Deutsch, 2016). Consult the UCSF *Guidelines* for further discussion and detailed algorithms on estradiol use in patients with significant venous thromboembolic event (VTE) risk factors and/or a personal or family history of VTE. The only absolute medical contraindication to estradiol use is an active estrogen-sensitive cancer, which would warrant a consultation with the patient's oncologist. In addition to estradiol, antiandrogens such as spironolactone or finasteride, which can block testosterone, may be used. Recommended dose ranges for spironolactone, finasteride, and dutasteride as well as information on the role of progesterone are available in the UCSF *Guidelines*. Progesterone may be helpful in improving breast tissue growth and shape and improvement in mood and is unlikely to have significant negative side effects (Deutsch, 2016).

GENERAL HEALTHCARE MAINTENANCE

For a more in-depth discussion of healthcare maintenance including cardiovascular risks, diabetes, bone health, sexual health, mental health, and aging see Fenway Health's *Medical Care of Trans and Gender Diverse Adults* (Thompson et al., 2021) as well as the UCSF *Guidelines*. In addition, see Table 25.5 for a guide on routine screening from prepuberty to adulthood. For another helpful long-term preventive care guide, see Sherbourne Health *Guidelines for Gender-Affirming Primary Care With Trans and Non-binary Patients* free online interactive tool and included tables whereby the clinician can click on the organ and access TGNB tailored screening guides specific to that part (www.rainbowhealthontario.ca/product/4th-edition-sherbournes-guidelines-for-gender-affirming-primary-care-with-trans-and-non-binary-patients).

Like many communities experiencing discrimination, transgender communities may have higher rates of tobacco, alcohol, and drug use due to the stress and violence experienced (Santos et al., 2014). It is important to provide TGNB-sensitive counseling and referrals. TGNB communities can also have an increased risk of sexually transmitted infections (STIs) potentially due to engagement in survival sex work, lack of access to safe sex methods including preexposure prophylaxis (PrEP) for HIV, and lack of access to affirming and TGNB-informed healthcare (Erickson-Schroth, 2022). Sexual health history questions need to be specific and focused. Asking patients if they have sex with men, women, or both does not specify whether the person is cisgender or TGNB and does not provide the information that is needed. Someone's gender does not indicate what body parts they have or how they use them. Krempasky et al. (2020) suggest sexual history questions that

TABLE 25.4 Expected Changes and Time Course of Feminizing Gender-Affirming Hormone Therapy[a]

FEMINIZING EFFECTS IN TRANSGENDER FEMALES[b]

EFFECT	ONSET	MAXIMUM
Redistribution of body fat	3–6 months	2–3 years
Decrease in muscle mass and strength	3–6 months	1–2 years
Softening of skin/decreased oiliness	3–6 months	Unknown
Decreased sexual desire	1–3 months	3–6 months
Decreased spontaneous erections	1–3 months	3–6 months
Male sexual dysfunction	Variable	Variable
Breast growth	3–6 months	2–3 years
Decreased testicular volume	3–6 months	2–3 years
Decreased sperm production	Unknown	>3 years
Decreased terminal hair growth	6–12 months	>3 years[c]
Scalp hair	Variable	–[d]
Voice changes	None	–[e]

[a]Estimates represent clinical observations: Toorians et al. (2003), Asscheman et al. (1988), and Gooren et al. (1985).
[b]The authors note that not all people using feminizing gender-affirming hormone therapy will necessarily identify as transgender females.
[c]Complete removal of male sexual hair requires electrolysis or laser treatment or both.
[d]Familial scalp hair loss may occur if estrogens are stopped.
[e]Treatment by speech pathologists for voice training is most effective.
Source: Adapted from Harris, M. S., Goodrum, B. A., & Krempasky, C. N. (2022). An introduction to gender-affirming hormone therapy for transgender and gender-nonbinary patients. Nurse Practitioner, 47(3), 18–28. https://doi.org/10.1097/01.NPR.0000819612.24729.c7

TABLE 25.5 Routine Screening Guide From Prepuberty to Adulthood for Transgender People[a]

	PREPUBERTY	EARLY PUBERTY (SEXUAL MATURITY STAGE 2 OR 3)	LATE PUBERTY (SEXUAL MATURITY STAGE 4 OR 5	ADULTHOOD
General transgender care	Establish rapport and provide nonjudgmental and confidential care.			
	Use patient's chosen name and pronouns as indicated.			
	Determine patient's and caregiver's goals for care.			
	Establish multidisciplinary team based on patient's needs and local resources; clinicians with expertise are preferred.			
	Detailed history: if clinically appropriate, explore the context of the patient's gender experiences, including psychosocial history for evidence of resilience (e.g., connectedness, positive social network) and risk (e.g., victimization, suicidality, isolation).			
	Assess for housing access, food availability, and financial or safety concerns.			
Mental health	Manage any mental health diagnoses or psychotropic medication use.			
	Consider referral for management of complex mental health diagnoses based on patient's needs; refer for comprehensive management of substance use disorder if present.			
	Facilitate relationships with family members or guardians, if allowed by the patient.			
	Gender exploration: an affirmative approach may be preferred to a supportive (or "wait and see") approach to prepubertal gender-diverse youth; care should be individualized with subspecialist support as available.			

(continued)

TABLE 25.5 Routine Screening Guide From Prepuberty to Adulthood for Transgender People[a] (continued)

	PREPUBERTY	EARLY PUBERTY (SEXUAL MATURITY STAGE 2 OR 3)	LATE PUBERTY (SEXUAL MATURITY STAGE 4 OR 5	ADULTHOOD
	Diagnosis of gender dysphoria or incongruence: consider referral to mental health professional with expertise in transgender care and proper use of the *Diagnostic and Statistical Manual of Mental Disorders* (5th ed.; APA, 2013).			
	Counseling and psychotherapy: consider referral to mental health professional with expertise in transgender care (and who is comfortable with lifespan development of transgender youth, if pertinent); encourage healthy exploration of gender identity and expression.			
Puberty suppression		Timely referral to pediatric endocrinologist or other clinician experienced in prescribing and monitoring gonadotropin-releasing hormone analog therapy		
		Prescribe gonadotropin-releasing hormone analogs		
		Surveillance: clinical, laboratory, and psychosocial monitoring; DEXA		
Specific gender affirmation care	Evaluate degree to which gender dysphoria or incongruence is persistent, consistent, and insistent.			
	Social affirmation: monitor for safety of affirmation environment and continued desire for affirmation.			
		Initiate or continue puberty induction; provide hormone therapy surveillance (generally after puberty suppression).		
		Bridge hormone prescriptions if in the process of referring.		
			Initiate or continue gender-affirming hormone therapy.	
			Hormone therapy surveillance: monitor for adverse effects clinically, with laboratory studies, and with DEXA; monitor for desired effects.	
			Gender-affirming surgery or other therapies: consider referral to surgeon experienced in transgender surgical techniques; consider referral for hair removal or vocal therapy.	
Reproductive health		Provide family planning counseling and contraceptives as indicated.		
		Screen for and treat sexually transmitted infection, counsel about safe sex practices, and prescribe pre- or postexposure prophylaxis as indicated for prevention of HIV infection.		
		Offer menstrual suppression (postmenarche only).		
		Consider referral to a reproductive endocrinologist for fertility preservation or artificial reproductive technology		
Preventive care	Cardiovascular disease screening: monitor blood pressure and weight, treat obesity, provide age- and risk-factor based screening for diabetes mellitus and hyperlipidemia, and counsel about tobacco cessation.			
	Cancer screening based on patient's current anatomy			
	Guideline-based bone mineral density screening			
	Age-appropriate and behavior-specific immunizations			
	No shading = Primary care clinicians may manage independently		*Shading = Consider referral, management, or comanagement*	

[a]Recommendations for interventions in this table may not be universally needed or desired and should be explored based on individual preferences; the clinician should tailor the history, physical examination, and subsequent referrals for each visit.
DEXA, dual-energy x-ray absorptiometry.
Source: Adapted from Klein, D. A., Paradise, S. L., & Goodwin, E. T. (2018). Caring for transgender and gender-diverse persons: What clinicians should know. American Family Physician, *98(11), 645–653. https://www.aafp.org/pubs/afp/issues/2018/1201/p645.html*

Box 25.1 Sexual Health Questions

- How do you identify your gender? What gender were you assigned at birth?
- What are your pronouns?
- Have you had any surgeries? (anatomic inventory)
- Do you have sex? (also inclusive of asexual patients)
  - If no: By choice or circumstance? Do you desire to have sex?
- What are the genders and bodies of your sexual partners? (not assuming monogamy)
  - How do you have sex with them?
  - Which body parts do you use?
  - Do you use toys?
- Do you use barriers for sexually transmitted infection prevention?
- Do you use anything for pregnancy prevention? Do you desire pregnancy now or in the future? What are your family building desires?
- Has anyone ever made you have sex when you didn't want to? Has anyone ever hit you or hurt you physically?
- What else about your sexual health and practices should we discuss to help keep you healthy?

Source: Adapted from Krempasky, C., Harris, M., Abern, L., & Grimstad, F. (2020). Contraception across the transmasculine spectrum. American Journal of Obstetrics and Gynecology, *222(2), 134–143. https://doi.org/10.1016/j.ajog.2019.07.043*

are inclusive of all patients, especially transgender communities, such as, "What are the genders and bodies of your sexual partners?" and "Which body parts do you use?" (Box 25.1).

The UCSF *Guidelines* note that evidence from several studies indicate that cardiovascular risk is unchanged among TGNB people using testosterone compared with nontransgender women. For transgender people on the feminine spectrum, studies have found increased morbidity and mortality risks from myocardial infarction and stroke compared with nontransgender men; however, these studies did not adjust for a number of risk factors including tobacco use, obesity, and diabetes (Deutsch, 2016).

The UCSF *Guidelines* indicate that transgender people should begin bone density screening at age 65 (Deutsch 2016). Screening between ages 50 and 64 should be considered for those with established risk factors for osteoporosis (Figure 25.1). Transgender people (regardless of sex assigned at birth) who have undergone gonadectomy and have a history of at least 5 years without hormone replacement should also be considered for bone density testing, regardless of age (Deutsch, 2016).

CANCER SCREENING

Cancer screening should follow anatomic screening recommendations rather than the gender of the patient. Focusing on nongendered body parts versus "women's" or "men's" cancer is incredibly important for informed care. It is important for healthcare providers to be aware of the need for transgender-specific screening for cancer based on the organs present,

hormone use, and gender-affirming surgery. As the primary care provider, it is important to be in communication with your patient's surgeon or help guide your patient in knowing what type of surgery is performed to make informed decisions on follow-up screenings needed.

Regarding breast/chest cancer screening, even after gender-affirming chest surgery for those on the masculine spectrum there may be residual breast tissue. Those who have not had chest or top surgery will require screenings based on guidelines for cisgender women. For transgender people on the feminine spectrum, mammograms are recommended once the person has been on feminizing hormone therapy for at least 5 to 10 years and is over the age of 50, with exceptions for other higher risk situations just as they are for cisgender women (Deutsch, 2016).

Peitzmeier et al. (2014) studied cervical cancer screening results from 233 transgender men and 3,625 female (cisgender) patients, reporting that transgender men were 8.3 times more likely to have inadequate samples when compared to female (cisgender) patients. The study suggested an association between testosterone and cervical cancer screening sample inadequacy. In addition to an increased incidence of unsatisfactory screening samples, transgender men also face many barriers in coming in for care that is typically gendered and therefore they may delay or not obtain care (Seay et al., 2017). As with all patients, this exam should be performed with sensitivity and with a trauma-informed approach. Providers may significantly improve collaboration with the patient by using nongendered, sensitive language and a patient-centered approach. Testosterone can also cause vaginal atrophy, making speculum exams more difficult; therefore, using a smaller speculum may be advisable.

Potter et al. (2015) developed recommendations to guide cervical cancer screening in transgender men that minimize emotional discomfort before, during, and after a pelvic examination; decrease physical discomfort during the examination; and explain how to adapt the cervical cancer screening sample collection to account for testosterone-induced anatomic changes. Recommendations include using a smaller speculum, short-term topical estrogen cream, and topical lidocaine (Peitzmeier et al., 2014; Potter et al., 2015). Cervical cancer screening for TGNB people with a cervix, including interval of screening and age to begin and end screening follows recommendations for nontransgender women as endorsed by the American Cancer Society, American Society of Colposcopy and Cervical Pathology (ASCCP), American Society of Clinical Pathologists, U.S. Preventive Services Task Force (USPSTF), and WHO (Deutsch, 2016).

TGNB people on the feminine spectrum who have had a vaginoplasty do not have a cervix. Patients who have had penile inversion vaginoplasty are recommended to have annual vaginal exams to evaluate for condyloma, skin cancers, or other concerns the patient may have (Deutsch, 2016).

Routine screening for endometrial cancer in TGNB people who are using testosterone is not recommended. Unexplained vaginal bleeding (in the absence of missed or changed dosing of testosterone) in a patient previously with testosterone-induced amenorrhea should be further evaluated following evidence-based guidelines (Deutsch, 2016). There is no evidence to suggest that TGNB people on testosterone are at increased risk for ovarian cancer (Deutsch, 2016).

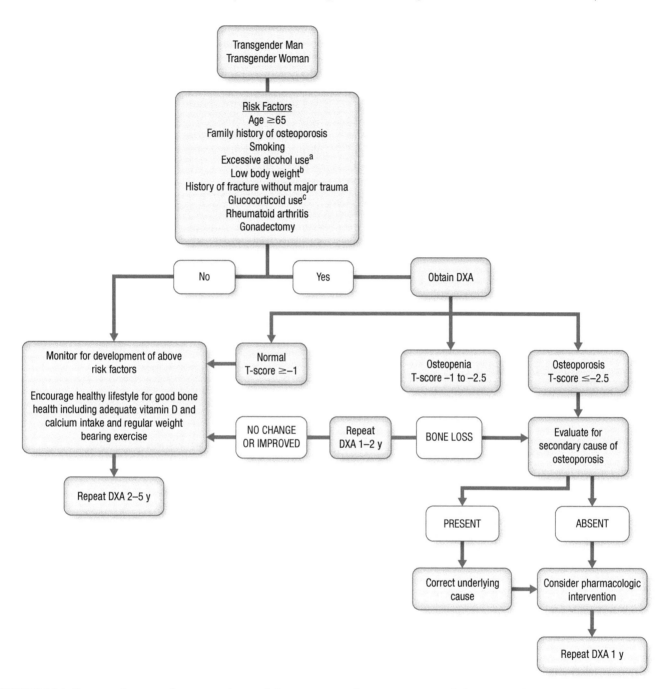

FIGURE 25.1 Suggested approach to screening and the treatment of osteoporosis in adult transgender patients.
DXA, dual-energy x-ray absorptiometry.
[a]Three or more drinks a day.
[b]Weighing less than 127 lb or a body mass index (BMI) of less than 20 kg/m.
[c]Prednisolone 5 mg/day or more for 3 months or more, current or past. Bone loss greater than least significant change.
Source: Adapted from Stevenson, M. O., & Tangpricha, V. (2019). Osteoporosis and bone health in transgender persons. Endocrinology and Metabolism Clinics of North America, 48(2), 421–427. https://doi.org/10.1016/j.ecl.2019.02.006

The USPSTF recommends against routine testicular cancer screening in people assigned male at birth (USPSTF, 2011). GAHT with estrogen can falsely lower the prostate specific antigen (PSA) blood test, which could mean the PSA screening test is less accurate in TGNB individuals on feminizing hormones than in cisgender men (Trum et al., 2015). Healthcare providers should follow TGNB-informed guidelines and recognize that TGNB people who have undergone vaginoplasty have a prostate anterior to the vaginal wall, and thus, a digital neovaginal exam examination may be more effective (Deutsch, 2016). It is important to note that the gender-affirming surgery of vaginoplasty does not involve removal of the prostate gland.

FERTILITY CARE

It is essential that prior to transition all TGNB people are counseled on fertility, as gender-affirming hormones and surgery can affect fertility options.

For TGNB people on the feminine spectrum, estrogen use can affect sperm production and may require a referral to sperm banking if the patient desires. TGNB people assigned female at birth may have a uterus and ovaries and be capable of achieving pregnancy. They also may engage in sexual activity that can achieve pregnancy. The degree to which testosterone may reduce risk for pregnancy is not known, although testosterone is considered a teratogen. People who were assigned female at birth and are on testosterone may get pregnant, even if they have amenorrhea (Krempasky et al., 2020). Evidence shows that amenorrhea is reversible when testosterone is discontinued, and pregnancies have been reported both during and after testosterone use (Deutsch, 2016). Finding TGNB-sensitive OB/GYN providers can be incredibly challenging. Using terms such as *pregnant people* instead of *pregnant women* can help create welcoming spaces.

In the *American Journal of Obstetrics and Gynecology* article on welcoming transgender and nonbinary clients, Stroumsa and Wu (2018) recommend helpful language to incorporate into practice (Table 25.6).

Patients at risk for pregnancy, based on current anatomy and sexual activity, should be counseled on contraceptive options. When conducting sexual healthcare for TGNB patients, exams should be conducted using trauma-informed techniques. No contraceptive methods, even those that contain estrogen and/or progesterone, are contraindicated due to testosterone use (Krempasky et al., 2020). When counseling patients on contraception use, it is important to consider factors that may affect gender incongruence such as chest tenderness, vaginal insertion, and privacy. Fertility preservation options for transgender men include oocyte cryopreservation, embryo cryopreservation, and ovarian tissue cryopreservation.

TABLE 25.6 Gender Inclusive Language for Sexual and Reproductive Healthcare

CURRENT PRACTICE	SUGGESTED ALTERNATIVE
Language	
Women's healthcare (providers, services, clinic, etc.)	Sexual and reproductive care
Well-woman examination	Annual examination, well-person examination, or Pap smear, pelvic examination
Breastfeeding	Breastfeeding or chestfeeding
Mother	Parent or gestational parent
Intake forms, EMRs, and history taking	
Address all patients as Ms. or Mrs.	Call patient in from the waiting room by last name only. Ask all patients: "How would you like me to address you?"
Questions about menstrual and obstetric history	Avoid assumptions about anatomy. Clarify whether the patient has a uterus. This approach is also more friendly for cisgender women who have had a hysterectomy and for intersex people.
Sexual history: "Are you sexually active with men, women, or both?"	Ask "Who do you have sex with?" "What anatomy (parts) do they have?" followed by appropriate questions regarding specific sexual practices, as needed.
Are you sexually active?	Acknowledge that there are many sexual practices that do not include penile-vaginal penetration. "Have you ever been sexually intimate in a way that included exchange of genital body fluids?" "Do you have oral or anal sex?" "Have you ever had vaginal (or front) penetration with a penis, finger, or toy?"
Sex marker: binary options (male or female)	Many EMRs now offer a preferred name and pronoun field. Use a two-step gender question: (1) what is your gender? Enable more than two options for people who identify as nonbinary, queer, or other; (2) what sex were you assigned at birth (i.e., on your original birth certificate)?
Visual cues	
Bathroom signage: men/women	Ensure at least one single-stall, nongender (or all-gender) bathroom that is accessible and easily identifiable.

EMR, electronic medical record.
Source: Adapted from Stroumsa, D., & Wu, J. P. (2018). Welcoming transgender and nonbinary patients: Expanding the language of "women's health." American Journal of Obstetrics and Gynecology, 219(6), 585.e1–585.E5. https://doi.org/10.1016/j.ajog.2018.09.018

GENDER-AFFIRMING SURGERY CARE

Gender-affirming surgery, like GAHT, can be lifesaving to transgender people. Although there are still many barriers to surgery, including cost and finding appropriate care, more health insurance programs in the United States are covering these medically necessary procedures. NPs should have knowledge about surgical options, surgery referrals, multidisciplinary surgery care, and support. Primary care providers would assist with preoperative clearance such as ensuring any health issues are stable, identifying support and any social issues, assessing expectations, and collaborating on pre- and postsurgery plans. It is important to be aware of what types of gender-affirming surgeries there are, how to assess for any complications that would warrant a referral to the surgeon, and what postoperative maintenance is needed. For example, after a vaginoplasty with the creation of a vaginal canal, the patient would need to self-dilate to maintain depth three to four times a day for the first several weeks and gradually this need decreases going forward. For those on the trans-feminine spectrum gender-affirming surgeries may include mammoplasty (breast augmentation), vaginoplasty (creation of a vagina with or without a vaginal canal), orchiectomy (removal of the testes), penectomy (removal of the penis), clitoroplasty (creation of a clitoris), vulvoplasty (creation of all parts of a vaginal except for the canal), and facial feminization surgery. Surgical options for transmasculine people include mastectomy often called chest surgery (removal of breast tissue), hysterectomy (removal of the uterus), oophorectomy (removal of ovaries), metoidioplasty (enlargement of the clitoris), phalloplasty (creation of a phallus with or without urethral lengthening), and scrotoplasty (creation of a scrotum). More information on each procedure, healthcare follow-up after the procedure, the role of the primary care provider, and managing complications are available at such references as UCSF *Guidelines* (Deutsch, 2016), *Trans Bodies Trans Selves* surgery chapter (Erickson-Schroth, 2022), considerations in gender-affirming surgery (Nolan et al., 2019), a review of gender affirmation surgery (Akhavan et al., 2021), and WPATH guidelines (WPATH, 2022).

FUTURE DIRECTIONS

Providers and staff should include their pronouns on their badges and when introducing themselves. All patients, not just those perceived to be transgender, should be asked for their chosen name, pronouns, sexual orientation, gender identity, and sex assigned at birth; this information should be documented in the electronic health record (Cahill & Makadon, 2014). Providers and staff should receive ongoing education regarding gender identity and transgender health (Deutsch, 2016). Unnecessarily gendered language should be avoided whenever possible (Krempasky et al., 2020).

Anatomy inventories are essential for care for all clients as they let healthcare providers know what body parts and internal organs clients have in order to conduct appropriate screenings. For example, a cisgender (nontransgender) woman who has had her breasts removed due to breast cancer or who has had a hysterectomy may not need the same screenings/health maintenance questions as a cisgender woman who has not had those procedures. This consideration is the same for transgender clients. It is helpful to remember that it is impossible to know the body parts, sexual activity, gender identity, and sexual orientation of any client unless the appropriate and sensitive questions are asked. Some electronic medical records can integrate an anatomy inventory to collect this information prior to healthcare visits in order to integrate the appropriate template, screening questions, and indications for laboratory testing. For example, a gendered template would not bring in a prompt to offer a pregnancy test or to ask about last menstrual period on a patient who is listed in the system as male, even though it may be medically necessary to their anatomy.

People assigned female at birth, including transgender and nonbinary people, may be in need of OB/GYN services offered to anyone who has a vulva, a vagina, or a uterus such as screening and treatment of STIs, vulvar care, cervical cancer screening, menstrual cycle management, contraception, prenatal care, breast/chest care, and fertility care (Stroumsa & Wu, 2018). People who were assigned male at birth, including transgender women and nonbinary people, may also need services within the scope of OB/GYN such as STI screening and treatment, contraception and fertility care, postoperative care of neovaginas (surgically created vaginas), and breast care (Stroumsa & Wu, 2018). Implementing inclusive language and informed clinical care recognizes the historical and current impact of gender-based discrimination on the healthcare of cisgender women and transgender populations and addresses these important health inequalities.

TRANSGENDER AND GENDER DIVERSE RESOURCES FOR PROFESSIONALS

Articles

- Klein, D. A., Paradise, S. L., & Goodwin, E. T. (2018). Caring for transgender and gender-diverse persons: What clinicians should know. *American Family Physician, 98*(11), 645–653.
- McDowell, A., & Bower, K. M. (2016). Transgender health care for nurses: An innovative approach to diversifying nursing curricula to address health inequities. *Journal of Nursing Education, 55*(8), 476–479. https://doi.org/10.3928/01484834-20160715-11

Books

- Erickson-Schroth, L. (Ed.). (2022). *Trans bodies, trans selves* (2nd ed.). Oxford University Press.
- Keuroghlian, A. S., Potter, J., & Reisner, S. L. (Eds.). (2022). *Transgender and gender diverse health care: The Fenway guide.* McGraw-Hill.

- Mukerjee, R., Wesp, L., Singer, R., & Menkin, D. (Eds.). (2021). *Clinician's guide to LGBTQIA+ care: Cultural safety and social justice in primary, sexual, and reproductive healthcare.* Springer Publishing Company.

Journals

- *International Journal of Transgender Health.* https://www.tandfonline.com/journals/wijt21
- *Transgender Health.* https://home.liebertpub.com/publications/transgender-health/634/overview

Websites/Links

- American College of Obstetricians and Gynecologists (ACOG) transgender healthcare:
  - ○ https://www.acog.org/education-and-events/creog/curriculum-resources/additional-curricular-resources/transgender-health-care
  - ○ https://www.acog.org/clinical/clinical-guidance/committee-opinion/articles/2021/03/health-care-for-transgender-and-gender-diverse-individuals
- *Creating equal access to quality healthcare for transgender patients: Transgender-affirming hospital policies.* https://www.lambdalegal.org/publications/fs_transgender-affirming-hospital-policies
- *Collecting gender identity and sexual orientation in electronic health records.* https://www.lgbtqiahealtheducation.org/wp-content/uploads/Collecting-Sexual-Orientation-and-Gender-Identity-Data-in-EHRs-2016.pdf
- *Creating a transgender health program at your health center.* https://www.lgbtqiahealtheducation.org/wp-content/uploads/2018/10/Creating-a-Transgender-Health-Program.pdf
- Guidelines for TGNB primary care/screenings/hormone protocols:

- ○ Callen-Lorde Community Health Center. https://callen-lorde.org/about
- ○ TransLine. https://transline.zendesk.com/hc/en-us/articles/229373288-TransLine-Hormone-Therapy-Prescriber-Guidelines
- ○ Sherbourne Health Center. https://www.rainbowhealthontario.ca/TransHealthGuide/index.html
- ○ *UCSF Transgender Care. Guidelines for the primary and gender-affirming care of transgender and gender nonbinary people* (2nd ed.). https://transcare.ucsf.edu/guidelines
- ○ *Fenway Health. The medical care of transgender persons.* www.lgbtqiahealtheducation.org/wp-content/uploads/COM-2245-The-Medical-Care-of-Transgender-Persons-v31816.pdf
- National LGBTQIA Health Education Center. https://www.lgbtqiahealtheducation.org
- National Organization of Nurse Practitioner Faculties. *Patient-centered transgender health: Toolkit for nurse practitioner faculty and clinicians.* https://cdn.ymaws.com/www.nonpf.org/resource/resmgr/files/transgender_toolkit_final.pdf
- *Quick guide to transgender primary care for the PCP.* https://www.hopkinsmedicine.org/center-transgender-health/_docs/TGD_GAHT_QUICK_GUIDE.pdf
- Transgender Medical Consultation Service:
  - ○ https://transline.zendesk.com/hc/en-us
  - ○ http://project-health.org/transline
- World Professional Association for Transgender Health. *Standards of care for the health of transsexual, transgender, and gender-nonconforming people.* www.wpath.org/publications/soc

REFERENCES

References for this chapter are online and available at https://connect.springerpub.com/content/book/978-0-8261-6722-4/part/part03/chapter/ch25

CHAPTER 26

Sexual Health Problems and Dysfunctions*

MEGAN R. MAYS

Sexuality is basic to the human condition, and people rate sexuality as an important quality-of-life issue. The Centers for Disease Control and Prevention (CDC) notes that the World Health Organization (WHO, 2006) defines *sexual health* as:

> a state of physical, emotional, mental and social well-being in relation to sexuality; it is not merely the absence of disease, dysfunction or infirmity. . . . Sexual health requires a positive and respectful approach to sexuality and sexual relationships, as well as the possibility of having pleasurable and safe sexual experiences, free of coercion, discrimination and violence. (WHO, 2006, p. 11)

Healthy sexual function with a partner nurtures the relationship, whereas sexual dysfunction may cause relationship disharmony with untoward repercussions to both partners. Healthy sexual functioning improves self-image and increases the motivation to take care of health concerns and adopt a healthier lifestyle. Studies suggest that less than 10% of providers initiated and included discussions about their patient's sexual health even though 60% of these providers felt that addressing sexual issues at a patient visit was important (Dyer & das Nair, 2013).

The clinician's role in assessing sexual dysfunction, initiating treatment, and making appropriate referrals is critical because sexuality is a vital quality-of-life issue; 43% of individuals ranked sexual health as highly important to their quality of life (Flynn et al., 2016). Moreover, gynecologic disease processes and therapeutic interventions can potentially affect sexual response.

NORMAL SEXUAL RESPONSE

Sexual Response Cycle

Various sexual response cycles were discussed in Chapter 19, Women's Sexual Health. These cycles have evolved from linear to circular models resulting in an updated version combining both the physical and mental influences on sexual response. Depending on the individual, their sexual response can alter between positive and negative depending on a multitude of factors such as stress, relationship, sleep, mood, or comfort.

Physiology of Normal Sexual Response

Although there are still gaps in the understanding of female sexual function, sex steroids and neurotransmitters in the central and peripheral nervous systems appear to play a significant role (Kingsberg et al., 2017) In the central nervous system (CNS), the neurotransmitter dopamine appears to modulate sexual desire. In addition, dopamine, along with norepinephrine, increases the sense of sexual excitement and the desire to continue sexual activity. Increasing levels of serotonin can diminish the effects of both dopamine and norepinephrine, whereas melanocortins, small protein hormones, may have a stimulatory effect on dopamine. Estrogen and testosterone function may, at least in part, be modulated by the effects of serotonin activity in the hypothalamus and associated limbic structures. Other hormones

---

*This chapter is a revision of the chapter that appeared in the second edition of this textbook, authored by Candi Bachour and Candace Brown, and we thank them for their original contribution.

also are involved in CNS modulation of sexual behavior. These include oxytocin, which may enhance sexual receptivity and orgasmic response. Conversely, the pituitary hormone prolactin negatively influences the sexual excitement phase and is inversely related to dopamine function (Kingsberg et al., 2017).

In the periphery, sex hormones are important mediators of genital structures and function (Kingsberg et al., 2017). Nitric oxide (NO) and vasoactive intestinal peptide (VIP) are implicated in engorgement of clitoral tissue following sexual stimulation; however, adequate levels of estrogen and free testosterone are needed in order for NO to stimulate vasocongestion. Peripheral serotonin has negative effects on vasocongestion, NO function, and sensation. Prostaglandin E and cholinergic fibers also induce vasocongestion.

Sexual arousal often has been equated with vaginal lubrication. This unconscious reflex organized by the autonomic nervous system in response to mental or physical stimuli that are recognized as sexual is only one aspect of sexual arousal. In addition to "genital arousal," some people may also experience cognitive arousal, or the feeling of being "turned on." Subjective sexual arousal is a product of the following components: mental sexual excitement—proportional to how exciting the individual finds the sexual stimulus and context; vulvar congestion—direct awareness (tingling, throbbing) is highly variable; pleasure from stimulating the engorging vulva; vaginal congestion—the individual's direct awareness is highly variable; pleasure from stimulating congested anterior vaginal walls and Halban's fascia; increased and edified lubrication—wetness usually is not directly arousing to the individual; vaginal nonvascular smooth muscle relaxation—the individual usually is unaware of this; pleasure from stimulating nongenital areas of the body; and other somatic changes—blood pressure level, heart rate, muscle tone, respiratory rate, and temperature. Measuring peripheral sex steroids has individual variability and makes measuring these peripheral sex steroids difficult regarding documenting the "hormonal factor" and decision-making on potential hormone treatments (Kingsberg et al., 2017).

SEXUAL DYSFUNCTION

As introduced in Chapter 19, Women's Sexual Health, there is considerable variation in how individuals rate the importance of sex, their idea of optimal sexual frequency, their preferred sexual practices, and the amount of stimulation required for arousal and satisfaction. It is important to note that although many people report sexual problems, the problem causes true distress in a smaller percentage of individuals. Worldwide, sexual dysfunction is reported as approximately 40% and increases with age (Shifren, 2018). What is less understood is the percentage reporting dysfunction and its correlation to personal distress. The PRESIDE study (Shifren et al., 2008) evaluated the prevalence of personal distress associated with sexual problems and is often cited as the foundational study. A 2017 Australian study with 2,020 women between the ages of 40 and 65 by Worsley and colleagues (2017) reported sexually related personal distress at 40.5%.

The criteria for diagnosis of female sexual dysfunction (FSD) is classified by the American Psychiatric Association's (APA) *Diagnostic and Statistical Manual of Mental Disorders (DSM)*. The *DSM* criteria for sexual dysfunctions have evolved throughout the years, reflecting the prevailing thinking of the time of publication. In the *DSM-IV* (APA, 1994), which was used until 2013, the diagnosis of a sexual dysfunction was based on the linear model of human sexual response proposed by Masters and Johnson (1966) and further developed by Kaplan (1974), with the idea that sexual desire was what led to the initiation of sexual activity. More recent research has questioned the validity of that model because of the strict distinction between different phases of arousal and the linear model proving to be inadequate to explain sexual behavior in participants (Ishak & Tobia, 2013). A movement away from the discrete and nonoverlapping phases of sexual function noted in the linear model toward a more circular model more representative of an individual's sexual response has been recently seen. The linear models have suggested that sexual response is the same for both cisgender male and cisgender female individuals and that desire always precedes arousal. Basson et al. (2000) nonlinear model of female sexual response recognizes that female sexual functioning is not as linear as male sexual functioning and is more complex. In this model, the individual is presumed to have motivations for sexual activity other than physical release. The decision to be sexual may come from a conscious wish for emotional closeness with a partner or as a result of seduction or suggestion from a partner. Sexual neutrality or being receptive to sexual activity rather than the initiation of sexual activity, is considered to be the normal variant of sexual functioning. This more updated framework for conceptualizing the female sexual response has led to several proposed changes in the diagnostic criteria of sexual dysfunction (Ishak & Tobia, 2013). The dual control model represents the net sum of mental and physical aspects of sexual function. Perelman's Sexual Tipping Point (STP) is considered a dual control model allowing a visual of the multitude of physical and psychosocial aspects affecting sexual response and dysfunction (Perelman, 2018). A benefit to the STP model is the visual illustration presenting all etiologic permutations of sexual balance, including "normal" sexual balance.

FSD may be lifelong (referring to a sexual problem that has occurred from the first sexual experience) or acquired (referring to a sexual problem that has developed after a time of relatively normal sexual function). FSD is further divided as situational (it is noted only in certain types of situations or stimulation or with certain partners) or generalized (it is not limited to certain situations, partners, or stimulation).

Multiple factors must be considered during the assessment of FSD:

- Partner factors such as the partner's health status or sexual dysfunction
- Relationship factors such as poor communication or discrepancies between partners' desire for sexual activity
- Individual vulnerability factors inclusive of a history of sexual or emotional abuse or the individual's poor body image

- Cultural or religious factors, which encompass an individual's attitude toward sexuality or inhibitions related to sexual activity and pleasure
- Medical factors that become relevant to prognosis and treatment

Under the *DSM-IV*, the classification of FSD was divided into four dysfunctions: (a) female desire disorders, including hypoactive sexual desire disorder and female sexual aversion disorder; (b) female sexual arousal disorder; (c) female orgasmic disorder; and (d) sexual pain disorders, including dyspareunia and vaginismus. In the revised *DSM-5* (APA, 2013), female sexual disorders are reclassified as (a) desire and arousal disorders, (b) genitopelvic pain/penetration disorder (inclusive of vaginismus and dyspareunia), and (c) female orgasmic disorder. Sexual aversion disorder has been removed from *DSM-5* because of the lack of supporting research (Ishak & Tobia, 2013). The separation of sexual dysfunction caused by a general medical condition from FSD, which is related to psychological causes, has also been removed, noting that most sexual dysfunctions are the result of both psychological and biological factors (Latif & Diamond, 2013). *DSM-5* sexual dysfunctions all require a minimum duration of 6 months, as well as a frequency of experiencing the disorder 75% to 100% of the time. Finally, for appropriate diagnosis, the disorder must cause "significant distress" (Ishak & Tobia, 2013).

Female Orgasmic Disorder

Female orgasmic disorder is characterized by marked delay in, infrequency of, or absence of orgasm and/or in markedly reduced intensity of orgasmic sensations. A wide variability in the type or intensity of stimulation that elicits orgasm has been shown in individuals. Furthermore, it has been found that subjective descriptions of orgasm are widely varied, which suggests that it is experienced in very different ways, both in various individuals as well as on different occasions by the same individual. For the diagnosis of female orgasmic disorder to be made, symptoms must be present for a minimum duration of approximately 6 months during approximately 75% to 100% of occasions of sexual activity. This criterion is used to distinguish between transient orgasm difficulties from more persistent orgasmic dysfunction. In addition, clinically significant distress must be present. If FSD symptoms are better explained by another mental disorder, a medical condition, or the effects of a substance/medication, then a diagnosis of FSD would *not* be made. If interpersonal factors, such as intimate partner violence, severe relationship distress, or other significant stressors are present, a diagnosis of female orgasmic disorder would also not be made.

Many individuals require adequate clitoral stimulation to reach orgasm, and in fact, a relatively small proportion of individuals report consistently experiencing an orgasm with penile–vaginal intercourse. An individual who experiences orgasm through clitoral stimulation but not with intercourse does not meet the criteria for the diagnosis of a sexual dysfunction. It is important to determine if difficulties with orgasm are the result of inadequate sexual stimulation, in which case education and care would be indicated but a diagnosis would not be made (APA, 2013).

Female Sexual Interest/Arousal Disorder

The diagnostic criteria for female sexual interest/arousal disorder includes lack of or significantly reduced sexual interest/arousal, as manifested by at least three of the following:

- Absent/reduced interest in sexual activity
- Absent/reduced sexual/erotic thoughts or fantasies
- No/reduced initiation of sexual activity and typical lack of response to a partner's attempts to initiate
- Absent/reduced sexual excitement/pleasure during sexual activity in 75% to 100% of sexual encounters
- Absent/reduced sexual interest/arousal in response to any internal or external sexual/erotic cues such as visual, written, or verbal cues
- Absent/reduced genital or nongenital sensations during sexual activity in 75% to 100% of sexual encounters

It is important to assess interpersonal context when assessing female sexual interest/arousal disorder. A "desire discrepancy," in which an individual experiences lower desire than the individual's partner would not be sufficient for diagnosing this disorder. For the criteria to be met, there must be absence or reduced frequency or intensity of at least three of the six listed indicators for a minimum duration of approximately 6 months. The minimum duration of 6 months is required in order to determine if the symptoms are a persistent problem indicative of dysfunction or a short-term change in sexual interest or arousal, which is common. In order for the diagnosis to be made, clinically significant distress must also accompany the symptoms. Distress may be a result of significant interference in an individual's life and well-being. A diagnosis would also not be made if a lifelong lack of sexual desire is better explained as one's self-identification as *asexual* (APA, 2013).

Sexual medicine experts continue to encourage the decisions around nomenclature for FSD to be more evidenced based. For example, The International Society for the Study of Women's Sexual Health (ISSWSH) revised its nomenclature in 2019 by defining the overarching category as female sexual arousal disorder (FSAD) and created two subtypes: female cognitive arousal disorder (FCAD) and female genital arousal disorder (FGAD) (Parish et al., 2019).

Genitopelvic Pain/Penetration Disorder

Tightening and tension, often involuntary, is what many providers term *vaginismus*. Historically, pain with penetration or intercourse has been termed *dyspareunia*. The combination of these two terms into genitopelvic pain/penetration disorder was a component of the *DSM-IV* to *DSM-5* transition. Of note, providers should be aware of the terminology, as many continue to use both vaginismus and dyspareunia as diagnoses. The decision to remove vaginismus was based on the conclusion that dyspareunia and vaginismus could not be reliably differentiated. This was due in part to a lack of empirical evidence supporting vaginismus as a "vaginal muscle spasm" as well as the fact that fear of penetration or pain is commonly found in descriptions of vaginismus (Parish et al., 2021).

Genitopelvic pain/penetration disorder is diagnosed by persistent or recurrent difficulties in one or more of the following:

- Vaginal penetration during intercourse
- Marked vulvovaginal or pelvic pain during vaginal intercourse or penetration attempts
- Marked fear or anxiety about vulvovaginal or pelvic pain in anticipation of, during, or as a result of vaginal penetration
- Marked tensing or tightening of the pelvic floor muscles during attempted vaginal penetration

Major difficulty in any one of these symptoms is sufficient to cause clinically significant distress. Therefore, a diagnosis can be made on the basis of marked difficulty in only one symptom dimension. All symptom dimensions must be assessed, however, as many individuals have more than one symptom.

Marked difficulty having vaginal intercourse or penetration can present as the ability to easily experience penetration in one situation such as tampon insertion or gynecologic examinations, but not in another such as intercourse. If pervasive, pain can cause complete inability to experience vaginal penetration in any situation. Marked pelvic or vulvovaginal pain during penetration attempts or vaginal intercourse indicates that pain occurs in different locations in the genitopelvic area. It is essential to assess the location as well as the intensity of pain. Pain may be characterized as occurring during initial penetration, affecting the vulva (described as "superficial pain"), or it can be felt further into penetration and thrusting, affecting the vagina and the pelvic floor muscles (described as "deep pain"). Pain may be provoked or occur only with stimulation, unprovoked, or spontaneous or occurs both with provocation and spontaneously. The pain can also persist for a period of time after intercourse has ceased or during urination.

Marked fear or anxiety about pelvic or vulvovaginal pain either in anticipation of or during vaginal penetration is common among individuals who have regularly experienced pain during sexual intercourse. This is a "normal" reaction and may lead to avoidance of sexual or intimate situations.

Marked tightening or tensing of the pelvic floor muscles with attempted penetration can vary from voluntary muscle guarding to reflexive-like spasm of the pelvic floor in response to fear, anxiety, or anticipation of pain.

Frequently, genitopelvic pain/penetration disorder is associated with other sexual dysfunctions because pain often results in decreased interest, arousal, and avoidance of intimacy. It is critically important to assess pain during the evaluation of any sexual dysfunction in order to determine the role it plays in other dysfunctions (APA, 2013).

Vulvodynia

Vulvodynia was first defined in 2003 with initial prevalence estimates at 8% of cisgender females in the United States, with more recent data estimating a prevalence around 16% (Loflin et al., 2019). According to Parish et al. (2021), vulvodynia is defined as pain in the vulvar area that has persisted for at least 3 months without a clear identifiable cause, is idiopathic pelvic or vulvar pain, or pain with penetrative sexual contact. In individuals who do seek medical care, their condition is often misdiagnosed because of a lack of knowledge among healthcare providers or because of inconsistent diagnostic criteria (Feldhaus-Dahir, 2011).

Generalized Vulvodynia

Torres-Cueco and Nohales-Alfonson (2021) outline three types of vulvodynia: Generalized, localized, and mixed. In all three types it is important to note that the vulvar structures are normal in appearance and often the etiology is elusive. Although some individuals are not able to decipher a trigger for their pain, many report an inciting factor such as having a yeast infection, starting an oral contraceptive (OC) or antibiotic, or sustaining a trauma or having surgery in their pelvic region (Goldstein et al., 2011).

Generalized vulvodynia (GVD) is typically described as a constant burning pain involving much of the vulva and often including the vulvar vestibule. In 2015, the International Society for the Study of Vulvovaginal Disease (ISSVD), the ISSWSH, and the International Pelvic Pain Society (IPPS) convened to align on the terminology of vulvodynia acknowledging the complexity of both the pathophysiology and presentation of vulvodynia. In 2019, the societies convened again to formulate a consensus publication providing 11 descriptors that were arranged into four groups. These four groups were location, onset, provocation, and temporal pattern.

Vestibulodynia

Vestibulodynia is the most common cause of pain with intercourse in premenopausal individuals. Often, *vestibulodynia* is best defined as localized vulvodynia and has been estimated to affect 15% in the gynecologic setting (Loflin et al., 2019). Vestibulodynia has been referred to by various names, including *vulvar vestibulitis syndrome, localized provoked vulvodynia,* and *provoked vestibulodynia* (Feldhaus-Dahir, 2011).

SEXUAL HEALTH CHALLENGES

Many health-related factors can affect sexual health. Experiencing illness and/or living with specific diseases or disorders, having surgery, becoming disabled, and using medications (both prescription and nonprescription) can have an impact on sexual health. There is a pervasive cultural bias implying that if an individual is disabled or sick, they are no longer a sexual person. Sexuality in the American culture is often only associated with young, healthy, able-bodied individuals. In addition to coping with feeling "different" from a sexual perspective, an individual with an illness or disability often struggles with changes in their body, self-perception, self-esteem, identity, and social and economic status (Foley et al., 2012).

Many diseases or health problems have the potential to affect desire, arousal, and orgasm. Similarly, a variety of drugs may affect sexual desire, arousal, and orgasm based on their neuroendocrine, neurovascular, or neurologic effects. Treatments that affect the vascular system or that produce nerve damage may also alter sexual function (Parish et al., 2021). Spinal cord injury, vascular damage, neurologic damage, and chemotherapy and other medications interfere with genital blood flow or alter feeling in the genitals and impede sexual arousal and orgasm. Spontaneous and responsive desire, orgasm, and arousal can be greatly affected by decreasing hormone levels, fatigue, depression, and pain that is often associated with chronic illness (Foley et al., 2012).

Diabetes can cause nerve damage or circulatory problems that cause alterations in sexual functioning. Individuals with type 1 and type 2 diabetes should be screened for sexual dysfunction as the risk is increased by factors of 2.27 and 2.49 in type 1 and 2 diabetes, respectively (Levin et al., 2016). Elevated blood glucose levels often lead to fatigue, resulting in decreased sexual interest. A decrease in vaginal lubrication is also common, and diabetic individuals have an increased prevalence of dyspareunia. A person with cardiovascular disease often has an overwhelming fear that sex will provoke another heart attack or stroke.

Cancer in an individual significantly affects their sexuality. In fact, it has been noted that >60% of female cancer survivors experience sexual dysfunction. Much of the research on cancer and sexuality has been done with breast cancer survivors; however, emerging literature in gynecologic cancers have reported similar incidences of sexual dysfunction (Valpey et al., 2019). Alterations in body image caused by surgery, menopause triggered by chemotherapy, hair loss, pain, and emotional stress make an individual with cancer more vulnerable to sexual problems. Sexual dysfunctions may result from surgery, radiotherapy, hormone therapy, or chemotherapy. Surgery, such as a mastectomy for breast cancer, or changes in the hormonal milieu, as in the case of an oophorectomy for ovarian cancer, influence a woman's sexuality because of direct anatomic changes. Oophorectomy causes an immediate depletion of estrogen in premenopausal individuals, resulting in early-onset menopause. This leads to symptoms of vaginal atrophy, compromised elasticity, and dryness, all of which can affect the ability of an individual to engage in sexual intercourse. Hysterectomy often results in direct anatomic changes to the vaginal vault, including fibrosis and vaginal shortening. Mastectomies in a person with breast cancer can affect body image and self-esteem, both of which can influence a woman's sexuality (Dizon et al., 2014). Selective estrogen receptor modulators (SERMs) such as tamoxifen and aromatase inhibitors, which decrease breast tissue exposure to estrogen, frequently can contribute to vaginal dryness, pruritus, and dyspareunia (Cakar et al., 2013). Cytotoxic agents cause fatigue, weakness,

nausea and vomiting, and altered body image from hair loss, all of which limit a woman's sexual arousal and interest (Dizon et al., 2014). Providers must be aware of the importance of sexuality for most individuals, and a diagnosis of cancer does not alter this.

People with disabilities, whether lifelong or acquired, experience significant challenges to their sexuality (Foley et al., 2012). Changes in physical appearance and changes in body image largely affect a woman's sexuality, both in self-concept and in partner responses. Researchers have found that individuals with more severe physical impairments experience more sexual depression, less sexual self-esteem, and less sexual satisfaction than those with mild or no impairment and that those with severe physical disabilities engage in sex less frequently. Specific physical effects of a given disability on sexual activity differ with the disability. Individuals with spinal cord injuries are generally not able to experience orgasm and experience diminished sensations at climax. They are able to experience sensuous feelings in other parts of their bodies and may discover new erogenous areas such as their necks, ears, or thighs. Individuals with disabilities must overcome the anger that is frequently present if their bodies do not return to their previous sexual function expectations. They must realign their expectations with their actual sexual capabilities in order to establish sexual satisfaction and health (Foley et al., 2012).

Many medications can alter sexual functioning and cause sexual dysfunctions, including decreased sexual desire, lack of sexual arousal, inadequate lubrication, and delayed or absent orgasm. These effects are summarized in Table 26.1, which lists medications associated with sexual dysfunction. Depending on the dosage and the individual's mental and physical state, it is not uncommon to see medications that decrease testosterone and dopamine production result in an individual's complaint of decreased sexual function (Clayton et al., 2018).

Having a disability or chronic illness does not mean that a woman's sexual life ends. A woman's sexual well-being is a quality-of-life issue, and it is necessary for providers to educate individuals with physical limitations about their sexuality, including counseling to build self-esteem and combat negative stereotypes. Providers need to give their patients "permission" to engage in sexual activities and suggest new activities or techniques in order for them to be able to have full and satisfying sex lives (Yarber et al., 2010).

TABLE 26.1 Medications That May Contribute to Sexual Dysfunction

Anticonvulsants	Phenytoin, primidone, carbamazepine
Cardiovascular medications	Amiodarone, beta-blockers, clonidine, digoxin, statins, methyldopa, hydrochlorothiazide, calcium channel blockers
Hormonal medications	Antiandrogens, combined hormonal contraceptives, tamoxifen, gonadotropin-releasing hormone agonists
Pain medications	Nonsteroidal anti-inflammatory drugs, opioids
Psychotropic medications	Serotonin reuptake inhibitors, serotonin and norepinephrine reuptake inhibitors, lithium, benzodiazepines, antipsychotics

Source: Adapted from Parish, S. J., Cottler-Casanova, S., Clayton, A. H., McCabe, M. P., Coleman, E., & Reed, G. M. (2021). The evolution of the female sexual disorder/dysfunction definitions, nomenclature, and classifications: A review of DSM, ICSM, ISSWSH, and ICD. Sexual Medicine Reviews, 9(1), 36–56. https://doi.org/10.1016/j.sxmr.2020.05.001

Sexual dysfunctions can occur with the use of substances such as alcohol, marijuana, and narcotics (American College of Obstetricians and Gynecologists [ACOG], 2019). As a result of popular culture and media images depicting thin, beautiful, and scantily clad individuals drinking, the belief that alcohol and sex go together is common. The belief that alcohol is a sexual enhancement is also a popular myth. Alcohol leads to disinhibition, causes decreased lubrication, dulls stimulation, and contributes to sexual risk taking. Similar to alcohol use, most recreational drugs interfere with libido and sexual functioning, including making orgasm difficult.

Sexually transmitted infections (STIs) are a significant health issue in the United States. In 2018, the prevalence of STIs was approximately 67.6 million. Risk factors for STIs in individuals include not using condoms with partners, using drugs or alcohol before intercourse, having multiple sex partners, and having concurrent partners. *Chlamydia infection*, trichomoniasis, genital herpes, and human papillomavirus infection accounted for 97.6% of all prevalent STIs (Kreisel et al., 2021).

Pathophysiology of Sexual Dysfunction

Research on the pathophysiology of sexual dysfunction has increased over the past decade. The largest amount of research on the anatomy of a cisgender female has been conducted on the vulva (mons pubis, clitoris and bulbs, labia majora, and labia minora). Sexual arousal encompasses both a physical and a mental state induced by multiple stimuli resulting in feelings of pleasure and desire. However, it is important to note that mental arousal can occur without genital physical changes and vice versa (Levin et al., 2016).

Etiology and Prevalence

The foundation for the etiology of sexual dysfunction sits in the brain. In the presence of sexual cues and stimuli, the inhibitory brain neuromodulators (the neurotransmitters opioids, serotonin, and endocannabinoids) are thought to be greater than the excitatory brain neuromodulators (the neurotransmitters dopamine, melanocortin, oxytocin, vasopressin, and norepinephrine).

Population surveys highlight the fact that cisgender female sexual disorders are highly prevalent. Comparison among countries is problematic because different definitions and methodologies are employed in different surveys. The most recent data highlight prevalence in relation to the amount of distress. Both psychological and relationship factors contribute to distress. Distressing problems related to desire, arousal, and orgasm affect 12% from adolescence to postmenopause (Parish et al., 2019).

Risk Factors

Numerous risk factors are associated with sexual dysfunction. Individuals may have certain medical conditions or take medications that place them at increased risk of sexual dysfunction. In addition, those individuals with a history of sexual or physical abuse and those with relationship difficulties are at increased risk. Finally, different cultural backgrounds, when there may be conflicts with personal or family values as well as societal taboos and inadequate education, place individuals at risk of sexual dysfunction.

MEDICAL CONDITIONS

Numerous medical conditions are associated with sexual dysfunction (Clayton et al., 2018; Table 26.2). Individuals with medical conditions such as depression, diabetes, cancer, and neurologic conditions such as spinal cord injury and multiple sclerosis are some of the most at-risk medical conditions for sexual dysfunction. Generally, a chronic medical condition that impairs blood flow could lead to sexual dysfunction.

Hormonal imbalances related to type 2 diabetes and its effects on the neurologic, psychological, and vascular health of the individual have been shown to cause sexual dysfunction. Diabetes prevalence continues to increase with a 2019 meta-analysis review of 25 studies and 3,892 individuals ages 18 to 70 years reporting the overall prevalence of sexual dysfunction in women with type 2 diabetes was 68.6% (Rahamian et al., 2019).

Gynecologic malignancies, specifically breast cancer, may cause sexual dysfunction. The adverse effects of cancer therapies are not limited to physiologic effects. Malignancies coexist with psychological and social difficulties and may impair self-image and decrease sexual desire. This issue is particularly important in conditions that may impair self-image, such as having a mastectomy or hair loss after chemotherapy.

Hormonal changes associated with menopause and aging, such as estrogen/androgen depletion, often cause important physical and psychological adverse effects on sexual function. Estrogen depletion often leads to dyspareunia, sleep disturbances, mood swings, and depression. The thinning of the vaginal epithelium, atrophy of the vaginal wall smooth muscle, and elevated pH changes in the vagina may ultimately

TABLE 26.2 Medical Conditions and Their Potential Impact on Sexual Function

CONDITION	DESIRE	AROUSAL	ORGASM	PAIN
Coronary artery disease		√		
Diabetes	√			
Depression	√	√	√	
Hypertension	√			
Metabolic syndrome	√	√	√	
Hypothyroid disorder		√	√	
Urinary incontinence	√	√		√
Malignancy and treatment	√	√	√	√
Vulvar conditions (lichen sclerosis, eczema, psoriasis)				√
Arthritis				√

√ indicates potential impact.
Source: Clayton, A. H., Goldstein, I., Kim, N. N., Althof, S. E., Faubion, S. S., Faught, B. M., Parish, S. J., Simon, J. A., Vignozzi, L., Christiansen, K., Davis, S. R., Freedman, M. A., Kingsberg, S. A., Kirana, P. S., Larkin, L., McCabe, M., & Sadovsky, R. (2018). The International Society for the Study of Women's Sexual Health process of care for management of hypoactive sexual desire disorder in women. Mayo Clinic Proceedings, 93(4), 467–487. https://doi.org/10.1016/j.mayocp.2017.11.002

result in vaginal dryness and pain during intercourse. Urogenital disorders, characterized by stress and/or urge incontinence (see Chapter 28, Perimenstrual and Pelvic Symptoms and Syndromes), may also affect an individual's level of comfort during sexual activity for fear of leakage.

MEDICATIONS ASSOCIATED WITH SEXUAL DYSFUNCTION

The most common medications associated with cisgender female sexual dysfunction are those containing serotonin (Parish et al., 2021). Parish and colleagues (2021) categorized medications predominantly causing specific sexual dysfunctions. The categories are outlined in Table 26.3.

In general, any antidepressants that interfere with serotonergic pathways (nonselective), such as SSRIs, or with acetylcholine pathways, such as tricyclic antidepressants, induce sexual dysfunction. In contrast, antidepressants that impact dopaminergic and (central) noradrenergic receptors, or selective hydroxytryptamine 5-HT_{1A} and 5-HT_{2C} receptors, are not likely to reduce sexual response. Therefore, those antidepressants least likely to interfere with sexual response include non-SSRI antidepressants, such as nefazodone (Serzone), mirtazapine (Remeron), bupropion (Wellbutrin), venlafaxine (Effexor, at doses of 150 mg or lower), duloxetine (Cymbalta), and buspirone (ACOG, 2019).

Other centrally acting medications, including psychoactive substances, such as antipsychotics, barbiturates, and benzodiazepines, and codeine-containing opiates may affect sexual function. Opinion varies as to whether anticonvulsants are associated with low sexual desire. Many individuals can take anticonvulsants for diseases other than epilepsy without experiencing sexual side effects. Anticholinergic agents, which interfere with acetylcholine function, such as antihistamines, also may impair sexual response (ACOG, 2019). Table 26.1 summarizes medications that can be contributing factors to sexual dysfunction.

Antihypertensives that penetrate the blood–brain barrier, such as beta-blockers and centrally acting antihypertensives, as well as diuretics, may reduce sexual desire. However, calcium channel blockers and angiotensin-converting enzyme (ACE) inhibitors are generally not considered to have sexual side effects. Other cardiovascular agents, such as antilipemics, may also induce sexual problems (ACOG, 2019).

Agents that interfere with the hypothalamic–pituitary–ovarian axis, such as gonadotropin-releasing hormone agonists, like leuprolide (Lupron), are likely to induce sexual problems. A subgroup of individuals using oral contraceptives reported low sexual desire, which may be caused by reduced free testosterone production and an increased serum level of sex hormone–binding globulin, which also may cause low sexual desire in some individuals receiving estrogen therapy. Progestins, such as medroxyprogesterone, may also induce sexual dysfunction by their negative effects on the mood. Some estrogen agonist/antagonists may have estrogen antagonistic activity in the vagina. Although, the above-mentioned hormones list potential negative sexual side effects, updated data reviewers report mixed positive and negative sexual side effects (Casado-Espada et al., 2019).

PSYCHOLOGICAL FACTORS ASSOCIATED WITH SEXUAL DYSFUNCTION

Several psychological factors can negatively affect sexual function. Relationship problems can interfere with the individual's interest in sexual expression and undermine the individual's enjoyment of sexual experiences. Cultural and religious background may affect how the individual views sexual activities, and interpersonal factors, such as depression, stress, substance use, or sexual trauma, can affect how the someone is able to interact and emotionally connect with others.

Interpersonal Factors

Low libido frequently accompanies individuals with major depression. An individual who reports mood changes, sleep disturbance, fatigue, decreased concentration, low self-esteem, reduced interest in activities, decreased energy and motivation, and appetite or weight changes may improve in sexual function if their depression is effectively treated (Box 26.1).

Individuals who are under tremendous stress often feel they do not have time to engage in sexual activity and may view it as just "another responsibility." Those who work full

TABLE 26.3 Categories of Medications That Cause Specific Sexual Dysfunctions

SEXUAL DYSFUNCTION	MEDICATIONS
Desire	Antihypertensives, anticonvulsants, antidepressants, antipsychotics
Arousal	Anticholinergics, antihistamines, antihypertensives
Orgasm	Primarily opioids and psychopharmacologic medications

Box 26.1 Psychological Causes of Female Sexual Dysfunction

Interpersonal

Depression/anxiety

Stress

Alcohol/substance abuse

Previous sexual or physical abuse

Relationship

Relationship quality and conflict

Lack of privacy

Partner performance and technique

Sociocultural

Conflict with religious, personal, or family values

Societal taboos

Inadequate education

Source: Adapted from Bachmann, G. A., & Avci, D. (2004). Evaluation and management of female sexual dysfunction. Endocrinologist, 14, 337–345. https://doi.org/10.1097/01.ten.0000146394.84092.1b

time, take care of children, and carry most of the responsibility for domestic activities may hold resentment toward their partner. In addition, assuming the role of "mother" and "wife" in heterosexual relationships may reduce the individual's feeling of being sexual, in both the individual's eyes and in those of the individual's partner. Increasing ways to reduce stress, such as increased partner assistance with responsibilities and having "date nights" may improve sexual response.

Although alcohol and other recreational substances may temporarily produce a "disinhibiting" effect on an individual who is anxious about sexual activity, and subsequently improve responsivity, chronic substance abuse impairs sexual function.

Other psychological factors commonly affect sexual response in individuals. These may include negative sexual experiences, including fear of a likely unsatisfactory or painful outcome; decreasing self-image; potent nonsexual distractions (e.g., baby); lack of physical privacy; feelings of shame; lack of education regarding sexual anatomy and physiology; embarrassment; partner sexual dysfunction; lack of safety from pregnancy and STIs; and fear of physical safety.

Relationship Factors

Perhaps the most common contributor to sexual dysfunction in individuals is a nonfunctional relationship with their partner. A variety of factors may contribute to this, including poor communication skills, infidelity, control issues, partner substance abuse, and parental conflicts. An individual will often seek sex therapy in order to improve the relationship, whereas if the individual and their spouse attended relationship therapy, their sexual function would most likely improve.

Lack of privacy, due to the presence of children or relatives living with a couple, may also affect an individual's comfort level in engaging in sexual activity. Additionally, any partner dysfunction can reduce an individual's motivation to be sexual. Commonly, this includes erectile dysfunction, premature ejaculation in their partners, and desire or orgasm difficulties in female partners.

Sociocultural Factors

Individuals who were raised in a very strict religious background, where sexual activity before marriage was considered wrong, may find it difficult to automatically transition into feeling sexual once they get married. If the individual received the message that sex was "dirty," that person may find it very difficult to think of it as an "act of love" in a committed relationship. Moreover, some cultures encourage an individual to have sex only as a function of performing "marital duties" and that a respectable individual should not enjoy the pleasures of sex. Finally, many people may not have received any education about sex, including basic knowledge of anatomy, and sexual response.

EVALUATION/ASSESSMENT
History

A comprehensive sexual history is the first step in establishing the diagnosis of a female sexual disorder. Sexual inquiry is aimed at exploring the areas of the individual's concerns, moving from general to more specific areas.

Box 26.2 Components of the Sexual History

History of present illness

Typical encounter

Current medications

Past medications

Current medications

Medical history

Social history

Psychiatric history

Family history

Developmental and sexual history

Relationship history

Stressors

Psychiatric examination

Mental status

Physical problems or limitations

Current diagnoses

Specifiers of the diagnosis (e.g., is it acquired or lifelong, situational, or generalized?)

Box 26.2 identifies the components of a thorough sexual history. Questions that are asked during the history of the present illness include chief sexual complaints (in the patient's own words) and eliciting information on the onset, duration, precipitating factors, and other sexual complaints. The clinician attempts to determine whether the symptoms are situational (occur in only one setting) or are generalized (present in all settings) and whether they are lifelong (have always been present) or acquired (there was a time when there was normal sexual functioning). The clinician determines the individual and their partner's explanation for the symptoms because patients often add significant insight into the cause of the problems. It is important to know why the individual is seeking treatment now, the amount of distress, and the individual's motivation for seeking treatment, as these factors may affect the individual's interest in and ability to follow the therapy plan. Information is elicited on the type of previous treatment and its success.

Individuals are asked, if they are comfortable, to describe a typical sexual encounter. This allows the person to "tell their story" and to feel heard. The typical encounter discussion evaluates all phases of sexual response (including desire, arousal, orgasm, and pain). The frequency and types of sexual activity are determined along with which partner initiates the activities. It is important to keep in mind that individuals often do not "initiate" sexual activity, rather their desire is more related to their "receptivity" to their partner. The significance of contextual factors, such as time of day, location, fatigue, privacy, atmosphere, and foreplay, are elicited. These factors can often be addressed by providing techniques in which to increase sexual stimulation. Fantasies can give information on sexual desire and normal sexual thoughts; however, they are often difficult to elicit at an initial interview and should not be prompted. It is preferable for the person to spontaneously disclose information about their sexual fantasies because it is important that the individual feels comfortable discussing these thoughts. Both the individual's and their partner's response to the symptoms are determined because they may involve misinterpretation and lead to communication difficulties.

Current medications are identified to determine any drug-induced sexual dysfunction. Past medications are recorded to determine previous response and assess if a change in medications is required.

A thorough medical history, including a history of illnesses, surgeries, and neurologic problems; head, eyes, ears, nose, and throat (HEENT) disorders; and endocrinologic, respiratory, cardiovascular, gastrointestinal, and genitourinary disorders, is obtained to determine illness-induced contributory factors. The woman's last menstrual period, childbirth history, date of last Pap smear, serum laboratory testing, mammogram, and bone density test are determined. Any history of allergies is identified in case a medication is prescribed. A personal and family history of illnesses such as hypertension, cardiovascular disease, cerebrovascular accidents, and cancer are ascertained, as prescribing hormone therapy will depend on these factors.

The psychiatric history includes any previous treatment, hospitalizations, and suicide attempts. The individual is questioned about previous or present psychotherapy, partners therapy, or sex therapy. Response to current and previous antidepressants is determined, as well as the presence of smoking, alcohol use, and substance use. A family history of psychiatric illness is also important in determining the presence of risk factors and in selecting proper antidepressants based on a family member's response.

Areas to be discussed during the family history include ethnicity, religion, parental interactions (demonstration of affection among family members and toward the woman), individual relationships with each parent (role modeling), and sibling relationships. Cultural factors, such as views of sexuality (premarital sex, masturbation, and sexual roles) and their negative connotations, are also assessed. Individuals who have been raised in strict religious settings may feel uncomfortable about having sex after marriage when it was unacceptable before marriage. They may also have inadequate sexual education. Individuals who have not observed parents who were affectionate, or who divorced early on, may not have had appropriate role models. Selection of mates may be based on maladaptive relationships with parental figures.

The development and sexual history include childhood, adolescent, and adult categories. Childhood history includes any losses, number of friends, family role, sexual knowledge, and sexual abuse. Early childhood experiences may have a long-term effect on self-esteem and comfort with one's sexuality. Adolescent areas include response to puberty, body image, masturbation, onset of sexual activity, and descriptions of dating and any rape. Poor body image may carry over into adulthood and affect a woman's ability to feel "sexy." Feelings of guilt about masturbation are elicited. Adult areas

cover college and occupations. A higher level of education may predict whether a woman will be a good candidate for individual therapies as described in the following discussion.

Relationship history concentrates on the current relationship, including partner description, conflicts, loss of trust or fidelity, communication problems, control issues, and intimacy. Conflicts often surround control issues, such as decisions regarding finances, parenting, and household responsibilities. It is important to determine whether the couple feels comfortable displaying nonsexual affection or if all types of affection have been abandoned. The number of children is identified and whether there are any conflicts regarding parenting. Previous relationships, including first major relationships and previous marriages and relationships (including lesbian, bisexual, and transgender relationships), are ascertained. Previous relationships can determine whether there is a pattern of choosing partners who are unlikely to be candidates for meaningful, long-term relationships, which may be addressed in individual counseling (see Chapter 19, Women's Sexual Health).

Any stressors are identified, such as relationship, work, illness, parenting, financial, and loss or deaths. Determining which stressors were present at the onset of sexual dysfunction can identify the relationship between these factors and the onset of sexual disturbance.

The psychiatric examination includes assessment of speech, thought process, judgment, insight, mood, and affect. The clinician determines whether the woman is euthymic, depressed, anxious, irritable, hypomanic, or labile. Mental status includes the woman's appearance, orientation, concentration, intellect, and memory (see Chapter 16, Genetics and Women's Health). These observational skills can determine the presence of a psychiatric disorder and its contribution to sexual symptoms.

Based on this information, the clinician will make an initial diagnosis and specify whether the condition is lifelong or acquired type, due to psychological or combined factors, and generalized or situational.

Physical Examination

Physical examination is crucial for diagnosing some but not all sexual disorders. In some instances, especially the initial meeting, a history and counseling visit can build comfort and reassurance for the patient. An example of a situation in which a physical exam is very beneficial is with chronic dyspareunia, for which a very careful genital examination is performed, especially of the introitus, because in most cases of dyspareunia, the pain is introital. Careful detailed inspection for vulvar atrophy or dystrophy or posterior fourchette scars (often facilitated by allowing the woman to see the examination using a mirror) and testing for allodynia around the hymenal edge with a cotton swab are needed. Resting vaginal tone and voluntary muscle contraction can be assessed approximately by the examining finger(s) and/or with the use of perineometry. Tenderness, often focal from pressing on the deep levator ani ring, can be checked along with pain and discomfort by palpating the uterus and adnexa. Fixed retroversion can be determined, along with any nodularity suggestive of endometriosis. Bladder and urethral sensitivity can be assessed by palpating the anterior vaginal wall (see Chapter 28, Perimenstrual and Pelvic Symptoms and Syndromes).

The role of the detailed physical examination for orgasmic disorder is less obvious when the disorder has been lifelong. Nevertheless, it can reassure the person to know that the results of their physical examination are normal. In cases of acquired female orgasmic disorder, especially in the presence of neurologic disease, the examination is important and requires additional neurologic testing. Cold sensation from the clitoris can be detected by using a cold water-based lubricant. This modality of sensory testing is clinically more relevant to orgasm potential than the use of touch. The motor aspect of the orgasm reflex (pudendal nerves S2 through S4) can be checked by asking the woman to voluntarily contract the muscles around the vagina or the anus or both.

Pelvic examinations for individuals with low libido or difficulty with arousal may have limited usefulness unless sexual pain is present. A general physical examination for acquired loss of desire or arousal is reasonable, although clues to any systemic illness usually would be found in the medical history.

On the other hand, pelvic examination and testing of vaginal pH and wet prep evaluation of vaginal secretions are helpful in eliminating common vaginal infections such as yeast, *Trichomonas*, and bacterial vaginitis infections. Vaginal, cervical, and vulvar swabs for culture may be indicated in individuals with chronic dyspareunia. Dyspareunia associated with vulvar atrophy is readily diagnosed during a pelvic examination.

DIFFERENTIAL DIAGNOSIS

The fourth International Consultation on Sexual Medicine (ICSM) convened in 2015 with over 300 sexual medicine experts to review and update classifications of female sexual dysfunctions. The consensus conference panel built on the existing framework of the WHO *International Classification of Disease-10* (*ICD-10*; WHO, 1994) and the *DSM-IV* of the APA (1994) and highlighted comparisons and contrasts between the *DSM-IV* and *DSM-5* (APA, 2013; Box 26.3) as well as the *ICD-10* and *ICD-11* (WHO, 2019). Of note, the *ICD-11* (WHO, 2019), which is the global standard for reporting health data, came into effect in 2022, and it is the first *ICD* edition to have a chapter dedicated to sexual health (Parish et al., 2021). An essential element of the *DSM-IV* and the newer *DSM-5* (APA, 2013) diagnostic system is the personal distress criterion, meaning that a condition is considered a disorder only if it creates distress for the individual experiencing the condition. The *DSM-5* version has removed the *DSM-IV* categories of sexual aversion *disorder* and sexual dysfunction due to a general medical *condition.*

Box 26.3 Female Sexual Dysfunction Categorized According to the *DSM-IV* and *DSM-5* Criteria

DSM-IV

- Sexual desire disorders (sexual desire/interest disorders)
  - Hypoactive sexual desire disorder
  - Sexual aversion disorder
- Sexual arousal disorder
- Orgasmic disorder
- Sexual pain disorders
  - Dyspareunia
  - Vaginismus
- Noncoital sexual pain disorders
- Sexual dysfunction due to a general medical condition
- Substance-induced sexual dysfunction
- Sexual dysfunction not otherwise specified
- Paraphilias
- Gender identity disorder

DSM-5 Changes

- Sexual desire disorder and sexual arousal disorder combined
  - Sexual interest arousal disorder (SIAD)
  - Sexual aversion removed
- Orgasmic disorder
- Sexual pain disorders (dyspareunia and vaginismus combined)
  - Genitopelvic pain/penetrative disorder
- Noncoital sexual pain disorders (sexual dysfunction due to a general medical condition removed)
- Gender dysphoria
  - Gender identity disorder removed

DSM-IV, Diagnostic and Statistical Manual of Mental Disorders, Fourth Edition; DSM-5, Diagnostic and Statistical Manual of Mental Disorders, Fifth Edition.
Source: Adapted from American Psychiatric Association. (1994). Diagnostic and statistical manual of mental disorders (4th ed.). American Psychiatric Publishing; American Psychiatric Association. (2013). Diagnostic and statistical manual of mental disorders (5th ed.). https://doi.org/10.1176/appi.books.9780890425596

Sexual Interest Arousal Disorder

As previously stated, hypoactive sexual desire disorder (HSDD) and FSAD have now been combined into one classification—sexual interest arousal disorder (SIAD). Due to SIAD being a newer disorder in the *DSM-5*, its prevalence is unknown; however, HSDD was reported in up to 31% of cisgender female individuals (Parish et al., 2021). SIAD criteria are met when an individual experiences at least three symptoms for at least 6 months, including lack of interest in sexual activity; reduced or absent fantasies and/or erotic thoughts; lack of initiation and receptivity to sexual activity; diminished pleasure during sexual activity; diminished or absent desire during a sexual encounter; and a reduction in sexual sensations both genital and nongenital structures (APA, 2013).

For both pre- and postmenopausal individuals, problems achieving adequate lubrication during sexual stimulation may be present; however, the prevalence of the problem is higher in the postmenopausal population. To date, lubrication as a clinical index has not had enough robust methods developed to use clinically (Levin et al., 2016).

Orgasmic Disorder

Orgasmic disorder is defined as the absence of reaching orgasm following sufficient sexual stimulation and arousal, which causes personal distress (ACOG, 2019). Studies of the general population and sex therapy clinic populations indicate that the prevalence of female orgasmic disorder ranges from 16% to 25% in Australia, Sweden, the United States, and Canada (McCabe et al., 2016).

This condition is usually further subdivided into either primary or secondary. Primary orgasmic disorder refers to a woman's inability to achieve an orgasm under any circumstances. A secondary orgasmic disorder most often refers to an inability to reach climax only during intercourse; orgasm can otherwise be achieved either with masturbation or during sexual foreplay. Inability to have orgasm via intercourse is common, occurring in approximately one third of individuals, and is only problematic if it distresses the woman. Trauma to pelvic nerves resulting from pelvic surgery or trauma to pelvic organs may be associated with this disorder. Implicit in this definition is an acceptance that a person does not have a release during their experience of arousal and this lack of release is distressing to the individual.

Sexual Pain Disorders

Dyspareunia is defined by experiencing one or more of the following symptoms: vaginal wall tightening, tension, pain, inability to accommodate penetration, burning with penetration, or intense fear of intercourse (ACOG, 2019). When looking at both pre- and postmenopausal populations, 10% to 20% of all women report pain during sexual activity (Caruso & Monaco, 2019). Like the other female sexual disorders, dyspareunia has both physical and psychological components. Individuals with previous sexual trauma or assault may experience pain during coitus in the absence of a physical cause. A lack of foreplay may result in sparse lubrication, which can lead to vaginal irritation. In addition to estrogen lack, several health conditions such as diabetes mellitus, scleroderma, and other connective tissue conditions increase the prevalence of coital pain. Vulvar vestibulitis and hymenal tags can cause localized pain during penetration that may be triggered by cotton swab probing during the gynecologic examination. Deep penetration pain may be the result of gynecologic problems, such as pelvic adhesions, pelvic inflammatory disease, ovarian disorders, and/or a retroverted uterus. Pathologic conditions involving adjacent structures such as bowel, bladder, and pelvic floor musculature may also cause deep penetration pain.

Vaginismus, similar to dyspareunia, is defined by experiencing one or more of the following symptoms: vaginal wall tightening, tension, pain, inability to accommodate penetration, burning with penetration, or intense fear of intercourse (ACOG, 2019). This definition has not been updated in over 100 years but has been removed from the *DSM-IV* and is not included in the *DSM-5*. Vaginismus, as well as dyspareunia, has been collapsed into a single diagnostic category—*genitopelvic pain/penetration disorder* per the new *DSM-5* classification system (APA, 2013).

Genitopelvic pain/penetration disorder criteria are met when a woman experiences difficulty with at least one of the following: vaginal penetration, pain with vaginal penetration, fear of vaginal penetration or fear of pain during vaginal penetration, or pelvic floor dysfunction (APA, 2013). This new *DSM-5* classification combines dyspareunia and vaginismus due to similarities between the two conditions. Due to the lack of research on this condition, this chapter reviews pertinent information on the conditions as separate entities.

DIAGNOSTIC STUDIES
Psychometric Tests

Several tools are available to screen for sexual dysfunction (Derogatis et al., 2020). As an initial assessment, the Brief Sexual Symptom Checklist is a short five-item self-report that is used as a preconsultation screening tool. A more detailed (19-item) questionnaire, the Female Sexual Function Index (FSFI), measures all dimensions of female sexual function. Other tools specifically target HSDD, such as the Decreased Sexual Desire Screener, a five-item self-report instrument for diagnosis of generalized acquired HSDD, and the Sexual Interest and Desire Inventory, which is clinician administered and evaluates the severity of HSDD. A more detailed self-report questionnaire, the Female Sexual Distress Scale, measures distress associated with female sexual dysfunction; the final item 13 specifically measures bother related to low sexual desire. These questionnaires have historically been used for research but use in clinical practice is increasing.

Laboratory Tests

If a medical etiology is implicated, laboratory values (complete blood count with differential [CBC + diff], complete metabolic panel [CMP], thyroid-stimulating hormone [TSH], cholesterol panel [high-density lipoprotein cholesterol, HDL-C; low-density lipoprotein cholesterol, LDL-C], follicle-stimulating hormone [FSH], estradiol, dehydroepiandrosterone sulfate [DHEA-S], serum sex hormone–binding globulin [SHBG], total and free testosterone) are in order. The need for performing a Pap smear and mammogram are determined, particularly if hormone therapy is being considered.

Other currently available laboratory investigations are of limited value. Estrogen status usually is detected by history and examination, although there may be occasions when assessment of estradiol levels is needed.

Testosterone levels are insensitive and inaccurate unless the dialysis method is used. However, when the history suggests that the concern is loss of androgen production, the testosterone level is assessed by the best method available to ensure that it is not high normal or high. It is more important to obtain either the free testosterone level or the percentage of free testosterone, rather than the total testosterone level, because SHBG binds with testosterone and the total testosterone level does not reflect the amount of testosterone free to act on androgen receptors. Parish and colleagues (2021) discuss the Global Position Statement, which included 10 societies that convened to recommend the most updated evidence-based screening and treatment options. This consensus panel recommends total testosterone as the best available measure, rather than free or bioavailable testosterone. Therapy goals should not target total testosterone. The main reasons to measure testosterone are (1) to exclude women with midrange to high values suggesting that the patient's symptoms are not associated the testosterone level and (2) for monitoring of androgen excess side effects (Parish et al., 2021).

However, the individual needs to be adequately estrogenized before testosterone therapy, and if the individual is naturally menopausal, progesterone is added to prevent endometrial hyperplasia in individuals who have a uterus.

When infertility or oligomenorrhea is present, prolactin levels are measured to account for low desire. When signs or symptoms of thyroid disease are present, TSH levels are measured.

TREATMENT/MANAGEMENT

Based on information gathered primarily during the history, the clinician will make an initial diagnosis and specify whether the condition is lifelong or acquired type, due to psychological or combined factors, and generalized or situational. The clinician will also identify an initial plan, such as requesting another patient visit, partner visit, or couple visit. If medical etiology is implicated, laboratory values are assessed (see Diagnostic Studies section). The clinician determines whether the woman would benefit from medications or if the individual needs to be referred to another professional.

Self-Management Measures

Providing information and education about normal anatomy, sexual function, and normal changes of aging, pregnancy, and menopause is vital. To enhance stimulation and eliminate routine, the clinician encourages use of erotic materials (videos and/or books); suggests self-pleasuring to maximize familiarity with pleasurable sensation; encourages communication during sexual activity; recommends use of vibrators; discusses varying positions, times of day, or places; and suggests making a "date" for sexual activity. Distraction techniques are also discussed, including encouraging erotic or nonerotic fantasy; recommending pelvic muscle contracting and relaxation (similar to Kegel exercise) with intercourse; and recommending use of background music and videos or television. The clinician recommends sensual massage, sensate-focus exercises (sensual massage with no involvement of sexual areas) where one partner provides the massage and the receiving partner provides feedback as to what feels good (aimed to promote comfort and communication between partners), and oral or noncoital stimulation, with or without orgasm. To minimize dyspareunia, the clinician recommends sexual positions including female superior or side lying for control of penetration depth and speed and use of lubricants, topical lidocaine, and warm baths before intercourse.

Psychological Treatment

There are many reasons for a reduction in sexual function, particularly desire, in couples who have been together for a long time. In general, the infatuation of courtship feeds the flames of desire; as the infatuation dies down, the intensity of the passion may diminish. Often, the fatigue and stress of work, child rearing, household duties, medical problems, and substance abuse may dampen sexual desire.

Psychological factors that reduce sexual desire after marriage are related to attitudes toward oneself, sex, and one's partner. For instance, self-doubts involving a sense of inadequacy or a fear of failure can carry over into sexual activities.

Some individuals whose physical appearance does not measure up to their ideal may feel ashamed or self-critical, and they may avoid sexual activities. An individual may dislike the size of their breasts or the shape of their thighs. Fearing that the individual does not appear as expected by mainstream society—that the individual lacks sex appeal—this individual may engage in a self-deprecation that interferes with the spontaneous expressions of their sexual drive.

Interpersonal problems between partners are a frequent source of trouble in an individual's sex life. One of the most obvious problems is a discrepancy in preferences—when, where, how, how long, and how often they have sexual activity. Conflicting desires about timing, frequency, or variety of sex activity can breed resentment, anxiety, or guilt. These unpleasant emotions can then interfere with their sexual contacts.

A medley of attitudes toward an individual's partner can encroach on their sexual feelings. For instance, if the individual believes that their partner is using them, does not care about their feelings, or is undeserving, the individual may experience an automatic inhibition of their sexual desire.

Many dysfunctional psychological thoughts can be corrected through cognitive therapy. Cognitive therapy focuses on how the individual and their partner perceive each other and the way they communicate, miscommunicate, or fail to communicate. The cognitive approach is designed to remedy distortions and deficits in thinking and communication. The essence of cognitive therapy consists of exploring with the individual and their partner their unrealistic expectations, self-defeating attitudes, unjustified negative explanations, and illogical conclusions. Cognitive therapy helps correct these negative thoughts, attitudes, and misinterpretations, and couples often find that their sexual desire can once again become active (ACOG, 2019).

Complementary and Alternative Medicine

HERBAL REMEDIES AND OVER-THE-COUNTER SUPPLEMENTS

The passage of the 1994 Food and Drug Administration (FDA) Dietary Supplement Health and Education Act (DSHEA) allowed for the expanded availability of androgenic substances. Androgenic dietary supplements do not require regulatory review and have thus not undergone formal trials for efficacy and safety. The most abundant steroid hormones in the body are dehydroepiandrosterone (DHEA) and its sulfate ester (DHEA-S). DHEA decreases with age, thus leading to the theory that DHEA supplementation may return sexual function to younger levels (Pluchino et al., 2015).

DHEA and androstenedione are the two major androgen supplements currently available, although there are a growing number of "pro-androgen" supplements being introduced to the marketplace either through the Internet or in stores without prescriptions. DHEA supplements have proved beneficial for some individuals with sexual dysfunction. The efficacy of oral DHEA supplementation has been controversial in part due to varying study length, measurement tools for evaluating positive response, and dose variation. In a 2014 study, Pluchino and colleagues (2015) studied early symptomatic premenopausal women taking 10 mg of oral DHEA daily showing an improved ability to orgasm in comparison to vitamin D. A subsequent review of 38 studies concluded DHEA supplementation had an overall positive outcome on sexual arousal, interest, orgasm, lubrication, and frequency of intercourse, specifically in the peri- and postmenopausal study participants (Peixoto et al., 2017).

Compounds that are made up of "generally recognized as safe" substances require no formal regulatory review. The following substances have limited evidence-based data and show strong placebo effect when participants are randomized. The first substance is L-arginine, which is often combined with other natural substances to enhance sexual function. Oral products that contain high doses of L-arginine need to be used with caution in individuals with histories of oral and/or genital herpes, due to a potentiating effect. In addition, ginseng is used with caution in individuals with poorly controlled hypertension. Additional studies have been performed to evaluate areas such as vaginal dryness, sexual dysfunction related to antidepressant use, and sexual desire. Some of the products studied are maca, ginseng, chasteberry, black cohosh, and red clover. Additional research is needed to establish more evidence-based data to support efficacy and safety of these supplements (Dording & Sangermano, 2018).

MECHANICAL DEVICES

The Eros-Clitoral Therapy Device, a small handheld mechanical device that increases blood flow to the clitoris, labia, and vagina by creating a vacuum over the clitoris, is the only FDA-approved mechanical device for the treatment of female sexual dysfunction. Clinical trials suggested that it improves genital sensation, lubrication, ability to experience orgasm, and sexual satisfaction (Billups et al., 2001). This device requires a prescription. The recommended use is three or four times a week, independent of sexual intercourse for tissue-conditioning effects or before intercourse. Eros therapy can be used as monotherapy or as adjunctive therapy such as with estrogen and/or testosterone therapy.

Pharmacotherapeutics

HORMONE THERAPY

Estrogen and androgen therapy may play a key role in the treatment of peri- and postmenopausal individuals. Estrogen therapy is helpful in maintaining vaginal wall elasticity, microbial flora, urinary continence, and a healthy pH (ACOG, 2019). However, estrogen therapy alone may not provide adequate relief of problems related to sexual function other than for dyspareunia and lubrication complaints.

As of 2021, the only country that has a government-approved testosterone product to treat HSDD in postmenopausal women is Australia. The Global Position Statement is the most comprehensive, evidence-based guideline to date providing clinical guidance on testosterone side effects, adverse effects and effects on mood, cognition, sexual function, cardiovascular health, and breast health (Parish et al., 2021).

Before starting testosterone therapy, clinicians need to establish a baseline of acne, hirsutism, and other androgenic signs and counsel individuals about potential androgenic changes. Baseline screening should include testosterone levels (free and total), estradiol levels, DHEA-S, fasting lipid profile, liver enzymes, mammography, and Pap smear (Phillips, 2000). In general, individuals with current or previous breast cancer, uncontrolled hyperlipidemia, liver disease, acne, or hirsutism should not receive testosterone therapy.

Initiate therapy as follows:

- Compounded testosterone vanishing cream
- Combination product (Covaryx or Covaryx HS, generic esterified estrogen and methyltestosterone, off-label testosterone gel [Testim])
- Testosterone gel (Testim) 1% (5 g/5 mL tube); apply 0.5 mL daily or every other day
- DHEA 25 mg taken orally at bedtime

Monitor symptoms and side effects throughout therapy. At 3 months, reevaluate androgen levels, DHEA-S, estradiol, fasting lipid profile, and liver enzyme levels. As treatment continues, taper therapeutic agents to lowest effective dose, review lipid levels and liver enzyme levels once or twice yearly, and perform routine Pap smear and mammography screenings (Phillips, 2020).

These treatment guidelines should be considered as recommendations. Individuals need to understand that there are no evidence-based protocols for androgen therapy and that testosterone is not approved by the FDA for the treatment of desire disorders in cisgender females before initiating therapy.

COMPOUNDED BIOIDENTICAL HORMONES

Compounded drugs are agents that are prepared, mixed, assembled, packaged, or labeled as a drug by a pharmacist. Unlike drugs that are approved by the FDA to be manufactured and sold in standardized dosages, compounded medications often are custom made for a patient according to a clinician's specifications. One category of compounded products is referred to as "bioidentical hormones," but there is confusion over what this term implies. Bioidentical hormones are plant-derived hormones that are biochemically similar or identical to those produced by the ovary or body. These preparations often come as injectables, oral capsules, or sublingual preparations. Compounded bioidentical hormonal therapies are not FDA approved and not recommended due to safety concerns and the potential for under- or overdosing (Pinkerton, 2020).

The steroid hormones most often compounded include dehydroepiandrosterone, testosterone, pregnenolone, and progesterone. Examples of compounded hormones include Biest and Triest preparations. The name Biest (biestrogen) commonly refers to an estrogen preparation based on a ratio of 20% estradiol and 80% estriol on a milligram-per-milligram basis. A similar preparation, Triest (triestrogen), usually contains a ratio of 10% estradiol, 10% estrone, and 80% estriol. It is important to note that these ratios are not based on each agent's estrogenic potency; rather, they are based on the milligram quantity of the different agents added (ACOG, 2012).

Currently, there is no scientific evidence to support claims of increased efficacy or safety for bioidentical hormones. Purchases of compounded hormones are not typically reimbursed by insurance companies. Additionally, the FDA has approved a bioidentical progesterone (micronized) and many forms of bioidentical estradiol, which are manufactured by pharmaceutical companies and available through traditional pharmacies.

SILDENAFIL (VIAGRA)

An elective inhibitor of phosphodiesterase 5 (PDE-5), sildenafil (Viagra) blocks the activity of PDE-5, causing the accumulation of $3′,5′$-cyclic guanosine monophosphate in the corpora cavernosa, which in turn leads to muscle relaxation (Fourcroy, 2003). Sildenafil has been prescribed to millions of individuals for erectile dysfunction and was the first investigated using controlled studies.

Older trials suggested that sildenafil may partially reverse sexual dysfunction in cisgender female participants with spinal cord injuries (Sipski et al., 2000) and improve arousal frequency, sexual fantasies, sexual intercourse, and orgasm (Caruso et al., 2001). Sildenafil also provides an improvement in vaginal lubrication and clitoral sensitivity (Kaplan, 1999). Additional clinical trials have found that sildenafil provides an improvement in sexual function of patients with antidepressant-induced sexual dysfunction in all genders (Shen et al., 1999). This finding was not supported by another clinical trial that reported sildenafil did not improve the sexual response among individuals with female sexual arousal disorder (Basson et al., 2002). Kingsberg and colleagues (2017) report more updated data on treatment with sildenafil for cisgender female sexual dysfunction is contradictory with the need for further efficacy data. The contradictory efficacy is likely related to the discordance between the participant's subjective measure versus genital measure of sexual response (Kingsberg et al., 2017).

However, sildenafil treatment is well tolerated, and no serious adverse effects have been reported in individuals. As with cisgender males, cisgender females who are using nitrates or have cardiovascular disease should not be prescribed PDE-5 inhibitors.

ANDROGENS

Phase 3 studies are being conducted using transdermal testosterone patches for treating naturally and surgically menopausal individuals with low sexual desire. Clinical trials have been contradictory as well as various professional society recommendations. For example, the North American Menopause Society recommends either oral or nonoral testosterone added to estrogen therapy can result in increased desire and improved sexual function. In contrast, the National Endocrine Society recommends against the use of testosterone for sexual dysfunction (Pluchino et al., 2015).

DOPAMINERGIC AGENTS

The use of dopaminergic agents was found to have a stimulatory effect on sexual behavior in some patients, more so lubrication than orgasm. Moreover, patients who received bupropion (Wellbutrin) for the treatment of SSRI-induced sexual adverse events reported experiencing an increase in sexual function, Dopamine appears to be a "prosexual" or "activating" neurotransmitter, while serotonin is an inhibitor (Kingsberg et al., 2017).

FLIBANSERIN

Flibanserin is a postsynaptic 5-HT_{1A} agonist and 5-HT_{2A} antagonist. In 2015, it was the first medication to receive FDA approval for the indication of premenopausal women with generalized hypoactive sexual desire disorder (Fisher & Pyke, 2017). These subtype receptors of serotonin are thought to be related to libido. Phase 3 trials have investigated the efficacy of flibanserin in treating low sexual desire in premenopausal individuals. Three large, randomized trials compared flibanserin and placebo, with 2,310 subjects randomized to flibanserin and 1,238 subjects randomized to placebo (Derogatis et al., 2012; Katz et al., 2013; Thorp et al., 2012). Improvements in desire were found in the number of satisfying sexual events, level of sexual desire on FSFI domain, and reduction of stress related to the low desire (Derogatis et al., 2012; Katz et al., 2013; Thorp et al., 2012). After a third review, the FDA approved flibanserin (Addyi) as the first FDA-approved treatment for HSDD (Gellad et al., 2015). Upon approval, because of hypotension and syncope when combined with alcohol, the drug was released with a risk evaluation and mitigation strategy (REMS) program requiring prescribers to be certified. In 2019, the FDA removed the alcohol ban recommendation and the REMS program for prescribers. Updated data report common side effects include dizziness, nausea, fatigue, and somnolence occur in approximately 10% of people taking flibanserin with a serious adverse event rate at less than 1% of people (Kingsberg et al., 2017).

α-MELANOCYTE-STIMULATING HORMONE

Findings indicate that effects on sexual dysfunction may be stimulated through melanocortin receptors in the brain. Bremelanotide was approved by the FDA in 2019 as the second FDA approved drug for premenopausal cisgender female individuals with hypoactive sexual desire disorder. The safety and efficacy in two phase 3 randomized placebo-controlled trials (RECONNECT trial) concluded that 1.75 mg subcutaneous injection 45 minutes prior to anticipated sexual activity showed significantly improved sexual desire in pre-menopausal women with hypoactive sexual desire disorder (Kingsberg et al., 2019).

α-ADRENOCEPTOR ANTAGONISTS

Phentolamine is a combined α_1- and α_2-adrenoceptor antagonist that was originally approved for the treatment of pheochromocytoma-induced hypertension and norepinephrine-related dermal necrosis (Fourcroy, 2003). The effects of oral phentolamine 40 mg daily were assessed in a placebo-controlled, pilot study of six postmenopausal individuals with lack of lubrication or subjective arousal during sexual stimulation (Rosen et al., 1999). Mild improvements in subjective (self-reported) arousal and objective (measured) changes in vaginal blood flow were observed. At the time of publication, studies to further evaluate phentolamine in cisgender female sexual function have not been conducted in over 15 years.

PROSTAGLANDINS

A 2017 review by Kingsberg and colleagues highlighted the mechanism of prostaglandins allowing relaxation of the arterial smooth muscle of the vagina resulting in an increase of vaginal secretions. Prostaglandin E_1 which is known as alprostadil, is the vasodilatory agent that has been evaluated in a few small studies. One of these was a placebo-controlled study of 79 postmenopausal individuals with sexual arousal disorders; the study investigated local application of the prostaglandin alprostadil at 100 mcg and 400 mcg and compared this to placebo. Alprostadil 400 mcg resulted in a significant improvement over placebo in genital tingling and lubrication associated with sexual arousal, and in subjective reports of sexual arousal and satisfaction with arousal following visual sexual stimulation (Heiman et al., 2006). The individuals receiving alprostadil 400 mcg reported significantly greater changes from the baseline of genital warmth, tingling, level of sexual arousal, satisfaction with sexual arousal, and sexual satisfaction than those receiving 100 mcg alprostadil or placebo.

TIBOLONE

Tibolone is a selective tissue estrogenic activity regulator (STEAR) that has not been approved by the FDA (Kingsberg et al., 2017). Tibolone has metabolites with estrogenic, androgenic, and progestagenic properties and randomized trials have shown improvement in sexual function for postmenopausal individuals receiving tibolone when compared to estradiol taken orally or transdermally (Kingsberg et al., 2017). Further studies are needed to assess the safety and efficacy of tibolone for treating female sexual dysfunction in postmenopausal individuals.

OSPEMIFENE

Up to 15% of individuals treated with estrogen therapy for dyspareunia do not have symptom relief and may need alternative treatment (McLendon et al., 2014). Ospemifene is the first FDA-approved medication for treating moderate to severe dyspareunia associated with vulvovaginal atrophy. Ospemifene (Osphena) is a selective estrogen receptor modulator (SERM) with estrogenic activity in the vagina, and no studies have shown significant effects on the endometrium or breasts (McLendon

et al., 2014; Wurz et al., 2014). To date, five phase 3 clinical trials have been conducted, which focused on efficacy, treatment for dyspareunia and vaginal dryness, and long-term safety and efficacy data. All studies included postmenopausal individuals ages 40 to 80 years, and the most common side effect was hot flushes (McLendon et al., 2014; Wurz et al., 2014). An extension study lasting a total of 52 weeks compared 30-mg and 60-mg doses to placebo and found no clinically significant adverse events (Simon et al., 2013). Ospemifene (60 mg daily) may be a safe alternative for treating dyspareunia due to atrophy in postmenopausal individuals who cannot or would prefer not to use a vaginal estrogen product.

Referrals

Typical reasons for referring a patient are listed in Box 26.4. In these instances, referral to a psychiatrist, psychologist, psychiatric nurse practitioner, sex therapist, or sexual medicine practice specialist may be in order. The best way to determine the location of a qualified certified sex therapist is to go to the website of the American Association of Sex Educators, Counselors, and Therapists (AASECT; www.AASECT.org).

Considerations for Special Populations

Different sexual concerns affect a woman during the reproductive life span. During childhood, sexual abuse may leave a permanent effect on an individual's sense of sexuality and trust in sexual partners. During adolescence, special concerns relate to their response to puberty, menstruation, and their body image.

A pregnant individual may avoid sexual activity due to fear of placing the fetus at risk, although there is little evidence to advise against coitus unless there are strong contraindications (MacPhedran, 2018). Childbirth also brings about a change in the sexual relationship. Dyspareunia and breastfeeding, in particular, may affect a woman's level of sexual

---

Box 26.4 Reasons to Refer an Individual With Sexual Complaints

If the individual has a complex history, including both physical and psychological symptoms

If the individual has not responded to traditional therapy (e.g., antidepressants)

If it appears there are major relationship issues (e.g., infidelity)

If there is a history of sexual abuse or domestic violence

If multiple medical conditions are present with coexisting medications

If the clinician does not have adequate knowledge in treating sexual disorders

If the clinician does not have adequate time or desire to treat sexual disorders

activity. Education by a clinician regarding pregnancy, childbirth, and lactation is essential in assisting couples through this rewarding, yet often stressful, period of their lives.

Postmenopausal individuals must cope with both physical and psychological changes that may affect their sexuality. Dyspareunia from vaginal atrophy, body image concerns, and attitudes about the appropriateness of sex may affect sexual activity.

Certain subgroups of individuals may feel alienated from sexuality as portrayed in the media. These include individuals from different cultural and ethnic backgrounds, those raised in restrictive religious environments, individuals in same gendered or nonbinary relationships, and individuals with physical disabilities. Transgendered individuals who have female genitalia and identify themselves as male or nonbinary may particularly suffer from societal discrimination. Counseling by a knowledgeable and nonjudgmental clinician is essential.

FUTURE DIRECTIONS

Many individuals experience sexual dysfunction. Medical conditions, psychosocial factors, medications, or a combination of factors can cause sexual dysfunction. A comprehensive history is always necessary and physical examination is needed in selective cases to identify the type and cause(s) of sexual dysfunction so that an effective management plan can be developed. Multiple management options exist, and in cases when the response is not satisfactory to the woman or the complexity level is high, referral to a specialist is warranted. Multiple new therapies are being evaluated that may be of use for individuals in the near future.

The alignment of professional societies on classifications and treatment options will ultimately serve the patient positively. One positive way this is happening is through the new *ICD-11* chapter that focuses on a unified classification of sexual health issues with the hope of reduced stigmatization and improved identification and treatment. This chapter, approved by the World Health Assembly in 2019, is available online for browsing at icd. who.int/browse11/I-m/en.

Additionally, the sexual response models have changed from linear to variable response models allowing for individuality and variability between mind and body. Ideally, this will move the education on sexual health models in the direction of the biopsychosocial models and remove some of the constraints between the mind–body split.

The COVID-19 pandemic has touched every aspect of life. Gleason and colleagues (2021) published survey results assessing sexuality behaviors during the first 6 months of the pandemic. Similar to other studies researching sexuality during the pandemic, themes of frequency, behaviors, and satisfaction were analyzed. Similarities were seen with small decreases in partnered sexual frequency, small decreases in sexual functioning, and small increases in solitary sexual frequency (Gleason et al., 2021). The long-term effect of the pandemic on mental health, personal relationships, and sexual intimacy needs to be a continued focus of research.

REFERENCES

References for this chapter are online and available at https://connect.springerpub.com/content/book/978-0-8261-6722-4/part/part03/chapter/ch26

CHAPTER 27

Vulvar and Vaginal Health[*]

DEBBIE T. DEVINE, SUSAN SALAZAR, AND VERSIE JOHNSON-MALLARD

Vaginal and vulvar issues related to abnormalities of dermatologic and anatomic origin can be neoplastic or non-neoplastic. Understanding both typical and atypical female genitalia is important in identifying and managing vulvar and vaginal problems for women and expands the clinician's previously established foundation of basic science, embryology, anatomy, infectious disease, genetics, physiology, and pathophysiology, as well as other fields of study. Regardless of gender identity, female anatomic structure should be assessed. It is appropriate to comprehensively label laboratory specimens (e.g., male with cervix) for accurate processing (American College of Obstetricians and Gynecologists [ACOG], 2021).

It is important to first consider anatomic and embryologic development because it can lead to a more intuitive understanding of disease. This is the case with müllerian abnormalities, such as vaginal septum or septate uterus. Once the developmental process is known, the malformations are recognized as missteps in development. This knowledge can also facilitate recollection of related issues that may require investigation, such as renal collecting system abnormalities in the case of uterine malformation. Knowledge of anatomic location is imperative to understanding the function of these structures (e.g., periurethral glands), and therefore, the goal of treatment is the return to normal function with a minimal possibility of untoward consequences.

EMBRYOLOGY AND ANATOMY

Development plays a crucial role in the histologic, anatomic, and functional nature of disease. Comprehension of the tissue's embryologic origin allows a more complete understanding of how and why disease develops and progresses, and how it can be effectively managed. Even with limited exposure to the specific clinical problem, observation, examination, and clinical correlation are greatly enhanced with good comprehension of anatomic development.

Anatomic variation becomes more intuitive when developmental processes are also understood, especially in the case of paramesonephric (müllerian) defects of the fallopian tubes, uterus, and vagina. Vaginal development progresses from both endoderm and ectoderm. The distal two thirds of the vagina is derived from the urogenital sinus ectoderm; (Koff, 1933). The proximal one third is derived from the paramesonephric ducts (Figure 27.1). In females, the paramesonephric ducts complete their development as the mesonephric (wolffian) ducts regress (Fu, 2002). Structures derived from these parallel ductal systems form either male or female internal reproductive organs based on the appropriate creation and recognition of genetic signals. Paramesonephric-derived structures include the fallopian tubes, uterus, cervix, and proximal third of the vagina.

External Features

Some features of the external genitalia can be difficult to appreciate on examination in healthy women. It can be difficult to locate specific epithelial glands until they become swollen, as with a cyst. Recognizing the normal locations of glands, folds, ducts, nerves, and other structures facilitates determination of the possible causes of problems. In the case of external anatomy, diagrams provide the most effective way both to display these features and to define the terms used in describing their location (Figures 27.1 and 27.2). Clinical terminology is used to follow a disease course or to describe a disease process to a colleague. This allows more specific localization of findings.

The mons pubis and labia majora are readily visible on inspection of the female genitalia. Both contain adnexal structures of hair and sebaceous glands. The perineal body between the vagina and anus lacks these structures. The

---

[*]This chapter is a revision of the chapter that appeared in the second edition of this textbook, authored by Robert Gildersleeve, and we thank him for his original contribution.

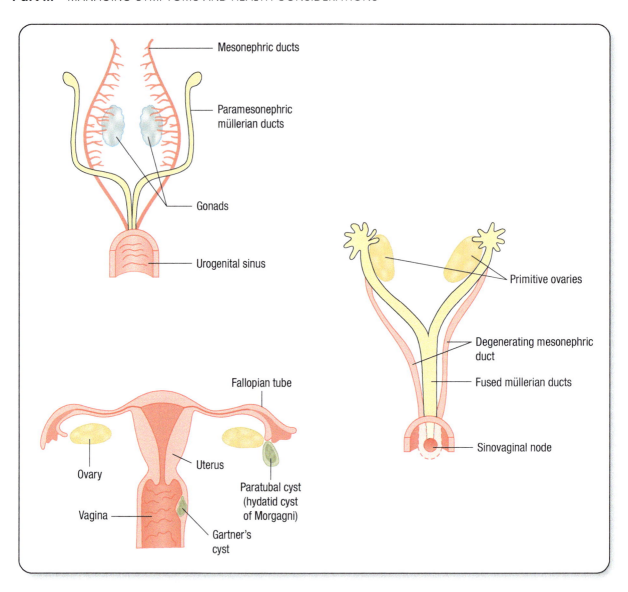

FIGURE 27.1 Embryologic development of ducts.
Source: Adapted from Kaufman, R. H., Faro, S., & Brown, D. (2004). Benign diseases of the vulva and vagina *(5th ed.). Elsevier Mosby.*

perineum (perineal body) is crucial to normal anatomic orientation of the vagina. It forms and maintains the outermost support structure for pelvic organs. Obstetric injuries to this area are frequently associated with loss of support and prolapse of the uterus, bladder, and rectum (Ashton-Miller & DeLancey, 2007; Maher & Baessler, 2006). On separation of the labia majora, the prepuce, clitoris, labia minora, and urethra become apparent. In Figure 27.2, note the location of Bartholin and Skene glands because they can play important roles in abnormalities. At the distal vagina (near the introitus or opening), the hymen or its remnants can be seen. The opening of the vagina is termed the introitus. Multiple anatomic variations are customary with most genital structures, especially the labia and hymen. There is rugation of the vagina. The most proximal portion of the vagina (nearest the cervix) is known as the fornix, which is further divided into lateral, anterior, and posterior fornices. The normal configuration of the closed vagina varies (Barnhart et al., 2006).

Some published studies have described the closed vagina as having an "H" (Figure 27.3) or butterfly shape (Fielding et al., 1996, 1998). This configuration is attributable to lateral support of the vagina from the pelvic sidewalls. Support defects are indicated by loss of rugation and protrusion of the vagina around the speculum from any direction. Examination is performed dynamically, moving the speculum so that defects can be seen along any surface. There are five surfaces of the vagina: apex, two sidewalls, anterior surface (bladder), and posterior surface (rectum). The apex is supported predominantly by the uterosacral and cardinal ligament complexes. The lateral sidewalls are attached to the arcus tendineus fasciae pelvis via endopelvic fibroelastic connective tissue. The anterior and posterior walls are composed of more fibroelastic connective tissue, forming a septum between the vagina and both the bladder and rectum, respectively (Ashton-Miller & DeLancey, 2007; Maher & Baessler, 2006).

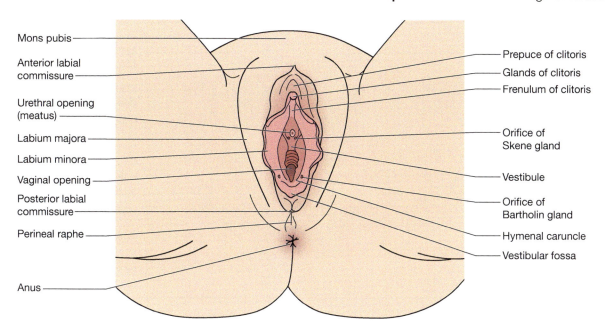

FIGURE 27.2 External female genitalia.
Source: Myrick, K., & Karosas, L. M. (Eds.). (2019). Advanced health assessment and differential diagnosis: Essentials for clinical practice. *Springer Publishing Company.*

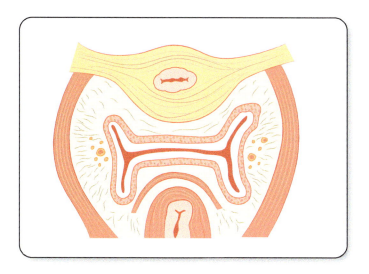

FIGURE 27.3 Cross section of vaginal shape, a crude H.

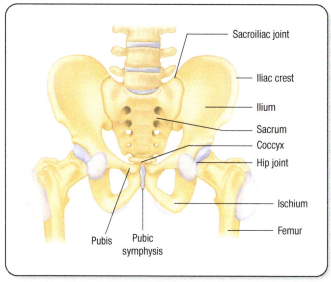

FIGURE 27.4 Pelvic bones.
Source: Myrick, K., & Karosas, L. M. (Eds.). (2019). Advanced health assessment and differential diagnosis: Essentials for clinical practice. *Springer Publishing Company.*

Internal Features

BONY STRUCTURES

The skeletal framework in which the female genitalia reside is composed of four bones: pubis, ilium, ischium, and sacrum (Figure 27.4; Netter, 2006; Standring, 2008; Katz et al., 2007). The pelvic outlet is bordered by the pubis anteriorly, the ilium and ischium laterally (the ischial tuberosities composing the most inferior portion), and the sacrum posteriorly. The pubis has a joint in the midline at the pubic symphysis. This can become markedly tender during pregnancy because the joint loosens and becomes more mobile, attributable to the effects of progesterone and the increasing pressure from the growing fetus. The iliac bones contain the femoral joints laterally. Their broad surfaces (also known as the alae, or wings) allow muscles of the back, legs, and abdomen to attach externally, and the anatomy of the pelvic floor to develop internally. The three-dimensional muscular structures of the pelvis and hip play an important role in both form and function of the pelvis. Although the spatial relationships are complicated to visualize, they are important because they impact sciatic pain, urinary stress incontinence, and pelvic organ prolapse, as well as other disorders.

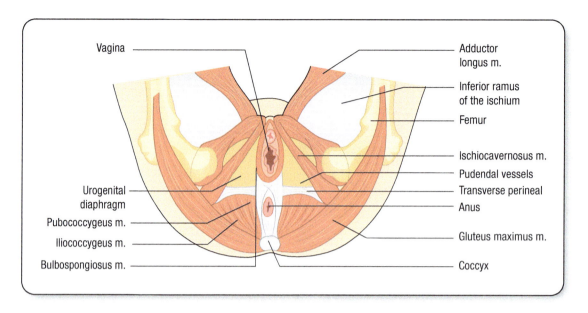

FIGURE 27.5 Pelvic triangle. m, muscle.
Source: Carcio, H. A., & Secor, R. M. (2015). Advanced health assessment of women: Clinical skills and procedures *(3rd ed.). Springer Publishing Company.*

The ischial tuberosities are the bony arcs on which body weight rests when sitting; they supply additional surface area for muscular attachment and add depth to the pelvis. The sacrum is the most inferior portion of the spine. An internally concave, arcing triangular shape, it forms the back wall of the pelvis. The sacral promontory is the ridge protruding anteriorly from the sacrum at the pelvic inlet, and is readily palpable in women of average weight. However, deep palpation can cause discomfort because of pressure on the abdominal structures, such as the abdominal aorta and large and small bowel.

MUSCULATURE

The musculature of the pelvis is relatively large and complex in its three-dimensional architecture. These muscles are described as superficial and deep muscles with the external vulva and vagina as the reference point. Viewed in lithotomy position, superficial muscles are those nearest the distal, or outermost, vagina (Figure 27.5). An alternative approach is to view the bowl of muscle that comprises the pelvic floor from inside the pelvis, which facilitates visualizing the relationships of pelvic organs internally (Figure 27.6).

Superficial muscles of the pelvis are between the skin and the urogenital diaphragm. The urogenital diaphragm is a triangular region bounded by the pubis anteriorly and the ischial tuberosities laterally. The muscles attach from the ischial tuberosities to the pubis. The bulbospongiosus muscles surround the vagina from the perineal body to the pubis. Transverse perineal muscles span from the perineal body to the ischial tuberosities laterally. Posteriorly, the perineal body comprises the external and internal anal sphincters (Figures 27.6 and 27.7; Netter, 2006; Standring, 2008; Katz et al., 2007).

The levator ani (levator plate) consists of four deep muscles that form the pelvic floor. These muscles extend from the pubis to the coccyx (pubococcygeus), form a hammock around the rectum initiating at the pubis (puborectalis), and then extend from the lateral pelvis to the sacrum (iliococcygeus and coccygeus). They create an elliptical gap through which the urethra, vagina, and rectum pass, known as the genital hiatus (Figure 27.8). These muscles function to keep the genital hiatus closed in healthy women. Defects attributable to age-related changes and obstetric trauma have been implicated in pelvic floor dysfunction. This can lead to urinary incontinence and pelvic organ prolapse, highlighting the importance of their anatomic function (Ashton-Miller & DeLancey, 2007; Maher & Baessler, 2006). Lateral support to the vagina is provided through attachments to the arcus tendineus fasciae pelvis, also known as "the white line" (Pit et al., 2003). This is located at the juncture of the lateral levator muscles and the medial aspect of the internal obturator muscle.

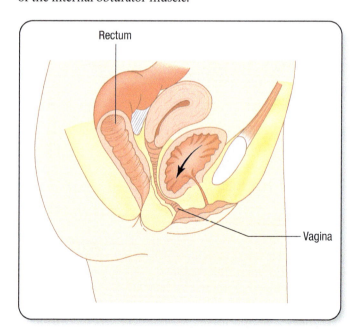

FIGURE 27.6 Pelvic viscera.
Source: Secor, R. M. C., & Fantasia, H. C. (2012). Fast facts about the gynecologic exam for nurse practitioners. *Springer Publishing Company.*

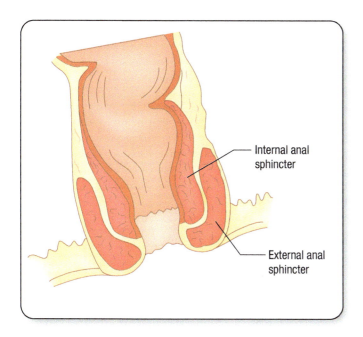

FIGURE 27.7 Anatomy of the anus and rectum.
Adapted from Wilson, S. F. (2005). Health assessment for nursing practice *(3rd ed.). Elsevier.*

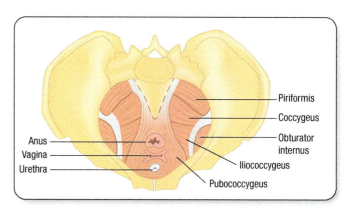

FIGURE 27.8 Pelvic floor musculature.
Source: Adapted from Gabbe, S., Niebyl, J., Simpson, J. L., Galan, H., Goetzl, L., Jauniaux, E., & Landon, M. (2007). Obstetrics: Normal and problem pregnancies *(5th ed.). Churchill Livingstone.*

INNERVATION

The vulva and vagina are predominantly innervated by the pudendal nerve (Figure 27.9). This nerve originates from S2 to S4 and provides motor and sensory supply to the majority of the vulva and lower vagina as well as the muscles of the anal sphincter, which form the posterior perineal body (Netter, 2006; Standring, 2008; Katz et al., 2007). Other prominent nerves include the ilioinguinal and posterior femoral cutaneous. The local dermatomes are illustrated in Figure 27.10. The vagina has two different sources of innervation, as would be expected considering embryologic development. The proximal one third of the vagina receives sympathetic (T11–L5) and parasympathetic innervation (S2–S4) from the uterovaginal and hypogastric plexuses, and the pudendal nerve innervates the distal two thirds (Figure 27.9 and Figure 27.11; Krantz, 1958).

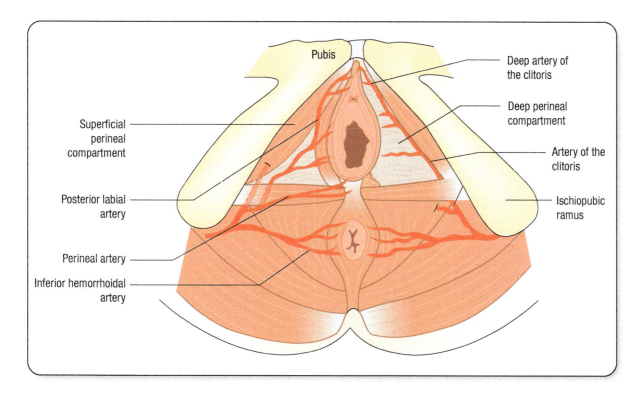

FIGURE 27.9 Vascular supply and innervation of the perineum.
Source: Adapted from Gabbe, S., Niebyl, J., Simpson, J. L., Galan, H., Goetzl, L., Jauniaux, E., & Landon, M. (2007). Obstetrics: Normal and problem pregnancies *(5th ed.). Churchill Livingstone.*

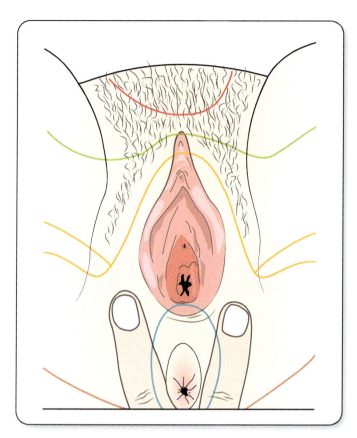

FIGURE 27.10 Vulvar dermatomes.

VASCULAR SUPPLY

The vascular supply to the lower genital tract is similar in anatomy to the nervous supply; hematologic and nervous supplies are tethered throughout the body as neurovascular bundles. The pudendal artery is a branch of the anterior division of the internal iliac artery. The distribution of the pudendal artery is the same as that of the pudendal nerve, serving nearly the entirety of the vulva, perineal body, and anus, as well as the distal vagina (Netter, 2006; Standring, 2008; Katz et al., 2007). The vaginal artery is a branch of the internal iliac artery and serves the remainder of the vagina (Figures 27.9 and 27.12).

BENIGN DISORDERS OF THE VAGINA

Considered anatomically, the vagina functions as both a sexual organ (a conduit allowing conception of pregnancy) and an obstetric organ (a conduit allowing for delivery). There is a broad range of anatomic variation, the parameters of which become more apparent with clinical experience. The length and shape of the labia minora, the development of the clitoris and its hood, the amount of fullness provided by adipose tissue in the labia majora, and the structure of the hymen all vary notably among typical women. A number of benign conditions can be recognized on inspection. Management for these conditions is based on the severity of the woman's symptoms.

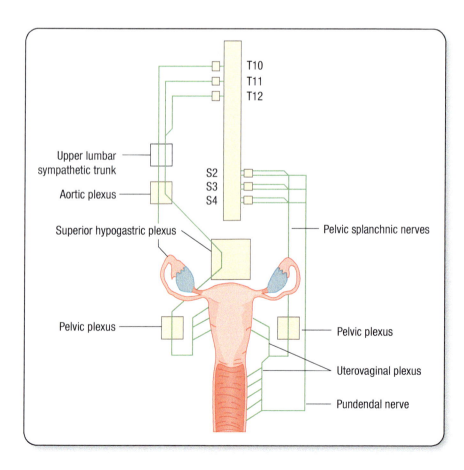

FIGURE 27.11 Innervation of internal genitalia.
Source: Adapted from Gabbe, S., Niebyl, J., Simpson, J. L., Galan, H., Goetzl, L., Jauniaux, E., & Landon, M. (2007). Obstetrics: Normal and problem pregnancies *(5th ed.). Churchill Livingstone.*

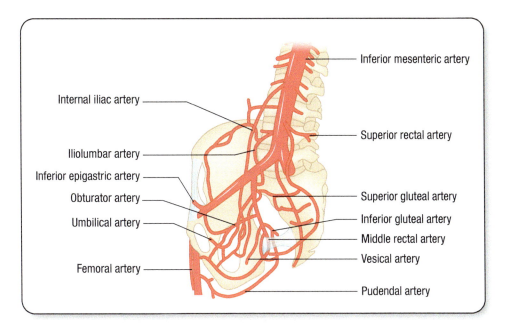

FIGURE 27.12 Vascular supply of pelvis.
Source: Adapted from Gabbe, S., Niebyl, J., Simpson, J. L., Galan, H., Goetzl, L., Jauniaux, E., & Landon, M. (2007). Obstetrics: Normal and problem pregnancies *(5th ed.). Churchill Livingstone.*

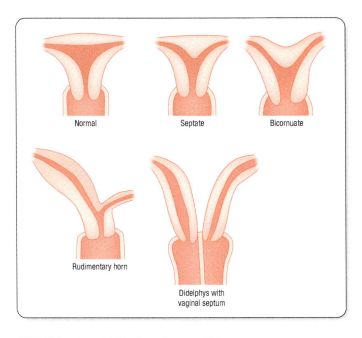

FIGURE 27.13 Müllerian abnormalities.
Source: Adapted from Fu, Y. S. (2002). Pathology of the uterine cervix, vagina, and vulva *(2nd ed.). Saunders.*

Thus, if not bothersome to the woman, treatment may not be necessary. Decisions regarding treatment follow the shared decision-making model that fully engages the woman.

Vaginal Septa

ETIOLOGY

Embryologic development of the vagina provides an explanation for the variety of septa that can occur. Transverse septa can arise from incomplete dissolution of the vaginal plate where the urogenital sinus tissue, derived from the ectoderm, meets the paramesonephric ducts, derived from the endoderm. Hematocolpos (an accumulation of blood in the vagina) can develop if the septum (or imperforate hymen) is complete enough to impede menstrual flow. Longitudinal septa are derived from incomplete fusion of the paramesonephric ducts. Instead of dissolution of the medial portions of the two paramesonephric ducts through a process called apoptosis, or programmed cell death, a persistent central wall dividing left from right, either in part or completely, develops. Longitudinal septa can occur anywhere through the uterus, cervix, or vagina. Longitudinal septa in the vagina are recognized as müllerian abnormalities (Figure 27.13), prompting further evaluation of the uterus, tubes, kidneys, and renal collecting systems. These müllerian abnormalities may have important implications for fertility, and can be associated with renal and urinary collecting duct abnormalities as well as cervicothoracic somite dysplasias (malformations of the vertebral bodies) in 15% to 30% of patients (Oppelt et al., 2006).

EVALUATION/ASSESSMENT

Vaginal septa commonly present in the adolescent population as amenorrhea or dysmenorrhea in those who have recently undergone menarche (Nazir et al., 2006). Complaints may include low abdominal pain, vaginal pain, or cramping without any vaginal blood loss. However, unusual presentations have been reported, such as the case of an adolescent girl with an inability to void (due to the vaginal and pelvic masses in a case of complicated müllerian abnormality; Kleinman & Chen, 2012). Septa can be visualized on examination as a sometimes tense, discolored, membranous bulge in the mid to upper vagina. Examination of the vagina is done carefully, or the presence of parallel vaginal canals can easily be overlooked, even when the clinician has been alerted to a previously identified anomaly. This is true of both speculum and digital examinations. In gynecology, frequently palpation is more sensitive than inspection.

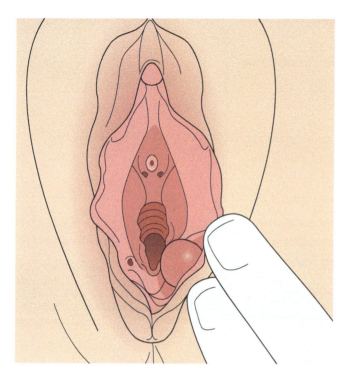

FIGURE 27.14 Bartholin duct cyst.
Source: Myrick, K., & Karosas, L. M. (Eds.). (2019). Advanced health assessment and differential diagnosis: Essentials for clinical practice. Springer Publishing Company.

TREATMENT/MANAGEMENT

Excision can be performed for complete resolution. It is notable that the pressure developed behind the septum can be considerable and can result in rather forceful extrusion of blood on incision. The pressure contained within the uterus and vagina helps to explain the symptoms described by patients in these instances. Additional investigation is indicated to assess the extent of the müllerian abnormality, which can be considerable and may involve multiple systems (Schutt et al., 2012). In the earlier case of the adolescent girl with trouble voiding, she was found to have Herlyn–Werner–Wunderlich syndrome, an unusual malformation of uterus didelphys, unilateral blind vaginal pouch, and ipsilateral renal agenesis (Kleinman & Chen, 2012).

Bartholin Duct Cyst

ETIOLOGY AND EVALUATION/ASSESSMENT

The Bartholin ducts typically drain into the vaginal introitus posterolaterally. They can become occluded, leading to Bartholin gland cyst, or infected, resulting in Bartholin gland abscess (Figure 27.14). Bartholin cysts are found in about 3% of asymptomatic women based on an MRI study (Berger et al., 2012). A Bartholin abscess has been found to be both mono- and polymicrobial and similar in constitution to normal vaginal flora. *Escherichia coli* were found to be the most common infectious agent in one study, though only 61% of cases were culture positive (Kessous et al., 2013).

TREATMENT/MANAGEMENT
Self-Management Measures

Cysts are best managed conservatively with frequent applications of warm compresses, soaking in a warm tub, and using sitz baths (Lashgari & Curry, 1995). These measures allow for dissolution of the blockage or spontaneous rupture and resolution of the cyst. Massage of the area may help with expression of accumulated fluid, which is tested for infection.

Surgical Intervention

If the cyst persists or becomes significantly symptomatic because of size or abscess formation, incision and drainage are indicated. Traditional management is stab incision after administration of local anesthetic at the introitus. Placement of the incision is near the hymenal ring to mimic the anatomic location of drainage as closely as possible. A Word catheter is inserted and maintained for at least 3 weeks (Word, 1968). This time frame allows adequate time for the epithelium to completely cover the newly created passageway. Recurrent cysts are treated with marsupialization, again at the vaginal introitus, not the vulvar epithelium. Marsupialization is the surgical creation of an outlet to the duct (Figure 27.15). The key feature of marsupialization is careful identification of the gland's epithelial

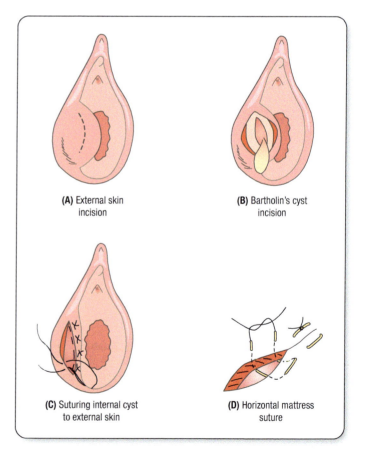

(A) External skin incision

(B) Bartholin's cyst incision

(C) Suturing internal cyst to external skin

(D) Horizontal mattress suture

FIGURE 27.15 Diagram of marsupialization.
Adapted from Kaufman, R. H., Faro, S., & Brown, D. (2004). Benign diseases of the vulva and vagina (5th ed.). Elsevier Mosby.

lining and suturing it to the epithelium of the vaginal introitus. Marsupialization ensures a continued avenue for drainage, making recurrent problems extremely unlikely, occurring in 10% or fewer cases (Blakey et al., 1966). Most marsupializations can be performed in the office using local anesthesia. However, an especially large cyst or abscess can be so painful that deep sedation or general anesthesia becomes necessary. The success of marsupialization and ablative techniques, such as carbon dioxide laser vaporization or alcohol sclerotherapy, makes complete excision of Bartholin gland unwarranted in almost all situations (Cobellis et al., 2006; Fambrini et al., 2008). Not only is it a painful, extensive, and difficult dissection, it can also be complicated by refractory hemorrhage or fistula (Zoulek et al., 2011). Systematic review has not identified a clearly superior method of management (Wechter et al., 2009); therefore, clinical discretion is employed. Broad-spectrum antibiotics are administered if cellulitis is present, taking into consideration that methicillin-resistant staphylococcal species were found in 64% of vulvar abscesses in one trial (Thurman et al., 2008).

Skene Duct Cyst

ETIOLOGY AND EVALUATION/ASSESSMENT

Less common than Bartholin duct cysts, Skene duct cysts are anterior and lateral in location, along the labia minora. Known also as the periurethral gland, providing an accurate description of its location, Skene gland can become occluded, leading to increasing pressure and swelling. This can elicit pain because of either tense tissue or infection. Differential diagnosis must also include urethral diverticulum, leiomyoma, vaginal wall inclusion cyst, urethral prolapse, urethral caruncle, and less commonly, malignancy or Gartner duct cyst (Tunitsky et al., 2012).

TREATMENT/MANAGEMENT
Self-Management Measures

Management is similar to that employed when treating Bartholin duct cysts. Attempts at nonsurgical resolution employ modalities such as warm compresses and soaking in warm baths as well as manual expression via massage. Expressed material is tested for infection.

Surgical Intervention

When the clinician is confident of the correct diagnosis or has been referred to a specialist for evaluation and management, surgical resolution may be appropriate. If self-management is not successful, or if pain is so prominent that conservative management is untenable, incision and drainage can be performed in the office setting after the administration of a local anesthetic (Hopkins & Snyder, 2005; Katz et al., 2007).

Mesonephric (Gartner) Duct Cyst

ETIOLOGY AND EVALUATION/ASSESSMENT

Gartner duct cysts are thin-walled, fluid-filled remnants of the incompletely reabsorbed mesonephros (Figure 27.1). In the male, the mesonephros would have formed the epididymis, and vestigial portions of this system in women can produce cystic structures in the lateral vagina, usually in the proximal two thirds. These can vary in depth, with some being found superficially. Although some Gartner cysts may be membranous in appearance, others may be palpable as soft, subtle distortions through an otherwise normal-appearing vaginal mucosa. These are usually 1 to 3 cm in diameter; however, they can be broader (Hopkins & Snyder, 2005; Katz et al., 2007). The vast majority of times, these cysts are asymptomatic, and treatment is not required. Rarely, they can produce dyspareunia, mechanical blockade (e.g., of tampons), or complaints of pain in the vagina. They can lead to symptoms and perhaps even urethral diverticula, which has been reported in pregnancy (Iyer & Minassian, 2013).

TREATMENT/MANAGEMENT

If intervention is needed, marsupialization is the preferred method (Binsaleh et al., 2007); however, anatomic location will determine the proper procedure to perform. Urethral diverticula are excised, for example.

Non-neoplastic Conditions

The distinction between non-neoplastic and neoplastic disease can be clarified by identifying the location of the changes on pathologic specimens. The term *histologic* refers to microscopically viewed tissue in an undisturbed orientation (such as a cervical biopsy). This is distinguished from *cytologic*, wherein a sampling of cells is viewed microscopically without the benefit of tissue structure (e.g., a smear of cervical cells). If the cellular changes are confined to their correct location in the tissue structure (usually by a basement membrane, Figure 27.16), the sample is considered non-neoplastic (benign). Alternatively, if cellular changes are apparent in tissues adjacent to or distant

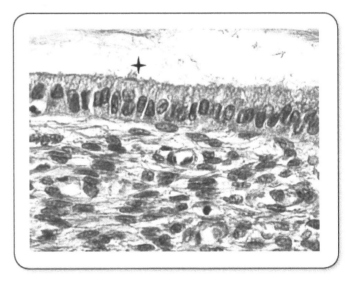

FIGURE 27.16 Normal histology of ectocervix.
Source: International Agency for Research on Cancer. (2023). Normal ectocervix. http://screening.iarc.fr/atlashisto_detail.php?flag=0&lang=1&Id=00003816&cat=B3

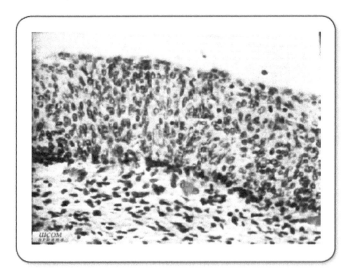

FIGURE 27.17 **Carcinoma in situ of the cervix.**
Source: https://screening.iarc.fr/atlashisto_detail.php?flag=0&lang =1&Id=00006993&cat=E2b

from the correct structural location, the specimen is considered to be neoplastic (malignant). For example, abnormal-appearing squamous epithelial cells that are contained by their basement membrane are non-neoplastic; they have not infiltrated the dermis (Figure 27.17). Once they have broken that barrier, however, they have become invasive, or malignant.

One entity that becomes unavoidable in dealing with non-neoplastic (and neoplastic) disease of the lower genital tract is human papillomavirus (HPV; ACOG, 2020b). HPV is discussed in detail in Chapter 32, Human Papillomavirus; however, a few points are emphasized here.

Some varieties of the more than 120 different types of HPV presently identified have been designated as high-risk type viruses. These are the types that are deemed causative of dysplasia of the cervix, vagina, and vulva (ACOG, 2020b). Dramatic accumulation and implementation of knowledge regarding the nature of HPV infection and the dysplasia it causes are currently underway. The results of initial inoculations of women in the general public using type-specific HPV vaccine are now being reviewed. Clinical trials have displayed nearly 100% efficacy in protecting against infection by these virus types (ACOG, 2020b). Among the four virus types covered by the quadrivalent vaccine are the most common high-risk types present today (HPV types 16 and 18). These two virus types are associated with almost 75% of cervical cancers. The vaccine is engineered to produce virus-like particles (VLPs), which stimulate recognition of the virus and initiate an immune response. The VLPs contain no genetic material, and thus cannot cause infection. Together with the VLPs for types 6 and 11, which prevents low-grade dysplasia and genital warts attributable to these viruses, the quadrivalent vaccine will hopefully reduce the incidence of cancer, just as it has proved to decrease the antecedent preinvasive diseases of the cervix, vagina, and vulva, as well as anal disease in homosexual men (Palefsky et al., 2011). Careful follow-up and epidemiologic studies will be required to measure the actual outcomes; however, optimism seems reasonable at the present time. Although pathologic conditions of the cervix will be most dramatically affected by this vaccine, it will also reduce vaginal and vulvar dysplasias.

VULVA/VAGINAL INTRAEPITHELIAL LESIONS
Etiology and Evaluation/Assessment

Vaginal intraepithelial neoplasia (VAIN) is analogous to cervical dysplasia; however, it is far less prevalent. Dysplasia in the lower genital tract is essentially a "field effect." Infection with HPV can lead to cellular changes in the epithelium of any genital tissue. Viral DNA can incorporate itself into cellular DNA and then alter cellular controls, creating a preinvasive condition. Lesions can be visualized within the vagina as whitened plaques on occasion; however, vaginal intraepithelial neoplasia is most frequently first detected as an abnormal Pap smear result with cervical cytologic screening. Although abnormalities are most commonly cervical, not all abnormal Pap smears will have a cervical origin; sampling of the cervix via spatula or brush cannot avoid the collection of epithelial cells from the vagina as well. The epithelia of the vagina and vulva have been similarly exposed to HPV and are therefore at risk of dysplastic change as well. The discrepant incidence of disease that occurs at the cervix is related to the special physiology of the squamocolumnar junction. Rapid turnover of cells in this region leads to the increased likelihood of abnormal growth. Dysplastic epithelial changes in the vagina progress slowly and are described similarly to those in the cervix. Low-grade infections, previously associated with either low- or high-risk HPV, are usually transient infections that may regress. High-risk HPV infections represent transformation that carries a risk of progression to invasive cancer being 2% to 12%. Presentation is most common with concurrent or preceding cervical dysplasia (cervical intraepithelial neoplasia [CIN]). Patients are largely asymptomatic; however, some do exhibit manifestations such as irritation, discharge, or bleeding.

Diagnostic Studies

Due to the lack of evidence-based screening strategies, identification most likely results with visual assessment confirmed by histopathology or from an abnormal cytologic smear. Cytologic smears are not site-specific; cells are collected from the vagina, ectocervix, endocervix, and possibly even the endometrium. Cytologic smears are interpreted by viewing cells without the benefit of the tissue structure surrounding them. Taken out of context, it is especially important to provide historical information to the pathologist to make evaluation more accurate and useful clinically. For example, all the following situations can alter the appearance of cells microscopically: the woman is postmenopausal, menstruating, or receiving estrogen therapy; the woman has a history of cervical dysplasia or cancer or has concurrent infection; or the sample is a smear of the vaginal apex after removal of the cervix. As stated previously, identification is most likely to occur because of an abnormal cytologic smear. Importantly, sampling of the vaginal apex in women who have undergone hysterectomy with a history of CIN II or greater remains important because VAIN II or greater will develop in as many as 7.4% of cases (Jhingran, 2022).

Once abnormal cytology has been discovered, colposcopic examination is used as the most effective means of investigating the extent of disease and selecting sites for biopsy. Shiller iodine stain is helpful in assessing the margins of the lesion. In women who have normal cervical colposcopy, special care is taken to view the proximal third of the vagina, where most vaginal lesions are located (Jhingran, 2022). Multifocal disease is the rule with VAIN. Thus, meticulous examination of the entire vaginal canal is imperative because skip lesions (islands of tissue abnormality in separate locations in the vagina) are frequently present (Disaia & Creasman, 2007). Biopsy sites are selected to include the most concerning locations. Local anesthesia, either topical or injectable, is used for vaginal biopsy procedures because they are significantly more painful than cervical biopsy procedures (Desaina & Creasman, 2007).

Treatment/Management

Management has taken many forms, including immunization with HPV vaccine, close clinical observation (for regression of low-grade lesions), surgical excision, topical chemotherapy, laser vaporization, and immunotherapy (Preti et al., 2022). Excision can be effective; however, the risk of vaginal stenosis (narrowing) is significant when areas of tissue are removed. Chemotherapy with 5-fluorouracil (5-FU) versus laser ablative therapy has shown comparable results. However, 5-FU can cause profound irritation when used for prolonged courses. There are numerous protocols attempting to minimize the caustic effects, with varying degrees of success. Basically, it still remains a fairly noxious, nonspecific treatment. Laser therapy can also be painful during the healing process. There are no perfect treatment options. However, the distribution of the laser's ablative effect is easier to control, which may limit the indiscriminant irritation of 5-FU contamination that is frequently external to the vulva. Imiquimod topical treatment has also shown promise when used in low-dose weekly treatments for 3 to 9 weeks (Preti et al., 2022). Imiquimod can also be associated with irritating symptoms but is well tolerated by most patients. Risk factors for recurrence following laser vaporization include age younger than 49 years and a disease classification of VAIN III (Kim et al., 2009).

Reports of the use of cavitational ultrasonic surgical aspiration (CUSA) are encouraging (Preti et al., 2022), albeit limited. This technology uses ultrasonic energy to lyse tissue via the generation of vacuoles within cells, and then aspirates the debris. There is a preferential destruction of cells with higher water content, therefore leaving vascular structures spared. It is effectively used in liver, neurologic, and gynecologic oncology surgeries because of this unique and desirable property. Treatments using CUSA have displayed lower recurrence rates (Preti et al., 2022). It also allows for easily directed effects with the handheld aspirator, leaving little collateral damage to surrounding tissues from thermal injury (Preti et al., 2022). Whatever treatment modality is selected, it is considered carefully with the woman because progression to invasive cancer is a possibility, especially with VAIN II and III lesions.

There is no clear consensus on follow-up regimens for VAIN treatment due to its low prevalence and therefore limited understanding of the natural history of the disease. Recent investigations have suggested that there is safety in annual cytology and colposcopy to follow affected patients as progression seems unlikely and resolution is very likely (Ao et al., 2022).

NEOPLASTIC VAGINAL DISEASE

Squamous Cell Carcinoma

ETIOLOGY AND RISK FACTORS

Cancer found in the vagina without clinical or histologic evidence of cervical or vulva cancer or a prior history is the strict definition of vaginal cancer per the International Federation of Gynaecology and Obstetrics (FICO). It is important to exclude other origins of cancer found in the vagina. True squamous cell carcinoma originating in the vagina is possible, but more frequently the vagina is the site of metastases from nearby pelvic organ cancer (uterus, endometrium, cervix, vulva) or from breast, kidney, or rectal cancer (Gurumurthy & Cruickshank, 2012). About 90% of primary vaginal cancers are of the subtype squamous cell and nearly two-thirds are HPV 16 related (Gurumurthy & Cruickshank, 2012). Although squamous cell carcinoma of the vagina is the most common form of vaginal cancer (approximately 85% of cases), malignancies of the vagina are extremely rare. The incidence of vaginal cancer is greater than that of vulvar cancer (Siegel et al., 2022; Jhingran, 2022). Vaginal cancer risk increases with age. Other risk factors include multiple sex partners, early intercourse before age 16 years, history of genital warts, and hysterectomy. Black and Hispanic women as well as women of Asian Pacific Island descent have both increased disease risk and decreased survival rates as compared to women of other ethnicities (Shah et al., 2009; Wu et al., 2008).

EVALUATION/ASSESSMENT AND DIAGNOSTIC STUDIES

Examination includes cytologic studies of the cervix and vagina in the event a lesion is not visible. Biopsy is imperative if lesions are seen. Promulgation could be via local invasion or via dissemination through the lymph-vascular space. Distribution to the paracolpos or pelvic organs can present with urinary tract symptoms if the lesion is located anteriorly. Similarly, posterior lesions can be symptomatic through the rectum; however, they are more commonly asymptomatic. Examination and investigation of metastasis do not overlook any of the possible sites of drainage.

A thorough physical examination is essential, noting location, gross morphology, sites of involvement, and dimensions of any visible palpable tumors. MRI is sensitive in detecting tumor size. PET/CT is the appropriate modality for assessing lymph node involvement or recurrence. Vaginal cancers are challenging to treat, and early detection is critical for early staging. Actively listening during all clinical encounters and intentional and strategic follow-up are key to early detection since no consensus exist on effective screening or effective regimens for treatment of vaginal cancer. As providers to women of all ages, please note that vaginal cancer is increasing in younger women mostly due to the increase in persistent HPV infection rates, especially in regions with high HPV prevalence.

TREATMENT/MANAGEMENT

Squamous cell carcinoma is managed according to staging of the tumor, as well as the health of the woman. There are circumstances when just surgical resection can be used, such as stage I disease of the proximal vagina. Surgery has a role that is limited and based on the proximity of the disease to other organs. Small stage I and II are defined as being contained to the upper posterior vagina. A radical hysterectomy and upper vaginectomy are treatment options. However, surgical intervention is contraindicated when the disease has metastasized or extended to the pelvic sidewalls. In these cases, pelvic exenteration (removing everything in the pelvis: bladder, reproductive organs, and rectum) would be ineffective. Decisions regarding treatment are individualized because no absolute consensus exists for all situations. In part, this may be due to the rarity of this disease entity. Radiation therapy is the treatment of choice in most patients (Jhingran, 2022). Chemotherapy plus radiation is most effective for stages II through IV, but radiation alone may be selected if chemotherapy is contraindicated. Radiation plus brachytherapy for treatment has shown favorable response (Meixner et al., 2021).

Survival is closely related to stage of disease Recurrence is a particularly disheartening occurrence; 80% recur within the first 2 years and 90% at 5 years (Jhingran, 2022). Follow-up after treatment includes visual inspection as well as cytology (Pap smear). For a person with stage I, the recommended scheduled surveillance is every 6 months for 2 years, then yearly for the remainder of their life. For all other stages, they would need to return every 3 months for 2 years, then every 6 months for 3 years, then annually if no recurrence.

Adenocarcinoma

ETIOLOGY

Adenocarcinoma of the vagina is also a rare entity; however, an increase in its incidence occurred in the generation following diethylstilbestrol (DES) use. DES was predominantly used during the 1940s and 1950s in high-risk pregnancies to reduce fetal loss, with some use continuing through the 1970s. Observant clinicians recognized the common history in a number of women identified with adenocarcinoma of the cervix and vagina, and DES was implicated as the causative factor (Herbst & Scully, 1970). DES-exposed women have approximately a 1% chance of developing a cervical or vaginal adenocarcinoma by age 24 years. Age of diagnosis heavily favors the early to mid-20s. Approximately 60% to 70% of cases of adenocarcinoma of the vagina during the late 20th century were associated with DES exposure. The incidence has dropped precipitously following the decline in the use of DES (shifted later in time by approximately 20 years). Adenocarcinoma has been noted to arise in the context of a variety of conditions (Lee et al., 2005; Tjalma & Colpaert, 2006). These represent rare occurrences and do not appear to indicate changing disease incidence; rather, they suggest heightened scrutiny and study of the disease. History of endometriosis is an example of a condition that can lead to the development of adenocarcinoma of the vagina, even after hysterectomy has been performed in postmenopausal women (Nomoto et al., 2010).

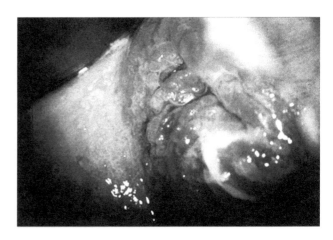

FIGURE 27.18 Vaginal adenosis.
Source: Hammes, B., & Laitman, C. J. (2003). Diethylstilbestrol [DES] update: Recommendations for the identification and management of DES-exposed individuals. Journal of Midwifery & Women's Health, 48(1), 19–29. https://doi.org/10.1016/s1526-9523(02)00370-7

EVALUATION/ASSESSMENT AND DIAGNOSTIC STUDIES

Carcinomas typically present with abnormal uterine bleeding in young women. Friable adenomatous tissue replacing more substantial squamous epithelium leads to irregular vaginal bleeding. Visual examination reveals the abnormal epithelium and prompts biopsy. Clinical findings include a glandular, velvety appearing vaginal epithelium, similar to vaginal adenosis (Figure 27.18), a "cock's comb" cervix (transverse ridges on the cervix), and hooding of the cervix by the anterior vagina. Biopsy is needed for diagnosis.

TREATMENT/MANAGEMENT

Management strategies include radical hysterectomy (removing much more of the supporting tissue lateral to the uterus [parametria] than standard hysterectomy), partial or complete vaginectomy, and radiation therapy. In very advanced disease, exenteration is a consideration. In very limited disease, it is possible to perform local excision and use limited radiation therapy to preserve function and fertility without a marked increase in recurrence risk (McNall et al., 2004). Referral to a gynecologic oncology specialist is necessary.

Melanoma

ETIOLOGY AND EVALUATION/ASSESSMENT

Melanoma is an extremely rare disease entity that can occur in the vagina. Melanoma has a remarkably poor prognosis in comparison to other vaginal cancers, with reported 5-year survival rates below 15% (Jhingran, 2022). Accumulation of data from the Surveillance, Epidemiology, and End Result (SEER) registry that identified about 200 patients with vaginal melanoma found 2- and 5-year survival rates of 24% and 15% (despite 46% of cancers diagnosed as stage 1; Kirschner et al., 2013). Presentation is most common with vaginal bleeding and/or mass (Jhingran, 2022; Gurumurthy & Cruickshank, 2012). Women over age 60 and White women are most at risk. These lesions are more common on the distal (closest to the introitus) anterior wall of the vagina (Jhingran, 2022).

TREATMENT/MANAGEMENT

Treatment can vary from exenteration (hysterectomy and vaginectomy) to wide local excision. Adjuvant therapies include radiation and chemotherapy. None of these is significantly effective with advanced disease.

Sarcoma

ETIOLOGY AND EVALUATION/ASSESSMENT

Sarcoma is also extremely rare and occurs more commonly in pediatric age groups than other gynecologic cancers, although the average age at diagnosis in the SEER registry data was 54 years. Of 4,000 vaginal cancers found over 22 years, 221 were sarcomas. Survival at 5 years was 89% for stage I disease and 47% for stage II disease, suggesting aggressive tumor behavior (Ghezelayagh et al., 2015). Diagnosis is made with the biopsy of suspicious lesions, typically a bulky lesion in the upper vagina. Types of sarcoma include leiomyosarcoma, rhabdomyosarcoma, mixed müllerian sarcoma, and endodermal sinus tumor, in decreasing order of frequency. Embryonal rhabdomyosarcoma (also known as sarcoma botryoides) is found in girls younger than 8 years of age. It is recognized because of its "bunch of grapes" appearance—a soft multiloculated mass occasionally protruding from the vagina. Leiomyosarcoma has been reported most commonly in the perimenopausal years.

TREATMENT/MANAGEMENT

Treatment is based primarily on conservation surgery (sparing the uterus and vagina) and, for embryonal rhabdomyosarcoma, chemotherapy. Survival rates in the pediatric age group can reach 90% in low-stage disease; however, metastatic disease will diminish survival rates to about 25% (Gurumurthy & Cruickshank, 2012; Jhingran, 2022).

BENIGN DISORDERS OF THE VULVA

Vulvar health continues to be a challenge for both patients and providers who assess, diagnose, and treat despite the challenge. Not doing so can have an overwhelming impact on women's overall health. Although vulvar health concerns are more common among the postmenopausal population, it is important not to dismiss concerns from women of all ages, as they are also impacted by these disorders. Because vulvar disorders are associated with signs and symptoms that resemble other disorders, a thorough medical history, physical examination including the vulva, and evaluation of vaginal fluid must be employed to elicit information not previously reported. This comprehensive approach not only allows women to openly speak about their concerns, but it also assists in building much needed trust and rapport with their provider, leading to faster, accurate diagnosis, treatment, and overall better health outcomes for all women dealing with disorder of the vulva.

The International Society for the Study of Vulvovaginal Disease (ISSVD) classified vulvar dermatoses based on histologic characteristics of disease state (ACOG, 2020a; Day et al., 2020; Stockdale & Boardman, 2018). Clinical diagnosis should not be based on biopsy results alone. In 2016, ISSVD updated their vulvar dermatoses classification to include categories. Within the categories, they placed the most common diagnosed vulvar disorders based on both pathologic and clinical data. Thus, although this current ISSVD recommendation, along with guidelines from ACOG and others, assists providers in developing a differential diagnosis that leads to timely and more accurate diagnosis and an individualized plan of care, it should not be all clinicians depend on before diagnosing or treatment women with vulvar dermatoses (ACOG, 2020a; Day et al., 2020; Rivera et al., 2022; Stockdale & Boardman, 2018). Despite having these resources available to assist in diagnosing vulvar disorders, incorporating the concerns of each individual woman dealing with disorders of the vulva is a must.

With experience and training, clinicians develop the capacity to recognize specific conditions and begin therapy regimens after completing a through physical examination and medical history review without the need of completing a biopsy or waiting for the results of one (Palacios, 2019; Rivera et al., 2022). When diagnosis is reached or high-risk lesions are highly suspected, creating and implementing therapeutic regimens that include short intervals of follow-up for assessment of disease resolution or effectiveness of therapy should not be delayed (Mauskar, 2021a; Rivera et al., 2022; Stockdale & Boardman, 2018). Biopsies, updated classifications, and guidelines such as the 2016 ISSVD terminology update (Bornstein et al., 2016) as well as other guidelines and recommendations are most useful in understanding diseases and their phenotypes, especially when a definite diagnosis is not reached, pathology results are delayed, and therapy has been initiated but the condition is not responding (ACOG, 2020a; Day et al., 2020). These tools should be used as needed without hesitation, they may provide timely diagnosis and treatment, leading to better health outcomes.

Vulvodynia

ETIOLOGY

Vulvodynia is considered a complex diagnosis characterized by continual vulvar pain lasting for a minimum of 3 months without a specific origin. Vulvar pain is typically localized to the vestibule, but it may also be diffused. Physical and visual investigation must be completed to rule out potential causes. Vulvar pain may be a result of yeast infection, sexually transmitted infections (STIs), injury, neoplasia, or side effects from medical procedures and medications. Despite resolution of original cause, due to the physiologic systems involved in vulvodynia (central nervous system pain pathways, pelvic floor musculature, and vestibular/vulva mucosa), pain is typically neurologic in nature and management must be specific to these pathways. Regardless of the impact vulvodynia has on overall health and quality of life, roughly 50% of persons afflicted request treatment, and when they do, the majority are misdiagnosed (Lewis et al., 2018; Palacios, 2019; Ringel & Iglesia, 2020; Stockdale & Boardman, 2018).

EVALUATION/ASSESSMENT

Persistent or recurring vulvovaginal manifestations may be difficult not only for the patients but also for healthcare practitioners when considering diagnosis and treatment. Once evaluation for potential triggers is completed, diagnosis is based on clinical assessment. Focus must be on the description of the pain (localized, generalized, provoked, spontaneous, or mixed). It is imperative to specifically ask when the symptoms began, how long does the pain last, where is the pain, what makes it worse or better, are symptoms related to the menstrual period, number of sexual partners, sexual activities, and whether there is any persistent or systemic illness that may contribute to the pain. In addition, a comprehensive physical exam must be included to confirm diagnosis of vulvodynia. Physical exam should include the cotton swab test. The cotton swab should create pressure in a circular fashion along the periphery of the vulvar vestibule, provoking pain even when gentle pressure is applied (Ringel & Iglesia, 2020; Stockdale & Boardman, 2018).

TREATMENT/MANAGEMENT

The complexity of the disease suggests that the treatment approach is multifaceted; no single treatment will work for all patients. Treatment needs to be understood as a process. Treatment starts with self-management, which includes easy adjustments in vulvar health (e.g., wear loose clothing, use mild soaps, and avoid any fragrances). Due to the complexity of vulvodynia, a multidisciplinary, multisystem approach or therapies (pelvic floor therapy, cognitive behavioral therapy, mindfulness-based stress reduction) may assist in the resolution of vulvar pain. Vulvodynia is considered neurologic in nature, which means oral agents (e.g., anticonvulsants, antidepressant), focusing on the central nervous system/pathways, and vaginal dilators (if constriction is confirmed) may need to be added to the physical and psychological therapies. These may be essential for patients suffering from severe localized vulvodynia without symptom improvement after physical, psychological, or oral therapies. Estrogen and or testosterone creams along with lidocaine ointment have not provided any evidence of efficacy and therefore should not be utilized to treat vulvodynia (Lewis et al., 2018; Palacios, 2019; Ringel & Iglesia, 2020; Stockdale & Boardman, 2018).

Lichen Sclerosus

ETIOLOGY AND EVALUATION/ASSESSMENT

Lichen sclerosus (LS) is considered a scarring inflammatory disorder, mostly affecting the vulva and anogenital area with documented cases affecting other parts of the body. LS is commonly related with the hypoestrogenic years of a woman's life as well as autoimmune disorders. Data reveal that women with LS are 30% more likely to also have an autoimmune disorder when compared to only 10% of those who do not have LS. Signs of autoimmune disorders have been found on the vulva, and in such cases these disorders are often mistakenly diagnosed as LS. Family history is particularly significant to explore since approximately another 30% had a positive family history of LS (Lee & Fischer, 2018; Nguyen & Corley, 2020; Stockdale & Boardman, 2018). Despite these statistics, and correlations, the exact origin of LS remains a mystery (Lee & Fischer, 2018; Nguyen & Corley, 2020; Rivera et al., 2022; Ringel & Iglesia; 2020; Spekreijse et al., 2020; Stockdale & Boardman, 2018). For those diagnosed with LS,

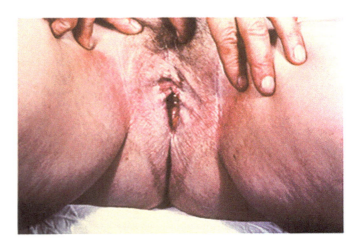

FIGURE 27.19 Lichen sclerosus.
Source: Gawlik, K. S., Melnyk, B. M., & Teall, A. M. (Eds.). (2021). Evidence-based physical examination: Best practices for health and well-being assessment. Springer Publishing Company.

typical symptoms may include, but are not limited to, pruritus, dyspareunia, burning, itching, scaring, abrasions, and sexual dysfunction. Presentation may be subtle or there may be no symptoms at all. Patients with LS are not only affected by physical challenges, but often endure mental health challenges, lifestyle disturbances, and disability (ACOG, 2020a; Mauskar, 2021b; Rees, 2021; Ringel & Iglesia, 2020; Rivera et al., 2022; Spekreijse et al., 2020). Available data show that approximately 1.7% of patients in one gynecology office are diagnosed with LS (Goldstein et al., 2005). This number is thought to be higher for the general population since 18% to 30% of women have no symptoms and therefore are not aware they have LS. Unfortunately, delay in diagnosis and treatment may lead to severe cases of LS and higher numbers of malignancy (ACOG, 2020a; Erni et al., 2021; Krapf et al., 2020; Lee & Fischer, 2021; Nguyen & Corley, 2020; Ringel & Iglesia, 2020; Spekreijse et al., 2020; Stockdale & Boardman, 2018).

The appearance of LS is unique to each individual and multifactorial. Thus, thorough examination of the external genitalia is imperative and the method of examination must be carefully individualized. Although presentation varies, affected areas are commonly described as being painful, and the skin looks inflamed, thin, crinkly, shiny (also described as parchment paper in appearance), white patchy, bleeding, thick, and fissured (Figure 27.19). Distribution is typically across the vulva, labia, and perineum, frequently extending to the perianal area. Often, diagnosis is made after inspection (Erni et al., 2021; Palacios, 2019; Ringel & Iglesia, 2020; Stockdale & Boardman, 2018).

TREATMENT/MANAGEMENT
Self-Management Measures

Self-care includes avoiding all possible irritants, which is extremely important for any woman who has lichen dystrophy or any other vulvar dystrophy. Several regimens are used (Box 27.1). It is important that the clinician employ a short interval for follow-up and reassessment. Incorporating practices that promote vulvar well-being is part of patient education and every treatment plan (ACOG, 2020a; Lewis et al., 2018; Nguyen & Corley, 2020; Stockdale & Boardman, 2018).

Box 27.1 Simple Perineal Care Regimen

Limit use of underwear whenever possible (air exposure is good).

When underwear is worn, use 100% cotton.

Do not use soaps, deodorants, or powders on the vulva (wash only with water; a gentle soap is used for the rest of the body; use only unscented toilet tissue and sanitary products).

Avoid abrading the skin (rinse after urination, pat the vulva dry with a soft cotton towel after voiding or bathing).

Avoid commercial vaginal lubricants.

TABLE 27.1 Suggested Clobetasol Treatment Regimen for Lichen Sclerosus

TIME PERIOD	FREQUENCY OF ADMINISTRATION
Weeks 1 to 6	Daily
Week 7: resolution (maintenance)	Two to three times per week

Pharmacotherapeutics

Empiric therapy is usually initiated based on clinical examination and biopsy when needing confirmation. Over the years with increased research and surveillance in this area, treatment of LS has evolved from testosterone and estrogen with the occasional low dose of corticosteroid when nothing else worked, to a consensus that high or medium potency corticosteroids (Table 27.1) such as clobetasol propionate 0.05%, triamcinolone acetonide 0.5%, desoximetasone 0.05%, and hydrocortisone butyrate 0.1% work and can be used as first line of treatment for LS. Data show that the benefits of these medications outweigh the risks of their use in the anogenital area when used based on the severity of the disease and the specific treatment plan is patient centered. Frequency of use is typically titrated down from daily to several times a week, to once a week, after weeks or months until symptom improvement is evident or an adverse reaction has occurred (ACOG, 2020a; Lewis et al., 2018; Nguyen & Corley, 2020; Stockdale & Boardman, 2018). Ointments are preferred over creams or other formulations because of the lower incidence of causing aggravation of disease. While complete resolution can be achieved, women will frequently have recurrent symptoms and require repeated courses of therapy or a combination of agents. Changing to a low potency steroid is advisable for maintenance therapy. Testosterone and estrogen should not be used to specifically treat LS due to the ineffectiveness in resolving or improving LS. Atrophy is less likely when using high or medium potency corticosteroid, if used appropriately. If atrophy becomes a concern, titration to a lower dose is recommended. Due to the high incidence of recurrence, lack of symptoms, or patients not seeking care in a timely manner, the need for surveillance and close follow-up

once treatment has begun, even if remission is obtained, must be understood by both the patient and provider (ACOG, 2020a; Lewis et al., 2018; Nguyen & Corley, 2020; Stockdale & Boardman, 2018). Calcineurin inhibitors are usually only used when topical steroid has failed as the first line of therapy. Other therapeutic regimens have been used without evidence of efficacy (ACOG, 2020a; Krapf et al., 2020; Stockdale & Boardman, 2018).

Other topical medications (immunosuppressive agents, immunomodulators), such as tacrolimus (Protopic) and pimecrolimus (Elidel), have been used, with 43% of patients in one study having resolution of LS by the 24th week of treatment (Lee & Fischer, 2018). Although those are promising outcomes, there may be a hypothetical concern, but nonetheless an important one. Local immunosuppressive medications may add to the risk for the development of vulvar cancer given the relationship of LS and squamous cell carcinoma as well as with the use of pimecrolimus therapy (Lee & Fischer, 2018). Laser (ablative) therapy may be helpful as an add-on therapy for those with hyperkeratotic disease but is not a replacement for topical corticosteroid (high, medium potency). While phototherapy effectiveness has been reported in treating anogenital LS, as well as the use of narrow-band UVB therapy as an add-on therapy to treat extragenital LSs, the question of safety has been raised concerning the relationship of LS and cancer and the increased risk that is present when using phototherapy (Lee & Fischer, 2018).

Hyperplastic Squamous Vulvar Conditions

ETIOLOGY, EVALUATION/ASSESSMENT, AND DIFFERENTIAL DIAGNOSIS

Conditions related to squamous overgrowth generally present with raised, whitened epithelium. Intense pruritus is a hallmark of change and may lead to the histologic changes of thickening and acanthosis (hyperkeratosis and thickened malpighian ridges, respectively). The most notable diagnosis among these is lichen simplex chronicus; however, other similar-appearing acanthotic dermatoses are possible. The patient's accompanying history may include insatiable itching. This pruritus may exacerbate, or even be the source of, the hyperplasia. Excoriations can result, complicating appearance as well as intensifying symptoms to include pain. Examination shows thickened whitened areas diffusely distributed over the vulva. Distribution tends to be on the labia majora, from clitoris to anus, bilaterally. Excoriations may be present as a result of the trauma of scratching.

TREATMENT/MANAGEMENT

In addition to self-care that employs a strict perineal regimen (Box 27.1), treatment consists of potent corticosteroids. Approximately 83% of women have exhibited complete resolution of disease using topical steroid, oral antipruritic, and vulva care (ACOG, 2020a). Investigation into alternative methods has been reported; however, topical ointments remain the preferred medication (ACOG, 2020a). Clinical resolution may require as long as 8 weeks; therefore, additional medication to mitigate pruritus, such as nonsedating antihistamines, is necessary.

Lichen Planus

ETIOLOGY

Lichen planus (LP) is considered an inflammatory disease affecting both typical skin and mucous membranes, thus making LP a multisystem disorder. Although its origin is not known, LP is thought to be an autoimmune disorder with T cell–mediated immunity disruption. As with LS, autoimmune diseases are also seen within the LP population. While the numbers of those with LP range between 1% and 2% of the overall U.S. population, LP mostly impacts women in the perimenopausal and menopausal stages of their lives (ACOG, 2020a; Stockdale & Boardman, 2018).

SYMPTOMS AND EVALUATION/ASSESSMENT

Presentation of LP varies depending on the severity of the disease and the affected area. LP typically presents with white, netlike patches, fernlike striae (Wickham striae), glossy purple pustules, dark pink genital lesions, inflammation, bleeding, scarring, and ulcerated areas. Other symptoms are pruritus, burning, pain, synechiae, and architectural changes. Unlike LS, LP is unlikely to present without symptoms. With tissue destruction, a copious malodorous discharge may be present. While the vulva may be the most common area of presentation, oral LP is seen in up to 75% in those with erosive vulvar LP, and for this reason, a comprehensive head-to-toe physical examination is imperative. Referral to a dental provider must be done with LP of the oral cavity (ACOG, 2020a; Day et al., 2020; Krapf et al., 2020; Stockdale & Boardman, 2018). Documentation of examination must be concise and descriptive including other disease (LS, autoimmune disease), site (color, shape, distinction), and features (appearance, margins, architectural changes). As with any other examination, thorough documentation of findings is needed to support diagnosis (ACOG, 2020a; Day et al., 2020; Krapf et al., 2020; Stockdale & Boardman, 2018).

TREATMENT/MANAGEMENT
Self-Management

Self-management begins with self-identification of any item responsible for irritating the affected areas. Incorporating practices that promote vulvar well-being must be part of patient education and every treatment plan (ACOG, 2020a; Nguyen & Corley, 2020; Lewis et al., 2018; Stockdale & Boardman, 2018).

Pharmacotherapeutics

Despite the increase in research and attention to this area of study, evidence remains scarce on a gold standard approach to grade or assess vulva diseases and an approach to treat LP. As with other inflammatory dermatoses, treatment is usually initiated based on clinical examination, impact of disease on patient's life, and biopsy of suspicious lesions or with lack of improvement with treatment. In addition, the experience of a provider along with the rapport with the patient might either facilitate or hinder the treatment implementation process (ACOG, 2020a; Krapf et al., 2020; Rivera et al., 2022; Stockdale & Boardman, 2018). The recommendation is to begin therapy with high to medium potency topical corticosteroids. Typically corticosteroids are used twice a day, with strength and frequency of use decreased as symptoms improve. Surveillance of symptom resolution and follow-up should be within 2 to 3 months after beginning therapy (ACOG, 2020a; Lewis et al., 2018; Nguyen & Corley, 2020; Stockdale & Boardman, 2018). Careful consideration should be given to the use of topical calcineurin inhibitors for patients with LP not responding to topical high or medium potency corticosteroid. Prior to the start of topical calcineurin inhibitors, it is important to provide patient education and review documentation of the Food and Drug Administration (FDA) black box warning of possible risk of malignancy related with these medications as well as the unidentified lasting safety profile (ACOG, 2020a). For those suffering from erosive LP extending to the vagina, intravaginal corticosteroids may be used as an adjunct to topical vulvar therapy. Patients using hydrocortisone acetate 25 mg suppositories intravaginally two times a day noted significant relief in burning, itching, pruritus, and vaginal discharge, as well as redness and tissue damage, although vaginal strictures did not change. As with LS, other therapeutic regimens have been used without evidence of efficacy (ACOG, 2020a; Krapf et al., 2020; Stockdale & Boardman, 2018).

Lichen Simplex Chronicus

ETIOLOGY

Lichen simplex chronicus (LSC) is a chronic inflammatory disorder of the skin, often confused with local atopic dermatitis. Persistent itching and constant scratching create scaling, or thick and leathery superficial skin lesions (lichenified plaques). As with the LS and LP, LSC's etiology is not known, but this skin disorder typically occurs in women in mid to late adult life, although it can happen at any age. Approximately, 65% to 75% of patients with LSC also suffer from allergic disorders (hay fever, asthma, childhood dermatitis). LSC of the vulva is approximately 10% to 35% of patients presenting to specialty clinics, which is thought to be approximately 0.5% of the U.S. population. Biopsy is typically not necessary for diagnosis as LSC can be diagnosed after a comprehensive history and physical exam. LSC has an uncommon relationship with malignancy (ACOG, 2020a; Stockdale & Boardman, 2018).

TREATMENT/MANAGEMENT

Patients complain of the inability to sleep at night due to scratching while asleep or being unable to stop once awake. The goal of treatment is to stop the immune response to irritants, thus stopping the itch-scratch cycle by identifying the cause of the problem (e.g., chronic yeast infection identified with culture). In addition, patient education should include measures to be taken by the patient to prevent and control symptoms through self-management and good anogenital hygiene by using 100% cotton unscented menstrual pads, silicone-based lubricants during intercourse, and only water when cleaning the vulva. Pharmacotherapy usually includes a medium or high potency topical corticosteroid ointment as well as an oral antipruritic if needed. Frequency of topical corticosteroid application may be once or twice a day. A 4-week follow-up from the start of treatment is recommended those using topical high potency corticosteroids. Strength of topical corticosteroids and how often they are used must be determined by the effect on LCS.

Strength and frequency must be decreased when adequate response has occurred, but not before, as response may be inadequate if strength and frequency are not sufficient. For those suffering from daytime itching or unable to take antihistamines (e.g., hydroxyzine) or calming agents (e.g., amitriptyline), selective serotonin reuptake inhibitors (e.g., fluoxetine, paroxetine, sertraline, or citalopram) may be considered as an adjuvant option. Relapse of disease is common, though remission is possible (ACOG, 2020a; Stockdale & Boardman, 2018).

Vulvar Squamous Intraepithelial Lesions

ETIOLOGY AND TERMINOLOGY

Terminology surrounding vulvar squamous intraepithelial lesions (LSIL, low-grade SIL of the vulva, or vLSIL) has played a significant role in diagnosis and treatment in past decades. Concerns over terminology mainly derived from the possibility of overdiagnosing and overtreating, and the possible consequences related to this. The goal of current terminology is to enhance pathologic precision and present the benign nature of LSIL (previously known as vulvar intraepithelial neoplasm I [VIN I]). LSIL is mostly related to HPV, more specifically low-risk HPV subtypes 6 and 11, which presents as genital warts (flat condylomata), and resolution is often spontaneous, thus posing a low to no risk for malignancy development (ACOG, 2020b; Bornstein, Bogliatto et al., 2016; Dockery & Soper, 2021; Garland et al., 2018; Huang & Lokich, 2022). Like precancerous disease of the cervix and vagina, LSIL is less common than cervical intraepithelial neoplasia (CIN), yet slightly more common than vaginal disease. Multiple sexual partners, cigarette smoking, history of STIs, and immunosuppression are risk factors associated with LSIL. LSIL and CIN may present simultaneously (Dockery & Soper, 2021; Huang & Lokich, 2022). The most affected age groups have traditionally been perimenopausal and menopausal women in the sixth decade of life, although the mean age at diagnosis has decreased, with increase in younger women as a probable result of the increase of high-risk HPV subtypes (Dockery & Soper, 2021; Eva et al., 2020; Huang & Lokich, 2022). High-grade squamous intraepithelial lesion (HSIL) was previously referred to as VIN II-III (also known as vulvar squamous dysplasia needing treatment). Since HPV disrupts both cellular and molecular levels (field effect), cancer of the vulva increases the likelihood of cervical dysplasia (Eva et al., 2020; Huang & Lokich, 2022). Those with vulvar dermatoses (differentiated vulvar intraepithelial neoplasia [dVIN, not HPV dependent], LS) are at greater danger of acquiring invasive carcinoma of the vulva (Dockery & Soper, 2021; Eva et al., 2020; Huang & Lokich, 2022). Current terminology should mimic that of cervical diseases using LSIL or HSIL. This nomenclature was adopted at a consensus conference attended by several professional organizations in 2015, the ISSVD being one (Bornstein, Goldstein et al., 2016; Bornstein et al., 2019; Radici et al., 2020).

SYMPTOMS, EVALUATION/ASSESSMENT, AND DIAGNOSTIC STUDIES

Presenting symptoms may include irritation, bleeding, pain, dyspareunia, and fissured areas, without resolution. Evaluation is systematic and precise. Findings can vary from

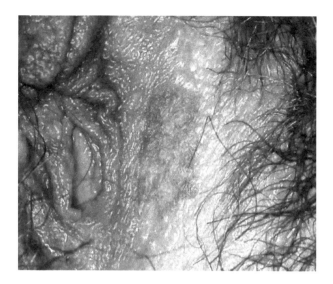

FIGURE 27.20 Vulvar intraepithelial neoplasia, hyperpigmented.

whitened areas to hypopigmented or hyperpigmented skin to reddened, pronounced, and hypopigmented or hyperpigmented skin (Figure 27.20). Abnormal tissue can be seen anywhere from the clitoral hood to the anus, most commonly in the inferior labia and perineum. Examination with colposcope is often useful in viewing impacted areas. Confirmation exists that acetic acid and toluidine blue enhance visualization of active lesions. Unfortunately, diagnosis of dVIN remains a challenge because all lesions look different and resemble other lesions as well as there not being a standardized assessment tool available. Consequently, large sections of atypical vulvar epithelium may appear, of which little warrants aggressive action. Therefore, acetic acid and toluidine blue are best in highlighting areas of greatest significance for which biopsy may support seriousness of disease. A cohesive approach of evaluation has yet to be acquired for HSIL, making a comprehensive history a crucial element, along with visualization during a regular gynecologic exam, or exam provoked by suggestive symptoms, resulting in biopsy of atypical areas. Palpation and visualization of lymph nodes, perianal area, and pubis must be included in the examination to identify possible lesions. Documentation of such requires anatomic location, whether the lesion is single or multifocal, whether edges are uniform or irregular, color, thickness, and if there are any unusual blood vessels noted (Dockery & Soper, 2021; Garland et al., 2018; Huang & Lokich, 2022).

TREATMENT/MANAGEMENT

Although it is a reasonable and common clinical practice to treat presumptively once for "yeast" or other infection (such as bacterial vaginosis), it is important to note that self-diagnosis is far from accurate and that continued "infection" may actually indicate VIN.

In addition to careful perineal care (Box 27.1), management is either via excision or by ablation (most commonly laser, cryotherapy, or even chemotherapy). Excision is preferable because it yields a surgical specimen that can be evaluated for invasive disease, thereby providing the opportunity to ensure no invasion following treatment (Penna et al., 2002).

To reduce the number of lesions reappearing, an extensive lesion removal is recommended and usually done for vulvar dysplasia. An atypical appearing lesion needs to be completely removed to avoid the chance of it returning. Though a well-defined compromise regarding the how wide a margin around a lesion should be when surgically removed, the side borders should be between 5 mm and 10 mm to reduce the chances of the lesion returning. When margins are negative, there is only a 15% to 17% chance of lesions returning as opposed to a 46% to 50% chance of lesions returning within 5 years if margins are positive. The likelihood of lesion return is higher for multifocal lesion and growth of HSILs in a different location. Negative margins for HSILs only decrease the chance for the lesion to return to the same site but it may grow in a different location of the vulva (Dockery & Soper, 2021; Huang & Lokich, 2022). A younger patient with an HPV-related multifocal VIN is a perfect patient for laser ablation management of the lesion because the danger of developing aggressive cancer in a healthy younger population is small. Older patients are best treated with surgical intervention. Low-risk genital warts can be managed with shallow vaporization as opposed to management of VIN, which must include deeper level of tissue reaching hair follicles for treatment to be effective (Dockery & Soper, 2021). Surgical management is typically reserved for HSIL and differentiated VIN (dVIN), which are considered high risk for development of aggressive cancer. While these options produce positive resolution, they are also painful as the tissue heals; painful scar tissue is possible and disfigurement can certainly occur (Dockery & Soper, 2021; Huang & Lokich, 2022).

Additional choices for treatments of VIN include topical therapy with immune-modulating agents and antiviral therapeutics. Imiquimod is an immune-modulating medication used on the vulva to create a focus of immune reaction of affected area. Release of cytokine adds effectiveness of natural killer cells to attack HPV-infected and oncogenic cells. Imiquimod has been approved for management of HPV-related condyloma or LSIL. Although it has not been approved for the management of HSIL, because of its 5% effectiveness on these lesions, it is used off label. Usual treatment plan is to apply imiquimod to each abnormal lesion sparingly three to five times each week on alternating days for 16 weeks. Side effects may include pain at location of application, swelling, vaginal discharge, redness of application site, and tissue destruction (Dockery & Soper, 2021; Huang & Lockich, 2022).

Although fluorouracil is an effective treatment option with high resolution of HSIL, it is infrequently utilized because the side effects (burning, pain, inflammation, edema, ulcerations) are not tolerated by patients. Fluorouracil produces chemical peeling of HSIL. Cidofovir is a nucleoside equivalent being tested to possibly manage HSIL. It works by stopping viral DNA polymerases. The recommended treatment dose is cidofovir 1% to affected area three times a week for 24 weeks. Documented findings suggest that cidofovir may be as effective as imiquimod. It is suggested that follow-up of HSIL and dVIN after treatment should be every 6 months for the first 2 years, then every year after that (Dockery & Soper, 2021; Huang & Lokich, 2022).

Special attention is to be given to individuals with HIV because of the greater danger of producing lower genital dysplasia because of the inability to get rid of HPV infections. A retrospective study found that 87% of 107 women with VIN who were HIV positive had cervical and vaginal dysplasia at the same time, as opposed to only 43% of patients without HIV. This finding requires more surveillance to assess for development of invasive carcinoma of the vulvar, cervix and vagina (Huang & Lokich, 2022).

NEOPLASTIC VULVAR DISEASE

Squamous Cell Carcinoma

ETIOLOGY

VIN is an abnormal overgrowth of cells in the basal layer of the vulvar epithelium, and it is the originator of squamous cell carcinoma (SCC), which is the most ubiquitous cancer impacting the vulva, accounting for 80% and 90% of vulvar cancers. The progression of SCC occurs through two conduits: HSIL or dVIN, which may be HPV dependent (hdVIN) or non-HPV dependent (nVIN). There is a direct correlation between HPV, smoking cigarettes, and HSIL, while LS or LP (inflammatory disorders) are precursors to hdVIN (Eva et al., 2020; Michalski et al., 2021). Women between ages 30 and 50 present with higher numbers of HSIL, while hdVIN is more often seen in women between 60 and 80 years old. The danger increases as women age, based on history of VIN, LS, delayed diagnosis, and not completing treatment plan. Data show there has been a considerable surge of hdVIN-related cancers and of vulvar SCC (0.55/100,000 from 1991 to 2000 to 0.83/100,000 from 2001 to 2016), and the majority of those affected are over age 50 (0.75/100,000 to 1.43/100,000). These numbers corroborate this rise in vulvar cancer because there is a higher load of HPV with a considerable rise in all hdVIN SCC. The numbers of nVIN SCC in women over 50 has drastically gone down from 2.53/100,000 to 1.62/100,000. The ratio of hdVIN SCC has risen from 25% to 51% (Eva et al., 2020; Michalski et al., 2021; Spekreijse et al., 2020).

SYMPTOMS, EVALUATION/ASSESSMENT, AND DIAGNOSTIC STUDIES

Symptoms may include itching that does not go away, pain, tenderness, bleeding (late stages), skin changes (color changes, thickening), warty lesions, or ulcers. Rarely, and equally reliant on the size and site of the lesion, SCC of the vulva can appear as pain with evacuation or micturition, discharge, or tenderness when seated. There are several influential histologic subsets of SCC: Verrucous SCC (exophytic warty growths that push into the dermis; Figure 27.21) presents with a small amount of irregularity, but lots of pale eosinophilic cytoplasm with low nuclear-to-cytoplasmic ratio), sarcomatoid (has morphologic structures of a sarcoma), showing malignant rod cells. Cancerous cells are organized in sheets, fascicles, or storiform pattern), and infiltrative (they are present as one cell or strings of cells spreading into the derma and hypodermic tissue. They can spread into the lymphatic system and reappear outside the excision's border. Radiation therapy must be contemplated as adjunct after the removal of an infiltrative

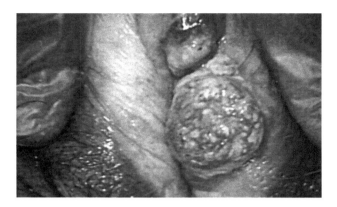

FIGURE 27.21 **Vulvar squamous cell cancer.**

tumor). Unfortunately, these symptoms are typically present long before someone presents for care, and it may be too late. Education is needed for both patient and provider regarding need for immediate action (Michalski et al., 2021). In past years, there has been substantial advances in diagnosing and treatment of vulvar cancers. This is important because delaying care, misdiagnosing, or inexperience in assessing or managing vulvar SCC may have consequences. The outcome and the overall health of those seeking care for what is perceived to be a vulvar malignancy is very much dependent mainly on a comprehensive history and physical examination with biopsy when necessary. Biopsy is a must for all questionable lesions, as well as lymphatics testing to confirm disease and staging. Most vulvar cancers progress from the labial skin because of the delay in seeking treatment or underdiagnosing. Vulvar cancer is easy to recognize due to the appearance of the lesion. In addition, if vulvar SCC is present, assessing the lymph nodes is of utmost importance. Generally, distribution is superficial to the ipsilateral inguinal femoral nodes and then deep to the obturator and pelvic iliac nodes. Rarely, deep nodes can be positive without evidence of disease at the superficial femoral nodes. Although ipsilateral dissemination is typical for most tumors that are lateral of midline, for example, in the mid-labia, tumors located near the clitoris or perineum can present with positive nodes to either side. Distant spread of disease is possible via a hematogenous route, most commonly arising in the lung (Eva et al., 2020; Michalski et al., 2021; Spekreijse et al., 2020). Staging methods have been put together by both the International Federation of Gynaecology and Obstetrics (FIGO) and the American Joint Committee on Cancer (AJCC) recommendations. FIGO and AJCC staging/grading system is centered on the main lesion (T), lymphatic system participation (N), and remote metastasis (M; TNM). As of 2021 FIGO has updated its staging criteria utilizing a new method. The new method examined newly analyzed information regarding cancer of the vulva to confirm the prognosis ability of staging at the time of publication. This update includes a new description for extent of infiltration; it utilizes the same description for lymph node metastasis used in cervical cancer, allowing results from partial imagery to be included into vulvar cancer staging. FIGO's updated staging for cancer of the vulva is a lot easier than previous modifications (Eva et al., 2020; Michalski et al., 2021; Olawaiye et al., 2021; Spekreijse et al., 2020).

TREATMENT/MANAGEMENT

Management of a suspicious cancerous lesion of the vulva begins with a comprehensive medical history and evaluation. Treatment of SCC typically involves multiple modalities (surgical and radiation). Chemotherapy or other systemic approaches are infrequently utilized. Quality of life must be considered since treatment may be extensive and overall quality of life and health will be greatly affected (Eva et al., 2020; Merlo, 2020; Michalski et al., 2021). Recommendations for management are delineated by the National Comprehensive Cancer Network (NCCN) and depends on stage of the disease. Stages I and II (early stage, no lymph node association). For localized lesions stage IA (≤2 cm, with ≤1 mm stromal involvement), the management options are a wide local excision (WLE), with 1- to 2-cm surgical borders. Data from clinical trials have not demonstrated any substantial evidence of reappearance in patients managed with WLE versus vulvectomy. Sentinel lymph node biopsy and lymphadenectomy are not mandatory for those with stage IA since the danger of lymph node invasion is small.

For stage 1B (>1 mm stromal involvement) or stage 2 (≤4 cm and tumor is 1 cm from the median line), the recommendations are WLE or a modified radical vulvectomy and ipsilateral sentinel node biopsy (SNB) or inguinofemoral lymph node removal since the danger of invasion goes up by 8%. If the tumor is within 2 cm of the median line, a WLE and removal of inguinofemoral lymph nodes from both sides are needed. When the lesion has locally progressed (stage 2 >4 cm and stage 3) and lymph nodes are positive, removal of the inguinofemoral lymph nodes should be completed; recommendations also call for chemotherapy and external beam radiation therapy focused on the main lesion with or without groin nodes. Data show the greatest indicator of local management is a 1-cm surgical border (Eva et al., 2020; Merlo, 2020; Michalski et al., 2021). Attempts to preserve the anatomy and structures are made; however, the main objective is removal of malignancy with as little chance of recurrence as possible.

Melanoma

ETIOLOGY AND EVALUATION/ASSESSMENT

Different from melanoma on other areas of the body that have been exposed to UV light, the etiology of vulvar melanoma is unclear. Mucosal melanomas are typically not greatly exposed to UV light and significant destruction. Melanoma of the vulva is uncommon, and the prognosis is not favorable. It makes up between 5% and 10% of vulvar cancers, placing it as the second most occurring cancer of the vulva. White women between ages 50 to 70 are the most afflicted by melanoma of the vulva. Lesions typically are found on the labia, and can emerge as nodules, papules, and macules with irregular margins and atypical colors, making it difficult to distinguish from a noncancerous lesion. For this reason, when doubts of cancer arise, a biopsy must be obtained. Those affected may complain of itching, pain, and bleeding, yet early tumors may present without symptoms. Diagnosis is commonly late, placing the 5-year survival rate between 10% and 63% (Eva et al., 2020; Merlo, 2020; Michalski et al., 2021).

TREATMENT/MANAGEMENT

In the past, radical vulvectomy was considered the standard practice for cancer of the vulva; however, morbidity is considerable for those undergoing this treatment. Over time, and with more evidence, wide local excision has become the standard of care for melanoma of the vulva because there is no evidence that having a radical vulvectomy decreases the chances of recurrence more than WLE. The NCCN recommends margins for melanoma in situ be 0.5 cm, melanoma with Breslow depth ≤2 mm with 1-cm borders, and melanoma with Breslow depth >2 mm with 2-cm borders. Despite WLE being the preferred treatment for melanoma of the vulva, staged removal could be an option in the future. The predictability of nodal spread has led to the evaluation of sentinel lymph node. Those with node involvement have the choice of lymph node removal or surveillance. While there is a rise in cancer-free survival, it does not enhance the total survival rate. Classification based on the AJCC for cutaneous melanoma are also applicable to melanoma of the vulva (Michalski et al., 2021; Wohlmuth & Wohlmuth-Wieser, 2021).

Traditionally, cutaneous melanoma has not responded to radiation; for this reason, adjunct radiation treatment is not recommended for melanoma of the vulva. Nevertheless, inseveral instances radiation therapy has been utilized as an adjunct, showing improved control of local cancer but not overall survival rate. Unlike radiation therapy, chemotherapy has not shown any increase in survival and therefore is not recommended in the management of melanoma of the vulva. No other treatment has shown significant evidence of overall survivability in patients with melanoma of the vulva and no other treatments are ecommended at this time (Eva et al., 2020; Merlo, 2020; Michalski et al., 2021).

Adenocarcinoma

ETIOLOGY AND EVALUATION/ASSESSMENT

Primary adenocarcinoma is an uncommon histologic variant of vulvar cancers. Although the majority of adenocarcinoma of the vulva originates from Bartholin glands, other adenocarcinomas reported include mammary gland adenocarcinoma, Skene gland adenocarcinoma, intestinal-type adenocarcinoma, and Paget disease. One study reported two cases with origin from high-risk HPV (subtype 16) adenocarcinoma (Chow et al., 2020; Nishio et al., 2021; Voltaggio et al., 2019). Most occur in postmenopausal women. Therefore, any enlargement in Bartholin glands in this population is treated with the utmost suspicion. Presentation can be with mass, dyspareunia, or ulceration. Because of the possible metastasis from the breast, a thorough physical examination including the breasts needs to be completed. High rates of lymph node involvement can occur, and distant metastasis is a distinguishable characteristic of adenocarcinoma (Chow et al., 2020; Maccio et al., 2021).

TREATMENT/MANAGEMENT

Surgical intervention (wide local excision or radical vulvectomy and inguinal lymphadenectomy) in combination with regional radiotherapy is the typical treatment modality. Chemotherapy is seldom used. Physiologic assessment of the sentinel lymph node is demonstrative of all additional lymph nodes in the region and physiologically, a negative sentinel node means no metastasis in the other adjacent nodes. Spread to regional lymph nodes significantly diminishes the likelihood of survival. The reason for adjuvant radiation therapy is to decrease the possibility of localized reappearance of disease and increase the overall survival rates. Because of the rarity of vulvar cancer, management outcomes are with no consensus on a specific treatment for adenocarcinoma of the vulva. The benefit of radiation therapy will be dependent on both the patient and the specifics of the individual tumor. Although chemotherapy is not endorsed to be used individually before or after surgery, it can be utilized along with radiation (chemoradiotherapy) alone or before surgery in patients with progressive tumors. These have demonstrated 5-year survival rates and thus represent reasonable treatment options for select patients. Minimally invasive methods, sentinel lymph node biopsy (standard treatment in chosen circumstances) versus removing inguinofemoral nodes, has considerably enhanced quality of life and decreased morbidity among patients with vulvar cancer (Kurita et al., 2019; Merlo, 2020; Nishio et al., 2021).

Basal Cell Carcinoma

ETIOLOGY AND EVALUATION/ASSESSMENT

Approximately 2% to 3% of vulvar cancer is basal cell carcinoma (BCC), mainly impacting women in their 70s, and presenting mostly on the labia majora. BCC has historically originated from basal cell nevus syndrome and exposure to UV light (questionable because of the location), with a small number said to arise from LS or extramammary Paget disease. Although presentation may vary, it is typically a disease that presents as a single pink or skin-colored lesion, but it may present on both sides of the labia, with symptoms such as bleeding, ulceration, pruritus, and/or pain. Historically most lesions are categorized as nodules and have exceptionally good outcomes (Furlan et al., 2020; Merlo, 2020; Michalski et al., 2021; Tan et al., 2019).

TREATMENT/MANAGEMENT

BCCs are managed with various approaches such as cryotherapy, imiquimod, radical vulvectomy (not used as often), WLE, or Mohs micrographic surgery (MMS). The high number of recurrences (10% to 25%) are perhaps due to partial removal of lesion or insufficient borders. For these reasons, MMS should be taken into consideration as it may facilitate enhanced overall outcomes for patients with BCC (Furlan et al., 2020; Merlo, 2020; Michalski et al., 2021; Tan et al., 2019).

Paget Disease

ETIOLOGY, EVALUATION/ASSESSMENT, AND DIAGNOSTIC STUDIES

Another condition that arises elsewhere in the body and occurs in the vulva is Paget disease. Characterized by erythematous, well-demarcated lesions along with areas of indurated, excoriated thickening, it presents with pruritus and pain in older women, remote from menopause; some may have no symptoms for years. Tumors may be complex and appear anywhere on the vulva. The main cause of the disease has not been truly identified, though one theory is that it arises from the mammary-like glands between the labia majora and labia minora (interlabial) sulci, perineum, or perianal region. The other proposition is that it originates from Toker cells (cytokeratin 7-positive clear cells). It can be associated with an underlying adenocarcinoma; therefore, it is important for the clinician to conduct the clinical examination with a level of suspicion and to perform adequate biopsy of the area, which may be an indication for fine-needle aspiration. Paget disease is inconsistent; it may be slow or rapid growing depending on clinical course it creates, and it may resemble other types of lesions, making it difficult to diagnose, postponing diagnosis an average of 2 years. After it infiltrates the dermis, it can rapidly progress through the lymph nodes or hematologic paths (Furlan et al., 2020; Merlo, 2020; Michalski et al., 2021; Tan et al., 2019).

TREATMENT/MANAGEMENT

Treatment is dependent on the type of lesion; primary lesions are treated with surgical removal (standard), despite there being a 12% to 58% reappearance of lesions irrespective of border status. CO2 laser ablation has been used successfully but may be related to extreme pain after the procedure and an elevated danger of reappearance. Topical 5% imiquimod cream has shown total resolution of extramammary Paget disease (EMPD). In addition, treatment with trastuzumab plus paclitaxel has shown success with lasting outcomes. Additional treatments that are used for primary Paget disease are adjuvant radiotherapy, photodynamic therapy, bleomycin, and 5-fluoroucacil, and adjuvant therapies (surgery followed by imiquimod or laser ablation) have provided different results depending on the lesion and overall patient history. Because secondary EMPD typically only impacts the epidermis, it is treated with either ablation or shallow excision, taking care of the entire lesion (Michalski et al., 2021; Tan et al., 2019).

Sarcoma

ETIOLOGY AND EVALUATION/ASSESSMENT

Sarcomas of the vulva are even more rare than cases of melanoma, BCC, and Paget disease. They may present with or without symptoms, which is the reason why they may be misdiagnosed, and treatment delayed. The labia majora is the most affected region. Sarcomas of the vulva mainly affect women of reproductive age. Outcome will be dependent on type, size, reappearance, time of diagnosis, timing, and type of treatment. Poor prognosis is attributable to early metastasis and rapid growth. There are several types of sarcomas of the vulva; proximal-type epithelioid sarcoma (PES) is characterized as having negative overall outcomes, whereas extraskeletal Ewing sarcoma (EES) has better outcomes, with a mean age of first diagnosis being 27.6 years (median: 26, range 10—52 years), which assists in the overall outcome of those impacted by this sarcoma. Other sarcomas such as rhabdomyosarcoma have also been identified. Sarcomas of the vulva are extremely rare, and more studies are needed to distinguish between all possible subtypes (Babu et al., 2020; Sundaram et al., 2018).

TREATMENT/MANAGEMENT

Due to the rarity of studies of sarcomas of the vulva, it is challenging to provide specifics regarding how any lesion will progress or how to best treat it. Sarcomas are mainly diagnosed through biopsy and histopathology. Management of PES includes WLE with proper border status. Management of these lesions remains a challenge. Despite established guidelines and recommendations, sarcomas of the vulva are managed like other soft tissue sarcomas (adjuvant radiotherapy and chemotherapy) with inadequate control and worse outcomes. For those affected by metastasis, management will be mainly palliative in nature. Timely diagnosis and adjuvant treatment may be necessary for better outcomes. Management of EES typically incorporates both surgical excision and chemotherapy. Radiation may enhance regional control. Standard chemotherapy agents include doxorubicin, vincristine, and cyclophosphamide, interchanging ifosfamide and etoposide. Once the maximum dose of doxorubicin is reached, antinomycin D will then be started. Outcomes are multifactorial dependent; therefore, timely referral, diagnosis, and treatment are imperative (Babu et al., 2020; Sundaram et al., 2018).

SPECIAL POPULATIONS AT RISK FOR VAGINAL AND VULVAR CANCERS

Many factors contribute to healthcare disparities, some of which are inherited, but many of which are social and have opportunities for improvement. The National Institutes of Health defines disparity as "differences in incidence, prevalence, mortality and burden of cancer and adverse related conditions that exist among specific populations" (Borrell & Vaughan, 2019).

Of the biological risks related to cancer outcomes, genetic predisposition to cancer cannot be altered, but as the science of cancer research evolves, screening for vulnerability and individualizing treatment based on one's genetics, should cancer develop, can reduce the burden that is borne with illness.

In the United States, race unfortunately has a very high impact on all epidemiologic measures of gynecologic neoplasia. The Centers for Disease Control and Prevention reports cancer statistics for White (Caucasian), Black (African American), Hispanic, and Asian American ethnic groups. Black men and women are more likely to die from cancer than any other racial group (Chatterjee et al., 2016). When examining specifically vaginal and vulvar cancers, Black women are more likely to present for care at a younger age, with advanced disease, and are less likely to receive treatment (Doddi et al., 2023). It is beyond the scope of this chapter to delve into all the factors related to healthcare racial inequality in the United States; the purpose is to provide the clinician with heightened awareness when caring for a woman of color.

The possibly modifiable determinants of cancer-related disease have been identified as:

1. Geographic (access to hospitals and specialized medical care from gynecology-oncologists, treatment variations from institutions)
2. Research-based discrepancies (lack of access/inclusion in clinical trials)
3. Socioeconomic and insurance status

Geographic access is defined as access to a gynecologist/oncologist provider and treatment center within 50 miles of residence; 81% of Americans reside in an urban or suburban area, which translates into a greater likelihood of medical center access. However, an adjunct to the risks associated with access is the volume of a particular cancer that institution treats per year. Low volume is defined as less than seven cases per year. Hospitals with low volume of vulvar and vaginal cancer diagnoses may not offer the most up-to-date treatment regimens (Chatterjee et al., 2016).

Disparities in care and outcomes are also affected from the input during the treatment research process. Geographic remoteness as well as minority status hinders the recruitment of diverse cohort participants. Those with logistic concerns or language barriers are not encouraged as much as others to join clinical trials. This limits access to treatment both immediately (not being able to join an ongoing study) and in the long term (results not necessarily effective for a minority).

Health insurance status and socioeconomic status can lead to disparities in cancer burden. Women who have Medicaid as opposed to Medicare or a private insurance are less likely to get surgery when treating vulvar and vaginal cancers. Lower socioeconomic status is associated with an increased rate of cancer and death, regardless of ethnicity. Persons with lower socioeconomic status have a higher likelihood of presenting with an advanced stage of cancer and are less likely to receive standardized treatment (Johnson et al., 2023; Kamat et al., 2023).

The final special population to be considered is transgender persons. ACOG (2021) reports that there are 1.4 million adults and 150,000 youths in the United States that report as transgender. In their committee statement, they support "any anatomical structure that warrants screening should be screened, regardless of gender identity." From a clinical perspective, providers need awareness about the individual for whom they are caring to offer the appropriate exam and screening.

As this situation applies to vaginal and vulvar cancers, the authors concentrate on transgender men (persons born biologically female but identify as male). These patients may be in any stage of gender affirmation transition. Some may not have used any testosterone or had any surgical procedures; some may have had removal of the breast tissue and pelvic female organs and/or closure of the vagina. The authors support the ACOG recommendations about screening anatomic parts that need screening. The evidence that is currently available does not show any increased risk for cancer from the use of testosterone. At this time, the current literature admits that the quality of available studies regarding this possible risk is low due to small sample sizes and less robust study designs.

Transgender persons are included in this disparity section due to reports of less access to care. Information gathered from studies reveals transgender persons perceive many barriers to appropriate healthcare such as cost of surgery and hormones, inadequate care from providers (knowledge deficit), and outward hostility and harassment. Transmen report more negative attitudes from providers than transwomen. Some transmen are uncomfortable with vaginal/cervical exams and thus are not getting regular screening. One study reported 50% of the respondents had not had a Pap screening in the past 4 years and 32% reported no Pap screening at all. Although hormone therapy does not increase one's risk for cancer, transgender persons have increased cancer-related factors such as tobacco use and alcohol abuse. Included with these related risks are early age at first intercourse, increased risk for HPV infections, more lifetime sexual partners, and decreased use of condoms (Stenzel et al., 2020).

As with all diseases, people present for care with inherited risks, modifiable risks, and lifestyle risks. Clinical excellence is achievable when current and future practitioners providing care to females customize the care for the population they serve by recognizing and incorporating strategies that target surveillance, detection, and treatment for those individuals based on sex and self-identifications.

FUTURE DIRECTIONS

There are numerous conditions that affect the health and well-being of the vulva and vagina. It can take years of practice for the clinician to recognize the conditions presented in this chapter and incorporate them into the lexicon of existing disease states. Initial conservative therapy is often reasonable, such as following a strict perineal care regimen; however, biopsy will be needed for clear diagnosis to guide management in many instances. Referral to a specialist is suggested when the woman's symptoms are not resolving, when diagnosis is uncertain, and when specialty care intervention is needed. Added research on less invasive diagnostic techniques and treatment modalities are ongoing and will shape the future of identifying and treating these conditions.

REFERENCES

References for this chapter are online and available at https://connect.springerpub.com/content/book/978-0-8261-6722-4/part/part03/chapter/ch27

CHAPTER 28

Perimenstrual and Pelvic Symptoms and Syndromes*

REGINA A. MCCLURE, JACQLYN C. SANCHEZ,[†] GRETCHEN E. SZYMANSKI,[†] AND ELIZABETH A. KOSTAS-POLSTON[‡]

Menstruation has a symbolic meaning within all cultures. Attitudes and beliefs about menstruation are culturally defined and typically handed down from mother to daughter. It is postulated that milestones experienced by women, such as menarche, pregnancy, and menopause, contribute to bodily based experiences that bring women in closer contact with the realities about their body to develop a language for talking about any illness (Charteris-Black & Seale, 2010). Socialization about menstruation contributes to individual appraisal of perimenstrual symptoms.

Well-woman examinations provide an excellent opportunity for healthcare providers to educate women about normal hormonal changes and remedies to ameliorate symptoms within the normal expectation. However, for some women, the hormonal changes associated with menstruation or uterine structural abnormalities bring extreme pain, emotional changes, and/or excessive blood loss that negatively influence their lives. This chapter provides an overview of the etiology, symptoms, evaluation, and management of abnormal uterine bleeding (AUB), amenorrhea, premenstrual syndrome, menstrual headaches, and dysmenorrhea.

FEDERATION OF GYNECOLOGY AND OBSTETRICS NOMENCLATURE AND PALM-COEIN CLASSIFICATION SYSTEM

The International Federation of Gynecology and Obstetrics (FIGO) systems for nomenclature of symptoms of normal and AUB in the reproductive years were designed to be flexible

and to be periodically reviewed and revised as needed (Munro et al., 2018). The latest revisions were published in 2018. The FIGO systems came about for a variety of reasons. For example, experts felt that the old FIGO nomenclature (e.g., dysfunctional uterine bleeding, menorrhagia, menometrorrhagia, metrorrhagia, oligomenorrhea) was not useful in helping clinicians delineate etiology and clinical management. Furthermore, terms were poorly defined and used inconsistently among healthcare providers in the United States and abroad. Regarding classification, experts determined that there existed a wide spectrum of potential causes of abnormal menstrual bleeding and that a new classification system would streamline research, education, and clinical care (Munro et al., 2018). For example, if a woman was diagnosed with endometrial hyperplasia and ovulation dysfunction with no other abnormalities, she would be categorized as AUB P_0 A_0 L_0 M_1-C_0 O_1 E_0 I_0 N_0. Recognizing that the full notation might be cumbersome, the full notation can be abbreviated: AUB – M;O (American College of Obstetricians and Gynecologists [ACOG], 2012). Although the new FIGO nomenclature and PALM-COEIN classification systems were announced a decade ago, many healthcare providers continue to use the old terminology. This chapter introduces and utilizes the new nomenclature and classification system (Figure 28.1).

MENSTRUAL CYCLE

In order to address abnormal perimenstrual conditions, it is important to first understand the normal menstrual physiology. Normal cyclic uterine bleeding is dependent

---

*This chapter is a revision of the chapter that appeared in the second edition of this textbook, coauthored with Candy Wilson, and we thank her for her original contribution.

[†]The opinions and assertions expressed herein are those of the author(s) and do not necessarily reflect the official policy or position of the U.S. Air Force, Department of Defense, or the U.S. government.

[‡]The opinions and assertions expressed herein are those of the author(s) and do not necessarily reflect the official policy or position of the Uniformed Services University or the Department of Defense.

Abnormal Uterine Bleeding (AUB)
- Heavy Menstrual Bleeding (AUB/HMB)
- Intermenstrual Bleeding (AUB/IMB)

PALM: Structural Causes
- **P**olyp (AUB-P)
- **A**denomyosis (AUB-A)
- **L**eiomyoma (AUB-L)
  - Submucosal Myoma (AUB-L_{SM})
  - Other Myoma (AUB-L_O)
- **M**alignancy & Hyperplasia (AUB-M)

COEIN: Nonstructural Causes
- **C**oagulopathy (AUB-C)
- **O**vulatory Dysfunction (AUB-O)
- **E**ndometrial (AUB-E)
- **I**atrogenic (AUB-I)
- **N**ot otherwise classified (AUB-N)

FIGURE 28.1 PALM-COEIN abnormal uterine bleeding classification.
Source: Adapted from Munro, M. G., Critchley, H. O. D., & Fraser, I. S. (2018). The two FIGO systems for normal and abnormal uterine bleeding symptoms and classification of causes of abnormal uterine bleeding in the reproductive years: 2018 revisions. International Journal of Gynecology & Obstetrics, 143(3), 393–408. https://doi.org/10.1002/ijgo.12666

on the complex interaction among the hypothalamus, the anterior lobe of the pituitary gland, and the ovaries. Increasing estrogen levels secreted by the follicles within the ovaries result in proliferation of the endometrium. Following ovulation, the corpus luteum continues to produce estrogen, but more importantly, the corpus luteum becomes the source of progesterone. Together these hormones stabilize the endometrium and prepare it for implantation of a blastocyst, should fertilization occur. If fertilization and implantation do not occur, the corpus luteum degenerates and the resulting drop in hormone levels leads to withdrawal bleeding. An intact coagulation pathway is also important in the regulation of normal menstruation. For example, deficiency of platelets or abnormal platelet function can result in profound changes in the menstrual cycle (e.g., heavy bleeding of longer duration). Usual menstrual flow begins every 24 to 38 days with regularity and lasts 4 to 8 days. Normal cycle length variation of 7 to 9 days is age dependent, and this variation is often expressed as ±4 days (Munro et al., 2018). The average volume of menstrual blood loss is less than 80 mL (Critchley et al., 2020). A structural menstrual history aids in the assessment of the patient.

ABNORMAL UTERINE BLEEDING

Definition and Scope

AUB originates from the uterine corpus and is a disturbance of the cyclic bleeding pattern of menstruation in nonpregnant reproductive-age women. AUB is a symptom, not a diagnosis, and the term is used to describe bleeding that falls outside population-based 5th to 95th percentiles for menstrual regularity, frequency, duration, and volume (Wouk & Helton, 2019). Altered menstrual patterns or volume of menses blood flow negatively affect quality of life (QOL) and contribute to financial loss, decreased productivity, poor health and well-being, and increased use of healthcare resources in premenopausal women (Wouk & Helton, 2019). The estimated prevalence of AUB in fertile age women is 10% to 30% and up to 90% in perimenopausal women (Belcaro et al., 2020). AUB may be acute or chronic and associated with heavy menstrual bleeding (HMB) or intermenstrual bleeding (IMB; Wouk & Helton, 2019; see Table 28.1).

HEAVY MENSTRUAL BLEEDING

HMB is the most common complaint of AUB (Singh et al., 2013) and is designated by the abbreviation AUB/HMB. Clinical definitions of HMB include the psychosocial aspect.

TABLE 28.1 Issues Affecting Quality of Life in Women With Abnormal Uterine Bleeding

ISSUE	DESCRIPTION
Irritation and inconvenience	Related irritation and inconvenience of unscheduled and/or heavy bleeding episodes
Bleeding-associated pain	Affected by severe cramping pain during heavy bleeding episodes
Self-conscious about odor	Concern that other people could be offended by perceived odor during menstrual bleeding
Social embarrassment	Embarrassing episodes involving staining clothing and/or furniture because of heavy flow or blood clots and/or unpredictable menstrual bleeding
Ritual-like behavior	Described routines and practices aimed at avoiding all possibilities of an embarrassing situation in which clothes could be stained in public: • Carry hygiene products at all times. • Try to anticipate/predict bleeding episode. • Avoid social activities. • Schedule activities according to availability and proximity to bathroom.

Source: Adapted from Matteson, K. A., Munro, M. G., & Fraser, I. S. (2011). The structured menstrual history: Developing a tool to facilitate diagnosis and aid in symptom management. Seminars in Reproductive Medicine, 29(5), 423–435. https://doi.org/10.1055/s-0031-1287666

HMB is defined as excessive menstrual blood loss that interferes with a women's physical, emotional, social, and material QOL (National Institute for Health and Care Excellence [NICE], 2021).

Chronic HMB (formerly known as *menorrhagia*) is defined as AUB that has occurred for 6 months, as compared with acute, which is defined as an episode of bleeding that can be emergent, requiring immediate intervention to prevent excessive blood loss. Intermenstrual bleeding (formerly known as *metrorrhagia*) is defined as spontaneous bleeding that occurs between menstrual periods and can be either cyclic or random (Munro et al., 2018). Terminology previously used to describe AUB was based on Greek and Latin words, leading to ambiguity in meaning and usage. Therefore, women's health experts recommended changing the terminology.

INTERMENSTRUAL BLEEDING

IMB refers to AUB that occurs at any time during the menstrual cycle other than during normal menstruation. According to the FIGO nomenclature, IMB is designated as AUB/IMB. It is often difficult to differentiate IMB from irregular, frequent periods. Similar to AUB/HMB, AUB/IMB is a symptom, not a diagnosis, and warrants follow-up evaluation (Table 28.2).

ETIOLOGY AND COMPONENTS OF PALM-COEIN CLASSIFICATION SYSTEM

Menstrual bleeding that causes a woman to alter her lifestyle or causes anxiety warrants a thorough history, assessment, and physical evaluation to determine the etiology and any indicated intervention(s), which should focus on improving her QOL as

TABLE 28.2 Symptoms of Abnormal Uterine Bleeding

CHARACTERISTIC	TERMINOLOGY (ABBREVIATION)	DESCRIPTION
Disturbances of heaviness of flow (patient determined)	Heavy menstrual bleeding (HMB) Heavy and prolonged menstrual bleeding (HPMB) Light menstrual bleeding	Excessive menstrual blood loss that interferes with a woman's physical, emotional, social, and material QOL; can occur alone or in combination with other symptoms Less common and is important to make a distinction from HMB as may have different etiologies and respond to different therapies Based on woman's complaint
Disturbances of regularity (normal variation ≤7–9 days)	Irregular menstrual bleeding (IrregMB)	A variation in menstrual regularity where the shortest to longest variation is 7–9 days, depending upon age (18–25 years ≤9 days; 26–41 years ≤7 days; 42–45 ≤9 days), and can also be expressed as ±4 days
Disturbances of frequency (normal every 24–38 days)	Absent menstrual bleeding (amenorrhea) Infrequent menstrual bleeding Frequent menstrual bleeding	No bleeding in a 90-day period Bleeding at intervals >38 days apart (one or two episodes in a 90-day period) Bleeding at intervals <24 days apart (more than four episodes in a 90-day period)
Disturbance of duration of flow (normal ≤8 days)	Prolonged menstrual bleeding	Describes menstrual blood loss that exceeds 8 days in duration
Irregular, nonmenstrual bleeding	Intermenstrual bleeding (IMB) Postcoital bleeding Premenstrual and postmenstrual spotting	Irregular episodes of bleeding, often light and short, occurring between otherwise fairly normal menstrual periods Bleeding postintercourse Bleeding that may occur on a regular basis for 1 or more days before or after the recognized menstrual period
Bleeding outside reproductive age	Postmenopausal bleeding (PMB) Precocious menstruation	Bleeding occurring more than 1 year after the acknowledged menopause Bleeding occurring before 9 years of age
Acute AUB	Acute AUB	An episode of bleeding in a reproductive-age woman, who is not pregnant, that is of sufficient quantity to require immediate intervention to prevent further blood loss
Chronic AUB	Chronic AUB	Bleeding that is abnormal in duration, volume, and/or frequency and has been present for most of the past 6 months

AUB, abnormal uterine bleeding; QOL, quality of life.
Source: Adapted from Munro, M. G., Critchley, H. O. D., & Fraser, I. S. (2018). The two FIGO systems for normal and abnormal uterine bleeding symptoms and classification of causes of abnormal uterine bleeding in the reproductive years: 2018 revisions. International Journal of Gynecology & Obstetrics, 143(3), 393–408. https://doi.org/10.1002 /ijgo.12666; Singh, S., Best, C., Dunn, S., Leyland, N., Wolfman, W. L., & Clinical Practice—Gynaecology Committee. (2013). Abnormal uterine bleeding in pre-menopausal women. Journal of Obstetrics and Gynaecology Canada: JOGC, 35(5), 473–479. https://doi.org/10.1016/S1701-2163(15)30939-7

opposed to focusing on blood loss. (ACOG, 2012; NICE, 2021). Pregnancy is the primary reason for AUB. Healthcare providers should consider gynecologic structural defects or systemic sources as possible causes of AUB, once pregnancy has been ruled out. FIGO developed a classification system that relates solely to assessment and management of nongestational AUB, and the system delineates the nine categories that cause AUB (Munro et al, 2018). This classification is known by the acronym PALM-COEIN: polyp (AUB-P), adenomyosis (AUB-A), leiomyoma (AUB-L), malignancy and hyperplasia (AUB-M), making up the PALM portion of the acronym; and coagulopathy (AUB-C), ovulatory disorders (AUB-O), endometrial (AUB-E), iatrogenic (AUB-I), and not otherwise classified (AUB-N), making up the COEIN portion of the acronym. PALM describes structural causes that can be identified by visualization and/or histopathology. COEIN describes nonstructural sources that are not defined by imaging or histopathology (Figure 28.1). The AUB-N category includes a spectrum of potential causes that may or may not be measured or defined by histopathology or imaging (Munro et al., 2018).

Polyps (AUB-P)

Polyps are hyperplastic overgrowths of endometrial glands, stroma, and blood vessels that project from the lining of the endometrium. They are identified and evaluated using transvaginal ultrasonography (US) and/or hysteroscopic examination. Saline infusion sonography enhances the view of the uterine cavity and is the gold standard for diagnosing polyps (Nijkang et al., 2019). Endometrial polyps are the most frequently observed pathologic finding in the uterus, and they can occur in both reproductive and postmenopausal age women. The majority of them are asymptomatic and usually discovered incidentally. However, as much as 50% of polyp cases do cause AUB and 35% contribute to infertility or pregnancy complications (Nijkang et al., 2019). For women with symptoms, the symptoms do not necessarily correlate with the size, location, and/or number of polyps present (Salim et al., 2011; Smith & Netter, 2008). While there is some potential for malignancy, approximately 95% of symptomatic polyps are benign, and the risk of malignancy is even lower in premenopausal years (Wouk & Helton, 2019). It is thought that polyps produce local inflammation, which in turn contributes to AUB and infertility (Nijkang et al., 2019). Though the exact cause remains unknown, genetic factors may contribute to the development of endometrial polyps. Risk factors for the development of endometrial polyps include age, hypertension, obesity, and tamoxifen use. Conflicting evidence exists as to whether increased estrogen and progesterone receptor concentrations contribute to the development of polyps. Small asymptomatic polyps (<1 cm) often resolve spontaneously, as compared with polyps that are 1.5 cm or greater, which may require medical and/or surgical intervention (Nijkang et al., 2019). Polyp regression may be associated with isolated events of HMB and cramping, followed by the resumption of normal menstruation (Yuksel et al., 2021).

Adenomyosis (AUB-A)

Adenomyosis is a benign condition of the uterus in which endometrial glands and stroma occur pathologically in the myometrium (Vannuccini & Petraglia, 2019). The incidence of adenomyosis ranges from 5% to 70% and its association with AUB is unclear (Wouk & Helton, 2019). One third of women with adenomyosis are asymptomatic, and those with symptoms may present with AUB, dysmenorrhea, dyspareunia, or infertility (Vannuccini & Petraglia, 2019). Traditionally this condition was attributed to women age 40 or older, multiparous, or with a history of cesarean section or other types of uterine surgery. However, recently, in addition to this traditional risk factor profile, due to improved imaging techniques, adenomyosis is more frequently diagnosed in young fertile-age women (Vannuccini & Petraglia, 2019). Vannuccini and Petraglia (2019) do note that despite the improvements in diagnostic tools the diagnosis of adenomyosis without hysterectomy remains difficult and unclear.

Leiomyomas (AUB-L)

Uterine leiomyomas (fibroids) are benign neoplasms that develop from uterine smooth muscle and can grow into enlarged pelvic masses that cause AUB and pelvic pain (Wouk & Helton, 2019). Age is the most common risk factor, with a lifetime risk in women older than 45 years being more than 60%. Leiomyomas are located on the uterus or cervix and any number of fibroids can be present at one time. The size and site influence the symptoms experienced. There are three types of fibroids based on location: intramural, serosal, and submucosal. The most common fibroid, intramural, develops within the myometrium. Serosal fibroids arise from the external surface of the uterus. Submucosal fibroids develop near the inner surface of the endometrium and are likely to cause HMB and infertility (Black et al., 2013).

The etiology of fibroids is unknown, but several correlates have been identified including African or Caribbean ethnicity, obesity, nulliparous, polycystic ovary syndrome (PCOS), late menopause, early menarche, hypertension, and a family history of fibroids (Giuliani et al., 2020). Hormone levels associated with pregnancy promote fibroid growth, whereas during menopause, when hormone levels decrease, fibroids tend to shrink. Fibroids can also undergo pathologic changes including hyaline degeneration, cystic degeneration, calcification, infection (abscess formation), and necrobiosis. Even though most leiomyomas are asymptomatic, approximately 30% of women will have severe symptoms such as AUB, anemia, pelvic pain and pressure, back pain, urinary frequency, constipation, or infertility. These severe symptoms require intervention (Giuliani et al., 2020).

Malignancy and Premalignant Conditions (AUB-M)

AUB-M includes both premalignant and malignant lesions. Even though the incidence of endometrial cancer increases with age, nearly 25% of newly diagnosed cases occur in women younger than 55 years old (Wouk & Helton, 2019). AUB is the *primary* symptom of endometrial neoplasia. Risk factors for atypical hyperplasia or endometrial cancer include advanced age, nulliparity with a history of infertility, obesity, polycystic ovaries, a family history of endometrial or colon cancer, and/or a history of tamoxifen use (Dunneram et al., 2019; Lee et al., 2020).

Coagulopathy (AUB-C; Systemic Disorders of Hemostasis)

Coagulopathy is defined as a spectrum of systemic hematologic disorders that impede the blood's ability to coagulate, potentially triggering AUB (Munro et al., 2018). One example of a coagulopathy that causes AUB is von Willebrand disease. Von Willebrand disease is a genetic hemorrhagic disorder caused by a missing or defective clotting protein (von Willebrand factor), which leads to impaired primary hemostasis (ACOG, 2013b). Approximately 13% of women who present with complaints of extended and extensive vaginal bleeding (AUB) will be diagnosed with von Willebrand disease (Munro et al., 2018). When collecting a thorough structured patient history, healthcare providers have a high probability of diagnosing bleeding disorders (see Box 28.1).

Ovulatory Disorders (AUB-O)

Ovarian dysfunction (formerly classified as *dysfunctional uterine bleeding* [DUB]) produces a progesterone deficient/estrogen dominant state that leads to the sustained proliferation of the endometrium but without the cyclic shedding induced by progesterone withdrawal (Wang et al., 2020). AUB-O often manifests as an irregular, often infrequent, and unpredictable menstrual flow that ranges from absent or minimal to heavy. Endocrine conditions (e.g., PCOS, uncontrolled diabetes mellitus, thyroid disorders, hyperprolactinemia) interfere with the hypothalamic–pituitary–ovarian (HPO) axis, and can lead to ovulatory dysfunction (ACOG, 2013c; Wouk & Helton, 2019). Wouk and Helton (2019) also list intense exercise or stress, and starvation (e.g., eating disorders) as additional causes of AUB-O. Gonadal steroids or drugs that affect dopamine metabolism, such

as phenothiazines and tricyclic antidepressants, may contribute to anovulation by raising prolactin levels (Munro et al., 2011). It is common for ovulation to be infrequent or absent during the first few years following menarche and during the perimenopause period and this irregularity does not necessarily denote underlying pathology (Wouk & Helton, 2019).

Endometrial Causes (AUB-E)

When a woman's ovaries are producing predictable and cyclic menstrual patterns, yet she is experiencing AUB, this is highly suggestive of an abnormality that resides in the endometrium (Wouk & Helton, 2019). The pathophysiology of endometrial dysfunction is not well understood and is likely due to vasoconstriction disorders, inflammation, or infections (Wouk & Helton, 2019). At present, there are no reliable diagnostic tests available for detection of abnormalities related to AUB-E and the diagnosis should not be made without excluding other causes (Wouk & Helton, 2019).

Iatrogenic Causes (AUB-I)

Gynecologic and nongynecologic interventions can be the source of AUB-I. Iatrogenic causes include contraceptive use (e.g., intrauterine devices/systems, medroxyprogesterone injections, progestin-only birth control pills, etonogestrel implants) and treatment with exogenous gonadal steroids (e.g., estrogens, progestins, androgens) and systemic agents that affect blood coagulation or ovulation. Abnormal bleeding (unscheduled) after initiation of a contraceptive method containing gonadal steroids is not unusual for the first 3 to 6 months. Anticoagulants and tricyclic antidepressants can cause AUB-I.

Not Otherwise Classified (AUB-N)

AUB-N is reserved for entities that are rare, or poorly defined and not well understood or studied (e.g., arteriovenous malformation [AVM]; Wouk & Helton, 2019). Complications related to undiagnosed pregnancy, genital tract trauma, foreign bodies in the reproductive tract, and cigarette smoking are thought to be possible sources of AUB-N (Black et al., 2013). This classification includes conditions such as AVMs and a lower segment or upper cervical isthmocele, which is uterine scar defect or cervical niche that is caused by previous cesarean delivery (Munro et al., 2018).

Risk Factors

Many of the risk factors were discussed in the earlier section. Women with AUB are more likely to be younger, White, and obese than women without AUB (Matteson et al., 2013). The family history, particularly the history of a woman's mother or sister, can provide great insight into potential cause(s) for AUB.

Symptoms

ACOG has suggested that healthcare providers use the menstrual cycle as a vital sign, differentiating between normal and abnormal menstrual bleeding (ACOG, 2015). Abnormal

---

Box 28.1 Structured History to Screen for Coagulopathies (AUB-C) or Disorders of Systemic Hemostasis

1. Heavy menstrual bleeding since menarche?

2. One of the following:
   - Postpartum hemorrhage?
   - Surgical-related bleeding?
   - Bleeding associated with dental work?

3. Two or more of the following symptoms:
   - Bruising once or twice a month?
   - Epistaxis once or twice a month?
   - Frequent gum bleeding?
   - Family history of bleeding symptoms?

Note: Consider coagulopathy testing for the following criteria: (a) heavy menstrual bleeding since menarche, (b) one item from Item 2, or (c) two or more items from Item 3.
Source: Munro, M. G., Critchley, H. O. D., & Fraser, I. S. (2018). The two FIGO systems for normal and abnormal uterine bleeding symptoms and classification of causes of abnormal uterine bleeding in the reproductive years: 2018 revisions. International Journal of Gynecology & Obstetrics, 143(3), 393–408. https://doi.org/10.1002/ijgo.12666

bleeding patterns often precipitate a visit to a healthcare provider's office for evaluation and workup. Symptoms of abnormal bleeding may include (a) bleeding heavier or for more days than normal, (b) leaking or soaking through clothing or having to change pads and/or tampons overnight, (c) bleeding between periods, (d) bleeding after intercourse, (e) spotting anytime in the menstrual cycle, and/or (f) bleeding after menopause (ACOG, 2012; Samuelson Bannow et al., 2021). Women who present with abnormal menstrual bleeding may also experience symptoms of anemia (e.g., fatigue, loss of concentration, headaches, easy bruising, restless legs, hair loss, and pica; Samuelson Bannow et al., 2021) and/or symptoms of thyroid, pancreas, or pituitary disorders. In all cases, it is important to determine whether the abnormal menstrual bleeding is of clinical significance.

Evaluation/Assessment

Diagnosis of AUB requires a detailed history, thorough physical examination, appropriate laboratory tests, and diagnostic imaging. Determination of laboratory and diagnostic imaging should be individualized.

MEDICAL HISTORY

A woman's medical history is perhaps the single most important tool used when evaluating AUB. Detailed information regarding intermenstrual intervals, duration of bleeding, volume, and the onset of abnormal menstrual bleeding can provide essential clues about possible etiology and can help guide determination of diagnostic imaging. When collecting a woman's medical history, it is important to consider other factors (e.g., age, weight, previous menstrual patterns, and other medical problems). Predictable cyclic menses every 24 to 38 days, even though heavy in nature, are generally associated with ovulation (Munro et al., 2018).

In contrast, ovarian dysfunctional bleeding is usually irregular and unpredictable, variable in amount and duration, and most often observed in adolescents and perimenopausal women as well as in obese women and those with PCOS. Regular cycles that are increasing in amount and/or duration of bleeding or chronic AUB/IMB superimposed on regular cycling may be associated with uterine structural lesions such as polyps or myomas (Singh & Belland, 2015). In reproductive-age women, AUB is often associated with pregnancy or complications of pregnancy such as abortion or miscarriage, abruption or subchorionic hemorrhage, and ectopic pregnancy (Wouk & Helton, 2019). If a woman presents with AUB/HMB from menarche or gives a history of frequent epistaxis or bleeding gums with brushing of teeth, or past episodes of excessive bleeding from trauma or surgery, she should be suspect for a coagulation disorder (Box 28.1; Munro et al., 2018). It is important to note that adolescents who present with a hemoglobin (Hb) of less than 10 g/dL and/or require a blood transfusion have an increased risk (20%–30%) for coagulopathy. Women with endometrial hyperplasia or adenocarcinoma often have a history of anovulation with long-term unopposed estrogen exposure. When obtaining a woman's medication history, it is important that the healthcare provider ask about prescription medications, over-the-counter (OTC) vitamins, and herbal remedies

that may contribute to or cause AUB (e.g., warfarin, heparin, nonsteroidal anti-inflammatory drugs [NSAIDs], hormonal contraceptives, gingko, ginseng, motherwort; ACOG, 2012).

Blood loss greater than 60 to 80 mL per menstrual cycle is typically associated with iron deficiency anemia (ACOG, 2010). A woman's subjective assessment of her menstrual blood loss may not correlate with laboratory analysis for the diagnosis of anemia but if it has a major impact on her QOL, the goal should be focused on improving this, as opposed to focusing on the actual amount of blood loss (NICE, 2021). The current recommendation for assessing the impact of AUB involves a two-part approach: a structured menstrual history and a symptoms impact element (Matteson et al., 2011; Table 28.3).

TABLE 28.3 Elements of a Structured Menstrual History

I. FOUR CRITICAL DIMENSIONS

1. Frequency	Absent (amenorrhea)	No bleeding
	Infrequent	>38 days
	Normal	24–38 days
	Frequent	<24 days
2. Regularity (shortest to longest cycle variation)	Normal or "regular"	≤7–9 days
	Irregular	≥8–10 days
3. Duration of flow	Normal	≤8 days
	Prolonged	>8 days

4. Volume assessment
- Number of menstrual products used per period
- Use of more than one menstrual product simultaneously
- Use of incontinence pads
- Frequency of changing menstrual products at times of heaviest flow
- Size and number of blood "clots"
- Soaking through/staining of clothing
- Frequency of changing menstrual products at night

II. DIAGNOSTIC MODULE

Ask questions and take a medical history to develop a list of possible diagnoses and finally the final diagnosis.

Structural abnormalities?[a]	Intermenstrual spotting?
	Postcoital bleeding?
	Pelvic pain (severity and treatment)?
	Pelvic pressure?
Underlying hemostatic disorder?[b,c]	
Ovulatory dysfunction?[d]	Bleeding regularity?
	Weight changes?
	Exercise habits?

(continued)

TABLE 28.3 Elements of a Structured Menstrual History *(continued)*

Endometrial dysfunction?[e]	Bleeding dimensions?
	History of gonorrhea, chlamydia infection, and/or PID?

III. SYMPTOM IMPACT MODULE

Incorporate questions that address menstrual bleeding that are meaningful to women (e.g., social embarrassment, fear of social isolation, missed work or school, and impaired QOL).

Bleeding questions
- Change in menstrual pattern
- Number of menstrual products (pads or tampons or both) on the heaviest day
- Frequency of menstrual products (pads or tampons or both) used at night
- Rate of change of products at time of heaviest flow
- Information about blood clots (size, quantity)

Social embarrassment
- Bleeding through clothes
- Bleeding onto furniture
- Bleeding onto sheets
- Bleeding through her clothes while not at home
- Need to change clothes when not at home

Fear of social embarrassment
- Questions about anxiety
- Questions about depression
- "I worry about . . ."

Avoidance behavior
- Missing work
- Changing social plans
- Canceling activities that require leaving the house
- Extra clothes at work
- Extra menstrual products at all times

[a]Targeted medical history → Polyps, hyperplasia, and cancer can be associated with intermenstrual spotting and postcoital bleeding; leiomyomas can be associated with increased pelvic pressure, urinary pressure, and constipation; and adenomyosis can be associated with pelvic pain.
[b]Consider incorporating a validated screening questionnaire.
[c]Targeted medical history → Severe infection, liver disease, leukemia. Women with a positive screen should be considered for further laboratory evaluation and referral to a hematologist.
[d]Targeted medical history → Thyroid disease, prolactin disorders, medications that can affect ovulation.
[e]Targeted medical history → Medication use (e.g., DMPA, oral contraceptive pills, tranquilizers, psychotropic medications, copper intrauterine device).
DMPA, Depo-medroxyprogesterone acetate; PID, Pelvic Inflammatory Disease; QOL, Quality of Life.
Source: Adapted from Matteson, K. A., Munro, M. G., & Fraser, I. S. (2011). The structured menstrual history: Developing a tool to facilitate diagnosis and aid in symptom management. Seminars in Reproductive Medicine, 29(5), 423–435. https://doi.org/10.1055/s-0031-1287666; Munro, M. G., Critchley, H. O. D., & Fraser, I. S. (2018). The two FIGO systems for normal and abnormal uterine bleeding symptoms and classification of causes of abnormal uterine bleeding in the reproductive years: 2018 revisions. International Journal of Gynecology & Obstetrics, 143(3), 393–408. https://doi.org/10.1002/ijgo.12666; Samuelson Bannow, B., McLintock, C., & James, P. (2021). Menstruation, anticoagulation, and contraception: VTE and uterine bleeding. Research and Practice in Thrombosis and Haemostasis, 5(5), e12570. https://doi.org/10.1002/rth2.12570

PHYSICAL EXAMINATION

A systematic approach to the physical examination is an important and necessary component of the initial assessment. Any time a woman presents complaining of significant vaginal bleeding, it is critical to evaluate her vital signs to establish whether immediate medical or surgical intervention is indicated. Acute AUB/HMB should be managed promptly (e.g., medication, blood transfusion) in order to stop the bleeding and reestablish hemodynamic balance (Benetti-Pinto et al., 2017). If hemodynamically stable, the woman's medical history will inform her physical examination. A head-to-toe assessment is required to help determine the cause for and the effects of the AUB. For example, obesity, hirsutism, acne, and acanthosis nigricans of the neck may be signs of PCOS and metabolic syndrome; and a thyroid nodule may be a sign of thyroid disease. Additionally, bruising and petechiae of the mucous membranes may be physical signs of a coagulopathy, such as von Willebrand disease or idiopathic thrombocytopenia. It is also very important for the healthcare provider to establish whether the AUB is uterine and not from another source (e.g., gastrointestinal [GI], genitourinary tract [GU]). A speculum examination should be performed to assess for cervical and/or vaginal lesions (Benetti-Pinto et al., 2017). Uterine size, shape, and consistency may indicate pregnancy as a source of AUB. A bimanual exam may be consistent with an enlarged uterus with irregular contours indicating the presence of uterine myomas, adenomyosis, or endometriosis, and the presence of uterine tenderness may indicate endometritis or pelvic inflammatory disease (PID).

Differential Diagnosis

Ovarian dysfunction is typically the source of AUB at the extremes of childbearing age groups (adolescents and perimenopausal women). Anovulatory menstrual patterns are sporadic in timing and volume and can be related to hormonal contraceptive use, pregnancy, and pelvic infection. Ovulatory patterns are usually predictable (within a few days) and typically increase in volume of blood loss over months or years. Ovulatory patterns of AUB include structural lesions and endometrial hyperplasia. The most common conditions to consider in the AUB differential diagnosis across a woman's life span are provided in Table 28.4.

Diagnostic Studies

LABORATORY TESTING

In reproductive-age women, it is always important to rule out pregnancy as a possible cause of AUB, even if the patient has had a tubal ligation or denies sexual activity. Cervical cytology to evaluate for cervical neoplasia as well as cervical cultures to rule out sexually transmitted infections (STIs) may also be indicated. If the healthcare provider suspects thyroid disease, thyroid function tests should be obtained (Singh et al., 2013). Hypothyroidism is commonly associated with AUB (ACOG, 2012).

Along with a structured medical and family history, a complete blood count and platelets are recommended to exclude anemia and thrombocytopenia. Furthermore, ACOG (2013b) recommends testing for von Willebrand disease in all patients (particularly adolescents) with excessive bleeding without any apparent cause, or with any bleeding that does not respond to medical treatment. Von Willebrand disease is the most common inherited blood disorder and

TABLE 28.4 Common Conditions in the Differential Diagnosis of Abnormal Uterine Bleeding by Age

AGE GROUP	DIFFERENTIAL DIAGNOSIS
13–18 years	Persistent anovulation because of immature/dysregulation of HPO axis Hormonal contraceptive use (often inconsistent use) Pregnancy Pelvic infection Coagulopathies Tumors
19–39 years	Pregnancy Structural lesions (e.g., leiomyomas or polyps) Anovulatory cycles (PCOS) Hormonal contraceptive use Endometrial hyperplasia Endometrial cancer (less common, but can occur)
40 years to menopause	Anovulatory bleeding because of declining ovarian function Endometrial hyperplasia or carcinoma Endometrial atrophy Leiomyomas

HPO, hypothalamic–pituitary–ovarian; PCOS, polycystic ovary syndrome.
Source: Adapted from American College of Obstetricians and Gynecologists. (2012). Practice bulletin no. 128: Diagnosis of abnormal uterine bleeding in reproductive-aged women. Obstetrics & Gynecology, 120*(1), 197–206. https://doi.org/10.1097/AOG .0b013e318262e320*

it is especially prudent to screen those adolescents with heavy bleeding onset at menarche for this coagulation disorder (ACOG, 2019). Consultation with a hematologist is recommended if a coagulation disorder is suspected. Coagulopathy laboratory testing includes (a) prothrombin time (PT), international normalized ratio (INR), and partial thromboplastin time (PTT), with fibrinogen and thrombin time being optional; (b) von Willebrand ristocetin cofactor activity; and (c) von Willebrand factor antigen, factor VIII (ACOG, 2019).

To establish ovulatory dysfunction as a cause of the AUB, basal body temperature evaluation and luteal phase serum progesterone levels should be evaluated to determine ovulatory status. A progesterone level greater than 3 ng/mL would be an indication that ovulation has occurred. The best time to test a woman's progesterone level is during the midluteal phase of her menstrual cycle (Munro et al., 2018). Determining the luteal phase of a menstrual cycle may be difficult in women diagnosed with AUB. Endometrial sampling, an expensive and invasive procedure that can establish whether the endometrium is secretory (indicating ovulation), is generally not necessary to determine ovulation. Once ovulatory dysfunction has been established, a thyroid-stimulating hormone (TSH) level should be evaluated to rule out thyroid disorders. A prolactin level should also be considered. If the prolactin level is elevated, it should be repeated as a fasting

blood test (ACOG, 2013c). Liver or renal function studies are only indicated in women with signs and symptoms or a current history of systemic disease.

DIAGNOSTIC TESTING
Ultrasonography and MRI

Transvaginal ultrasonography (TVUS) should be the first-line imaging modality for women presenting with AUB (Munro et al., 2018). In adolescents, transabdominal ultrasonography (TAUS) may be more appropriate (ACOG, 2012). For premenopausal women, US should be performed between days 4 and 6 of the menstrual cycle (ACOG, 2013c). The use of TVUS for evaluation of a woman's endometrial echo-complex thickness is helpful when determining which women should undergo endometrial sampling. When ruling out polyps as the source of a woman's AUB, TVUS may not be an effective screening tool as small polyps may be undetectable. TVUS criteria for findings that may be consistent with adenomyosis (AUB-A) include (a) asymmetrical thickening of uterine walls, (b) intramyometrial cysts and/or hyperechoic islands, (c) fan-shaped shadowing of the myometrium, (d) myometrial echogenic subendometrial lines and buds, (e) translesional vascularity, and (f) irregular or interrupted junctional zone (Vannuccini & Petraglia, 2019). However, even with these criteria, it is important for healthcare providers to note that there is no consensus on the definition and classification of lesions, making a clear diagnosis of adenomyosis difficult and unclear (Vannuccini & Petraglia, 2019). TVUS may help to differentiate ovulatory abnormal menstrual bleeding from anatomic causes, but if images are inconclusive, then more sensitive imaging techniques are recommended such as hysteroscopy and/or sonohysterography (Munro et al., 2018). MRI may be utilized in instances in which vaginal access is difficult (e.g., adolescents, virginal women), and it may be superior to other methods of imaging for measuring submucosal leiomyomas or differentiating adenomyosis from leiomyomas (Munro et al., 2018). Munro et al. (2018) caution clinicians to balance the use of MRI with the awareness of its cost and lack of access within many healthcare systems.

Saline Infusion Sonohysterography

Excessive menstrual bleeding associated with myomas usually correlates with the location and size of a myoma. Intramural myomas that obstruct the uterine vasculature contribute to excessive cyclic bleeding. Saline infusion sonohysterography (SHG) assists in the diagnosis of discrete uterine abnormalities such as submucosal fibroids (Munro et al., 2018). SHG involves infusion of sterile saline through a small catheter into the uterine cavity (ACOG, 2013c). This diagnostic test allows for precise assessment of the endometrial cavity, to include measurements of the thickness of the endometrium. An endometrial lining measuring 4 mm or less has a greater than 99% negative predictive value for endometrial cancer (ACOG, 2018a). In premenopausal woman, the thickness count of their endometrium will vary depending on the timing of the US and the woman's menstrual cycle. During the proliferative phase, the thickness can range from 4 to 8 mm as compared with the secretory phase, when it may range from 8 to 14 mm (ACOG, 2013c).

Aspiration Biopsy and Dilation and Curettage

Healthcare providers should consider obtaining endometrial tissue samples from women with a family history of hereditary nonpolyposis colorectal cancer syndrome, also known as Lynch syndrome, as they have a significantly increased lifetime risk of developing endometrial cancer (Munro et al., 2018). As postmenopausal bleeding (PMB) is the *most common presenting symptom* for endometrial carcinoma, any bleeding after 12 months of complete amenorrhea warrants immediate evaluation. There are two procedures used to obtain endometrial tissue for histologic evaluation: aspiration biopsy (e.g., endometrial biopsy) and dilation and curettage (D&C; ACOG, 2012). Aspiration biopsy of the endometrium should be performed in women 40 years of age and older presenting with AUB. Moreover, aspiration biopsy should be performed in women in all age groups with a history of 2 to 3 years of untreated, anovulatory bleeding, especially if they are obese and/or have not responded to medical treatment (Fritz & Speroff, 2011). Endometrial tissue is collected by using a straw-like device with a plunger that the healthcare provider gently pulls back on after they gently insert into the uterus. Pulling back on the plunger creates a suction, which allows for collection of the endometrial sample. Before inserting the catheter, using sterile technique, the healthcare provider measures the depth of the uterus to avoid perforation. Endometrial aspiration is an office procedure that requires no or minimal analgesic or anxiolytic medication. In anticipation of this procedure, women may be counseled to take OTC NSAIDs, as directed by the manufacturer. A blinded biopsy provides 100% specific and positive predictive value (PPV); however, they have a low sensitivity for detecting polyps and leiomyomas (ACOG, 2013c). Therefore, if an endometrial biopsy is negative and the woman's AUB persists and/or the endometrial biopsy specimen is considered inadequate, then further diagnostic testing is indicated (e.g., hysteroscopy; ACOG, 2018a). Women should be referred for further evaluation if:

- There is a history of repeated or persistent irregular or intermenstrual bleeding, or if risk factors for endometrial carcinoma are present.
- Cervical cytology is abnormal.
- Pelvic examination is abnormal.
- There is significant pelvic pain unresponsive to simple analgesia.
- There is failure of first-line treatment after 6 months. (Black et al., 2013)

Aspiration biopsy and surgical D&C have been shown to be equally successful in diagnosing endometrial pathologies (Gungorduk et al., 2014), and aspiration biopsy may be preferred over D&C because it is less invasive (ACOG, 2013c). However, endometrial biopsy may miss localized thickening of the endometrium, and only sonohysterography can differentiate focal pathologies from diffuse, uniform thickening (ACOG, 2012).

Hysteroscopy-Directed Endometrial Sampling

Although an invasive procedure, hysteroscopy with guided biopsy is the *gold standard* for diagnosis of intrauterine pathology (e.g., endometrial polyps; Bittencourt et al., 2017). Hysteroscopy permits full visualization of the endometrial cavity and endocervix and is useful when verifying the diagnosis and when less invasive procedures such as aspiration biopsy, TVUS, and SHG are inadequate (ACOG, 2013c). Targeted biopsy samples collected via hysteroscopy improve the sensitivity of endometrial cancer diagnosis to 99.5% (ACOG, 2013c). Hysteroscopy can be performed in the office or operating room (ACOG, 2013c).

Treatment/Management

MEDICAL MANAGEMENT
Acute AUB

The method of treatment for acute AUB depends on clinical stability, overall acuity, suspected etiology of the bleeding, desire for future fertility, and underlying medical problems (ACOG, 2013a). Management of acute AUB is targeted at controlling the episode of heavy bleeding and reducing menstrual blood loss in future menstrual cycles. Intravenous (IV) conjugated equine estrogen is the only Food and Drug Administration (FDA) approved treatment for acute AUB. In situations of acute AUB, surgical management may be the choice of treatment, although medical management is the preferred initial treatment.

A category of drug therapy that is an effective treatment for chronic AUB is antifibrinolytic drugs, and they have been shown to reduce bleeding by 30% to 55% (ACOG, 2013a). These medications work by blocking the breakdown of fibrin. Tranexamic acid is an antifibrinolytic that has been shown to reduce bleeding in surgical patients, and its use (oral or intravenous) is recommended for acute AUB as it is likely effective for these patients as well (James et al., 2011). Additionally, intrauterine tamponade with a 26F Foley catheter infused with 30 mL of saline solution appears to successfully control bleeding (Benetti-Pinto et al., 2017).

Once hemodynamically stable, multiple, long-term treatment options are available for use. Hormonal management is the recommended, first-line medical treatment. In addition to IV conjugated equine estrogen, combined oral contraceptives (COCs; monthly or extended cycling), progestin therapy (oral or intramuscular), the levonorgestrel intrauterine system, tranexamic acid, and NSAIDs are all recommended therapies. Medical therapy using COCs or cyclic progesterone therapy is the mainstay of treatment for ovulatory dysfunctional bleeding. Healthcare providers should add progestin or transition women who have received IV conjugated equine estrogen to COCs. Long-term unopposed estrogen therapy is contraindicated as it increases a woman's risk of endometrial hyperplasia and carcinoma. Contraindications to hormone therapy must be considered before prescribing. Healthcare providers should consult the *U.S. Medical Eligibility Criteria for Contraceptive Use 2016* (Curtis et al., 2016) to determine which women are eligible for treatment with hormone therapy. It is important to remember that estrogen-containing contraceptives are contraindicated for women older than 35 who smoke or who have a history of thromboembolic disease. Progesterone hormonal options are ideal for these women.

A shared treatment goal with realistic expectations that includes discussion about anticipated side effects improves a woman's satisfaction and the likelihood of her continuation of treatment. It is also important for the healthcare provider to remember that unless the underlying problem is corrected, similar episodes of AUB are likely to recur (ACOG, 2013a; Fritz & Speroff, 2011).

A hematologist should follow women with known or newly diagnosed coagulopathies. Desmopressin has been shown to be effective in treating acute AUB in women with von Willebrand disease. Desmopressin can be administered via intranasal inhalation, intravenously, or subcutaneously (Kadir et al., 2005). Desmopressin is contraindicated in women with massive hemorrhage who are receiving IV fluid resuscitation as it may result in fluid overload (James et al., 2011). What is more, fluid retention and hyponatremia have been linked to desmopressin therapy (James et al., 2011). In women with von Willebrand disease, treatment with recombinant factor VIII and von Willebrand factor may be required to control severe hemorrhage (ACOG, 2013b). Because of the known effect on platelet aggregation and other interactions with drug therapies that might affect liver function and the production of clotting factors, women with known bleeding disorders or platelet function abnormalities should avoid NSAIDs (Kadir et al., 2005).

Chronic AUB

COMBINED HORMONAL TREATMENTS

The amount of abnormal bleeding that a woman is experiencing along with an assessment of her complete blood count (CBC) will determine her initial treatment regimen. On determination of hemodynamic stability, a low-dose, monophasic oral contraceptive may be used (one pill twice daily). Bleeding should markedly slow or stop within 24 to 48 hours, although the treatment regimen should continue for 5 to 7 days. If the woman presents with mild anemia, iron therapy (dietary intake and/or iron supplementation) is needed in conjunction with the low-dose contraceptive. If the woman presents with severe anemia, the healthcare provider should consider inpatient management to allow for IV high-dose estrogen and possible blood transfusion (ACOG, 2013a).

To prevent heavy withdrawal bleeding on discontinuation of this twice-daily regimen, the woman can take the COC daily until the package of pills is completed. Withdrawal bleeding can be expected within a few days after the last active pill. A maintenance therapy of a low-dose COC should be prescribed and initiated. Over time, COCs have been shown to reduce menstrual blood flow by 40% to 50% in women, and the effectiveness is increased by extended cycle or continuous COC regimens because the overall total number of bleeding episodes is reduced (ACOG, 2010).

Occasionally, women who are taking COCs on a regular basis may experience AUB, such as irregular bleeding. Once the healthcare provider has confirmed that the irregular bleeding is not because of missed pills, they may consider changing the COC formulation to one with a higher progestational and androgenic effect, with lower estrogen. It can take up to 3 months to determine if the change in COC formulation was effective in resolving the irregular bleeding.

Although it has not been studied for effectiveness in resolving AUB, combined estrogen-progestin contraception with either the vaginal ring (NuvaRing) or the transdermal patch (Ortho Evra) has also been determined to be appropriate for maintenance therapy (Singh et al., 2013; Vasudeva et al., 2018). Extended cycling and continuous use of oral contraceptives, the contraceptive patch, or the vaginal ring all appear to have reduced both the amount of blood loss per cycle and the number of bleeding episodes per year when compared with regular, monthly regimens with a pill-free week allowing for a withdrawal bleed (Singh et al., 2013).

NONSTEROIDAL ANTI-INFLAMMATORY DRUGS

There is a progressive increase in levels of prostaglandins in the endometrium throughout the menstrual cycle, with very high concentrations noted in the menstrual endometrium. NSAIDs inhibit prostaglandin synthesis via the inhibition of the enzyme cyclooxygenase. Although the exact mechanism of action is not understood, it appears that the end effect is a reduction of menstrual blood loss, when compared with placebo. The most commonly used NSAIDs are naproxen (550 mg, orally, on the first day of menses; then 275 mg daily thereafter) and mefenamic acid (500 mg, three times daily for 5 days). Treatment should be initiated 1 day before the onset of menses and continue for 3 to 5 days or until bleeding stops (Singh et al., 2013). Both naproxen and mefenamic acid have been shown to decrease blood loss by approximately 10% to 52% (Wouk & Helton, 2019). Although helpful, NSAIDs do not appear to be as effective as tranexamic acid, danazol, or the levonorgestrel-releasing intrauterine system (LNG-IUS; Benetti-Pinto et al., 2017). Contraindications to NSAIDs include hypersensitivity, preexisting gastritis, and peptic ulcer disease (Benetti-Pinto et al., 2017; see Table 28.5).

PROGESTIN-ONLY METHODS

Progestin-only methods are available for women who prefer nonestrogen methods or have a contraindication to combined hormonal contraceptives. After a thorough workup and confirmation of the source of the AUB, the healthcare provider should consider the LNG-IUS as a possible means of AUB treatment. The LNG-IUS is a progestin-releasing intrauterine system/device that has two FDA-approved indications: (1) as a method of contraception, and (2) for the treatment of AUB/HMB. This 32-mm device administers 20 mcg of levonorgestrel (LNG) daily to the endometrium, resulting in endometrial atrophy, thereby reducing mean uterine vascular density. Systemic side effects are minimal because of the low concentration of LNG that is absorbed into the systemic circulation (0.4—0.6 nmol/L). The LNG-IUS is FDA approved for 5 years of continuous, intrauterine use for the treatment of AUB/HMB. Studies have suggested that women who have an LNG-IUS inserted have similar bleeding outcomes as women who have had an endometrial ablation (Singh et al., 2013). In the first few months after insertion, many women reported intermenstrual spotting, but the spotting was resolved after a few months with up to 80% of women becoming amenorrheic by 1-year postinsertion (Singh et al., 2013). The LNG-IUS is more effective than oral medication at reducing menstrual flow. The majority of women using the LNG-IUS will

TABLE 28.5 NSAIDs and COX-2 Inhibitors Commonly Used for Primary Dysmenorrhea

DRUG	TRADE NAME	RECOMMENDED DOSAGE
Ibuprofen	Advil, Motrin	400 mg every 4–6 hours
Naproxen	Aleve	220 mg every 8–12 hours
Naproxen	Anaprox	Initially 550 mg, then 550 mg every 12 hours or 275 mg every 6–8 hours
Naproxen	Naprelan	1 g once daily
Naproxen	Naprosyn	Initially 500 mg, then 500 mg every 12 hours or 250 mg every 6–8 hours
Diclofenac	Cataflam	50 mg every 8 hours
Meclofenamate	Meclomen	50–100 mg every 4–6 hours for up to 6 days starting with menstrual flow
Mefenamic acid	Ponstel	Initially 500 mg, then 250 mg every 6 hours (take with food)
Celecoxib	Celebrex	Initially 400 mg, then 200 mg twice daily

COX-2, cyclooxygenase-2; NSAIDs, nonsteroidal anti-inflammatory drugs.

ultimately experience amenorrhea and are more satisfied with and continue this form of treatment compared with progesterone-only pills (ACOG, 2010). Side effects reported included intermenstrual bleeding and breast tenderness (ACOG, 2010). Healthcare providers should consider the LNG-IUS as a first-line therapy for appropriate candidates with AUB that is not associated with anatomic abnormalities of the uterus. The 3-year LNG-IUS contraceptive, a smaller system/device measuring 28 mm, releases 14 mcg of LNG daily. This smaller device is not FDA approved for AUB/HMB.

Some women prefer not to use the intrauterine system and instead opt for another type of progesterone therapy. Women who chose an oral progestin agent for menstrual control and contraception must be counseled about the importance of taking the pill at the same time each day. It is important to note that few women experience reduced menstrual blood loss when using the progesterone-only pill (POP) for contraception (Singh et al., 2013).

Injected progestin, depo-medroxyprogesterone acetate (DMPA), is both a contraceptive and has been used to treat AUB/HMB. DMPA works by suppressing ovulation and ovulatory steroidogenesis, thereby reducing the estrogen-mediated stimulation of the endometrium, leading to endometrial atrophy (Singh et al., 2013). During the first few months of treatment, women can expect unpredictable and irregular spotting and bleeding. Approximately 50% of women will experience amenorrhea by 1 year of continued use (Wouk & Helton, 2019). Other side effects include breast tenderness, nausea, weight gain, mood disturbances, and a small reduction in bone mineral density that reverses once the medication has

been discontinued. Healthcare providers should use caution when using DMPA in women with a history of depression.

ESTROGEN THERAPY

When AUB/HMB is associated with a thin, denuded endometrium, as seen in adolescent girls and perimenopausal women, treatment should include high-dose estrogen therapy. High-dose estrogen therapy successfully stops heavy bleeding by promoting endometrial growth to cover the fragile, denuded endometrial surfaces. Estrogen is given either IV or orally, depending on the amount of abnormal menstrual bleeding. IV conjugated estrogen (Premarin) 25 mg is given every 4 hours until the menstrual bleeding subsides. If high-dose oral therapy is administered, 1.25 mg conjugated estrogen or 2 mg micronized estradiol is given by mouth, every 4 to 6 hours for 24 hours, then tapered to a once-daily dose for 7 to 10 days (Benetti-Pinto et al., 2017). Both regimens are effective means for stopping bleeding and should be followed by treatment with either a progestin or COC for the purpose of stabilizing the endometrium and providing a regular menstrual cycle (Benetti-Pinto et al., 2017). High-dose estrogen is contraindicated in women with a history of thrombosis and/or with a family history of spontaneous thromboembolism (ACOG, 2013a).

DANAZOL

Danazol, a derivative of testosterone, has been shown to be effective in reducing heavy menstrual blood loss, but the androgenic side effects (e.g., weight gain, acne, hirsutism) tend to be an issue for most women. Danazol inhibits ovarian steroidogenesis through suppression of the pituitary–ovarian axis and reduces blood losses by up to 80%. The prescribed regimens range between 100 mg and 400 mg daily, in divided doses. Danazol and gonadotropin-releasing hormone agents (GnRH) agonists have considerable side effects, and it is important for the provider to weigh the benefits of the medications against the cost and frequent side effects; these medications are often used for only short periods of time until more definitive long-term options are available, such as surgery (Benetti-Pinto et al., 2017).

GONADOTROPIN-RELEASING HORMONE AGONISTS

GnRH agents suppress pituitary secretion of follicle-stimulating hormone (FSH) and luteinizing hormone (LH), creating a hypoestrogenic, menopausal-like state. Cessation of menstruation usually occurs within 3 to 4 weeks after administration. GnRH agonist treatment has most commonly been used to treat the symptomatology associated with adenomyosis, leiomyomas, or endometriosis, or as pretreatment before surgery for abnormal menstrual bleeding. GnRHs can be administered intramuscularly, subcutaneously, or intranasally. Menopausal symptoms such as hot flashes and vaginal dryness are common side effects. The most significant disadvantage to GnRH agonists is rapid bone demineralization that increases the risk of osteoporosis. Because of this serious side effect, it is recommended that treatment be limited to no more than 6 months (Singh et al., 2013). Another disadvantage of GnRH therapy includes the possibility of regrowth of previously treated uterine leiomyomas once therapy has been discontinued (Black et al., 2013).

ANTIFIBRINOLYTICS

Women with AUB/HMB have elevated endometrial levels of plasminogen activators with more local fibrinolytic activity as compared with women with normal menstrual loss. Antifibrinolytics cause a degradation of blood clots. They have been shown to be effective in reducing blood flow volume by 30% to 55% (ACOG, 2013a). The primary issue with antifibrinolytic use is the associated GI side effects as well as increased risk of intermenstrual bleeding. The use of antifibrinolytic therapy is contraindicated in women with a personal medical history of thromboembolism or renal failure (Benetti-Pinto et al., 2017; Wouk & Helton, 2019).

SURGICAL MANAGEMENT

The need for surgical treatment is based on a woman's hemodynamic stability, severity of bleeding, contraindications to hormonal management, a failed response to medical management, and underlying medical conditions (ACOG, 2013a). Surgical interventions include D&C, myomectomy, endometrial ablation, uterine artery embolization, and hysterectomy. Surgical intervention is chosen based on the hemodynamic stability of the woman and her desire for future fertility. Uterine artery embolization, endometrial ablation, and hysterectomy are surgical options that have been shown to successfully control acute AUB when medical treatments have failed (Benetti-Pinto et al., 2017).

Operative Hysteroscopy

In cases in which structural abnormalities are the cause of acute AUB, surgical procedures such as hysteroscopy with D&C, polypectomy, and/or myomectomy may be indicated. Operative hysteroscopy is primarily used to treat intracavity lesions such as submucosal fibroids and endometrial polyps (Salim et al., 2011). This is a quick, safe, and effective outpatient procedure. It is important to remember that D&C without hysteroscopy is inadequate for evaluation of uterine disorders and has been shown to reduce abnormal bleeding only temporarily (Bettocchi et al., 2001). Surgical intervention for polyps is usually reserved for polyps greater than 1 cm; smaller polyps often spontaneously regress and may only require watchful waiting as a treatment option (Nijkang et al., 2019).

Myomectomy, or removal of intramural or subserosal uterine leiomyomas (fibroids), is the procedure of choice for women who have symptomatic leiomyomas and wish to preserve their fertility. The type of surgical procedure chosen (e.g., hysteroscopy, laparoscopy, or laparotomy) is dependent on the number, size, and location of the leiomyomas. Leiomyomas recur more than 50% of the time when multiple fibroids are removed (Giuliani et al., 2020).

Uterine Artery Embolization

Uterine artery embolization is another treatment option for symptomatic leiomyomas (including heavy bleeding). This is a minimally invasive procedure whereby, using local anesthesia, a small catheter is inserted through the femoral artery and then guided into the uterine artery through x-ray imaging. The uterine artery is then occluded with embospheres, polyvinyl alcohol particles, coils, or gel foam, resulting in necrosis and shrinkage of the leiomyoma(s). Uterine artery embolization is not recommended for large leiomyomas or in women who desire to retain their fertility.

Hysterectomy

As a last resort in women who do not respond to medical treatment, hysterectomy (the definitive treatment for controlling heavy bleeding) may be necessary. The procedure can be performed vaginally, laparoscopically, or abdominally depending on the woman's diagnosis and the etiology of the AUB. Hysterectomy is a major procedure that requires hospitalization and several weeks of recovery, and is associated with significant morbidity and even death.

Endometrial Ablation

Endometrial ablation should be considered only as a last resort and in cases in which the woman does not desire future fertility. Furthermore, it is critical to rule out endometrial carcinoma as the cause of the acute AUB before performing an endometrial ablation. Endometrial ablation is a less invasive procedure and an alternative to hysterectomy for treatment of AUB. Several ablation techniques are available including thermal balloon, circulated hot fluid, cryotherapy, radiofrequency electrosurgery, and microwave energy. These newer technologies treat the endometrial cavity globally rather than ablating the endometrium section by section, as was done with rollerball electrosurgery or laser. Randomized controlled trials (RCTs) indicate that endometrial ablation has been associated with positive patient satisfaction, even without the occurrence of amenorrhea, following the procedure (Singh et al., 2013). As a result, bleeding is controlled in 87% to 97% of women and more than 80% require no additional surgery for up to 5 years after ablation (Singh et al., 2013). When preparing the patient for ablation, it should be emphasized that the goal of the procedure is to reduce menstrual bleeding and not to induce amenorrhea (see Box 28.2).

SELF-MANAGEMENT

Options for self-management of AUB are dependent on etiology. Lifestyle changes may be helpful (e.g., exercise, weight loss, stress management). Women who are overweight or obese may experience an improvement or cessation of

---

Box 28.2 Recommended Preoperative Checklist for Global Endometrial Ablation

- Document failure, refusal, or intolerance to medical management.
- Confirm that patient does not desire future pregnancy.
- Establish a plan for contraception.
- Exclude endometrial hyperplasia or malignancy with a tissue sample.
- Perform adequate endometrial imaging to exclude a lesion that would preclude the use of global endometrial ablation.

Source: Adapted from Sharp, H. T. (2006). Assessment of new technology in the treatment of idiopathic menorrhagia and uterine leiomyomata. Obstetrics & Gynecology, 108*(4), 990–1003. https://doi.org/10.1097/01.AOG.0000232618.26261.75*

their symptoms with as little as a 10- to 15-lb weight loss (www.acog.org/Patients/FAQs/Polycystic-Ovary-Syndrome -PCOS). Regular exercise is one means for weight loss. Women with diabetes should be counseled on the importance of maintaining their blood sugar levels in normal range.

INTEGRATIVE MEDICINE

Although acupuncture is used for various gynecologic concerns, research on AUB and fibroids is limited (Smith & Carmady, 2010; Zhang et al., 2010). In one study, acupuncture was proved effective in reducing the size of one patient's myoma, resulting in resolved anemia and a subsequent pregnancy (Habek & Akšamija, 2014). In an animal model study, researchers reported improved ovarian function in rats with induced PCOS who were later treated with electroacupuncture (Maliqueo et al., 2015).

In a meta-analysis of 38 RCTs, treatment with Guizhi Fuling Formula (consisting of five herbs—*Ramulus Cinnamomi, Poria, Semen Persicae, Radix Paeoniae Rubra* or *Radix Paeoniae Alba,* and *Cortex Moutan*) reduced uterine fibroids when used either alone or with mifepristone. To date, no serious adverse events have been reported. It should be noted, however, that the authors of the meta-analysis reported the methodologic quality of the RCTs as poor overall (Chen et al., 2014).

AMENORRHEA

Definition and Scope

Amenorrhea is the absence or cessation of menstruation and can be further defined as primary or secondary, depending on the woman's presentation. Primary amenorrhea is defined as no menses by age 13 years associated with the absence of the development of secondary sexual characteristics, or no menses by age 15 years even in the presence of normal secondary sexual characteristics (Waller & Pantin, 2019). Secondary amenorrhea is defined as the absence of menses for a period of three cycles with a history of normal menstruation, or 6 months in a woman with previously irregular menstruation (Waller & Pantin, 2019). There are many underlying diseases and disorders that can result in amenorrhea (Box 28.3).

Etiology

The usual cause of amenorrhea is physiologic (e.g., pregnancy, lactation). In the case of lactation, milk production relies on a rise in prolactin, which inhibits GnRH release, thereby preventing normal ovarian stimulation. On cessation of lactation, menses typically return within weeks (Black et al., 2013). There are numerous causes for amenorrhea, and many are rare.

Primary amenorrhea is often caused by chromosomal irregularities that lead to ovarian insufficiency (e.g., Turner syndrome) or anatomic abnormalities (e.g., müllerian agenesis). Disorders arising from the hypothalamus, anterior pituitary, ovary, and genital tract make up the pathologic causes of amenorrhea. Pathologic causes of secondary amenorrhea most commonly are the result of PCOS, hypothalamic amenorrhea, hyperprolactinemia, or primary ovarian insufficiency.

HYPOTHALAMIC DISORDERS

Impairment of the GnRH pulsatile secretion occurs from reversible conditions such as weight loss–related amenorrhea, stress-related amenorrhea, and exercise-related amenorrhea. In these conditions, a *functional hypothalamic amenorrhea* (FHA) results, which is characterized by low or normal levels of FSH and LH, normal prolactin levels, normal imaging of the pituitary fossa, and low estrogen.

Regular menstruation requires an endocrine balance and is dependent on healthy weight parameters with healthy levels of fat storage. The two body states that can affect the menstrual status include unhealthy weight loss (loss of body weight of 10%–15% typically seen in aggressive calorie-restrictive diets) and strenuous physical training (e.g., athletes). The sequelae of such a high-intensity exercise regimen may result in an unhealthy state known as the *female athlete triad.* The prevalence is unknown as athletic women may not present with the three criteria: (a) disordered eating, (b) amenorrhea, and (c) osteoporosis (Chamberlain, 2018; Matzkin et al., 2015).

PITUITARY DISORDERS

High prolactin levels from pituitary disorders can cause secondary amenorrhea. About 40% of prolactin-secreting tumors originate in the anterior pituitary. One third of women with this type of tumor complain of galactorrhea. Antidopaminergic effects from medications can cause an elevation in prolactin levels, thereby leading to amenorrhea. These medications include phenothiazines, antihistamines, butyrophenones, metoclopramide, cimetidine, and methyldopa.

In rare circumstances, severe obstetric hemorrhage and subsequent hypotension can permanently damage the anterior pituitary. This rare necrosis of the anterior pituitary is referred to as Sheehan syndrome. Sheehan syndrome may be a source of secondary amenorrhea.

OVARIAN DISORDERS

Genetic syndromes, autoimmune disorders, ovary removal or destruction, and neoplasms commonly precipitate ovarian disorders. Premature ovarian failure (POF) is defined as the cessation of ovarian function before the age of 40 years. POF is characterized by amenorrhea and an increase in gonadotropin levels that result in a hypoestrogenic state. POF affects approximately 1% of all women and is usually nonreversible. Turner syndrome is the most common genetic syndrome associated with POF. Autoimmune disorders, such as systemic lupus erythematosus (SLE) and myasthenia gravis (MG), cause autoimmune oophoritis. Although extremely rare (occurs in only approximately 4% of women), it can lead to POF. Other causes of amenorrhea include surgical removal, destruction by radiation, and/or infection of the ovaries. Although ovarian neoplasms are rare, in such cases, excessive levels of estrogen and testosterone are produced.

Box 28.3 Major Causes of Amenorrhea

Disorders of the Outflow Tract

Congenital

  Complete androgen resistance

  Imperforate hymen

  Müllerian agenesis

  Transvaginal vaginal septum

Acquired

  Intrauterine synechiae (Asherman syndrome)

  Cervical stenosis

Primary Ovarian Insufficiency

Congenital

  Gonadal dysgenesis (other than Turner syndrome)

  Turner syndrome or variant

Acquired

  Autoimmune destruction

  Chemotherapy

Pituitary Disorders

Autoimmune disease

Cocaine

Cushing syndrome

Empty sella syndrome

Hyperprolactinemia

Infiltrative disease (e.g., sarcoidosis)

Medications

  Antidepressants

  Antihistamines

  Antihypertensives

  Antipsychotics

Opiates

Other pituitary or central nervous system tumor

Prolactinoma

Sheehan syndrome

Central Nervous System Disorders (Hypothalamic Causes)

Eating disorder

Functional (overall energy deficit)

Gonadotropin deficiency (e.g., Kallmann syndrome)

Infection (e.g., meningitis, tuberculosis, syphilis)

Malabsorption

Rapid weight loss (any cause)

Stress

Traumatic brain injury

Tumor

Endocrine Gland Disorders

Adrenal disease

Adult-onset adrenal hyperplasia

Androgen-secreting tumor

Chronic disease

Constitutional delay of puberty

Cushing syndrome

Ovarian tumors (androgen producing)

Polycystic ovary syndrome (multifactorial)

Thyroid disease

Physiologic Causes

Breastfeeding

Contraception

Exogenous androgens

Menopause

Pregnancy

Source: Adapted from Seppä, S., Kuiri-Hänninen, T., Holopainen, E., & Voutilainen, R. (2021). Management of endocrine disease: Diagnosis and management of primary amenorrhea and female delayed puberty. European Journal of Endocrinology, 184(6), R225–R242. https://doi.org/10.1530/eje-20-1487

POLYCYSTIC OVARY SYNDROME

PCOS affects 5% to 10% of childbearing-age women and is associated with approximately 75% of all anovulatory disorders causing infertility. Often women will complain of light or infrequent periods. On US, a woman's ovaries may appear enlarged and contain many small fluid-filled structures just under the ovarian capsule, which are often not *true* cysts. The polycystic ovary has an increased ovarian stroma, which may lead to abnormal endocrine properties. Although approximately 25% of women will have PCOS-appearing ovaries on US, only a small percentage will develop true PCOS.

Women with PCOS have elevated pituitary and ovarian hormone levels, specifically, an abnormally elevated LH level and absence of the LH surge. Estrogen and FSH levels are often normal and because of alterations in the feedback process, the result is an increased LH/FSH ratio. Ovarian secretion of testosterone, androstenedione, and dehydroepi-androsterone (DHEA) is also elevated, and prolactin levels, too, are elevated.

Pathogenesis of PCOS

The cause of PCOS is unknown; however, there is evidence pointing to both genetic predisposition and lifestyle. The hallmark signs of PCOS are abnormalities in androgen biosynthesis and insulin resistance. Insulin resistance lends itself to obesity and hyperlipidemia, both of which increase the risk of a woman developing a noninsulin-dependent diabetes and metabolic syndrome.

The ovary produces the primary androgens, testosterone and androstenedione, whereas the adrenal glands produce DHEA. In the case of a woman with PCOS (abnormalities in androgen biosynthesis and insulin resistance), the production of androgens is significantly increased by insulin and insulin-like growth factors. This production cannot be suppressed by adrenal steroids; however, it can be suppressed by GnRH agonists.

PCOS is clinically diagnosed by inclusion of two of the following three criteria: (a) light and/or irregular menses, or amenorrhea; (b) on examination, physical evidence of hyperandrogenism; and (c) cystic-appearing ovaries on US.

UTERINE CAUSES

Scarring of the endometrium resulting from trauma and/or infection, leading to the development of endometrial adhesions, can also cause amenorrhea. This condition is known as Asherman syndrome. Asherman syndrome is often caused by severe postpartum hemorrhage that requires dilation and sharp curettage, resulting in some endometrial damage and adhesions.

HIDDEN MENSTRUATION

Cervical stenosis can obstruct or block menstrual flow, leading to amenorrhea. Stenosis can occur from infection as well as surgical procedures (e.g., D&C, elective abortions), which lead to an obstruction of the outflow tract. Hidden menstruation can also be caused by an imperforate hymen and transverse vaginal septum (Seppä et al., 2021).

Risk Factors

As with many other perimenstrual symptoms and syndromes, risk factors for amenorrhea depend on etiology. The defining characteristic in determining differentials and final diagnosis(es) is whether the woman has ever experienced menstruation. As with any form of AUB, a detailed history of a woman's medical and family history is warranted as often there is a genetic predisposition.

Symptoms

Amenorrhea is the absence or cessation of menstruation. Menstruation usually begins within 2 years of thelarche, or breast budding. As an aside, although most adolescents begin menstruating by 16 years of age, the onset of puberty has fallen substantially across the developed world. This is attributed to improved nutrition and access to preventive health services

(Bellis et al., 2006). Secondary amenorrhea occurs in women who have previously experienced menstruation yet have not menstruated for at least 6 months. It is important for healthcare providers to consider amenorrhea as a symptom of a systemic condition. As such, evaluation and assessment of the woman experiencing amenorrhea are critical.

Evaluation/Assessment

A thorough history and physical examination is the first step when working up a woman presenting with amenorrhea.

HISTORY

The amenorrheic woman's history should include information regarding her growth and development, specifically changes of puberty such as breast development and pubic hair growth. The beginning of breast development signals estrogen stimulation. She should be asked about physical and emotional signs of cyclic hormonal changes (e.g., breast tenderness, mood changes). Cyclic abdominal pain may be a sign of outflow tract obstruction such as an imperforate hymen. It is also important to inquire about eating habits, exercise patterns, changes in body weight, drug use, prescription medications, current or previous acute or chronic illnesses, and presence of emotional stress, as well as to conduct a comprehensive family history. Changes in hair growth, skin, and/or frequency of headaches should be noted. Headaches, if associated with galactorrhea and visual disturbances, may indicate a pituitary tumor (Russ et al., 2021).

PHYSICAL EXAMINATION

In the majority of cases, the physical examination is normal, but occasionally it may provide additional clues that point to the possible cause of the woman's amenorrhea. Anthropomorphic measurements, or the growth chart, may substantiate a delay in menses as just a constitutional delay of growth and puberty. An elevated body mass index (BMI), especially if associated with truncal obesity, may be a sign of PCOS or Cushing disease. Furthermore, skin changes such as acanthosis nigricans, acne, and hirsutism also suggest PCOS, whereas purple striae suggest Cushing disease. Tanner staging will provide insight. Breast development is an excellent indictor of ovarian estrogen production. Dysmorphic features, such as a webbed neck, widely spaced nipples, or short stature, may indicate Turner syndrome. When examining the breasts, any galactorrhea should be noted. If only a vaginal pouch is present with absent or sparse pubic hair, androgen insensitivity syndrome (AIS) should be considered, whereas the same findings with normal pubic hair may be suggestive of müllerian agenesis (congenital absence of a vagina and abnormal or absent uterine and fallopian tube development). It is important to note that breast development is normal with both AIS and müllerian agenesis (Fulare et al., 2020; Herlin et al., 2020).

Differential Diagnosis

ANATOMIC ABNORMALITIES

Müllerian agenesis, a congenital malformation, is a common cause of primary amenorrhea. It is manifested in women with normal breast and pubic hair development, with no visible vagina, and other congenital malformations such as defects in the urinary tract and fused vertebrae. Imperforate hymen and a transverse vaginal septum may obstruct menstrual flow, yet women may experience cyclic premenstrual changes and complain of pelvic pain. In women presenting with müllerian agenesis, the physical examination will be consistent with a normal vaginal opening, shortened vagina, no cervix, and a palpable bloody mass (hematocolpos).

In rare instances, AIS, testicular feminization or male pseudohermaphroditism will cause amenorrhea. Women with AIS will have normal breast development, sparse or absent pubic and axillary hair, and a blind vaginal pouch. Furthermore, they may have 5-alpha-reductase deficiency, which is characterized by partially virilized genitalia. Laboratory analysis of serum testosterone will be consistent with what a normal value would be in a male. This is because of the contrast in genotype and phenotype (gonadal sex = male, contrasting phenotype = female). Women with this syndrome should be referred to a specialist for follow-up care.

Cervical os stenosis may occur following cervical procedures. Symptoms include worsening dysmenorrhea or prolonged light staining or spotting after menses. Amenorrhea can occur on rare occasions. US evaluation may reveal a hematometra (blood retained in the uterus).

Secondary amenorrhea is a symptom of Asherman syndrome. This syndrome is iatrogenic; it is caused by uterine instrumentation during gynecologic or obstetric procedures that in turn cause intrauterine adhesions that obstruct or obliterate the uterine cavity. Administering an estrogen/progesterone challenge test in a woman with Asherman syndrome will result in no withdrawal bleeding.

PRIMARY OVARIAN INSUFFICIENCY

Ovarian disorders can cause primary or secondary amenorrhea. Primary ovarian insufficiency is characterized by follicle depletion or dysfunction that leads to impaired ovarian function. Ovarian insufficiency is diagnosed in women younger than 40 years of age with a history of amenorrhea or light, infrequent periods and elevated FSH measured on two separate occasions, 1 month apart. Women who desire fertility should be referred to a reproductive endocrinologist, early in their medical care, for counseling regarding egg donation or in vitro fertilization (IVF). Approximately 5% to 10% of women diagnosed with ovarian insufficiency conceive and deliver a pregnancy. Hormone therapy may be indicated to help reduce vasomotor symptoms experienced because of ovarian insufficiency. Healthcare providers should consider prevention of osteoporosis by prescribing weight-bearing exercises, supplemental calcium (1,200 mg/daily), and vitamin D (800 IU/daily).

Primary ovary insufficiency has been attributed to chromosomal abnormalities, fragile X permutations, autoimmune disorders, radiation therapy, and chemotherapy. For example, Turner syndrome has unique physical characteristics including a webbed neck, a low hairline, cardiac defects, and lymphedema. Women who present with short stature and amenorrhea are suspect for Turner syndrome and so should undergo genetic testing (e.g., karyotype analysis). An endocrinologist and/or genetics counselor may need to be consulted. A genetic counselor will complete a family history consisting of a three-generation pedigree and will appropriately counsel and recommend further genetic testing that may be warranted. Autoimmune disorders should be evaluated by determining thyroid function and adrenal autoantibodies.

HYPOTHALAMIC AND PITUITARY CAUSES

For proper functioning, the ovaries require hormonal stimulation from the hypothalamus and pituitary gland. Stress, weight loss, excessive exercise, and/or disordered eating negatively influence the function of the HPO axis, thereby decreasing ovarian function, which leads to a reduction in the availability of estrogen. As a result, laboratory tests will reveal low or low-normal levels of serum FSH, LH, and estradiol. However, these results can fluctuate. Women with a reduced calorie intake should be evaluated for eating disorders, fad diets, and malabsorption syndromes (e.g., celiac disease). Treatment involves nutrition support and education. A bone density measurement may be necessary to evaluate a woman's bone health. It may be necessary to prescribe OTC calcium and vitamin D supplements. Although COCs will restore regular menses, they will not correct bone loss or protect bone health. Bisphosphonates are not helpful in this population of women.

Diagnostic Studies

A pregnancy test should be the first step in the laboratory evaluation. The most common cause of secondary amenorrhea is pregnancy. After ruling out pregnancy, the healthcare provider should collect a CBC and comprehensive metabolic panel. The workup for amenorrhea is a three-step process.

STEP ONE

This step includes a serum prolactin level, TSH, FSH, and a progestational challenge test (Table 28.6). If the woman's history or physical examination is suggestive of a hyperandrogenic state, consider ordering a serum free and total testosterone, and DHEA concentration. If galactorrhea is present, imaging of the sella turcica may be indicated, particularly if the prolactin level is elevated (Box 28.4).

Although hypothyroidism is an infrequent cause of amenorrhea, it is easy to diagnose, and menstrual cycles resume promptly with thyroid hormone replacement therapy. The purpose of the progestational challenge test is to evaluate the level of endogenous estrogen present as well as to assess for any outflow tract abnormalities. A withdrawal bleed should occur within 2 to 7 days after conclusion of the challenge test. A positive bleed indicates the presence of a reactive

TABLE 28.6 Progestational Challenge Test and Estrogen/Progestin Challenge Test

DRUG	DOSING	DURATION
Parenteral progesterone in oil	200 mg, intramuscularly	Single dose
Micronized progesterone	300 mg, orally	Daily for 5 days
Medroxyprogesterone acetate (Depo-Provera)	10 mg, orally	Daily for 5 days

Box 28.4 Causes of Galactorrhea

Prolactin-secreting pituitary tumor

Medications

    Phenothiazine derivatives

    Opiates

    Diazepam

    Tricyclic antidepressants

    Amphetamines

Hypothyroidism

Excessive estrogen (e.g., oral contraceptives)

Nipple stimulation

Thoracotomy scars

Cervical spinal lesions

Herpes zoster

Stress

Hypothalamic lesions

Other prolactin-secreting tumors (e.g., lung and renal tumors; uterine leiomyoma)

Severe renal disease

Source: Adapted from Atluri, S., Sarathi, V., Goel, A., Boppana, R., & Shivaprasad, C. (2018). Etiological profile of galactorrhoea. Indian Journal of Endocrinology and Metabolism, 22(4), 489–493. https://doi.org/10.4103/ijem.IJEM_89_18.

endometrium and a functioning outflow tract. A diagnosis of anovulation is confirmed if a woman's prolactin and TSH levels are normal. If galactorrhea is not present, no further evaluation is necessary. No withdrawal bleeding indicates either an outflow tract abnormality or inadequate estrogen stimulation of the endometrium.

STEP TWO

Step two of the diagnostic workup involves administering a second round of the estrogen/progestin challenge test (Table 28.6). In the absence of a withdrawal bleed, a validating second estrogen/progestin challenge is recommended. After the second test, the woman will have either a withdrawal bleed or not. No withdrawal bleeding indicates an outflow tract abnormality. US is indicated to determine if a uterus is present; an MRI or laparoscopy of the pelvis may be necessary for confirmation of the diagnosis. In women with a normal uterus, but an imperforate hymen or a transvaginal septum, outflow tract obstruction may be confirmed as the cause. A positive withdrawal bleed indicates a problem with either the HPO axis or the ovary.

STEP THREE

During step three, the gonadotropin assay (FSH and LH) is drawn and sent for laboratory analysis. There should be a delay of 2 weeks between the conclusion of step two and the beginning of step three, as administration of the estrogen/progestin challenge test may cause an artificial alteration in gonadotropin levels. Elevated FSH (>20 IU/L) and LH (>40 IU/L) suggest ovarian dysfunction, whereas normal or low levels of FSH (<5 IU/L) and LH (<5 IU/L) suggest a pituitary or hypothalamic abnormality. When the gonadotropin levels are found to be elevated, they are repeated to confirm that they are not transient. In the case of normal or low levels of gonadotropins, MRI of the sella turcica is indicated to rule out a pituitary tumor. A normal MRI indicates a hypothalamic cause of amenorrhea. It is important to note that all women younger than the age of 30 years diagnosed with ovarian dysfunction based on elevated gonadotropins must be further evaluated with a karyotype. The presence of mosaicism (an individual with at least two cell lines such as 45,X/46,XY) with a Y chromosome requires removal of the gonads because of a significant increase in the risk of malignancy.

Elevated gonadotropins associated with amenorrhea and hypoestrogenism may indicate a menopausal state. On average, menopause occurs at 50 years of age and is a result of depletion of ovarian follicles. Menopause that occurs before the age of 40 years is considered to be POF. As with menopause, POF places a woman at risk of osteoporosis and heart disease. POF has also been associated with autoimmune disorders and endocrinopathies, such as hypothyroidism, but in many cases the cause is unknown (ACOG, 2014a). Other less common autoimmune disorders include Addison disease and diabetes mellitus. A fasting glucose and antibodies testing for 21-hydroxylase should be included in the woman's workup. POF may also be the result of alkylating chemotherapy and radiation of the pelvic area. Approximately 50% of women diagnosed with POF experience intermittent ovarian function. As such, elevated gonadotropins are not always indicative of infertility status, and conception remains a possibility.

Normal or low FSH and LH levels along with normal imaging studies is consistent with hypothalamic amenorrhea. This is a diagnosis of exclusion and is associated with suppression of GnRH below its critical range and disruption in the normal HPO axis. The most common causes for this type of amenorrhea are excessive weight loss (frequently associated with an eating disorder), strenuous exercise, and/or stress. A rare cause of hypothalamic amenorrhea is an inherited genetic disorder, Kallmann syndrome. This syndrome results in deficient secretion of GnRH and is also associated with anosmia (inability to smell; Kim et al., 2019).

Additional evaluation includes US to determine whether there are any anatomic reproductive abnormalities. If a pituitary tumor is suspected, MRI should be conducted (Junsanto-Bahri, 2019).

Treatment/Management

MEDICAL MANAGEMENT

Treatment should be directed at the cause of a woman's amenorrhea and individualized to meet her needs. A woman desiring to achieve pregnancy will be managed differently from a woman wanting only to reestablish a normal menstrual cycle or needing hormone therapy (HT) for symptoms of hypoestrogenism.

For women with PCOS, oral contraceptives or cyclic administration of progestational agents will establish regular withdrawal bleeding and help to maintain a normal endometrium. Oral contraceptives also have the additional benefit of lowering free testosterone levels, thereby decreasing the symptoms of hyperandrogenism. For women with insulin resistance, insulin-sensitizing agents (e.g., metformin) have been shown to improve ovulatory function. Still others may desire conception and need induction of ovulation in order to conceive.

Patients with POF may need HT to address vasomotor symptoms and to prevent osteoporosis. If the amenorrhea is associated with an eating disorder, weight gain generally restores normal menstruation. In many cases, women with severe eating disorders will require the intervention of a psychologist or psychiatrist who specializes in the management of these conditions. Women diagnosed with conditions such as hyperprolactinemia or outflow tract abnormalities must be referred to specialists for treatment and management (e.g., endocrinologist, surgeon).

SELF-MANAGEMENT

If amenorrhea is confirmed to be a symptom of PCOS, protecting the woman's endometrium from hyperplasia by establishing regular menstrual cycles, treating her androgenic signs and symptoms, and decreasing her insulin resistance are all of critical importance. If she is overweight or obese, weight-reduction strategies may be helpful in restoring normal menstruation, decreasing insulin resistance, and lowering androgen levels. If the woman's amenorrhea is a symptom of the female athlete triad, she will need to be counseled on eating healthy meals withsufficient calories and calcium to maintain healthy bone mass. Women with PCOS who experience hirsutism and acne may benefit from visiting an aesthetician to improve healthy skin. Topical OTC acne products and a skin care regimen should be discussed, and a referral provided to a dermatologist as needed.

INTEGRATIVE MEDICINE

Women with chronic health complaints are higher users of integrative techniques; however, there is limited evidence regarding efficacy. Furthermore, integrative treatments are often cost prohibitive. Although limited, various treatments for PCOS have been reported. For example, in one study (Lim et al., 2019), acupuncture was used to treat PCOS. In a comprehensive review article, herbal medicine treatments for PCOS appeared to be beneficial for improving amenorrhea, ovulatory function, lipid metabolism dysfunction, obesity, and insulin resistance (Moini Jazani et al., 2019).

PREMENSTRUAL SYNDROME AND PREMENSTRUAL DYSPHORIC DISORDER

Definition and Scope

PREMENSTRUAL SYNDROME

Dr. William Dewees of the University of Pennsylvania first identified premenstrual syndrome (PMS) in 1843. During that time, PMS was referred to as the *melancholies of menstruation.*

Dewees theorized that the uterus controlled the female body and was able to modify disease (Taylor, 2005). The exact cause of this highly complex, psychoneuroendocrine disorder remains unclear. ACOG (2015) defines the period that occurs approximately 5 days before menstruation and ends a few days after menstruation starts and is accompanied by physical and psychological symptoms as PMS. PMS symptoms negatively affect a woman's QOL. Women who have PMS may experience changes in body perception, a decrease in self-confidence, social isolation, and disrupted interpersonal relationships (Abay & Kaplan, 2019). Approximately 85% of women experience one or more PMS symptoms before and/or during menses. It is estimated that of these women, approximately 30% to 40% meet the criteria for PMS (Danis et al., 2020). While over 150 PMS symptoms have been reported, the most common behavioral and psychological symptoms are mood swings, depression, irritability, anxiety, crying, social withdrawal, difficulty concentrating, and forgetfulness (Danis et al., 2020). The most common physical symptoms are fatigue, bloating, weight gain, acne, breast tenderness, changes in appetite/food cravings, edema, headache, and GI upset (Danis et al., 2020; Box 28.5). Differentiating PMS from other conditions poses challenges as many symptoms overlap. However, Danis et al. (2020), the International Society for Premenstrual Disorders (iapmd.org), ACOG (2014b), and the *Diagnostic and Statistical Manual of Mental Disorders* (5th ed.; American Psychiatric Association [APA], 2013) agree on the following set of diagnostic criteria for PMS:

- The woman must be ovulating.
- The woman experiences a constellation of disabling physical and/or psychological symptoms that appear in the luteal phase of her menstrual cycle.
- The symptoms improve soon after the onset of menses.
- There is a symptom-free interval before ovulation.
- There is prospective documentation of symptoms for at least two consecutive cycles.
- The symptoms are sufficient in severity to affect activities of daily living and/or important relationships.

Evaluation/Assessment

There are two components to diagnosing PMS. The first is one of exclusion; the healthcare provider must rule out other medical and psychiatric etiologies. The second component is evidence via a woman's completed calendar that supports true modulation of symptoms severe enough and impairing her QOL. It is critical that the calendar be generated prospectively for 2 to 3 calendar months. Several symptom diary charts are available to aid in the timing of the symptoms of PMS (Danis et al., 2020). Healthcare providers, through collection of a careful history, physical examination, and laboratory testing, should be able to rule out medical and psychiatric diagnoses.

PREMENSTRUAL DYSPHORIC DISORDER

From 3% to 8% of women suffer from premenstrual dysphoric disorder (PMDD), a more severe form of PMS, with significant impairment in a woman's individual, family, social, and occupational activities (Rajic & Varela, 2018). This disorder is

Box 28.5 Commonly Reported Symptoms and Diagnostic Criteria for Premenstrual Syndrome[a]

Physical Symptoms

Food cravings

Bloating and weight gain

Swelling of hands and feet

Fatigue

Gastrointestinal symptoms

Headache

Breast engorgement and tenderness

Abdominal cramps

Psychosocial Symptoms

Anxiety

Depression

Hostility

Irritability

Panic attacks

Paranoia

Violence toward self or others

Social withdrawal

Angry outbursts

Crying spells

Poor concentration

[a]Premenstrual syndrome can be diagnosed if (1) a woman reports at least one of the physical symptoms and psychosocial symptoms during the 5 days leading up to her menses for three menstrual cycles; (2) symptoms are relieved within 4 days of the onset of menses, without recurrence until at least cycle day 13; (3) symptoms are present in the absence of any pharmacologic therapy, hormone ingestion, or drug or alcohol use; (4) symptoms occur reproducibly during prospective recording of two menstrual cycles; and (5) the woman exhibits identifiable dysfunction in social, academic, or work performance.
Source: American College of Obstetricians and Gynecologists. (2014). Premenstrual syndrome. In Guidelines for women's health care: A resource manual *(4th ed., pp. 607–613). Author; Chandru, S., Indusekhar, R., & O'Brien, S. (2011). Premenstrual syndrome. In R. W. Shaw, D. Leusley, & A. Monga (Eds.),* Gynaecology *(4th ed., pp. 391–404). Elsevier.*

Box 28.6 Diagnostic Criteria for Premenstrual Dysphoric Disorder

At least five symptoms must be present in the luteal phase of the menstrual cycle, improve within a few days after the onset of menses, and be minimal or absent in the week following menses.

1. One or more of the following symptoms must be present:

   - Marked affective lability (mood swings, feeling suddenly sad or tearful, or increased sensitivity to rejection)
   - Marked irritability, anger, or increased interpersonal conflicts
   - Marked depressed mood, feelings of hopelessness, or self-deprecating thoughts
   - Marked anxiety, tension, or feelings of being keyed up/on the edge (or both)

2. One or more of the following symptoms must additionally be present (making for a total of five symptoms when combined with symptoms for aforementioned Item 1):

   - Decreased interest in usual activities (work, school, and friends)
   - Difficulty concentrating
   - Lethargy, easy fatigability, or marked lack of energy
   - Marked change in appetite, overeating, or food cravings
   - Hypersomnia or insomnia
   - Sense of being overwhelmed or out of control
   - Physical symptoms (breast tenderness, swelling, joint or muscle pain, bloating, weight gain)

Symptoms are described as follows:
Symptoms should be documented by prospective daily ratings during at least two symptomatic cycles.
Symptoms are associated with clinically significant distress or interference with woman's social, academic, or work performance, or relationships with others.
The symptoms are not an exacerbation of symptoms of another disorder (major depressive disorder, panic disorder, persistent depressive disorder, or personality disorder).
The symptoms are not attributable to the physiologic effects of a substance (pharmacologic therapy, hormone ingestion, or drug or alcohol use).
Source: Adapted from American College of Obstetricians and Gynecologists. (2017). Committee opinion no. 705: Mental health disorders in adolescents. Obstetrics & Gynecology, 130*(1), e32–e41. https://doi.org/10.1097/AOG.0000000000002160; American Psychiatric Association. (2013). Diagnostic and statistical manual of mental disorders (5th ed.). https://doi.org/10.1176/appi.books.9780890425596*

a worldwide phenomenon and is not influenced by geography or culture (Rajic & Varela, 2018). PMDD is defined by the APA (APA, 2013) as the "cyclic recurrence of severe, sometimes disabling changes in affect—such as mood lability, irritability, dysphoria, and anxiety—that occur in the luteal phase of a woman's menstrual cycle and subside around or shortly thereafter the onset of menses" (ACOG, 2013). The primary distinction between PMS and PMDD is that the symptoms of PMDD are severe and interfere with a woman's ability to function, comparable with other mental disorders (e.g., major depressive episode, general anxiety disorder; see Box 28.6). Women with PMDD have a 50% to 78% lifetime risk for

psychiatric disorders to include: major depression, seasonal affective disorder, dysthymic disorder, generalized anxiety disorder, and suicidality (Rajic & Varela, 2020).

Etiology

The etiologies of PMS and PMDD are not known. Although estrogen and progesterone levels have been found to be normal in women with PMS and PMDD, it has been postulated that there may be an underlying neurobiological vulnerability to normal fluctuations of these hormones (ACOG, 2015). There is also speculation that women with PMDD have impaired production of ALLO, a progesterone metabolite, or impaired sensitivity to GABA during the luteal phase (Dilbaz & Aksan, 2021). It has also been postulated that hormonal fluctuations are associated with impaired serotonin functioning and result in dysregulation of mood, eating, cognition, and sleep behaviors (Rajic & Varela, 2018). Brain imaging has revealed that women with PMDD show enhanced reactivity to the amygdala, which processes emotional and cognitive stimuli during the luteal phase (Rajic & Varela, 2018). While a definitive etiology has been difficult to define, researchers do know that many medical and psychiatric disorders can be exacerbated during the luteal phase and may mimic the signs and symptoms of PMDD, making this a diagnosis of exclusion (Dilbaz & Aksan, 2021).

Risk Factors

Although PMS and PMDD affect reproductive-age women, those with severe symptoms tend to be in their late 20s to mid-50s (Abay & Kaplan, 2019). Sociocultural factors influence a woman's experiences with menstruation. Interestingly, reported symptoms of PMS vary according to geographic location, marital status, parity, education, and occupation (Dilbaz & Aksan, 2021). For example, women in Western cultures may have been socialized to expect uncomfortable symptoms before menstruation. There is also a relationship between menstrual symptoms experienced by mothers and daughters, as well as between sisters, suggesting that responses to menstruation may be learned (Abay & Kaplan, 2019). Other risk factors for the development of PMDD include smoking, lower educational level, history of traumatic events, anxiety disorders, and higher daily stressors (Dilbaz & Aksan, 2021).

Symptoms

More than 150 symptoms have been attributed to PMS and PMDD (Danis et al., 2020). Symptoms vary in character and intensity from woman to woman and may differ in the same woman from cycle to cycle. Symptoms include, but are not limited to, depression, angry outbursts, irritability, crying spells, anxiety, confusion, social withdrawal, poor concentration, insomnia, breast tenderness, food cravings, bloating and weight gain, headaches, swelling of hands and feet, fatigue, GI symptoms, and abdominal pain. It is important for healthcare providers to note that depression and anxiety disorders are the most common conditions that overlap with PMS and PMDD. Determining whether depression and anxiety are symptoms of PMS and/or PMDD or separate conditions will be guided by a woman's medical history. For example, the healthcare provider should inquire as to whether the symptoms of depression and anxiety are present all month, as well as whether or not symptoms are more pronounced just before and during menstruation. The key to diagnosis of PMS and PMDD is the timing of the symptoms and not the symptoms themselves.

Differential Diagnosis

Any condition that results in cyclic mood or physical changes should be included in the differential diagnosis of PMS and PMDD. Several different diagnoses are considered when working a woman up for PMS and/or PMDD. According to Rajic and Valera (2018), there are seven major categories of diagnoses:

1. **Neurologic disorders:** Epilepsy, migraine headache, menstrual headaches
2. **Psychiatric disorders:** Major depressive disorder, anxiety, dysthymic disorder, panic disorder, personality disorder, substance abuse, bulimia
3. **Endocrine disorders:** Hypothyroidism, hyperthyroidism, hypoglycemia, diabetes
4. **Blood disorders:** Anemia
5. **Gynecologic disorders:** Physiologic ovarian cyst, pelvic inflammatory disease, endometriosis, perimenopause, chronic pelvic pain, early menopause
6. **Musculoskeletal disorders:** Arthralgia, arthritis, fibromyalgia
7. **GI disorders:** Irritable bowel syndrome, Crohn disease, functional bowel disorder

The diagnosis of PMS or PMDD is based on exclusion of any of these conditions.

Diagnostic Studies

The diagnosis of PMS or PMDD is not easy, nor can it be made in one office visit. What is more, women often present with symptomology because they have seen their mother or sister suffer from symptoms of PMS or PMDD. On completion of her premenstrual symptom diary (2–3 consecutive months), the woman will follow up with her healthcare provider. Although there are no recommended laboratory tests or diagnostic imaging, the healthcare provider should run a variety of tests for ruling out other pathology. For example, a chemistry profile, CBC, and TSH may be part of the initial testing. Further testing will be based on the woman's history and physical examination. PMS and PMDD are most often diagnoses of exclusion.

Treatment/Management

The overall goals of treatment for either PMS or PMDD are to reduce symptoms, restore normal function, and optimize the woman's overall health. The approach to treatment is based on the specific symptom or constellation of symptoms and their severity. In most cases, treatment options should be approached in a four-step process:

1. **Training and counseling:** Creating awareness, self-screening of symptoms, lifestyle changes (adequate sleep, regular exercise, smoking cessation, communications, dietary changes, stress management)
2. **Nonpharmacologic treatments:** Cognitive behavioral therapy, complementary and alternative treatments (calcium, vitamin D, magnesium, agnus castus, acupuncture)
3. **Pharmacologic treatment:**
   Symptomatic treatment: NSAIDS, diuretics
   Nonhormonal treatment: Selective serotonin reuptake inhibitors (SSRIs; fluoxetine, paroxetine, sertraline); consider anxiolytic agents for women who don't respond to SSRIs

Hormonal treatment: Ovulation suppression with combined oral contraceptives (first line: COC containing drospirenone, 24/4), estrogen (patches/gels) combined with progestins as appropriate, GnRH analogs, danazol

4. **Surgical treatment:** Oophorectomy, laparoscopic hysterectomy with bilateral salpingo-oophorectomy (Abay & Kaplan, 2019)

SELF-MANAGEMENT MEASURES

The first self-management measure that a woman newly diagnosed with PMS or PMDD should be counseled about is lifestyle change. It is critical that the woman understand the importance of her role in managing symptoms. Lifestyle changes include diet and physical activity. The strongest evidence for effective PMS interventions includes calcium supplementation, the use of the diuretic spironolactone, COCs that contain drospirenone (an analog of spironolactone), and cognitive behavioral therapy (CBT; Rajic & Valera, 2018). Drug therapy should be considered for women with severe symptoms and/or those with symptoms who fail to respond or do not respond well to supportive therapy. SSRIs, the recommended initial drug of choice, have been found to be very effective when treating PMS (Abay & Kaplan, 2019). Treatment with anxiolytic alprazolam is also effective in women whose symptoms are not relieved by any of the aforementioned treatment interventions.

Diet and Exercise

For women with mild to moderate PMS and PMDD, lifestyle changes, such as regular aerobic exercise, three to four times a week, particularly during the luteal phase of the menstrual cycle, and nutritional changes (reducing caffeine, salt, alcohol; a diet rich in complex carbohydrates) may be helpful. Although the evidence supporting these interventions comes from epidemiologic studies rather than randomized trials, there is little risk or cost to the woman, and anecdotal experience has shown that when used as an adjunct, they decrease the severity of symptoms in some women (Rajic & Varella, 2018).

Vitamin and Mineral Supplements

Dietary supplements have been studied in RCTs with conflicting results. Calcium as a nutritional supplement has shown the most promise. It appears to improve mood as well as several somatic symptoms such as water retention, food cravings, fatigue, and pain. Research indicates that imbalances in calcium regulation and subsequent deficiency may be responsible for premenstrual symptoms (Danis et al., 2020). An added benefit of calcium is improvement of bone density. For treatment of PMS, calcium 1,200 mg by mouth daily is recommended (Danis et al., 2020).

The role of vitamin B_6 (pyridoxine), a cofactor in serotonin and dopamine metabolism, in the treatment of PMS is unclear. It is thought that vitamin B_6 has the ability to raise levels of serotonin, norepinephrine, histamine, dopamine, and taurine (Danis et al., 2020). Vitamin B_6 in doses of up to 100 mg/day may be of modest benefit in relief of PMS symptoms. Vitamin B_6 can also be found in a wide variety of foods including fortified cereals, beans, meat, poultry, fish, and some fruits and vegetables. It is important to counsel women about the danger associated with exceeding vitamin B_6 supplementation of 100 mg/day, specifically symptoms of peripheral neurotoxicity. It is recommended to discontinue supplemental vitamin B_6 if no improvement in symptomology is observed.

Researchers have reported mixed results for treatment with magnesium and vitamin E (Danis et al., 2020). Studies have shown superior efficacy for essential fatty acids that contain linoleic acid, gamma-linoleic acid, oleic acid, and vitamin E in improving PMS when compared with placebo (Nevatte et al., 2013). Data do not support the benefit of evening primrose oil. It appears to be most beneficial for cyclic mastalgia (Danis et al., 2020).

Mind/Body Therapies

Mind/body therapies (MBTs) are based on the emerging scientific evidence that thoughts and feelings affect normal physiology as well as physical health with the goal to disrupt negative, destructive thought patterns (Dilbaz & Aksan, 2021). Women learn how to cope with premenstrual symptoms, including stress. Mind/body approaches vary widely and include interventions such as psychotherapy (e.g., individual counseling, psychoeducational group therapy), massage, reflexology, hypnotherapy, biofeedback, guided imagery, yoga, and relaxation training. Most of the evidence regarding mind/body approaches for PMS is limited, but since many of these methods teach coping strategies for reducing stress or increasing relaxation, there is still strong rationale for including them in the treatment of PMS (Girman et al., 2003). This therapy may benefit by reframing negative and irrational thinking and increasing coping skills.

Psychoeducational group therapy may be especially helpful. This is a unique opportunity for women to not only learn about their disorder, but to be afforded the opportunity to meet with other women who share similar experiences. This shared experience has been shown to reduce the sense of isolation that many women who suffer from PMS feel. Over time, many women are empowered by the support and their increased knowledge about PMS and, as a result of therapy, develop new behaviors and strategies to help reduce symptoms of PMS (Association of Reproductive Health Professionals, 2008; Nevatte et al., 2013).

Complementary and Alternative Medicine

Referral to an acupuncturist may be appropriate, as acupuncture may provide some relief from symptoms. Some research suggests that acupuncture shows promise, though not definitive, in ameliorating PMS symptoms (Cho & Kim, 2010; Jang et al., 2014; Kang et al., 2011). True acupuncture techniques are tailored to the individual woman's need and therefore make interventional research design more challenging. Jang et al. (2014) reported in their systematic review that acupuncture and herbal medicine reduced symptoms by 50%. Pain-relieving modalities such as transcutaneous electrical nerve stimulation (TENS) and interferential therapy may also be used to reduce physical symptoms related to PMS/PMDD (Kirthika et al., 2018).

HERBAL PREPARATIONS

Chasteberry (*Vitex agnus-castus*) is used by medical herbalists to treat female hormonal disorders and is considered a hormone modulator (British Herbal Medicinal Association [BHMA], 1996). This herb has been reported to improve PMS symptoms when taken daily (20 mg/day). A recent meta-analysis concluded that extracts from agnus-castus were not superior to SSRIs or oral contraceptives for management of PMS/PMDD symptoms; however, it was suggested that there was a possible benefit over use of other minerals for this indication (Danis et al., 2020). Another study involving 1,542 women with PMS reported 33% of the patients had total relief of symptoms with an additional 57% reporting partial relief (Taylor et al., 2006). German health authorities have approved the use of chasteberry for PMS, irregularities of the menstrual cycle, and mastodynia (breast pain/tenderness). Chasteberry is contraindicated in pregnancy and during lactation. Agnolyt, a commercially available chasteberry, has few reported side effects and is sold in most health food stores. No evidence of improvement in PMS symptoms has been reported when using other herbal preparations (e.g., black cohosh, ginko biloba, kava, or oil of evening primrose; BHMA, 1996). It would follow that St. John's wort (*Hypericum peforatum*), because of its SSRI-like effects, would be a logical choice for treating PMS symptoms. The use of St. John's wort in women with PMS has yet to be studied using an RCT study design. It is important that healthcare providers note that St. John's wort Induces enzyme systems, such as cytochrome P450, which when activated, increases the rate at which many drugs are cleared from the bloodstream, thereby reducing their efficacy.

PHARMACOTHERAPEUTICS
Hormonal Therapy

Hormonal therapy can improve physical symptoms by suppressing ovulation and reducing hormonal fluctuations (Abay & Kaplan, 2019). These fluctuations can lead to psychological symptoms in susceptible women. Some have postulated that within the central nervous system (CNS) is a mechanism that determines susceptibility. For this reason, it has been proposed that eliminating the menses, using hormonal contraception, for example, is often effective. Contraceptives that contain drospirenone and ethinyl estradiol have been FDA approved for the treatment of PMDD in women who choose to use an oral contraceptive as their method of contraception (Rajic & Varela, 2018). Current research does not support the use of older generation COCs or progesterone alone in management of PMS (Abay & Kaplan, 2019). GnRH analogs have generally reduced both physical and psychological symptoms; however, because of their negative effects on bone density, use for longer than 6 months is not recommended (Abay & Kaplan, 2019). GnRH agonists and surgical oophorectomy have also been shown to be effective in treating women with PMS. (Abay & Kaplan, 2019).

Selective Serotonin Reuptake Inhibitors

For women with severe PMS or PMDD, SSRI pharmacotherapy should be considered. Numerous RCTs have shown that almost all SSRIs are superior to placebo in improving premenstrual emotional and physical symptoms (Abay & Kaplan, 2019). A low threshold for initiating therapy for women with severe cases of PMDD should be utilized due to their elevated suicide risk. A study by presented by Shams-Alizadeh et al. (2018) on suicidality reported that women with PMDD were significantly more likely to report suicidal ideation (37.4%), plans (19.1%), and attempts (16.2%) compared with women with PMS (22%, 7.6%, and 7.4%, respectively); therefore, it is vitally important not to delay treatment in acute cases (Osborn et al., 2020). SSRIs are the first-line choice for management of severe PMS/PMDD. The effect of SSRI therapy is rapid, with symptom improvement generally seen within 24 to 48 hours. This differs from the treatment of depression or anxiety, where it may take 4 to 6 weeks to see the maximum effect suggesting a different mechanism of action for the treatment of symptoms of PMS or PMDD. Benefits of intermittent SSRI therapy include fewer adverse side effects and less cost to the woman. Intermittent therapy can be started at the beginning of the luteal phase of the menstrual cycle (e.g., 2 weeks before the expected menstrual period) or on the first day that the woman experiences her initial symptoms. With either regimen, the drug is discontinued within 1 to 3 days after the first day of menses. In a meta-analysis, intermittent SSRI dosing was found to be less effective than continuous dosing (Shah et al., 2008). Other antidepressants, such as clomipramine (Anafranil) and venlafaxine (Effexor), are considered second-line therapies for PMS or PMDD and are less well tolerated (Dilbaz & Aksan, 2021). Alprazolam (Xanax), a short-acting benzodiazepine, with anxiolytic and antidepressant properties, has been shown to be more effective that placebo, but should be used with caution because of the risk of tolerance and dependence. SSRIs are generally well tolerated but may be associated with side effects such as GI symptoms (nausea), insomnia, fatigue, and drowsiness, (Abay & Kaplan, 2019). These side effects generally resolve within a few weeks after initiation and may not be much of an issue given the recommended short-term, intermittent dosing. Long-term, continuous dosing may be associated with decreased libido and delayed orgasm (Abay & Kaplan, 2019). SSRI therapy will most likely be necessary through menopause. Some women will experience a recurrence of symptoms when discontinuing the SSRI. It is important to note that although there are a number of successful therapeutic interventions available for the treatment of PMS and PMDD, they by no means replace the healthcare provider–female patient relationship.

MENSTRUAL MIGRAINES

Definition and Scope

Migraines are largely a female disorder. Several female reproductive milestones correlate with a change in migraine frequency or type, thereby implicating sex hormones in the pathogenesis of migraines (Ornello et al., 2021). While migraines occur three to four times more frequently in women than in men, it has been noted that migraine prevalence is the same in men and women prior to the onset of puberty (Ornello et al., 2021). There are two subtypes of menstrual migraines: (1) pure menstrual migraines, migraines that occur only during menstruation, and (2) menstrual-related migraines, which occur regularly with menstruation, but can also occur during other days of the month (Xu et al., 2020). The International Classification of Headache Disorders (ICHD-3 beta) provides diagnostic criteria for the two most common menstrual-related headaches: migraine without aura and menstrual-related migraine without aura (Headache Classification Committee of the International Headache Society, 2013). Menstrual migraines can occur from estrogen fluctuations, either from a naturally occurring menstrual cycle or from the withdrawal of exogenous progestogen provided by COCs or cyclic hormone therapy, or it may be related to perimenopausal hormonal fluctuations, which make management strategies differ (Headache Classification Committee of the International Headache Society, 2013). Collaboration with a neurologist is appropriate and encouraged in women with ongoing menstrual migraines.

Etiology

Throughout the reproductive years, menstruation is one of the most significant events related to the occurrence of migraine attacks. The greatest incidence is during the 5-day window that begins 3 days before onset and continues through the first 3 days of menstruation. Migraines without aura appears to be associated with estrogen withdrawal, whereas migraine with aura is associated with high estrogen levels. Differences may be related to a woman's ability to metabolize estrogens, or to a polymorphism in her genes encoding for sex hormones, their receptors, or metabolites of the hormonal pathways (Ornello et al., 2021).

Estrogen and progesterone influence the pain-processing networks and the endothelium involved in the pathology of migraine (Ornello et al., 2021). These hormones are present in the CNS by passively crossing the blood–brain barrier. Estrogens affect the cellular excitability of the cerebral vessels. Furthermore, there are interrelationships between estrogens and brain neurotransmitters such as serotonin, norepinephrine, dopamine, and endorphins. Estrogen increases serotonergic tone. Peak estrogen levels are associated with a significant decrease in magnesium levels that affects the N-methyl-D-aspartate (NMDA) channel opening (Ornello et al., 2021). Prostaglandins also play a role in the development of menstrual migraine. Systemic circulation of prostaglandins can lead to throbbing headache, nausea, and vomiting. Estrogen facilitates the glutaminergic system, thereby potentially enhancing neural reactivity, which in turn is modulated by progesterone (Martin, 2018).

Risk Factors

Menstrual-related migraine has repeatedly been found to be longer in duration, more disabling, and less responsive to acute therapy (Maasumi et al., 2017). Studies have shown that some women may experience their first migraine with the initiation of COCs. In women with a history of migraines, COC use may cause a worsening of frequency and severity, or no change in migraine occurrence. In COC users, migraines are more likely to be worse during the pill-free week (Calhoun, 2018). Menstrual migraine is often comorbid with other conditions such as dysmenorrhea, irregular cycles, ovarian cysts, endometriosis, heavy menstrual bleeding, and thyroid dysfunction (Albay & Tütüncü, 2020).

Symptoms

Migraines are typically unilateral, pulsating in quality with moderate to severe pain, and interfere with a woman's QOL. Often, the headache is aggravated by light (photophobia) or sounds (phonophobia). Typically, headaches last 4 to 72 hours and last longer than a migraine with aura. Attacks of menstrual migraine (MM) are more often associated with nausea and vomiting as compared with nonmenstrual headaches without aura (Ornello et al., 2021). It has been long established that there is a strong correlation between PMS and MM. Auras are described as visual, sensory, or speech disturbances. Visual symptoms are described as flickering lights, spots, or lines and/or negative features such as loss of vision. Sensory symptoms can include positive features, such as pins and needles, and/or negative features such as numbness. Auras usually occur within 60 minutes before headache onset (Mathew et al., 2013).

Evaluation/Assessment

Gathering a thorough medical history is the first step in the assessment of a woman presenting with migraine headache. It is important to assess if migraines occur at other times than just during menstruation. Women who suffer with migraines without aura tend to have attacks that last longer in duration and are accompanied by nausea as compared with women with nonmenstrual migraines (Vetvik et al., 2015). When evaluating and assessing women with migraines, healthcare providers should pay special attention to the woman's vascular and neurologic examination (Table 28.7). Wippold et al. (2023) refer to the mnemonic *SNOOP* when assessing and examining a patient. This mnemonic helps to triage patients who present with emergent cases:

- *Systemic* symptoms, illness, or condition (e.g., fever, weight loss, cancer, pregnancy, immunocompromised state including HIV)
- *Neurologic* symptoms or abnormal signs (e.g., confusion, impaired alertness)
- *Onset* that is new or sudden
- *Other* associated condition or features (e.g., head trauma, illicit drug use, or toxic exposure; headache awakens patient from sleep, headache is worse with Valsalva maneuver or is precipitated by a cough, exertion, or sexual activity)
- *Previous* headache history with headache progression or change in attack frequency, severity, or clinical features

Differential Diagnosis

Several diagnoses could be added to a working differential diagnosis list for a chief complaint of migraine. Researchers have reported characteristics of stress-related anxiety or depression in women who suffer with migraines without aura (Parashar et al., 2014). Perimenopause may trigger MM due to the frequent fluctuations in estrogen characteristic of this phase of a female life (Ornello et al., 2021). Tension-type headaches can occur at any time during the month

TABLE 28.7 History and Examination for the Chief Complaint of Menstrual Migraine

HISTORY	PHYSICAL EXAMINATION
Age at onset	Obtain blood pressure and pulse
Aura or prodromal symptoms	Assess for bruit at neck, eyes, and head
Frequency of headaches	Palpate the head, neck, and shoulders
Location and radiation of pain	Assess temporal and neck arteries
Associated symptoms	Palpate the spine and neck muscles
Family history of migraines	Cranial nerve assessment
Precipitating and relieving factors	
Ability to engage in activities with migraine	
Ask about relationship between food and alcohol	
Previous treatment and response to treatment	
Any recent change in vision	
Any recent trauma	
Changes in sleep, exercise, weight, or diet	
Changes in method of birth control	
Association with environmental triggers	
Effects of menstrual cycle and exogenous hormones	

Source: Adapted from Wippold, F. J., II, Whealy, M. A., & Kaniecki, R. G. (2023). Evalution of headache in adults. UpToDate. http://www.uptodate.com/contents /evaluation-of-headache-in-adults

irrespective of menstrual cycle, present bilaterally with a pressing or tightening quality, are not aggravated by routine physical activity, and do not accompany nausea, vomiting, or photophobia (Headache Classification Committee of the International Headache Society, 2013). Sinus congestion accompanying menstruation can precipitate sinus pressure and headache. Any new onset of headache should be worked up for a number of possible serious disorders.

Diagnostic Studies

The diagnostic workup for a new-onset menstrual migraine is the same as with any other new-onset headache. Women presenting with a positive *SNOOP* assessment should be triaged into an emergent care category. The choice for brain imaging is MRI, as it is more sensitive in the detection of edema, vascular lesions, and other intracranial pathology. When there is concern that the woman has presented with a thunderclap headache (a severe and sudden onset headache), a CT scan can also be performed. A thunderclap headache is often a symptom of subarachnoid hemorrhage (SAH), which is associated with a very high mortality rate. Should a person survive SAH, they are usually left with a high degree of morbidity and residual impairment. Laboratory analysis will be guided by a woman's physical examination and the healthcare provider's working differentials. It is common, especially in cases of new-onset headache, for a lumbar puncture and CSF analysis and testing to be conducted.

Treatment/Management

Women who experience migraines only during menstruation respond more positively to hormone prophylaxis (Headache Classification Committee of the International Headache Society, 2013) as compared with those with nonmenstrual-related migraines (Maasumi et al., 2017). Treatment is triaged into three levels of care: (1) acute treatment during the attack, (2) prevention, during the menstrual window, and (3) daily preventive treatment used throughout the month (Maasumi et al., 2017).

SELF-MANAGEMENT

Not all women experience the same triggers that can induce a migraine. Notable migraine triggers include stress, lack of sleep or jet lag, food additives, alcohol, odd or strong smells, hunger or dehydration, highly caffeinated beverages, medication overuse, bright lights and loud sounds, changes in weather, hormones, physical activity, and foods. Avoiding triggers such as the weather is impractical and can become restrictive. What is more, healthcare provider recommendation to avoid triggers is not evidence based. Rather, some have suggested that healthcare providers counsel women to *cope with* rather than *avoid* triggers, as avoidance may further sensitize women to headache precipitating factors (Hoffman & Recober, 2013). Avoiding triggers can become a significant stressor. Healthcare providers should individualize patient recommendations and women with menstrual headaches should use common sense when balancing trigger avoidance and coping strategies (Hoffman & Recober, 2013). Referring the patient with ongoing symptoms of menstrual migraine is encouraged.

INTEGRATIVE MEDICINE

Acupuncture is performed routinely for the prevention and treatment of migraines, while physical therapy and mindfulness have seen an increase in popularity in recent years (Wells et al., 2019). There is limited existing evidence regarding the relationship between vitamin supplementation and decrease in migraine incidence. Riboflavin is also thought to be effective in treating migraines (Wells et al., 2019). There is ongoing research examining whether melatonin, vitamin B_6 with folic acid, vitamin D, omega-3 butterbur, and feverfew also play a role in treatment (Wells et al., 2019).

PHARMACOTHERAPEUTICS

Regardless of whether menstrual or nonmenstrual-related migraine, treatment strategies are the same, with the addition of miniprophylaxis and hormonal manipulation for treatment of menstrual migraines (Ornello et al., 2021). There are three general treatment strategies for menstrual migraine management: acute, miniprevention (before and during), and long-term prevention. Women with irregular cycles are not good candidates for miniprevention strategies because of the unpredictability of their menses (Calhoun, 2018). One strategy for women with irregular cycles is to have the woman use basal body temperature or to use an ovulation predictor kit to evaluate when ovulation will occur.

Nonsteroidal Anti-Inflammatory Drugs

NSAIDs are the oldest class of migraine treatments that effectively block prostaglandin synthesis by inhibiting the enzyme cyclooxygenase, enhancing adrenergic transmission by increasing norepinephrine release and suppressing inflammation that decreases central sensitization (Martin, 2018). NSAIDs initiated 5 to 7 days before the onset of menstruation may decrease or eliminate the migraine (Martin, 2018).

Triptans

Triptans are effective short-term prophylactic treatment for menstrual migraine (Martin, 2018). The triptans are selective serotonin receptor agonists that interfere with migraine pathogenesis.. The three most commonly used triptans are frovatriptan, naratriptan, and zolmitriptan. Triptans have been found to be more effective than placebo in preventing menstrual migraines and reduce their frequency (when treating 5 to 7 days before the onset of menstruation). Triptans and other adjunctive therapies, such as NSAIDs, estradiol, and topiramate, are thought to increase the effectiveness by reducing or aborting menstrual migraines (Martin, 2018; Ornello et al., 2021).

Hormonal Therapies

The use of COCs may have differing effects on menstrual migraines. COCs are contraindicated in women who experience migraine attacks with aura due to an elevated stroke risk (Nappi et al., 2022). For some women, menstrual migraine may present for the first time with the initiation of COCs due to the degree of estrogen withdrawal (Nappi et al., 2022). In this case, COCs should be discontinued.

Migraine Without Aura

There are several approaches to providing a sustained level of estrogen throughout the month by prescribing supplemental estradiol (e.g., hormonally active pills, transdermal application using a menstrual suppression strategy). These approaches are associated with overall reduction in migraine severity and frequency. Estrogen supplementation that can also be provided during menstruation includes (a) oral, (b) gel, or (c) patch (moderate to high dose) delivery systems (Nappi et al., 2022). It is also reasonable to trial continuous dosing COCs (low dose) to eliminate the hormone-free period, thus reducing likelihood of MM (Nappi et al., 2022).

Migraine With Aura

According to the *U.S. Medical Eligibility Criteria for Contraceptive Use 2016*, prescribing considerations for women with migraines are delineated by those with and without aura (Curtis et al, 2016). COCs should *not* be prescribed for women suffering from migraine with aura as they may lead to further vascular risk such as stroke and SAH. The ideal treatment for migraine with aura is a nonhormonal method, with the copper intrauterine device (IUD; a long-acting reversible contraception [LARC] method) preferred.

DYSMENORRHEA

Definition and Scope

Dysmenorrhea is the most common gynecologic condition among reproductive-age women and occurs in 50% to 90% of menstruating women (ACOG, 2018b). Dysmenorrhea is an underdiagnosed condition consisting of painful menstruation. It often goes undiagnosed because many women dismiss the symptoms as a normal part of menstruation. More than one half of women who menstruate have some pain for 1 to 2 days each month (ACOG, 2020). Although mild discomfort during menstruation is widely experienced by most women, actual dysmenorrhea is cyclic pain that prevents normal activity and requires medication (ACOG, 2020). The pain is characterized as cramping or *labor-like* pain that begins with or just before the onset of menses and generally lasts for 2 to 3 days. The pain may be experienced in the lower abdomen and lower back and may radiate into the inner aspects of the thighs. There are two types of dysmenorrhea. An excess of prostaglandins leading to painful uterine muscle activity causes primary dysmenorrhea. Primary dysmenorrhea is associated with ovulatory cycles and does not usually occur until later in adolescence. It is estimated that 14% to 26% of adolescents have pain severe enough to cause them to miss school and work (ACOG, 2020). Secondary dysmenorrhea is caused by a disorder of the reproductive tract (e.g., adenomyosis, endometriosis, PID, cervical stenosis, leiomyomas, and polyps); secondary dysmenorrhea tends to get worse over time (ACOG, 2020). Transgender individuals experience dysmenorrhea at the same rates as cisgender individuals; however, they are often underdiagnosed (Shim et al., 2020).

Etiology

Primary dysmenorrhea is caused by excessive secretion of uterine prostaglandins, specifically prostaglandin $F_{2\alpha}$ ($PGF_{2\alpha}$), released from the endometrium during the menses. $PGF_{2\alpha}$ induces uterine contractions that can lead to uterine hypoxia. During the luteal phase of the menstrual cycle, declining levels of progesterone cause lysosomes to release a phospholipase enzyme, which in turn hydrolyzes cell membrane phospholipids to generate arachidonic acid. Arachidonic acid serves as a precursor for the synthesis of prostaglandins.

Prostaglandin synthesis is mediated by two isoforms of cyclo-oxygenase (COX-1 and COX-2), enzymes that convert arachidonic acid to several metabolites, including $PGF_{2\alpha}$. Higher concentrations of $PGF_{2\alpha}$ have been found in the menstrual fluid of women with dysmenorrhea (ACOG, 2020). Intensity of menstrual cramps has been found to be directly related to the amount of $PGF_{2\alpha}$ released. The association between $PGF_{2\alpha}$ and dysmenorrhea is supported by three observations: (1) in anovulatory cycles without dysmenorrhea, menstrual fluid concentration of prostaglandins is not elevated; (2) intravenous injection of $PGF_{2\alpha}$ causes uterine cramps and pain; and (3) medications that inhibit prostaglandin secretion relieve dysmenorrhea (ACOG, 2020). $PGF_{2\alpha}$ can also cause nausea, vomiting, diarrhea, headache, and dizziness, symptoms that are frequently associated with primary dysmenorrhea. Along with $PGF_{2\alpha}$, the uterus also produces prostaglandin E_2 (PGE_2), which has been implicated as a cause of primary menorrhagia, as it is a potent vasodilator and inhibitor of platelet aggregation (Saei Ghare Naz et al., 2020).

Risk Factors

The scope and risk factors of primary dysmenorrhea are not fully understood. The most widely accepted reason of primary dysmenorrhea is the overproduction of uterine prostaglandins. Risk factors that are associated with primary dysmenorrhea include higher BMI, extreme ends of the reproductive years, and nulliparity. Menstrual and family history include early age of onset of menses, longer and heavier menstrual flow, and family history of dysmenorrhea. Lifestyle behaviors that have been linked to primary dysmenorrhea include smoking and alcohol consumption. The copper IUD may also be associated with increased menstrual pain, whereas the LNG-IUS tends to decrease menstrual pain. The most common causes of secondary dysmenorrhea have accompanying AUB associated with endometriosis, adenomyosis, or fibroids.

Symptoms

Primary dysmenorrhea usually begins early in the reproductive years and has a clear and predictable pattern, beginning before or at the start of menstruation. The pain typically lasts 8 to 72 hours and is most severe on the first day of menstruation. Systemic symptoms include nausea, vomiting, diarrhea, fatigue, and insomnia because of the pain (Ferries-Rowe et al., 2020). Secondary dysmenorrhea is often caused by endometriosis, but other causes include adenomyosis, leiomyomas, infection, cervical stenosis, ovarian cysts, and PID. The initiation of the pain pattern can start at any time, but typically presents 6 to 12 months after menarche when adolescents begin having ovulatory cycles and is often accompanied by AUB/HMB or AUB/IMB (ACOG, 2018b).

Evaluation/Assessment

HISTORY

Primary dysmenorrhea is a diagnosis of exclusion. A complete history and physical examination are needed to make an accurate diagnosis. A thorough history should include questions to determine when the pain occurs, how the patient treats the pain, if there are associated symptoms, how contraceptives affect the pain, and if the pain becomes more severe over time (ACOG, 2020). The onset of primary dysmenorrhea in close proximity to menarche and the timing of the pain in relationship to the menses are key diagnostic features of primary dysmenorrhea. A contraceptive history should be obtained to rule out if an IUD, for example, may be the cause of menstrual pain. The onset of pain is typically the first day of menses; pain peaks in severity during the first 2 days of the menstrual cycle, and then decreases thereafter. Patients may also experience nausea, vomiting, diarrhea, and headache during these painful episodes.

A detailed medical history should reveal symptoms related to underlying gynecologic abnormalities, in turn informing the etiology of a woman's secondary dysmenorrhea. A woman diagnosed with adenomyosis, leiomyomas, or polyps may present with AUB/HMB with combined dysmenorrhea (Bernardi et al., 2017). Pelvic heaviness or changes in abdominal shape may suggest large leiomyomas or intra-abdominal neoplasia, whereas infection is usually associated with chills, malaise, and fever. Secondary dysmenorrhea accompanied by report of infertility raises the possibility of endometriosis or chronic PID (Bernardi et al., 2017).

PHYSICAL EXAMINATION

The physical examination of a symptomatic woman with dysmenorrhea is directed at discovering possible causes (Bernardi et al., 2017). Primary dysmenorrhea can only be diagnosed when the physical examination does not reveal pelvic diseases or other gynecologic abnormalities. Assessment may reveal generalized pelvic tenderness focused more in the area of the uterus than the adnexa, no palpable abnormalities of the uterus, and no abnormalities on speculum or abdominal examination (Ferries-Rowe et al., 2020). In some instances, diagnostic imaging may be indicated to rule out pelvic abnormalities and definitively diagnose primary dysmenorrhea.

The physical examination of patients with secondary dysmenorrhea varies depending on the causative pathology. Leiomyomas may cause pelvic asymmetry or irregular enlargement of the uterus. Findings on bimanual exam usually include an irregular-shaped mobile uterus that is nontender, with either a firm or rubbery solid consistency that may be palpable abdominally (Smith & Kaunitz, 2021). Although adenomyosis can only be definitively diagnosed by histologic examination, physical examination may reveal a uterus that is tender, symmetrically enlarged, and "boggy" (Smith & Kaunitz, 2021). Endometriosis should be suspected when there are painful nodules in the posterior cul-de-sac and restricted motion of the uterus. If infection is suspected, a cervical culture should be collected and sent for ruling out STIs (*Neisseria gonorrhoeae* and *Chlamydia trachomatis*). More invasive procedures, such as laparoscopy, may be needed to make a confirmatory diagnosis.

Differential Diagnosis

In most cases, the final diagnosis can be reached by careful history and physical examination; in some instances, a diagnostic laparoscopy may be needed for histologic confirmation. Conditions to consider include processes outside the uterus (e.g., endometriosis, tumors, adhesions, and nongynecologic causes), those within the myometrium (e.g., adenomyosis, myomas), and conditions within the endometrium (e.g., myomas, endometrial polyps, infection, IUDs, cervical stenosis). When the patient continues to experience pain between menstrual periods, these conditions may be the source of her chronic pelvic pain.

Treatment/Management

The goal of treatment is to reduce the menstrual pain so that the woman's health and QOL improve. Once dysmenorrhea has been diagnosed, approaches to treatment and management include pharmacologic, nonpharmacologic, and surgical interventions.

INTEGRATIVE MEDICINE

Magnesium has been used to relieve primary dysmenorrhea, although the ideal dose, type of magnesium (e.g., magnesium oxide, magnesium carbonate), and dosing regimen have not been clarified. Vitamin D showed a significant improvement in reported menstrual pain when taking 50,000 IU orally once per week (Saei Ghare Naz et al., 2020). Vitamin E in various dosages has been shown to reduce menstrual pain more effectively than placebo (Saei Ghare Naz et al., 2020). This same systemic review/meta-analysis showed improvements in dysmenorrhea with use of zinc, vitamin B_1, and vitamin K injection, although the evidence for efficacy is limited (Saei Ghare Naz et al., 2020).

Although there is no solid evidence to support this, several studies support the use of exercise as a way to reduce the severity of dysmenorrhea. A recent study showed that high-frequency TENS is more effective for relieving menstrual pain when compared with the placebo group (Elboim-Gabyzon & Kalichman, 2020). Acupuncture has been shown to be somewhat effective in alleviating dysmenorrhea (ACOG, 2018b). There is not enough evidence to recommend herbal and dietary therapies for dysmenorrhea, but many home remedies may provide a certain level of relief for some women.

PHARMACOTHERAPEUTICS

Acetaminophen and NSAIDs are the most commonly prescribed medications for treatment of primary dysmenorrhea. When taken as prescribed, they are often very effective in providing pain relief. NSAIDs reduce pain by inhibiting prostaglandin synthesis and by their direct CNS analgesic effect. They reduce the number of prostaglandins that the body makes and lessen their effect. For optimal efficacy, it is best to start NSAIDs 1 to 2 days before the anticipation of the onset of menses/pain, as their effectiveness for treating pain appears to decrease once menses has begun. Women are counseled to take both medications *as needed,* although if pain control is poor, the woman may benefit from regularly scheduled doses. Because of a long-standing history of safety and efficacy, OTC availability, and relative low cost, NSAIDs have become the treatment of choice for primary dysmenorrhea. Although adverse side effects occur infrequently with intermittent use of NSAIDs, healthcare providers should be aware that there is always that possibility, and in such cases therapy should be discontinued. Women with coagulopathies, asthma, aspirin allergy, liver damage, peptic ulcer disease, or stomach disorders should not take NSAIDs (ACOG, 2020).

Cyclooxygenase inhibitors (COX-2 inhibitors), such as celecoxib, have been found to be effective in treating dysmenorrhea, although no studies have shown they are any better than naproxen. In the recent past, COX-2 inhibitors were becoming the NSAIDs of choice because of their specific and targeted action to treat dysmenorrhea. However, because of serious health and safety concerns, including life-threatening cardiovascular and GI adverse effects, they now are rarely used (Beckmann et al., 2014).

COCs containing estrogen and progestin can be used to treat dysmenorrhea in women who do not desire childbearing and who may not be able to tolerate NSAID therapy. By suppressing ovulation and stabilizing estrogen and progesterone levels, COCs lower the level of endometrial prostaglandins and reduce spontaneous uterine activity. COCs can be taken cyclically in the traditional 28-day schedule, or for more extended periods of time allowing for longer intervals between menses (ACOG, 2018b). Often dysmenorrhea can be completely eliminated by the continuous use of hormonal contraceptives (Beckmann et al., 2014). Hormonal contraceptives, as long as not contraindicated, may be given for more than 6 to 12 months. Many women continue to experience pain-free menses even after discontinuation of hormonal treatment. The pill, the patch, and the vaginal ring are options, along with progestin-only methods like the DMPA injection or an implantable intrauterine system (LNG-IUS). Oral contraceptives and NSAIDs are known to have a synergistic effect on menstrual pain caused by primary dysmenorrhea (ACOG, 2018b). They can be taken together or alone to achieve pain relief.

Women who do not respond to acetaminophen, NSAID, and/or hormonal contraceptive therapy should be reevaluated for abnormalities associated with secondary dysmenorrhea. For conditions such as adenomyosis and when the woman wishes to preserve fertility, a definitive treatment plan may not be an option. Instead, a symptomatic treatment plan of analgesics or menstrual cycle modification may be most appropriate (Beckmann et al., 2014). Transgender individuals have the same treatment options as discussed here, and many start with NSAIDS and oral contraceptives (Shim et al., 2020). Transgender individuals have also seen improvement in dysmenorrhea with testosterone treatment (Shim et al., 2020). More studies on this population are needed as limited studies and data are currently available.

SURGICAL THERAPY

In women who do not respond to medical therapies, surgery may be indicated for definitive treatment. The type of surgical procedure is dependent on the underlying cause of pain as well as if fertility is desired. Laparoscopic uterosacral ligament division and presacral neurectomy have been a purposed treatment option, although this is considered a conservative surgical therapy. There is, however, insufficient evidence to recommend either at this time (ACOG, 2018b). A partial or total hysterectomy may eventually be required for treatment of adenomyosis, endometriosis, or residual pelvic infection that has not been responsive to medical treatments or even conservative surgical therapies.

FUTURE DIRECTIONS

The menstrual cycle is a natural process for women. However, cyclic changes or structural anomalies can produce ill-effects and negatively impact women's lives. Management of the disorders covered in this chapter is an evolving science. Early recognition through genetic identification can tailor patient management of these conditions.

REFERENCES

References for this chapter are online and available at https://connect.springerpub.com/content/book/978-0-8261-6722-4/part/part03/chapter/ch28

CHAPTER 29

Urologic and Pelvic Floor Health Problems

RICHARD S. BERCIK AND CHERRILYN F. RICHMOND

Urologic and pelvic floor health problems, including issues such as prolapse, urinary incontinence (UI), interstitial cystitis (IC), and urinary tract infections (UTIs), can significantly reduce quality of life (QOL) for women and transgender men with female organs. Accurate identification and management are critical to prevent untoward sequelae and to sustain high QOL. (In this chapter, *woman* and *women* are used as general terms to include all persons with a vagina and uterus.)

PELVIC ORGAN PROLAPSE

Pelvic relaxation disorders (also referred to as pelvic organ prolapse [POP]) is the term used to describe clinical manifestations of damaged or weakened support mechanisms in the female pelvis. POP includes disorders of the anterior vaginal compartment (cystocele and urethrocele), the posterior vaginal compartment (rectocele), the apical compartment (uterus or posthysterectomy vaginal vault), the rectovaginal space (enterocele), and the perineum (Weber et al., 2001).

Women who experience POP have symptoms that can be mild to severe and can alter their QOL. Evaluation of the problem, degree of bother, and possibilities for management are individualized for each woman.

Etiology

An understanding of the anatomy of pelvic support is essential to understanding POP and its management. Pelvic organ support is maintained by a combination of pelvic musculature and connective tissue. The uterosacral and cardinal ligaments comprise mostly smooth muscle, vascular elements, and loosely organized collagen fibers and are responsible for uterine and apical support. They merge with the ring of pericervical fascia either posteriorly (uterosacral) or laterally (cardinal). These are the main structures of uterine support as the round ligaments do not contribute in any significant way to uterine support (DeLancey, 1994). The anterior endopelvic fascia extends distally from the pericervical ring to the

perineal membrane and laterally to the arcus tendineus fascia pelvis (ATFP; Weber & Walters, 1997). The lateral margin of the vagina is attached to the sidewall at the ATFP, which extends from the ischial spine anteriorly to the pubovesical ligament (DeLancey, 1994). Anterior compartment prolapse can occur either from defects in these attachments (paravaginal defect) or disruption of the vaginal muscularis (central cystocele; Ashton-Miller & DeLancey, 2007).

Posteriorly, a true fascial layer has been identified between the rectum and vagina; this layer has been identified not only in adult cadavers, but also in newborns and is derived from mesenchymal differentiation (Ashton-Miller & DeLancey, 2007). Posterior prolapse results from defects in this layer, which can occur laterally, centrally, or in combination. Enteroceles form because of a defect in the superior portion of this layer (Lukacz & Luber, 2002; Segal & Karram, 2002). The levator muscle complex is also integral to maintaining pelvic organ support. Composed of the puborectalis, pubococcygeus, and iliococcygeus muscles, this complex forms a sheet of muscular support for the pelvic viscera (Ashton-Miller & DeLancey, 2007; DeLancey et al., 2007). This structure extends from pelvic sidewall to sidewall and encircles the urethra, vagina, and rectum, establishing the genital hiatus. Enlargement of the genital hiatus occurs during vaginal childbirth, and while it will often approach predelivery diameters postpartum, residual changes persist after delivery. With aging, time, abdominal pressures, and hypoestrogenic conditions, the levator is prone to further loss of tone and resultant pathologic widening of the genital hiatus. When this occurs POP often results, as connective tissue support can no longer compensate for levator muscle weakness.

Definition and Scope

Prevalence of POP disorders increases with age. As the population older than 65 years continues to increase so will the demand for the evaluation and management of POP. Approximately 200,000 women undergo more than 300,000 inpatient procedures for POP in the United States each year, and one in nine American women will have a surgical procedure for POP or UI throughout their lifetime (Schulten et al., 2022).

POP was generally considered a disorder that occurred in White, parous, postmenopausal women; however, these preconceptions have been proved false. Although POP affects all women, exact incidence is difficult to establish because the dividing line between normal parous support and POP is difficult to define. Some degree of descent occurs in most women who have experienced vaginal childbirth, and yet most of these women have no symptoms.

Pelvic organ relaxation is commonly seen in about 50% of parous women; 40% of women age 45 to 85 years can have stage 2 prolapse (Schulten et al., 2022). Formal graded pelvic examinations (pelvic organ prolapse quantification [POPQ]) performed on a population of gynecologic patients revealed that 2.6% of the women had stage 3 prolapse (within 1 cm of introitus) and none had stage 4 prolapse (Drutz & Alarab, 2006; Table 29.1). Disparities have historically been reported regarding the prevalence of POP with higher rates among White and Hispanic groups compared to Black cohorts. These findings have been challenged by studies showing no difference among groups when prolapse is diagnosed by physical examination (Sears et al., 2009).

The rate of vaginal vault prolapse after hysterectomy is reported to range from 0.5% to 1.5% (Swift et al., 2005). Aging of the population will further increase the number of women affected; it has been estimated that by the age of 80 years, approximately 11% of the female population will have had a corrective procedure for either POP or UI (Swift et al., 2005).

In 1999, the International Continence Society published a consensus statement on standardizing terminology related to lower urinary tract function (Weber et al., 2001). In general, POP is defined as descent of the pelvic structures to a degree that interferes with organ function, causes distress (emotional or physical) to the patient, creates a life-threatening condition, or significantly interferes with everyday activity. POP is described by the location of key anatomic structures, in relation to fixed points such as the ischial spines and the hymenal ring. Physical examination is the main tool to describe the affected segments and the points of maximal prolapse. Terms such as cystocele, rectocele, and enterocele are avoided because of their lack of descriptive quality.

Preferably, terms such as *anterior vaginal wall*, *posterior vaginal wall*, *vaginal apex*, and *genital hiatus* are used in conjunction with standardized measurements. Nine specific points or measurements are the components of the POPQ. Listed here are the pelvic relaxation disorders (with their previously used terminology).

ANTERIOR VAGINAL WALL PROLAPSE

Anterior vaginal wall prolapse (previously referred to as cystocele) is the inferior and ventral displacement of the anterior vaginal wall (and possibly bladder) caused by an anterior pelvic support defect. This may be because of a midline (central) defect in the vesicovaginal connective tissue or a lateral (paravaginal) defect, which involves a detachment of the vagina from the ATFP.

HYPERMOBILE URETHRA

Hypermobile urethra (previously referred to as urethrocele) is a significant downward rotation (more than 35 degrees) of the distal anterior vaginal wall caused by a defect in the suburethral connective tissue and pubourethral (pubovisceral) ligaments.

APICAL VAGINAL PROLAPSE

Apical vaginal prolapse (previously referred to as enterocele) results in uterine prolapse, or if the uterus is absent, vaginal cuff prolapse. A defect in uterosacral and cardinal ligament support (type I) is thought to be the mechanism for this prolapse.

POSTERIOR VAGINAL WALL PROLAPSE

Posterior vaginal wall prolapse (previously referred to as rectocele) is the ventral and superior displacement of the posterior vaginal wall (and possibly the distal rectum and anus) caused by a defect in the rectovaginal connective tissue.

Risk Factors

Gender, aging, body mass index (BMI), and childbirth are the most significant risk factors for POP. Prolonged labor followed by cesarean delivery does not protect a woman from pelvic relaxation (Schulten et al., 2022). Nulliparity protects against POP only until menopause. As nulliparous women progress further beyond menopause, the incidence of POP continues to rise and probably equals that of a parous female at age 75 years (Richter, 2006). Twenty percent of the Women's Health Initiative population had some degree of POP (Jelovsek et al., 2007).

Modifiable risk factors include weight, smoking status, avoidance of constipation, and maintaining good physical conditioning. Therefore, it is possible for lifestyle interventions to reduce the lifetime risk for POP. These interventions include avoiding constipation, avoiding chronic heavy lifting, avoiding chronic coughing associated with smoking, maintaining a healthy weight, and maintaining the strength of the striated muscles of the pelvic floor. Examples of nonmodifiable factors include congenitally acquired connective tissue abnormalities, aging, and menopause (Jelovsek et al., 2007; Nieminen et al., 2003; Nygaard, Bradley, et al., 2004; Tegerstedt et al., 2006).

TABLE 29.1 Stages of Pelvic Organ Prolapse	
Stage 0	No prolapse
Stage 1	The most distal portion of the prolapse is more than 1 cm **proximal to** the hymen
Stage 2	The most distal potion of the prolapse is **beyond** stage 1, but not yet stage 3
Stage 3	The most distal portion of the prolapse protrudes **more than 1 cm distal to** the hymen, but not yet stage 4
Stage 4	Complete eversion of the vaginal walls and/or the cervix protrudes

Symptoms

Symptoms of POP are varied and at times nonspecific. Usually, symptoms are related to the degree of prolapse and the predominant compartment affected (Santaniello et al., 2007). Patients with vaginal prolapse often do not complain of any symptoms until the prolapse has progressed to stage 3 (i.e., the leading point of prolapse is within 1 cm of the vaginal introitus). At this point, patients often complain of a vaginal protrusion or bulge first noticed while bathing (Burrows et al., 2004; Digesu, Chaliha, et al., 2005).

Stages 1 and 2 prolapse may have few to no symptoms. At this stage, the leading point of prolapse is not yet 1 cm beyond the hymenal ring. Early symptoms of stages 1 and 2 prolapse include lower back pain, pelvic heaviness or fullness, vaginal pain, and pain during intercourse. Urinary complaints may include urinary urgency, hesitancy, and UI or anorgasmia during sexual activity. Rectal frequency and urgency alternating with bouts of constipation are common. In general, symptoms worsen with increased physical activity and/or prolonged standing (Drutz & Alarab, 2006; Richter et al., 2007).

Stage 3 prolapse consists of the leading point of prolapse to be more than 1 cm beyond the hymenal ring but not yet completely prolapsed. At this point, patients will often complain of being able to feel the organs descending into or beyond the vagina. Often patients are unable to engage in sexual activity at this point. There is difficulty using tampons and pain with sitting or prolonged walking as the vaginal protrusion progresses. Symptoms of obstructive urination often worsen at this stage so that incomplete bladder emptying, postvoid dribbling, excessive straining to void, or the need to manually reduce the prolapse to void (digital splinting) might arise. Similarly, symptoms associated with obstructive defecation might be problematic at this point. Constipation, rectal straining, and need to digitally splint to defecate can occur (Drutz & Alarab, 2006; Kahn et al., 2005; Mouritsen & Larsen, 2003; Swift et al., 2005; Weber & Richter, 2005). Symptoms associated with this stage are often quite distressing to the patient, prompting the patient to seek treatment.

Stage 4 prolapse consists of complete prolapse of one or more vaginal components. After hysterectomy this consists of complete vaginal eversion with enterocele. Pain is often present because of mucosal drying, erosion, and ulceration combined with persistent rubbing of the prolapse as the patients perform everyday activity. Symptoms of obstructive voiding worsen so that urinary retention is usually present. Advanced cases may result in urinary retention with urethral obstruction or ureteral blockage resulting in hydroureter, hydronephrosis, and subsequent renal damage. These patients may require an indwelling bladder catheter or learn to perform clean intermittent self-catheterization (CISC). Urinary infection risk is increased and at times urosepsis may be the presenting symptom.

Women with advanced POP often do not complain of UI. They may have a normal urethral continence mechanism, but also may have occult stress incontinence (also labeled potential or masked stress urinary incontinence [SUI]). This occurs because urethral kinking increases urethral resistance leading to obstruction, which then masks an incontinent urethral mechanism. Recent data indicate that this may occur in as many as 33% of patients with advanced POP (Burrows et al., 2004; Davis & Kumar, 2005).

Evaluation/Assessment

HISTORY

In addition to obtaining a history regarding symptoms of urinary, defecatory, and sexual dysfunction, a complete history is needed to determine possible medical comorbidities. Measures of the impact of symptoms on the patient's QOL also must be completed.

Obstetric history, including a review of pregnancies and deliveries, is essential. It includes route of delivery, number of deliveries, length of labor and second stage, birth weights, operative deliveries, episiotomy with or without laceration, and presence of any postpartum incontinence (anal and urinary). If applicable, a thorough review of perimenopause and menopause-related symptoms and history is completed. Specifically, time since the last menstrual period, a timeline of menopause-related symptoms and problems associated with vaginal atrophy (e.g., pain, dryness, discharge, and dyspareunia) are considered. The medical history must be complete and specifically address the presence of diabetes, any neurologic disorders, changes in mental status, and medications. Surgical history with specific questions regarding hysterectomy (route and indication), oophorectomy, any vaginal surgery, and prior surgery for POP and/or UI must also be complete. Social history includes caffeine and alcohol intake, occupation, marital status, sexual activity, and living environment. The last item, living environment, is particularly important for the geriatric patient; for example, physical obstruction to bathroom facilities is problematic. Finally, family history with attention to POP, urinary or fecal incontinence, collagen diseases, and early menopause should be documented.

Many patients with POP do complain about UI. In general, detecting UI by history has a high sensitivity but low specificity. It is further complicated by the fact that 10% to 30% of patients with stress UI also have overactive bladder UI. In patients with pure stress UI symptoms, 65% to 90% will have stress UI on urodynamic testing. If urge incontinence, enuresis, and sensory urgency are present, 80% to 85% will have overactive bladder identified on urodynamic testing (Helström & Nilsson, 2005; Fitzgerald & Brubaker, 2002; Reena et al., 2007). History information to obtain is listed in Box 29.1.

PHYSICAL EXAMINATION

The physical examination includes a general examination to identify any undiagnosed cardiac, pulmonary, gastrointestinal, or other disorders. Pelvic examination includes close inspection of the vulva and vagina with attention to potential epithelial lesions (see Chapter 27, Vulvar and Vaginal Health). Any ulcers or suspicious lesions should be biopsied. Evaluation of the genital hiatus (introitus) is done both at rest and with straining. Note the thickness of the perineal body and look for a "dovetail" sign indicating a nonintact external anal sphincter. During the digital rectal examination assess external anal sphincter tone (four grades; see Box 29.2).

Box 29.1 History Information for Urinary Incontinence

Severity

1. How often do "accidents" occur?
2. Do you leak urine when you cough, laugh, or sneeze?
3. Do you wear pads/protection?
4. If yes, how many pads per day?
5. Does this problem interfere with your social life or work?

Infection, Malignancy

1. Do you have a history of bladder or kidney infections?
2. Do you have pain or discomfort on urination?
3. Have you ever had blood in your urine?

Voiding Dysfunction

1. Is the urine stream slow or intermittent?
2. Do you have to strain to get the urine out?
3. After urination, do you have dribbling or a sensation that your bladder is still full?

Urge/Detrusor Instability

1. Do you ever have an uncomfortable need to rush to the bathroom to urinate?
2. If yes, do you ever have an "accident" before you reach the toilet?
3. How many times during the day do you urinate?
4. How many times do you get up from sleep to urinate?
5. When in a hurry or under stress, do you feel an urgent need to urinate?
6. Have you had any episodes of wetting the bed?
7. Do you ever have leakage during intercourse?

Box 29.2 Sphincter Tone Grading

1. No squeeze felt
2. Squeeze felt minimally around finger
3. Squeeze felt less than 50% finger circumference
4. Squeeze felt more than 50% finger circumference and held for longer than 2 seconds

A focused neurologic examination is performed, including evaluation of sensory function of the sacral dermatomes, perineal area, and the lower extremities. Motor function of the lower extremities, including extension and flexion of the hip, knee, and ankle, and inversion/eversion of each foot are also assessed. Be sure to check the patellar and ankle reflexes, as well as the bulbocavernosus reflex (contraction of external anal sphincter noted when stroking of the labia majora or clitoris [also referred to as the "anal wink"]).

The speculum examination focuses on vaginal support. Inspect the lateral vaginal fornices looking for obliteration of sulci, indicating a paravaginal defect. Note the presence or absence of vaginal rugae. Smooth vaginal epithelium points to a fascial defect in that area. Split speculum examination, using only the posterior blade, is very helpful in determining what compartment is prolapsing. Depression of the posterior wall aids inspection of the anterior compartment and splinting a prolapsed anterior vaginal wall will allow for visualization of a posterior defect. Bimanual pelvic examination includes assessment of levator tone both at rest and with contraction. During rectal examination, palpation of the anal sphincter is done to determine any defects. Additionally, the patient is asked to contract the anal sphincter to assess tone (Box 29.2).

The examiner must determine the point of maximal prolapse for each vaginal compartment. This can be done in several ways. Traction may be applied at the point of prolapse; this is only possible with uterine prolapse. Examining the patient while she stands and bears down (Valsalva maneuver) will usually confirm the full extent of prolapse. This is readily performed by having the patient place one foot on a low stool while the examiner palpates the vaginal walls during the maneuver. It is helpful to have the patient confirm that the extent of the protrusion seen by the examiner is as extensive as that which she has experienced. The patient may use a small handheld mirror to view the protrusion during this process. This examination is especially important if the supine examination is not consistent with the woman's history.

The International Continence Society approved a standard system to measure POP. The POPQ system evaluates nine measurements (see Box 29.3).

The POPQ system has many advantages. It is easily learned, is a standardized approach using the introitus as a reference point, and is reproducible from observer to observer (Chiarelli et al., 1999; Kelly, 2003). While evaluating the prolapse, clinicians should, at a minimum, measure the points along the anterior wall, the posterior wall, and the cervix that prolapse the furthest. The reference for these points is the hymenal ring, which is considered "zero" location. Points proximal to the hymen are designated negative, while those beyond the hymen are positive. For example, a cervix that advances to 1 cm proximal to the hymen is at −1 position,

Box 29.3 Pelvic Organ Prolapse Quantification Measurements

1, 2. Two along the anterior wall
3, 4. Two along the posterior wall
   5. Location of the cervix (or cuff if uterus is absent)
   6. Location of the posterior fornix
   7. Size of the genital hiatus
   8. Thickness of the perineal body
   9. Total vaginal length

while if it were 3 cm beyond the hymen, the prolapse would be designated +3. Points of maximal prolapse for the anterior and posterior vaginal walls can also be so documented. These measurements provide a standard system to quantify the degree of prolapse (Muir et al., 2003; Weber et al., 2001).

Diagnostic Studies

LABORATORY EVALUATION

Urinalysis and culture and sensitivity to rule out UTI are performed on all patients. Consider blood urea nitrogen (BUN), creatinine, estimated glomerular filtration rate (eGFR), calcium, and glucose if there is any suspicion of renal compromise. Urine cytology is performed for patients older than 50 years of age who have irritative bladder symptoms (e.g., urgency, frequency) or hematuria with a negative urine culture. Cytology has a sensitivity of 40% to 50% and specificity greater than 90%. Referral for cystoscopy is indicated for acute onset of irritative symptoms without infection, positive cytology, or unexplained hematuria with a negative culture. Microscopic hematuria with three or greater red blood cells (RBCs) per high power field on a properly collected specimen should be investigated (Ghibaudo & Hocke, 2005).

CLINICAL TESTING

All patients should be screened for UTI, have their postvoid residual urine volume (PVR) measured, and have simple cystometric studies done. The PVR is measured within 15 minutes of voiding (measure voided volume). This can be done by bladder catheterization or by using a dedicated ultrasound unit configured for bladder volume measurement. There is no mutually agreed on volume that constitutes an abnormal PVR. Most investigators agree that less than 50 mL is normal and that greater than 200 mL is abnormal. The International Continence Society (ICS) states that the PVR should be less than 25% of the total bladder volume (PVR/PVR+ voided volume less than 0.25; Chiarelli et al., 1999; Helström & Nilsson, 2005; Mouritsen, 2005).

Simple cystometric evaluation includes retrograde filling of the bladder in 50-mL increments with room temperature saline. This can be done with a 50-mL irrigation syringe and catheter. To perform a simple cystometry, after the patient has voided and the volume has been recorded, place the patient in the supine position. The patient is then catheterized and the PVR noted. The catheter is left in place and a 60-mL bulb syringe is attached to the end of the catheter. Remove the bulb from the top of the syringe and begin filling it with 50 mL of fluid. Record the volume at which the patient first has the sensation of bladder filling (S1), the first urge to void (S2), and the maximum volume of filling that the patient can tolerate (S3). Look for sudden elevation of the fluid level in the syringe that may indicate bladder spasm. Normal ranges for S1, S2, and S3 are 90 to 150 mL, 200 to 300 mL, and 300 to 600 mL, respectively. Once the bladder is full, have the patient cough and observe for stress incontinence. If negative, repeat this maneuver while reducing any anterior prolapse to identify occult stress incontinence. The clinician should be careful to avoid urethral compression while doing this. Finally, measuring voiding time and voided volume is a simple way to screen for voiding disorders. Average flow should be greater than 10 mL/sec. Reduced flow rates may indicate a voiding dysfunction, which is an indication for follow-up, complex, multichannel, urodynamic studies.

URODYNAMICS

Urodynamic testing is not necessary in all patients; however, in certain situations it can be particularly helpful. When occult UI is identified and surgical correction is planned for presumed stress UI, it is important to confirm with urodynamic testing which type of incontinence is present. This ensures that surgery is appropriate. Conversely, it can be useful to repeat urodynamics postoperatively if surgical correction has failed to diagnose new reasons for incontinence. Urge symptoms may be exacerbated postoperatively because of manipulation of the bladder. Alternatively, nerve injury could contribute to a neurogenic component of urinary voiding dysfunction. The desire to understand the etiology of incontinent episodes is also sufficient indication for urodynamic testing.

There are multiple components of urodynamic testing. Cystometry is the study of bladder pressures and volumes during both the filling and storage phases. A simple office version (see simple cystometry described earlier) or a computerized multichannel cystometry can be performed. Indications for multichannel cystometry are found in Box 29.4.

A pressure flow study evaluates bladder function by correlating pressure and flow during voiding. This study (also referred to as a cystometrogram [CMG] uroflow) is helpful when evaluating voiding dysfunction.

Uroflowmetry is the study of urinary flow rates. A normal urinary stream should rise quickly and steadily. Flow should then be maintained at a constant rate for a period, followed by a brisk and not abrupt decline in flow. Simple uroflow can be done by measuring the voiding time and voided volume to obtain an average flow rate. This rate should be greater than 10 mL/sec for females older than 65 years and 12 mL/sec for woman of ages 45 to 65 years. Maximum flow (Qmax) can be obtained by electronic (complex) uroflow measurements and

---

Box 29.4 Indications for Multichannel Cystometry

1. Mixed incontinence symptoms
2. Symptoms of overactive bladder not responsive to therapy
3. Inconclusive simple cystometry results
4. Recurrent incontinence
5. Neurologic signs/symptoms
6. Urinary retention
7. Continuous leakage
8. Low-volume stress urinary incontinence (UI) or workup before surgery for UI
9. Previous radiation therapy or radical surgery
10. Previous anti-incontinence surgery

should be 20 to 35 mL/sec. Complex uroflow is indicated if symptoms of obstructed voiding are present or simple uroflow is abnormal.

Electromyography (EMG) measures the muscle activity of the external urethral sphincter using surface or needle electrodes placed close to or into the sphincter. EMG may be helpful when evaluating women with neurogenic bladder, but it does not add significant information for routine evaluation of UI.

A urethral pressure profile is necessary to determine the presence or absence of intrinsic sphincter deficiency (ISD). A urodynamic pressure catheter is pulled through the urethra from the bladder neck to the urethral meatus, and the urethral pressures are continuously recorded. Alternatively, urethral pressures can be measured in the lumen at rest, during coughing or straining, and during voiding. Urethral closure pressure (UCP) is urethral pressure minus vesical pressure. UCP less than 20 cmH_2O indicates ISD while greater than 30 cmH_2O is considered normal.

IMAGING STUDIES

In general, imaging studies are not clinically indicated for POP. One exception is stage 4 anterior prolapse or complete vaginal eversion (Barber et al., 2000; Jelovsek et al., 2007; Ross, 1996). In such instances, ureteral obstruction with consequent hydroureter and/or hydronephrosis can occur. Renal sonography or intravenous pyelography can identify this consequence of advanced prolapse and are indicated if the renal indices (serum BUN and creatinine) are elevated. Although both static and dynamic MRI techniques, including defecography, have been used to evaluate POP, no normative values for these studies have been determined, and therefore, the International Continence Society does not consider their use essential. MRI defecography may be helpful when clinical symptoms and clinical examination do not correlate.

QOL ASSESSMENTS

Using validated QOL questionnaires provides pre- and post-treatment measures. Examples of these QOL tools include the Pelvic Floor Distress Inventory (PFDI), Pelvic Floor Impact Questionnaire (PFIQ), and the Prolapse Quality of Life Questionnaire (P-QOL; Barber, 2007; Digesu, Khullar, et al., 2005; Jelovsek & Barber, 2006; Ross, 1996). These tools can be time consuming and may not be applicable in general practice. Short versions of several of these tools have been developed and validated; they can be used in clinical practice. The PFDI-20 consists of 20 questions and the PFIQ-7 consists of seven questions. Both tools are valid and reliable; they are used to assess the effects of pelvic relaxation on QOL in women (Barber et al., 2006). The PISQ-12 (Female Sexual Function Index and the Sexual History Form 12) has been demonstrated to accurately measure the effect of POP on the patient's sexual function (Price et al., 2006).

Multiple studies have documented the effects of POP on the patient's perceived QOL. It is no surprise that POP negatively affects QOL, sexual function, and perceived body image (Barber et al., 2005). More advanced prolapse affects sexual and bowel function more than urinary function. Patients with stage 2 prolapse report more distress related to UI than patients with stages 3 and 4 prolapse. Patients with posterior vaginal prolapse report higher overall distress,

especially as related to bowel function and fecal incontinence (Fitzgerald et al., 2007). Apical vaginal prolapse (cervix and uterus, or vaginal apex if uterus is absent) has more effect on sexual function and dyspareunia than either the anterior or posterior compartment defects. Finally, patients with more advanced prolapse are more likely to feel self-conscious and less likely to feel physically attractive, sexually attractive, or feminine (Barber et al., 2005).

Treatment consists of both nonsurgical and surgical modalities. Nonsurgical treatment includes behavioral modification, pelvic floor muscle therapy (PFMT), medications (antimuscarinic, beta agonist), and pessary use. When prolapse is severe enough to cause urinary obstruction, ureteral compromise, vaginal erosion, or severe vaginal infection, treatment is mandated. Otherwise, the patient's comfort, preferences, and QOL are factored into any treatment plan.

Treatment is generally dictated by symptoms and/or functional impairment. When overactive bladder (OAB) symptoms, such as urinary frequency, urgency, and urge incontinence, are very bothersome, treatment for these symptoms is reasonable. The American Urological Association (AUA) OAB pathway guidelines are in Table 29.2 and Figure 29.1 (AUA, 2019; Lightner et al., 2016). Table 29.3 shows medications available for OAB treatment.

PELVIC FLOOR MUSCLE THERAPY

PFMT is often recommended to women with stage 1 and 2 vaginal prolapse. PFMT involves a concentrated exercise regimen of 6 to 12 weeks led by either a knowledgeable and appropriately trained physical therapist, nurse practitioner, or other appropriate staff member. This exercise regimen involves instructing the patient in the correct methods to isolate and contract the muscles of the pelvic floor. Although PFMT will not reverse anatomic derangements, it may alleviate many of the symptoms of POP including urinary/fecal urgency, frequency, and incontinence (Jelovsek & Barber, 2006; Kammerer-Doak, 2009). Multiple observational studies have indicated subjective relief for patients

TABLE 29.2 American Urological Association OAB Pathway Guidelines

FIRST-LINE TREATMENT (WELK ET AL., 2020)	SECOND-LINE TREATMENT INCLUDES MEDICATIONS	THIRD-LINE TREATMENT
Fluids management Bladder training Timed voiding Fluid management PMFT	See Table 29.3	Percutaneous tibial neurostimulation (PTNS) Botox injections into the bladder. Interstim sacral neuromodulation

OAB, overactive bladder; PFMT, pelvic floor muscle therapy.
Source: Lightner, D. J., Agarwal, D., & Gormley, E. A. (2016). The overactive bladder and the AUA guidelines: A proposed clinical pathway for evaluation and effective management in a contemporary urology practice. Urology Practice, 3(5), 399–405. https://doi.org/10.1016/j.urpr.2016.01.004; Welk, B., & McArthur, E. (2020). Increased risk of dementia among patients with overactive bladder treated with an anticholinergic medication compared to a beta-3 agonist: A population-based cohort study. BJU International, 126(1), 183–190. https://doi.org/10.1111/bju.15040

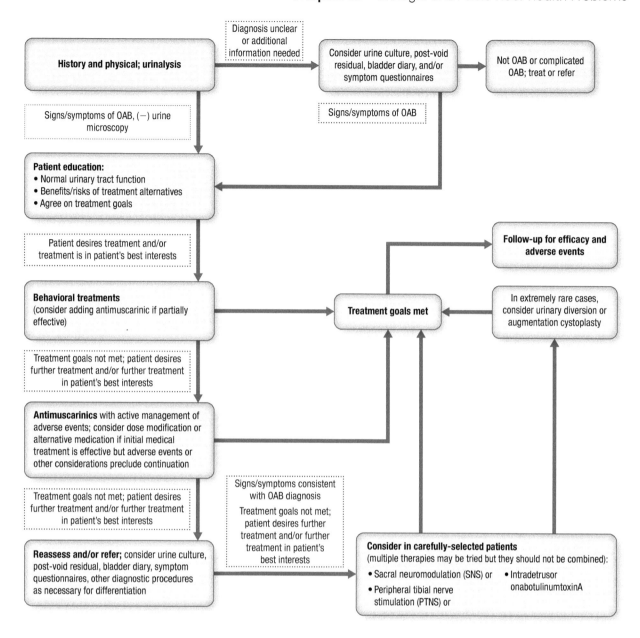

FIGURE 29.1 Diagnosis and treatment algorithm: American Urological Association guideline on non-neurogenic overactive bladder in adults.
Source: American Urological Association. (2019). Diagnosis and treatment of non-neurogenic overactive bladder (OAB) in adults: AUA/SUFU guideline. https://www.auanet.org/guidelines-and-quality/guidelines/overactive-bladder-(oab)-guideline

treated with PFMT (Blackwell, 2003; Bruch & Schwandner, 2004; Goode et al., 2003; Lagro-Janssen et al., 1994; Lamers & van der Vaart, 2007; Rosenbaum, 2007). Pelvic floor muscle rehabilitation (PFMR) and electrical stimulation (ES) therapy and/or pessary therapy are indicated measures if a woman's QOL is affected and she does not wish to have surgery, desires to delay surgery, had surgery that was not effective, is not a good candidate for surgery, or wishes to have more children (Jelovsek & Barber, 2006). A randomized trial for stage 1 and 2 POP indicated that PFMR may actually improve the anatomic derangement and reduce the degree of prolapse in nearly half of the patients undergoing treatment (Sampselle, 2003).

PELVIC FLOOR MUSCLE REHABILITATION AND ELECTRICAL STIMULATION

The pelvic floor musculature provides support to maintain the position and function of the pelvic organs. When weakened, it loses its ability to adequately support these structures. In addition, sphincters that surround the urethra and anus also lose strength and tone and may not close tight enough to prevent leakage. This often occurs with activities that increase intra-abdominal pressure. PFMR is targeted toward the levator ani, which consists of the pubococcygeus, the puborectalis, the ileococcygeus, and the coccygeus muscles. Strengthening of these muscle groups is an integral part of PFMR/ES (Hagen et al., 2006, 2009; Jelovsek & Barber, 2006).

TABLE 29.3 Medications Available for OAB Treatment

DRUG	MECHANISM OF ACTION	DOSING	COMMON SIDE EFFECTS
Trospium	Nonselective anticholinergic	20 mg BID	Dry mouth/eyes, constipation, Possible ↑ dementia risk
Oxybutynin	Nonselective anticholinergic	5–10 mg BID or TID	Dry mouth/eyes, constipation, Possible ↑ dementia risk
Tolterodine	Nonselective anticholinergic	1–2 mg BID	Dry mouth/eyes, constipation, Possible ↑ dementia risk
Fesoterodine	Nonselective anticholinergic	4 or 8 mg daily	Dry mouth/eyes, constipation, Possible ↑ dementia risk
Darifenacin	Selective, M3 receptors	7.5 or 15 mg daily	Dry mouth/eyes, constipation, Possible ↑ dementia risk
Solifenacin	Selective M2, M3 receptors	5 or 10 mg daily	Dry mouth/eyes, constipation, Possible ↑ dementia risk
Mirabegron	β3-adrenergic receptor agonist	25 or 50 mg daily	Headache, nausea, HTN, UTI
Vibegron	β3-adrenergic receptor agonist	75 mg daily	Headache, nausea, HTN, UTI
Botulinum toxin	Inhibits detrusor (blocks ACh)	100 U, 200 U	Urinary retention
Desmopressin	Antidiuretic effect (ADH)		Headache, nausea, flushing
Vaginal estrogen	Unknown		Headache, vaginal bleeding

ACh, acetylcholine; ADH, antidiuretic hormone; BID, twice a day; HTN, hypertension; TID, three times a day; UTI, urinary tract infection.

The muscle fiber type is determined by the nerve fiber supplying it. Slow-twitch striated muscle fibers (tonic, type 1) sustain activity, whereas fast-twitch striated muscle fibers (phasic, type 2) are involved in bursts of activity. In asymptomatic women, the pelvic floor muscles are approximately 30% fast-twitch fibers and 70% slow-twitch fibers. A muscle contraction must be:

- Greater than that of its ordinary everyday activity to increase in force
- Longer lasting to increase the endurance capability

A digital, vaginal examination helps the provider determine the degree of muscle levator ani strength and is recorded and graded as in noted Table 29.4.

The exercise program will consist of squeezing and holding the levator ani muscle contraction. The average mmHg pressure generated and the maximal time in seconds for maintaining a contraction for each patient is determined at baseline and recorded as the baseline contractile strength and time. The goal for these intervals is to hold each contraction for 10 seconds and then to relax the muscle for 10 seconds. However, in patients who are unable to hold the contraction for 10 seconds at baseline, the study is performed using their baseline contractile time in seconds. Patients perform squeeze–hold–relax repetitions until fatigue of the muscle is noted (fatigue is defined as not being able to hold the contraction for the baseline time in seconds or a drop from the peak contraction strength). Once a patient's muscle begins to fatigue, the patient is instructed to perform two additional

TABLE 29.4 Muscle Strength Scale

STRENGTH	DESCRIPTION
None	No discernible muscle contraction, pressure and/or displacement of examiner's finger
Flicker	1/5: Trace but instant contraction <1 second, very slight compression of examiner's finger
Weak	2/5: Weak contraction or pressure with or without elevation/lifting of examiner's finger, held for >1 second but <3 seconds
Moderate	3/5: Moderate contraction or compression of examiner's finger with or without elevation/lifting of finger, held for at least 4 to 6 seconds, repeated three times
Firm	4/5: Firm contraction with good compression of examiner's finger with elevation/lifting of finger toward the pubic bone, held for at least 7 to 9 seconds, repeated four to five times
Strong	5/5: Unmistakably strong contraction and grip of examiner's finger with posterior elevation/lifting of finger, held for at least 10 seconds, repeated four to five times

repetitions for their home therapy. This exercise program is used to develop strength and endurance (instructions for doing Kegel exercises are available at www.webmd.com/women/tc/kegel-exercises-topic-overview), under visual video computerized observation and instruction by the provider with a PFMR unit. The patient's maximum pelvic muscle strength contraction for the endurance exercise is measured in mmHg.

The patient is either able or not able to contract and relax muscles when instructed. An appropriate or inappropriate response will be obtained. The contractions will be graded as nonexistent, weak, moderate, or strong, and the average contraction will be measured in mmHg and time (in seconds) of duration. With the patient performing the directed squeezing and relaxing of the pelvic floor muscles, the duration of contraction (in seconds) and the number of repetitions are recorded.

The patient is encouraged through detailed and explicit instruction on how to perform and improve the pelvic floor muscle contraction function. Fast-twitch exercises are done to decrease urinary urges and prevent leakage. With this exercise, the fast-twitch or short muscle fibers are strengthened. The patient's maximum pelvic muscle strength contraction for fast-twitch exercise is measured in mmHg. The average strength of the fast-twitch contraction is measured if the short muscle fiber develops weak, moderate, or strong amplitude.

The next portion consists of electrical stimulation. The vaginal probe is kept in the vagina, and electrical stimulation is initiated for stress UI patients; 50 Hz are used for 15 minutes, with a pulse of 5 seconds on and 5 seconds off. A similar pattern is used for urge UI and OAB patients, except that a frequency of 12.5 Hz is selected. The stimulation regimen used is an alternating 50 Hz and 12.5 Hz every other week for mixed UI. The electrical stimulation level is measured in uV (electrical activity)/mA (milliamps). Toleration of the stimulation is evaluated because electrical stimulation will be maintained during therapy based on the patient's tolerance. Management of the patient involves instructing her to continue the prescribed exercise at home. For home therapy, the patient is prescribed exercise repetitions based on their endurance and muscle fatigue. All patients need to do exercises three times per day, 7 days per week in a sitting, standing, and lying position.

Pelvic muscle rehabilitation with electrical stimulation (PMFR/ES) can also be used to treat women with OAB/urge incontinence, stress urinary incontinence, or mixed urinary incontinence (Richmond et al., 2016).

The COVID-19 pandemic suspended mostly all outpatient clinic appointments, leaving many patients without care for symptoms that affected their daily QOL. Research identified efficacy in providing PMFR via explicit instruction describing how to squeeze and lift the pelvic floor correctly. This virtual environment was used via video/telehealth, phone, postal mail, and internet pathways (Carlin et al., 2021). Women who used the various virtual pathways during the pandemic had significant improvement in QOL compared to women who had face-to-face intervention (da Mata et al., 2021).

NEUROLOGIC STIMULATION THERAPY

ES devices to treat UI are taught to stimulate the pelvic muscles indirectly via electrodes, vagina sensor or probe, and acupuncture needle or directly such as intravesical stimulation implant. This therapy can be used in combination with Kegel exercises or alone.

ES is typically used in PFMR to stimulate the pelvic nerves to enhance the contractile response. ES works via the model of neuromodulation, which remodels the neuronal reflex loop by stimulating afferent nerve fibers of the pudendal nerve that influence this reflex loop. By this method of inhibiting bladder reflex contraction and using high-intensity stimulus for a short duration (15 minutes), the bladder spasm is reduced or the detrusor muscle is "calmed." ES has also been shown to strengthen the pelvic muscle and structural support of the urethra and the bladder neck. It is hypothesized that combining therapy with PFMR and ES together will provide patients with an optimal combination for improving UI symptoms.

Intone

Intone is a prescriptive medical device that provides noninvasive treatment for OAB/mixed UI. The device combines Kegel exercises and electrical stimulation via voice-guided instruction to be used at home. It requires 12 minutes of therapy per day for about 3 months. The insertion unit can be inflated in the vagina for a snug fit to accommodate different size vaginal calibers. The sensor within the insertion unit measures pelvic muscle strength. The stimulation unit in the device uses biphasic waveforms to ensure patient comfort and to prevent skin irritation, alternating between 12 Hz and 50 Hz (Barber et al., 2007).

Leva

Leva is a digital health intravaginal home device that has an app and a intravaginal sensor probe embedded with MEMS (micro electromechanical system) that allows real time information of pelvic muscle maximal squeeze during pelvic muscle exercises or the technique of Kegel exercises (Bohorquez et al., 2020).

Eiltone

Eiltone is another at-home device that has electrodes to provide ES to the perineal tissue for stress UI. The electrodes are attached to the woman's underwear and she can manually control the intensity of the stimulation (Kolb et al., 2019).

Percutaneous Tibia Nerve Stimulation

Percutaneous tibia nerve stimulation (PTNS) or neuromodulation is the stimulation of nerves that enervate the bladder indirectly. The theory of neurologic stimulation therapy is that stimulation of the nerves can stimulate pelvic muscle contractions and/or detrusor contractions. The initial studies of neurologic stimulation therapy focused on the sacral nerve. Although sacral nerve stimulation can improve the symptoms of incontinence, the procedures to implant these devices are somewhat invasive. Therefore, PTNS was developed. This procedure delivers retrograde access to the sacral nerve plexus via electrical stimulation of the posterior tibial nerve. PTNS involves a needle electrode being inserted into the posterior tibial nerve at the medial malleolus of the ankle to a depth of 3 to 4 cm. The electrode is then connected to a handheld nerve stimulator, which sends an electrical impulse to the nerve. This nerve impulse is then transmitted to the sacral plexus, which regulates the control of bladder and pelvic floor muscles. The maximum treatment intensity is determined by slowly increasing the stimulus until the patient's great toe begins to curl. The level at which the patient's toe curls is determined to be the maximum intensity for treatment. The most common side effects are local and related to placement of the electrode. They include minor bleeding and bruising, mild pain, tingling, and inflammation of the skin. To date there have been no serious adverse events reported in any of the observational studies or clinical trials evaluating PTNS. In the clinical trials, which have systematically assessed adverse effects, overall rates of bruising, bleeding, discomfort, and leg tingling have been low, although not all studies have reported the exact percentages (Davis et al., 2012; Guralnick et al., 2015; Peters et al., 2013).

PESSARY THERAPY

Pessary therapy is an integral part of the management of POP (Dannecker et al., 2005; Kincade et al., 2005). Pessaries are especially helpful for women who are medically unable to undergo surgery or wish to avoid a surgical procedure. Pessaries are made of silicone, soft plastic, rubber, and clear plastic and may have a bendable, metal form, which allows contouring for the patient's anatomy. Most modern pessaries are made of silicone as this material is less likely to discolor, less likely to fracture from repeated cleaning, and seems to be less allergenic than rubber.

Indications include the need for vaginal support, UI, and incompetent cervix in pregnancy. Pessaries are often chosen when a patient has medical comorbidities rendering surgery dangerous or the patient desires an alternative to surgery. Pessaries may also be used preoperatively to identify occult UI or to hasten healing of atrophic, inflamed, or eroded vaginal epithelium before surgery.

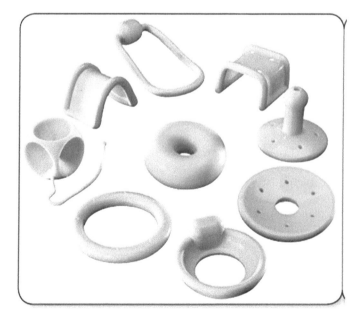

FIGURE 29.2　Pessaries are available in a wide variety of configurations and sizes. Clinicians should be familiar with at least one type of pessary used to treat each stage of pelvic organ prolapse.

Pessary fitting is accomplished through trial and error. Figure 29.2 shows many of these devices. In general, the type of pessary used is determined by the stage of prolapse, the main compartment affected, and the size of the genital hiatus (introitus). Active pelvic or vaginal infections must be treated before pessary use. If significant vaginal atrophy or epithelial drying or erosion is present, then a course of vaginal estrogen will be required before pessary placement.

For stage 1 or 2 prolapse, the following devices may be used: (a) ring (with or without support); (b) dish (with or without urethral bolster); and (c) Hodge (with or without support). The ring and dish pessaries are placed in a manner like diaphragm placement. One edge is placed under the symphysis pubis and the other edge in the posterior fornix. These pessaries are often not retained in the patient who has had a total hysterectomy. Once placed, the ring and dish pessary should rest in the anterior compartment of the vagina. For this reason, they are both very helpful for anterior vaginal wall prolapse (cystocele). Both pessaries are usually easy for a patient to remove and reinsert. The Hodge pessary requires advanced knowledge for proper placement. It usually has one edge resting behind the cervix with the other edge against the perineum. The Hodge is often difficult for a patient to remove and reinsert on her own.

Stage 3 anterior and apical prolapse may be treated by the dish or ring; however, these devices are often not retained and larger volume pessaries are needed. Examples of the larger pessaries are the donut and Gellhorn devices. The donut pessary has a much thicker, rounded edge and occupies more space within the vagina than the ring or dish. This donut is helpful when the introitus is very wide. Because of its size, the donut precludes sexual activity and therefore sexually active patients need to learn how to remove and reinsert the device. Insertion is generally accomplished by aligning the long axis of the device with the introitus and with steady firm pressure (and lubrication) placing the pessary into the distal vagina. Once in the vagina, the provider rotates the pessary 90 degrees and advances it into the proximal portion of the vagina.

The Gellhorn device is T-shaped and has a flat discoid section with a stem. The stem can range between 2 and 4 cm and the disc between 1 and 3 inches. This pessary is meant to have the disc against the upper apex or cervix and the stem against the perineum. It is inserted by aligning the flat disc vertically against the introitus and then slowly pushing it into the distal vagina. Once proximal to the hymen, the device is rotated so that the stem is facing the provider. The device is then further inserted into the upper vagina. Once in place, the provider must ensure that the disc does not cause undue pressure against the vaginal epithelium. A finger should be easily inserted between the pessary and the vaginal wall along the entire 360 degrees of the disc. This device generally precludes sexual activity because it is quite difficult for a patient to remove and reinsert (Kaaki & Mahajan, 2007).

Stage 4 prolapse usually requires larger volume pessaries. The donut and Gellhorn pessaries may be attempted. When these are not retained, a cube or inflatoball pessary may be used. The first pessary is cube shaped and has concavities on each surface so that it will create suction to stay in place. It is compressible so that its volume can be reduced for insertion by squeezing together its sides. Once in the vagina, it will expand slightly and stay in place. The provider must be sure that the device does not cause pressure to the vaginal epithelium. The cube pessary is difficult for a patient to remove.

The inflatoball pessary has the advantage that it can be inflated and deflated for insertion and removal. This allows a patient with advanced prolapse to remove the device at night and for sexual activity. The device comes with a bulb similar to that in a sphygmomanometer, which attaches to a stem with a valve. The deflated ball is placed into the vagina and the patient inflates it until it is retained and is comfortable. The valve is opened for deflation and removal. Ideally, a patient will remove this device every night and reinsert in the morning. This will help to prevent vaginal infection and erosion.

After fitting, the patient remains in the office to ambulate and ensure retention of the pessary. This may prevent repeat visits for the patient for whom the initial device is too small or not the right shape. The patient should also demonstrate the ability to void before leaving. When appropriate, the patient should be instructed on how to remove and reinsert the device. The patient should return within 1 week so the provider can examine the vagina for any signs of irritation, erosion, or infection. At this and subsequent visits, the provider must carefully look for signs of excess pressure against the vaginal walls, such as erosion, laceration, or granulation tissue. The device must also be inspected to be sure it is intact. Vaginal irrigation with iodine or chlorhexidine gluconate may be used if secretions are excessive. Once pessary therapy is established, regular visits at 2- to 3-month intervals are recommended, although this interval can be extended up to 6 months for patients who are not experiencing a pessary- related complication (Miceli et al., 2020; Thys et al., 2020). Unless contraindicated, a maintenance schedule of vaginal estrogen therapy inserted intravaginally using an applicator is instituted to prevent erosion of the vaginal epithelium (Cundiff et al., 2007; Nygaard, Bradley et al., 2004; Powers et al., 2006). With larger pessaries, or when a patient does not regularly remove the device, it is common for the patient to develop a malodorous vaginal discharge caused by a change in the bacterial environment of the vagina. Commonly, anaerobic bacteria may overgrow the normal flora. In these instances, intermittent use of antibiotic vaginal creams (e.g., metronidazole- or clindamycin-containing preparations) inserted using an applicator may be used for patient comfort.

Complications associated with pessary use include vaginal discharge and odor, vaginal bleeding, urinary retention, constipation, and rarely vaginal fistula because of erosion into a proximate organ (Dannecker et al., 2005). A recent survey of 104 pessary users showed that 70% of the women were satisfied or more than satisfied with pessary therapy and 20% were unable to continue pessary use, mostly because of repeated expulsion of the pessary (Powers et al., 2006). The patient should be informed to notify the provider immediately should they develop vaginal bleeding, abdominal pain, urinary or bowel retention, or signs of UTI. The most common reasons for discontinuing pessary use include a persistent vaginal discharge, worsening UI, pain, recurrent vaginal erosions, failure to provide support, and inability to retain the pessary in the vagina.

During the COVID-19 pandemic, most patients who were scheduled for 3-month maintenance pessary checks were unable to be seen in the clinic for their scheduled appointment. When they were able to have their pessary checks at their rescheduled in-person clinic appointment at 6 months, no increase in vaginal irritation, pain, or discharge was noted (Thys et al., 2020).

PHARMACOTHERAPEUTICS

Local vaginal estrogen therapy applied with an applicator is a mainstay of therapy in the postmenopausal patient who has no contraindication to its use. Increased vascularity and collagen content of the vaginal mucosa may explain diminution of symptoms in women with early-stage vaginal prolapse (Bernier & Jenkins, 1997; Hanson et al., 2006; Maito et al., 2006; North American Menopause Society, 2007). Local estrogen therapy is generally prescribed with pessary usage to reduce the risk of erosion of the vaginal mucosa. Added vaginal lubrication and moisture may aid in the placement and removal of a pessary. Local estrogen therapy may increase the biomechanical strength of vaginal tissue and, while not reversing anatomic derangement, does ameliorate many of the symptoms caused by early-stage POP (Castelo-Branco et al., 2005; Suckling et al., 2006).

Vaginal estrogen preparations are available as creams, suppositories, or an estradiol-impregnated silicone ring placed in the vagina. When using either a cream or suppository form, it is common to have a short period of treatment induction followed by a maintenance schedule. With use of the ring, no induction schedule is employed, and the ring is simply placed intravaginally for up to 90 days (Hsu et al., 2005).

A typical initial schedule of cream would be to place 1.0 to 2.0 g of conjugated equine estrogen (CEE) cream (Premarin) or 2.0 to 4.0 g of estradiol vaginal cream (Estrace) in the vagina nightly for 1 to 4 weeks. After repeat vaginal examination, a maintenance schedule would usually employ 0.5 to 1.0 g of CEE or 1.0 to 2.0 g of estradiol cream one to two times per week. A similar schedule may be used with estradiol vaginal suppositories (Vagifem). Although the absorption of estrogen into the bloodstream is much less with vaginal preparations than with oral or transdermal products, the clinician must pay attention to the same precautions and contraindications associated with systemic use (Dezarnaulds & Fraser, 2003; Maito et al., 2006; Weber et al., 1995). Pregnancy, undiagnosed vaginal bleeding, active liver disease, porphyria, an active thromboembolic disorder or a past thromboembolic disorder associated with estrogen use, an estrogen-sensitive malignancy (e.g., breast, endometrium), or prior hypersensitivity to estrogen are all absolute contraindications to estrogen use. Relative contraindications include history of thromboembolic disorder not associated with pregnancy or estrogen use, prior history of estrogen-sensitive neoplasm, gallbladder disease, benign hepatic adenoma, and untreated hypertension or diabetes.

Patients are typically placed on therapy for 3 to 6 months. Long-term maintenance treatment may be needed, especially if a pessary is used. In those cases, regular monitoring at 3- to 6-month intervals is necessary and should include endometrial biopsy if abnormal uterine bleeding occurs. All forms of vaginal estrogen performed similarly when comparing efficacy to relieve symptoms of atrophy; however, the estradiol ring may cause fewer side effects such as abnormal bleeding and breast pain and a lower likelihood of endometrial hyperplasia (Hsu et al., 2005). Multiple studies revealed greater ease of use and patient satisfaction with the estradiol ring than with vaginal cream (Hsu et al., 2005).

SURGICAL MANAGEMENT

Surgery for POPpelvic organ prolapse includes vaginal, abdominal, and laparoscopic (with or without robotic technology) procedures (often in combination). Surgery often involves correction of multiple physical problems. Anterior and apical problems can be approached through one of the previously mentioned routes, while posterior defects are usually corrected via the vaginal route. The aim of surgery is to relieve symptoms, restore normal function, and create a durable repair (Carlström et al., 1982; Martin et al., 1984). White and Hispanic groups report prolapse more frequently than Black groups and more often choose surgical options for treatment (Alas et al., 2016). Black women who undergo prolapse surgery have a longer hospital stay with higher rate of morbidity (Shah et al., 2007).

Repair of Anterior Defects

Proper correction of a cystocele depends on identification of the defect causing the prolapse. As previously mentioned, defects may be central or lateral (paravaginal). The standard anterior colporrhaphy with midline plication of endopelvic connective tissue is a vaginal procedure that only corrects a central defect. Unfortunately, recurrence of anterior prolapse is common and may be as high as 40% for standard colporrhaphy (Maher et al., 2007). Paravaginal repair attempts to reattach the lateral vagina to the ATFP and can be completed either abdominally (most common), laparoscopically, or vaginally. Laparoscopic and vaginal paravaginal defect repairs require advanced surgical skills and can be quite difficult to complete. The long-term success of paravaginal repair is not known (American College of Obstetricians and Gynecologists, 2019). When both central and lateral defects exist, the surgeon and patient face a difficult dilemma (Diez-Itza et al., 2007).

Complications of anterior colporrhaphy include failure (20%–50%), infection (3%–5%), de novo urgency-frequency syndrome (5%–25%), de novo dyspareunia (2%–9%), vaginal stenosis, and urinary retention or incontinence (Antosh et al., 2021; Maher et al., 2007; Morse et al., 2007). Complications of paravaginal defect repair also include urgency-frequency syndrome, urinary retention, and possible recurrent posterior prolapse.

In the past 15 years, surgical mesh augmentation for the correction of anterior defects was introduced for anterior vaginal repair. Initial reports described short-term failures of the mesh (2 years) as low as 5%. Mesh exposure occurs in 3% to 9% of patients and is generally easily managed (Kisby & Linder, 2020). Symptoms include vaginal discharge and bleeding. Most exposures are reversed with local estrogen treatment alone. If not, then excision of exposed mesh with reapproximation of the vaginal epithelium is easily accomplished (Daneshgari et al., 2006; de Tayrac et al., 2006; Maher & Baessler, 2006; Naumann & Kolbl, 2006; Sergent et al., 2007).

Repair of Vaginal Apical Prolapse

Surgical procedures for vaginal apical prolapse include abdominal, vaginal laparoscopic, or combined approaches. The "gold standard" of therapy is the abdominal sacral colpopexy (Moen, 2004; Weber & Richter, 2005). This procedure has the lowest long-term failure of all procedures described with a success rate (no apical prolapse) of 78% to 100%. The mean reoperation rate for POPpelvic organ prolapse for this procedure is 4.4% (Salomon et al., 2004). As an abdominal procedure, it entails longer operative time, lengthier hospitalization, higher blood loss, and higher rates of bowel and ureter complications than procedures completed through the vaginal approach. Long-term complications include UI, voiding dysfunction, and erosion of vaginal mucosa overlying mesh material (mesh erosion). Sacrocolpopexy using laparoscopic and robotic surgery techniques has been introduced to avoid the problems associated with the abdominal approach. The results of patients with 2 to 5 years of follow-up demonstrate efficacy (Hilger et al., 2003; Klauschie et al., 2009; North et al., 2010; Nygaard, McCreery et al., 2004). These procedures are as durable as their abdominal counterparts.

Vaginal approaches for the surgical correction of apical prolapse have usually entailed either a sacrospinous ligament fixation or uterosacral ligament suspension (which may also be done laparoscopically) to secure the vaginal apex into the hollow of the sacrum. Both procedures may be done either at the time of hysterectomy or for posthysterectomy vault prolapse. The long-term success rates of these procedures generally are lower than abdominal or laparoscopic approach apical support surgeries. These procedures generally require less postoperative analgesia, a shorter hospital stay, and less recovery time than the abdominal approach (Carlström et al., 1982; Dietz et al., 2007; Maher et al., 2004; Misraï et al., 2008; Patel et al., 2009; Weber & Richter, 2005).

Repair of Posterior Defects

The traditional vaginal approach to posterior defects involves the midline plication of the rectovaginal connective tissue. Although recurrence is less common than with anterior procedures, dyspareunia may occur in as many as 38% of the patients undergoing these procedures. In the past 10 years, a "site-specific" repair has gained favor for correction of posterior defects. This repair involves the identification and repair of specific problems in the rectovaginal fascia. These problems may occur in multiple configurations and the repair should succeed in repairing all problems while reattaching the fascia to the perineal body. To date, no studies have confirmed long-term superiority of either approach (Abramov et al., 2005; Karram et al., 2001; Paraiso et al., 2006; Silva et al., 2006).

Obliterative Procedures

Partial and complete colpocleisis procedures involve the partial or complete obliteration of the vaginal cavity. Partial colpocleisis (LeFort procedure) involves denuding large sections of the vaginal epithelium followed by suturing together the anterior and posterior vaginal walls. This is often done in combination with an anti-incontinence procedure, levator plication, and/or perineorrhaphy. Complete colpocleisis removes the vaginal epithelium in its entirety. Recurrence rates range from 0% to 10%. These procedures are reserved for older patients who do not wish to retain vaginal function and/or whose medical comorbidities preclude an extensive reparative procedure (Ghielmetti et al., 2006; Glavind & Kempf, 2005; Hullfish et al., 2002; Wheeler et al., 2005).

COMPLICATIONS ASSOCIATED WITH VAGINAL MESH PROCEDURES

In 2008 and then again in 2011, the U.S. Food and Drug Administration (FDA) released two bulletins regarding possible complications associated with the use of mesh in pelvic floor surgery. The alerts essentially dealt with vaginal approach procedures using mesh for both prolapse and UI treatment. Subsequent to these alerts there has been a rapid increase in product liability lawsuits surrounding these procedures. A partial list of the conditions associated with these devices is provided in Box 29.5. In 2016 the FDA reclassified all vaginal mesh devices as class III, the highest risk group. This change in classification required postmarket studies to evaluate device safety. In 2019 the FDA ordered the manufacturers of all remaining surgical mesh products indicated for the transvaginal repair of POP to stop selling and distributing their products in the United States (FDA, 2019). Nevertheless, patients with implanted devices can potentially develop complications going forward. When evaluating patients with these conditions or symptoms who have had a vaginal mesh procedure for either prolapse or incontinence, it is imperative to document the timeline and severity of these conditions as they relate to prior surgeries. The examination should document specific locations of vaginal/genital pain, tenderness, visible mesh, bands or tightness in the vagina, and muscular pain or tightness. The provider might consider referral to a physician or center with expertise in treating mesh complications.

Box 29.5 Complications Associated With Vaginal Mesh Procedures

Dyspareunia

Partner dyspareunia

Pelvic pain

Voiding dysfunction, for example, urinary incontinence, urinary retention, overactive bladder

Mesh erosion/exposure

Bladder injury

Rectal injury

Infection

Vaginal discharge

Vaginal bleeding

Recurrent urinary tract infection/cystitis

Recurrent vaginitis

Neuralgia

Pudendal nerve damage

Obturator nerve damage

Groin pain

FUTURE DIRECTIONS

POP is quite common and affects millions of women. POP includes a variety of conditions, and symptoms may range from none to total vaginal prolapse with urinary/fecal obstruction. The clinician should systematically approach the patient to determine the extent of anatomic derangement, the level of functional impairment, and the appropriate management strategies for the patient. The woman's expectations and desires must be factored into all treatment decisions. A realistic description of any treatment success must be relayed to the woman so that she can make a truly informed decision. Future study is aimed toward identifying procedures that are less invasive and have greater long-term success.

PAINFUL BLADDER SYNDROME/ INTERSTITIAL CYSTITIS

Painful bladder syndrome/interstitial cystitis (PBS/IC) is a disorder characterized by bladder pain of variable severity, lasting over a protracted period. It can affect women or men and is more common in women. The diagnosis and treatment of PBS/IC are controversial, like they are for other enigmatic medical conditions of unknown origin that are difficult to treat.

Definition and Scope

Definitions of PBS/IC have widely varied widely over the past few decades and are continuing to evolve. Before 2002, IC was defined in research settings according to the criteria of the National Institute for Diabetes and Diseases of the Kidney (NIDDK); however, the NIDDK criteria were too restrictive for general use, so in 2002 the ICS published new recommendations for definition of the painful bladder disorders (Abrams et al., 2002; MacLennan et al., 2000). The ICS defines PBS as a clinical syndrome (i.e., a complex of symptoms) consisting of "suprapubic pain related to bladder filling, accompanied by other symptoms, such as increased daytime and nighttime frequency in the absence of proven infection or other obvious pathology" (Abrams et al., 2002, p. 170 Oravisto, 1975; Wein et al., 2010). By comparison, the term "*interstitial cystitis*" is reserved for patients who have PBS symptoms and who also demonstrate both classic cystoscopic and histologic characteristics during bladder hydrodistentsion (Tomaszewski et al., 2001).

The International Society for the Study of Bladder Pain Syndrome (ESSIC) proposed another system. The diagnosis of bladder pain syndrome (BPS), distinct from PBS, is based on the presence of pain related to the urinary bladder and accompanied by at least one other urinary symptom. Diseases that cause similar symptoms need to be excluded, and cystoscopy with hydrodistention and biopsy (if indicated) should be performed. The ESSIC suggests avoiding the term IC, and instead using the term BPS, followed by a grade denoting severity of cystoscopic appearance and severity of biopsy findings (if performed; van der Merwe et al., 2008). Further refinement of terminology is likely during the coming years.

Because of variable diagnostic criteria, reported prevalence rates for PBS/IC vary widely. Population-based studies report prevalence rates of 10 to 865 cases per 100,000 women (Clemens, Meenan, O'Keeffe Rosetti, Brown, et al., 2005; Clemens, Meenan, O'Keeffe Rosetti, Gao, et al., 2005). A survey of participants in the U.S. Nurses' Health Studies suggested a prevalence of 52 to 67 cases per 100,000 women (Curhan et al., 1999). The prevalence of physician-diagnosed PBS/IC in a managed care population was 197 cases per 100,000 women and 41 per 100,000 men, but the prevalence of PBS/IC symptoms in the same population was much higher, at 11% of women and 5% of men (Clemens, Meenan, O'Keeffe Rosetti, Brown, et al., 2005; Clemens, Meenan, O'Keeffe Rosetti, Gao, et al., 2005).

The estimated clinical prevalence is highest in reports by researchers who believe that many, or even most, women with chronic pelvic pain may actually have IC, as well as those who think that many men with lower urinary tract symptoms or prostatitis also may have IC and those who use somewhat nonspecific symptom questionnaires to make the diagnosis (Clemens, Meenan, O'Keeffe Rosetti, Brown, et al., 2005; Clemens, Meenan, O'Keeffe Rosetti, Gao, et al., 2005; Jones & Nyberg, 1977; Nickel et al., 2005). The true prevalence of PBS/IC will only be established when agreement is reached about diagnostic criteria and a gold standard is available for its diagnosis.

Etiology

Little is known about the etiology and pathogenesis of PBS/IC. Ongoing and future research will likely demonstrate that patients currently grouped together under the umbrella diagnosis of PBS/IC actually suffer from several distinct conditions with distinct etiologies. Several pathogenic mechanisms have been proposed to explain the clinical phenomena, and it is accepted that any of several inciting factors may lead to the clinical manifestation of PBS/IC.

Many studies have documented that patients with IC have urothelial changes present in bladder biopsies (Graham & Chai, 2006; Hurst et al., 1996; Slobodov et al., 2004). Importantly, it is not known whether these urothelial changes represent primary or secondary phenomena (i.e., whether the bladder changes are secondary to another process that is yet unrecognized). These changes include altered bladder epithelial expression of HLA class I and II antigens, decreased expression of uroplakin and chondroitin sulfate, altered cytokeratin profile (toward a profile more typical of squamous cells), and altered integrity of the glycosaminoglycan (GAG) layer (Graham & Chai, 2006; Hurst et al., 1996; Slobodov et al., 2004). In addition, the expression of interleukin 6 and P2X3 ATP (adenosine triphosphate) receptors is increased, and activation of the nuclear factor-kB (*NFkB*) gene is enhanced (Graham & Chai, 2006; Hurst et al., 1996; Slobodov et al., 2004).

The GAG layer normally coats the urothelial surface and renders it impermeable to solutes; thus, defects in this layer may allow urinary irritants to penetrate the urothelium and activate the underlying nerve and muscle tissues (Parsons, 2007). This process may promote further tissue damage, pain, and hypersensitivity. Bladder mast cells may also play a role in the propagation of ongoing bladder damage after an initial insult.

Antiproliferative factor (APF) may also have a pathogenic role in the generation of PBS/IC symptoms. APF is a glycopeptide that is produced by the urothelium of IC patients, but not by control subjects without IC (Mouritsen & Larsen, 2003). APF may affect urothelial activity through altered production of growth factors and other proteins involved in urothelial growth and function.

It is likely that neurologic upregulation with central sensitization and increased activation of bladder sensory neurons during normal bladder filling plays a role in the generation and maintenance of PBS/IC symptoms (Nazif et al., 2007). This increased sensitivity may be present in the bladder itself or may be because of increased activity and new pathways within the central nervous system. Animal models suggest that hypersensitivity in bowel and other pelvic organs may be responsible for sensitization of the bladder (Ustinova et al., 2006). Similar alterations in neural pathways may be responsible for the tenderness that is present in PBS/IC patients. It is also possible that the increase in visceral (bladder) sensitivity is secondary to a primary somatic injury that has sensitized central pathways that overlap with afferents from the bladder.

Risk Factors

Studies have consistently found that PBS/IC is more common in women, with a female/male ratio typically reported as 4.5 to nine females to one male (Ashton-Miller & DeLancey, 2007; DeLancey et al., 2007; Swift et al., 2005). The mean age of diagnosis is probably about 42 to 45 years, although symptoms have been recognized in children (Close et al., 1996; Koziol et al., 1993). A greater concordance of IC among monozygotic than dizygotic twin pairs suggests a genetic susceptibility to IC (Warren et al., 2001).

In a population-based study, PBS/IC was associated only with depression in men. In women, it was associated with depression, history of UTIs, chronic yeast infections, hysterectomy, and use of calcium channel blockers or cardiac glycosides. Use of thyroid medications or statins showed an inverse association (Hall et al., 2008).

Symptoms

The presentation of PBS/IC is variable, but there are many common clinical features. All patients with PBS/IC have pain, which is associated with bladder filling and/or emptying, and usually accompanied by urinary frequency, urgency, and nocturia (Bogart et al., 2007; O'Leary et al., 1997; Teichman & Parsons, 2007). The pain that is thought to be of bladder origin is usually described as being suprapubic or urethral, although patterns such as unilateral lower abdominal pain or low back pain with bladder filling are common. The severity of pain ranges from mild burning to severe and debilitating.

Increased urinary frequency arises because the pain of bladder filling is partially or completely relieved by voiding, so patients prefer to maintain low bladder volumes. Clinically, it is useful to ask patients why they void frequently to help distinguish PBS/IC from other causes of frequency. As an example, patients with OAB syndrome void frequently to avoid urinary urge incontinence, whereas in PBS/IC they void frequently to avoid discomfort.

Affected patients may also describe chronic pelvic pain that is distinct from their bladder pain, as well as other ongoing, distinct pain symptoms. These patients often carry several diagnoses, such as irritable bowel syndrome (another visceral pain syndrome), dysmenorrhea, endometriosis, vulvodynia, migraine, or fibromyalgia. They may also describe exacerbation of their PBS/IC symptoms during times when other pain symptoms are at their worst (e.g., "flares" of PBS/IC when irritable bowel syndrome is symptomatic).

The character of symptoms may vary from one day to the next in a single patient. Exacerbation of PBS/IC symptoms may occur after intake of certain foods or drinks (e.g., strawberries, oranges, beer, and coffee), or during the luteal phase of the menstrual cycle, during stressful times, or after activities such as exercise, sexual intercourse, or being seated for long periods of time (e.g., a plane trip; Koziol, 1994).

In severe disease, urinary frequency of as many as 60 voids daily may occur, with associated disruptions of daytime activities and sleep (Koziol, 1994). Patients may describe sitting on the toilet for hours at a time in order to let urine dribble from their bladders more or less continuously so that bladders remain as empty as possible to minimized pain. Associated disruption of home and work life, avoidance of sexual intimacy, and chronic fatigue and pain predictably result in some degree of worsening of QOL in all affected patients. In surveys, 50% of patients reported being unable to work full time, 75% described dyspareunia, 70% reported sleep disturbance, and 90% reported that PBS/IC affected their daily activities (Koziol, 1994).

Most patients describe symptoms that are of gradual onset, with worsening of discomfort, urgency, and frequency over a period of months (Koziol, 1994). A smaller subset of patients describes symptoms that are severe from their onset. Symptoms of PBS/IC begin suddenly, with some patients able to name the exact date on which symptoms began. In other patients, symptoms begin after an apparently uncomplicated UTI or surgical procedure, episode of vaginitis or prostatitis, or after a trauma, such as a fall onto the coccyx. In hindsight, these "sentinel events" have often been empirically diagnosed and treated, and usually are themselves somewhat enigmatic (Koziol, 1994).

Evaluation/Assessment

A thorough history and physical examination of patients with PBS/IC is of critical importance in making a diagnosis and planning treatment. Identifying and clarifying symptoms often can assist with ruling out other possible differential diagnoses and will provide information to guide the treatment plan. On observation, many patients will be tearful and appear fatigued and/or depressed. Variable tenderness of the abdominal wall, hip girdle, soft tissues of the buttocks, pelvic floor, bladder base, and urethra is almost universally present, probably because of sensitization of afferent nerve fibers in the dermatomes (thoracolumbar and sacral) to which the bladder refers.

In some women, adequate speculum and bimanual examination cannot be conducted because of exquisite tenderness of the pelvic tissues. Pelvic ultrasound can be helpful for assessing the pelvic organs in these patients. It is important to remember that allodynia (perception of non-noxious stimuli, such as light touch, as being noxious or painful; Koziol, 1994) can be present in any patient who has been in chronic pain. Allodynia may make it impossible to perform an adequate pelvic examination in the awake patient. In this situation, clinicians may choose to begin empiric treatment for PBS/IC, and to defer full examination until either symptoms have improved to the point where examination is possible, or until symptoms have not responded to usual therapies and the diagnosis must be revisited.

DIFFERENTIAL DIAGNOSIS

Several diseases and conditions have symptoms like PBS/IC. They may be ruled out, diagnosed instead of IC, or found to be coexistent (Box 29.6).

Diagnostic Studies

To diagnose PBS/IC, diseases that cause similar symptoms must be ruled out (see Box 29.6). Urine culture and urinalysis are performed to test for bacteria and signs of infection. A cystoscopy with hydrodistention, performed under general anesthesia, is the standard diagnostic procedure for PBS/IC. The bladder is filled to capacity with water (commonly) or gas. This allows for examination of the epithelium with a small, telescopic fiberoptic camera or scope that is inserted through the urethra to the bladder. Glomerulations (tiny hemorrhages that are the telltale sign of IC) are revealed only while the bladder is distended. These hemorrhages are present in 95% of IC cases (Graham & Chai, 2006; Hurst et al., 1996; Slobodov et al., 2004; van de Merwe et al., 2008).

Box 29.6 Diagnoses to Consider in the Differential Diagnosis of Painful Bladder Syndrome/Interstitial Cystitis

Bladder stones (urolithiasis)

Carcinoma of the bladder in situ

Gynecologic disorders (endometriosis, ectopic pregnancy, fibroids, ovarian tumor)

Inflammation of the bladder (caused by chronic low-grade bacterial cystitis, cyclophosphamide cystitis, tuberculosis cystitis, radiation cystitis)

Kidney disease (renal tuberculosis)

Neurologic disorders (multiple sclerosis)

Pelvic floor dysfunction

Prostatitis (men)

Sexually transmitted infections (e.g., genital herpes, *Chlamydia* infection)

Surgical adhesions

Urethrocele (bladder hernia into the vagina) or cystocele (tissue growth around the urethra)

Urinary tract infection

Less frequently, epithelial ulcerations (Hunner's ulcers), lesions, and scars are found (Tomaszewski et al., 2001). Hunner's ulcers are indicative of PBS/IC, though hydrodistention is not needed to see them. A biopsy is performed to distinguish between ulcers and cancer and to evaluate the presence of mast cells, which are sometimes seen in abundance in PBS/IC-affected bladders. Some PBS/IC sufferers do not have epithelial glomerulations or ulcers. Cystoscopy may also reveal bladder stones, which can cause symptoms similar to those in PBS/IC.

Cystoscopy and hydrodistention are performed under anesthesia because distending the bladder of a PBS/IC sufferer is painful and otherwise causes urgent urination. Hydrodistention may also have therapeutic effects. Some patients repeat the procedure occasionally as treatment for PBS/IC because it may temporarily alleviate pain and pressure.

CYSTOSCOPY

Cystoscopy is not mandatory and is performed at the discretion of the clinician. In the United States, it is usually reserved for patients with hematuria (gross or microscopic) or with symptoms that raise suspicion for other processes. As an example, synthetic mesh is frequently used for urologic and gynecologic surgery, and mesh erosion into the lower urinary tract has become an increasingly important cause of urinary symptoms. When a patient has a history of pelvic surgery that predates their symptoms, it is important to use cystoscopy to exclude the presence of foreign body in the lower urinary tract.

HYDRODISTENTION

Hydrodistention of the bladder is not required for diagnosis or treatment of PBS/IC, although strong opinions are voiced on both sides of this issue (Fall & Peeker, 2006; Ottem & Teichman, 2005). When used, patients are placed under anesthesia and the bladder is filled with water or saline until 70 cmH$_2$O pressure is reached, usually at a bladder volume that is far greater than the awake capacity of the patient (e.g., 1,000 mL). This bladder dilation is maintained for several minutes, and then the dilating fluid is released.

POTASSIUM SENSITIVITY TEST

The potassium sensitivity test (PST) has also been proposed by some researchers as useful for diagnosis of PBS/IC (Barber, 2007; Hohlbrugger & Riedl, 2001; Parsons, 2005a); PST is not recommended for routine use because its results are nonspecific for PBS/IC (Hanno, 2005). During this test, 40 mL sterile water is instilled into the bladder, and note is made of any associated pain. The bladder is drained and then filled with 40 mL of 0.4 M potassium chloride; a finding of increased pain during this second fill is considered indicative of bladder hypersensitivity and suggestive of PBS/IC.

SYMPTOM SCALES

Some centers use symptom scales to aid in diagnosis of PBS/IC; however, in practice, use of these scales adds little to the ability to make a diagnosis and thus use is not widespread. Symptom scales can be useful in the monitoring of clinical progress after diagnosis. Three such scales are the O'Leary–Sant IC Symptom and Problem Index (Propert et al., 2006),

the Pelvic Pain and Urgency/Frequency (PUF) patient symptom scale (Propert et al., 2006), and the University of Wisconsin Interstitial Cystitis Scale (Goin et al., 1998).

Treatment/Management

NONSPECIFIC THERAPIES

The following components are part of all treatment programs.

Psychosocial Support

Psychosocial support is an integral part of the treatment of any chronic pain disorder. Patients may benefit from identification of a support person within the clinical practice whom they may contact as needed. They may benefit from pain support groups such as the Interstitial Cystitis Association (www.ichelp.org) or the Interstitial Cystitis Network (www.ic-network.com). Referral to a mental health clinician with expertise in support of patients with chronic illness may be helpful as well.

Pain Specialist

Referral to specialists in pain management should be considered if the full range of pain management options are not available within the practice.

Treatment of Comorbid Conditions

Depression is common in patients with chronic pain and may impede treatment success. Referral for mental health evaluation may be useful when there is any suspicion that depression is present.

Acute genitourinary disorders (e.g., UTI, vulvovaginitis) can exacerbate PBS/IC symptoms and need to be addressed promptly. Other disorders associated with visceral pain also require treatment because sensitization of any viscera probably results in increased bladder sensitivity. Thus, it is critically important to treat concomitant inflammatory bowel disease (Crohn disease, ulcerative colitis, and diverticulitis), irritable bowel syndrome, dysmenorrhea, and/or endometriosis. As PBS/IC patients often carry more than one of these diagnoses, treatment decisions can be complex, and collaboration with other medical professionals is usually necessary.

Avoidance of Activities Associated With Flares

Patients frequently note that some exercises or recreational activities, sexual activities, or body positions seem to worsen their bladder symptoms. Others note that some foods or beverages are troublesome. These factors should be avoided until symptoms are resolved, at which time they may be reintroduced. Some practitioners strongly recommend the highly restrictive IC diet (DeLancey, 1994), but its benefit has never been studied, and in practice, most patients with food sensitivities are already aware of them and have already excluded them from their diet.

Behavioral Therapy

Behavioral therapy forms the cornerstone of all treatment packages. It includes avoidance of exacerbating activities and some form of a timed voiding reeducation protocol to expand functional bladder capacity. Such protocols are critical because frequent voiding leads to diminished functional bladder capacity (possibly because of shrinkage of smooth muscle, similar to diminished stomach capacity after fasting or after chronic intake of smaller amounts of food).

A typical bladder reeducation protocol involves teaching patients to "void by the clock" rather than voiding when they feel an urge to do so. For example, a patient who is currently voiding every half an hour is asked to void only on the hour during the daytime (drills are not typically continued through the night), whether they feel the need to void or not, and not to void more frequently than the prescribed interval. This voiding interval is continued for a full week, and if patients are successful at that voiding interval, it is increased. This might result in the prescription of a voiding interval of 90 minutes for the second week, of 2 hours for the third week, 2.5 hours for the fourth week, and 3 hours for the fifth week. Other similar bladder retraining therapies are widely used because they are inexpensive, without side effects, and universally available.

Specific Therapies

Because the exact cause of PBS/IC is poorly understood, there are several approaches to care that are based on various theories of the cause.

UROTHELIUM THERAPIES

Clinicians who favor the theory that urothelial abnormalities are responsible for symptoms often use therapies directed at the urothelium. These therapies include the following.

Pentosan Polysulfate Sodium

Pentosan polysulfate sodium (PPS) is the only oral medication approved by the FDA for treatment of IC. The approved dose is 100 mg three times daily, although off-label treatment using 200 mg twice daily is clinically common (Erickson et al., 2006; Sant et al., 2003). PPS is a protein that is supposed to be filtered by the kidneys and appear in the urine so that it can reconstitute the deficient GAG layer over the urothelium. In fact, only a tiny proportion of the drug is absorbed by the gastrointestinal tract and excreted in the urine (Erickson et al., 2006). Urinary levels in patients who respond to treatment are not significantly different from the levels in patients for whom the therapy is not effective (Erickson et al., 2006; Sant et al., 2003).

A systematic review of randomized trials assessing pharmacologic treatments of PBS/IC found that PPS was more effective than placebo in overall improvement of patient-reported symptoms (pain, urgency, frequency) but the magnitude of effect was modest (Dimitrakov et al., 2007). There was considerable heterogeneity in the studies that addressed this question. The FDA recently announced side effects related to eye health, specifically macular degeneration (Pearce et al., 2018).

Intravesical Heparin and Lidocaine

Some clinicians recommend intravesical instillations of heparin and/or lidocaine, PPS, and sodium bicarbonate in various nonstandardized drug cocktails. No controlled studies of these therapies exist. As an example, use of a solution consisting of 40,000 U of heparin, 8 mL of 2% lidocaine, and 3 mL of 8.4% of sodium bicarbonate to reach a total fluid volume of 15 mL instilled into the bladder has been described as effective, with more than 80% of patients experiencing good remissions after 2 weeks of three treatments per week (Parsons, 2005b). Similar solutions have been recommended for use in patients with severe symptoms as a "rescue" intervention (Peeker et al., 2000; Perez-Marrero et al., 1988). Patients can be taught to perform the instillations themselves at home.

Intravesical Dimethyl Sulfoxide

Dimethyl sulfoxide (DMSO) was approved by the FDA for use in IC in 1997 based on data from one uncontrolled clinical trial. The action of DMSO is thought to be nonspecific, including anti-inflammatory, analgesic, smooth muscle relaxing, and mast cell inhibiting effects (Peeker et al., 2000; Perez-Marrero et al., 1988). Treatment involves bladder catheterization with instillation of 50 mL DMSO weekly for 6 to 8 weeks, followed by 50 mL every 2 weeks for 3 to 12 months. Small, randomized trials initially suggested benefit; however, adverse effects, including pain and significant exacerbation of symptoms, limited its use (Peeker et al., 2000; Perez-Marrero et al., 1988). DMSO is currently less commonly used than in the past, because other, less painful treatments have become available.

Hydrodistention

Hydrodistention is usually used as a diagnostic aid for PBS/IC. It has also been used as a treatment because some patients report prolonged relief of symptoms after the procedure, possibly because of disruption of sensory nerves within the bladder wall. One uncontrolled study reported a positive effect in 35 of 50 patients (70%) who underwent 30 minutes of hydrodistention and another reported that hydrodistention followed by bladder training reduced flares related to menses and sexual intercourse in 80% of 361 patients (Dunn et al., 1977; Hsieh et al., 2008; Yamada et al., 2003). Others have reported improvement in only 40% of patients (Dunn et al., 1977; Hsieh et al., 2008; Yamada et al., 2003).

When there is benefit, it is usually short-lived; many patients experience worsening of their symptoms after hydrodistention. Thus, many clinicians feel that the risk:/benefit ratio of hydrodistention therapy is not appropriate for their patients. It may be appropriate to reserve use of repetitive therapeutic hydrodistention for patients who generally obtain significant and prolonged relief. Risks of hydrodistention include bleeding (from ruptured vessels) and, rarely, rupture of the bladder wall.

Intravesical Botulinum Toxin

The use of intravesical botulinum toxin for treatment of PBS/IC is controversial and is not approved by the FDA (Kuo & Chancellor, 2009). Investigation into this therapy is based on the ability of botulinum toxin to modulate sensory neurotransmission. Initial results regarding symptom relief with botulinum are promising; however, this therapy is also associated with chronic urinary retention. The need for catheterization would be particularly devastating for a patient with a painful bladder.

In the only randomized trial ($n = 67$) to evaluate this treatment, suburethral injection of botulinum toxin (100 or 200 U) followed by hydrodistention was compared with hydrodistention alone (Kuo & Chancellor, 2009). Successful treatment (based on multiple measures) was found in significantly more patients treated with botulinum toxin plus hydrodistention versus hydrodistention alone at 12-month (55% vs. 26%) and 24-month follow-up (30% vs. 17%). However, the rate of complications in the botulinum groups was concerning. Use of 200 U of botulinum toxin was decreased to 100 U after 1 year because of adverse reactions in nine of 15 patients (e.g., urinary retention, severe dysuria) and these complications were found in more patients treated with 100 U botulinum than with hydrodistention alone (five of 29 vs. one of 23; Kuo & Chancellor, 2009).

NEUROMODULATION THERAPIES

Proponents of the theory that PBS/IC represents a neurologic hypersensitivity disorder tend to favor use of neuromodulation treatments. These include the following.

Amitriptyline

Medications used to treat other pain syndromes are commonly used for IC patients. Amitriptyline is commonly prescribed for relief of PBS/IC symptoms. In Germany, one trial randomly assigned 50 subjects with IC to amitriptyline or placebo (IC was defined according to NIDDK criteria; Wein et al., 2010). Subjects were treated for 4 months with a self-titration protocol that allowed them to escalate drug dosage by 25 mg increments weekly to a maximum of 100 mg. Amitriptyline use resulted in greater improvement in symptom scores than placebo. In addition, significantly more subjects taking amitriptyline rated their satisfaction with treatment as being "good" or "excellent" (63%) than those given placebo (4%). However, only 42% of patients in the amitriptyline group experienced more than a 30% decrease in symptom score, suggesting that benefits are modest. An open-label study of the long-term use of amitriptyline in 94 patients followed for a mean of 19 months reported similar results (van Ophoven & Hertle, 2005). Almost one half of patients rated satisfaction with treatment as "good" or "excellent" and designated themselves as being "moderately" or "markedly" improved. However, about one third dropped out of the study after a mean treatment period of 6 weeks, with nonresponse to treatment being the primary reason for dropout. Side effects of amitriptyline include sedation, dry mouth, and weight gain. A National Institutes of Health–sponsored randomized trial comparing behavioral therapy to amitriptyline-plus-behavioral therapy for treatment of PBS is ongoing (Hassani et al., 2022).

Side effects of amitriptyline include anticholinergic effects, sedation, weight gain, orthostatic hypotension, and conduction abnormalities.

Gabapentin

In an uncontrolled study, 21 patients with refractory genitourinary pain were treated with gabapentin at a dose of 300 to 1,200 mg/day (Sasaki et al., 2001). About one half of the patients reported reduction in pain, including five of eight patients who had a diagnosis of IC. Anecdotal reports also suggest that pregabalin can be effective for pain relief in PBS/IC, but no formal studies support its use.

Electrical Stimulation Therapy

Several reports support treatment of PBS/IC symptoms with implanted sacral neuromodulation (e.g., InterStim device, Medtronic Inc., Minneapolis, MN; Comiter, 2003; Peters & Konstandt, 2004; Peters et al., 2007; Zabihi et al., 2008). This device is FDA approved for treatment of urinary urgency and frequency, but not specifically for treatment of PBS/IC (Comiter, 2003; Peters et al., 2007; Peters & Konstandt, 2004; Zabihi et al., 2008). The device consists of an implanted lead that lies along a sacral nerve root (usually S3) and is attached to an implanted pulse generator. An uncontrolled study from a single center described 17 patients diagnosed with IC according to NIDDK criteria who received InterStim implants and were followed for an average of 14 months (Nygaard, McCreery et al., 2004). Mean daytime and nighttime voiding frequencies decreased from 17 and nine to four and one, respectively. Average pain rating decreased from 5.8/10 at baseline to 1.6/10 (Nygaard et al., 2004). Another case series documented "moderate" or "marked" improvement in pain in 20 of 21 IC patients (NIDDK criteria) during 1 year of follow-up (Nieminen et al., 2003).

InterStim is a costly procedure; adverse events include surgical site infections and pain, and repeat surgery for revisions at the lead or pulse generator site(s) is common. The sacral neuromodulation lead can be placed either along the sacral nerve root (most common) or to stimulate the pudendal nerve. A randomized crossover trial compared the efficacy of leads placed at these two sites in 22 patients with IC/PBS. The pudendal placement was chosen as the "better" lead in 77% of patients (Jelovsek et al., 2007).

Another study reported results after placement of bilateral neuromodulation leads to simultaneously stimulate bilateral sacral nerve roots S2 through S4 (Santaniello et al., 2007). Among 30 patients, 77% responded initially to this therapy and 42% reported at least 50% improvement in symptoms at a minimum of 6-month follow-up. In this study, there was a 22% removal rate because of infection or malfunction (Comiter, 2003; Peters et al., 2007; Peters & Konstandt, 2004; Zabihi et al., 2008).

A less expensive and noninvasive alternative to sacral nerve stimulation is percutaneous posterior tibial nerve stimulation (Peters et al., 2010). One study reported guardedly positive results after tibial nerve stimulation was applied twice weekly in 18 patients with IC/PBS: eight (44%) experienced benefit from the treatment (Zhao et al., 2008).

SOMATIC THERAPIES

Proponents of the theory that bladder symptoms are caused or maintained by somatic (body wall) abnormalities favor somatic therapies. At present, physical therapy is the only somatic therapy in routine use.

Physical Therapy

Treatment of the somatic abnormalities in PBS/IC patients is not within the scope of training of most physical therapists, even those who are skilled in treatment of UI. Resolution of the tender points, trigger points, connective tissue restrictions, and muscular abnormalities of the soft tissues requires specialized training in pelvic soft tissue manual manipulation and rehabilitation. The therapist may also suggest that manual therapy treatments be supplemented by heat or ice treatments.

The effectiveness of myofascial physical therapy for treatment of PBS/IC was illustrated by a randomized trial in which 50% of patients reported they were moderately or markedly improved after a course of targeted treatments, while only 7% of control subjects who received global massage therapy reported improvement (Burrows et al., 2004). The duration of this response after completion of therapy remains to be established. Several case series have also described symptom relief from manual physical therapies (Fitzgerald et al., 2009; Oyama et al., 2004; Weiss, 2001). As an example, one study reported that 70% of IC patients who were treated with manual physical therapy to the pelvic floor tissues for 12 to 15 visits experienced moderate to marked improvement (Fitzgerald et al., 2007). Another study of 21 women with IC and associated pelvic floor hypertonicity demonstrated decreased symptom scores after 5 weeks of pelvic floor massage (Richter et al., 2007). A second randomized trial of physical therapies for treatment of PBS/IC is currently ongoing (Richter, 2006).

MAST CELL THERAPY

Proponents of the theory that mast cells play a critical role in the development and/or maintenance of IC symptoms favor therapies directed at mast cells and allergic phenomena (Sant et al., 2003; Theoharides et al., 2001). These include the following.

Hydroxyzine and Cimetidine

Until recently, the antihistamine hydroxyzine was a mainstay of IC treatment, with an initial dosing of 10 mg in the evening (Keay et al., 2003; Sant et al., 2003; Theoharides, 1994), increasing to 50 to 100 mg daily as needed. However, a randomized controlled trial found hydroxyzine had no benefit over placebo (Keay et al., 2003; Sant et al., 2007). Two small studies suggested benefit of treatment with cimetidine, an H2-receptor blocker, but clinical experience has not generally supported these smaller studies, and cimetidine is not commonly used (Seshadri et al., 1994; Thilagarajah et al., 2001).

Montelukast

The presence of leukotriene D4 receptors in human detrusor myocytes and increased urinary leukotriene E4 in patients with IC and detrusor mastocytosis suggest that cysteinyl-containing leukotrienes may have a role as proinflammatory mediators in this disease (Reena et al., 2007). One small study of 10 women with IC (NIDDK criteria) and detrusor mastocytosis received a single dose of montelukast daily for 3 months (Bouchelouche et al., 2001). After 1 month of montelukast treatment, there was a statistically significant decrease in 24-hour urinary frequency, nocturia, and pain that persisted during the 3 months of treatment. After 3 months, 24-hour urinary frequency decreased from 17.4 to 12 voids, nocturia decreased from 4.5 to 2.8 voids, and pain decreased from 46.8 to 19.6 mm on a visual analog scale. No side effects were observed during treatment. Further investigation of this modality is required.

Dimethyl Sulfoxide

See the previous discussion under Intravesical Dimethyl Sulfoxide.

IMMUNOMODULATORY TREATMENTS

There is interest in exploring immunomodulatory treatments for PBS/IC.

Cyclosporine A

In one trial, 64 patients were randomized in a 1:1 ratio to 1.5 mg/kg cyclosporine A twice daily or 100 mg PPS three times daily for 6 months (Ustinova et al., 2006). Cyclosporine A was superior to PPS in all clinical outcome parameters measured: micturition frequency in 24 hours was significantly reduced (-6.7 ± 4.7 vs. -2.0 ± 5.1 times) and the clinical response rate (according to global response assessment) was significantly higher for cyclosporine than for PPS (75% vs. 19%). Adverse effects of cyclosporine A include hair growth, gingival hyperplasia, paresthesias, abdominal pain, flushing, and muscle pain (Sairanen at al., 2005).

Bacillus Calmette–Guérin

Although intravesical instillation of bacillus Calmette–Guérin (BCG) triggers a variety of local immune responses and has an acceptable safety profile, it has not provided significantly greater relief of IC symptoms than placebo in randomized trials (Mayer et al., 2005; Teichman & Parsons, 2007).

GUIDED IMAGERY

One randomized study suggests benefit from the use of guided imagery for treatment of IC/PBS symptoms (Carrico et al., 2008). For 8 weeks, twice daily for 25 minutes, a group of women either listened to a guided imagery recording or rested. Significantly more women responded to treatment in the guided imagery group (45% vs. 14%).

Emerging Treatment Options

Three therapies are emerging as possible options for women with IC/PBS. Phosphodiesterase-5 inhibitor preventing mast cell degranulation has been associated with a success rate of about 63%. Cannabinoids have demonstrated analgesic and anti-inflammatory properties and have been studied in many chronic pain conditions. Hyperbaric oxygen therapy used to increase oxygen delivery to hypoxic urothelial tissue may be of value (Colemeadow et al., 2020).

CYSTITIS

Acute cystitis refers to infection of the bladder, which is one component of the lower urinary tract system and includes the urethra.

Definition and Scope

Cystitis is inflammation (-itis) in the bladder (cyst-), usually caused by bacteria entering through the urethra. UTIs are a serious health problem affecting millions of people each year. Infections of the urinary tract are common—only respiratory infections occur more often. UTI incidence is about 0.5 among young women and 0.7 in postmenopausal women (annual incidence per person/year; Li & Leslie, 2023).

Etiology

Women are especially prone to UTIs for reasons that are poorly understood. One woman in five develops a UTI during her lifetime. The most common bacteria causing uncomplicated UTI in women is *Escherichia coli*, followed by Enterobacteriaceae, *Proteus mirabilis*, *Klebsiella pneumoniae*, and *Staphylococcus saprophyticus*.

The key elements in the urinary system are the kidneys. The kidneys remove liquid waste from the blood in the form of urine, keep a stable balance of salts and other substances in the blood, and produce a hormone that aids the formation of red blood cells (RBCs). The ureters carry urine from the kidneys to the bladder. Urine is stored in the bladder and emptied through the urethra. The average adult passes about 1.5 quarts of urine each day. The amount of urine varies, depending on the fluids and foods a person consumes. The volume formed at night is about half that formed in the daytime.

Symptoms

Common symptoms reported in women with a UTI include a frequent urge to urinate and a painful, burning feeling in the bladder area or urethra during urination. Some will report malaise, myalgias, and urinary pain even when not urinating. Uncomfortable pressure above the pubic bone is common as is the complaint of passing only a small amount of urine despite a strong urge to urinate. The urine may look milky or cloudy, even reddish if blood is present. Pyelonephritis may be present in women with fever, flank pain, nausea, or vomiting.

Evaluation/Assessment

The history provides strong data in favor of a UTI. Physical examination may reveal suprapubic tenderness. Flank pain may be present in women with pyelonephritis.

Differential Diagnosis

The differential diagnoses in women who present with symptoms suggestive of UTI includes IC, pyelonephritis, and sexually transmitted infections.

Diagnostic Studies

Often an office dipstick urine test showing positive leukocytes and positive nitrates confirms a UTI. If results are equivocal, or a woman has a UTI within 1 month of a prior UTI, culture and sensitivity tests are useful to identify the exact pathogen so that appropriate antibiotic therapy can be selected.

Treatment/Management

The mainstay of UTI treatment is antibiotic therapy. Antibiotics are selected based on the pathogenic bacteria. In the absence of a culture, antibiotic therapy is selected based on the most common bacterial causes of UTI and includes trimethoprim/sulfamethoxazole, fosfomycin, nitrofurantoin, cephalexin, and ciprofloxacin. Knowledge of resistant bacteria in the community is important as trimethoprim/sulfamethoxazole has become ineffective because of antibiotic resistance in many communities.

In women with significant urinary tract pain on urination, use of phenazopyridine (Pyridium) can be helpful until the antibiotic has eradicated the causative bacteria. It is important to warn women that this medication will change the color of their urine to an orange red color.

Complementary medicine options such as cranberry and vitamin C are thought to be helpful by some patients; however, data supporting their use are lacking.

UTI prevention measures such as wiping front to back, urinating when the urge is present (not "holding it"), wearing cotton underwear, and hydrating well are also important.

Recurrent Urinary Tract Infections

Recurrent UTIs are more common in women and are frequently defined as two or more episodes in the last 6 months or three or more episodes in the last 12 months (Hooton, 2012; Nicolle et al., 2005). In a primary care setting, 53% of women above the age of 55 years and 36% of younger women report a UTI recurrence within 1 year. Recurrent UTI can be managed with methenamine (Hiprex) 1 g with vitamin C 500 mg twice a day, as first-line treatment (Aydin et al., 2015), then low-dose preventive antibiotic therapy after evaluation to ensure that no mechanical urinary system concerns are present (Hooton, 2012; Nicolle et al., 2005).

FUTURE DIRECTIONS

Treatment of urinary and pelvic floor problems in women has evolved tremendously over the past few decades. As science continues to identify new methods for therapy, resolution of these problems that negatively affect QOL for women will be simpler and less invasive, providing options for women that are not available today.

Health disparities remain high regarding knowledge of risk factors and treatment options of UI and POP among racially and ethnically diverse women. As an example, Black women were less likely to know that childbirth is a risk factor for POP and UI compared to White women (Mandimika et al., 2015). Educational programs and further research to identify methods to close this disparity are needed.

REFERENCES

References for this chapter are online and available at https://connect.springerpub.com/content/book/978-0-8261-6722-4/part/part03/chapter/ch29

CHAPTER 30

Sexually Transmitted Infections*

JOYCE D. CAPPIELLO AND MAUREEN BOARDMAN

Sexual relations are a natural and healthy part of a woman's life and should be free of infection (Hatcher et al., 2018). However, sexually transmitted infections (STIs) are a substantial health challenge in the United States (Workowski et al., 2021). Preventing, diagnosing, and treating STIs has become even more challenging as rates increase with more severe infections (Hatcher et al., 2018; Workowski et al., 2021). STIs include a variety of clinical syndromes and infections caused by pathogens that can be acquired and transmitted through sexual activity. This chapter covers STIs and introduces STI sequelae as the most common health problems in the United States today.

DEFINITION AND SCOPE

The CDC estimates that 26 million new STIs occur every year in the United States with almost half occurring among young people ages 15 to 25 years (Workowski et al., 2021). The most recent estimates from the CDC show that 20% of the U.S. population or one in five people had an STI on any given day in 2018. Rates of curable STIs in the United States are the highest among developed countries and are higher than rates in some developing countries (Workowski et al., 2021). Individuals with an STI are often undiagnosed regardless of whether they are symptomatic or asymptomatic and are a significant risk for the spread of infection. More than one in two Americans will contract an STI during their lifetime (Workowski et al., 2021).

ETIOLOGY

STIs cause pain and suffering, place heavy demands on healthcare services, and account for more than $16 billion in yearly healthcare costs (Workowski et al., 2021). The human costs are equally overwhelming. A cervical cancer diagnosis, living with chronic pelvic pain, or experiencing a preterm delivery or stillbirth can cause prolonged grief and distress. Couples faced with a diagnosis of infertility because of STIs may require invasive diagnostic procedures and assisted reproductive technology such as in vitro fertilization.

RISK FACTORS

STIs are a group of contagious diseases. The risk of transmission is from person to person by close intimate contact. The organisms causing STIs include a wide variety of microorganisms—bacteria, viruses, spirochetes, protozoans, and obligate intracellular organisms that infect the mucosal surfaces of the genitourinary tract—as well as ectoparasites (organisms that live on the outside of the body such as lice) and the dozens of clinical syndromes that they cause (Workowski et al., 2021). The common STIs in people with a vagina are chlamydia infection, human papillomavirus (HPV) infection, gonorrhea, herpes simplex virus type 2 (HSV-2) infection, syphilis, hepatitis B virus (HBV) infection, and HIV infection (Workowski et al., 2021).

In the past, public health efforts aimed at the control of gonorrhea and syphilis; however, more recently, when it appeared that these diseases were controlled, the concern focused on other diseases, including infection with chlamydia, HSV, HPV, and HIV. Unfortunately, this shifting of focus does not mean that gonorrhea and syphilis are no longer concerns. In recent years, increases in the number of primary, secondary, and congenital syphilis; chlamydia infection; and gonorrhea and drug-resistant strains of gonorrhea have become increasingly more common (Workowski et al., 2021). Recent CDC data show between 2015 and 2019 there was almost a 30% increase in cases of chlamydia infection, gonorrhea, and syphilis. The highest increase was in syphilis diagnosis in newborns, which almost quadrupled. In the

---

*This chapter is a revision of the chapter that appeared in the second edition of this textbook, authored by Catherine Ingram Fogel, and we thank her for her original contribution.

United States, STIs are among the most common infections and are a potential threat to an individual's immediate and long-term health and well-being (Workowski et al., 2021).

IMPACT OF SEXUALLY TRANSMITTED INFECTIONS

Although, historically, STIs were considered to be symptomatic illnesses usually infecting all genders, women and children have the most severe symptoms and sequelae of these diseases. STIs have a greater and more long-lasting impact on women's health than on men's health. STIs in women and children are associated with multiple severe complications and death (Table 30.1).

Reproductive Health Concerns

Pelvic inflammatory disease (PID), a preventable complication of some STIs, such as chlamydia infection and gonorrhea, is a serious threat to reproductive capabilities. More than 1 million people every year experience an episode of PID (Workowski et al., 2021). At least 25% who have had PID experience long-term sequelae, including pelvic abscesses, chronic pelvic pain, dyspareunia, and ectopic pregnancy because of partial tubal scarring and blockage, tubal infertility, increased need for reproductive tract surgery, and recurring PID (Workowski et al., 2021). Among person with PID, tubal factor infertility is the most common cause of infertility accounting for 30% of female infertility in the United States. Only half of those people have been previously diagnosed with PID (Tsevat et al., 2017).

Women who have had PID are six to 10 times more likely to have an ectopic pregnancy compared with women who have not. Ectopic pregnancy occurs in about 2% of all pregnancies and is a significant cause of pregnancy-related death (Workowski et al., 2021). Approximately 10% of all pregnancy-related deaths are attributed to ectopic pregnancy (Anderson et al., 2004). Ectopic pregnancy also substantially increases the risk of tubal-factor infertility. In contrast, STIs rarely cause infertility in men.

TABLE 30.1 Consequences of Sexually Transmitted Infections for Women and Children

HEALTH CONSEQUENCES	WOMEN	CHILDREN
Cancers	Cervical cancer Vulva cancer Vaginal cancer Anal cancer Liver cancer T-cell leukemia Body cavity lymphoma	Liver cancer as adult
Reproductive health problems	Pelvic inflammatory disease Infertility Spontaneous abortion Tubal scarring	
Pregnancy-related problems	Ectopic pregnancy Preterm delivery Premature rupture of membranes Puerperal sepsis Postpartum infection	Stillbirth Neonatal death Prematurity Low birth weight Conjunctivitis Pneumonia Neonatal sepsis Hepatitis, cirrhosis Hepatitis B virus infection Neurologic damage Laryngeal papillomatosis Congenital abnormalities
Neurologic problems	Human T-lymphotropic virus-associated myelopathy (paralysis) Neurosyphilis	Cytomegalovirus-, herpes simplex virus-, and syphilis-associated neurologic problems
Other health consequences	Chronic liver disease Cirrhosis Disseminated gonococcal infection Septic arthritis Tertiary syphilis (cardiovascular and gumma)	Chronic liver disease Cirrhosis

Source: Adapted from Workowski, K. A., Bachmann, L. H., Chan, P. A., Johnston, C. M., Muzny, C. A., Park, I., Reno, H., Zenilman, J. M., & Bolan, G. A. (2021). *Sexually transmitted infections treatment guidelines, 2021.* MMWR Morbidity and Mortality Weekly Report Recommendations and Reports, 70(4), 1–187. https://doi.org/10.15585/mmwr.rr7004a1

Adverse Pregnancy Outcomes

STIs may cause acute complications for pregnant people and their offspring. Pregnant people may transmit the infection to their newborn, infant, or fetus through vertical transmission (through the placenta before delivery, during vaginal birth, or after birth through breastfeeding) or horizontal transmission (close physical or household contact). Some of the complications associated with an STI experienced by pregnant people can include spontaneous abortion, stillbirth, premature rupture of membranes, and preterm delivery. Vaginal and cervical STI infections during pregnancy can lead to inflammation of the placental or fetal membranes, resulting in maternal fever during or after delivery, wound and pelvic infections after cesarean section, and postpartum endometritis. Sexually transmitted pathogens that have serious consequences tend to be more serious, potentially life-threatening health conditions in the fetus or newborn. Damage to the brain, spinal cord, eyes, and auditory nerves are of concern with STIs in the fetus and the infant. For example, severe, permanent central nervous system manifestations or fetal or neonatal death can occur with congenital syphilis. Currently, all transmission of HIV to infants in the United States is attributable to mother-to-infant transmission. Ophthalmia neonatorum occurs when infants are exposed to vaginal gonorrheal or chlamydial infections during delivery and, if untreated, can result in corneal ulcers and blindness (Workowski et al., 2021).

Cancer-Related Consequences

HPV infections are highly prevalent in the United States, especially among young, sexually active women (Workowski et al., 2021). Furthermore, persistent infection of some types can cause cancer and genital warts. HPV types 16 and 18 account for approximately 70% of cervical cancer worldwide and HPV types 6 and 11 account for 90% of genital warts (Workowski et al., 2021). Cervical cancer is the second most common cancer among women worldwide, and about 95% of cervical cancers are associated with 10 to 15 HPV subtypes. People with HPV infection of the cervix are 10 times more likely to develop invasive cervical cancer than women without HPV (Lei et al., 2020). HIV infection may increase the risk that HPV infection will progress to cervical, vaginal, vulvar, and anal cancers.

Increased HIV Risk

A synergistic relationship exists between HIV and STIs (Looker et al., 2017). The inflammation or disruption of genital mucosa that occurs with ulcerative and inflammatory STIs is a risk factor for contracting HIV during a sexual encounter (Looker et al., 2017). People with vaginas with genital ulcer diseases or gonococcal or chlamydial cervicitis have an estimated to be two- to fourfold increase of HIV acquisition (Workowski et al., 2021).

Preventing, identifying, and managing STIs are essential components of women's healthcare. APRNs and certified nurse midwives, referred to as clinicians in this chapter, play an essential role in promoting reproductive and sexual health by counseling patients about STI risk, encouraging sexual and other risk-reduction measures, incorporating education regarding STI disease prevention in their nursing practice,

and being current on management strategies. By doing so, clinicians can assist people in both avoiding STIs and in living better with the sequelae and chronic infections of STIs (see Table 30.1).

TRANSMISSION OF SEXUALLY TRANSMITTED INFECTIONS

The chance of contracting, transmitting, or developing complications from HIV and STIs depends on multiple biological, behavioral, social, and related risk factors. However, most individuals are reluctant to discuss sexual health issues openly because of the biological and social factors associated with these infections. Microbiological, hormonal, and immunologic factors influence individual susceptibility and transmission potential for STIs. These factors are partially influenced by an individual's sexual practices, substance use, and other health behaviors. Health behaviors, in turn, are influenced by socioeconomic factors and other social factors. In general, the prevalence of STIs tends to be higher in those who are unmarried, young (ages 15–35 years), and living in urban areas (Workowski et al., 2021).

Biological Factors

Biological factors place women at a greater risk than men for acquiring STIs and for suffering more severe health consequences associated with STIs (Workowski et al., 2021); for example, the risk of a woman contracting gonorrhea from a single act of intercourse is 60% to 90%, whereas the risk for a man is 20% to 30%. Men are two to three times more likely to transmit HIV to women than the reverse. The vagina has a large amount of genital mucous membranes exposed and an environment more conducive to infections than the penis. Moreover, the risk for tissue trauma is greater during vaginal intercourse for women than for men. The cervix, particularly the squamocolumnar junction/transformation zone and endocervical columnar epithelial cells, is most susceptible to HIV; however, the virus can invade the vaginal epithelium as well.

More than 50% of bacterial and 90% of viral STIs are asymptomatic and are likely to go undetected in women. If or when symptoms develop, they may be confused with those of other diseases not transmitted sexually. The frequency of asymptomatic and unrecognized infections can lead to delayed diagnosis and treatment, chronic untreated infections, and complications. It can be more challenging to diagnose STIs in a woman because the anatomy of her genital tract makes clinical examination more complicated. Lesions inside the vagina and in the cervix are not readily seen. The normal vaginal environment (warm, moist, enriched medium) is ideal for infection.

Age and gender influence an individual's risk for an STI; specifically, young women (age 20–24 years) and female adolescents (15–19 years) are more susceptible than are their male counterparts (Workowski et al., 2021). STIs tend to occur at a younger age in females than in males. Compared with women before menopause, female adolescents and young women are more susceptible to cervical infections, such as chlamydial infections and gonorrhea, and HIV because of the ectropion of the immature cervix and resulting in the larger exposed surface of cells unprotected by cervical mucus. As women age, the cells eventually recede into the inner cervix. Postmenopausal women also are at increased risk because of thin vaginal and cervical mucosa. Pregnant women also have higher rates of cervical ectropion.

Other biological factors that increase a woman's risk for acquiring, transmitting, or developing complications of certain STIs include vaginal douching, risky sexual practices, and the use of hormonal contraceptives. The risk for contracting the infections that lead to PID is increased with vaginal douching. Sexual practices such as anal intercourse, sex during menses, and "dry sex" (inserted vaginal sex without sufficient lubrication) may predispose a woman to acquire an STI. Such sexual practices may cause bleeding and tissue trauma that facilitate invasion by pathogens. Although normal vaginal flora may confer nonspecific immunity, younger and postmenopausal women may be at greater risk of acquiring HIV because of a thinner vaginal epithelium and increased friability, thus providing direct access to the bloodstream. The use of hormonal contraceptives can be a risk factor secondary to the fact that people using hormonal contraceptives to protect against pregnancy often fail to use a barrier method to prevent STIs. Oral contraceptives appear to protect against PID but may increase the risk of lower genital tract chlamydial infection.

Social Factors

Preventing the spread of STIs and HIV is difficult without addressing individual and community issues that have a tremendous influence on prevention, transmission, and treatment of these diseases. Societal factors such as poverty, lack of educational opportunities, racial inequity, and inadequate access to healthcare indirectly increase the prevalence of STIs and HIV in risk populations (Prather et al., 2016).

Persons with the highest rates of many STIs are often those with the poorest access to healthcare, and health insurance coverage influences if and where a individual obtains STI services and preventive services. Suppose a socioeconomically disadvantaged person perceives themself to be at risk for an STI. In that case they may not practice protective behaviors if survival is an overarching concern or if other risks appear to be more threatening or imminent. The need to secure shelter, food, clothing, safety for self and children, and money may override concerns about preventive health and prevent individuals from changing risky behaviors.

Social Interactions and Relationships

STIs are the only illnesses whose spread is directly related to the human urge to share sexual intimacy and reproduce. Because intimate human contact is the typical vehicle of transmission, sexual behavior is a critical risk factor for preventing and acquiring STIs. The gender-power imbalance and cultural proscriptions sometimes associated with sexual relationships can make it difficult for individuals to protect themselves from infection (Opara et al., 2021; Park et al., 2016).

An individual may be dependent on an abusive partner or a partner who places them at risk by their risky sexual behaviors. The risk of acquiring STIs or HIV infection is high among physically and sexually abused individuals. Intimate partner violence is associated with the lack of sexual protection (Orchowski et al., 2020). Additionally, fear of physical harm and loss of economic support hamper an individual's efforts to enact protective practices. Furthermore, prior and current abuse are strongly associated with substance abuse, increasing the risk of contracting an STI.

An individual's risk of acquiring an STI is determined not only by their actions but by their partner's risky behavior. Although prevention counseling customarily includes recommending that women identify the partner at high risk because of drugs and medical factors and also determine their sexual practices, this advice may be unrealistic or culturally inappropriate in many relationships. Many women who identify themselves as lesbian have had intercourse with a man by choice, force, or necessity.

Societal Norms

Cultural and religious attitudes regarding appropriate sexual behaviors affect risk at the individual and community levels. Relationships and sexual behavior are regulated by cultural norms that influence sexual expression in interpersonal relationships. Power imbalances in relationships are the product of and contribute to maintaining traditional gender roles. As long as traditional gender norms define the roles for sexual relationships with men having the dominant role in sexual decision-making, negotiating condom use by women will remain difficult (Opara et al., 2021; Tarzia & Hegarty, 2021). Cultural barriers also may impede the use of condoms. Gender roles in both Latina and Black women make it difficult for them to suggest using condoms to a partner (Gimenez-Garcia et al., 2018; Opara et al., 2021).

Recognition of Risk

Lack of a perception of risk is given as a reason for not using sexual protective practices. Younger individuals may incur more STIs because they have less knowledge of reproductive health, less effective skills in communicating and negotiating with their partners about safer sex practices, and more barriers to access to healthcare services. Taking risks is a universal human element. In the throes of passion, people can make unwise sexual decisions.

Substance Use

Substance use (alcohol and illicit drugs) is associated with an increased risk of HIV and STIs (Murali & Jayaraman, 2018), and STI rates are higher in areas where rates of substance abuse are high. People who use drugs are at a higher risk for HIV and STI because of drug-related and sexual transmission (Murali & Jayaraman, 2018). For example, cocaine and heroin use has paralleled trends in syphilis, gonorrhea, and HIV infection. There are several possible reasons for this association, including social factors, such as poverty and lack of educational and economic opportunities, and individual factors such as risk taking and low self-efficacy. In addition to the risk from sharing needles, use of illicit drugs and alcohol may contribute to the risk of HIV infection by undermining cognitive and social skills, thus making it more challenging to engage in HIV-protective actions. Depression and other psychological problems and or a history of sexual abuse are associated with substance abuse and thus contribute to risky behaviors (Murali & Jayaraman, 2018). Being impaired by illicit drugs and thus being unable or unwilling to clean drug paraphernalia can be a pervasive barrier to protective practice. Moreover, drug use may occur in settings where persons participate in sexual activities while using drugs. Many people who use cocaine routinely engage in high-risk sexual behaviors that place them at high risk of HIV and other bloodborne STIs secondary to sexual impatience caused by the stimulant effect of cocaine (Johnson et al., 2017). Finally, individuals who use illicit drugs may be at a higher risk because of exchanging sex for drugs or money, resulting in a higher number of sexual partners and sexual encounters.

Past and current physical, emotional, and sexual abuse characterize the lives of many, if not most, drug-using women (Imtiaz et al., 2016). For women who have experienced violence, use of alcohol and drugs can become a coping mechanism by which they self-medicate to relieve feelings of anxiety, depression, guilt, fear, and anger stemming from the violence (Imtiaz et al., 2016).

Cultural and religious attitudes and beliefs also affect healthcare services. The loss of support for safer sex education programs in favor of an abstinence-only program does not protect adolescents. Abstinence-only programs have been proved ineffective in multiple studies and often result in higher teen pregnancy and STI rates (Santelli et al., 2017). Unfortunately these educational programs do not stop teenagers from having sex nor do they teach them how to have sex safely.

SPECIAL POPULATIONS

Incarcerated Women

Incarcerated women experience STI/HIV infection at a rate 13 times greater than women in the general population (Workowski et al., 2021). This heightened risk is because of a unique confluence of factors, including histories of sex work, substance abuse, experienced violence, mental illness, concurrent partners, and infection with other STIs (Workowski et al., 2021). Additionally, before incarceration, many women had limited access to medical care. Women 35 years and younger in juvenile and adult detention facilities have higher rates of chlamydial infection and gonorrhea than nonincarcerated females in the community (Workowski et al., 2021). Furthermore, syphilis rates are considerably higher in adult incarcerated women than in nonincarcerated females (Workowski et al., 2021). In short-term correctional facilities (jails and juvenile detention facilities), retention rates are short (often 48 hours), and as a result, treatment completion may be less than optimal. Furthermore, the mobility of this population in and out of the community increases the risk for further infections.

The current CDC STI screening recommendation is that all women 35 years and younger in correctional facilities should be screened for chlamydia and gonorrhea. Universal syphilis screening should be conducted on the basis of the local area and institutional prevalence of primary, secondary, and early latent syphilis (Workowski et al., 2021).

Women Who Have Sex With Women

Women who have sex with women (WSW) are a diverse group with variations in sexual identity, sexual behaviors, sexual practices, and risk behaviors (Workowski et al., 2021). Some WSW, particularly younger women and adolescents and women who have sex with both men and women, may be at increased risk for STIs and HIV (Workowski et al., 2021). The percentage of WSW who have a history of an STI is three times as higher in WSW who have a history of heterosexual intercourse than in those who have not. A landmark study from 1999 reported that 75% of women who identified as lesbian had a history of intercourse with men and of that group, 66% reported having unprotected intercourse with men (Diamant et al., 1999). Therefore, obtaining a thorough and complete sexual history is imperative. WSW exclusively also risk exposure to trichomoniasis, gonorrhea, chlamydia, genital herpes, HPV, hepatitis C (HCV), syphilis, and HIV and should be screened for these infections (Petti, 2018). HPV transmitted through skin-to-skin contact, is common in WSW, and sexual transmission of HPV also occurs among female sex partners (Workowski et al., 2021). Examples of specific questions to include in the health history are: Are you having sex with males, females, both or another?

- Are you having sex with males, females, both, or another?
- Do you participate in oral-to-vaginal contact with your partner(s)?
- Do you participate in finger-to-vaginal or anal contact with your partner(s)?
- Do you use sex toys (vibrators, strap-on penis, pelvic balls)?
- Do you share these with your partner(s)?
- Do you participate in oral-to-anal contact with your partner(s)?
- Do you use barrier protection with female partners (gloves during digital-genital sexual activities, condoms with sex toys, and latex or plastic barriers [e.g., dental dams])?

Effective screening requires that clinicians and their patients have open and comprehensive discussions of sexual and behavioral risks beyond sexual identity. It is also essential that clinicians understand their comfort level to have open, candid discussions regarding sexual practices and behaviors.

PREVENTION

Preventing infection (primary prevention) is the most effective way of reducing the adverse consequences of STIs for women, their partners, and society. Prevention and control of STIs are based on five major strategies:

- Accurate risk assessment, education, and counseling of persons at risk on ways to avoid STIs through changes in sexual behaviors and use of recommended prevention services
- Preexposure vaccination of persons at risk for vaccine-preventable STIs
- Identification of an asymptomatically infected person(s) with STIs

- Effective diagnosis, treatment, counseling, and follow-up of infected persons
- Evaluation, treatment, and counseling of sex partners of persons who are infected with an STI (Workowski et al., 2021)

Prompt diagnosis and treatment of current infections (secondary prevention) also can prevent personal complications and transmission to others. Primary prevention of STIs begins with changing those behaviors that place persons at risk for infection. Moreover, treatment of infected individuals is a form of primary prevention of spread within the community in that it reduces the likelihood of transmission of STIs to sexual partners (Workowski et al., 2021). Furthermore, the key to real progress in STI prevention is the coordination of prevention programs for unintended pregnancy and HIV with those for other STIs because all are the consequences of unprotected sexual activity. Risk factors for STIs and HIV are summarized in Box 30.1.

Education

Educational efforts, both population-based and individual gender and culture-specific and at an appropriate literacy level, are essential to STI control. Educational messages about specific infections, personal protective practices, and communication skills should be delivered in age-appropriate, culturally sensitive, appealing formats.

Individual Counseling

With the advent of HIV and other chronic viral STIs, individual counseling is critical. As chronic infections have emerged, the role of treatment with cure has lessened, and the need

---

Box 30.1 Risk Factors for STIs and HIV

People who are at an increased risk of contracting STIs and HIV include those:

- Who have unprotected vaginal, anal, or oral intercourse
- Who have more than one sex partner
- Who use alcohol or illicit drugs during sexual activity
- With high-risk sex practices, including fisting, oral–anal contact, anal intercourse
- Who share sex toys and douching equipment
- Who share needles or other drug-use paraphernalia
- Who have partners who are bisexual men who also have sex with other men
- With a previous history of a documented STI or HIV infection
- With partners who have a previous history of STIs or HIV
- Involved in the exchange of sex for drugs or money
- Who live in areas with a high STI/HIV incidence or prevalence
- Whose initiation of sexual activity was at an early age

STI, sexually transmitted infection.
Source: Adapted from Workowski, K. A., Bachmann, L. H., Chan, P. A., Johnston, C. M., Muzny, C. A., Park, I., Reno, H., Zenilman, J. M., & Bolan, G. A. (2021). Sexually transmitted infections treatment guidelines, 2021. MMWR Morbidity and Mortality Weekly Report Recommendations and Reports, 70(4), 1–187. https://doi.org/10.15585/mmwr.rr7004a1

---

for risk-reduction counseling has increased. Person-centered counseling should be a standard component of STI care regardless of where provided in the healthcare system. Counseling skills characterized by respect, compassion, and a nonjudgmental attitude toward all patients are essential to obtaining a complete sexual risk history and counseling individuals effectively about prevention. These specific techniques are effective in providing prevention counseling:

- Using open-ended questions (e.g., "What has your experience with using condoms been like?")
- Using understandable language (e.g., "Have you ever had a sore or a scab on your private parts or lips?"), normalizing language (e.g., "Some of my patients tell me that it is hard to use a condom every time they have sex. How has it been for you?")
- Reassuring the person that treatment is provided regardless of consideration, such as the ability to pay, language spoken, or lifestyle (Workowski et al., 2021)

Assurances of confidentiality are equally important in providing effective risk reduction counseling. Prevention messages should include descriptions of specific actions to avoid acquiring or transmitting STIs and should be tailored to the individual, with attention given to specific risk factors (Workowski et al., 2021). Examples include advice to refrain from sexual activity if the person has STI-related symptoms and to vaccinate against HPV and hepatitis B.

Safer Sex Practices

Counseling that encourages abstinence from sexual intercourse is critical during STI treatment, for individuals whose partner is being treated for an STI, and for persons wanting to avoid all possible consequences of sex (e.g., STIs, HIV, and unintended pregnancies). Alternatively, involvement in a mutually monogamous relationship with an uninfected partner also eliminates risk of contracting an STI. For someone beginning a mutually monogamous relationship, screening for common STIs for both the person and their partner before beginning a sexual relationship is advised to decrease the risk for future transmission of asymptomatic STIs (Workowski et al., 2021). However, when neither of these options is realistic, the clinician must focus on other, more feasible measures.

An essential component of primary prevention is counseling individuals regarding safer sex practices, including knowledge of their partner, reducing the number of partners, low risk sex, and avoiding the exchange of body fluids. No aspect of prevention is more important than knowing one's partner. Reducing the number of partners and avoiding partners who have had many previous sexual partners decreases a person's chance of contracting an STI. Discussing each new partner's previous sexual history and exposure to STIs will augment other efforts to reduce risk. Caution that, in any sexual encounter other than a mutually monogamous relationship, safer sex measures are always advisable, even when partners insist otherwise. It is critical to negotiate condom use if the person is unsure about their partner's sexual history.

When used correctly and consistently (Box 30.2), male latex condoms are highly effective in preventing sexual transmission of HIV infection and can reduce the risk for other STIs (gonorrhea, chlamydia, and trichomonas; see Box 30.1). Condoms are

Box 30.2 Suggestions on How to Use a Male Condom

Use new condoms every time you perform any vaginal, anal, and oral sex (try flavored).

- Open the package carefully to avoid damage.
- Do not unroll before placing it on the penis.
- Gently press out air at the tip before putting it on.
- Put it on when the penis is erect.
- Unroll to cover the entire erect penis.
- If it tears or comes off in the vagina, stop immediately and withdraw; put on a new one before you continue.
- After ejaculation and before the penis gets soft, withdraw the penis and the condom together.
- Hold on to the rim as you withdraw so nothing spills.
- Gently pull the condom off the penis.
- Discard in waste containers.
- Do not flush down the toilet.
- Never reuse condoms.

more effective in preventing infections transmitted by fluids from mucosal surfaces (gonorrhea, chlamydia, trichomonas, and HIV) than those transmitted by skin-to-skin contact (e.g., HSV, HPV, syphilis, chancroid) as condoms do not cover all exposed skin surfaces. Furthermore, by limiting lower genital infections, condoms may also reduce PID risk (Workowski et al., 2021). Rates of latex condom breakage during sexual intercourse and withdrawal are low (about two condoms per 100 condoms used) in the United States (Workowski et al., 2021). Nonlatex condoms (e.g., those made of polyurethane) can be substituted for persons with latex allergies (Workowski et al., 2021) to prevent pregnancy. However, nonlatex condoms can have pores up to 1,500 nm in diameter, which is more than 10 times the diameter of HIV and more than 25 times the diameter of HBV. They also have higher rates of breakage and slippage than do latex condoms. The failures of condoms to protect people against STI transmission or unintended pregnancy are usually the result of inconsistent or incorrect use rather than from condom breakage. The U.S. Food and Drug Administration (FDA) has approved the first condom specifically to prevent STIs during anal sex (FDA, 2022).

Laboratory studies have demonstrated that the female condom, a lubricated polyurethane sheath with a ring on each end inserted into the vagina, is an effective mechanical barrier to viruses, including HIV and semen (Workowski et al., 2021). Furthermore, clinical studies have documented its effectiveness in protecting from recurrent trichomonas infection. If used consistently and correctly, the female condom should reduce the risk of contracting or transmitting an STI (Box 30.3).

The selection of a contraceptive method has a direct impact on STI risk. Many individuals view condoms first, and perhaps only, as a method of contraception. People who have another method of birth control, such as sterilization or hormonal contraceptives, are less likely to use condoms. The effectiveness of contraceptive methods against STIs, including HIV, is summarized in Table 30.2. The contraceptive methods that are most protective against STIs are not the most effective pregnancy prevention methods. For example, condoms are the most protective method against STIs and HIV but are not the most effective method in preventing pregnancy. The use of dual protection to prevent pregnancy and STIs is critical. Because it is unclear how many individuals understand the need for dual protection, clinicians can play an important role in counseling women in this regard and in the importance of other risk-reduction practices (see Table 30.3).

Until recently, people were counseled to use spermicides—specifically nonoxynol-9 (N-9)—with condoms to prevent HIV and other STIs. Research has found no significant reduction in the risk of HIV and STIs with the addition of N-9 spermicide to condom use. Furthermore, there is some evidence of harm disruption of genital or rectal epithelium, slightly higher rates of urogenital gonorrhea, and an increased risk for bacterial urinary tract infections in women who are nonoxynol-9 users (Workowski et al., 2021; Hatcher et al., 2018). At this time, no proven topical antiretroviral agents exist for the prevention of HIV (Workowski et al., 2021).

The risk of HIV transmission through ingestion of sexual secretions is not known definitively; however, a few HIV cases have been linked to transmission through oral sex (Workowski et al., 2021). HBV and HCV can rarely be spread through saliva, and HSV type 1 (HSV-1) and HSV type 2 (HSV-2), syphilis, gonorrhea, and chlamydia can be spread through oral sex. Therefore, individuals should use barriers such as dental dams, male unlubricated condoms cut in half, or non-microwaveable Saran wrap when engaging in cunnilingus, plus unlubricated condoms for fellatio helps reduce risk.

Cultural barriers also may impede the use of condoms. Latinx gender roles make it difficult for Latina women to suggest using condoms to a partner (Morales-Alemán & Scarinci, 2016).

Clinicians can suggest strategies to enhance condom negotiation and communication skills. Suggesting that someone talk with their partner about condom use when removed from sexual activity may make it easier to bring up the subject. Role-playing possible partner reactions and alternative responses can be helpful. Asking a person who appears particularly uncomfortable to rehearse how they might approach the topic is useful, particularly when a person fears their partner may be resistant. The clinicians might suggest someone begin by saying, "I need to talk with you about something that is important to both of us. It's hard for me and I feel embarrassed but I think we need to talk about safe sex." If someone is able to sort out their feelings and fears before talking with their partner(s), they may feel more comfortable and in control of the situation. The person can be reassured that it is natural to be uncomfortable and that the hardest part is getting started. Clinicians should help their clients clarify what they will and will not do sexually because it is easier to discuss it if they are clear. The clinicians can remind patients that their partner may need time to think about what has been said and pay attention to their partner's response. If the partner seems to be having difficulty with the discussion, the person may need to slow down and wait a while. If the partner resists safer sex, the patient may wish to reconsider the relationship. In addition, if a patient indicates fear for their safety after suggesting condom use, the clinicians must provide resources for prevention of violence and emphasize that personal safety is paramount.

People who have been diagnosed with an STI also need prevention counseling. Both partners need treatment for

Box 30.3 Female Internal Condoms

What Are Female Condoms?

Female condoms are made of very thin polyurethane.
Prelubricated
No spermicides
Made of plastic
May be used with oil-based lubricants

Where Do They Go?

Female condoms are placed in a vagina to line it and prevent sperm entering the cervix.
If used perfectly, they can be as effective as other barrier contraceptives.
If used in conjunction with hormonal contraceptives, IUDs, and other barrier methods, condoms are even more effective.

What Are the Advantages of Female Condoms?

- The person is in control of their contraception.
- Female condoms can protect against infections.
- You can put a female condom in any time before sex.

What Makes Them Less Effective?

- If the penis touches the vagina or area around it before a female condom is inserted
- If the condom splits
- If the female condom gets pushed too far into the vagina (the open end must stay outside the vagina during sex)
- If the penis enters the vagina outside the condom

How to Use Female Condoms

A new packet will have full instructions, including diagrams.

1. Check if it is new and check the use-by date.

2. You can put one in when you are lying down, squatting, or have one leg on a chair (like using a tampon, find the position that suits you best).

3. Take it out of the packet with care (fingernails and rings can tear polyurethane).

4. Hold the closed end of the condom and squeeze the inner ring (at the closed end) between your thumb and middle finger. If you keep your index finger on the inner ring too, it will help to keep it steady.

5. With your other hand, spread the outer and inner lips (labia), which are the folds of skin around your vagina. Push the squeezed ring into the vagina and as far up as you can (about a long-finger length). Now put your index finger or both your index and middle fingers inside the open end of the condom, until you can feel the inner ring at the top. Push the inner ring at the top as far as you can into your vagina. (You will be able to feel the hard front of your pelvis—pubic bone—just in front of your fingers if you curve them forward a bit.)

6. The outer ring should be close against the outside of your vagina (vulva).

7. The female condom is loose fitting, so it is a good idea for the woman to help guide the penis into the ring. It will move about a bit during sex, but you will be protected from pregnancy and most infections as long as the penis stays inside the condom.

How to Remove Female Condoms

Take hold of the outer ring (the open end), and give it a twist to trap any semen inside it. Pull it out gently.

What to Do With Used Female Condoms

Never reuse a female condom. Wrap it up in a tissue and throw it in a trash bin. Do not put it in the toilet.

TABLE 30.2 Effectiveness of Contraceptives Against Sexually Transmitted Infections

Contraceptive Method	Bacterial Infection	Viral (Including HIV) Infection
Condoms	Reduces risk; most protective in preventing infections transmitted by fluids	Protective
Sterilization	No protection	No protection
Vaginal spermicides with nonoxynol-9	Not effective in preventing cervical gonorrhea, chlamydia infection[a,b]	No protection, possibly increased risk[a,c]
Diaphragm, cervical cap	Modest protection against cervical infection (gonorrhea, chlamydia, trichomoniasis)	Questionable
Oral contraceptives	No known protection	Not protective
Implantable/injectable contraceptives	Not protective	Not protective
Intrauterine device	Associated with pelvic inflammatory disease in first month after insertion[c]	No protection
Natural family planning	No protection	No protection

[a]Efficacy in receptive and anal intercourse is unknown for most condoms. Data for the newer condom specifically designed for anal intercourse has a higher efficacy rate than traditional condoms.
[b]Frequent use is associated with genital lesions, which may be associated with an increased risk of HIV transmission.
[c]Likely to be caused by microbial contamination at insertion.
Source: Adapted from Hatcher, R., Kowal, D., Nelson, A., Trussell, J., Cwiak, C., Carson, P., Policar, M., Edelman, A., Aiken, A., & Marrazzo, J. (2018). Contraceptive technology (21st ed.). Managing Contraception; U.S. Food and Drug Administration. (2022, February 23). FDA permits marketing of first condom specifically indicated for anal intercourse. https://www.fda.gov/news-events/press-announcements/fda-permits-marketing-first-condom-specifically-indicated-anal-intercourse; Workowski, K. A., Bachmann, L. H., Chan, P. A., Johnston, C. M., Muzny, C. A., Park, I., Reno, H., Zenilman, J. M., & Bolan, G. A. (2021). Sexually transmitted infections treatment guidelines, 2021. MMWR Morbidity and Mortality Weekly Report Recommendations and Reports, 70(4), 1–187. https://doi.org/10.15585/mmwr.rr7004a1

TABLE 30.3 Sexual Behavior and Levels of Risk

SAFEST	LOW RISK	POSSIBLE RISK	HIGH RISK
Behavior Abstinence Self-masturbation Mutual monogamy (both partners monogamous and no high-risk activities) Hugging, touching, massaging[a] Dry kissing Mutual masturbation Drug abstinence **Prevention** Avoid all drug and sexual high-risk behaviors	**Behavior** Wet kissing Vaginal intercourse with condom Fellatio interruptus Urine contact with intact skin **Prevention** Avoid exposure to any potentially infected body fluids Consistently use latex or polyurethane condoms	**Behavior** Cunnilingus Fellatio Mutual masturbation with skin breaks Anal intercourse with condom **Prevention** Avoid anal intercourse Use dental dam, unlubricated male condom cut in half, female condom, or plastic wrap with cunnilingus Use latex gloves with masturbation	**Behavior** Unprotected anal intercourse Unprotected vaginal intercourse Unprotected oral–anal contact Vaginal intercourse after anal intercourse without a new condom Fisting Multiple sex partners Sharing sex toys, needles or other drug paraphernalia, or douching equipment **Prevention** Avoid exposure to potentially infected body fluids Consistent condom use with vaginal and anal intercourse Avoid anal penetration If having anal penetration, use condom with intercourse, latex glove with hand penetration Avoid oral–anal contact Do not share sex toys, drug paraphernalia, or douche equipment Clean needles and drug paraphernalia with bleach and water before and after use

[a]Assumes no breaks in the skin.
Source: Adapted from Center for Disease and Control and Prevention. (2023). Sexual risk behavior: Youth engage in sexual risk behaviors. https://www.cdc.gov/healthyyouth/sexualbehaviors; Fogel, C. J. (2016). Sexually transmitted infections. In K. D. Schuiling & F. K. Likis (Eds.), Women's gynecologic health (2nd ed., pp. 485–530). Jones & Bartlett; Workowski, K. A., Bachmann, L. H., Chan, P. A., Johnston, C. M., Muzny, C. A., Park, I., Reno, H., Zenilman, J. M., & Bolan, G. A. (2021). Sexually transmitted infections treatment guidelines, 2021. MMWR Morbidity and Mortality Weekly Report Recommendations and Reports, 70(4), 1–187. https://doi.org/10.15585/mmwr.rr7004a1

their infection and counseling to avoid reinfection. Key aspects to emphasize for people already infected include:

- Responding to infection suspicion by obtaining appropriate assessment promptly
- Taking oral medications as directed
- Returning for follow-up tests when applicable
- Encouraging sex partners to obtain examination and/or treatment when indicated
- Avoiding sexual exposure while infectious
- Preventing future exposure by practicing protective practices
- Confidentiality

COVID-19 Pandemic and Sexually Transmitted Infections

Prior to the COVID-19 pandemic, STIs were increasing in the United States and Europe. One study from Spain reported that since the start of the COVID-19 pandemic the number of STI reported cases was 51% less than expected. The sharpest decrease was for chlamydia diagnosis, which decreased by 72%, and the smallest decrease was for syphilis diagnosis which decreased by 22% (Sentis et al., 2021). The decline in diagnosis is thought to be multifactorial, including fears of COVID-19 infection, socioeconomic impacts such as job loss, insurance coverage disruptions, disruptions to healthcare in general and STI testing services in particular, and decreased sexual activity may have led to reduced actual and/or perceived rates of risk. Reduced access to testing and diagnoses may have led some people to spread infection unwittingly.

The COVID-19 pandemic worsened an already stretched system for STI diagnosis and treatment in the United States. According to one survey as of January 2021 approximately one-third of state and local STI program staff continued to be deployed to assist with COVID-19 response efforts. Another recent report on STIs by the National Academies of Sciences, Engineering, and Medicine (2021) articulates how the COVID-19 pandemic uncovered the lack of investment in our public health preparedness structure. However, as clinics and medical offices reopen, infection rates are again on the rise. The expected postpandemic rebound in STI/HIV rates will require a robust response from our overstressed public health system (Ogunbodede et al., 2021).

SCREENING AND DETECTION

Clinicians are responsible for educating their clients regarding the signs and symptoms of STIs. Opportunities for education and screening include times when a individual comes in for a well-person examination, seeks contraception, obtains preconceptual care, or comes to a healthcare provider for prenatal care. Clinicians also must ensure that clients know where and how to obtain care if they think they might have contracted an STI. A critical first step to detecting STIs is for clinicians to routinely and regularly obtain STI histories from their patients. Ask specific questions during the health history. The questions in Box 30.4 help shape a risk assessment and STI history tailored to the cultural and social context of a patient's life and the prevalence of various STIs in a specific geographic area. Key aspects of obtaining an STI history include assurances of confidentiality and a nonjudgmental attitude. The history must be conducted privately, ideally with the person fully clothed. Begin history taking with a rationale for why the questions are asked and reinforce the importance of sexual health as a part of total health. Risk assessment depends on a person's willingness to self-identify risk factors seen as socially unacceptable or stigmatizing. Some people may prefer to complete a written questionnaire rather than reveal risk factors directly to a clinician. Consider using a previsit, online questionnaire using questions similar to those given in the sexual-risk history. All pregnant people must be screened for gonorrhea, syphilis, chlamydia, HIV, and HBV. Prenatal screening is discussed in each specific infection section.

Evaluation

People diagnosed with an STI should be asked to identify and notify all exposed partners. General procedures for screening, treating, and reporting specific STIs are discussed in the next sections. In addition to safe sex practices, prevention is available for HPV and hepatitis A and B. Vaccinations are key for prevention. Preexposure prophylaxis (PrEP) is available for individuals at risk for HIV. Local health departments have listings of available clinics to treat STIs.

CARING FOR A PERSON WITH A SEXUALLY TRANSMITTED INFECTION

Individuals may delay seeking care for STIs because they may be asymptomatic or unaware that they have an infection, the concept of an STI is not part of their thinking, they have privacy concerns, or have limited access to healthcare services. In this age of widespread and often sensational media publicity about STIs, they may fear the social stigma. When an individual is diagnosed with an STI, their reactions may range from acceptance to hurt, disbelief, anger, or concern. These reactions may vary with the expectations in the individual's subculture and personal experience. Treatments for all genders are discussed as women's health clinicians often treat a patient's partner. The CDC updates STI guidelines approximately every 5 years. The most recent guidelines are available from the CDC with mobile for both android and iOS platforms (www.cdc.gov/std/treatment-guidelines/toc.htm). The full citation for the new guidelines is in the reference list (Workowski et al., 2021).

Assessment

STI assessment and prevention counseling should be interactive and individually focused using client-centered language and motivational interviewing skills. The CDC has simple advice for providers: Talk, Test, Treat. The "talk" part of this advice is the most challenging for many providers. When sexual history taking is included as part of each routine health history, providers become comfortable with the pertinent questions.

The diagnosis of an STD is based on integrating relevant history, physical exam, and laboratory data. A comprehensive and specific history is essential for accurate diagnosis (Box 30.4). Information should be collected nonjudgmentally, avoiding assumptions of sexual preference. All partners should be referred to as partners and not by gender. Begin with open-ended questions that might elicit information that otherwise would be missed; these can be followed with symptom-specific questions and relevant history. Specific areas to include are the reason why the individual has sought care; symptoms; a sexual history, including a description of the date and type of sexual activity; number of contacts;

Box 30.4 Risk Screening: The Five Ps

Facilitate rapport and ask permission: for example, "I ask all patients a few questions about their sex life to assess any risk for sexually transmitted infections. May I ask you some questions?"

1. Partners
   - Are you currently having sex of any kind?
   - What is the gender(s) of your partner?
     ○ Many providers use the phrasing of "Are your partners men, women, or both?" Consider changing the phrasing to "men, women, both, or another" OR
     ○ Describe body parts instead of gender: "Do your partners have penises, vaginas, or both?"
   - Tell me about any new sex partners you have had since your last visit (if the patient has previously been seen in the practice).
   - If you haven't established the sexual orientation and gender identity of the individual, ask:
     ○ What do you consider yourself to be?
     ○ What is your current gender identity?
     ○ What sex were you assigned at birth, as shown on your original birth certificate?
2. Practices
   - To understand any risk for STIs, I need to ask more specific questions about the kind of sex you have had recently.
   - What kind of sexual contact do you have or have you had?
     ○ Do you have vaginal sex, meaning penis in vagina sex?
     ○ Do you have anal sex, meaning penis in the rectum/anus sex?
     ○ Do you have oral sex, meaning mouth on penis/vagina?
3. Protection from STIs
   Try using normalizing language, for example, "Some of my patients have difficulty using a condom with each act of sex. How is it for you?"
4. Past history of STIs
   - Have you ever been tested for STIs and HIV? If yes, how long ago and what was the result?
   - Have you ever been diagnosed with an STI in the past?
   - Have any of your partners had an STI?
   Additional questions for identifying HIV and hepatitis risk:
   - Have you or any of your partner(s) ever injected drugs?
   - Is there anything about your sexual health that you have questions about?
5. Pregnancy intention
   - Do you think that you would like to have (more) children in the future?
   - How important is it to you to prevent pregnancy (until then)?
   - Are you or your partner using contraception or practicing any form of birth control?
   - Would you like to talk about ways to prevent pregnancy?
6. Plus: The National Coalition for Sexual Health suggests adding a sixth question to the standard five Ps. Although the information may or may not be pertinent to an STI assessment, the information will help you discuss overall sexual health with patients. See Chapter 19, Women's Sexual Health, for further discussion of the sixth P.
   - Pleasure
   - Problems
   - Pride

STI, sexually transmitted infection.
Source: Adapted from U.S. Preventive Services Task Force. (2020). Hepatitis C *virus infection in adolescents and adults:* Screening. *https://www.uspreventiveservicestaskforce.org /uspstf/recommendation/hepatitis-c-screening; U.S. Preventive Services Task Force. (2021).* Chlamydia and *gonorrhea:* Screening. *https://www.uspreventiveservicestaskforce.org /uspstf/recommendation/chlamydia-and-gonorrhea-screening; Workowski, K. A., Bachmann, L. H., Chan, P. A., Johnston, C. M., Muzny, C. A., Park, I., Reno, H., Zenilman, J. M., & Bolan, G. A. (2021). Sexually transmitted infections treatment guidelines, 2021. MMWR Morbidity and Mortality Weekly Report Recommendations and Reports, 70(4), 1–187. https://doi.org/10.15585/mmwr.rr7004a1*

whether contact with someone who recently had an STI; and potential sites of infection (mouth, cervix, urethra, and rectum). Pertinent medical history includes anything that will influence the management plan: history of drug allergies, previously diagnosed chronic illnesses, and general health status. A menstrual history, including the date of the individual's last menstrual period, must always be obtained to rule out pregnancy. Certain medications used to treat STDs are contraindicated in pregnancy. All adults and adolescents from ages 13 to 64 should be tested at least once for HIV.

When indicated, an HIV-oriented systems review should be conducted (see Chapter 31, Women and HIV/AIDS, for further detail). Follow up on any positive answers regarding symptoms to elicit information about onset, duration, and specific characteristics, such as color, amount, and consistency of discharge. Base screening recommendations on anatomy. For example, if the individual has a cervix, follow the guidelines for cisgender women for screening. Consider infection screening of the rectal area if the individual is having anal intercourse.

The CDC and the U.S. Preventive Services Task Force (USPSTF) make recommendations for screening based on age and population. Screening discussions should be based on shared clinical decision-making between the individual and the clinician. Screening discussions include applicability to their lives, privacy matters, how and when results will be provided, and what needs to be reported to the public health department (see Box 30.4):

- **All adults and adolescents from ages 13 to 64** should be tested for HIV and hepatitis C at least once. The USPSTF recommends screening for hepatitis C starting at age 18 (USPSTF, 2020c).
- **All sexually active people with a vagina** <25 years old should be tested for gonorrhea and chlamydia annually.
- **People with a vagina** ≥25 years and older with risk factors such as new or multiple sex partners or a sex partner who has an STI should also be tested for gonorrhea and chlamydia annually.
- **All pregnant people** should be tested for syphilis, HIV, hepatitis B, and hepatitis C starting early in pregnancy and chlamydia and gonorrhea, if indicated. Repeat testing as needed.
- **All sexually active people with penises who have sex with people with penises should be:**
  - Tested at least annually for syphilis, chlamydia, and gonorrhea. Those with multiple or anonymous partners should be tested more frequently (e.g., every 3 to 6 months).
  - Tested at least once a year for HIV and may benefit from more frequent HIV testing (e.g., every 3 to 6 months).
  - Tested at least annually for hepatitis C, if living with HIV.
  - The USPSTF has a draft recommendation (A rating) to test all asymptomatic, nonpregnant adolescents and adults who are at increased risk for syphilis infection (Adapted from Workowski et al., 2021; National Coalition for Sexual Health, n.d.)

If sexual assault is suspected, a sexual assault forensic exam by a trained healthcare professional is necessary to collect DNA evidence. Most outpatient offices are not equipped to conduct a forensic exam and must refer to an ED.

The physical examination begins with careful visualizing of the external genitalia, including the perineum. Note any erythema, edema, distortions, lesions, or trauma from scratching, sexual activity, sports activity, or injury. Palpation can locate areas of tenderness. The most common STIs, chlamydia infection and gonorrhea, can be diagnosed with a patient-collected vaginal swab or urine screen. Assess the vagina and cervix for edema, thinning, lesions, abnormal coloration, trauma, discharge, and bleeding during the speculum examination. Assess for vaginal secretion and odor. Lesions should be evaluated and cultures obtained when appropriate. When collecting specimens, lubricate the speculum with water as artificial lubricants may interfere with testing accuracy for some lab studies. Reassure that every effort will be made to make the speculum examination as comfortable as possible. Assess for

vaginal discharge and the characteristics of the cervix. Self-swabs may be sufficient and preferred by the individual (Doshi et al., 2008). If indicated for further assessment of symptoms, perform a bimanual exam. Appropriate laboratory studies will be suggested, in part, by the history of individual risk factors, symptoms, community prevalence, physical examination results, and national screening standards. Point-of-care (POC) STI testing may be available at some clinics. Once someone is tested, make sure they know how to access test results.

Treatment

An individual with a STI will need support in seeking care at the earliest stage of symptoms. Counseling about STIs is essential for (a) preventing new infections or reinfection; (b) increasing adherence with treatment and follow-up; (c) providing support during treatment; and (d) assisting individuals in discussions with their partner(s). Provide time for questions and shared decision-making. Individuals should be given a brief description of the disease in a language that they can understand. This description should include modes of transmission, incubation period, symptoms, infectious period, and potential complications. Thorough, careful instructions about medications must be provided, verbally and in writing, as this is a time of high anxiety for many individuals, and they may not be able to hear or remember the information. Side effects, benefits, and risks of the medication should be discussed. Suggest comfort measures that decrease symptoms. Many booklets on STIs are available, or the clinician may wish to develop literature specific to the practice setting.

In general, advise individuals to refrain from intercourse until all treatment is finished to prevent reinfection. If this has not been done already, all individuals who have contracted an STI should be taught safer sex practices. Urge individuals to continue condom use to prevent recurring infections, especially if they have had an episode of PID or have new partners. The CDC recommends retesting at 3-month intervals after treatment for new chlamydia, gonorrhea, or syphilis infections. Partner services include an in-person visit to assess and treat, notifying partner(s) directly (with patient permission), or expedited partner treatment (EPT). Expedited partner therapy is the clinical practice of treating sex partners of individuals diagnosed with chlamydia or gonorrhea by giving a prescription or the actual medication to the patient to give to their partner. Check local state laws prior to engaging in EPT. As of this writing, 46 states allow EPT, with the remaining four potentially allowing the practice (Division of STD Prevention, 2021a). Written material about the infection, symptoms, treatment, and side effects should be provided to both partners.

Preexposure vaccination is an important prevention strategy. Hepatitis B vaccination is recommended for all unvaccinated persons sexually active with more than one person. Both Hepatitis A and B vaccinations are recommended if the person injects drugs, has chronic liver disease, has HIV, or has hepatitis C. If homeless, hepatitis A vaccination is also recommended. Administer HPV vaccination to all individuals at 11 to 12 years of age (or as young as 9 years) through age 26. From ages 26 to 45, assess the risk benefit of the vaccine with the individual. Antiretroviral medications, either daily or monthly, are available for HIV prevention, called preexposure prophylaxis (PrEP). Pre- and postexposure prophylaxis for HIV is discussed in Chapter 31, Women and HIV/AIDS.

Addressing the psychosocial component of STIs is essential. Learning that one has an STI may be upsetting; knowledge of an STD may unsettle a sexual relationship. Remember that an individual may be afraid or embarrassed to tell their partner, ask their partner to seek treatment, or admit sexual practices, and may be concerned about confidentiality or the threat of violence from the partner. Support the individual in whatever manner they need.

Offering literature and role-playing situations may also be of assistance. Clinicians who take time to counsel their clients on how to talk with their partner(s) can improve adherence and case finding. Accurate identification and timely reporting of STIs are integral components of successful infection control efforts and assessing morbidity trends. All states require that gonorrhea, chlamydia, syphilis, chancroid, and HIV/AIDS cases are reported to public health officials. The reporting of other STIs varies from state to state. Reporting can be provider based, lab based, or both. Clinicians are legally responsible for knowing the reporting mechanism in their state and in their practice and for informing patients of reporting requirements. The individual should be assured that the information reported to and collected by health authorities is maintained in strictest confidence; in most jurisdictions, reports are protected by statute from subpoena. Most public health departments trace contacts with exposure to syphilis, HIV/AIDS, and hepatitis but do not have the resources to conduct contact tracing for chlamydia and gonorrhea. In the case of chlamydia and gonorrhea, the clinician must discuss and manage contact tracing with their patient.

The following sections outline the treatments for specific STIs following CDC guidelines. When available, they also delineate self-care measures and preventive strategies.

CERVICITIS

Cervicitis is characterized by two major diagnostic signs: (1) a purulent or mucopurulent endocervical discharge and (2) sustained endocervical bleeding easily induced by gentle passage of a cotton swab in the cervical os. Either or both may be present. However, cervicitis is frequently asymptomatic. Some people complain of intermenstrual bleeding and postcoital bleeding. When a cause of cervicitis is determined, it is typically chlamydia or gonorrhea. Cervicitis can occur with trichomoniasis and genital herpes (primary HSV-2) infections (Workowski et al., 2021). Because cervicitis may be a sign of upper genital tract infection, anyone with a new episode of cervicitis should be assessed for PID, tested for chlamydia and gonorrhea, and assessed for bacterial vaginosis (BV) and trichomoniasis.

Chlamydia Infection

Chlamydia trachomatis infection is the most frequently reported bacterial infectious disease in the United States, and its prevalence is highest in persons age 24 years or younger (Workowski et al., 2021). Sequelae from chlamydial infection include PID,

ectopic pregnancy, and infertility. Acute salpingitis, a form of PID, is the most serious complication of chlamydial infections and is a major etiologic factor in the subsequent development of tubal-factor infertility, ectopic pregnancy, and chronic pelvic pain. Chlamydial infection of the cervix causes inflammation resulting in microscopic cervical ulcerations and thus may increase the risk of acquiring HIV infection. Chlamydia infection in pregnancy has been associated with premature rupture of the membranes, preterm birth, stillbirth, and low-birth-weight infants. Maternal chlamydial morbidity includes an increased risk of postabortion endometritis salpingitis, and postpartum endometritis. Neonatal chlamydial infections result from perinatal exposure to the mother's infected cervix during birth, involving the eye's mucous membrane, oropharynx, urogenital tract, and rectum. Conjunctivitis usually develops 5 to 12 days after delivery in 20% to 50% of exposed infants. Chlamydia is also a common cause of subacute, afebrile pneumonia in infants ages 1 to 3 months (Workowski et al., 2021).

ASSESSMENT AND DIAGNOSIS

Annual screening of all sexually active people with vaginas who are age 25 years and younger is recommended, as is a screening of older people with vaginas at increased risk for infection, including those who have a new sex partner, multiple sex partners, a partner with concurrent partners, or a partner with an STI (USPSTF, 2021). A sexual risk history should always be done and may indicate more frequent screening for some individuals. The clinician should inquire about any symptoms. Although usually asymptomatic, some people may experience spotting or postcoital bleeding, mucoid or purulent cervical discharge, increased urinary frequency, or dysuria. Cervical spotting and bleeding result from inflammation and erosion of the cervical columnar epithelium. Occasionally, individuals report lower abdominal pain and dyspareunia.

All pregnant people should be routinely screened for chlamydia at the first prenatal visit. Additionally, screening for chlamydia should be done in the third trimester (36 weeks) if at increased risk. First trimester screening might prevent the adverse effects of chlamydia during pregnancy; however, evidence for adverse effects in pregnancy is minimal, and when screening is done only early during the first trimester, an extended period exists for acquiring infection before delivery (Workowski et al., 2021).

Public health screening measures focus on women, who bear the burden of the long-term effects. Screening programs have not focused on young men because of feasibility and cost effectiveness, although screening should be considered in high-risk populations such as in STI clinics, teen clinics, and correctional facilities. The USPSTF give an I (Insufficient) rating for preventive screening of men (2021), although this guidance is primarily for low-risk individuals and public health screening programs. Diagnostic testing is always necessary if someone is symptomatic or high risk.

Nucleic acid amplification tests (NAAT) for chlamydia have sensitivities well above 90% with specificity >99% (Papp et al., 2014). A vaginal swab is the most efficacious sampling. Self-collected vaginal specimens are equivalent in sensitivity and specificity to clinician collected swabs and may be preferred by the patient (Doshi et al., 2008). An endocervical swab is acceptable when a pelvic examination is indicated.

Chlamydia testing can be ordered on a liquid-based cytology specimen, although test sensitivity is slightly less. First-void urine samples can be used if vaginal or endocervical testing is unacceptable to the individual. There is a high prevalence of reinfection in people with vaginas who have had chlamydia infections in the preceding several months, usually from reinfection by an untreated partner. Because reinfection rates are high and the risk of complications increases, clinicians should advise all people with vaginas, especially adolescents, with a chlamydial infection to be rescreened 3 months after treatment (Workowski et al., 2021). In men, urine NAAT testing is the first-line testing. For men who cannot provide a urine specimen, a provider-collected or patient self-swab of the ureteral meatus is acceptable. The FDA has approved some brands of NAAT testing for oropharyngeal and rectal testing in both males and females. Self-collected oropharyngeal and rectal swabs have been shown to be as effective as clinician swabbing (Berry & Stanley, 2017; Dize et al., 2016; Doshi et al., 2008).

TREATMENT

The CDC 2021 guidelines have changed recommendations to include doxycycline 100 mg orally twice a day for 7 days as first-line therapy for chlamydia (Workowski et al., 2021). Alternative regimens include azithromycin 1 g orally in a single dose or levofloxacin 500 mg orally once daily for 7 days. Doxycycline is more effective for treating rectal chlamydial infection. There is a concern that anyone with a vagina, even if not engaging in anal intercourse, may have contamination to the rectal area. If not treated with the more efficacious doxycycline, the rectal infection may be a source of autoinoculation for the vaginal area. Oropharyngeal infection may also respond better to doxycycline. The CDC does not currently recommend routine screening of the oropharyngeal site. Erythromycin is no longer recommended as an alternative therapy due to the significant gastrointestinal complaints, which affect treatment adherence. Advise treated individuals to refrain from sexual intercourse for 7 days and until their sex partners are treated. Anyone who tests positive for chlamydia is likely at risk for other STIs. Test for gonorrhea, syphilis, and HIV, and perform other testing if indicated. Repeat testing is advised at 3 months, not because of concern about treatment failure but because of reinfection from untreated partners or exposure to a new, infected partner.

Treating pregnant people usually prevents neonatal transmission. Doxycycline is contraindicated in the second and third trimesters of pregnancy because of the risk of tooth discoloration. In pregnant individuals, first-line therapy is azithromycin 1 g in a single dose with amoxicillin 500 mg orally three times a day for 7 days as an alternative therapy. Test of cure is indicated at 4 weeks after treatment in pregnant individuals but not before. NAAT testing for chlamydia may remain positive for up to 4 weeks. Retest again in the third trimester or at the time of delivery in high-risk individuals. Partners of infected individuals should be retested near the end of their partner's pregnancy. Untreated chlamydia exposes the neonate to conjunctivitis and to pneumonia. See STI treatment guidelines for neonatal treatment regimens (www.cdc.gov/std/treatment-guidelines/STI-Guidelines-2021.pdf, p. 68; Workowski et al., 2021). Individuals with a chlamydia infection and a concurrent HIV infection should be treated with the same regimen used for HIV-negative patients.

Gonorrhea

Gonorrhea is probably the oldest communicable disease in the United States and is the second most commonly reported communicable bacterial disease. The latest CDC figures estimate over 600,000 cases reported in 2019. Rates increased 92% from 2009 to 2019. Rates are higher among males than females; however, the rate increase has been documented in all people (Division of STD Prevention, 2021b).

Common sites of gonococcal infection in people with a vagina are the endocervix (primary site), urethra, Skene's and Bartholin's glands, and rectum. The main complication of gonorrheal infections is PID and subsequent infertility; pelvic abscess or Bartholin's abscess may also occur. Gonococcal infections in pregnancy potentially affect both mother and infant. Pregnant people with cervical gonorrhea may develop salpingitis in the first trimester. Perinatal complications of gonococcal infection include spontaneous septic abortion, premature rupture of membranes, preterm delivery, chorioamnionitis, neonatal sepsis, intrauterine growth retardation, and maternal postpartum sepsis. Endometritis after elective abortion or chorionic villus sampling procedures may also occur. Amniotic infection syndrome manifested by placental, fetal, and umbilical cord inflammation following premature rupture of the membranes has been associated with gonorrheal infections during pregnancy. Disseminated gonococcal infections (DGIs) are a rare complication (0.5%–3%) of untreated gonorrhea. DGI occurs in two stages: the first stage is characterized by bacteremia with chills, fever, and skin lesions and is followed by stage two, during which the patient experiences acute septic arthritis with characteristic effusions, most commonly of the wrists, knees, and ankles (Star & Deal, 2004).

ASSESSMENT AND DIAGNOSIS

Up to 80% of people with a vagina are asymptomatic; when symptoms are present, they are often less specific than the symptoms in people with a penis. As with chlamydia, the recommendation is to screen all those with a vagina younger than age 25 on an annual basis and age 25 and older if at increased risk. Increased risk is defined as having a new sexual partner, more than one sexual partner, or a sex partner with other partners or STI.

Vaginal discharge is usually minimal or absent, although a few individuals may have a purulent, irritating endocervical discharge. Menstrual irregularities may be the presenting symptom, or people with a vagina may complain of chronic or acute pelvic or lower abdominal pain or more prolonged, more painful menses. Unilateral labial pain and swelling may indicate Bartholin's glands infection, and periurethral pain and swelling may indicate inflamed Skene's glands. Infrequently, dysuria, vague abdominal pain, or low backache prompts someone to seek care. Later symptoms may include fever (possibly high), nausea and vomiting, joint pain and swelling, or upper abdominal pain (liver involvement). Gonococcal rectal infection may occur following anal intercourse. Individuals with rectal gonorrhea may be completely asymptomatic or, conversely, experience severe symptoms with profuse purulent anal discharge, rectal pain, and blood in the stool. Rectal itching, fullness, pressure, and pain are also common symptoms, as is diarrhea. Gonococcal pharyngitis may appear similar to viral pharyngitis; some individuals will have a red, swollen uvula and pustule vesicles on the soft palate and tonsils similar to streptococcal infections. Diffuse vaginitis with vulvitis is the most common form of gonococcal infection in prepubertal girls. There may be few signs of infection, or vaginal discharge, dysuria, and swollen, reddened labia may be present.

Given that gonococcal infections are often asymptomatic, they cannot be diagnosed reliably by clinical signs and symptoms alone. When symptoms are present in people with a vagina, they typically are less specific than those seen in people with a penis. NAAT testing with vaginal swabs is preferred for vaginas and first-void from penises. NAAT tests can be used to swab the oropharyngeal and rectal areas. Check the product inserts for each NAAT manufacturer for sensitivity, specificity, and collection methods for oropharyngeal and rectal testing. As with chlamydia testing, patient-collected specimens are acceptable. Cultures and Gram stains can be used for testing but are less available in many offices. Cultures offer the advantage of antimicrobial susceptibility testing, which cannot be performed from NAAT tests and thus are preferred if there is a concern of treatment failure. A test for gonorrhea should be done at the first prenatal visit. A repeat culture should be obtained in the third trimester for at-risk pregnant people or if living in areas with high prevalence (Workowski et al., 2021).

TREATMENT

Gonorrhea, although first identified in the late 1800s, was not effectively treated until the development of penicillin in the 1940s. Overuse of penicillin led to resistance, necessitating a switch to quinolones. Over time, resistance again developed, with a switch to cephalosporins. The previous CDC guideline recommended dual therapy; however, the concern of microbiome damage and effect on other pathogens lowered the benefits of dual therapy. The current guideline recommends single therapy with a dosing increase and a recommendation for dosing based on weight: ceftriaxone 500 mg IM (intramuscular) in a single dose for persons weighing <150 kg or 1 g for a person weighing ≥150 kg (or 330.7 lb). This regimen is effective against urogenital and rectal infections. Pregnant people need treatment with ceftriaxone 500 mg IM in a single dose. Pharyngeal gonococcal infections are challenging to treat and may act as transmission and antibiotic resistance reservoirs. If a concurrent chlamydia infection is identified, add doxycycline 100 mg twice a day for 7 days. Whenever possible, administer medications on site. Advise individuals to abstain from sexual intercourse for 7 days and have all sex partners treated. If an individual has an allergy to ceftriaxone, consult with an infectious disease specialist. All individuals diagnosed with gonorrhea should be tested for chlamydia, syphilis, and HIV, and should undergo other tests as indicated.

Persons treated for uncomplicated urogenital or rectal infections do not require a test of cure. If the individual had a positive oropharyngeal infection, follow up in 7 to 14 days, ideally using culture as NAATs may be falsely positive in this time frame. Antimicrobial testing, if needed, can be done from the culture. Retest all positive individuals (from any site) in 3 months. Persons are more likely to return if a follow-up

appointment is made at the time of the initial treatment. See partners for an evaluation or arrange expedited partner treatment. In some states, pharmacists can administer the injection. Treatment failure is suspected if symptoms do not respond in 3 to 5 days. If a clinician is concerned about a treatment failure, they should consult with a local health department or infectious disease specialist or utilize the National Network of STD Clinical Prevention Training Centers Clinical Consultation online service (www.std.uw.edu/page/site/clinical-consultation). Complications of gonorrhea, although infrequent, include disseminated infection. Symptoms may include petechiae or pustules, polyarthralgia, tenosynovitis, or oligoarticular septic arthritis. Rarely, endocarditis, meningitis, or perihepatitis occur. Treatment includes consultation with an infectious disease specialist, hospitalization, and ceftriaxone I g IV (intravenous) every 24 hours. Partners must be treated.

In pregnancy, screening and treatment are the best tools for preventing neonatal gonococcal infections. If the neonate is exposed to a mother's infected cervix during birth, symptoms usually occur 2 to 5 days later. Gonococcal ophthalmia neonatorum and sepsis are significant sequelae. Ocular prophylaxis with erythromycin 0.5% ointment for all newborns <24 hours after birth is recommended, rated grade A (Acceptable), which is the highest rating (USPSTF, 2019) to prevent blindness. Infants with gonococcal ophthalmia should be hospitalized and assessed for signs of disseminated infection (sepsis, arthritis, meningitis). A single dose of ceftriaxone 25 to 50 mg/kg IV or IM is adequate for gonococcal conjunctivitis (Workowski et al., 2021). Mothers of infants who have a gonococcal infection and the mother's sex partners should be assessed and treated.

PELVIC INFLAMMATORY DISEASE

PID is a spectrum of inflammatory disorders of the upper female genital tract, including any combination of endometritis, salpingitis, tubo-ovarian abscess, and pelvic peritonitis. Sexually transmitted pathogens or bacterial vaginosis pathogens cause 85% of cases (Brunham et al., 2015; Mitchell et al., 2021). Most PID results from an ascending spread of microorganisms from the vagina and endocervix to the upper genital tract. This spread most frequently happens at the end of or just after menses. Several factors facilitate the development of an infection: the os is slightly open; the cervical mucus barrier is absent, and menstrual blood is an excellent medium for growth. PID also may develop following an abortion, pelvic surgery, or delivery. Each year, more than 2 million people with vaginas in the United States have an episode of symptomatic PID. Risk factors include a younger age of sexual debut because of greater biological vulnerability, a higher number of lifetime vaginal sex partners, and a prior history of STIs (Kreisel et al., 2017).

PID causes major medical complications. Short-term consequences include acute pelvic pain, tubo-ovarian abscess, tubal scarring, and adhesions. Long-term complications include an increased risk (12%–16%) of infertility, ectopic pregnancy, chronic pelvic pain, dyspareunia, and recurrent episodes of PID (Brunham et al., 2015). Because chlamydia-associated PID is more commonly asymptomatic, it results in tubal obstruction from delayed diagnosis or inadequate treatment. PID unrelated to STI can be caused by anaerobic and aerobic enteric bacteria: group B streptococcus, *Escherichia coli, Bacteroides fragilis, Campylobacter,* or respiratory pathogens such as *Haemophilus influenzae, Streptococcus pneumoniae,* group A streptococcus, and *Staphylococcus aureus.* Postoperative pelvic peritonitis, pregnancy-related infections, trauma-related pelvic infections, and secondary infections can also present similarly to STI-related PID (Workowski et al., 2021). Because PID may be caused by various infectious agents and encompasses a wide variety of pathologic processes, the infection can be acute, subacute, or chronic with a wide range of symptoms. All people who are diagnosed with acute PID need testing for HIV, gonorrhea, and chlamydia, and should undergo other tests as indicated.

Assessment and Diagnosis

Diagnosis of acute PID is difficult because the symptoms of PID vary and the most common signs and symptoms can occur in urinary, gastrointestinal, or reproductive tract problem (Hillier et al., 2021). Symptoms may mimic other disease processes, such as ectopic pregnancy, endometriosis, ovarian cyst with torsion, pelvic adhesions, inflammatory bowel disease, or acute appendicitis. Table 30.4 contains detailed information on diagnosing PID.

History taking must be comprehensive. Menstrual history helps establish the relationship of onset of pain to menses and identifying any variations from normal in the cycle. Other relevant history includes recent pelvic surgery, delivery, dilation of the cervix, abortion, recent intrauterine device (IUD) insertion (within the past 3 weeks), purulent vaginal discharge, irregular bleeding, and a prolonged or heavier menstrual period. A thorough sexual risk history should also be obtained, including current or most recent sexual activity, number of partners, and method of contraception, and will assist in identifying a possible increased risk for STD exposure. Intestinal and bladder symptoms are important to review. People may report various symptoms ranging from minimal pelvic discomfort to dull cramping and intermittent pain or severe, persistent, and incapacitating pain. Pelvic pain usually develops within 7 to 10 days of menses, remains constant, is bilateral, and is most severe in the lower quadrants. Pelvic discomfort is exacerbated by Valsalva maneuver, intercourse, or movement. Anyone with acute PID also may complain of intermenstrual bleeding. Symptoms of an STD in a partner(s) also should be noted.

vital signs are obtained, and a complete physical examination is performed. A fever of 102°F or more is characteristic. Physical examination reveals adnexal tenderness, with or without rebound, and exquisite tenderness with cervical movement. Pelvic tenderness is usually bilateral. There may or may not be a palpable adnexal swelling or thickening. Fever and peritonitis are more characteristic of gonococcal PID than PID caused by other organisms, which are more likely to be "silent."

Subacute PID is far less dramatic, with a great variety in the severity and extent of symptoms. Symptoms are so mild and vague that a person may ignore them. Symptoms that suggest subacute PID are chronic lower abdominal pain, dyspareunia, menstrual irregularities, urinary discomfort,

TABLE 30.4 Diagnostic Criteria for PID Screening and Management

The sensitivity of clinical diagnosis is only 65% to 90%. Because of the potential consequences of PID, even patients with minimal findings need treatment.

DIAGNOSIS/ MANAGEMENT	FINDINGS/RECOMMENDATIONS
Diagnosis/Screening Presentation Exam findings	Pelvic or lower abdominal pain Cervical motion tenderness Uterine tenderness Adnexal tenderness
Additional diagnostic criteria	Oral temperature >38.3°C (>101°F) Abnormal cervical mucopurulent discharge or cervical friability Abundant numbers of WBCs seen on saline microscopy of vaginal fluid
Office-based testing	Always rule out pregnancy Microscopy NAAT testing for chlamydia, gonorrhea If available, NAAT testing for *Mycoplasma genitalium* HIV screening Syphilis testing
Laboratory confirmation	*Neisseria gonorrhoeae, Chlamydia trachomatis,* or *M. genitalium*
Additional testing	Pelvic imaging consistent with PID (TVUS, CT, MRI) Laparoscopic abnormalities Histologic evidence of endometritis via biopsy
Management General approach	Maintain a low threshold of suspicion for the diagnosis and treatment of PID.
Outpatient management: patients with mild to moderate PID can tolerate oral medications and are expected to adhere to therapy	Ceftriaxone 500 mg for individuals <150 kg or 1 g for individuals ≥150 kg IM with Doxycycline 100 mg bid × 14 days orally with Metronidazole 500 mg orally bid × 14 days
Hospital management	See CDC guidelines

bid, twice a day; CDC, Centers for Disease Control and Prevention; IM, intramuscular; NAAT, nucleic acid amplification test; PID, pelvic inflammatory disease; TVUS, transvaginal ultrasound; WBCs, white blood cells.
Source: Data from Brunham, R. C., Gottlieb, S. L., & Paavonen, J. (2015). Pelvic inflammatory disease. New England Journal of Medicine, 372(21), 2039–2048. https://doi.org/10 .1056/NEJMra1411426; Centers for Disease Control & Prevention (2021). Pelvic Inflammatory disease (PID). https://www.cdc.gov/std/treatment-guidelines/pid.htm; Workowski, K. A., Bachmann, L. H., Chan, P. A., Johnston, C. M., Muzny, C. A., Park, I., Reno, H., Zenilman, J. M., & Bolan, G. A. (2021). Sexually transmitted infections treatment guidelines, 2021. MMWR Morbidity and Mortality Weekly Report Recommendations and Reports, 70(4), 1–187. https://doi.org/10.15585/mmwr.rr7004a1

low-grade fever, low backache, and constipation. Abdominal examination usually reveals no rebound tenderness; there is slight adnexal tenderness with cervical movement, and cervical or urethral discharge, often purulent, may be present.

Most people with PID have either mucopurulent cervical discharge or evidence of white blood cells (WBCs) on microscopic evaluation of saline preparation of vaginal fluids (wet prep). Essential laboratory studies are a complete blood count with differential, erythrocyte sedimentation rate (highest in chlamydial infections), and cervical cultures for gonorrhea and chlamydia. Laboratory data are useful only when considered in conjunction with symptoms and physical examination findings.

Clinical diagnosis of PID is imprecise; nevertheless, most diagnoses of PID are clinical because laparoscopy and biopsy are too expensive and invasive to be practical screening tools. Because delay in diagnosing and treating PID is associated with severe sequelae, the Workowski et al. (2021) guidelines established new minimum criteria for beginning treatment. The CDC recommends a "low threshold for diagnosing PID" because of the risk of damage to reproductive health. The 2021 guidelines recommend empiric treatment of PID if one or both of two minimum criteria are present and if no other cause(s) of the illness can be identified: (1) uterine or adnexal tenderness or (2) cervical motion tenderness (Workowski et al., 2021). Furthermore, consider a diagnosis of PID in a woman with any pelvic tenderness and any sign of lower genital tract inflammation.

Treatment

Perhaps the most critical nursing intervention for PID is prevention. Primary prevention would be education in avoiding the acquisition of STIs, whereas secondary prevention involves preventing a lower genital tract infection from ascending to the upper genital tract. Instruct people in self-protective behaviors, such as practicing safer sex and using barrier methods. Also important is detecting asymptomatic gonorrheal and chlamydial infections through routine screening. Partner notification when an STI is diagnosed is essential to prevent reinfection. If treating in the outpatient setting, see the individual for follow-up within 3 days. If no clinical improvement has occurred, the next step is hospitalization. All individuals with a PID diagnosis should be retested at 3 months. PID risk with IUD use generally occurs within 3 weeks of insertion. If an individual acquires PID after this time period, treat the PID and do not remove the IUD. Consider IUD removal only if the woman does not respond to therapy within the 72-hour window. Pregnant people with PID should be hospitalized and treated with antibiotics because of the high risk for preterm delivery and maternal morbidity (Workowski et al., 2021).

Health education is central to the effective management of PID. Clinicians should explain to individuals the nature of the disease and encourage them to comply with all therapy and prevention recommendations, emphasizing the necessity of taking all medication, even if symptoms disappear. Assess for any financial issues for filling prescriptions or lack of transportation for follow-up appointments. The importance of follow-up visits should be stressed. Counsel individuals to refrain from sexual intercourse until treatment is completed. Provide contraceptive counseling and suggest barrier methods for STI prevention. Individuals with PID may be acutely ill or may experience long-term discomfort. Pain in itself is debilitating and is compounded by the infectious process. The potential or actual loss of reproductive capabilities is closely tied to sexuality, body image, and self-concept. Part of the clinician's role is to help a patient adjust their self-concept to fit into reality and to accept alterations in a way that promotes health.

ULCERATIVE GENITAL INFECTION

Syphilis

Syphilis, one of the earliest described STIs, is a systemic disease caused by *Treponema pallidum*, a motile spirochete. The disease is characterized by periods of active symptoms and symptomless latency. It can affect any tissue or organ in the body. Transmission occurs by entering the subcutaneous tissue through microscopic abrasions during sexual intercourse. The highly contagious disease can also be transmitted through kissing, biting, or orogenital sex. Primary and secondary syphilis rates have increased, particularly in men having sex with men, partners of men having sex with men, and heterosexual populations. Much of the rise in cases seen is directly attributable to illicit drug use, the exchange of sex for drugs or money, reduction in the resources for syphilis control programs, and rising poverty rates. Rises in cases of congenital syphilis have paralleled syphilis rates in pregnancy. Transplacental transmission may occur at any time during pregnancy; the degree of risk is related to the number of spirochetes in the maternal bloodstream. Congenital syphilis rates are increasing, with 1,870 cases in 2019 with almost 100 cases of syphilitic stillbirths (preventable with effective and robust public health measures in place). Clinicians need to be diligent in identifying and treating pregnant people at risk for syphilis. The most common missed syphilis prevention opportunity in pregnancy was (1) lack of timely follow-up after a positive test, and (2) lack of prenatal care and thus lack of opportunity for testing (Division of STD Prevention, 2021b).

Syphilis has historically been called "the Great Pretender" as its symptoms can look like many other conditions. Clinicians must maintain a high degree of consideration of syphilis for their differential diagnosis list. The infection manifests itself in distinct stages with different symptoms and clinical manifestations (Table 30.5). Primary syphilis is characterized by a primary lesion, a chancre that often begins as a painless papule at the inoculation site and then erodes to form a painless, shallow, indurated, clean ulcer several millimeters to centimeters in size. The chancre is loaded with spirochetes and is most commonly found on the genitalia, although other sites include the cervix, perianal area, and mouth. Secondary syphilis is characterized by a widespread, symmetrical maculopapular rash on the palms and soles and generalized lymphadenopathy; order syphilis testing with any unexplained dermatologic eruption including alopecia. The infected individual may experience fever, headache, and malaise. Condylomata lata (wartlike infectious lesions) may develop on the vulva, perineum, or anus. If untreated, the patient enters a latent phase that is asymptomatic for most individuals. Without treatment, approximately one third of patients will develop tertiary syphilis. Cardiovascular (chest pain, cough), dermatologic (multiple nodules or ulcers), skeletal (arthritis, myalgia, myositis), or neurologic (headache, irritability, impaired balance, memory loss, tremor) symptoms can develop in this stage. Neurologic, ocular, or otic involvement can occur at any stage of syphilis. A neurologic examination should be performed in all patients diagnosed with syphilis. A comprehensive neurologic exam

TABLE 30.5 Stages of Syphilis

DIAGNOSTIC FEATURE	PRIMARY	SECONDARY	EARLY LATENT	LATE LATENT	TERTIARY
Time after exposure	9–90 days	6 weeks to 6 months	3–12 months	More than 1 year	Years
Duration	Weeks	Weeks	Less than 2 years	More than 1 year	Variable
Infectious	Yes	Yes	No	No	Yes
Clinical symptoms	Chancre Multiple or atypical anogenital lesions	Skin lesions; papular rash of soles and palms; patchy alopecia; condyloma; symptoms of systemic illness (fever, malaise, anorexia, weight loss, headache, myalgias, generalized lymphadenopathy)	No symptoms at this stage	No symptoms at this stage	Cardiovascular (aortitis, coronary vessel disease) Gumma skin lesions Late neurologic complications (e.g., tabes dorsalis, general paresis)
Laboratory changes	Dark-field serology[a] often negative or rising titers VDRL and FTA-ABS	Dark-field exam positive; peak antibody titers Seroconversion of FTA-ABS or MHA-TP positive CSF abnormal in up to 50% of women Proteinuria	Falling VDRL/RPR titers	Falling VDRL/RPR titers	Laboratory evidence of serologic, CSF, or direct pathology testing

[a]Dark-field serologic testing is only useful when examining moist lesions of primary syphilis.
CSF, cerebrospinal fluid; FTA-ABS, fluorescent treponemal antibody absorption; MHA-TP, microhemagglutination assay for Treponema pallidum; RPR, rapid plasma reagin.
Source: Data from New York City Department of Health and Mental Hygiene, & New York City STD Prevention Training Center. (2019). Diagnosis, management and prevention of syphilis: An update and review. https://www.nycptc.org/x/Syphilis_Monograph_2019_NYC_PTC_NYC_DOHMH.pdf; Spach, D., & Ramchandani, M. (2021). National STD curriculum: Syphilis overview. https://www.std.uw.edu/cu; Workowski, K. A., Bachmann, L. H., Chan, P. A., Johnston, C. M., Muzny, C. A., Park, I., Reno, H., Zenilman, J. M., & Bolan, G. A. (2021). Sexually transmitted infections treatment guidelines, 2021. MMWR Morbidity and Mortality Weekly Report Recommendations and Reports, 70(4), 1–187. https://doi.org/10.15585/mmwr.rr7004a1

should include testing of cranial nerves, nuchal rigidity, motor function, sensation, deep tendon reflexes, coordination, and balance. Individuals with a diagnosis of syphilis plus ocular, otic, or neurologic symptoms require cerebrospinal fluid (CSF) testing. With ocular or otic findings, a referral to ophthalmology for a slit-lamp examination and evaluation by an otolaryngologist or audiologist is warranted.

SCREENING AND DIAGNOSIS

Dark-field examination and direct fluorescent antibody tests of lesion exudates or tissue provide a definitive diagnosis of early syphilis. Diagnosis is dependent on serology during latency and late infection. Any test for antibodies may not be reactive in the presence of early active infection because it takes time for the body's immune system to develop antibodies to any antigens. A presumptive diagnosis is possible using two serologic tests: nontreponemal and treponemal. Nontreponemal antibody tests such as the Venereal Disease Research Laboratory (VDRL) or rapid plasma reagin (RPR) tests are used as screening tests; they are relatively inexpensive, sensitive, moderately nonspecific, and fast. False-positive results are not unusual with these tests, particularly with conditions such as acute infection, autoimmune disorders, malignancy, pregnancy, and drug addiction or after immunization or vaccination. The FDA issued an advisory in December 2021 warning of false-positive results with specific RPR tests after COVID-19

vaccination (FDA, 2021). Both qualitative and quantitative nontreponemal testing can be performed. With quantitative testing, serial dilutions of serum specimens are used to define the amount of nontreponemal antibodies present. Each dilution represents a twofold change. Thus, a change of two dilutions means a fourfold change. When comparing results over time, a fourfold change in an RPR/VDRL titer represents a clinically significant change. Treatment of primary syphilis usually causes a progressive decline to a negative RPR/VDRL within 2 years. In secondary, latent, or tertiary syphilis, low titers persist in about 50% of cases after 2 years. Rising titers (a fourfold change) indicate relapse, reinfection, or treatment failure. The treponemal tests, fluorescent treponemal antibody absorption test and microhemagglutination assays for antibodies to *T. pallidum,* are used to confirm positive results. Test results in early primary or incubating syphilis may be negative as seroconversion usually takes place 6 to 8 weeks after exposure.

Given that serologic testing may not confirm infection in the very early stages, a very high degree of clinical suspicion must be maintained. Consultation with the local public health department or infectious disease specialist is warranted. Treponemal antibody tests frequently remain positive for life regardless of treatment or disease activity; therefore, treatment is monitored by the titers of the VDRL or RPR test. Sequential serologic tests should be obtained using the same testing method (VDRL or RPR), preferably by the same laboratory (see Table 30.5).

Tests for concomitant STIs, including HIV, should be performed. All pregnant people should be screened for syphilis at the first prenatal visit and in the late third trimester for high-risk patients. Some states also mandate screening of all patients in the third trimester and/or at delivery. If a pregnant, laboring individual has not had prenatal care nor screening for syphilis, screen them in labor. No infant should be discharged from the hospital without the syphilis serologic status of its mother having been determined at least once during pregnancy.

TREATMENT

Parenteral penicillin G is the preferred drug for treating patients with all stages of syphilis (Table 30.6). It is the only proven therapy widely used for patients with neurosyphilis, congenital syphilis, or syphilis during pregnancy. Intramuscular benzathine penicillin G (2.4 million units IM once) is used to treat primary, secondary, and early latent syphilis. Individuals who have had syphilis for more than a year (late latent or tertiary stage) require weekly treatment of 2.4 million units of benzathine penicillin G for 3 weeks. Individuals treated for syphilis may experience a Jarisch–Herxheimer reaction. This is an acute febrile reaction to the toxins given off by treponemes when killed rapidly by treatment; the reaction occurs within 24 hours after treatment with penicillin and is characterized by fever up to 105°F, headache, myalgia, and arthralgia that lasts 4 to 12 hours (Workowski et al., 2021). Supportive measures such as acetaminophen may be helpful.

Although doxycycline and tetracycline are alternative treatments for penicillin-allergic individuals, both tetracycline and doxycycline are contraindicated in pregnancy. Pregnant people should, if necessary, receive skin testing, be desensitized and treated with penicillin (Workowski et al., 2021). They should be advised to contact their pregnancy provider for additional testing in the second trimester or later for a sonogram evaluation of their fetus. Pregnant people treated in the second half of pregnancy who experience a Jarisch–Herxheimer reaction are at risk of preterm labor and delivery or fetal distress.

Quantitative nontreponemal serologic tests are repeated at 6, 12, and 24 months. The individual should be advised to practice sexual abstinence until treatment is completed, all evidence of primary and secondary syphilis is gone, and serologic evidence of a cure is demonstrated. Advise the individual to notify all partners who may have been exposed and that the disease is reportable. Preventive measures should be discussed. PrEP is indicated for patients currently diagnosed with syphilis if they are sexually active and not in a monogamous relationship with a recently tested HIV-negative partner.

Genital Herpes Simplex Virus Infection

Unknown until the middle of the 20th century, genital herpes is one of the most common STIs in the United States, especially for people with vaginas, who contract it far more often than people with penises. Over 572 million new infections are reported annually (Kreisel et al., 2021). Genital herpes is a chronic viral disease characterized by a painful vesicular eruption of the skin and mucosa of the genitals. Two types of HSV can cause genital herpes: HSV-1 and HSV-2. HSV-2 is usually transmitted sexually and HSV-1 nonsexually. Historically HSV-1 was more commonly associated with gingivostomatitis and oral labial ulcers (fever blisters) and HSV-2 with genital lesions; both types are not exclusively associated with the respective sites.

Although HSV infection is not a reportable disease, CDC estimates over a half million new cases of genital infections annually (Kreisel et al., 2021). As with most STIs, most new cases occur in individuals between 15 and 34 years of age, and prevalence is higher with more than one sexual partner. Most persons infected with HSV-2 have not had the condition diagnosed, and as a result, many genital herpes infections are transmitted by persons who are unaware that they have the infection or are asymptomatic.

An initial herpetic infection (primary genital herpes) characteristically has systemic and local symptoms and lasts about 3 weeks. People with vaginas generally have a more severe clinical course than do men. Flu-like symptoms with fever, malaise, and myalgia appear initially about a week after exposure, peak within 4 days, and subside over the next week. Multiple genital lesions develop at the site of infection,

TABLE 30.6 Treatment of Syphilis in Women

STAGE OF DISEASE	NONPREGNANT, OLDER THAN 18 YEARS OF AGE	PREGNANT	LACTATING
Primary, secondary, early latent disease Late latent or unknown duration disease	Benzathine penicillin G 2.4 million units IM single dose Benzathine penicillin G 7.2 million units total, administered as three doses 2.4 million units IM each at 1-week intervals	Penicillin G 2.4 million units IM once Benzathine penicillin G 7.2 million units total, administered as three doses 2.4 million units each at 1-week intervals No proven alternatives to penicillin in pregnancy Pregnant women who have a history of allergy to penicillin should be desensitized and treated with penicillin.	Benzathine penicillin G 2.4 million units IM once
Penicillin allergy	Doxycycline 100 mg orally four times per day for 28 days or tetracycline 500 mg orally four times per day for 28 days[a]		

[a]Use only with close clinical follow-up.
IM, intramuscular.

Source: Adapted from Workowski, K. A., Bachmann, L. H., Chan, P. A., Johnston, C. M., Muzny, C. A., Park, I., Reno, H., Zenilman, J. M., & Bolan, G. A. (2021). Sexually transmitted infections treatment guidelines, 2021. MMWR Morbidity and Mortality Weekly Report Recommendations and Reports, 70(4), 1–187. https://doi.org/10.15585/mmwr.rr7004a1

usually the vulva; other common sites are the perianal area, vagina, and cervix. The lesions begin as small painful blisters or vesicles that become "unroofed," leaving ulcerated lesions. Individuals with primary herpes often develop bilateral tender inguinal lymphadenopathy, vulvar edema, vaginal discharge, and possibly severe dysuria. Ulcerative lesions last 4 to 15 days before crusting over. New lesions may develop up to the 10th day of infection. Herpes simplex viral cervicitis also is common with initial HSV-2 infections; the cervix may appear normal or be friable, reddened, ulcerated, or necrotic. A heavy, watery to purulent vaginal discharge is common. Extragenital lesions may be present because of autoinoculation. Urinary retention and dysuria may occur secondary to autonomic involvement of the sacral nerve root.

Recurrent HSV infections commonly present with only local symptoms. Systemic symptoms are usually absent, although the characteristic prodromal genital tingling is common. Recurrent lesions are unilateral, less severe, and usually last 7 to 10 days without prolonged viral shedding. Lesions begin as vesicles and progress rapidly to ulcers. Very few individuals with recurrent disease have cervicitis.

SCREENING AND DIAGNOSIS

The risk profile for herpes is less clear-cut than in other STIs, and screening for asymptomatic people is not recommended. Diagnosis of genital herpes can be difficult because the typical painful, multiple vesicular, and ulcerative lesions associated with HSV may be absent in many infected persons. Although a clinical diagnosis of genital herpes is both insensitive and nonspecific, a careful history provides much information when diagnosing herpes. A history of exposure to an infected person is key, although infection from an asymptomatic individual is possible; a history of having viral symptoms, such as malaise, headache, fever, or myalgia, is suggestive. Local symptoms, such as vulvar pain, dysuria, itching or burning at the site of infection, and recurrent painful genital lesions that heal spontaneously are suggestive of HSV infections. The clinician should ask about an earlier history of primary infection, prodromal symptoms, vaginal discharge, dysuria, and dyspareunia. The clinician should assess for inguinal and generalized lymphadenopathy and elevated temperature during the physical examination. The entire vulvar, perineal, vaginal, and cervical areas should be carefully inspected for vesicles or ulcerated or crusted areas. A speculum examination may be challenging for the patient because of the extreme tenderness associated with herpes infections.

Although a diagnosis of herpes infection may be suspected from the history and physical examination, it should be confirmed by laboratory studies. Type-specific HSV NAATs can distinguish between HSV-1 and HSV-2. Recurrence and subclinical shedding are less common for HSV-1 and may give some consolation for the patient with a HSV-1 type lesion. The sensitivity of any testing is best if the specimen is taken during the vesicular stage of the disease; the culture sensitivity declines rapidly as lesions begin to heal. In a primary infection, viral shedding is prolonged, and the HSV is more easily isolated.

Although testing lesions is the preferred diagnostic approach, type-specific serology based on glycoprotein G1 and G2 is available. False-negative results are frequent in the early stages of infection. Results are most reliable after 12 weeks from

the time of initial infection. The enzyme immunoassay glycoprotein G type-specific tests commonly used has poor positive predictive value for HSV-2 and poor negative predictive value for HSV-1 (Agyemang et al., 2017). Until more accurate testing is available, consider using a Western blot to confirm HSV serologic testing. Immunoglobin M (IgM) and G (IgG) serology tests are type-specific, less accurate, and not recommended. HSV polymerase chain reaction (PCR) cultures are reserved for CNS and systemic infections such as meningitis, encephalitis, and neonatal herpes (Workowski et al., 2021). POC glycoprotein serologic testing is available. Interpretation of serology tests with HSV-1 results can be difficult without an accurate history and clinical examination. An individual may have HSV-1 antibodies from oral HSV acquired in childhood. Some of such infections are asymptomatic.

All pregnant people should be screened by history for genital herpes. The risk to a neonate is low (>1%) among people with a history of recurrent herpes; antiviral treatment can be instituted the last 4 weeks of pregnancy for further protection (Pasternak & Hviid, 2010; Stone et al., 2004). If a person acquires genital HSV in the second trimester, consult with an infectious disease or maternal-fetal specialist. If genital HSV is acquired late in pregnancy, the risk of transmission to the newborn is as high as 30% to 50%. All persons in labor should be screened and examined for risk of recent HSV acquisition. A cesarean section will reduce transmission to the neonate if a newly acquired infection is present. In discordant couples where the male partner has a documented history of HSV, and the pregnant person does not, the pregnant person will reduce risk by abstaining from oral sex (if partner has HSV-1) and vaginal sex during the last trimester (if partner has HSV-2). While the CDC does not recommend serologic testing for screening all pregnant people, serology may be useful in discordant couples. All newborns with neonatal herpes need prompt attention from a pediatric infectious disease specialist.

TREATMENT

All persons experiencing an initial episode of genital HSV should be treated to decrease symptoms. Ideally, antiviral therapy should be started as soon as 72 hours after lesions develop or soon after. However, antiviral therapy should be offered beyond this time frame to any individual with ongoing development of new lesions or significant symptomatology. Oral antiviral therapy decreases the duration and severity of disease by days to weeks in primary cases. Antiviral drugs do not eradicate the latent virus and do not affect subsequent risk, frequency, or severity of recurrence after the drug is stopped. Provide a prescription for an antiviral agent so that people can self-initiate medication at the first sign of a recurrence. Although counseling should occur at the initial visit, a follow-up visit, when the person is not in pain, is helpful for discussing episodic versus suppressive therapy and reinforcing strategies for reducing and or preventing HSV transmission.

Three antiviral medications provide clinical benefit for genital herpes: acyclovir, valacyclovir, and famciclovir (Workowski et al., 2021). Treatment recommendations are given in Table 30.7. It is suggested to see patients on suppressive therapy on an annual basis to discuss the need for continued

TABLE 30.7 Treatment of Genital Herpes in Women

NONPREGNANT, OLDER THAN 18 YEARS OF AGE	PREGNANT	LACTATING
Primary infection: Acyclovir 400 mg orally three times per day for 7–10 days or Valacyclovir 1 g orally twice a day for 7–10 days or Famciclovir 250 mg orally three times a day for 7–10 days Treatment may be extended if healing is incomplete after 10 days of therapy. **Recurrent infection:** Acyclovir 800 mg orally three a day for 5 days or Acyclovir 800 mg orally two times per day for 2 days or Valacyclovir 500 mg orally twice a day for 3 days or Valacyclovir 1 g orally once a day for 5 days or Famciclovir 125 mg orally twice daily for 5 days or Famciclovir 1 g orally twice a day for 1 day or Famciclovir 500 mg once, followed by 250 mg twice daily for 2 days **Suppression therapy:** Acyclovir 400 mg orally twice per day or Valacyclovir 500 mg orally once daily (>10 recurrences annually) or Valacyclovir 1 g orally once a day (>10 recurrences annually) or Famciclovir 250 mg orally twice a day	Acyclovir 400 mg orally three times a day or Valacyclovir 500 mg orally twice a day Suppressive treatment recommended starting at 36 weeks with history of recurrent genital herpes.	Acyclovir, valacyclovir, or famciclovir therapy are believed to be safe in lactation.

Source: Adapted from Workowski, K. A., Bachmann, L. H., Chan, P. A., Johnston, C. M., Muzny, C. A., Park, I., Reno, H., Zenilman, J. M., & Bolan, G. A. (2021). Sexually transmitted infections treatment guidelines, 2021. MMWR Morbidity and Mortality Weekly Report Recommendations and Reports, 70(4), 1–187. https://doi.org/10.15585/mmwr.rr7004a1

therapy. The number of recurrences diminishes over time, whether on antiviral therapy or not. The current antiviral medications are safe to use for suppressive therapy; one study confirmed long-term safety and efficacy after 20 years (Tyring et al., 2002). Acyclovir is considered safe in pregnancy and during breastfeeding (Briggs, 2017).

Less data are available on valacyclovir or famciclovir but they are thought to be safe. Rarely is hepatitis seen with HIV infection in pregnant people. In any pregnant person with fever and unexplained severe hepatitis, disseminated HSV infection should be considered, and empiric acyclovir IV started immediately pending test results (Workowski et al., 2021; see Table 30.7).

Home comfort measures include warm sitz baths; keeping lesions dry with a hairdryer on a cool setting; patting dry rather than rubbing dry with toilet paper; wearing cotton underwear and loose clothing; using drying aids such as Burrow's solution, oatmeal baths, or Domeboro solution; or applying cool, wet black tea bags to lesions. Acetaminophen or ibuprofen will help relieve pain and systemic symptoms associated with initial infections. Because the mucous membranes affected by herpes are very sensitive, any topical agents should be used with caution. Ointments containing cortisone should be avoided and occlusive ointments may prolong the course of infections.

Counseling and education are critical components of the nursing care of people with herpes infections. Information regarding the etiology, signs, symptoms, sexual and perineal transmission, methods to prevent transmission, and treatment should be provided. The clinician should explain that each person is unique in their response to herpes and emphasize the variability of symptoms. People should be helped to understand when viral shedding and thus transmission to a partner is most likely, and that they should refrain from sexual contact from the onset of prodrome until complete healing of lesions. Condom use will reduce, although not eliminate, the risk of transmission.

The clinician should explain the role of precipitating factors in the reactivation of the latent virus and recurrent episodes. Stress, menstruation, trauma, febrile illnesses, and chronic illness trigger genital herpes. Individuals may wish to keep a diary to identify stressors. Suggestions for stress reduction therapy, yoga, or meditation classes may be made. The emotional impact of contracting herpes is considerable. Media publicity regarding this disease can make receiving a diagnosis of genital herpes a devastating experience. At diagnosis, many emotions may surface—helplessness, anger, denial, guilt, anxiety, shame, or inadequacy. People need to be allowed to discuss their feelings and may need help in learning to live with this infection. Herpes can affect sexuality, sexual practices, and current and future relationships. Individuals may need help in raising the issue with partner(s) or with future partners.

Chancroid

Chancroid or soft chance is a bacterial infection of the genitourinary tract caused by the gram-negative bacteria *Haemophilus ducreyi*. The prevalence of chancroid has declined in the United States, and when an infection does occur is usually associated with sporadic outbreaks. Worldwide, chancroid also appears to have declined, though infection still occurs in some regions of Africa and the Caribbean (Workowski et al., 2021). Because chancroid is a genital ulcer, it is a risk factor in the transmission and acquisition of HIV infection. The primary way chancroid is acquired is through sexual contact; trauma or abrasion is necessary for the organism to penetrate the skin. Chancroid is characterized by a rapidly growing ulcerated lesion formed on the external genitalia. The incubation period is usually 3 to 10 days but may be as long as 3 weeks.

Typically, the patient presents with a history of a painful macule on the external genitalia, which rapidly changes to a pustule and then to an ulcerated lesion. Autoinoculation of fingers or other sites occasionally occurs. The patient may develop enlarged unilateral or bilateral enlarged inguinal nodes known as buboes. After 1 to 2 weeks, the skin overlying the lymph node becomes erythematous, the center becomes necrotic, and the node becomes ulcerated.

ASSESSMENT AND DIAGNOSIS

Definitive diagnosis of chancroid is difficult because the organism must be identified on a special culture media that is not used routinely. A probable diagnosis can be made based on the presence of painful ulcers, the appearance of the ulcer(s), and lymphadenopathy consistent with chancroid; syphilis is excluded by either dark-field microscopy, NAAT, or serology, and HSV testing of the ulcer is negative (Workowski et al., 2021). Gonorrheal, chlamydia, and HIV testing should be done at the time of diagnosis.

TREATMENT

The recommended treatment for chancroid includes azithromycin 1 g orally single dose or ceftriaxone 250 mg IM single dose or ciprofloxacin 500 mg orally twice a day for 3 days or erythromycin base 500 mg orally three times a day for 7 days (Workowski et al., 2021). Uncircumcised and HIV-infected individuals do not respond as well to treatment. No adverse effects of chancroid on pregnancy outcome or the fetus have been reported.

Patients should be reexamined 3 to 7 days after beginning therapy. If treatment is successful, there should be symptomatic improvement within 3 days of starting therapy and objectively within 7 days after therapy. If no clinical improvement is seen, the clinician should consider whether the diagnosis is correct; the patient is coinfected with another STI; the patient is infected with HIV; the treatment was not used as recommended; or the strain causing the infection is resistant to the prescribed antimicrobial agent (Workowski et al., 2021). It should be noted that it may take more than 2 weeks for complete healing of the ulcers to occur. All sexual partners who have had sexual contact within 10 days preceding the onset of symptoms with a person diagnosed with chancroid should be evaluated regardless of symptoms.

Two other genital ulcerative diseases occur. Granuloma inguinale (donovanosis) is rarely seen in the United States, but clinicians working globally should include it in their differential diagnosis of genital ulcer disease. Lymphogranuloma venereum (LGV) is seen in rectal exposure among people with vaginas or MSM. The most common presentation is proctocolitis, which can mimic inflammatory bowel disease, although asymptomatic cases have been reported. As with chancroid, laboratory testing is not widely available. A presumptive diagnosis can be made if proctocolitis (bloody discharge, tenesmus, ulceration), severe inguinal lymphadenopathy with bubo formation, a genital ulcer in which other infections have been ruled out, or a *C. trachomatis* NAAT is noted at the symptomatic site. Treatment is doxycycline 100 mg twice a day for 21 days. See Workowski et al. (2021) guidelines for further details.

DISEASES CHARACTERIZED BY VAGINAL DISCHARGE

Vaginal discharge and itching of the vulva and vagina are among the most common reasons a woman seeks help from a clinician. Indeed, more people complain of vaginal discharge than any other gynecologic symptom. Vaginal discharge resulting from an infection must be distinguished from normal secretions. Normal vaginal secretion or leukorrhea is clear to cloudy in appearance and may turn yellow after drying; the discharge is slightly slimy, nonirritating, and has a mild, inoffensive odor. Normal vaginal secretions are acidic, with a pH range of 3.8 to 4.2. The amount of leukorrhea present differs with phases of the menstrual cycle, with more significant amounts occurring at ovulation and just before menses. Leukorrhea also increases during pregnancy. Normal vaginal secretions contain lactobacilli and epithelial cells. People who have adequate endogenous or exogenous estrogen will have vaginal secretions. Vaginitis, an inflammation of the vagina characterized by an increased vaginal discharge containing numerous WBCs, occurs when the vaginal environment is disturbed by a microorganism (see Table 30.8) or by a situation that allows the pathogens that are found normally in the vagina to proliferate. Factors that can disturb the vaginal environment include douches, vaginal medications, antibiotics, hormones, contraceptive preparations (oral and topical), stress, sexual intercourse, and changes in sexual partners. Vulvovaginitis or inflammation of the vulva and vagina may be caused by vaginal infection; copious amounts of leukorrhea, which can cause maceration of tissues, and chemical irritants, allergens, and foreign bodies may produce inflammatory reactions. BV, vulvovaginal candidiasis (VVC), and trichomoniasis are the most common causes of abnormal vaginal discharge. Vaginal irritants, not sexually related, can cause allergic reactions and symptoms. Allergens are mentioned as part of a differential diagnosis of vaginal complaints. As part of a comprehensive history taking, ask about the use of over-the-counter products, feminine sprays and deodorants, new toiletry products, perfumed toilet tissue and soaps, changes in laundry soaps, fabric softener, body soaps, new sex toys, and lubricants.

Trichomoniasis

The most prevalent vaginitis (nonviral) worldwide is caused by *Trichomonas vaginalis*. Although it is not a reportable disease, it is estimated that 3.7 million persons worldwide have had the infection (Alcaide et al., 2016).

Highest infection rates are seen in women younger than 40 years of age, STI clinic patients, and incarcerated women. Trichomoniasis is caused by *T. vaginalis*, an anaerobic one-celled protozoan with characteristic flagella. The organism lives in the vagina, urethra, Bartholin's and Skene's glands in vaginas, and prostate gland. It is transmitted during vagina–penis intercourse. Although most trichomoniasis is asymptomatic, typical symptoms include yellowish to greenish, frothy, mucopurulent, copious, malodorous discharge. Inflammation of the vulva, vagina, or both may be present, and the woman may complain of irritation and pruritus.

TABLE 30.8 Conditions Characterized by Vaginal Discharge

DIAGNOSTIC FEATURE	NORMAL DISCHARGE	TRICHOMONIASIS	BACTERIAL VAGINOSIS	VULVOVAGINAL CANDIDIASIS
Sexually transmitted infection	No	Yes	No	No
Vaginal pH	3.8–4.2	>4.7	>4.5	<4.5 (usually normal)
Wet prep	Normal flora	With normal saline: delay results in drying and loss of characteristic shape of protozoan	With saline solution: positive for clue cells, decreased lactobacilli	With potassium hydroxide (KOH): pseudohyphae with yeast buds
Discharge	White/clear Thin/mucoid	Malodorous, copious, frothy or nonfrothy, thin or thick, white/yellow–green/gray Often asymptomatic	Thin, homogeneous, grayish white, adherent, coats the vaginal walls	Thick white, curd-like; cottage cheese–like, adherent
Amine odor (KOH "whiff" test)	Normal body odor	Unpleasant smell may be present	Present (fishy)	None/yeasty, musty odor
Vulvular pruritus	No	Soreness rather than itching, swelling, redness; burning and soreness of thighs and perineum	Mild if present at all	Yes, swelling, excoriation, redness
Genital ulceration	No	No	No	Skin may crack in severe cases
Pelvic pain	No	Yes, in severe cases; severe pelvic pain with tender inguinal lymph nodes	No	No
Dysuria	No	Yes	Occasionally	Severe cases
Dyspareunia	No	Yes	Occasionally	Occasionally
Main patient complaint	No	Excessive discharge, dysuria, vaginal irritation, dyspareunia, postcoital bleeding	May be asymptomatic discharge, bad odor, possibly worse after intercourse; may report suprapubic pain	Itching/burning, discharge
Risk of pelvic inflammatory disease	No	May develop	Yes	No

Source: Adapted from Carcio, H. A., & Secor, R. M. (2015). Advanced health assessment of women: Clinical skills and procedures (3rd ed.). Springer Publishing Company; Workowski, K. A., Bachmann, L. H., Chan, P. A., Johnston, C. M., Muzny, C. A., Park, I., Reno, H., Zenilman, J. M., & Bolan, G. A. (2021). Sexually transmitted infections treatment guidelines, 2021. MMWR Morbidity and Mortality Weekly Report Recommendations and Reports, 70(4), 1 -187. https://doi.org/10.15585/mmwr.rr7004a1

Dysuria and dyspareunia are often present. Typically, the discharge worsens during and after menstruation. The cervix and vaginal walls will often demonstrate the characteristic "strawberry spots" or tiny petechiae, and the cervix may bleed on contact. In severe infections, the vaginal walls, cervix, and occasionally the vulva may be acutely inflamed. Vaginal trichomoniasis is associated with a two- to threefold increase in HIV acquisition. Adverse pregnancy outcomes include premature rupture of the membranes, preterm delivery, and low birth weight (Workowski et al., 2021). In people with HIV, trichomoniasis is associated with an increased risk for PID (Workowski et al., 2021).

ASSESSMENT AND DIAGNOSIS

The external genitalia should be observed for excoriation, erythema, edema, ulceration, and lesions. A speculum examination always is done, even though it may be very uncomfortable for the woman; relaxation techniques and breathing exercises may help the woman with the procedure. Any of the classic signs may be present on physical examination. The pH is elevated. The NAAT test is highly sensitive and can detect up to three to five times more *T. vaginalis* infections than wet-mount microscopy (Workowski et al., 2021); however, it is expensive and may not be widely available. The culture of a woman's vaginal secretions is another method of diagnosis with a sensitivity of 75% to 96% (Workowski et al., 2021). A readily available and inexpensive test diagnosing trichomoniasis is microscopic evaluation of wet prep of genital secretions; however, the sensitivity is low (51%–65%) in vaginal specimens (Workowski et al., 2021). Although Pap smear results frequently include reports of trichomonads, accuracy is low, and it is not considered diagnostic. However, the presence of *T. vaginalis* on a Pap smear should trigger further, more accurate testing. NAAT testing includes clinician-collected vaginal swabs, endocervical swabs, female urine specimens and liquid Pap smear specimens with higher sensitivity and specificity than wet mount. Rapid office-based testing POC testing, approved for clinician and patient collection, has higher sensitivity and specificity than wet mount. None of these tests are approved to use with males. Because trichomoniasis is an STI, gonorrhea, chlamydia, syphilis, and HIV testing should be considered once the diagnosis is confirmed.

TREATMENT

Treatment reduces symptoms and signs of *T. vaginalis* infection and might reduce transmission. The recommended treatment for people with vaginas is metronidazole 500 mg twice a day for 7 days. Male partners are treated with metronidazole 2 g orally in a single dose. Metronidazole is an antiprotozoal and antibacterial agent. Tinidazole 2 g orally in a single dose is more expensive but has fewer gastrointestinal side effects and has the same or somewhat better coverage (Nailor & Sobel, 2007).

Metronidazole was previously contraindicated in the first trimester of pregnancy; however, multiple studies and meta-analyses have not demonstrated a consistent association between metronidazole use and teratogenic or mutagenic effects in offspring (Sheehy et al., 2015). Symptomatic pregnant people should be treated with 2 g orally in a single dose. Treatment of pregnant people with asymptomatic trichomoniasis is not indicated because data have not demonstrated that this strategy effectively prevents preterm delivery (Workowski et al., 2021). Metronidazole is secreted in breast milk. Although several reported case series have found no evidence of adverse effects in infants exposed to metronidazole in breast milk, some clinicians advise deferring breastfeeding for 12 to 24 hours after maternal treatment (National Center for Biotechnology Information, n.d.). The Drugs and Lactation Database (LactMed) contains information on drugs and other chemicals to which the breastfeeding mothers may be exposed (National Center for Biotechnology Information, n.d.).

Side effects of metronidazole are numerous, including sharp, unpleasant metallic taste in the mouth, furry tongue, central nervous system reactions, and urinary tract disturbances. When oral metronidazole is taken, the client is advised not to drink alcoholic beverages to avoid a risk of severe abdominal distress, nausea, vomiting, and headache. Metronidazole can cause gastrointestinal symptoms regardless of whether alcohol is consumed and can also darken urine. A Norwegian literature review found that the warning regarding alcohol and metronidazole appears to be based on laboratory experiments and individual case studies with a high likelihood that the adverse effects were caused by either single agent but not from the combination of the two (Fjeld & Raknes, 2014). The FDA continues to recommend avoiding alcohol while using metronidazole.

People with trichomoniasis need to understand the sexual transmission of this disease. The individual should know that the infection may be asymptomatic, perhaps for several months, and that it is not possible to determine when infection occurred. People should be informed of the necessity for treating all sexual partners and helped with ways to raise the issue with their partner(s). A 3-month follow-up with retesting is recommended. Current sexual partners should be evaluated or provided EPT.

Bacterial Vaginosis

BV—formerly called nonspecific vaginitis, *Haemophilus vaginitis*, or *Gardnerella vaginitis*—is the most common type of vaginal discharge or malodor in childbearing people; however, the majority of those with BV are asymptomatic. BV is a clinical syndrome in which normal H_2O_2-producing lactobacilli are replaced with high concentrations of anaerobic bacteria (*Prevotella* sp., *Mobiluncus* sp., *Gardnerella vaginalis* (Workowski et al., 2021). With the proliferation of anaerobes, the level of vaginal amines is raised, and the normal acidic pH of the vagina is altered. Epithelial cells slough, and numerous bacteria attach to their surfaces (clue cells), causing a polymicrobial biofilm. When the amines are volatilized, the characteristic fishy odor of BV occurs. The cause of the microbial alteration is not entirely understood, although it is associated with menses, a new sex partner, more than one sexual partner, douching, lack of condom use, HSV-2 infection, and depletion of lactobacilli. BV is rarely found in people with vaginas who have never been sexually active. BV is not considered an actual STI; it is considered a risk factor for acquiring STIs. BV infection has been implicated in miscarriage, chorioamnionitis, premature rupture of fetal membranes, preterm birth, postpartum or postabortion endometritis, and postpartum complications in the infant (Workowski et al., 2021). Because the association is not clear and treatment of BV has not shown to decrease premature birth rates, the USPSTF does not recommend screening all pregnant people for BV (rated Grade D = discourage) but does give an I (insufficient evidence) rating for screening people at increased risk of preterm birth (USPSTF, 2020a). BV increases a woman's risk of acquiring STIs and HIV infection and transmitting HIV infection.

ASSESSMENT AND DIAGNOSIS

A careful history may help distinguish BV from other vaginal infections if the person is symptomatic but must be followed by a physical examination. Reports of fishy odor and increased thin vaginal discharge are most significant, and report of increased odor after intercourse is also suggestive of BV. The previous occurrence of similar symptoms, diagnosis, and treatment should be asked about because some people may experience repeated episodes, repeated antibiotic use, douching, or life stresses.

A speculum examination is done to inspect the vaginal walls and cervix.

Clinical diagnosis is based on the Amsel criteria (Amsel et al., 1983):

- Vaginal pH >4.5
- Homogeneous white, gray, or yellow milky discharge
- Release of an amine (fishy) odor after addition of 10% potassium hydroxide (KOH) solution to the vaginal fluid (whiff test)
- Presence of clue cells on saline microscopy

At least three of the preceding four criteria must be met. Equipment needed includes a microscope, vaginal pH paper, saline, and KOH for POC testing. Several commercial POC tests are available for use when microscopy is unavailable.

TREATMENT

Treatment is recommended if there are symptoms. The benefits of treatment are to relieve vaginal symptoms and signs of infection. Other potential benefits of treatment are reduction in risk of acquiring chlamydia, gonorrhea, HIV, and HSV-2 infections.

Treatment of sexual partners has not been beneficial in preventing recurrent BV infections although clinical trials are ongoing. Recurrent BV is common. Off-label treatment includes a longer initial course of metronidazole to 7 to 10 days, followed by compounded boric acid suppositories 600 mg vaginally for 21 days followed by metronidazole vaginal gel 2%, one application twice weekly for 4 to 6 months (Reichman et al., 2009).

Vulvovaginal Candidiasis

ASSESSMENT AND DIAGNOSIS

Candida species, usually *Candida albicans,* cause VVC. VVC symptoms are typically pruritus, soreness, dyspareunia, occasionally thick vaginal discharge, and occasionally dysuria. The most cost-effective diagnosis is microscopy with saline and KOH 10% preparations. The KOH prep is more likely to demonstrate budding yeast, hyphae, and pseudohyphae than the saline. The diagnosis is made by history, clinical presentation, microscopy, and culture, if necessary.

TREATMENT

There are many over-the-counter (OTC) and prescription vaginal creams for treatment. The shorter course therapies of 1 to 3 days are effective and preferred by people over the longer 7-day courses. One oral agent, fluconazole 150 mg in a single dose, is available and may be preferred over vaginal products by many individuals. Oral fluconazole is advantageous for people using condoms as the vaginal products are oil-based and may weaken latex condoms. Only topical agents are recommended in pregnancy. Most partners do not need treatment but it is considered if a partner has penile balanitis. There is a lack of evidence for routine treatment of female-to-female partners (Muzny et al., 2014).

ECTOPARASITIC INFECTIONS

Ectoparasitic infections are defined as infestations by parasites that live on, or burrow into, the surface of their host's epidermis. Most ectoparasites are arthropods, defined as invertebrates (without a backbone), with an exoskeleton (skeleton on the outside with a shell made of chitin for structural support). Individuals with pediculosis pubis or scabies usually seek care because they notice lice or nits on their pubic hair or because of pruritus. Pediculosis pubis is caused by the parasite *Phthirus pubis* and is usually transmitted by sexual contact. Diagnosis is made by clinical observation. One of the legitimate uses of ivermection is as an alternative treatment for pediculosis pubis as resistance is growing to the commonly prescribed permethrin and pyrethrin.

Scabies

Scabies is caused by the mite *Sarcoptes scabiei,* which causes itching. Scabies among adults is usually sexually acquired while scabies among children is usually not. To establish the diagnosis, the clinician should identify burrows, mites, eggs, or the mites' feces on the skin either through observation, adhesive tape test, skin scrapings (low sensitivity), or dermoscopy (Abdel-Latif et al., 2018). Permethrin 5% cream is a topical treatment or oral ivermectin may be prescribed.

HEPATITIS

Hepatitis is an acute, systemic viral infection. This section discusses the sexual transmission of hepatitis A, B, and to some extent, C. Vaccinations to hepatitis A and B are key to prevention. Although vaccination to hepatitis A and B are part of routine childhood immunization schedules, more than 30 states have been affected by hepatitis A outbreaks since 2016. Outbreaks are seen primarily among people who use drugs and people who are homeless. Progress on hepatitis prevention has stalled in many states plus the increased opioid epidemic has fueled infections. Rates are highest in the age group most impacted by the opioid crisis, the 20- to 40-year-old age group (Jalal et al., 2020). This group also a high rate of concurrent STIs. Hepatitis B and C are have contributed to the increased rates of liver cancer seen in the United States.

Hepatitis A

Hepatitis A is the most common form of hepatitis, a mild, self-limited disease characterized by flu-like symptoms with malaise, fatigue, anorexia, nausea, pruritus, fever, and upper right quadrant pain; usually, there are no chronic sequelae to infection. Hepatitis A virus (HAV) infection is primarily acquired through a fecal–oral route by ingestion of contaminated food—particularly milk, shellfish, or polluted water—or person-to-person contact. HAV risk is higher in MSM, persons injecting drugs, children and employees in day care centers, people experiencing homelessness, international travelers, or those in close contact with an international adoptee. As with other enteric infections, HAV is transmitted from person to person during sexual activity, likely through the fecal–oral route. Unlike other persons with STIs, HAV-infected persons are infectious for only a brief period of time.

DIAGNOSIS

Diagnosis is not made on clinical findings alone and requires serologic testing. The presence of the IgM antibody is diagnostic of acute HAV infection. The IgM antibody is detectable 5 to 10 days after exposure and can remain positive for up to 6 months. Because HAV infection is self-limited and does not result in chronic infection or chronic liver disease, treatment is usually supportive. Individuals who become dehydrated from nausea and vomiting or who have fulminating hepatitis A may need to be hospitalized. Medications that might cause liver damage or metabolize in the liver should be used with caution. No specific diet or activity restrictions are necessary. Immunoglobulin (Ig) or immune-specific globulin is indicated for any pregnant person exposed to HAV to provide passive immunity through injected antibodies. Perinatal transmission of HAV has not been demonstrated. Two products are available to prevent hepatitis A: hepatitis A vaccine and Ig for IM administration. Inactivated hepatitis A vaccines are available in the United States in a two-dose series (0, 6 months) and induce protective immunity in virtually all adults following the second dose. A combined vaccine for hepatitis A and B is available, administered on a 0-, 1-, or 6-month schedule with effectiveness equal to the monovalent vaccine. All household contacts should receive Ig. When administered before or within 2 weeks after exposure to HAV, Ig is 85% effective in preventing HAV. Persons in the following groups who are likely to be treated in STI clinics should be offered the HAV vaccine: all women who have sex with MSM; MSM, people using drugs (both injecting and noninjecting drugs); and persons with chronic liver disease.

Hepatitis B

Hepatitis B virus (HBV) is a bloodborne pathogen transmitted primarily by exposure to infectious blood or less frequently by body fluids (e.g., semen, saliva). HBV is more infectious than HIV and hepatitis C virus. The highest concentrations are in blood, with lower concentrations in other body fluids, including wound exudates, semen, vaginal secretions, and saliva. Chronically infected persons can transmit the infection and are at 15% to 25% increased risk for premature death from cirrhosis or hepatocellular carcinoma. Perinatal transmission does occur; however, the fetus is not at risk until it comes in contact with contaminated blood at delivery. Rates have been relatively stable over the past decade, with any rate decline likely stalled by the opioid epidemic. Rates are almost twice as high in males as females (Division of Viral Hepatitis, 2021).

Factors considered to place a person at risk for HBV are those associated with STI risk in general (history of more than one sexual partner, history of frequent STIs, IV drug use if sharing needles). Other non-STI factors that increase risk are associated with blood contact (e.g., public safety workers exposed to blood in the workplace or healthcare workers who are not vaccinated) and persons born in a country with a high incidence of HBV infection. Individuals who share needles, are incarcerated, or had tattoos in unsanitary situations are also at risk.

HBV infection is asymptomatic in up to one third of infected persons. Symptoms of HBV infection are similar to those of HAV: arthralgias, arthritis, lassitude, anorexia, nausea, vomiting, headache, fever, and mild abdominal pain. Later, the patient may have clay-colored stools, dark urine, increased abdominal pain, and jaundice.

ASSESSMENT AND DIAGNOSIS

The role of the clinician is to operationalize the national strategy to eliminate hepatitis B:

- Universal screening of pregnant people for HBV surface antigen (HBsAg) during each pregnancy
- Screen all HBsAg-positive pregnant people for HBV DNA to guide the use of maternal antiviral therapy during pregnancy.

- Refer for case management of HBsAg-positive mothers and their infants.
- If working in the acute care setting:
  - All infants born to infected mothers should be provided immunoprophylaxis, including hepatitis B vaccine and hepatitis B immune globulin, within 12 hours of birth.
  - Ensure routine vaccination of all infants with the hepatitis B vaccine series, with the first dose administered within 24 hours of birth. (Workowski, 2021)

Any person who tests positive for HBsAg needs counseling and education about modes of transmission; prevention of HBV transmission to their personal and family contacts; substance abuse treatment, if appropriate; and referral for further medical evaluation for chronic disease. If pregnant, the person will have perinatal concerns (e.g., HBsAg-positive mothers can breastfeed) that should be addressed.

Physical examination includes inspecting the skin for rashes, inspecting the skin and conjunctivae for jaundice, and palpating of the liver for enlargement and tenderness. Weight loss, fever, and general debilitation should be noted. If the HBsAg is positive, further laboratory studies are needed: HIV testing should be done. Interpretation of testing for hepatitis B is complex. See the CDC's Interpretation of Hepatitis B Serologic Test Results (CDC, n.d.).

TREATMENT

There is no specific treatment for hepatitis B. Recovery is usually spontaneous in 3 to 16 weeks. Individuals should be advised to rest, increase their fluid intake, and avoid medications that are metabolized in the liver, including drugs and alcohol. People with a definite exposure to hepatitis B should be given hepatitis B immunoglobulin IM in a single dose as soon as possible, preferably within 24 hours after exposure (Workowski et al., 2021). Usually, pregnancies complicated by acute viral hepatitis are managed on an outpatient basis. The Workowski et al. (2021) recommends routine vaccination of all newborns and older children at high risk for HBV infection.

Hepatitis C

Hepatitis C is the most common bloodborne disease in the world, with an estimated 2.4 million individuals infected (low estimate; Division of Viral Hepatitis, 2021). Sexual transmission of hepatitis C virus (HCV) can occur but the virus is not easily transmitted through sex. Shedding of HCV in the semen and rectum of men with HIV infection has been documented (Foster et al., 2017; Turner et al., 2016). Positive HIV status likely increases HCV transmission (Garg et al., 2013). Heterosexual transmission of HCV was very rare in 500 discordant couples over 3 years (Dodge & Terrault, 2014).

Lab testing is straightforward: screening with an anti-HCV antibody test. If positive, follow up with a PCR test for HCV RNA to identify chronic HCV infection. As a clinician, order an HCV test if a person has abnormally high liver function tests. The average time to seroconversion is 4 to 10 weeks; anti-HCV can be detected among approximately 97% of people by 6 months after exposure. In chronic HCV infection, 10% to 20% may develop liver cirrhosis within two to three decades. Most people are asymptomatic and thus are a source of transmission to others. The USPSTF (2020c) recommends screening asymptomatic adults (including pregnant persons) ages 18 to 79 years without known liver disease at least once in their lifetime. Persons who inject drugs need testing more frequently. The current standard treatment for HCV is oral direct-acting antiviral (DAA) regimens (without interferon). There are not sufficient data to treat pregnant or lactating people with DAA therapy.

FUTURE DIRECTIONS

STIs are among the most common health problems of people in the United States and worldwide. People with vaginas experience a disproportionate amount of the burden associated with STI infections, including infertility complications perinatal infections, poor pregnancy outcomes, chronic pelvic pain, and genital tract neoplasms. Additionally, these infections interfere with one's lifestyle and cause considerable emotional and physical distress. Clinicians can support people to negotiate healthy, positive sexual relationships through accurate, safe, sensitive, and supportive care. Clinicians should be aware that STI knowledge is constantly increasing and changing with new and improved prevention, diagnostic, and treatment modalities. The STI guidelines were updated in 2021 and should be part of the clinician armamentarium (Workowski et al., 2021). Furthermore, clinicians must be aware of the state's policies, recommendations, and guidelines in which they practice, which also may change frequently. Expedited partner treatment is now within the standard of care in most states.

POC testing is available, although more rapid and straightforward tests are needed. Patient-collected specimens are now common in many practices. Clinicians need to be aware of the comparable accuracy of self-collected specimens and offer this approach to improve the patient experience. Opt-out screening is the recommended approach in routine practice. Telehealth will continue to be the future of healthcare and expand STI services. A telehealth approach can support self-testing and patient-collected specimens linked to pharmacies or retail clinics for onsite injections, especially in rural areas. STI express clinics can provide ready access walk-in testing and treatment in more populated areas, expand clinic

hours, and target at-risk groups (National Academy of Public Administration, 2019). Unfortunately, funding for such clinics has declined. Investment is needed in communities that have been traditionally underserved to reduce health disparities and address structural racism to strengthen STI prevention and management. Reducing the burden of STIs must be multifactorial, not solely focusing on individual counseling and behavior. Our public health network must be strengthened. STI surveillance, research, and services were underfunded prior to the pandemic and now are even more so. Strategies at the federal, state, and local level should be supported to eliminate insurance and payment obstacles (National Academies of Sciences, Engineering, and Medicine, 2021), expand public health infrastructure, and ensure that all healthcare students receive education in STI health promotion and prevention.

More research is needed for STI vaccine research and development and concurrent research on effective strategies to promote vaccine uptake. STI risk reduction interventions focused on behavior change, such as increasing condom use and decreasing the number of sexual partners, have not curbed the increasing STI rate. Research that focuses on an STI-PreP is urgently needed. Preliminary research is investigating doxycycline as a possible pre- or postexposure prophylaxis for syphilis, gonorrhea, and chlamydia and should be expanded (Treatment Action Group [TAG], 2019). A vaginal gel for women, an STI-PreP, is also in the research pipeline (TAG, 2019). Specific and ongoing research must focus on drug-resistant gonorrhea. Affordable, oral alternatives to intramuscular ceftriaxone treatment are needed, such as zoliflodacin (TAG, 2019; Taylor et al., 2018).

Sexual health discussions and screening in primary care are critical for a holistic approach, recognizing sexual health as a component of overall health and wellness. Although the clinician must understand the risk assessment and management of STIs, the clinician must also endeavor to change the STI paradigm from disease-oriented care to emphasizing sexual health as an essential component of overall health.

REFERENCES

References for this chapter are online and available at https://connect.springerpub.com/content/book/978-0-8261-6722-4/part/part03/chapter/ch30

CHAPTER 31

Women and HIV/AIDS*

RASHEETA CHANDLER AND CRYSTAL CHAPMAN LAMBERT

In the summer of 1981, the Centers for Disease Control and Prevention (CDC, 1981) reported the occurrence of clusters of several rare illnesses—*Pneumocystis carinii* pneumonia, *Mycobacterium avium intracellulare*, cryptosporidiosis—and tumors (Kaposi sarcoma, non-Hodgkin lymphoma) in homosexual and bisexual men in California and New York. This was the beginning of the AIDS pandemic and represented a medical mystery that was solved with the identification of a single infectious agent destroying the immune system of infected persons: human immunodeficiency virus (HIV). Initially, HIV infection appeared to be associated with homosexual activities, but symptoms of the syndrome were identified in a woman within 2 months of the earliest reports of the disease in men. It soon became clear that heterosexual activity and direct blood contact could also transmit the virus. The first female AIDS case was reported to the CDC in July 1982, and, within the first year of the epidemic, women partners of infected hemophiliacs, female intravenous (IV) drug abusers, and women partners in heterosexual relationships were diagnosed with AIDS. Early misunderstanding of the nature of transmission of HIV led researchers and the medical community to grossly underestimate the numbers of women who were or would become infected with HIV.

DEFINITION AND SCOPE

The term *diagnosis of HIV infection* is defined as HIV infection regardless of stage of disease, referring to all persons with the diagnosis (CDC, 2015a). HIV infection and AIDS have spread rapidly throughout the world, affecting millions of persons and resulting in millions of deaths. For the year 2019, the CDC estimated that 1,189,700 persons age 13 years and older were living with HIV in the United States (CDC, 2021b). From the years 2015 to 2019 HIV diagnoses decreased by 9% in the United States compared to previous years, 36,801 individuals being diagnosed with HIV in 2019 (CDC, 2022b). Among these new diagnoses, 69% were

among men who had sex with men, 23% were among heterosexual men and women, and 7% were among individuals who inject drugs (CDC, 2022b). The age demographic with the highest rate of new HIV diagnoses was 25- to 34-year-olds, followed by 13- to 24-year-olds (CDC, 2022b). Black/African American and Hispanic/Latinx people are disproportionately reported to be affected by HIV with higher incidence rates compared to their White counterparts. In 2019, Black/African American people reportedly accounted for 42% (15,305) of new HIV diagnoses despite making up only 13% of the population (CDC, 2022b). Hispanic/Latinx individuals reportedly accounted for 29% (10,494) of new HIV diagnoses despite making up 18% of the population (CDC, 2022b). Among women, the estimated number of new HIV infections remained stable from the years 2014 to 2018 (CDC, 2022a).

SOCIAL CONTEXT

Deeply ingrained social and cultural forces that tend to devalue women, and particularly poor women of color, perpetuated the tendency for HIV and AIDS to be underdiagnosed in women, resulting in the delay of treatment. HIV infection was long considered to be a men's disease and more specifically a disease of homosexual men. However, most new HIV diagnoses in women are attributed to unprotected heterosexual sex (CDC, 2019b).

Very few diseases in history have had the level of stigma that accompanies an HIV diagnosis. Many persons with HIV choose to keep their diagnosis a secret from family, friends, and coworkers. Although this means that they must hide clinic visits, medications, and HIV-related illnesses, they may feel this is preferable to experiencing the stigma that accompanies the diagnosis. Persons with HIV may face dissolution of important relationships when and if the diagnosis becomes known. Nurse practitioners can assist patients in identifying supportive others who can be helpful as the patient adapts

---

*This chapter is a revision of the chapter that appeared in the second edition of this textbook, authored by Catherine Ingram Fogel, and we thank her for her original contribution.

to the diagnosis and antiretroviral therapy (ART) when initiated. Nurse practitioners should respect the patient's decisions about disclosure of the diagnosis (CDC, 2015a).

The woman may also want to make explicit her wishes regarding end-of-life care by establishing advance directives and entrusting a friend or family member with power of attorney in the event she becomes incapacitated. Nurse practitioners can be useful in explaining the meanings of various levels of advanced care and the implications of aggressive care in advanced HIV disease and AIDS. Young women with children may want more aggressive therapies and interventions than older women whose children are grown. This is a personal decision based on a variety of considerations, including spiritual and theological issues. Nurse practitioners must be careful not to make assumptions about what is desirable and appropriate for each woman.

Nurse practitioners can help patients reframe their understanding of HIV, particularly in terms of understanding it as a chronic disease that can be managed, rather than the "death sentence" it once was before the advent of effective ART. When a woman learns of her HIV diagnosis, she may become severely depressed, with numerous psychosocial implications particularly, as an HIV diagnosis is associated with substantial stigma. Furthermore, patients who are not aware of treatment options may equate HIV with fatalism. At the beginning of the pandemic, researchers and scientists sought to identify the mechanism of infection and to seek a cure. In the ensuing two decades, scientists have identified the means of infection, although a cure remains elusive. However, in contrast to the early days of the epidemic, when HIV infection typically meant premature death from AIDS-related complications, a diagnosis of HIV infection now means a less certain trajectory toward AIDS and death. With improved antiviral therapy, HIV infection in many people has evolved into a treatable chronic infection. Intervening early with patients who are newly diagnosed by providing adequate counseling and education regarding their HIV diagnosis is critical. When counseling newly diagnosed patients, an emphasis should be placed on the capability of patients living long healthy lives due to effective ART. Although many patients who are newly diagnosed are able to positively adjust to their diagnosis and require minimal intervention, many newly diagnosed patients may experience prolonged periods of distress, anger, frustration, guilt, fear, and anxiety (Chipphindale & French, 2001). Such challenges and difficulties with coping may persist due to difficulties in discussing a positive HIV diagnosis with family and peers, stigma and discrimination associated with HIV, loss of social support, feelings of isolation, and difficulties in accessing mental health services may contribute to adverse mental health outcomes among individuals who are newly diagnosed with HIV (National Institutes of Health [NIH], 2021a). Numerous studies have noted that individuals living with HIV experience higher rates of depression and mood disorders; thus, it is imperative to conduct mental health screenings for patients at each visit, and to provide referrals to a mental health specialist as needed (Bhatia & Munjal, 2014; Tran et al., 2019). Nurse practitioners are in a unique position to understand the multiplicity of factors and issues that face persons with HIV. Awareness of these factors can enhance nursing interventions to improve both physical and mental health and the long-term health outcomes for their HIV-positive patients.

In the course of their practice, most APRNs will likely have occasion to provide care for women infected with HIV. Although AIDS is a long-term sequela of unchecked viral replication and immune system damage with its attendant infections, the more salient effect of the HIV epidemic on advanced nursing practice is the management of patients chronically infected with this virus, not those who have developed AIDS. For many women, HIV infection is treated as a chronic condition, and it may never progress to AIDS. Therefore, this chapter addresses the issues more closely associated with management of HIV infection rather than AIDS.

Untreated HIV disease progresses relentlessly. In untreated patients, the time between HIV infection and the development of AIDS ranges from a few months to 17 years, with the median interval without treatment being 10 years (Glaubius et al., 2021; Migueles & Connors, 2010). The rate of disease progression in an individual is determined by interactions between the host (the infected person), the virus, and the environment. The clinical goal is to minimize viral replication by determining the particular combination of ARTs, health-related behaviors, and psychosocial support needed to sustain a woman's health, limit the number of acute illness episodes related to HIV, and prevent mother-to-child transmission.

EPIDEMIOLOGY OF HIV

Early in the epidemic, HIV infection and AIDS were diagnosed in relatively few women, although current knowledge suggests that many women were infected but were not diagnosed (CDC, 2007; Workowski et al., 2015). The growing number of women living with HIV/AIDS is a dominant feature of the AIDS epidemic; approximately one of every four people living with HIV in the United States is a woman (HIVinfo, 2021a). Additionally, an increasing number of women living with HIV/AIDS are older than 50 years. Although the increase can be explained in part by AIDS-delaying benefits of combination ART—thus women infected early in life are now being diagnosed with AIDS later in life—it may also be associated with women being infected later in life and being overlooked because of the assumption that older women are not as sexually active. Women who were married for 20 or more years and subsequently divorced have found themselves single again and have begun having sex (Kalibala et al., 2016; Minkin, 2016).

Of the total 36,400 new HIV infections in the United States in 2018, 18% (6,700) were among women (CDC, 2022a). HIV diagnoses among women have declined in recent years; however, women of color, particularly Black women, are reportedly disproportionately affected by HIV/AIDS. Although annual HIV infections remained stable among Black women from 2014 to 2018, the rate of new HIV infections among Black women is 13 times that of White women and four times that of Latina women (HIV.gov, 2022). HIV infection is currently the sixth leading cause of death for Black women ages 20 to 44 years (CDC, 2016). Furthermore, the U.S. age-adjusted death rate of all Black women with HIV is roughly 15 times higher than that of the total number of HIV-infected women (CDC, 2015c).

In the United States, the HIV/AIDS epidemic is not evenly distributed throughout the states. The South currently accounts for an estimated 51% of all new HIV cases annually although 38% of the U.S. population lives in the region (CDC, 2019c). In 2017, the South had a significantly higher proportion of new HIV diagnoses compared to all other regions in the United States combined (CDC, 2019c). Generally, HIV/AIDS cases are concentrated in urban areas with states containing major metropolitan areas reporting higher rates of HIV/AIDS with Miami, Orlando, and Atlanta being the most heavily burdened metropolitan areas (CDC, 2015b, 2019a, 2022c). The states with the highest number of individuals living with an HIV diagnosis are Florida, California, Texas, Georgia, New York, North Carolina, Illinois, New Jersey, Pennsylvania, and Ohio (Kaiser Family Foundation, 2021).

Women are more likely to be diagnosed at younger ages than men, with the majority (77%) of women with AIDS diagnosed between the ages of 25 and 44 years, indicating that many were infected at a young age. In 2010, almost 2,000 girls and young women age 13 to 24 years were diagnosed with a new HIV/AIDS infection (CDC, 2019b). The CDC recommends that each state and U.S. territory conduct HIV case surveillance in addition to ongoing AIDS case surveillance. Early in the epidemic, AIDS surveillance data were adequate to allow public health officials to understand and evaluate the impact of the illness and to make programmatic decisions regarding prevention efforts. However, the widespread use of effective ART has diminished the numbers of AIDS cases, even though the numbers of persons infected with HIV have increased. Therefore, it has become necessary for the CDC to recommend expanded HIV case surveillance to monitor the epidemic and shape policy, prevention, and care services in response to surveillance data.

This is particularly important for women with HIV, because women tend to be underrepresented in AIDS surveillance data, as are ethnic minorities. HIV case surveillance is likely to reflect the epidemic in women earlier than AIDS data, which may be reported late in the disease after treatment failure or the onset of serious immunocompromised and health sequelae. The CDC has recommended HIV case surveillance rather than AIDS prevalence reports alone as it can provide a more realistic, useful estimate of the resources needed for patient care and services (Workowski et al., 2015).

NATURAL HISTORY AND HIV DISEASE PROGRESSION

The human immune system functions to protect the body from invasion by a variety of types of microbes and tumor cells. The immune system comprises two arms: humoral immunity, which is involved with antibody production, and cellular immunity, which is affected largely through cytotoxic T cells. Central components of the cellular arm of the immune system are macrophages and CD4+ T cells.

HIV is a retrovirus that specifically targets CD4+ T cells, binding to the cell surface protein known as the CD4+ receptor (Hessol et al., 2005). The virus affects the cells two ways: first, the absolute numbers of these cells are depleted; second, the function of the remaining cells is impaired, resulting in a gradual loss of immune function. Progressive depletion of CD4 cells in peripheral blood is the hallmark of advancing HIV disease (Hessol et al., 2005). Unimpeded, HIV can destroy up to 1 billion CD4 cells per day. In addition to its aggressive destruction, HIV is genetically highly variable, mutating with apparent ease.

Untreated HIV infection is a chronic illness that progresses relentlessly through several characteristic clinical stages. AIDS, the end point of HIV infection, results from severe immunologic damage, loss of effective immune response to specific opportunistic pathogens, and tumors. AIDS is diagnosed when one of these specific infections or cancers occurs or when CD4 cell levels are less than 200/mm^3.

HIV STAGING AND PROGRESSION

There is a brief period, typically 5 to 10 days after acquiring HIV, when no laboratory markers can detect the virus. This period is referred to as the eclipse period. Following HIV infection, approximately half of individuals will develop transient nonspecific symptoms that resemble flu-like symptoms (e.g., headache, fever, fatigue, malaise, lymphedema, rash). This period is referred to as acute HIV infection in which detection of HIV RNA or p24 antigen is present before the development of antibodies (Miller et al., 2010). During this period, individuals have a significantly high risk of transmitting HIV due to elevated HIV RNA levels (Miller et al., 2010; NIH, 2021b; Pilcher et al., 2004).

Untreated HIV infection causes a wide range of symptoms and clinical conditions reflecting the level of immunologic injury and other predisposing factors. Certain conditions tend to occur at the same time and at specific CD4 cell counts. Staging systems for HIV disease facilitate clinical evaluation and therapeutic intervention, help to determine individual level of infirmary, and provide information with which to make diagnoses. The most widely used system for classifying HIV infection and AIDS in adults and adolescents in industrialized countries was developed by the CDC. When a patient has been diagnosed with HIV, clinicians need two important pieces of data in planning appropriate therapies and in estimating the patient's prognosis: (1) how far the disease has progressed already and (2) how fast the disease is progressing. The CD4+ count provides a clue as to how far the disease has progressed, whereas the viral load provides a clue as to the rate of progression. Clinically, these data are more relevant to direct appropriate care than are strict categories of illness in which individuals may or may not receive the best care tailored to their own particular state of illness or relative health. However, stages of HIV disease described in general terms are clinically relevant (Table 31.1).

TABLE 31.1 Stages of HIV Infection

Acute infection	Virus establishes itself in the body; acute HIV syndrome (viral flu-like syndrome) occurs within 2–4 weeks of exposure to HIV. Characterized by fever, swollen glands, rash, muscle and joint aches and pains, and headaches. May last for several weeks. May become transiently immunocompromised. Takes 6–12 weeks for immune system to produce antibodies. Newly infected individual's blood may not test positive; however, individual may be highly contagious.
Clinical latency	Viral load stabilizes. Period of clinical latency with few or no symptoms; however, viral replication in lymphoid tissues continues. The individual is relatively symptom free but may have transient episodes of HIV-related infections. Women may be prone to aggressive cervical dysplasia. If on ART, clinical latency may last for several decades because the treatment helps keep the virus in check. For those not on ART, the clinical latency stage lasts an average of 10 years, although some may progress through this stage faster.
AIDS	CD4$^+$ count <200. The immune system is badly damaged and individual is vulnerable to opportunistic infections such as PCP. Individuals can respond to aggressive ART. CD4$^+$ count <50. Individual is severely ill with extensive organ involvement, aggressive neoplasia (Kaposi sarcoma), wasting disease syndromes, severe disseminated infections such as *Mycobacterium tuberculosis* and extrapulmonary histoplasmosis. Death occurs with vascular collapse and organ failure.

ART, antiretroviral therapy; PCP, Pneumocystis pneumonia.
Source: Centers for Disease Control and Prevention. (2014). Revised surveillance case definition for HIV infection—United States, 2014. Morbidity and Mortality Weekly Report. https://www.cdc.gov/mmwr/preview/mmwrhtml/rr6303a1.htm?s_cid=rr6303a1_e

TABLE 31.2 Myths and Facts About HIV Transmission

MYTH	FACT
HIV is transmitted through casual contact.	HIV is not transmitted through everyday, casual contact, including shaking hands and sharing eating utensils, even when living in close contact.
HIV is transmitted through insect bites.	There is no evidence of HIV transmission through bloodsucking or biting insects, including mosquitoes, flies, ticks, and fleas.
Donating or receiving blood is risky in the United States.	There are numerous safeguards to the U.S. blood supply, including only allowing persons with clean bills of health to donate, drawing blood with sterilized needles, and performing nine screening tests on all donated blood to ensure a safe blood supply.
Pets and other animals can carry HIV and transmit the virus to people.	Humans are the only animal that can harbor HIV. Some animals do carry similar viruses that can cause immune disease in their species; however, these cannot be transmitted to humans.
HIV can be transmitted through tears, sweat, and saliva.	Saliva, sweat, tears, and urine either carry no HIV or contain quantities too small to result in infection.

Source: Derose, K. P., Griffin, B. A., Kanouse, D. E., Bogart, L. M., Williams, M. V., Haas, A. C., Flórez, K. R., Collins, D. O., Hawes-Dawson, J., Mata, M. A., Oden, C. W., & Stucky, B. D. (2016). Effects of a pilot church-based intervention to reduce HIV stigma and promote HIV testing among African Americans and Latinos. AIDS and Behavior, 20(8), 1692–1705. https://doi.org/10.1007/s10461-015-1280-y; Mwamwenda, T. S. (2016). Myths and misconceptions about global HIV/AIDS: University students in Zimbabwe. Transylvanian Review, 24(6). https://doi.org/10.21506/j.ponte.2018.11.15

Initially, women appeared to have a more rapid progression of illness than men and to present with different opportunistic infections. However, current data suggest that the incidence and distribution of HIV-related illnesses are similar in men and women except for Kaposi sarcoma, which is seen more often in men, and the gynecologic manifestations of HIV. In general, predictors of the rate of HIV disease progression and survival among women are the same as those in men. CD4 cell count depletion and higher HIV ribonucleic acid (RNA) level are strong predictors of a woman's progression and survival.

TRANSMISSION

Virtually all cases of HIV are transmitted by three primary routes: sexual, parenteral (blood-borne), and perinatal. Rates of transmission from the infected host to the uninfected recipient vary by mode of transmission and specific circumstances of transmission (Hessol et al., 2005). Because HIV is a relatively large virus, has a short half-life in vitro, and only lives within primates, it is not transmitted through casual contact (i.e., hugging or shaking hands), by surface contact (e.g., toilet seat), or from insect bites. Myths and misconceptions about HIV transmission are found in Table 31.2.

Sexual Activity

The most common mode of transmission involves depositing HIV on mucosal surfaces, especially genital mucosa (Landovitz, 2016). Sexual transmission of HIV occurs through male-to-female, female-to-male, male-to-male, and female-to-female sexual contact. Receptive anal and vaginal intercourse appears to have the greatest risk of infection; however, insertive anal or vaginal intercourse also is associated with HIV infection. The majority (72%) of HIV infections in women occur through unprotected heterosexual intercourse (HIVinfo, 2021b). A much smaller percentage of HIV-infected women report having had sex with women; however, most of these had other risk factors, including injection drug use and sex with men who were infected or who had risk factors of infection (CDC, 2015c). Female-to-female transmission of HIV is exceptionally rare, with documented cases occurring primarily through acts that may result in vaginal trauma such as sharing sex toys without condoms or digital play with fingers with cuts or sharp nails (CDC, 2015c; Kwakwa & Ghobrial, 2003; Workowski et al., 2015). However, assuming that a woman is of very low risk for HIV because she has an expressed sexual preference for women overlooks the fact that many lesbians have a history of sexual intercourse with men or may have other risk factors for HIV infection (Lacombe-Duncan, 2016; Lunn et al., 2017). Therefore, their HIV risk should also be comprehensively assessed.

Parenteral Route

HIV can reach a person's infectable cells via infected blood or blood products, most commonly through injection drug use, but also via razor blades or tattoo needles. In 2005, approximately 26% of cases of HIV/AIDS in women occurred through injection drug use (CDC, 2012, 2019b).

HIV also can be transmitted from person to person through transfusion of blood or blood products; however, strict standards regarding testing of blood and blood products before administration have reduced the risk of exposure to HIV through this route. Once the presence of HIV was recognized in the blood supply in the early 1980s, very strict standards for donors regarding behavioral risk factors were set and testing of donor blood was initiated. Since the institution of these standards, the risk of exposure to HIV through blood and blood product administration is negligible.

Vertical (Perinatal) Route

Perinatal transmission of HIV can occur in utero, during labor and delivery, or postpartum through breastfeeding. Transmission rates vary by maternal stage of disease, use of ART, duration of ruptured membranes, and breastfeeding (Workowski et al., 2015).

Occupational Transmission

Occupational transmission of HIV to healthcare providers is extremely rare. As of date, only 58 cases of occupational HIV transmission have occurred in the United States (CDC, 2019a). Direct inoculation of HIV via needlestick injury imposes a risk of infection of 0.3% (3 in 1,000) to healthcare workers (Workowski et al., 2015). Casual contact with patients, even those known to be HIV positive, has not been determined to increase one's risk of acquiring HIV. To prevent HIV transmission in the workplace, healthcare workers must assume that blood and all body fluids from all patients are potentially infectious; therefore, standard precautions should be used in caring for all patients to minimize the risk of exposure and infection by HIV and other infectious agents (CDC, 2019a). Standard precautions include adequate hand hygiene, the use of personal protective equipment (PPE), safe handling of needles and sharps, respiratory hygiene, safe injection practices, use of sterile instruments and devices, and ensuring environmental surfaces are clean and disinfected (CDC, 2018; Table 31.3).

FACTORS FACILITATING TRANSMISSION

Transmission of HIV infection can be influenced by several factors, including characteristics of the infected host and the recipient, as well as the amount and infectivity of the virus itself.

Standard precautions synthesize the major features of blood and body fluid precautions (designed to reduce the risk of transmission of blood-borne pathogens) and body substance isolation (BSI; designed to reduce the risk of transmission of pathogens from moist body substances) and applies them to all patients receiving care in hospitals, regardless of their diagnosis or presumed infection status. Standard precautions apply to (a) blood; (b) all body fluids, secretions, and excretions except sweat, regardless of whether they contain visible blood; (c) nonintact skin; and (d) mucous membranes. Standard precautions are designed to reduce the risk of transmission of microorganisms from both recognized and unrecognized sources of infection in hospitals. Use standard precautions, or the equivalent, for the care of all patients.

Infectivity of the Host

There is an association between the amount of virus circulating in the blood and the risk of transmitting HIV. Transmission is more likely to occur when viral replication is high during the initial stage of infection and in the advanced stages of HIV disease. Individuals with high viral loads are more likely to transmit HIV to their sexual partners, persons with whom they share drug paraphernalia, and their offspring. Furthermore, viral load has been found to be the chief predictor of heterosexual transmission risk of HIV-1 (Herbeck et al., 2016). Regular adherence to ART is critical in reducing viral load and achieving viral suppression. Viral suppression occurs when HIV RNA level is so low that it cannot be detected with a lab test and is therefore referred to as an undetectable viral load. The CDC defines an undetectable viral load as having less than 200 copies of HIV per millimeter of blood; however, this number may vary depending on the lab test that is used (e.g., certain lab machines have a lower limit of detection and can detect HIV RNA levels down to 50 copies/mL). Achieving an undetectable viral load is key to ensuring good health among individuals living with HIV, and it significantly reduces the risk of HIV transmission. Individuals who achieve an undetectable viral load have effectively no risk of transmitting HIV to an HIV-negative partner through sex (CDC, 2022d). Individuals who are nonadherent with their ART and who are virologically uncontrolled have a higher risk of experiencing adverse health outcomes and opportunistic infections in addition to having a significantly higher risk of transmitting HIV to HIV-negative partners.

Transmission of HIV increases through sexual contact among individuals with preexisting sexually transmitted infections (STIs) and when sexual trauma occurs (e.g., genitoanal injury; CDC, 2022e; Ghosh et al., 2013). Circumcision has been found to reduce HIV transmission among

TABLE 31.3 Standard Precautions for HIV Prevention	
Hand hygiene	1. Wash hands after touching blood, body fluids, secretions, excretions, and contaminated items, even if gloves are worn. Wash hands immediately after gloves are removed, between patient contacts, and when otherwise indicated to avoid transfer of microorganisms to other patients or environments. It may be necessary to wash hands between tasks and procedures on the same patient to prevent cross-contamination of different body sites. 2. Use a plain (nonantimicrobial) soap for routine handwashing. 3. Use an antimicrobial agent or a waterless antiseptic agent for specific circumstances (e.g., control of outbreaks or hyperendemic infections), as defined by the infection control program.
Gloves	Wear gloves (clean, nonsterile gloves are adequate) when touching blood, body fluids, secretions, excretions, and contaminated items. Put on clean gloves just before touching mucous membranes and nonintact skin. Change gloves between tasks and procedures on the same patient after contact with material that may contain a high concentration of microorganisms. Remove gloves promptly after use, before touching noncontaminated items and environmental surfaces, and before going to another patient, and wash hands immediately to avoid transfer of microorganisms to other patients or environments.
Mask, eye protection, face shield	Wear a mask and eye protection or a face shield to protect mucous membranes of the eyes, nose, and mouth during procedures and patient care activities that are likely to generate splashes or sprays of blood, body fluids, secretions, and excretions.
Gown	Wear a gown (a clean, nonsterile gown is adequate) to protect skin and to prevent soiling of clothing during procedures and patient care activities that are likely to generate splashes or sprays of blood, body fluids, secretions, or excretions. Select a gown that is appropriate for the activity and amount of fluid likely to be encountered. Remove a soiled gown as promptly as possible, and wash hands to avoid transfer of microorganisms to other patients or environments.
Patient care equipment	Handle used patient care equipment soiled with blood, body fluids, secretions, and excretions in a manner that prevents skin and mucous membrane exposures, contamination of clothing, and transfer of microorganisms to other patients and environments. Ensure that reusable equipment is not used for the care of another patient until it has been cleaned and reprocessed appropriately. Ensure that single-use items are discarded properly.
Environmental control	Ensure that the hospital has adequate procedures for the routine care, cleaning, and disinfection of environmental surfaces, beds, bedrails, bedside equipment, and other frequently touched surfaces, and ensure that these procedures are being followed.
Linens	Handle, transport, and process used linens soiled with blood, body fluids, secretions, and excretions in a manner that prevents skin and mucous membrane exposures and contamination of clothing and that avoids transfer of microorganisms to other patients and environments.
Occupational health and blood-borne pathogens	1. Take care to prevent injuries when using needles, scalpels, and other sharp instruments or devices; when handling sharp instruments after procedures; when cleaning used instruments; and when disposing of used needles. Never recap used needles or otherwise manipulate them using both hands or use any other technique that involves directing the point of a needle toward any part of the body; rather, use either a one-handed "scoop" technique or a mechanical device designed for holding the needle sheath. Do not remove used needles from disposable syringes by hand, and do not bend, break, or otherwise manipulate used needles by hand. Place used disposable syringes and needles, scalpel blades, and other sharp items in appropriate puncture-resistant containers, which are located as close as practical to the area in which the items were used, and place reusable syringes and needles in a puncture-resistant container for transport to the reprocessing area. 2. Use mouthpieces, resuscitation bags, or other ventilation devices as an alternative to mouth-to-mouth resuscitation methods in areas where the need for resuscitation is predictable.
Patient placement	Place a patient who contaminates the environment or who does not (or cannot be expected to) assist in maintaining appropriate hygiene or environmental control in a private room. If a private room is not available, consult with infection control professionals regarding patient placement or other alternatives.

Source: Centers for Disease Control and Prevention. (2015). Universal precautions for the prevention of transmission of HIV and other blood borne infections. https://www.cdc.gov/infectioncontrol/basics/standard-precautions.html

heterosexual men; however, although circumcised men have a lower risk of acquiring HIV than do those who are uncircumcised, circumcision does not appear to decrease risk of transmission to a woman and may increase the risk if sexual activity is resumed before the circumcision wound is completely healed.

Susceptibility of Women

Women are biologically more vulnerable to HIV infection than men for several reasons. Sexual transmission of HIV is two to four times more efficient from male to female than from female to male (Workowski et al., 2015) because HIV in semen is in higher concentrations than in cervical and vaginal infections and because the vaginal area has a much larger mucosal area of exposure to HIV than does the penis. Certain characteristics of an uninfected woman may increase her likelihood of infection. Age and female anatomy are directly related to HIV transmission risk. Younger women have increased exposure of vaginal and cervical columnar epithelium, known to be a risk factor in the transmission of other STIs. Pregnant women also have an increased exposure of columnar epithelium. This tissue is associated with endocervical inflammatory cells and can bleed more easily during intercourse. Normal vaginal flora may confer nonspecific immunity, and data suggest that women with bacterial vaginosis are at increased risk for HIV seroconversion (Workowski et al., 2015). Both younger and postmenopausal women may be at greater risk for acquiring HIV because of a thinner vaginal epithelium, resulting in increased friability and risk of trauma during intercourse, thus providing direct access to the bloodstream (HIVinfo, 2021a; CDC, 2015d).

The integrity of the tissues of the female lower genital tract also influences HIV transmission risk. Trauma during intercourse, STI-related inflammation or cervicitis, cervical dysplasia, and an STI ulcer or chancre increase susceptibility to HIV infection. Any activity or condition that disrupts the tissues of the vagina may predispose a woman to infection with HIV. This includes the use of highly absorbent tampons, which are associated with vaginal desquamation with long-term use. Furthermore, higher rates of HIV transmission should be expected in sexual assault cases when trauma to the genital area occurs. Cases of domestic violence and sexual abuse also have been identified as important correlates of HIV in women (Chakraborty, 2016).

Sexual activity during menstruation may increase a woman's risk of acquiring HIV (CDC, 2019b). Similarly, the disruption of tissues through receptive penile–anal intercourse provides a highly efficient means of HIV transmission. Some contraceptive methods (e.g., barrier methods) may decrease HIV transmission; however, others may afford no protection or increase the risk of transmission (HIVinfo, 2021a). The effect of hormonal contraception on viral shedding is unclear, and these agents may interact with antibiotics and antiretrovirals (Dong et al., 2023). Although some research findings suggest that oral contraceptive use increases the risk of cervical ectopy and thus the risk of infection, others do not find this to be the case after adjusting for behavioral risk factors (CDC, 2019b). Use of the vaginal and rectal microbicide nonoxynol-9 provides no protection against HIV acquisition and may even increase susceptibility to infection because of mucosal barrier disruption, particularly with frequent use (Hatcher et al., 2011).

Douching, which is not recommended, can destroy the protective lactobacilli of the vagina and may increase a woman's susceptibility to bacterial vaginosis, STIs (gonorrhea, chlamydia, trichomonas), and HIV (Hatcher et al., 2011). Douching has no scientific rationale, dries out the vagina, traumatizes vaginal mucosa, and makes it more susceptible to tears. In addition, douching after sexual intercourse can push infectious agents further into the genital system, increasing the likelihood of infection. Douching is pointless and should be discouraged.

RISK FACTORS FOR HIV

Unlike many viruses that are easily transmitted through the air, water, food, and/or casual contact, HIV transmission usually requires risky behaviors. Common risky behaviors in women include vaginal, anal, and oral sex without a condom or vaginal barrier, concurrent partners, numerous lifetime partners, substance use or abuse, and a history of intimate partner violence. However, these behaviors do not occur in a vacuum, and biological, behavioral, psychological, demographic, and sociocultural factors all affect the likelihood and consequences of these behaviors (Workowski et al., 2015).

Cultural and religious attitudes and beliefs also affect healthcare services. The loss of support for safer sex education programs in favor of an abstinence-only model does not protect adolescents. Teens who pledge to remain a virgin until marriage have the same, if not higher, rates of STIs than those who do not commit to abstinence (Bordogna et al., 2023; Woolweaver et al., 2023). In response to these findings, a more pragmatic abstinence-plus or "ABC" message based on harm-reduction principles has been instituted. The message is Abstinence, Be faithful for married couples or those in committed relationships, and use a Condom for individuals who are or put themselves at risk of HIV infection.

Biological Factors

Heterosexual transmission of HIV is 12 times more likely from men to women (Derose et al., 2016). A number of biological factors make HIV transmission easier or more difficult. These include the presence of STIs, tissue/ membrane vulnerability, viral load, and anatomic characteristics (see Susceptibility of Women section).

A person's biological sex (i.e., female, male) as well as the social roles associated with biological sex (gender) influence other risk factors of HIV/AIDS. For example, women are more likely to acquire HIV through heterosexual sexual activity than men because of their anatomy. Similar rates of exposure through heterosexual contact are seen in White (65%), Black (74%), and Hispanic (69%) women (Workowski et al., 2015). HIV can be transmitted through receptive oral sex with ejaculation. Any condition that interrupts the integrity of oral tissues, including periodontal disease, increases the risk of HIV transmission in this manner.

Demographic Characteristics

Demographic factors such as gender, ethnicity, and age shape HIV risk behaviors and influence social networks, making it more or less likely that an individual who engages in risky behaviors will associate with persons who are HIV positive.

In the United States, most new AIDS cases, persons living with AIDS, and the majority of AIDS deaths are reported among racial and ethnic minorities. Black/African American and Hispanic/Latina women are disproportionally reported to have HIV compared with women of other races/ethnicities (CDC, 2019b). Furthermore, HIV-infected Black/African American and Hispanic/Latina people are more likely than infected White people to be uninsured, have less access to antiretroviral drugs, and lack access to healthcare (Workowski et al., 2015). Closely connected to ethnicity and race is socioeconomic status, one of the most powerful predictors of health and illness. Ethnicity may also be associated with certain contextual factors. Specific factors for Black/African American women include the gender-ratio imbalance and historical and personal victimization.

Social Factors

Factors such as poverty, lack of education, social inequity, and inadequate access to healthcare indirectly increase the prevalence of HIV in at-risk populations. Communities with the highest rates of HIV are often those with the poorest access to healthcare, and health insurance coverage influences if and where a woman has access to care and whether she can afford antiretroviral medications. Many women, even if they perceive themselves to be at risk of contracting HIV, may not be able to practice protective behaviors if survival is an overarching concern or if there are other risks that appear to be more threatening or imminent. Survival concerns, such as secure shelter, food, safety for self and children, and money may override any concerns about protecting a woman's own health (Workowski et al., 2015).

Recognition of Risk

Beliefs and misconceptions about personal risk can increase an individual's risk of getting HIV infection. A woman who believes she has no risk factors for contacting an STI—including HIV—is unlikely to practice any risk-reducing behaviors. In addition, persons who believe they are not at risk of HIV infection are more apt to have risky behaviors. Younger women may be at higher risk because they have less knowledge of reproductive health, less skill in communicating and negotiating with their partners about risk-reduction practices, and more barriers to access to healthcare services. Taking risks is a universal human element. In the throes of passion, people can make unwise sexual decisions. Furthermore, safer sex is not always perceived to be the most enjoyable sex.

Personality Characteristics

Personality characteristics, such as low self-esteem, feelings of low self-efficacy, impulsivity, narcissism, tendency to take risks, and tendency to seek out new sensations are related to sexual risk behaviors. Furthermore, women with a sense of low self-efficacy and lack of self-confidence may be unable to negotiate safer sex practices. Coping strategies, such as high-risk sexual behaviors or drug and alcohol use to relieve or escape stress, can increase personal risk of HIV infection.

Social Interactions and Relationships

Because intimate human contact is a common vehicle of HIV transmission, sexual behavior in the context of relationships is a critical risk factor for preventing and acquiring HIV. Cultural and religious attitudes regarding appropriate sexual behaviors affect risk at the individual and community

levels. Relationships and sexual behaviors are regulated by cultural norms that influence sexual expression in interpersonal relationships. Often women are still socialized to please their partners and to place men's needs and desires first; thus, they may find it difficult to insist on safer sex behaviors. Traditional cultural values associated with passivity and subordination may diminish the ability of many women to adequately protect themselves.

Power imbalances in relationships are the product of and contributors to the maintenance of traditional gender roles that identify men as the initiators of and decision-makers about sexual activities and women as passive gatekeepers. As long as traditional gender norms define the roles for sexual relationships as men having the dominant role in sexual decision-making, negotiating condom use by women will remain difficult. Additionally, cultural norms define talking about condoms as implying a lack of trust that runs counter to the traditional gender norm expectations for women (Maman et al., 2000). Women sometimes do not request condom use because of a need to establish and maintain intimacy with partners. Research has demonstrated that women at risk of HIV place significant importance on and investment in their heterosexual relationships and that these dynamics have an impact on the women's risk taking and risk management. Urging women to insist on condom use may be unrealistic, because traditional gender roles do not encourage women to talk about sex, initiate sexual practices, or control intimate encounters.

A woman who is dependent upon an abusive male partner or a partner who places her at risk by his own risky behaviors is at higher risk for contracting HIV than are women who are not dependent (Hutchison et al., 2023; Nabayinda et al., 2023). The risk of acquiring HIV infection is high among women who are physically and sexually abused. Past and current experiences with violence—particularly sexual abuse—erode women's sense of self-efficacy to exercise control over sexual behaviors, engender feelings of anxiety and depression, and increase the likelihood of risky sexual behaviors (Chakraborty, 2016). Additionally, fear of physical harm and loss of economic support hamper women's efforts to enact protective practices. Furthermore, past and current abuse is strongly associated with substance abuse, which also increases the risk of contracting an STI.

The risk of acquiring an STI is determined not only by the woman's actions, but by her partner's as well. Although prevention counseling customarily includes recommending that women identify the partner who is at high risk because of drugs and medical factors and also determine his sexual practices, this advice may be unrealistic and/or culturally inappropriate in many relationships. Women who engage in sexual activities with other women only may or may not be at risk of infection. Many women who identify themselves as lesbian have had intercourse with a man at one time by choice, by force, or by necessity or may have used drugs and shared drug paraphernalia such as needles.

Behavioral Risks

Any behavior that increases a woman's contact with bodily fluids of another person increases the likelihood of HIV transmission. During sexual activity, infected blood, semen, vaginal fluids, and anal fluids can enter the uninfected woman's body through cuts, tears, and lesions on the penis or labia and in or on the vagina or anus. Cuts and tears are more likely to occur during forced or rough sex, anal sex, dry sex, or when women are very young and their cervixes are not fully developed and thus more likely to rip or tear during sex (Sathe et al., 2016).

Substance Use

Drug and alcohol use is associated with increased risk of HIV (CDC, 2019b). Sharing unclean drug paraphernalia—particularly needles and syringes—increases the risk of HIV transmission, particularly in areas where there is a high incidence of HIV infection among drug users. For example, in many areas, crack use parallels trends of HIV infection. Among several possible reasons for this association are social factors such as poverty and lack of educational and economic opportunities and individual factors such as risk taking and low self-efficacy. In addition to the risk from needle sharing, use of drugs and alcohol may contribute to the risk of HIV infection by undermining cognitive and social skills, thus making it more difficult to engage in HIV-protective actions. Furthermore, depression and other psychological problems and a history of sexual abuse are associated with substance abuse and thus contribute to risky behaviors. Being high and thus not able to clean drug paraphernalia can be a pervasive barrier to protective practice. Furthermore, drug use may take place in settings where persons participate in sexual activities while using drugs. Cocaine abusers have demonstrated higher levels of sexual risk behaviors than other addict populations. Finally, women who use drugs may be at higher risk because of the practice of exchanging sex for drugs or money and high numbers of sexual partners and encounters (Chakraborty, 2016; Deslauriers et al., 2023; Dickson et al., 2023).

Past and current physical, emotional, and sexual abuse characterizes the lives of many, if not most, drug-using women (Chakraborty, 2016; Klevens et al., 2016). For women who have experienced violence, the use of alcohol and drugs can become a coping mechanism by which they self-medicate to relieve feelings of anxiety, depression, guilt, fear, and anger stemming from the violence. Women's drug use is strongly linked to relationship inequities and some men's ability to mandate women's sexual behavior. Sexual degradation of women is described as an intimate part of crack cocaine use.

PREVENTION

Primary prevention of HIV infection through condom use, reduction of risky sexual behaviors, using clean syringes and injection equipment, and using preexposure prophylaxis (PrEP) are effective methods in reducing the risk of HIV transmission (CDC, 2021a). Secondary prevention through the diagnosis, counseling, and treatment of HIV/AIDS infection can prevent disease progression and complications for individuals and can reduce transmission to others. (Readers are referred to Chapter 30, Sexually Transmitted Infections, for a discussion of primary prevention of STIs, including HIV.)

Preexposure Prophylaxis for HIV Prevention

Primary prevention through condom use is an effective method of reducing HIV risk. However, in certain cases women may not have control over sexual health decisions and condom use, which can necessitate the need for female-controlled methods such as PrEP. PrEP currently is available in two forms that are approved for women. The most frequently used form is a daily pill consisting of tenofovir disoproxil fumarate (TDF)/emtricitabine (FTC), which is also referred to by the brand name Truvada. Truvada is a daily pill first approved in 2012 with data indicating that when taken consistently; it reduces the risk of contracting HIV in 93% of high-risk individuals (CDC, 2019b) and HIV-negative men and transgender women who had sex with men (Grant et al., 2014). More recently, the long-acting injectable cabotegravir (Apretude) as an intramuscular injection has been approved for HIV prevention among women (U.S. Food and Drug Administration [FDA], 2021). Prior to initiating Apretude, an oral lead-in dose may be used for approximately 1 month followed by single injections given 1 month apart for 2 consecutive months. Injections should then be continued every 2 months thereafter (FDA, 2021).

PrEP is recommended as one preventive option for adult heterosexually active men and women who are at substantial risk of contracting HIV. It is also recommended for adult injection drug users (IDU) at risk of HIV and heterosexually active women whose partners are known to have HIV. Before prescribing PrEP, acute and chronic infection with HIV must be excluded by patient history and HIV testing immediately. Women who are on Truvada for PrEP should have follow-up visits every 3 months to provide HIV testing, medication adherence counseling, behavioral risk-reduction support, and side effect assessment. Additionally, women should be seen at 6 months and every 6 months thereafter to assess renal function and test for bacterial STIs (Smith et al., 2014). Women on Apretude must follow-up based on dosing schedule as indicated here. There are significant secondary benefits associated with use of PrEP including frank discussion about sex and risk and increased attention to screening, prevention, and treatment of STIs (Grossman, 2017).

Types of HIV Tests

Beginning in 1985, HIV has been perhaps most associated with antibody testing, either for determination of serostatus or screening blood and tissue donations (Bennett, 2006). HIV infection is diagnosed by serologic tests to detect antibodies against HIV-1 and HIV-2 and by virologic tests that detect HIV antigens (p24 antigen) or RNA. Initial testing for HIV should be done with either a fourth-generation or fifth-generation antigen/antibody combination immunoassay that can detect HIV-1 and HIV-2 antibodies along with HIV-1 p24 antigen. If a positive result is obtained with an antigen/antibody combination immunoassay, an antibody immunoassay that differentiates HIV-1/HIV-2 should be conducted. Rapid HIV tests are available to allow clinicians to make a preliminary diagnosis of HIV infection in 30 minutes; however, they can produce negative results in recently infected individuals

Box 31.1 Indications for HIV Testing

- Physical symptoms consistent with HIV-related illness
- History of multiple sexual partners
- History of crack cocaine, cocaine, or methamphetamine use
- History of injection drug use
- History of sex with an HIV-positive person or one suspected to be HIV positive
- History of sex with an intravenous drug user
- History of a direct inoculation with HIV from an occupational exposure (e.g., operating room, ED)
- Social history that includes injection drug use or illicit drugs such as crack cocaine
- Pregnancy
- History of intimate partner violence
- Tattoos or body piercing

Source: From Centers for Disease Control and Prevention. (2022). HIV basics. *https://www.cdc.gov/hiv/basics/index.html*

because they become reactive later than conventional laboratory-based serologic assays (Workowski et al., 2015). The specific recommendations for testing for HIV infection are found in Box 31.1.

The standard of practice for HIV diagnostic testing requires two tests on the same sample to be reactive for a person to be considered HIV positive. When an individual shows HIV antibodies on two or more serologic tests, an independent, highly specific supplemental test—commonly the HIV-1/HIV-2 antibody differentiation assay, Western blot test, or indirect immunofluorescent-antibody assay—is used (Workowski et al., 2015). The Western blot test is less sensitive than the enzyme-linked immunosorbent assay (ELISA) test, but rarely is there a false-positive result, and therefore it is used for confirming the ELISA test.

HIV Testing Guidelines

HIV testing is a serious matter with several social, ethical, and psychological implications, in addition to the obvious healthcare issues. Certain persons have histories or clinical indications that warrant HIV testing (Box 31.1). Counseling for risk factors will help healthcare providers determine the relative risk of a patient for HIV. Testing for HIV is recommended and should be offered to all women seeking evaluation for and treatment of STIs (Workowski et al., 2015).

The first guidelines for HIV testing were issued by the U.S. Public Health Service in 1987. In 1993, the CDC expanded the guidelines to include hospitalized patients and individuals receiving healthcare as outpatients in acute care settings. An important component of these guidelines was HIV counseling and testing as a priority prevention strategy for at-risk persons regardless of the healthcare setting. The CDC expanded current guidelines to recommended anonymous testing, which allowed persons to find out their status while minimizing their concern that their identities could be revealed.

The most recent recommendations for HIV testing in primary care settings were released in 2015 (Workowski et al., 2015). Specific recommendations include the following:

- HIV screening is recommended for all persons seeking evaluation or treatment for STIs. Testing should be done at the time of an STI diagnosis in populations at high risk of HIV infections.
- HIV testing must be voluntary and free from coercion. Persons should not be tested without their knowledge.
- Opt-out HIV screening (notifying the individual that the HIV test will be performed, unless she declines) is recommended in all healthcare settings.
- Specific signed consent for HIV testing should not be required. General informed consent for medical care is considered sufficient to encompass informed consent for HIV testing.
- Use of antigen/antibody combination tests are encouraged unless persons are unlikely to receive their results.
- Preliminary positive-screening tests for HIV infection must be followed with additional testing to definitively establish the diagnosis.
- Providers should be alert to the possibility of acute infection and perform antigen/antibody immunoassay or HIV RNA in conjunction with an antibody test.
- Persons suspected of recently acquired HIV infection should be immediately referred to an HIV clinical care provider.

Although a negative antibody test usually indicates that a person is not infected, these tests cannot exclude a recent infection. A patient with a negative test who is at very high risk of contracting the virus should be retested 3 to 6 months after the initial baseline test. A person with a specific exposure to HIV—for example, in an occupational setting or via unprotected sexual contact with a person known to have HIV—should be tested serially: first, at the time of the exposure to determine the baseline serologic status, and then at 3- and 6-month intervals until seroconversion is determined or the person remains seronegative for 1 year.

HIV Counseling

Researchers found that interactive client-centered counseling can reduce risk behaviors and the incidence of new STIs (Workowski et al., 2015) The impact of counseling and testing is likely to be greatest for HIV-positive individuals, because the information gained could be used to avoid transmitting HIV to others (Workowski et al., 2015). Although prevention counseling is desirable for all persons at risk of HIV, it is recognized that counseling may not be feasible in all settings.

Although prevention counseling is no longer required as a part of the HIV screening programs in healthcare settings, it is strongly encouraged for all persons at high risk of HIV. It is also recommended that easily understood informational materials should be available in the languages of the persons using the healthcare services.

State laws vary regarding disclosure of a positive diagnosis for HIV to persons other than the patient, such as spouses or sexual contacts. Healthcare providers must be aware of the regulations governing their practice and should inform the patient of these regulations before testing, so that the patient can be fully informed as to the social and legal implications of a positive test. For many women, partner notification may make her vulnerable to abuse and violence in the event she is HIV positive.

Box 31.2 lists the issues that should be addressed in counseling a patient seeking HIV testing. All women seeking HIV testing should also be tested for hepatitis B. The posttest visit can be stressful for the patient, regardless of the results; therefore, test results should be disclosed as soon as possible in the visit, because the patient may be very anxious regarding the outcome. If the results are positive for HIV, the woman must be given time to accept the message and to react emotionally as needed. She must assimilate a lot of information at the time of this visit. Allowing her to express her feelings before discussing issues related to partner notification, treatments, and other issues may help her to take in some of the important information that must be conveyed at this time.

Seropositive patients must understand that, although they may exhibit no signs or symptoms of HIV disease, they are still infectious and will be for life. Basic information regarding minimizing transmission risk must be relayed to the patient at this time. A specific goal is to minimize the risk of transmission of the virus to others; therefore, the woman needs to understand immediately the implications of her HIV seropositivity in terms of transmission risk. Furthermore, APRNs must assess the newly diagnosed HIV-positive patient's need for further psychological and emotional supportive services.

Box 31.2 HIV Test Counseling

- Explain the meaning and implications of negative and positive test results and the meaning of indeterminate results.
- Discuss HIV risk reduction, including behaviors specific to the woman being tested.
- Inform the woman of state-mandated reporting requirements.
- If relevant, explain anonymous versus confidential testing.
- Determine the woman's support system and coping and stress management strategies that may be enlisted based on test results.
- Arrange for a return visit to discuss test results.

Source: Centers for Disease Control and Prevention. (2021). HIV surveillance supplemental report: Estimated HIV incidence and prevalence in the United States, 2015–2019 (Vol. 26, No. 1). http://www.cdc.gov/hiv/library/reports /hiv-surveillance.html; Centers for Disease Control and Prevention. (2021). HIV prevention. https://www.cdc.gov/hiv/basics/prevention.html; Fogel, C. I., & Black, B. (2008). Sexually transmitted infections, including HIV: Impact on women's reproductive health. March of Dimes.

TREATMENT PLANNING

HIV treatment or ART is recommended for all persons with HIV and should be initiated early to reduce risks of mortality, morbidity, and HIV transmission. A plan for treatment must be developed. Often this requires a referral to an infectious disease healthcare setting that can provide expert care for the individual. Unless the provider is familiar with HIV management, there is likely to be an interval between diagnosis and treatment decisions. However, the goal is to minimize the time between HIV diagnosis and treatment by starting ART immediately, also known as rapid ART initiation. Rapid ART initiation may not be appropriate for every patient, so the provider should refer to the current HIV management guidelines. If there is a delay in linkage to HIV care, it is appropriate to offer the women emotional and psychological support as well as education about HIV. In addition, this is the time to begin the discussion regarding who must be told about her infection and to begin to integrate behaviors that are required to minimize her risk of transmitting the virus to others.

The impact of HIV on future childbearing is an important consideration in counseling women with HIV. Many women with HIV are diagnosed during their childbearing years. They must be given adequate information regarding vertical transmission and treatment during pregnancy to make informed decisions regarding their pregnancy. The decision to become pregnant or to forgo future childbearing should be made only when the woman is fully informed regarding HIV and pregnancy. The risk for perinatal transmission of HIV can be reduced with the use of antiretroviral treatment. With treatment the risk of transmitting HIV to a neonate can be reduced to less than 1% with antiretroviral treatment and obstetric intervention, including cesarean section at 38 weeks' gestation if the HIV RNA level is >1,000 copies/mL and not breastfeeding (Panel on Treatment of HIV-Infected Pregnant Women and Prevention of Perinatal Transmission, 2012). Pregnant women with HIV should be linked to comprehensive HIV medical and psychosocial care as well as prenatal and postpartum care (Andrews et al., 2018).

Many women are diagnosed with HIV at a slightly older age than are men (CDC, 2021b). Furthermore, the prevalence of HIV is higher in African American or Hispanic women, and factors contributing to this disparity include oversampling, poverty, lack of health insurance, limited access to care, discrimination, and racism (Agénor et al., 2021; Bosh et al., 2021; Relf et al., 2019; Scott et al., 2023). Thus, a comprehensive plan of care that takes into consideration the multiplicity of stressors that women with HIV experience has a greater chance at making a healthy impact on their lives.

TREATMENT OF HIV IN WOMEN

Women with undiagnosed HIV often seek care for routine gynecologic services including treatment for candidiasis, which presents an opportunity to recommend HIV testing. Recurrent vulvovaginal candidiasis is one common symptom of HIV infection in women, and treatment is the same for a woman with or without HIV (CDC, 2021c). Furthermore, prevalence rates for vulvovaginal candidiasis are higher in women with

HIV, and symptoms can be worse in those with deteriorating immune function (CDC, 2021c). In addition, some gynecologic infections and conditions affect women with HIV differently than women without HIV. Women with HIV are also more likely than women without HIV to have abnormal cervical cytology and human papillomavirus infection, which have results in the development of cervical cancer screening guidelines for women with HIV (Moscicki et al., 2019). Other common infections such as pelvic inflammatory disease, genital herpes, and bacterial vaginosis can be more severe and difficult to treat in women with HIV compared to women without HIV; thus, refer to the special considerations section of the STI treatment guidelines (Cameron et al., 2020; CDC, 2021c). While not all women seeking gynecologic services for conditions such as recurrent vaginal candidiasis and abnormal cervical cytology have HIV infection, providers should consider testing undiagnosed women who are experiencing similar symptoms and assessing immune function in women with HIV.

Individuals with a new diagnosis of HIV infection should be informed about (a) the importance of prompt linkage to HIV care and what to expect when they begin healthcare of HIV infection, and (b) the effectiveness of HIV treatments, as well as the goal of treatment including reduced risk of HIV transmission and mortality (Panel on Antiretroviral Guidelines for Adults and Adolescents, 2022). The care of a person with HIV should be supervised by an expert in HIV and/or infectious diseases. All women newly diagnosed with HIV should undergo an extensive medical history review, physical examination, and laboratory evaluation. The initial encounter should be nonjudgmental and focus on establishing rapport. The medical history (Table 31.4) should include inquiries related to sexual behaviors, STIs, and chronic illnesses unrelated to but affected by HIV and its treatments, such as heart disease and diabetes mellitus. The history also should include inquiries about illnesses and conditions associated with immunosuppression, such as tuberculosis; herpes zoster and genital herpes; acute and chronic skin disorders, such as fungal infections and molluscum contagiosum; severe and repeated episodes of vaginal candidiasis; diarrhea associated with various fungi or bacteria; and frequent bouts of pneumonia and sinusitis (Panel on Antiretroviral Guidelines for Adults and Adolescents, 2022; Thompson et al., 2021). The presence or frequency of these infections not typically found in persons with normal immunologic status may help pinpoint the time of infection. In addition, women with HIV should be asked about their gynecologic and obstetric history, including birth control method and plans for future childbearing.

The physical examination for patients with HIV should be very thorough. Vital signs should be carefully monitored, especially temperature and weight. The wide-scale and subtle effects of HIV on various body systems require careful examination, especially of the mouth, eyes, skin, lungs, heart, lymph nodes, abdomen, genitourinary system, rectum, and nervous system. HIV may cause subtle or obvious changes in each of these systems. Clinical abnormalities in these systems will give the practitioner evidence of the level of immune system compromise in the patient with HIV. In addition, certain laboratory tests (Table 31.5) should be included in the initial examination of the woman with HIV. In addition, all patients should be tested for tuberculosis initially and annually

TABLE 31.4 Medical History for Women With HIV

TOPIC	SPECIFIC POINTS TO ADDRESS
HIV diagnosis	Date/year of first test; reason for being tested; mode of transmission
HIV treatment history	Nadir CD4 count; most recent and highest viral load Specific antiretroviral treatment history including prior resistance testing, reasons for regimen changes
Sexually transmitted infections and other infection history	Syphilis; gonorrhea; herpes simplex; pelvic inflammatory disease; anogenital warts; tuberculosis; hepatitis A, B, or C; prior vaccinations; history of chickenpox or shingles
Obstetric and gynecologic history	Pregnancies and their resolution, menstrual disorders, anovulation, perimenopause, uterine fibroids or polyps, abnormal vaginal discharge, cancer, genital tract infections
Other medical diagnoses	Hypertension, type 2 diabetes mellitus, cardiovascular disease, premalignant or malignant conditions, thyroid disease
Sexual practices	Condom use; other birth control methods; number of current partners; sexual activity with men, women, or both; history of transactional sex for drugs or money; history of anal sex
HIV-associated signs and symptoms	Bacterial pneumonia, thrush, severe headache, midline substernal discomfort with swallowing, visual changes including flashes of light, floaters, or visual field deficits
Mental health history	Past and current problems, evidence of depression (change in appetite, trouble sleeping, loss of interest in usual activities, anhedonia)
Family history	Age and health of children, including HIV tests if done; HIV in other family members; hypertension; type 2 diabetes; cardiovascular disease; malignancy
Medications	Prescription and over the counter; history of and attitude toward regular medication use; use of complementary and alternative therapies; drug allergies
Social history	Place of birth, where raised, who woman has lived with, child care responsibilities, housing status, history of interpersonal violence, education and occupational history, travel history, substance use or abuse, illicit drug use
Sources of support	Who has the woman told of her diagnosis, and what were their reactions? Does she have friends and family members she can talk to? Does she have a job? Does she have health insurance?
Patient education	

Source: Panel on Antiretroviral Guidelines for Adults and Adolescents. (2022). *Guidelines for the use of antiretroviral agents in adults and adolescents with HIV. Department of Health and Human Services.* https://clinicalinfo.hiv.gov/sites/default/files/guidelines/documents/adult-adolescent-arv/guidelines-adult-adolescent-arv.pdf; Thompson, M. A., Horberg, M. A., Agwu, A. L., Colasanti, J. A., Jain, M. K., Short, W. R., Singh, T., & Aberg, J. A. (2021). Primary care guidance for persons with human immunodeficiency virus: 2020 update by the HIV Medicine Association of the Infectious Diseases Society of America. *Clinical Infectious Diseases, 73*(11), e3572–e3605. https://doi.org/10.1093/cid/ciaa1391

TABLE 31.5 Baseline HIV Laboratory Tests

Serology	• HIV antibody testing • CD4 T lymphocyte count (T cell or CD4 cell count) • Plasma HIV RNA (viral load) • Genotypic resistance testing (testing may not be successful for patients with an HIV RNA level or viral load of ≤100 copies/mL) • HLA B*5701 in patient being considered for abacavir therapy • Complete blood count, including white blood cell count and differential • Chemistry panel, including liver and renal function • Lipid profile • Syphilis • Varicella-zoster virus if no history of chickenpox or shingles; immunity to measles, mumps, and rubella in persons born in 1957 or after • Toxoplasmosis IgG, cytomegalovirus IgG, and cryptococcal antigen if the patient is symptomatic or CD4 count <100 copies/mL • Hepatitis A, B, C
Specimen	• Urinalysis • Pap smear (cervical and anal specimens) • Chlamydia test (urine or vaginal specimens as well as rectal and oropharyngeal if patient engaging in anal or oral intercourse) • Gonorrhea test (urine or vaginal specimens as well as rectal and oropharyngeal if patient engaging in anal or oral intercourse) • *Trichomonas* test (urine and vaginal specimens) • Human papillomavirus assay
Other	• Screening for *Mycobacterium tuberculosis* using a tuberculin skin test or an interferon-γ release assay • Pregnancy testing • Glucose-6-phosphate dehydrogenase

IgG, immunoglobulin G; HLA, human leukocyte antigen.
Source: Panel on Antiretroviral Guidelines for Adults and Adolescents. (2022). Guidelines for the use of antiretroviral agents in adults and adolescents with HIV. Department of Health and Human Services. https://clinicalinfo.hiv.gov/sites/default/files/guidelines/documents/adult-adolescent-arv/guidelines-adult-adolescent-arv.pdf; Thompson, M. A., Horberg, M. A., Agwu, A. L., Colasanti, J. A., Jain, M. K., Short, W. R., Singh, T., & Aberg, J. A. (2021). Primary care guidance for persons with human immunodeficiency virus: 2020 update by the HIV Medicine Association of the Infectious Diseases Society of America. Clinical Infectious Diseases, 73(11), e3572–e3605. https://doi.org/10.1093/cid/ciaa1391

thereafter (Panel on Antiretroviral Guidelines for Adults and Adolescents, 2022; Thompson et al., 2021).

General clinical findings in women with HIV are similar to those found in men, with the exception of a high frequency of reproductive tract disorders, including cervical dysplasia and refractory vaginal candidiasis (CDC, 2021a). Women with HIV should have an initial Pap smear to test for the presence of cervical dysplasia and it should be repeated at least yearly thereafter. After three consecutive Pap test results are normal, subsequent Pap tests should be performed every 3 years (Panel on Antiretroviral Guidelines for Adults and Adolescents, 2022). Cotesting (Pap test and HPV test) is recommended for women with HIV who are 30 years of age or older (Panel on Antiretroviral Guidelines for Adults and Adolescents, 2022). In comparison to the population of women without HIV, women with HIV should undergo cervical cancer screening throughout their lifetime (Panel on Antiretroviral Guidelines for Adults and Adolescents, 2022). Some women will require Pap smears more frequently based on initial findings and gynecologic history. For women with cervical dysplasia, referral may be made for follow-up with a specialist for gynecologic management for colposcopy and treatment.

The management of lower genital tract neoplasia represents a specific treatment issue in the care of women with HIV. Women with HIV are at risk of developing lower genital tract neoplasia, particularly as the HIV disease progresses and the woman becomes increasingly immunocompromised. Cervical intraepithelial neoplasia and invasive cervical cancer can be persistent and progressive and difficult to manage effectively in women with HIV. Women with these conditions should be referred to a gynecologist or gynecologic oncologist for management.

Appropriate vaccinations will be offered based on patient history and lab findings. Common vaccinations include yearly influenza immunizations, pneumococcal immunizations, human papillomavirus, and the hepatitis A and hepatitis B series, as indicated.

Based on the patient's history and physical exam and the laboratory findings, the healthcare team will devise a plan of follow-up care. Decisions related to the initiation of ART, chemoprophylaxis against opportunistic infections, and follow-up evaluation may be deferred until all test results are received if the patient appears to be generally healthy at the time of the initial examination. Patients who are obviously immunocompromised with signs and symptoms of AIDS-related illness or opportunistic infection at the time of initial evaluation may be treated presumptively, with further refinements and changes in treatments possible at the time all laboratory data are reviewed.

Two specific lab values that shape treatment decisions in persons with HIV are the viral load (HIV-1 RNA) and the CD4 count. With increasing emphasis in HIV care on maintaining viral load levels at an undetectable level, these lab values are important in ascertaining appropriate ART (Table 31.6) and adherence to the medication regimen. The CD4 count is an important tool in assessing the overall status of the immune system. Also known as helper T cells, CD4 cells signal other immune system cells to fight infection. Depletion of these cells is the hallmark of advancing HIV disease.

Antiretroviral Therapy

ART is the use of HIV medications to treat HIV infection. Effective ART involves using a combination of medications that slow viral replication, but ART does not eliminate HIV infection. The goals of ART are (a) to prolong the length and quality of life; (b) to reduce HIV-related morbidity and mortality; (c) maximal, durable suppression of viral load; (d) restoration and/or preservation of immunologic function; and (e) to prevent HIV transmission (Panel on Antiretroviral Guidelines for Adults and Adolescents, 2022; Thompson et al., 2021).

There is a rationale for beginning ART before symptom onset to prevent immunosuppression. Further therapy must be continuous to prevent viral replication. Benefits and risks exist in initiating ART in treatment-naïve, asymptomatic patients (see Table 31.6) that must be considered before the initiation of ART. The risks and benefits of treatment of asymptomatic patients must be weighed carefully on a case-by-case basis to determine the appropriate course for any patient. The decision to initiate treatment in an asymptomatic patient must balance several competing factors that influence risk and benefit.

TABLE 31.6 Benefits and Risks of Antiretroviral Therapy

Benefits	• Prolonged duration and quality of life • Control of viral replication and reduction of viral load • Prevention of progressive immunosuppression by control of viral load • Delayed progression of clinical disease and progression to AIDS • Decreased inflammation • Decreased risk of resistant virus • Decreased risk of viral transmission
Risks	• Reduction of quality of life from adverse drug effects, including headaches, occasional dizziness, weight gain, bone loss, and more serious ones such as swelling of the mouth and tongue as well as liver and kidney damage • Drug interactions with other medications, including HIV medicines • Limitations of future options for therapy if drug resistance develops in current agents • Potential for transmission of drug-resistant virus • Limitation of future drug choices because of the development of resistance • Potential long-term toxicity of therapy • Unknown duration of effectiveness of current therapies

Source: Panel on Antiretroviral Guidelines for Adults and Adolescents. (2022). Guidelines for the use of antiretroviral agents in adults and adolescents with HIV. Department of Health and Human Services. https://clinicalinfo.hiv.gov/sites/default/files/guidelines/documents/adult-adolescent-arv/guidelines-adult-adolescent-arv.pdf; Thompson, M. A., Horberg, M. A., Agwu, A. L., Colasanti, J. A., Jain, M. K., Short, W. R., Singh, T., & Aberg, J. A. (2021). Primary care guidance for persons with human immunodeficiency virus: 2020 update by the HIV Medicine Association of the Infectious Diseases Society of America. Clinical Infectious Diseases, 73(11), e3572–e3605. https://doi.org/10.1093/cid/ciaa1391

Box 31.3 AIDS-Defining Illnesses

- CD4$^+$ count below 200 cells/mm^3
- Candidiasis, esophageal, tracheal, bronchial, or pulmonary
- Cervical cancer, invasive
- Coccidioidomycosis, disseminated or extrapulmonary
- Cryptococcosis, extrapulmonary
- Cryptosporidiosis with diarrhea for more than 1 month
- Cytomegalovirus of any organ other than liver, spleen, or lymph nodes
- HIV encephalopathy
- Herpes simplex infection: chronic ulcers of more than 1 month's duration; or bronchitis, pneumonitis, or esophagitis
- Histoplasmosis, disseminated or extrapulmonary
- Isosporiasis with diarrhea for more than 1 month
- Kaposi sarcoma
- Lymphoma, Burkitt, immunoblastic, primary central nervous system
- *Mycobacterium avium* complex or *Mycobacterium kansasii*, disseminated or extrapulmonary
- *Mycobacterium*, other or unidentified species, disseminated or extrapulmonary
- *Pneumocystis* pneumonia
- Pneumonia, recurrent bacterial with more than two episodes in 12 months
- Progressive multifocal leukoencephalopathy (PML)
- *Salmonella* septicemia
- Toxoplasmosis of internal organ or brain
- Wasting syndrome caused by HIV

Source: Panel on Antiretroviral Guidelines for Adults and Adolescents. (2022). Guidelines for the use of antiretroviral agents in adults and adolescents with HIV. Department of Health and Human Services. https://clinicalinfo.hiv.gov/sites/default/files/guidelines/documents/adult-adolescent-arv/guidelines-adult-adolescent-arv.pdf; Centers for Disease Control and Prevention. (1992). 1993 revised classification system for HIV infection and expanded surveillance case definition for AIDS among adolescents and adults. MMWR Morbidity and Mortality Weekly Report Recommendations and Reports, 41(RR-17), 1–19. https://www.cdc.gov/mmwr/preview/mmwrhtml/00018871.htm

ART is recommended for all persons with HIV. All patients initiating ART must receive thorough education and counseling regarding this decision. Patients must be fully informed and willing to initiate therapy; therefore, providers must assess the patient's readiness to begin ART. Although this seems to be an obvious consideration in any therapeutic regimen, it is of particular importance in initiating ART. The patient must be reasonably likely to adhere to the regimen as prescribed, although no patient should automatically have ART withheld based on behaviors that some may assume are associated with a likelihood of nonadherence (Panel on Antiretroviral Guidelines for Adults and Adolescents, 2022). Thorough patient education and counsel and ongoing follow-up counsel and support increase the likelihood of effective adherence to ART.

While ART is recommended for all persons with HIV, persons with the following conditions should start ART immediately: pregnancy, advanced HIV disease (AIDS), HIV-related illnesses and coinfections, and early HIV infection (the first 6 months after infection). All patients who show signs of HIV disease progression should be offered ART. These signs can include thrush, wasting, unexplained fever for more than 2 weeks, and symptoms of opportunistic infection. Any patient with AIDS-defining criteria (Box 31.3) should be offered ART. Initiating ART can improve immune function/recovery, potentially improve treatment outcome for opportunistic

infection, and reduce HIV transmission (Panel on Antiretroviral Guidelines for Adults and Adolescents, 2022). For most patients with opportunistic infection ART should be initiated before or at the same time as diagnosis of the infection; however, two exceptions are cryptococcal and tuberculous meningitis, which may warrant a delay before initiation of ART. Providers should consult a specialist and refer to the Panel on Antiretroviral Guidelines for Adults and Adolescents (2022).

Specific Antiretroviral Therapy

The development of effective ART represents a significant scientific achievement in controlling HIV and prolonging survival. A caveat is necessary before discussing ART in the treatment of HIV infection: The research and development of new therapies and the testing of different combinations of therapies can quickly change the state of the science. APRNs are encouraged to use reliable sources (e.g., the CDC, U.S. Department of Health and Human Services, and the National

Institutes of Health) available on the Internet for the most current recommendations and practices in HIV care.

Highly active antiretroviral therapy (HAART) consists of two or more antiretroviral agents used in combination to try to decrease an individual's plasma viral load to an undetectable level. Issues to be considered when choosing an antiretroviral regimen include (a) the patient's preferences, daily routines, and social support as they influence her ability to adhere to a particular regimen; (b) the side effects of the medications, including evaluation of the patient's other medical conditions that may increase the risk of certain adverse effects; (c) any drug interactions with other medications the woman may be taking; (d) pregnancy status or desire to become pregnant; and (e) HIV lab tests such as CD4 count, HIV viral load, and resistance test results (Panel on Antiretroviral Guidelines for Adults and Adolescents, 2022). Currently, eight classes of antiretroviral medications are available, but we will discuss six classes: nucleoside reverse transcriptase inhibitors (NRTIs), non-nucleoside reverse transcriptase inhibitors (NNRTIs; e.g., efavirenz, delavirdine, and nevirapine), protease inhibitors (PIs; e.g., atazanavir, darunavir, lopinavir), integrase strand transfer inhibitors (INSTIs), a CCR5 antagonist (e.g., maraviroc), and fusion inhibitors (e.g., enfuvirtide; Panel on Antiretroviral Guidelines for Adults and Adolescents, 2022). NRTIs and NNRTIs work by disrupting the work of reverse transcriptase. Reverse transcriptase is an enzyme that changes the virus's chemical genetic message into a form that can be easily inserted inside the nucleus of an infected cell. This process occurs early in the viral replication cycle. Reverse transcriptase inhibitors interrupt the duplication of genetic material necessary for the virus to replicate. PIs work inside infected cells late in the HIV-replication process. After HIV has infected a cell, it continues relentlessly to replicate itself. However, the newly produced genetic material, in the form of long chains of proteins and enzymes, is functional only after these long chains have been cut into shorter pieces by the HIV enzyme protease. By inhibiting the function of protease, PIs reduce the number of new infectious copies of HIV. INSTIs work by disrupting the work of the integrase enzyme. Integrase combines HIV's DNA with the DNA of the host's cell. INSTIs are an important class of antiviral medications that are currently in the forefront of treatment options.

Preferred initial therapies consist of two NRTIs plus an INSTI (e.g., bictegravir/emtricitabine/tenofovir alafenamide or dolutegravir/abacavir/lamivudine) and one INSTI plus one NRTI (e.g., dolutegravir plus lamivudine; except in persons with a viral load >500,000; Panel on Antiretroviral Guidelines for Adults and Adolescents, 2022). Refer to the Guidelines for the Use of Antiretroviral Agents in Adults and Adolescents with HIV for a more detailed list of initial combination regimens for treatment-naïve persons. Preferred alternatives consist of two NRTIs plus an NNRTI or a PI boosted by cobicistat or ritonavir. Combination ART medications work together effectively to reduce the circulating viral load. With two different points of disruption of the replication cycle, concurrent use of these medications represents the best hope of managing HIV infection as a chronic illness.

ART medications have demonstrated a high level of effectiveness in reducing viral load in persons who are adherent. Optimal adherence to ART can be challenging for some

persons with HIV as a result of several multilevel factors (e.g., stigma, mental health issues, and lack of access to care, health insurance, transportation, and social support). Poor adherence can result in detectable viral load, virologic failure, and ultimately drug resistance. Managing persons with resistance is complex and may require consultation with an HIV expert. Disparities are well documented. Compared to other persons with HIV, women with HIV have lower viral suppression rates (CDC, 2023). Disparities are even more evident among Black or African American women with HIV with lower rates of adherence and viral suppression compared to the White and Hispanic female counterparts (Geter et al., 2019). Reasons for poor adherence and viral suppression among Black/African American women include stigma, discrimination, lack of child care and transportation, limited access to care, and low levels of resilience (Geter et al., 2019). Intense patient counseling to ensure maximal adherence to HAART is one crucial component of care for persons with HIV to prevent development of resistant virus and to maximize viral suppression. Identifying barriers and implementing evidence-based strategies to address social and structural barriers are also important components of care to maximize viral suppression.

Patients on ART may have other chronic conditions requiring medications and frequent monitoring of lab values. For any patient for whom ART is initiated, the interactions between HIV medications and other medications the patient takes regularly must be examined. Furthermore, scheduling of medications to minimize untoward interactions is a critical component of care for these patients.

Occupational and nonoccupational postexposure prophylaxis (PEP) with ART is recommended for people who are HIV-negative who have an exposure to HIV during sex, persons who were sexually assaulted, persons who shared needles or other equipment to inject drugs, and healthcare workers exposed through a needlestick injury or cut with a contaminated object, contact of a mucous membrane or nonintact skin with potentially infectious material or body fluids, or prolonged exposure (several minutes or more) of intact skin to potentially infectious materials (Workowski et al., 2015). PEP must be started within 72 hours after an exposure and taken daily for 28 days. Clinicians should consult an expert prior to starting ART for PEP. Clinicians may contact the National Clinician Consultation Center for PEP consultation (CDC, 1992).

Adherence to Antiretroviral Therapy

Adherence to ART is crucial. A critical nursing challenge is to teach and counsel persons with HIV in adhering to the prescribed medication regimen. Failure to adhere to an ART protocol results in a rapid increase in viral load with concurrent immune system damage. The likelihood of developing AIDS is directly related to viral load. Simply, the presence of more virus means more immune system damage and a worsening ability to fend off aggressive opportunistic infections.

The development of ART-resistant strains of virus is a primary concern in treatment failure and represents a serious sequela of nonadherence. Cross-resistance among treatment options limits the availability of effective therapy. Furthermore, the transmission of resistant strains complicates therapies for treatment-naïve patients, who may have few options available from the onset of the infection. Patients who fail to follow their ART regimen as prescribed face the risk of developing a resistant strain of virus. The danger of nonadherence is dual: First, an increased viral load with a resistant virus is an alarming clinical situation associated with a poor outcome for the patient. Second, additional treatments for opportunistic infections, with their concomitant side effects, will be necessary as symptoms of advancing disease manifest themselves.

Nurse practitioners have a distinct role in the preparation of patients as they begin ART. Effective nursing care must take into consideration the following issues related to the initiation of a treatment protocol that demands careful adherence:

- *What is the patient's understanding of HIV?* Nurse practitioners in settings that see HIV patients regularly may take for granted that patients have a more thorough understanding of HIV than they really do. With much of the knowledge about HIV filtered through rumor, innuendo, and incomplete or misleading media reports, patients may be woefully lacking in substantive knowledge of their disease. Recent developments in ART have allowed the healthcare professional to understand HIV as a chronic and manageable disease; however, this understanding has not reached all segments of the public. Emphasizing the chronic rather than fatal nature of the infection may help patients to reframe their understanding of the illness. Basic to the establishment of an effective nursing care plan is the thorough assessment of the patient's understanding of the disease, including its meaning to the patient.

- *Can the patient understand how the medications are to be taken?* The patient may have a limited ability to understand the issues surrounding ART and adherence. It is incumbent on the nurse practitioner to ensure that the patient or the patient's caregiver understands the importance of taking the medications as ordered. The nurse practitioner may have to be creative in devising charts, journals, pill boxes, or other reminders for the patient and the caregiver to enhance the chances of successful adherence.

- *What is the patient's daily schedule, and how does ART fit into the schedule?* The nurse practitioner must consider shift work, sleep–wake patterns, mealtimes, and family responsibilities in assisting the patient in establishing a medication schedule to which the patient can adhere. If is it clear that the patient is likely to fail in following a complex schedule of medications in the context of a busy and active life, the nurse should consult with the physician or nurse practitioner in identifying alternative medications that may be more suitable for the patient. For example, the nurse or nurse practitioner can assess if the patient is eligible to switch to a single-tablet regimen.

- *Are there any social constraints on the patient related to taking ART?* ART represents the constant presence of HIV, an incurable infection that is fraught with social implications in addition to its health implications. Some persons find that the frequent reminder of the infection through taking ART is onerous and psychologically painful, lessening the likelihood of long-term adherence.

Many women keep their HIV infection a secret from their closest family members and friends. The presence of ART medications in the home increases the risk that someone will discover the patient's diagnosis. The patient must be counseled about that possibility and encouraged to think about the social implications if the HIV is discovered.

Beginning ART represents a small step in going public with the diagnosis. The patient must understand that the pharmacist filling the prescriptions will know the patient's diagnosis. The patient may prefer to have prescriptions filled in a place that is likely to offer more anonymity, such as a hospital pharmacy, HIV clinic pharmacy, or a discount store pharmacy with a high volume of business. Finances may be an important consideration for the patient, who may have to seek outside sources of funds to enable the purchase of ART.

The goal for nurse practitioners is always the same; patients will adhere to their ART schedules as evidenced by decreasing and ultimately nondetectable viral loads, maintaining that level for as long as possible. Simply handing a patient several prescriptions for expensive medications requiring complicated schedules and having a number of uncomfortable and potentially serious side effects is likely to result in treatment failure. Nurse practitioners are in a unique position to make a substantial positive impact on the lives of persons living with HIV by spending time in careful assessment, planning, intervening, and goal setting.

Prevention of Opportunistic Infections

In the 40 years since the identification of HIV/AIDS, great improvements have been made in the prevention of opportunistic infections that ravaged the earliest victims of the HIV pandemic. Increasingly, aggressive use of ART has helped in maintaining the immune systems of persons with HIV, reducing the need for routine chemoprophylaxis against opportunistic infections. Furthermore, infections such as *Pneumocystis* pneumonia (PCP), toxoplasmosis, and other bacterial diseases have been effectively prevented in patients requiring chemoprophylaxis. A single daily dose of double-strength trimethoprim-sulfamethoxazole (Septra, Bactrim) has reduced the incidence of PCP, toxoplasmosis, and bacterial infections (Panel on Antiretroviral Guidelines for Adults and Adolescents, 2022). This is a particularly useful medication because it is effective, generally well tolerated, simple to take, and inexpensive. However, for those who are sensitive to or allergic to trimethoprim-sulfamethoxazole, dapsone is an effective alternative.

Persons with HIV should follow some specific, although not overly restrictive, guidelines regarding minimizing exposure to potential sources of opportunistic infection. For women who are likely to be managing the care of the home and children, understanding how to preserve and maintain her own health while fulfilling her household and parenting obligations is very important. Nurse practitioners should counsel women in basic good hygiene practices that can minimize the risk of many exposures. These practices include:

- Thorough handwashing with water and soap after toileting, after assisting children in toileting, and at intervals throughout the day. Paper towels in the bathroom provide a more sanitary means of drying hands than a hand towel that stays damp and may be used by others.

- Minimizing exposure to animal or human waste by using disposable gloves. This includes wearing disposable gloves when doing yard work and when changing a baby's diaper.
- Drinking water only from sources known to be dependable and clean; avoiding ingestion of water from lakes, rivers, and recreational swimming pools.
- Avoiding contact with animals in specific circumstances:
  - Pets younger than 6 months old (increased likelihood of exposure to parasites)
  - Any animal with diarrhea
  - All reptiles: turtles, lizards, snakes, iguanas (risk of salmonella exposure)
  - Situations that may expose the patient to bird droppings
- Treating cats with special care:
  - Adopting cats that are more than 1 year old (risk of exposure to bacteria and parasites)
  - Daily cleaning of litter box, preferably by a person without HIV
  - Keeping the cat indoors, not allowing the cat to hunt
  - Avoiding cat scratches or bites and washing scratches or bites thoroughly and immediately
  - Controlling fleas on cats
- Avoiding raw or undercooked eggs, poultry, meat, or seafood, and preventing cross-contamination by using separate kitchen utensils and cutting boards when processing these foods. Cutting boards should be thoroughly scrubbed after each use. Careful kitchen and cooking practices can decrease greatly the risk of foodborne infection.

In addition, HIV-positive patients should be counseled to consult with a healthcare provider before traveling to developing countries that may result in exposure to opportunistic pathogens. The CDC website (https://wwwnc.cdc.gov/travel) provides travelers with up-to-date information regarding endemic diseases and recommendations regarding vaccinations before travel.

Basic health practices, such as family planning (Table 31.7), adequate sleep and rest, good nutrition, exercise, smoking cessation, and avoidance of stress should not be overlooked in counseling HIV-positive persons. Family planning choices and possible birth control options should be discussed. Vertical transmission and medical interventions should be addressed. Seven to 8 hours of sleep a night is ideal for most adults. This amount may be difficult to achieve; however, nurse practitioners can assist the patient in developing a sleep schedule that allows adequate rest. Principles of good nutrition apply to persons with HIV and, in fact, are especially necessary to provide adequate vitamins, minerals, electrolytes, and protein. Persons with HIV who are significantly under- or overweight should be encouraged to improve their nutritional status through support groups, nutritional counseling, or other means of weight management. Persons with a high intake of alcohol should be counseled to decrease their intake, because alcohol does not have any significant nutritional value, can interfere with vitamin absorption, and contains excess calories. Furthermore, chronic alcohol abuse can exacerbate liver problems. It is important to note

TABLE 31.7 Contraception for Women With HIV

METHOD	BENEFITS	DISADVANTAGES
Male condom	Protects against STIs and HIV; protects partner	Partner cooperation required
Female condom	Protects against STIs and HIV; protects partner	Partner cooperation helpful
Oral contraceptive	Effective when used consistently	Some HIV medications may reduce the effectiveness of hormonal contraceptives No HIV protection for partner No STI protection Risk of cervical ectopy Possible interaction with antibiotics and antiretrovirals
Depo-Provera injection	Effective Limited compliance needed	No STI protection No HIV protection for partner
Intrauterine device	Effective	No HIV protection for partner No STI protection
Diaphragm	Effective Female controlled	Leave in 6–8 hours after ejaculation May increase risk of urinary tract infection
Patch	Avoids first-pass metabolism Easy to use	No STI protection No HIV protection for partner
Tubal ligation	One-time procedure Permanent	No STI protection No HIV protection for partner

STIs, sexually transmitted infections.
Source: HIV.gov. (2023). Recommendations for the use of antiretroviral drugs during pregnancy interventions to reduce perinatal HIV transmission in the United States. *https://clinicalinfo.hiv.gov/en/guidelines/perinatal/whats-new; Cotter, A., Potter, I. E., & Tessler, N. (2006). Management of HIV/AIDS in women. In J. Beal, J. J. Orrick, & K. Alfonso (Eds.),* HIV/AIDS primary care guide *(pp. 533–546). Crown House.*

that excessive alcohol intake will impair one's ability to make good judgments regarding health and sexual behaviors and to adhere to the ART regimen.

Exercise improves muscle tone and cardiovascular health and reduces stress—all important factors in maintaining a state of health. HIV-positive persons should be encouraged to engage in some form of exercise on a regular basis. Nurse practitioners can assist the patient in identifying simple means of increasing activity, even if the patient is somewhat debilitated or reluctant to engage in regular workouts. Walking is a simple form of exercise that is within the abilities of most persons and can be incorporated into one's daily routine with little effort.

Patients should be encouraged and supported in their efforts to stop smoking. In addition to the well-documented negative effects of smoking on health, the propensity of

HIV-positive persons to pulmonary infections makes smoking cessation imperative. Nurse practitioners should be cognizant of the difficulty of stopping smoking and support any efforts the patient makes to decrease the number of cigarettes per day. However, the nurse practitioner is also in an excellent position to help the patient find therapies, group support, and other means to stop smoking.

Stress reduction plays an important role in health maintenance. Nurse practitioners can assist patients in identifying changeable stressors and in developing strategies to decrease overall stress. Many persons with HIV have significant social stressors related to poverty and other sociocultural issues that may be difficult to ameliorate. Nurse practitioners can help these patients understand management of their HIV infection to lessen the effects of HIV on their lives. An important nursing intervention, then, is to help HIV patients understand the chronic, manageable aspects of the infection. Careful planning with patients in terms of making regular clinic visits, initiating and adhering to an ART regimen, and improving general health behaviors can be an effective means of reducing some of the HIV-related stresses for these patients.

SPECIAL POPULATIONS

Women With HIV of Childbearing Age

Special considerations must be taken into account when managing HIV in women of childbearing age. The goals of their treatment include improving overall health and quality of life, minimizing disease progression, minimizing unwanted pregnancies, preventing heterosexual transmission, and avoiding prescribing medical treatments with teratogenic potential. Comprehensive reproductive and sexual health counseling are essential for women with HIV. There are benefits and drawbacks of various contraceptives. Some HIV medications may reduce the effectiveness of hormonal contraceptives (see Table 31.7). Barrier methods are necessary for HIV and STI prevention. The effect of hormonal contraceptives on viral shedding is not clear, and the bioavailability of ethinyl estradiol in hormonal contraceptives may be significantly reduced by some antiretroviral medications, including ritonavir, cobicistat, or ritonavir-boosted protease inhibitors. Women using oral contraceptive methods, an intrauterine device, or tubal ligation should be counseled to use a barrier method as well to reduce the risk of contracting an STI or transmitting HIV or an STI to her partner. It is essential that APRNs be aware of the drug interactions between oral contraceptives and ART, because some of the interactions may compromise the effectiveness of either the contraceptive method by lowering oral contraceptive drug levels (e.g., nevirapine, ritonavir) or lowering the effectiveness of the ART (Panel on Antiretroviral Guidelines for Adults and Adolescents, 2022). Clinicians should refer to Recommendations for the Use of Antiretroviral Drugs During Pregnancy and Interventions to Reduce Perinatal HIV Transmission in the United States (HIV.gov, 2023).

HIV in Pregnancy

Childbearing in women with HIV is a complex issue to be addressed carefully and thoroughly by clinicians working with this population. Reproduction is a major life activity and refusing to help someone based solely on their HIV status is considered illegal discrimination. Couples with HIV or serodiscordant couples should not be denied assisted reproductive techniques based solely on their seropositive status (Chambers et al., 2021; Jaideep et al., 2021).

Preconception counseling for women known to have HIV is an important means of optimizing maternal health before pregnancy. Elements of preconception counseling for women with HIV should include appropriate contraceptive methods to reduce unintended pregnancy; safer sex practices; avoidance of alcohol, illicit drug use, and cigarette smoking; risk factors of perinatal transmission and effective strategies to reduce and prevent transmission; and potential effects of HIV on pregnancy and maternal health (Panel on Antiretroviral Guidelines for Adults and Adolescents, 2022). Elements to be considered in providing care to women with HIV considering pregnancy include avoiding antiretroviral agents with a potential for teratogenicity, achieving and sustaining suppressed HIV-1 RNA, evaluating the need for prophylaxis or preconception immunizations (influenza, pneumococcal, hepatitis B), optimizing nutritional status and folic acid supplementation, evaluating for opportunistic infections and initiating appropriate treatments or prophylactic regimens, screening for psychiatric and substance abuse disorders and domestic violence, standard genetic and reproductive health screening, and planning for pediatric and perinatal consultation (Panel on Antiretroviral Guidelines for Adults and Adolescents, 2022).

Protection of the health of the pregnant woman and the fetus is the primary therapeutic goal in all prenatal and perinatal care, and this goal is the same for all women regardless of their HIV status. For women with HIV, minimizing the risk of vertical transmission is an additional therapeutic goal. Without intervention, HIV is effectively transmitted from mother to child. Before antiretroviral prophylaxis use, vertical transmission rates ranged from 13% to 32% in industrialized countries. Transmission can occur at any time during a pregnancy; however, without any prevention measures, most transmission occurs during the intrapartum period (HIV.gov, 2023). Factors affecting vertical transmission are found in Table 31.8. Perinatal transmission of HIV to the fetus has decreased significantly in the past decade to less than 1% in the United States because of the prophylactic administration of antiretroviral prophylaxis to pregnant women in the prenatal and perinatal periods. Healthcare providers should follow the same guidelines used for women who are not pregnant (CDC, 2022a). During labor, women take HIV medicines to reduce the risk of mother-to-child transmission. The newborn infant then receives HIV medicines from birth up to 6 weeks of life, beginning within 6 hours after birth (Panel on Treatment of HIV-Infected Pregnant Women and Prevention of Perinatal Transmission, 2012). Breastfeeding is not recommended in the United States (Panel on Treatment of HIV-Infected Pregnant Women and Prevention of Perinatal Transmission, 2022).

TABLE 31.8 Factors Affecting Vertical HIV Transmission

DISEASE-RELATED FACTORS	MATERNAL HEALTH AND SOCIAL FACTORS	OBSTETRIC FACTORS	INFANT FACTORS
Maternal HIV-1 RNA (plasma and genital tract) Maternal CD4$^+$ count Viral genotype and phenotype Viral resistance mutations	Clinical stage STIs during pregnancy Vitamin A deficiency Ongoing intrauterine device Tobacco and substance use Multiple sexual partners during pregnancy	Duration of ruptured membranes Chorioamnionitis from use of invasive antenatal procedures Mode of delivery	Prematurity Breastfeeding Developing immune system Gastrointestinal factors

STIs, sexually transmitted infections.
Source: Amin, O., Powers, J., Bricker, K. M., & Chahroudi, A. (2021). Understanding viral and immune interplay during vertical transmission of HIV: Implications for cure. Frontiers in Immunology, 12, 757400. https://doi.org/10.3389/fimmu.2021.757400

Use of ART during pregnancy involves two aims: (1) improve maternal health and (2) reduce mother-to-child transmission. As with nonpregnant women, decisions regarding therapy initiation and selection should be based on standard clinical criteria, applicable to all adults with HIV. Balancing potentially conflicting needs of mother and infant health may be challenging because data regarding the safety, efficacy, and pharmacokinetics of ART in pregnancy may be limited, particularly with newer drugs. Women who are pregnant or considering pregnancy must be counseled regarding the potential short- and long-term risks and benefits associated with antiretroviral management strategies. Clinicians should refer to Recommendations for Use of Antiretroviral Drugs During Pregnancy (Panel on Treatment of HIV-Infected Pregnant Women and Prevention of Perinatal Transmission, 2012).

Before the widespread use of HAART, elective cesarean was routinely recommended as the preferred delivery method for women with HIV. Whether cesarean delivery continues to be the optimal method of delivery today, given that current transmission rates are very low and multiagent chemoprophylaxis is the norm, has not been established (Panel on Treatment of HIV-Infected Pregnant Women and Prevention of Perinatal Transmission, 2012). The Panel on Treatment of HIV-Infected Pregnant Women and Prevention of Perinatal Transmission (2012) advise that women with HIV-1 RNA greater than 1,000 copies/mL in the third trimester should be counseled regarding the potential benefits of elective cesarean delivery.

Breastfeeding has been implicated in the transmission of HIV. The current recommendation is that HIV-positive mothers in the United States formula-feed their infants to avoid possible transmission of the virus (Panel on Treatment of HIV-Infected Pregnant Women and Prevention of Perinatal Transmission, 2012). However, in developing countries, women may not have access to safe alternatives to breast milk for their infants.

Mothers face the difficult issue regarding guardianship of their children in the event of their death. Women with HIV are more likely to be poor and may have limited financial and social support. A single mother may have little or no contact with the father of her children, or he may be a poor candidate for parenting the children full-time. Making choices regarding her children's welfare may be difficult at best, and impossible if she has severely limited familial or social support. She may face the possibility that her children will be placed into foster care if she becomes very ill or dies. Nurse practitioners

can assist HIV-infected mothers in expressing fear and grief over this possible, if not likely, scenario. Furthermore, nurse practitioners can assist the woman in seeking community services dedicated to managing the legal affairs of persons with HIV if those services are available. HIV case managers at the local level can also assist HIV-infected women in making decisions about the eventual care of their children. Women who address this issue early after their diagnosis may feel relieved that the issue of guardianship is resolved and formalized.

Incarcerated Women

Incarcerated women are 15 times more likely to be HIV infected than women in the general population because the behaviors for which they are incarcerated place them at higher risk (CDC, 2015a, 2015c). They are often victims of substance abuse including injection drugs, have partners who are IDUs, have experienced intimate partner violence, or have been forced to have unprotected sex and/or trade sex for food or housing. Often, they have few or no marketable job skills, have little or no access to HIV prevention methods, and are afraid to ask their partners to use protection.

Prevention challenges include a lack of awareness about HIV and lack of resources for HIV testing and treatment in prisons. Although prisons are more likely to have HIV programs, most incarcerated individuals are detained in jails (Workowski et al., 2015). Most jail inmates are released within 72 hours and the rapid turnover in jail populations contributes to a lack of testing and connection with treatment. Additionally, inmate concerns regarding privacy and fear of stigma lead to a lack of disclosure of high-risk behaviors.

Transgender Women

Persons who are transgender identify as a gender that is not the same as the sex assigned to them at birth. Transgender women identify as women but were born with male anatomy. Transgender women account for 2% of HIV infection in the United States and most new infections are among Black/African American transgender women and transgender women living in the U.S. South (CDC, 2021a). Transgender persons are more likely to access care when services are provided in a gender-affirming environment (e.g., use of chosen name and pronoun). Providers caring for transgender women should have knowledge of their patients' current anatomy and patterns of sexual behavior before counseling them about STI/HIV prevention. For transgender women with HIV, clinicians should provide comprehensive care based on the personalized needs of the individual.

SUMMARY

HIV is associated with multifaceted dimensions of morbidity, mortality, and societal costs that are often disproportionately experienced by women and their infants. The need for prevention is critical, and nurse practitioners must assume a primary role in helping women decrease risky behaviors and increase protective practices as well as HIV testing.

FUTURE DIRECTIONS

To decrease the burden of HIV on women, screening, early detection, and treatment are essential. Again, nurse practitioners are a first-line defense in providing these services. Finally, treatment of HIV can lessen the impact of the disease. Education and counseling are essential to ensure that women obtain the maximum benefit from treatment.

REFERENCES

References for this chapter are online and available at https://connect.springerpub.com/content/book/978-0-8261-6722-4/part/part03/chapter/ch31

CHAPTER 32

Human Papillomavirus

Elizabeth A. Kostas-Polston,[*] Versie Johnson-Mallard, and Naomi Jay

ANOGENITAL HUMAN PAPILLOMAVIRUS–RELATED DISEASE

There was a time when our understanding of the human papillomavirus (HPV) and its role in anogenital disease was limited. The discovery of the Pap smear 75 years ago by Dr. George Papanicolaou led to the subsequent discovery made by Dr. Harald zur Hausen regarding HPV as *the* necessary cause of cervical cancer and other anogenital diseases. Clinical evidence supporting cervical cancer screening guidelines—perhaps the most successful cancer screening model in the United States (National Cancer Institute [NCI], 2014)—have helped to make great strides in our understanding of the natural history of HPV, its association with sexual transmission, and the role it plays in anogenital disease and cancer. HPV infection may lead to disease and cancer in primarily anogenital sites (e.g., cervix, vulva, vagina, anus, and penis). HPV has more recently been associated with oropharyngeal and other head and neck diseases and cancer. This chapter focuses on anatomic sites where HPV infection wreaks much of its havoc in women, namely, the cervix and the anus.

Definition and Scope

According to the Centers for Disease Control and Prevention (CDC), HPV infection is the most common sexually transmitted infection (STI) in the United States (CDC, 2015, 2021). It is estimated that in 2015 there were 79 million individuals in the United Stated infected with HPV. It is estimated that each year in the United States approximately 37,300 new cases of HPV-related cancers are diagnosed (CDC, 2021). Additionally, 14 million people will become infected yearly with HPV (CDC, 2015, 2021). In fact, it is postulated that greater than 90% of sexually active individuals will develop an HPV infection during their lifetime (CDC, 2015; Chesson et al., 2014).

HPV-associated morbidity includes external genital warts (EGWs) and cancer precursors. Cancer precursors may lead to HPV-associated cancer. A necessary requisite for transformation to occur (from a precursor to carcinoma) is persistent infection, which is not a common occurrence (~10% persistence; CDC, 2021). The female anatomic sites infected by HPV and leading to carcinogenesis are provided in Table 32.1.

Etiology

Once cervical cancer was the leading cause of cancer death in U.S. women until cervical cancer screening was initiated as standard for women. It is widely accepted that HPV infection is the cause of almost all cases of precancerous and cancerous lesions of the cervix. There are more than 200 genotypes of HPV, of which 14 genotypes are associated with cervical cancer (high-risk oncogenic genotypes 16, 18, 31, 33, 35, 39, 45, 51, 52, 56, 58, 59, 66, and 68; NCI, 2022). The more than 200 genotypes include low-risk or nononcogenic types that often cause benign changes and mild cellular abnormality, and the high-risk or oncogenic types that have the potential to cause neoplasia and cancer. Although most HPV cases are subclinical, present no physical symptoms, and clear spontaneously within 2 years, others develop into benign papilloma or malignant cancers (Markowitz et al., 2014). HPV 16 and HPV 18 are particularly of interest, as 70% of HPV-associated cervical cancers are associated with at least one of the two strains (Uyar & Rader, 2014).

HPV infection is epidemic, but cancer is a rare occurrence; the infection is usually transient and clears as a result of an individual's immune response (Moscicki et al., 2012). Progression to cancer occurs when an HPV infection with a high-risk HPV type persists over time. Persistent infection is defined as the detection of the same HPV type two or more times within a given interval of time.

The HPV type affects both the likelihood of persistence and the risk of progression to precancer. HPV 16 persists

---

[*]The opinions and assertions expressed herein are those of the author(s) and do not necessarily reflect the official policy or position of the Uniformed Services University or the Department of Defense.

TABLE 32.1 U.S. Annual Human Papillomavirus Cancer Cases in Women: Anatomic Site

LOCATION	CASES IN WOMEN
Oropharynx	2,300
Cervix	11,100
Anus	4,700
Vulva	2,900
Vagina	700
Total	**21,700**

Source: Adapted from Centers for Disease Control and Prevention. (n.d.). How many cancers are linked with HPV each year? Retrieved July 8, 2023, from https://www.cdc.gov/cancer/hpv/statistics/cases.htm

longer than other types and also is especially carcinogenic, with a risk of cervical intraepithelial neoplasia (CIN)-3 of 40% at 5 years (Moscicki et al., 2006). High-risk HPV can cause neoplastic changes of other lower genital tract sites (e.g., vagina, vulva, anus, and penis) as well as nongenital sites (e.g., oral cavity, esophagus, and oropharynx). We still have much to learn about the impact of oncogenic HPV in the carcinogenesis of nongenital cancers.

HUMAN PAPILLOMAVIRUS TYPES

The most common anogenital low-risk (nononcogenic) HPV types are 6 and 11 (which cause 90% of genital warts), and types 40, 42, 43, 44, 53, 54, 61, 72, 73, and 81. Most low-risk HPV infections clear spontaneously within the first year after infection; however, some may take up to 2 years to clear. As previously mentioned, high-risk (oncogenic) HPV genotypes are associated with cervical neoplasia and cancer. HPV 16 is most commonly associated with cervical high-grade squamous intraepithelial lesions (HSIL) and invasive cancers. Although women infected with HPV 16 are at greater risk for developing cervical HSIL, most HPV 16 infections will not develop into abnormal cellular changes. HPV 18 is most commonly associated with cervical adenocarcinoma. This type of cervical cancer is more difficult to detect on cytology because it occurs in the upper portion of the endocervical canal. For the same reason, it is also more difficult to detect adenocarcinoma using colposcopy-directed biopsies.

Risk Factors

Many decades of data support that HPV is a skin cell virus and is transmitted through skin-to-skin contact (Hogenwoning et al., 2003; Manhart & Koutsky, 2002; Winer et al., 2006). It is important for healthcare providers to remember that there is no way to determine when or by whom an individual was infected with HPV.

Clinical Presentation

In most cases, HPV infection is transient and has no clinical manifestations or sequelae. In cases of condylomata acuminata (genital warts), lesions may be visible. However, it is important for healthcare providers to note that this may not always be the

case. Condylomas develop because of exposure to HPV types 6 and 11, which are low risk or nononcogenic, and may appear as flat, fleshy, or exophytic; cauliflower-like in appearance; and/or pink or hyperpigmented lesions in either squamous epithelium and/or on mucous membranes (Hogenwoning et al., 2003; Manhart & Koutsky, 2002; Winer et al., 2006).

Most often, HPV infection is detected through cervical cancer screening—specifically, because of an abnormal Pap smear or positive, high-risk HPV DNA test, which is now considered the primary screening tool for cervical cancer prevention.

Evaluation and Assessment

Collecting a thorough medical and sexual health history is the first step in evaluating risk. Smoking and the use of immunosuppressive medications, for example, significantly increase the likelihood of HPV infection persistence. Inquiring as to whether an individual has a history of abnormal cervical cytology and treatment is also an important data gathering point. The healthcare provider must become proficient and comfortable when conducting a complete sexual history. Sexual health history questions are sensitive and may be perceived to be invasive by the woman. Healthcare provider sensitivity is needed.

Physical Examination

GENITAL LESIONS

Although usually benign, genital warts are highly infectious. As a result, infection with HPV types 6 and/or 11 creates a significant amount of morbidity and healthcare costs related to treatment. Furthermore, a diagnosis of genital warts, especially in younger women, often carries with it psychological distress. Women with extensive disease are likely to have an alteration in the integrity of their immune system. This can be seen during times of pregnancy, when a woman's immune response is physiologically altered; if the HIV status of a woman changes; or if a woman begins smoking. Smoking carries a significant risk for persistent or recurrent HPV disease. Genital warts may be self-limiting and clear on their own, or may clear as a result of treatment. The development of new warts is not necessarily indicative of new infection or even reinfection, but rather may be caused by active disease that develops as a result of a persistent HPV infection.

Occasionally, a lesion with the appearance of a genital wart may be cancerous. In order to avoid missing a rare diagnosis of verrucous carcinoma or squamous cell carcinoma, healthcare providers should biopsy all atypical lesions and send for histologic evaluation. Missing such a diagnosis would be detrimental by leading to a delay in treatment, thereby leading to needless morbidity or even death.

Differential Diagnosis

Disease caused by HPV infection, unless an overt genital wart, does not usually cause visible changes that can readily be noted on inspection and physical examination. It is important to differentiate a woman's normal anatomy from physical changes that may suggest HPV infection or disease.

Physical findings which may suggest current infection or disease include all of the following:

- Micropapilliferous and microfilamentous changes of the micropapillomatosis labialis
- Skin tags, hymenal remnants
- Raised pigmented red, dark, or white, or cauliflower-like lesions on the external genitalia
- Nevi
- Dermatoses (e.g., lichen sclerosus)
- Melanomas
- Molluscum contagiosum
- Verrucous carcinoma

CERVICAL CANCER

In 2023, it is estimated that 13,960 new cases of cervical cancer will be diagnosed in American women. Further, it is estimated that 4,310 women will die in the United States due to cervical cancer (American Cancer Society [ACS], 2023). These statistics are most unfortunate as cervical cancer is a *preventable* and *curable* cancer. What is more, most of the women who will succumb to cervical cancer have never undergone cervical screening. In fact, the National Breast and Cervical Cancer Early Detection Program (NBCCEDP) has put into place strategies to help low-income, uninsured, and underinsured women gain access to timely cervical cancer screening and diagnostic services. The goal of cervical cancer screening is to identify high-grade disease early and treat for the purpose of preventing the development of cervical cancer.

Cervical Cancer Screening

The overall goal of cervical cancer screening is to identify disease early and with certainty before cervical precancerous disease develops into cancer. Cervical cancer screening is guided by two principles: (1) risk stratification—identifying who is at risk and what their risk is; and (2) disease stratification—identifying who will actually benefit from intervention. This goal is accomplished by (a) identifying, treating, and surveilling high-grade cervical cancer precursors (cervical HSIL), thereby reducing a woman's risk of developing invasive cancer; and (b) avoiding unnecessary treatment or overtreatment of benign and transient HPV infections and cancer precursor lesions that most likely will regress. Loop electrosurgical excision procedure (LEEP) and cold knife conization (CKC) are associated with adverse obstetric outcomes, which include preterm delivery and perinatal death (Khan & Smith-McCune, 2014). Currently, international and U.S. national cervical screening guidelines differ (see Table 32.2). More and more, primary HPV testing plays a more important role in cervical cancer screening as it is significantly more sensitive in detecting high-grade cervical dysplasia than cytologic specimens collected on a Pap smear. At the time of print of this edition, the U.S. Preventive Services Task Force (USPSTF) cervical screening guidelines were "under revision for updates."

Diagnostic Tests

There are FDA (U.S. Food and Drug Administration)-approved screening tests available for use when screening for cervical cancer: cytology alone (conventional Pap smear or liquid-based Pap smear) and/or high-risk (HR) HPV DNA testing (Cobas HPV test, APTIMA HPV Assay, Hybrid

TABLE 32.2 Cervical Cancer Screening Guidelines

The American Cancer Society - www.cancer.org/cancer/cervical-cancer/detection-diagnosis-staging/screening-tests/hpv-test.html	- The preferred test for cervical cancer screening for women ages 25–65 years is primary HPV testing - Because some HPV tests are approved by the FDA as part of a cotest, primary HPV testing may not be an option. In those instances, a cotest every 5 years or a Pap test every 3 years is recommended

The U.S. Preventive Services Task Force (USPSTF)
www.uspreventiveservicestaskforce.org/uspstf/recommendation/cervical-cancer-screening
 	
Endorsed by:
The American College of Obstetricians and Gynecologists (ACOG)
www.acog.org/clinical/clinical-guidance/practice-advisory/articles/2021/04/updated-cervical-cancer-screening-guidelines
The American Society for Colposcopy and Cervical Pathology (ASCCP)
www.asccp.org/screening-guidelines
Society of Gynecologic Oncology (SGO)
- www.sgo.org/news/sgo-endorses-acog-new-practice-advisory-of-uspstf-cervical-cancer-screening-recommendations
	- Ages 21–29
	   ○ Cytology alone every 3 years
	- Ages 30–65
	   ○ Cytology alone every 3 years, or
	   ○ FDA-approved primary HR HPV testing alone every 5 years
	   ○ Cotesting (HR HPV testing and cytology) every 5 years
	- Ages ≥66
	   ○ No screening after adequate negative prior screening results

World Health Organization
- https://www.who.int/publications/i/item/9789240040434
	- General population of women:
	   ○ Primary screening method is HPV DNA detection, beginning at age of 30, with regular testing every 5–10 years
	   ○ HPV DNA detection in a screen, triage and treat approach starting at the age of 30 years with regular screening every 5 to 10 years
	- Women living with HIV: HPV DNA detection in a screen, triage and treat approach starting at the age of 25 years with regular screening every 3 to 5 years

FDA, Food and Drug Administration; HPV, human papillomavirus; HR, high risk.

TABLE 32.3 Human Papillomavirus (HPV) DNA Tests Approved by the Food and Drug Administration

TEST	PURPOSE	INTENDED USE
Cobas HPV test (Roche Molecular Systems)	Identifies DNA from 14 high-risk genital HPV types commonly associated with cervical cancer	• Provides information about a woman's risk for developing cervical cancer • In women ≥30 years of age or women ≥21 years of age with borderline cellular results to assess indication for follow-up and/or diagnostic procedures
APTIMA HPV Assay (Gen-Probe)	Identifies RNA from 14 high-risk genital HPV types commonly associated with cervical cancer	• Provides information about a woman's risk for developing cervical cancer • Used for women ≥30 years of age or any age with borderline cytology results to determine any need for follow-up procedures
Hybrid Capture 2 High Risk HPV DNA test (Digene)	Identifies genetic DNA from HPV in cervical cells	• Detection of high-risk HPV (HR HPV) • Follow-up test when a Pap smear is mildly abnormal
Cervista HPV HR and Genfind DNA Extraction (Hologic)	Identifies DNA from 14 high-risk genital HPV types commonly associated with cervical cancer	• Determines a woman's risk for developing cervical cancer
Cervista HPV 16/18 (Hologic)	Identifies HPV genotypes 16 and 18 in cervical samples	• Determines a woman's risk for developing cervical cancer • Used for women ≥30 years of age or any age with borderline cytology results to determine indication for any follow-up procedures

Source: Adapted from LabCE. (n.d.). FDA-approved HPV tests. https://www.labce.com/spg761630_fda_approved_hpv_tests.aspx

Capture 2 High Risk HPV DNA test, and Cervista HPV HR and Genfind DNA Extraction, or Cervista HPV 16/18). Recommended screening modalities are as follows: cytology alone, HR HPV DNA testing alone, and finally cotesting using both cytology and HR HPV DNA testing (Table 32.3).

CERVICAL CYTOLOGY

Historically, cervical cytology has been the mainstay of cervical cancer prevention screening. Cervical cytology consists of two collection methods: conventional Pap (exfoliated cells are smeared onto a slide and fixed with preservative) and liquid-based thin layer (exfoliated cells are collected using an endocervical brush and then transferred into a liquid preservative). Most healthcare providers use liquid-based cytology as its sensitivity is greater when compared with conventional cytology. Liquid-based cytology is often most preferred as it allows for reflex HPV testing as well as gonorrhea and chlamydia testing. Regardless of method, a low-grade squamous intraepithelial lesion (LSIL) cytology triages many women into a low-risk category. An LSIL cytology result is typically translated to be an active HPV infection, of which most are self-limiting. In contrast, HSIL cytology identifies women who are at the greatest risk of developing an invasive cancer. Treatment of this cancer precursor is indicated to prevent transformation into invasive cancer.

HUMAN PAPILLOMAVIRUS DNA TESTING

We have identified HPV as a necessary cause of cervical cancer. What is more, women infected with HPV types 16 and 18 have a 10-fold increased risk of developing cervical cancer (Khan et al., 2005). HPV DNA testing uses advanced molecular biological methodologies for the detection of high-risk HPV. It is important that healthcare providers only use HPV DNA tests that are approved by the FDA.

COTESTING

Cotesting with cervical cytology and HPV DNA testing has been shown to increase sensitivity, thereby increasing early detection rates. An increased sensitivity translates into greater clinical confidence in the lengthening of screening intervals. In turn, lengthening screening intervals allows for transient HPV infection clearance and minimizes opportunities to overtreat.

Positive HPV DNA testing allows for risk stratification and identification in women who, for example, cytology alone was reported as normal. In these cases, a woman with a negative cytology result and a positive high-risk HPV result will require additional evaluation (e.g., colposcopy). When requesting an HPV DNA test, the healthcare provider may also request HPV genotyping (either at initial collection or after the HPV DNA test results are reported). Positive HPV types 16 and 18 genotyping results help guide the healthcare provider in further stratifying a woman's risk of developing a cancer precursor and invasive cancer.

Treatment and Management

CONDYLOMATA ACUMINATA (GENITAL WARTS)

Although the primary purpose for treating EGWs is cosmetic, it is not uncommon for individual's to experience psychological and emotional distress related to learning of their diagnosis and also side effects associated with treatment, for example, skin irritation, mild pain and mild pruritus, and reddening of the skin. For this reason, it is important for the healthcare provider to establish a trusting relationship, establish good communication, educate, and when indicated, refer for psychological evaluation (Lawrence et al., 2009; Nahidi et al., 2018).

During pregnancy, when it is physiologically normal for an individual's immune system to be suppressed, shifts in hormone levels may cause preexisting genital warts to proliferate.

TABLE 32.4 Treatment Regimens for Genital Warts

<table>
<tr><th colspan="2" style="text-align:center">RECOMMENDED REGIMENS FOR EXTERNAL GENITAL WARTS</th></tr>
<tr>
<td>Patient self-applied</td>
<td>*Podofilox* 0.5% solution or gel
Imiquimod 5% cream
Sinecatechins 15% ointment</td>
</tr>
<tr>
<td>Healthcare provider administered</td>
<td>*Cryotherapy* with liquid nitrogen or cryoprobe; repeat applications every 1–2 weeks
TCA or BCA 80%–90%
Surgical removal either by scissor excision, shave excision, curettage, or electrosurgery</td>
</tr>
<tr><th colspan="2" style="text-align:center">ALTERNATIVE REGIMENS (MORE SIDE EFFECTS, LESS DATA ON EFFICACY)</th></tr>
<tr>
<td>Recommended regimen for cervical warts</td>
<td>For those with exophytic cervical warts, a biopsy evaluation to exclude high-grade SIL must be performed before treatment is initiated. Management of exophytic cervical warts should include consultation with a specialist.</td>
</tr>
<tr>
<td>Recommended regimens for vaginal warts</td>
<td>*Cryotherapy with liquid nitrogen.* The use of a cryoprobe in the vagina is not recommended because of the risk for vaginal perforation and fistula formation.
TCA or BCA 80%–90% applied to warts. A small amount should be applied only to warts and allowed to dry, at which time a white frosting develops. If an excess amount of acid is applied, the treated area should be powdered with talc, sodium bicarbonate, or liquid soap preparations to remove unreacted acid. This treatment can be repeated weekly, if necessary.</td>
</tr>
<tr>
<td>Recommended regimens for urethral meatus warts</td>
<td>*Cryotherapy with liquid nitrogen*</td>
</tr>
<tr>
<td>Recommended regimens for anal warts</td>
<td>*Cryotherapy with liquid nitrogen (perianal only)*
TCA or BCA 80%–90% applied to warts (intra- or perianal). A small amount should be applied only to warts and allowed to dry, at which time a white frosting develops. If an excess amount of acid is applied, the treated area should be powdered with talc, sodium bicarbonate, or liquid soap preparations to remove unreacted acid. This treatment can be repeated weekly, if necessary.
Combination of liquid nitrogen and TCA may allow for more rapid regression
Office-based ablation with electrocautery
Surgical removal (for extensive warts)</td>
</tr>
</table>

BCA, bichloroacetic acid; SIL, squamous intraepithelial lesion; TCA, trichloroacetic acid.
Source: Adapted from Centers for Disease Control and Prevention. (n.d.). Genital HPV infection: Basic fact sheet. *http://www.cdc.gov/std/hpv/stdfact-hpv.htm*

In cases in which EGWs begin to grow, surgical removal and sometimes cesarean section may be indicated (in rare cases when they obstruct the birth canal). The recommended period of gestation for treatment is around 32-weeks' gestation. Post-treatment, obstetric patients should be monitored as recurrence may occur. During pregnancy, EGWs are to be treated as per CDC recommended treatment guidelines (see Table 32.4). Treatment of genital warts includes both healthcare provider–administered and patient-administered therapies. When contemplating a treatment plan, healthcare providers should consider all of the following: genital wart size, number, location, morphology, woman's choice, healthcare provider experience, convenience, and adverse effects.

Increasing Severity of Squamous Intraepithelial Lesions and Treatment Modalities

Two treatment modalities are used to address the increasing severity of SIL: ablative therapy and excisional therapy.

ABLATIVE THERAPY

This treatment modality includes the use of cryotherapy and laser vaporization. When performing cryotherapy or laser vaporization, it is important to note that no surgical specimen will be available for histologic testing. For this reason, many healthcare providers prefer using excisional therapies. Advantages of cryotherapy include ease to perform in an outpatient setting, minimal healthcare provider training, affordability, and minimal long-term fertility issues. Significant cramping and watery, malodorous vaginal drainage for up to 3 weeks are the most commonly reported disadvantages to cryotherapy. Laser vaporization is also readily performed in the outpatient setting with minimal risk to the individual. The most common reason this procedure is not preferred by healthcare providers has to do with the necessary additional training and the additional cost of the equipment. Women tolerate laser vaporization well, and often receive some type of sedative prior to the procedure to help with any discomfort/pain and to minimize patient movement during the procedure. The biggest advantage of laser vaporization is the precision at which the tissue/area of concern is destroyed.

EXCISIONAL THERAPY

Excisional therapy includes LEEP and CKC biopsy. The result of these procedures is a tissue specimen, which is sent to pathology for histologic evaluation and diagnosis. Individuals are most often treated with a local anesthetic during these procedures and with nonsteroidal anti-inflammatory medication for postprocedure cramping. Vaginal bleeding and discharge are common and may last for up to 2 weeks. Thermal artifacts are evident on the margins of a specimen, and care must be taken by both the healthcare provider and pathologist to ensure that the margins are clear; this indicates that there is evidence that no high-grade lesions were missed during the procedure. Typically, a CKC biopsy procedure is typically performed when there is evidence and concern for an increased possibility of invasive cancer. The biggest advantage of a CKC procedure versus a LEEP procedure has to do with the fact that the biopsy specimen collected via CKC will not have undergone any thermal damage to the tissue margins. Because more tissue is collected during a CKC procedure, the individual is at greater risk for developing acute bleeding, and long-term cervical stenosis and cervical insufficiency, which may lead to, for example, premature delivery.

Current Approaches to Cervical Cancer Prevention

Current approaches to cervical cancer prevention include (1) HPV vaccination, (2) cervical cancer screening, (3) follow-up evaluation using colposcopy and cervical biopsy, and (4) treatment for biopsy-confirmed high-grade cervical cancer precursors. Approaches 2 and 4 have previously been discussed. In the following section, we discuss HPV vaccination as a means of prevention.

Human Papillomavirus Vaccination

Since 2017, the 9-valent vaccine is the only HPV vaccine available in the United States (KFF Women's Health Policy, 2021). Unfortunately, uptake of the vaccine in the United States continues at less than hoped-for rates. As of 2019, only 54% of women and less than 49% of men in the recommended age groups had received all recommended doses. Decreasing persistent HPV infection rates, disease, and cancer burden will be achieved if HPV cancer prevention vaccine uptake increases through the implementation of interventions that are successful at improving vaccine uptake. Widespread, HPV cancer prevention vaccination will sharply reduce genital warts and anogenital cancers; cervical, vaginal, vulvar, and anal dysplasia and cancer; and EGWs.

The Advisory Committee on Immunization Practices (ACIP) recommends routine vaccination at age 11 to 12 and may begin as early as age 9 years (Meites et al., 2016). The vaccine is most effective at early age before exposure to the HPV through sexual activity and provides antibody levels equivalent to those who received three doses of the HPV vaccine. The HPV vaccination is also recommended as catchup for females ages 13 to 26 years and for males ages 13 to 21 years, for those who have not been previously vaccinated, or who have not completed the three-dose vaccine series. Males age 22 to 26 years may be vaccinated. In October 2018, the FDA approved the expanded use of the 9-valent HPV vaccine in individuals ages 27 to 45. It is recommended that individuals ≥27 years of age, and up to 45, together with their healthcare provider, determine risk for new HPV infection acquisition through shared decision-making to determine benefit of vaccine uptake (American College of Obstetricians and Gynecologists [ACOG], 2020). See Table 32.5 for the 9-valent vaccine schedule.

HUMAN PAPILLOMAVIRUS VACCINE UPTAKE AND THE FIGHT AGAINST CANCER IN AMERICA

In 2012, the President's Cancer Panel determined that low rates of adolescent HPV vaccine uptake were a threat to America's progress against cancer (President's Cancer Panel, 2014). At that time, the CDC estimated that increasing current low vaccination rates up to 80% (a *Healthy People 2020* target) would prevent an additional 53,000 future cervical cancer cases in the United States in adolescent girls 12 years old or younger over the course of their lifetimes (CDC, 2013). Barriers to vaccine uptake were identified. They included (a) missed clinical opportunities, (b) misinformation, (c) mistrust, (d) lack of knowledge, (e) insufficient access and/or system gaps, and (f) cost concerns (President's Cancer Panel, 2014). In an effort to address these barriers, the Panel recommended three critical goals that must be achieved to increase HPV vaccine uptake in the United States. The overall goal is completion of the vaccine series by all vaccine-eligible adolescents for whom the vaccine is not contraindicated. Critical goals include the following: (a) reduce missed clinical opportunities to recommend and administer the vaccines; (b) increase parents', caregivers', and adolescents' acceptance of the vaccine; and (c) maximize access to HPV vaccination services (President's Cancer Panel, 2014).

MISSED CLINICAL OPPORTUNITIES

Often, adolescents receive other recommended vaccines during well-child visits, but not HPV vaccines. Healthcare providers should strongly encourage HPV vaccination whenever other vaccines are administered and healthcare organizations should use electronic health records and immunization information systems to avoid missed opportunities for HPV vaccination. Precounseling patients to expect mild local discomfort after inoculation is a reinforcer of vaccine safety. Mild local discomfort is not a cause for alarm, nor an adverse event. Healthcare providers should not test for HPV DNA before vaccination and pregnancy testing is not recommended. The HPV vaccination is safe during breastfeeding. There is no need to revaccinate individuals who previously completed some but not all the vaccine series. Healthcare providers should recommend HPV vaccination as early as possible in children and adolescents with a history of child abuse.

Although, overall, the United States is experiencing an uptake of HPV vaccination, there remain socioeconomic disparities in the United States. These disparities are seen in adolescents living at or above the poverty level as well as in those living in rural America, as they are less likely to participate in well-child visits (CDC, 2023). Participating in few well-child visits results in fewer opportunities for healthcare providers to recommend and administer the vaccine.

KNOWLEDGE, ATTITUDES, AND BELIEFS

Parental and caregiver knowledge, attitudes, and beliefs affect whether children receive any vaccine, including HPV vaccines. Most parents believe that vaccines protect their children from potentially life-threatening diseases, but some refuse one or more recommended vaccines based on concerns, such as safety. The most important predictor of vaccination in the clinical setting is a strong recommendation

TABLE 32.5 Human Papillomavirus Vaccine Schedule in the United States

9-VALENT HPV VACCINE

Manufacturer	Merck & Co., Inc.
Target age	9-years[a] 11–12 years target age[b] 13–26 years as catch up[c] 27–45 years in some women
Sex	Boys and girls
HPV genotypes	6, 11, 16, 18, 31, 33, 45, 52, 58

SCHEDULE

9–14 years	15–26 years	27–45 years
If vaccinated before age 15, two doses are needed; 0 (baseline) and 6–12 months. The 6-month interval is critical for adequate immune titers. If the interval between doses is <5 months, a third dose is recommended.	Three doses are needed at 0 (baseline), 1–2 months, and 6 months after the first dose. If unvaccinated by age 26 years and younger, start the series.	Licensed for men and women. Recommended for those not in committed monogamous relationships, recently diagnosed with an STI.

[a]Included in the adolescent immunizations platform.
[b]Target age as part of the adolescent immunization platform.
[c]Catchup period regardless of sexual activity, prior exposure to HPV, and/or sexual orientation.
HPV, human papillomavirus; STI, sexually transmitted infection.
Source: Adapted from American College of Obstetricians and Gynecologists. (2020). ACOG Committee Opinion Summary, No. 809: Human papillomavirus vaccination. Obstetrics & Gynecology, 136(2), 435–436. https://doi.org/10.1097/AOG.0000000000004001

from a healthcare provider. Failure of healthcare providers to strongly recommend HPV vaccines, as well as a lack of parental understanding of HPV vaccine safety and efficacy, has contributed to poor HPV vaccine uptake.

Maximizing Access to Vaccination Services

In an effort to maximize HPV vaccine uptake in the United States, settings other than traditional healthcare provider offices should be considered for vaccine administration. Schools and pharmacies are two examples of promising alternative settings.

SPECIAL POPULATIONS

Access to HPV vaccinations, screening, testing, and management for women in rural and underresourced communities is disparate (NCI, n.d.). This is particularly true in communities of color where disproportionately higher incidence, and morbidity and mortality related to cervical cancer are experienced (Buskwofic et al., 2020). The death and 5-year survival rates for cervical cancer among minority women is lower when compared to White women. Regardless of race, ethnicity, socioeconomic status, geographic location, sexual activity or sexual orientation, or prior exposure to HPV, vaccination coverage should be intentional nationwide. Researchers have suggested that once primary HPV testing becomes widely available and accessible to rural communities and communities of color, cervical cancer rates will decrease (Johnson et al., 2020). Cytology-based self-screening can also improve cervical cancer screening leading to decreased disparity that continue to plague rural, underresourced communities of color.

Vaccination during pregnancy is not recommended, although the HPV vaccine does not appear to be associated with risk for fetal defects. If the HPV vaccine series is not completed or is interrupted due to pregnancy, there is no need to restart the vaccine series after pregnancy. Messaging to parents regarding vaccination of their children should be intentional and consistent regardless of the sex of the child. Sexual orientation is not a concern but female reproductive organs in transgender individuals should be a concern. Following the dosing schedule is crucial for ensuring adequate immune titers. HPV vaccine is not associated with early onset of sexual activity or increased incidence of STIs.

Males age 22 to 26 years may have a completed HPV vaccination. Additionally, MSM and immunocompromised individuals through age 26 years may be vaccinated (Ault, 2007).

Future Directions

The best approach to cervical cancer prevention is continued education, screening, and prevention. The more that healthcare providers recommend HPV vaccination, the greater the uptake in vaccination, resulting in the continued decline of HPV infection and disease prevalence. Thanks to improved technologies for biomedical analysis, how we screen women for cervical cancer is ever evolving. Vaccine development and self-sampling are also pushing the ticket for the many choices women have regarding cancer-vaccine prevention. HPV vaccines are cancer-prevention vaccines. Healthcare providers must make it a priority to not miss opportunities for HPV cancer vaccine education, administration, and prevention.

The 9-valent vaccine is indicated for prevention of cervical, vulvar, vaginal, anal, oropharyngeal, and other head and neck cancers; penile cancer in males; and EGWs in individuals. In 2019, the ACIP expanded HPV vaccination to include individuals 27 to 45 years of age to receive the vaccine through shared decision-making with their healthcare provider.

ANAL HUMAN PAPILLOMAVIRUS–RELATED DISEASE

Definition and Scope

HPV is associated with a spectrum of abnormal changes in the anal canal, including infection with the virus, its associated lesions, anal LSIL, HSIL, and anal cancer. Anal cancer itself is rare. In 2021, there were an estimated 9,090 new cases in the United States and 1,430 deaths (NCI, 2021). Although the incidence rate is approximately 2.0 per 100,000 in women and men, the incidence is increasing annually at a rate of 2.1%, and in women the incidence has doubled since the mid-1970s (NCI, 2021). There are identified populations considered at increased risk for anal cancer. The highest risk population is men who have sex with men (MSM) living with HIV (LWH), with anal cancer rates estimated to be 85 per 100,000, although rates as high as 131 per 100,000 have been reported (Clifford et al., 2021), surpassing the highest rates of cervical cancer for any other group. Women identified as high risk for anal cancer include women with a history of gynecologic HSIL and cancer, and those who are immunocompromised. Current anal cancer rates in women LWH are reported as high as 30 per 100,000 (Silverberg et al., 2012). There are elevated rates of anal cancer in other immune-suppressed populations as well. Increases in anogenital cancers of up to 100-fold were reported in the mid-1980s in solid organ transplant recipients (Blohmé & Brynger, 1985; Penn, 1986). This is believed to be a result of the iatrogenic effect of immunosuppressive medications. More recent data also showed elevated incident rates of anal (11.6) as well as vulvar cancer (20.3) in a study analyzing data from the U.S. Transplant Cancer Match (Madeleine et al., 2013). Similar data have been reported in studies analyzing transplant registries in Italy and Denmark (Busnach et al., 1993; Sunesen et al., 2010). The risk increased after 2 years, with an average diagnosis of a cancer in the fourth or fifth year following transplant (Madeleine et al., 2013) and the incidence was 50 per 100,000 10 years post-transplant (Clifford et al., 2021). Elevated risks for anal cancer are also found in patients on long-term steroid therapy for conditions such as systemic lupus erythematosus (Dreyer et al., 2011), and Crohn's disease (Sunesen et al., 2010). Finally, the association of gynecologic cancers with anal canal disease has been well documented. In an early study, nearly 13% of women with a history of vulvar cancer had anal cancer, and a total of 47.5% had HPV-associated lesions (Ogunbiyi et al., 1994). Elevated risks for anal cancer have been documented in women with a history of cervical, vaginal, or vulvar HSIL, and/or cancer (Chaturvedi et al., 2007; Jiménez et al., 2009; Saleem et al., 2011). In summary, though rare, for certain at-risk women, anal cancer rates far exceed rates for cancer of the cervix.

Etiology

ANAL HUMAN PAPILLOMAVIRUS AND SQUAMOUS INTRAEPITHELIAL LESION

While anal cancer is rare, both HPV infection and HPV-associated anal lesions are common. The prevalence of HPV infection ranged from 4% to 22% among women in the general population compared with 23% to 36% in women with a history of gynecologic HPV-associated disease. In women LWH, the prevalence was as high as 85% (Stier et al., 2015). The incidence is consistently higher in women LWH versus women not LWH; 76% of women LWH were HPV positive as compared with 42% of those not LWH (Palefsky et al., 2001).

RISK FACTORS

Risk factors include the presence of cervical HPV, CD4 less than 200 in women LWH, smoking, and concurrent or a history of perianal and/or vulvar warts (Stier et al., 2015). A reported history of anal intercourse and higher number of lifetime sexual partners was associated with HPV prevalence in some, but not all studies (Castro et al., 2012; Kojic et al., 2011). HPV persistence is a known risk factor for the development of cervical HSIL, although less studied in the anal canal. The average clearance of anal HPV infection was reported at 5 months in one study (Goodman et al., 2008), and the majority of anal HPV had cleared by 3 years in another study (Moscicki et al., 2014). Persistence was associated with immunosuppression (Suardi et al., 2014) and recent anal sexual activity, as well as persistent cervical HPV infection (Moscicki et al., 2014).

The incidence of anal LSIL or HSIL has been measured by cytology, histology, or a composite of the two, by which the highest grade of disease was reported. Histology results usually are based on anoscopy or high-resolution anoscopy (HRA), considered the most accurate means for determining presence or absence of either LSIL or HSIL. However, in many studies, HRA was provided only to subjects with abnormal cytology or a convenience sample subset of those that followed up with a referral for HRA following abnormal cytology. Some studies do not distinguish LSIL separately from HSIL, thereby inflating the incidence of SIL but not providing clarity regarding the risk of the anal cancer precursor lesion.

As a screening test, anal cytology, like cervical, is not a reliable indication of the grade of disease and its low sensitivity means many patients with disease will have false-negative results. Fortunately, this is not problematic in a slow-developing disease such as HPV-associated lesions, as repeated screening tests, over time, will eventually test positive in someone with a persistent lesion. False-positive cytology is considered rare and therefore a positive cytology requires referral for higher level evaluation. For anal disease, like cervical, the gold standard is colposcopy-directed biopsy with HRA.

There are few studies that evaluated all subjects with HRA. In cohorts that were nonimmunocompromised, the incidence of anal SIL ranged from 4% to 20%, and anal HSIL ranged from 2% to 9% (ElNaggar & Santoso, 2013; Heráclio et al., 2011; Jacyntho et al., 2011; Koppe et al., 2011; Likes et al., 2013; Santoso et al., 2010; Tatti et al., 2012). In comparison, a single study of 31 women LWH, all referred for HRA, reported 52% SIL and 26% HSIL (Tatti et al., 2012). A more recent study of women LWH who all underwent HRA as a screening study reported anal HSIL rates of 27% (22% to 33%; Stier et al., 2020).

These data, however, may provide low estimates and reflect the overall inexperience of this relatively new practice. Healthcare providers with at least 10 years of HRA experience report anal HSIL in more than 40% of immunocompromised women, or in those women with a history of gynecologic HSIL or cancer (unpublished personal data). Unlike the cervical literature, longitudinal natural history studies are not yet available for anal disease. Finally, the heterogeneity of the data is difficult to synthesize and to statistically analyze, underscoring the need for continued research.

ETIOLOGY OF ANAL CANAL HUMAN PAPILLOMAVIRUS–ASSOCIATED DISEASE

The cervix has served as a hypothetical model for anal cancer screening because of biological similarities between the anus and the female genital tract. Both the cervix and anus have a squamocolumnar junction (SCJ) where squamous epithelium borders columnar epithelium, inducing a transformation zone in which normal metaplasia occurs. The dynamic process of metaplasia is conducive to the development of an abnormal transformation or dysplasia, and both LSIL and HSIL frequently occur here. The SCJ is only appreciated with HRA similar to its identification on the cervix with a colposcope.

The same strains of HPV affect the anus and genital tract, including the low-risk types associated with LSIL and the high-risk types associated with HSIL and cancers (Williams et al., 1994). The high-risk strain HPV 16 is found in a greater percentage of anal cancers (77%) than cervical (51%; Steinau et al., 2013). Anal LSIL and HSIL lesions are morphologically similar to their respective cervical lesions, and HSIL is known to be the cancer precursor lesion in both sites (Berry et al., 2014). The natural history of cervical HSIL and cancer are better characterized because of decades of research. There are compelling data supporting a similar natural history development for anal cancer (Berry et al., 2004; Kreuter et al., 2010; Watson et al., 2006).

Screening programs for anal cancer, based on the cervical model, have been proposed and initiated in many communities. The successful conclusion of the Anal Cancer HSIL Outcome Research (ANCHOR) trial has shown that anal cancer can also be prevented by identification and treatment of anal HSIL, just like the cervix (Palefsky et al., 2022).

ANAL CANCER SCREENING

The goal of anal cancer screening, like cervical cancer screening, is primarily to identify anal HSIL allowing for targeted treatment of these lesions, thereby preventing progression to cancer. As noted earlier in the general population, anal cancer is rare. However, there are special populations that are at higher risk; thus, healthcare providers focus their attention on these populations. Most anal cancer screening programs are targeting MSM LWH. Additionally, elevated rates of anal cancer are found in specific populations of women, including those who are immunocompromised and those with a history of lower genital tract HSIL and cancers. Healthcare providers can consider including these women considered at risk in anal cancer screening programs as well.

SCREENING TOOLS

Techniques for evaluation of the cervix have been adapted for anal canal disease. These include validation of anal cytology (Palefsky et al., 1997), HPV DNA testing (Palefsky et al., 2001), and HRA (Jay et al., 1997). HRA requires the use of a colposcope and colposcopic techniques for evaluation of the anal canal (Jay et al., 1997). The screening modality is dependent on available resources. HRA remains a relatively young field and there are few Centers of Excellence or trained healthcare providers across the United States. Therefore, anal cytology should only be provided if there is a referral source for abnormal results. If HRA is not available, consideration should be given to alternative options (see sections on Digital Anal Rectal Examination and Anal Cytology). The aim of anal cancer screening is to identify individuals with potential HSIL for evaluation with HRA, who can then be treated and followed with the overall goal of preventing progression to anal cancer. In high resource settings, screening would include anal cytology and digital anal rectal examination (DARE) with referral to HRA for abnormal findings, including cytological results greater than atypical squamous cells of undetermined significance (ASC-US) cytology, or to a surgeon in the absence of HRA for abnormal DARE findings.

ANAL CYTOLOGY AND HISTOLOGY

Anal cytology and histology are classified with the same taxonomy as the cervix and genital tract, now unified using the newer Lower Anogenital Squamous Terminology (LAST) system (Darragh et al., 2013). The sensitivity of anal cytology ranges from 69% to 93% and specificity from 32% to 59%, similar to cervical cytology (Chiao et al., 2006). False-positive cytology results are rare, and the positive predictive value of abnormal cytology has been reported as 96% for the presence of any lesion in HIV-positive MSM (Cranston et al., 2007). Cytology results are not predictive of the level of dysplasia and will commonly underestimate the actual severity of disease. As much as 50% of ASC-US cytology will result in a finding of HSIL on HRA (Jay et al., 2012). This is true regardless of an individual's risk. Therefore, it has become common practice to refer any abnormal cytology for follow-up HRA (e.g., ≥ ASC-US) provided there are adequate referral resources.

Human Papillomavirus Testing

Although frequently incorporated into research studies, HPV testing is not FDA approved for the anal canal. Its utility may be similar to approved tests developed for the cervix, and eventually may help guide practice decisions. Occasionally, HPV testing is used, without clinical evidence, for its negative predictive value. For example, in women who have been treated for anal cancer, a negative HPV test might indicate the need for less frequent, follow-up HRA examinations. There is growing interest in the utility of specific high-risk HPV types such as HPV 16 for anal canal screening. Sensitivity and specificity of HPV 16 for anal HSIL was 75% and 85%, respectively, in one recent study (Ellsworth et al., 2021). Potentially, a woman with a HR HPV 16 positive result, would be triaged for HRA.

HIGH-RESOLUTION ANOSCOPY

HRA, like cervical colposcopy, requires advanced training, which can be obtained in courses provided by specialized professional organizations (e.g., the International Anal Neoplasia Society). However, all healthcare providers should have an understanding of abnormalities that require referral to a specialist providing HRA. These include abnormal clinical findings as well as abnormal cytology. Clinical findings that would prompt referral to an HRA-trained healthcare provider include grossly evident perianal disease such as warts, lesions, erosions, atypical appearing hemorrhoids, and/or vulvar disease that extends to the perianus. In these cases, it is important to determine if intra-anal disease is present as well. HRA allows the trained healthcare provider to determine if microscopic lesions are present in addition to the macroscopic findings. Persistent symptoms, such as bleeding, pain, and pressure, that cannot be explained by a clinical examination may be better evaluated by HRA or, if unavailable, by a colorectal surgeon. Abnormal findings on the DARE should also prompt referral. These would include a mass, pain with palpation, and a hemorrhoid or wart that is hard or painful or does not resolve with common interventions.

The HRA examination itself is a relatively short procedure generally lasting no longer than 15 to 20 minutes. The examination is usually well tolerated with only minor discomfort caused by the pressure of the anoscope on the sphincter. The evaluation includes thorough examination of the anus and perianus using a small anoscope, which is inserted into the anus, along with application of acetic acid and Lugol's solutions to highlight potential lesions. As most women referred for HRA have documented abnormal cytology, they should expect that biopsies will be done. Biopsies are not generally painful as there are no pain nerve endings in the anal canal. Perianal biopsies, however, do require local anesthesia. Following HRA, individuals may experience minor bleeding with bowel movements for a few days.

TREATMENT AND MANAGEMENT ALGORITHMS

Algorithms for triage to HRA following abnormal anal cytology, similar to those considered standard of care for cervical screening, are not yet established for anal canal disease. The newer triage protocols for cervical cytology, including less frequent screening and incorporation of HPV DNA testing, have not been validated for anal canal disease. In part, this is caused by the high prevalence of anal HSIL in populations considered at risk and therefore cannot be compared with cervical screening programs targeted at the general population of women. However, the essential principle is the same and an abnormal cytology should be referred for HRA (e.g., anal colposcopy). Different healthcare centers may establish

different guidelines for triage to HRA and treatment until standards of care are adopted (Figure 32.1).

Evaluation and Assessment

MEDICAL AND SEXUAL HEALTH HISTORY

All women should be evaluated with an HPV-focused medical and sexual reproductive history of the entire genital tract. The woman's reported medical and sexual history will help the healthcare provider determine whether a woman (a) is considered high risk and should be offered anal cytology, (b) needs a DARE (although this exam should be included in routine annual care regardless of history of symptoms), and/or (c) requires referral for HRA. For the anus specifically, it is important to ascertain whether the woman has had prior diagnoses such as anal warts, SIL, and/or cancer, and/or whether she has a prior or current history/diagnosis of hemorrhoids, fissures, fistulas, and/or abscess. The healthcare provider should collect information on any treatment(s) and response(s) to treatment(s). While collecting a woman's medical and sexual health history, current symptoms such as bleeding, pain, irritation, and pruritus should be documented. Document the presence of symptoms present with anal intercourse (voluntary or coerced), including frequency, duration, and if symptoms are stable or worsening over time. A history of immunosuppression, steroid medications, and smoking or other tobacco use is also important to note, because they may play a role in persistent HPV disease, a necessary cause of anal cancer (Daling et al., 1992). Finally, inquire whether there are new, severe, or persistent diarrhea, constipation, urgency, and/or any changes in bowel patterns or incontinence as part of a woman's medical and sexual history. Healthcare providers should be aware that these questions are sensitive and women may be reluctant to discuss them.

WHAT TO LOOK FOR

The hallmarks of anal cancer include pain and bleeding. It is important to ascertain whether or not these symptoms are new, persistent, or worsening over time. Early or microinvasive cancers may present with only minor symptoms or none at all and may be an incidental finding during a hemorrhoidectomy or DARE. Vague symptoms such as minor pressure or a sudden change in bowel habits may indicate that a mass is developing. Once a cancer is established, the onset of symptoms may be sudden (e.g., bleeding with bowel movements) or subclinical (e.g., mistaken for a fissure or hemorrhoid).

DIGITAL ANAL RECTAL EXAMINATION

The most important service that can and should be provided by any healthcare provider is the DARE. The common story described by many anal cancer survivors is that despite complaining of discomfort and/or bleeding for months and sometimes years, no one looked or palpated, and they were told it was "just a hemorrhoid." All hemorrhoids should be evaluated by both observation and palpation. Hemorrhoids are not hard (unless thrombosed, which also requires referral for treatment). It is important that healthcare providers remember that an atypical presentation or persistent symptoms in a presumed hemorrhoid that do not resolve with common,

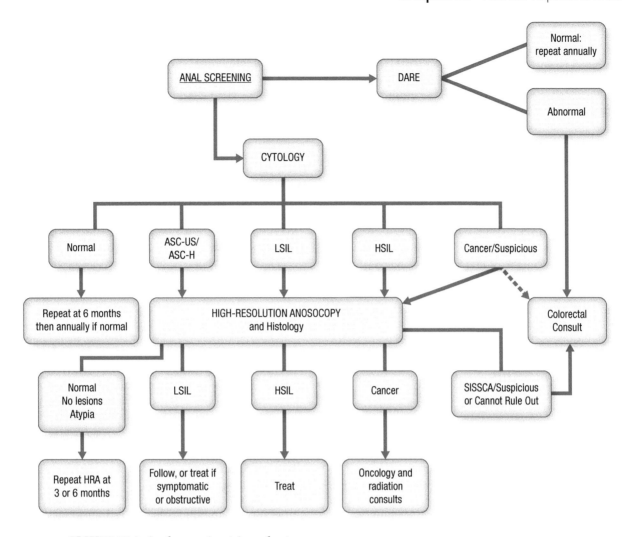

FIGURE 32.1 Anal screening triage chart.
(Many centers provide high-risk HPV cotesting, though it is not FDA approved for anal canal screening.) ASC-US/ASC-H, atypical squamous cells of undetermined significance/atypical squamous cells, cannot rule out high-grade squamous intraepithelial lesion; DARE, digital anal rectal examination; FDA, U.S. Food and Drug Administration; HPV, human papillomavirus; HRA, high-resolution anoscopy; HSIL, high-grade squamous intraepithelial lesion; LSIL, low-grade squamous intraepithelial lesion; SISSCA, superficially invasive squamous cell carcinoma of the cervix.
Source: Adapted from Donovan, B., Franklin, N., Guy, R., Grulich, A. E., Regan, D. G., Ali, H., Wand, H., & Fairley, C. K. (2011). Quadrivalent human papillomavirus vaccination and trends in genital warts in Australia: Analysis of national sentinel surveillance data. Lancet Infectious Diseases, 11(1), 39–44. https://doi .org/10.1016/S1473-3099(10)70225-5; Paavonen, J., Jenkins, D., Bosch, F. X., Naud, P., Salmeron, J., Wheeler, C. M., Chow, S. N., Apter, D. L., Kitchener, H. C., Castellsague, X., de Carvalho, N. S., Skinner, S. R., Harper, D. M., Hedrick, J. A., Jaisamrarn, U., Limson, G. A., Dionne, M., Quint, W., Spiessens, B., . . . Dubin, G. (2007). Efficacy of a prophylactic adjuvanted bivalent L1 virus-like-particle vaccine against infection with human papillomavirus types 16 and 18 in young women: An interim analysis of a phase III double-blind, randomized controlled trial. Lancet, 369(9580), 2161–2170. https://doi.org/10.1016/S0140-6736(07)60946 5

short-term interventions should be referred for HRA or to a colorectal surgeon for follow-up evaluation. In summary, the DARE should be used as a screening tool for detection of anal cancers, rather than precancers. When done correctly, it may detect early cancers (Nyitray et al., 2020). This simple assessment should be a standard part of an annual physical or when a woman presents with symptoms of anal pain, bleeding, or unusual pressure.

Other findings that may require referral to a specialist include fissures, fistula openings, pruritus ani, and dermatologic findings. Unfortunately, women sometimes become accustomed to persistent symptoms that can be easily resolved with the correct intervention (which sometimes is beyond our scope of practice). Treatments and interventions can be offered, but it is suggested that the healthcare provider have a low threshold for referral if symptoms do not resolve or improve within a short time frame (e.g., 1 month).

GROSS EVALUATION OF THE PERIANUS

Healthcare providers are accustomed to evaluating the cervix, vagina, and vulva with gross visualization and are competent to diagnose and treat conditions such as genital warts, molluscum contagiosum, herpes, and simple dermatologic conditions. Persistent disease that does not resolve with standard treatment requires referral to the appropriate specialist. With proper education and training, perianal evaluation and a simple anoscopy can be incorporated into the physical examination of the woman. Gross evaluation will assess for atypical findings, including warts, changes in skin contour or color, redundant tissue or anal tags, hemorrhoids, fissures, ulcerations, denuded epithelium, or rashes. Visualized abnormalities should be queried for any accompanying symptoms such as pruritus, bleeding, discomfort, or pain. If the patient has peripheral neuropathy or is on pain medication for other healthcare problems, they may have decreased anal sensation and may not report pain or discomfort. The healthcare provider should also assess for the extension of any abnormalities to or from the vulva and perineum or into the anal canal. Warts may seem typical in appearance, but consideration should be given to providing a biopsy for histologic confirmation, especially if there are any atypical qualities such as fissure, ulceration, bleeding, or pigmentation changes. If a healthcare provider is uncertain, consultation with a specialist should be considered.

External Genital Warts

More commonly, women may present with condylomata or EGWs, with estimates as high as 120 cases per 100,000 person-years in women. Although these data include all EGWs (Hoy et al., 2009), anal warts are rarely reported separately. EGWs are found most frequently in younger women age 20 to 24 (Hoy et al., 2009). While genital warts are benign, the diagnosis and treatment can have substantial economic and psychological impact on the individual. Presenting symptoms include raised lesions, discrete or clustered, that may be pruritic or bleed. Treatment is similar to treatment of vulvar warts (see Table 32.4).

ANAL CYTOLOGY

Following visual inspection, anal cytology can be performed and cells collected, if indicated, based on a woman's risk factors for potential anal HPV-associated disease. If a referral source for abnormal cytology is available, annual anal cytology can then be provided to women considered in high-risk groups (e.g., immunosuppression of any etiology, those with a history of gynecologic HSIL or cancer). The anal cytology collection always precedes a DARE or insertion of an anoscope.

With minimal training, anal cytology specimens can be collected by any licensed healthcare provider. Patients should be instructed to avoid douching, using enemas, or inserting anything into their rectum a minimum of 24 hours before the exam. Fewer cells exfoliate from the anus and this will increase the yield of cells for cytologic evaluation. Healthcare providers should monitor their results for adequacy; the unsatisfactory rate should be maintained at less than 3%. Applying additional pressure, longer contact with the anal walls (compared with the cervical specimen collection), and longer agitation of the swab in the collection medium will all help improve the satisfactory rate of anal cytology. Depending on insurance coverage, the healthcare provider can request HPV cotesting. At this time, it is not recommended to do primary HPV testing for the anal canal.

Anal Cytology Steps

1. The individual can be placed in any position that provides adequate visualization of the anal opening (e.g., left or right lateral or lithotomy).
2. Use a synthetic swab (e.g., Dacron or polyester) moistened with tap water. Avoid use of a cytobrush, which is unnecessarily uncomfortable.
3. Insert the swab approximately 3 to 4 cm into the anus; this will ensure that cells are collected from the distal rectum to the anal verge. If initial resistance is encountered, change the position or angle of the swab and reinsert. It may be helpful if the individual retracts the upper buttock while lying in a lateral position.
4. Gently, but with pressure, rotate the swab in a slow circular motion. This will ensure sampling from all aspects of the anal canal. The swab should be in contact with the anal mucosa with more pressure and more time compared with cervical cytology collection.
5. Women have shorter anal canals, and the anal SCJ may be just within the verge; therefore, be certain to maintain pressure and continue rotating the swab even as the tip of the swab is nearly out of the canal.
6. Agitate the swab in the liquid medium for at least 30 seconds, or if using conventional slides preserve the exfoliated cells quickly to avoid air-dried artifacts.

Following the visual assessment and cytology collection, the DARE should be performed. This should be done annually or more frequently if needed. The DARE emphasizes palpation of the anal walls rather than just the distal rectum (as with a digital rectal examination [DRE]). Abnormal thickening, hard masses, and bright red bleeding evidenced on exam should be referred for HRA or, if unavailable, to simple anoscopy.

DARE INSTRUCTIONS

1. Mix a small amount of 2% to 5% lidocaine gel or cream into K-Y Jelly. Use this mixture to lubricate the gloved finger.
2. Gently insert a gloved and lubricated finger slowly into the rectum.
3. Apply firm pressure on the external sphincter, allowing it to relax before advancing into the rectum.
4. Once inside the rectum, carefully palpate the entire circumference. Beginning in the distal rectum, feel the mucosa over the internal sphincter and the walls of the distal anal canal.
5. Palpate for warts, masses, ulcerations, fissures, and focal areas of discomfort or pain with palpation.
6. Complete the examination by performing a perianal sweep noting any thickening or areas of hardness, particularly in relation to any redundant tags or hemorrhoids.
7. Correlate findings with a visual inspection of the perianus.

TREATMENT

EGWs can be managed by most primary care providers with either provider- or patient-applied methods; provider-applied treatments include liquid nitrogen and trichloroacetic acid, or ablation with electrocautery. Patient-applied methods for warts include imiquimod 5%, podofilox 5%, or sinecatechins 15%. Although any of these can be very successful and more tolerable than ablation, a particular therapy may work better than another for any individual, and healthcare providers should consider changing therapy if there is no response within a reasonable time frame. Treatment for perianal HSIL or intra-anal LSIL, including condylomata or HSIL, is best managed by a specialist trained in HRA. The majority of these can be managed with in-office ablative treatment including cryotherapy (for external only), trichloroacetic acid (for small lesions only) and electrocautery for more extensive presentations. The trained healthcare provider determines whether the burden of disease is amenable to an in-office procedure or requires referral to a colorectal surgeon. Patients should be aware that all treatments aim to locate visible evidence of HPV-associated lesions and that we cannot treat the underlying virus. In time, and with more research, there may be systemic or topical therapies that both eliminate lesions and target the virus.

SUMMARY

HPV infection is a sexually transmitted infection that usually clears itself, but in some cases, it persists. Individuals with persistent HPV infections are triaged into a higher-risk stratification and surveilled for the development of cancer precursors or transformation of cells into cancer. Historically, the Pap smear has been the go-to screening test. Recently, primary HPV testing is gaining favor as the method for primary cervical cancer screening because it has proved to be more sensitive at detecting high-grade cervical dysplasia. However, not every woman who is HPV positive will develop cervical cancer. The challenge is to determine the best triage option to identify which HPV-positive woman is truly at risk for developing cervical cancer and would benefit most from colposcopy. At the time of printing of this edition, updated cervical screening guidelines are expected from the USPSTF. This is important as in the past, the USPSTF guidelines have been endorsed by major U.S. professional organizations. We anticipate that those organizations, too, will update their recommendations.

Populations of women who are at risk of anal HPV-associated pathology have been identified and healthcare providers should have a heightened awareness to include the anus and perianus for clinical evaluation. Prevention is the best "treatment strategy" for anal cancer and requires using a screening model similar to that used for cervical disease. In 2010, the FDA added prevention of anal intraepithelial neoplasia (AIN) and anal cancer in both men and women as an approved indication for the HPV vaccine. It is hoped that this will have an impact on the natural history of anal HSIL and cancer for future generations.

REFERENCES

References for this chapter are online and available at https://connect.springerpub.com/content/book/978-0-8261-6722-4/part/part03/chapter/ch32

CHAPTER 33

Gynecologic Cancers*

ZAHRA AMIRKHANZADEH BARANDOUZI AND LYNDA LEE LAPAN

WOMEN'S EXPERIENCE WITH GYNECOLOGIC CANCER

Women's experience with cancer of the gynecologic tract can be life threatening and involves dramatic changes in their lives and lifestyles. There are multiple areas in which primary care providers can have a positive impact on the woman's experience with the prevention, diagnosis, treatment, and survivorship of a gynecologic malignancy. This chapter identifies areas in which primary providers of women's healthcare can have a major positive influence on women's knowledge of, and experience with, gynecologic cancer.

IMPORTANCE OF PRIMARY CARE RELATED TO GYNECOLOGIC CANCERS

In providing primary care to women and individuals with female reproductive health organs, the APRN plays an important role by enhancing cancer patients' quality of life while decreasing healthcare cost (Campbell et al., 2020). The APRN is both an educator and an advocate. From prevention, screening, diagnosis, treatment, survivorship, and end of life, both education and advocacy are essential for optimal outcomes.

Education

Primary prevention of gynecologic cancers begins with education. This may be the education of the patient about their anatomy, normal physiologic function, and normal variations that are not a concern. It may also include education of the patient about prevention (promotion of healthy lifestyle and vaccination), screening, risk factors, and warning signs of cancer. Additionally, the APRN may be involved in educating

parents, schools, religious communities, cultural groups, healthcare organizations, and government bodies regarding the prevention needs of the patients in their care. This can be achieved by training APRNs using competency-based education to prepare them for critical thinking and incorporating research findings to enhance patient outcomes.

Education for the patient with a gynecologic cancer regarding the next steps in their care, including seeking specialist providers, the urgency of obtaining treatment, the expected diagnostic and treatment modalities that they may encounter, and even the need for routine healthcare during and after their cancer diagnosis is essential. Education on expected side effects, using coping tools, and shared decision-making throughout treatment are integral roles of the nurse. Also, an APRN can educate the patient on the importance of follow-up care after treatment to detect a secondary cancer or recurrence. This will enable the patient to have some sense of knowledge and control in an otherwise unfamiliar and fearful life situation.

Advocacy

The APRN plays an important role as a patient advocate across the span of the disease spectrum from prevention through survivorship. They can identify gaps in oncology patient care and establish roles specific to an organization, clinical care setting, and an individual practitioner to better serve cancer patients. Advocacy for health education, easy access to a broad range of women's healthcare services, the availability of affordable healthcare, involvement in multidisciplinary cancer care treatment, and providing all care in a way that is respectful of the person continue to be the role of the APRN (Campbell et al., 2020; Murphy & Mollica, 2016).

False assumptions by healthcare providers regarding women's awareness of their bodies may limit the ability to effectively assess and examine a genital concern until it is past the point of primary treatment. Women, girls, and

---

*This chapter is a revision of the chapter that appeared in the second edition of this textbook, authored by Barbara J. Silko and Leslie J. Heron, and we thank them for their original contribution.

others with female reproductive organs often lack adequate knowledge of their own body and its functioning. They may be unaware of what to anticipate about normal age-related body changes, from puberty to menopause. If they are not sure what is "normal," they may be unable to identify normal versus abnormal states. Awareness of their bodies may be limited by individual, family, religious, societal, and cultural norms. Access to education about their bodies may be limited by financial, geographic, cultural, religious, and societal barriers. There may be limited access to books, education opportunities, healthcare providers, or types of healthcare services that are required. Personal history of physical, psychological, or sexual abuse may create fear and hesitation to seek care. Social stigma regarding the words used for female genitals, and an assumption that the use of these words is discouraged or shameful in general conversation, may also prevent individuals from clearly speaking their concerns.

ACCESS TO AND USE OF WOMEN'S HEALTH SERVICES

Socioeconomic and Geographic Risk Factors

Women, as a population, are at greater socioeconomic risk, resulting in multiple disadvantages to accessing healthcare services (American Psychological Association [APA], 2015). In 2015, women with a high school diploma and postgraduate degrees were paid 80% and 74% of what their male peers were paid respectively (APA, 2015). Women are more likely to be single parents and/or unpaid caregivers to family and community members. In 2013, the U.S. Census Bureau reported that there were about 15 million female heads of household, compared to 5 million male heads of household in the United States (Vespa et al., 2013). From 1990 to 2019, the female heads of household increased from 17.6% to 22.6% (Goodman et al., 2021). Working longer hours, or more than one job, to meet their economic needs places limits on the amount of time women must access healthcare, especially during regular business hours. Although the education gap has been decreased between women and men over the last 3 decades, the median income of households headed by women is $20,000 lower than those headed by men (Goodman et al., 2021). With limited child care options, women may need to bring children into the examination room with them for healthcare visits. This may be a deterrent to seeking a women's health (pelvic) examination. Women heads of households are less likely to have disposable income to spend on healthcare and are more likely to use those healthcare dollars for the care of their children rather than on themselves. Longer life expectancy for women compounds socioeconomic risk by limiting funds available for healthcare needs in old age.

In addition to socioeconomic issues, geography plays a role in access to healthcare. Women living in rural areas frequently commute long distances to access routine healthcare services. If there is a gynecologic concern requiring a specialist for diagnosis or treatment, the woman may need to travel as far as another state to obtain care. Up to 14.8 million women nationwide have difficulty with access to care centers that specialize in gynecologic cancers (Shalowitz et al., 2015). Limited access to gynecologic and oncologic specialized care may lead to delayed detection, misdiagnoses, incorrect chemotherapy or surgeries, incomplete treatment protocols, and limited follow-up after oncology treatment.

Social Stigma of Sexual Activity

Social stigma around sexual activity limits access to preventive and diagnostic gynecologic services. Parents may decline immunization against human papillomavirus (HPV) for their child due to worry of promoting promiscuity or denial that their child will eventually be sexually active and therefore will be at risk of contracting HPV. Stigma that presenting to the clinic with any gynecologic concern might imply having been sexually active and worry that symptoms might be related to a sexually transmitted infection (STI; World Health Organization [WHO], 2022) may delay access to care for single and partnered women. A new onset of gynecologic symptoms may also imply sexual activity with multiple partners, or infidelity in a long-term relationship, leading to delayed evaluation of symptoms. There is lack of clarity regarding symptoms of STIs versus gynecologic cancers, time from exposure to symptom occurrence with HPV infection, low-risk versus high-risk HPV, and even with screening guidelines for gynecologic examinations and Pap testing (Lemieux, 2010).

Sexual Minorities

Lesbian, bisexual, and gender nonconforming women statistically present later for gynecologic concerns, including gynecologic cancers. Self-perception that routine gynecologic care is unnecessary if one is not seeking contraception, discomfort with the potential for discrimination by healthcare providers and staff, and decreased socioeconomic status all limit access to care (Carroll, 2015). There may be decreased sharing and trust in provider–patient interactions due to earlier visits with providers who were insensitive or uneducated around the needs of sexual minorities.

Many factors put this population at increased risk for gynecologic cancers. These include falsely assumed low risk for STI exposure, even though up to 90% of women who have sex with women report sex with a man at some point in their lifetime, and a greater than 30% prevalence of HPV in women who have sex with women (Carroll, 2015). They are at increased risk of sexual victimization over their lifetime yet may avoid both the medical and legal systems due to the fear of stigmatization. Gender nonconforming women may not feel engaged with their genitals and may not report if there are changes in tissues or menstrual patterns. There is also a correlation of increased risk for gynecologic cancers with increased body mass index (BMI), smoking, and alcohol intake, all which have been statistically associated with lesbian, bisexual, and transgender populations (Carroll, 2015; Flemmer et al., 2012). Also, bisexual and lesbian women may not follow up on routine healthcare for low rate of health insurance coverage and negative experience with a healthcare provider (American Cancer Society, 2021).

Religious and Cultural Factors

In many cultures and religions, women are discouraged from discussing gynecologic issues or being aware of their genitals. Information is passed down from one generation to the next, limiting new information regarding risks and symptoms of gynecologic cancers. There may be shame and a risk of being an outcast for seeking knowledge outside family or religious boundaries. Arranged marriages, marriage contracts, the importance placed on both virginity at marriage and on an ability to produce children all may impact women's patterns of seeking gynecologic care.

For non-English-speaking women, language barriers create yet another layer of risk for missed diagnosis of gynecologic conditions. Limited comfort with an unfamiliar or foreign medical system may delay access to care, and miscommunication may limit understanding of diagnosis, treatment, and referrals. The use of interpreters can assist in these situations but is not always a complete solution. Patients may not feel comfortable speaking freely if the interpreter is a family member; a male; a part of, or not a part of, their specific community or religion; or speaking a different dialect. These women frequently have compounded barriers, including lower socioeconomic status, transportation issues, limited knowledge of where or how to access care, and potentially, fear of accessing care due to undocumented residency.

Conclusion

APRNs have a unique and vital opportunity to educate and advocate for the women in their care. Socioeconomic, sexual, religious, cultural, and other societal risk factors may limit trust of, and access to, gynecologic care. Knowledge and awareness of sociocultural risk factors will assist the primary care provider to effectively negotiate their patient interactions for gynecologic concerns.

DEFINITION AND SCOPE OF GYNECOLOGIC CANCERS

The risk for and incidence of gynecologic cancers are dependent on which of the gynecologic organs is affected. There are five major organs or sites for malignancy in the female genital tract: the vulva, vagina, cervix, uterus, and the ovary/fallopian tube/primary peritoneum (Centers for Disease Control and Prevention [CDC], n.d.-a). Cancer in each separate gynecologic organ is diagnosed uniquely, and therefore, the cancer treatment will vary by primary organ site. Women's experiences of the diagnosis and the treatment of their gynecologic cancer are likely to be related to the physical effects of the treatment as well as the emotional elements of having cancer of a female organ.

OCCURRENCE, DIAGNOSIS, AND TREATMENT OF THE CANCERS OF THE FEMALE GENITAL TRACT BY SITE

Vulvar Cancer

INCIDENCE/PREVALENCE

In the United States, the estimated new cases of vulvar cancer were 6,330 in 2021 (National Cancer Institute [NCI], 2022; see Table 33.1). Vulvar cancer constitutes approximately 6% of the cancers in female reproductive organs and 0.7% of all cancers in women (American Cancer Society, 2022). The vulva refers to the external genital tissue that surrounds the clitoris, urethra, and vaginal opening (introitus), and extends from the midline of the clitoral hood, around the vaginal opening to the perirectal tissue. Often referred to as the labia majora and labia minora, the vulva serves to protect the structures of the urethra and introitus and is also capable of expanding and stretching significantly to allow for vaginal childbirth. The vulva is primarily a structure made of layers of skin and glandular tissue. Most vulvar cancers affect the epithelium or skin and therefore are treated similarly to other skin cancers of the body. The vulvar skin cells at risk for malignancy include squamous epithelial cells, basal cells, and melanin cells. Most vulvar cancers are squamous cell carcinomas (Elkas et al., 2016). Squamous cell vulvar carcinomas may be related to underlying vulvar dystrophies, or more often may be related to HPV infection. Women may harbor or carry HPV for many years without a detectable lesion, though sometimes they may report that they had genital warts/lesions in the past. If the virus is present and active, and the woman's immune system or genital skin is compromised, it may be a trigger for the virus to become more virulent, causing cellular skin changes. More rare vulvar cancers include melanomas, basal cell carcinomas and glandular or adenocarcinomas, and sarcomas. Combined, these rarer vulvar cancers make up only approximately 10% of all vulvar cancers (Elkas et al., 2016).

TABLE 33.1 Incidence of Gynecologic Cancers by Organ Site in the United States

ORGAN SITE	ANNUAL INCIDENCE
Vulva	6,330 cases
Vagina	8,870 cases
Cervix	14,100 cases
Uterus	65,950 cases
Ovary	19,880 cases

Source: Adapted from American Cancer Society. (2022). Cancer facts & figures, 2022. https://www.cancer.org/research/cancer-facts-statistics/all-cancer-facts-figures/cancer-facts-figures-2022.html Cancer.net, Cancer Facts and Figures (2022).

SYMPTOMS

Symptoms of vulvar dysplasia, a precancerous lesion, can be a visible or a palpable lesion, or it can be an area of persistent itching, burning, or pain. The most common symptom is prolonged itching or pain in the vulva. Sometimes, women will report that they have noted a lump or bump that has persisted over time. Based on the vague symptoms and their location these lesions are frequently initially treated as a benign condition, such as a candidal infection or lichen sclerosus. However, if an irritating condition is related to either dysplasia or neoplasia, it will not get better with the treatment for either of those presumed benign etiologies. If women present with persistent symptoms that do not improve with topical over-the-counter or prescription treatments, the primary provider needs to perform a thorough examination of the vulvar skin, with a biopsy of any suspicious-looking areas. The skin may be erythematous, or whitish gray in appearance, and sometimes an ulcerative area is present. If there is a squamous invasive malignancy, the provider may note a nodular firm area at the site of the irritation, as this invasive carcinoma will infiltrate the lymphatic tissues, forming a mass, and will have potential to metastasize. Also, in some cases, women may experience painful urination, discharge, and bleeding that is not related to menstrual blood (Cancer.net, 2022i).

There are several rare types of vulvar cancers. Vulvar basal cell skin cancers resemble basal cell malignancies of other skin areas. They are typically pink, with raised edges, with a characteristic appearance of irritation, sometimes called a "rodent" lesion (Elkas et al., 2016). These lesions are usually well demarcated and do not invade deeply into the lymphatic tissue, and thus they do not typically metastasize. However, basal cell carcinomas may be associated with abnormal skin lesions in other areas of the body, and thus dermatology referral for a total body evaluation might be warranted. Other rare types of precancerous vulvar lesions affect glandular cells. These glandular dysplasias of the vulva are known as nonmammary Paget lesions. These noninvasive neoplasms become inflamed and roughened in appearance, and typically, women will report intense itching and irritation at the site of the lesion. The risk for recurrence is high in women with vulvar Paget disease, and thus, regular surveillance and follow-up are necessary (Fanning et al., 1999) with biopsy of any suspicious area. The Bartholin gland in young women may become inflamed from an infectious process, but after age 40 years these glands rarely enlarge. Any woman older than 40 years presenting with an enlarged painful Bartholin glandular process should undergo a thorough evaluation with biopsy to ensure that malignancy is ruled out.

Melanoma is the second most common malignancy affecting vulvar tissue (Elkas et al., 2016). Women with vulvar melanoma may have symptoms similar to those of other vulvar cancers such as itching, pain, a lump, and discharge or bleeding (American Cancer Society, 2018a). As with melanomas in other parts of the body, vulvar melanomas are aggressive and must not be ignored. If a woman presents with a new or persistent skin discoloration that is dark blue, dark brown, or nearly black, this should be thoroughly evaluated and biopsied. Early diagnosis with biopsy and referral for surgical excision is the best chance for cure from any melanomatous lesion.

RISK FACTORS

Risk factors for vulvar cancers include, but are not limited to, older age, smoking history, HPV infection, immune system deficiency, precancerous condition/vulvar intraepithelial neoplasia, and lichen sclerosus (American Cancer Society, 2018b). Age is a risk factor, as about 85% of all vulvar cancers are diagnosed in women older than 50 years of age (Elkas et al., 2016). HPV-related skin changes of the vulva can be a risk factor for squamous cell vulvar cancer (CDC, n.d.-b). The use of tobacco increases HPV-related premalignant changes of the vulva (Elkas et al., 2016). Women who have autoimmune disorders, HIV, or who are on any chronic immunosuppressive medications are at an increased risk for HPV-related vulvar disease (CDC, 20n.d.-b). Vulva precancerous conditions (e.g., vulvar intraepithelial neoplasia, Paget disease) can enhance a person's risk of developing vulvar cancer (Cancer.net, 2022h). A benign chronic vulvar condition called lichen sclerosus may also increase a woman's risk for vulvar dysplasia or cancer (Cooper et al., 2015). The various cell types of vulvar cancer may have different predisposing risk factors. Vulvar squamous epithelial cells are the most likely cells to be affected by either premalignancy or malignancy. The squamous cells of the vulva serve as the first line of defense and are thus often affected by skin irritants or viruses. A common potential threat to vulvar tissue is HPV (International Agency for Research on Cancer [IARC], 2007). Multiple strains of HPV exist, and many are benign. However, there are several strains of HPV that are considered high risk, and these have the potential to cause precancerous changes in the skin, which may lead to cancer if undetected and/or untreated (CDC, n.d.-b; Table 33.2). Skin-to-skin contact during sexual activity may expose a woman to HPV. HPV may be present but may go undetected, as often as there may be no visible or palpable lesion. Healthy intact tissue of the vulva is normally able to ward off the skin-damaging effects of HPV, and women can be sexually active without any symptoms of HPV exposure. However, for some high-risk HPV types, it is harder for the body to resist infection with HPV, and genital lesions may arise. Vulvar squamous cell carcinomas are associated with strains 6, 11, 16, 18, and 33 (IARC, 2007).

TABLE 33.2 HPV Strains and Their Association With Gynecologic Organs

HIGH-RISK HPV STRAINS	GYNECOLOGIC SITE THAT MAY BE AFFECTED
16, 18, 31, 33, 35, 39, 45, 51, 52, 56, 58, 59, 66	Cervix
6, 11, 16, 18, 33	Vulva
16, 18	Vagina

HPV, human papillomavirus.
Source: Adapted from International Agency for Research on Cancer. (2007). Human papillomaviruses. IARC Monographs on the Evaluation of Carcinogenic Risks to Humans, 90. *https://monographs.iarc.fr/ENG/Monographs/vol90/mono90.pdf*

TABLE 33.3 Vulvar Cancer Stages

Stage I	Cancer confined to vulva; tumor has not spread.
Stage II	Tumor is of any size and has spread to nearby organs but it has not spread to lymph nodes.
Stage III	Cancer has spread to nearby tissue (anus, vagina, urethra) and/or lymph nodes of one side of body but there are no distant metastases.
Stage IV	Cancer has spread to the upper part of the vagina or upper part of the urethra or to a distant part of the body.

Source: Adapted from Cancer.net. (2022). Vulvar cancer: Stages. https://www.cancer
.net/cancer-types/vulvar-cancer/stages

DIAGNOSIS AND TREATMENT

Diagnosis of vulvar cancer is dependent on pathologic confirmation from a biopsy. The primary care provider can perform a punch biopsy of the suspicious area or make a referral to a gynecologic colleague for biopsy. The pathologist will make a diagnosis of a particular type of vulvar cancer. The patient should be referred to a gynecologic oncologist for further evaluation and planning for treatment.

Staging of vulvar cancer involves clinical examination and sometimes imaging (CT scans to detect enlarged lymph nodes) may be needed in planning for appropriate treatment (Table 33.3).

Treatment may include one or more modalities, such as surgery alone, radiation alone, or surgery plus radiation and/or chemotherapy. Precancerous lesions are treated with surgical management, either CO_2 laser or surgical excision or a combination thereof. If there is no evidence of invasive disease and surgical margins are clear, a woman has an excellent prognosis for survival but will need close surveillance. Invasive vulvar cancers are treated with surgical excision with possible lymph node dissection for staging and treatment. Survival rates from invasive vulvar cancers are based on the histologic type of vulvar cancer and the stage of the disease at the time of diagnosis. The 5-year survival rate for women with early-stage vulvar cancer is 86%, whereas for those with advanced-stage vulvar cancers that spread to distant nodes and/or organs, the survival rate is 20% and they have a higher risk of cancer recurrence (Cancer.net, 2023e). Women with a diagnosis of vulvar carcinoma will need close gynecologic surveillance for several years after treatment is completed.

Vaginal Cancer

INCIDENCE/PREVALENCE

Vaginal cancer is the rarest of gynecologic cancers. In 2021, 8,180 women in the United States were diagnosed with vaginal cancer (Cancer.net, 2023d). The vagina refers to the canal or tube that leads from the external vulvar tissue to the upper genital organs (cervix, uterus, ovaries, and fallopian tubes). Vaginal cancer can originate in the outermost layer of vaginal skin, called squamous cell cancer, or the deeper glandular tissue, called adenocarcinoma. There are several rare types of vaginal cancer including melanoma (Frumovitz et al., 2010)

and clear cell carcinoma, which may occur in women whose mothers took the drug diethylstilbestrol (DES) to prevent miscarriage (prescribed from 1940s up to the early 1970s; Verloop et al., 2000).

RISK FACTORS

Many risk factors are associated with vaginal cancer. These risks include age greater than 50 years, HPV infection, history of precancerous lesions of the cervix or vagina, cigarette smoking, previous radiation therapy in the vaginal area (Cancer.net, 2021e), exposure to DES in utero, and altered immune system (Karam et al., 2022).

SYMPTOMS

Vaginal cancer may present as a symptom of an unusual vaginal discharge or discomfort in the pelvic or vaginal area. Frequently, women present with symptoms of irritation or burning inside the vagina. Women with vaginal cancer also commonly describe symptoms of pain and/or bleeding with intercourse as well as difficulty or pain during urination. The vaginal mucosal skin may be discolored, abraded, or ulcerated and may be friable on examination. These women may have pain in their back or swelling in the legs and abnormal bowel function (Cancer.net, 2021f).

DIAGNOSIS AND TREATMENT

As with vulvar cancers, the diagnosis of a vaginal cancer is made by examination and biopsy of the visibly or palpably abnormal vaginal tissue. Biopsy can be done in the office with a punch or a Tischler instrument. Treatment of vaginal cancers is determined by the stage of the cancer (Table 33.4). Preinvasive or early-stage vaginal cancer may be treated with laser surgery or surgical excision. Advanced-stage vaginal cancers may be treated with chemotherapy and/or radiation plus chemotherapy (Shah et al., 2009).

Cervical Cancer

INCIDENCE

Cervical cancers at one time were a common gynecologic cancer. Better screening has resulted in earlier detection of precancerous changes of the cervix, which has resulted in fewer diagnoses of invasive cervical cancer. Despite the decline in cervical cancer diagnosis, there were still approximately 14,100 women diagnosed with cancer of the cervix in 2020 in the United States (Cancer.net, 2023a). The cervix refers to the most external portion of the uterus; it is the mouth of the uterine body. Only the outermost part of the cervix of the

TABLE 33.4 Vaginal Cancer Stages

Stage I	Tumor is confined to the vaginal surface.
Stage II	Tumor invades the wall of the vagina.
Stage III	Cancer spreads to pelvic lymph nodes or pelvic wall.
Stage IV	Cancer spreads to bladder, rectum, or beyond pelvis.

Source: Adapted from Cancer.net. (2021). Vaginal cancer: Stages. https://www.cancer
.net/cancer-types/vaginal-cancer/stages

uterus is visible/palpable on clinical pelvic examination. The cervix contains both squamous and glandular cells, and cancer can affect either type of cell. The most external cells of the cervix are called the ectocervical cells, made up of squamous cells, and the most common cervical cancer is squamous cell carcinoma. Glandular cells line the interior portion of the cervix, and these endocervical cells may develop an endocervical adenocarcinoma. Pap smears, which are a screening test for abnormal cells of the cervix, are ideally able to screen for both ectocervical and endocervical abnormalities. There are several rare cervical cancers, including neuroendocrine, small cell, and glassy cell carcinomas. These rare cancers are aggressive and usually very fast growing, and prompt referral to gynecologic oncology is important.

SYMPTOMS

Symptoms of cervical cancer may or may not be present. Sometimes, cervix cancer is found when a woman has an abnormal Pap smear, and the workup demonstrates cancer on pathology analysis. Other times the woman with cervix cancer will present for evaluation of new symptoms, such as pain or bleeding/spotting with intercourse. A woman may report abnormal menstrual pattern with intermenstrual bleeding or prolonged menstrual bleeding, bleeding after intercourse/pelvic examination/douching, or bleeding after menopause (Cancer.net, 2022b). Cervical cancer may be identified when a woman presents with a persistent foul-smelling vaginal discharge. Women with an advanced cervical cancer may also present with unexplained changes in bowel or bladder habits; unexplained pain in the pelvis, hips, back, or flank areas; or unilateral leg swelling and/or pain.

RISK FACTORS

Risk factors for cervical cancer are typically categorized according to the type of cancer that is detected. Squamous cell carcinomas are the most common of all cervix cancers and these are highly associated with HPV infection, early coitarche, multiple sexual partners, cigarette smoking, altered immune status, herpes, exposure to DES, and low socioeconomic status. Cervical adenocarcinomas, which are the second most common type of cervical cancers, account for approximately 15% to 20% of all cervix cancers (Cancer.net, 2023a). These glandular cell abnormalities are typically a more aggressive or faster growing abnormality. Risk factors for adenocarcinomas of the cervix include HPV infection and past birth control pill usage.

DIAGNOSIS AND TREATMENT

Guidelines for cervix screening have changed with advances in research on HPV. Primary and gynecologic care providers for women will want to consult with the published Pap smear guidelines to determine when to begin, and how often to obtain, screening Pap smears, and how to follow-up on the results (Lemieux, 2010; Limmer et al., 2014; Saslow et al., 2012; Table 33.5). Abnormal or atypical Pap smears may be followed clinically, or may require a referral for a colposcopy, where the cervix can be evaluated under magnification to look for abnormal skin and vessel changes (American College of Obstetricians and Gynecologists [ACOG], 2012). The clinician performing the colposcopies will be able to provide

TABLE 33.5 Guidelines for Pap Smear Screening Among General Population

AGE GROUP	RECOMMENDATION FOR SCREENING
Women younger than 21 years	No Pap smear
Women 21–29 years old	Screening with Pap cytology alone every 3 years
Women 30–65 years old	Screening with cytology every 3 years or FDA-approved primary hrHPV testing alone every 5 years or cotesting (hrHPV and cytology) every 5 years
Women older than 65 years	No screening if no abnormal cytology (CIN 2+) in past 20 years
Posthysterectomy	No screening cytology if no history of abnormal cytology (CIN 2+); if prior abnormal cytology (CIN 2 or 3 or cancer), will need long-term surveillance after hysterectomy

CIN, cervical intraepithelial neoplasia; FDA, Food and Drug Administration; hrHPV, high-risk human papillomavirus.
Source: Adapted from American College of Obstetricians and Gynecologists. (2021). *Updated cervical cancer screening guidelines. https://www.acog.org/clinical/clinical -guidance/practice-advisory/articles/2021/04/updated-cervical-cancer-screening -guidelines; Saslow, D., Solomon, D., Lawson, H. W., Killackey, M., Kulasingam, S., Cain, J., Garcia, F. A., Moriarty, A. T., Waxman, A. G., Wilbur, D. C., Wentzensen, N., Downs, L. S., Spitzer, M., Moscicki, A. B., Franco, E. L., Stoler, M. H., Schiffman, M., Castle, P. E., Myers, E. R., & ACS-ASCCP-ASCP Cervical Cancer Guideline Committee. (2012). American Cancer Society, American Society for Colposcopy and Cervical Pathology, and American Society for Clinical Pathology Screening Guidelines for the Prevention and Early Detection of Cervical Cancer. CA: A Cancer Journal for Clinicians, 62(3), 147–172. https://doi.org/10.3322/caac.21139*

a thorough evaluation of the cervical appearance and an opportunity for biopsy of any abnormal tissue. Precancerous cervical lesions can be effectively treated with noninvasive surgery, which can result in the prevention of cervix cancer. However, the woman treated for a precancerous lesion of the cervix requires a long-term close surveillance to ensure early detection of subsequent abnormal Pap results (Fields, 2013). According to the current guidelines, women with precancerous cervical changes will need to be examined for many years after the treatment is completed (Feldman et al., 2023; Perkins et al., 2020; Saslow et al., 2012; Wang et al., 2023).

Diagnosis of cervical cancer is based on the clinical findings of the pelvic examination and cervical biopsies. Neither Pap smears nor HPV testing are a diagnostic tool, although a Pap smear may detect an abnormality of the cervix, which in turn will lead to a more thorough investigation of the cervix, including HPV testing, biopsy, or molecular testing of the tumor (Cancer.net, 2022a) to determine if there is a high-risk HPV present or a precancerous or cancerous lesion of the cervix (Wright et al., 2011). If the biopsy confirms a cervical cancer, the stage of the cancer is based on the findings of the cervical lesion on pelvic examination and using x-ray, CT, MRI, and/or PET scan to get a picture of the inside of body (Cancer.net, 2022a; Table 33.6). Early-stage cancers are confined to the cervix and are smaller than 4 cm. Advanced stages of cervical cancer are based on whether the tumor has spread to surrounding tissues, such as the vaginal walls, the rectum, or the bladder (Cancer.net, 2023a).

TABLE 33.6 Cervical Cancer Stages

Stage I	Cancer has spread to the deep cervix lining but has not spread beyond the uterus.
Stage II	Cancer has spread beyond the uterus to nearby areas such as the vagina or adjacent tissue but is still in the pelvis; there is no spread to lymph nodes.
Stage III	Cancer has spread to the pelvic sidewall or distal or lowest part of the vagina.
Stage IV	Cancer has invaded bladder or rectum, and spread to distant parts of the body.

Source: Adapted from Cancer.net. (2022). Cervical cancer: Introduction. http://www .cancer.net/cancer-types/cervical-cancer/introduction; Cancer.net. (2022). Cervical cancer: Stages. https://www.cancer.net/cancer-types/cervical-cancer/stages

Treatment of cervical cancer may involve surgery alone for an early-stage cancer. The surgery for cervix cancer is a radical hysterectomy that includes surgery to remove the uterus and cervix, as well as the surrounding parametrial tissue of the vagina that could be at risk for a cancer spread. Targeted therapy is another approach that targets specific cancer tissue. If the tumor is larger than 4 cm or if there is evidence of spread of the cancer beyond the cervix, the cancer will be treated with radiation therapy with or without radiosensitizing chemotherapy. In case of recurrence or spread of cancer, immunotherapy to boost the body's immune system will be used during or after chemotherapy Sometimes, a patient with an advanced cervical cancer will have a surgical lymph node sampling to reduce the amount of tumor burden and/or to help in designing the radiation field for treatment (Cancer.net, 2022c). Cancer of the cervix that has spread beyond the pelvis will be treated with systemic chemotherapy.

Uterine Cancer

INCIDENCE

The most common of all gynecologic cancers is cancer of the uterus. The uterus, also called the womb, has various functions, including menstruation, pregnancy, labor, and delivery (Ameer et al., 2021). The uterus is typically a small pear-shaped organ, but when it is supporting a pregnancy, the uterus can enlarge to accommodate a full-term pregnancy and may occupy a large portion of the pelvis. The uterus is made up of three tissue layers, including perimetrium/serosa (the thin outer layer), myometrium (the middle muscle layer), and endometrium (the inner lining composed of functional and basal endometrium; Ameer et al., 2021). Cancers of the uterus can affect either the endometrium or the myometrium. In 2021, 66,570 women in the United States were diagnosed with uterine cancer (Cancer.net, 2021b, 2023c). The endometrium, which comprises the inner lining or glandular portion of the uterus, is the area most often affected by cancer, and these endometrial adenocarcinomas account for more than 80% of all uterine cancers (Cancer.net, 2021b). A small percentage of endometrial cancers are a rare, serous carcinoma. The second type of uterine cancer affects the myometrium, or outer muscle portion of the uterus, and they are referred to as sarcomas. Uterine sarcomas account for 2% to 4% of all uterine carcinomas (Cancer.net, 2021b).

SYMPTOMS

Women with endometrial cancer frequently present with postmenopausal spotting or bleeding. Perimenopausal or premenopausal women may report a sudden change in their menstrual cycle, such as very heavy or prolonged menstrual periods. Uterine cancer may also present as a feeling of pain, congestion, pressure, or cramping in the pelvis with or without bleeding.

RISK FACTORS

Risk factors for uterine cancer vary depending on where the uterine cancer originates. Several risk factors may increase the risk for endometrial carcinomas (Crosbie et al., 2010). Women older than 50 years are at a higher risk of endometrial cancer than younger premenopausal women (Cancer. net, 2021b). White women have higher incidence of uterine cancer than women of other races/ethnicities. However, Black women and Hispanic women have higher risk of developing aggressive tumors. Postmenopausal hormone therapy may increase a woman's risk for endometrial cancer (Grady et al., 1995; Jaakkola et al., 2011; Zang et al., 2014). Obesity is associated with endometrial cancer (Crosbie et al., 2010; Engel, 2014). Diabetes, which is associated with obesity, can increase risk of uterine cancer. A personal history of breast cancer, colon cancer or ovarian cancer and/or a family history of uterine or colon cancer may place a woman at an increased risk for uterine/endometrial cancer (Lancaster et al., 2015). Previous exposure to radiation therapy in the pelvic area may increase the risk of uterine cancer. Diet containing high animal fat is another risk factor for uterine cancer (Cancer.net, 2021c). Stromal or myometrial tumors are rare and are not associated with particular risk factors.

DIAGNOSIS AND TREATMENT

Various tests exist to find and diagnose uterine cancer. A Pap test during pelvic examination and/or transvaginal ultrasound can be used as tests to suggest uterine cancer. Definitive diagnosis of uterine cancer is made based on biopsy of the uterus either through an in-office endometrial biopsy or by intraoperative dilation and curettage (D&C) of the endometrial tissue. Once the biopsy has confirmed a neoplasm, which can range from preinvasive to invasive carcinoma, the woman should be referred to a gynecologic oncologist for evaluation and planning for treatment. Depending on the pathology and presenting symptoms, imaging—either a pelvic ultrasound, MRI, or a CT scan of the chest/abdomen/pelvis—may be necessary to formulate a treatment plan (Cancer.net, 2021a).

Treatment options for uterine cancer depend on cancer type, cancer stage, and the woman's age and desire to maintain fertility (Cancer.net, 2021d). Treatment for endometrial precancers and cancers almost always involves surgery. The type of surgery may depend on the level of abnormality diagnosed on the biopsy, and how much of the uterus and surrounding tissues are involved based on the imaging. Young women with precancers or low-grade neoplasms who are still interested in pursuing pregnancy may have the opportunity

TABLE 33.7 Uterine Cancer Stages

Stage I	Cancer is confined to uterus lining, invading less than one half of lining thickness.
Stage II	Cancer has spread from uterus to cervix.
Stage III	Cancer has spread from uterus to pelvis, such as lymph nodes.
Stage IV	Cancer invades rectum or bladder, groin lymph nodes, or spreads from pelvis to distant part of body, such as lung.

Source: Adapted from Cancer.net. (2021). Uterine cancer: Introduction. http://www
.cancer.net/cancer-types/uterine-cancer/introduction; Cancer.net. (2021). Uterine
cancer: Stages and grades. http://www.cancer.net/cancer-types/uterine-cancer/stages
-and-grades

for conservative treatment. This conservative management may involve a therapeutic D&C to remove all the abnormal endometrial tissue; then the woman is placed on hormonal management to reverse the process. She is monitored frequently and if the hyperplasia and/or atypia do not recur, she may be allowed to pursue a pregnancy. However, if the woman has completed childbearing when she is diagnosed with an endometrial neoplasm, she will likely be counseled to undergo hysterectomy for definitive management. If there is a true invasive endometrial cancer the treatment is surgical removal of the uterus (including the cervix) and the fallopian tubes/ovaries. The disease is staged based on the pathology results (Table 33.7). Early-stage low-grade neoplasms may be treated by surgery alone. Higher grade neoplasms or advanced-stage disease noted at the time of the initial workup will be treated with a full staging surgery, which would include complete hysterectomy, removal of the bilateral fallopian tubes/ovaries, and dissection of the pelvic and para-aortic lymph nodes, followed by an adjuvant treatment, which may include radiation therapy or therapies using medications such as chemotherapy, hormone therapy, targeted therapy, and immunotherapy (Cancer.net, 2021d).

Cancers of the Ovary/Fallopian Tube/Primary Peritoneum

INCIDENCE/PREVALENCE

The ovaries are in the pelvis on either side of the uterus. The fallopian tubes connect the ovaries to the uterus and play a role in the transport of the eggs released from the ovaries to the uterus. The epithelial surface of the ovary, the inner epithelium of the fallopian tubes, and the lining of the pelvis are all made up of cells known as müllerian cells. These cells arise from fetal gonadal stem cells (Dubeau, 2008). These müllerian cells in any of the sites can develop epithelial carcinoma. The disease is identified based on where it originates, such as ovarian, fallopian tube, or primary peritoneal carcinoma. All these carcinomas tend to behave similarly, and thus their treatment is similar. For simplicity, the term ovarian cancer will be used to refer to any of these cancers. Ovarian cancer affected 21,410 women and caused 13,770 deaths in the United States in 2021 (Cancer.net, 2022e, 2023b). Epithelial

ovarian cancers are the most common type of ovarian cancers, and these typically affect women older than 50 years of age (Cancer.net, 2022e). Another rare type of ovarian cancer, which is called a germ cell tumor, arises from within the ovarian egg or yolk sac. These tumors most often arise in young women 10 to 29 years old (Billmire et al., 2004) and may be called a dermoid or teratoma. Germ cell tumors may be benign or malignant. Malignant germ cell tumors are diagnosed and treated with surgery alone or by a combination of surgery with chemotherapy. Sex cord stromal tumors are a rare type of ovarian cancer that develops in the connective tissue cells. Over 90% of stromal tumors are called granulosa cell tumors, which are usually treated with surgery (Khosla et al., 2014). The last type is fallopian tube cancer, which begins in a fallopian tube, and most of them are serious cancers (Cancer.net, 2022e).

SYMPTOMS

Ovarian cancer is most often detected after it has spread to an advanced stage (Andersen et al., 2008). The symptoms of ovarian cancer may be vague, and it is important to monitor symptoms if they present more than a few weeks for further follow-up. The symptoms include fatigue, pressure or discomfort or a sense of feeling full, menstrual irregularities, swelling in the pelvis or abdomen, vaginal discharge, constipation, back/pelvic/abdominal pain, and indigestion (Cancer.net, 2022e), or the symptoms may be more pronounced, such as significant pain or discomfort, bowel or bladder dysfunction, or even increased abdominal distention from a buildup of fluid in the pelvis. Occasionally, the symptoms of neoplasm may be specific to one area, such as unilateral pelvic pain. Presenting symptoms of primary peritoneal tumors may be abnormal distention related to the accumulated pelvic fluid known as ascites (Urban et al., 2003). Frequently, the woman with pelvic ascites describes symptoms of increased waist size, feeling full too fast (early satiety), and/or chronic sense of bloating (Slatnik & Duff, 2015). Primary and gynecologic providers are encouraged to discuss and assess any unusual pelvic symptoms and to work up persistent, unexplained symptoms for evaluation (Goff et al., 2004, 2012).

RISK FACTORS

Risk factors associated with ovarian cancer include age (particularly over 50), obesity (specifically in early adulthood), family history, genetics, ethnicity (women of North American, Northern European, or Ashkenazi Jewish descent), having a diagnosis of breast cancer, having a diagnosis of endometriosis, using hormone replacement therapy, and a certain reproductive history (started menstrual periods earlier than 12 years old, never being pregnant, unexplained infertility, started menopause later than 51 years old; Cancer.net, 2022e, 2022f; Lacey et al., 2006). Women with a strong family history of ovarian or breast cancer, or family history of cancer of the gastrointestinal (GI) tract (colorectal, stomach, pancreas, or liver) may wish to undergo genetic counseling and possible genetic testing (Pennington & Swisher, 2012). Risk factors for malignant ovarian germ cell tumors have not been clearly identified, though there is a higher risk among individuals with germ cell XY chromosomes combined with androgen insensitivity syndrome (Cancer.net, 2022e).

DIAGNOSIS AND TREATMENT

Most ovarian cancers are diagnosed when a woman presents with symptoms of an abnormal feeling in the pelvis. Due to vagueness of symptoms associated with ovarian cancer, the disease is often not detected until it is in its advanced stage, and thus it is often called "the silent killer" (Andersen et al., 2008). Early-stage ovarian cancers may be detected on a routine screening pelvic bimanual examination if there is nodularity or a firm mass on palpation. Women undergoing pelvic imaging for the workup of infertility may have an abnormality of their ovary and this may prompt referral to a gynecologic oncologist and result in an early-stage diagnosis. Pelvic ultrasound ordered to evaluate the adnexal structures may show a cystic or solid component within, or adjacent to, the ovary or fallopian tube. Women who are still ovulating may have ovarian follicular cysts with their cycle, and these may be enlarged and causing discomfort. Serial, short-interval follow-up ultrasound exams and repeat cancer antigen 125 (CA-125) testing can be helpful in monitoring these ovarian cystic masses to ensure that they resolve with time. However, postmenopausal women, who no longer menstruate, should have small ovaries without cysts; thus, any cystic or solid mass in or near the ovary of an older woman should be evaluated by a gynecologic oncologist. A blood test of the tumor marker CA-125 may be obtained to determine if it is elevated to help in planning for management of a pelvic mass (Bast et al., 2005). CT scan, MRI, PET, biopsy, and molecular testing of the tumor are other ways of diagnosing ovarian cancer (Cancer.net, 2022d).

Treatment of ovarian cancers typically involves multiple modalities, including surgery and systemic therapy using medications, including chemotherapy, targeted therapy, immunotherapy, and hormone therapy. Dependent on the cancer stage, women with ovarian cancer may receive one type of systematic therapy or combination of different types of systematic therapy (Cancer.net, 2022g). Women will have a preoperative staging CT scan of the chest, abdomen, and pelvis to evaluate the pelvic structures, the lymph nodes of the pelvis and along the midline, and the omentum. If there is evidence of a significant amount of disease outside the pelvis at the time of the staging CT scan, the gynecologic oncologist may recommend initial treatment with three to four cycles of chemotherapy to reduce the disease volume and then take her to surgery to achieve optimal surgical results. Many women with ovarian cancer will undergo surgery first for debulking to reduce the burden of the tumor load to a very small residual volume, and then will receive chemotherapy to treat any remaining microscopic disease (Bristow et al., 2002). The success of placing the woman into remission after chemotherapy is positively influenced by the ability of the surgeon to reduce the disease to a volume of less than a centimeter at the completion of the surgery (Bristow et al., 2002). The staging is calculated based on where the disease is identified by imaging as well as the pathology results of the surgery (Table 33.8). The patient and her gynecologic oncologist will set up a plan

TABLE 33.8 Ovarian Cancer Stages

Stage IA	Cancer is confined to one ovary or one fallopian tube.
Stage IB	Cancer involves both ovaries or both fallopian tubes.
Stage IC	Cancer of ovary or fallopian tube and pelvic washings are positive for malignant cells.
Stage IIA	Cancer of ovary has spread to uterus or fallopian tube.
Stage IIB	Cancer of ovary or fallopian tube has spread to other tissues within the pelvis.
Stage III	Cancer has spread to the peritoneum outside the pelvis and/or to lymph nodes in the retroperitoneum behind the abdomen.
Stage IV	Cancer invades organs outside the abdominal area such as spleen, liver, lungs.

Source: Adapted from Cancer.net. (2022). Ovarian, fallopian tube, and peritoneal cancer: Stages and grades. http://www.cancer.net/cancer-types/ovarian-cancer/stages-and-grades

for treatment, which may include observation alone for stage I disease, versus stage II to III and IV diseases, which are treated with chemotherapy delivered either through an intravenous method or a combination of intravenous and intraperitoneal method (Cancer.net, 2022e).

PRIMARY CARE CONSIDERATIONS IN THE TREATMENT AND MANAGEMENT OF GYNECOLOGIC CANCERS

Screening and Diagnosis of Gynecologic Cancers

Nurses are educated in patient assessment beginning in nursing school and continue to augment and refine this skill with continued education and professional growth in caring for patients over their career. When nurses enter advanced practice education, assessment skills are cultivated into a more highly developed and expanded repertoire of skills. Moving into the field of primary care allows the APRN an opportunity to bring this expanded skill set to an ever-changing population of patients with diverse and unexpected healthcare needs. Staying alert to key findings with each patient, from history to physical examination, will prevent missed diagnoses and build trust in the patient–provider relationship (Boxes 33.1 through 33.3).

Care of the Whole Person

Women facing gynecologic cancers continue to have responsibilities to themselves as well as their family, workplace, and community. Ask if there are family members or support persons whom she would like invited into medical visits. Assess

Box 33.1 Key Components of Symptom Analysis: What Not to Miss in Primary Care

- Unexplained change in menstrual bleeding pattern
- Any postmenopausal bleeding or spotting
- Unusual vaginal discharge
- Persistent vulvar/perineal discomfort or itching
- Incomplete or no HPV vaccination
- History of abnormal Pap smears, as well as history of any evaluations and interventions in assessment and treatment of the same
- Pain and/or bleeding from sexual activity
- Family history of gynecologic, gastrointestinal, genitourinary cancers, or melanoma
- After two office visits with persistent concern for abdominal or pelvic pain that has not resolved in more than 2 to 4 weeks, with or without treatment, further assessment and workup are warranted, including pelvic examination, pelvic ultrasound, and possible lab work.

HPV, human papillomavirus.

Box 33.2 Key Components of a Gynecologic Physical Examination: What Not to Miss in Primary Care

- Perform a thorough abdominal exam, noting any nodularity, mass, firmness, or discomfort with examination.
- Evaluate lymphadenopathy in the inguinal regions and left supraclavicular nodes.
- Inspect all external genital structures with pelvic exam.
- Evaluate any skin lesions or discolorations with special attention to palpable thickened, nodular, or plaque-like lesions.
- Inspect vaginal tissues by gentle rotation of the speculum to allow for visualization of the superior and inferior vaginal tissue for any skin discoloration, lesions, or ulcerations.
- Palpate for thickened or nodular areas on bimanual examination.
- Evaluate the size, shape, and density of pelvic organs. Rectovaginal exam can help assess the deep posterior pelvis for any mass or nodularity of the rectovaginal septum.

Box 33.3 Key Diagnostic Studies: What Not to Miss in Primary Care

- Pap smear, HPV testing and typing
- Follow the American Society for Colposcopy and Cervical Pathology (ASCCP) Management Guidelines for any Pap smear, HPV, and cytology results. The ASCCP issues guidelines on management of abnormal cancer screening results. The ASCCP has an app that can be downloaded which walks the clinician through determining evidence-based next steps.
- Biopsy, or referral for biopsy, of any abnormal looking area of the vulva or vagina
- Ultrasound of the pelvis (transvaginal) to evaluate uterine endometrial stripe (thickness) or any endometrial lesion if there is abnormal vaginal bleeding
- Endometrial biopsy for abnormal bleeding pattern, including any postmenopausal spotting or bleeding. Endometrial cancer can still be present even if the endometrial stripe is less than 4 mm, depending on the histology of endometrial cancer. An ultrasound exam alone does not rule out endometrial cancer.
- If the cervix looks abnormal, refer for colposcopy and biopsy; a Pap test is not diagnostic.
- Ultrasound of the pelvis (transvaginal) if there is concern for persistent pelvic pain and/or palpable mass or "fullness" on examination

HPV, human papillomavirus.

Fertility Preservation

The suspicion of gynecologic cancer leads rapidly to extensive testing, biopsy, often surgery, diagnosis, staging, and adjuvant or neoadjuvant treatment. With every additional intervention, there is the possibility of disrupting fertility. Assessing the desire for future childbearing is recommended for any patient of childbearing age but becomes an essential assessment when there is the possibility of a gynecologic malignancy. This conversation needs to happen with the gynecologic oncologist at the time of initial consultation, so the oncologist can partner with the woman in offering fertility-sparing treatment options, if available, and provide evidence for potential risks and benefits of each option, as well as referral to a reproductive endocrinologist. Fertility preservation needs to be addressed before any treatment with the potential to affect fertility, including surgical biopsy, surgery, chemotherapy, and radiation exposure. Become familiar with the reproductive endocrinologists in your area or region and be ready to urgently refer a woman with a potential gynecologic cancer. Fertility preservation techniques may or may not be appropriate to initiate, but this decision needs to be made by the woman herself. Alternative fertility options available after treatment will also be reviewed by the reproductive endocrinologist, allowing the woman to understand the full range of options available to her, including adoption.

the woman's physical, psychosocial, and spiritual needs and participate in shared decision-making interventions to meet the woman's needs. Supporting women with identified needs creates an environment of trust, helps to ensure needs are met, and allows the woman the time and ability to focus on the things that bring joy in her life. Partner with the woman to journey in her cancer experience with her, assuring her of the supports available to her and her family.

Communication

To more fully provide coordination of care with the woman's other healthcare providers, it is prudent for the oncology provider to send office notes to include plan, progress, and outcomes; inpatient hospitalizations; summaries of care; and survivorship plans. If this does not happen, it may be necessary for other offices to request these documents from the oncology team or medical records. Doing so will keep everyone informed regarding the woman's oncology care and will provide some data to know if primary care or specialty care assistance might be helpful. Symptom management related to the oncologic diagnosis is typically treated by the oncology team. Chronic and acute medical conditions unrelated to oncology are typically treated by the primary care team. Primary care can also be a resource in additional community resources and support services.

PROMOTING PREVENTION OF GYNECOLOGIC CANCERS IN PRIMARY CARE

Role of the APRN

APRNs, in their role as both educator and advocate, have an opportunity to assist patients in health promotion across the life span. Prevention of gynecologic cancers begins with role modeling body acceptance and providing a safe environment for women to address genital concerns. Educating parents and children on the timely administration and lifesaving potential of cancer-preventing vaccines begins when the child is still in elementary school (Table 33.9). Encouraging girls to have a portion of their well-child visit alone with their healthcare provider will set the expectation of their wellness visit being a safe opportunity to share information and concerns. Providing open and unbiased education regarding normal form and function

of the genitals, sexuality, physical and psychological safety, and ways of avoiding STIs sets the stage for comfort and trust with healthcare providers. This trust will promote scheduling timely routine health screenings, willingness to ask questions, and comfort in seeking early consultation for any woman's health concern.

Risk Factors for Gynecologic Cancers

Some risk factors cannot be prevented. Genetic predisposition, in utero exposures to toxins, as well as aging, for example, are out of our direct control. Educating women regarding these risks can assist them in seeking care without delay if they have a concern. Each area of the gynecologic tract has its own risk factors that can be prevented or attenuated. Advanced practice providers can advocate for lifestyle changes and educate women on risk reduction.

VULVAR

Increased risk: Cigarette smoking; HPV infection; vulvar or cervical intraepithelial neoplasia; prior history of cervical cancer; vulvar lichen sclerosis; immunodeficiency syndromes; northern European ancestry (Berek & Karam, 2022)

Decreased risk: No exposure to tobacco/nicotine; safer sex practices; timely vaccination with HPV vaccine (NCI, 2022)

VAGINAL

Increased risk: Smoking (Karam et al., 2022); early age at time of first intercourse (Karam et al., 2022); multiple lifetime sexual partners (Karam et al., 2022); DES exposure in utero; HPV exposure through unprotected sexual contact; repeated HPV exposure through multiple partners; lack of HPV vaccination; history of abnormal Pap cytology

Decreased risk: Regular gynecologic surveillance; routine management of abnormal Pap cytology; timely vaccination with HPV vaccine

CERVICAL

Increased risk: HPV infection (Frumovitz, 2022); low socioeconomic status (Frumovitz, 2022); immunosuppression (Frumovitz, 2022); smoking (Frumovitz, 2022); genetics (Frumovitz, 2022); family history of pelvic cancers; DES exposure in utero; alcohol intake; HPV exposure through unprotected sexual contact; repeated HPV exposure through multiple partners; lack of HPV vaccination; history of abnormal Pap cytology; lack of management for abnormal Pap cytology; exposure to other STI or sexual assault; cervical trauma; pelvic radiation; lack of HPV vaccine

Decreased risk: No exposure to tobacco/nicotine; safer sex practices; timely vaccination with HPV vaccine; regular surveillance with pelvic examination and Pap smear to evaluate for abnormal cytology; circumcised males (Frumovitz, 2022)

TABLE 33.9 Vaccine Options for Gynecologic Cancer Prevention

HPV VACCINE	HPV STRAIN TARGETED
Human papillomavirus bivalent vaccine (Cervarix)	16, 18
Human papillomavirus quadrivalent vaccine (Gardasil).	6, 11, 16, 18
Human papillomavirus 9-valent vaccine (Gardasil)[a]	9 6, 11, 16, 18, 31, 33, 45, 52, 58

[a]Presently, in the United States, the only vaccine available is the 9-valent.
HPV, human papillomavirus.
Source: Data from Cox, J. T., & Palefsky, J. M. (2022). *Human papillomavirus vaccination.* UpToDate. https://www.uptodate.com/contents/human-papillomavirus-vaccination

ENDOMETRIAL

Increased risk: Family history of pelvic and colorectal cancers; age older than 50 years; increased estrogen exposure, such as in obesity, polycystic ovary syndrome, nulliparity, unopposed estrogen replacement, early menarche, late menopause, and use of postmenopausal tamoxifen (Halla, 2022)

Decreased risk: Lower estrogen states, including multiparity, late menarche, early menopause, oral contraceptive use, levonorgestrel-releasing intrauterine device (IUD), and combination estrogen and progesterone hormone replacement therapy

OVARIAN

Increased risk: Aging; early menarche or late menopause; genetic factors; nulliparity; endometriosis; asbestos; pelvic radiation. Fertility drugs without pregnancy; prolonged use of hormone replacement with sequential estrogen and progesterone; ovarian cysts; pelvic and colorectal cancers are controversial risk factors (Chen & Berek, 2022).

Decreased risk: Regular surveillance by a healthcare provider; oral contraceptives; tubal ligation; hysterectomy and salpingo-oophorectomy; breastfeeding; and parity (Chen & Berek, 2022)

GENETIC TRAITS AND TESTING FOR GYNECOLOGIC CANCERS

Genetic Risk Factors

Ovarian cancers were previously thought to be random in occurrence. With the advances made in unraveling the genetics of diseases, many, though the minority, of ovarian cancers have been found to be associated with genetic traits identifiable in testing for specific genetic mutations. Genetic causes have been found for cervical, uterine, endometrial, and ovarian cancers. Although there are many genetic traits and syndromes, three are most frequently associated

with gynecologic cancers: breast cancer (*BRCA*) gene 1 or 2, hereditary nonpolyposis colorectal cancer (Lynch syndrome), and Peutz–Jeghers syndrome (Table 33.10).

Genetic Counseling and Testing

Genetic counseling is a process to evaluate and understand a family's risk of an inherited medical condition. A genetic counselor is a healthcare professional with specialized training in medical genetics and counseling (National Society of Genetic Counselors, www.nsgc.org).

Women with gynecologic malignancies should be referred for genetic counseling for any of the following circumstances: those with a personal or family history of breast, colon, or endometrial cancer in women younger than 50; ovarian cancer; microsatellite instability (MSI) high endometrial cancer; as well as multiple cancers in an individual or family (Mahon, 2016). Red flags for hereditary risk include the following: diagnosed with cancer before the age of 50; diagnosis of more than one cancer; family with multiple members having a cancer diagnosis; and diagnosis of a rare cancer (Mahon, 2016). It is imperative to assess and update the woman's and her family's medical history annually to be better able to identify the development of potential hereditary risk (Mahon, 2016). Women without these indications, but who have had a gynecologic cancer not fitting the risk profiles outlined earlier in this chapter may also benefit from genetic counseling.

Genetic counseling can help identify if a patient's cancer is hereditary, which can help inform cancer treatment (Mahon, 2016). In addition, it helps inform the patient's family, if disclosed by the patient, of potential risk allowing for testing and informing of potential risk-reducing strategies (Mahon, 2016). Genetic testing is not always appropriate once the assessment has taken place. Genetic testing is best done on the person who has had cancer; when that is not possible, testing can be done on other family members. With new knowledge regarding genetics, and ever-expanding genetic testing possibilities, returning to a genetic counselor may be recommended for women with high-risk family histories but inconclusive findings, or positive findings with unknown significance. There are many medical, ethical, and financial considerations involved in genetic counseling and testing, and they are covered in Chapter 16, Genetics and Women's Health.

TABLE 33.10 Genetic Traits Associated With Gynecologic Cancers

TYPE OF CANCER	*BRCA1* OR *BRCA2* MUTATION	LYNCH SYNDROME	PEUTZ–JEGHERS SYNDROME
Cervical			X
Uterine			X
Endometrial		X	
Ovarian/fallopian	X	X	X
Primary peritoneal	X		

SURVEILLANCE RECOMMENDATIONS FOR GYNECOLOGIC CANCERS

High-Risk Patient Surveillance

Women with a strong family history of cancer of the breast, uterus, or ovary should be referred for genetic counseling. The genetic counselor may recommend genetic testing, which includes evaluation for various genetic variants based on the specific family's cancer history. Surveillance recommendations will be made depending on history as well as genetic testing results.

Women with hereditary nonpolyposis colorectal cancer (Lynch syndrome) are at increased risk for ovarian and/or endometrial cancer, as well as colon cancer, and will need to have a judicious screening and prevention plan of care in place. Present screening recommendations for uterine and ovarian cancer are as follows: Biannual pelvic exam starting at age 25; annual to biannual transvaginal ultrasound, as well as CA-125 testing (Mahon, 2016). Prevention strategies include consideration of oral contraceptives for chemoprevention, as well as prophylactic hysterectomy and bilateral salpingo-oophorectomy upon completion of childbearing, or at age 35 or over (Mahon, 2016).

Surveillance of the Cancer Survivor

Women who have been diagnosed and treated for a gynecologic malignancy will need close surveillance after the completion of treatment. Surveillance guidelines from the Society of Gynecologic Oncology (SGO; Salani et al., 2017) should be followed for the most up to date surveillance guidelines. Women should be followed by their gynecologic oncologist. The surveillance guidelines from SGO (Salani et al., 2017) will advise on when and if surveillance can be shared in an alternating fashion between the gynecologic oncologist and a benign provider, and when and if care can be resumed by a benign provider.

There are three overarching principles of surveillance. Surveillance will depend on the stage of disease and risk of recurrence (Salani et al., 2017). In addition, the most efficacious approach to surveillance includes review of systems, thorough physical exam, as well as education on signs and symptoms typical of a recurrence (Salani et al., 2017). Data support against routine use of imaging and cytology. Imaging may be used when there is clinical suspicion of disease recurrence (Salani et al., 2017).

Vulvar and Vaginal Cancer Posttreatment Surveillance

Per SGO, the woman with high-risk disease, defined as advanced stage or high-risk histology, should have surveillance exams and be followed by the gynecologic oncologist for more than 5 years out from completion of therapy (Salani et al., 2017). Women with low-risk disease should be followed by the gynecologic oncologist until 2 to 5 years out from completion of therapy; at that time care can be provided by a generalist (Salani et al., 2017). There is insufficient evidence to support routine use of radiographic imaging; However, if there is suspicion for recurrent disease a CT or PET/CT scan may be useful (Salani et al., 2017). A Pap/cytologic test can be considered on a yearly basis; The data do not support cytology utilization to determine a recurrence but cytologic testing may have a value in detecting neoplasia of the genital tract and in patients who are immunocompromised (Salani et al., 2017).

Women with vulvar and vaginal dysplasia (precancerous conditions) will require close surveillance for several years. Surveillance should include a thorough examination of the vulva, vagina, and cervix every 3 months for the first year after treatment, and then, if there is no recurrence, visits can be extended to every 6 months for several years (Salani et al., 2017). Pap smears may be indicated yearly for evaluation of the lower genital tract, though this may vary based on whether the patient has undergone earlier hysterectomy and/or whether she has had an earlier abnormal Pap smear (Salani et al., 2017).

The provider will need to follow the algorithm for abnormal Pap smear follow-up based on the most current ACOG guidelines for Pap surveillance (Khan, 2023; Perkins et al., 2021).

Cervical Cancer Posttreatment Surveillance

Per SGO, the woman with high-risk disease, defined as advanced stage or high-risk histology, should have surveillance exams and be followed by the gynecologic oncologist until more than 5 years out from completion of therapy (Salani et al., 2017). Women with low-risk disease should be followed by the gynecologic oncologist until 2 to 5 years out from completion of therapy; At that time care can be provided by a generalist (Salani et al., 2017). There is insufficient evidence to support routine use of radiographic imaging; however, if there is suspicion for recurrent disease a CT or PET/CT scan may be useful (Salani et al., 2017). A Pap/cytology test can be considered on a yearly basis; The data do not support cytology utilization to determine a recurrence but cytologic testing may have a value in detecting neoplasia of the genital tract and in patients who are immunocompromised (Salani et al., 2017).

Endometrial Cancer Posttreatment Surveillance

Women diagnosed with early-stage endometrial cancer are often treated with surgery alone. Per SGO, the woman should be followed by the gynecologic oncology provider until the woman is more than 5 years out from time of completion of primary therapy or is 2 to 5 years out with low-risk endometrial cancer (Salani et al., 2017). Physical exams in the surveillance setting must include a speculum, pelvic, and rectovaginal exam with each surveillance visit (Salani et al., 2017). Pap smears are not required after hysterectomy for endometrial cancer (Salani et al., 2017). Advanced-stage endometrial cancers will be treated with both surgery and adjuvant treatment, such as radiation therapy and/or chemotherapy.

Ovarian Cancer Posttreatment Surveillance

Per SGO, the woman should be followed by the gynecologic oncology provider until the woman is more than 5 years out from completion of initial therapy (Salani et al., 2017). Physical exam in the surveillance setting must include a speculum, pelvic, and rectovaginal exam with each surveillance visit (Salani et al., 2017). The surveillance visit will also include a thorough review of systems. CA-125 value is elevated in about 80% of cases in women with ovarian cancer (Salani et al., 2017). There should be an open decision-making conversation with the patient about potential benefits and risks of CA-125 monitoring (Salani et al., 2017). Imaging should not be routinely conducted and should be saved for concerns of recurrence by symptoms, exam findings, or rising CA-125 (Salani et al., 2017). When there is a concern for recurrence, the CT scan obtained should be of the chest, abdomen, and pelvis (Salani et al., 2017). For those women who do not have an elevated CA-125 level at diagnosis, there should be a decision-making conversation with the patient about potential benefits and risks of imaging (Salani et al., 2017).

SYMPTOM MANAGEMENT DURING TREATMENT FOR GYNECOLOGIC CANCER

Managing Treatment-Related Symptoms

Most patients undergoing cancer treatment will be under the direct care of their oncology team and will have treatment-related symptoms managed by their gynecologic oncologist, or radiation oncologist if receiving radiation, including the immediate postradiation treatment symptoms. In some cases, such as in more rural areas, patients may seek assistance from their primary care provider. It is always appropriate to request chart notes and treatment information from the oncology team for coordination of care. Reaching out to the oncology team for assistance with symptom management and wellness during cancer treatment will assure that the patient is receiving the most appropriate treatment, that treatments will not interfere with oncology agents, and that therapies are not being duplicated. The Oncology Nursing Society (ONS) offers a breadth of evidence-based practice guidelines for symptom management as well as practice (www.ons.org/ons-guidelines).

PAIN

Pain may be due to surgery, the cancer itself, or side effects from treatment, such as peripheral neuropathy from taxane and platinum agents or radiation therapy. Acute surgical pain needs to be addressed by the gynecologic oncologist. Surgical pain after a hysterectomy and bilateral salpingo-oophorectomy (BSO) can most often be managed with ibuprofen, acetaminophen, and sparing doses of an opiate analgesic. Cancer-related pain management may require escalating doses of opioid pain medicines and is not routinely managed in primary care. If the woman is requiring opioids for cancer-related pain, it is important that there be one provider managing opiate prescribing. It is imperative there be demonstrated good stewardship of opiate prescribing, including a risk assessment and consent. Opiate analgesics are often just one pharmaceutical intervention for treating cancer pain, and other adjuvant medications should be considered depending on the type of pain. For example, anticonvulsants such as gabapentin, pregabalin, or tricyclic antidepressants are helpful in treating neuropathic pain. Corticosteroids are helpful in treating bone pain. In addition, a referral to a palliative care service when a woman has an advanced-stage cancer is also appropriate. Offering referrals for complementary therapies, such as massage, reflexology, acupuncture, reiki, meditation, and hypnosis can assist the patient with pain management and will not interfere with cancer treatments.

NAUSEA

Nausea and other gastrointestinal (GI) symptoms may be due to chemotherapy, inflammation from radiation, ascites, or tumor burden. There are guidelines for management of chemotherapy-induced nausea and vomiting from the National Comprehensive Cancer Network (NCCN) and American Society of Clinical Oncology (ASCO). These guidelines recommend antiemetics based on the emetogenic potential of the antineoplastic agent(s). The goal is prevention of nausea and vomiting, and the regimens often call for scheduled dosing in addition to taking antiemetics as needed at home.

HOT FLASHES

Hot flashes, also called vasomotor symptoms, during gynecologic cancer treatment are caused by the disruption in estrogen production that occurs with surgery, chemotherapy, or radiation of the reproductive organs. Some women who have already gone through age-related menopause report a recurrence of hot flashes with cancer treatment. Treatment with supplemental estrogen is most often contraindicated with gynecologic malignancies and treatments. Supportive care with acupuncture, acupressure, layered clothing, fans, as well as stress reduction techniques, such as breathing exercises and meditation, are effective for many women. If environmental strategies are ineffective, treatment with a selective serotonin reuptake inhibitor (SSRI) may provide significant relief of hot flashes.

RADIATION DERMATITIS

The most common radiation-related skin condition is radiation dermatitis. Pruritus, pain, edema, erythema, dryness, and even blistering may occur. Encourage patients to use cool to lukewarm water and gentle soaps without fragrance for washing, to wear loose-fitting, light cotton clothing, and to avoid direct sun exposure. Topical corticosteroids, aloe, and fragrance-free moisturizers can be used over intact skin. Topical antibiotics may be used on open or peeling areas. Antioxidant supplements may protect cancer cells as well as healthy cells, thereby limiting the therapeutic effect of radiation, and should be avoided. Radiation oncology typically manages these acute skin toxicities.

MUCOSITIS

Mucositis is another condition that can be caused by radiation and chemotherapy. Mucositis can affect the mucosa of the mouth, esophagus, genitals, intestines, and rectum. Soft, bland foods, cool or lukewarm beverages, and supportive care with pain-relieving mouthwashes may be helpful. It is important to avoid most commercial mouthwashes as many contain alcohol or harsh ingredients. Using a mouthwash of salt water with baking powder can help to make the oral cavity less acidic and thereby helps to minimize mucositis. Mucositis may be more severe, and there is an increased risk of secondary infection when radiation is combined with chemotherapy. Contact the oncology team for assistance if mucositis is severe, if eating or elimination is affected, or if there are signs or symptoms of infection.

FATIGUE

Fatigue is a prevalent side effect reported by cancer patients and cancer survivors alike. Fatigue is multifactorial and may be caused by cancer itself, cancer treatments, side effects from medications such as antiemetics to mitigate side effects, and the emotional response to cancer, among others. Cancer-related fatigue is treated symptomatically the way non-cancer-related fatigue is treated, but it does not rebound or reverse as easily. Activity, appropriate periods of rest, supportive nutrition and hydration, and stress reduction are essential for fatigue management. Daily exercise is to be encouraged, even if only slow walking, stretching, or gentle yoga is tolerated. Realistic time management allowing for balance of activity and rest is encouraged for fatigue management during and after active cancer treatment. Prescription stimulant and nonstimulant medications can also be considered.

SYMPTOM MANAGEMENT FOR SURVIVORS OF GYNECOLOGIC CANCER

Cancer Survivorship

NCCN prints standards of survivorship care among other oncology groups (NCCN, 2022). It is a long-held belief that survivorship starts at the moment of diagnosis and continues for the duration of the person's life, regardless of disease state. Standards of survivorship include the following tenets: prevention and screening for new and recurrent cancers; prevention, assessment, and treatment of late effects from cancer and treatment; surveillance; coordination of care between providers; and planning for ongoing survivorship care (NCCN, 2022).

More people than ever before are surviving cancer. With advances in prevention, screening, detection, treatment, and research, cancer survivors numbered an estimated 16.9 million in the United States as of January 2019 (NCI, 2020). That number is expected to increase to 26.1 million by 2040 (NCI, 2020), with approximately 8%, or 1.3 million of those being survivors of cervical, uterine, or ovarian cancers (NCI, 2020). An estimated 75.8% of current cancer survivors are aged 60 years and older in the United States at this time (NCI, 2020).

The National Coalition for Cancer Survivorship (NCCS) conducted the 2021 State of Survivorship Survey including 1,104 cancer survivors from a representative sample of patients by age, race, region, and gender (NCCS, 2021). Data demonstrate there are substantial disparities in the equity and access to oncology care with a disproportionate effect on young adult, female, Hispanic/Latinx, and lower income (NCCS, 2021). In addition, those with metastatic disease have different priorities in care, especially in the arena of quality of life (NCCS, 2021).

Documents called treatment summaries and survivorship care plans are created with the intent of providing a summary of treatment, as well as information on potential long-term and late effects of that treatment, risk surveillance, lifestyle recommendations, and resources for cancer survivors and their nononcology healthcare providers.

Transition to a Shared Care Model

While actively on cancer treatment, patients look to their oncology team for much of their care. Even though the oncology provider will see the survivor back for surveillance and monitoring, even for many years after treatment, they do not provide primary care. Cancer survivors need to understand what care is offered by the oncology provider and what care is given by the primary care provider. It is common in practice to find patients do not have a primary care provider, and patients need to be encouraged to establish care with a primary care provider, understanding this may be a lengthy process because of often closed practices or long wait times in open practices to establish primary care. Over time, some patients will become lost to follow-up for any care, as they are released from the care of their oncologist but do not return to primary care. Cancer survivors are frequently not up to date on routine age-related health screenings, preventive interventions such as immunizations, or monitoring of chronic conditions, such as hypertension, due to this loss of connection to primary care during and after cancer treatment. It is important to assess if women are participating in health maintenance, including immunizations and management of chronic health conditions, cancer prevention screenings, and maintenance of healthy lifestyle interventions.

As primary care providers, APRNs continue providing care to their patients during and after cancer treatment, promoting a shared care model with the oncology team. Advocating for communication with the oncology team throughout active treatment, and with a treatment summary and survivorship care plan at the end of treatment will build trust and confidence in this shared care model. By educating patients regarding the need to maintain a connection with primary care and educating them regarding symptom management during and after treatment, APRNs will be ready to assist patients as they transition off active treatment.

Physical Symptom Management

LONG-TERM AND LATE EFFECTS

Cancer treatments can cause acute, long-term, and late effects. Acute symptoms are addressed by the oncology team and resolve shortly after treatment ends (see Managing Treatment-Related Symptoms, discussed earlier). Long-term effects begin during the treatment phase and persist after treatment ends. Fatigue and peripheral neuropathy are classic long-term effects. Late effects may not be evident for years after treatment ends. Cardiomyopathy, osteoporosis, and secondary cancers are a few examples of known late effects. Some effects, such as peripheral neuropathy, may completely resolve over time, while others, such as infertility, will not. Some effects, such as cardiomyopathy and metabolic syndrome can be prevented or attenuated with lifestyle measures.

Long-term and late effects are dependent on the type of treatment, total dose or exposure, and targeted region of cancer therapy. Table 33.11 demonstrates common long-term and late effects from cancer treatments.

TABLE 33.11 Long-Term and Late Effects of Cancer Treatment by Body System			
AFFECTED AREA	**SURGERY**	**RADIATION**	**CHEMOTHERAPY**
Vision/eye			Dry eyes
Oral/teeth			Dry mouth, dental carries
Cardiac	Lower extremity edema and varicosities	Pelvic and lower extremity lymphedema	Cardiomyopathy, congestive heart failure, hypertension, hyperlipidemia
Respiratory			Restriction, cough, pulmonary fibrosis
Gastrointestinal	Adhesions, changes to bowel function	Colitis, proctitis, chronic nausea	Colitis, irritable bowel syndrome, nausea, food intolerances
Hepatic		Altered liver function	Altered liver function
Urologic	Adhesions, incontinence, urinary urgency and/or frequency	Altered kidney function, urinary incontinence, urgency and/or frequency, cystitis, secondary cancer	Altered kidney function, cystitis, hematuria
Pelvis	Infertility, adhesions, incontinence, lymphedema	Infertility, adhesions, incontinence, lymphedema, atrophic vaginitis, dyspareunia	Infertility, atrophic vaginitis, dyspareunia
Musculoskeletal	Adhesions	Osteoporosis, adhesions, contractures, myalgia, arthralgia	Myalgia, arthralgia
Skin	Adhesions	Adhesions, secondary cancers	Dry skin, urticaria, rash, palmar plantar erythrodysesthesia
Endocrine	Infertility, menopause	Infertility, menopause, hypothyroidism, fatigue	Metabolic syndrome, infertility, fatigue, menopause, thyroid dysfunction especially with immunotherapies
Neurologic	Pain, nerve injury	Pain, paresthesia, fatigue	Tinnitus, pain, peripheral neuropathy, fatigue, cognitive dysfunction

Systematic Treatment of Symptoms

Treatment of reversible long-term and late effects begins with symptomatic and supportive care. Adequate rest, nutrition, hydration, and exercise are routinely the best measures for all body-system symptom management after cancer treatment. Primary care providers will need to assess underlying issues that may interfere with a woman's ability to manage the long-term effects after cancer treatment. The primary provider will want to look for factors that affect the woman's ability to acquire adequate sleep, such as anxiety; that affect her ability to maintain adequate nutrition and hydration, such as nausea; or that may affect her ability to exercise, such as pain or fatigue. Identifying and treating these underlying issues will help move her toward self-management and a sense of control in her adjustment after active treatment.

VISION/ORAL

Dry eyes can be treated with lubricating drops or artificial tears. Dry mouth is reduced by staying well hydrated, although this may not be fully effective. There should be assessment for gum recession and dental caries, and if indicated, primary providers will want to encourage and promote routine dental care with a dental professional.

CARDIAC/RESPIRATORY

Cardiac and respiratory late effects are best managed with awareness, prevention, and early recognition and treatment. A progressive exercise program, potentially guided by a physical therapist, and use of compression garments can prevent or stabilize lymphedema and assist with edema and varicosities. Exercise and a heart healthy diet can prevent hypertension, hyperlipidemia, and help delay or attenuate atherosclerosis, cardiomyopathy, and congestive heart failure. Exercise assists with respiratory restriction and symptoms of fatigue. Smoking cessation is essential, and prevention of respiratory illness with COVID-19, pneumonia, and influenza vaccines is recommended. Careful cardiovascular and respiratory evaluation, to include lipid, blood pressure, and vascular evaluation, is encouraged with an annual wellness examination.

GASTROINTESTINAL

GI symptoms caused by adhesions may be symptomatically improved with massage and yoga, but the adhesions are not reversible without surgical intervention, which in turn will cause more adhesions. Constipation, loose stools, fecal incontinence, and colitis symptoms often respond to soluble fiber and probiotics. Dietary changes, stress reduction strategies, and acupuncture may also be successful in addressing these conditions. For women with radiation-induced colitis, colorectal surgery is commonly involved in the scope and management for the colitis. If liver function tests remain abnormal and do not trend to normal range at the end of cancer treatment, referral to gastroenterology is indicated.

PELVIC AND GENITOURINARY

Pelvic symptoms of incontinence, adhesions, and pain are in part evaluated and managed with assistance from gynecologic oncology, urogynecology, urology, and pelvic floor physical therapy. These symptoms may be reduced with pelvic floor physical therapy, core exercises, and massage therapy. Atrophic vaginitis after treatment for gynecologic cancers may be managed with vaginal moisturizers and lubricants. After open decision-making with the patient on potential risks and benefits, in some situations vaginal estrogen may be utilized. In some situations, vaginal estrogen may be contraindicated, and often, but not always, hormone replacement is contraindicated. Consult with the treating gynecologic oncologist when considering estrogen therapy for a woman with a gynecologic malignancy. Nonestrogen vaginal moisturizers and lubricants are also available, and these products can be used independently or in conjunction with estrogen products, if not contraindicated, to assist with both function and comfort of vulvar and vaginal tissues. Dyspareunia related to hormone deficiency or radiation-induced vaginal atrophy can be managed in part with pelvic floor physical therapy, consistent use of a well-lubricated vaginal dilator, or penetrative coitus with a water-based lubricant three or more times a week. In addition, a small amount of viscous lidocaine may be added to water-based lubricants for use with the vaginal dilator and penetrative intercourse as well. Counseling may be helpful if there is posttraumatic stress, persistent pelvic pain, or body image or sexuality concerns after gynecologic cancer treatments. Altered kidney function, hematuria, interstitial cystitis, and other conditions may require the assistance of a urologist.

SKELETAL

Osteoporosis is a risk with both radiation exposure and reduction in estrogen production. Prevention with resistance exercise, adequate dietary and/or supplemental calcium, and supplemental vitamin D is advised. A bone density (dual-energy x-ray absorptiometry [DEXA]) examination and vitamin D level is recommended at the completion of cancer treatment to assess baseline risk status. Follow-up at least yearly with assessment of exercise participation and calcium and vitamin D intake. For abnormal DEXA scan results consider referral to endocrinology for evidence-based interventions and consideration of repeat DEXA scans, depending on baseline study results and treatment interventions for bone health. Myalgia, arthralgia, adhesions, and weakness can be addressed with physical therapy, massage, acupuncture, nutrition, exercise, and topical anesthetic use such as a lidocaine patch for comfort.

INTEGUMENT

Dry skin, skin sensitivity, urticaria, and rash are common after cancer treatments. Routine use of fragrance-free moisturizers and gentle soaps is often enough to reduce symptoms. After radiation exposure, cancer survivors are at increased risk for various skin cancers in their radiation field. Sunscreen use and avoiding prolonged direct sun exposure are encouraged. Dermatologic evaluation of the radiation field is recommended and may be needed for evaluation and treatment of other skin conditions after cancer treatments. Hair loss in the radiation field may be permanent.

ENDOCRINE

Radiation, chemotherapy including immunotherapy, surgery, and treatment modalities such as aromatase inhibitors all contribute to endocrine effects (Gebauer et al., 2019). Endocrine changes with cancer treatments may be acute, such as surgical menopause, or late, such as osteoporosis. Symptomatic management of hot flashes, osteoporosis risk, and fatigue, as outlined earlier, assists with acute and long-term effects.

INFERTILITY

Infertility is highly likely, but is not always an outcome of radiation and/or chemotherapy exposure, depending on the treatment field and doses provided. A very small amount of radiation to the ovaries will result in ovarian failure. Avoidance of pregnancy for 1 full year after cancer treatment is recommended, and contraception is advised if there is the potential for pregnancy. A fertility evaluation, which includes ultrasound evaluation of the reproductive organs, laboratory evaluation of hormone levels, physical examination, and a consultation with a reproductive endocrinologist, is recommended if the survivor of gynecologic cancer is interested in childbearing, and this should occur before treatment has commenced to most fully explore potential interventions and procedures if fertility is desired. The support of a mental health counselor or support group may be helpful if there is a sense of grief around loss of fertility.

PAIN

Symptom management of postcancer pain includes interventional procedures, massage, physical therapy, acupuncture, acupressure, guided imagery, hypnosis, meditation, exercise, counseling, and distraction. Medications, such as anti-inflammatories, non-narcotic pain relievers, muscle relaxants, antidepressants, anticonvulsants, and opiate pain relievers may be appropriate for some patients. It is good to remember that this pain may be temporary or chronic, and treatments need to be monitored and reassessed for appropriateness over time. Referral to a pain management specialist is recommended if assistance is needed for chronic pain management or if interventional procedures may be beneficial in relieving pain. There also can be consideration for referral to a palliative medicine service in managing chronic pain.

NEUROPATHY

Peripheral neuropathy decreases after cancer treatment but may not ever fully resolve, interfering with sensation, comfort, and even function. Excellent supportive care assists in symptom reduction over time. Massage, acupuncture, nutritional support, and exercise are effective in the reduction of symptoms for many cancer survivors. Physical and occupational therapy may be needed if balance concerns create a fall risk for survivors with persistent lower extremity neuropathy or if function of the digits/hands is affected.

COGNITIVE DYSFUNCTION

Cognitive dysfunction, often referred to as "chemo brain," is common in cancer survivors, but a specific cause is yet to be determined, though there are likely multiple etiologies involved. Reports of cognitive dysfunction range from mild, intermittent word finding concerns to complete memory blocks. Inability to organize and prioritize tasks may alter the ability to return to previous employment, especially for those who need optimal cognition to safely perform job tasks, and for whom decreased short-term memory may severely alter the ability to remember or learn new skills. As with other survivorship symptoms, supportive care and time generally improve cognitive function. Compensatory devices, such as keeping appointment reminders in a notebook or cell phone, mapping the route and list of errands to run, and having a routine for work-related tasks can be helpful. If cognitive dysfunction persists or impacts performance and quality of life at work or home, referral for neuropsychological evaluation is indicated.

Psychological Symptom Management and Support

It is normal for the cancer survivor to be afraid of cancer recurrence and experience a sense of living with uncertainty. Reassurance that this is normal, and reduces over time, may be all your patient needs to move forward. Encourage her to discuss her feelings of worry with family, friends, counselors, and support groups of other cancer survivors. If worry begins to interfere in functioning, or there are signs of posttraumatic stress disorder, referral for counseling is indicated. Depression, anxiety, posttraumatic stress disorder, insomnia, body image concerns, and relationship issues are all common after cancer treatment. These may be transient or persistent; they may be situational or global. Careful assessment of the cancer survivor at each visit will allow for early intervention and appropriate management. Supportive care with support groups, counseling, and cognitive behavioral therapy may need to be augmented with medications for anxiety, depression, or insomnia. Exercise, yoga, meditation, hypnosis, acupuncture, and massage all have shown demonstrable impact on mental health for cancer survivors. Referral for a sleep medicine evaluation may be indicated if the cancer survivor reports persistent fatigue, insomnia, or disordered sleep–wake cycles after treatment.

SEXUAL HEALTH

The impact on intimacy and sexual health can be profound in the survivor of a gynecologic cancer. Relationship roles may have shifted during treatment to more of a caregiver–patient relationship than that of an intimate couple. Fear of pain, altered body image, and feeling that the genital area is no longer sensual, or a source of pleasure, and even perhaps displeasure is common after gynecologic cancer treatment. Encourage communication between partners; suggest they explore other ways of expressing intimacy; offer help with vaginal moisturizers, sexual lubricants, and hormone replacement as appropriate (see Symptom Management, discussed earlier); and make referrals for counseling as needed.

For nonpartnered women, reentering the dating arena poses additional stressors with body image concerns, fear of rejection, and emotional vulnerability. Support groups as well as counseling can be helpful to address these issues. Providers certified by the American Association of Sexuality Educators, Counselors, and Therapists (aasect.org) can be especially helpful to address issues of intimacy and sexuality after cancer.

SPIRITUAL DISTRESS

Spiritual distress, including feelings of doubt, guilt, shame, hopelessness, questioning the meaning of the illness in their life, fear, and questioning one's relationship with one's deity in cancer survivors are well documented. Feeling in conflict with, or abandoned by, family, friends, or community is common. Questioning faith and trying to find meaning after cancer can lead to a sense of hopelessness and spiritual struggle. Many cancer survivors find that talking with a professional chaplain, a trusted religious or spiritual advisor, or a therapist about these issues is helpful. Being able to "give back," through volunteering or paid work with organizations helping various populations in need, is often therapeutic for management of spiritual distress.

Returning to work, inability to return to work, resuming routine activities of daily living, finding assistance with care needs, lack of control, and the financial burden of medical costs are all stressors related to cancer survivorship without easy solutions. Advanced care planning discussions, including encouraging completion of documents, such as living wills and durable power of attorney for healthcare, can assist cancer survivors to have a feeling of control over end-of-life issues. Assisting patients with referrals to community agencies, filling out Family and Medical Leave Act (FMLA, 1993) or disability paperwork, and advocating for social services are all within the role of the APRN.

Wellness and Lifestyle Management

Exercise, nutrition, hydration, sleep, stress management, and mental and spiritual wellness contribute to healthy cancer survivorship. Lifestyle management, including addressing substance use, relationship issues, and finding meaning promote healthy coping. Supportive care with routine health maintenance visits, surveillance for cancer recurrence, and preventive healthcare services promote early detection and treatment for physical and mental health issues. Education and advocacy for healthy lifestyle management for the gynecologic cancer survivor is well within the scope of the APRN.

END-OF-LIFE CONSIDERATIONS

Not all cancer patients become long-term cancer survivors. As noted at the beginning of this chapter, many women will present late for evaluation of pelvic symptoms, will have limited warning symptoms, or were previously not appropriately assessed and managed upon presentation for the gynecologic cancer rendering a late or misdiagnosis and will present for care to gynecologic oncology with late-stage or metastatic disease. The primary care provider frequently has a long-standing relationship with the patient and may be looked to for information and advice on end-of-life care. Advance knowledge regarding resource availability in the community for end-of-life care will assist in directing the patient with confidence to the appropriate resources.

Palliative care services are becoming more available, in both inpatient and outpatient settings. Palliative care providers can assist with management of symptoms such as pain, fatigue, and spiritual distress. Unlike hospice, palliative care may be pursued during active cancer treatment (Mo et al., 2021). It is now optimal to refer to palliative care at the beginning of the disease trajectory. As the woman and her family move forward on the disease trajectory and reach a place of palliation of symptoms, and then end-of-life care, the relationship with the interdisciplinary palliative care team has been well established and embedded as care team members, and goals of care and symptom management have been provided for over the long haul. The palliative care team continues to be embedded in care with end-of-life services, often in conjunction with community resources if the patient stays at home or in the community. Hospice becomes available to patients who are no longer seeking disease-targeted treatments (Mo et al., 2021), have an estimated prognosis of 6 months or less, and who wish to focus on relief of symptoms and end-of-life care. Hospice, like palliative care, assists with symptom management—pain, fatigue, mobility issues, altered nutrition status, establishing and revising goals of care, establishing and revising advance directives, but not while under treatment for disease-ameliorating intent. Patients and healthcare providers often believe that these services are only helpful at the very end of life. Both palliative care and hospice focus on function and quality of life and can assist the patient and family with staying comfortable, functional, and in control of their symptoms for long periods of time and have been shown to dramatically improve symptoms and distress throughout the course of the disease (Mo et al., 2021). Knowing how, and when, to access and refer to these services in the community can make a dramatic difference in the quality of life for the woman with cancer and her family members.

There is the potential for significant distress for the woman and her family as the end of her life approaches. She may be afraid to ask about resources for symptom management, end-of-life issues, funeral services, and may not have previously arranged to have a durable power of attorney (DPOA) for healthcare decisions. She may not have had a safe place or opportunity to discuss her end-of-life wishes, distress, and fears. As an APRN, you may be the one addressing these issues and providing support for the woman at the end of life, as well as for her family. Knowledge of referral sources for counselors, legal assistance, funeral services, and supportive care services in the community is an essential skill set to have for these situations. Continuing to educate and advocate for patients at the end of life, making referrals, and providing direct care brings full circle the role of the APRN.

FUTURE DIRECTIONS

There are technological advances in the areas of genetic screening, genomics, molecular medicine, biomarkers, and biological agents in the news headlines. Vaccines for both cancer prevention and treatment are in development. Cancer survivorship is being recognized as a specific phase of cancer care, and there are more people surviving cancer than ever before. With an ever-expanding number of primary care patients having cancer as part of their past medical history, cancer is rapidly becoming a chronic medical illness being managed in the primary care and oncology settings.

REFERENCES

References for this chapter are online and available at https://connect.springerpub.com.

ADDITIONAL READING

An additional reading list for this chapter is online and available at https://connect.springerpub.com/content/book/978-0-8261-6722-4/part/part03/chapter/ch33

CHAPTER 34

Menopause*

Ivy M. Alexander, Annette Jakubisin-Konicki, Amanda M. Swan, Jessica L. Palozie, and Jenna LoGiudice

The stages of menopause consist of a progression of physical and psychological processes identified as perimenopause, menopause, and postmenopause. Premature menopause caused by surgical removal of ovaries, ovarian failures, or other circumstances has an impact on a person's life that is frequently not addressed by either the person or the medical profession. Attitudes toward menopause are culturally based. Current cultural views of menopause vary; some view it as "mental balance" and enhanced personal freedom, while others see menopause as a loss of culture, health, and social status (Stanzel et al., 2017).

Although now more widely viewed as a natural life stage, negative attitudes about menopause were common in developed countries where youth is valued. Postmenopausal people were depicted as "irritable and cranky," and as sexless, useless, or crazy. In a study of Mexican and American college students, participants from both countries defined a postmenopausal woman as "old *and* irritable" (Marvan et al., 2008, p. 678). Anthropologists studying menopause found that symptoms vary between cultures; in some cultures, there are no words to describe some menopause-related symptoms such as "hot flashes" (HFs) or even menopause itself (Sievert, 2014). Some ethnic groups describe speaking of menopause as a "private matter," saved for those of their own race and gender (Dillaway et al., 2008). Other societal attitudes have viewed discussion of menopause as "taboo" (Edwards et al., 2021).

Male perceptions of menopause have rarely been explored; however, one study of British men found that sharing the responsibility for being in a relationship was common, including when the women partners were experiencing menopause. Many men described a joint endeavor and the importance of prioritizing the women's well-being. Others described feeling redundant and helpless, and unable to be supportive (Liao et al., 2015).

Historically, Western societies medicalized menopause, concentrating on pharmaceuticals, including hormone replacement therapy (now called hormone therapy, HT), antidepressants, and other medications to relieve symptoms. "The introduction of the first synthetic replacement hormone in 1938 led to the construction of menopause as a 'hormone deficiency disease'" (Newhart, 2013, p. 366). As early as 1966, Wilson described menopause as "an estrogen deficiency" and touted HT to provide youth, beauty, and sexuality for postmenopausal women (Wilson et al., 1966). Currently, there is less use of synthetic HT and an increased interest in managing symptoms with lifestyle changes and using biologically identical hormone therapy (BHT) if necessary. While BHT is synthesized in a laboratory, some women reported selecting it over pharmaceutical or synthetic HT because they believed BHT provides effective symptom management, is safer than HT, and is individualized. Conversely, reasons against using BHT included uncertainty of therapy safety, aversion to conjugated estrogens, and lack of trust of the medical system (Thompson et al., 2017). Although reduced estrogen production is the main biological etiology and pharmaceuticals, HT or BHT, are one way to address it, we know that menopause encompasses many more transformations.

For many, the transition to postmenopause (TPM) is associated with changed perceptions of health, family, and social situations and presents an opportunity to reevaluate one's life and reaffirm their desire to improve and maintain their health (Alexander et al., 2003; Kaufert et al., 1998). The importance of health during and following the TPM is receiving greater attention in part because of the increasing number of people living through and past menopause. Because of the increased life span, a full one third of one's life is lived after menopause. According to the 2019 U.S. Census, 48,913,000 women were between 50 and 74 years of age and in total 61,180,000 were between 50 and 85 years of age (U.S. Census Bureau, 2019). As the population ages, the unique health needs during postmenopause are becoming better understood as natural changes.

Adjustment to postmenopause is reported to incorporate both an emotional and psychological adaptation to the loss of fertility and perceived changes in appearance and health. Shifting beliefs and attitudes related to the biological adjustments occur as more years pass after menopause (Dasgupta & Ray, 2017). The heightened attention to health during and

---

*This chapter is a revision of the chapter that appeared in the second edition of this textbook, coauthored with Seja Jackson, Devangi Ladani, and Lauren Vo, and we thank them for their original contribution.

following menopause is also related to the changes in health risks that are associated with midlife. The natural alterations in the hormonal milieu that accompanies menopause and other natural aging processes increase risk for heart disease, bone loss, diabetes, obesity, and various types of cancer. As estrogen and progesterone levels decline, menopause-associated symptoms are more likely and may prompt one to seek healthcare. These consultations provide a unique opportunity to assist with symptom management as well as to provide evaluation and education about other midlife health risks.

Harris (2008) recommends a holistic model to optimize care at midlife with recognition that community, sociocultural, and sociopolitical contexts can support or disable positive aging (Harris, 2008). Harris encourages learning from those who have already made the journey through menopause to optimize the opportunities to strengthen body, mind, and spirit. Contemporary perspectives continue to adjust to better understand antecedents that influence experiences and care needed at midlife and beyond.

A note about language: The authors attempt to use inclusive language throughout this chapter. The need to accurately represent data from research often requires the use of terms such as *woman* and *women* as few data are available that represent the experiences of the midlife transition and postmenopause among individuals who do not identify as female. The term *female* is used when describing a person who was born with a uterus and ovaries and is not taking gender affirming HT.

DEFINITION AND SCOPE

Menopause is technically identified as a point in time following 12 consecutive months of amenorrhea occurring in response to normal physiologic changes in the hypothalamic–pituitary–ovarian (HPO) axis (Table 34.1; North American Menopause Society [NAMS], 2019). These changes result in fewer follicles developing in the ovary during each menstrual cycle throughout the TPM, which encompasses the 2 to 10 years preceding the final menstrual period (FMP) and the 12 months of amenorrhea immediately before menopause. The follicles that develop during the perimenopausal period are less sensitive to follicle-stimulating hormone (FSH), and ovarian production of estradiol, progesterone, and androgens declines. In addition, there is a reduction in circulating antimüllerian hormone (AMH) and inhibin B, both of which help to restrain follicular growth causing accelerated follicle atresia (Hansen et al., 2008). Together, these changes cause alterations in the normal negative feedback system that causes hypothalamic production of gonadotropin-releasing hormone (GnRH) in response to elevated estrogen and progesterone levels, allowing FSH and luteinizing hormone (LH) production by the anterior pituitary to continue. Over time, follicle production in the ovaries ceases, estrogen and progesterone hormone levels remain low, FSH and LH levels remain high, and menstruation ceases altogether. Although the term *postmenopausal* is commonly applied after menopause, the postmenopausal period technically refers to the first 5 years after menopause. Hormonal fluctuations are common during

TABLE 34.1 Terms and Definitions Used With Menopause

TERM/ABBREVIATION	DEFINITION/COMMENT
Perimenopause	Period preceding final menstrual period by 8–10 years, usually occurring between 48 and 55 years of age, associated with many symptoms of menopausal transition attributable to fluctuating hormone levels. Also encompasses the 12 months following FMP (see Box 34.1).
Menopause	Point in time occurring 12 consecutive months after natural cessation of menses; average age in North America is 51 years.
Postmenopause	Period following menopause, commonly associated with symptoms attributable to waning estrogen and progesterone levels
HRT	Hormone replacement therapy; older term now replaced by preferred term, hormone therapy (HT) or menopausal hormone therapy (MHT)
HT	Hormone therapy; term encompasses ET, EPT, ETT, estrogen + bazedoxifene; preferred term for accurate communication; use urged by NAMS
MHT	Menopause hormone therapy
BHRT	Biologically identical hormone replacement therapy
ET	Estrogen therapy
EPT	Estrogen-progestogen therapy
ETT	Estrogen-testosterone therapy

FMP, final menstrual period; NAMS, North American Menopause Society.
Source: Adapted from The North American Menopause Society. (2019). Menopause practice: A clinician's guide (6th ed.). Author.

this period. The average age for natural menopause in North America is 51, with most experiencing it between 48 and 54 years of age (NAMS, 2019).

ETIOLOGY

Reduced levels of estrogen and progesterone are largely responsible for the menopause-related symptoms that women experience (NAMS, 2019). Alpha and beta estrogen receptors have been identified; these receptors have different affinities for the three different forms of endogenous estrogen (estrone, estradiol, estriol). Both types of receptors are located throughout the body—in the brain (cognitive and vasomotor centers), heart, skin, eyes, gastrointestinal tract,

Box 34.1 Menopause From Causes Other Than Natural Aging

- *Primary ovarian insufficiency* (POI) or *premature ovarian failure* (POF) is transient or permanent loss of ovarian function in women younger than 40 years. It is usually associated with other health problems such as genetic anomalies, autoimmune disorders, or metabolic disturbances, as well as pelvic surgery, radiation, or chemotherapy. Further assessment is appropriate if a woman younger than 40 years of age misses three or more consecutive menstrual cycles.
- *Induced menopause* results from surgical removal of both ovaries (bilateral oophorectomy) or ablation of ovarian function from chemotherapy, medications, or radiation. Fertility and menstruation cease abruptly following surgical menopause, and symptoms can be quite severe because of the sudden cessation of ovarian hormone production and subsequent abrupt drop in circulating estrogen levels. For women who experience induced menopause following ablative therapies, fertility and menstruation may continue for several months until they finally cease.
- *Premature menopause* occurs before the age of 40 years and frequently follows the same pattern as natural menopause including the permanent cessation of menstruation and fertility.
- *Early menopause* occurs in women between the ages of 40 and 45 years and about 5% of women are affected.
- *Temporary menopause* can occur at any age if normal ovarian function is interrupted and then resumes. Temporary menopause can be medication induced, related to a disease process, or idiopathic.

Source: Adapted from The North American Menopause Society. (2019). Menopause practice: A clinician's guide (6th ed.). *Author.*

vascular system, urogenital tract, breast tissue, and bone. Similarly, progesterone receptors are located throughout the body—in the pituitary, vasomotor, and hypothalamic areas in the brain; vascular tissues and heart; lung; pancreas; bones; and breasts and reproductive organs. When the hormone levels fluctuate and decline, estrogen and progesterone receptors remain unbound, resulting in symptoms, such as vaginal dryness and HFs. As a result of the different affinities of receptors located throughout the body and among women, symptoms are individualized.

Although the perimenopausal transition sounds like a smooth process, it is anything but smooth for many women. Hormonal levels can fluctuate widely, causing abrupt changes that lead to many of the symptoms women experience. These fluctuating hormone levels explain in part why some women have wide variations of symptoms, being asymptomatic some days and manifesting severe symptoms on other days. Hormonal fluctuations are caused by multiple factors, including the reduced number of functioning ovarian follicles.

Interestingly, women continue to produce both estrogen and androgens after menopause (NAMS, 2019). Estrone (E1), the weakest estrogen, is the primary estrogen found in postmenopausal women. It is produced by adipose tissue conversion of androstenedione secreted by the adrenal glands (95%) and the ovaries and by estradiol metabolism (5%).

Following menopause, the ovaries cease to produce functional follicles. However, the hilar and corticostromal cells of the ovarian stromal tissue are steroidogenic and continue to produce significant levels of both testosterone and androstenedione. In postmenopausal women, circulating levels of androstenedione are about half those of their premenopausal counterparts. In contrast, circulating testosterone levels are relatively constant in pre- and postmenopausal women, partially attributable to the effects of high FSH levels, which stimulate ovarian stromal tissue to increase testosterone production. Dehydroepiandrosterone (DHEA), produced primarily in the adrenals, and DHEA-S, a sulfated metabolite of DHEA, levels decline with natural aging but have been shown to temporarily increase in the late TPM. The physiologic significance of this remains unclear (McConnell et al., 2012). Aromatization of DHEA, testosterone, and androgen to estrone and estradiol does increase with age. Overall, androgen metabolism is more heavily affected by the aging process than by the decline in ovarian function associated with menopause (NAMS, 2019).

In biological females, androgens are responsible for sexual sensation, libido, and motivation to pursue sexual activity, as well as for maintaining muscle and bone strength. Testosterone exists in both bound and unbound forms (NAMS, 2019). Circulating unbound or free levels of testosterone constitute approximately 2% of the total testosterone that exists in a female's body. The rest of the circulating testosterone binds to either sex hormone binding globulin (SHGB) or albumin. Higher SHBG levels (as seen when oral estrogen therapy [ET] is used) can reduce free testosterone levels. Conversely, lower levels of SHBG (a condition that can occur with hypothyroidism and obesity) can increase free testosterone levels (NAMS, 2019). Although total testosterone levels are usually fairly constant in postmenopause, free levels might increase or decline slightly in some. Multiple factors besides natural aging can cause menopause (see Box 34.1; NAMS, 2019).

FACTORS AFFECTING THE TIMING OF MENOPAUSE

Although all who are biologically predisposed and live long enough will experience menopause, predicting age for menopause is difficult. Gene mutation and statistical models have had minimal success in predicting the onset of menopause or risk of early menopause (Hefler et al., 2006; Huber et al., 2006). However, there is some correlation with the age when a mother or older sister experienced it (Bentzen et al., 2013; Cramer et al., 1995). There are substantial differences in age of menopause between geographical areas.

Multiple factors that may affect the age of menopause have been studied: age at menarche, height, body mass index (BMI), weight change, exercise participation, level of education, parity, breastfeeding, diet, nicotine use (Lujan-Barosso et al., 2018), alcohol consumption, and oral contraceptive use (Choi et al., 2017; Ding et al., 2020; InterLACE Study Team, 2019). Although there is no unequivocal evidence that any of these factors have a significant effect on the timing of menopause, smoking has emerged as having a fairly consistent correlation with earlier menopause by approximately 1.5 years (Butts et al., 2014; Sapre & Thakur, 2014). Initially, obesity and smoking were premised to link with early menopause. However, smoking and being underweight have been linked with early menopause (Mishra et al., 2019). Similarly, changes in menstrual cycling (e.g., cycle length, amount of bleeding, and 60- or 90-day periods of amenorrhea) suggest a shorter length of time to the FMP (Gracia et al., 2005; Harlow et al., 2006). Heavy bleeding was associated with fibroids or obesity (Harlow, 2018). The data gathered by the U.S.-based Study of Women's Health Across the Nation (SWAN) suggest that several variables together may be useful in predicting the FMP, such as age, irregular menstrual cycling, serum hormone levels, and smoking (Gold et al., 2013). Many studies (Butts et al., 2014; Chen et al., 2014; Lu et al., 2010; Spencer et al., 2013) examine the effect of genetics on onset of menopause, and more than 17 (He & Murabito, 2014) specific genetic markers are associated with earlier onset.

Ethnicity could also affect the timing of menopause. The Multiethnic Cohort Study (Henderson et al., 2008) revealed that Hispanic women, especially those born outside the United States, experienced significantly earlier menopause than White women. Black women experienced menopause at the same age as White women, and Japanese women experienced significantly later menopause. Conversely, a longitudinal analysis as part of the SWAN study (Gold et al., 2013) found that, like with many health issues, racial and ethnic differences are no longer statistically significant once socioeconomic, lifestyle, and health variables are controlled. This supports the finding that social determinants of health are more strongly related to age at menopause than ethnicity or race alone. Body size may also play a role in the timing of menopause, possibly because adipose tissues store androstenedione and convert it to estrogen.

SYMPTOMS

Despite the negative press often associated with the TPM, it is a normal life stage and normalizing the experience may be beneficial. Hormonal fluctuations can cause distressing symptoms that may negatively affect quality of life (QOL; NAMS, 2019). However, for some, the transition is essentially silent. Approximately one third experience little or no menopause-related symptoms. Another one third may experience mild symptoms that are only bothersome on occasion. The final one third may have moderate to severe symptoms that can interfere with daily activities and sleep, leading to disruptions in work performance and causing moodiness or irritability.

Every person presenting with symptoms suggestive of the TPM should be carefully assessed as there is a wide variation in the experience for individuals. Common symptoms are listed in Box 34.2.

The severity of the symptoms experienced may vary. Generally, symptoms begin during the years prior to the FMP and slowly increase in severity over time (NAMS, 2019). Irregular menses are often the first sign of hormonal changes associated with the TPM. Such changes may include alterations in flow or cycle length, missed periods, and increased or newly developing premenstrual symptoms. The most common menopause-associated symptoms are vasomotor symptoms (VMS; including HFs and night sweats) and vaginal dryness. The frequency, severity, and incidence of VMS are highest for 5 to 7 years after menopause; however, many women continue to experience HFs for several more years (Tepper et al., 2016).

VMS are the most common menopause-related symptom, affecting 60% to 80% during the TPM and postmenopause (NAMS, 2019; Thurston & Joffe, 2011). Several risk factors for VMS have been identified in large-scale studies but only a few have strong enough associations to be considered predictive. These include socioeconomic factors, obesity, and cigarette smoking. The SWAN, which included a racially and ethnically diverse population, found that those who reported difficulty paying for basic needs were more likely to report VMS compared to others (Gold et al., 2006). SWAN also found that increased abdominal adiposity and higher body fat percentages were associated with higher odds of reporting VMS (Thurston, Sowers, Chang, et al., 2008). Interestingly, the connection between obesity and increased VMS seems to be strongest in earlier stages of the TPM. In contrast, obesity has been associated with fewer reported VMS during postmenopause (Gold et al., 2017). Smoking cigarettes has consistently been shown to increase the risk of VMS; there seems to be a dose-response relationship between pack-years and risk of VMS (Jenabi & Poorolajal, 2015).

Most experience VMS as an intense heat sensation, beginning at the head and moving down the body or beginning at the feet and moving upward. Some have a prodromal sensation. VMS cause a measurable increase in skin conductance and temperature and may or may not be accompanied by sweating. The heat sensation is often followed by a decrease in core body temperature, sometimes causing a chill, which can be exacerbated with sweating. Some also experience flushing of the upper chest and face (hot flushes). Night sweats are defined as HFs that occur during sleep and are a common manifestation of VMS. The etiology of VMS remains unclear and multiple mechanisms are likely involved. VMS have been associated with a surge in the LH level. Because of a narrowing of the thermoneutral zone, small changes in core body temperature may precipitate VMS, sweating, or chills when the core body temperature rises above or falls below the thermoneutral thresholds (Freedman & Blacker, 2002).

Sleep problems are also common during the TPM. Some sleep changes are related to aging: they are an overall reduced need for sleep (8 hours per night initially and ~7 hours as the person ages), more frequent periods of brief arousal, and less time spent in sleep stages III (early deep sleep) and IV. Night sweats can further interrupt sleep (NAMS, 2019). Sleep

Box 34.2 Menopause-Related Symptoms

Acne

Anxiety/nervousness

Arthralgia

Asthenia

Cognitive changes

Cystitis, recurrent

Depression

Dizziness

Dry eyes

Dry skin and hair

Dyspareunia

Dysuria

Fatigue

Forgetfulness

Formication

Frequent urinary tract infection (UTI)

Genitourinary burning

Headache

Hirsutism/virilization

Hot flashes/flushes

Insomnia

Irregular menstrual bleeding

Irritability/mood disturbances

Mastalgia

Myalgia

Night sweats

Nocturia

Odor

Palpitations

Paresthesia

Periodontal inflammation

Poor concentration

Postcoital bleeding

Reduced libido

Skin dryness/atrophy

Sleep disturbances

Stress urinary incontinence[a]

Thinning hair/female pattern hair loss (FPHL)

Urinary frequency

Urinary urgency

Vaginal atrophy

Vaginal dryness

Vaginal/vulvar irritation

Vaginal/vulvar pruritus

Vaginal discharge

Vaginitis, recurrent

[a]Data are inconclusive.
Source: Adapted from The North American Menopause Society. (2019). Menopause practice: A clinician's guide (6th ed.). Author.

loss causes fatigue and has been associated with stress; headache; depression; poor work, home, or school functioning; diabetes; hypertension; emotional lability; irritability; and difficulty with reasoning, concentrating, and remembering (Centers for Disease Control and Prevention [CDC], n.d.).

Cognition and memory problems are common in the TPM, although some research suggests these changes may not be related to menopause (Woods et al., 2000). Sleep interruptions and increased stress with resultant increased cortisol levels can interfere with cognition and memory. Depression and anxiety can contribute to slower processing speed (Greendale et al., 2009). Additionally, studies have demonstrated the positive correlation between normal estrogen levels and improved memory, cognition, and cerebral blood flow (Hogervorst et al., 2004; Resnick et al., 1998; Shaywitz et al., 2003). Even with adequate sleep and relatively low levels of stress, some have difficulties with concentration and memory during the TPM; however, some studies suggest that they return to baseline after menopause (Greendale et al., 2009).

The genitourinary syndrome of menopause (GSM) is a group of signs and symptoms associated with decrease in estrogen and other gonadal steroids, resulting in changes to the labia, introitus, vagina, clitoris, bladder, and urethra (NAMS, 2019). Urogenital changes will affect all biological females during the TPM and after. However, urogenital changes are not bothersome to all. Atrophy of the vaginal epithelium can cause vaginal dryness and dyspareunia, and can predispose a person to urinary incontinence and recurrent urinary tract infections (UTIs). After menopause, microtears during intercourse and atrophic genital tissues can increase vulnerability to infection (NAMS, 2019). In the past, falling estrogen levels leading to urethral atrophy were believed to increase the likelihood of urinary incontinence, but studies have not supported this (Grodstein et al., 2004). Factors that have been associated with urinary incontinence include age, diabetes mellitus, hysterectomy, obesity, weight gain, parity, and depression (NAMS, 2019). Although midlife changes may predispose a person to urinary incontinence, it is never normal and is evaluated and treated accordingly (see Chapter 29, Urologic and Pelvic Floor Health Problems).

Other normal changes of aging can negatively affect sexual function (NAMS, 2019). With aging, vaginal secretion production decreases and more time is needed during sexual activity to achieve adequate vaginal lubrication. Vaginal dryness (Dennerstein et al., 2000), atrophy, and superficial dyspareunia (Versi et al., 2001) increase progressively as menopause gets closer and afterward. Vaginal elasticity, rugae, pigmentation, and superficial cell numbers all decline, leading to petechiae and even bleeding following minor trauma such as intercourse or other forms of sexual activity (NAMS, 2019). The risk for vaginal infection increases because of the increased vaginal pH resulting from reduced numbers of lactobacilli. Vulvar collagen and adipose tissues atrophy, further increasing the likelihood of dyspareunia. Libido may also decline. These changes, combined with possible relationship concerns, partner sexual difficulties, and/or reduced sexual activity may lead to reduced interest in sex (Dennerstein et al., 2001). Regardless of the causes of sexual dysfunction or dyspareunia, patients often find the subject difficult to broach. Clinicians should ask about sexual satisfaction and function and remain open to the fact that sexual expression takes many forms (see Chapter 19, Women's Sexual Health and Chapter 26, Sexual Health Problems and Dysfunctions).

Skin and hair changes are also frequently associated with menopause. As estrogen levels decrease, unbound estrogen receptors in the skin and normal changes of aging lead to a reduction in number of collagen fibers, degree of elasticity, skin thickness, glycosaminoglycans levels, and skin vascularity. Collagen loss of 30% occurs in the first 5 years of postmenopause, with an average loss of 2.1% per year (Brincat et al., 1987). Skin dryness and hair changes, such as increased coarseness, thinning hair on the head, and increased body hair, especially at the nares or ear canals, are common.

Menopause-related symptoms may be affected by cultural or ethnic background. In the SWAN study, the number of psychosomatic symptoms (e.g., headache, moodiness, and palpitations) was highest among White and Hispanic women (Avis et al., 2001). However, the presence and severity of VMS (e.g., sweats, HFs) were highest among Black women (Gold et al., 2000, 2006). Interestingly, VMS reports increased among all ethnicities as women progressed from premenopause to early and then late perimenopause (Gold et al., 2006). Vaginal dryness was more common among Black and Hispanic women. Hispanic women were more likely than White women to report urine leakage, heart racing or pounding, and forgetfulness. Sleeping difficulty was reported by White women more than any other group (Gold et al., 2000). In the Women's Health Initiative (WHI) trials, baseline data indicated the prevalence of urogenital symptoms (e.g., dryness, discharge, irritation, itching, and dysuria) was higher among Hispanic women (Pastore et al., 2004). The level of bother from some symptoms may also be higher among different ethnic groups. For example, Black women reported high bother from night sweats and sleep changes, vaginal and body odor, moodiness, "rage," weight gain, and irritability (Alexander et al., 2003). Asian women reported more problems with joint stiffness and pain, especially in the back, shoulders, and neck (Gold et al., 2000). The frequency, intensity, and bother from specific symptoms may be related to genetic, cultural, or environmental effects.

EVALUATION/ASSESSMENT

Evaluation of a patient presenting with symptoms suggestive of menopause includes a comprehensive personal and family history focusing on their unique experience of symptoms and symptom combinations, a complete physical examination, and selective diagnostic studies to determine the true cause of the symptoms.

History

Given the extensive list of possible choices in the differential diagnosis for the various symptom combinations associated with menopause, the approach to the history must be comprehensive. Symptoms suggestive of menopause may vary in duration and severity. Foundational longitudinal studies such as the SWAN (El Khoudary et al., 2019) identified clinical manifestations of the TPM. Findings from these studies were used to establish the Stages of Reproductive Aging Workshop (STRAW). STRAW is a gold standard reproductive aging staging system (Bacon, 2017), which clearly identifies the varied signs and symptoms associated with this transition (Gracia & Freeman, 2018). Health questionnaires are available to assist clinicians in reviewing the history of menopause-related symptoms such as the Greene Climacteric Scale (Greene, 1976) and the Menopause Health Questionnaire developed by the NAMS (2023).

The history of presenting illness includes information on the presence and severity of symptoms associated with the TPM (Box 34.2). Further information on the onset, frequency, and severity of each of the symptoms and the menstrual cycle will inform the clinician about the progression in the TPM.

The medication history includes review of any current or past use of hormonal contraceptives. Long-acting contraceptives may induce amenorrhea and limit the use of amenorrhea as an indicator of becoming postmenopausal. Both prescription and over-the-counter (OTC) treatments used for menopause-related symptoms are noted, including the duration of use, effect, any side effects experienced, and why they are no longer being used. Allergies or sensitivities to hormonal contraceptives are noted as this may influence treatment options (Goodman et al., 2011).

The gynecologic history includes information on age of menarche, typical menses patterns during the reproductive years, and what is currently being experienced. Many report increasing intermenstrual interval changes as they get closer to menopause (Harlow et al., 2012). All gynecologic-related problems and surgeries are reviewed and documented. Notations of the dates of screenings, such as cervical cytology testing and mammogram, are listed.

The obstetric history includes any pregnancy history including total number of pregnancies, full-term births, premature births, abortions, and living children. The age at the first pregnancy and any pregnancy-related complications are included. The sexual history is reviewed in a nonjudgmental manner facilitating an environment that encourages the patient to share their practices and any concerns or issues. Questions that address the five areas of sexual functions that change during the TPM are (1) decline in sexual desire, (2) decreased sexual activity, (3) diminished sexual responsiveness, (4) dyspareunia, and (5) a partner with sexual function concerns.

The past medical history includes a review of any existing health problems, focusing on identifying established cardiovascular disease (CVD), previous cancers, obesity, or osteoporosis as these have implications for postmenopause. Note factors related to induced menopause such as hysterectomy, chemotherapy, or radiation therapy (Goodman et al., 2011). The surgical history includes both gynecologic and other surgeries.

Family history is reviewed and maternal age at onset of menopause is noted if known as there may be a correlation (Bentzen et al., 2013; Forman et al., 2013). The presence and age of onset is documented for family members with gynecologic or breast cancers, CVD, diabetes mellitus, or osteoporosis.

Social history includes behaviors and activities that may influence health and disease risk. Sleep patterns and concerns are documented as well as the current level of physical activity. Identify and note stressors and supports, recreational drug use, present or past tobacco use, alcohol consumption, occupation, and relationship status as these may have implications for health status, QOL, and ability to access care. Mood changes or mood disorders are reviewed keeping in mind that those having experienced hormone-related mood issues before menopause are more likely to experience mood-related issues during the TPM (Freeman et al., 2014). Other health-related behaviors (nutrition, stress management, caffeine intake, etc.) are also identified with a goal of identifying modifiable risk factors that may reduce the frequency and severity of menopause-related symptoms and improve overall health (Butts et al., 2012).

Physical Examination

The comprehensive physical examination is geared to identify health risks as well as other potential causes of symptoms. Include the vital signs of heart rate, blood pressure (BP), height, weight, BMI, waist circumference, and oxygen saturation as well as the results of breast and pelvic examinations.

Significant bone loss occurs at the beginning of postmenopause and slows later (see Chapter 35, Osteoporosis). Documenting maximum adult height with current height will allow for assessment of bone loss; loss of height greater than 1.5 inches is suspect for vertebral compression fractures and thus osteoporosis (Nasto et al., 2012). Assessment of weight allows calculation of BMI stratifying the weight-associated health risk if the BMI is elevated. Waist circumference measurements of 35 inches or greater are indicative of central adiposity, which has been associated with the risk of coronary heart disease, hypertension, dyslipidemia, and type 2 diabetes mellitus in women (see Chapter 43, Cardiovascular Disease in Women, and Chapter 44, Endocrine-Related Problems).

A clinical breast examination is a low-risk endeavor, though no longer recommended as an evidence-based approach to reducing breast cancer mortality (American College of Obstetricians and Gynecologists [ACOG], 2017). The pelvic examination may reveal changes associated with decreasing estrogen levels: thinning hair distribution; thinning of the epithelium at the introitus and into the vagina;

and bladder, rectal, or uterine descensus may be observed as evidence of decreased pelvic support (see Chapter 29, Urologic and Pelvic Floor Health Problems). Patients presenting with dyspareunia may be sensitive to gentle pressure distal to the hymen. The internal examination includes direct visualization of the cervix and cervical cytology and sexually transmitted infection (STI) screenings, if appropriate. High levels of vaginal pH obtained from the vaginal sidewall suggest low estrogen levels. The internal reproductive organs are assessed during bimanual pelvic examination noting any pain, masses, size, and location of each. The benefit of a digital rectal examination is not clear given the current colonoscopy screening recommendations.

Differential Diagnosis

Several different health problems or the use of medications, drugs, or alcohol can mimic symptoms commonly associated with menopause and are considered in the differential diagnosis (Table 34.2; NAMS, 2019).

TABLE 34.2 Sample Differential Diagnosis for Menopause-Related Symptomatology

DIAGNOSIS	SYMPTOMS SIMILAR TO PERIMENOPAUSE/MENOPAUSE
Adenomyosis, endometriosis, fibroids, ovarian cysts, ovarian tumors, pregnancy, spontaneous abortion, uterine polyps	Menstrual changes, menorrhagia, worsening PMS
Anemia	Cognitive changes, fatigue
Anovulation, pregnancy	Amenorrhea, irregular bleeding
Arrhythmias	Fatigue, palpitations
Arthritis	Joint aches/pain
Depression	Anxiety, fatigue, insomnia, irritability, moodiness, sleep disturbances
Diabetes	Fatigue, HFs/heat intolerance, lack of energy
Hypertension	Headaches, HFs/heat intolerance
Hyperthyroidism	Heat intolerance, insomnia, irritability, nervousness, sleep disturbance
Hypothyroidism	Cognitive complaints, dry skin, fatigue, sleep disturbances, weight gain
Infections (fever, HIV, influenza, STIs, tuberculosis, viral illnesses)	Cystitis symptoms, dyspareunia, fatigue, vaginitis, vasomotor symptoms
Vulvar dystrophy	Dyspareunia, vaginal atrophy

HFs, hot flashes; PMS, premenstrual syndrome; STIs, sexually transmitted infections.
Source: Adapted from The North American Menopause Society. (2019). Menopause practice: A clinician's guide (6th ed.). Author.

DIAGNOSTIC STUDIES

The most accurate way to diagnose natural menopause is the clinical absence of a menstrual period for 12 consecutive months together with age and symptoms indicative of the TPM (Box 34.2). Serum FSH testing is not recommended for determining perimenopausal or menopausal status. FSH levels are too variable and may unexpectedly return to normal, causing a rise in estrogen levels that may trigger the LH surge that prompts ovulation (NAMS, 2019). If the clinical picture is not clear, selected testing for conditions that commonly cause symptoms suggestive of menopause (Table 34.2) may be appropriate, such as thyroid-stimulating hormone (TSH) levels and blood glucose or hemoglobin A1c.

TREATMENT/MANAGEMENT

Menopause management focuses on control of symptoms and reduction of health risks. Several approaches are used: self-management measures such as lifestyle changes, complementary and alternative medicine (CAM), HT, and nonhormonal prescription medications. It is important to discuss the various symptom treatment options available and encourage active involvement in the decision-making process.

Often several diagnoses are present to contend with simultaneously, such as diabetes, hypertension, and perimenopause. Control of concomitant medical problems may also reduce menopause-related symptoms to the point that they no longer affect QOL.

Self-Management Measures

DIETARY CHANGES

Several food substances have been associated with increased frequency or severity of HFs: caffeine (cold and hot beverages, other substances that contain caffeine such as chocolate), sugar (especially refined sugars), alcohol, and spicy foods (Alexander et al., 2003). Women are counseled to avoid or use these substances moderately if they perceive that they cause VMS.

Extra water ingestion is also recommended to replace the added insensible fluid lost through sweating. Drinking extra water, especially cold water, has been reported to reduce discomfort with sweating and HFs, as well as to minimize other symptoms such as dry skin (Alexander et al., 2003). Water intake of at least six to eight 8-oz glasses each day is recommended. Women who experience nocturia are counseled to ingest most of their daily water in the morning to reduce nighttime wakening for urination. Only when bathroom access may be limited is moderate restriction of water intake warranted for women who experience urinary incontinence (NAMS, 2019).

Phytoestrogens found in foods such as soybeans, hops, flaxseeds, fruits, vegetables, legumes, and whole grains have been proposed to decrease VMS due to their weak estrogenic effects, but a meta-analysis did not find a strong association (Roberts & Lethaby, 2014). The Women's Study for the Alleviation of VMS (Barnard et al., 2021) found that a low-fat, vegan diet with daily soybean intake was associated with a significant decrease in VMS frequency and severity. A Western diet high in sugar and dietary fat was associated with an increased risk of VMS while a Mediterranean diet was negatively associated with VMS (Herber-Gast & Mishra, 2013). Further studies are warranted to determine the best dietary approach or other approaches to decreasing VMS during the TPM.

VITAMINS, MINERALS, AND DIETARY SUPPLEMENTS

Many turn to vitamins, minerals, and dietary supplements to reduce menopause-related symptoms and midlife health risks. While nutrients should ideally be obtained from a healthy diet, the use of a multivitamin/mineral supplement may be appropriate for some populations including those eating limited diets, individuals with poor absorption, and those with known nutritional deficiencies. Multivitamins have not been shown to prevent cancer or CVD and should not be taken for these purposes (Fortmann et al., 2013).

Vitamin A may be beneficial in the prevention of several cancers including breast cancer (Fulan et al., 2011); however, studies in postmenopausal women have suggested that too much vitamin A in the form of retinol can increase the risk of hip fracture (Wu et al., 2014). This may be due to vitamin A's ability to trigger osteoclasts and interfere with vitamin D. Calcium and vitamin D are critical for maintaining bone strength and preventing osteoporosis (LeBoff et al., 2022) and thus are especially recommended at midlife. High levels of homocysteine are associated with osteoporotic fracture, CVD, cerebrovascular accident, and Alzheimer disease. The B vitamins (folate, B_6, and B_{12}) are known to reduce homocysteine levels and the U.S. diet often lacks sufficient fruits and vegetables, which are high in B complex vitamins (Fairfield & Fletcher, 2002; van Meurs et al., 2004). Thus, a B-complex or multivitamin containing B vitamins may be appropriate for some. Magnesium deficiency is widespread in the United States (U.S. Department of Health and Human Services, 2015) and low magnesium may be associated with an increased risk for bone loss. Magnesium supplementation may be beneficial in those at increased risk of magnesium deficiency, such as those with Crohn disease, celiac disease, diabetes mellitus, alcoholism, or a history of gastric bypass surgery. A diet containing magnesium-rich foods such as vegetables, fruits, legumes, and whole grains should be encouraged (NAMS, 2019). Omega-3 fatty acid supplements in a randomized trial showed no efficacy for VMS management (Cohen et al., 2014); however, a more recent meta-analysis suggested that omega-3 fatty acid supplementation may decrease night sweats (Mohammady et al., 2018). Omega-3 polyunsaturated fatty acids can reduce triglyceride levels, which are associated with increased CVDs.

See the discussion under Isoflavones in the section on Complementary and Alternative Medicine for information on dietary soy and supplements.

EXERCISE

Regular aerobic exercise is recommended for maintaining cardiovascular health, reducing the risk for osteoporosis and falls (LeBoff et al., 2022), and moderating glucose metabolism and weight gain. Regular aerobic exercise has also been shown to reduce the severity of menopause-related symptoms such as depression, forgetfulness, and sleep disturbances (Afonso et al., 2012) and to improve QOL among postmenopausal women (NAMS, 2019; Reed et al., 2014). Lower levels of physical activity have been associated with increased frequency of menopause-related symptoms, particularly sleep disturbances, forgetfulness, soreness or stiffness, and heart racing or pounding (Gold et al., 2000). Interestingly, exercise has not been shown to decrease VMS (Sternfeld et al., 2014); however, the other benefits of exercise may serve to indirectly decrease VMS.

Emphasizing the benefits of regular exercise may serve as a motivator to continue or begin an exercise program. Persons older than 50 years need to be evaluated before initiating a new exercise regimen to rule out any underlying CVD (see Chapter 43, Cardiovascular Disease in Women). The American Heart Association recommends 150 minutes per week of moderate-intensity exercise such as brisk walking, 75 minutes per week of vigorous exercise, or a combination equal to both to decrease risk of CVD (Mosca et al., 2011). Small amounts of exercise are also beneficial, and beginning at even 10 or 20 minutes per day is a reasonable recommendation for starting a new exercise program.

ENVIRONMENT AND CLOTHING CHANGES

The goal for clothing and environmental changes is to minimize core temperature changes to reduce VMS such as sweating or shivering. Wearing layered clothing that can be easily removed when room or air temperatures rise and using breathable fabrics, such as linen or cotton, help to reduce HF triggers. Wearing high-neck or turtleneck shirts; tight clothing or clothing that does not allow for air circulation; extra layers, such as full-length stockings, girdles, or slips; and fabrics that do not absorb sweat, such as silk or polyester, are avoided. Wicking fabrics that dry quickly, such as those designed for exercising, can help to pull moisture away from the body when sweating does occur. There are pajamas designed specifically for reducing discomfort from night sweats. Using these fabrics can reduce nighttime sleep disruptions attributable to night sweats.

Environmental adjustments can also reduce HF triggers. Circulating air with an open window or room fan, or both, and keeping the room temperature cool are beneficial, especially at night, because core temperature tends to rise under blankets and sheets while sleeping. Using sheets and blankets made of breathable fabrics to allow for air movement can reduce HF triggers at night. Similarly, using fabrics with imbedded Thermocules can be helpful. Based on space travel temperature regulation technologies, Thermocules are embedded into fabrics used for mattresses, pillows, mattress pads, and sleepwear, and absorb excess body heat. Stored heat is released when the body cools, thus helping to maintain a steady temperature. Ingesting cold beverages or foods to reduce the core body temperature can also be beneficial, though supporting data are lacking (Alexander et al., 2003; NAMS, 2019).

VAGINAL LUBRICANTS AND MOISTURIZERS

Both lubricants and moisturizers can help to reduce the discomfort and dyspareunia experienced because of vaginal atrophy. Water-based, nonhormonal lubricants are readily available OTC at pharmacies and grocery stores or can be purchased online and include products such as Astroglide, K-Y Personal Lubricant, Liquid Silk, and YES Personal Lubricant. Lubricants are typically used before or during sexual activity and are most beneficial for reducing vaginal dryness and thereby increasing comfort and pleasure. Oil-based and silicon-based products are also available and may be preferable to some. It is important to know that oil-based products can cause the breakdown of diaphragms and condoms. This is especially important for anyone who may be at risk for pregnancy or those at risk for STIs. An exception is vitamin E oil, which is nonirritating, does not interfere with condom or diaphragm function, and is safe for application directly to the vaginal walls.

More severe dryness that causes discomfort when walking or sitting is best managed using long-acting vaginal moisturizers such as K-Y Silk-E and Replens. Compared with lubricants, moisturizers help to replenish and sustain fluids in the epithelial cells of the vaginal walls and provide longer lasting relief. Moisturizers can be especially beneficial for women who have daily discomfort; in addition, moisturizers are preferable because they support a normal vaginal pH and are therefore effective in reducing the likelihood of vaginitis (NAMS, 2019).

Lubricants or moisturizers that contain fragrances, flavors, warming agents, or other additives may cause irritation or vaginitis and should be used with caution. Other products that may cause irritation due to chemical additives include toilet tissue, soaps, tampons, powders, or perfumes. Douching increases dryness and infection risks by removing normal vaginal flora and altering the vaginal pH (NAMS, 2019).

SLEEP AIDS

If HFs, night sweats, or other menopause-related symptoms are causing sleep disruption, then treating the symptoms will usually restore normal sleeping patterns. HT or nonhormonal medications can assist with HFs and night sweats. Less severe HFs may be managed with lifestyle modifications and improved sleep hygiene. However, sleep disturbances are often related to other etiologies than menopause-related symptoms; in these cases, a more general approach is appropriate (see Chapter 15, Healthy Practices: Sleep).

If stimulants are identified as potential problems, then avoidance of alcohol, caffeine, and other stimulants can help to restore normal sleep patterns (NAMS, 2019). Alcohol can have an initial sedative effect; however, it frequently causes sleep pattern disruptions after falling asleep such as rebound awakening and fragmented sleep. Because stimulant effects from caffeine can last more than 20 hours, complete elimination is recommended. To provide relief from common caffeine withdrawal side effects, such as headache, it is preferable to slowly reduce caffeine intake by substituting a caffeine-free beverage in increasing amounts over 1 month. Nicotine also increases sleep latency and causes reduced overall duration of sleep; thus, smoking cessation is encouraged. Regular exercise and yoga (Afonso et al., 2012) can improve sleep quality and reduce sleep latency. Timing of exercise is critical, as exercising too close to bedtime can act as a stimulant and increase sleep latency (NAMS, 2019; see Chapter 14, Healthy Practices: Physical Activity).

Sleep-restriction therapy or sleep retraining can be helpful for those with short duration of sleep (NAMS, 2019). Before initiation of a sleep-retraining program, the current average number of sleep hours per night is determined. This time is subtracted from the desired morning rising time to identify when bedtime should be. After successfully (i.e., 95% of time) achieving this sleeping goal, the bedtime is moved back by 0.5 to 1 hour. This pattern is repeated gradually until sleep is sustained for the desired amount of time most nights. For the program to be successful, *all* stimulants and sleep medications must be avoided, and the patient must remain awake (no napping) except for the specified sleep hours. For example, if they are sleeping 4 hours at night and need to rise at 6:30 a.m. for work, they should go to bed at 2:30 a.m. and rise at 6:30 a.m. each day. They continue with this pattern until they are sleeping the full 4 hours 95% of the time. When this goal is reached, they change bedtime to 2:00 a.m. After they are sleeping the 4.5 hours for 95% of the time, bedtime is changed to 1:30 a.m. This pattern is continued until they are sleeping the desired number of hours. Education also includes the normal amount of sleep needed (NAMS, 2019; see Chapter 15, Healthy Practices: Sleep).

Regardless of the underlying cause for sleep disruption, sleep hygiene is an important part of the management plan (NAMS, 2019). Good sleep hygiene will reduce sleep latency and nocturnal wakening. Sleep hygiene practices cue the brain that it is time to sleep, prompting the brain's reticular activating system (RAS), which controls sleep-wake functions, to assume control. Just like children, adults sleep best when they follow a familiar and soothing routine before sleep. This is especially important during the TPM because sleep disruptions are so common. Bedtime routines that signal the mind for sleep might include grooming and relaxing activities. Activities that are stimulating are avoided just before bedtime, especially for those who have extended sleep latency. Reserving the bedroom for only sleep and sexual activity can further increase positive environmental triggers for sleep (see Chapter 15, Healthy Practices: Sleep).

There are limited data on the nonprescriptive remedies of melatonin or sedative botanicals for the treatment of sleep disorders. However, melatonin may be beneficial for reducing sleep latency (NAMS, 2019).

SMOKING CESSATION

Smoking is linked to increased morbidity and mortality risks, particularly for CVD, cancer, bone loss, earlier age of menopause, and a higher prevalence of several menopause-related symptoms (NAMS, 2019). Several approaches can assist women with smoking cessation, the most important of which is a clinician recommendation to stop smoking. Smoking cessation may mediate menopause-related HFs (Smith et al., 2015) and reduce the risk of developing dementia (Williams et al., 2010).

TECHNIQUES FOR STRESS MANAGEMENT

Stress is an identified trigger for menopause-related symptoms (Alexander et al., 2003). Stress is also linked to poor sleep and may cause moodiness or depression outside of the mood changes and sleep disruption that often accompany the TPM. At midlife, many women face multiple sources of stress, encompassing their work life, home life, relationships, and personal health (see Chapter 9, Midlife Women's Health).

Stress management techniques may be helpful and should be tailored to the individual, as different people perceive different activities as relaxing. Some common activities that support relaxation include meditation, yoga, reading, journaling, prayer, regular exercise, massage, tai chi, a warm bath, deep or paced breathing, or seeking support from friends or family members. CAM therapies have been shown to provide sleep benefits (Frame & Alexander, 2013). Biofeedback and progressive muscle relaxation have not been shown to change HFs significantly. Paced respiration had been associated with significantly reducing HFs (Freedman & Woodward, 1992; Irvin et al., 1996); however, in a recent randomized trial the use of paced respirations was not found to be any better at reducing HF bother, interference, frequency, or severity (Sood et al., 2013). Some report that effective management or avoidance of stress minimizes HF intensity and frequency (Alexander et al., 2003). Deep breathing for relaxation and HF reduction can be done by inhaling over a count of four, holding the breath over a count of seven, and exhaling slowly over a count of nine. Mindfulness-based stress reduction has shown some reduction in the intensity of HFs and bother, but was not statistically significant (Carmody et al., 2011), whereas both cognitive behavioral therapy (Hunter, 2014) and hypnosis (Elkins et al., 2013) significantly reduced HF frequency and bother. Yoga has been shown to reduce VMS, joint pain, fatigue, and sleep disturbances, and increase QOL among postmenopausal breast cancer survivors (Reed et al., 2014).

ACTIVITIES FOR MEMORY FUNCTION ENHANCEMENT

Although some decline in mental function is normal with aging, many experience more abrupt, bothersome cognitive changes that they associate with menopause. Most cognitive changes at midlife, such as difficulty remembering and concentrating, are related to poor sleep patterns or high stress levels. However, hormonal changes may also play a role. Brain structures involved in learning and memory such as the hippocampus and prefrontal cortex are high in estrogen receptors. Several studies have suggested modest declines in processing speed and memory in late perimenopause and postmenopause when compared to premenopause (Greendale et al., 2009, 2010). Cognitive problems can also be associated with numerous medical problems. Thus, a comprehensive assessment should be completed to identify the most likely cause of the cognitive changes before a treatment plan is determined.

Lifestyle-based activities worth implementing that may help memory or potentially protect against dementia include remaining active both physically and mentally, maintaining an extensive social network, increasing dietary intake of omega-3 fatty acids, following a Mediterranean style diet, reducing CVD risk factors (Lehert et al., 2015; Sydenham et al., 2012), keeping alcohol intake to a moderate level, and not smoking (Williams et al., 2010). These activities, though not confirmed with rigorous studies, do have observational data linking them to better memory. Evidence does not support the use of HT to improve cognitive function during postmenopause (Espeland et al., 2013; Gleason et al., 2015; Henderson & Popat, 2011; Henderson et al., 2016).

Establishing routines may help with memory, for example, storing keys and accessories in the same location, noting appointments and important events in a calendar, and keeping an easily accessible list so that shopping needs and tasks can be monitored. Storing paper and pens at the bedside to note thoughts during the night can alleviate stress and may reduce nighttime awakenings. Attending to sleep hygiene and using relaxation methods can also improve memory. Keeping the mind actively engaged by participating in stimulating mental activities can also help retain cognitive function.

Complementary and Alternative Medicine

Use of CAM for menopause-related symptom management is increasing (NAMS, 2019). Because many patients do not report CAM use, it is critical that clinicians ask about the use of these modalities. CAM therapies may provide reductions in VMS, assist with improving sleep, and reduce moodiness (NAMS, 2019).

ISOFLAVONES

Isoflavones are manufactured from plants that have both non-estrogenic and estrogenic properties. They are found in foods, such as red clover and soy, and in commercially manufactured OTC products and are converted to estrogenic compounds in the intestines. Because isoflavones can weakly bind with systemic estrogen receptors, particularly beta receptors, they are frequently called phytoestrogens and have been studied extensively for managing HFs. Red clover and soy extracts also bind with progesterone and androgen receptors (Beck et al., 2003). Results from studies evaluating isoflavone efficacy on HF reduction have been contradictory. Genestein was identified as a compound that deserves further investigation due to its potential for benefit (Roberts & Lethaby, 2014). In a comparison of the most recent randomized, blinded, comparative clinical trials, the review found soy isoflavonids to be no more effective than a placebo (Chen et al., 2015). In a Cochrane review continuous use for up to 1 year of phytoestrogens was noted to be safe (Lethaby et al., 2013), but long-term use (5 years or longer) of soy phytoestrogens may increase the risk for endometrial hyperplasia (Unfer et al., 2004). A systematic review from 2019 found soy isoflavones to be significantly more effective in reducing the frequency and severity of HFs than placebo and more effective in attenuating lumbar spine bone mineral density loss but found no conclusive effect on vaginal dryness or other urogenital symptoms (Chen et al., 2019). The major challenge in comparing study outcomes was the heterogencity of the various studies.

HERBAL PRODUCTS

Many herbal preparations are used for managing menopause-related symptoms (Table 34.3). Clinical studies evaluating the efficacy and safety of herbal remedies are increasing, especially for HFs. Herbal products, such as black cohosh, ginseng, and Chinese herbs, are also commonly utilized for symptomatic management during the menopausal transition. Most studies of these herbs have shown that they are unlikely to alleviate menopausal symptoms. Additionally, because herbal preparations are generally identified as dietary supplements, they are not held to the same Food and Drug Administration (FDA) regulations as are prescription medications or other OTC products, leading to concerns regarding purity and consistency. Product strength and use may also differ depending on the preparation (e.g., extract vs. tincture vs. poultice).

Many herbs are packaged in combination products or in Chinese herbal mixtures, sometimes making it difficult to determine the specific products that are being used. Women need to be asked specifically if they are using any of these products, because herbal products can interact with both other herbs and prescription medications.

POLLEN EXTRACTS

Pollen extracts have been investigated over the last 15 years as a nonhormonal supplement used daily to reduce menopause-related symptoms. Though earlier studies lacked sufficient clinical significance, a 2019 study demonstrated a significant decrease in menopause-related symptoms after 12 weeks, with the most impact being a reduction of sleep disturbances by approximately 50% and HF by 48% (Fait et al., 2019). The main action of the pollen extracts has been generation of oxygen free radicals and inhibiting reuptake of various neurotransmitters including serotonin (Genazzani et al., 2020).

BIOIDENTICAL OR "NATURAL" HORMONES

Many women request "natural" hormones for menopause-related symptom management. "Natural" hormones are mistakenly believed by many women to cause fewer side effects and to demonstrate higher safety than pharmaceutically manufactured hormones (Alexander, 2006). However, all commercially available hormones are manufactured. Furthermore, the term *natural* refers to substances with primary components derived from animal, plant, or mineral sources, which encompasses all pharmaceutically manufactured hormones as well. Many women also mistakenly believe that "natural" hormones are identical to the hormones produced in a woman's body (Stanczyk et al., 2021).

In contrast, *bioidentical* hormones are manufactured hormones that are chemically identical to those produced by a woman's body. Often, women who request natural hormones are actually interested in bioidentical products. Several bioidentical hormones (e.g., 17β-estradiol, estriol, estrone, and micronized progesterone) are FDA-approved prescription products; others are available from compounding pharmacies.

Compounded estrogen products such as Bi-Est or Tri-Est can be prescribed. These topical creams are used for vasomotor and vaginal atrophy symptoms. Estriol vaginal cream can also be prescribed through a compounding pharmacy. Tri-Est (estradiol, estrone, estriol) and Bi-Est (estradiol and estriol) are often advertised only identifying the estriol content, which is misleading. However, both Bi-Est and Tri-Est contain enough estradiol (usually 0.25 to 0.5 mg) to also require use of progesterone for endometrial protection in those with an intact uterus (Gaudet, 2004). Advertisements by compounding companies were known to frequently imply that their products were safer than pharmaceutical grade hormones. The FDA acted against these companies to stop

TABLE 34.3 Herbal Therapies for Menopause-Related Symptoms[a]

PRODUCT	USUAL DOSAGE[b]	PURPOSE IN MENOPAUSE	COMMENTS
Black cohosh (*Cimicifuga racemosa*)	20 mg twice a day (proprietary standardized extract)	• Vasomotor symptoms	• Research evidence controversial; some data show beneficial effects close to that of estrogen for HF relief, and other data show no benefit • Safety for use greater than 6 months not established • Can potentiate antihypertensives • Multiple products and formulations available • Wide variations in product ingredients, purity, and extraction processes • Product labels frequently recommend much higher doses • Rare cases of hepatitis reported • Side effects rare, usually intestinal upset, dizziness, headache, hypotension, painful extremities; more common with higher doses
Chaste tree berry (*Vitex agnus-castus*)	Effective dose unknown; hard to find standardized extract	• Menstrual irregularity	• No data on relief of menopause-related symptoms • More popular in Europe than United States; approved in Germany for PMS, mastalgia, and menopause-related symptoms • Often found in combination products • Side effects rare, usually headache, intestinal upset
Dong quai (*Angelica sinensis*)	Two capsules two to three times a day; usually in combination products	• Gynecologic conditions	• Research found no benefit for menopause-related symptoms • Widely used in Asia • Used in Chinese herb combinations; Chinese *material medica* cautions not to give alone • A "heating" herb, can cause red face, HFs, sweating, irritability, or insomnia • Contains coumarin derivatives, contraindicated in those taking warfarin • Can cause photosensitivity, hypotension, anticoagulation, and possibly has carcinogenicity properties
Evening primrose oil (*Oenothera biennis*)	3–4 g daily in divided doses	• HFs • Mastalgia	• No benefit for menopause-related symptoms • Potentiates risk for seizure if taken by person with seizure disorder or person taking phenothiazines and other medications that lower seizure threshold • Side effects include diarrhea and nausea
Ginkgo (*Ginkgo biloba*)	40–80 mg three times a day of standardized extract	• Memory changes	• Insufficient research on safety and efficacy • Memory changes often related to sleep disturbances; menopausal sleep disturbances frequently related to HFs, stress • Side effects include intestinal distress, hypotension; chronic use has been linked with subarachnoid hemorrhage, subdural hematoma, and increased bleeding times
Ginseng (*Panax ginseng*)	1–2 g of root daily in divided doses	• General "tonic" • Improved mood, fatigue	• Little to no benefit to menopausal symptoms; benefits well-being, general health, and depression • Heavily adulterated • Can cause uterine bleeding, mastalgia • Contraindicated in women with breast cancer and in women who are also taking monoamine oxidase inhibitors, stimulants, or anticoagulants; may potentiate digoxin and others (multiple drug interactions) • Side effects include rash, nervousness, insomnia, hypertension
Kava (*Piper methysticum*)	150–300 mg of root extract daily in divided doses	• Irritability • Insomnia	• Little data available to support use • Banned in several countries because of hepatotoxicity; thus not recommended • Contraindicated with depression • Side effects include GI discomfort, impaired reflexes and motor function, weight loss, hepatotoxicity, rash
Licorice root (*Glycyrrhiza glabra*)	5–15 mg of root equivalent daily in divided doses	• Menopause-related symptoms	• No data supporting relief of HFs • Found in many Chinese herb mixtures • High doses can lead to primary aldosteronism, cardiac arrhythmias, cardiac arrest • Contraindicated in presence of hepatic or renal disease, diabetes, hypertension, pregnancy, hypertonia, hypokalemia, or arrhythmia, or when taking diuretics
Passion flower (*Passiflora incarnata*)	3–10 g daily, divided doses	• Sedative	• Mixed results in sleep improvement • Menopausal sleep disturbances frequently related to HFs, stress

Pollen, purified (PureCyTonin, Serelys, Femal, Femalen, Femelis Meno, Menolesse, Sansage, and Relizen)	160 mg daily, 320 mg daily	• Vasomotor symptoms, HFs, sleep disturbances	• Menopausal sleep disturbances frequently related to HFs, stress • Nonestrogenic alternative for managing symptoms associated with menopause. • Does not interfere with tamoxifen as it does not inhibit CYPD26
St. John's wort (*Hypericum perforatum*)	300 mg three times a day (standardized extract)	• Vasomotor symptoms • Irritability • Depression	• No data supporting vasomotor relief • Research findings support use for depression; there are no clinical trials for menopause • Often combined with black cohosh for menopause symptom treatment • Interferes with metabolism of many medications that are metabolized in liver; affects cytochrome P450 enzymes (e.g., estrogen, digoxin, theophylline); reduces INR levels; not to be used concomitantly with antidepressants, monoamine oxidase inhibitors, or immunosuppressants • Side effects include photosensitivity, rash, constipation, cramping, dry mouth, fatigue, dizziness, restlessness, insomnia
Valerian root (*Valeriana officinalis*)	300–600 mg of aqueous extract 0.5 to 1 hour before bed (insomnia); 150–300 mg every morning and 300–400 mg every evening aqueous extract (anxiety)	• Sedative • Antianxiety	• Research showed improvement in sleep and depression/mood scales • Used for insomnia in intermittent dosing, for anxiety with chronic dosing • Side effects include headache, uneasiness, excitability, arrhythmias, morning sedation, GI upset, cardiac function disorders (with long-term use)
Wild yam (*Dioscorea villosa*)	Unknown	• Menopausal symptoms	• Research showed no benefit to menopausal symptoms • Products claim that creams are converted to progesterone; however, human body cannot convert topical or ingested wild yam into progesterone • Wild yam is used as main ingredient in some products to manufacture progesterone in laboratory; these products have demonstrated some efficacy • Many preparations have been adulterated with undisclosed steroids that may cause potential harm and therefore are not recommended for use

[a]See prescribing reference for full information on doses, side effects, contraindications, and cautions.
[b]Dosages vary and frequently differ according to form (e.g., drops, essential oil, liquid extract, standardized extract, tincture).
GI, gastrointestinal; HFs, hot flashes; INR, international normalized ratio; PMS, premenstrual syndrome.
Source: Adapted from Kargozar, R., Azizi, H., & Salary, R. (2017). A review of effective herbal medicines in controlling menopausal symptoms. Electron Physician, 9(11), 5826–5833. https://doi.org/10.19082/5826; Peng, W., Adams, J., Sibbritt, D. W., & Frawley, J. E. (2014). Critical review of complementary and alternative medicine use in menopause: Focus on prevalence, motivation, decision-making, and communication. Menopause, 21(5), 536–548. https://doi.org/10.1097/GME.0b013e3182a46a3e

false advertisement claims for unsupported efficacy, safety, and superiority that are misleading to women and clinicians (FDA, 2008).

PROGESTERONE CREAM

OTC progesterone creams are available (e.g., Pro-Gest, PhytoGest, MenoBalance, and Endocreme). Progesterone content in these creams varies from less than 2 mg to greater than 700 mg per ounce. Progesterone creams can be prescribed through compounding pharmacies. These creams are considered dietary supplements. Thus, FDA regulations for prescription medications do not apply, and there are concerns about concentration and purity.

Although some women would like to use progesterone cream to avoid the potential systemic effects of oral progesterone, data do not support the use of progesterone creams for endometrial protection in women taking systemic ET (Stanczyk et al., 2021). Pharmacokinetic studies of progesterone topical creams showed only about 10% of the progesterone was detected in serum (Zava et al., 2014). Transdermal progesterone cream does have some efficacy for reducing HFs (Prior, 2018) and may be a more frequently used option in the future.

ACUPUNCTURE

Acupuncture is a widely recognized modality for pain relief and relaxation. Meta-analyses of published acupuncture studies found a lack of convincing evidence to support the use of acupuncture for HF management (Ee et al., 2017; Johnson et al., 2019). However, a clinically significant reduction in the primary outcome of HF and improvement in other menopause-related symptoms such as day-and-night sweats, sleep problems, and emotional symptoms was identified more recently (Lund et al., 2019). Despite these controversial findings, acupuncture is a safe, well-accepted form of CAM and may be acceptable to women who prefer nonhormonal treatments for menopause-related symptoms. The relaxation and any placebo effects experienced with acupuncture may reduce HFs enough to provide benefit for some; however, there are not enough data to recommended it for treating VMS at this time (NAMS, 2019).

Pharmacotherapeutics

HORMONE THERAPY

HT, consisting of ET, estrogen-progestogen therapy (EPT), or estrogen with bazedoxifene, remains the most effective strategy for managing moderate to severe VMS and vaginal symptoms associated with menopause (NAMS, 2019, 2022). HF severity is defined by the individual according to its effect on their QOL (NAMS, 2019, 2022).

Multiple different estrogen compounds are available (Table 34.4). Estrogens have differing dose equivalencies and target tissue responses. Preparations for estrogen include systemic (oral, patch, cream, gel, spray, vaginal ring) and local (vaginal cream, tablet, or ring) delivery systems. Except for the 0.5- and 0.1-mg versions of the vaginal Femring, local vaginal ET has little effect on systemic estrogen levels and is not indicated for VMS. Rather, local therapy is used for managing symptoms of vaginal atrophy (NAMS, 2019, 2022). Estrogens are FDA approved for relief of moderate to severe VMS and vaginal atrophy.

In the postmenopausal person with a uterus, either progesterone or bazedoxifene, a selective estrogen receptor modulator (SERM), is used to protect against developing endometrial hyperplasia or adenocarcinoma when ET is used (Table 34.4; NAMS, 2019, 2022). Progesterone is occasionally used alone (off-label) for VMS management if estrogen is not tolerated or is contraindicated.

When considering HT for menopause-related symptom management, all contraindications, side effects, and cautions (Table 34.5) are first carefully reviewed. The patient's personal and family histories are evaluated to identify possible risk factors or contraindications. The patient must be engaged in the decision and comfortable with the use of HT. The known risks and benefits, as well as the unanswered scientific questions about HT, are openly discussed. Results from the Heart and Estrogen/Progestin Replacement Study (HERS; Grady et al., 2002; Hulley et al., 1998, 2002) and WHI (Anderson et al., 2004; Heiss et al., 2008; Rossouw et al., 2002; Shumaker et al., 2003) trials indicate that HT may increase risks for CVD, stroke, thromboembolism, breast cancer, and dementia (Alexander, 2012). The possibility that these risks are lower for those who are in early postmenopause are also reviewed (Grodstein et al., 2006; Hsia et al., 2006; Rossouw et al., 2007; Salpeter et al., 2004). The controversies that surround the relationship between HT and breast cancer and dementia are also discussed. Some studies demonstrate protective effects against dementia with HT (Bagger et al., 2005; Craig et al.,

2008; Zandi et al., 2002) and others show increased risks (Shumaker et al., 2003). Breast cancer risk likely increases after 3 to 5 years of EPT use (Chlebowski et al., 2009; Li et al., 2008; NAMS, 2019, 2022; Rossouw et al., 2002) and may return to baseline after cessation (Chlebowski et al., 2009; Coombs, Taylor, Wilcken, & Boyages, 2005; Coombs, Taylor, Wilcken, Fiorica, & Boyages, 2005; Heiss et al., 2008). Additionally, epidemiologic data identifying fluctuating rates of breast cancer following the decline in HT use (Alexander, 2011; Clarke et al., 2006; Ravdin et al., 2007) and the reduced rates of mammography screenings (Breen et al., 2007; Meissner et al., 2007) are reviewed. Finally, it is important to discuss the possibility of mammographic changes while taking HT; for example, increased breast density may obscure detection of an early breast cancer lesion or mammogram abnormalities may lead to unnecessary biopsy (Chlebowski et al., 2008). There are no data identifying an increased risk of breast cancer with estrogen + bazedoxifene. NAMS notes that bazedoxifene may reduce the risk for breast cancer because bazedoxifene is a SERM (NAMS, 2019, 2022).

QOL benefits from HT are also considered. Many describe a decline in QOL with the TPM (NAMS, 2019, 2022). If menopause-related symptoms are bothersome and negatively affecting QOL, then HT may be an appropriate option. In addition to relief of VMS and vaginal atrophy, HT is known to preserve skin thickness and reduce the appearance of wrinkles (Brincat, 2000); reduce sleep latency and insomnia and increase rapid eye movement (REM) sleep (Antonijevic et al., 2000; Schiff et al., 1980); improve mood (Soares et al., 2001); improve sexual function (Cayan et al., 2008); decrease colon cancer incidence; and maintain bone strength, reducing the possibility of osteoporotic fractures (Rossouw et al., 2002).

If a person is an appropriate candidate for HT and elects to use it for symptom management, they are counseled about the possible regimen combinations and methods of delivery. ET is prescribed only to those who do not have an intact uterus. EPT can follow several different patterns. One option is the continuous combined (CC-EPT) method in which a progestogen is taken daily with estrogen, either in the same tablet or pill or as a separate oral medication such as with creams or gels. An alternative to this method is the pulsed regimen in which estrogen is taken every day and the progestin dose is "pulsed" by taking estrogen and progestin for 2 consecutive days, then estrogen only for 1 day, then both estrogen and progestin for 2 consecutive days in a repeating pattern. Both the CC-EPT and pulsed regimens will reduce or remove withdrawal bleeds over time. The pulsed regimen was developed to provide similar benefits as CC-EPT with fewer progestogen-related side effects. However, breakthrough bleeding is more common when the pulsed regimen is used. In the combined sequential (CS-EPT) method, estrogen is taken daily, and the progestogen is added for 12 to 14 days of the month, often starting on the first day of the month. When this method is used, a withdrawal bleed will usually occur following completion of the progestogen. This sequence is repeated monthly. Some prefer to take the progestogen for only 3 or 4 months of the year. This will reduce side effects of progestin and the frequency of withdrawal bleeds and does reduce the risk of endometrial overgrowth and cancer; however, it is not as effective as the

TABLE 34.4 Selective Hormone Therapy Products[a]

TYPE	PRODUCT NAME (MANUFACTURER)	ACTIVE INGREDIENT	DOSAGE
Estrogens, oral	Estrace; generics	Estradiol	0.5 mg, 1 mg, or 2 mg once daily
	Menest	Esterified estrogens	0.3 mg, 0.625 mg, 1.25 mg, or 2.5 mg once daily
	Generic	Estropipate	0.75 mg, 1.5 mg, or 3.0 mg once daily
	Premarin	Conjugated estrogens (formerly conjugated equine estrogens)	0.3 mg, 0.45 mg, 0.625 mg, 0.9 mg, or 1.25 mg once daily
Estrogens, transdermal	Generic	Estradiol	0.025 mg, 0.0375 mg, 0.05 mg, 0.06 mg, 0.075 mg, or 0.1 mg daily Change patch twice weekly Apply to lower abdomen or upper outer buttocks
	Climara; generic	Estradiol	0.025 mg, 0.0375 mg, 0.05 mg, 0.06 mg, 0.075 mg, or 0.1 mg daily Change patch weekly Apply to lower abdomen or upper outer buttocks
	Divigel	Estradiol	0.1% gel packet 0.25 mg/d, 0.5 mg/d, 0.75 mg, 1.0 mg/d, 1.25 mg Apply one packet to thigh daily
	Elestrin	Estradiol	0.06% gel pump 0.87 g per pump of gel delivers 0.52 mg of estradiol daily Apply gel once daily to upper arm
	Estrasorb cream	Estradiol	2.5% (4.35 mg/1.74 g/packet) emulsion/lotion 8.7 mg to skin daily Two packets rubbed into thighs every morning for more than 3 minutes
	EstroGel	Estradiol	0.06% gel 1.25 g per pump of gel delivers 0.75 mg of estradiol daily Apply gel once daily to arm from shoulder to wrists
	Evamist	Estradiol	1.7% solution 90 mcg/L spray delivers 1.53 mg of estradiol daily Start with one spray daily; increase to two to three sprays as needed One spray once daily to forearm
	Menostar	Estradiol	0.014 mg daily Change patch weekly Apply to lower abdomen FDA approved for osteoporosis prevention; recent study also showed efficacy for HF relief
	Minivelle, Vivelle-Dot; generics	Estradiol	0.025 mg, 0.0375 mg, 0.05 mg, 0.075 mg, or 0.1 mg daily Change patch twice weekly
Progestogens, oral	Aygestin	Norethindrone acetate	2.5 mg to 10 mg daily continuously or on set cycle schedule Used for those with intact uterus taking estrogen
	Camila; generics	Norethindrone	0.35 mg Off-label use
	Prometrium	Micronized progesterone	200 mg at bedtime continuously or on set cycle schedule Used for those with intact uterus taking estrogen Contains peanut oil
	Provera; generics	Medroxyprogesterone acetate (MPA)	2.5 mg, 5 mg, or 10 mg daily continuously or on set cycle schedule Used for those with intact uterus taking estrogen

(continued)

TABLE 34.4 Selective Hormone Therapy Products[a] *(continued)*

TYPE	PRODUCT NAME (MANUFACTURER)	ACTIVE INGREDIENT	DOSAGE
Combination estrogens + progestogens, oral	Activella	Estradiol + norethindrone acetate	0.5/0.1 mg or 1.0/0.5 mg once daily (continuous combined)
	Angeliq	Estradiol + drospirenone	0.5/0.25 mg or 1/0.5 mg once daily (continuous combined)
	Fyavolv	Ethinyl estradiol + norethindrone acetate	2.5 mcg/0.5 mg or 5 mcg/1 mg once daily (continuous combined)
	Prefest	Estradiol 3 tabs then estradiol + norgestimate 3 tabs	1 mg × 3 days alternating with 1 mg/0.9 mg × 3 days, once daily sequentially
	Premphase	Conjugated estrogens (14 tabs), then conjugated estrogens + MPA (14 tabs)	0.625 mg, then 0.625 mg/5 mg Once daily sequentially
	Prempro	Conjugated estrogens + MPA	0.3 mg/1.5 mg once daily; 0.45 mg/1.5 mg once daily; 0.625 mg/2.5 mg once daily; or 0.625 mg/5 mg once daily Taken daily (continuous combined)
Combination estrogens + progestogens, transdermal	Climara Pro	Estradiol + levonorgestrel	0.045 mg/0.015 mg daily Change patch once weekly Apply to lower abdomen Continuous combined regimen
	CombiPatch	Estradiol + norethindrone acetate	0.05 mg/0.14 mg or 0.05 mg/0.25 mg daily Change patch twice weekly Apply to lower abdomen; rotate sites Use in rotation with estradiol patch to provide sequential progestogen, or daily as continuous combined regimen
Combination estrogens + bazedoxifene, oral	Duavee	Estrogens, conjugated + bazedoxifene	0.45 mg/20 mg once daily
Estrogens, vaginal creams	Estrace Vaginal	Micronized estradiol-17β	0.01% cream, 1 g = 0.1 mg of estradiol 2–4 g daily for 1–2 weeks; then taper as symptoms tolerate
	Premarin Vaginal	Conjugated estrogens (formerly conjugated equine estrogens)	0.625 mg per 1 g cream 1–2 g daily for 1–2 weeks; then taper to lowest effective dose
Estrogens, vaginal tablets	Vagifem	Estradiol	10 mcg tab 1 tab vaginally daily for 2 weeks; then taper to lowest effective dose
Estrogens, vaginal rings	Estring	Micronized estradiol-17β	7.5 mcg delivered in 24 hours Replace vaginal ring every 3 months
	Femring	Estradiol acetate	0.05 mg delivered in 24 hours or 0.1 mg delivered in 24 hours Start with 0.05 mg/day ring Replace vaginal ring every 3 months Effective for both systemic vasomotor symptoms and local vulvovaginal symptoms
Progestogens, vaginal gel	Crinone	Progesterone	4%, 8% vaginal gel Off-label use
	Prochieve	Progesterone	4%, 8% vaginal gel Off-label use

IUS	Mirena	Levonorgestrel	52 mg IUS
			Ensure not pregnant
			Off-label use
			Provides local progesterone to prevent endometrial hyperplasia and cancer
			5-year use

[a]See prescribing reference for full information on doses, side effects, contraindications, and cautions; use lowest effective dose for shortest time possible; progestogen is needed for any woman with an intact uterus who is using estrogen (oral, patch, cream, gel, systemic ring, and possibly for vaginal products) to prevent endometrial hyperplasia and cancer.
HF, hot flash; IUS, intrauterine system; MPA, medroxyprogesterone acetate.
Source: Adapted from ePocrates. (n.d.). Computerized pharmacology and prescribing reference (updated daily). *www.epocrates.com*

monthly dosing pattern. Breakthrough bleeding is common for all forms of EPT in the first several months following initiation of therapy. It will decrease over time, and with the CC-EPT method bleeding often will cease completely. The cyclic regimen is another CS-EPT option, in which estrogen is taken alone on days 1 to 11 and together with the progestogen on days 12 to 21 of the month. This method is rarely used because of the frequency of rebound symptoms that occur during the withdrawal bleed period (days 22 to 28) when no hormones are taken. If rebound symptoms are not experienced, then tapering the HT is considered. Estrogen + bazedoxifene is administered in a continuous pattern of one combined tablet daily. Progestogen administered through an intrauterine system (e.g., Mirena; Mirena PI; labeling.bayerhealthcare.com/html/products/pi/Mirena_PI.pdf) can be considered for off-label endometrial protection in those who are taking ET and who prefer not to use or cannot tolerate oral progestogens.

Although progestogen therapy (PT) can be used alone for menopause-related symptom management, this is uncommon because EPT generally provides better symptom relief and progestogen-only use is off label. For those who cannot take estrogen, PT using Megace (megestrol), a progestogen used for breast cancer treatment, or injectable medroxyprogesterone acetate (Depo-Provera) might be considered (Loprinzi et al., 2006). However, other alternatives to HT may be equally effective and are also considered and discussed.

HT is available in multiple routes of delivery. Oral products are available as tablets, pills, coated tablets, and timed-release tablets. All orally ingested hormones are rapidly metabolized to estrone in the liver. Although maximum serum concentrations are achieved in approximately 6 hours and a steady state is present in about 1 week, it may take up to 6 weeks for symptom control to manifest because circulating hormones bind slowly to unbound hormone receptors.

Transdermal products are available as patches, sprays, creams, and gels. The hepatic first-pass effect is largely avoided when transdermal administration is used. As a result, lower doses of hormones can be used and clotting risks may be reduced (ePocrates, n.d.; NAMS, 2019, 2022). Otherwise, transdermal hormones generally carry the same risks and benefits as oral products (ePocrates, n.d.; NAMS, 2019, 2022). Although often more costly than oral products, this route of administration is ideal for women with a history of thrombosis, high triglyceride levels, hypertension, or other chronic diseases. Transdermal administration, especially with patches, tends to provide more constant hormone levels than oral administration.

Vaginal hormones are available in creams, tablets, and rings. As with the transdermal products, they largely avoid the hepatic first-pass effect; in addition, for women with underlying chronic disease or history of thrombosis, they are considered safer than oral methods. Although they carry the same overall risks and benefits as oral products, most vaginal products work locally in the vagina and are the preferred treatment option for women with primary symptoms attributable to atrophic vaginitis. Very low doses, such as 10 mcg, can be effective (NAMS, 2019, 2022). Femring does have systemic properties, is effective for both VMS and vaginal atrophy, and may require use of a progestogen.

Injectable hormones are available in formulations intended to provide relatively immediate or prolonged effects. Injectable hormones that provide relatively immediate effects are most often used for treating bleeding or protecting pregnancy. Some forms of contraception (see Chapter 21, Fertility Self-Management and Shared Management) and HT are also available in longer-acting injectable forms. The HT formulations rapidly provide steady serum levels and remain effective over a period of approximately 1 month. As with other methods of delivery, receptor binding and thus symptom control may take up to 6 weeks.

When initiating HT, NAMS (2019, 2022) recommends starting with a low dose of estrogen. Some will require higher doses to achieve adequate symptom control. Efficacy is determined by monitoring symptoms and dose is titrated to the lowest possible effective dose.

Different side effects may be experienced depending on the type of estrogen or progesterone being taken. Trying different types to determine which products are most acceptable is appropriate and often necessary. Similarly, some will determine that the delivery method initially selected is not agreeable and may need to be changed.

Clinicians provide anticipatory guidance regarding normal HT side effects and management strategies (Table 34.5). Many attribute HT with weight gain; however, research provides evidence that HT does not increase body weight. Rather, it assists in preventing the weight increase and abdominal adiposity associated with midlife (NAMS, 2019,

2022). HT also helps to prevent diabetes, which affects more women as they age (NAMS, 2019, 2022). A follow-up appointment approximately 1 to 2 months after HT is initiated provides an opportunity to reevaluate symptoms, answer questions, and reiterate patient education. Dose adjustments can be made at this time if symptoms are not at an acceptable level.

TABLE 34.5 Common Hormone Therapy Side Effects and Management Strategies[a]

SIDE EFFECT	MANAGEMENT STRATEGY
Alopecia, extra hair growth	• Consider changing estrogen. • Consider changing progestogen.
Abdominal bloating, cramping, flatulence	• Advise avoiding grapefruit and grapefruit juice. • Advise ingesting six to eight 8-oz glasses of water daily. • Change to low-dose transdermal estrogen. • Consider adding a low-dose diuretic. • Consider reducing progestogen dose, changing to alternate progestogen, or using micronized progesterone.
Bleeding, spotting (vaginal)	• Ensure the HT is taken at same time each day. • Educate that breakthrough bleeding is common with continuous combined EPT during first few months of therapy. • Consider changing to a different HT or reducing dose. • If bleeding begins after the first few months of continuous combined EPT, evaluate using ultrasound and/or endometrial biopsy.
Breast changes, tenderness	• Advise reducing salt, peanuts, chocolate, and caffeine ingestion. • Advise wearing a supportive bra. • Consider changing progestogen. • Consider reducing or changing estrogen. • Consider use of evening primrose oil.
Chloasma/ malasma	• Ensure use of sunscreen daily. • Advise wearing a wide-brimmed hat or visor to shield face.
Depression, mood changes	• Ensure that sleep is adequate. • Ensure that daily water intake is adequate. • Assess for stress and stress management. • Advise limiting salt, alcohol, and caffeine consumption. • Consider changing or reducing progestogen. • Consider changing to a continuous combined EPT regimen.
Dry eyes, intolerance of contact lenses	• Advise avoiding antihistamines. • Advise avoiding smoke. • Advise adequate water intake. • Consider referral to discuss change in contact lenses. • Recommend reduced wearing time for contact lenses. • Recommend use of ophthalmic lubricating drops or rewetting drops for contact lens wearers.
Elevated blood pressure	• Advise avoiding alcohol. • Advise avoiding/discontinuing (if applicable) smoking. • Advise regular exercise. • Advise limiting salt intake. • Advise weight loss if BMI is >25 kg/m^2. • Advise adequate water intake. • Assess for stress and stress management. • Ensure that antihypertensives are being taken correctly. • Consider reducing, changing, or discontinuing estrogen. • Monitor blood pressure; if consistently elevated, consider discontinuing HT.
Elevated blood glucose levels, glucose intolerance	• Ensure consistently following diet and exercising. • Consider adjusting diabetes medication(s). • Consider reducing estrogen.
Fluid retention	• Advise ingesting six to eight 8-oz glasses of water daily; consider adding lemon for a natural diuretic effect. • Advise regular exercise. • Consider adding a low-dose prescription diuretic or herbal diuretic. • Consider changing to transdermal estrogen patch, gel, or cream. • Consider reducing or changing progestogen.
Gastrointestinal upset, nausea, vomiting	• Advise taking hormones with meals. • Ensure adequate daily water intake. • Consider changing or reducing estrogen. • Consider changing or reducing progestogen. • Consider changing to transdermal estrogen.
Loss of libido	• Consider adding testosterone (off-label use). • Assess sexual function, social factors, and relationship; make recommendations (see Chapter 19, Women's Sexual Health and Chapter 29, Urologic and Pelvic Floor Health Problems).
Headache or migraine aggravation	• Advise limiting salt, caffeine, and alcohol use. • Assess for stress and stress management (see Chapter 12, Mental Health and Chapter 40, Mental Health Challenges). • Ensure adequate daily water intake. • Consider change to continuous combined EPT regimen to reduce hormone fluctuations. • Consider change to transdermal estrogen. • Consider decreasing estrogen and/or progestogen.
Rash	• Ensure that patch is applied over clean, dry area. • Ensure that patch location is rotated. • If urticaria develops, stop medication and assess for allergic response.

[a]See prescribing reference for full information on side effects, cautions, and contraindications for estrogen, progestogens, and testosterone hormone therapy products. EPT, estrogen-progestogen therapy; HT, hormone therapy; BMI, body mass index.
Source: Adapted from ePocrates. (n.d.). Computerized pharmacology and prescribing reference (updated daily). www.epocrates.com; *The North American Menopause Society. (2019).* Menopause practice: A clinician's guide *(6th ed.). Author.*

The need for HT is reevaluated at least annually; if symptom control is still necessary, then HT may be continued for the shortest period possible. If symptoms are well controlled using a specific dose, then reducing the dose to determine if symptom control continues is appropriate. Some will have symptoms for a few years, whereas others continue with moderate to severe symptoms for many years (NAMS, 2019, 2022). The decision to discontinue HT is made collaboratively with the patient and based on their individual risks, needs, and QOL. The discussion on discontinuation of HT needs to include the newest findings from ongoing research regarding cardiovascular, breast cancer, and venous thromboembolic event risks. (NAMS, 2019, 2022).

NONHORMONE PRESCRIPTION MEDICATIONS

Although ET, EPT, and estrogen + bazedoxifene are superior for VMS management (NAMS, 2019, 2022), those who are unwilling or unable to take hormones may benefit from using alternative prescription options (Table 34.6). These may be added to lifestyle changes and/or some CAM therapies. Many of the studies evaluating efficacy of nonhormonal oral prescription medications for HF management were conducted with breast cancer survivors who were experiencing HFs. Clinicians need to consider whether the results apply to those who have not had breast cancer and also whether treatment options need to be tailored because some nonhormonal medications may interfere with breast cancer therapies (NAMS, 2019, 2022).

Considerations for Special Populations

Because hormonal fluctuations and ovulation are possible, perimenopausal persons with a uterus who engage in sexual intercourse with males can become pregnant. Almost half (45%) of all pregnancies are unintended (Guttmacher Institute, 2019). Although data specifying unintended pregnancy rates among perimenopausal women are lacking, the CDC reported that 2.7 abortions were performed for every 1,000 women over age 40 years between 2010 and 2019 (Kortsmit et al., 2021). Thus, it is important to discuss contraception with perimenopausal persons who may become pregnant (see Chapter 21, Fertility Self-Management and Shared Management).

Premature or temporary menopause (see Box 34.1) causes early loss of fertility and potentially more severe symptoms than natural menopause. There is a higher risk for osteoporosis and CVD because of the comparatively earlier reduction in estrogen and progesterone. Other significant health concerns may arise related to underlying disease processes (NAMS, 2019, 2022). Likewise, menopause generally occurs earlier following hysterectomy, most likely attributable to the reduced circulation to the remaining ovaries following surgical interruption of the uterine blood supply, which also partially feeds the ovaries.

TABLE 34.6 Nonhormonal Pharmacologic Options[a] for Vasomotor Symptom Management

CATEGORY	DRUG	DOSAGE[a]	COMMENT[a]	COMMON SIDE EFFECTS[a]	CONTRAINDICATIONS[a]
Anticonvulsants	Gabapentin (Neurontin)	Initial dose 300 mg/day Increase at 3- to 4-day intervals to 300 mg three times daily as needed	Avoid abrupt cessation Effective in two out of two trials	Ataxia, dizziness, fatigue, somnolence	No antacids within 2 hours of use Alcohol potentiates CNS depression
Antihypertensives	Clonidine	0.05–0.1 mg twice daily	Available as a patch Less effective than SSRIs/SNRIs or gabapentin Avoid abrupt cessation	Agitation, arrhythmias, constipation, dizziness, drowsiness, dry mouth, hypotension, impotence, insomnia, myalgia, nausea, orthostatic hypotension, rash, urticaria, weakness	Antagonized by tricyclic antidepressants Potentiates CNS depressants
	Methyldopa and Bellergal		Not recommended because of toxicity		
Breast cancer agent (progestin)	Megestrol (Megace)	20 mg daily (divided doses)	May increase insulin requirements	Asthenia, chest pain, decreased libido, dyspepsia, edema, fever, hyperglycemia, hypertension, insomnia, intestinal disturbance, rash, urinary frequency, weight gain	Use with caution in women with diabetes or history of thromboembolic disease

(continued)

TABLE 34.6 Nonhormonal Pharmacologic Options[a] for Vasomotor Symptom Management (continued)

CATEGORY	DRUG	DOSAGE[a]	COMMENT[a]	COMMON SIDE EFFECTS[a]	CONTRAINDICATIONS[a]
SSRIs/SNRIs[b]	Fluoxetine (Prozac)	Start at 20 mg/day Titrate up as needed	Avoid abrupt cessation Monitor weight	Anorgasmia, asthenia, GI upset, reduced libido, somnolence, insomnia, sweating	Avoid concomitant use of MAO inhibitors or thioridazine Use with caution with warfarin Avoid use with alcohol Use with caution in women with diabetes, diseases that affect metabolism, or heart disease
	Paroxetine (Brisdelle)	7.5 mg/day	Only SSRI with FDA approval for treatment of HFs Avoid abrupt cessation	See fluoxetine	
	Desvenlafaxine (Pristiq)	Start at 50 mg/day Titrate up to max dose of 400 mg/day as needed	Avoid abrupt cessation	See fluoxetine	
	Venlafaxine (Effexor XR)	Start at 37.5 mg/day Titrate up as needed	Avoid abrupt cessation	See fluoxetine	

[a]See prescribing reference for full information on doses, side effects, contraindications, and cautions; except for paroxetine 7.5 mg (Brisdell), use of these products for vasomotor symptom relief is off-label; efficacy for HF management with these products is less than that with estrogen.
[b]Effective in four out of six trials in meta-analysis.
CNS, central nervous system; FDA, Food and Drug Administration; GI, gastrointestinal; HFs, hot flashes; MAO, monoamine oxidase; SNRI, serotonin-norepinephrine reuptake inhibitor; SSRI, selective serotonin reuptake inhibitor.
Source: Adapted from ePocrates. (n.d.). Computerized pharmacology and prescribing reference (updated daily). *www.epocrates.com; The North American Menopause Society. (2019).* Menopause practice: A clinician's guide (6th ed.). *Author.*

FUTURE DIRECTIONS

Much has been learned about managing menopause-related symptoms over the past several decades. Landmark research studies have clarified risks and benefits of HT, nonhormonal therapy, and various CAMs for managing menopause-related symptoms, and the importance of maintaining a high QOL has been underscored. Current research is evaluating various other methodologies, such as alternative hormones, novel nonhormone therapies, other CAM therapies, and unique delivery options, to evaluate their effectiveness in mitigating VMS while retaining a strong safety profile for health. These new therapies are likely to provide important relief in the future.

REFERENCES

References for this chapter are online and available at https://connect.springerpub.com/content/book/978-0-8261-6722-4/part/part03/chapter/ch34

CHAPTER 35

Osteoporosis*

IVY M. ALEXANDER, MATTHEW WITKOVIC, KARA VIGNATI, AND DANIELA LAROSA KARANDA

Osteoporosis (OP) is the most common bone disease in humans, representing a major public health problem (Sarafrazi et al., 2021; LeBoff et al., 2022; North American Menopause Society [NAMS], 2021). Fracture attributable to OP is a significant health problem that affects all genders, especially those experiencing menopause (LeBoff et al., 2022; NAMS, 2021). As estrogen and progesterone levels fall, bone strength also declines.

OP is a disorder of the skeletal system characterized by a reduction in bone strength and increased risk for fracture (Camacho et al., 2020; Sarafrazi et al., 2021; LeBoff et al., 2022; NAMS, 2021). Low bone mass (LBM; previously identified as osteopenia) is like OP except that there is a lesser amount of bone lost. Two factors contribute to bone strength: bone mineral density (BMD) and bone quality. BMD refers to the thickness and volume of the bone. Bone quality refers to the bone architecture, mineralization, rate of turnover, and accumulated damage (Camacho et al., 2020; LeBoff et al., 2022; NAMS, 2021). BMD is easily measured using densitometry testing such as the dual-energy x-ray absorptiometry (DXA). Bone quality is more difficult to assess as simple measurement devices are not readily available.

OP is a silent condition in that it is not evident until a fracture occurs or kyphosis is recognized. Even with fracture, OP is often missed. For these reasons, national organizations have initiated programs to increase awareness and recommend prevention early in life as well as routine screening to identify and manage bone loss before fractures occur. The goal for preventing, identifying, and managing OP is to prevent fractures, which are associated with extensive negative sequelae.

A note about language: The authors attempt to use inclusive language throughout this chapter. The need to accurately represent data from research sometimes requires the use of specific terms such as *woman* and *women*. Additionally, because bone remodeling is greatly influenced by endogenous female or male hormones, the terms *female* and *male* are used to represent biological sex when appropriate. Bone remodeling in a transgender person who does not take gender-affirming hormone therapy (GAHT) or a nonbinary person is the same as that in persons of the same biological sex. Bone remodeling is thought to remain stable across the lifespan for transgender persons who do take GAHT since the endogenous decreases in hormones are overridden by their exogenous GAHT.

DEFINITION

OP is defined by BMD at the hip or lumbar spine that is 2.5 or more standard deviations below the mean BMD of a young adult reference population. When the score is compared to the average young adult reference population matched by sex and ethnicity, the score is referred to as a *T-score* (*Alexeeva* et al., 1994). OP is a skeletal disorder characterized by a loss of bone matrix and reduced bone integrity and strength. It predisposes patients to an increased risk for fracture (Dolan & Walsh, 2022). OP is a risk factor for fracture, just as hypertension is a risk factor for stroke. The disease causes over 2 million fractures annually in the United States, exceeding the combined number of new cases of breast cancer, myocardial infarction, and prostate cancer (LeBoff et al., 2022). Fracture incidence is projected to increase to approximately 3.2 million annually by the year 2040 (LeBoff et al., 2022).

Primary OP is due to bone loss related to age, gender, family history, and other factors. Bone loss accelerates in females with the decline of estrogen and progestogen hormones after menopause. One large modifiable risk factor for OP is nutritional deficiency including low intake of calcium, vitamin D, dietary protein, and fruits and vegetables, or high consumption of alcohol. Other modifiable risk factors include a sedentary lifestyle, low body mass index (BMI), cigarette smoking, stress, and air pollution. Nonmodifiable risk factors include history of falls, older age, sex, White ethnic background, prior fractures, and genetic predisposition (Pouresmaeili et

---

*This chapter is a revision of the chapter that appeared in the second edition of this textbook, coauthored by Emily Miesse, and we thank her for her original contribution.

al., 2018). Among postmenopausal persons, low BMD at the femoral neck (T-score of −1.0 or below) is found in 10% of Black Americans, 16% of Mexican Americans, and 21% of White Americans. More than 20% of postmenopausal persons have prevalent vertebral fractures (VFs). In the United States, as many as 8 million females and 2 million males have OP (Lindsay & Cosman, 2018), and more than 40 million people have bone mass levels that increase their risk for contracting OP.

Secondary OP results from medical conditions or pharmacologic treatments that hinder attaining peak bone mass and/or interfere with bone turnover or predispose to accelerated bone loss (Camacho et al., 2020; LeBoff et al., 2022; NAMS, 2021). Secondary causes of OP include chronic use of some medications, especially corticosteroids, as well as an array of conditions that interfere with bone modeling or remodeling such as hypogonadism, hyperparathyroidism, chronic liver disease, inflammatory diseases, renal disease, cardiovascular disease, diabetes mellitus, and dementia (Pouresmaeili et al., 2018).

OP affects approximately 10 million U.S. adults, and about 43 million more have LBM (Sarafrazi et al., 2021; Lindsay & Cosman, 2018). LBM is defined as a BMD T-score of −1.0 to −2.5, meaning the person's BMD is between 1 and 2.5 standard deviations below that of an average young person of the same sex and ethnicity. Despite the high prevalence of OP and LBM, only a small fraction of these cases are diagnosed and treated (Camacho et al., 2020; LeBoff et al., 2022; Lindsay & Cosman, 2018; NAMS, 2021).

OP and LBM increase a person's risk for fracture (Camacho et al., 2020; LeBoff et al., 2022; Lindsay & Cosman, 2018; NAMS, 2021). At age 50, the lifetime risk of developing fractures is estimated to be 40% to 50% for White U.S. females (Camacho et al., 2020; LeBoff et al., 2022; NAMS, 2021). The lifetime risk for a hip fracture is estimated at 6% among American Blacks, 14% among American Hispanics, and 17% among American Whites. Yearly incidence of OP-related fracture is projected to increase by 68% by 2040 (Camacho et al., 2020; LeBoff et al., 2022; NAMS, 2021).

The real concerns related to bone loss are related to fracture. OP-related fractures are often associated with devastating sequelae. Hip fracture conveys extraordinary morbidity and mortality outcomes. Up to one out of every four patients die in the year following a hip fracture (25% mortality rate), 25% need long-term (nursing home) care, and half (50%) never return to their prefracture level of mobility. Hip fractures are also associated with an increased incidence of deep vein thrombosis (DVT) and pulmonary embolism (PE; Lindsay & Cosman, 2018). VFs frequently cause substantial acute and chronic pain, loss of height, and kyphosis. Kyphosis can advance to restrict movement, interfere with gastrointestinal and other abdominal organ function, and limit lung capacity (Camacho et al., 2020; LeBoff et al., 2022; NAMS, 2021). Physical disability and inability to enjoy previous activities add to the burden of the disease by causing isolation and depression, factors that can increase risks for additional bone loss and falls through inactivity.

Enormous costs result from OP-related fractures, both personally and economically. Annual costs of $57 billion are projected to exceed $95 billion by 2040. The current annual financial toll accounts for hospital admissions (currently over 432,000), long-term care facility admissions (over 180,000), and around 2.5 million outpatient healthcare visits (NAMS, 2021).

ETIOLOGY

Peak bone mass is usually attained by about age 30 years (Camacho et al., 2020; LeBoff et al., 2022; NAMS, 2021). When peak bone mass is achieved, bone remodeling continues. Osteoclast cells secrete enzymes that digest bone and create microscopic holes, called resorption cavities, along the surface of the bone. Osteoblasts then migrate to the surface and secrete collagen to fill the resorption cavities with newly formed osteoid material. The osteoblasts are eventually replaced with lining cells, and the process repeats. Bone formation and remodeling are regulated by multiple endocrine and hormonal mechanisms. During childhood, when bone mass increases rapidly, osteoblasts act independently and in response to growth hormones. However, in adulthood, osteoblasts act in response to osteoclast activity and functional load stress that is exerted on bone, such as the stress caused by physical exercise. LBM and OP are caused when the normal processes of bone remodeling are unbalanced and resorption rates exceed bone formation, resulting in reduced bone quality and strength (Camacho et al., 2020; LeBoff et al., 2022; NAMS, 2021).

Primary OP is associated with aging for both females and males. It affects females more than males because of the rapid increase in bone loss that accompanies the decline in estrogen and progesterone levels during the transition to postmenopause (TPM; Camacho et al., 2020; LeBoff et al., 2022; NAMS, 2021). The rate of bone turnover and bone loss accelerates during the 3- to 5-year span preceding menopause. On average, bone loss of 2% occurs annually during the 1 to 3 years prior to menopause and over 5 to 10 years after, resulting in bone loss of 10% to 12% across the TPM (Camacho et al., 2020; LeBoff et al., 2022; NAMS, 2021).

Secondary OP is bone loss caused by disease processes or medications (Box 35.1) that interfere with the normal process of bone formation (Camacho et al., 2020; LeBoff et al., 2022; NAMS, 2021). Secondary OP can affect males or females at any age and may be considered if the *Z-score* identified on a DXA scan is low. Z-score compares the patient BMD to that of the average same-aged reference population matched by sex and ethnicity. Low Z-scores may also be seen in females or males who never achieved peak bone mass levels when growing up. Fracture risk is also affected by disease processes or medications that increase risk for fracture (Box 35.1).

RISK FACTORS

Some risk factors for OP can be controlled; others cannot (Box 35.2). Risk factors for fracture and falls are distinct from the risk factors for bone loss (Box 35.3).

Box 35.1 Medications[a] and Medical Conditions[a] Associated With Bone Loss or Increased Fracture Risk

Medications Associated With Bone Loss or Increased Fracture Risk

Aluminum-containing antacids (e.g., Amphojel, Maalox, Mylanta)

Androgen deprivation therapy

Anticoagulants (unfractionated heparin)

Anticonvulsants (e.g., carbamazepine [Carbatrol, Tegretol], divalproex [Depakote], phenobarbital, phenytoin [Dilantin], valproate [Depacon])

Aromatase inhibitors

Barbiturates

Cholestyramine (e.g., Questran)

Chemotherapy/immunosuppressors (e.g., methotrexate [Trexall])

Cytotoxic agents

Glucocorticosteroids (e.g., prednisone [Deltasone, Sterapred])

Gonadotropin-releasing hormone (GnRH) agonist or antagonist

Immunosuppressive agents

Insulin with hypoglycemia

Lithium (e.g., Eskalith, Lithobid)

Medroxyprogesterone acetate intramuscular injection (e.g., Depo-Provera)

Methotrexate

Parenteral nutrition

Proton pump inhibitors (PPIs, e.g., rabeprazole [AcipHex], esomeprazole [Nexium], lansoprazole [Prevacid], omeprazole [Prilosec])

Selective norepinephrine-reuptake inhibitors (SNRIs, e.g., duloxetine [Cymbalta])

Selective serotonin reuptake inhibitors (SSRIs, e.g., citalopram [Celexa], sertraline [Zoloft])

SGLT2 inhibitors (gliflozins)

Tamoxifen (premenopausal for breast cancer)

Thiazolidinediones (e.g., pioglitazone [Actos], rosiglitazone [Avandia])

Thyroid hormone (in excess; e.g., levothyroxine [Levoxyl, Levothroid, Synthroid])

Warfarin (e.g., Coumadin)

Medical Conditions Associated with Bone Loss or Increased Fracture Risk

Alcoholism

AIDS/HIV

Bone disorders (e.g., acromegaly, ankylosing spondylitis, osteogenesis imperfecta, posttransplant bone disease)

Chronic liver disease, cholestatic liver disease, primary biliary cirrhosis

Chronic renal failure, end-stage renal disease, renal tubular acidosis

Connective tissue diseases (e.g., lupus, multiple sclerosis, rheumatoid arthritis, sarcoidosis)

Depression

Eating disorders (e.g., anorexia nervosa, vitamin D deficiency, calcium deficiency, obesity)

Endocrine disorders (e.g., diabetes [type 1, type 2], gonadal insufficiency [primary, secondary], hypercortisolism [e.g., Cushing syndrome], hyperparathyroidism, hyperthyroidism, hypothyroidism [overtreated], thyrotoxicosis)

Gastrointestinal disorders (e.g., celiac disease, malabsorption syndromes, gastrectomy, gastric bypass surgery, inflammatory bowel disease, pancreatic disease)

Genetic disorders (e.g., cystic fibrosis, Gaucher disease, hemochromatosis, hypophosphatasia, Klinefelter syndrome, Marfan syndrome, osteogenesis imperfecta, sickle cell, thalassemia, Turner syndrome)

Hematologic disorders (e.g., hemophilia, leukemia)

HIV/AIDS

Liver disease, chronic, cirrhosis

Neuromuscular disorders (muscular dystrophy, paraplegia, quadriplegia, proximal myopathy)

Prolonged immobility

Renal disease, chronic

Respiratory disorders (e.g., cystic fibrosis, chronic obstructive pulmonary disease)

Rheumatologic disease

Seizure disorders (e.g., epilepsy)

[a]Representative list, not exhaustive.

Source: Adapted from Camacho, P. M., Petak, S. M., Binkley, N., Diab, D. L., Eldeiry, L. S., Farooki A, Harris, S. T., Hurley, D. L., Kelly, J., Lewiecki, E. M., Pessah-Pollack, R., McClung, M., Wimalawansa, S. J., & Watts, N. B. (2020). American Association of Clinical Endocrinologists/American College of Endocrinology clinical practice guidelines for the diagnosis and treatment of postmenopausal osteoporosis—2020 update. Endocrine Practice, 26(Suppl. 1), 1–46. https://doi.org/10.4158/GL-2020-0524SUPPL; *LeBoff, M. S., Greenspan, S. L., Insogna, K. L., Lewiecki, E. M., Saag, K. G., Singer, A. J., & Siris, E. S. (2022). The clinician's guide to prevention and treatment of osteoporosis.* Osteoporosis International, 33(10), 2049–2102. https://doi.org/10.1007/s00198-021-05900-y; *North American Menopause Society. (2021). Management of osteoporosis in postmenopausal women: The 2021 position statement of the North American Menopause Society.* Menopause, 28(9), 973–997. https://doi.org/10.1097/GME.0000000000001831

SYMPTOMS

OP itself is asymptomatic. A person cannot tell that their bones are losing density. OP may be recognized when a person loses 1.5 inches in height (usually due to silent or painless VFs) or due to the pain associated with a clinically evident fracture related to the bone loss (Cosman et al., 2014).

Kyphosis, usually due to VFs, causes a permanently stooped appearance and may be first noted when there is a documented loss of height (Camacho et al., 2020; LeBoff

Box 35.2 Osteoporosis Risk Factors

Potentially Modifiable Risk Factors

Amenorrhea (caused by eating disorder or excessive exercise)

Body weight less than 127 lb, body mass index less than 21 kg/m²

Chronic diseases (see Box 35.1)

Cigarette smoking (active or passive)

Falls

Frailty

Low estrogen level (e.g., menopause)

Medications (see Box 35.1)

Nulliparity

Poor nutrition (e.g., excessive vitamin A, excessive alcohol or caffeine intake, excessive soda intake, excessive sodium intake, inadequate calcium/vitamin D intake, protein deficiency)

Sedentary lifestyle/immobility

Nonmodifiable Risk Factors

Advanced age

Dementia

Delayed puberty

Endocrine disorders (Cushing syndrome, thyrotoxicosis, diabetes mellitus)

Family history of osteoporosis

Female gender

First-degree relative with history of fracture

Fracture history (fracture at 40–45 years or older is associated with an increased risk for osteoporosis)

Genetic factors (variations in or absence of genes that regulate protein receptors or enzymes needed for bone development)

Race (Caucasian and Asian women at greatest risk, then Hispanic and African American)

Source: Adapted from Camacho, P. M., Petak, S. M., Binkley, N., Diab, D. L., Eldeiry, L. S., Farooki A, Harris, S. T., Hurley, D. L., Kelly, J., Lewiecki, E. M., Pessah-Pollack, R., McClung, M., Wimalawansa, S. J., & Watts, N. B. (2020). American Association of Clinical Endocrinologists/American College of Endocrinology clinical practice guidelines for the diagnosis and treatment of postmenopausal osteoporosis—2020 update. Endocrine Practice, 26(Suppl. 1), 1–46. *https://doi.org/10.4158/GL-2020-0524SUPPL; LeBoff, M. S., Greenspan, S. L., Insogna, K. L., Lewiecki, E. M., Saag, K. G., Singer, A. J., & Siris, E. S. (2022). The clinician's guide to prevention and treatment of osteoporosis.* Osteoporosis International, 33(10), 2049–2102. *https://doi.org/10.1007/s00198-021-05900-y; North American Menopause Society. (2021). Management of osteoporosis in postmenopausal women: The 2021 position statement of the North American Menopause Society.* Menopause, 28(9), 973–997. *https://doi.org/10.1097/GME.0000000000001831*

Box 35.3 Risk Factors for Falls and Fracture[a]

Evaluated in the FRAX Algorithm

Age (especially older than 65 years, fracture risk doubles with each 7–8 years after age 50 years)

Body mass index (BMI) less than 21 kg/m²

Current smoking

Femoral neck raw bone mineral density (BMD) in g/cm²

Gender (female sex at greater risk than male sex)

Glucocorticoid use

Ingestion of three or more units of alcohol per day

Parent history of hip fracture (increases risk ~130%)

Personal prior fracture (risk for future fracture doubles)

Rheumatoid arthritis

Secondary osteoporosis

Selected Other Risk Factors

Depression/anxiety/decreased cognitive function

Environmental (poor lighting, trip hazards, etc.)

Frailty

History of falls, fainting, off balance

Impaired mobility

Low vitamin D levels

Neurologic disease

Neuropathy, especially lower extremities

Orthostatic hypotension

Poor vision

Sedentary lifestyle

Use of medications or substances that cause drowsiness, dizziness, lightheadedness, or imbalance; use of multiple medications

Vertigo

Weakness

[a]Risk factors have variable influences on fracture or fall risk. In the FRAX algorithm, all variables except age, height, weight, and gender are binary (entered as yes/no). This limits the weighting of some variables that would carry a higher risk for fracture if values were entered on a continuum. For example, a woman with a history of two prior fractures and taking 30 mg of oral steroid daily is at greater risk than a woman with one prior fracture who is taking 5 mg of steroid daily. The FRAX does calculate fracture risk using all the variables noted in the upper half of Box 35.3; therefore, the presence of multiple risks in one person is recognized.

FRAX, fracture risk assessment.

Source: Adapted from Camacho, P. M., Petak, S. M., Binkley, N., Diab, D. L., Eldeiry, L. S., Farooki A, Harris, S. T., Hurley, D. L., Kelly, J., Lewiecki, E. M., Pessah-Pollack, R., McClung, M., Wimalawansa, S. J., & Watts, N. B. (2020). American Association of Clinical Endocrinologists/American College of Endocrinology clinical practice guidelines for the diagnosis and treatment of postmenopausal osteoporosis—2020 update. Endocrine Practice, 26(Suppl. 1), 1–46. *https://doi.org/10.4158/GL-2020-0524SUPPL; LeBoff, M. S., Greenspan, S. L., Insogna, K. L., Lewiecki, E. M., Saag, K. G., Singer, A. J., & Siris, E. S. (2022). The clinician's guide to prevention and treatment of osteoporosis.* Osteoporosis International, 33(10), 2049–2102. *https://doi.org/10.1007/s00198-021-05900-y; North American Menopause Society. (2021). Management of osteoporosis in postmenopausal women: The 2021 position statement of the North American Menopause Society.* Menopause, 28(9), 973–997. *https://doi.org/10.1097/GME.0000000000001831*

et al., 2022; NAMS, 2021). Kyphosis also causes the rib cage to slump downward. With progression of bone loss, the ribs eventually come to rest on the ischial spines, thus minimizing thoracic and abdominal cavity space for organs. This restriction frequently leads to gastrointestinal problems, such as gastric reflux, anorexia, and constipation, and to respiratory disorders, such as shortness of breath (Camacho et al., 2020; LeBoff et al., 2022; NAMS, 2021). Self-image can also be negatively affected because of body changes and difficulty in finding clothing that fits properly over the kyphotic hump.

EVALUATION/ASSESSMENT

Office assessment for OP includes a thorough history to identify personal and familial risk factors for bone loss. Possible causes of secondary OP (Box 35.3) are also investigated through history and physical examination to identify any negative effects on bone health that can be eliminated or reduced (Camacho et al., 2020; LeBoff et al., 2022; NAMS, 2021).

History

Gathering information that will enable risk stratification and identification of potential secondary causes for OP is critical when taking a history. Medications used and health habits such as diet and exercise, smoking, and daily alcohol consumption are all important in understanding risk and determining nonpharmacologic treatments (Boxes 35.1 and 35.2). Uncovering symptoms suggestive of systemic conditions that cause OP (e.g., hyperthyroidism) or increase risks for fracture or falls is also essential (Boxes 35.1, 35.2, and 35.3). Noting nonmodifiable risk factors such as age, ethnicity, history of fractures, and family history will help in determining if DXA scanning is needed earlier than standard age-related screening. Using the fracture risk assessment (FRAX) algorithm scale will help quantify these risk factors (Camacho et al., 2020; LeBoff et al., 2022; NAMS, 2021).

A comprehensive risk assessment for falls is completed, especially in those with established OP, including hearing or vision impairments, neurologic status, and other medical problems or medications that may increase fall risk (Box 35.3).

Physical Examination

The physical examination includes assessment for physical risk factors, such as low BMI (less than 21 kg/m²) or body weight (less than 127 lb), kyphosis, tooth loss, or spinal tenderness; signs of low estrogen levels; signs of thyroid abnormalities; and clues to other secondary causes for OP. Height is measured accurately using a stadiometer, not taken via patient report. Reductions in height can be an important first clue for painless (or silent) VFs (Camacho et al., 2020; LeBoff et al., 2022; NAMS, 2021). Fall risk can also be assessed by observing gait when the patient is entering or leaving the room. If there is concern for falls, Romberg and orthostatic blood pressure readings can provide additional information.

VFs can be painless; however, they are often associated with significant pain (Camacho et al., 2020; LeBoff et al., 2022; NAMS, 2021). VFs can be caused by normal activities of daily life, such as bending forward to pick up an item. The anterior edge of a vertebral bone crumbles in response to the increase in pressure exerted while bending forward, and changes into a wedge shape. Over time, having multiple wedge-shaped bones on top of one another, instead of the usual square/cube shape, forces the spine to curve forward, causing kyphosis.

DIFFERENTIAL DIAGNOSIS

The diagnosis of OP is based on DXA results, physical exam findings, and laboratory results. A clinical diagnosis of OP is made when the patient has a low-trauma fracture of any type. A low-trauma fracture is a fracture sustained from relatively minor force, such as a fall from a standing height or less. Differentiating primary from secondary OP is important because some causes of secondary OP may be treatable and may rectify the bone loss. For example, a person with BMD test results that indicate OP may have disorders other than OP, such as osteomalacia or multiple myeloma, which may be treatable once identified. If serum calcium level is low, the cause needs to be identified and treated before an antiresorptive agent is administered, because it may exacerbate the problem. If vitamin D levels are low, replacement is necessary.

OP can be missed in patients who sustain a low-trauma fracture. Recognition of OP is critical as medications and a multidisciplinary approach to management are most effective (Camacho et al., 2020; LeBoff et al., 2022; NAMS, 2021).

DIAGNOSTIC STUDIES

DXA is the gold standard for screening and diagnosing OP (Camacho et al., 2020; LeBoff et al., 2022; NAMS, 2021). Radiation is used to measure central BMD at the hip and lumbar spine areas. Peripheral DXA is also available; however, central DXA is the standard for diagnosing and monitoring BMD (Camacho et al., 2020; LeBoff et al., 2022; NAMS, 2021; U.S. Preventive Services Task Force [USPSTF], 2018). Laboratory testing is needed to screen for secondary causes of OP (Camacho et al., 2020; Fitzgerald, 2022; LeBoff et al., 2022; NAMS, 2021). Quantitative computed tomography (QCT) can also be used to evaluate central BMD. QCT is especially useful in evaluating patients with osteoarthritis because it is less likely to detect osteophytes, which can falsely increase BMD measures identified with DXA.

Other methods for evaluating bone density include peripheral DXA, single-energy x-ray absorptiometry (SXA), peripheral QCT, radiographic absorptiometry (RA), peripheral quantitative ultrasound (QUS), and radiogrammetry. QUS done at the calcaneus is often used at health fairs as it is housed in a small unit often on wheels and therefore easily moved. These methods are not used to diagnose OP;

however, they may alert a person that their peripheral BMD is low and prompt them to seek central DXA testing. OP can also be incidentally identified on x-ray studies. However, it is apparent on x-ray images only if there is bone loss of 30% to 40%; x-rays are not used to diagnose OP. When bone loss is identified with noncentral measures, the patient is referred for DXA. See Box 35.4 for the recommendations for DXA screening.

DXA results for BMD are reported as T-scores and Z-scores (Camacho et al., 2020; LeBoff et al., 2022; NAMS, 2021). The T-score indicates the number of standard deviations the patient's BMD falls above or below that of a young adult, sex- and ethnic-matched norm. The World Health Organization determined classifications for T-score results (*Alexeeva* et al., 1994; Table 35.1). The Z-score indicates the number of standard deviations the BMD is above or below the mean for an age-, sex-, and ethnic-matched cohort. The Z-score is most often used for diagnosing bone loss in children or young adults, and can be helpful in identifying secondary OP. When the Z-score is low, it indicates either that the BMD is lower than the age cohort due to secondary OP causes or that peak bone mass was not achieved in young adulthood (Camacho et al., 2020; Fitzgerald, 2022; LeBoff et al., 2022; NAMS, 2021).

Box 35.4 Recommendations for DXA Screening

- All females 65 years old or older
- Females younger than age 65 years (postmenopausal or transitioning to postmenopause) who have clinical risks for OP identified with screening
- Individuals who sustain a fracture after age 50 years
- Individuals who have a clinical condition or take medications that are associated with bone loss or decreased bone mass

DXA, dual-energy x-ray absorptiometry; OP, osteoporosis.
Source: Adapted from LeBoff, M. S., Greenspan, S. L., Insogna, K. L., Lewiecki, E. M., Saag, K. G., Singer, A. J., & Siris, E. S. (2022). The clinician's guide to prevention and treatment of osteoporosis. Osteoporosis International, 33(10), 2049–2102. https://doi.org/10.1007/s00198-021-05900-y

TABLE 35.1 World Health Organization T-Score Classifications

T-SCORE RESULT	INTERPRETATION
At or above −1.0	Normal
−1.0 to −2.5	Osteopenia
At or below −2.5	Osteoporosis
At or below −2.5 with low-trauma fracture(s)	Severe or established osteoporosis

Source: Adapted from Alexeeva, L., Burkhardt, P., Christiansen, C., Cooper, C., Delmas, P., Johnell, O., Johnston, C., Kanis, J. A., Lips, P., Melton, L. J., Meunier, P., Seeman, E., Stepan, J., 3rd, & Tosteson, A. (1994). Assessment of fracture risk and its application to screening for postmenopausal osteoporosis (WHO Technical Report Series 843). https://apps.who.int/iris/handle/10665/39142.

Before a diagnosis of OP is confirmed, even with DXA results of −2.5 or below, a comprehensive history, physical examination, and laboratory studies are needed to identify possible causes of secondary OP or contraindications to medications (Camacho et al., 2020; LeBoff et al., 2022; NAMS, 2021). Initial laboratory testing should include complete blood count, albumin, calcium (albumin adjusted), renal function tests, phosphorus, magnesium, liver tests, 25(OH)-vitamin D, and parathyroid hormone (PTH), depending on the clinical picture. Additional testing to consider includes serum protein electrophoresis, serum immunofixation, serum free kappa and lambda light chains, thyroid-stimulating hormone with reflux free thyroxine (T4), tissue transglutaminase antibodies, IgA (immunoglobulin A) levels, iron, ferritin, homocysteine, prolactin, tryptase, bone turnover markers (BTMs), 24-hour urinary creatinine and calcium, and urinary histamine, protein electrophoresis (UPEP), and free cortisol (LeBuff et al., 2022; NAMS, 2021).

Biochemical BTMs are not used to diagnose OP. They are serum markers that have been used in research to evaluate fracture risk and treatment response. BTMs reflect osteoclast bone resorption activity (C-terminal telopeptide of type 1 collagen) or osteoblast activity for bone formation (procollagen type 1 N-terminal propeptide or alkaline phosphatase [bone-specific]). BTMs are not currently recommended for routine use to evaluate patients with OP (LeBoff et al., 2022; NAMS, 2021).

The FRAX, launched by the University of Sheffield (www.shef.ac.uk/FRAX) in 2008, uses data about 11 different risk factors as well as femoral neck BMD to provide added information to support clinical decision-making for initiating medication therapy, especially among those with osteopenia (see Pharmacotherapeutics section).

TREATMENT/MANAGEMENT

OP management begins early in life with recommendations about diet and exercise tailored to develop full peak bone mass as a young adult and continues with the goal of preventing bone loss at midlife. Once bone loss has occurred, the goal continues focusing on prevention of further bone loss as well as fracture prevention. Strategies for maximizing peak bone mass and bone loss prevention include changes in diet, use of supplements, and an exercise program that includes both weight-bearing and resistive activities. Fall prevention and use of pharmacotherapeutics are the mainstays of fracture prevention. Referral to a specialist is warranted when patients do not respond to first-line pharmacotherapeutics or when comorbid disease makes management complicated.

Self-Management

DIET AND SUPPLEMENTS

OP prevention needs to start early in life by ingesting a diet rich in calcium, vitamin D, and minerals, which are necessary to achieve peak bone mass. Maintaining adequate intake of both calcium (Table 35.2) and vitamin D (800–1,000 U/day)

TABLE 35.2 Daily Calcium Recommendations for Females at Various Ages

AGE	DAILY CALCIUM RECOMMENDATION (MG)
Birth to 6 months	200
6–12 months	260
1–3 years	700
4–8 years	1,000
9–13 years	1,300
14–18 years and pregnant or lactating	1,300
19–50 years and pregnant or lactating	1,000
51–70 years **>70 years**	1,200 **1,000** **1,200**

Source: Adapted from Ross, A. C., Manson, J. E., Abrams, S. A., Aloia, J. F., Brannon, P. M., Clinton, S. K., Durazo-Arvizu, R. A., Gallagher, J. C., Gallo, R. L., Jones, G., Kovacs, C. S., Mayne, S. T., Rosen, C. J., & Shapses, S. A. (2011). The 2011 report on dietary reference intakes for calcium and vitamin D from the Institute of Medicine: What clinicians need to know. Journal of Clinical Endocrinology and Metabolism, 96(1), 53–58. https://doi.org/10.1210/jc.2010–2704

remains necessary with aging and throughout postmenopause. Supplementation is often needed to increase the 600 to 700 mg of calcium ingested by women over 50 in a typical diet (Ross et al., 2011).

Although UV sunlight exposure to bare skin can synthesize vitamin D, this is not the recommended modality to obtain adequate levels of vitamin D, both because of the increased risk for skin cancer and because of variables that interfere with a consistent amount of vitamin D production. Thus, supplementation or ingestion of vitamin D–fortified foods is recommended. Individuals with low serum 25-(OH)vitamin D levels (less than 30 ng/mL) may require supplementation (Camacho et al., 2020; LeBoff et al., 2022; NAMS, 2021).

Other dietary considerations include minimizing ingestion of soda and caffeinated beverages. Caffeine intake should not exceed four cups of coffee per day as caffeine limits intestinal calcium absorption (Coronado-Zarco et al., 2019). The phosphorus in soda and the caffeine in other beverages may interfere with bone formation and remodeling processes if consumed in very high quantities. More important, for most people, is that frequent ingestion of these beverages can replace ingestion of calcium-rich milk, posing a greater harm to developing and maintaining bone strength. Adequate amounts of phosphorus are needed; however, phosphorus intake must be balanced because either excessive or insufficient amounts can interfere with bone formation. Adequate citric acid, protein, and fiber are also needed for proper bone formation. Excessive protein or fiber intake can interfere with normal intestinal absorption of calcium. Alcohol consumption should be limited to two drinks per day as three or more drinks per day may be associated with an increased fracture risk (Camacho et al., 2020; LewBoff et al., 2022; NAMS, 2021).

Although supplementation with adequate amounts of calcium and vitamin D is important for general health, there is limited evidence that calcium, vitamin D, or calcium with vitamin D combinations will alone provide a reduction in fracture risk (American College of Obstetricians and Gynecologists' Committee on Clinical Practice Guidelines–Gynecology, 2021; Barrionuevo et al., 2019). Calcium and vitamin D from dietary sources, and supplementation when dietary sources do not meet recommended daily intakes, should be initiated in conjunction with other OP treatment modalities in those with a high risk of fracture (Camacho et al., 2020; Eastell et al., 2019; LeBoff et al., 2022; NAMS, 2021). Calcium from dietary sources is preferred over supplements; however, calcium intake from dietary sources is frequently below the recommended dietary allowance. Furthermore, individuals with lactose intolerance may not tolerate dairy products that are richest in calcium, making supplementation necessary (Camacho et al., 2020; LeBoff et al., 2022; NAMS, 2021). The recommended dietary allowances (RDAs) for calcium are based on elemental calcium, the amount of calcium that is absorbed from a food or supplement and used in the body. To promote adequate absorption, doses should be spaced and not exceed 500 to 600 mg per dose (Coronado_Zarco et al., 2019). Most supplements now list elemental calcium levels on their labels; therefore, determining the amount of calcium that is absorbed is straightforward. Taking 1,000 mg of calcium supplement daily was not associated with increased risks for cardiovascular disease or stroke in the Nurses' Health Study (Paik et al., 2014). However, increased calcium doses may increase kidney stone risk and may increase cardiac risk at higher doses (NAMS, 2021). Several different types of calcium supplements are available (Table 35.3).

EXERCISE

Establishing an active lifestyle early in life and maintaining it throughout the older years is crucial to encourage normal bone formation and slow bone loss. The effects of exercise on bone are site specific because osteoblast activity increases locally in response to load stress caused by exercise (e.g., walking supports bone density in the hips, lower spine, and legs; hand weights benefit the arms and wrists; and overhead weights benefit the shoulders, upper arms, wrists, and upper spine; Camacho et al., 2020; LeBoff et al., 2022). Weight-bearing, resistance, and balance exercises are recommended (Camacho et al., 2020; LeBoff et al., 2022). Physical activity in which bones and muscles work against gravity, such as walking, are considered weight-bearing exercises (Cosman et al., 2014). Other examples of weight-bearing exercises include jogging, dancing, and lifting weights. Resistance training includes activities such as water aerobics, cycling, and yoga. When severe OP is present, exercises that compress forces on the spine, such as forward bending, trunk rotation, or lifting heavy weights, should be avoided to minimize fracture risk (Camacho et al., 2020). In addition to improving bone strength and providing overall fitness, exercise helps women maintain their balance, and thus reduces fall risk. Exercise and activities that carry a high risk for falls are also discouraged in women with established OP.

TABLE 35.3 Calcium Supplements

TYPE	BRAND NAMES	COMMENTS
Calcium carbonate	Caltrate, Os-Cal, Tums, Viactiv, others	• Available in liquid, chewable tablet • Needs to be taken with food; needs acidic environment for absorption • Not a good choice for women taking proton pump inhibitors because of lowered gastric acidity, even with meals • Often causes flatulence, constipation; can minimize these symptoms if taken in combination with magnesium • May contain lead if made from bone meal, dolamite, or oyster shell; concern mainly for children, pregnant or lactating women
Calcium citrate	Citracal	• Available in liquid, tablet, and chewing gum forms • Can be taken with or without food; easily absorbed and not affected by acid level
Calcium phosphate tribasic	Posture	• Can be taken with or without food; absorption not affected by acid level • Usual formulation added to calcium-fortified drinks
Calcium gluconate	Various	• Less frequently used • Usually combined with calcium carbonate in vitamin or mineral supplement products
Calcium glubionate Calcium lactate	Calcionate Ridactate	• Liquid form • Less frequently used Less bioavailability and taken three times a day before meals

Source: Adapted from Camacho, P. M., Petak, S. M., Binkley, N., Diab, D. L., Eldeiry, L. S., Farooki A, Harris, S. T., Hurley, D. L., Kelly, J., Lewiecki, E. M., Pessah-Pollack, R., McClung, M., Wimalawansa, S. J., & Watts, N. B. (2020). American Association of Clinical Endocrinologists/American College of Endocrinology clinical practice guidelines for the diagnosis and treatment of postmenopausal osteoporosis—2020 update. Endocrine Practice, 26(Suppl. 1), 1–46. https://doi.org/10.4158/GL-2020-0524SUPPL; Drugs.com. (n.d.). *Calcium supplement oral, parenteral advanced patient information. https://www.drugs.com/cons/calcium-acetate.html; LeBoff, M. S., Greenspan, S. L., Insogna, K. L., Lewiecki, E. M., Saag, K. G., Singer, A. J., & Siris, E. S. (2022). The clinician's guide to prevention and treatment of osteoporosis.* Osteoporosis International, 33(10), 2049–2102. https://doi.org/10.1007/s00198-021-05900-y; North American Menopause Society. (2021). *Management of osteoporosis in postmenopausal women: The 2021 position statement of the North American Menopause Society.* Menopause, 28(9), 973–997. https://doi.org/10.1097/GME.0000000000001831

SMOKING CESSATION

Avoiding or quitting smoking to maximize peak bone formation and prevent bone loss is crucial (Camacho et al., 2020; Cosman et al., 2014; National Institutes of Health [NIH], 2017). Smoking has adverse effects on skeletal health, may increase osteoporotic fracture risk, and is detrimental to general health (Camacho et al., 2020; Coronado-Zarco et al., 2019). Patients should be counseled about the negative effects of tobacco use and supported for cessation efforts.

FALL PREVENTION

Fall prevention becomes more important in those with established bone loss who are at increased risk for fracture. A home assessment is done to determine and remedy the presence of environmental hazards including loose rugs, stairs, uneven floors and grounds, pets, or exposed cords. Poor lighting and cluttered walkways can increase fall risk, especially at night. Some patients can conduct this assessment and rectify problems themselves. In other instances, clinicians, community-based providers, or family members need to intervene. Sedating medications, such as narcotics, benzodiazepines, and alcohol, should be avoided as they can increase fall risk. Vision and hearing exams should be part of routine health maintenance. Consultation occupational or physical therapy can assist with in-home evaluations and targeted interventions to improve balance and decrease fall risk (American College of Obstetricians and Gynecologists' Committee on Clinical Practice Guidelines–Gynecology, 2021).

Complementary and Alternative Medicine

MASSAGE, RELAXATION THERAPIES, AND CHIROPRACTIC MANIPULATION

Massage may indirectly benefit bone strength because it can relax and assist in muscle flexibility, potentially increasing exercise tolerance. Chair massage is performed with caution because forward bending in those with established OP potentially increases the risk of VFs. Massage does not usually provide enough force to cause fracture with established OP and may provide relaxation that assists with pain reduction.

Other complementary and alternative medicine (CAM) modalities that enhance and encourage relaxation such as aromatherapy, yoga, and meditation may be helpful for pain management in those with OP fractures. Chiropractic manipulation techniques are modified by skilled chiropractors to avoid injury or fracture of weak bones. Some chiropractors do not perform manipulations on those with OP; instead, they counsel patients about dietary needs and safe exercise techniques.

There is an abundance of research supporting yoga as treatment for OP. Yoga is safe and inexpensive and includes both weight-bearing and non-weight-bearing modalities. Yoga has also been demonstrated to improve balance (Motorwala et al., 2016).

BOTANICALS AND ACUPUNCTURE

Research evaluating the use of isoflavones to improve bone density has provided conflicting results. Although some have shown moderate benefit in preventing bone loss after menopause, they are not recommended for postmenopausal OP management or prevention (Camacho et al., 2020; NAMS, 2021).

Treatment results for OP with acupuncture have been mixed. Acupuncture is more often used in combination with Chinese herbs for OP in the practice of traditional Chinese medicine (TCM; Guillaume, 1992). Acupuncture (warm acupuncture and tuina acupuncture) is recognized by some as effective treatment for OP (Pan et al., 2018). Tuina is another type of acupuncture used in China for OP treatment. TCM notes benefits for blood stasis and kidney function related to OP through acupuncture effects that nourish immune and nerve system function, promote blood circulation, alleviate pain and spasm, and dredge the meridian channel (Dong et al., 2018; Pan et al., 2018).

Herbs that might be used for OP management are intended to boost estrogen levels, such as cypress, black cohosh, sage, licorice, and ginseng. Data on efficacy of herbs for BMD are lacking, and generally herbs do not demonstrate robust benefits (Leung & Siu, 2013).

Pharmacotherapeutics

Several prescription medications are available for OP management (Table 35.4). Prescription medications are recommended to treat OP in postmenopausal persons in guidelines published by the Bone Health and OP Foundation (LeBoff et al., 2022), NAMS (2021), and the American Association of Clinical Endocrinologists (AACE; Comacho et al., 2020). The focus of medication for treating OP is to reduce the risk for fracture and subsequent sequelae. NAMS (2021) also recommends prescription medications to prevent OP in their guidelines. The goal for preventive therapy is to stop postmenopausal

---

TABLE 35.4 Prescription Medications for Osteoporosis Treatment or Prevention[a,b]

MEDICATION	FDA-APPROVED USE AND DOSE	CONSIDERATIONS
Alendronate (Fosamax)	Prevention: 5 mg by mouth daily or 35 mg by mouth weekly Treatment: 10 mg by mouth daily or 70 mg by mouth weekly	• Before any food ingestion, take oral doses in morning with 8 oz plain water, remain upright, and ingest no food or drink for at least 30–60 minutes • Take oral doses 2 hours before antacids/calcium • Caution with oral forms if upper gastrointestinal disease present; clinical association with dysphagia, esophagitis, or ulceration • Beneficial effects may last for years after medication is discontinued • Fosamax Plus D: combined bisphosphonate and vitamin D3 in a single tablet taken weekly • IV ibandronate and zoledronic acid are not associated with gastrointestinal side effects: no limitations on timing dose around food, water, calcium, or medication intake • Osteonecrosis of jaw (ONJ), exposed bone in mouth for >3 months with nonhealing lesions, has been associated with high-dose IV bisphosphonate therapy among individuals with cancer-related bone disease (2%–10%); cancer patients with dental problems, gum injury, oral bony abnormalities, or taking medications that interfere with healing; and, in very rare cases, healthy individuals with similar risk factors who are taking bisphosphonates for osteoporosis (incidence estimated at 0.001%–0.002%). Consider stopping therapy for 2–3 months if invasive dental procedures are required and resume after healing is complete; encourage usual dental care (e.g., cleaning, fillings, crown work).
Alendronate + cholecalciferol (Fosamax Plus D)	Treatment: 70 mg plus 2,800 U of vitamin D3 or 70 mg plus 5,600 units of vitamin D3 in combined tablet by mouth weekly	
Risedronate (Actonel)	Prevention: 5 mg by mouth daily; 35 mg by mouth weekly; or 150 mg by mouth monthly Treatment: immediate-release: 5 mg by mouth daily; 35 mg by mouth weekly; 150 mg by mouth monthly Treatment: delayed-release: 35 mg by mouth weekly	
Ibandronate (Boniva)	Prevention: 150 mg by mouth monthly Treatment: 150 mg by mouth monthly; 3 mg IV every 3 months	
Zoledronic acid (Reclast)	Prevention: 5 mg IV every 2 years (24 months) Treatment: 5 mg IV yearly (12 months)	
Calcitonin (calcitonin salmon nasal; Miacalcin)	Treatment: 200 IU of intranasal spray daily (calcitonin salmon nasal) or 100 IU subcutaneously every other day (Miacalcin)	• Usually administered as nasal spray • Alternate nares for nasal spray • Most often used for analgesic effect on acute pain resulting from vertebral compression fractures
Denosumab (Prolia)	60 mg subcutaneously every 6 months	• Administered by a healthcare professional • Calcium and vitamin D needed • Contraindicated with hypocalcemia • May increase risk for infection • ONJ has been reported

(continued)

TABLE 35.4 Prescription Medications for Osteoporosis Treatment or Prevention[a,b] *(continued)*

MEDICATION	FDA–APPROVED USE AND DOSE	CONSIDERATIONS
Estrogen[b] (Alora, Climara, Estrace, Estraderm, Menest, Menostar, Premarin, Vivelle, Vivelle-Dot)	Prevention: doses and routes vary	• Also effective in alleviating most symptoms related to menopause (even Menostar, which has a very low dose and was shown to effectively reduce severity and frequency of hot flashes in a 2007 study) • Available in several forms (e.g., pills, patch, ring, cream, gel)
Estrogen–progestin combination products[b] (Activella, Climara Pro, FemHRT, Prefest, Premphase, Prempro)	Prevention: doses and routes vary	• Use for 2 to 3 years immediately following menopause; may provide some beneficial effects on bone health after discontinuation
Estrogens conjugated/bazedoxifene (Duavee)	Prevention: 1 tab by mouth daily (0.45 mg estrogen, conjugated/20 mg bazedoxifene	• Also approved for menopause-related vasomotor symptom management (no progestogen needed if intact uterus)
Genistein + citrated zinc bisglycinate + cholecalciferol (Fosteum Rx)	Prevention: 1 capsule twice daily (each capsule contains 27 mg of genistein, 20 mg of citrated zinc bisglycinate, 200 IU of cholecalciferol)	• Medical food • Meets FDA standards for GRAS (generally recognized as safe) • Not recommended if taking hormone therapy, estrogen agonist–antagonists
Raloxifene (Evista)	Prevention: 60 mg by mouth daily Treatment: 60 mg by mouth daily	• May cause hot flashes • Not recommended if taking ET or EPT • Also approved for prevention of breast cancer in women at high risk for invasive breast cancer
Teriparatide (recombinant human PTH 1–34) (Forteo)	Treatment (high fracture risk): 20 mcg subcutaneously daily; two courses of 2 years of therapy in lifetime	• Usually second line unless very high risk for fracture • Most effective when used sequentially following antiresorptive and antiresorptive resumed following PTH
Abaloparatide (Tymlos)	Treatment: 80 mcg subcutaneously daily, 24 months cumulative use	
Romosozumab (Evenity)	Treatment: 210 mg subcutaneously monthly, 12 months	

[a]See prescribing reference for full information on doses, side effects, contraindications, and cautions. Combining therapies is uncommon and generally initiated only by an osteoporosis specialist because of potential side effects, including frozen bone syndrome—a condition in which bone turnover is suppressed to the point that bone quality declines despite increasing bone density, creating increased risk for fracture.
[b]Lowest effective dose is used; the FDA recommends considering nonestrogen osteoporotic agents when ET/EPT use is solely for the purpose of osteoporosis prevention.
EPT, estrogen-progestogen therapy; ET, estrogen therapy; FDA, U.S. Food and Drug Administration; IV intravenous; PTH, parathyroid hormone.
Source: Adapted from Camacho, P. M., Petak, S. M., Binkley, N., Diab, D. L., Eldeiry, L. S., Farooki A, Harris, S. T., Hurley, D. L., Kelly, J., Lewiecki, E. M., Pessah-Pollack, R., McClung, M., Wimalawansa, S. J., & Watts, N. B. (2020). American Association of Clinical Endocrinologists/American College of Endocrinology clinical practice guidelines for the diagnosis and treatment of postmenopausal osteoporosis—2020 update. Endocrine Practice, 26(Suppl. 1), 1–46. https://doi.org/10.4158/GL-2020-0524SUPPL; *ePocrates. (n.d.). Computerized pharmacology and prescribing reference (updated daily).* https://www.epocrates.com/; *LeBoff, M. S., Greenspan, S. L., Insogna, K. L., Lewiecki, E. M., Saag, K. G., Singer, A. J., & Siris, E. S. (2022). The clinician's guide to prevention and treatment of osteoporosis.* Osteoporosis International, 33(10), 2049–2102. https://doi.org/10.1007/s00198-021-05900-y; *North American Menopause Society. (2021). Management of osteoporosis in postmenopausal women: The 2021 position statement of the North American Menopause Society.* Menopause, 28(9), 973–997. https://doi.org/10.1097/GME.0000000000001831

bone loss before skeletal architecture damage progresses to the point of increased risk for fracture. Medications approved for OP prevention and treatment are included in Box 35.5.

The FRAX algorithm was developed to identify 10-year fracture probabilities to assist in determining best practices for initiating medication therapy among patients with T-score BMDs in the LBM range (Camacho et al., 2020; LeBoff et al., 2022; NAMS, 2021). The FRAX algorithm is accessible online (www.shef.ac.uk/FRAX) and initially was developed for use in patients who are naïve to OP pharmacotherapy. It is specific to country and in the United States is also categorized according to ethnicity. Ten-year fracture risk probability for hip fracture and any major osteoporotic fracture (e.g., forearm, hip, humerus, or vertebrae) is calculated using 10 risk factors for fracture (Box 35.3) and the femoral neck BMD. The calculated FRAX fracture probabilities are now printed on BMD DXA results in the United States. Eight of the variables are dichotomous, and thus limit the ability to fully specify calculations to individuals. Additionally, the use of ethnicity as a risk factor has been called into question. Despite these limitations, FRAX does identify level of risk across populations well. Its ability to identify risk for a single person is more limited (Camacho et al., 2020; LeBoff et al., 2022; NAMS, 2021). The U.S. FRAX algorithm adapted to clinical scenarios provides the basis for clinical recommendations for initiating medication therapy among those with LBM (Box 35.5; Camanche et al., 2020; LeBoff et al., 2022; NAMS, 2021). Another online FRAX tool, called QFracture, was released in 2009 and updated in 2016. It may have some improved discrimination over FRAX; however, it was based on data from England and Wales and is only applicable to these patient populations (Hippisley-Cox & Coupland, 2009).

Box 35.5 Recommendations for Initiating Medication Therapy to Treat Bone Loss/Osteoporosis

Medication therapy is recommended for postmenopausal persons if:

1. The T-score BMD at the femoral neck, spine, or hip is −2.5 or below

2. A hip fracture or vertebral fracture is sustained (regardless of BMD T-score)

3. The BMD T-score is −1 to −2.5 (LBM) **AND**

    a. A fracture of the pelvis, hip, or distal forearm is sustained

    OR

    b. The FRAX 10-year risk for major OP-related fracture is ≥20% or hip fracture is ≥3%

4. Multiple fractures are sustained (not at femoral neck, spine, hip)

BMD, bone mineral density; FRAX, fracture risk assessment; LBM, low bone mass; OP, osteoporosis.
Source: Adapted from Camacho, P. M., Petak, S. M., Binkley, N., Diab, D. L., Eldeiry, L. S., Farooki A, Harris, S. T., Hurley, D. L., Kelly, J., Lewiecki, E. M., Pessah-Pollack, R., McClung, M., Wimalawansa, S. J., & Watts, N. B. (2020). American Association of Clinical Endocrinologists/American College of Endocrinology clinical practice guidelines for the diagnosis and treatment of postmenopausal osteoporosis—2020 update. Endocrine Practice, 26(Suppl. 1), 1–46. https://doi.org/10.4158/GL-2020-0524SUPPL; LeBoff, M. S., Greenspan, S. L., Insogna, K. L., Lewiecki, E. M., Saag, K. G., Singer, A. J., & Siris, E. S. (2022). The clinician's guide to prevention and treatment of osteoporosis. Osteoporosis International, 33(10), 2049–2102. https://doi.org/10.1007/s00198-021-05900-y; North American Menopause Society. (2021). Management of osteoporosis in postmenopausal women: The 2021 position statement of the North American Menopause Society. Menopause, 28(9), 973–997. https://doi.org/10.1097/GME.0000000000001831

Several medication therapies are currently approved by the Food and Drug Administration (FDA) for OP management, which includes both prevention and treatment. These medications work by modulating—either inhibiting or activating—bone metabolism. There are two general categories among these medications. Antiresorptive or antiremodeling agents are in the first category and include bisphosphonates, estrogens, estrogen agonists/antagonists (EAAs; formerly known as selective estrogen receptor modulators [SERMs]), tissue selective estrogen complex, RANKL (receptor activator of nuclear factor kappa-B ligand) inhibitor, and calcitonin (rarely used). These medications maintain or increase BMD and reduce fracture risk primarily by inhibiting bone resorption and have some effects on bone formation. Specifically, they inhibit osteoclast function, thus reducing bone resorption and increasing bone density by allowing osteoblast activity to surpass osteoclast activity. However, they do not repair or improve trabecular bone disruptions that occur with OP. In the second category are osteoanabolic agents including PTH and analog of PTH-related peptide. The mechanism of action of anabolic agents is to increase osteoblast activity and

thereby stimulate formation of new bone. They improve bone structure (both trabecular and/or cortical) and increase BMD significantly, which reduces fracture risk more quickly than the antiresorptives. Also available is the fully human monoclonal antibody to sclerostin, which has a novel mechanism to act with both antiresorbtive and osteoanabolic properties. Finally, one other prescription agent, a medical food, is available. Medical foods meet the FDA standard for GRAS, which means "generally regarded as safe." Fosteum Plus meets this standard and includes a combination of genistein (an isoflavone that is purified from soy), vitamin D, and zinc (www.fosteumplus.com/assets/pdfs/prescribing-information/fosteum-pi.pdf). Studies evaluating Fosteum show that it does improve BMD; however, no data on fracture rates are available.

Agent selection for initial treatment is guided by BMD T-score and fracture risk level prior to treatment (Table 35.5). First-line therapies for persons with high risk include those that have demonstrated efficacy for reducing spine, hip, and nonvertebral fractures and include denosumab, zoledronate, alendronate, and risedronate (Camacho et al., 2020; LeBoff et al., 2022; NAMS, 2021).

DXA testing is used to monitor efficacy of OP or LBM treatment. DXA testing is done every 1 to 2 years until stability is achieved, and then every 3 years. Patients should be treated to meet target outcomes of BMD total hip T-scores between −2.0 to −1.5. BMD has been demonstrated as an effective surrogate marker for fracture risk; as BMD rises, fracture risk falls. If goal T-score is not met, consider changing therapy (e.g., from bisphosphonate to RANKL inhibitor) or initiating sequential therapy with an osteoanabolic agent or human monoclonal antibody to sclerostin (Camacho et al., 2020; LeBoff et al., 2022, NAMS, 2021). Referral or consultation is appropriate prior to changing or initiating second-line medications for clinicians who are not managing OP on a regular basis.

In those with normal bone mass at baseline, repeat DXA testing is done in 5 years. Repeat testing is done earlier if the patient's risk factors for OP change (Camacho et al., 2020; LeBoff et al., 2022; NAMS, 2021).

Considerations for Special and Minoritized Populations

Temporary secondary bone loss can affect persons receiving Depo-Provera injections for contraception and during pregnancy and lactation when calcium is leached from the bone. Bone mass usually reverts to prepregnancy and pre-Depo-Provera levels following birth, cessation of breastfeeding, or discontinuation of Depo-Provera. A low-dose estrogen patch can be prescribed to preserve bone mass for those using Depo-Provera while they are taking the medication. Increasing calcium intake before pregnancy and maintaining appropriate calcium intake during pregnancy and lactation are critical (Ross, 2011).

In 2020, Vyas et al., published a paper that proposed eliminating the use of algorithms that make guideline recommendations based on race. Given data that demonstrate disproportionate risks for bone loss and OP among varied ethnic groups, use of algorithms like FRAX continues. However, clinicians must consider other factors that pose risks to patients— – considerations must include existing health

TABLE 35.5 Selection of Initial Medication for Osteoporosis Based on Fracture Risk

FRACTURE RISK LEVEL	SUGGESTED CRITERIA	FIRST-LINE MEDICATIONS
Very high	• Prior fractures: recent, multiple, while on OP medication, while taking medications that cause bone loss • T-score: very low, e.g., <−3.0 • Falls: high risk or prior injuries • Fracture probability: very high, e.g., FRAX major OP >30%, hip >4.5%	Osteoanabolic, human monoclonal antibody to sclerostin
High	• T-score: demonstrates OP, ≤−2.5 • Fracture: possibly parent, one prior fracture at earlier age, or not high probability on FRAX • Falls: not at increased risk	RANKL inhibitor, bisphosphonate
Moderate	• T-score: demonstrates LBM with elevated FRAX, or demonstrates OP • No other risk factors	Bisphosphonate, estrogen agonists/antagonists, estrogen*, tissue-selective estrogen complex*

*For OP prevention, used for those also experiencing menopause-related vasomotor symptoms.
FRAX, fracture risk assessment; LBM, low bone mass; OP, osteoporosis; RANKL, receptor activator of nuclear factor kappa-B ligand.
Source: Adapted from Camacho, P. M., Petak, S. M., Binkley, N., Diab, D. L., Eldeiry, L. S., Farooki A, Harris, S. T., Hurley, D. L., Kelly, J., Lewiecki, E. M., Pessah-Pollack, R., McClung, M., Wimalawansa, S. J., & Watts, N. B. (2020). American Association of Clinical Endocrinologists/American College of Endocrinology clinical practice guidelines for the diagnosis and treatment of postmenopausal osteoporosis—2020 update. Endocrine Practice, 26(Suppl. 1), 1–46. https://doi.org/10.4158/GL-2020-0524SUPPL; LeBoff, M. S., Greenspan, S. L., Insogna, K. L., Lewiecki, E. M., Saag, K. G., Singer, A. J., & Siris, E. S. (2022). The clinician's guide to prevention and treatment of osteoporosis. Osteoporosis International, 33(10), 2049–2102. https://doi.org/10.1007/s00198-021-05900-y; North American Menopause Society. (2021). Management of osteoporosis in postmenopausal women: The 2021 position statement of the North American Menopause Society. Menopause, 28(9), 973–997. https://doi.org/10.1097/GME.0000000000001831

disparities and co-morbidities faced by certain populations, specifically Black, Asian, and Hispanic people. Culturally competent healthcare interventions must be provided that address their health concerns and reduce disparities. The International Osteoporosis Foundation and the American Society for Bone and Mineral Research have recommendations to better address OP management for various populations (Kanis et al., 2020). The clinician's role is to diagnose, treat, manage, and provide education. Importantly, informing minoritized populations of both modifiable and non-modifiable risks of fracture and bone loss (Kanis et al., 2020). isare critical for patients to be able to make informed decisions about their lifestyle activities and treatment.

FUTURE DIRECTIONS

Bone health is a critical issue across the lifespan. Attending to building maximum bone mass during childhood and young adulthood will provide a strong foundation for fracture prevention with aging. Bone loss during midlife is managed for all through diet, supplementation, and exercise. The FRAX algorithm can assist with providing some information on who may benefit from pharmacologic therapy. Multiple pharmacotherapeutic options are available, making it realistic to tailor a medication plan for an individual. Future research is evaluating new delivery methods for existing pharmacotherapeutics as well as additional pharmacotherapeutic agents for bone health.

REFERENCES

References for this chapter are online and available at https://connect.springerpub.com/content/book/978-0-8261-6722-4/part/part03/chapter/ch35

CHAPTER 36

Pregnancy Decision-Making and Supportive Care*

KATHERINE SIMMONDS AND JOYCE D. CAPPIELLO

Throughout history, people have employed various techniques and technologies to prevent or increase their chances of becoming pregnant (Schneider & Schneider, 1995). For many, deciding when to become pregnant is crucial to their sense of personal well-being (Frost & Lindberg, 2013; Klann & Wong, 2020). For some, an unwanted or mistimed pregnancy can threaten their or their family's survival; for others, failure to achieve a pregnancy can lead to shame, ostracization, and in some cases, even death. People's decisions about whether, when, and how to become—or not become—pregnant are unique, and central to their very existence and identities.

In this chapter, we focus on how clinicians can support people who present for healthcare related to a pregnancy diagnosis. Before describing some approaches and best practices for clinical care in this area, we provide an overview of pertinent terms, concepts, and demographic data. In addition, because it is common among health researchers and clinicians to classify pregnancies as "intended" or "unintended," we briefly describe the debate that has emerged about this dichotomous categorization of pregnancy. Though we do use the terminology of intent to describe epidemiologic trends, we acknowledge the concept is deeply flawed and useful only at the population level, if at all. Because most clinical care takes place between clinicians and individuals, this chapter focuses primarily on interventions at this level.

Finally, a few words about language and guiding frameworks for this chapter. First, we recognize that language about gender and sex is in flux, and this is likely to continue to change in the future. In this chapter, we strive to use currently accepted gender-neutral terms (e.g., people with the capacity for pregnancy, they/them/theirs); however, given that much of the available research uses binary categories with respect to sex/gender (female/male, women/men), we repeat these terms when reporting on findings of a given study. Second,

in considering the care of people who are deciding about, presenting for care, and engaging in actions related to a pregnancy, we ascribe to the tenets of reproductive justice and principles of trauma-informed care. For more about these frameworks, see Chapter 21, Fertility Self-Management and Shared Management, and Chapter 22, Preconception Counseling. While full discussion is beyond the scope of this chapter, clinicians are encouraged to learn about and incorporate these frameworks into their clinical practice as they care for people experiencing pregnancy.

DEFINITIONS AND EPIDEMIOLOGY

Demographers and public health researchers define unintended pregnancy as "a pregnancy that is mistimed, unplanned, or unwanted at the time of conception" (Centers for Disease Control and Prevention [CDC], 2021). Within this framework, if a person did not want to become pregnant at the time they did or at any time in the future, the pregnancy is considered "unwanted." If they wanted to become pregnant at some point in the future but *not* at the time they did, it is classified as "mistimed."

Large-scale population surveys like the National Survey of Family Growth (NSFG) and the Pregnancy Risk Assessment Monitoring System (PRAMS) are the most commonly cited sources of data on unintended pregnancy in the United States. According to the NSFG, 38% of all pregnancies were unintended in the years from 2017 to 2019, continuing a general trend of decline observed over the past few decades that has largely been attributed to increases in use and efficacy of contraception (Finer & Zolna, 2016). *Healthy People 2030* has established a goal of further decreasing the proportion of unintended pregnancies in the United States to 36.5% (Office of Disease Prevention and Health Promotion, 2020).

---

*This chapter is a revision of the chapter that appeared in the second edition of this textbook, coauthored with Lisa Stern, and we thank her for her original contribution.

Disparities in Unintended Pregnancy

Unintended pregnancy rates vary by select geographic, personal, and population characteristics. Globally, 48% of pregnancies are estimated to be unintended (Samankasikorn et al., 2019); however, this figure obscures wide variations in rates from country to country as well as intranationally. Overall, unintended pregnancies are more frequent in low- as compared to high-income countries, a reflection of global inequities in access to sexual and reproductive health services. Similarly, geographic disparities in unintended pregnancy rates are present within the United States, with states in the South tending to have the highest rates. In 2019, Mississippi (47.1%) and Florida (42.1%) had the highest proportions overall, while Vermont (20%) and New Hampshire (20.8%) were lowest (America's Health Rankings, 2019). Economic factors and insurance coverage are partial explanations for these observed variations across states.

At the population level, unintended pregnancy has been associated with certain demographic and socioeconomic factors. According to the NSFG, women with low incomes and living in poverty, and those who are not married—especially those who live with their partner—experience disproportionate rates of unintended pregnancy. Racial and ethnic disparities are also evident: Black and Hispanic women are more likely than White women to have unintended pregnancies. Education and age are also factors, as women without a high school degree, and those between ages 18 and 24 are more likely to experience unintended pregnancies than those who attend or graduate from college or are age 25 or older (Finer & Zolna, 2016). Intimate partner violence and reproductive coercion have also been implicated as contributors to disproportionately higher rates of unintended pregnancy (Samankasikorn et al., 2019).

Social determinants of health, including income inequality and racism, underlie disparities in unintended pregnancy. Encouraging people to individually plan for pregnancy is an inadequate response for overcoming the effects of structural forces on health outcomes, including those related to reproduction. Social and reproductive justice offers a framework for clinical care providers to contextualize unintended pregnancy and promote the health of individuals, families, communities, and populations. Nursing scholars have called for a public health approach to unintended pregnancy that broadens the focus beyond individual patient encounters and toward access to high-quality, evidence-based sexuality education and broad preventive health services that empower people and their families to attain healthy pregnancy outcomes (Taylor et al., 2010). For people who do become pregnant, high-quality, accessible obstetric and abortion services are essential.

Clinicians and public health experts play an important role in advocating for public policies that increase access to healthcare and health education, decrease racism and other forms of oppression, and enhance the economic power of women, transgender, and gender nonbinary people. Although this chapter—intended for a clinical audience—focuses primarily on clinical interventions at the individual level, to truly advance reproductive justice, structural barriers to reproductive healthcare must be dismantled and health equity must be broadly promoted (Klann & Wong, 2020).

Outcomes and Clinical Implications of Unintended Pregnancy

Excluding miscarriages, 42% of unintended pregnancies in the United States ended in abortion, and 58% in live births, reflecting a continuing downward trend in the abortion rate since its peak in the 1980s (Finer & Zolna, 2016). Over the past 30 years, abortions have declined in United States, although an 8% upswing has been noted from 2017 to 2020 (Guttmacher Institute, 2022a). Globally from 2015 to 2019, an estimated 61% of unintended pregnancies ended in abortion, a rise of approximately 10% from previous years (Bearak et al., 2020). In pregnancies that end in live births, children may go on to be raised by biological or adoptive parents, or within kinship networks.

Studies of the relationship between pregnancy intent and maternal and child health outcomes have yielded mixed results in the past; however, the results of the first prospective, longitudinal study of women who did and did not receive an abortion as requested produced informative data. The Turnaway Study found that women receiving an abortion did not experience harm to their health and well-being (Biggs et al., 2017), but being denied an abortion resulted in worse financial, health, and family outcomes (Foster, Ralph et al., 2018). Being denied an abortion had serious implications for the child, with higher rates of poor maternal bonding and living in poverty (Foster, Biggs et al., 2018), while existing children experienced negative developmental and socioeconomic consequences (Foster, Raifman et al., 2018).

Although it is difficult to obtain precise numbers, approximately 18,000 to 20,000 domestic-born infants were adopted in the United States (0.5% of annual births; Sisson, 2022). Clinicians need to be prepared to provide unbiased information, decision support, and referrals about each of these options to patients who present with an initial positive pregnancy test. General information and resources as well as principles and specific techniques for fulfilling this clinical role are discussed later in this chapter.

ISSUES IN THE MEASUREMENT OF UNINTENDED PREGNANCY

Intention is a complex and highly subjective concept. In order to enhance the validity and stability of the measure of pregnancy intent, typically researchers have not asked directly whether a pregnancy was intended or unintended, but rather posed a series of related questions (Klerman, 2000). In the NSFG, women were asked about each pregnancy they have had as to whether they wanted to have a baby at the time they conceived; further questions were then based on this initial response (Hayford & Guzzo, 2016). This retrospective approach to measurement of pregnancy intention is problematic; survey participants are asked about their desire to have become pregnant *before* it occurred, but many are responding months or even years after its occurrence. This leads to potential recall bias, which threatens the validity of the findings (Joyce et al., 2002). Additionally, substantial evidence has demonstrated that people's views on intent may change over time, even during the course of a pregnancy (Aiken et al., 2015; O'Donnell et al., 2018; Rocca et al., 2019).

Recently, greater interest in men's role in pregnancy decision-making has emerged. Although the initial survey upon which the NSFG is based (known as the Indianapolis Survey) attempted to capture pregnancy intent by querying married, heterosexual couples, most subsequent studies have only engaged female participants. However, in recent years more researchers have sought to understand men's attitudes toward pregnancy and the relationship to outcomes (Guzzo & Hayford, 2020; Lee et al., 2018; Li et al., 2022).

Though public health has long assumed the position that unintended pregnancy is a problem, recent research suggests some people may not view pregnancy planning as meaningful, feasible, or a priority. Rather, many women express feelings of ambivalence about pregnancy or regard it as something that "just happens" (Arteaga et al., 2019; Hernandez et al., 2020; O'Donnell et al., 2018). Some suggest this supports a need for more widespread preconception planning, while others argue it reveals misplaced assumptions underlying the framework of pregnancy "intention" or "planning." Regardless of an individual's personal stance on pregnancy intention or planning, upholding and promoting reproductive decision-making that includes high-quality comprehensive reproductive health services as part of a full spectrum of patient-centered healthcare is an established responsibility of clinical care providers (Klann & Wong (2020).

ASSESSMENT

All clinicians who provide care to people of reproductive age must be prepared to assess whether a patient desires a given pregnancy. In her seminal guide to pregnancy options counseling, Baker (1995) describes three distinct but related types of patient encounters clinicians may be involved in: (1) pregnancy testing; (2) pregnancy options counseling; and (3) abortion counseling. In the first, a person may suspect pregnancy but seek confirmation or, less commonly, are unaware they may be pregnant until the clinician suggests the possibility. In either case, the clinician proceeds with a pregnancy test, physical examination (if indicated), and delivery of test results (discussed later). If assessment confirms the person is pregnant, the clinician engages in the second type of encounter, pregnancy options counseling. In other cases, a person may present for care already certain they are pregnant but seeking education and counseling about their options. Suggested steps for clinicians for such visits are discussed in the section in this chapter on pregnancy options counseling. Finally, some people present for care with a confirmed pregnancy and have already decided how they want to proceed. In those cases, the clinical visit may just be to initiate desired service (abortion or prenatal care) or to obtain a referral. Abortion counseling is provided when a person has decided to end their pregnancy but is seeking support and information about this option specifically. This type of counseling is discussed further in the section on abortion. Approaches to self-sourcing and self-managing abortion outside the formal health system are also discussed.

History

As with all patient encounters, obtaining a relevant history is the first step when assessing a person who might be or knows they are pregnant. Beginning the visit with open-ended questions to determine why they have come in often

reveals important information about the possibility of pregnancy as well as their feelings about it. If a reproductive age person reports symptoms commonly associated with early pregnancy, such as nausea, breast tenderness, fatigue, irregular vaginal bleeding, and/or amenorrhea, the clinician should rule out the possibility of pregnancy by asking for additional information about sexual activity and contraceptive use. In some clinical encounters, a patient's presenting complaint may have nothing to do with pregnancy, but the possibility emerges during a review of systems or routine evaluation for another issue (e.g., before ordering x-rays or as part of a preoperative examination).

If a person indicates they suspect or are already sure they are pregnant, eliciting additional information can yield important data to inform clinical assessment and management. For example, recent unprotected vaginal-penile intercourse may have prompted the visit, but it may be too early for a pregnancy test (if less than 7–10 days from fertilization). If a person is not currently seeking pregnancy and had unprotected sex less than 120 hours (5 days) ago, the clinician should recommend emergency contraception (see Chapter 21, Fertility Self-Management and Shared Management). If the sexual encounter was between 4 and 5 days prior to the visit, ulipristal acetate (Ella), or—if the patient is interested in and eligible for long-acting reversible contraception—a Copper-T intrauterine device (IUD; Paragard) can be offered, as these methods are more effective than levonorgestrel-containing methods.

Before proceeding with a pregnancy test, the clinician should confirm the first day of the patient's last menstrual period (LMP) and if it was normal (usual amount of flow, duration, etc.) in order to accurately determine the estimated gestational age (EGA) of the pregnancy. If the LMP is unknown or unsure, a pelvic examination and/or ultrasound can be performed to establish the gestational age. Patient reports of any spotting, bleeding, pain, or other early pregnancy warning signs also warrant further evaluation (see Chapter 23, Prenatal Care and Anticipating Birth, for further discussion). Screening for intimate partner violence and reproductive coercion should be a standard component of assessing patients for pregnancy.

If a patient reports a positive home pregnancy test, the clinician should determine if they have already decided whether to continue or end the pregnancy, or if they would like additional information or counseling. Nobel et al. (2022) found that patients with a positive pregnancy test were more likely to report a positive experience if their provider discussed all their options. If a patient indicates they have made their decision, the clinician can assist them with obtaining desired services; if they are unsure about their decision or need additional information, education and counseling about their options is the next step.

Physical Examination and Diagnosis

If a patient's history suggests pregnancy is possible, a qualitative, immunometric urine test for human chorionic gonadotropin (hCG) should be performed. The clinician may also decide to perform a physical examination including a pelvic examination, ultrasound, and/or a quantitative beta-hCG test based on the patient's history and clinical presentation. The presence of probable signs of pregnancy on physical exam, including Chadwick (bluish hue of the vagina and cervix), Goodell (softening of the cervix), and Hegar (softening of the uterine isthmus) signs, as well as enlargement of the uterus, can contribute to a diagnosis of pregnancy; however, these signs may not be present in early pregnancy or may be too subtle for the clinician to detect. Physical examination findings should correlate with pregnancy test results and EGA; any discrepancy warrants further investigation, including review of the menstrual and gynecologic history to confirm accuracy of the LMP. If a discrepancy persists, a quantitative hCG and/or transvaginal ultrasound are typically the next steps in management (see Chapter 22, Preconception Counseling).

MANAGEMENT

Providing Pregnancy Test Results

Once pregnancy has been ruled out or confirmed, the patient should be informed. Use of neutral language, such as "the pregnancy test is positive, which means you are pregnant" is recommended. If the pregnancy test is negative, possible reasons for the result should be explained to the patient, including that it may be too early for the test to be positive or that they are not actually pregnant. If review of the menstrual and sexual history reveal it may be too early for a positive result, the patient can be instructed to repeat the test in 1 to 2 weeks. When performed correctly, 98% of people will have a positive test result within 7 days of implantation (Baldwin & Edelman, 2018). With immunometric tests, the type used in most clinical settings, false negative results are possible, but extremely rare. These rare false negatives are associated with elevated lipids, high immunoglobulin levels, and low serum protein associated with severe kidney disease. If a clinician doubts the accuracy of a negative result, they can order a quantitative beta subunit radioimmunoassay (Baldwin & Edelman, 2018).

Following a negative pregnancy test, if a person does not want to become pregnant and anticipates future sexual activity that could lead to pregnancy (i.e., with a person with a penis), the clinician should initiate a discussion about contraceptive options, including a review of previous methods used, what has or has not worked for the person in the past, and about their desire for future pregnancies. Using a shared decision-making approach, together the patient and clinician can establish a contraceptive plan that includes follow-up.

If the pregnancy test is positive, or pregnancy is otherwise confirmed, the clinician needs to determine the EGA and relay it to the patient, as it may be a factor in their decision about how to proceed, and in what options are available to them. This is discussed further in the next section, which focuses on providing pregnancy options counseling.

Pregnancy Options Counseling

After confirming pregnancy or delivering a positive pregnancy test result, the clinician must determine whether a patient wants or needs additional information and support about the

options available to them. As previously mentioned, Noble et al. (2022) studied 14 family planning clinics in the southern United States and found patients' satisfaction with care was higher when all options were discussed by the provider. This study offers evidence that people prefer to receive complete, unbiased information from providers so they can make fully informed decisions about their reproductive options.

Though every patient encounter should be tailored to the individual, Simmonds et al. (2022) suggest four general steps for delivering options counseling: (1) explore how the patient feels about the pregnancy, including assessing their knowledge and providing education about each option; (2) help identify support systems and assess for risks; (3) assist with decision-making as needed; and (4) provide or refer for desired service. Each of these steps are discussed next.

EXPLORE FEELINGS

Pregnancy can precipitate an abrupt change in a person's life, relationship(s), living arrangements, financial stability, or self-concept. Baker (1995) suggests that for some, it may represent a crisis and lead to uncomfortable emotions or physical symptoms that interfere with a person's ability to function. Awareness of these possibilities can help a clinician deliver nonjudgmental, patient-centered care.

Asking open-ended questions such as "How do you feel about the pregnancy (or pregnancy test result)?" at the start of a visit can help the pregnant person feel comfortable sharing their concerns and experience. Finding out if they have considered or have already made up their mind about how to proceed allows the clinician to assess their decision-making process, as well as understanding available options. Some patients will report they have already decided, while others may not have decided yet; some may not feel comfortable sharing their thoughts with the clinician. Nondirective statements that indicate support for a person's decision—no matter what it is—can help create an environment in which they feel comfortable expressing their emotions and asking questions. For example, the clinician can say, "I want to be sure you know what all your options are, and I'll help you get good care no matter what you decide about the pregnancy." It is important to ascertain whether a person understands their options, particularly those from certain vulnerable populations (such as adolescents or people who have recently immigrated to the United States). Because of stigma associated with abortion and adoption, clinicians need to assess patients' knowledge about these options in particular. The 2022 Supreme Court decision (*Dobbs v. Jackson Women's Health Organization*, 2022) has blocked access to abortion for many people in the state where they reside, and some may not be aware that abortion is still legally available in other states. See the section on abortion in this chapter for further discussion of these barriers.

Some individuals may need time to accept a new or confirmed diagnosis of pregnancy. Clinicians should allow the time to reflect before discussing options or making specific plans; some individuals may prefer to do this outside the clinical setting, in which case a follow-up plan should be established. Follow-up can consist of a telephone call or return visit when further counseling and education can be delivered, or simply a confirmation that the person decided and knows how to arrange the next step of their care. Social and economic barriers that could interfere with follow-up, such as adolescents who do not plan to tell their parent or guardian that they are pregnant or a person with unstable housing, should be taken into consideration when establishing the follow-up plan.

If a patient is ready and wants to discuss options, the clinician can proceed with counseling and education. In order to provide high-quality care, it is essential for clinicians to be current in their knowledge about available resources pertinent to all of the options (childrearing, adoption, abortion), as well as the legal landscape. Assessing a patient's baseline knowledge and perceptions about each option can be accomplished by asking a question such as "Tell me, what you have heard about adoption/abortion?" or "Do you have any questions about what it would be like to be a parent/place a child for adoption/have an abortion?" Strategies and tools for assisting people with decision-making are discussed in the following paragraphs.

IDENTIFY SUPPORT SYSTEMS AND ASSESS FOR RISK

In addition to discussing feelings about the pregnancy and, if the patient desires, providing education about their options, the clinician should inquire about their support systems and assess risk for violence or other personal harm that could be further exacerbated by the pregnancy. Asking if they have told others they are or might be pregnant can provide insight into the patient's relationships and help identify those who may need more support, including additional follow-up or referral for social/mental health services. All people should be screened for risk of violence, abuse, or coercion at some point during a pregnancy options counseling visit. Reproductive coercion, at the intersection of violence and reproductive health, is a specific form of gender-based, intimate partner violence (Basile et al., 2021). Reproductive coercion encompasses contraceptive coercion, pregnancy coercion, and abortion coercion. For some, reproductive coercion may result in pregnancy, and/or be an important factor in their decision-making, as partners, parents, or other influential people in their social network may exert excessive pressure or control regarding the decision. These situations can be ethically and legally complex in clinical practice. Resources to assist with identifying and managing such cases are available for clinicians (American College of Obstetricians and Gynecologists [ACOG], 2013). If coercion seems to be a factor in a person's pregnancy decision-making, additional counseling and follow-up are warranted. (See Chapter 42, Gender-Based Violence and Women's Health, for further discussion.

ASSIST WITH DECISION-MAKING

Many people who know or strongly suspect they are pregnant may have already decided how they would like to proceed before presenting for clinical care; others may seek information or decision support from a clinician before making their final decision. For a person who has not decided how to proceed, it is important to contextualize their decision in relation to the gestational age of the pregnancy, and include education that early entry into prenatal care and early abortion are advised because they are both associated with better health outcomes. Furthermore, clinicians need to inform patients that abortion can be logistically difficult or impossible to obtain at advanced gestational ages, and that a delay in decision-making may preclude this option altogether.

For people who are unsure whether to continue a pregnancy or have an abortion, tools to assist with decision-

TABLE 36.1 Resources for People and Providers on Abortion in the Post–Roe Era

ADOPTION		
Open Adoption & Family Services	www.openadopt.org	Prochoice, child-centered open adoptions including ongoing and lifelong services.
All-Options	www.all-options.org	Peer-based talk line to discuss pregnancy options or past/current experiences with abortion, adoption, parenting, infertility, or pregnancy loss.
Pregnancy Options Workbook	www.pregnancyoptions.info /pregnant.htm	A guide for those facing a pregnancy decision.
LEGAL/POLICY ISSUES		
If/When/How	www.reprolegalhelpline.org	Helpline to answer questions about legal rights with self-managed abortion.
Guttmacher Institute	www.guttmacher.org/state-policy /explore/overview-abortion-laws	Abortion laws by state.
Center for Reproductive Rights	https://reproductiverights.org/maps /abortion-laws-by-state	Abortion laws by state.
Kaiser Family Foundation	www.kff.org/womens-health-policy/ issue-brief/interactive-how-state-policies-shape-access-to-abortion -coverage	State policies on abortion coverage in Medicaid, private insurance, and Affordable Care Act (ACA) Exchange Plans.

(continued)

TABLE 36.1 Resources for People and Providers on Abortion in the Post-Roe Era *(continued)*

LEGAL/POLICY ISSUES

Reproductive Rights.gov	https://reproductiverights.gov	U.S. Department of Health and Human Services website with accurate, up-to-date information about access to and coverage of reproductive healthcare and resources.

INFORMATION ON SELF-MANAGED ABORTION PILLS

Plan C	www.plancpills.org	Provides information on how to access abortion pills online for self-managed abortions depending on your state.
Miscarriage + Abortion Hotline	www.mahotline.org	Proabortion clinicians with years of experience in caring for miscarriage and abortion provide advice on self-managing a miscarriage or abortion, do not provide medications.
Ineedana	www.ineedana.com/about	Provides information on closest clinics, parental consent laws, abortion funds plus other financial resources and telehealth or abortion pills by mail if allowed in your state.
Aid Access	https://aidaccess.org/en	An online source of abortion pills from outside the United States, provided by trained clinicians.
Reprocare Healthline	https://abortionhotline.org	Anonymous healthline provides peer-based emotional support, medical information, information on abortion funds, and referrals to people having self-managed abortions at home with pills.

FINANCIAL RESOURCES FOR ABORTIONS

National Network of Abortion Funds	https://abortionfunds.org	Network of >80 organizations with goal to remove financial and logistical barriers to abortion access; for example, assistance with paying for abortion, support such as transportation, child care, translation, doula services, and housing if traveling to get an abortion.

POSTABORTION SUPPORT

Connect & Breathe	www.connectandbreathe.org/about.html	Peer-based, postabortion nonjudgmental talk line.
Exhale	https://exhaleprovoice.org	Peer-based talk line for nonjudgmental support after abortion.
Abortion Resolution Workbook	www.pregnancyoptions.info	*Free download of Abortion Resolution Workbook: A Guide for Those Seeking Emotional and Spiritual Resolution.*

RESOURCES FOR CLINICIANS

Abortion Provider Toolkit	https://aptoolkit.org	The Toolkit helps clinicians compile evidence to support the integration of early abortion care into their practice: (1) documenting education, knowledge, and training, (2) utilizing clinical and professional standards/competencies to provide safe care, and (3) understanding roles of state and national professional organizations and state licensing boards.
Values Clarification Workshop Curriculum (RHAP)	www.reproductiveaccess.org/resource/values-clarification-workshop	Two-hour curriculum for healthcare staff who want to explore their attitudes and beliefs regarding issues surrounding abortion.
The Safety and Quality of Abortion Care in the United States (2018)	https://nap.nationalacademies.org/read/24950/chapter/1	The National Academies of Sciences, Engineering, and Medicine confirmed the safety and quality of abortion care in the United States, concluding "advanced practice clinicians (physician assistants, certified nurse-midwives, and nurse practitioners) can safely and effectively provide medication and aspiration abortions."
Society of Family Planning Interim Clinical Recommendations: Self-managed abortion	www.smfm.org/publications/442-sfp-interim-clinical-recommendations-self-managed-abortion	Expert clinical guidelines
National Abortion Federation Clinical Policy Guidelines for Abortion Care, 2022	https://prochoice.org/providers/quality-standards	Expert guidelines for clinician-provided procedural and medication abortion.

making may be helpful. See Table 36.1 for a list of resources developed for use during a clinical visit or given to a patient to use after the visit. Another suggested strategy to support decision-making is to have the pregnant person make a list of pros and cons of each option. The Ottawa Personal Decision Guide is an evidence-supported, theory-based tool that has been designed to help patients with making health or social decisions (O'Connor et al., 2015). Though there are no published studies on its use among people facing a pregnancy decision, it may be a helpful aid in pregnancy options counseling. The Reproductive Health Access Project (2022c) has also developed a model for options counseling with people who are ambivalent about pregnancy.

PROVIDE DESIRED SERVICE OR REFER TO APPROPRIATE PROVIDER

The final step of a pregnancy options counseling visit is establishing a plan with the pregnant person for obtaining desired care. If a patient is not ready to make their decision, a plan for follow-up should be discussed that considers their current EGA. Timely initiation of prenatal or abortion care should be encouraged, as this is considered standard of care. If a person is considering adoption, referral to a social worker or agency that can provide accurate information and supportive counseling about this option is recommended. See Table 36.1 for adoption resources.

Depending on state-level APRN scope-of-practice regulations, type of certification, and clinical protocols, some clinicians may be able provide the services a patient desires (prenatal care and/or abortion), while others may need to refer to another provider or facility. Given the dynamic nature of abortion policy at the time of this writing, readers are directed to the section on abortion in this chapter for further discussion of providing or referring for this option. With appropriate education and certification, many primary care clinicians are able to provide routine prenatal care. Personal preference and availability of services in a particular area, as well as insurance plans or public assistance programs, may influence the type(s) of clinician (e.g., midwife, obstetrician, other) a patient selects for their prenatal and delivery care provider.

Clinicians who do not or cannot provide a patient with the pregnancy-related service(s) they seek must refer to another provider or site. Developing relationships with individual providers and/or referral sites can give clinicians better understanding of the setting and quality of care delivered, which may be helpful when referring patients, especially for allaying anxiety that may arise when there is a break in continuity of care.

Once a decision and plan of care have been made, the pregnancy options counseling encounter is over. Unless a clinician will also provide the subsequent prenatal or abortion care, a person may not return until they resume routine primary care. As with other referrals, if the patient will be obtaining services in a different facility, it is the referring providers' responsibility to assist with securing an appointment, verify they were successful in accessing services in a timely manner, and follow up to determine satisfaction with care.

SPECIAL CONSIDERATIONS WHEN PROVIDING OPTIONS COUNSELING

Clinicians may experience conflicts between their personal feelings and professional responsibilities when providing care to a person who has recently discovered they are pregnant or are deciding whether to continue or end a pregnancy. Regardless of personal beliefs, health professionals are bound to uphold patient rights to autonomy and deliver care that is respectful and nonjudgmental by professional codes of ethics. The American Nurses Association (ANA) Code of Ethics for Nursing With Interpretive Statements (ANA, 2015) is one such guiding document. Although health professionals have certain rights to refuse to provide care that violates their personal beliefs, if a patient faces a life-threatening situation, or is otherwise at risk of not receiving needed care, conscientious objection cannot be invoked. Conversely, Harris (2012) suggests that some clinicians may choose to invert this concept of conscience, and instead use it to assert their *willingness* to provide certain types of care, such as abortion.

Ideally, before providing options counseling, clinicians should engage in a process of values clarification to reflect on how their personal beliefs about parenting, adoption, abortion, and related reproductive health issues may influence their interactions with patients. Tools and workshops to assist healthcare providers in exploring these personal and professional intersections have been developed. If a clinician's personal values threaten or interfere with delivery of unbiased, nondirective counseling or referrals, the patient's care should be transferred to another provider. Every effort should be made to minimize delays and limit burdens to patients in obtaining care from another provider. The political landscape surrounding abortion in the United States demands clinicians to engage in a new level of reflection in considering their role in upholding patients' reproductive autonomy.

ABORTION

Induced abortion—or the practice of ending a pregnancy before viability—has been practiced throughout history and across cultures. Extensive historical and anthropological evidence indicates induced abortion has been practiced for thousands of years with a variety of means. Sociologist Carole Joffe asserts that in times and places when abortion has been forbidden, people have continued to seek it, and a culture of illegal provision has proliferated (Joffe, 2009).

Until about 1880, abortion was legal in the United States. After that time, most states banned it, except to save the life of the mother. In 1973, following the U.S. Supreme Court ruling on the case of *Roe v. Wade*, the decision to end a pregnancy "before viability" became a constitutionally protected right. Before that ruling, many people still had abortions (estimates range from 200,000 to 1.2 million per year), including through legal channels in some cases, but more often by self-induction, underground, or "back alley" providers, as well as traveling outside the continental United States for services (Steinkopf-Frank, 2019). As a result, many people died from sepsis, hemorrhage, or other complications from abortions that were poorly performed. In 1930, 18% of maternal deaths in the United States were attributed to induced abortion. By 1965, the absolute number of abortion-related deaths had dropped considerably (to less than 200 per year), largely as a result of the discovery of antibiotics in the 1940s. Rates for abortion deaths are now <0.01% (National Center for Health Statistics, 2016).

Globally, unsafe abortion continues to be a major cause of maternal morbidity and death, especially in countries where abortion is illegal or highly restricted. Between 2010 and 2014 (the most recent data available), an estimated 25.1 million unsafe abortions took place worldwide (Ganatra et al., 2017).

As of June 24, 2022, abortion in the United States is no longer a constitutionally guaranteed, legal right, but rather has been returned to each state to determine (*Dobbs v. Jackson Women's Health Organization,* 2022). At this time, total abortion bans and heavy restrictions have been enacted in approximately half of the states; in others, the right to abortion has been codified into state law. An exhaustive discussion of abortion-related legislation is beyond the scope of this chapter; however, it is essential for clinicians to stay apprised of both state and national abortion laws and regulations in order to provide accurate information to patients about their legal rights and support them in obtaining desired and needed services. A number of reliable sources for up-to-date information on state and national abortion legislation and policy are available, including the Guttmacher Institute (2022), the Center for Reproductive Rights (reproductiverights .org/maps/abortion-laws-by-state), and the Kaiser Family Foundation (www.kff.org/womens-health-policy/issue-brief /interactive-how-state-policies-shape-access-to-abortion-coverage).

In addition to state level legal restrictions, a number of other factors may determine whether or not a person can obtain an abortion. These include provider availability, geographic location, transportation, insurance coverage, economic resources, and other social determinants of health. Because geographic disparities in access are now very stark, most southeastern and midwestern states have banned or heavily restricted abortion (refer to Table 36.1 for current information about the legal status of abortion in different states). Traveling to an abortion provider is excessively burdensome for many people given the time and expense it entails; for some, these obstacles may be insurmountable. Medication abortion, either with supervision from a healthcare provider or procured and "self-managed" outside the formal health system, can increase access for some people.

In addition, other economic factors impact access to abortion. In 2020, the median cost for a first trimester procedural abortion was $575, $560 for an early medication abortion. The cost of an abortion after the first trimester is higher (median $895) and increases with gestational age (Upadhyay et al., 2022). Prior to the June 2022 Supreme Court ruling, most people having an abortion in the United States paid out of pocket (Jerman et al., 2016). Among those with private insurance, 61% reported they still paid out of pocket (Jerman et al., 2016). A 2020 study found this level of unplanned healthcare expenditure would be financially catastrophic for households earning the state's median income in 39 states (Zuniga et al., 2020).

The Hyde Amendment prohibits the use of federal funds for abortion except in cases of life endangerment, rape, or incest. As of this writing, 16 states allow use of state Medicaid funds to cover abortion, while 33 and the District of Columbia do not (Guttmacher Institute, 2022a). South Dakota goes further, prohibiting use of federal funds except in cases of life endangerment. State policies regarding insurance coverage for abortion also vary across private, health insurance marketplace, and public employee plans. Some aim to ensure coverage, while others seek to block the use of insurance to cover abortions. In the wake of the *Dobbs* June 2022 Supreme Court ruling, questions about insurance coverage for people who must now travel out of state for an abortion are an emerging area of policy activity and legal debate. Given this shifting landscape, for the most current information readers are referred to the resources previously mentioned. In sum, before the recent Supreme Court overturning of *Roe v. Wade,* many people needed financial support to obtain an abortion; this situation is anticipated to be even more acute as many people will now need to travel significant distances to access abortion services; this will also lead to delays in care, with associated increases in cost. Abortion funds have been established to help individuals pay for services and related expenses, including transportation and lodging. See Table 36.1 for information about abortion funds.

Other factors, including lack of reliable information, intimidation by protesters, stigma, and violence directed toward abortion providers, also create barriers to abortion. Education and support from clinicians can help those navigating these challenges. In states where abortion remains legal and nurse practitioners, midwives, and/or physician assistants are permitted to provide medication and/or aspiration abortion, these clinicians may be able to help alleviate provider shortages by incorporating this service into their clinical practice, discussed further later in this chapter.

Incidence

Overall, the abortion rate in the United States steadily declined since 1980, when it was at its peak of 29.3 per 1,000 women age 15 to 44 years (Jones & Kooistra, 2011). However, a recent analysis indicates a change in this 40-year trend, with an observed 8% increase in the number of abortions that occurred between 2017 and 2020. According to this study, 930,160 abortions took place in the United States in 2020, a rate of 14.4 per 1,000 women age 15 to 44 years, up from 2017 when it was 13.5 per 1,000, the lowest rate observed since abortion became legal across the nation (Jones, Philbin et al., 2022). During the same period, fewer pregnancies occurred and the total number of births in the United States decreased by 6%, indicating that a larger proportion of pregnant people chose to have an abortion. It is unknown whether these trends will persist. Of note, abortions that occurred outside the U.S. healthcare system, either through self-management or other nondomestic services, were acknowledged as one factor that may have contributed to this observed decline in the rate. Although accurate data are elusive, estimates are that approximately 7% of all of U.S. women reported having attempted self-managed abortion in their lifetime (Ralph et al., 2020). See discussion of abortion self-management later in this chapter.

By age 45, approximately one in four women in the United States will have an abortion, making it one of the most common healthcare procedures in the country (Jones & Jerman, 2016). According to the most current CDC surveillance data, 92.7% of abortions in the United States occurred before 13 weeks' gestation, and most (79.3%) below 9 weeks' gestation; less than 1% took place after 21 weeks' gestation. Over half of all abortions were among people in their 20s, and most (85.5%) were never married (Kortsmit et al., 2021).

People of all economic levels, ages, races, ethnicities, gender identities, and religions have abortions; however, notable disparities in rates have been observed, mirroring trends in unintended pregnancy (discussed previously), though with some variations. Overall, abortion is disproportionately concentrated among people who are poor; 75% of those who had abortions in 2014 had incomes less than 200% of the federal poverty level. People identified as Black were also more likely to end a pregnancy with an abortion than those identified as White or Hispanic (Jerman et al., 2016). Dehlendorf et al. (2013) assert that variations in abortion rates should be interpreted within the larger sociocultural context in which people live, work, engage in sexual activity, use contraception, and make decisions about whether and when to have children.

Studies about why people decide to have an abortion have identified multiple interrelated personal, social, economic, and health-related factors. A synthesis of studies from around the world found socioeconomic concerns to be the most commonly cited reason, and that many people report multiple reasons for their decision (Chae et al., 2017). In addition to financial constraints, other common reasons for having an abortion included pregnancy timing or not wanting another child, partner issues, and interference with life opportunities (Chae et al., 2017). Notably, most people who have abortions (59%) in the United States have given birth at least once (Jerman et al., 2016).

Assessment and Management

The *Dobbs* Supreme Court decision in 2022 to return regulation of abortion to the states has profound implications for assessment and management of a person seeking an abortion. Current laws in the state where a person resides and where they present for care critically impact the management plan. When providing care to a patient seeking an abortion, a clinician's role includes providing information about which methods are possible based on the gestational age of the pregnancy, legality, availability of services in the state, their medical and social history, preferences, and financial resources. As part of the abortion care team, a clinician may provide decision-making support and the abortion itself, depending on the method selected and the laws and regulations in the state. In states where abortion remains legal, a clinician who cannot or decides not to provide abortions is expected to refer patients to an alternative provider or site. Care coordination and follow-up, which includes helping patients make appointments, secure financial resources, arrange child care and/or transportation, and successfully navigate other logistic challenges to obtain the service, is also a responsibility of

the clinical team. In states where abortion is banned altogether or is severely restricted, clinicians need to be aware of legal constraints on their practice related to advising and referring for services within or outside the state (see Table 36.1).

Postabortion care is discussed later in this chapter. The aim of the following section is to provide a general overview of abortion methods to help clinicians in providing accurate, unbiased patient education and counseling. For clinicians who decide to provide abortion care beyond counseling and education, additional training is necessary. State laws and practice regulations vary as to whether nurse practitioners, nurse midwives, and physician assistants are permitted to provide procedural and/or medication abortion without physician oversight, discussed further in the following sections.

Abortion Methods

Because most abortions in the United States take place before 13 weeks' gestation (Kortsmit et al., 2021), this section focuses primarily on the methods most commonly used in early pregnancy; those used later in pregnancy are only discussed briefly. There are two general approaches to early abortion. In this chapter, we use the term *procedural abortion*, also referred to as *aspiration abortion*, when referring to the method that involves removal of a pregnancy by applying suction to the uterine cavity. The term *surgical abortion* has been abandoned as it is not considered patient-friendly and because it situates the skill within the domain of physicians. The term *aspiration* can be confusing for patients; therefore, we prefer the term *procedure* as it better conveys the actual nature of what an abortion entails. Sharp curettage is no longer recommended as an adjunct to procedural abortion as evidence has mounted against its safety and acceptability to patients (World Health Organization [WHO], 2018, 2022).

The second approach, *medication abortion* (also referred to as *medical abortion*, *abortion with pills*, or sometimes *chemical abortion*), is now widespread in the United States. Medication abortion now accounts for 54% of all abortions up to 10 weeks of pregnancy in the United States (Jones, Nash et al., 2022). Early abortions are most often performed or initiated in an ambulatory setting, which is both safe and cost effective. In sites where medication and aspiration abortion are offered, efforts are made to keep cost roughly equivalent, so this does not drive patients' decision between the two methods. With the COVID-19 pandemic, telehealth provision of medication abortion has become more available and been recommended by WHO (Chong et al., 2021; WHO, 2022). In rare cases, a patient may have a complicating medical condition that requires their abortion to be performed in a hospital setting, which increases cost.

PROCEDURAL ABORTION

A typical visit for an outpatient abortion begins with review of the patient medical and social history, laboratory tests (urine pregnancy test as indicated, hemoglobin, Rh factor if 12 weeks or greater), and counseling that includes discussion of the procedure and obtaining informed consent. This may be followed by a focused physical examination including pelvic, and if indicated by history or physical examination, screening for vaginitis, sexually transmitted infections, and/or cervical cancer. In some settings, ultrasound exam is routinely performed to confirm intrauterine pregnancy and gestational age, and rule out uterine anomalies, twin pregnancy, or other potentially complicating conditions. After these preliminary steps, if no contraindications have been detected, the procedure can be initiated.

The first step of a procedural abortion is addressing patient comfort. Pain can be alleviated through a number of pharmacologic and nonpharmacologic interventions. Local anesthesia in the form of a paracervical block is considered a standard of care worldwide (Ayegbusi et al., 2021). Most settings in the United States offer additional options for relief of pain and anxiety, ranging from minimal to deep sedation administered by mouth or parenterally. Ipas, a leading international nongovernmental organization that specializes in abortion care, recommends the following interventions for pain relief during early abortions: (1) a combination of paracervical block and preprocedure nonsteroidal anti-inflammatory drugs (NSAIDs; acetaminophen is not effective for this purpose); (2) additional measures such as narcotic analgesics and anxiolytics if needed; (3) intravenous sedation, if available. General anesthesia is not routinely recommended for pain management in early procedural abortions (Ipas, 2021b, p. 1). In addition, suggested nonpharmacologic strategies to reduce pain during the procedure include respectful staff; a clean environment; ensuring confidentiality; verbal support; and presence of family, friends, and supportive staff (Ipas, 2021b; National Abortion Federation [NAF], 2022). In some settings, abortion or "full-spectrum" doulas are available to support women undergoing abortion (May, 2022-).

Prophylactic pain management is followed with cervical dilation, which can be achieved in one of several ways including by inserting progressively larger dilators into the cervical opening (os) immediately before the procedure or administering vaginal or oral misoprostol (a prostaglandin analog) several hours earlier. Another technique more commonly used in later abortions involves placing osmotic dilators into the os several hours to a day before the procedure to slowly dilate the cervix.

After the cervix is adequately dilated, the provider introduces a cannula into the uterine cavity. This is attached to an electric or manual vacuum aspirator that creates suction, causing the endometrial lining in which the pregnancy, or "products of conception" (POC), is embedded to separate from the uterine wall. Typically, the POC are examined to ensure that the pregnancy has been successfully and completely removed before the patient is discharged from the facility. Some facilities also send the POC to an offsite lab for pathologic evaluation, though this is not considered necessary (NAF, 2022). The entire procedure—from dilation through uterine evacuation—is typically complete within several minutes.

Procedural abortion has low rates of morbidity and mortality, making it among the safest of medical procedures (Creanga et al., 2017; Jatlaoui et al., 2019). In the United States, the overall mortality rate for all abortions (early–late) is approximately 0.7 death per 100,000 procedures (Zane et al., 2015). Complications following procedural abortion may include infection (0.17%), incomplete abortion or retained tissue, (0.37%) hemorrhage (<1%), continuing pregnancy, cervical laceration or uterine perforation, hematometra, and pain (Taylor et al., 2017).

Strategies to reduce risk of infection include prescribing preprocedure prophylactic antibiotics (NAF, 2022) and instructing patients to avoid douching and sexual activity involving vaginal penetration following the procedure. Evidence to support recommendations against tub bathing, swimming, and use of tampons is lacking; however, these proscriptions are still commonly advised.

In addition to providing guidance about possible complications, relaying accurate information about the long-term safety of abortion is important when providing abortion counseling. There is no evidence that early abortion increases risks of infertility, ectopic pregnancy, spontaneous abortion, birth defects, or preterm or low-birth-weight delivery with future pregnancies (National Academies of Sciences, Engineering, and Medicine [NASEM], 2018). Extensive studies and reviews have concluded there is no link between abortion and breast cancer (ACOG, 2021; Tong et al., 2020), nor any other type of cancer. Among people with unplanned pregnancies, those who have abortions have no greater risk of subsequent mental health problems than those who carry the pregnancy to term (Biggs et al., 2017; Collaborative for Reproductive Equity, 2021; Major et al., 2009; Steinberg et al., 2014). Conversely, Foster and colleagues (2015) found that being denied a wanted abortion was associated with a higher risk of experiencing adverse psychological outcomes in the short term than having an abortion.

Generally, most people are eligible for procedural abortions. Certain conditions, such as cervical stenosis, uterine anomalies, or morbid obesity can make aspirating the uterus challenging, and may require a more experienced provider. Other medical conditions, such as asthma, hypertension, and coagulopathies may also require special preparations for the service to be delivered safely. In rare cases, such as severe cardiac disease, an abortion may need to be performed in a hospital rather than outpatient setting. However, given the greater risks associated with pregnancy and childbirth compared to abortion, there are essentially no absolute contraindications to procedural abortion other than absence of informed patient consent.

Immediately following a procedural abortion, patients are typically monitored for 30 to 90 minutes to ensure they are clinically stable before discharge. During this time, aftercare, warning signs (Box 36.1), and instructions about who to contact in case any of these arise are typically reviewed. Patients who are Rh negative and were ≥12 weeks pregnant receive RhoGAM if it was not already administered during the visit. Routine follow-up is not necessary (NAF, 2022; WHO, 2022); nevertheless, clinicians must be prepared to provide routine postabortion care as well as to assess for complications, as some patients may present for this type of care. This is discussed further in the section on postabortion care. One potential benefit of a postabortion visit is that it can provide an opportunity for a patient to reflect on their abortion experience in a supportive environment.

Box 36.1 Postabortion Warning Signs and Self-Care Instructions

Following an abortion, all patients should be given information about who to contact in case of emergency and instructions about warning signs.

Warning Signs

- Temperature greater than or equal to 100.4°F
- Chills
- Foul-smelling discharge
- Persistent/increasing abdominal pain
- Bleeding: saturating more than one pad an hour for 2 hours, or twice as much as a heavy period

Other Self-Care Instructions

- Rest immediately after the abortion, and for up to 24 hours if possible.
- If strenuous exercise or heavy lifting causes an increase in bleeding, reduce the activity for several days.
- Avoid use of alcohol or drugs that could interfere with noticing complications.
- Abstain from vaginal penetration for at least 1 week. Use contraception as soon as resuming vaginal-penile intercourse to avoid pregnancy.
- Change pads/tampons frequently.
- Do not douche.
- Take all prescribed medications as directed.
- Take ibuprofen (400–800 mg every 4–8 hours) or acetaminophen (up to 1,000 mg every 4 hours) for pain as needed. Heating pads/hot water bottles and massage can also help to relieve pain.
- Pregnancy symptoms should resolve within a week after the abortion. If they do not, contact the provider. Do not perform a pregnancy test, as it may be positive even if no longer pregnant.

Source: Adapted from National Abortion Federation. (2022). Clinical policy guidelines for abortion care. https://prochoice.org/wp-content/uploads/2022-CPGs.pdf

MEDICATION ABORTION

Medication abortion refers to administration of pharmaceutical agents to intentionally disrupt a pregnancy. In the United States, the most common method of medication abortion involves the use of mifepristone (Mifeprex) in combination with misoprostol. Mifepristone is an "anti-progestin" (prostaglandin E1) that blocks the activation of receptors by endogenous progesterone. When taken by a person in early pregnancy, it causes the endometrial lining in which the pregnancy sac is embedded to separate from the underlying decidua. This endometrial and pregnancy tissue is eventually expelled from the uterus, a process that can be accelerated with misoprostol, a prostaglandin that promotes uterine contractions. Misoprostol has been widely available as an agent for gastric ulcer prevention without significant side effects. Methotrexate (also administered in combination with misoprostol) and misoprostol-only are alternative pharmacologic approaches for inducing early abortion; however, compared to mifepristone, these regimens are somewhat less effective (Raymond et al., 2019). Mifepristone combined with misoprostol is the most widely used method for medication abortion in the United States, and therefore is the main focus of this section.

Medication abortion is Food and Drug Administration (FDA)-approved for use up to 70 days of pregnancy (10 weeks) in the United States. Currently, mifepristone is regulated under the FDA Risk Evaluation and Mitigation Strategy (REMS) program, which, among other restrictions, requires that patients receive the medication at a healthcare facility. During the pandemic this restriction was lifted to allow telehealth provision and use of mail order pharmacies; this change was made permanent in December 2021 (FDA, 2021). Other than mail order pharmacies, however, mifepristone cannot be dispensed by retail pharmacies. After completing a prescriber agreement with the manufacturer, clinicians can order mifepristone directly from the manufacturer to dispense from a clinical setting. In December 2021, the FDA added a special certification requirement for pharmacies that dispense mifepristone. At the time of this writing, much is still unknown about this certification requirement or if it will expand pharmacy access to retail pharmacies.

In a study of more than 30,000 people with pregnancies of up to 64 days efficacy of medication abortion (mifepristone and misoprostol) was compared with procedural abortion. Medication abortion was found to be 99.6% effective versus 99.8% for procedural abortions. The medication abortion group had a slightly higher risk of continuing pregnancy, persistent pain or bleeding, or both compared to aspiration procedures (2.1% vs. 0.6%). Overall, major adverse rates were very low. Efficacy rates were not affected by gravidity, parity, or body mass index (Ireland et al., 2015).

Misoprostol alone has not been widely prescribed in the United States due to its lower efficacy rate (93%–97%) compared to mifepristone/misoprostol; however, it is the most prescribed abortion method worldwide (WHO, 2018). Use of misoprostol in self-managed medication abortion is widely credited for the global declines in maternal morbidity and mortality rates (WHO, 2018). Raymond and colleagues (2019) conducted a systemic review of the use of misoprostol alone in the first trimester. They found misoprostol alone to be effective and safe in the first trimester although further research is needed to refine the dosage and efficacy late in the first trimester. In addition, the different routes of misoprostol administration (buccal, sublingual, and vaginal) as well as the side effects were acceptable to users, and the ability to predict timing of the bleeding was reported as the best feature of taking medicines at home (WHO, 2018). The standard recommended regimen for pregnancies <12 weeks is 800 µg of misoprostol administered by vaginal, sublingual, or buccal routes.

For pregnancies of gestational age >12 weeks (84 days), the recommended method is 400 µg of misoprostol administered vaginally, buccally, or sublingually every 3 hours until the pregnancy tissue has passed. In the WHO 2018 guidelines for pregnancies >12 weeks, the maximum number of doses and the interval between dosing was removed. Rather, healthcare providers are advised to consider repeat doses of misoprostol until a successful abortion is achieved (WHO, 2018, 2022, p. 68). Letrozole, a drug used to treat breast cancer in postmenopausal women, in combination with misoprostol is another safe and effective option for medication abortion that was added to the 2022 WHO guidelines. Recommended dosing is letrozole 10 mg orally daily for 3 days followed by misoprostol 800 µg sublingually on the fourth day. This approach is not yet common among providers in the United States. In general, routine prescription of prophylactic antibiotics is not recommended with medication abortion. Pain medication such as nonsteroidal anti-inflammatory agents should be offered (WHO, 2021).

The delivery of abortion services was disrupted by the COVID-19 pandemic, as with all healthcare services. Staff shortages due to quarantining, school closures, travel restrictions, and higher cost all affected the provision of services. A number of state legislatures took advantage of this situation to enact further abortion restrictions (see Guttmacher Overview State Abortion Laws website for more information [www.guttmacher.org/state-policy/explore/overview-abortion-laws]; Guttmacher Institute, 2022a, 2022b; Roberts et al., 2020). As delivery of health services pivoted to telehealth, this practice was facilitated by the lifting of federal and state insurance restrictions; abortion became part of this widespread trend. A study of the safety of telemedicine medication abortion provision compared to in-person provision during the pandemic found similar efficacy rates (99.2% vs. 98.1%) and low rates of major complications (0.02 vs. 0.04%), respectively (Aiken et al., 2021).

Regardless of the medication regimen used, it is important for individuals considering medication abortion to understand it is a process that involves several steps. As with procedural abortion, the first steps in a medication abortion involve reviewing the person's medical and social history, providing appropriate counseling, including obtaining informed consent, and performing laboratory testing. Because medication abortion is more effective in the first trimester, confirmation of gestational age is critical, and a positive pregnancy test is a standard of care. Menstrual history and uterine sizing by physical examination are acceptable, evidence-based approaches for confirming gestational age (Bracken et al., 2011). According to the NAF Clinical Practice Guidelines (2022), ultrasound exam is not required before providing a first trimester abortion. If performed, a limited ultrasound exam for pregnancy dating includes a full scan of the uterus in both the transverse and longitudinal planes to confirm the pregnancy is intrauterine; evaluation for number of embryo(s) or fetus(es); and measurement and evaluation of pregnancy landmarks such as yolk sac or/or cardiac activity to document gestational age. If indicated to assess for possible ectopic pregnancy, evaluation of the adnexa and cul-de-sac should be performed or referral to an appropriate provider for this purpose should be made (NAF Clinical Practice Guidelines, 2022, pp. 13–14). Following preabortion evaluation, if no contraindications are detected the primary abortifacient medication can be administered on site or via telehealth. Because mifepristone is currently the most common drug used for medication abortion in the United States, only this method will be discussed further in this chapter.

The current FDA-approved dosage for mifepristone to end early pregnancy is 200 mg orally followed by misoprostol 800 µg (four pills) administered buccally 24 to 48 hours later (FDA, 2021). Follow-up with a healthcare provider 7 to 14 days later is advised. Evidence supports many variations to the FDA-approved regimen, and many abortion providers use these alternative approaches. While an exhaustive discussion of the benefits and limitations of each of these variations is beyond the scope of this chapter, several are highlighted here.

In the United States, at-home administration of misoprostol is standard practice. Timing of administration has been studied extensively, and a number of approaches have been found to be equivalent in terms of efficacy (Creinin & Grossman, 2014). Evidence supports self-administration of misoprostol between 6 and 72 hours after mifepristone (Schaff et al., 2000). Few people of reproductive age have contraindications to mifepristone/misoprostol abortion. Contraindications include a previous allergic reaction to mifepristone or misoprostol, inherited porphyria, chronic adrenal failure, or known or suspected ectopic pregnancy (Ipas, 2021a). With other serious/unstable health conditions such as bleeding disorders, heart disease, or severe anemia precautions should be taken. In addition, mifepristone should be used cautiously in people with severe, uncontrolled asthma or long-term corticosteroid therapy. If an IUD is in place, it must be removed prior to initiating the abortion (Ipas, 2021a). Data on the effects of mifepristone and misoprostol on infants who are breastfeeding are limited. Current recommendations do not recommend interrupting breastfeeding after a single dose of 200 mg of mifepristone. The extremely low levels of misoprostol in breast milk are also not known to cause any adverse effects; therefore, special precautions are not needed (National Library of Medicine, 2006). If a patient is not comfortable with this approach, they may pump and discard breast milk for several days. LactMed is part of the National Library of Medicine's (NLM) Toxicology Data Network (TOXNET), a database of drugs and dietary supplements that may affect breastfeeding. All data are derived from the scientific literature and fully referenced. The LactMed app can be downloaded for free.

Most people begin bleeding between 1 and 3 hours after administration of misoprostol. For the majority, bleeding peaks after 4 to 6 hours, coinciding with expulsion of the pregnancy from the uterus. Bleeding then usually slows but continues, with a mean duration of 14 to 17 days and a range of 1 to 69 days. Typically, bleeding is heaviest during the first day after misoprostol use. It is considered excessive if the person soaks more than two thick sanitary pads for 2 consecutive hours at any point during the abortion process (FDA, 2016, p. 5). Patients who do not experience bleeding can take an additional dose of misoprostol or undergo uterine aspiration to complete the abortion (FDA, 2016, p. 4). Cramping is expected with medication abortion. Intensity ranges widely; for most people, cramps tend to be strongest when the bleeding is heaviest. NSAIDs are suggested either prophylactically or at time of cramping for pain management. Acetaminophen is not recommended unless the person cannot tolerate NSAIDs. Narcotics have not been found to relieve pain during medication abortion (Ipas, 2021b; WHO, 2022). Nonpharmacologic methods, such as heating pads, adhesive heat pads, and relaxation techniques, can provide relief for some people. In addition to bleeding and cramping, nausea, vomiting, and diarrhea are common with misoprostol use; vaginal administration may reduce these side effects (Kulier et al., 2011). Evidence supports vaginal, buccal, or sublingual routes for administration of misoprostol (NASEM, 2018; WHO, 2022), although the FDA only lists buccal (FDA, 2016). The pharmacokinetic, efficacy, and side effect profiles of each of these routes vary (Soon et al., 2016; NAF, 2022). To lessen nausea, some providers routinely prescribe an antiemetic for prophylactic use before administration of misoprostol.

As part of self-care during and after a medication abortion, individuals are instructed to monitor their bleeding and pain and to look for signs of infection (fever, foul odor); any abnormalities should be reported to the provider (see Box 36.1). Contraceptive counseling, education, and provision are standard components of a medication abortion visit. As with procedural abortion, return to fertility following medication abortion is rapid. For this reason, individuals who do not want to become pregnant again are encouraged to initiate contraception promptly (within 7 days) after the abortion if they anticipate resuming sexual activity that could lead to pregnancy. The U.S. Selected Practice Recommendations for Contraceptive Use (CDC, 2016) feature guidance for providers about when to initiate use of specific methods based on established evidence-based criteria about how to be reasonably certain a person is not pregnant. In general, hormonal methods, including implants, can be started immediately after mifepristone has been taken (Park et al., 2016; Raymond Weaver, Tan et al., 2016; Raymone, Weaver, Louie et al., 2016), and IUDs can be inserted as soon as the gestational sac has been expelled (Sääv et al., 2012; Shimoni et al., 2011).

Risks and complications associated with medication abortion are similar to those with procedural abortion, absent those that result from uterine instrumentation (cervical laceration, uterine perforation) and anesthesia. In the early 2000s, several cases of *Clostridium sordellii* infection, which can cause fatal toxic shock, were observed among people who had undergone medication abortion (Aultman et al., 2021). *C. sordellii* has been noted in miscarriage, childbirth, aspiration, and other nonpregnancy-related events. The CDC continues to monitor all *C. sordellii* infections, and this complication was one of the rationales for the FDA's REMS program to include mifepristone. Less severe uterine infections are also possible, though are uncommon (Taylor et al., 2017).

Excessive bleeding is another possible complication of medication abortion. Acute hemorrhage or prolonged excessive bleeding can lead to decreases in hemoglobin severe enough to warrant treatment, including uterine aspiration or, rarely, transfusion. One death due to hemorrhage following medication abortion has been reported in the United States (Aultman et al., 2021). A chart review of 233,805 patients having a medication abortion used the marker of requiring a blood transfusion to identify the incidence of hemorrhage, calculated at 0.05% (Cleland et al., 2013).

After taking the medications, patients are instructed to contact the abortion provider if they experience any signs or symptoms of complications, including absence of bleeding or other signs that the pregnancy tissue has passed. Routine follow-up between several days and 2 weeks after the abortion is commonly recommended; however, this may be via telehealth. Some providers may make the follow-up visit optional as long as the patient experiences expected symptoms and agrees to follow up with any questions or concerns (Reproductive Health Access Project, 2022b).

While ultrasound exam is routinely performed in some settings, clinical history or, if warranted, physical examination and/or quantitative hCG testing are evidence-based alternatives that may be used to confirm completion of the abortion. Urine pregnancy tests assessing completion of medication abortion have also been found to be safe, effective, and acceptable (Schmidt-Hansen et al., 2020) and may be especially useful when providing care to patients who live in remote areas, and when care is delivered through telehealth.

Early Abortion Counseling: Procedural Versus Medication

Clinicians may encounter patients who have decided to end an early pregnancy but are unaware or unsure of what their options are. Some people may hold beliefs about abortion based on inaccurate information relayed by friends, family members, or media sources. As with pregnancy options counseling, the clinician's role in abortion counseling is to provide an overview of available methods, correct misinformation, support decision-making, and ultimately provide the desired service or, alternatively, an appropriate referral. For people who are eligible for either medication or aspiration abortion, counseling can include comparing the two approaches, providing information about where each can be obtained, and supporting the patient's selection of a method (Table 36.2). The Reproductive Health Access Project (2021a) has created a useful patient fact sheet (available in English and Spanish) comparing the two early abortion options as a patient decision aid.

Self-Managed Abortion

INCIDENCE

The term *self-managed abortion* has recently emerged to describe when a person takes actions to end a pregnancy outside the formal healthcare system. It includes the self-sourcing of medications, which is a well-known phenomenon throughout the world (Moseson et al. 2020). The 2022 WHO Abortion Care Guidelines state that it is possible for people to manage the medication abortion process on their own, and that this should not automatically be considered a "last resort" option or the result of a nonfunctioning health system, but rather recognized as a potentially empowering approach that some people may prefer (WHO, 2022, 3.6.2).

A global scoping review identified eight subsets of self-managed abortion: ingestion of plants and herbs, physical

TABLE 36.2 Comparison of Procedural and Medication Abortion

MEDICATION ABORTION	PROCEDURAL ABORTION
Some contraindications, including gestational age limit (typically <11 weeks in United States)	Rare contraindications
Avoids a procedure	Procedure
Takes place over several days. Typically involves in-office or telehealth visit (which may be asynchronous).	Requires only one visit to complete abortion; follow-up visit optional.
Involves heavy bleeding; some bleeding may persist for several weeks after medication taken.	Bleeding is generally light after procedure.
Person may feel they have more control.	Provider has high level of control during the procedure.
Abortion occurs at home (greater privacy).	Abortion occurs in clinic, office, or hospital setting (less private).
Efficacy 98%–99%	Efficacy 99%
Self-management options outside the healthcare system exist.	Self-management is not an option

Source: Adapted from Reproductive Health Access Project. (2022). Mifepristone/misoprostol abortion care protocol. https://www.reproductiveaccess.org/resource/medication -abortion-protocol/2022-06-mifepristone_protocol_final-3; Reproductive Health Access Project. (2022). Early abortion options. https://www.reproductiveaccess.org/resource /early-abortion-options

trauma, intrauterine trauma, alcohol and drug use, ingestion of toxic substances, and other drugs and mixtures followed by misoprostol alone and mifepristone and misoprostol (Moseson et al., 2020). The review also found that the most likely sources of information about self-managed abortion were the internet, family and friends, nonclinical people, and safe abortion hotlines or groups (Moseson et al., 2020). People chose self-management for many reasons including privacy, perceptions about safety and ease of self-management, knowing others who had self-managed, and avoidance of anticipated negative treatment by clinicians (Moseson et al., 2020).

This section focuses primarily on self-managed abortion with pills. A study by Aiken et al. (2018) found that women chose self-managed abortion because of the high cost of care, barriers to access (long distances to care, lack of transportation, difficulty finding information), waiting periods, or ultrasound requirements, or because they wanted privacy. A 2020 study found that in a 10-month period the organization Women on Waves, an international virtual abortion service (www.womenonwaves.org), received over 6,000 requests for medication abortion from the United States; 76% came from states with the most legal restrictions (e.g., Mississippi; Aiken et al., 2020). Aiken asserts that self-managed abortion has shifted from previously conceived as people inserting a sharp object into their uterus or ingesting toxic substances to the present-day use of mifepristone and/or misoprostol-alone obtained on the internet. A 2020 national sample estimated that 900,000 to 1.3 million people of reproductive age in the United States had experience with self-managed abortion (Ralph et al., 2020). Acknowledging underreporting, the researchers estimated that up to 7% of U.S. women will use self-managed abortion methods over their lifetime. The number of individuals choosing to self-manage their abortion with pills is expected to rise since the Supreme Court overturned the 50-year-old *Roe v. Wade* (1973) decision, eliminating the federal constitutional right to abortion (*Dobbs v. Jackson Women's Health Organization*, 2022). As self-managed abortion increases, innovative methodologies will be critical to obtaining accurate data about rates, as accurate abortion statistics are important for policy making and planning for clinical services.

ACCESS

Given the dramatically shifting abortion policy landscape in the United States, many online sources of abortion pills are emerging. As of this writing, Plan C (www.plancpills.org) is one organization that serves as a clearinghouse for up-to-date information on access to medication abortion for people and healthcare providers. Many other organizations are forming to provide access in states where abortion is banned or heavily restricted (Baker, 2022). Individuals are advised to take precautions to protect their privacy when searching for information about abortion online. Search engines and apps specifically designed to prevent data tracking (e.g., VPNs, DuckDuckGo, Euki) are available, and it is likely more will be forthcoming in the future. The Digital Defense fund (digitaldefensefund.org/ddf-guides/abortion-privacy) is an organization that has developed information specifically for people about abortion and digital privacy issues. This is a rapidly evolving area of legal policy; clinicians are advised to seek the most current available information from reliable information sources to protect themselves and patients. See Table 36.1 for a list of additional organizations and information sources on self-managed abortion, digital privacy, and abortion policy.

Clinicians have clinical encounters with people who are at various stages of self-managing an abortion. It is important to recognize that self-management may present legal risks to people who pursue this option for ending an unwanted pregnancy (Jenkins et al., 2021). As with many issues in healthcare, clinicians may hold a range of feelings about self-managed abortion, from believing that it is a safe option, is risky, or should occur only within the formal healthcare system (Baldwin et al., 2022; Kerestes et al., 2019). Professional ethics oblige clinicians to provide nonjudgmental and compassionate care, and adherence to HIPAA (Health Insurance Portability and Accountability Act) privacy, regardless of personal beliefs. According to legal experts, no existing laws mandate reporting of self-managed abortion to law enforcement or vital statistics (clinicians are only required to report the abortions they provide; Harris & Grossman, 2020). Reporting could lead to unnecessary criminalization of a person who self-managed their abortion. Implicit and explicit bias may lead some clinicians to report people who are marginalized more readily to law enforcement (Verma et al., 2022).

People may limit the information they provide to a healthcare provider; if a clinician has sufficient information to appropriately provide care for a patient about their chief concern(s), further questioning in not necessary and may protect an individual from prosecution. Spontaneous miscarriage and self-managed abortion can present similarly, and management is the same. A symptom-focused history can yield sufficient information to care for a patient without querying about the cause of the pregnancy loss (Harris & Grossman, 2020). Generally, it is legal for clinicians to provide *information*; however, offering healthcare *advice* or referring patients to a particular source to access medications for a self-managed abortion may carry legal risks in certain states. As of this writing, some professional clinician groups have issued position statements in support of the decriminalization of self-induced abortions (ACOG, 2017; American Medical Association [AMA], 2018); others have denounced the 2022 Supreme Court decision on *Dobbs v. Jackson Women's Health Organization* (American Academy of Nursing, 2022; American College of Nurse-Midwives, 2022; ANA, 2022; Association of Women's Health, Obstetric and Neonatal Nurses, 2022; Nurse Practitioners Women's Health, 2022).

Later Abortion

Currently in the United States, two general approaches are used for abortions that take place after 14 to 16 weeks' gestation: dilation and evacuation (D&E) and labor induction. A brief overview of these methods is provided in this section.

Regardless of method, abortions after the first trimester have low rates of complications and mortality; however, this risk increases exponentially with advancing gestational age, and consequently, gestational age has been found to be the largest risk factor for abortion-related mortality (NASEM, 2018). Although there has been a general trend toward earlier abortions in the United States with two thirds occurring at 8 weeks or earlier (Guttmacher Institute, 2019), people continue to have abortions after the first trimester. A number of individual and structural causes, including logistical factors, such as difficulty finding a provider, traveling long distances, problems with child care; emotional factors, such as difficulty deciding and fear of having an abortion; late discovery of pregnancy; and financial barriers contribute to delays in obtaining services (NASEM, 2018).

DILATION AND EVACUATION

D&E is the most common method for second trimester abortions in the United States. Studies have shown that compared to labor induction, D&E is both safer and better for the psychological health of patients (NASEM, 2018). Labor

induction abortion is infrequently used, accounting for approximately 2% of all abortions after 14 weeks (Jatlaoui et al., 2019), and carries a slightly higher complications rate than D&E (Bryant et al., 2011).

As with procedural abortion, D&E is accomplished by dilating the cervix and applying suction to the uterine cavity to remove the endometrial lining and POC. In later gestations (beyond 15–16 weeks), forceps may also be used. D&E requires more cervical dilation than procedures performed at earlier gestations; this process is often carried out with osmotic dilators. Alternatively, or in addition, prostaglandins can be given to achieve dilation, while minimizing trauma to the cervix. Although mechanical dilation can be used, risks of hemorrhage, cervical tear, or unsuccessful uterine evacuation increase with this approach.

D&E can be performed in an outpatient setting but is more commonly performed in a hospital than first trimester abortions. Regardless of setting, preoperative assessment and counseling are carried out and informed consent is obtained before the procedure. In the United States, clinical standards include universal ultrasound after 14 weeks EGA to ensure accurate pregnancy dating, which allows for appropriate cervical dilation as well as compliance with laws pertaining to gestational age limits for abortion (NAF, 2022). In addition to a paracervical block, pain relief options may include light sedation, or if desired, general anesthesia. Although D&E is similar to procedural abortion, it is a lengthier procedure, requiring more skill to perform. As previously discussed, risks of serious morbidity and mortality increase with gestational age and causes of such complications are the same as with abortions performed earlier in pregnancy.

Postoperative care after D&E is generally the same as with earlier abortions. Immediately after the procedure, women are monitored for complications and provided with education about self-care, signs and symptoms of complications, and contraception. A routine follow-up visit is generally advised several weeks after completion of the procedure.

POSTABORTION CARE

As the availability of abortion providers declines, primary care clinicians may be expected to provide routine follow-up care, as well as manage complications. This section provides an overview of current recommendations and guidelines for postabortion care.

When abortions are performed safely, the risk of complications is very low (NASEM, 2018). As a result, the need for routine follow-up after abortion has been questioned. Although standard practice has been to recommend routine follow-up 2 to 3 weeks after a procedural abortion, studies as early as 2004 asserted that there is limited evidence to support this practice (Grossman et al., 2004). The authors noted that routine follow-up visits did not typically reveal complications that people could not be taught to identify themselves. Furthermore, the recommended timing for routine follow-up is not well-suited for detecting the most severe potential complications. associated with abortion. People may have difficulty returning to a provider for a myriad of logistical reasons—distance and transportation to healthcare sites, child care issues, work constraints, and language barriers (ACOG, 2021). The NAF Guidelines do not require routine postprocedure follow-up (NAF, 2022). Patients can be given instruction on self-monitoring and how to report complications; for those who desire it, a telehealth follow-up or an in-person visit can be arranged. Some people may benefit from an in-person or telehealth appointment for reassurance that the procedure was complete without lingering side effects. The postabortion visit can be a time for patients to reflect on their abortion experience and gain closure.

For those who do opt for an in-person visit, clinicians have the opportunity to assess physical and emotional well-being, provide contraceptive counseling and management, and address other identified reproductive or general health needs. At the start of the visit, the clinician should review the abortion experience by asking the person how they have been feeling since the procedure, and if they experienced any complications during or since that time. Some people may have a record from the abortion provider and/or a pathology report if a procedural abortion was performed. If needed, the medical record may be requested from the abortion provider. The clinician should ask about bleeding patterns, pain, signs and symptoms of infection or continuing pregnancy, and emotional state since the abortion. The APA has refuted the claim that abortion leads to mental health problems (Abrams, 2023); a preponderance of research has found the predominant emotion people report after an abortion is relief (Rocca et al., 2020). Offering support, and—for any who need it—a referral for counseling, is an important aspect of the postabortion visit.

In addition to vital signs, a clinician may decide to perform a physical examination including speculum and bimanual examination to assess for signs of infection (purulent discharge, soft, tender uterus, fever), excessive bleeding, ongoing pregnancy, or retained POC (bleeding, uterus not well involuted) as part of a routine postabortion visit. Screening for sexually transmitted infections, vaginitis, and cervical dysplasia may also be clinically warranted. Routine performance of a pregnancy test is generally not advised in women who report resolution of pregnancy symptoms, as it may be positive for up to 4 to 8 weeks after an abortion due to lingering hCG and the high sensitivity of pregnancy tests (Cappiello et al., 2011). Ultrasound imaging is not required to assess postprocedure efficacy in early abortion. Given the low rate of complications, most postabortion assessments are routine and without significant findings.

Postabortion Contraception

Contraception is often a major focus in a postabortion visit. In order to be truly patient-centered when addressing contraceptive desires and needs, clinicians must be aware of their own biases, and respect that patients may not share their values and views about pregnancy, contraception, and abortion. Cansino and colleagues (2018) found that more than 70% of women wanted a method of birth control at their postabortion appointment; however, only 30% felt they needed contraceptive counseling, as they already knew what method they wanted. A patient-centered approach begins with asking the patient if they want to discuss contraception, and if they already have a method they would like to use or learn more about. In addition, offering a similar discussion about contraception during the preabortion counseling can preempt the need for a follow-up visit to provide contraception (Lohr et al., 2018; Roe et al., 2018). Because ovulation may occur as early as 8 days after an abortion (mean: 21–29 days), contraceptive counseling, selection, and provision either at the previsit (often via telephone), at the time of the procedure, or at the postvisit is advised. Clinicians should assess contraceptive acceptability, side effects, and adherence, and establish a patient-centered management plan that takes these factors into account. Most types of contraception can be initiated immediately after an abortion is complete; evidence supports same-day initiation of IUDs, implants, and injectables as an effective strategy for decreasing subsequent pregnancies in the year following an abortion (Nippita & Paul, 2018). If a person does not start or resume use of a method after an abortion, asking about the reasons can help to inform a contraceptive plan that effectively addresses their needs and preferences. Also, if a person has resumed sexual activity that could lead to pregnancy, the clinician must determine whether there is a risk for a repeat pregnancy. Emergency contraception can be taken at any time after an abortion if it is indicated. Readers are referred to the previously mentioned resource, the CDC's Selected Practice Recommendations for Contraceptive Use (2016), for detailed information about initiating/resuming use of contraception following abortion.

Assessment and Management of Postabortion Complications

Occasionally, a person may present to a primary care clinician with concerns or complications following a procedural or medication abortion. In such cases, referring the patient back to the provider or setting where the abortion was performed is recommended. If this is not feasible or desirable, a primary care clinician may be able to manage the case independently, or in consultation with the abortion provider or another qualified healthcare provider. In a California study of nearly 20,000 patients, the rate of serious or major adverse events was rare (0.06%) with the majority of adverse events due to retained POC (0.37%), failed attempt (0.15%), and postabortion infection (0.17%; Taylor et al., 2017). A brief review of possible complications and general information about management of complications follows.

BLEEDING

Following procedural abortion, women experience a wide range of bleeding patterns, from none to moderate amounts for a week or longer. Aftercare and warning signs regarding bleeding are typically reviewed following the procedure (see Box 36.1). Although difficult to quantify, suggested measures for determining if bleeding is excessive include saturating a sanitary pad in less than an hour for 2 consecutive hours, or bleeding twice as heavily as with normal menstrual flow. Passing clots is also common after an abortion (NAF, 2022). Using pads can make observing bleeding easier. Once bleeding has slowed, tampons (or menstrual cups) may be used (NAF, 2016). People may resume activities of daily living immediately after an abortion. If strenuous activity leads to increased bleeding, it should be avoided for several days (NAF, 2016).

Some patients may contact their primary care clinician with concerns about bleeding after an abortion. In-person assessment may be warranted to ensure that the amount is not excessive and the patient is stable. Checking for signs of orthostatic hypotension, as well as a hemoglobin or hematocrit to evaluate hematologic stability, and a pelvic exam to assess amount and source of bleeding are appropriate. Management will depend on the degree of blood loss, and may include iron supplementation, intravenous therapy, or rarely, transfusion. In addition to excessive bleeding, some patients may report persistent bleeding after an abortion. The clinician must determine whether this is normal or could be due to infection, ongoing pregnancy (including ectopic), retained POC, or another cause unrelated to the abortion, such as a sexually transmitted infection. Treatment is based on the cause. People who initiate a hormonal method of contraception following abortion can also experience persistent bleeding or spotting. Ruling out other possible causes can support the diagnosis of vaginal bleeding due to exogenous hormone use.

People who do not have bleeding but report increasing pain or cramps following a procedural abortion may be experiencing hematometra. This uncommon complication is caused by a blood clot or multiple clots accumulating in the uterus, which prevents blood flow through the cervix. Typically, hematometra occurs immediately or within hours after the procedure, and is not likely to arise after the patient has left the facility where the abortion was performed. Management typically involves reevacuation of the uterus.

Menses typically resumes 4 to 6 weeks after an abortion. Failure to menstruate can indicate a repeat pregnancy. If repeat or continued pregnancy has been ruled out and hormonal contraception is not affecting bleeding patterns, if the person usually has their menses every 4 to 6 weeks, referral to a gynecologist is indicated.

INFECTION

Although the risk of postabortal infection is low, estimated at 0.17% (Taylor et al., 2017), in the United States many providers routinely prescribe prophylactic antibiotics on the day of the procedure to prevent infection (NAF, 2022). Patients who call or present with fever >100.4°F, chills, severe or persistent pelvic pain, body aches, or general malaise should be evaluated for this complication. Signs and symptoms of infection typically emerge within 48 to 96 hours after the procedure. Pelvic tenderness and an elevated white blood cell count are likely. Screening for sexually transmitted infections should be performed, and broad-spectrum antibiotics administered promptly to prevent serious sequelae, such as infertility, chronic pelvic pain, and sepsis. Treatment can be oral, but if the patient fails to respond within 48 to 72 hours, parenteral therapy should be initiated.

ONGOING PREGNANCY

Following procedural abortion, <0.15% of people may experience persistent pregnancy symptoms (Taylor et al., 2017). However, though pregnancy symptoms usually resolve

within a week after an abortion, hCG may be detectable for up to 8 weeks. For this reason, patients should be instructed not to perform a home pregnancy test after an abortion. Those who report persistent pregnancy symptoms (e.g., nausea, breast tenderness) need to be assessed for continued pregnancy which can be attributed to a number of factors including the pregnancy was not successfully disrupted because it was very small, was outside the uterus (ectopic), a uterine anomaly interfered with removal, more than one gestation was present, or the provider was inexperienced. In most settings the uterine aspirate is evaluated to verify the presence of pregnancy tissue to identify those at risk of these complications. If ectopic pregnancy is suspected, a plan for close follow-up must be established that includes instructing the patient about warning signs. If ongoing pregnancy (including ectopic) is suspected, serial quantitative hCGs and/or ultrasound scans are warranted. Ideally, the abortion provider should manage this care, but it may be carried out by or in consultation with the primary care provider. Ultimately, management depends on the clinical diagnosis. If an ongoing pregnancy is detected and verified as intrauterine, the patient may opt to repeat the procedure or continue the pregnancy. Ectopic pregnancy should be managed according to current standards of clinical care.

RETAINED TISSUE

Another uncommon (0.37% in first trimester abortions) but possible complication following abortion is retained tissue in the uterus (Taylor et al., 2017). Individuals with retained tissue may experience lower abdominal pain or cramps and persistent bleeding including clots. Accompanying infection is rare unless large amounts of tissue are present. On exam, the uterus may feel somewhat enlarged and soft. Ultrasound often reveals heterogeneous material in the uterus that is indistinguishable from blood clots. If the amount of tissue present is small and the patient prefers to avoid a repeat uterine aspiration, watchful waiting is an appropriate management option.

Recommendations for management of an incomplete abortion are the same as with retained tissue following miscarriage. Options for pregnancies <14 weeks include expectant management (allowing more time for the expulsion of pregnancy tissue); administration of misoprostol 400 μg sublingually, vaginally, or buccally for pregnancies <14 weeks, or every 3 hours until tissue is passed for pregnancies ≥14 weeks; or uterine aspiration (WHO, 2022). With medication abortion, all patients are informed about the possibility of a failed or incomplete abortion and that due to the potential teratogenicity of misoprostol uterine evacuation may be warranted.

APRNS AS ABORTION PROVIDERS

Numerous studies have demonstrated that, with appropriate training, nurse practitioners, midwives and physician assistants (hereafter collectively referred to as advanced practice clinicians, or APCs) are safe, effective providers of early abortion care who are acceptable to patients (Barnard et al., 2015). Indeed, based on the available evidence, the NASEM recognized APCs along with OB-GYN, family, and other physicians as capable of providing both medication and aspiration abortion in their report on the Safety and Quality of Abortion in the United States (NASEM, 2018). A number of professional organizations, including the American Academy of Physician Assistants, American College of Nurse Midwives, American College of Obstetricians and Gynecologists, American Medical Women's Association, American Public Health Association, National Abortion Federation, National Association of Nurse Practitioners in Women's Health, Nurses for Sexual and Reproductive Health, and Physicians for Reproductive Choice and Health have also issued statements in support of this role for APRNs (ACOG, 2014; Taylor et al., 2018).

To determine whether an APC can legally provide abortions in a specific state, both abortion laws and regulations regarding their practice must be considered. At this time (2022), 13 states and the District of Columbia allow APCs to provide both medication and procedural abortion; seven states permit them to provide medication abortion. The other 30 states either have physician-only laws that expressly prohibit any clinician who is not a physician from providing abortion or other legal or regulatory barriers to APC provision of abortion (Guttmacher Institute, 2022c). APCs interested in providing abortion as part of their practice are advised to gather information about current, relevant state laws and regulations, seek professional support including support from state or national organizations familiar with the nuances of abortion-related laws and regulations, and seek appropriate training. The Abortion Provider Toolkit is a comprehensive resource for clinicians seeking to incorporate abortion into their practice (Taylor et al., 2018).

Personal beliefs and considerations may also influence clinicians' decisions about whether to incorporate abortion into their clinical practice. Resources for health professionals have been developed to clarify their personal values about abortion in the context of professional roles and responsibilities. Regardless of personal beliefs, facilitating access to abortion services is a professional responsibility for all clinicians. As discussed previously in the section on options counseling, clinicians are bound by professional ethical codes to respect patients' rights and autonomy, including with regard to abortion. Although health professionals may refuse to participate in abortion care provision, personal beliefs should never obstruct or present an undue burden to patients who are seeking abortion. If a clinician must refer a patient to another provider or facility for abortion-related services, every effort should be made to ensure it does not lead to untimely delays or lower quality of care provided. In the post-*Roe* era, referring patients to providers in other states due to legal restrictions presents additional challenges that may require providers to provide education and logistic support that exceeds previous expectations. Alternately, some states are codifying clinician protections into law to strengthen and protect clinicians' ability to provide telehealth abortions in states where abortion is illegal (Commonwealth of Massachusetts, 2020). The legal ramifications of this approach are unknown as of this writing.

SPECIAL CONSIDERATIONS IN PROVIDING PREGNANCY DECISION SUPPORT AND ABORTION CARE

As discussed in this chapter, the diagnosis of a pregnancy can stir a wide range of responses and emotions for the person experiencing this major reproductive life event. Given the shifting policy landscape in the United States following the June 2022 Supreme Court decision in *Dobbs v. Jackson Women's Health Organization*, access to the full range of options when faced with an unwanted or mistimed pregnancy is no longer a constitutionally guaranteed right. For people who are already marginalized or vulnerable in our society due to their economic status, age, race, ethnicity, educational level, geographic location, gender identity, disability status, citizenship, or other identities, this new reality will further exacerbate existing disparities in their ability to access reproductive services and realize their reproductive health and desires. This new era demands clinicians to engage in advocacy efforts that center the reproductive health needs of those who are at the margins.

SUMMARY

Clinicians who care for people of reproductive age are responsible for providing pregnancy and abortion care that is patient centered, ethically sound, nonjudgmental, unbiased, equitable, and trauma informed. To that end, clinicians must be prepared to provide pregnancy testing, options counseling, and direct services for continuing or ending a pregnancy, or to refer patients to providers who are qualified to deliver these services. As self-managed abortions increase due to state restrictions on abortion care, clinicians must be aware of the legal environment in their state. Medication abortion is safe whether clinician-provided or patient-managed. Routine follow-up care for those with complications is within the scope of practice of primary care clinicians. Ensuring that care provided is accurate, compassionate, and nonjudgmental is paramount and requires clinicians to engage in a process of continuing education and self-reflection. Our patients deserve no less.

REFERENCES

References for this chapter are online and available at https://connect.springerpub.com /content/book/978-0-8261-6722-4/part/part03/chapter/ch36

CHAPTER 37

Infertility

Rachel Oldani Bender and Elizabeth A. Kostas-Polston

Infertility is rapidly becoming a routine evaluation often performed by the APRN. As such, having a solid foundation and resources to turn to will be invaluable in practice. The purpose of this chapter is to give an overview of fertility evaluation and treatments, as well as the many ethical and psychological dilemmas that may be encountered when caring for the client and their family. Infertility should be treated systematically, and care should be standardized throughout all practices. The American Society for Reproductive Medicine (ASRM) serves as an invaluable resource for healthcare providers and provides invaluable information on reproductive, evidence-based practice guidelines.

DEFINITION AND SCOPE

The American College of Obstetricians and Gynecologists (ACOG) defines infertility as not having become pregnant after 1 year of having regular sexual intercourse without the use of birth control, or after 6 months in women older than 35 years (ACOG, 2022). A woman is considered to have primary infertility if she has never achieved pregnancy after regular, unprotected, and well-timed intercourse (ACOG, 2022). A woman who has previously experienced a pregnancy and who then is unable to conceive again or who experiences repeated pregnancy loss is known to have secondary infertility. The probability of a woman conceiving within one menstrual cycle is known as *fecundability* (ACOG, 2022). By age 24 years, a woman reaches her maximum fertility potential, with declining rates beginning at age 32 and more rapidly after age 37 (Faddy et al., 1992). Today, the average age at which many women deliver their first child in the United States has increased. Between 1990 and 2019, the first-time birth rate for women age 35 to 39 years was 53% and for ages 40 to 44 years it was 12% (Martin et al., 2021).

Infertility is not specifically a female issue; thus, both sexual partners should be evaluated simultaneously for factors impairing fertility, if possible. It is important to remember that recognition, evaluation, and treatment of infertility are highly stressful for most couples.

PREVALENCE

The National Survey of Family Growth (NSFG) study included interviews of 12,279 women ages 15 to 44 years to estimate the prevalence of infertility in the United States. Infertility was determined if a woman reported continuous cohabitation during the previous 12 months or more, had intercourse each month with no use of contraception, and had not become pregnant (Chandra et al., 2013). In 2002, 10% of women of childbearing age desired infertility counseling and in 2015 this was updated to state that impaired fecundability was noted in 13.8% of women ages 15 to 49 years old (Martinez et al, 2018).

ETIOLOGY

Approximately one third of infertility is caused by male factors, one third by female factors, and one third by a combination of factors in both partners. Overall, 20% of infertility cases are unexplained (Practice Committee of the ASRM, 2013). Each month or menstrual cycle, a woman has a 20% chance of becoming pregnant. Over 1 year, the cumulative pregnancy rate is 85% (ASRM, 2012). According to the National Center for Health Statistics of the Centers for Disease Control and Prevention (CDC), in the United States, the number of married women age 15 to 44 years who have difficulty getting pregnant or carrying a baby to term has increased from 24.2% (2011–2013; CDC, n.d.-a) to 26.8% (2015–2019: CDC, n.d.-c). A woman's fertility peaks between the late teens and the late 20s, and subsequently begins to decline. A woman's risk for miscarriage increases beginning age 30 years (Practice Committee of the ASRM, 2013). Almost one in five women in the United States now has her first child after 35 years of age. With declining fertility, one third of the women face fertility issues (ASRM, 2012). Although it is often recommended that women seek evaluation after 12 months of unexplained infertility, in older women, the ASRM recommends seeking earlier evaluation and treatment (as early as 6 months of unprotected coitus).

Ovulation Disorders

WORLD HEALTH ORGANIZATION CLASSIFICATION

The World Health Organization (WHO) classifies ovulation disorders into three categories.

WHO Class 1, hypogonadotropic hypogonadal anovulation, occurs in approximately 5% to 10% of infertile couples. Low or low–normal follicle-stimulating hormone (FSH) levels and low estradiol levels are the result of decreased hypothalamic secretion of or pituitary response to gonadotropin-releasing hormone (GnRH; WHO, 1992). Functional hypothalamic amenorrhea (FHA), caused by an excessively low body mass index (BMI) or extreme exercise, is an example of a WHO Class 1 ovulation disorder. In FHA, it is believed that there is a decrease in the pulsatile GnRH secretion. The abnormal release of GnRH causes a decrease in endogenous gonadotropins. In turn, this results in the absence of a luteinizing hormone (LH) surge and absence or abnormal development of follicles, resulting in anovulation and decreased estradiol concentrations (Gordon, 2010; Gordon et al., 2017).

WHO Class 2, normogonadotropic normoestrogenic anovulation, is the most common type of disorder of ovulation. It occurs in approximately 75% to 80% of infertile couples. Normal amounts of gonadotropins are secreted; however, the FSH levels during the follicular phase are low (WHO, 1992). Polycystic ovary syndrome (PCOS) is an example of a WHO Class 2 ovulation disorder. PCOS can often be treated with behavioral changes (ASRM, 2014b). Weight loss, improved nutrition, and exercise are the recommended first-line therapy. Insulin-sensitizing agents help in improving the body's response to insulin, thereby working to restore normal insulin levels. Metformin (Glucophage), an antihyperglycemic, reduces insulin and androgen levels. According to the ASRM, clomiphene citrate (a selective estrogen receptor modulator) or letrozole (a nonsteroidal aromatase inhibitor) are both recommended as first-line treatment for women diagnosed with PCOS, followed by injectable gonadotropins (ASRM, 2014b; Spaan et al., 2016).

WHO Class 3, hypergonadotropic hypoestrogenic anovulation, is estimated to occur in approximately 5% to 10% of couples experiencing infertility. In women with WHO Class 3 ovulatory disorders, there is an absence of follicular development due to premature ovarian failure (POF) or gonadal dysgenesis (WHO, 1992). POF or primary hypogonadism is the cessation of ovarian function and elevation of serum FSH before age 40 years. POF affects 1% of women and can happen as early as the teenage years. In POF, the ovaries cease to function and, thus, menstrual cycles become irregular and eventually stop (ASRM, 2014a).

RISK FACTORS

The literature has identified many risk factors for infertility, both modifiable and unmodifiable (Boxes 37.1 and 37.2). According to leading experts, smoking, alcohol consumption, and weight are modifiable risk factors that can impact both male and female fertility (Practice Committee of the ASRM, 2012; CDC, n.d.-b). Other risk factors for infertility include advanced maternal age and chronic diseases such as diabetes, hyper- or hypothyroidism, lupus, arthritis, hypertension, or asthma, all of which increase in prevalence as a woman ages

Box 37.1 Causes of Infertility in Females

- Problems with ovulation
  - Follicle-stimulating hormone/luteinizing hormone
  - Polycystic ovary syndrome
  - Luteal phase defect
  - Premature ovarian failure
  - Thyroid disease
  - Pituitary disease
- Problems with reproductive organs
  - Fallopian tube pathology
  - Endometriosis
  - Cervical disease
  - Uterine abnormality or pathology
- Genetic syndromes
  - Sheehan syndrome
  - Kallmann syndrome
  - Turner syndrome
  - Hypothalamic hypogonadotropic anovulation
- Immunologic causes
  - Antibodies
- Unknown causes

Box 37.2 Causes of Infertility in Males

- Abnormal sperm production or function because of undescended testicles
- Obstruction of the reproductive tract
- Varicocele (enlarged veins in the testes)
- Ejaculatory disorders
- Genetic defects
- Diabetes
- Infections
- Sexually transmitted infections (e.g., chlamydia, gonorrhea)
- HIV infection
- Immunologic
- Sperm antibodies
- Tobacco/marijuana consumption

(CDC, n.d.-b). We further discuss some of the risk factors for infertility in the following sections.

Advanced Maternal Age

There is an inverse relationship between female age and oocyte quality and quantity. Research shows that after the age of 35 years, there is an increased risk of genetic abnormalities as well as spontaneous abortion (ASRM, 2012; Practice Committee of the ASRM, 2015a; Chandra et al., 2013; Mosher &

Pratt, 1991). In the United States, the mean age of first-time mothers increased from 24.9 to 26.3 years between 2000 and 2014 (Mathews & Hamilton, 2016). This increase is caused by a reduction in teen pregnancy as well as societal trends (e.g., education, career), which have led many women to delay childbearing into their 30s or 40s (Crawford & Steiner, 2015). Women older than 35 years of age experience a decrease in fertility by approximately 30%. Furthermore, as a woman ages, there is a decrease in ovarian reserve, quality of oocyte, and regularity of ovulation, thus increasing the risk of pregnancy loss.

BEHAVIORAL RISK FACTORS
Tobacco

Both active and passive smoking reduce female and male fertility (Practice Committee of the ASRM, 2012). In women, smoking increases the risk for infertility and natural menopause occurring before the age of 50 years (Hyland et al., 2016). Chemicals in cigarettes accelerate egg loss and decrease reproductive function by interfering with the ability of ovarian cells to make estrogen. This leads to an increase in susceptibility of the oocytes to genetic abnormalities (Practice Committee of the ASRM, 2012). Furthermore, smoking has been linked to decrease in the quality of sperm, leading to decreased quantity and motility and increased abnormal morphology (ASRM, 2012; Caserta et al., 2013; Kovac et al., 2015; Practice Committee of the ASRM, 2012). Clients should be counseled about the risks of smoking in relation to not only infertility but also long-term morbidity and premature mortality (Practice Committee of the ASRM, 2012).

Marijuana

Marijuana use in the United States increased from 4.1% to 9.5% between 2001 and 2013 (National Institutes of Health [NIH], 2015). The literature has begun to explore the association between marijuana use and fertility in men. Initial results have demonstrated that chronic marijuana use is associated with poor semen quality (Gundersen et al., 2015). For example, anandamide, a well-studied endocannabinoid, has been shown to decrease the mobility of sperm at higher doses (Fronczak et al., 2012).

Alcohol

Although it is well known that no amount of alcohol is safe at any given time during pregnancy, the impact of alcohol on female fertility is unknown. It has been postulated that any effects of alcohol on fertility are probably dose-dependent, but no studies dictate any safe amounts. Although some literature has shown no association between alcohol consumption and fertility, other studies reported an increased risk of infertility with alcohol consumption (Rossi et al., 2016). In males, the impact of alcohol consumption and fertility is also ambiguous. While some literature has suggested that moderate drinking in males does not impact reproductive health (Burgo et al., 2015; Jensen, Gottschau et al., 2014; Jensen, Swan et al., 2014; Mikkelsen et al., 2016), other literature suggests that moderate habitual alcohol consumption is associated with decreased semen quality (Jensen, Gottshau et al., 2014; Jensen, Swan et al., 2014). Furthermore, the literature has suggested that heavy alcohol consumption has

deleterious effects on sperm concentration, semen volume, and sperm motility (Sadeu et al., 2010).

Caffeine

To date, the relationship between caffeine consumption and infertility remains ambiguous. While some studies have shown that caffeine consumption may increase the risk of infertility in males (Wesselink et al., 2016), others have reported no association (Homan et al., 2007). The association between caffeine and infertility may be confounded as some literature suggests that a particular type of caffeine may affect fertility. For example, Wesselink et al. (2016) reported that caffeinated tea was slightly correlated with infertility in women and that caffeinated soda and energy drinks were associated with infertility in males. Currently, although the association remains unknown, women who are pregnant or who are trying to conceive are recommended to limit their caffeine consumption to less than or equal to 200 mg each day (equivalent to one 12-ounce cup of coffee; March of Dimes, n.d.).

Weight

Women with a BMI of 25 kg/m^2 or greater, or of 20 kg/m^2 or less, can experience hormonal imbalances, which may lead to ovulatory dysfunction (CDC, n.d.-b). These women include those with eating disorders (e.g., anorexia nervosa, bulimia) and those on very low-calorie diets. The lack of important nutrients, such as vitamin B$_{12}$, zinc, iron, and folic acid, may also result in fertility issues in women. Women who are underweight and have very low body fat, either due to eating habits or exercise, are more likely to experience irregular menstruation and infertility. Females with decreased body fat or those who are underweight can experience oligomenorrhea or irregular menstrual cycles, leading to decreased fertility treatment success rates and an increased risk of spontaneous abortion (ACOG, 2013, 2014; CDC, 2014).

Weight can play a major role in a female's ability to ovulate. Ovulatory dysfunction can occur in both underweight and obese women (ACOG, 2013; CDC, 2014). Counseling regarding the benefits of regular exercise and a healthy diet should be completed (ACOG, 2013; CDC, 2014). According to the CDC, *obesity* is defined as a BMI of 30 or higher. In obese women, increased amount of adipose tissue causes increased aromatization of androgens to estrogens, and decreased levels of sex hormone–binding globulin (SHBG), which causes increased free estradiol and testosterone, and increased insulin resistance, resulting in ovarian stromal stimulation–producing androgens (ACOG, 2013, 2014; CDC, 2014). Improved ovulatory function and pregnancy rates are seen with a 5% to 10% weight loss in obese Clients. Clients with a BMI of less than 19 should be referred for close management and counseling (Practice Committee of the ASRM, 2015a).

Stress

Couples who are being treated for infertility experience stress (Mental Health Professional Group [MHPG], 2023). Stress has not been proved to cause infertility; however, it can affect the autonomic nervous, endocrine, and immune systems; change hormone levels; and interfere with ovulation (MHPG, 2023; Homan et al., 2007). With each passing menstrual cycle, it is important for the healthcare provider to address stress in couples hoping for a pregnancy. This is important because there is some evidence that increased stress level negatively affects, for example, the outcome of fertility treatment and also a couple's decision to discontinue fertility treatments (Brandes et al., 2009).

Sexually Transmitted Infections

In 2021, 1.64 million cases of chlamydia infection and 710,151 cases of gonorrhea were reported in the United States (CDC, 2023a). Often, sexually transmitted infections (STIs) can be asymptomatic and cause long-term sequelae in men and women. Pelvic inflammatory disease (PID) in women and epididymitis in men are often caused by an untreated STI. Depending on the severity of inflammation, effects can be devastating for women, resulting in scarring of the fallopian tubes, which can cause blockage, pelvic adhesions, spontaneous abortions, and ectopic pregnancies (CDC, n.d.-d).

COVID-19 Vaccine

As of January 9, 2021, no data have been found to show that the COVID-19 vaccine negatively impacts male or female fertility. According to the ACOG all pregnant and lactating women should be offered the COVID-19 vaccine. This is due to the known safety and efficacy of the vaccines and to the known risk of more severe disease if contracted during this time. The Society for Maternal-Fetal Medicine has recommended that pregnant women have access to the currently approved Pfizer COVID-19 vaccine. The American Society of Reproductive Medicine (ASROM), American College of Obstetricians and Gynecologists (ACOG), and the Society for Maternal-Fetal Medicine (SMFM) fully support COVID vaccination in women planning to conceive, undergoing fertility treatment, or for those currently pregnant (ACOG, 2023a).

HEALTH ASSESSMENT

Completion of a thorough history and physical examination is an important first step that will be used by the healthcare provider to determine an appropriate plan of care for a client's infertility workup and diagnostic testing. The ASRM website offers the most current guidelines regarding optimal evaluation of the infertile female and infertile male (www.asrm.org).

Infertile Females

MEDICAL AND SURGICAL HISTORY

A complete health history, including family, medical, surgical, allergy, social, and reproductive history, should be obtained from both partners. A systematic review of all body systems should be performed. Special attention should be given to a proven history of fertility in either partner, and details of pregnancy and delivery can aid in guiding the healthcare provider. Duration of infertility, previous evaluation and treatment(s), and menstrual cycle history (including cycle length and characteristics) should be discussed. Previous history of STIs, history of PID, abnormal cervical cytology and histology, and all treatment(s) should be noted. Furthermore, the

healthcare provider should be sure to rule out, either by history or testing, thyroid dysfunction, galactorrhea, hirsutism, pelvic and/or abdominal pain, dysmenorrhea, and dyspareunia (Practice Committee of the ASRM, 2015a, 2015b). Completing a comprehensive medical history is critical. It is important to identify changes in body weight as well as calculate a woman's BMI. A woman's physical activity history should be obtained. Excessive physical activity could result in low body fat composition, which can interfere with ovulation. Finally, it is important to identify, evaluate, and treat any underlying health issues as conception and pregnancy can further challenge a woman's overall health and well-being.

Finally, it is important to treat both members of a couple with fertility issues. It is critical that the healthcare provider not label one partner as having fertility issues. Instead, the healthcare provider should objectively complete the history, physical examination, and any indicated diagnostic tests, as necessary, addressing both members of the couple. The couple should be interviewed together and separately, allowing for confidentiality (e.g., history of past relationships).

GYNECOLOGIC HISTORY

An in-depth review of a woman's gynecologic history should be completed. A description of her menstrual cycle, including age of menarche, length of cycle, duration, and flow, as well as any pain associated with past menstrual cycles, should be ascertained. It is important to note any history of skipped periods, intracycle spotting, or irregular menstrual cycles. Irregular menstrual cycles are classified as less than 24 days or greater than 35 days. If an irregular menstrual cycle is described by the woman, further evaluation is needed to assess for ovulatory dysfunction (Practice Committee of the ASRM, 2015a, 2015b).

Contraception history (e.g., type of contraception, length of use, date of discontinuation) is an important part of the initial history. Return of fertility, based on contraception, should be discussed with the woman to improve realistic expectations. A complete documentation is needed regarding past pregnancies, including gestational age, mode of delivery, spontaneous/therapeutic abortions, complications, and outcomes (Practice Committee of the ASRM, 2015a, 2015b). Sexual history should include number of lifetime partners, history of STIs, and timing of intercourse. It is imperative to document the timing and frequency of intercourse, related to ovulation, as per the couple. Any previous fertility treatments, pelvic/abdominal surgeries, and cervical procedures (e.g., loop electrosurgical excision procedure [LEEP], cold knife cone [CKC] biopsies) should be disclosed (ASRM, 2014a, 2018).

SOCIAL HISTORY

Employment history should be obtained to determine if there are any potential exposures to toxic chemicals. Often employment can also cause a separation of the couple. Distance interferes with regular, unprotected intercourse. Disclosure of tobacco consumption, alcohol, and drug use is *essential*.

FAMILY HISTORY

Significant family history that should be obtained includes history of infertility, POF, recurrent pregnancy loss, endometriosis, thyroid disease, cancer, and endocrine or genetic problems (Practice Committee of the ASRM, 2015a, 2015b).

PHYSICAL ASSESSMENT

A thorough head-to-toe physical assessment, including pelvic examination, should be completed. Physical examination should be focused on assessing signs for potential causes of infertility. The healthcare provider should calculate BMI and distribution of fat; extremes are associated with decreased fertility (Practice Committee of the ASRM, 2015c). Disproportional abdominal fat can be correlated with increased insulin resistance and may lead to a diagnosis of PCOS (ASRM, 2014b; Practice Committee of the ASRM, 2015c). Body shape and development or underdevelopment of secondary sex characteristics should be noted to rule in or out hypogonadotropic hypogonadism or Turner syndrome. The presence of thyroid abnormalities, galactorrhea, hirsutism, acne, and male pattern baldness may point to endocrinopathies such as hyper/hypothyroidism, hyperprolactinemia, PCOS, or adrenal disorder. Pelvic examination should include evaluation of the adnexa and posterior cul-de-sac for masses or tenderness, possibly suggesting PID or endometriosis. The vagina and cervix should be inspected for normality to rule out müllerian anomaly, infection, or cervical factors. The uterus should be palpated for enlargement, nodularity, irregularity, and lack of mobility, suggesting a uterine anomaly, leiomyoma, endometriosis, and pelvic adhesion disease (Practice Committee of the ASRM, 2015a).

Infertile Males

HISTORY

The medical history in the male is focused on identifying systemic conditions that could impact fertility (Practice Committee of the ASRM, 2015b). Similar to the female history, the male reproductive history should be documented. Age of puberty, history of erectile dysfunction, undescended testicles, illness resulting in high fevers, mumps, trauma to the genital area, and exposure of the groin to radiation and infection (epididymitis, prostatitis, urinary tract infections, and purulent discharge from the penis) should be noted (Practice Committee of the ASRM, 2015b). Medical history should be obtained to rule out factors such as diabetes, which can cause impotence and retrograde ejaculation or hypertension. It is important to note that many hypertensive medications can cause impotence. Thus, the importance of a complete list of medications taken is evident (Practice Committee of the ASRM, 2015b). Surgical history should include any hernia repairs, testicular/pelvic floor surgery, varicocele repair, and vasectomy/vasectomy reversal. Family history should be obtained to rule out genetic or endocrine conditions. If further evaluation is needed, referral to a urologist is recommended (Practice Committee of the ASRM, 2015b).

PHYSICAL ASSESSMENT

Semen analysis is performed as a first step in the assessment of the infertile couple. Evaluation of the male begins with a semen analysis (Cooper et al., 2010; Practice Committee of the ASRM, 2015b). It is an easy, noninvasive test, and 2 to 3 days of abstinence, before collection, is optimum. Semen can be collected by means of masturbation into a specimen container or via intercourse with the use of a special semen collection condom that is chemical free so as not to interfere with sperm viability (Cooper et al., 2010; Practice Committee of

the ASRM, 2015b). The specimen should be taken to the laboratory for semen analysis within 1 hour of ejaculation. Sperm volume, concentration, motility, morphology, pH, and cellularity are evaluated. The sperm parameters that have been suggested to predict male fertility include a sperm count of 48 million/mL, sperm motility greater than 63%, and sperm morphology greater than 12% normal forms, set by strict criteria for evaluation (Cooper et al., 2010; Practice Committee of the ASRM, 2015b; WHO, 2010). Healthcare providers must proceed with caution, though, as there is evidence suggesting that some men with an optimal semen analysis may be infertile, while those with a suboptimal analysis may be fertile. Hence, semen analysis alone has not proved to be a powerful discriminator when evaluating male infertility (Cooper et al., 2010; Guzick et al., 2001; Practice Committee of the ASRM, 2015b; WHO, 2010). Clients with semen analyses that do not fall within normal laboratory reference ranges should be referred to a urologist for further testing, including endocrine evaluation, postejaculatory urinalysis, ultrasonography (e.g., transrectal, scrotal), and specialized clinical tests on semen and sperm (e.g., quantification of leukocytes, antisperm antibodies, sperm viability, and DNA fragmentation tests; Cooper et al., 2010; Practice Committee of the ASRM, 2015b). Genetic screening may also be warranted and may include (a) testing for cystic fibrosis gene mutations, (b) karyotypic chromosomal abnormalities (e.g., Klinefelter syndrome, inversion, and balanced translocations), (c) Y-chromosome microdeletions, and (d) chromosome aneuploidy (Cooper et al., 2010; Guzick et al., 2001; Practice Committee of the ASRM, 2015b).

MANAGEMENT OF INFERTILE COUPLES

Diagnostics

Testing should be performed simultaneously on both members of the couple. The approach should be systematic, focusing on the processes previously identified during health assessment. As with all diagnostics, testing should begin with the least invasive and move to more invasive. Preconception evaluation may be done at this time as it can be used for diagnostic and therapeutic counseling. Preconception evaluation includes blood type and Rh, rubella status, cystic fibrosis screening, chlamydia and gonorrhea screening, and Pap smear collection. Diagnostic testing is divided into three categories: (a) semen analysis, (b) ovulatory function and reserve, and (c) tubal patency (Practice Committee of the ASRM, 2015a, 2015b).

1. *Semen analysis.* Semen analysis is used to determine whether or not there is a male factor attributed to the couple's infertility. Sperm quantity, motility, and morphology are measured. Proper sperm collection is critical. The specimen should be collected within 2 hours of drop off after abstaining from ejaculation for 2 to 3 days and must be maintained at body temperature. On ejaculation, the specimen should be collected in a sterile container. Once the specimen has arrived in the laboratory, the sperm is *washed* and the ejaculate is separated (e.g., prostaglandins and seminal fluid). This procedure concentrates the amount of motile sperm by

removing cellular debris (Practice Committee of the ASRM, 2020). If a male factor is suspected, referral for evaluation by a urologist is recommended.

2a. *Assessment of ovulatory function.* Forty percent of infertility in women is attributable to ovulatory disorders (Mosher & Pratt, 1991). Of those women who regularly menstruate, approximately 95% to 98% experience ovulatory cycles. Nonovulatory cycles are usually the cause for irregular menstrual cycles and, thus, require further evaluation. A laboratory assessment of ovulation should be performed in women who do not have grossly abnormal menstrual cycles (Practice Committee of the ASRM, 2015a). A mid-luteal-phase progesterone level will establish ovulation approximately 1 week before the expected menses. A progesterone level greater than 3 ng/mL is consistent with ovulation (Practice Committee of the ASRM, 2015a).

Ovulation predictor kits (OPKs) are another reliable method to monitor and measure amount and level of LH in urine, which begins to rise approximately 12 to 24 hours before ovulation (McGovern et al., 2004). OPKs improve intercourse timing as they are used to prospectively predict ovulation and allow for planning versus basal body temperature, which predicts ovulation retrospectively (McGovern et al., 2004). Daily ultrasound exams used to follow the development and eventually the disappearance of a follicle (most accurate method of documenting ovulation), and endometrial biopsy (provides information about the secretory changes of the endometrium) are too expensive or invasive to use for routine diagnostic assessment of ovulation. Clients requiring this level of diagnostic testing should be referred to a reproductive endocrinologist (RE; ASRM, 2018; Practice Committee of the ASRM, 2015a).

2b. *Assessment of ovarian reserve.* Decreased ovarian reserve refers to decreased oocyte quality, quantity, or reproductive potential. Many screening tests are utilized; however, there is *no highly reliable, single test* used for predicting pregnancy potential. Ovarian reserve can be assessed by measuring FSH and estradiol (E_2) on cycle day 2 or 3. FSH values greater than 10 to 20 IU suggest decreased reserve and deceased fertility potential, while FSH values less than 20 IU are predictive of a decrease in fertility (Practice Committee of the ASRM, 2015a).

Tarun et al. (2004) conducted a meta-analysis in which the clomiphene citrate challenge test (CCCT) and basal FSH were used to determine the ovarian reserve. In their study, basal FSH serums were measured on cycle days 2, 3, or 4. Clomiphene citrate 50 to 100 mg was given on days 5 to 9 of the menstrual cycle, with a basal FSH obtained on days 3 and 10. The FSH response to the stimulation of the ovary, due to the clomiphene, determines the ovarian function. The test is considered abnormal if the FSH is found to be elevated on either day, which is translated into a poor prognosis of fertility (Tarun et al., 2004). The CCCT is costlier than a single, basal FSH level and is associated with greater inconvenience and potential side effects. Overall, the study concluded that basal FSH and CCCT were statistically similar in predicting the fecundability of a woman. However, having a "normal" result was less valuable (meaning that it did not guarantee that the woman could conceive); whereas an "abnormal" result was significantly valuable (meaning that it nearly guaranteed that pregnancy will not occur without medical intervention; Tarun et al., 2004). These diagnostic tests should be performed in women with suspected POF or early menopause.

Present-day use of CCCT has decreased as serum antral follicular count (AFC) and antiMüllerian hormone (AMH) markers for ovarian reserve are less time-consuming and are sensitive in predicting ovarian response (Practice Committee of the ASRM, 2015a). Antral follicles are immature follicles on the ovary measuring 2 to 10 mm in diameter. Transvaginal ultrasound is performed on cycle days 2 and 4 to measure the antral follicle counts by calculating the number of antral follicles on both ovaries. An antral follicle count between 4 and 10 is considered a low result and can be correlated with decreased ovarian reserve. Despite being a good predictor of ovarian reserve, AFC is a weak predictor of oocyte quality, response to artificial reproductive technology, or pregnancy outcome (Hsu et al., 2011).

AMH is secreted by the small (less than 8 mm) preantral and early antral follicles (Dewailly et al., 2014). Because AMH is determined by the preantral and early antral follicles, the primordial follicle pool is being measured and, therefore, is theoretically the best biochemical marker of ovarian function. AMH gradually declines as the woman ages and the primordial pool declines. AMH is undetectable at menopause (Hsu et al., 2011). It is believed that AMH may play an especially important role when determining fertility potential and the need for possible cryopreservation in special patient populations, such as cancer patients and those with a history of ovarian injury either from radiation or surgery. AMH is used in in vitro fertilization (IVF) to measure the number of oocytes to be retrieved after stimulation, or to diagnose ovarian hyperstimulation (Dewailly et al., 2014). AMH levels are laboratory dependent and healthcare providers should reference their own laboratory's reference range.

3. *Assessment of uterine cavity and tubal patency.* As discussed earlier in this chapter, testing should progress from least to most invasive. Therefore, assessment of the uterine cavity and tubal patency should be performed only after the confirmation of ovulation and evaluation of semen analysis. Evaluation of the uterine cavity and tubal patency can be done through hysterosalpingography (HSG), ultrasound, sonohystogram, hysteroscopy, and laparoscopy. An HSG is performed by a physician and/or radiologist under fluoroscopy. The procedure highlights tubal patency or occlusion as well as uterine cavity abnormalities. A history of PID is most often the cause of tubal occlusion (Coppus et al., 2007). Uterine abnormalities that can be diagnosed (but not treated) include uterine septum, polyps, and submucosal myomas. HSG can be used to diagnose proximal or distal tubal occlusion, salpingitis isthmica nodosa, and rule in or out tubal structure abnormality (Practice Committee of the ASRM, 2015a).

HSGs are performed in the midfollicular phase of the cycle—approximately 2 to 3 days after menstrual flow has stopped (Wass et al., 2014). Ideally, HSGs are scheduled before an intrauterine insemination (IUI) or induction of ovulation in cases of unexplained infertility, as studies show that the performance of an HSG increases fertility in subsequent months (Panchal & Nagori, 2014; Practice Committee of the ASRM, 2015a, 2020). Pain and cramping can be controlled with a mild analgesic or prostaglandin synthesis inhibitor, administered orally, approximately 30 to 40 minutes before the HSG (Practice Committee of the ASRM, 2015a). It is important to note that HSG cannot be performed if there is tenderness palpated on bimanual exam (Practice Committee of the ASRM, 2015a). HSG has clear diagnostic value; however, whether there is a true therapeutic value remains controversial (Practice Committee of the ASRM, 2015a). It is generally thought that HSG increases fertility potential by opening the tubes from the mechanical lavage of the dye, dislodging mucus plugs, and breaking down peritoneal adhesions. It is believed that HSG may also stimulate the cilia within the lumen of the tubes, thereby increasing the transit time of the oocyte (Panchal & Nagori, 2014; Practice Committee of the ASRM, 2015a).

Transvaginal ultrasonography is used as an initial evaluation in detecting uterine or ovarian abnormalities (Practice Committee of the ASRM, 2015a). If an abnormality is found or suspected on HSG or ultrasound, a sonohysterogram should be performed. Sonohysterography uses transvaginal ultrasonography and injection of saline into the uterine cavity for the examination of the uterus. The uterine cavity is then highlighted on ultrasound and there is greater sensitivity in the ability to differentiate between fibroids that are submucous versus intramural fibroids (Practice Committee of the ASRM, 2015a).

Some types of uterine pathology (e.g., uterine polyps, fibroids, septa) require direct visualization inside the uterus for diagnosis and treatment. For such pathology, hysteroscopy can be performed (Panshy et al., 2006). During a hysteroscopy, a small tool-operative hysteroscope is placed through the cervix into the uterine cavity. The uterine cavity is filled with a warm, lactated Ringer solution to enhance visualization and facilitate treatment. The patient is given local anesthesia and sedation or may be placed under light general anesthesia (Panshy et al., 2006).

Asherman syndrome is a gynecologic disorder that involves changes in menstrual pattern due to intrauterine adhesions most often secondary to dilatation and curettage (D&C) and infections of the endometrium (e.g., PID; National Organization for Rare Disorders [NORD], 2021). Treatment of Asherman syndrome is performed either with hysteroscopy or a combination of laparoscopy and hysteroscopy (NORD, 2021).

Unexplained Infertility

Peritoneal factors, endometriosis, and/or adnexal adhesions must be considered when all other diagnoses have been ruled out. As the healthcare provider begins to rule out diagnoses based on the patient's history, physical examination, and diagnostic evaluation, this information, in itself, is not sufficient for diagnosis (Practice Committee of the ASRM, 2015a). For example, in the most severe stages of endometriosis (stages 3 and 4), ultrasonography may be able to identify an endometrioma, but again, it is not diagnostic (Bulletti et al., 2010). Direct visualization is required to make a diagnosis of endometriosis or adnexal adhesion during laparoscopy (Bulletti et al., 2010; Hsu et al., 2010). However, mild endometriosis (stages 1 and 2) has minimal impact on fertility. Most women who have significant adnexal adhesions or stage 3 and 4 endometriosis will have risk factors such as pelvic pain, previous pelvic infection or surgery, or an abnormal HSG (Bulletti et al., 2010). Laparoscopy is indicated for these select individuals when treatment of disease may provide benefit to potential fertility. It is not used routinely for evaluation of infertility (Practice Committee of the ASRM, 2015a), and there is no existing evidence to support superior results related to its use in the treatment of endometriosis (Bulletti et al., 2010). For cases of failed laparoscopic treatment and/or failed medical treatment, assisted reproductive technology (ART), technology used to achieve pregnancy (e.g., fertility medication, artificial insemination [IVF]) is appropriate as the next step to enable fertility (ASRM, 2018).

Unexplained infertility (UI) is a *definition of exclusion* made in the presence of a normal assessment of ovulation, evaluation of uterotubal function, and semen analysis. The incidence of UI is about 30% in infertile couples (Nardo & Chouliaras, 2015). Because of the nature of UI, treatment is usually targeted at ovulation induction on clomiphene citrate or FSH combined with IUI or ART. In the event of failure, gamete intrafallopian transfer (GIFT), IVF, and/or IVF with intracytoplasmic sperm injection (ICSI) must be discussed with the couple (Guzick et al., 1998).

TREATMENT AND MANAGEMENT

Treatment of Oligomenorrhea or Anovulation

Oligomenorrhea and anovulation can lead to infertility. Oligomenorrhea is light or infrequent menstruation, whereas anovulation is the failure of the ovary to release ova over a period (ACOG, 2023b). There are three categories of medications that are used to treat oligomenorrhea and anovulation. These medications are targeted for inducing ovulation.

CLOMIPHENE CITRATE (CLOMID)

This oral medication is a selective estrogen receptor modulator (SERM) with both estrogen antagonist and agonist properties, thus increasing gonadotropin release. Clomiphene citrate is indicated only for the treatment of WHO Class 2 ovulation disorders (Legro et al., 2014). Treatment typically begins on cycle day 5, and continues through day 9, with Food and Drug Administration (FDA)-approved dosages ranging from 50 to 150 mg/day (Legro et al., 2014). Approximately 50% of women will ovulate on 50 mg of clomiphene citrate (Practice Committee of the ASRM, 2017). The dosage can be increased in subsequent cycles, up to 100 mg daily, for 5 days in women who fail with 50 mg (Practice Committee of the

ASRM, 2017). The maximum dose is 200 mg daily, for 5 days (Practice Committee of the ASRM, 2017); however, close following of follicular development is needed at this dosage range. Referral to an RE specialist should be considered if a couple fails to achieve conception (Practice Committee of the ASRM, 2017).

Ovulation can be determined with home OPKs, serum midluteal phase progesterone levels, or serial ultrasound exams measuring follicular development. The reported side effects include vasomotor flushes and abdominal discomfort (because of ovarian stimulation), breast tenderness, nausea, vomiting, nervousness, insomnia, and visual symptoms (Practice Committee of the ASRM, 2017). Symptoms do not appear to be dose dependent. The patient should be informed that a fairly common side effect of clomiphene citrate therapy is the antiestrogenic effect on the uterus and cervix. This effect can result in a decrease in the quantity and quality of cervical mucus, as well as a thinning of the endometrium (Practice Committee of the ASRM, 2017).

The success rate of ovulation induction with clomiphene therapy is approximately 80% and the pregnancy success rate is approximately 30%—with most of the pregnancies occurring in the first three ovulatory cycles. There is a less than 10% chance for multiple gestations, and should it occur, most multiple gestations will result in a twin gestation (Practice Committee of the ASRM, 2012). There is no association with clomiphene therapy and increased congenital abnormalities. To date, there has been no correlation between ovarian stimulation and increased risk for endometrial or colorectal cancer (ASRM, 2014b).

AROMATASE INHIBITORS

Aromatase inhibitors (AIs) are most widely used for the treatment of breast cancer and prevention of recurrence. In regard to infertility, AIs have been proved to be effective when treating women with WHO Class 2 ovulatory disorders (those women who have failed to respond to clomiphene or those who have a thin endometrium; Practice Committee of the ASRM, 2017). The mechanism of action for AIs is the inhibition of aromatase (Practice Committee of the ASRM, 2017). If given during early follicular development, AIs prevent the usual negative feedback from estradiol on the hypothalamopituitary axis, thus causing an increase in gonadotropin release by the pituitary (primarily FSH; Legro et al., 2014). Their administration is typically done in doses between 2.5 and 5 mg/day, cycle days 3 and 7 (Practice Committee of the ASRM, 2017).

Their overall side effects are well tolerated, but can include hot flashes, nausea, vomiting, and leg cramps (Practice Committee of the ASRM, 2017). There are advantages to using AIs instead of clomiphene for induction of ovulation. When using AIs, there is a reduced number of follicles produced, thus decreasing the risk of multiples during gestation. Furthermore, AIs have a shorter half-life (50 hours vs. days), resulting in less antiestrogenic effect on the endometrium and cervical mucus (Legro et al., 2014). Studies have shown that the resulting pregnancy rates may be higher, and with fewer miscarriages, with AI use as compared to clomiphene citrate (Legro et al., 2014). AIs have been proved equally safe when compared to clomiphene citrate (Practice Committee of the ASRM, 2017).

GONADOTROPINS

Follicular development is induced in women who are anovulatory or who are being treated with ART by gonadotropins. Agents include recombinant, FSH, or human menopausal gonadotropins combined with FSH and LH. There are many different protocols that are available and vary based on healthcare provider experience and evidence. Success rates, which range from 20% to 60%, are determined by the woman's age and fertility. Management of gonadotropins requires specialized laboratory and radiological availability. Therefore, because of the highly specialized nature of follow-up, management extends well beyond the scope of a primary healthcare provider's scope (ASRM, 2012; Practice Committee of the ASRM, 2017).

Gonadotropin-Releasing Hormone Analogs

GnRH agonists bind to the GnRH receptors that are located in the pituitary. This binding effect causes an initial rise in both FSH and LH (known as the *flare effect*), but with continued binding, downregulation of the GnRH occurs, causing suppression of the pituitary gonadotropin release, thereby preventing the LH surge and ovulation (Practice Committee of the ASRM, 2017). GnRH antagonists competitively bind to the GnRH receptors located in the anterior pituitary, suppressing the LH surge and, thereby, preventing ovulation (Practice Committee of the ASRM, 2017). GnRH agonists and antagonists are used simultaneously with AIs or gonadotropin ovulation induction to control ovulation and allow for more follicular development in the ovary during one stimulation cycle. Studies show that cycles that involve the use of GnRH agonists or antagonists have higher success rates (Practice Committee of the ASRM, 2017).

Human Chorionic Gonadotropin

Human chorionic gonadotropin (hCG) stimulates the LH surge that causes ovulation at midcycle (Practice Committee of the ASRM, 2017). The molecular structure of hCG is identical to that of LH, and therefore, it can "trigger" ovulation if given exogenously. hCG is given 32 to 38 hours before the desired ovulation time. Healthcare providers should note that a pregnancy test will be falsely positive if taken 10 days or less after hCG administration (Practice Committee of the ASRM, 2017).

INTERVENTIONS FOR INFERTILITY

Intrauterine Insemination

IUI is theoretically grounded in the belief that the likelihood of fertilization is increased when a large number of sperm are placed high in the reproductive tract. The procedure involves the placement of motile, concentrated sperm directly into the uterine cavity (Practice Committee of the ASRM, 2020). In order for IUI to be performed (a) a woman's cycle must be ovulatory; (b) there must be at least one patent fallopian tube; (c) an adequate number of sperm must be available at hand; and (d) there can be no suspicion or evidence of cervical, uterine, or pelvic infection (Practice Committee of the ASRM, 2020). Although most women experience cramping, IUI is usually well tolerated. IUI is known to increase the likelihood of pregnancy when used in conjunction with clomiphene and gonadotropins (Practice Committee of the ASRM, 2017).

DONOR INSEMINATION

Some diagnoses require insemination with donor sperm. Indications for donor insemination (DI) include azoospermia, low sperm count, abnormal sperm motility/morphology, absence of testes and/or vas deferens, antisperm antibodies, and previous vasectomy (Guzick et al., 2001; WHO, 2010). Couples may also choose to use DI when (a) there is a personal or family history of genetic disease or birth defect, (b) an individual is serodiscordant for sexually transmitted viruses (Sauer et al., 2009), (c) the patient is a woman without a male partner (ASRM, 2015), and/or (d) an individual has hemolytic disease. Donors are blood typed and screened for STIs, cytomegalovirus, Tay-Sachs disease, thalassemia, and sickle cell disease. Donor matching is performed to ensure compatibility in donor and female patient characteristics. More and more, IVF and ICSI are the choice of treatment because of successful conception rates, as compared to DI (Practice Committee of the ASRM, 2020). There have been no studies that show an increase in spontaneous abortion or birth defect rates when compared with spontaneous conception (Practice Committee of the ASRM, 2020).

Assisted Reproductive Technologies

ART is a complex procedure that is usually conducted by an RE specialist (ASRM, 2018). This section is a brief overview of the procedure and is presented through the lens of patient counseling. As such, a discussion on the technique/procedure and follow-up is limited. ART now consists of a conglomerate of all techniques involved with the direct retrieval of oocytes from the ovary. These technologies have expanded exponentially over the last 10 years. They include (a) GIFT, (b) zygote intrafallopian transfer (ZIFT), (c) IVF, and (d) ICSI. Sperm aspiration techniques include (a) testicular sperm extractions (TESE) and (b) microsurgical epididymal sperm aspiration (MESA; ASRM, 2018). In 2018, the live birth rate for each ART cycle initiated by age was 13.2% for women aged 41-42 years as compared to 55.1% for women younger than 35 years of age (Lee & Zhang, 2022).

OOCYTE RETRIEVAL

Serial measurements of follicular development with transvaginal ultrasound and serum estradiol are used to monitor ovarian stimulation. Once determined by a RE that retrieval is necessary, a transvaginal, ultrasound-guided aspiration technique is used. Oocyte retrieval takes approximately 30 minutes and is performed approximately 34 to 36 hours after hCG (trigger) administration (ASRM & Society for Assisted Reproductive Technology [SART], 2013). Although bleeding and/or infection are noted complications, they are uncommon (ASRM & SART, 2013; Spaan et al., 2016).

PRESERVATION OF EMBRYOS

The preservation of embryos has become a great concern given the ability to aspirate multiple follicles during retrieval. The ASRM promotes singleton gestation, reduction of twin gestations, and the elimination of high-order multiple gestations (≥3 fetuses). In support of this, guidance was developed to assist both clinicians and patients in determining the number of cleavage-stage embryos or blastocysts transferred (Practice Committee of the ASRM & SART, 2021). In patients determined to have a favorable prognosis, guidance for transfer of a euploid embryo should be limited to one (regardless of patient age). In patients 39 to 40 years of age, no more than three untested cleavage-stage embryos or 2 blastocysts should be transferred. Patients 41 to 42 years of age should not receive more than four untested cleavage-stage embryos or three blastocysts (Practice Committee of the ASRM & SART, 2021). Unused extra embryos can be cryopreserved for later use. However, because of the delicate nature of embryos, only two thirds survive the freezing and thawing process. Of those that do survive, a significant increase in success rate is noted as the "durability" of the embryo is proven (Practice Committee of the ASRM & SART, 2021).

GAMETE INTRAFALLOPIAN TRANSFER

GIFT is a modified version of IVF. This procedure is indicated for couples without fallopian tube pathology and a normal sperm count. During GIFT, oocytes are retrieved from the ovaries and the washed sperm laparoscopically placed directly into the fallopian tubes using a transfer catheter (ASRM, 2018). Individuals may choose GIFT over IVF (e.g., religious beliefs) as GIFT relies on the body's biological processes to produce a pregnancy (ASRM, 2018).

ZYGOTE INTRAFALLOPIAN TRANSFER

ZIFT is a variation of GIFT with distinct differences: (a) fertilization occurs in vitro, after oocyte retrieval from the ovaries; (b) ejaculated or surgically retrieved sperm are washed and approximately 50,000 sperm are placed around each (ASRM, 2018); and (c) the fertilized egg, a zygote, is then transferred into the fallopian tubes laparoscopically. The goal is to achieve fertilization naturally. ZIFT procedures constitute approximately 1% of total ART (ASRM, 2018).

IN VITRO FERTILIZATION

To date, 99% of all ART is performed using IVF (ASRM & SART, 2013). Since its introduction in the United States in 1981, IVF has grown exponentially. According to archives, more than 500,000 babies were born in the United States as a result of ART (GIFT, ZIFT, IVF, or a combination) between 1985 and 2007 (ASRM & SART, 2013). By 2011, 36% of all fresh, nondonor ART cycles resulted in pregnancy and 29% resulted in a live birth (Sunderam et al., 2015). In the general population, and as a result of advances in ART, a single IVF cycle now has a higher fecundability (29%) as compared to a natural conception cycle (27.7%; Luke et al., 2012). The average cost of an IVF cycle in the United States is $12,000; medications run an additional $3,000 to $5,000 (Sunderam et al., 2015). Couples with the following diagnoses qualify for IVF: failed conservative therapy, male factor infertility, multifactorial infertility, tubal endometrial factor infertility, advanced maternal age, declining ovarian reserve or ovarian failure (requiring donor eggs), uterine factor (requiring surrogacy), genetic abnormalities, and history of recurrent miscarriage (ASRM, 2018; Practice Committee of the ASRM & SART, 2021).

ADVANCED TECHNIQUES FOR HARVESTING SPERM

Sperm Aspiration

Viable sperm is attainable for men diagnosed with azoospermia (no sperm), low-motility sperm, or dead sperm through sperm aspiration (Guzick et al., 2001). If a blockage develops in the male reproductive tract, causing sperm to be trapped in the epididymis, obstructive azospermia occurs. If there is impaired/nonexistent sperm production, nonobstructive azospermia is diagnosed. In either obstructive or nonobstructive azoospermia, ICSI must be used to facilitate fertilization and aspiration (Practice Committee of the ASRM, 2015b). The following is a discussion about the three, sperm-harvesting techniques used to obtain sperm from men with obstructive azospermia.

MICROSURGICAL EPIDIDYMAL SPERM ASPIRATION

Sperm can be aspirated using the MESA technique in men who have a congenital absence of the vas deferens or have had a vasectomy. Minimal complications are noted and MESA is considered safe when performed by a provider specialized in microsurgery (Practice Committee of the ASRM, 2015b).

TESTICULAR SPERM EXTRACTION

Men who have nonobstructive azoospermia can have TESE performed. During TESE, testicular tissue is removed and sperm is retrieved from within the seminiferous tubules. This can also be an alternative option for men with obstructive azospermia (ASRM, 2018; Practice Committee of the ASRM, 2015b). Freezing and storing can be used to preserve sperm that can be used for a later date (as with other aspiration techniques; ASRM, 2018; Practice Committee of the ASRM, 2015b).

INTRACYTOPLASMIC SPERM INJECTION

ICSI is indicated in cases of severe male factor infertility. With ICSI, a mature sperm (single) is isolated and injected directly into the oocyte with the use of a microneedle in an attempt to attain fertilization. Fertilization rates, using ICSI, are approximately 50% to 80% (ASRM, 2018; Practice Committee of the ASRM, 2015b).

OOCYTES AND GENETICS

Preimplantation Genetic Diagnosis

Preimplantation genetic diagnosis (PGD) is a reproductive technology used with an IVF cycle. Specifically, the procedure involves removing a cell from an IVF embryo for genetic testing before transferring the embryo to the uterus. PGD can also be used for prenatal aneuploidy screening and the diagnosis of chromosomal abnormalities (e.g., translocations, inversions; ACOG, 2023c; Genetics & IVF Institute, n.d.). For example, when one of the parents is a known translocation carrier, PGD testing helps to reduce the risk of spontaneous abortion. The ASRM does not recommend the use of PGD for the purpose of sex selection or any nonmedical reason as it poses an ethical dilemma (Ethics Committee of the American Society for Reproductive Medicine, 2015).

Oocyte Donation

Using donated oocytes can be a highly effective infertility treatment for women (a) who are older than 35 years, (b) have experienced POF, (c) are younger and have failed to achieve a pregnancy with IVF using their own oocytes, and/or (d) with poor-quality oocytes (ASRM & SART, 2021). The success rate of oocyte donation is approximately 55% (ASRM & SART, 2021; CDC, 2015a; Ethics Committee of the American Society for Reproductive Medicine, 2013c). The selection criteria for gamete donors are narrow. They include women (a) younger than 28 years, and (b) who meet established criteria (e.g., physical, medical, and psychological health; ASRM & SART, 2021).

With oocyte donation, the partner's sperm is used to fertilize the oocyte. The fertilized embryo is then placed into the recipient. The recipient is then given medication to enhance the endometrium to ensure adequate lining, ideally less than 6 mm (ASRM & SART, 2021). As per any IVF protocol, only one or two embryos are placed and extra embryos are frozen to be used, as needed, for future cycles (ASRM & SART, 20213b). Concern about gamete donation, compensation, and informed consent among other ethical dilemmas are addressed by the ASRM and are found in a committee opinion labeled, *Recommendations for Gamete and Embryo Donation: A Committee Opinion* (ASRM & SART, 2021).

MENTAL HEALTH AND WELL-BEING OF THE INFERTILE COUPLE

The mental health of the couple is equally important for healthcare providers to address during fertility therapy. In cases of infertility, conception cannot be controlled, and if the couple is unable to achieve pregnancy, it is often internalized by the couple as a *failure*. Together, the loss of control of one's reproductive capabilities and this sense of failure can make for the *perfect storm* that can lead to anger, sadness, despair, jealousy of others, and depression. Healthcare providers must address the couple's mental health. For example, it is not uncommon for men to feel that they cannot be sad as they have to be strong for their female partner. Counseling is often needed to guide the couple through grief, encourage communication and healing, and to avoid resentment, which is often directed at the other partner. As with other causes of grief-filled experiences, couples and individuals find solace and comfort when surrounded by those with similar life experiences. RESOLVE, an infertility support group, offers counseling, group meetings, and anonymous online support. There are local chapters across the United States. Meetings are held regularly addressing support through infertility and/or loss. The link to the RESOLVE website is www.resolve.org.

Society views conception through sexual intercourse as an intimate exchange between two individuals. ART and infertility remove the intimacy and spontaneity of procreation, making it purposeful, calculated, and technical. Male partners often feel pressured to "perform." Conception is now a medical therapy or treatment. Using therapeutic communication, couples can be reassured that they are not alone in their discomfort and are allowed the space to express their feelings (e.g., resentment toward the process).

It is important for the healthcare provider to be sensitive and empathetic to possible triggers that may negatively impact the infertile couple. For example, holidays, baby showers, Mother's and Father's Day celebrations, and pregnancy announcements from friends can cause undue stress and add more burden to the already burdened couple. Screening tools are available to aid the healthcare provider when screening for depression. Healthcare providers must assess for stress. The following questions can be used to assess stress and depression in couples challenged with infertility (Domar et al., 2015):

- Do you feel uncomfortable being around pregnant women and/or children/babies?
- Do you find that you try to avoid situations where there may be pregnant women and/or small children/babies?
- Is your sexual relationship very satisfying, satisfying, or dissatisfying? If dissatisfying, do you feel that your infertility has led to a negative impact on your sex life?
- Do you only make love during the fertile times of your cycle?
- Do you feel that you and your partner mostly agree about how to proceed with infertility treatment?
- Do you feel that your partner is sympathetic and supportive of you?
- How is your mood? How have you been feeling? Are you able to enjoy your usual activities?
- Are you worried? Do you have difficulty concentrating or sleeping? Are you restless?
- Has your appetite changed?

The need to provide infertile couples with a safe place to express their feelings, both as a couple and individually, cannot be overstated. Some couples do not feel comfortable sharing their infertility with others, and can hold all emotions inside, concealing their journey. Couples must be allowed to cry, yell, scream, mourn, grieve, and to be frustrated. Healthcare providers can refer couples to trained therapists well versed in infertility.

REPRODUCTIVE TECHNOLOGIES AND ETHICS

Reproductive technology is increasingly gaining the public's attention. What was previously considered rare is now becoming normalized. Women and couples are seeking care before attempting pregnancy, concerned that they are infertile. Healthcare providers must ensure that they are using a systematic, clinical approach when caring for individuals with infertility. Sensitivity to cost and avoidance of undue procedures are important. If the prognosis for conception is poor, realistic expectations should be shared with the woman and/or couple. It is critical to portend a false sense of hope. Fertility centers must be transparent and give full disclosure as to

their success rates before treatment (Ethics Committee of the American Society for Reproductive Medicine, 2012a).

Because of the high cost of fertility treatments, family gamete donors/surrogates are becoming more popular. Counseling must be strongly recommended to avoid ethical and moral dilemmas (Ethics Committee of the American Society for Reproductive Medicine, 2012b). However, consanguineous gamete donations from a first-degree relative is unacceptable and goes against medical advice because of an increased risk of birth defects (Ethics Committee of the American Society for Reproductive Medicine, 2012b). Because of the sensitive nature, couples must consider if their resulting children will be informed of the method of their conception. If disclosure to the child is desired, when should the child be told? How much information should be shared with the child? When is the right time for disclosure? All parties should agree in advance to avoid misinformation, misunderstanding, hurt feelings, and anger. The ultimate decision rests with the parent(s) (Ethics Committee of the American Society for Reproductive Medicine, 2013b).

The determination of what to do with unused embryos poses another dilemma. Should they be donated to couples unable to fertilize embryos, or should they be used for embryonic stem cell research (Ethics Committee of the American Society for Reproductive Medicine, 2013a)? Since the introduction of IVF, this question has prompted conflicting options. According to the ASRM Ethics Committee, it is considered ethically acceptable to use unused embryos for embryonic stem cell research if that research is likely to yield beneficial information that improves human health. Such research should be conducted with supreme respect for the embryo(s).

Compensation for gamete donation/surrogacy is referred to earlier in the chapter; however, it is important to note that this also poses an ethical dilemma. PGD used for the purpose of gender selection and family balancing is unethical (Practice Committee of the ASRM, 2015a). Most fertility centers do not offer PGD unless it is used for the purpose of screening for X-linked disorders (Ethics Committee of the American Society for Reproductive Medicine, 2015).

As discussed earlier in the chapter, selection criteria for gamete donation are extensive. The donor's health history should be available should unforeseen circumstances arise. Ethical questions may arise once genetic information is made available. Should the donors be notified of genetic disorders found? Should the offspring be informed of new diagnoses that could potentially negatively impact their health (Ethics Committee of the American Society for Reproductive Medicine, 2013b)? These questions remain unanswered. Counseling is critical throughout the entire PGD process.

FERTILITY CONSIDERATIONS FOR SPECIAL POPULATIONS

Cancer Survivors

Fertility preservation and reproduction are a major concern in cancer patients (ASRM, 2014a). Improvement in cancer therapies has led to a decrease in morbidity and mortality rates. It is not unusual for many women, ages 20 to 49 years, diagnosed with cancer, to have excellent (5–10 years) survival times (ASRM, 2014a). Successful treatment in younger patients may lead to reduced fertility; this varies and is dependent on the age at diagnosis as well as the type of cancer and treatment. Before the initiation of cancer treatment, and if damage to the reproductive organs is unavoidable, cryopreservation of gametes, embryos, and/or gonadal tissue may be suggested by the healthcare provider. Techniques for freezing oocytes and ovarian tissue should be considered. Individuals who have their gametes, embryos, and/or tissues cryopreserved and stored must provide very specific directions for future disposition (ASRM, 2014a). Another issue to consider is whether the offspring of these patients are at an increased risk of congenital abnormalities, chromosomal defects, or cancer—as a result of any cancer treatment(s) or effects from ART. No significant increases in congenital malformations or cancer in the resulting offspring have been demonstrated (ASRM, 2014a). Infertility after cancer certainly can increase the likelihood of stress, loss, and anger (ASRM, 2014a).

LGBTQ+ Family Building Through Artificial Reproductive Technology

As the science of reproductive technology evolves, so too do options for the LGBTQ+ community to bear children. According to data collected by the UCLA School of Law in 2018, there were 114,000 same-sex couples raising children in the United States. Of these, 25% were female same-sex couples and 8% were male same-sex couples. Thirty-seven percent of LGBTQ+ adults had a child at some point in their life. Currently, 68% of same-sex couples raising children are also a biological parent. Twenty-five percent of transgender individuals are parents (Amato et al., 2021). The aforementioned technologies can be used in many different circumstances depending on the individual couples' needs. However, healthcare discrimination and access to technologies create barriers for many families. A multidisciplinary approach is best to serve this community to the fullest, and healthcare professionals need to be aware of the common psychological, legal, and practical issues that LGBTQ+ patients face (Amato et al., 2021).

SUMMARY

When caring for the infertile couple, the goals of the healthcare provider are to (a) conduct a complete medical investigation, (b) treat abnormalities, (c) educate a couple as to their treatment choices, and when appropriate, (d) refer the couple to support services in the case of adoption. Advances in infertility treatment are occurring rapidly and it is challenging for the primary healthcare provider to stay abreast of the most advanced and appropriate treatment regimens for couples with fertility issues. The ASRM Practice Committee has established evidence-based guidelines to assist healthcare providers with best clinical practice recommendations (Practice Committee of the ASRM, 2015a, 2015b). Finally, the far-reaching social and psychological impact on couples experiencing infertility should not be minimized.

REFERENCES

References for this chapter are online and available at https://connect.springerpub.com/content/book/978-0-8261-6722-4/part/part03/chapter/ch24

CHAPTER 38

High-Risk Childbearing*

Heather S. Hubbard[†], Monica A. Lutgendorf[‡], and Stephanie N. Shivers[†]

The significant increase in maternal morbidity and mortality in the United States over the last few decades is alarming. More than 80% of maternal deaths in the United States are preventable (Centers for Disease Control and Prevention [CDC], 2022). This chapter on high-risk childbearing focuses on the factors that indicate a pregnancy is high risk and includes a comprehensive overview of the most common high-risk maternal and fetal conditions. In each factor, the epidemiology and prevalence, risk factors, diagnosis, and management are provided.

This content is meant to assist with anticipatory guidance to providing safe competent care to pregnant women. Evidence-based diagnostic studies and suggested management plans based on current national protocol/guidelines are also presented. This chapter concludes with professional recommendations.

HIGH-RISK PREGNANCY FACTORS

The development of a human being is complex and can be affected by many factors including the environment, genes, and exposures. The underlying etiology and timing of the exposure can affect the risk to the fetus and its development. Questions often arise regarding medications (including topical medications and over-the-counter medications, vitamins, and supplements) and exposures in pregnancy and while breastfeeding. Current information including resources for health professionals, patient information sheets and information about ongoing studies open for enrollment are available from the nonprofit Organization of Teratology Information Specialists (OTIS) at www.mothertobaby.org.

TERATOGENESIS AND EXPOSURES

Epidemiology and Prevalence

The background risk for having a baby with a birth defect is 3% to 5%. Teratology is the study of congenital anomalies, their etiology, and mechanisms of disease. Teratogens irreversibly alter the growth, structure, or function of the developing fetus. Teratogens can include medications, viruses, chemicals, and environmental factors. The principles of teratology relate to placental transfer of the agent, which depends on molecular weight, ionization and fat solubility, and pH. Potential effects on the fetus are related to the gestational age at exposure, route of administration, drug absorption, dose, maternal serum levels, maternal and placental clearance, genotype of the mother and fetus, and the method and time of testing (Buhimschi & Weiner, 2009). Many drugs have not been studied in pregnancy and have limited information on potential effects and safety. Thus, it is also important to consider maternal benefit from therapies, and ensure mothers taking necessary medications are on effective doses to ensure maternal benefit.

---

*This chapter is a revision of the chapter that appeared in the second edition of this textbook, authored by Marianne T. Stone-Godena, and we thank her for her original contribution.
[†]The opinions and assertions expressed herein are those of the author(s) and do not necessarily reflect the official policy or position of the Uniformed Services University or the Department of Defense.
[‡]The opinions and assertions expressed herein are those of the author(s) and do not necessarily reflect the official policy or position of the U.S. Air Force, Department of Defense, or the U.S. government.

Management

Risk assessment and management of pregnant or lactating women includes a thorough assessment of the maternal medication use or exposure, an assessment of ongoing exposure or benefit from a particular medication, and an individualized approach to recommendations for continued treatment. An assessment of the risks, benefits and alternatives should be conducted to determine the best course for each patient. The Reprotox resource provides summary information on the effects of medications and chemical agents on fertility, pregnancy, and lactation, and is available at www.reprotox.org.

PRENATAL SCREENING AND TESTING OPTIONS

Epidemiology and Prevalence

Population studies have reported a prevalence of chromosome abnormalities of 43.8/1,000 births. For the common trisomies, the prevalence was 23/10,000 births for trisomy 21 (Down syndrome), 5.9/10,000 births for trisomy 18 (Edward syndrome), and 2.3/10,000 births for trisomy 13 (Patau syndrome). Sex chromosome trisomies had a prevalence of 2/10,000 births, and 45,X (Turner syndrome) had a prevalence of 3.3/10,000 births (Wellesley et al., 2012). The incidence of chromosome abnormalities is higher in early gestation as it is a significant contributor to miscarriage, and the incidence of chromosome abnormalities increases with increasing maternal age, though all patients may be affected. The risk of having an affected child at the age of 20 is 1 in 1,250, and this risk increases to 1 in 86 at the age of 40 (American College of Obstetricians and Gynecologists [ACOG], 2020c).

Risk Factors

An increased risk of chromosome abnormalities is present with advancing maternal age, parental translocations, and prior affected pregnancies; such abnormalities may be detected during screening ultrasound exams or positive serum or cell-free DNA screening. Although there is increased risk of chromosome anomalies with advancing maternal age, pregnant persons of all ages should be offered the option for screening, diagnostic testing, or no testing/screening in early pregnancy (ACOG, 2020c).

Diagnosis

Prenatal testing should be discussed with all pregnant persons with the final decision for screening, diagnostic testing, or no testing to be based on the patient's values, beliefs, and desires for information balanced with the testing limitations and potential risks. The options for prenatal testing include screening (serum screening with or without nuchal translucency [NT] ultrasound or cell-free DNA screening) and diagnostic testing. Diagnostic testing gives patients an answer about whether their baby will have a chromosomal condition, while screening provides information on whether there is an increased chance of having a child affected by a condition. Provider counseling should focus on the risks and benefits of the procedures and how patients may choose to use the information from testing so that they may make a fully informed decision. Importantly, prenatal testing cannot identify all abnormalities in pregnancies, and there is a wide range of severity and clinical presentations for many conditions that cannot be predicted by genetic testing (ACOG, 2016a).

Screening testing may be performed in the first trimester, second trimester, or both, and can include ultrasound and/or laboratory tests. If patients desire screening, a single approach should be selected. Multiple simultaneous screening tests are not recommended. Adequate pretest and posttest counseling is important, and timely communication of both positive and negative screening results is important. *Cell-free DNA screening* may be performed at any time in the pregnancy after 9 to 10 weeks' gestation. The test analyzes cell-free DNA in the maternal blood, which is a mixture of maternal DNA and fetal DNA from apoptosis of placental trophoblasts. The detection rate for Down syndrome is 99%, and the test also screens for trisomy 18 (98% detection rate) and trisomy 13 (99% detection rate) as well as sex chromosome aneuploidies. The combined false-positive rate of the test is 0.13% (ACOG, 2020c). Though the test performs well for the common trisomies, false-negative and false-positive results can occur, and diagnostic testing (chorionic villous sampling [CVS], amniocentesis, or postnatal cord blood) is recommended for confirmation of results (ACOG, 2020c). Cell-free DNA tests that return with low fetal fraction have an increased rate of chromosome anomalies of approximately 3%. These patients should be offered diagnostic testing and counseling with maternal–fetal medicine or genetics counselors.

First trimester screening includes blood analytes with or without an NT ultrasound. The NT ultrasound is performed in the first trimester with a crown–rump length between 38–45 mm and 84 mm, which is between 10 and 14 weeks of gestation (ACOG, 2020c). The NT is a fluid-filled space on the back of the fetal neck. An enlarged NT (greater than 3 mm) is associated with fetal aneuploidy and structural anomalies such as congenital heart defects. Serum analytes include serum beta-human chorionic gonadotropin (β-hCG), pregnancy-associated plasma protein A (PAPP-A), and alpha-fetoprotein (AFP) levels. The risk estimate for trisomies 13, 18, and 21 are calculated using the analytes and maternal factors of age, aneuploidy history, weight, race and number of fetuses, and NT measurement (ACOG, 2020c).

Combined first and second trimester screening with integrated, sequential, or contingent screening provides a higher detection rate than one-step first or second trimester screening. *Integrated screening* includes a first trimester NT ultrasound with first trimester serum analytes followed by second trimester serum analytes with a single result in the second trimester. The detection rate is 96% for trisomy 21, with a 5% false-positive rate. If NT ultrasound is not available or not technically feasible, a *serum integrated screen* may be performed, with a detection rate for trisomy 21 of 88% with a 5% false-positive rate. *Stepwise sequential screening* includes an NT ultrasound and first trimester serum analytes with an initial risk assessment provided to the patient in the first trimester. If the first trimester screen is below the laboratory cutoff for positive screens, the patient receives the first trimester result, and completes second trimester screening to receive a final risk estimate. The detection rate for trisomy 21 is 95% with a false-positive rate of 5%. *Contingent screening* assigns risk as high, intermediate, or low based on the first trimester screening, with those at high risk offered additional testing with either cell-free DNA screening or diagnostic testing. Those at intermediate risk complete second trimester screening with a final aneuploidy risk calculation. The detection rate for trisomy 21 is 88% to 94% with a 5% false-positive rate.

Second trimester screening with the *quadruple marker screen* is performed between 15 and 22 weeks, and gives a risk assessment for trisomy 21, trisomy 18, and open fetal defects (spina bifida and gastroschisis). Serum analytes include hCG, AFP, dimeric inhibin A (DIA), and unconjugated estriol (uE3), which is combined with maternal factors of age, aneuploidy history, weight, race, number of fetuses and the presence of diabetes to give a risk assessment. The detection rate for trisomy 21 is 81% with a false-positive rate of 5%.

A short educational video for patient counseling is available at www.youtube.com/watch?v=-vIJGFWJquk. Such video education improves patients' knowledge and decreases testing and decisional conflict and decisional regret regarding testing (Stortz et al., 2021). All patients should be offered a second trimester ultrasound (typically performed between 18 and 22 weeks) as a screening for fetal structural defects regardless of their choice for aneuploidy screening, diagnostic testing, or no testing.

Diagnostic testing determines whether a specific genetic condition is present in the fetus. This is accomplished prenatally with either CVS or amniocentesis, or postnatally using neonatal blood. CVS is performed between 10 to 13 weeks' gestation by obtaining placental villi through transabdominal or transcervical sampling of the placenta (ACOG, 2016a). The procedure-related loss rate is estimated to be 0.22%, with the incidence of failed cell culture, amniotic fluid leakage, or infection less than 0.5% (ACOG, 2016a). The benefit to CVS is the earlier gestational age at which results are available. Amniocentesis is typically performed between 15 and 20 weeks' gestation, though it can be performed at later gestational ages. Amniocentesis involves removing a sample of amniotic fluid under ultrasound guidance. The procedure-related loss rate is approximately 0.1% to 0.3%, and the rate of minor complications such as vaginal spotting or amniotic leakage is approximately 1% to 2%, and failed cell culture occurs in 0.1% (ACOG, 2016a).

The available tests for prenatal genetic diagnosis include conventional karyotype, which can detect chromosomal abnormalities >5–10 Mb; chromosomal microarray, which can detect copy number variants >50–200 kb; and molecular DNA testing for genetic mutations present in a family or suspected based on ultrasound findings. Pretest and posttest counseling is recommended (ACOG, 2016a).

Management

Management depends on the final diagnosis as well as the patient's values, beliefs, and desires. Prenatal diagnosis allows patients to end a pregnancy early or continue the pregnancy with planning for postdelivery care. Specialized counseling including maternal–fetal medicine subspecialists and genetic counseling can be particularly helpful in cases with abnormal or complex testing results.

CARRIER SCREENING

Epidemiology and Prevalence

Carrier screening is genetic testing performed in individuals who do not have a specific disease condition but may be carriers of allele variants that may be associated with the condition in their offspring. Carrier screening and counseling should be offered to all pregnant persons, ideally prior to pregnancy as this allows patients to learn about their reproductive risk and consider all their reproductive options. Patients may decline any or all carrier screening. If patients are found to be a carrier for a genetic condition, their relatives are also at risk of carrying the same mutation. Their reproductive partner should be offered testing to obtain more information that could inform reproductive outcomes, and if both partners are carriers of a genetic condition, genetic counseling should be offered. Prenatal diagnosis and advanced reproductive technologies to decrease risk to an affected offspring should be discussed (ACOG, 2017a). Concurrent screening of both the patient and their partner is suggested if there are time constraints for decisions regarding prenatal diagnostic evaluation (ACOG, 2017a).

Risk Factors

Risk factors for inherited conditions depend on the condition in question and the patient's family history. A family history should be obtained for the patient and their reproductive partner, including ethnic background and any known consanguinity. If there is a positive family history of a specific genetic condition, genetic counseling should be offered. In these cases, genetic test results of the affected family member are helpful to screen the patient to ensure testing covers the familial mutation.

Diagnosis

Screening for spinal muscular atrophy and cystic fibrosis are recommended for all women who are considering pregnancy or are currently pregnant (ACOG, 2017a). Fragile X premutation carrier screening is recommended for women with a family history of fragile X–related disorders or intellectual disability suggestive of fragile X syndrome or unexplained ovarian insufficiency or elevated follicle-stimulating hormone level before age 40 and who are considering pregnancy or are currently pregnant. Screening for Tay-Sachs disease should be offered if either member of the couple is of Ashkenazi Jewish, French-Canadian, or Cajun descent, or with a family history consistent with Tay-Sachs disease and considering pregnancy or during pregnancy. A number of autosomal recessive conditions are more common in individuals of Ashkenazi Jewish (Eastern European and Central European) descent, and those individuals should be offered carrier screening for Canavan disease, cystic fibrosis, familial dysautonomia, and Tay-Sachs disease. Additional screening may be considered for the following disorders as well: Bloom syndrome, familial hyperinsulinism, Fanconi anemia, Gaucher disease, glycogen storage disease type I, Joubert syndrome, maple syrup urine disease, mucolipidosis type IV, Niemann-Pick disease, and Usher syndrome. Screening for hemoglobinopathies is accomplished with a complete blood count with red blood cell indices prior to pregnancy or in early pregnancy. Hemoglobin electrophoresis should be performed if there is concern for a possible hemoglobinopathy with a low mean corpuscular hemoglobin (MCH) or mean corpuscular volume (MCV) or based on ethnicity (African, Mediterranean, Middle Eastern, Southeast Asian, or West Indian descent).

Management

Carrier screening for a particular condition should be performed only once in a lifetime, with results documented in the medical record. Decisions to rescreen with newer or more expanded panels should be undertaken with the advice of a genetics professional (ACOG, 2017a). Prenatal carrier screening does not replace newborn screening. Patients with negative screening should be informed of these results as well as the low residual risk of having an affected child (either due to de novo mutations or mutations not screened for with the carrier panel). For couples in which both patient and their partner are carriers for a genetic condition, genetic counseling should be offered. The counseling should cover the disease condition, outcomes and options for prenatal diagnosis with amniocentesis or chorionic villous sampling, and advanced reproductive technologies to decrease risk to an affected offspring. Patients may choose to decline prenatal diagnostic testing and complete postnatal diagnostic testing on neonatal cord blood after delivery.

INTIMATE PARTNER VIOLENCE IN PREGNANCY

Epidemiology and Prevalence

Violence during pregnancy is more common than gestational diabetes, neural tube defects, and preeclampsia. *Intimate partner violence* (IPV) is defined as physical violence, sexual violence, stalking, and psychological aggression by a current or former intimate partner. Pregnancy is associated with increased risk with escalating severity and frequency of violence (Lutgendorf, 2019). The prevalence of IPV in pregnancy is between 4% and 20%, and IPV has been associated with adverse outcomes including miscarriage, bleeding, preterm birth, stillbirth, low birth weight, and neonatal death. Violence can also extend to other family members, and witnessing violence is a risk factor for abusive relationships as an adult. IPV is also a risk factor for homicide, and women are killed by an intimate partner at twice the rate of men and are most at risk after separation or leaving a violent relationship. Homicide during pregnancy or the postpartum period is a leading cause of pregnancy-associated death, with 3.62 homicides per 100,000 live births during pregnancy or within 1 year postpartum (Wallace et al., 2021).

Risk Factors

IPV can affect all pregnant persons, and routine screening is recommended in pregnancy for all pregnant persons. Individual risk factors include younger age, short-term relationships, intellectual disability, chronic mental illness, limited education, low socioeconomic status, Indigenous status, and drug or alcohol use disorder. Relationship risk factors include separated relationship status, marital disagreements, poor parenting practices, poor or disparate educational levels, negative attitudes toward women, a history of abuse or witnessing IPV as a child, and having other sexual partners. Community risk factors include high levels of crime, poverty and unemployment, low social cohesion, lack of opportunities, and lack of social services for IPV victims. Social risk factors include gender inequality, devaluation of women, cultural acceptance of IPV, and social or religious support of IPV and laws against divorce (Lutgendorf, 2019). Pregnancy risk factors include late presentation for prenatal care, unintended pregnancy, and being unhappy about the pregnancy.

Diagnosis

Screening for IPV is recommended in pregnancy at the initial obstetric visit, each trimester, and postpartum. IPV screening during pregnancy can be conducted with surveys such as the Abuse Assessment Screen (Soeken et al., 1998; Wiist & McFarlane, 1999). The Abuse Assessment Screen is a five-item questionnaire validated for screening during pregnancy, with a sensitivity of 93%, specificity of 55% to 99%, and a positive predictive value of 33% and a negative predictive value of 97% (Lutgendorf, 2019). When screening it is important to make sure the patient is alone, and that it is safe to talk. Screening with the abuser present could lead to escalation of violence. Providers should disclose any mandatory reporting requirement (state dependent) and are always required to report suspected child abuse or if there is threat of imminent harm to another individual. Compliance with reporting requirements generally includes civil and criminal immunity. Framing questions are helpful to initiate the conversation and introduce the topic, and can include: "Because intimate partner violence has so many effects on health, I now ask all my patients about it." If patients answer "no" to screening questions, you can follow up: "I see you answered no to questions about feeling unsafe with your partner. I want you to know that if anything like this does ever come up, this is a safe place to talk about it and get help."

Management

Because of the cycle of violence includes periods of calm and making up, and blaming of the patient for "causing" abuse, it can be difficult for patients to recognize their experiences as abuse, and many patients will leave their abusers seven to 10 times before leaving for the last time. If patients respond affirmatively to being abused, clinicians should acknowledge the trauma and provide education and support. Clinicians should emphasize the fact that the patient is not responsible for the abuse. They should help patients establish a plan and assess the safety of the patient and their children and others living with them. Is there a risk of escalation of violence? Are there weapons in the home? Remember, the decision to take action can be a long and difficult process for the patient experiencing abuse. Clinicians should document all screening, including "no" responses, and if concerns for abuse exist, these should be documented as well. Patient statements, history, timelines, examinations, symptoms, imaging, and lab tests should also be documented, as well as referrals for services and law enforcement notification (ACOG, 2005). Resources for patients and clinicians are available at:

National Coalition Against Domestic Violence (online tool for patients to create a safety plan): www.ncadv.org

National Domestic Violence Hotline (trained counselors and help with safety planning and crisis intervention): 1-800-799-SAFE, www.ndvh.org

Futures Without Violence (posters, brochures, and safety planning cards): www.futureswithoutviolence.org

Epidemiology and Prevalence

Overall, about 15% of clinically recognized pregnancies result in miscarriage. Recurrent pregnancy loss (miscarriage) is defined as two to three consecutive pregnancy losses prior to 20 weeks' gestation and affects 1% to 2% of women (Ford & Schust, 2009).

Risk Factors

Causes of recurrent pregnancy loss include genetic factors such as parental chromosomal abnormalities; uterine anatomic abnormalities; antiphospholipid antibody syndrome; untreated diseases such as diabetes and hypothyroidism; immunologic abnormalities; infections; and environment. Despite a thorough evaluation, up to 40% to 50% of cases will remain unexplained.

Diagnosis

The evaluation of patients with recurrent pregnancy loss includes paternal karyotype for both parents; uterine cavitary evaluation with a hysterosalpingography, hysteroscopy, or saline infusion sonohysterography; TSH evaluation; and testing for insulin resistance, antiphospholipid antibody syndrome with anticardiolipin antibody (IgG/IgM), lupus anticoagulant, and beta-2-glycoprotein antibody (IgG/IgM; Ford & Schust, 2009). A diagnosis of antiphospholipid antibody syndrome requires a clinical feature (recurrent early pregnancy loss, adverse pregnancy outcome of stillbirth after 20 weeks or early delivery for fetal growth restriction or preeclampsia at less than 34 weeks, or venous or arterial thrombosis) and persistent elevated antiphospholipid antibodies in medium to high titers on two occasions at least 12 weeks apart (ACOG, 2012).

Management

Management depends on the outcome of the evaluation. For patients with thyroid disease, treatment should be initiated with thyroid hormone replacement. Parents with abnormalities on karyotype evaluation should receive genetic counseling to discuss reproductive risk and outcomes. Patients with uterine cavitary anomalies should be evaluated by specialists in gynecology and obstetrics for discussion as to whether the identified anomalies could be contributing to pregnancy loss and possible treatment options. Patients with antiphospholipid antibody syndrome should receive a baby aspirin and prophylactic anticoagulation with low-molecular-weight heparin in early pregnancy to improve outcomes.

This chapter describes the most common maternal conditions that complicate pregnancy. Preexisting chronic diseases and disorders account for the largest proportion of maternal morbidity and maternal death. Advanced maternal age is more closely examined at the beginning of the chapter and the chapter ends with psychiatric disorders in pregnancy, which are rising at an alarming rate.

Epidemiology and Prevalence

Women of advanced maternal age (AMA), defined as age 35 and older, accounted for 17% of all births in 2018 in the United States. Pregnancy loss from all etiologies is greater among women of AMA, thought to be largely related to the increased risk for aneuploidy. Ectopic pregnancy risk is four to eight times greater in AMA due to more likely exposure to multiple partners, pelvic infection, tubal pathology, and oocyte transportation delay (Attali & Yogev, 2021). In addition to the obvious risk to the pregnancy, ectopic pregnancy can result in significant maternal morbidity and death.

AMA is associated with increased risk of chronic diseases including asthma, chronic hypertension, diabetes mellitus, metabolic syndrome, cancer, renal disease, and autoimmune disease. AMA is also associated with placental abnormalities and labor and delivery complications (Attali & Yogev, 2021).

Uterine leiomyoma, a common uterine neoplasm, is found with increasing frequency in women in their 30s and 40s and in up to 3.9% of all pregnant women. Uterine leiomyomata are independently associated with miscarriage, placental abruption, dysfunctional labor, intrauterine growth restriction, fetal malpresentation, and cesarean delivery. Obstetric complications are greater if the leiomyoma is larger than 3 cm (Qidwai et al., 2006).

Risk Factors

Common predictors for AMA birth include desire for pregnancy, history of live birth, insurance, income, education level, race and ethnicity, marital status, and urban dwelling. Women who have six or more live births are 17 times more likely to have a child in AMA. Unwanted pregnancy rates are 1.9 times higher in women of AMA (Maloney et al., 2021).

Diagnosis

A woman is considered AMA if she will be 35 or older at the time of delivery. Women age 40 and older are at an even greater risk for maternal morbidity and death and have a twofold increased risk for congenital malformations and birth defects in their offspring (Attali & Yogev, 2021).

Management

Evaluation and treatment for chronic diseases in pregnant women of AMA is essential. Prenatal care of AMA patients includes more frequent visits, education on risks, offering aneuploidy screening, fetal anatomy ultrasound by a perinatologist, and close monitoring of fetal well-being and growth. Many aspects of AMA are covered throughout this chapter.

HYPERTENSION

Epidemiology and Prevalence

Chronic hypertension in pregnancy is determined by hypertension occurring before 20 weeks of gestation. The prevalence of chronic hypertension in pregnancy is 1.5% and has increased significantly in recent decades with the highest increase among Black women. Severe, uncontrolled chronic hypertension in pregnancy is associated with an increased maternal risk of renal failure, pulmonary edema, cerebrovascular accidents, preeclampsia, placental abruption, cesarean delivery, postpartum hemorrhage, and gestational diabetes (ACOG, 2019a). Fetal risks include intrauterine growth restriction, low birth weight, preterm delivery, congenital anomalies, perinatal death, and stillbirth (ACOG, 2019a).

Risk Factors

Advanced maternal age, obesity, and Black ethnicity are risk factors for chronic hypertension. Underlying renal, vascular, and endocrine disorders increase the risk for chronic hypertension.

Diagnosis

Chronic hypertension in pregnancy is generally defined as a systolic blood pressure of 140 mmHg or greater and/or a diastolic blood pressure of 90 mmHg or greater on two occasions at least 4 hours apart. A faster determination can be made if the blood pressure is in the severe range, which includes readings at or greater than 160 mmHg systolic and/or 110 mmHg diastolic (ACOG, 2019a).

Management

Specific tests are recommended for pregnant women with chronic hypertension. Due to the effect of chronic hypertension on the heart and kidneys, the evaluation includes the following lab tests: serum aspartate aminotransferase, alanine aminotransferase, serum creatinine, serum electrolytes, blood urea nitrogen, complete blood count, and either a urine protein/creatinine ratio or 24-hour urine total protein and creatinine. A baseline EKG is ordered. Common oral antihypertensive agents used to treat chronic hypertension in pregnancy include labetalol, nifedipine, methyldopa, and hydrochlorothiazide (ACOG, 2019a).

DIABETES

Epidemiology and Prevalence

During pregnancy, human placental lactogen secreted by the placenta acts on insulin receptor sites binding them, raising circulating levels of maternal glucose. Prepregnant maternal weight and weight at term are noted to increase with age. Glucose impairment increases at all ages with increasing weight. Pancreatic B cell function and insulin sensitivity fall with age, and the incidence of gestational and overt diabetes increases.

Approximately 14.9 million U.S. women have diabetes mellitus (ACOG, 2018c). Pregestational diabetes is prevalent in 1% to 2% of pregnancies (ACOG, 2018c). Pregestational diabetes includes type 1 and type 2 diabetes mellitus. Type 1 diabetes mellitus is an autoimmune disease involving the destruction of pancreatic B cells, whereas type 2 diabetes mellitus is caused by insulin resistance and obesity (ACOG, 2018c). Most pregnant women with type 1 diabetes mellitus are managed by a perinatologist. The combination of age, obesity, and pregnancy increases the likelihood of overt and gestational diabetes from 3% of the random obstetric population to 12% of women older than 40 years and 20% of women older than 50 years (ACOG, 2018c). The complications of diabetes in pregnancy include an increased risk for congenital anomalies, preeclampsia, induction of labor, fetal macrosomia, and cesarean delivery (ACOG, 2018c).

Risk Factors

All pregnant women are at risk for gestational diabetes mellitus (GDM). However, there are ethnic risk factors seen in a greater prevalence among Hispanic, Black, Native American, and Asian women (ACOG, 2018c). GDM has been increasing in incidence as the rates of obesity have risen in the United States (ACOG, 2018c). Women with a prior history of GDM are also at increased risk (ACOG, 2018c).

Diagnosis

Since 1973, the universal screening for GDM is the 1-hour 50-g oral glucose tolerance test (OGTT; ACOG, 2018b). Early screening is recommended for all pregnant women with risk factors; all others should be screened at 24 to 28 weeks of gestation (ACOG, 2018b). Pregnant women with an abnormal 1-hour OGTT are tested with a 3-hour diagnostic 100-g

OGTT, and if two or more of the 3-hour OGTT values are abnormal, GDM is diagnosed (ACOG, 2018b).

Management

The goal of managing pregestational diabetes and GDM is to keep glucose levels within normal ranges in order to reduce risks for preeclampsia, negative neonatal outcomes, and birth complications. Upon diagnosis, nutritional therapy begins as well as blood glucose surveillance four times daily. The glucose log includes once after fasting and 1 or 2 hours after each meal. A consistent and complete glucose log provides the best basis for targeted management decisions to improve glycemic control. Lifestyle changes, which include a focus on a healthy diet, regular physical exercise, and keeping a good glucose log, are the only interventions shown to improve pregnancy outcomes in women with GDM (Martis et al., 2018). When indicated, pharmacologic treatments include the standard therapy of insulin and off-label use of oral antidiabetic medications such as metformin and glyburide (ACOG, 2018b).

OBESITY

Epidemiology and Prevalence

Obesity in pregnancy is associated with pregnancy loss and congenital anomalies. Antepartum complications include gestational diabetes, obstructive sleep apnea, nonalcoholic fatty liver disease, cardiac dysfunction, proteinuria, and preeclampsia. Bariatric surgery is a treatment option that has dramatically increased. More than 80% of procedures are performed in females with one half occurring during the reproductive age. Pregnancy complications following bariatric surgery include nutritional deficiencies and gastrointestinal dysfunction (ACOG, 2009). Delivery complications include cesarean delivery, failed trial of labor, endometrial infection, wound rupture, and venous thrombosis (ACOG, 2021a). The prevalence of obesity in U.S. women of reproductive age is 39.7% (ACOG, 2021a).

Risk Factors

Obesity has increased over the last few decades in the United States with variance noted among ethnic groups. Non-Hispanic Black women have the highest prevalence of obesity (56.9%), compared to Hispanic (43.7%), non-Hispanic White (39.8%), and non-Hispanic Asian women (17.2%; ACOG, 2021a).

Diagnosis

Obesity is defined by a body mass index (BMI) of 30.0 or greater. Obesity is classified by the World Health Organization as class I (BMI 30.0–34.9), class II (BMI 35.0–39.9), and class III (BMI 40 or greater).

Management

The target total weight gain goal for all obese pregnant women is 11 to 20 lb. Weight loss medications should be avoided. Regular exercise is beneficial for moderating weight gain.

Early screening for gestational diabetes and antenatal fetal surveillance are also recommended. Consultation with anesthesia should be considered for obese pregnant women with obstructive sleep apnea due to the increased risk for complications including sudden death (ACOG, 2021a).

THYROID DISEASE

Epidemiology and Prevalence

In a normal pregnancy, there is an increased demand on the thyroid gland. Maternal thyroid abnormalities can be confused with the physiologic thyroid changes in pregnancy. Increased production of thyroid hormones, human chorionic gonadotropin, renal iodine excretion, and thyroxine-binding proteins influence thyroid function tests (Panda et al., 2018). Thyroid disease in pregnancy is associated with preeclampsia, intrauterine growth restriction, and preterm delivery. Fetal complications of maternal thyroid disease include neonatal intensive care admission, macrosomia, and low birth weight (Sitoris et al., 2020).

Hypothyroidism is prevalent in 1% of pregnancies. Subclinical hyperthyroidism is found in 1.7% of pregnant women and has not been associated with adverse outcomes to the pregnant woman or fetus. Neither a national nor international consensus has been reached to support routine screening for thyroid disease in pregnancy (Jouyandeh et al., 2015).

Risk Factors

Screening for thyroid disease is recommended in pregnant women with a personal or family history of thyroid disease, thyroid abnormalities on examination, or type 1 diabetes mellitus (ACOG, 2020b).

Diagnosis

Diagnosis of thyroid disease in pregnancy is based on levels of TSH and thyroid hormones (free thyroxine [T4], total triiodothyronine [T3]). Typically, the thyroid hormones are tested based on a TSH level outside the normal pregnancy range.

Management

Hyperthyroidism is treated with thioamides, either propylthiouracil or methimazole, depending on thyroid hormone levels and the trimester of pregnancy. Treatment of hypothyroidism with T4 replacement therapy is based on the TSH level and the trimester of pregnancy. The TSH level is checked regularly to ensure a euthyroid state. Rare, but life-threatening, a thyroid storm and thyrotoxic heart failure require prompt evaluation and treatment in an ICU (ACOG, 2020b).

CARDIOVASCULAR DISEASE

Epidemiology and Prevalence

Cardiovascular disease includes congenital heart disease and acquired heart disease. Factors contributing to an increase in cardiovascular disease in pregnancy includes women with congenital heart disease in the childbearing years and advanced maternal age (Elkayam et al., 2016). Cardiovascular disease represents a significant proportion of maternal morbidity and death. Common presentations include heart failure and arrhythmia; less common are aortic dissection and myocardial infarction (Ruys et al., 2013). Approximately 1% to 4% of U.S. pregnancies are complicated by cardiovascular disease each year (ACOG, 2019b).

Risk Factors

Risk factors for cardiovascular disease in pregnancy include African American race, maternal age over 40, obesity, hypertensive pregnancy disorders, chronic hypertension, history of GDM, obstructive sleep apnea, history of preterm delivery, family history of heart disease, and cardiotoxic drug exposure. The presence of any of these risk factors should alert the healthcare provider to the increased risk of cardiovascular disease in pregnancy. More than a quarter of maternal deaths could be prevented by proper recognition of these risk factors (ACOG, 2019b).

Diagnosis

Patients with an acute coronary syndrome present with typical symptoms of chest pain or shortness of breath or atypical symptoms of vomiting, reflux, or diaphoresis, which can be difficult to distinguish from normal pregnancy symptoms. The California Improving Health Care Response to Cardiovascular Disease in Pregnancy and Postpartum toolkit algorithm is used for assessment and to determine whether symptoms require reassurance, nonemergent evaluation, or prompt evaluation by a pregnancy heart team (Hameed et al., 2023). In addition to vital signs and physical exam, evaluation for cardiac abnormalities includes EKG, chest x-ray, echocardiogram, and 24-hour to 48-hour or longer EKG monitoring (ACOG, 2019b).

Management

The World Health Organization provides specific guidance for pregnancy care and delivery location based on a pregnancy risk classification for women with preexisting cardiovascular disease. A comprehensive, multidisciplinary team of advanced skilled practitioners ensures cardiology evaluation and follow-up as well as delivery in a healthcare center with high-risk cardiac condition expertise (ACOG, 2019b).

RESPIRATORY DISORDERS

Epidemiology and Prevalence

Asthma is caused by chronic airway inflammation and is the most common respiratory disorder in pregnancy. Asthma is also the most common chronic disease in pregnancy, prevalent in 4% to 8% of U.S. pregnancies (ACOG, 2008a).

Risk Factors

Pregnant women with asthma often have multiple comorbid conditions such as hypertension, depression, anxiety, obesity, GDM, and rhinitis. Exacerbations of asthma during pregnancy are associated with viral infections and comorbidities (Murphy, 2022).

Diagnosis

A complete physical examination is recommended at the beginning of pregnancy to include auscultation of the heart and lungs. Symptoms of asthma include wheezing, cough, chest tightness, and difficulty breathing. Prompt evaluation of asthma symptoms includes vital signs with pulse oximetry. The physical exam should observe for any signs of cyanosis in the skin, lips, nail beds, or eyes.

Management

Well-controlled moderate asthma is associated with healthy maternal and fetal outcomes. Maintaining adequate oxygenation to the fetus by preventing maternal hypoxic episodes is essential. Management includes objective lung function measurement with peak flow readings and regular monitoring of asthma symptoms every 4 to 6 weeks. Pregnant women with asthma are educated to avoid or control asthma triggers, including smoking cessation. Vaccination is recommended for influenza and COVID-19 (Murphy, 2022).

Individualized pharmacologic therapy is based on the frequency and severity of asthma symptoms. Inhaled short-acting beta-2-agonists are the preferred rescue therapy for asthma symptoms and should be prescribed to all pregnant women with asthma. If a good response does not occur with home treatment, seeking prompt medication attention is critical. A stepwise approach to manage persistent asthma symptoms is preferred and includes low-dose inhaled corticosteroids and long-acting beta-2-agonists (ACOG, 2008a).

PSYCHIATRIC DISORDERS

Epidemiology and Prevalence

Psychiatric disorders are associated with poor obstetric outcomes. Depression increases the risk for preterm delivery and gestational hypertension. Pregnant women with posttraumatic stress disorder (PTSD) are at greater risk for ectopic pregnancy, pregnancy loss, preterm labor, preterm delivery, and excessive fetal growth. Preterm delivery and placental abnormalities are associated with schizophrenia. Pregnant women who receive outpatient psychotherapy or take anticonvulsant medications are at higher risk for pregnancy complications (Kang-Yi et al., 2017). Depression occurs in 44% of high-risk pregnancies (Tsakiridis et al., 2019). Nine percent of pregnant women meet the criteria for major depressive disorders (ACOG, 2018a).

Substance use disorders include abuse of alcohol, tobacco, stimulants, opioids, cannabis, cocaine, hallucinogens, and sedatives. In a sample of nearly 3 million inpatient pregnancy hospitalizations, pregnant women with a substance use disorder were three times more likely to have psychiatric comorbidities (anxiety, depression, attention deficit hyperactivity disorder [ADHD], manic episode, bipolar disorder, and schizophrenia; Keller et al., 2023). Substance use is a strong risk factor for a pregnancy-associated death due to accidental overdose (Bronson & Reviere, 2017). Opioid use in pregnant women has risen along with the skyrocketing use in the general population, with 22% of women filling an opioid prescription during pregnancy in a study of Medicaid programs in 46 states (Desai et al., 2014).

Suicide is a leading cause of maternal death and accounts for 20% of postpartum deaths (Chin et al., 2022). Suicidal behavior and self-harm are associated with low-birth-weight infant, preterm delivery, placental abruption, premature rupture of membranes, and postpartum hemorrhage (Zhong et al., 2019). Prevalence of suicidal ideation occurs in 2% to 5% of pregnant women and up to 10% of pregnant veterans (Chin et al., 2022).

Risk Factors

Health disparities are a strong risk factor for psychiatric disorders in pregnancy, particularly in Black and Hispanic racial groups and women of low socioeconomic status. However, White women are more likely to die from suicide or an accidental overdose. Other risk factors include chronic pain conditions and history of physical and sexual abuse (Mangla et al., 2019).

Diagnosis

The most common screening tool for psychiatric disorders in pregnancy is the Edinburgh Postnatal Depression Scale (EPDS). The American College of Obstetricians and Gynecologists (2018c) recommends screening for depression and anxiety at least once during pregnancy. Anxiety and insomnia are common symptoms (ACOG, 2018a). Pregnant women with suicidal ideation should be closely followed. Mental health consultation is recommended to ensure appropriate diagnosis and treatment.

Management

The use of psychotropic medications involves a discussion of risks between the pregnant woman and her healthcare provider. All the known psychotropic medications cross the placenta and are present in amniotic fluid. The Food and Drug Administration (FDA) reports the risk of teratogenesis of all psychotropic medications and provides information that can be used to counsel patients on treatment options. Other electronic resources that assist healthcare providers in psychotropic medication decision-making in pregnancy include Reprotox developed by the Reproductive Toxicology Center (www.reprotox.org) and the Teratogen Information System (TERIS; depts.washington.edu/terisweb). Single medication use is favored over multiple medication use. The use of selective serotonin reuptake inhibitors (SSRIs) has shown limited evidence of teratogenic effects and transient neonatal complications when used late in pregnancy. The use of psychotropic medications in pregnancy is considered with the risk of relapse of psychiatric conditions (ACOG, 2023a).

PREGNANCY CONDITIONS

Specific conditions that occur in pregnancy are described in this section. While not all inclusive, the most common pregnancy conditions are addressed.

Alloimmunization Rh

EPIDEMIOLOGY AND PREVALENCE

Red blood cells (RBCs) are covered with a variety of proteins called antigens. The antigens are divided into groups. One of the best-known groups is the Rh. There are three alleles (variations) in the Rh factor group: Cc, D, and Ee. The D allele of the Rh factor, the most clinically relevant, is found on the RBC membranes in most people. Those with this antigen are called Rh positive. Those without this antigen are known as Rh negative. If the fetus has a different Rh factor from the mother, any mixing of fetal and maternal blood can stimulate an immune reaction from the mother.

RISK FACTORS

Fetal blood cell production begins within a few weeks of conception. When a fetus of an Rh-negative mother is carrying antigens of the CDE (Rh) system and the mother has no antibodies, she can become sensitized or alloimmunized to her fetus and produce immunoglobulin G (IgG) anti-D antibodies that readily cross the placenta, bind to fetal RBCs, and are ultimately destroyed by the fetal spleen. The initial antibody response to the D antigen can take up to 6 months, so immunization during a first pregnancy is uncommon. However, if untreated, about 20% of women will become sensitized at the time of birth (de Haas et al., 2015).

Subsequent pregnancy of an Rh-positive fetus will result in a rapid secondary immunologic response in days, not months. The spleen rapidly destroys RBCs, which affects fetal organs, interferes with placental perfusion, and can result in hydrops fetalis. This process is known as hemolytic disease of the newborn (HDN) or hemolytic disease of the fetus. Infants born with HDN demonstrate pallor, jaundice that begins within 24 hours after delivery, unexplained bruising or petechiae, tissue swelling (edema), respiratory distress, seizures, lack of normal movement, and poor reflex response.

DIAGNOSIS

Prenatal determination of maternal blood type, Rh status, and antibody screening is a standard of care in most industrialized nations at the initial prenatal visit. If antibodies are present, they are measured as a titer. A titer greater than 1:4 is considered sensitized. Although the majority of alloimmunization occurs in response to the D Rh, there are other non-Rh groups that can be associated with HDN.

MANAGEMENT

The groups Kell, Kidd, and MNS account for a small percentage of HDN and the treatment is very similar, but there is no current preventive strategy. ABO incompatibility is also a source of hemolysis but is rarely severe and when present with Rh incompatibility reduces the risk of immunization to about 5% (de Haas et al., 2015).

For the unsensitized woman, obtain the blood type and Rh of the father of the baby, if available. If it is unknown or Rh positive, the woman should receive Rh immunoglobulin (IgG) at various points in the pregnancy. If there is no bleeding during pregnancy, a 300-mcg dose of Rh IgG at 27 to 28 weeks is adequate to cover up to 15 mL of fetal RBCs, which may mix with maternal blood for the next 12 weeks. If there is first trimester bleeding, a smaller dose of Rh IgG may be administered. If there is bleeding, or risk of bleeding, as from an amniocentesis or abdominal trauma, the full 300-mcg dose should be administered. After birth, the newborn blood type will be available and if it is Rh⁺, Du⁺, the woman should receive another dose of Rh IgG within 72 hours of birth (ACOG, 2017c).

A sensitized woman during her initial sensitized pregnancy should have the blood type and Rh of the father if not already known and the father is available. An antibody titer will be obtained on the mother during the first prenatal visit. If the titer is less than 1:16, the woman may be followed collaboratively between the APRN and a collaborating physician. Titers will be repeated every 2 to 4 weeks depending on gestation and levels of dilution (ACOG, 2017c).

If the titer on the initial prenatal visit is greater than 1:16, the woman's care will be per physician management and will include periodic assessment of amniotic bilirubin levels. As RBCs are being destroyed by the fetal spleen, the RBC pigment is released and can be detected as bilirubin in the maternal amniotic fluid. If an antibody titer is greater than 1:16, fetal blood typing may eliminate the need for more invasive testing. Fetal blood type can be obtained through a process called percutaneous umbilical blood sampling (PUBS) in which a small amount of blood is taken directly from the fetal umbilical cord under ultrasonographic guidance. If the fetal blood type is determined to be Rh negative, no further evaluation is necessary. If the fetus is Rh positive and the maternal antibody titer is greater than 1:16, the fetal bilirubin can be followed by periodic PUBS procedures, or more commonly, the bilirubin will be measured indirectly by spectrophotometric analysis of the amniotic fluid obtained during amniocentesis. If the titer surpasses 1:32 for the first time after 27 to 28 weeks, usually the fetus can grow safely to term with the periodic amniotic fluid analyses and concomitant ultrasonographic evaluation of the fetus for hydrops. Hydrops fetalis is a condition of severe edema in fetal tissue. As RBCs are destroyed in the fetus, anemia develops and subsequently hypoproteinuria. Hypoproteinuria causes a drop in the colloidal osmotic pressure and blood is pushed from the vasculature into the tissue. Organs including the heart, liver, and spleen are unable to compensate. The heart experiences high output failure; fluid collects in the heart, lungs, and abdomen (ascites). The changes are seen ultrasonographically as an enlarged heart, liver, and spleen. The placenta becomes thickened. Edema is even observed subcutaneously in the fetal scalp (de Haas et al., 2015).

Subsequent sensitized pregnancies are followed similarly but with surveillance beginning earlier and occurring more often based on the changes during the previous affected pregnancy. Changes in the bilirubin concentration of the amniotic fluid are plotted on a graph called a Liley curve with certain values being associated with no to minimal disease (zone 1), higher numbers with moderate disease, and highest numbers (above zone 2 to 3) indicating severe disease and the need for immediate intervention in the form of fetal transfusion or delivery.

Multiple Gestation

EPIDEMIOLOGY AND PREVALENCE

Pregnancies of multiple gestation were on the rise for more than 30 years (1980–2014) in both the United States and worldwide. In recent years, in the United States, that rate has stabilized and is on a slight decline. As of 2019 an estimated 3% of all live births in the United States were twin gestations and 0.09% were attributed to triplet or higher-order births (ACOG, 2021b; Martin et al., 2021). Worldwide data are challenging to collect and are unreliable in some areas; however, of the 112 countries with sound data collection processes the rate of twinning was an estimated 1.2% between 2010 and 2015. This is a 25% increase in the global rate, which was estimated at 0.9% in the early 1980s (Monden et al., 2021). Dizygotic (DZ) twins account for approximately 70% of all spontaneous twin gestations whereas monozygotic (MZ) twins account for the other 30%. Rates of DZ twins vary by population (Chasen, 2021), while MZ twins occur in approximately 1 in 250 spontaneous pregnancies with the prevalence increasing significantly due to in virto fertilization (1 in 50) or ovulation induction (1 in 25; Lewi, 2020).

RISK FACTORS

Risk factors for multiple-order births are almost exclusively associated with DZ twins, also known as fraternal or nonidentical twins. The only certain risk factor for MZ or identical twins is assisted reproductive technology (ART) (Lewi, 2020). ART is the most significant risk factor for DZ twins as well and is directly associated with the increasing worldwide prevalence. Other risk factors include increasing maternal age, race, geographic location, increasing parity, family history, maternal height and weight, and diet (Chasen, 2021). While some of these are also shared risk factors for infertility and thus the reason for utilization of ART, it is important to note that some, such as maternal age, are also risk factors for spontaneous twinning (ACOG, 2021b). A retrospective analysis conducted by Adashi and Gutman (2018) of more than 238 million U.S. births between 1949 and 2016 concluded that delayed childbearing is an independent risk factor for multiple-order births. Black and white women ages 35 to 39 in the pre-ART era (prior to 1971) were two- to threefold more likely to have a multiple-order birth than women ages 15 to 19.

SYMPTOMS AND DIAGNOSIS

There are no early pregnancy symptoms that are exclusive to multiple gestation. Women may, however, anecdotally report that they experienced an array of early pregnancy symptoms to a more severe degree (nausea, vomiting, constipation, exhaustion). If not diagnosed in the first trimester, other symptoms such as a large for dates uterus or fetal movements consistent with more than one baby may be reported.

Diagnosis of multiple gestation pregnancies is most commonly achieved with ultrasound evaluation. ACOG and the Society for Maternal-Fetal Medicine (SMFM) recommend ultrasound screening in the first trimester for dating purposes and again in the second trimester for anatomy evaluation (ACOG, 2017b). Multiple gestation pregnancies are ideally diagnosed in the first trimester, giving the care team and family the greatest opportunity to provide optimal prenatal care. At the time of diagnosis, it is important to establish the number of fetuses, gestational age, chorionicity, and amnionicity. An experienced bedside sonographer may be able to establish all of these details with the first ultrasound; in other cases the patient may need to be referred for a formal first trimester scan.

Chorionicity and amnionicity are most accurately evaluated in the first trimester but after the seventh week of gestation. Chorionicity refers to the number of placentas whereas amnionicity refers to the number of amniotic sacs. DZ twins are almost exclusively dichorionic/diamniotic (di/di), each twin having its own placenta and amniotic sac. Ultrasound findings supporting the diagnosis include early visualization of distinctly separate placentas/amniotic sacs, presence of a triangular projection of tissue arising from the intertwin membrane of fused-appearing placentas (often called the lambda sign), a thickened intertwin membrane with four distinct layers, and identification of fetuses of opposing sex. MZ twins can be either monochorionic/diamniotic (mono/di) or monochorionic/monoamniotic (mono/mono). Mono/di twins are composed of a shared single placenta with two separate amniotic sacs. Diagnostic ultrasound findings include a thin intertwin membrane and abutted amniotic sacs that form a 90-degree angle with the placenta. Contrary to the di/di lambda sign, this is often referred to as the "T" sign. Mono/mono twins share a single placenta and amniotic sac. Diagnostic ultrasound findings include an absent intertwin membrane, a single yolk sac, intertwined umbilical cords and/or fetal parts and conjoined fetal parts (Chasen, 2021). Higher-order pregnancies are composed of various combinations of chorionicity and amnionicity that are similar to that of twin gestations.

At initial diagnosis it is also important to identify the fetuses in a way that will allow for continuity of future evaluations. The presenting fetus (closest to the cervix) has classically been referred to as fetus A, and while this nomenclature system may work, it is also possible that another system may be more accurate (sex, anatomic findings, etc.) or need to be used given variations in placentation and fetal positioning.

MANAGEMENT

Twin and higher-order pregnancies are, in many ways, managed similarly to singleton pregnancies. Many of the basic antenatal care principles including dating confirmation, genetic screening, monitoring weight gain, nutrition and exercise education, offering supplementation, screening for anatomic abnormalities, screening for diabetes and beta streptococcus, among others, are still applicable (with some

varied recommendations) to multiple gestation pregnancies. Adequate weight gain is essential to decreasing the risk for preterm birth and improving birth weights while excessive weight gain increases the risk for pregnancy-induced hypertensive disorders and cesarean birth. Women who are pregnant with twins and have a normal prepregnancy BMI should gain approximately 37 to 54 lb. Maintaining an active lifestyle with regular exercise is essential in all pregnancies. Limitations should be individualized considering prepregnancy routine, gestational age, and complications (Chasen, 2022). Dietary needs are increased in multiple-order pregnancies and, as such, all women should be placed on additional supplementation and offered a nutrition consult. Table 38.1 outlines many of these basic recommendations for managing twin pregnancies.

All twin and higher-order pregnancies are at risk for many complications; in fact, nearly all known pregnancy complications occur at higher rates in these pregnancies. Fetal growth restriction, congenital anomalies, preterm birth, pregnancy-induced hypertensive disorders, and GDM are among the more common disorders requiring evaluation and treatment. As such, they require, at minimum, comanagement with an obstetrician and referral to a perinatologist. Adequate antenatal care is critical to recognition of complications and includes routine visits, regular interval growth scans, and antepartum fetal testing.

Other complications are specific to twin pregnancies and can be categorized based on chorionicity and amnionicity. Monochorionic twins are at particularly increased risk for twin-twin transfusion syndrome, twin anemia polycythemia sequence, selective fetal growth restriction, and twin reversed arterial perfusion syndrome. Monoamniotic twins are at risk for intertwin cord entanglement and conjoined twins (Chasen, 2021). These complications are likely to be diagnosed, monitored, and treated by a perinatologist.

Delivery route and timing are individualized based on complications, chorionicity and amnionicity, and fetal presentation. An obstetrician should be readily available at the time of delivery and involved in the delivery planning. Delivery often occurs in the operating room regardless of the intent for a vaginal delivery. This allows for an expedient transition to cesarean section if complications arise. Adequate staffing to provide separate neonatal resuscitation teams for each fetus is also essential.

PRETERM LABOR AND BIRTH

Epidemiology and Prevalence

Clinical concern for preterm labor (PTL) and impending preterm birth (PTB) is the most prevalent reason for hospitalization in the antenatal period (ACOG, 2016c). In 2020, 10.09% of all births in the United States were preterm with early preterm (less than 34 weeks) accounting for 2.7% and late preterm (34–36 weeks) accounting for the other 7.4% of PTBs (Osterman et al., 2022). It is estimated that approximately 50% of these births were preceded by PTL (ACOG, 2016c). Worldwide, the prevalence of PTB ranges from 5% to 18% and is impacted by

TABLE 38.1 Twin Pregnancy Recommendations

Weight Gain Goal:
BMI
<18.5—No data
18.5–24.9—37–54 lb
25.0–29.9—31–50 lb
≥30.0—25–42 lb

First Trimester Recommendations

Consultation: Obstetrician, maternal-fetal medicine, nutrition, others as indicated
Supplementation: 1 prenatal vitamin (PNV), 1,500 mg calcium, 1,000 IU vitamin D, 400 mg magnesium, 15 mg zinc, 300–500 mg docosahexaenoic acid/eicosapentaenoic acid (DHA/EPA), 1 mg folic acid, 500 mg vitamin C, 400 mg vitamin E, 81 mg aspirin (preeclampsia prevention)
Lab analysis: Routine prenatal labs, ferritin, folate/vitamin B_{12}, early glucose, vitamin D, genetic screening

Second Trimester Recommendations

Consultation: Ongoing as indicated
Supplementation: 2 PNV, 2,500 mg calcium, 1,000 IU vitamin D, 800 mg magnesium, 30 mg zinc, 300–500 mg DHA/EPA, 1 mg folic acid, 500 mg vitamin C, 400 mg vitamin E, 81 mg aspirin (preeclampsia prevention)
Lab analysis: As indicated to evaluate symptoms and follow up abnormalities

Third Trimester Recommendations

Consultation: Ongoing as indicated
Supplementation: 2 PNV, 2,500 mg calcium, 1,000 IU vitamin D, 800 mg magnesium, 30 mg zinc, 300–500 mg DHA/EPA, 1 mg folic acid, 500 mg vitamin C, 400 mg vitamin E, 81 mg aspirin (preeclampsia prevention)
Lab analysis: Complete blood count, ferritin, glucose screen, otherwise as indicated to evaluate symptoms and follow up abnormalities

both race and ethnic background (Mandy, 2022). In the United States, 14.3% of non-Hispanic Black, 9.8% of Hispanic, and 9.1% of non-Hispanic White infants were born preterm (Osterman et al., 2022). Accounting for 70% of neonatal deaths, PTB is the leading contributor to neonatal death (ACOG, 2016c).

Risk Factors

Many risk factors are tied to PTB, the most significant of which are a history of PTB, preterm premature rupture of membranes (PPROM), and a shortened cervix (ACOG, 2021c). Risk factors for PTB include history of prior PTB, genetics (women born preterm, first-degree relative born preterm), race, age (increased at extremes), history of cervical or transcervical procedures (cold knife cone biopsy, loop electrosurgical excision, dilation and curettage, dilation and evacuation), uterine malformations (congenital and acquired), chronic medical conditions (hypertension, renal disease, diabetes, pathologic anemia, certain autoimmune diseases), history of sudden infant death syndrome in a prior infant, ART, multiple gestation, vaginal bleeding in early pregnancy, short cervix, dilated cervix, preterm labor, infection (chorioamnionitis, bacteriuria, periodontal disease, sexually transmitted infections, bacterial vaginosis, colonization with group B streptococci, persistent human papillomavirus type 16/18, malaria), short interval pregnancies, cigarette smoking, substance abuse, inadequate dietary nutrition, weight (malnourished and morbid obesity), short stature, stress, poor prenatal care, fetal conditions (male sex, some congenital anomalies, growth restriction; ACOG, 2021c; Robinson & Norwitz, 2022).

Diagnosis

Deliveries occurring between 20 weeks 0 days and 36 weeks 6 days are preterm. Most PTBs (70%–80%) are spontaneous and can be attributed to PTL (40%–50%), PPROM (20%–30%), and in rare cases, cervical insufficiency alone. The other 20% to 30% are induced due to maternal–fetal conditions in which the risks of continued pregnancy outweigh the risk of delivery (Robinson & Norwitz, 2022).

Management

It is often difficult to determine if PTL will result in PTB as labor may resolve (30% of cases) and even in cases of hospitalization women often (50% of cases) give birth at term. Attempts to delay delivery should be of benefit to the fetus with the goal of preventing poor neonatal outcomes. Both suspected proximity to delivery as well as gestational age of the fetus impact the management of PTL (ACOG, 2016c).

PTL occurring between 23 weeks and 36 weeks 6 days accompanied by high suspicion of delivery within 7 days is an indicator for maternal corticosteroid administration. Attempts to delay labor may be indicated in certain clinical scenarios as these steroids aid in fetal lung maturity and the reduction of neonatal morbidity and mortality risks. Corticosteroids commonly used include two doses of betamethasone 12 mg intramuscular (IM) given 24 hours apart or four doses of dexamethasone 6 mg IM given 12 hours apart (ACOG, 2016c; Crowther et al., 2019; McGoldrick et al., 2020). In cases of PPROM without PTL, administration of steroids is also indicated. For women who re-present in labor, a rescue dose of steroids is indicated if less than 34 weeks and previously treated more than 14 days prior. In some settings a rescue course may be considered as soon as 7 days from the prior administration. There is insufficient evidence to recommend rescue steroids if greater than 34 weeks or in cases of PPROM (ACOG, 2016c).

Uterine contractions and associated cervical change are anticipated predictors of PTB and as such there may be some benefit to the utilization of tocolytics. There is no substantial evidence that tocolytics directly impact neonatal outcomes; however, they can be used to delay delivery and are thought to be effective for approximately 48 hours. The goal of use should be to allow for administration of antenatal corticosteroids, and potentially stabilize for transport to a tertiary medical center with a neonatal intensive care unit (NICU) capable of providing for the newborn. They should not be used for spontaneous PTL in previable fetuses and should be reserved for viable fetuses up to 34 weeks' gestation. First-line agent selection varies based on several factors including gestational age and include cyclooxygenase inhibitors, calcium channel blockers, and beta-adrenergic receptor agonists (ACOG, 2016c; Simhan & Caritis, 2022). Indomethacin, a cyclooxygenase inhibitor, and nifedipine, a calcium channel blocker, are two of the preferred first-line treatments as they have a lower maternal side effect profile, are successful at delaying delivery for 48 hours, and have been shown to positively impact rates of neonatal mortality and respiratory distress syndrome (Simhan & Caritis, 2022). Indomethacin is the medication of choice between 24 and 32 weeks (Simhan & Caritis, 2022) as calcium channel blockers and beta-adrenergic receptor agonists are generally avoided with coadministration of magnesium sulfate, a fetal neuroprotective agent (ACOG, 2016c). Nifedipine is recommended as a first-line treatment if indomethacin must be avoided and in pregnancies at 32 to 34 weeks' gestation (Simhan & Caritis, 2022).

Magnesium sulfate has several roles in obstetric management and has been used in the past as a tocolytic agent and currently in eclampsia prevention. In cases of PTL it serves a different purpose: fetal neuroprotection. In cases of PTL before 32 weeks when suspicion of PTB is high its use is associated with reduced incidence of cerebral palsy.

Antibiotic therapy in women without signs of infection and with intact membranes has not been found to improve neonatal outcomes and as such is not recommended as routine therapy. Women with unknown group B streptococcus status should receive prophylaxis with an appropriate agent in progressing PTL (ACOG, 2016c).

Maternal lifestyle limitations such as bed rest, sedation, avoiding intercourse or orgasm, and increasing hydration have not been proved to be effective at preventing or treating PTL. Although progesterone administration may have a role in PTB and PTL prevention, it is not considered an effective treatment for acute PTL (Simhan & Caritis, 2022).

Progesterone treatment for PTL and PTB prevention has been controversial in recent years. Initial studies showed a significant statistical reduction (by approximately one third) in recurrence of PTB when given weekly IM progesterone injections during a subsequent pregnancy. As a result of this study women with a prior spontaneous singleton PTB were counseled to begin hydroxyprogesterone caproate (17-OHPC) weekly starting between 16 and 20 weeks and continuing until the 36th week of pregnancy. More recent data collected from the PROLONG trial, a randomized, double-blind study of 1,740 women, found no statistical difference in the rate of recurrent PTB, putting into question the efficacy of treatment (ACOG, 2021c). The EPPPIC meta-analysis, which included data from the PROLONG study in addition to 30 other trials, evaluated 11,644 women at risk for PTB due to prior history or with a short cervix (<25 mm) and the use of various progesterone preparations as well as no treatment. This analysis concluded that progesterone does reduce the risk (though not statistically significant) for PTB before 34 weeks and a specific preparation (IM or vaginal) could not be recommended over another. Evidence for vaginal progesterone use was the most consistent, and as such the authors concluded it may be most beneficial in women with a short cervix without a prior spontaneous PTB. Current SMFM and ACOG guidelines endorse shared decision-making with full disclosure of the data when considering treatment and counseling patients on 17-OHPC or vaginal progesterone use for prevention of recurrent PTB. The use of vaginal progesterone in the prevention of PTB in women without a prior history and with a shortened cervix is recommended by SMFM (ACOG, 2021c; EPPPIC Group, 2021; SMFM, 2021).

GESTATIONAL HYPERTENSION, PREECLAMPSIA, HELLP, ECLAMPSIA

Epidemiology and Prevalence

Hypertensive disorders of pregnancy are a leading cause of maternal morbidity and death and include gestational hypertension and preeclampsia. Preeclampsia is a disease in pregnancy of hypertension with proteinuria and/or multiple organ edema. Preeclampsia occurs primarily in primiparous women at the extremes of their childbearing years. Preeclampsia has increased by 25% in the United States since 1987 and complicates up to 8% of pregnancies. Hypertensive disorders are attributed to 16% of maternal deaths (ACOG, 2020a).

A complication of pregnancy involving coagulation defects and microthrombi was first described in 1892 (Barton & Sibai, 2004). In 1982, Dr. Louis Weinstein first coined the acronym HELLP for this syndrome consisting of *h*emolysis, *e*levated *l*iver enzymes, and *l*ow *p*latelets (thrombocytopenia; Weinstein, 1982). Considered by some to be a severe form of preeclampsia, by others to be a mild form of disseminated intravascular coagulation (DIC), the precise pathogenesis of all three entities is unknown. They may be separate diseases with some common pathways or they may be extreme variations of one another (Barton & Sibai, 2004). A leading investigator of HELLP, Dr. Baha Sibai, estimates the incidence of HELLP at 1/1,000 pregnancies in the general population (Table 38.2). He further estimates that approximately 10% to 20% of women with severe preeclampsia or eclampsia develop HELLP but up to 20% of women with HELLP are diagnosed without the preeclampsia criteria of proteinuria and hypertension. This lack of association with preeclampsia seems to be especially true with postpartum onset of HELLP (Sibai et al., 1993). The timing of HELLP is slightly different from that of preeclampsia in that preeclampsia is relatively rare in the second trimester and postpartum period.

The incidence of HELLP rises with advancing gestation, peaking in late third trimester. The peak occurrence of HELLP is mid-third trimester. Approximately 30% of the time, HELLP is not noted until the postpartum period, most commonly within the first 48 hours after birth, but occasionally up to 7 days after birth (Table 38.3; Barton & Sibai, 2004; Sibai et al., 1993). Preeclampsia has been diagnosed as late as 6 weeks postpartum but the overall incidence of postpartum onset preeclampsia is 5%.

Like preeclampsia, HELLP is a disease of endothelial dysfunction and vasospasm. Whether the endothelial dysfunction is the cause or effect of vasospasm is not known. What is known is this dysfunction untreated results in microangiopathic hemolysis, destruction of RBCs from narrowing or obstruction of small vessels, which can be observed on a peripheral smear as schistocytes, spherocytes, and other abnormally shaped RBCs. Microangiopathic hemolysis is also associated with an elevated indirect bilirubin, decreased haptoglobin, and elevated lactic acid dehydrogenase levels. The damage occurs chiefly in the liver and kidneys, though the heart, lungs, and brain may also be affected. Sibai's group found the degree of cellular damage could not be directly correlated with the lab abnormalities or the clinical picture (Sibai, 1990). As the elevated liver enzymes portion of the acronym HELLP implies, some degree of liver damage is inherent in the disease. The liver enzyme abnormalities are not specific to HELLP, and other diseases, especially acute fatty liver of pregnancy, must be excluded. Liver enzyme abnormalities are generally higher with HELLP and jaundice occurs much later in HELLP (Padden, 1999).

TABLE 38.2 Epidemiology of HELLP Versus Preeclampsia

FACTOR	HELLP	PREECLAMPSIA
Incidence	0.2%–0.6% all pregnancies	5%–7% all pregnancies
Parity	Multiparous	Nulliparous
Age	>25 years	<20 and >40 years
Ethnicity	More Caucasian	More African American
Genetics	Family history	Family history
Incidence postpartum onset	30%	5%
Predisposing comorbidities	Previous history Antiphospholipid antibody syndrome	Diabetes Multiple gestation Chronic hypertension Antiphospholipid antibody syndrome
Occurrence rates of HELLP in subsequent pregnancies	17%–29%	20% if severe preeclampsia
Occurrence of preeclampsia in subsequent pregnancies	43%–50%	2.5%–10%

HELLP, hemolysis, elevated liver enzymes, and low platelets.
Source: Sullivan, C. A., Magann, E. F., Perry, K. G., Roberts, W. E., Blake, P. G., & Martin, J. N. (1994). The recurrence risk of the syndrome of hemolysis, elevated liver enzymes, and low platelets (HELLP) in subsequent gestations. American Journal of Obstetrics and Gynecology, 171(4), 940–943. https://doi.org/10.1016/s0002-9378(94)70063-x

TABLE 38.3 Timing of HELLP and Preeclampsia by Week of Gestation

WEEKS AT ONSET	HELLP (%)	PREECLAMPSIA (%)
<20	3	<1
24–27	11	5
27–36	50	10 at <34 weeks
36+	15	78.5
Postpartum	30	5.4

HELLP, hemolysis, elevated liver enzymes, and low platelets.
Source: Sibai, B. M., Ramadan, M. K., Usta, I., Salama, M., Mercer, B. M., & Friedman, S. A. (1993). Maternal morbidity and mortality in 442 pregnancies with hemolysis, elevated liver enzymes, and low platelets (HELLP syndrome). American Journal of Obstetrics and Gynecology, 169(4), 1000–1006. https://doi.org/10.1016/0002-9378(93)90043-i

Risk Factors

It is estimated about half of the women with HELLP have a risk of renal involvement and up to 20% experience acute renal failure with DIC. Coagulopathy, if present, is a late sign of HELLP syndrome, though some authors speculate all patients with HELLP have an underlying coagulopathy that remains subclinical because the woman is delivered before becoming fulminant or because laboratory tests have not been fully explored. Most women will have normal coagulation studies (Padden, 1999). In pregnancy onset HELLP, once the fetus is delivered, even severe renal involvement typically resolves (Weinstein, 1982). However, HELLP syndrome with postpartum onset is associated with greater risk for pulmonary edema and renal failure (Sibai et al., 1993).

Diagnosis

Women with high blood pressure and proteinuria may or may not have symptoms preceding the signs that give them a diagnosis of preeclampsia. When preeclampsia is diagnosed first, clinicians are more alert for complications and HELLP syndrome may be more readily recognized. In some women, HELLP symptoms occur without hypertension and the condition is initially misdiagnosed. Patients with HELLP often present with general malaise of a few days duration. Gastrointestinal disturbances in the form of epigastric pain and nausea and vomiting are common. Some women experience a headache as well. This combination of symptoms may be interpreted initially as flu or other illness or in the case of postpartum onset might be attributable to exaggerated postpartum sensations.

Physical assessment often provides less information than patient history. The liver may be enlarged or tender to palpation. A liver capsule hematoma may cause pain referred to the shoulder. If preceded by preeclampsia, central edema of the face, abdomen, and sacrum may be noted and deep tendon reflexes may be brisk. A ruptured liver capsule can cause rapid abdominal distention and shock. Rarely, less than 5% of the time, jaundice is evident (ACOG, 2020a). As HELLP has overlapping symptoms with many other diseases, diagnosis is often based on timing of symptoms and history and less often based on laboratory studies (see Box 38.1).

Management

Gestational hypertension and preeclampsia are managed similarly with weekly follow-up and laboratory evaluation as well as recommend delivery at 37 0/7 weeks' gestation. Severe features may necessitate an earlier delivery. Eclampsia is managed in the hospital setting with a focus on seizure prevention and management, patient safety, and delivery as quickly as possible.

HELLP syndrome is most appropriately managed by a physician, preferably in a tertiary care center. Deterioration in maternal or fetal status can occur rapidly. The fetus is assessed, and the mother stabilized, then transported to the hospital. There is no place for home management of HELLP syndrome. The woman is maintained on left lateral bed rest with intravenous hydration, careful monitoring of blood pressure

Box 38.1 Diagnosis of HELLP: Supportive Laboratory Testing

1. Liver test abnormalities cannot predict the clinical severity of the disease, complications, or recovery; they support the diagnosis. The transaminases aspartate aminotransferase (AST) and alanine aminotransferase (ALT) will be moderately elevated and lactic acid dehydrogenase will be markedly elevated. Elevated liver enzymes are thought to result from obstruction of the hepatic blood flow by fibrin deposits, leading to periportal necrosis.
2. The most sensitive marker for HELLP is the platelet count, which is markedly to severely depressed.
3. Hemoglobin and hematocrit may be in the normal range but abnormal cells will be noted on the peripheral smear.
4. A mildly elevated indirect bilirubin may be noted.
5. D-dimer may be positive in the presence of an abnormally high level of fibrin degradation products. It indicates significant clot (thrombus) formation and breakdown in the body, but it does not tell the location or cause. In women with preeclampsia this test is predictive of who will develop HELLP. The D-dimer will be positive before coagulation studies change.
6. Prothrombin time and partial thromboplastin time are usually normal
7. HELLP, hemolysis, elevated liver enzymes, and low platelets.

and fluid balance, preferably in a tertiary care center. While a diagnosis is being established and if conservative management is appropriate, laboratory markers should be followed. Classification of severity of HELLP syndrome that is based on laboratory markers may be useful in directing management. The use of corticosteroids compared to placebo in the treatment of HELLP syndrome showed no difference in the risk of maternal morbidity or mortality, only an improved platelet count; therefore, there is insufficient evidence for the use of corticosteroids in HELLP syndrome (Woudstra et al., 2010). The treatment of choice for HELLP is to expedite birth within 48 hours of diagnosis, even if the fetus is premature. Maternal liver function can decline rapidly and the risk for DIC is high.

Postpartum hemorrhage (PPH) is a common sequela of HELLP. However, prophylactic blood transfusion is usually not necessary if vaginal birth is anticipated, unless the platelets fall below 25,000/mm^3. Transfusion does not reduce the risk of PPH or accelerate the rate of platelet recovery. Vaginal delivery is not contraindicated. Cesarean section should be performed for the same indications as for all women. For patients undergoing cesarean section, transfusion is considered when platelets decline below 50,000/mm^3. More than half of patients with HELLP will receive some form of blood product, most often postpartum (ACOG, 2020a).

Women with HELLP should be screened for antiphospholipid antibodies. There are no known preventive measures for HELLP, though calcium and aspirin supplementation have been studied. The woman may have permanent liver damage, which may require a transplant or can be fatal. When counseling the woman for future pregnancy, it is important to strike a balance between conveying the risk for future pregnancies with a sense of optimism. The woman should be encouraged early in the pregnancy to make plans for who will watch her older child(ren) should she become ill again; if she works, she might advise her employer she is at risk for preterm delivery. A transdisciplinary approach is essential for the recovery and future health of women who experienced the difficult diagnoses of preeclampsia, HELLP syndrome, and eclampsia.

FETAL CONDITIONS

The next section of this chapter is focused on fetal conditions indicating a high-risk pregnancy. Findings on fetal ultrasound can determine the plan of care and inform the level of care for pregnancy management and delivery. This section concludes with the very sad and unfortunate outcome of stillbirth, which is more prevalent in high-risk pregnancies.

Fetal Ultrasound and Prenatal Diagnosis

EPIDEMIOLOGY AND PREVALENCE

Obstetric ultrasound is commonly used in prenatal care for confirmation of fetal viability with the presence of cardiac activity, as well as identification of fetal presentation and assessment of fetal well-being and pregnancy complications and screening for fetal anomalies (ACOG, 2016c). The background risk for having a baby with a birth defect is 3% to 5% in all pregnancies. A standard obstetric ultrasound examination evaluates fetal presentation and number, amniotic fluid volume, cardiac activity, placental location, fetal biometry and anatomic survey with assessment of maternal cervix and adnexa if technically feasible (ACOG, 2016c). The sensitivity of ultrasound in the detection of fetal anomalies varies, with overall sensitivity of 40%, ranging from 15% to 80% (Levi, 2002). Higher detection rates have been reported at tertiary centers and centers with higher training and expertise of the ultrasound operators. Other factors such as maternal obesity and fetal positioning can affect detection rates of fetal anomalies on ultrasound. Thus, the benefits and limitations of ultrasound in the detection of fetal anomalies should be discussed with patients (ACOG, 2016c).

Risk Factors

Risk factors for fetal anomalies depend on the condition, the background rate of anomalies, and the patient's personal and family history. Conditions present in families with familial recurrence may be seen with increased frequency depending on the inheritance. A thorough family history for the patient and their reproductive partner, with additional genetic counseling and/or specialized and more detailed ultrasound examinations for specific conditions, is recommended and may aid in the detection of anomalies. A specialized ultrasound examination is recommended when there is an increased risk of fetal anomalies based on the history, laboratory results (such as aneuploidy screening tests), or suspected findings on the standard ultrasound screening examination.

Diagnosis

Diagnosis of fetal anomalies is accomplished with ultrasound, with the limitations noted previously. Additional information can be obtained through the use of prenatal diagnostic procedures such as chorionic villous sampling and amniocentesis, and additional imaging adjuncts such as fetal MRI may also be used.

Management

Depending on the condition, in utero fetal therapy may be an option for some conditions. Examples include in utero repair of open myelomeningocele (Adzick et al., 2011) and laser therapy for twin-twin transfusion syndrome (Akkermans et al., 2015). Thus, timely identification and referral of these and other conditions are important. Ongoing sonographic surveillance of fetal conditions depends on the specific condition in question and is guided by gestational age and fetal prognosis in collaboration with maternal-fetal medicine subspecialists.

Fetal Growth Restriction

EPIDEMIOLOGY AND PREVALENCE

Fetal growth restriction is defined as overall fetal growth less than the 10th percentile or abdominal circumference less than the 10th percentile for gestational age. This condition occurs in up to 10% of pregnancies and is associated with significant neonatal morbidity and mortality (SMFM, Martins et al., 2020a). There is an increased rate of stillbirth, acidosis, NICU admission, and prematurity. Additionally, long-term effects on health include metabolic programming, cardiac remodeling, and long-term neurodevelopmental impairment (SMFM, Martins et al., , 2020a). The risk for adverse outcomes increases with decreasing growth percentiles.

RISK FACTORS

Risk factors for fetal growth restriction include a prior history of fetal growth restriction, maternal medical conditions such as hypertension and diabetes, fetal anomalies and chromosomal aneuploidies, infections (such as cytomegalovirus [CMV] infection and toxoplasmosis), and exposures to alcohol and drugs.

DIAGNOSIS

The diagnosis of fetal growth restriction is made with ultrasound assessment of fetal growth less than the 10th percentile or abdominal circumference less than the 10th percentile for gestational age. A detailed ultrasound assessment is recommended to search for possible fetal or chromosomal anomalies. Patients should be offered fetal diagnostic testing including chromosomal microarray testing if a fetal anomaly or polyhydramnios is suspected or if isolated unexplained fetal growth restriction is suspected at less than 32 weeks' gestation. Generally serologic screening for CMV and toxoplasmosis is not recommended unless there are risk factors or ultrasound findings that increase suspicion. In patients who choose diagnostic testing with amniocentesis, polymerase chain reaction testing for CMV is recommended on the amniocentesis specimen. However, it should be noted that the prevalence of CMV in cases of fetal growth restriction is low, and there is a lack of effective antenatal interventions for CMV.

MANAGEMENT

Once the diagnosis is made, pregnancies are followed with serial ultrasound examinations including umbilical artery doppler assessments. Umbilical artery doppler exams assess the impedance to blood flow in the fetal component of the placental unit, and an abnormal umbilical artery doppler finding is a pulsatility index (PI), resistance index (RI), or systolic-to-diastolic (S/D) ratio greater than the 95 percentile for gestational age or absent or reversed end-diastolic velocity. Abnormal umbilical artery waveforms reflect uteroplacental insufficiency and can be used to appropriately time delivery. Absent and reversed end-diastolic flow reflect uteroplacental deterioration and increased rates of perinatal morbidity. For patients with increased resistance of severe fetal growth restriction below the 3rd percentile, umbilical artery doppler assessments should be performed weekly. For absent end-diastolic flow, umbilical artery dopplers should be performed two or three times per week, and for reversed end diastolic flow, patient should be admitted, receive corticosteroids for fetal maturation, and undergo umbilical artery dopplers two or three times per week and cardiotocography at least one or two times per day. Once diagnosed, fetal growth should also be assessed every 2 to 4 weeks. Delivery is recommended at 38 to 39 weeks in patients with normal umbilical artery dopplers and fetal growth between 3rd and 9th percentiles. Delivery is recommended at 37 weeks for increased resistance and/or fetal growth at <3rd percentile. Delivery is recommended at 33 to 34 weeks for absent end-diastolic flow and at 30 to 32 weeks for reversed end-diastolic flow. Earlier delivery may also be indicated for other maternal or fetal indications (SMFM, Martins et al., 2020a).

Hydrops Fetalis

EPIDEMIOLOGY AND PREVALENCE

Hydrops fetalis is associated with pathologic fluid collection in the fetal soft tissues and cavities. The condition is caused by RBC alloimmunization (immune hydrops) and other causes (nonimmune hydrops). Nonimmune hydrops is associated with various other conditions, commonly cardiovascular disorders, chromosomal abnormalities, hematologic abnormalities, structural fetal anomalies, complications of multiple gestation, infection, and placental abnormalities (SMFM et al., 2015). With the development of Rh(D) immune globulin, the prevalence of Rh(D) alloimmunization has decreased, and nonimmune hydrops now accounts for 90% of cases of hydrops with a prevalence of 1 in 1,700 to 3,000 pregnancies (SMFM et al., 2015). The underlying pathophysiology relates to an imbalance in the regulation of fluid movement between the fetal vascular and interstitial spaces, with an increase in interstitial fluid production or decreased lymphatic return caused by various conditions.

RISK FACTORS

Risk factors for nonimmune hydrops include fetal cardiovascular anomalies, which account for about 20% of cases; chromosomal anomalies; and hematologic anomalies. Additional risk factors include fetal anomalies, twin-to-twin transfusion syndrome, congenital infections, placental abnormalities, fetal tumors, fetal anemia (from alloimmunization or hemoglobinopathies, fetomaternal hemorrhage, hemolysis, parvovirus infection, or RBC aplasia), metabolic disorders, and a prior pregnancy affected by hydrops (SMFM et al., 2015).

DIAGNOSIS

Hydrops fetalis is diagnosed with ultrasound findings of two or more abnormal fluid collections in the fetus, including ascites, pleural effusions, pericardial effusion, and generalized skin edema (skin thickness >5 mm). Other ultrasound findings include thickened placenta (≥4 cm in the second trimester and ≥6 cm in the third trimester) and polyhydramnios.

MANAGEMENT

Evaluation and management include an antibody screen (indirect Coombs test) to verify that the process is nonimmune, a detailed ultrasound of the fetus and placenta, fetal echocardiography, middle cerebral artery Doppler to assess for anemia, and fetal karyotype and microarray to assess for genetic causes. The recommended treatment and prognosis will depend on the underlying etiology of hydrops and the gestational age of the fetus (SMFM et al., 2015). Such management and decisions will be undertaken in collaboration with maternal–fetal medicine subspecialists.

ABNORMAL PLACENTATION (CESAREAN SCAR PREGNANCY, PLACENTA ACCRETA SPECTRUM)

Epidemiology and Prevalence

Cesarean scar pregnancy occurs when an early pregnancy implants in the scar from a prior cesarean delivery. This can have significant maternal risk and challenges related to diagnosis and management. It is estimated to occur in 1:1,800 to 1:2,656 pregnancies (SMFM, Miller et al., 2020b). Placenta accreta spectrum is diagnosed with pathologic placental adherence to the uterine myometrium. It is further classified as placenta increta (when placental tissue invades into the myometrium) and placenta percreta (when placental tissue invades through the myometrial serosa and into surrounding structures). Severe and life-threatening maternal hemorrhage can occur at delivery, particularly with attempts to remove the placenta. The incidence of placenta accreta is increasing, with recent reports as high as 1:272 births.

Risk Factors

Risk factors for cesarean scar pregnancy and placenta accreta include a history of prior cesarean delivery and prior uterine procedures. The pathogenesis of cesarean scar pregnancy is thought to be similar to that for placenta accreta. With implantation of the pregnancy in the fibrous scar tissue, there is an increased risk of uterine dehiscience, placenta accreta, and hemorrhage as the cesarean scar pregnancy progresses (SMFM, Miller et al., 2020b). The risk for placenta accreta spectrum also increases with increasing numbers of prior cesarean deliveries and with associated placenta previas. Placenta accreta spectrum occurs in 3% of women with a placenta previa and no prior cesarean deliveries, and in women with a prior cesarean delivery and a placenta previa, the rates of placenta accreta are 3%, 11%, 40%, 61%, and 67% for the first through fifth cesarean delivery, respectively (Silver et al., 2006). Other risk factors for placenta accreta spectrum include placenta previa, other uterine surgeries or curettages, and Asherman syndrome (SMFM, Miller et al., 2020b).

Diagnosis

Ultrasound is the primary imaging modality, though adjunctive imaging with MRI can be helpful at times. Transvaginal ultrasound is the optimum imaging modality, and ultrasound criteria include an empty uterine cavity and endocervix with the placenta, gestational sac, or both imbedded in the hysterotomy scar, and a triangular or rounded gestational sac that fills the scar or "niche" with a thin or absent myometrial layer between the gestational sac and the bladder and a prominent vascular pattern in the area of the cesarean scar with an embryonic or fetal pole, yolk sac, or both. However, not all of these criteria are observed in every case (SMFM, Miller et al., 2020b). The diagnosis of placenta accreta spectrum on ultrasound includes the finding of multiple vascular lacunae within the placenta, loss of the hypoechoic retroplacental lucency between the placenta and the myometrium, decreased retroplacental myometrial thickness (<1 mm), abnormalities of the uterine serosa and bladder interface, and extension of the placenta into the uterine myometrium, serosa, or bladder (SMFM, Miller et al., 2020b). Color flow Doppler may also demonstrate abnormal vascularity.

Management

There is limited information on the natural history of cesarean scar pregnancies, though there is a high rate of severe complications in the second and third trimesters of pregnancy. Cesarean scar pregnancies have resulted in live births, though with associated placenta accreta, cesarean hysterectomies, and massive hemorrhage at delivery. Because of these risks, expectant management is not recommended for cesarean scar pregnancies, and pregnancy termination is generally advised with confirmation of the diagnosis (SMFM, Miller et al., 2020b). Generally, management of placenta accreta spectrum involves a scheduled cesarean delivery at 34 to 35 + 6/7 weeks' gestation with planned hysterectomy. Careful surgical planning and multidisciplinary planning is recommended due to the increased risk for hemorrhage and massive transfusion.

Delivery should take place at a tertiary care center with adequate resources for complicated surgery and massive transfusion. Prenatal diagnosis allows early identification and complex surgical planning with improved outcomes.

OTHER ULTRASOUND FINDINGS: PLACENTA PREVIA, VASA PREVIA, VELAMENTOUS CORD INSERTION, MARGINAL CORD INSERTION

Epidemiology and Prevalence

Placenta previa is defined as placental implantation that overlays or abuts the cervical os (SMFM & Gyamfi-Bannerman, 2018). The incidence ranges from 5% to 20% on second trimester ultrasound, with a decrease to 0.3% to 0.5% at term. Placenta previa has been associated with bleeding in pregnancy, classically painless vaginal bleeding. *Vasa previa* occurs when fetal vessels course in the membranes overlying the cervical os or in close proximity (within 2 cm of the cervical os). This occurs in 1 in 2,500 pregnancies with an increased incidence after resolution of placenta previa, cases of succenturiate placental lobes (in which vessels communicating between the lobes can overlie the cervix), and cases of velamentous cord insertion. *Velamentous cord insertion* is a condition in which the umbilical cord vessels insert on the placental membranes and traverse unprotected by Wharton's jelly to insert on the placenta. This occurs in approximately 1% of singleton pregnancies and has been associated with increased risk of fetal growth restriction, preterm labor, placental abruption, vasa previa, abnormal fetal heart rate patterns, and retained placenta (Sepulveda et al., 2003). *Marginal cord insertion* occurs when the placental cord insertion inserts 2 cm or less from the placental edge. Marginal cord insertion has been associated with fetal growth restriction, and both marginal and velamentous cord insertions have been associated with an increased risk of hemorrhage in the third stage of labor and the need for manual removal of the placenta (Ebbing et al., 2015).

Risk Factors

Risk factors for placenta previa include advanced maternal age, multiparity, prior cesarean delivery, multifetal gestation, and smoking (SMFM & Gyamfi-Bannerman, 2018). Risk factors for vasa previa include resolved placenta previa, velamentous cord insertion, succenturiate placental lobe, in vitro fertilization, and multiple gestation.

Diagnosis

The diagnosis of these conditions is made with ultrasound, with increased accuracy in differentiation with the use of transvaginal ultrasound (SMFM & Gyamfi-Bannerman, 2018). Perinatal morbidity and mortality associated with vasa previa can be decreased with prenatal diagnosis and transvaginal ultrasound with color Doppler assessment of the lower uterine segment recommended in cases of resolved placenta previa to exclude vasa previa.

Management

Management depends on the clinical presentation and gestational age. For persistent placenta previa at term, delivery is recommended at 36 + 0/7 to 37 + 6/7 weeks for patients who are stable and without bleeding or other pregnancy complications (SMFM & Gyamfi-Bannerman, 2018). For patients with active ongoing hemorrhage in the late preterm period, stabilization and delivery are recommended. Complications from vasa previa include fetal hemorrhage, exsanguination, and death if fetal vessels rupture. The goal is to deliver prior to rupture of membranes while minimizing the risk of iatrogenic prematurity (SMFM Publications Committee et al., 2015). Thus, in cases of vasa previa management includes antenatal corticosteroids at 28 to 32 weeks, consideration for preterm hospitalization at 30 to 34 weeks, and delivery is recommended between 34 and 37 weeks' gestation via planned cesarean delivery (SMFM Publications Committee et al., 2015). Emergent delivery is recommended for any patient with late preterm bleeding due to a known vasa previa.

STILLBIRTH

Epidemiology and Prevalence

Stillbirth (fetal death) occurs in approximately 1 in 160 deliveries in the United States, approximately 5 or 6 per 1,000 deliveries (ACOG et al., 2020). It is defined as the delivery of a fetus with no signs of life (breathing, heartbeat, pulsation of the umbilical cord, or movements of voluntary muscles). Suggested criteria for reporting include fetal deaths at 20 weeks or greater if gestational age is known or a weight greater than 350 g if the gestational age is not known.

Risk Factors

Risk factors for stillbirth include non-Hispanic Black ethnicity, nulliparity, advanced maternal age, obesity, pregestational diabetes and other comorbid medical conditions, chronic hypertension, smoking, alcohol use, assisted reproductive technology to conceive, multiple gestation, male fetal sex, and a past history of stillbirth (ACOG, 2023b). Patients of non-Hispanic Black ethnicity have a stillbirth rate twice that of other ethnicities (MacDorman & Gregory, 2015). The stillbirth rate of twin pregnancies is 2.5 times greater than for singletons (approximately 14 per 1,000 live births), and the risk increases with increasing gestational age and monochorionic versus dichorionic pregnancies. The stillbirth rate for triplet and higher-order multiples is even higher at 30 per 1,000 live births (MacDorman & Gregory, 2015). Patients with a past obstetric history of preterm birth, fetal growth restriction, or preeclampsia are at increased risk of stillbirth in a subsequent pregnancy with 1.7- to twofold increased risk (ACOG, 2023b). Patients with a prior stillbirth have an odds ratio of 4.83 for a recurrent stillbirth (Lamont et al., 2015). Patients with pregestational diabetes have a two- to fivefold increased risk of stillbirth, those with chronic hypertension have a two- to fourfold increased risk of stillbirth, and those with other conditions such as lupus, obesity, and chronic renal disease have an increased risk of stillbirth, for which antenatal fetal surveillance is recommended (ACOG, 2023b). The rate of stillbirth increases after 39 weeks with a relative risk of 2.9 at 41 weeks and 5.1 at 42 weeks (SMFM, 2020). Fetal growth restriction is associated with a significant increased risk of stillbirth with risk increasing for lower growth percentiles (ACOG, 2023b). Genetic and chromosomal abnormalities, infections, and umbilical cord events are also associated with stillbirth (ACOG, 2023b).

Diagnosis and Management

A stillbirth is diagnosed with ultrasound and the absence of fetal cardiac activity. This is often confirmed with two separate examiners. Upon diagnosis emotional support is provided to the patient and their family. The essential components of a stillbirth evaluation include a fetal autopsy or examination; gross and histologic examination of the placenta, umbilical cord, and membranes; and a genetic evaluation. Maternal evaluation includes a thorough maternal medical and obstetric history and family history with a three-generation pedigree, with particular attention to recurrent pregnancy losses, individuals with developmental delay or structural anomalies, consanguinity, and a history of cardiac arrhythmias and sudden cardiac death. Additional maternal assessment should include fetomaternal hemorrhage (Kleihaur-Betke or flow cytometry test as soon as possible after the diagnosis) and evaluation for antiphospholipid antibody syndrome (laboratory evaluation for lupus anticoagulant, immunoglobulin G and immunoglobulin M for both anticardiolipin and beta-2-glycoprotein antibodies; if positive, confirmatory repeat testing is recommended in 12 weeks). In cases of preterm labor, PPROM, or chorioamnionitis further investigations for infectious causes may also be undertaken (ACOG, 2023b).

Delivery of the stillborn fetus may be accomplished by induction of labor or dilation and evacuation in the second trimester (if an experienced healthcare provider is available), though this may limit the efficacy of autopsy and may preclude the patient and family from seeing and holding the fetus. There is an increased risk for needing a dilation and curettage for placental removal after induction in the second trimester. Thus, the risks and benefits of each mode of delivery should be discussed with the patient and their family, with shared decision-making to determine the optimal method for delivery on an individualized basis.

In subsequent pregnancies, patients who have experienced a stillbirth have a 2.5 times increased risk of recurrence, 18 to 22 per 1,000 births. This risk may be higher based on the underlying etiology or contributions to the prior stillbirth, and for many cases, the etiology is unknown or unexplained (ACOG, 2023b). A careful review of relevant original medical records and documentation of the prior stillbirth, placental pathology, autopsy, and other evaluations should be completed. Antepartum surveillance should be conducted for maternal specific conditions such as diabetes and hypertension, and for patients with previous stillbirth antepartum surveillance is recommended once or twice weekly beginning at 32 weeks or 1 to 2 weeks prior to the gestational age of the previous stillbirth. Timing of delivery should be individualized, with consideration of the increased risk of neonatal admission with respiratory complications for deliveries less than 39 weeks; however, significant maternal anxiety in the setting of a prior stillbirth may warrant an early term delivery between 37 + 0/7 and 38 + 6/7 weeks gestation with appropriate education, counseling, and acceptance of neonatal risks in the early term period (ACOG, 2023b).

PROFESSIONAL CONSIDERATIONS

This chapter describes the high-risk pregnancy factors and specific maternal and fetal conditions of high-risk pregnancies that contribute to maternal morbidity and mortality. The APRN is a key member of the transdisciplinary team needed to treat high-risk pregnancies. APRNs are particularly useful in reducing barriers to care in rural communities. Collaboration, consultation, and communication are paramount to improving the health of pregnant women and their babies.

REFERENCES

References for this chapter are online and available at https://connect.springerpub.com/content/book/978-0-8261-6722-4/part/part03/chapter/ch38

CHAPTER 39

Intrapartum and Postpartum Care*†‡

Alyssa Davis Larsen, Kady Frye, Rachel Cox, Rebeccah Dindinger, and Brittany Jessica Hannigan

No matter how much an expectant parent and their clinician/s prepare and plan, birth is a spontaneous, unpredictable event. Furthermore, the care provided to a patient during the intrapartum and postpartum periods has the potential to affect a patient for the rest of their life. This chapter focuses on the care rendered to a patient during the life-altering event known as childbirth.

INTRAPARTUM CARE

The intrapartum period is the period of care received during labor and delivery or childbirth. Specifically, the intrapartum period begins with the onset of labor and ends at the completion of the third stage of labor.

Labor and Delivery

LABOR

The antenatal, intrapartum, and postpartum healthcare provider's knowledge of the normal physiologic changes that occur during labor, delivery, and postpartum is essential when managing the care of a patient during childbirth. Intrapartum providers in hospitals are most often certified nurse-midwives (CNMs), certified nurse anesthetists (CRNAs), and medical doctors (MDs) with a certification in obstetrics. The role of the women's health nurse practitioner (WHNP) as an intrapartum healthcare provider mostly occurs in triage units, education, and sometimes management of labor but not delivery (in most states). However, all healthcare providers must be familiar with the assessment and management of labor and possible delivery of the antenatal client in an emergency situation. The cause of labor is not implicit; diagnosis of labor is based on clinical judgment and has no clear-cut, explicit, agreeable starting point (Kobayashi et al., 2017). If a patient is admitted before active labor, they are at increased risk for obstetric intervention. If the healthcare provider fails to diagnose labor, the patient is at risk for a medically unattended birth, which increases the risk of complications for the patient and neonate.

The initiation of human parturition is affected by a course of speculated causes involving changes in the maternal uterus and fetoplacental hormonal stimulation. Labor is the presence of uterine contractions of adequate intensity, frequency, and duration to convey consistent, progressive effacement and/or dilation of the cervix. Labor is divided into three phases. The first phase of labor, known as the latent phase, occurs when uterine contractions are becoming coordinated and lasts until onset of the active phase. Once cervical dilation is 6 cm, the laboring patient is usually entering the active phase, which is illustrated by organized, strong contractions and the most rapid changes in cervical dilation as plotted against time (Hanley et al., 2016). The active phase of labor includes both an increased rate of cervical dilation and, ultimately, descent of the presenting fetal part.

On the contrary, Braxton Hicks contractions are weak, irregular contractions, and can occur for weeks before the onset of actual labor, resulting in no progressive cervical change. The transformation of the uterus from calm to active contraction remains a conundrum. Some shared theories include fetal maturation, cervical ripening, and stretching of the uterus. Other theories deserve further explanation, such as a shift in estrogen and progesterone levels, and uterine sensitivity to oxytocin and the inflammatory process.

---

*This chapter is a revision of the chapter that appeared in the second edition of this textbook, authored by Heather Dawn Reynolds, Allison McCarson, Lilyan Kay, and Meredith Goff, and we thank them for their original contribution.
†The opinions and assertions expressed herein are those of the author(s) and do not necessarily reflect the official policy or position of the Uniformed Services University or the Department of Defense.
‡The opinions and assertions expressed herein are those of the author(s) and do not necessarily reflect the official policy or position of the U.S. Air Force, Department of Defense, or the U.S. government.

Physiology of Labor

ESTROGEN AND PROGESTERONE SHIFT

Estrogen and progesterone, as well as several other hormones, play an important role in maintaining pregnancy. During pregnancy, these hormones increase sevenfold as compared to a nonpregnant patient. Elevated estrogen levels in pregnancy have significant effects on the maternal cardiovascular system, liver protein synthesis, and the uterus itself. These effects include an increase in various aspects, such as binding proteins and clotting factors, uterine blood flow, and sodium retention, and a decrease in vascular resistance. Estrogen stimulates uterine growth, increases the blood supply to the uterine vessels, and increases uterine contractions near term. It also aids in the development of the glands and ducts in the breasts in preparation for lactation. These are all necessary in the maternal adaptation to pregnancy and can have a profound effect on pregnancy. During the last 6 weeks of pregnancy, there is a rapid increase in estrogen levels, causing a change in the ratio between estrogen and progesterone before the onset of labor.

Progesterone synthesis, initially occurring in the corpus luteum, takes place in the placenta following the seventh week of pregnancy. Progesterone induces changes in the endometrium that are required for implantation; these levels must be maintained for the pregnancy to progress. This hormone acts to relax the smooth muscles of the uterus, preventing spontaneous abortion; however, withdrawal of progesterone in early pregnancy results in spontaneous abortion. Progesterone also plays a role in changes that occur in immune function during pregnancy to prevent rejection of the fetus or placenta as foreign antigens (Chan et al., 2002; Druckmann & Druckmann, 2005). A drop in the ratio between progesterone and estrogen has been thought to signal the onset of labor. Progesterone withdrawal, the most frequently recognized model of labor initiation, is thought to interrupt the myometrium or the smooth core tranquil state, resulting in uterine contractions (Chan et al., 2002; Druckmann & Druckmann, 2005).

OXYTOCIN

Oxytocin, a cyclic nonapeptide (a peptide made up of nine amino acids) biochemically similar to vasopressin, is synthesized as a large precursor peptide in the paraventricular and supraoptic nuclei of the hypothalamus. This precursor peptide, which undergoes cleavage during its transport to the posterior pituitary, is stored in association with another protein, neurophysin, in granules in the nerve terminals located in the posterior pituitary (Chan et al., 2002; Druckmann & Druckmann, 2005). In response to peripheral stimuli from the cervix and vagina, the neurophysin–oxytocin complex is released from the storage granules into the plasma in a pulsatile fashion. Once in the plasma, the oxytocin–neurophysin complex dissociates and oxytocin becomes a free molecule, able to bind to its receptors in myometrial, endometrial, and amnion cells.

The role of oxytocin in the regulation of uterine myometrial contractility is well documented. Myometrial oxytocin receptor sites increase by almost 200% during pregnancy, reaching their peak in early labor. This rise in oxytocin receptivity and stimulation of prostaglandin release in the uterus are thought to mediate contractions, which transform the uterus from quiescent to active contractions (Chan et al., 2002; Druckmann & Druckmann, 2005). It is known that the frequency of oxytocin cyclic pulses increases during spontaneous labor, reaching maximal frequency during the second and third stages of labor. This increased oxytocin production is probably necessary for the expulsive efforts needed for the birth of the baby and placenta (Chan et al., 2002; Druckmann & Druckmann, 2005). However, uterine contraction pressures and cervical dilation do not correlate with peripheral plasma oxytocin levels, so it remains unclear what role oxytocin plays in the initiation of parturition.

INFLAMMATORY PROCESS

It has been suggested that a major proportion of genes (e.g., interleukin 8 [IL-8], manganese superoxide dismutase, and metalloproteinase-9) upregulated during labor is associated with inflammatory-immune pathways of the lower segment of the myometrium (Chan et al., 2002). Another theory purports a mild proinflammatory state with increased IL-6 levels and may prime neonatal neutrophils to maximize their antibacterial potential (Chan et al., 2002). Labor at term or early onset labor could potentially boost neutrophil numbers by delaying apoptosis without excessive neutrophil activation or tissue damage.

As noted, many aspects of labor are not clearly understood. However, the regulation of uterine activity by progesterone, estrogen, and oxytocin appear to hold a role in parturition. However, just as the mechanism for the initiation of labor is not yet determined, the precise onset of labor is not readily discernible. A challenge is presented when a patient's self-diagnosis of labor does not coincide with clinical diagnosis and time of admission to hospital (Hanley et al., 2016).

Assessment

SIGNS OF LABOR

Standard signs of labor are painful contractions resulting in cervical dilatation of at least 5 cm, which progressively changes; an increase in bloody show; and spontaneous rupture of membranes. Patients and healthcare providers struggle with identifying the *right time* to make the transition to the healthcare facility with complete accuracy (Gross et al., 2006). Teaching patients when to transition from home to hospital includes instructions about the timing, frequency, duration, and strength of contractions and status of the amniotic membranes.

Patients are encouraged to report to their clinician the following signs of labor: regular uterine contractions that increase in frequency, intensity, and duration; spontaneous rupture of membranes; and/or bloody show. These preliminary signs may or may not lead to cervical change. Patients who wait too long to seek medical assistance increase their risk for an unattended birth at home or birth en route to the healthcare facility. On the other hand, premature admission to the labor and delivery unit may result in an increased risk of obstetric intervention, epidural anesthesia, and/or cesarean delivery (Hanley et al., 2016). A critical point of assessment for the clinician is to be open to the varied types of unique experiences patients may be having and actively listen to their concerns (Slade et al., 2003). The clinician can accomplish this by explaining to patients the range of normal while also adding that there is not just one *right way* to identify labor or to define it (Slade et al., 2003). Any patient reporting leaking of vaginal fluids or suspicion for rupture of membranes should be encouraged to seek medical care to rule out or confirm the suspicion of ruptured membranes. The function of labor contractions is to dilate the cervix and move the fetus through the birth canal. In both nulliparous and multiparous patients, dilation from 4 to 5 cm can take up to 6 hours, and it can take over 3 hours to go from 5 cm to 6 cm. After 6 cm, progress of labor can be plotted using graphs with an expectation of 0.5 to 0.7 cm/hour dilation for nulliparous patients and 0.5 to 1.3 cm/hour for multiparous, which is considered normal labor progression (Zhang et al., 2010).

The strength of contractions varies with the stage of labor, state of the cervix, exogenous oxytocin administration, and pain medication. The strength of contraction is assessed by observation of the patient, palpation of the fundus, and use of an internal pressure transducer.

When the evaluation of contractions is difficult due to various factors (e.g., body habitus) or when the response to oxytocin is unclear, intrauterine pressure catheters may be beneficial. The intrauterine pressure of the uterus during a contraction is reported in Montevideo units (MVUs). To calculate MVUs, choose a 10-minute period, subtract the baseline pressure of each contraction in the period from the peak of each contraction, then calculate the sum of those numbers. The use of MVUs for evaluation of contraction strength varies by institutional protocol and may not be used in all areas of the United States. Caution must be taken when using intrauterine pressure monitoring as a substitute for one-on-one nursing care during labor.

Healthcare providers who manage labor are concerned with fetal size, lie, presentation, attitude, position, station, and pelvis. The fetal head attempts to accommodate the birth canal through a process known as the cardinal movements of labor. These movements are engagement, descent, flexion, internal rotation, extension, external rotation, and expulsion. Engagement is the arrival of a fetal presenting part below the pelvic inlet, at or below the ischial spines, and is determined by palpation of the fetal head in relation to the ischial spines. Descent is the downward passage of the presenting part through the pelvis. Ideally, the fetus is in a cephalic presentation, with a completely flexed fetal head descending through the pelvis. The presenting part rotates anteriorly or posteriorly as it passes through the pelvis, resulting in the widest axis of the fetal head lining up with the widest axis of the pelvis. Once the head is in line with the pelvis, it descends to the level of the introitus and extension occurs. The fetal head delivers and the fetal torso rotates as the body of the fetus is delivered (expulsion). Cardinal movements are described as passive actions synchronized with contractions and maternal pushing.

Stages of Labor

The indication of active labor is generally signified with regular uterine contractions with cervical dilation of 6 cm or greater; this is also commonly the accepted criteria for admission to a labor and delivery unit in many institutions. The onset of active versus latent labor is usually arbitrarily assigned based on subjective reports. Being decisive as to when a patient is in true labor can be challenging even for the most experienced healthcare provider. A goal for the healthcare provider is to avoid the temptation to admit a patient in the latent phase of labor in order to relieve their pain or soothe their fear. A mutual understanding of the diagnosis of labor can be exasperating for both the patient and healthcare provider.

STAGE ONE

Stage one of labor consists of three phases: latent, active, and transition. This stage of labor is marked by psychological and physical changes; it consists of distention of the lower uterine segment and ends with full dilation of the cervix. Anxiety and fear of personal injury and fetal injury are the most commonly verbalized psychological concerns and vary from patient to patient. A patient experiencing excessive anxiety produces increased catecholamine secretions, which make their brain perceive physical pain that is out of proportion to the physiologic stimulus. Physical change is the consequence of mechanical stretching of cervical tissue and pressure on adjacent structures surrounding the vagina and distention of the pelvic floor as the fetus descends into the pelvis. The physical changes associated with the first stage of labor can last 12 to 14 hours as the cervix thins and dilates.

Latent Phase

During the latent phase, a patient or their support person may call the office or hospital to report regular, somewhat uncomfortable contractions, which may be described as lower back pain. This phase of labor is usually marked by slow, progressive change. Contractions usually increase in frequency, duration, and intensity of discomfort. The patient may note an increase in bloody show as well as experience a spontaneous rupture of amniotic membranes.

The most frequently asked question directed at the healthcare provider during the latent phase is, when should I go to the hospital? The healthcare provider should instruct the patient to seek medical care when their contractions are approximately 3 to 5 minutes apart; when their contractions become progressively stronger, longer, and more uncomfortable (e.g., can't walk or talk through contractions); or immediately if their amniotic membranes rupture. During this phase, anticipatory guidance regarding labor and pain management options becomes more important to the patient. Education is most effective, with the inclusion of family along with the laboring patient. The family member or support person is encouraged to provide emotional support to the laboring patient. The use of complementary therapies (e.g., back rubs, baths, meditation) may assist with discomfort during this phase.

Active Phase

As the patient's cervical dilation progresses from 6 to 8 cm (the active phase of labor), they will report more intense discomfort (King & Pinger, 2014). The fetus continues to descend into the pelvis, contributing to the patient's increased discomfort, which often results in a request for greater pain management—such as an epidural.

Admission is ensured with the onset of painful, regular uterine contractions resulting in progressive cervical effacement and/or dilatation. Full evaluation of the laboring patient includes fetal presentation, position, uterine contraction pattern and strength, fetal heart rate (FHR) pattern, and evaluation of the patient's prenatal record.

Transition

Transition (8–10 cm of cervical dilation) is the period when the patient experiences the strongest, most frequent contractions, commonly marked by a transition to high anxiety and fear of losing control (even in the previously calm, cooperative patient). The laboring patient may exhibit nausea with vomiting, shivering, and shaking; all of which are normal during labor.

STAGE TWO

The second stage of labor begins with full cervical dilatation (10 cm) and ends with the delivery of the infant. This stage varies from a few minutes to a few hours. A fetus with a large presenting diameter may increase the mean duration of stage two. If the second stage exceeds 3 hours without an epidural or 4 hours with an epidural in a nulliparous patient, it is considered to be a prolonged second stage of labor. In a multiparous patient, the second stage is considered prolonged if labor exceeds 2 hours without an epidural, or 3 hours with an epidural (Kopas, 2014; Spong et al., 2012).

A patient in this stage may report rectal pressure and an involuntary urge to bear down with contractions. The healthcare provider may note an increase in bloody show and rapid fetal descent as the laboring patient responds to the urge to push.

STAGE THREE

Time from delivery of the infant to separation and expulsion of the placenta is the third stage of labor. Following delivery of the fetus, the upper segment of the uterus retracts rapidly. Separation of the placenta then occurs due to the shrinking of the site and the area of attachment. The placenta is forced down into the lower uterine segment and as the abdominal muscles and diaphragm contract, the placenta is then expelled through the vagina. The mechanism of action behind this separation is a decrease in placental site, a decrease in intrauterine pressure, formation of a line of cleavage in the decidua, and formation of a retroplacental clot. Bleeding from the newly uncovered implantation site continues until the placenta is expelled. The placenta can be expelled through either the Schultze mechanism or the Duncan mechanism.

The Schultze mechanism is used when the placenta separates from the central area to the margins with inversion, causing the fetal side to present first. With the Duncan mechanism, the placenta separates from the margins to the center and the maternal side is presented first. Placental separation is marked by the lengthening of the umbilical cord, a gush of blood from the vagina, and a globular shape of the fundus. After the expulsion of the placenta, the maternal and fetal surfaces, as well as the umbilical cord, should be inspected for intactness and abnormalities. The placenta usually weighs about one seventh of the neonatal weight. The fetal surface is shiny, and the maternal surface consists of cotyledons (each cotyledon consists of a main stem of chorionic villus). The normal appearance of the umbilical cord consists of three vessels (two arteries and one vein) and usually measures 50 to 60 cm in length. The cord should be inserted far from the margin on the fetal surface of the placenta and should have a coiled pattern.

If the placenta does not separate spontaneously or copious bleeding occurs, an abnormal implantation must be considered. Such an abnormal invasion of the placental villi to the uterine wall can be a life-threatening condition (Wiedaseck & Monchek, 2014). Placenta accreta occurs when the placental villi abnormally adhere to the myometrium, with partial or complete absence of the decidua basalis. Placenta increta occurs when the placental villi embed deeply into the muscular walls of the uterus. Placenta percreta occurs when the placenta penetrates through the entire uterine wall and attaches to the bladder or other organs. This diagnosis may require advanced medical intervention or surgery and can lead to the necessity of a peripartum hysterectomy.

A previous cesarean delivery is associated with more significant risk for placenta accreta, placenta previa, uterine rupture, injury to internal organs during surgery, excessive blood loss, need for hysterectomy, and maternal death. Uterine scarring secondary to previous cesarean delivery may lead to abnormal trophoblast invasion and subsequent placenta accreta (Hundley & Lee-Parritz, 2002). Approximately 50% of pregnancies complicated by placenta accreta are in patients who have had a previous cesarean section; the risk increases with each subsequent cesarean delivery, reaching a rate of more than 60% in patients with greater than three cesarean deliveries (Hundley & Lee-Parritz, 2002).

Management of Labor

STAGE ONE

Maintaining adequate uterine contractions, monitoring for cervical progression, evaluation of fetal descent, as well as monitoring maternal and fetal well-being is the focus of this stage of labor (Box 39.1). If spontaneous contractions fail to affect progressive cervical dilation or descent of the fetus, artificial stimulation of uterine contractions with oxytocin augmentation should be considered. If not already ruptured, an amniotomy may also be performed to augment labor or to facilitate internal monitoring. Measures such as massage, controlled breathing, baths, and previously established epidurals can be used to facilitate comfort and relaxation during this phase of labor (Impey et al., 2000; Slade et al., 2003).

STAGE TWO

During stage two, the healthcare provider focuses on fetal descent and well-being. If an unexpected birth occurs outside the hospital, the healthcare provider needs to be prepared with an emergency delivery kit and appropriate supplies (Box 39.2).

Before any invasive management interventions during the second stage, the healthcare provider should consider reassessment of the maternal pelvis, cervix, expulsive forces, and the fetus for size, position, and presentation. Maternal position for pushing and birth have shifted with the transition to hospital birth and increased assisted vaginal delivery with forceps. In recent decades, after the shift of childbirth to the hospital, the lithotomy position has become the norm for the second

Box 39.1 Summary of ACOG Recommendations for Labor Management

- Counsel patients that upright positions (walking, standing, sitting, kneeling) may shorten the duration of the first stage of labor and decrease risk of cesarean and operative vaginal birth.
- It is beneficial for patients and their newborns to have continuous support during labor.
- Although active management of labor may shorten labor in nulliparous patients, it has not consistently been shown to reduce the rate of cesarean delivery.
- Amniotomy may be used to enhance progress in active labor but may increase the risk of maternal infection.
- Data support pushing at the start of the second stage of labor for nulliparous patients with an epidural. Risks of delayed pushing include infection, hemorrhage, and neonatal acidemia.

ACOG, American College of Obstetricians and Gynecologists.
Source: American College of Obstetricians and Gynecologists. (2019). ACOG Committee Opinion No. 766: Approaches to limit intervention during labor and birth. Obstetrics & Gynecology, 133(2), e164–e173. https://doi.org/10.1097/AOG.0000000000003074

Box 39.2 Emergency Delivery Kit

Towels, sheets, and blankets

Neonatal hat

Sterile gloves

Sterile scissors

Oxytocin

Intravenous infusion start kit (optional)

Syringes

22-gauge, 1-inch needles

Alcohol wipes

Bulb syringe

Cord clamps (2)

Kelly clamps

Methylergonovine (Methergine)

1,000 mL lactated Ringer's solution (optional)

Source: McFarlin, A. (2019). The emergency department management of precipitous delivery and neonatal resuscitation. Relias Media. https://www.reliasmedia.com/articles/144422-the-emergency-department-management-of-precipitous-delivery-and-neonatal-resuscitation

stage of labor. Evidence suggests that the lithotomy or a supine position increases the risk for FHR abnormalities and fewer spontaneous vaginal deliveries. The upright position, either sitting or squatting, is optimal for fetal descent with a lateral or hands–knees position for decreased lacerations during birth (Kopas, 2014). When bearing down efforts are not reflexive or spontaneous, coaching may be needed. Directed pushing, or

coaching, should be considered an intervention; it is the most common management of the second stage of labor. Directed pushing methods are conducted with the patient in a lithotomy position while holding their breath and pushing for 10 seconds. Spontaneous pushing has been found to be safer for both mom and fetus, but if guidance is needed, encourage the laboring patient to push instinctively with three to four focused pushes of less than 6 seconds with each contraction. There are a variety of ways to encourage a patient to push; however, the paramount method is what works best for them.

If the patient has not attended childbirth classes or does not have a coach, they should be encouraged to do what comes naturally and to follow their body's urge (Bloom et al., 2006). Patients may choose to squat, stand, kneel, or sit on the toilet. The patient may also use a squatting bar or birthing ball. Other than in the Western culture, patients rarely choose to push while lying in bed.

STAGE THREE

Management of the third stage of labor includes clamping of the umbilical cord, delivery of the placenta, and evaluation of the maternal status to include close assessment for postpartum hemorrhage (PPH). There have been many documented studies that show the benefits of delayed umbilical cord clamping, including increasing neonatal iron stores and preventing anemia in both full-term and preterm infants. The incidence of hyperbilirubinemia requiring phototherapy increases slightly with delayed cord clamping, so it is important to consider the resources for treatment. It is recommended to delay cord clamping for 30 to 60 seconds after birth in vigorous term and preterm infants (American College of Obstetricians and Gynecologists [ACOG], 2020b; McDonald et al., 2013).

Active management of the third stage of labor is recommended for reduction of the risk of severe PPH. This active management of the third stage includes the administration of oxytocin immediately following fetal delivery, gentle cord traction, and uterine massage (Begley et al., 2019). Several maneuvers can be used to deliver the placenta and should be considered if the placenta has not separated after 20 to 30 minutes. The Brandt–Andrews maneuver is used frequently to assist with the delivery of the placenta. The abdominal hand secures the uterine fundus to prevent inversion and downward traction is exerted on the umbilical cord with the other hand. Another method is the Crede maneuver, by which the cord is fixed with the lower hand and the uterine fundus is secured while traction is exerted upward using the abdominal hand.

Retained products of conception will contribute to continued uterine bleeding, in which case manual uterine exploration should be considered to remove any retained products of conception. Oxytocin should be given intravenously as an initial bolus dose then a continuous maintenance infusion for a minimum of 4 hours. If intravenous (IV) access is not available, and oxytocin is given intramuscularly, this route will take 3 to 5 minutes to stimulate contraction of the uterus (Association of Women's Health, Obstetric and Neonatal Nurses [AWHONN], 2021a).

The average blood loss during a vaginal delivery is 500 mL. A loss of more than 1,000 mL during the first 24 hours following a vaginal or cesarean delivery is defined as PPH, though an even lower blood loss in a patient with anemia can result in hemodynamic instability. PPH was traditionally a subjective diagnosis based on estimated blood loss (EBL). This is problematic as, in many instances, the amount of bleeding is underestimated due to the fact that blood is mixed with amniotic fluid and is often absorbed in linens and towels used during labor and delivery (Magann & Lanneau, 2005). More recently, some hospitals have introduced methods to quantitatively assess blood loss by weighing and measuring output. This is thought to increase accuracy in EBL, leading to faster treatment of patients with acute blood loss anemia and hemodynamic instability from PPH. After the delivery of the placenta, assessment should also include a thorough evaluation of the labia, perineum, cervix, and vagina for lacerations.

Obstetric Interventions

The most frequent obstetric interventions performed during labor are induction or augmentation of labor with cervical ripening, oxytocin, amniotomy, and cesarean section. As previously mentioned, oxytocin is used to stimulate labor and to differentiate functional uterine disorders from dystocia, which are frequently caused by four abnormalities (Fraser et al., 1993):

- Expulsive forces (e.g., contractions)
- Conditions, position, or development of the fetus (e.g., large for gestational age, malpresentation)
- Maternal bony pelvis (e.g., cephalopelvic disproportion [CPD])
- Other factors such as soft tissue dystocia

CERVICAL RIPENING

Cervical ripening can be used when there is an indication for induction, but the cervix is unfavorable (determined by Bishop score). This can soften, thin, and dilate the cervix, resulting in a reduction in failed induction rates and induction to delivery time. Common methods used include mechanical dilators, such as a Foley catheter or double balloon device, and pharmacologic agents, such as synthetic prostaglandin E1 (PGE1) and prostaglandin E2 (PGE2). There is not sufficient evidence to assess whether mechanical methods versus prostaglandins are more effective for decreased vaginal delivery time. However, compared to oxytocin alone, mechanical induction methods are associated with a decreased cesarean delivery rate. Additionally, prostaglandins increase the likelihood of vaginal delivery within 24 hours of induction, but do not decrease the rate of cesarean delivery (ACOG, 2009).

AMNIOTOMY

An amniotomy is frequently performed to induce or augment labor or to facilitate internal monitoring. For patients in spontaneous labor or patients who have slowed labor progress, amniotomy with oxytocin augmentation has shown to reduce labor duration by approximately 1 hour. Amniotomy alone has not been shown to have any significant difference in outcomes (ACOG, 2019b).

Internal Monitoring

Some patients may require internal monitoring to gather additional information required for decision-making. An intrauterine pressure catheter (IUPC) is placed through the vagina into the uterine cavity and is used to measure contractions with more precision and accuracy than an external monitor. This is especially useful when oxytocin is being used for induction and no labor progress is being made. Inserting an IUPC can give a clearer picture of the strength and adequacy of contractions. An IUPC is also used when an amnioinfusion is indicated.

A fetal spiral electrode (FSE) is another internal monitor that is used in patients who require closer monitoring of the FHR or when FHR cannot be detected accurately with external monitoring. FSEs can also provide limited information about some types of arrhythmias but is not a diagnostic tool. Internal monitoring is invasive and slightly increases risk for infection, so it should be used based on clinical need (Lyndon & Wisner, 2021).

OXYTOCIN

Oxytocin is a medication used for induction and augmentation of labor. The goal of oxytocin use is to strengthen uterine contractions, effecting cervical change and fetal descent, while simultaneously avoiding uterine tachysystole and fetal compromise. The role oxytocin plays in the initiation of labor is unclear; however, its role in establishing labor is better understood. In addition, the contractile response of the uterine myometrium to oxytocin is to some extent predictable; the higher concentration of receptors to the uterine fundus increases the response of synthetic oxytocin.

Oxytocin protocols vary according to institutional policy. Common protocols include starting infusion at 1 to 2 mU/min and increasing by 1 to 2 mU/min every 30 to 60 minutes. The half-life of oxytocin is approximately 10 to 12 minutes and to reach physiologic steady state, three to four half-lives are needed; therefore, 30 minutes is the earliest recommended time for increasing in order to assess the full effect of dosage. It is recommended to use the lowest dose of oxytocin needed to achieve adequate labor in order to reduce the risk of tachysystole. If the dosage reaches 20 mU/min, consider reevaluating the clinical situation (Lyndon & Wisner, 2021; Simpson, 2020).

Laboring patients are usually not restricted to staying in bed during an oxytocin infusion. Issues regarding whether to be on bed rest or not during oxytocin administration have centered around a laboring patient's increased risk for uterine tachysystole (historically monitored with continuous fetal monitoring). With the advent of ambulatory fetal monitoring capability, many institutions now allow a laboring patient to freely move about during oxytocin administration.

RISK FACTORS

Tachysystole is a major potential risk of oxytocin and is defined as more than five contractions in 10 minutes, averaged over a 30-minute window (Robinson & Nelson, 2008). Tachysystole may occur without corresponding FHR abnormalities, but should be treated in the same way, as it can result in decreased oxygenation to the fetus.

The risk for uterine rupture increases with tachysystole and is particularly increased if the patient has an earlier history of uterine surgery. Other risks associated with exogenous oxytocin use include maternal water intoxication, hypotension, and with prolonged use (such as with a long and difficult labor induction), postpartum uterine atony and subsequent hemorrhage. Water intoxication, though relatively rare, should be considered in the differential diagnosis of laboring patients with acute changes in mental status or seizures (Ophir et al., 2007).

In the presence of tachysystole, immediate discontinuation of the oxytocin infusion, increasing IV fluids, and positioning the patient in a lateral position usually result in a quick termination of tachysystole and potential fetal distress (Raghuraman et al., 2021; Robinson & Nelson, 2008). However, if the problem persists, the maintenance IV fluids should be increased and a subcutaneous dose of terbutaline can be given. Terbutaline is a beta-adrenergic receptor agonist that causes relaxation of the smooth muscle of the uterus and therefore can be useful as a tocolytic. However, terbutaline is not without side effects, including jitteriness, increased heart rate, tremors, headaches, dizziness, and very rarely, increased blood sugar and seizures (Smith & Merrill, 2006). If tachysystole is prolonged and results in ominous signs of fetal distress, a prompt cesarean section is often indicated.

OPERATIVE VAGINAL INTERVENTIONS

Operative obstetric vaginal delivery interventions include vacuum extraction and forceps-assisted deliveries. Operative vaginal delivery procedures are only appropriate after complete dilation. They may be indicated for prolonged second stage of labor, fetal compromise, or maternal exhaustion or compromise. Potential maternal risks associated with the use of these techniques include soft tissue damage, PPH, thromboembolic events, puerperal infections, and wound infections. Potential risks to the neonate include bruising, lacerations, cephalohematoma, retinal hemorrhage, and brachial plexus palsy.

EPISIOTOMY

There are no specific situations that warrant an episiotomy; therefore, a provider must make the decision based on clinical considerations. Restrictive episiotomy versus routine episiotomy reduces the risk for maternal complications, such as severe perineal trauma and healing complications (ACOG, 2019b).

Mediolateral episiotomy is associated with fewer anal sphincter lacerations than midline episiotomy. Midline (also known as median) episiotomy increases perineal laceration length as well as incidence for sphincter disruption. Midline episiotomy over mediolateral episiotomy preference varies according to the station and position of the presenting part in addition to the experience of the healthcare provider (Macleod & Murphy, 2008). Mediolateral episiotomies are associated with higher blood loss than midline and some studies have demonstrated higher pain scores.

Fetal Monitoring

Electronic fetal monitoring (EFM) was made available in the United States around the 1960s. Fetal compromise has been associated with changes in the baseline FHR, repetitive decelerations, and prolonged decreased variability of the FHR noted during fetal monitoring. EFM was projected to improve perinatal outcome, possibly associated with fetal acidosis. However, false-positive results have led to increased surgical intervention without the expected decline in neonatal morbidity and mortality. The goal of EFM is to prevent severe fetal/neonatal acidemia with minimal unnecessary intervention. Intrapartum fetal assessment can be performed using intermittent or continuous fetal monitoring.

Intermittent monitoring is accomplished with the use of a handheld Doppler—an external transducer or, in low-resource settings, a fetoscope held against the maternal abdomen. Continuous monitoring can be accomplished using an external transducer, held in place by an elastic belt on the patient's gravid abdomen or an internal monitor applied as an electrode attachment to the fetal scalp. The internal monitor requires the cervix to be dilated and amniotic membrane to be ruptured. The decision as to the method of fetal monitoring may vary among stage of labor, institution, and healthcare provider. Interpretation of fetal monitoring patterns includes notation of baseline rate and variability, presence or absence of accelerations, presence of periodic or episodic decelerations in reference to contractions, depth of deceleration, length of deceleration, and trends in patterns, including frequency and duration of contractions.

ASSESSMENT

EFM can be classified in three categories: category I, II, and III. Category I is considered normal and indicates a well-oxygenated fetus. No specific action is required based on a category I tracing. Category II is considered indeterminate. These tracings require continuous monitoring and reevaluation. Category III is abnormal and indicates significant risk for fetal metabolic acidemia. This requires immediate action and expedited delivery if not resolved (Lyndon & Wisner, 2021). EFM should be used as a screening tool for fetal distress. The reporting or recording of fetal monitoring patterns must be inclusive of baseline rate and variability, presence or absence of accelerations, periodic or episodic decelerations, and trends and patterns, and should include frequency and duration of contractions to adequately evaluate fetal well-being and tolerance of labor. It is important that gestational age be considered in the explanation of the pattern. Note that a lack of agreement in visual interpretation of FHR patterns and definitions exists. Fetal monitoring is a procedure performed in 99% of labors occurring in a hospital; however, more research is needed to substantiate the efficacy of EFM (Lyndon & Wisner, 2021). There is no complete agreement concerning guidelines for clinical management of, or interpretation of, category II FHR patterns using EFM. This lack of agreement may delay or prevent clinical intervention for interpretation of fetal monitoring.

COMPLICATIONS IN LABOR

Pain Management

Coping with labor pain represents both a physiologic and psychological challenge to the patient (Smith et al., 2006). Uterine contraction, dilation of the cervix, and stretching of the pelvic floor are the contributing factors to labor pain. Patients may fear that their inability to control themselves during labor may cause harm to their unborn child. Also, if a patient chooses to use pain medication, an additional fear may be complications for themselves. The uncertainty of labor (including the length of time that pain will be experienced, as well as the uncertainty of how strong contractions will get) can lead to increased anxiety in the laboring patient as well as the inability to cope as labor progresses.

The healthcare provider aims to reduce the amount of pain a laboring patient experiences during childbirth by informing them of interventions available, including: parenteral medications, epidural, and nonpharmacologic interventions (e.g., the use of a doula or other support person to coach relaxation and breathing techniques, imagery, acupressure, therapeutic touch, biofeedback, and hypnosis). The use of complementary alternative therapies is increasing due to support by professional organizations such as state boards of nursing.

Complementary and Alternative Therapies

Complementary and alternative medicine (CAM), a group of diverse medical and healthcare systems, practices, and products that are not considered part of conventional medicine, is recognized by the National Institutes of Health and specifically by the National Center for CAM (Table 39.1). Published research supports CAM therapies as safe. In labor and delivery, complementary and alternative therapies, such as the use of doulas, Lamaze techniques, and guided imagery have been shown to reduce the use of pharmaceuticals and epidurals (Cyna et al., 2004).

DOULAS

Ideally, a patient in labor receives one-on-one professional nursing support and care. In reality, the amount of labor support provided is directly related to the availability of staff and patient acuity. Charting, monitoring, medication distribution, high numbers of patients, and low numbers of staff may leave very little time to provide emotional, spiritual, and physical care to the laboring patient. Continuous support by a doula has resulted in reduced cesarean section rates, decreased oxytocin augmentation, shortened duration of labor, and decreased negative maternal perceptions about their delivery (Bohren et al., 2017). Therefore, prenatal care visits should include education about other options for support, such as a doula or other support person.

Traditionally, doulas are women assisting patients and their partners during active labor and immediately postpartum, providing continuous comfort measures. These paraprofessionals assist patients and their partners to carry out their birth plans. The assistance is accomplished by facilitating communication among the patient, their partner, and the healthcare provider. Doulas have no medical or clinical care responsibilities, and their skill set focuses on providing emotional, spiritual, and physical support during labor and delivery. These skilled persons are not friends, family, or relatives, but rather birth assistants. Doulas usually utilize a fee-for-service contract, although some doulas do volunteer their services. Doulas may be trained and apply national standards set forth by their professional organization, DONA (Doulas of North America) International (Steel et al., 2015). Standards include knowledge related to the physiology of labor, the stages of labor, comfort measures, and breastfeeding techniques (Steel et al., 2015). Doulas use imagery, massage, and acupressure to minimize fear and anxiety for the laboring patient. Access to doula services is, however, limited by location, affordability, and insurance coverage.

PREPARED CHILDBIRTH CLASSES

Another form of CAM is active involvement in prepared childbirth classes. Various types of childbirth classes are available, such as the Bradley Method, hypnobirthing, birthing from within, and the most common, Lamaze International. Lamaze is a childbirth education program focused on teaching patients to trust their ability to give birth with minimal medical interventions (Wu et al., 2021). Patients are taught breathing and muscle relaxation techniques (Wu et al., 2021). Patients may present with a birth plan requesting limited intervention including: no restrictions on eating and drinking during labor, the avoidance of IV fluids, no continuous EFM unless absolutely medically necessary, and freedom of movement (DeBaets, 2017; Javernick et al., 2021). The requests of the laboring patients may challenge the medical model and may require discussion on an individual basis (DeBaets, 2017).

GUIDED IMAGERY

Guided imagery is a cognitive activity that focuses on the mind–body connection to decrease pain (Kaplan & Cevik, 2021). The thought is to engage a laboring patient's mind with

TABLE 39.1 Five Domains of CAM

TYPE	EXAMPLES
Alternative medical systems	Homeopathic, naturopathic, Chinese medicine, and Ayurveda medicine
Mind–body medicine	Support groups, biofeedback, Lamaze, cognitive behavioral therapy, meditation, prayer, mental healing, art, music and dance therapies
Biological-based therapies	Herbs, foods, vitamins
Manipulative and body-based therapies	Chiropractic or osteopathic manipulation, massage
Energy therapies	Biofeedback (qigong, reiki, healing touch) Bioelectromagnetic (pulsed fields, magnetic fields, alternating current or direct current fields)

CAM, complementary and alternative medicine.
Source: Data from Smith, C. A., Collins, C. T., Cyna, A. M., & Crowther, C. A. (2006). Complementary and alternative therapies for pain management in labour. Cochrane Database of Systematic Reviews, 2006(4), CD003521. *https://doi.org/10.1002/14651858.CD003521.pub2*

breathing and deep relaxation techniques so that the awareness of the pain from the contraction is reduced. Guided imagery has been shown to decrease anxiety and pain in labor (Kaplan & Cevik, 2021). Catecholamine response decreases as the laboring patient becomes less anxious, resulting in an increased uterine blood flow and decreased muscle tension. Pain tolerance increases even more when the laboring patient's thoughts are guided to pleasant experiences with an end point in relaxation.

HYPNOSIS

Hypnosis is a psychological intervention that reduces awareness of external stimuli and increases response to suggestions (Madden et al., 2016). Suggestions can be in the form of verbal and nonverbal communication that results in noticeable spontaneous changes in perception, mood, or behavior. The therapeutic communication of medical hypnosis is directed at the laboring patient's subconscious (Madden et al., 2016). Patients can be taught self-hypnosis, which can be an adjunct to facilitate and enhance other analgesics for the purpose of reducing labor pain. Hypnosis in childbirth may decrease the use of analgesia but current evidence does not show any significant impact on epidural use or vaginal delivery rate (Madden et al., 2016).

ACUPRESSURE AND THERAPEUTIC TOUCH/MASSAGE

Acupressure is the application of finger pressure or deep massage to the traditional acupuncture points on the hands, feet, and ears or energy flow lines to reduce labor pain (Schlaeger et al., 2017). Therapeutic touch/massage is effective to manage labor pain, lower anxiety, and lower agitation. There are three main goals of therapeutic touch: (1) reduction of pain and anxiety, (2) initiation of relaxation, and (3) stimulation of the healing process (Pinar & Demirel, 2021).

Therapeutic touch/massage therapy can be taught quickly and effectively at the bedside to a friend, family member, or significant other. Laboring patients who receive therapeutic touch/massage have been shown to have shorter labors and less postpartum depression (Pinar & Demirel, 2021). However, not every patient desires to be touched during contractions, and therefore, techniques must be individualized.

AROMATHERAPY

Aromatherapy oils and/or lotions are often used in conjunction with massage. Popular essential oils for use in labor include lavender or jasmine, mixed with a carrier oil or lotion. Inhalation of lavender aroma has been shown to decrease labor pain (Kazeminia et al., 2020). Peppermint oil can be used to decrease nausea and vomiting (Amzajerdi et al., 2019). A few drops of an essential oil (ginger or lemongrass) to hydrotherapy baths can also promote relaxation. When applied during back massage, ginger oil can decrease pain during active labor (Azizi et al., 2020). Hence, guidelines for use of oils in late pregnancy and labor need to be followed according to institutional policy.

HYDROTHERAPY

Another technique frequently used in the first stage of labor is hydrotherapy (laboring in water). To accommodate a laboring patient's request for hydrotherapy, some hospitals have added oversized showers and jetted tubs to their labor units. Although literature to support hydrotherapy is limited, researchers agree that hydrotherapy does not cause harm to the patient or fetus. Hydrotherapy appears to assist with decreasing pain and anxiety in the first stage of labor and decreases the use of regional anesthesia without differences in complication or delivery rates (Cluett et al., 2018). The goal of managing labor pain without causing harm to the patient or fetus can be met by using complementary and alternative pain control methods.

Epidural Analgesia

Another intervention for controlling labor and surgical pain is epidural analgesia. Epidurals have been shown to be effective and safe and are the most commonly used method of pain control in the United States. Small doses of epidural or spinal opioids alone or combined with low doses of local anesthetics have been shown to not affect the well-being of the neonate at birth (Capogna & Camorcia, 2004). The process consists of medications, such as ropivacaine and levobupivacaine, with the addition of an opioid administered through a catheter into the epidural space. During and after the placement of an epidural, the laboring patient must be monitored closely for hypotension and fetal bradycardia, both of which are commonly associated with an epidural. These complications can often be resolved by maternal position change and hydration. Epidural analgesia is also associated with maternal fever, postepidural headache, decreased sensation for pushing, inability to ambulate, potential need for urinary catheterization, and narcotic use in labor (Cluett et al., 2004).

Perineal Trauma

Perineal trauma, or genital tract injury, occurs in 53% to 79% of all vaginal births (ACOG, 2018c). Most perineal trauma is a first- or second-degree laceration. Factors contributing to an increased risk of severe perineal lacerations include poor maternal nutrition, untreated vaginal infections, and uncontrolled expulsion of the fetus. The occurrence of third- or fourth-degree tears is relatively rare and is associated with forceps-assisted delivery, vacuum-assisted delivery, and midline episiotomy. Long-term risk of fecal incontinence, fecal urgency, and/or sexual dysfunction is associated with third- and fourth-degree laceration (ACOG, 2018c).

Lacerations may occur with or without an episiotomy. Some interventions used during labor and birth to minimize the risk of perineal trauma include pushing in the lateral position, upright, and on hands and knees; delivery of the fetal head between contractions; warm compresses; and flexion/counter pressure to slow birth of the fetal head. Prenatal perineal massage with sweet almond oil, evening primrose oil, or other vegetable-based oil for 5 to 10 minutes daily from 34 weeks until delivery (particularly in nulliparous patients) is a protective perineal intervention that can promote elasticity of the perineum (ACOG, 2018c).

MANAGEMENT

Attention should be focused on signs of infection and hemorrhoids during the first few hours to days postdelivery. Monitor the patient for elevated temperature (which could indicate infection of the genitourinary tract). Cool packs of ice or gel applied to the perineum in the immediate postpartum period after a vaginal delivery can help treat pain, edema, and prevent the development of edema or a hematoma, and provides comfort (Petersen, 2011). The laceration or episiotomy site should be free of heat, drainage, or redness. The acronym REEDA can be used as a reminder that the site should be assessed for redness (R), edema (E), ecchymosis (E), discharge (D), and approximation (A). Sutures, used for homeostasis and to approximate tissue, may or may not be visible or palpable.

Assess the postpartum patient's pain level and encourage them to empty their bladder. Encourage warm or cool sitz baths and benzocaine spray to promote pain control and healing. If hemorrhoids are present, offer witch hazel pads and stool softeners, and instruct the patient to increase their fluid and fiber intake. Stool softeners may also be helpful the first few weeks following delivery in the case of a third- or fourth-degree laceration. Kegel exercises should be encouraged to strengthen perineal tone once soreness has decreased and healing of the perineum has occurred.

Cesarean Section

Cesarean delivery is the most common surgical procedure in females in the United States. It accounted for 32.0% of all births in the United States from 2016 to 2018 (Matsuo et al., 2021). Cesarean section carries risks of infection, pelvic structure injury, and potential for blood transfusion. An increase in elective cesarean delivery has stimulated debate in the medical community. In a committee opinion published in January 2019, ACOG did not recommend elective cesarean delivery, but supports a planned vaginal delivery in the absence of medical indications. ACOG recommendations to assist with counseling and decision-making stipulate elective cesarean deliveries should not occur before 39 weeks' gestation (ACOG, 2019a). Patients elect cesarean delivery to reduce a perceived risk of maternal pelvic organ prolapse, urinary and fecal incontinence, pelvic floor dysfunction, avoidance of anxiety and the pain of labor, fear of pelvic exam, and anxiety due to loss of control (Jenabi et al., 2020).

Cesarean delivery can be a lifesaving intervention for the fetus when the pregnancy is complicated by HIV, active herpes, fetal malpresentation, macrosomia, multiple gestation, fetal structural abnormalities, cord prolapse, placental abruption, and fetal distress as noted via FHR monitoring. In emergent situations, such as fetal distress, ACOG recommends incision within 30 minutes of the decision to undertake emergency cesarean section. Even so, the time from decision to incision exceeds 30 minutes in one third to one half of pregnant patients experiencing cesarean sections for nonreassuring FHR tracing.

LABOR DYSTOCIA

Labor dystocia is an idiom used to suggest abnormal labor caused by ineffective expulsive forces of the uterus (power); the position, size, or presentation of the fetus (passenger); and the maternal pelvis or soft tissues (passage). A leading cause of operative vaginal and cesarean delivery and any accompanying complications has been attributed to labor dystocia (ACOG, 2014). Any combination of these factors may result in mechanical problems with the passage of the fetus

through the birth canal. The *International Statistical Classification of Diseases (ICD-10)* coding for labor dystocia includes the diagnoses of prolonged stages of labor, abnormalities of forces of labor (contractions), obstructed labor due to malposition or malpresentation of fetus, or obstructed labor due to maternal pelvic abnormality (World Health Organization [WHO], 2016). A lack of correspondence between the size of the maternal pelvis and the fetal head that results in arrest of fetal descent is termed *dystocia secondary to cephalopelvic disproportion* (Althaus et al., 2006). However, the clinical diagnosis of dystocia cannot be made until the completion of the latent phase of labor and the initiation of active labor (an increased rate of cervical dilatation and descent of fetus), to include an adequate trial of labor. Clinical diagnosis of dystocia, or active phase labor abnormalities, as defined by ACOG's 2014 Obstetric Care Consensus, includes the protraction (slower than normal) or arrest (complete cessation of progress) of labor over time. The diagnosis of arrest of dilation is suggested not to be made prior to 6 cm of dilation (ACOG, 2014).

Many maternal and fetal characteristics may play a role in labor dystocia (see Box 39.3). Other factors labeled as *potentially contributing* to a diagnosis of labor dystocia include hospital admission before active labor has been established (<5–6 cm dilated), induction of labor, use of epidural analgesia, and lack of labor support (King & Pinger, 2014; Lowe, 2007).

For a diagnosis of labor dystocia, the provider should assess and document all the following:

- Cervical dilation at 6 cm or greater
- Ruptured membranes
- No cervical change despite:

Box 39.3 Factors Contributing to Labor Dystocia

Maternal Factors

Nulliparous patient

Age older than 35 years

Height less than 5 feet

Pregnancy weight gain more than 35 lb

Emotional distress and fear

Fetal Factors

Fetal weight more than 4,000 g

Occipitoposterior position

Breech presentation

Infection/sepsis

Fetal station above zero with active labor

Source: Lowe, N. K. (2007). A review of factors associated with dystocia and cesarean section in nulliparous women. Journal of Midwifery & Women's Health, 52(3), 216–228. https://doi.org/10.1016/j.jmwh.2007.03.003

- ○ 4 hours or more of adequate uterine contractions—more than 200 MVUs measured via intrauterine pressure catheter
- ○ 6 hours of inadequate uterine contractions with oxytocin administration

HYPOTONIC LABOR

Dysfunctional labor can be the result of abnormal uterine activity. This can be categorized as hypotonic or hypertonic labor. Hypotonic labor is present when contractions are occurring with normal frequency, but the peak pressure is too low to achieve cervical dilation or descent of the fetus. Although effective contractions can vary in strength from patient to patient, MVUs less than 200 is generally the considered criterion for a diagnosis of hypotonic labor. This type of labor dysfunction usually occurs during the active phase of labor when contractions have been previously established, but then diminish in frequency and strength.

Management

Interventions that can be used for hypotonic labor include rest, ambulation, artificial rupture of membranes, and if no improvement is evident in 1 to 2 hours, labor augmentation with oxytocin.

HYPERTONIC LABOR

Hypertonic labor is characterized by either a high uterine resting tone or by frequent, uncoordinated contractions. This is sometimes referred to as uterine irritability. The contractions will often be perceived by the laboring patient as very strong yet will not cause dilation of the cervix. It is important to rule out placental abruption and chorioamnionitis when this type of labor pattern occurs as this irritability can be a direct result of these issues. Hypertonic labor typically occurs during the latent phase of labor and can be associated with precipitous labor.

Management

This dysfunctional labor pattern can be managed with oxytocin administration in an attempt to establish a more regular, adequate contraction pattern. In contrast to this intervention, analgesia and/or sedation may be used in an effort to cause relaxation of the uterus and then subsequently a new trial of labor can be initiated.

PRECIPITOUS LABOR

Precipitous labor is defined as labor that progresses from start to delivery of an infant in less than 3 hours. Precipitous labor should not be confused with precipitous delivery, which can occur after a labor of any length, and can occur in or out of the hospital or birth center, when a trained assistant is not present for the delivery. Complications that can occur as a result of precipitous labor and delivery include uterine rupture, cervical lacerations, severe perineal lacerations, and hematomas of the vagina or vulva.

MALPRESENTATION/MALPOSITION

The most common fetal presentation is the vertex of the fetal head. Malpresentations are all presentations of the fetus, other than vertex, and can include complete breech, frank breech, footling or double footling breech, or transverse lie. Although complete or frank breech presentations can sometimes be delivered vaginally, it is up to the discretion of the healthcare provider who will take into consideration pelvimetry, absence of macrosomia, and a flexed fetal head.

By contrast, fetal malpositions are abnormal presentations of the vertex fetal head (in reference to the occiput) relative to the maternal pelvis. This includes most commonly the occiput posterior (OP) position. Spontaneous rotation of the fetal head occurs in approximately 90% of cases during the labor process (Simkin et al., 2005). If this rotation does not occur, arrested labor can result as the head does not rotate and descend further into the pelvis. Furthermore, delivery in these cases may be complicated by perineal tears or extension of an episiotomy. Other malpositions that must be addressed are brow presentation, face presentation, chin anterior or posterior presentation, and compound presentation. Each of these presentations are managed differently depending on the individual circumstances (Simkin et al., 2005).

Management

One of the most commonly used interventions to encourage the rotation of the fetus from the OP position is to help the laboring patient get into an open knee–chest position, with their head resting on the bed and hips flexed to greater than 90 degrees. This position tilts the pelvis forward with the inlet lower than the outlet. This allows gravity to encourage the unengaged fetal head to move out of the pelvis and to reposition more favorably toward the occiput anterior position (Simkin et al., 2005). The knee–chest position may also offer relief to patients who are experiencing back labor secondary to laboring with a fetus in the OP position. Lastly, manual rotation of the fetal head may be considered prior to operative vaginal delivery or cesarean delivery (ACOG, 2014).

BREECH PRESENTATION

Over recent years, there has been a trend toward performing cesarean deliveries for breech presentation, and subsequently the number of healthcare providers experienced in breech vaginal deliveries has declined. Cesarean deliveries, however, are not without risk for patient and baby. Decision aids such as booklets or audio-CDs have been found to be an effective, useful, and acceptable adjunct to standard counseling about management options for breech presentation (Nassar et al., 2007; Tiran, 2004). During the last weeks of prenatal visits, when breech presentation is persistent, this information has been shown to be effective in helping a pregnant patient make an informed decision regarding their delivery options (Tiran, 2004).

Management

Research findings reflect that pregnant patients who reviewed decision aids reported feeling significantly more informed and experienced less uncertainty (Nassar et al., 2007). If the pregnant patient wishes to avoid cesarean section when the fetus is in breech, there are several nonsurgical options that may be useful. An external cephalic version can be attempted to turn the fetus to a vertex position so vaginal delivery can be attempted. This is generally done with the aid of ultrasound and tocolytics in order to relax the uterine smooth muscle so the fetus can be manipulated by placing manual pressure on the abdomen to guide the fetus into a vertex position. In addition to this method, various alternative techniques can be used to encourage breech fetuses to spontaneously turn to a vertex position. These methods include pelvic tilt, light, music, the Webster technique, moxibustion, acupressure, homeopathics such as *Pulsatilla*, and herbs such as Bach's Bougainvillea Essence (Tiran, 2004).

Twin Gestation

In the United States, twin (and multiples) gestation has increased in part due to assisted reproductive technology, and increasing maternal age at conception when it is more likely to occur naturally. Although the incidence of twinning has increased, risks associated with twin pregnancy (including during labor and birth) remain greater than with a singleton pregnancy.

RISK FACTORS

A multiple gestation pregnancy has a significantly increased risk of preterm delivery and associated fetal and neonatal complications. The average duration of pregnancy in twins is 35.0 weeks. Patients with multifetal gestations also have an increased incidence of hypertensive disorders of pregnancy, anemia, hemorrhage, cesarean delivery, and postpartum depression.

ASSESSMENT

Chorionicity should be established by ultrasonography as early in pregnancy as possible, ideally in the first trimester or early second trimester, due to the increased risks associated with monochorionic pregnancies. Serial ultrasound exams throughout the pregnancy are commonly performed to assess for fetal anomalies, amniotic fluid, placentation, fetal growth, and position of the presenting fetus. Antepartum fetal testing may also be considered toward the end of pregnancy to monitor fetal well-being (ACOG, 2021b).

MANAGEMENT

The choice of augmentation, induction, vaginal delivery, or cesarean section is influenced heavily by ultrasonographic confirmation of fetal position, gestational age, and experience of the clinician performing the delivery. ACOG (2021b) recommends patients with monoamniotic twin gestations be delivered by cesarean to avoid umbilical cord complications; however, in diamniotic twin gestations, vaginal delivery may be considered if greater than 32 weeks gestation and the presenting fetus is vertex. Due to uterine overdistention and increased incidence of anemia in twin gestations, there is a greater risk for atony and PPH (Cruikshank, 2007). High-dose, IV oxytocin infusion should be considered, as well as methylergonovine and prostaglandin analogs (such as hemabate and misoprostol) and should be readily available for administration in cases of continuous, immediate postpartum bleeding.

Shoulder Dystocia

Shoulder dystocia, a component of labor dystocia, can have serious consequences and cause major concern and even fear among healthcare providers. Shoulder dystocia is frequently unpredictable and has been linked with PPH and neonatal death (Gherman et al., 2006). Other common complications include higher degree perineal lacerations, and neonatal brachial plexus injuries and fractures of the clavicle and humerus (ACOG, 2017a). Shoulder dystocia occurs infrequently and represents a size discrepancy between the fetal shoulders and the pelvic inlet, resulting in the failure of delivery of the fetal shoulder (usually the anterior shoulder). The risk for shoulder dystocia increases when truncal rotation does not occur.

RISK FACTORS

Shoulder dystocia is largely unpredictable with about half occurring in fetuses of average gestational size. There are associated factors, the most prominent of which is higher birth weight. Fetal weight greater than 5,000 g in pregnant patients without diabetes and greater than 4,500 g in pregnant patients with diabetes is a common denominator connecting maternal and fetal risk for shoulder dystocia (Athukorala et al., 2007). Infants of diabetic patients experience shoulder dystocia at an increased rate over nondiabetic patients because of the distribution of the fetal weight. Higher birth weight (fetal macrosomia and large for gestational age) is common among infants of diabetic patients, therefore increasing their risk of shoulder dystocia (Athukorala et al., 2007). History of shoulder dystocia in a prior pregnancy significantly increases the risk of recurrence in subsequent pregnancies. Other proposed risk factors have provedn to be poor predictors of the occurrence of shoulder dystocia, further contributing to its unpredictable nature (ACOG, 2017a).

MANAGEMENT

Up to 42% of shoulder dystocia is reported to be correctable using the McRoberts maneuver as an initial step for the disimpaction of the shoulder during a vaginal delivery. This maneuver is performed by sharply flexing the maternal thighs onto the abdomen. It results in a straightening of the maternal sacrum relative to the lumbar spine, consequently increasing the mean angle of inclination between the symphysis pubis and sacral promontory (Gherman et al., 2006).

Calling for pediatric support is important during shoulder dystocia, an emergency in which fetal hypoxia-acidosis is common (Crofts et al., 2006; Kovavisarach, 2006). Although shoulder dystocia is not a soft tissue issue, an episiotomy may allow the fetal rotational maneuvers to be performed and create more room for attempted delivery of the posterior arm. Suprapubic pressure is usually given before or with the McRoberts maneuver. Pressure is directed posteriorly in an attempt to force the anterior shoulder under the symphysis pubis. Other maneuvers include:

- **Delivery of the posterior arm:** Pressure should be applied at the antecubital fossa in order to flex the fetal forearm. The arm is subsequently swept out over the infant's chest and delivered over the perineum. Rotation of the fetal trunk to bring the posterior arm anterior is sometimes required. Grasping and pulling directly on the fetal arm, as well as application of pressure onto the midhumeral shaft, should be avoided because bone fracture may occur.

- **Woods corkscrew maneuver:** Abduct the posterior shoulder by exerting pressure onto the anterior surfaces of the posterior shoulder.
- **Rubin maneuver:** Pressure is applied to the posterior surface of the most accessible part of the fetal shoulder to effect shoulder adduction.
- **All fours maneuver (also known as the Gaskin maneuver):** Have the patient roll from their existing position onto their hands and knees. The downward force of gravity or favorable change in pelvic diameters produced by this technique may allow disimpaction of the fetal shoulder (Kovavisarach, 2006).
- The Zavanelli maneuver is reserved when all attempts at correction of the shoulder dystocia have failed. The goal of the maneuver is to replace the fetus into the pelvis, relieving the impaction while preparing for cesarean delivery. This maneuver is accomplished by the reversal of the cardinal movements of labor with manual replacement of the fetal vertex into the vagina. There are significant maternal and neonatal complications inherent in this procedure.
- Fundal pressure is not a maneuver believed to alleviate shoulder dystocia and is discouraged from practice in the United States. This technique has been associated with an increased risk of Erb palsy and thoracic spinal cord injury in the neonate. Fundal pressure may further impact the anterior shoulder behind the symphysis pubis (Gherman et al., 2006).

A contemporary approach to preparing personnel for a shoulder dystocia is simulation training. As with cardiopulmonary resuscitation, shoulder dystocia simulation drills provide repeated practice and acquisition of the aforementioned techniques, improving clinical performance of these maneuvers and reducing the incidence of medical negligence (Maslovitz et al., 2007).

ACOG recommends a cesarean delivery be considered for an estimated birth weight of greater than 5,000 g in nondiabetic patients, and greater than 4,500 g in those with diabetes, as a prevention to avoid shoulder dystocia. The decision to perform a cesarean delivery for labor dystocia should be made based on clinical assessment of the patient, the fetus, and the skills of a trained obstetrician (ACOG, 2017a; Crofts et al., 2006).

Nuchal Cord

Nuchal cord, a common fetal complication, can be associated with an increased risk of variable decelerations, acidemia, meconium-stained amniotic fluid, and emergency cesarean section. The degree of tightness of the umbilical cord around the fetal neck has been found to correlate to the degree of fetal distress. A moderately tight cord around the fetal neck may impair cephalic venous blood flow and a very tight nuchal cord may compromise the umbilical circulation and produce systemic hypoxia, hypercapnia, acidemia, and ultimately fetal death.

Meconium-stained amniotic fluid is another common occurrence seen in infants with nuchal cord. Meconium passed by the fetus in labor is often interpreted as a sign of fetal distress or compromise. The risk of fetal compromise is greater when meconium accompanies a nuchal cord. Conversely, the presence of clear amniotic fluid can be an unreliable sign of fetal well-being (Greenwood et al., 2003).

CONSIDERATIONS FOR SPECIAL POPULATIONS

Teen Intrapartum Care

Young maternal age carries with it much pregnancy risk. Being a pregnant young teen has been linked to low birth weight, preterm labor, fetal growth restriction, and infant mortality (McCracken & Loveless, 2014). Pregnant teens have a higher prevalence of anemia, eclampsia, and preeclampsia than pregnant patients between the ages of 20 and 34 years. The risk of intrapartum stillbirth among teens younger than 15 years of age has also been found to be about three times that of older adolescents (Wilson et al., 2008). Therefore, intrapartum fetal surveillance and supportive labor care are important contributions to a positive labor and delivery outcome for the younger teen.

Regardless of the outcome of the pregnancy, teens are at greater risk for repeat pregnancies and sexually transmitted infections than their older counterparts. Safe sex and reproductive education should be a priority with teens during the immediate postpartum period to help prevent close interval pregnancy (McCracken & Loveless, 2014). Long-acting reversible contraception (LARC) may be a good option for these patients, but patients should be counseled on all contraceptive options (McCracken & Loveless, 2014). In addition, teenage patients are more likely to experience postpartum depression and have limited social support; screening and treatment for postpartum depression are critical to positive outcomes for both the teen parent and newborn (McCracken & Loveless, 2014).

Pregnant Athletes

Most professional athletes continue to work out during their pregnancy. Current data show that athletic patients are likely to have term, average-sized infants and may even have an enhanced labor and delivery experience due to their physical fitness (Duncombe et al., 2006). Due to their rigorous regimen and their focus on a healthy lifestyle, these patients may prefer CAM methods of managing labor pain. Many times, these patients seek medical advice to identify any potential risk to themselves or their unborn fetus in reference to continued vigorous exercise during pregnancy and any potential effects at delivery. The ACOG (2020a) Committee Opinion on exercise during pregnancy and during the postpartum periods recommends that the average patient can perform moderate exercise for 30 minutes a day, 7 days a week, and that athletes can remain active during pregnancy but should modify their usual exercise routines as indicated by their healthcare provider. Patients should be instructed not to initiate a vigorous exercise program during the first trimester of pregnancy and limit themselves to moderate exercise a few times a week with medical supervision (Duncombe et al., 2006).

Care of Gender-Diverse Patients

Not all persons who give birth identify as female and care of these patients during labor and the postpartum period requires additional consideration. The use of patient-chosen language, whether gender-affirming or gender-neutral, is important to maintaining trust and confidence in the perinatal care team (Roosevelt et al., 2021). There is not a universal set of correct terminology that will be preferred by every patient, but incorporating the individual's desired terminology for their self, parenting role, and body parts can help to prevent distress due to being misgendered (Hahn et al., 2019; Roosevelt et al., 2021). Providing trauma-informed patient-centered care is particularly beneficial due to increased risk of domestic violence for gender-diverse persons and feelings of dysphoria related to physical changes of pregnancy (Roosevelt et al., 2021).

Gender identity is not an independent risk factor for pregnancy or postpartum complications (Hahn et al., 2019; Roosevelt et al., 2021). Intrapartum care for this population may include limiting cervical exams, use of appropriate pronouns, and utilizing gender neutral terms such as parental heart rate versus maternal heart rate (Hahn et al., 2019). A high rate of elective cesarean deliveries occurs in this population, as some patients perceive vaginal birth as disturbing (Garcia-Acosta et al., 2019). Postpartum contraception should be discussed, as testosterone is not a reliable form of ovulation suppression (Roosevelt et al., 2021).

Lactation care in the postpartum period should focus on the desires of the patient, whether it is to feed human milk or to dry up the milk supply. Allow the birthing parent to choose their desired terminology for infant feeding, whether it is breastfeeding, chest feeding, or human milk feeding (Hann et al., 2019).

Not all patients will want to lactate, and some may have had chest masculinization procedures, which limit milk production. Birth parents may opt to restart testosterone therapy, which interferes with milk production (Garcia-Acosta et al., 2019). Binding the chest, or a history of binding the chest, can lead to an increased risk of mastitis (Garcia-Acosta et al., 2019). In addition to transmasculine patients, parents who identify as transfeminine may be able to lactate through use of the domperidone and breast stimulation with an electric pump (Reisman & Goldstein, 2018), though the literature supporting this is limited.

Racism

In the United States, there are disparities in maternal and infant outcomes for Black patients, compared to their White counterparts (Chambers et al., 2021). Black patients are more likely to have severe complications, fewer breastfeeding resources, and poor pain control (AWHONN, 2021b). inequities persist across socioeconomic status and education, leading to a focus on examining bias to provide safer care. Examining implicit bias in the provision of perinatal care, with the understanding that knowledge, language, and action matter when ensuring care is free from racism and bias (AWHONN, 2021b).

Summary

The healthcare provider's knowledge of antenatal, intrapartum, and postpartum physiology is essential in managing the care of a patient and their unborn child. Healthcare providers who manage labor are concerned with two patients and the safety of both during the course of labor and delivery. Recognizing aberrancies in physiology and pathophysiology of labor and birth and developing an alternative plan of care are critical to ensure the safety and well-being of the laboring patient and their neonate.

POSTPARTUM CARE

The postpartum period begins immediately at birth and extends for up to 12 weeks. This period is a time of great change. What is more, it is also a time of great vulnerability: the patient's health and recovery; the need to acquaint themselves with the infant's needs; if they elect, the need to establish lactation; figuring out where the spouse or partner fit in; and the list goes on. Healthcare providers play an integral role in supporting the newly delivered birth parent and their family to take in all these changes, which impact the family from delivery and beyond.

During the postpartum period, which is also known as the puerperium, patients and their families adapt physically, psychologically, and socially to the changes that have taken place following birth. Commonly, this transition is defined as lasting from 6 to 12 weeks, and it is described as a return to the normal, nonpregnant state (Gabbe et al., 2007). In order to address more acute issues and to close the gap in care often noted after delivery for the postpartum patient, care shouldn't wait until the traditional time of 6 weeks; new recommendations for ongoing individualized care should be reestablished at the 3-week mark and continue as needed through the 12th week (ACOG, 2018a). The postpartum period begins after the delivery of the placenta, with the first hour being referred to as the fourth stage of labor. Although seemingly anticlimactic, it is a crucial juncture calling for vigilance on the part of caregivers. During this first hour, the new birth parent and their infant are monitored closely for a number of physiologic risks, including maternal PPH or respiratory distress in the newborn. During this time, caregivers need to address the patient's comfort needs in addition to providing assistance to the family with bonding with the newborn.

The first 24 hours after birth is referred to as the *immediate postpartum period*, whereas the second day through the first week is called the *early postpartum period*. The term *late postpartum period* refers to the secosecond through 12twelfth weeks. Although some sources claim that these designations are arbitrary, it is worth noting that a number of disparate cultures practice postpartum rituals that entail 40-day periods of seclusion for new parents and babies (Hundt et al., 2000; Kim-Godwin, 2003;0) (see Box 39.4).

Physical Changes of the Postpartum Period

BREASTS

By the end of pregnancy, each breast has gained nearly 1 lbone pound in weight as a result of increased fat, myoepithelial cells, connective tissue, electrolytes, water retention, and

Box 39.4 Cultures That Practice 40 Days of Postpartum Seclusion

Non-Western cultures in which the 40th day has cultural significance include the following:

Palestinian Bedouin

Jordanian

Lebanese

Egyptian

Ancient Hebraic (according to Leviticus 12)

Indian

Mexican American

Source: Hundt, G. L., Beckerleg, S., Kassem, F., Abu Jafar, A. M., Belmaker, I., Abu Saad, K., & Shoham-Vardi, I. (2000). *Women's health custom made: Building on the 40 days postpartum for Arab women.* Health Care for Women International, 21(6), 529–542. https://doi.org/10.1080/07399330050130313; Kim-Godwin, Y. S. (2003). *Postpartum beliefs and practices among non-Western cultures.* American Journal of Maternal/Child Nursing, 28(2), 74–78. https://doi.org/10.1097/00005721-200303000-00006

the hypertrophy of blood vessels. Blood flow to the breasts nearly doubles, which ensures perfusion of the enlarged, lobular structures of the alveolar milk ducts. Colostrum may be secreted at varying times during pregnancy up until the first 2 to 3 days postpartum, and this is followed by transitional and then full milk. Before mature milk comes in, the growth of blood vessels, lymphatics, alveoli, and the further enlargement of the lobules may cause a painful hardening of the breasts known as engorgement. This condition is less likely to occur if the patient is able to breastfeed early and often. The transition to mature milk may be accompanied by low-grade fever; however, significant temperature elevation (e.g., greater than 38°C or 100.4°F) warrants further assessment to identify symptoms (e.g., erythema and tenderness in a wedge shape of one breast, systemic myalgias) that may suggest mastitis (Amir & the Academy of Breastfeeding Medicine Protocol Committee [ABMPC], 2014).

After the delivery of the placenta, the hormones estrogen and progesterone diminish, while prolactin is secreted by the anterior pituitary gland; this in turn stimulates the breasts to secrete colostrum. In response to the stimulus of the infant's suckling, the patient's posterior pituitary gland secretes oxytocin, which stimulates the contractile tissue around the milk ducts and the alveoli, a process known as the *letdown reflex.* Oxytocin also continues to stimulate uterine contractions, preventing PPH (Lee, 2007). Thus, breastfeeding serves an important physiologic function for the birth parent as well as the baby, particularly during the period immediately following delivery.

UTERUS

Immediately after delivery, the uterus decreases to about half of the size that it was before labor (e.g., the size that it was at ~20 weeks' gestation) and weighs about 2 lb. The uterine fundus is palpable at or just below the level of the umbilicus, although the exact location may vary with factors such as the patient's

habitus and the baby's size. For each postpartum day after delivery, the fundus normally descends approximately one fingerbreadth below the umbilicus. By the end of the first week, the uterus reduces in size to a weight of approximately 1 lb. The fundus is palpable just above the pubic symphysis, which is approximately the size that it was at 12 weeks' gestation. The fundus is usually not palpable after 10 days postpartum.

Strong coordinated contractions of the uterus allow involution to occur. The primiparous uterus tends to remain contracted, whereas multiparous patients experience contractions at intervals; these cause *after-pains,* which tend to escalate in severity with higher parity and with breastfeeding. After-pains may last for 2 to 3 days, and they can be relieved with the application of heat to the lower abdomen. Nonsteroidal anti-inflammatory drugs (NSAIDs) may be taken safely if necessary, or narcotic analgesics may be given in the event of cesarean delivery.

The sudden decompression and diminished size of the uterus after the baby's birth causes the placenta to shear off and deliver. When this occurs, the uterine muscle, the placental site, and the adjacent arterial muscle walls all contract vigorously to ensure hemostasis and to prevent hemorrhage.

CERVIX

Pregnancy- and birth-induced changes to the cervix, including hypervascularity, any lacerations that occurred during the birth, and ecchymosis, normally resolve by 6 weeks, while edema and hyperplasia of the cervical glands may last for up to 3 months. Small amounts of lateral tearing to the cervix commonly occur during delivery, at the completion of involution the parous cervical os is changed, appearing as a horizontal slit rather than the characteristically small, round opening of the nulliparous cervical os.

Profound changes also take place within the cervix at the cellular level. Ahdoot et al. (1998) found that 50% of patients diagnosed with high-grade cervical dysplasia prenatally had markedly improved condition after vaginal delivery. Although these findings have been replicated by some investigators (Strinić et al., 2002), others have failed to find a significant association between pregnancy and improved cervical cytology (Kaneshiro et al., 2005).

LOCHIA

The vaginal discharge following birth, which is called lochia rubra, contains blood and epithelial cells as well as the superficial layer of the deciduas (e.g., the lining of the uterus). This red, menses-like flow diminishes in quantity after several hours and lasts for 2 to 3 days. As the blood diminishes in proportion to the serous component, the discharge becomes reddish brown and is called lochia serosa, which continues for 3 to 6 weeks. From the 10th day on, the discharge may become yellowish white ias a result of an increase in leukocytes; at this point it is called lochia alba. Meanwhile, between the 10th day and the 8th week, a new endometrial lining is generated from the decidua basalis (e.g., the deep layer of the uterine lining).

PLACENTAL INVOLUTION

As the process of uterine involution progresses, the placental site undergoes its own involution process. As the outer layer of the decidua is shed with the lochia, the surrounding margins draw downward and the endometrium is regenerated from the decidua basalis underneath. This process is normally complete by the 6th week postpartum.

VAGINA AND PERINEUM

The distended vaginal wall, which has been stretched and smoothed out during the birth process, returns to its rugated and contracted state by the third week postpartum, although it does not go back to its previous size. The extent to which the voluntary muscles of the pelvic floor regain their tone will depend on a variety of factors: parity, nutritional status, the size of the baby, the type of delivery, and the degree to which the birth parent has exercised their pelvic floor muscles (e.g., performed Kegel exercises). Changes to the appearance of the vaginal introitus result from tears of the hymenal tags that occur during delivery; these form remnants known as carunculae myrtiformes.

Severe stretching or laceration of the vagina or perineum can lead to relaxation and decreased pelvic support, the prolapse of the pelvic organs, and, eventually, problems with incontinence. The management of the perineum at the time of delivery has consequences for the integrity of the pelvic floor musculature postpartum. In the past, prophylactic episiotomy had been widely believed to preserve pelvic muscle function and to prevent perineal laceration. However, episiotomy is associated with more perineal pain, trauma, and long-term complications, and is no longer recommended routinely (Hartmann et al., 2005; WHO, 2018).

Antenatal perineal massage performed one to two times per week beginning at 35 weeks' gestation is an evidence-based intervention that has been demonstrated to prevent birth-related trauma to the perineum, including episiotomy (Beckmann & Garrett, 2006). Pelvic floor physical therapy (PFPT) is a low-cost, highly effective intervention for the treatment of pelvic floor dysfunction, which occurs in 46% of patients within the first 6 weeks after birth. Recommendations are for pregnant patients to start pelvic floor exercises during pregnancy and the postpartum period to prevent and treat pelvic floor disorders (Wallace et al., 2019).

Assessment

The thorough assessment of the perineum can be ensured by using the acronym REEDA, which will help the clinician to remember to look for redness, ecchymosis, edema, discharge, and wound approximation. This systematic assessment will reveal problems such as infection, hematoma, dehiscence of repair, excessive bleeding, and hemorrhage (Kindberg et al., 2008).

Management

Postpartum care includes the application of ice packs for 20-minute periods for the initial 24 hours. Thereafter, either warm or cold sitz baths may be recommended. A randomized trial demonstrated no difference in REEDA score with the use of heat or cold on the perineum during the first 24 hours postpartum (Hill, 2006). However, cold sitz baths are more effective in reducing edema and hematoma formation and provide more effective pain relief by causing local vasoconstriction and decreasing nerve conduction and muscle spasm (Gabbe et al., 2007; Ramler & Roberts, 1986). Never-

theless, cold therapy may not be acceptable in some cultures that believe that the loss of blood during birth creates a cold state in the body, which would necessitate the provision of warmth postpartum.

Pharmacotherapeutics

Patients should be involved in shared decision-making, allowing a more individualized pain management plan of care. Participating in shared decision-making has proved effective in decreasing opioids prescribed for patients after a cesarean birth. A stepwise multimodal approach should be taken for both vaginal and cesarean deliveries. Nonopioid medications such as NSAIDs and acetaminophen should be used as first-line agents, followed by low-dose and low-potency analgesics (ACOG, 2021a). Alternating acetaminophen and NSAIDs on a set schedule provide analgesic coverage and reduce the need for opioids. If this regimen proves inadequate for pain control, low-dose, low-potency, and short-acting doses of opioids can be prescribed at the lowest dose tolerated in addition to the NSAID and acetaminophen, such as codeine, morphine, tramadol, hydrocodone, and oxycodone. Combination NSAID-opioids and acetaminophen-opioids should be avoided to prevent unintentional medication toxicity and excess exposure to opioids. Ibuprofen is effective orally or rectally, and it is safe during lactation. A Cochrane Review of rectal analgesia for pain from perineal trauma after delivery points out that 50% of the medication bypasses the liver and thus results in faster and more effective pain relief than oral medication. This meta-analysis identified rectal analgesia with NSAIDs as an effective means of analgesia postpartum (Hedayati et al., 2003). In the event of a fourth-degree laceration necessitating repair of the rectal sphincter, suppositories are not given. Oral NSAIDs are appropriate and stool softeners and avoidance of constipation or straining of any kind is important. Although previous guidance has suggested to avoid the use of NSAIDs with patients diagnosed with hypertensive disorders in pregnancy, newer studies have shown support in NSAID use as a first-line agent for all postpartum patients, including patients with hypertensive disorders (ACOG, 2021a).

HORMONES
Ovarian Function

Ovarian function is suppressed in lactating patients and it typically returns around 6 months postpartum. Estrogen and progesterone levels are diminished, while prolactin levels rise in response to the stimulus of breastfeeding, thus increasing the secretion of milk. Therefore, giving supplementation reduces the prolactin secretion needed to develop an adequate milk supply.

The postpartum suppression of ovulation is determined to a large extent by the frequency and duration of breastfeeding and whether there is exclusive breastfeeding or supplementary feeding with formula, which diminishes the amenorrheic properties of lactation (Kennedy & Visness, 1992). Maternal nutritional status has also been shown to significantly affect the resumption of ovulation postpartum. Patients with a lower body mass index (BMI) have been shown to consistently remain amenorrheic longer after birth, regardless of breastfeeding behavior, child nutritional status, and child age, suggesting that maternal nutritional status has an effect that is independent of breastfeeding behavior (Peng et al., 1998).

The hypoestrogenic state of the puerperium is extended in lactating patients. The elevation in prolactin leads to a decreased libido and the thinning and dryness of the vaginal mucosa; this, in addition to healing vaginal and perineal trauma, may contribute to frequent complaints of dyspareunia and sexual dysfunction postpartum (Henderson & MacDonald, 2004).

POSTPARTUM THYROIDITIS

The thyroid gland, which increases in size and function during pregnancy, returns to its normal size by 12 weeks postpartum. Thyroid hormones normally return to prepregnancy levels by 4 weeks postpartum. Postpartum thyroiditis occurs up to 12 months after birth and may include hypothyroid or hyperthyroid dysfunctions. A small percentage of patients, approximately 5% to 10%, experience transient autoimmune thyroiditis. Diagnosis may be difficult as it presents as vague symptoms and usually develops months after birth. Patients experiencing symptoms such as palpitations, fatigue, weight loss, irritability, or heat intolerance as well as a small goiter may be experiencing the hyperthyroid or thyrotoxic phase; symptoms are usually mild and last a few months. The second phase, overt hypothyroidism, happens around usually 4 to 8 months after birth; symptoms again are vague and nonspecific such as constipation, fatigue, and depression. Serum thyroid-stimulating hormone (TSH) is the gold standard for testing thyroid function; if abnormal, a free thyroxine (T4) test should be performed. Patients without significant thyroid history, symptoms, or abnormal thyroid levels should not receive routine antithyroid peroxidase antibody testing due to lack of evidence supporting improved pregnancy outcomes with thyroid hormone replacement for these antibodies. Risk factors include type 1 diabetes, previous thyroid problems, and a family history of thyroid disease or autoimmune disease. Routine testing isn't necessary given the thyroid gland may enlarge during pregnancy by up to 30%; research has not shown identifying and treating patients with subclinical hypothyroidism improves fetal neurocognitive function or pregnancy outcomes. Patients who are asymptomatic with a slightly enlarged thyroid wouldn't require further testing; however, a significant goiter or prominent thyroid nodules would warrant further assessment and closer follow-up. Most patients diagnosed with postpartum thyroiditis will have resolved spontaneously. About one third of these patients go on to develop permanent hypothyroidism (ACOG, 2020d). Further testing and consultation with a specialist are recommended by the American Thyroid Association. Medication management should be closely monitored and adjusted to the levels of free T4 for hyperthyroidism and total triiodothyronine (T3) in hypothyroidism.

MUSCULOSKELETAL AND DERMATOLOGIC CHANGES
Striae Gravidarum

The distention of the pregnant abdomen causes the rupture of the elastic fibers in the skin and stretches the broad and round ligaments. These anatomic changes may result in a soft and flaccid abdomen and striae gravidarum, which are purple or dark-brown lines (depending on the patient's skin color) that may appear on the abdomen, breasts, and buttocks. These will eventually fade; however, they will not disappear completely. Two herbal creams have been shown to have some beneficial effect in minimizing striae. One cream contained the active ingredients vitamin E, essential fatty acids, panthenol, hyaluronic acid, elastin, and menthol. The second cream contained tocopherol, collagen-elastin hydrolysates, and *Centella asiatica*. The active ingredients in both creams can be difficult to obtain (Young & Jewell, 1996). Although a Cochrane Review reported no adverse effects from these interventions, other researchers have noted that no studies have addressed the safety of these herbs or the many others that are commonly used during pregnancy (Ernst, 2002; Tunzi & Gray, 2007).

Diastasis Recti

The separation of the abdominal muscles may persist following delivery, which results in a condition called diastasis recti. Berg-Poppe et al. (2022) found it occurs in 35% to 60% of patients in the immediate postpartum period. This can be described by the number of fingerbreadths that the healthcare provider can fit between the abdominal muscles as the supine patient reaches their arms forward and lifts their head, neck, and shoulders; this number diminishes over time as the muscles come back together. Ultrasound is the most reliable diagnostic method; however, palpation is also sufficient (Berg-Poppe et al., 2022). Recovery is helped with the use of abdomen-strengthening exercises, specifically when targeting deep core muscles such as the transverse abdominis muscle. Exercises that increase intra-abdominal pressure should be avoided. Exercises may begin as soon as the patient is able to after 6 weeks postpartum.

HAIR

During pregnancy, scalp hair generally thickens as a result of a decrease in the progression of hair growth from the anagen phase (e.g., the "growing" stage) to the telogen phase (e.g., the "resting" stage; Elling & Powell, 1997; Wong, 1996). This telogen phase persists during 1 to 5 months postpartum. During the postpartum period, the loss of scalp hair beyond this 1- to 5-month period is fairly common and is called telogen effluvium. Telogen effluvium usually ends within 15 months postpartum; however, the scalp hair may never regain its prepregnancy thickness (Winton & Lewis, 1982).

BONE DENSITY

Following delivery and lactation there is a temporary decrease in bone mineralization (Karlsson et al., 2005). Lactating parents require the additional intake of calcium, although calcium needs are met with the reabsorption of maternal skeletal calcium and a decrease in the excretion of calcium by the kidneys. Lactating patients are likely to experience a decrease in bone density, losing as much as 7% of their bone mass by 9 months of continued breastfeeding (Laskey & Prentice, 1999). However, this demineralization is reversible after weaning has occurred (Karlsson et al., 2005).

WEIGHT LOSS

With delivery comes weight loss as a result of the birth of the baby, the placenta, amniotic fluid, and blood loss, normally resulting in a loss of 10 to 13 lb at the time of birth (Gabbe et al., 2007). Further diuresis accounts for an additional 4 to 7 lb lost during the first week postpartum. Although 28% of birthing patients return to their prepregnancy weight by 6 weeks postpartum, most remain about 3 lb heavier, and have increased waist-to-hip ratios. Multiparous patients tend to retain more weight than primiparous patients. Birthing parents who gain more than 35 lb during their pregnancy remain an average 11 lb heavier (Gabbe et al., 2007).

CARDIOVASCULAR SYSTEM

Although the plasma volume increases by about 1,200 mL by the third trimester, it diminishes by about 1,000 mL as a result of blood loss immediately after delivery. By the third day postpartum, it has again increased by 900 to 1,200 mL as a result of the shift of extracellular fluid into the vascular space. Normally, a rise in systolic and diastolic blood pressure of about 5% occurs during the first 4 days postpartum (Henderson & MacDonald, 2004). After delivery, there is a sudden increase in venous return, because the newly emptied uterus no longer impedes blood flow from the extremities. This results in an abrupt rise in cardiac output, which causes bradycardia. Cardiac output returns to its prelabor value 1 hour after delivery and to its prepregnancy levels between 2 and 4 weeks after delivery (Gabbe et al., 2007).

There is four to five times higher risk of venous thromboembolism (VTE) during pregnancy as well as during the postpartum period, with VTE being a leading cause of maternal death in the United States (ACOG, 2018b). The three conditions that predispose birthing patients to VTE are referred to as Virchow's triad: increased occurrence of vascular endothelial injury, a hypercoagulable state, and venous stasis (Burrows et al., 2004; Greer, 1999). VTE occurs twice as frequently during the postpartum period as it does during pregnancy, specifically the first few weeks following birth (ACOG, 2018b; Nisenblat et al., 2006; Simpson et al., 2003). The single most important risk factor for VTE is patient history of thrombosis; there is a three to four times higher risk of recurrent VTE in pregnancy. There is vascular injury at the placental site during labor, delivery, and the postpartum period that contributes to vascular endothelial injury. Throughout pregnancy, there is a progressive increase in clotting factors I, II, VII, VIII, IX, and X; this, in combination with an increase in fibrinogen and platelets and a decrease in fibrinolytic activity and free protein S, contributes to the hypercoagulable state of pregnancy that persists during the postpartum period (Beck et al., 2005; Marik & Plante, 2008). Patients with inherited thrombophilic disorders, such as factor V Leiden and prothrombin gene mutations, may be at increased risk for VTE during pregnancy (Gerhardt et al., 2000; Tsu, 2004). Of the patients who have had VTE in pregnancy or postpartum, 20% to 50% had thrombophilia (ACOG, 2018b). Pulmonary embolism (PE) is more likely to occur during the postpartum period than the antepartum period, although deep vein thrombosis (DVT) occurs more frequently during the antepartum period (Beck et al., 2005; Heit et al., 2005). Another population-based study found that the VTE event of DVT in the postpartum population occurred four times more frequently than in the antenatal population (Greer, 1999). The incidence of VTE was increased fourfold among patients who delivered via cesarean section as compared with patients who delivered vaginally. Other risk complications such as autoimmune diseases, preeclampsia, hypertension, heart disease, PPH, sickle cell disease, and obesity also increase the risk of VTE, especially for a patient recovering from a cesarean birth (ACOG, 2018b).

KIDNEYS AND URINARY TRACT

The normal pregnancy-induced increase in renal plasma flow begins to fall during the third trimester; however, it takes 1 to 2 years to return to prepregnancy levels. Both the increased glomerular filtration rate (GFR) and the consequent rise in creatinine clearance rates that occur during pregnancy return to normal by 8 weeks postpartum. In response, blood urea nitrogen (BUN) also resumes its prepregnant level by 1 week postpartum (Gabbe et al., 2007). Urinary incontinence occurs in 34% of postpartum patients. When done later in pregnancy, patients who performed pelvic floor physical therapy (PFPT) noted to have lower risk of urinary incontinence at 3 to 6 months postpartum in comparison to patients who did not participate in antepartum PFPT (Wallace et al., 2019). Urinary tract infection (UTI) is discussed further under Complications in the section titled Urinary Tract Infection and Pyelonephritis.

METABOLISM, FLUIDS, AND ELECTROLYTES

In addition to the substantial blood and fluid loss that are sustained during labor and delivery, an additional 3.5 L of fluid are lost during the first 6 weeks postpartum. Although the total amount of sodium diminishes, its serum concentration increases as the loss of fluid surpasses it, and plasma potassium also rises. This results in a net increase of serum cations and anions and thus an increased plasma osmolality and a decreased serum chloride level as the serum bicarbonate level increases.

By the second postpartum day, fatty acids return to their normal concentration in the blood, whereas cholesterol and triglycerides take 6 to 7 weeks to return to their prepregnant levels. Both fasting and postprandial blood glucose levels decline after birth, dropping to their lowest levels on the second and third days postpartum and then increasing back up to prepregnant levels. This has important implications for the interpretation of blood sugar tests and insulin requirements during the first week postpartum. As recommended by ACOG (2018a), all gestational diabetic patients should have a fasting glucose serum or 75-g 2-hour glucose tolerance test (GTT) performed to further assess if blood glucose management is required postpartum.

Postpartum Complications

A heightened focus on preventing postpartum complications should be at the forefront for providers. A shift from the traditional timeline for follow-ups to more personalized and closer interval visits may decrease the rate of postpartum morbidity and mortality. There is a drastic increase; more than half of pregnancy-related maternal deaths occur after the infant is born. Complications from hypertensive disorders also require closer follow-up, given one half of postpartum strokes occur within 10 days of hospital discharge (ACOG, 2018a).

The incidence of postpartum complications is related to the mode of delivery: there are fewer complications associated with vaginal birth than with cesarean section delivery (Burrows et al., 2004). Cesarean section delivery is associated with an increased risk for infection, hemorrhage, VTE, anesthetic complications, and a longer and more painful recovery (Greer, 1999; Liu et al., 2007). After cesarean section delivery, maternal and neonatal complications exist for future pregnancies as well (Beck et al., 2005; Galyean et al., 2009).

ASSESSMENT AND MANAGEMENT AFTER CESAREAN SECTION

Postoperative care after cesarean section delivery is similar to care after other abdominal surgeries; however, it also encompasses the myriad needs that are common to all patients who have just given birth (Hundt et al., 2000). For some patients, a cesarean section delivery represents the loss of a hoped-for birth experience or even a personal failure. It is important to allow the birth parent to have time to talk about their birth experience soon afterward and then again, several weeks postpartum.

Physical care is directed at detecting, preventing, and treating potential complications, which include hemorrhage, infection, thrombosis, pneumonia, and complications of anesthesia. Early ambulation and fluid intake may help to prevent some of the more common complications.

POSTDURAL PUNCTURE HEADACHE

Postdural puncture headaches, which are also known as spinal headaches, may occur after spinal anesthesia or after epidurals that have inadvertently become spinals. Spinal fluid leaks from the dural space through the puncture site into the extradural space, which causes a headache that immediately improves when the patient is supine. An epidural blood patch with the patient's own blood is the most effective treatment; it provides immediate relief for most patients (Ahmed et al., 2006; Reamy, 2009).

POSTPARTUM HEMORRHAGE

Excessive postpartum blood loss is the greatest cause of maternal death worldwide, responsible for up to 150,000 deaths per year. It is estimated that one patient dies every 4 minutes from PPH, most often as a result of primary or early PPH, which occurs within the first 24 hours after birth (ACOG, 2017b). As defined by ACOG's reVITALize program, a PPH is the cumulative blood loss greater than or equal to 1,000 mL or blood loss with hypovolemic symptoms within 24 hours after birth, for a vaginal or cesarean birth. This newer definition should not negate the need for awareness, assessment, and interventions for blood loss of greater than 500 mL after vaginal deliveries. It is important to note that signs of hypovolemia such as hypotension and tachycardia are later signs and do not present until significant blood loss, up to 25% of total blood volume, has occurred (ACOG, 2017b). Therefore, earlier recognition and frequent assessment are paramount in prevention and management of PPH.

The estimation of postpartum blood loss (EBL) is notoriously inaccurate and can delay recognition and management of PPHs. When using EBL, providers tend to grossly under-estimate in larger blood loss and overestimate in lower blood loss. Utilizing quantitative blood loss (QBL) calculations can significantly improve the accuracy and give real-time blood loss (ACOG, 2019c; AWHONN, 2021c). QBL is an objective measurement that utilizes a standardized approach to calculate blood loss and can facilitate earlier identification of both PPH and patients at risk for developing PPH. QBL is calculated by subtracting the dry weight of items being weighed in grams from the wet or bloodied weight of those items. One gram is equivalent to 1 mL of blood. Root cause analysis (RCA) for maternal mortality consistently shows EBL misses or delays the diagnosis and treatment of PPHs. Waiting until a severe blood loss is suspected to start calculating blood loss as a standard of practice only adds to the cycle of delayed identification and treatment (AWHONN, 2021c). A PPH bundle utilizing QBL improves patient outcomes by refining team awareness of emergencies, highlights the necessity for earlier uterotonics and additional resources, and decreases instances of blood transfusions and additional interventions (ACOG, 2019c; AWHONN, 2021c).

PPH occurs when there is a malfunction of one of the processes that control bleeding after birth, commonly called the "4 Ts": tone, tissue, trauma, and thrombin. The most common of these is tone, or uterine atony, which accounts for 75% to 85% of the cases of early PPH. Risks for atony include the over distention of the uterus caused by macrosomia, multiple gestation, fibroids, or polyhydramnios; uterine muscle fatigue caused by prolonged, rapid, or augmented labor; uterine infection; or a full bladder interfering with the ability of the uterine muscles to contract (Lowdermilk et al., 2000; Tsu, 2004). Tissue refers to retained fragments of placental tissue or membranes that may result in hemorrhage and may necessitate uterine exploration and removal of the retained tissue. Retained placenta occurs when there is abnormal placental adherence to the uterine wall, which occurs with placenta accreta and placenta percreta. These conditions are more common in pregnancies after cesarean section delivery as a result of the abnormal development of the placenta, which takes place over the site of the hysterotomy scar. PPH caused by trauma is most commonly a result of genital tract laceration after a vaginal birth or the extension of a uterine incision during cesarean section delivery; infrequent causes include uterine rupture or inversion. The least frequent cause of hemorrhage is abnormalities of coagulation (e.g., thrombin), which may preexist or be acquired during pregnancy (see Box 39.5).

Interventions to prevent or decrease the incidence of PPH have received international attention; the most effective of these is active management of the third stage of labor. Recommended by international obstetric and midwifery organizations, active management of the third stage consists of the administration of uterotonics immediately before or within 1 minute of the birth of the baby, controlled cord traction to deliver the placenta, and the massage of the uterine fundus immediately after the delivery of the placenta (AWHONN, 2021a). During the immediate postpartum period, attention is focused on detecting, preventing, and managing uterine atony. After delivery, the uterine fundus should be firm, midline, and approximately reaching the level of the umbilicus. As noted previously, it may be slightly higher or lower,

Box 39.5 Risks for and Associated Factors of Postpartum Hemorrhage

Uterine atony

Overdistended uterus

Macrosomia

Multiple gestation

Polyhydramnios

Fibroids

Blood clots

Prolonged labor (first stage, second stage)

Labor induction

Parity (nulliparity, grand multiparity)

Medications (e.g., tocolytics [magnesium sulfate, oxytocin])

Anesthesia

Ethnicities/race (e.g., Hispanic, Asian)

Pathology

Hypertensive disorders

Infection (chorioamnionitis)

Diabetes mellitus

Prolonged rupture of membranes

Internal monitoring

Lacerations (perineal, cervical, or vaginal)

Operative delivery (i.e., forceps, vacuum, or cesarean section delivery)

Precipitous delivery

Retained/history of retained placenta

Uterine rupture

History of previous postpartum hemorrhage

Abnormal adherence of placenta

Placenta accreta

Placenta percreta

Hematoma (may have signs of shock without visible blood loss)

Traumatic delivery

Source: Dunn, P. M. (2005). Ignac Semmelweis (1818–1865) of Budapest and the prevention of puerperal fever. Archives of Disease in Childhood, Fetal and Neonatal Edition, 90(4), F345–F348. https://doi.org/10.1136/adc.2004.062901; Ende, H., Lozada, M., Chestnut, D., Osmundson, S., Walden, R. L., Shotwell, M. S., & Bauchat, J. R. (2021). Risk factors for atonic postpartum hemorrhage: A systematic review and meta-analysis. Obstetrics & Gynecology, 137, 305–323. https://doi.org/10.1097/AOG.0000000000004228; Katz, V. L. (2007). Postpartum care. In S. G. Gabbe, J. R. Niebyl, J. L. Simpson, H. L. Galan, L. Goetzl, E. R. M. Jauniaux, & M. B. Landon (Eds.), Obstetrics: Normal and problem pregnancies (5th ed.). Churchill Livingstone.

depending on the size of the baby, the habitus of the birth parent, and the number of hours postpartum. The lochia should not be in excess of a normal menses; soaking through one or more large perineal pads per hour is abnormal. If the fundus is deviated to the side or if the bladder itself is palpable, the patient is either helped to void or is catheterized. The uterus is then reassessed and the fundus firmly massaged while the uterus is stabilized with the other hand above the symphysis. Fundal massage usually causes the atonic uterus to contract, which results in a noticeable decrease in the amount of vaginal bleeding (Hofmeyr et al., 2008; Mousa & Alfirevic, 2007). Assessments should be performed every 15 minutes for the first 2 hours of recovery, with a measured or quantified cumulative blood loss (AWHONN, 2021b). If bleeding continues after fundal massage, other sources of bleeding need to be considered. The perineum, vagina, and cervix are examined for lacerations. If no lacerations are found, retained fragments of placenta or membrane should be considered. Coagulation disorders are the least common cause, and most are known before the onset of labor (Anderson & Etches, 2007; Miller et al., 2004).

In cases of uterine atony, if active management of the third stage of labor has not been performed or if excessive bleeding persists after fundal massage, uterotonics are indicated. Oxytocin is the uterotonic of choice both for the active management of the third stage and as the first-line treatment of PPH. It can be given IV or IM, has a rapid onset of action, and has few side effects. It causes rhythmic uterine contractions, which constrict the spiral arteries in the myometrium, thereby decreasing blood flow. IV oxytocin is preferable to IM injection. For IV administration, an initial bolus followed by a maintenance rate over a minimal time period of 4 hours is recommended (AWHONN, 2021a). If excessive bleeding persists after oxytocin administration, additional medications are given. Methergine, which is an ergot alkaloid, is the usual second-line choice. Its IM administration causes a sustained contraction of the uterine muscle; however, it is contraindicated in patients with elevated blood pressure. If bleeding continues to be excessive, prostaglandins are given (Tsu, 2004). These uterotonics require skill for administration, and some also require refrigeration, which can present important limitations when caring for patients in developing countries. Recently, there has been an effort to identify uterotonics that may be more appropriate for areas of the world in which access to skilled birth attendants capable of giving injections may be limited. Misoprostol is an inexpensive and stable prostaglandin analog that is administered in tablet form. It may be given orally, rectally, or sublingually, and has been found to be effective for decreasing postpartum blood loss, although it has more side effects than the more commonly used uterotonics. Side effects that are commonly associated with prostaglandin use (e.g., fever, chills, nausea, vomiting, diarrhea, pain from uterine contractions) appear to be dose related (Blum et al., 2007; Geller et al., 2006; Hofmeyr et al., 2009; Vivio & Williams, 2004).

Tranexamic acid (TXA), an antifibronolytic agent, when used prophylactically in cesarean deliveries and early in PPHs has proved effective in reducing maternal morbidity and mortality. The World Maternal Antifibrinolytic (WOMAN) Trial was a double-blind, placebo-controlled randomized control trial in multiple centers and multiple countries that blazed the trail for early treatment utilizing TXA in PPH to reduce maternal deaths caused by bleeding, especially when given within 3 hours of birth or onset of PPH (Shakur et al.,

2010). The laparotomy rate was significantly reduced and there were substantial ICU cost savings. Based on its findings, ACOG, Royal College of Obstetrics and Gynecology, and WHO support and highly recommend use of TXA in the early treatment of PPH (ACOG, 2017b; Sudhof et al., 2019).

If uterotonics fail to control PPH, providers must consider other interventions. Balloon tamponade, such as a Bakri balloon, can be inserted inside the uterus to provide compression to improve uterine atony; the balloon is inflated with up to 500 mL of fluid. The Bakri balloon has a drainage port to allow for blood to drain and to be measured. Uterine packing with gauze may also be used; however, caution must be taken to ensure packing has been properly counted. It may be helpful to have the patient wear a bracelet to inform providers and staff of the retained foreign objects. Surgical interventions such as uterine compression sutures, uterine artery embolization, laparotomy, or hysterectomy may be necessary if all other measures fail (ACOG, 2017b).

PPH algorithms and treatment pathways should be utilized on labor and delivery units for quick reference during PPH emergencies. An example to reference is ACOG's Obstetric Hemorrhage Bundle and Checklist. These should outline the stages of PPH and the appropriate interventions used in each stage to include steps, resources, team actions, and medications. Information on massive transfusion protocols should also be addressed. A helpful tool in preparedness for PPH is the utilization of a PPH cart—a recommended instrument in the ACOG Safe Mother Initiative for Obstetric Hemorrhage Bundle (https://www.acog.org/community/districts-and-sections/district-ii/programs-and-resources/safe-motherhood-initiative/obstetric-hemorrhage).

LATE PPH

Although most hemorrhages take place within the first 24 hours after birth (and most of these occur within the first 4 hours), "late" PPH can also occur. Late or secondary PPH is defined as excessive bleeding that occurs more than 24 hours and up to 12 weeks postpartum in about 1% of postpartum patients (ACOG, 2017b); it most typically begins 1 to 2 weeks after delivery. Common causes are infection, retained products of conception, and subinvolution of the uterus, which occurs when there is a failure of the uterine muscle, the placental site, or the adjacent arterial muscle walls to contract adequately to ensure hemostasis. When assessing the quality and quantity of bleeding in patients days or weeks after delivery, it is important to remember that a lesser yet steady amount of bleeding may appear deceptively insignificant relative to the more extensive bleeding that occurs at the time of birth; however, if this type of bleeding continues over time, it will result in significant blood loss. Diagnosis and management may include transvaginal ultrasound and curettage, if necessary; broad-spectrum antibiotics; and uterotonics (Dunn, 2005; Lausman et al., 2008).

LACERATIONS

If uterotonics and fundal massage successfully firm the uterus and bleeding still continues, the most likely cause is laceration of the vagina or cervix. A laceration of the perineum, periurethral area, or labia would likely be visualized and repaired by the healthcare provider at the time of delivery; however, a deep sulcus (vaginal) or cervical laceration may be missed. Identifying lacerations requires careful inspection with adequate visualization and pain control for the patient, and this inspection may be difficult if the laceration is deep and if the field is obscured by bleeding. It is crucial to summon expert help without delay, because severe blood loss can occur rapidly and is controllable only by the repair of the laceration.

HEMATOMA

On rare occasions, trauma to the soft tissue during delivery may cause lacerations to blood vessels in which significant hidden blood loss occurs and results in a hematoma. Most of these lacerations occur after an operative vaginal delivery with forceps or vacuum or after an episiotomy. The symptoms of hematoma of the vulva or, less commonly, of the vagina are pain, swelling, bruising, a palpable mass, and signs of shock (if blood loss is great enough). Vulvar hematomas will eventually become visible as they increase in size; however, vaginal hematomas may not be visible. If hemodynamically stable, the patient with a vulvar or vaginal hematoma may be followed with observation, ice packs, and analgesia for symptomatic relief, and an indwelling urinary catheter, if necessary. If hemodynamically unstable, the hematoma may need to be excised, drained, and packed with a drain left in, depending on the size of the hematoma. Retroperitoneal hematoma is a rare yet serious complication of cesarean section delivery that must be surgically repaired (Miller et al., 2004).

POSTPARTUM FEVER

The accepted definition of postpartum febrile morbidity is an oral temperature of 38°C (100.4°F) or more on any two of the first 10 days postpartum (exclusive of the first 24 hours). A temperature elevation of up to 38°C (100.4°F) during the first 24 hours after delivery or of up to 39°C (102.2°F) for 24 hours after the patient's milk comes in may be a normal finding. Fever after the first 24 hours postpartum or fever that is unrelated to breast engorgement is most often the result of infection and requires further evaluation to identify the source.

ENDOMETRITIS

Postpartum endometritis occurs after 1% to 3% of vaginal births and is up to 10 times more frequent after a cesarean birth. It is caused by the contamination of the uterine lining by vaginal organisms, which may include group A or B streptococci, *Chlamydia trachomatis*, *Neisseria gonorrhoeae*, *Mycoplasma hominis*, or *Ureaplasma urealyticum*, the prevalence of which vary depending on the population. Postpartum endometritis may be a continuation of amnionitis that began during labor. A long labor, prolonged rupture of the membranes, multiple vaginal examinations, invasive monitoring, and forceps or vacuum extraction are all risk factors for this condition (Faro, 2005; French & Smaill, 2004).

In the past, puerperal fever was commonly spread by obstetricians and medical students who neglected to wash their hands between pelvic examinations or after handling cadavers. Ignaz Semmelweis, a 19th-century Hungarian physician, after studying the puerperal fever rate in two clinics, observed that patients in the clinic attended by midwives, as well as patients who were unattended at birth, were more likely to survive and had lower rates of fevers than patients who were delivered by doctors or medical students. Semmelweis deduced that handwashing by healthcare providers would improve the chances of a patient's survival. This discovery became the basis for infection control in all areas of healthcare. Even today, proper hand hygiene is emphasized as an important tool for the prevention of postpartum infection (French & Smaill, 2004; Maharaj, 2007).

The clinical diagnosis of postpartum endometritis is based on the presence of fever and uterine tenderness. Other signs include abdominal tenderness, foul-smelling lochia, and leukocytosis. Symptoms most frequently occur within 48 hours of delivery; a later onset of symptoms may present as a late PPH caused by the subinvolution of the uterus (Faro, 2005). A combination of gentamicin and clindamycin is the gold standard for the initial treatment of postpartum endometritis to cover the broad range of possible causative organisms. If this regimen is ineffective for resolving fever and other symptoms within 3 days, further workup is warranted to assess for the adequacy of antibiotic levels, the presence of resistant organisms, or another etiology of maternal fever. Further treatment is critical, because the progression of the infection can lead to life-threatening complications, such as peritonitis, sepsis, and abscess (Faro, 2005).

URINARY TRACT INFECTION AND PYELONEPHRITIS

A number of factors contribute to the development of UTIs during the postpartum period: decreased bladder tone that leads to urinary stasis, incomplete emptying of the bladder, the introduction of bacteria with pelvic examinations and catheterizations, and the prevalence of asymptomatic bacteriuria in pregnancy. *Escherichia coli* is the causative bacteria in 80% to 90% of cases. If left untreated, pyelonephritis may develop into a more serious infection that is characterized by fever, chills, flank pain, nausea, vomiting, and costovertebral angle tenderness (French & Smaill, 2004). UTI and pyelonephritis are treated with the use of appropriate antibiotic therapy. Some patients with pyelonephritis require IV support for fluid management as a result of the associated nausea and vomiting.

MASTITIS

Postpartum mastitis is the inflammation of the breast associated with lactation characterized by fever and flu-like symptoms, pain that is most often unilateral, erythema, warmth, and possibly a streaked appearance to the breast (Amir & ABMPCThe Academy of Breastfeeding Medicine Protocol Committee, 2014). More commonly seen in primiparous patients, it is associated with milk stasis, poor latch, maternal stress, fatigue, rapid weaning and cracked nipples, which allow for the entry of bacteria (Amir & TABMPC, 2014). This is differentiated from the generalized engorgement and temperature elevation that sometimes occurs with the onset of mature milk production around the third or fourth day postpartum. Conservative treatment for mild symptoms consists of bed rest, increased intake of fluids, the application of warm compresses, and the emptying of the breast either by the suckling of the infant or a breast pump. However, some patients may be acutely ill and require antibiotics. If the patient does not respond to antibiotics, breast

milk cultures and drug sensitivities may need to be performed (Amir & TABMPC, 2014).

POSTPARTUM WOUND INFECTION

Infection of an episiotomy or perineal laceration after a vaginal delivery is suspected in postpartum patients who complain of perineal pain, swelling, and erythema. If the infection appears superficial, it may be treated with sitz baths and analgesia. Deeper infections may require surgical exploration and drainage and can then be allowed to heal by secondary intention. Wound infection is more commonly seen after a cesarean section delivery and occurs in up to 16% of patients. Risk factors include obesity, length of surgery, amount of blood loss, and presence of chorioamnionitis. The risk is significantly decreased by the administration of perioperative antibiotics; additional antibiotics may need to be given postoperatively to those patients who do develop a wound infection (French & Smaill, 2004).

VENOUS THROMBOEMBOLISM

Pregnancy and the postpartum period are hypercoagulable states, thereby increasing the risk for DVT and PE. This is most likely a protective mechanism that evolved to decrease a patient's risk of excessive bleeding after childbirth. Cesarean section delivery, obesity, increased parity, and advanced maternal age further increase this risk, with cesarean section delivery being associated with up to 75% of all fatal thromboembolic events. DVT is characterized by a unilateral redness (most often the left leg), tenderness, swelling of the calf or thigh, and a positive Homans sign. If DVT is suspected, compression ultrasonography is indicated to confirm the diagnosis. Because levels of D-dimer increase during pregnancy, this is less useful as a diagnostic test (ACOG, 2018b; Marik & Plante, 2008; Whitty & Dombrowski, 2002). Patients with undiagnosed DVT have an increased risk of PE; therefore, prompt diagnosis and treatment are critical. Classic signs and symptoms include leg swelling, tachycardia, tachypnea, and dyspnea. Immediate medical attention is required (Whitty & Dombrowski, 2002). Early ambulation and the use of compression stockings during the postpartum period may decrease risk. Emphasis should be placed on applying compression stockings on cesarean patients prior to surgery. After the condition is diagnosed, management consists of anticoagulation, with low-molecular-weight heparin as the anticoagulant of choice. It's important to note low-molecular-weight and unfractionated heparin are safe to use when breastfeeding since they do not accumulate in breast milk, nor do they inflict any anticoagulant effect on the infant. A postpartum anticoagulation regimen should last at least 6 weeks, with changes made appropriately to the patient's clinical status. Providers should implement and utilize VTE risk assessment tools to increase awareness and decrease poor outcomes for at-risk patient populations (Payne, 2021).

PERIPARTUM CARDIOMYOPATHY

Postpartum hemodynamic stresses make this an extremely high-risk time for patients with preexisting heart disease. In addition, postpartum or peripartum cardiomyopathy (PPCM) is a rare form of congestive heart failure that affects one in 4,000 to one in 10,000 birth parents, with 5% to 10% of patients dying or requiring a cardiac transplant by 1 year postpartum (ACOG, 2019e). PPCM is the onset of left ventricular dysfunction (e.g., an ejection fraction [EF] of less than 45%; severe cases of left ventricular ejection fraction [LVEF] at less than 30%) during the last month of pregnancy or within 5 months of delivery in an otherwise previously healthy person. The most common time frame for diagnosis is the first month postpartum. PPCM cannot be fully explained by other etiologies, and its cause is still not completely understood (Davis et al., 2020; Pearson et al., 2000). Some studies suggest autoimmune disorders, viral myocarditis, and nutritional deficiencies may be contributing causes. However, newer studies note the breakdown of the nursing hormone prolactin, which in turn can cause vascular and myocardial dysfunction (Davis et al., 2020). Risk factors for PPCM are gestational hypertension, preeclampsia, advanced patient age, multiples gestation, and a personal history of PPCM; the rate of recurrence with a previous patient history is approximately 20% (ACOG, 2019e). A meta-analysis of 979 cases of PPCM in 22 studies found hypertension and preeclampsia have been strongly connected to PPCM, with 37% of patients also having hypertensive disorders and 22% diagnosed with preeclampsia (Davis et al., 2020). Providers should recognize and advocate for their non-Hispanic Black patients experiencing any symptoms of PPCM; this particular patient population is disproportionately noted to have increased incidence, as much as 40% (Davis et al., 2020), as well as a lower recovery rate for complete myocardial recovery (ACOG, 2019e).

Many cases go undiagnosed or are misdiagnosed due to some symptoms experienced by patients in the last month of pregnancy. Heart failure (HF) is a common presenting feature of PPCM. Patients often experience edema, shortness of breath, fatigue, arrhythmias, chest discomfort, or palpitations (ACOG, 2019e; Davis et al., 2020). Postpartum patients who present with marked fluid retention may be misdiagnosed as having had excessive IV fluids administered during delivery (Task Force on the Management of Cardiovascular Diseases During Pregnancy of the European Society of Cardiology, 2003). For patients who present with symptoms before delivery, delivery is planned as soon as possible (Pearson et al., 2000; Task Force on the Management of Cardiovascular Diseases During Pregnancy of the European Society of Cardiology, 2003). An echocardiogram is the most reliable test for diagnosis. Lab tests, such as brain natriuretic peptide (BNP), are usually slightly elevated in patients with preeclampsia and are significantly elevated in PPCM. Cardiologists should be consulted and patients should be referred to a higher level of care with appropriate resources (ACOG, 2019e; Davis et al., 2020).

Many of the standard pharmacologic therapies for HF (e.g., loop diuretics, spironolactone, angiotensin-converting enzyme [ACE] inhibitors, and angiotensin II receptor blockers [ARBs]) are contraindicated in pregnancy; however, these medications are safe and are recommended to use for postpartum patients (Davis et al., 2020). Additionally, newer recommendations by the American College of Cardiology (ACC) state the addition of the experimental dopamine agonist bromocriptine may improve myocardial recovery for postpartum patients by blocking the pituitary release of prolactin (ACOG, 2019e; Davis et al., 2020). Due to the increased risk for developing left ventricular throm-bus, notably in patients with an LVEF less than 30%, and an overall higher risk for thromboembolism in PPCM patients, anticoagulation therapy is advised by the American Heart Association (AHA). Low-molecular-weight heparin is safe to use in pregnancy and lactating postpartum patients (Davis et al., 2020). PPCM is the most common cause of cardiogenic shock, making up to 60% of cases of cardiogenic shock in patients during pregnancy or early postpartum period. Temporary mechanical cardiac support may be necessary.

The prognosis is dependent on improvement in left ventricular function. According to the North American Registry Investigations of Pregnancy-Related Cardiomyopathy, patients with an initial LVEF >30% had a full myocardial recovery 90% of the time (ACOG, 2019e). However, if left ventricular dysfunction persists, patients may need to remain on medication and treatments indefinitely. For patients with LVEF <50%, subsequent pregnancies should be discouraged. Patients with improved LVEF of >50% should have detailed counseling for contraception and close follow-up for subsequent pregnancies to include routine labs, echocardiograms, stress tests, and multidisciplinary consults (Davis et al., 2020).

Psychosocial Issues

Even the arrival of the most hoped-for infant creates a stressful period of disequilibrium within the family while its members adjust to their new roles. On the basis of her observations of postpartum patients during the 1960s, Rubin developed her classic theory on the nature of the new mother's evolving psyche. During the somewhat narcissistic *taking in* phase that immediately follows birth, the postpartum patient is primarily concerned with their own physical needs. This is followed by *taking hold*, when they gradually transfer their attentions onto their infant, and then the *letting go* phase occurs. During letting go, the patient finally becomes comfortable in their new role as mother (Davidson et al., 2007). Since the late 20th century, this paradigm has been challenged by nurse researchers, who have applied social science's tests of validity and found the theory to be lacking (Ament, 1990; Martell, 1996). Rubin's work laid an important foundation during a time when the transition to new motherhood was poorly understood. Current social and cultural norms have shifted since Rubin's work, and the birth experience in America has been transformed. Patients may no longer have the chance to take in before it is time to briefly take hold and then let go. Thus, although these experiences may no longer be distinct phases, the theory sheds important light on the transitions and emotions that new parents experience.

POSTPARTUM PSYCHIATRIC DISORDERS

Public awareness of the prevalence and importance of postpartum emotional disorders has grown during recent years, primarily because of high-profile cases in the media, some of which have involved celebrities or resulted in catastrophic outcomes. A direct result of this attention has been the passage of both state and federal legislation to support research and mandate education for healthcare providers about postpartum depression. Nevertheless, postpartum psychiatric problems often remain undetected. Postpartum psychiatric disorders are commonly divided into three categories.

Baby Blues

Baby blues is a transient condition characterized by mild depressive symptoms such as sadness, crying, unstable mood, depression, anxiety, insomnia, and confusion (Ntaouti et al., 2020). These symptoms typically develop within 2 to 3 days of delivery and resolve by 2 weeks postpartum (O'Hara & Wisner, 2014). This condition is considered benign and self-limiting and is experienced by approximately 39% of postpartum patients (Rezaie-Keikhaie et al., 2020).

Postpartum Depression

This is a more serious condition, with symptoms similar to the nine depressive symptoms used to diagnose major depressive episodes that occur outside the postpartum period (Hoertel et al., 2015). Therefore, the criteria to diagnose postpartum depression are the same as those used to diagnose nonpuerperal major depression and are a minimum of five of the following symptoms: depressed mood, diminished interest in activities, significant weight loss or gain, insomnia or hypersomnia, psychomotor agitation or retardation, fatigue or loss of energy, feelings of worthlessness or guilt, decreased concentration or indecisiveness, and/or thoughts of death, suicidal ideation, or a suicide attempt (American Psychiatric Association, 2013). These symptoms typically develop between 1 and 3 weeks postpartum but can occur up to 1 year postpartum (ACOG, 2021c). Postpartum depression affects approximately 13% to 19% of postpartum patients (O'Hara & McCabe, 2013).

Posttraumatic Stress Disorder

Posttraumatic stress disorder occurs in 4% of the general population in the first postpartum year, with estimates up to 18.5% in high-risk groups (e.g., those with history of sexual trauma, high-risk pregnancy, complicated delivery; Yildiz et al., 2017). While available data are not robust in this area, it has been noted that risk factors include subjective distress in labor, obstetric emergencies, infant complications, lack of support during labor and delivery, psychological difficulties in the pregnancy, and other previous traumatic experiences (Andersen et al., 2012).

Postpartum Psychosis

This condition is related to severe depression and is characterized by delusions. It is more likely to occur among patients with bipolar disease, particularly those with a family history of postpartum psychosis. Although the condition is relatively rare, postpartum psychosis is an extremely dangerous condition with a high risk of infanticide and suicide, and of recurrence with future pregnancies. This condition requires immediate emergency hospitalization (Haessler & Rosenthal, 2007). Postpartum psychosis occurs in 0.89 to 2.6 per 1,000 postpartum patients (VanderKruik et al., 2017).

POSTPARTUM DEPRESSION

It is crucial that patients and their families be made aware of the signs of postpartum depression as they can mimic the normal transient mood changes that follow delivery (e.g., baby blues) or the normal signs of postpartum fatigue. Postpartum depres-

Box 39.6 Antenatal Risks for Postpartum Depression

Lack of social support

Low self-esteem

Life stressors, including child care stress

Fatigue

Prenatal depression

Prenatal anxiety

Poor marital relationship

History of depression

Difficult infant temperament

"Baby blues"

Low socioeconomic status (e.g., financial problems with housing or income)

Single marital status

Unplanned or unwanted pregnancy

Age younger than 20 years

Medically indigent

Comes from a family of six or more children

Separated from one or both parents during childhood or adolescence

Received poor parental support and attention during childhood

Had limited parental support during adulthood

Has poor relationship with partner

Is dissatisfied with the amount of education

Shows evidence of past or present emotional problems

Source: Beck, C. T. (2008). State of the science on postpartum depression: What nurse researchers have contributed—Part 1. American Journal of Maternal/Child Nursing, 33(2), 121–126. https://doi.org/10.1097/01. NMC.0000313421.97236.cf; Hanretty, K. P. (2003). Obstetrics illustrated (6th ed., p. 341). Churchill Livingstone; Katz, V. L. (2007). Postpartum care. In S. G. Gabbe, J. R. Niebyl, J. L. Simpson, H. L. Galan, L. Goetzl, E. R. M. Jauniaux, & M. B. Landon (Eds.), Obstetrics: Normal and problem pregnancies (5th ed.). Churchill Livingstone.

sion has profound consequences for the children of affected parents; their social and psychological development is jeopardized as a result of their birth parent's diminished ability to interact or provide needed stimulation. Particularly in developing countries, a parent's postpartum depression is likely to lead to the malnutrition and poor health of their children. Antenatal risks for postpartum depression are identified in Box 39.6.

ETIOLOGY AND IMPORTANT FACTORS OF POSTPARTUM DEPRESSION
Hormones and Stress Response

Levels of ACTH and corticotropin-releasing hormone (CRH) have been found to be increased among postpartum patients who are depressed, thus indicating an altered stress response

(Jolley et al., 2007). There is evidence that the hormones of breastfeeding have a protective effect against stress (Groer et al., 2002); therefore, promoting breastfeeding antenatally is an important strategy for preventing postpartum depression, particularly in patients who are at increased risk for postpartum depression.

Transcultural Factors

Although cross-cultural studies have found that postpartum depression occurs in disparate cultures throughout the world, it varies widely in prevalence and with regard to its associated risk factors. Some risks are common across cultures, such as poverty, a history of depression, a history of multiple miscarriages, and an unemployed or absent father of the baby. However, in parts of the world in which sons are valued over daughters (e.g., Turkey, India), the incidence of postpartum depression is higher among patients who have daughters. Although the incidence of postpartum depression in Western societies has been estimated to be between 13% and 19%, the worldwide incidence is anywhere from close to 0% to as high as 60% (Halbreich & Karkun, 2006; O'Hara & McCabe, 2013). In societies in which stoicism is valued and mental illness is stigmatized, patients may be disinclined to disclose feelings of depression. In cultures in which female family members are there to take care of the baby's siblings and household tasks, where patients are given the support they need during the postpartum period, the rates of depression are significantly lower. Even when the condition exists, its roots are not perceived to be based in the biologic medical model, and thus the concept of its diagnosis and treatment as a disease may be incongruous with local customs (Halbreich & Karkun, 2006).

Considering the risk factors that are common to cultures throughout the world, it is clear that postpartum depression is a socially mitigated phenomenon. Poverty, single parenthood, and bearing a daughter in a place and time when it is considered a shameful misfortune are not biologically based phenomena. Even so, the puerperium is a time during which susceptible individuals experience a uniquely stressful situation that is potentiated by particular coexisting factors.

Assessment

Although birth parents traditionally are not seen by their obstetric healthcare provider until 4 to 6 weeks after delivery, ACOG (2018a) recommends that all patients have contact with their obstetric provider within the first 3 weeks postpartum, ongoing care as needed, and a comprehensive postpartum visit by 12 weeks postpartum. Home visits by nurses or doulas are also known to be helpful to new parents. These visits are also cost effective in that they reduce the number of newborn hospital readmissions (Paul et al., 2004).

The initial assessment within 3 weeks postpartum provides the opportunity to make a number of critical assessments, including screening for depression. In addition, the U.S. Preventive Services Task Force (USPSTF) and the American Academy of Pediatrics (AAP) recommend screening the birth parent at infant well visits, with AAP extending its recommendation to screen parents at every well visit through 6 months (Rafferty et al., 2019). Administering the Edinburgh Postpartum Depression Scale (EPDS), which is a well-validated

10-question instrument, is the most frequently used method of screening patients for depression during their postpartum visits (ACOG, 2018a). Patients who score greater than or equal to 11 on the EPDS have a positive screen (Levis et al., 2020). These patients should be evaluated for immediate safety and then referred with an appropriate level of urgency to psychiatric clinicians for diagnosis and treatment (Cox et al., 2014). If emergent care is not necessary, the patient is given information about crisis intervention resources should the need arise before their appointment date. They are also screened for other possible causes of depression, such as hypothyroidism. A thorough discussion of the issue of sleep deprivation is crucial, because it may be related to depression both as a contributing factor and as an effect. Pregnant patients and their families are made aware of the signs of postpartum depression and given crisis referral information, which is reinforced before discharge from the hospital. Concrete plans for help at home and support after discharge are ensured for patients who are at risk for postpartum depression.

COMPLEMENTARY AND ALTERNATIVE MEDICINE

The quality of the research on therapies for postpartum depression has been low to moderate over the past 20 years. Chow et al. (2021) found that antidepressants and telecommunication therapy are the most effective treatments for postpartum depression. Traditional Chinese herbal medicine was also shown to be effective and could be considered as an option for postpartum patients looking for a therapeutic alternative to conventional therapies. The efficacy of physical exercise, hormonal therapies, and cognitive behavioral therapy as treatments for postpartum depression are of uncertain signification and warrant more research.

PHARMACOTHERAPEUTICS

Breastfeeding patients with postpartum depression should weigh the risks and benefits of antidepressant medications with their healthcare provider, including risks of untreated depression and of infant exposure to the medication through breast milk. Selective serotonin reuptake inhibitors (SSRIs) are commonly prescribed, as they are generally thought to be compatible with breastfeeding (Stewart & Vigod, 2016). For patients who initiated antidepressants prior to delivery, it is reasonable to continue prescribing the same dose postpartum. For patients who initiate antidepressants after delivery, medication management is similar to that for those being treated for depression in the general population. If a patient was on an antidepressant prior to pregnancy, stopped during pregnancy, and wants to resume the same antidepressant postpartum, the target dose should be the dose that was effective at treating their depression prior to pregnancy (Deligiannidis et al., 2014). Prescribing one antidepressant at a higher dose is preferred over a combination of antidepressants at lower doses (Payne, 2021).

Changes in Low-Risk Obstetric Care

THE DECLINE OF THE DELIVERY ROOM AND THE NEWBORN NURSERY

Birth and postpartum care have evolved from the sterile operating room type of delivery involving a recovery room to birth rooms and postpartum care floors. In most instances, the parent–infant dyad is together in the same room and cared for by the same nurse. The newborn nursery is only used for assessing newborns and for caring for infants whose parents require special postpartum care themselves.

LENGTH OF HOSPITAL STAY

The typical hospital postpartum stay ranges from 48 hours for a vaginal delivery to 96 hours for a cesarean delivery. A shorter stay may be considered if certain maternal and infant criteria are met. Maternal criteria include normal vital signs, labs results received and addressed (including drug screen, if collected), RhoGAM injection given to the patient (if indicated), the color and amount of lochia are appropriate, the uterus is firm, urine output is adequate, surgical wounds are normal for current stage of healing, the patient is able to walk and pain is under control, the patient is able to eat and drink, and postpartum follow-up has been scheduled. Postpartum teaching should have been completed for both parent and baby, and the parent should be able to recognize deviations from normal and how to respond to signs of danger. The parent should demonstrate readiness to care for themselves and their baby and should have received information on postpartum activity, exercise, common discomforts, and relief measures. Support persons should be identified and available to assist for the first few days after discharge. The infant should have met all criteria for discharge as well (AAP & ACOG, 2012).

THE FAMILY MEDICAL LEAVE ACT

Unlike other countries in the industrialized world, the United States does not have a national paid maternity or paternity leave program. However, job protection and continuation of benefits (without pay) are protected for up to 12 weeks under the federal Family and Medical Leave Act of 1993 (FMLA), as well as numerous state laws. The application of this protection is limited to workers with more than 1 year of employment at a company with more than 50 employees. Because of these eligibility criteria, only about 60% of workers in the United States are eligible, often leaving low-income families unprotected (Klerman et al., 2014). If there are pregnancy or postpartum complications that require longer than 12 weeks of leave, leave may be able to be extended under the Americans With Disabilities Act (Equal Opportunity for Individuals With Disabilities, 2016).

Medical Concerns Before Hospital Discharge

The patient is offered a rubella vaccine before discharge if they are found to be nonimmune during their prenatal care. If they are Rh negative, the results of the RhoGAM workup are evaluated, and the birth parent is given Rh immunoglobulin (e.g., RhoGAM) within 72 hours of delivery if the baby is Rh positive to prevent Rh isoimmunization. During the winter season, the flu vaccine is also offered. None of these preventive measures are contraindicated for breastfeeding parents.

Rest and Recovery After Delivery

Fatigue is an expectation during the puerperium, and factors such as multiple gestation and complicated, high-risk, or operative deliveries may cause even greater fatigue. Many patients and their families are neither prepared for the level of exhaustion that they experience nor the length of time that it lasts. Interventions include breastfeeding while side lying rather than sitting, which has been shown to be effective for reducing postpartum fatigue (Troy, 2003). After delivery, the new parent is counseled to sleep when the baby sleeps and wake with the baby for feedings. They are encouraged to arrange for help at home with household chores and other children for the first several weeks so that they have time to recover physically and to bond with the baby. Family and friends are asked to help with household chores rather than infant care. Patients who are recovering normally may gradually increase their activity levels, both inside and outside the home, as tolerated. Exercise is effective for preventing depression of any kind, including postpartum depression.

Sexuality

Patients and their partners are counseled so they are prepared for the normal changes related to sexuality that occur during the months and sometimes years after delivery that are caused by a number of factors. Dyspareunia may occur as a result of perineal trauma suffered during birth, particularly if lacerations, episiotomy, forceps, or vacuum extraction were involved. It may also occur as a result of the changes in hormone levels postdelivery, especially those that are associated with breastfeeding. Diminished estrogen levels in relation to progesterone and decreased levels of androgens result in less lubrication, thinning of the vaginal mucosa, and diminished libido. Additionally, exhaustion and emotional lability come with being the parent of a newborn. For some breastfeeding patients and their partners, it is difficult to accept the breasts as a mode of nourishing a child, while in another setting they are sexual organs. Rest, support, vaginal lubricants, taking things slowly, open communication, and a considerate partner are essential. A vaginal estrogen cream can be prescribed if over-the-counter lubricants are insufficient for treatment of atrophic vaginal tissue, which may occur during lactation (Gabbe et al., 2007). Desire discrepancy between partners around the birth of a child, as well as the new parent's understandable preoccupation with their baby, have been major challenges in relationships throughout the ages.

Contraception

Counseling the postpartum patient about contraceptive options takes into account religious, cultural, and personal beliefs as well as the desired method of infant feeding and any medical contraindications. Breastfeeding patients should avoid estrogen-containing birth control methods for 4 to 6 weeks postpartum, as they may affect milk supply (ACOG, 2023). Progesterone-only methods include intrauterine device (IUD), implant, shot, and pill form. Hormone-free methods include the copper IUD, barrier methods (e.g., spermicides, condoms, sponges, diaphragms, and cervical caps), and surgical sterilization.

Patients who are not breastfeeding may ovulate within a few weeks postpartum; however, hypercoagulability of the postpartum period extends to 3 weeks after birth, thereby increasing the risk of VTE (ACOG, 2019d, 2023). Due to this increased risk, combined contraceptives are contraindicated during the first 21 days postpartum. Patients with additional VTE risk factors are advised to not start using combined contraceptives during the first 42 days postpartum (ACOG, 2019d). Progesterone-only methods may be started earlier, with various progesterone-only methods offered before the woman is discharged from the hospital. For patients who desire long-term contraception, the IUD may be a good option whether the patient is breastfeeding or not. This type of device is inserted either immediately postpartum, or, more typically, at or after the 6-week postpartum visit. Although it is possible to insert the IUD after the placenta has been delivered, this presents a greater risk for the expulsion of the device (ACOG, 2023). For exclusively breastfeeding with amenorrhea, the lactational amenorrhea method (LAM) of birth control may be the patient's method of choice for birth control for up to 6 months postpartum (or until menses has returned). The patient must breastfeed at least every 4 hours during the day and every 6 hours during the night. It is unclear whether or not pumping decreases this method's effectiveness (ACOG, 2023).

Diet

Dietary concerns of recently delivered birth parents frequently center around their desire to lose weight. This needs to be balanced with nutritional needs, particularly if they are breastfeeding, in which case they are counseled to consume at least 1,800 calories per day. An adequate intake of nutrients, particularly fluids; calories from a balance of protein, vegetable, and fruit sources; fats; vitamins; and minerals are essential for establishing an adequate milk supply, the replacement of fluids and blood, and wound healing after delivery. The patient should be counseled to eat foods rich in protein, iron, and calcium, and to continue to take prenatal vitamins and an iron supplement if they have been anemic or experienced a large blood loss. Iron deficiency anemia can contribute to the fatigue of the postpartum period, thus increasing the challenges of recovery, breastfeeding, and newborn care. Fiber intake is also important to prevent constipation, which can be quite painful if the patient had a perineal repair. Patients must be followed closely if they had a fourth-degree repair, with referral for any difficulty with bowel movements.

Exercise

There are no absolute contraindications to exercise after a normal vaginal delivery; healthy patients can gradually resume prepregnancy exercise routines as they regain strength. A patient may start with head raises for abdominal muscles, Kegel exercises, and walking. Heavy lifting and high impact exercise is discouraged until much later because excessive exercise during the early postpartum period may increase the risk for hemorrhage. Activity is modified in the event of cesarean section since stress on the abdomen needs to be avoided until clearance is obtained from the healthcare provider. Maternal weight loss does not influence infant growth, provided the patient has adequate caloric and fluid intake to produce sufficient breast milk. A review of diet and exercise for postpartum weight loss found that diet alone as well as diet plus exercise led to postpartum weight loss without compromising breastfeeding; exercise alone did not lead to weight loss (Amorim-Adegboye et al., 2007).

Newborn Care

New parents' early postpartum educational priorities range from basic infant care to normal development. A multiparous patient should be assessed for basic knowledge as well as their awareness of changes in care that may have occurred since the birth of their last child. The healthcare provider should assess the patient's level of knowledge, family support, as well as the new parent's readiness and ability to take in information. It is also important to consider what has transpired during labor and delivery, because patients who have experienced prolonged or difficult labors or operative deliveries may take longer to bond with their infants and experience difficulty doing so.

Research suggests that parents play an important role in the development of the newborn's physical, cognitive, emotional, and social growth. The four key factors that have been identified as integral to this development are healthy attachment, responsive care, protection from harm, and breastfeeding (Bryanton & Beck, 2010). An excellent method for teaching and assessing parents' knowledge, beliefs, and practices regarding infant care and for observing parents' interactions with their infants is to include them when performing the newborn examination. Adolescent parents in particular will benefit from this experience, because they can be taught the basics of newborn care. The ability of the baby to actively interact with the environment, the infant's sleep–wake cycles, and the newborn's individual temperament should be discussed in concrete terms (Davidson et al., 2007).

SAFETY
Sleep Safety

Infant sleep practices are influenced by ethnic, social, economic, and other factors, including the method of infant feeding. There is a strong relationship between breastfeeding and bed sharing. Patients who choose to bed share with their infants need to be informed about safe sleep practices, as the AAP (2016) does not recommend cosleeping. Safe sleep practices include placing the baby on a firm, flat surface (e.g., no waterbeds or couches) in a supine position, with the bedding tucked in tightly (e.g., no pillows, stuffed animals, quilts, duvets, or comforters). There should be no spaces in which the infant's head could become trapped (e.g., between the bed and a headboard or a wall). Placing the baby on a firm mattress on the floor away from a wall may be a safe alternative. Having an infant sleep in the same room as their parents, without cosleeping, appears to be protective against sudden infant death syndrome (SIDS; Academy of Breastfeeding Medicine Protocol Committee, 2008; Box 39.7).

Newborns need to be kept warm; however, it is equally important that parents not overdress their infants. In particular, heavy blankets and soft or furry bedding (e.g., lambskin) are hazardous and have been associated with an increased risk of SIDS. It is therefore essential that healthcare providers

Box 39.7 Safe Sleeping Instructions

Always put a baby to sleep on their back.

Baby should have their own sleep space, a firm mattress in their own crib or bassinet, close to parents or caregivers.

Do not place pillows, stuffed animals or blanket rolls in the crib.

Do not smoke in a house with a baby.

Breastfeeding reduces a baby's risk of sudden infant death syndrome.

Consider offering pacifier for naps and bedtime.

Source: American Academy of Pediatrics. (2016). SIDS and other sleep-related infant deaths: Updated 2016 recommendations for a safe infant sleeping environment. Pediatrics, 138(5), e20162938. https://doi.org/10 .1542/peds.2016-2938

assess whether new parents have adequate heating or cooling available in their homes upon discharge. If they do not, the healthcare provider should arrange for social services to evaluate the home situation before discharging newly delivered parents and infants. New families must be provided with safe sleep instructions.

Car Safety

All infants are discharged from the hospital in federally approved, rear-facing infant car seats that are correctly installed in the back seat. Therefore, staff need to be trained to ensure the car seat is sized appropriately to the infant and is not recalled or expired.

Social Support: Home Visits

Knowledge of community resources or the ability to refer to social service agencies is essential for healthcare providers who work with postpartum families. Postpartum home visiting programs that make use of nurses and paraprofessionals have demonstrated significant positive effects on a number of health outcomes. The rate of hospital readmissions of infants for jaundice and dehydration was reduced by one such program, and indicators of positive family and mental health outcomes among parent–child dyads were still present at 2-year follow-up assessments in another. These included the parent's sense of mastery, improved parent–child interactions, increased child spacing, and improved child development (Meyer et al., 2001).

Discharge Instructions

Discharge teaching includes verbal and written instructions about the following (Box 39.8):

- Follow-up appointments for parent and baby
- Danger signs, including a fever of more than 38°C (100.4°F); painful urination; lochia that has become heavier than a period (lochia is usually lighter after cesarean section delivery); a reddened or tender area of the breast accompanied by flu-like symptoms; thigh or calf pain with redness and tenderness; separation

Box 39.8 Postpartum Discharge Instructions

Follow-Up Appointments

Maternal: Routinely in 4 to 6 weeks; may be sooner as needed

Infant: Routinely in 2 weeks; may be sooner as needed

Activity

Rest for first 2 to 4 weeks

Ask visitors and relatives to help with other children, household chores, and errands

Sudden Infant Death Syndrome Prevention

Pacifier use should not be stopped suddenly during the first 26 weeks of life

Safe sleep environment: the crib should meet safety regulations, and no pillows, soft bedding, or toys should be used

Bed sharing increases risk with a parent who smokes, drinks, or takes certain drugs or medications

Maternal Danger Signs

Sudden or persistent blood loss

Faintness or dizziness

Fever, chills, abdominal pain, and foul-smelling lochia

Headaches and visual disturbances

Red or painful area of the leg or breast

Persistent or severe feelings of depression

Chest pain, difficulty breathing

Infant Danger Signs

Jaundice (worsening or new onset) or pale stools

Diarrhea or constipation

Lack of wet diapers

Excessive or inconsolable crying

Fever of more than or equal to 38°C (100.4°F)

Source: Data from Demott, K., Bick, D., Norman, R., Ritchie, G., Turnbull, N., Adams, C., Barry, C., Byrom, S., Elliman, D., Marchant, S., McCandlish, R., Mellows, H., Neale, C., Parkar, M., Tait, P., & Taylor, C. (2006). Clinical guidelines and evidence review for post natal care: Routine post natal care of recently delivered women and their babies. National Collaborating Centre for Primary Care; Royal College of General Practitioners.

of the wound or redness or oozing at the wound site; and abdominal pain that increases in severity or that is unrelieved by prescribed pain medication

- Seeking care for severe depression or the patient's inability to care for themself or their baby; seeking help if they have thoughts of harming themselves or others
- Functional systems in place for help after hours and for families that may require the services of a language interpreter

SUMMARY

The postpartum patient has many concerns to address, including their own health, bonding with and nurturing their baby, and caring for other family members. They need careful assessment and support in meeting their extra nutritional requirements as well as in their need to obtain restorative rest. Rest is important to properly recover from labor and delivery and to facilitate the demanding physiologic processes of involution, lochia discharge, breastfeeding, and caring for the newborn. They are monitored for postpartum complications and provided with extensive education for recognizing problems in addition to having a thorough understanding of how to care for both themselves and their newborn.

REFERENCES

References for this chapter are online and available at https://connect.springerpub.com/content/book/978-0-8261-6722-4/part/part03/chapter/ch39

CHAPTER 40

Mental Health Challenges

DEBORAH ANTAI-OTONG

The prevalence of psychiatric disorders in women and other minoritized gender persons seen in primary care settings is high, especially for anxiety, major depression, substance use, and eating disorders. Approximately 20% to 30% of all women experience at least one psychiatric disorder during a given year (Kessler et al., 2005). Even more concerning is the exceptionally higher rate of psychiatric disorders in women of childbearing age (Kessler et al., 2005). Situations in which people lack autonomy, independent income, decision-making power, and locus of control make managing stressful situations difficult and increase vulnerability to psychiatric conditions.

The COVID-19 epidemic has had a dramatic effect on worldwide mental health of women and other minoritized gender persons. During the pandemic current data indicate a higher incidence of major depression and anxiety disorders, eating disorders, and intimate partner violence, particularly among younger persons (Holmes et al., 2020; Piquero et al., 2021). The higher incidence of mental health problems in women and minoritized gender persons is attributed to social distancing, home quarantine and forced cohabitation, high levels of stress, uncertainty, and exacerbation of psychiatric disorders (Parvar et al., 2022). Complex neurobiological, immunologic, genetic, cultural, and psychosocial factors contribute to psychiatric disorders in women. Female gender is a powerful constitutional determinant of mental health that interacts with individual characteristics, including age, race, ethnicity, gender identity, reproductive transition, developmental stage, personality traits, self-worth, and strengths. The concurrence of hormonal and reproductive transitions and biological factors in women's lives increase the risk for mood and anxiety disorders during various reproductive events, such as postpartum and perimenopausal depression (Hong et al., 2021; Soares, 2019; Zuberi et al., 2021). Social influences, which include environmental and sociocultural factors, life events, history of abuse, family dynamics, socioeconomic and educational status, and access to equitable and gender-centered healthcare, are equally linked to women's as well as other minoritized gender persons' well-being and mental health (Slavich, 2020).

Mental healthcare described in this chapter is intended to include cisgender women, transgender women, transgender men, and gender-nonbinary persons. The terms *patient, people,* and *person* are used to include all of these individuals.

The terms *woman* and *women* often could include all of these persons, but data are lacking on the larger population of minoritized gender persons in many instances. Therefore, *woman* and *women* are used here to include cisgender women and nonbinary persons identified as female at birth and not taking hormone therapy.

MENTAL HEALTH DISORDERS

Definition and Scope

Women are twice as likely as men to experience depressive and anxiety disorders, particularly posttraumatic stress disorder PTSD; (Kessler et al., 2017; Slavich & Sacher, 2019). A disproportionate number of women and minitorized gender persons experience trauma. Precipitating events associated with mental health problems include rape, deployment and combat-related stressors, other sexual assaults, intimate partner violence (IPV), history of childhood physical and/or sexual abuse, or being threatened with a weapon. Common consequences associated with experiencing violence include development of depression, PTSD, anxiety and/or substance use disorders (SUDs) during pregnancy and the postpartum period, as well as negative effects on children and adolescents exposed to environmental violence (Rosado et al., 2021; Thompson et al., 2022). For example, persons exposed to psychological IPV were more likely to suffer from PTSD than control subjects (Rosado et al., 2021). In addition, suicide risk and gastrointestinal (GI) conditions are commonly associated with psychosocial stressors.

The prevalence of eating disorders varies with sampling and evaluation methodology. The lifetime estimates from the *Diagnostic and Statistical Manual of Mental Disorders* (5th ed.; *DSM-5*; American Psychiatric Association [APA], 2013) for women diagnosed with anorexia nervosa, bulimia nervosa, and binge eating disorder are 0.8%, 2.3%, 3.5%, respectively. Disordered eating or eating disorders are more common in older adolescents and young women and uncommon in men.

A common myth about eating disorders is that they are limited to middle- and upper-middle-class White women. Although some studies suffering from population selection bias limitation support this myth, other studies indicate that the incidence of eating disorders is similar across ethnic and racial groups and that culturally sensitive interventions must be implemented to reduce the risk of eating disorders among vulnerable and minoritized populations (Ruchkin et al., 2021). Disordered eating is found to have a high co-occurrence with other psychiatric disorders such as anxiety, mood, substance use, and personality disorders. The mortality rate in this population has not improved during the past decade (Ruchkin et al., 2021; van Hoeken & Hoek, 2020). Thus, inquiring about symptoms of disordered eating in persons of all races and ethnicities is necessary to ensure accurate diagnosis and appropriate management to reduce morbidity and mortality.

Access to timely and appropriate healthcare also challenges people with mental health problems. It is widely documented that many patients with a mental health problem receive mental healthcare from a primary care clinician rather than a mental health clinician. Growing concerns about the complexity of mental healthcare and provision of integrated mental health services in primary care practice remains a challenge because of the importance of timely monitoring and, in some cases, the need to collaborate with mental health clinicians. Primary care clinicians must bridge the gap and work with mental health and physical health services to develop collaborative approaches for managing mental health problems for patients. Regardless of where a person enters the healthcare system, clinicians must recognize and value the unique biological and psychosocial makeup that increases risk for mental health problems and need for individualized interventions.

Etiology and Risk Factors

Mental health is influenced by one's capacity to cope with the daily stress of living, establish and maintain meaningful relationships, tolerate frustration and anxiety, and contribute to society. The diathesis-stress theory suggests that psychosocial, neurobiological, and genetic factors; sex hormones; cultural, economic, and healthcare disparities; and environmental influences as well as personality traits together modulate stressful events and vulnerability to psychiatric disorders (Lombardo, 2021). Furthermore, researchers posit that alterations in neurobiological processes, particularly the hypothalamic–pituitary–adrenal (HPA) axis, demonstrate a significant role in the diathesis of suicide (Lombardo, 2021). These complex factors play principal roles in the development of psychiatric disorders and have implications for treatment considerations. Reproductive events mediated by psychosocial stressors and complex underpinnings predispose women to psychiatric disorders.

GENETIC VULNERABILITY

Major depression, anxiety, substance use, and eating disorders appear to be more heritable in women than men, and are associated with interactions between biological, genetic, hormonal, and psychosocial factors (Bandelow et al., 2022). Family and twin studies correlate genetic vulnerability to psychiatric disorders, seemingly particularly higher in women with personality disorders (e.g., borderline personality disorder) and a history of childhood adversity, stress, or

trauma (Lombardo, 2021). Genetics also predispose women to early-onset, coexistent psychiatric conditions, including alcohol misuse, panic disorder (PD), lifetime overall anxiety disorders, and recurrence of major depression (Lombardo, 2021; Salminen et al., 2021; Thompson et al., 2022). Explanations for genetic risk factors associated with psychiatric conditions involve alterations in serotonin transporter (5-HTT), less functional s-allele transporters, and tryptophan depletion (Lewis et al., 2020; Thompson et al., 2022).

The extent to which genetic and environmental factors contribute to stress-induced mental health problems may also be based on the context of environmental risk factors and neurobiological vulnerabilities (Lewis et al., 2020; Salminen et al., 2021; Thompson et al., 2022). Given women's sensitivity and vulnerability to psychosocial stressors and higher incidence of early childhood and other trauma exposure, the diathesis-stress model suggests that anxiety and mood disorders are mediated by genetic and neurobiological vulnerabilities as well as psychosocial stressors. The diathesis-stress model can guide therapeutic interventions, such as pharmacologic interventions that target both genetic and biological underpinnings (serotonin receptor sites), to reduce symptoms and strengthen coping skills.

BIOCHEMICAL FACTORS

Alterations in complex brain regions and neurocircuitry pathways contribute to variability in thought processing, behavior, and mood—hallmark features of mood and anxiety disorders. Serotonin and its metabolite, cerebrospinal fluid (CSF) 5-hydroxylindoleacetic acid (5-HIAA), and tryptophan depletion are widely accepted as biological markers of major depressive disorders. Lower CSF serotonin levels are implicated in women with severe major depression (Salminen et al., 2021; Thompson et al., 2022). Neurotransmitters are target sites for antidepressant medications, particularly those that enhance serotonergic levels and norepinephrine. Increased CSF 5-HIAA levels have also been found in women with co-occurring major depression and PD and implicate increased serotonin release and greater serotonin metabolism and/or decreased 5-HIAA clearance. Co-occurring psychiatric conditions, such as borderline personality disorder (BPD), PTSD, and major depression, are associated with serious psychiatric disorders, increased rates of disability and mortality, and poor treatment outcomes (Kessler et al., 2017; Thompson et al., 2022).

NEUROIMAGING ALTERATIONS

Findings from neuroimaging studies involving psychiatric disorders point to alterations in three brain regions: the medial prefrontal cortex, amygdala, and hippocampus. For instance, in PTSD, dysregulation of the amygdala and prefrontal cortex appear to contribute to the exaggerated physiologic responses to stimuli such as startle response, hypervigilance, avoidant behaviors, and increased heart rate and blood pressure (Ginty et al., 2019). Similar findings were discovered in persons with BPD, who often suffer from childhood trauma and PTSD (Sarkheil et al., 2020). Data from these studies also demonstrated abnormalities in the frontal-amygdala circuitry, namely, hypometabolism and decreased volume (Sarkheil et al., 2020). Alterations in the medial prefrontal cortex are associated with poor impulse control, emotional instability, maladaptive coping behaviors, and suicide and self-injurious behaviors—core features of BPD and individuals with eating disorders. Selective serotonin reuptake inhibitor (SSRI) antidepressants are effective in treating major depression and aggressive impulsive behaviors, which are commonly found in persons with BPD. The efficacy of these agents is their stabilizing effect of prefrontal cortex metabolism on impulsive behaviors commonly found in individuals with BPD and PTSD (Sarkheil et al., 2020).

NEUROENDOCRINE FACTORS

Alterations in the HPA axis are often linked to medical and psychiatric conditions. Depression and anxiety disorder have long been linked to abnormalities in the HPA axis (Ginty et al., 2019; Sarkheil et al., 2020). Converging data using combined dexamethasone (DEX) and corticotropin-releasing hormone (CRF) demonstrated marked dysregulation in the HPA axis in persons with unipolar and bipolar depression (Sarkheil et al., 2020). These data confirmed earlier findings implicating the role of neuroendocrine factors in the genesis of depression and other psychiatric conditions.

Prolonged stress reaction is also implicated in mood, anxiety, and medical disorders (e.g., breast and ovarian cancers, Alzheimer disease, premature aging; Hwang et al., 2020; Ji & Wang, 2020). Prolonged stress produces alterations in hippocampal function, inflammatory responses, and structure in animal models, an effect mediated primarily by increased glucocorticoids and limited neurogenesis. These findings are consistent with MRI studies of individuals with PTSD who had reduced hippocampal volume and deficits in memory and cognition. Hormonal changes are likely to occur during reproductive transitions (Hwang et al., 2020). Antidepressants play a key role in the modulation of serotonin transmission by mediating stress-regulating processes in those with PTSD and major depression (Ginty et al., 2019). These agents enhance neurogenesis and neuroprotection, increase hippocampal volume, and improve cognitive and memory function.

REPRODUCTIVE TRANSITIONS

The reproductive cycle has been implicated in the pathogenesis of psychiatric disorders in women and is associated with dysregulation of ovarian steroids. Estrogen is widely distributed to receptors in the brain and believed to modulate dopamine, norepinephrine, and acetylcholine neurotransmitters involved in mood and cognition. Hyperactivity of the HPA in women is linked to depression and believed to play a regulatory role in sex hormones. Greater emphasis has centered on the serotonin–estrogen connection in the modulation of mood and cognition, although the significance of this relationship is unclear. Estrogen's unique relationship with serotonin has spurred robust interest, mainly because serotonin is well studied, clearly connected with regulation of mood, and a primary target for pharmacologic treatment of unipolar depression (Hwang et al., 2020).

Premenstrual dysphoric disorder (PMDD) is a good example of the interrelationship among estrogen–serotonin, neuroendocrine factors, and the genesis of mood disorders. Although the precise cause of PMDD continues to be studied, most evidence suggests dysregulation in neuroendocrine, hormonal, or serotonergic neurocircuitry. Abnormal serotonergic transmission and the efficacy of SSRIs further strengthen the premise of this neurotransmitter effect in the pathogenesis and treatment of mood and anxiety disorders (Hwang et al., 2020; Slavich & Sacher, 2019). Use of gender-affirming hormone therapy (GAHT) is not associated with this effect, presumably because GAHT doses are consistent and do not wax and wane over a cycle as endogenous hormones do in women.

ENVIRONMENTAL AND ADVERSE LIFE STRESSORS

Stressful life events increase vulnerability to mood and anxiety disorders (Lombardo, 2021). However, not all persons who experience life stressors develop mood and anxiety disorders. Emerging models posit that the effect of adverse life events is modulated by the person's repertoire of coping skills, quality of support systems, and personality style. Heightened levels of perfectionism, low self-esteem, and perceived ineffectiveness are common traits in persons with eating disorders and concomitant mood disorders. In addition, family and twin study results implicate genetic vulnerability in women contributing to adverse life events and susceptibility to psychiatric illness (Lombardo, 2021; Rosado et al., 2021).

Psychosocial stressors contribute to depressive and anxiety disorders, and the nature of stress itself is a significant risk factor for mental health problems. Women often face significant stressors such as the demands of single parenthood, childrearing, and caring for aged parents. Lack of close and meaningful relationships, low self-esteem, low confidence, interpersonal violence, and marital discord further overburden coping skills. Psychosocial stressors and adverse life events must be thoroughly evaluated to determine their effects on current complaints, experience, adaptation, level of danger to self and others, functionality, and quality of life.

Diverse Sexual Minority Stress

Currently there is a paucity of research that highlights disparities and stress among diverse sexual minorities (e.g., lesbian, transgender, bisexual, nonbinary, genderqueer) populations across racial and ethnic populations. According to results from the 2015–2018 National Survey on Drug Use and Health, a lack of openness about sexual identity contributed to disparities and psychosocial stress and risk of psychiatric disorders, SUDs, and suicide risk (Kelly et al., 2021; Motmans et al., 2019; Rodriguez-Seijas et al., 2019). Black and Hispanic LGBTQ+ women were more likely to experience these issues than White LGBTQ+ women (Schuler et al., 2019). Implications from these findings emphasize the importance of gleaning a greater understanding of the patient's experiences and coping responses to discrimination about their sexual identity and gender preferences.

CULTURAL AND ETHNICITY INFLUENCES

Demographic changes that have occurred in recent decades in the United States are shifting certain populations from minority to majority. This shift strengthens the importance of addressing and valuing the needs of diverse populations. A growing body of evidence demonstrates that persons from various cultural and ethnic backgrounds experience discrimination, insensitivity, lack of knowledge about their religious and cultural practices, and poor access to mental healthcare. Assessing and addressing the mental health needs of underserved and marginalized populations must be a priority for all clinicians. Clinicians must recognize their explicit and implicit biases and prejudices that affect their perception of the patient's symptoms, health practices, and treatment responses, as well as the patient's definition of wellness. This process offers an opportunity to establish meaningful and quality relationships, display empathy, and provide culturally and linguistically sensitive mental healthcare. A failure to employ these approaches is likely to place a patient at a greater risk of poor clinical outcomes, adversely impact the clinician–patient relationship and result in inappropriate mental healthcare (Moreno & Chhatwal, 2020).

Evaluation/Assessment

HISTORY AND SYMPTOMS

Persons with psychiatric conditions typically seek help from their primary care clinician, presenting with complaints of somatic problems such as fatigue or sleep disturbances. In these situations, it is imperative to ask about reasons for seeking treatment at this time, determine what has resolved somatic complaints in the past, and identify recent stressors. Clinicians must understand the basic concepts of diagnosing and treating patients who present with mental health problems. The diagnosis of psychiatric disorders is determined by the quality of the interview, the level of clinical expertise with psychiatric evaluation, patient history, and patient motivation to change.

A successful comprehensive interview is built on establishing a therapeutic relationship in which the clinician displays empathy, genuine interest, respect, and competence (Box 40.1; Antai-Otong, 2008, 2009). An extensive chronology of mood changes, if any, during hormonal events, such as menstrual cycles, pregnancy, postpartum, and menopause, must be

Box 40.1 Key Components of a Successful Comprehensive Interview

Assuring adequate time to perform a psychiatric and physical evaluation

Eliciting the patient's symptoms, experience, and level of distress

Consulting or collaborating with a mental health professional when appropriate

Developing a patient-centered treatment plan, based on client preferences, wishes, gender, culture, and ethnicity

Source: Antai-Otong, D. (2009). Psychiatric emergencies: How to accurately assess and manage the patient in crisis *(2nd ed.). Professional Educational Systems.*

Box 40.2 Data Collected in a Systematic Comprehensive Psychiatric History

Reasons for seeking treatment

- Chief complaint—use patient's own words, that is, "I am depressed and can't sleep"
- Duration of symptoms and patient's goals or need to address psychiatric symptoms

Current stressors or significant changes the past 6 to 12 months

Strengths; quality of support system (marital status, significant other, friends, community); interests, preferences, and values pertaining to healthcare

Sociocultural needs; spiritual and religious beliefs

Attitude concerning weight, shape, and eating, and associated psychiatric symptoms

History of current symptoms and chronology of remissions and exacerbation

- Description and severity of current symptoms—sleep disturbances, altered mood and anxiety states, hallucinations, delusions, cognitive deficits

Chronology of psychiatric history/treatment, including exposure to antipsychotic agents, medication side effects, response; most recent periods of stability and episodes when symptoms produced severe distress and impaired function

Family history of psychiatric problems, including eating disorders

Current medications, including OTC drugs, vitamins, herbs, or complementary therapies

Allergies or serious or distressful adverse drug reactions

Present and past general medical history and responses to previous treatment

Significant personal history—coping styles

Recent/past hospitalizations, surgeries

Current health status, last physical examination, diet

Trauma exposure—rape, military, natural disaster, witness to violence, bullying

Inquire and assess for emotional and physical signs of IPV

Legal history—past and present charges, arrests, incarceration, parole or probation, DUI charges

History of abuse and/or violence

Substance abuse/dependence history (illicit, licit), treatment, dual diagnosis (concurrent psychiatric and substance use disorder)

Review of systems; focused medical history

Functional, occupational, psychosocial status

Relevant military history (e.g., combat, noncombat; military sexual trauma); discharge status

DUI, driving under the influence; IPV, intimate partner violence; OTC, over the counter.
Source: Antai-Otong, D. (2008). Psychiatric nursing: Biological and behavioral concepts (2nd ed.). Thomson Delmar Learning.

obtained. Systematic data collection and synthesis of a number of topics are important (Box 40.2).

PHYSICAL EXAMINATION

Patients with psychiatric symptoms must receive a diagnostic evaluation to develop a differential diagnosis of a psychiatric and/or medical disorder. Routine data from vital signs, neurologic evaluation, signs of abuse or self-injurious behaviors (e.g., bruises, rashes, cuts, and punctures), functional status, and nutritional status provide relevant information needed to make a differential diagnosis. Symptoms of eating disorders often manifest as serious medical conditions that require immediate management and stabilization. Throughout both the history and physical examination, the clinician observes carefully to complete a mental status examination and identify any signs of dysfunction (Table 40.1).

Differential Diagnosis

Standardized psychiatric rating scales provide useful screening tools to both identify psychiatric conditions and monitor response to treatment. They can be specific or comprehensive and measure internal experiences, such as depression, and external observable behaviors. Rating scales quantify mental status, behavior, and relationships with others and society. Data collected from these tools provide baseline information and an objective strategy to monitor treatment efficacy. Because of the time involved in using various structured tools, most mental health clinicians and primary care clinicians may opt to use diagnostic criteria listed in the *DSM-5* (APA, 2013). The *DSM-5* is a nonaxial classification system that is based on diagnostic assessment presented in *International Statistical Classification of Diseases and Related Health Problems* (10th ed., *ICD-10; World Health Organization, 2016)* diagnoses (formerly Axes I, II, and III; APA, 2013). This section includes mental health diagnosis and relevant medical conditions (APA, 2013). Axis IV (formerly psychosocial stressors) has been replaced with a World Health Organization (WHO) Disability Assessment Schedule (WHODAS) score, whereas Axis V (formerly referred to as global level of functioning [GAF]) has been deleted from

DSM-5. The WHODAS classification evolves from the International Classification of Functioning, Disability and Health (ICF) for use in vast medical and healthcare settings (APA, 2013). Thus diagnostic assessment of a psychiatric disorder includes relevant medical condition(s) and relevant specifier(s) together with the WHODAS score.

Psychiatric emergency refers to a severe disturbance of mood, thought, or behavior that requires immediate medical and psychiatric attention. Specific presentations and management for common psychiatric problems are presented in the following separate sections (Antai-Otong, 2009).

Diagnostic Studies

The following diagnostic and laboratory studies are frequently needed: serum chemistry profile; liver and renal function panels (particularly for those receiving GAHT); serum electrolytes; urinalysis; complete blood count (CBC); platelet count; erythrocyte sedimentation rate (ESR); thiamine, vitamin B_{12}, and folate levels; vitamin assay (in those with signs of eating disorders); fasting glucose, thyroid panel; comprehensive metabolic profile; pregnancy test for women of reproductive age and nonbinary and transgender men who can become pregnant, even if use of contraception is reported; blood and urine cultures; toxicology screens; ideal body weight (Webb et al., 2020) and EKG.

Treatment/Management

Treating psychiatric disorders in primary care requires evidence-based practice and use of best practices guidelines. Collaboration with a mental health clinician offers expertise, decision support, and additional resources to manage mental healthcare. For example, although patients suffering from major depression are commonly treated in primary care settings, the concurrent risk of suicide and other life-threatening behaviors must always be evaluated and managed. Failing to recognize worsening symptoms or assess suicide risk during brief primary care appointments may have dire consequences. The collaborative model provides greater resources (e.g., education about mental health) and decision support and

TABLE 40.1 Mental Status Function Examination: Key Points to Note During the History and Physical Examination

ASSESSMENT CATEGORY	EVALUATION POINTS
General	• Appearance—hygiene, grooming, appropriateness of attire (e.g., wears warm clothing during cold weather) • Approximate age—based on general appearance • Gender identity, gender expression • Level of distress • Responses to questions • Facial expression, posture, and gait • Attentiveness to details and understanding of the interview • Eye contact—consider cultural and ethnicity influences • Overt behavior and psychomotor activity—restlessness, pacing, irritability • Attitude—cooperative, distant, uncooperative, distrustful, or suspicious • Mode of arrival—alone, with significant other, friend
Mood and affect	• Mood—internal and subjective pervasive or sustained emotion • Affect—present emotional responsiveness; note range, intensity, and stability • Blunted—severely decreased feeling tone • Restricted—minimal intensity of feeling tone • Flat—absence of emotional feeling tone • Appropriate versus mood incongruence—whether mood appropriately reflects what is being discussed
Speech	• Quality • Fluency • Articulation • Accent • Rate—rapid during the manic phase of bipolar disorder, anxiety • Spontaneity—may be reduced in person who is in shock from recent trauma exposure, depression • Pressured—normally found in bipolar disorder, manic episode • Rambling—may occur during psychosis or mania • Hesitant—often occurs during depression or psychosis • Mumbled—may occur with psychosis, paranoia, or suspiciousness • Loud—may indicate hearing disturbances or indicate anger or agitation
Perceptual and sensory function	• Hallucinations—based on internal stimuli • Illusions—based on misinterpretation of external stimuli, such as a shadow for a person • Circumstances of hallucinations or illusions (i.e., stress, falling asleep) • Content of hallucinations or delusions
Thought processes (thought organization and flow of ideas)	• Loose associations (unrelated, disconnected)—associated with psychosis • Flight of ideas (rapid thinking-connected and related)—usually indicates mania or psychosis • Racing thoughts, tangentiality, and circumstantiality—commonly found in bipolar disorder I, manic episode
Thought content	• Delusions—false beliefs, which are not shared by a person's culture and cannot be substantiated with rational explanations. They are *very real* to the patient. Types of delusions include persecutory, grandiose, somatic, and jealousy. • Preoccupations • Obsessions • Paranoia • Phobias • Suicidal/homicidal ideations • Ideas of reference
Sensorium and cognition	• A systematic evaluation of cognitive function, including: • Level of consciousness • Orientation • Attention • Concentration • Memory
Insight	• Understanding of illness and motivation to adhere to treatment recommendations
Impulsivity	• Degree and appropriateness in which client is able to control impulses
Judgment	• Degree and appropriateness of decision making, assessed by asking "what if" questions

Source: Antai-Otong, D. (2008). Psychiatric nursing: Biological and behavioral concepts (2nd ed.). Thomson Delmar Learning; Antai-Otong, D. (2009). Psychiatric emergencies: How to accurately assess and manage the patient in crisis (2nd ed.). Professional Educational Systems.

improves clinical outcomes for women with mental health problems. The COVID-19 pandemic has prompted clinicians to explore and adopt various technologies, using secure and safe venues to provide mental health services to clients and strengthen collaboration between mental health and primary care providers. Telehealth and tele-mental health have provided continuity of care and, in some cases, reduced no-show rates (Adepoju et al., 2022) Most psychiatric disorders require both pharmacologic and psychotherapeutic interventions. The decision to initiate psychotropic medications in the primary care setting must include consideration of severity of illness and associated level of functioning, history of response, safety of medication (lethality in overdose), side effects (short term and long term), medication interactions, coexisting disorders, cost (affordability), patient preferences, and reproductive events including pregnancy and lactation.

More severe psychiatric disorders, such as acute or exacerbation of psychiatric conditions (e.g., schizophrenia, PTSD, generalized anxiety disorder [GAD], bipolar-manic episode, drug-induced psychosis, postpartum psychosis, or acute suicidal ideations and behaviors), are best treated by a psychiatric clinician. Psychiatric emergencies are best treated in emergency settings to ensure patient and staff safety. Thus, in emergency presentations—such as those requiring immediate psychiatric and medical interventions or those where the patient complains of physical distress and mood or anxiety disorders—referral by primary care clinicians to an emergency facility is appropriate.

ANXIETY DISORDERS

Definition and Scope

Anxiety disorders affect an estimated 18% or 40 million Americans each year and occur in women twice as often as in men (Kessler et al., 2005; Roest et al., 2021; Zuberi et al., 2021). Anxiety disorders tend to run in families and often go unrecognized and undertreated in primary care (Kessler et al., 2012). According to the National Comorbidity Replication Survey, the lifetime prevalence of anxiety disorders is 28.8%, mood disorders is 20.8%, and substance abuse is 14.6% (Kessler et al., 2005). The median age of onset for anxiety disorders is 11 years (Kessler et al., 2005). Findings from the National Comorbidity Replication Survey (Cougle et al., 2009) demonstrated that social anxiety, PTSD, GAD, and PD were predictors of suicidal ideation. Further analyses of these data indicated that women with all four anxiety disorders had a greater risk of suicidal ideation or suicide attempts when compared with men, whose risks increased with PTSD and PD (Cougle et al., 2009). Anxiety disorders are pervasive, disabling, and generally coexist with mood and other psychiatric disorders. Women tend to present with co-occurring mood and personality disorders, variables that adversely affect treatment outcomes. The prevalence of and lasting effects from anxiety has prompted the U.S. Preventive Services Task Force (USPSTF) to recommend routine screening for anxiety among children ages 8 to 18 years and draft recommendations to recommend screening all adults, including those over age 65 years (USPSTF, 2022a, 2022b).

Etiology

Anxiety disorders are caused by a multitude of factors as described previously. Additional specific factors are specified in the following sections addressing specific diagnoses.

Treatment/Management

Documented poor treatment outcomes in primary care settings relate to the numerous physical complaints that dominate a patient's concerns and obscure complaints of anxiety-related symptoms; beliefs, knowledge, and attitudes toward mental health services; realities of time constraints and competing demands placed on primary care clinicians to quickly assess, treat, and monitor treatment response; and clinician's lack of knowledge about current psychiatric treatment guidelines (Kessler et al., 2012). Even those who are accurately diagnosed with anxiety disorders in primary care settings have gaps in the continuum of care they receive as evidenced by poor adherence to medication, inadequate follow-up and monitoring, and rare exposure to effective evidence-based psychotherapies, such as cognitive behavioral therapy (CBT; Beck et al., 1985). Growing evidence indicates the effectiveness of CBT in the treatment of postpartum depression (PPD). Similarly, a recent randomized controlled study of postmenopausal women who met criteria for poor quality sleep demonstrated improved sleep scores and quality of sleep among those who participated in internet-based CBT. Researchers concluded this was an effective and cost-efficient approach to manage sleep disturbances during postmenopause (Abdelaziz et al., 2021).

SELF-MANAGEMENT MEASURES

Patients can benefit from various self-management measures including stress management, relaxation techniques, sleep hygiene, yoga, meditation, digital self-help, face-to-face videoconferencing, mindfulness, and deep-breathing exercises to aid in their management of anxiety.

COMPLEMENTARY AND ALTERNATIVE MEDICINE

Referral to a mental health clinician is imperative and provides a patient with access to various psychotherapeutic interventions such as CBT. CBT is an empirically based, time-limited psychotherapy approach that has demonstrated effectiveness in the treatment of vast psychiatric disorders and SUDs, including depression and anxiety disorders. This structured approach centers on the interface among thoughts (cognitions), emotions (feelings), and behaviors. The success of this approach is often enhanced by a holistic and interdisciplinary approach that involves the nurse psychotherapist, patient, and primary care provider. Through various structured activities, such as homework assignments, the patient actively develops adaptive problem-solving and coping behaviors. Homework assignments can help challenge anxiety-provoking thoughts and feelings and substitute these for realistic and positive thoughts and adaptive coping behaviors. Typically, there are weekly sessions for 6 to 12 weeks, although longer treatment demonstrates greater improvement.

PHARMACOTHERAPEUTICS

Because of the biological nature of anxiety and mood disorders, some patients may not benefit from the sole treatment of CBT and require pharmacologic interventions depending on the severity and debilitation associated with their illness. Specific agents used in various types of anxiety disorders are delineated in the following sections.

Considerations for Special Populations

PREGNANCY AND ANXIETY DISORDERS

Anxiety disorders and presenting with an anxiety disorder during pregnancy can have deleterious effects on both the pregnant person and the fetus. Evidence implicates pregnancy as one of the most stressful and emotional periods in a person's life. Biological factors associated with increased estrogen and progesterone levels, coupled with psychosocial stress and anxiety about personal health and health of the developing fetus and associated lifestyle risks, increase the possibility of anxiety, mood disorders, and exacerbating pre-existing psychiatric conditions.

Early screening for anxiety disorders during pregnancy and the postpartum period are critical to identifying persons at risk and initiating appropriate interventions to reduce harm to the pregnant person and child (Bandelow et al., 2022). The aim of treatment during pregnancy and the postpartum period is to employ interventions to minimize toxic exposure to the pregnant person and the child. The high co-occurrence of major depression with GAD and panic attacks warrants concern and further evaluation. Left untreated, anxiety disorders increase the risk of harm to the developing child including preterm birth, low birth weight, and attention deficits (Bandelow et al., 2022). The high incidence of anxiety disorders during pregnancy and potential long-term effects on the pregnant person, infant, and family make it critical to discuss holistic and empirically based treatment options. Empirically based treatment options include antidepressants, CBT, and relaxation techniques (Bandelow et al., 2022

Panic Disorder

ETIOLOGY

PD, one of the most debilitating and costly anxiety disorders, is associated with high co-occurrence with depression, physical symptom burden, functional impairment, suicide risk, and increased use of healthcare services. Women are twice as likely as men to present with PD with or without agoraphobia. Symptoms occur suddenly "out of the blue," are repeated with no warning, and can result in alcohol or substance abuse, depression, and social and occupational impairment (APA, 2013). Women are more likely than men to present with multiple somatic complaints.

EVALUATION/ASSESSMENT AND SYMPTOMS

PD is separate from agoraphobia and is a distinct anxiety disorder (APA, 2013). Clinical features of PD generate substantial distress and fearfulness, which are often mistaken for medical conditions, such as "having a heart attack" or fears of "going crazy," mainly because of autonomic arousal and heightened anxiety level. Patients with PD often present in EDs complaining of chest pain, dizziness, heart palpitations, diaphoresis, and intense anxiety. Agoraphobia refers to anxiety about being in open places or situations in which escape is embarrassing or difficult (e.g., standing in line or crowds or traveling over a bridge). Anxiety-provoking situations are usually avoided or tolerated. In the latter situation, patients experience intense anxiety and distress or choose to be accompanied by a friend or family member. First symptoms of PD are rare during childhood. Symptoms usually occur during adolescence or early adulthood and often follow a chronic and remitting course (APA, 2013).

Normally panic attacks emerge rapidly, within minutes, and can occur from a calm state or an anxious state. They typically reach a peak within 10 minutes of increasingly worse intensity, and generate feelings of doom and gloom. Normal duration is 20 to 30 minutes, and rarely 1 hour. Attacks tend to occur two to three times a week. Clinicians must inquire if the panic attack was expected (generated by a stressful situation) or unexpected. Unexpected panic attacks are classic symptoms of PD. A question about the focus on anxiety or fear is equally significant in distinguishing PD from other anxiety disorders. A lack of focus is also common in PD. Mental status examination during the attack reveals difficulty speaking, memory deficits, and stammering. Loss of control and sense of helplessness often generate depression during the attack. Symptoms abate quickly or gradually with a sense of exasperation. During a panic attack at least four of the following symptoms occur:

- Palpitations, pounding heart, or accelerated heart rate
- Sweating
- Trembling or shaking
- Sensations of shortness of breath or smothering
- Feelings of choking
- Chest pain or discomfort
- Nausea or abdominal distress
- Feeling dizzy, unsteady, lightheaded, or faint
- Chills or heat sensations
- Paresthesias
- Derealization (feelings of unreality) or depersonalization (being detached from oneself)
- Fear of losing control or "going crazy"
- Fear of dying (APA, 2013)

Culture-specific symptoms (e.g., tinnitus, neck soreness, headache, uncontrollable screaming or crying) may be seen but should not count as one of the four required symptoms.

DIFFERENTIAL DIAGNOSIS

The first concern is to rule out potentially life-threatening medical illness such as a heart attack or endocrine disorders (e.g., hyperthyroidism) or drug/alcohol intoxication or withdrawal. Diagnosis of PD using *DSM-5* criteria (APA, 2013) can be complicated because of physical symptoms that are manifested and obscure co-occurring psychiatric disorders. It should be determined whether some other anxiety disorder might be the cause of the panic attacks; if they are associated with a specific type of situation, disorders to consider are social anxiety disorder, a specific phobia, obsessive-compulsive disorder, PTSD, and separation anxiety disorder.

In PD, it is likely that at least one of the attacks has been followed by (1) persistent concern about additional panic attacks or their consequences and/or (2) a maladaptive change in behavior related to the attacks, such as behavior designed to avoid them (APA, 2013).

TREATMENT/MANAGEMENT

Clinical findings from the physical examination are critical in treating PD along with reassuring the patient that they are not dying or "going crazy." Presenting data from the physical examinations, such as a normal EKG and standard diagnostic laboratory studies, provides objective data concerning the symptoms.

Once a definitive diagnosis of PD is confirmed, treatment options are discussed to develop a plan of care that considers gender-specific factors, preferences, co-occurring psychiatric and medical conditions, and cultural considerations. In general, two approaches to treatment are available: pharmacotherapy and psychotherapy. Effective treatment outcomes are associated with combined therapies.

Complementary and Alternative Medicine

Persons with PD should be referred to a qualified mental health clinician for psychotherapy, such as CBT, to address distorted cognitions that generate anxiety. Relaxation and deep-breathing exercises are also useful in controlling the physiologic response to anxiety-provoking situations.

Pharmacotherapeutics

Primary care clinicians may prescribe pharmacotherapeutics to manage the biological basis of anxiety disorders in collaboration with a mental health clinician who provides psychotherapy.

Acute Management

Benzodiazepines offer rapid, limited relief for acute panic attacks by reducing the frequency and intensity of an attack (Sadock et al., 2019). Benzodiazepines are contraindicated in persons with a history of SUD and must be used cautiously during pregnancy. Although benzodiazepines were the mainstay treatment of anxiety disorders and have been extensively studied, concerns about potential for dependence, cognitive impairment, and abuse, particularly with long-term use, challenge clinicians to use these medications sparingly and carefully monitor for signs of dependence. Alprazolam, a common high-potency benzodiazepine used to treat PD, has been linked to a discontinuation syndrome after regular dosing of only 6 to 8 weeks' duration. Slowly tapering these agents, particularly after chronic use, reduces discontinuation syndrome. Suggestions for tapering depend on the patient, duration of treatment, and medication potency and half-life. For instance, alprazolam must be decreased by 0.5 mg/week; faster tapering increases the risk of seizures and

delirium (Sadock et al., 2019). Agents with a long half-life (e.g., clonazepam) have a propensity to cause impaired daytime sleepiness or "hangover," but they require less frequent dosing and may be more useful in acute and maintenance treatment. Shorter half-life agents (e.g., alprazolam) carry a higher risk of withdrawal and rebound between doses and require frequent dosing. Apart from the potential for dependence and abuse, additional side effects are few such as sedation, fatigue, and confusion. Side effects are usually managed with dose adjustment. As confusion and disorientation are especially common in older adults, these agents should be used cautiously in this age group.

Some patients find it comforting to carry a dose or two with them in the event they have an attack. The association and conditioning of ending the attack with a benzodiazepine is often helpful in allaying anxiety. It also offers control over an anxiety-related situation and their physiologic responses, and thus empowers them to self-manage their condition.

Antidepressants: Maintenance Treatment

Antidepressants have demonstrated efficacy in the treatment of panic attacks and mitigating anticipatory and avoidance behaviors, which are core symptoms of PD. They are also effective for treating coexisting major depression. SSRIs (Table 40.1) are generally well tolerated and should be considered first-line treatment for PD (Bandelow et al., 2022; Garakani et al., 2020; Sadock et al., 2019). Therapeutic effects have been observed in 1 to 2 weeks. Initially, these agents may increase anxiety. SSRIs must not be taken within 14 days of other antidepressant agents, such as monoamine oxidase inhibitors (MAOIs) and *Hypericum perforatum* (St. John's wort), because of serious drug interactions. Careful patient education about desired and adverse effects along with the time required to reduce anxiety is imperative.

In addition to SSRIs, selective norepinephrine reuptake inhibitors (SNRIs) and dual-acting antidepressants, such as venlafaxine (regular or extended release), should also be considered for maintenance treatment. Venlafaxine is a potent inhibitor of both serotonin and norepinephrine and a weak inhibitor of dopamine. These medications are safe, well tolerated, and effective for preventing relapse in outpatients with PD and in treating major depression (Bandelow et al., 2022; Garakani et al., 2020). SSRIs have proven efficacy in treating women with PD and/or co-occurring major depressive illness (Bandelow et al., 2022; Garakani et al., 2020).

Starting doses of antidepressants should be low and gradually titrated up until efficacy is achieved (Table 40.2). The starting dose of medications used to treat PD is usually one-half the starting dose used to treat depression. Age-related changes and medical conditions should also be considered when deciding the initial dose. Normally, 4 to 6 weeks are necessary to achieve a therapeutic response and patients should continue taking the medication for at least 12 months (Bandelow et al., 2022; Sadock et al., 2019). Follow-up and close monitoring are important to evaluate for response, side effects, and suicide risk and any needed medication adjustment.

SSRIs and SNRIs cannot be discontinued abruptly as this may precipitate a withdrawal syndrome. The syndrome is primarily associated with paroxetine and SSRIs with short

TABLE 40.1 Common Major Side Effects Associated With SSRIs

SYSTEM	POTENTIAL EFFECTS
CNS	• Headaches (most common), activation of mania or hypomania, hyperkinesia, aggressive reactions • Insomnia • Anxiety, nervousness, dizziness • Fatigue, sedation • Fine tremor • Akathisia (primarily with fluoxetine) • Nocturnal bruxism • Concentration disturbances, lightheadedness
GI	• Nausea (most common), vomiting • Diarrhea (especially sertraline; normally abates after 10–14 days, reduced by food) • Weight gain
Cardiovascular	• Palpitations • Hot flashes
Endocrine/metabolic	• Induced syndrome of inappropriate secretion of antidiuretic hormone (SIADH) • Elevated prolactin levels
Genitourinary	• Sexual dysfunction • Decreased libido • Orgasmic disturbances
Respiratory	• Rhinitis • Cough • URI
Musculoskeletal	• Asthenia • Myalgia
Miscellaneous	• Fever • Fatigue • Taste disturbances

CNS, central nervous system; GI, gastrointestinal; SSRIs, selective serotonin reuptake inhibitors; URI, upper respiratory infection.
Source: Adapted from American Psychiatric Association. (2013). Diagnostic and statistical manual of mental disorders (5th ed.). https://doi.org/10.1176/appi.books.9780890425596; Gelenberg, A. J., Freeman, M. P., Markowitz, J. C., Rosenbaum, J. F., Thase, M. E., Trivedi, M. H., & Van Rhoads, R. S. (2010). Practice guideline for the treatment of patients with major depressive disorder (3rd ed.). American Psychiatric Association; Bandelow, B., Werner, A. M., Kopps, I., Rudolf, S., Wiltink, J., & Beutel, M. E. (2022). The German Guidelines for the treatment of anxiety disorders: First revision. European Archives of Psychiatry and Clinical Neuroscience, 272(4), 571–582. https://doi.org/10.1007/s00406-021-01324-1; Sadock, M. S., Ahmad, S., & Sadock, V. A. (2019). Kaplan and Sadock's pocket handbook of clinical psychiatry (6th ed.). Wolters Kluwer.

TABLE 40.2 Suggested Dosing for Antidepressants Used to Treat Panic Disorder

ANTIDEPRESSANT	STARTING DOSE PER DAY	MAINTENANCE DOSE PER DAY
Fluoxetine	5–10 mg	20 mg
Paroxetine	5–10 mg	20–40 mg
Paroxetine CR	12.5 mg	25 mg
Citalopram	10 mg	20–40 mg
Escitalopram	5 mg	10–20 mg
Sertraline	12.5–25 mg	50–200 mg
Nefazodone	100–200 mg BID	300–600 mg
Bupropion-SR- IR XR	150 mg 100 mg BID 150 mg	450 mg 300 mg (divided 150 mg) 450 mg
Venlafaxine	37.5 mg	75 mg once daily
Desvenlafaxine	50 mg	50–400 mg
Duloxetine	40–60 mg	60 mg
Levomilnacipran	40 mg	Up to 120 mg
Vortioxetine	10 mg	20 mg
Vilazodone	10 mg	20–40 mg
Mirtazapine	15 mg	15–45 mg

BID, twice a day.
Source: Adapted from American Psychiatric Association. (2013). Diagnostic and statistical manual of mental disorders (5th ed.). https://doi.org/10.1176/appi.books.9780890425596; Gelenberg, A. J., Freeman, M. P., Markowitz, J. C., Rosenbaum, J. F., Thase, M. E., Trivedi, M. H., & Van Rhoads, R. S. (2010). Practice guideline for the treatment of patients with major depressive disorder (3rd ed.). American Psychiatric Association; Bandelow, B., Werner, A. M., Kopps, I., Rudolf, S., Wiltink, J., & Beutel, M. E. (2022). The German Guidelines for the treatment of anxiety disorders: First revision. European Archives of Psychiatry and Clinical Neuroscience, 272(4), 571–582. https://doi.org/10.1007/s00406-021-01324-1; Sadock, M. S., Ahmad, S., & Sadock, V. A. (2019). Kaplan and Sadock's pocket handbook of clinical psychiatry (6th ed.). Wolters Kluwer.

Adrenergic Receptor Antagonists (Alpha-Adrenergic Blockers)

The off-label use of adrenergic receptor antagonists for anxiety disorders continues to be explored. Initial findings from agents used to treat acute and chronic symptoms of stress-related anxiety support the efficacy of these agents in reducing physiologic aspects of anxiety, sleep disturbances, nightmares, and memory consolidation, particularly with PTSD (Hoskins et al., 2021). These results were inconsistent in some veteran populations. A 26-week randomized controlled study of veterans with chronic PTSD demonstrated a poor response to prazosin. Researchers attributed a lack of improvement to selection bias of veterans with stable PTSD symptoms (Raskin et al., 2018).

Propranolol and other beta blockers suppress acute biological symptoms of panic attacks such as racing heart, palpitations, and sweating. Major side effects associated with these

half-lives; patients must be warned not to stop the medication abruptly. Hallmark features of this syndrome include dizziness, especially with head motion, dry mouth, rebound anxiety, sleep disturbances, headaches, and cognitive disturbances. It is time-limited and symptoms abate spontaneously in 3 weeks. This syndrome is associated with daily dosing of at least 6 weeks (Sadock et al., 2019). When discontinued, it should be gradually tapered over a 2- to 3-week period (Sadock et al., 2019). Long-acting SSRIs, such as fluoxetine, are less likely to precipitate this syndrome.

agents include reduced blood pressure, bradycardia, drowsiness, and depression. They should be avoided in patients with a history of asthma or congestive heart failure.

CONSIDERATIONS FOR SPECIAL POPULATIONS

Benzodiazepines should not be prescribed during pregnancy as they freely cross the placenta, accumulate in fetal circulation, and have teratogenic properties (e.g., cleft palate). They are present in breast milk at sufficient levels to produce adverse effects in the newborn. The precise effects on the newborn continue to be researched; however, they are metabolized slowly in the newborn and can accumulate.

Generalized Anxiety Disorder

SCOPE AND ETIOLOGY

GAD is among the most common psychiatric conditions, affecting 8% to 10% of the general population, and is more prevalent in women than in men (APA, 2013). The 12-month prevalence of GAD varies from 2% to 9% and even higher in primary care settings (Kessler et al., 2012). An estimated 8% of all primary care visits are patients with GAD of whom a large percentage experience co-occurring major depression (Kessler et al., 2008; Ruscio et al., 2017). Comparable findings were noted in a cross-sectional comparison of the epidemiology of GAD across the globe. Prevalence varied extensively across countries and the lifetime prevalence of GAD was 3.7%; 12-month prevalence of 1.8% with higher incidence in high- income countries (5.0%) and lower incidence in low-income countries (1.6%) (Ruscio et al., 2017). Similar to other anxiety disorders, GAD usually begins in childhood and continues throughout adulthood. It is highly heritable and often coexists with other anxiety and mood disorders. Major depression is the most common co-occurring psychiatric condition in women with GAD (Bandelow et al., 2022; Kessler et al., 2005; Ruscio et al., 2017). PD has been found in 25% of those with GAD because of overlapping symptoms (Kessler et al., 2005). Twin studies suggest a shared genetic vulnerability to anxiety disorders, including GAD and major depression (Bandelow et al., 2022; Showraki et al., 2020).

EVALUATION/ASSESSMENT

Persons with GAD typically complain of excessive worrying about everyday life, muscle tension, headaches, and exaggerated attentiveness. Clinically, they exhibit free-floating anxiety, unfocused anxiety, and are overly anxious. Cognitive vigilance often manifests as irritability and agitation. Similar to other anxiety disorders, symptoms are chronic, disabling, and involve extensive healthcare utilization, particularly in primary care settings. Chief complaints are usually somatic: headaches, GI disturbances, and sleep disturbances (APA, 2013; Bandelow et al., 2022).

DIFFERENTIAL DIAGNOSIS

Differential diagnosis is based on findings from physical and psychiatric evaluation, including the mental status examination and diagnostic physical exam workup. Because of the high prevalence of co-occurrence, depression, other anxiety disorders, and SUDs must be ruled out. The *DSM-5* criteria include all of the following major symptoms of GAD (APA, 2013):

- Excessive worrying that occurs more days than not for at least 6 months, major focus on everyday issues, such as children, work, and home
- Difficulty controlling the worry
- Anxiety associated with three of more of the following:
  ○ Restlessness, on edge, keyed up
  ○ Irritability
  ○ Easily fatigued
  ○ Difficulty concentrating
  ○ Muscle tension
  ○ Sleep disturbances—difficulty falling or staying asleep or nonrestorative sleep
- Does not meet criteria for other anxiety disorders
- Symptoms significantly interfere with usual activities
- Symptoms are not associated with an underlying medical condition or substance induced

TREATMENT/MANAGEMENT

Early diagnosis, appropriate treatment, collaboration with mental health clinicians, and adherence to treatment offer hope to patients suffering from GAD. In the case of coexisting major depression, treatment involves antidepressants and anxiolytic agents such as buspirone. When there is evidence of active or past alcohol use disorder or other SUDs, patients must be referred for evaluation and treatment for SUDs and subsequently treated for GAD and co-occurring psychiatric disorders.

Pharmacotherapeutics

SSRIs and novel antidepressant medications (e.g., venlafaxine, venlafaxine CR, mirtazapine, and buspirone) have demonstrated efficacy in the treatment of GAD (Bandelow et al., 2022; Garakani et al., 2020; Sadock et al., 2019). Treatment considerations for patients presenting with GAD are similar to those used to manage PD. Venlafaxine is also effective in treating comorbid major depression and social anxiety disorder (SAD), formerly known as social phobia. Dosing for venlafaxine or venlafaxine CR is titrated up gradually based on reduction of target symptoms of muscle tension, sleep disturbances, restlessness, agitation, and concentration disturbances (Garakani et al., 2020; Sadock et al., 2019). Side effects associated with venlafaxine are similar to the central nervous system (CNS), GI, and sexual side effects caused by SSRIs. Excessive diaphoresis and elevated blood pressure may also occur.

Buspirone has anxiolytic and mild serotonergic properties and has proven efficacy in the treatment of GAD and concomitant major depression (Bandelow et al., 2022). Its low potential for tolerance, abuse, or dependency makes it an excellent option for those in which tolerance and addiction are concerns (Sadock et al., 2019). Buspirone also produces minimal cognitive deficits and can be used in those with a history of substance-related disorders. Major disadvantages include the length of time to produce anxiolytic effects (i.e., 2–4 weeks) and the need for regular use to reduce anxiety (versus as needed use with benzodiazepines). Common side effects associated with buspirone include headaches, dizziness, lightheadedness, nervousness, and GI disturbances. Because this agent affects dopamine receptors, there is a risk of extrapyramidal side effects, especially when combined with antipsychotic agents. Hypomania and mania have been observed, primarily in older adults who do not meet criteria for bipolar disorder. Safety in pregnancy or lactation is not established (Bandelow et al., 2022)

Social Anxiety Disorder

DEFINITION, SCOPE, AND ETIOLOGY

The lifetime prevalence of SAD is about 12.1% (Kessler et al., 2005; Ruscio et al., 2008). Social phobia is an anxiety disorder characterized by extreme fear and phobic avoidance of social and performance situations and associated with reduced quality of life (APA, 2013). It may be associated with PD and GAD. More than 50% of people with SAD have coexisting major depression (Kessler et al., 2005; Ruscio et al., 2008). This potentially disabling anxiety disorder occurs more frequently in women than in men, particularly among adolescents, and appears to diminish throughout the life span. Fears in women tend to be more generalized about social concerns compared to men.

EVALUATION/ASSESSMENT AND SYMPTOMS

In general, persons with SAD express fear and sensitivity to criticism from others associated with social or performance situations, such as public speaking, resulting in distress and functional impairment (APA, 2013). People with SAD tend to experience and avoid social situations in which they feel inept or judged harshly.

DIFFERENTIAL DIAGNOSIS

Co-occurring psychiatric conditions, such as PD, GAD, major depression, and SUDs may make it difficult to distinguish symptoms from SAD. A comprehensive physical and psychiatric evaluation is needed to rule out underlying medical conditions. *DSM-5* criteria for SAD are as follows (APA, 2013):

- there is a persistent and exaggerated fear of social situations in which the person is exposed to possible scrutiny by others.
- Exposure to feared social situations evokes intense anxiety.
- The person recognizes the fear is unreasonable or excessive.
- The person avoids the feared social situations or endures them with significant distress and anxiety.
- Avoidance of social situations interferes significantly with the person's social, occupational, academic, and interpersonal relationships.
- Symptoms persist for at least 6 months.
- Symptoms are not related to underlying general medical conditions or SUDs.

TREATMENT/MANAGEMENT

Treating patients with anxiety and co-occurring major depression and other psychiatric disorders challenges clinicians in all practice settings to conduct a comprehensive psychiatric and physical examination to determine an accurate diagnosis and treatment. Collaboration with a mental health clinician is necessary to further evaluate and determine overall mental health needs, including suicide risk. Integrated treatment models include pharmacologicl and psychotherapeutic interventions.

Pharmacotherapeutics

SSRIs, SNRIs, and other novel antidepressants are effective in managing SAD or social phobia. Mirtazapine is effective in treating SAD because it enhances serotonergic function distinct from reuptake inhibition by disinhibiting the norepinephrine activation, thus ultimately increasing serotonergic transmission (Bandelow et al., 2022; Sadock et al., 2019). These properties allow mirtazapine to allay anxiety and sleep disturbances and increase appetite. It is also a potent histamine-1 (H_1) receptor blocker.

Major side effects associated with mirtazapine include somnolence, dry mouth, weight gain, and constipation. It may also increase liver enzyme levels and produce reversible blood dyscrasias (e.g., agranulocytosis) requiring a CBC with differential at baseline and for monitoring. Because of this side effect, this medication is not used during pregnancy or lactation.

Obsessive-Compulsive Disorder

DEFINITION, SCOPE, AND ETIOLOGY

The prevalence of obsessive-compulsive disorder (OCD) is approximately 1.6% (APA, 2013; Zuberi et al., 2021). Although the treatment of this complex anxiety disorder should occur in mental health settings, it is important for the primary care clinician to recognize its prevalence and major symptoms in order to make a provisional diagnosis and refer. OCD affects women and men equally and is highly heritable. Depression commonly coexists with OCD and heightens the risk of poor outcomes, suicide, and substance abuse. OCD tends to have a sudden onset following a stressful event, such as a pregnancy, sexual assault, or significant loss.

EVALUATION/ASSESSMENT AND DIFFERENTIAL DIAGNOSIS

Characteristically, the patient recognizes that their behaviors are unreasonable, but they have difficulty controlling impulses or ritualistic behaviors to allay anxiety generated by obsessions. Patients with OCD often seek treatment for physical problems and, because of embarrassment and secrecy about irrational behaviors and thoughts, they seldom mention them during encounters with primary care clinicians. Diagnosis is seldom made until 5 or 10 years after onset, making it difficult to treat this chronic condition. Questions about ritualistic or compulsive behaviors must be asked. *DSM-5* clinical features of OCD include obsession(s), compulsion(s), or both (APA, 2013):

- *Obsessions*—Recurrent persistent thoughts, impulses, or images that produce anxiety and distress
- *Compulsions*—Repetitive behaviors or mental acts performed in response to obsessions

And each of the following (APA, 2013):

- The person recognizes that the compulsions or obsessions are unreasonable.

- Obsessions or compulsions disrupt the person's normal activities, cause significant distress, or take a great deal of time.
- Compulsions or obsessions exceed the focus of any other Axis I disorder the person may have.
- Symptoms cannot arise from an underlying medical condition or be induced by substances.

TREATMENT/MANAGEMENT

Major challenges for primary care clinicians are the patient's reluctance to adhere to medications and resistance to accepting a referral to a mental health clinician for psychotherapy to address underlying issues associated with OCD symptoms and behaviors (Del Casale et al., 2019). Collaboration with a mental health clinician is imperative.

Pharmacotherapeutics

Antidepressants used to treat other anxiety conditions extend to OCD. The first-line approach is to start with an SSRI or clomipramine, a tricyclic antidepressant. Clomipramine is the first drug approved by the Food and Drug Administration (FDA) for treatment of OCD. Studies indicate that using combination exposure therapy and clomipramine may be superior to monotherapy with clomipramine (Del Casale et al., 2019). Improvement is seen in 2 to 4 weeks and symptoms may continue to abate over 4 to 5 months. Primary side effects of clomipramine include dry mouth, sedation, seizures, significant weight gain, and cardiac arrhythmias. Before prescribing clomipramine, routine screening for seizures and cardiovascular disease is necessary because of its cardiotoxic properties and seizure risk (Del Casale et al., 2019; Sadock et al., 2019).

Fluvoxamine, an SSRI, is also approved for OCD (Del Casale et al., 2019). The side effect profile is the same as that for other SSRIs (Table 40.1) except it has numerous drug–drug interactions. Higher doses need to be divided for twice daily dosing (Sadock et al., 2019).

Posttraumatic Stress Disorder

SCOPE, ETIOLOGY, AND RISK FACTORS

PTSD affects about 7.7 million American adults; however, it can occur at any age (APA, 2013). Women are twice as likely to develop PTSD as men because of the increased life-span likelihood of being a survivor of violence (APA, 2013; Kessler et al., 2017). Women are 4.9 times as likely to experience violence before the age of 25 years as men and are more likely to report co-occurring major depression and anxiety disorder (Kessler et al., 2017). The growing number of women deployed during the Iraq, Afghanistan, and other wars exposes them to additional stressors (e.g., military sexual trauma [MST]) and the risk of PTSD. Although PTSD is not an inevitable consequence of trauma exposure, 10% of women who experience trauma develop this psychiatric disorder (APA, 2013). Women diagnosed with PTSD usually have experienced or witnessed an overwhelming, life-threatening traumatic event that generates fear, anxiety, horror, disbelief, and self-blame (Chung & Breslau, 2008). Trauma exposure is most likely to occur among survivors of rape, childhood trauma, military warfare and confinement, physical assault, IPV, or threats of harm (APA, 2013).

EVALUATION/ASSESSMENT

The *DSM-5* (APA, 2013) definition of PTSD has undergone considerable changes. Primary changes include the removal of emotional reactions to trauma exposure as part of Criterion A. Manifestations of PTSD symptoms vary among individuals. Depending on the nature of the trauma and when it occurred (acute vs. chronic symptoms), it is imperative to accept and believe the woman's perception of the event, avoid pressing for details to avoid retraumatization, express genuine concern, and use a nonjudgmental approach. Support and safety are principal interventions following acute trauma exposure. Inquire about recent stressors and be mindful of the difficulty the patient may have in sharing the experience. Fears of not being believed or understood are common barriers to sharing a painful emotional experience. Clinicians must be able to distinguish normal stress reactions from PTSD. Health education about normal stress reactions is critical to "normalizing" the patient's feelings, thoughts, and behaviors.

Most persons with PTSD present immediately following the attack for injury evaluation or later with somatic complaints such as fatigue and sleep problems. They may express difficulty going out at night because of concerns about personal safety. Their mental status examination may reveal hypervigilance and that they are easily startled; however, findings are individual and depend on the acuteness and nature of the event and availability of quality support. Based on their mental status examination, it is vitally important to evaluate and understand the nature of their distress and precipitating stressors.

A person with a history of trauma-related anxiety, such as MST and/or rape trauma syndrome, may appear calm or distraught or in a "state of shock" (e.g., dissociation) and have difficulty believing what happened to them and/or providing details about the event. They must have time to respond to questions. For persons presenting later with somatic symptoms, asking about a history of trauma may be the first indication they suffered an unresolved traumatic event.

Routine screening for IPV or other trauma exposure events, especially in women of childbearing age and other minoritized gender persons, is recommended by some professional organizations. Clinicians must be cognizant of state laws governing how to report IPV and work with local agencies to ensure patient and family safety.

DIFFERENTIAL DIAGNOSIS

A comprehensive psychiatric evaluation, physical examination, and diagnostic studies provide the basis for determining what to consider in the differential diagnosis. *DSM-5* criteria for PTSD include all of the following (APA, 2013):

- Exposure to an overwhelming traumatic or stressful event that threatens life/personal integrity or causes intense fear, horror, or helplessness
- The traumatic event is persistently reexperienced in one or more of the following:
  - Nightmares or distressing dreams of the event
  - Autonomic arousal when exposed to trauma reenactment
  - Intrusive repeated reliving the event; flashbacks, intense emotional distress when exposed to trauma reenactment

○ Physical or psychological distress to cues/reminders of the event
- Persistent avoidance of the stimuli linked to the traumatic event (not present before the event) as evidenced by three or more of the following related to the trauma:
  ○ Inability to remember important aspects of the event
  ○ Avoiding people, places, and objects
  ○ Inability to recall important aspects of the trauma
  ○ Feelings of detachment or distance from others
  ○ Reduced interest in activities
  ○ Avoiding thoughts and reminders of the event
  ○ Foreshortened perspective of own future, no self-view for future
- Persistent symptoms of arousal such as:
  ○ Decreased sleep
  ○ Increased anger outbursts, agitation
  ○ Hyperarousal
  ○ Hypervigilance
  ○ Exaggerated startled response
- Duration of symptoms lasts more than 4 weeks
- Causes marked distress or impairment in functional abilities

TREATMENT/MANAGEMENT

Treatment considerations for PTSD must be individualized and target underlying symptoms and behaviors. Patients must be offered referral to a mental health clinician and encouraged to participate in psychotherapeutic approaches, including CBT and relaxation techniques, trauma-focused therapies, eye movement desensitization and reprocessing (EMDR), and/or meditation, and maintain continuity with their clinicians.

Complementary and Alternative Medicine

Trauma-related symptoms can be ameliorated using several interventions: supportive counseling; CBT, or other therapies from a mental health clinician; education about normal stress reactions; learning and using simple stress-reduction exercises, such as deep breathing, sleep hygiene, and muscle relaxation; and participation in support groups to normalize reactions and receive ongoing support.

Pharmacotherapeutics

First-line treatment of PTSD is with SSRIs and novel antidepressants (Stein et al., 2013). Maintenance treatment of PTSD with SSRIs improves the psychiatric and clinical outcome of patients with the disorder and prevents relapse and symptom exacerbation (Garakani et al., 2020; Hoskins et al., 2021).

Adrenergic-antagonist agents, such as prazosin, reveal promising results in the treatment of physiologic and hyperarousal features of PTSD (Hoskins et al., 2021) and in preventing presynaptic norepinephrine receptors and reducing cortisol-mediated memories. They may also prevent consolidation of traumatic memories and fear conditioning 2 to 3 months post-trauma (Hoskins et al., 2021). Emerging evidence further indicates the efficacy of novel medications such as glutamate N-methyl-D-aspartate (NMDA) receptor antagonists (e.g., ketamine, cannabinoids) and CRH receptor antagonists in the treatment of PTSD (Garakani et al., 2020). Esketamine (FDA approved) has a rapid onset when dosed intravenously or as a nasal spray and is used following trauma for treatment-resistant depression (TRD) and PTSD. It is thought to dampen the expression (intensity) of fear. Major side effects of esketamine include GI disturbances, dissociation, dizziness, and lightheadedness that are more likely to occur in women than men (Jones et al., 2020). Results of preliminary findings are inconsistent and longitudinal and larger studies are needhed (Garakani et al., 2020). Medications used in the treatment of PTSD are largely determined by co-occurring psychiatric disorders, SUDs, and medical conditions and personal preferences.

CONSIDERATIONS FOR SPECIAL POPULATIONS

Exposure to trauma in pregnancy poses a unique danger to mother and child and is associated with a disproportionately high rate of PTSD. IPV remains a leading cause of death and is the second most common injury-related death during pregnancy (Centers for Disease Control and Prevention [CDC], 2019; Wallace et al., 2020). Assaults during pregnancy generally occur in the abdomen and to the unborn child. High-risk factors associated with IPV and murder during pregnancy are being younger than age 20 years and receiving late or no prenatal care. Consequences of IPV during pregnancy include risk of depression, suicide, and substance-related disorders (CDC, 2019; Wallace et al., 2020).

A history of violence is common before the pregnancy and frequency increases during pregnancy. It is imperative to inquire or assess for IPV at all primary care visits. Besides pregnancy, women of childbearing age are at the greatest risk of trauma exposure, accounting for a lifetime range of 10.4% to 13.8% (CDC, 2019).

MOOD DISORDERS ACROSS THE LIFE SPAN

Similar to the prevalence seen in most anxiety disorders, women are at a substantially higher risk for developing mood disorders than men. Some women may be more emotionally and physically sensitive during reproductive cycles and thus more vulnerable to mood disorders. Reasons for this disparity are poorly understood; however, fluctuating changes in female hormone levels across the life span may have a direct or indirect influence on mood. Clinicians should routinely screen women for mood disorders and collaborate with mental health clinicians to implement evidence-based treatment when appropriate to promote optimal functioning, reduce suicide risk, and improve quality of life.

Major Depressive Disorder

SCOPE AND ETIOLOGY

Lifetime prevalence of major depression in women (21.3%) is twice as common as in men (12.7%; Kessler et al., 2005). This ratio has been documented worldwide and among diverse ethnic groups. One possible explanation is mood changes that correlate with reproductive and cyclic hormonal changes. Although cyclic hormonal changes are more noticeable during the childbearing years, they also occur during peri- and postmenopause (Wu et al., 2020).

It is interesting to note that despite the high prevalence of mood and anxiety disorders in women, until a decade ago or so, the inclusion of women of reproductive ages was limited or prohibited during early clinical trials. Although most epidemiologic studies include a preponderance of women, there is a lack of consistent data that distinguish gender-related interactions. Gender differences may play a vital role in the clinical manifestations of depression, namely, its course, chronicity, and co-occurring psychiatric disorders (APA, 2013). Recent data indicate these earlier assertions were inconsistently found in women. However, treatment considerations that include psychopharmacology and psychotherapeutic approaches must be person-centered and based on the patient's needs, informed decision-making, developmental stage, and presenting symptoms.

EVALUATION/ASSESSMENT

A comprehensive medical and psychiatric examination is necessary to differentiate major depression from medical and other psychiatric conditions. Queries and evaluation of mood changes that parallel hormonal changes, such as menstruation, pregnancy, postpartum, and peri- and postmenopause, provide invaluable data concerning treatment and management.

DIFFERENTIAL DIAGNOSIS

Of particular importance is ruling out conditions such as hypothyroidism and certain cancers, such as pancreatic, that may manifest as depression, to ensure an accurate diagnosis and appropriate treatment. Co-occurring anxiety disorders complicate treatment and are associated with poor treatment outcomes and chronicity. *DSM-5* diagnostic criteria for major depression include persistent symptoms for at least 2 weeks, a change from prior functioning, *either* a depressed mood *or* loss of interest in things that were once pleasurable, *and* five of the following (APA, 2013):

- Depressed or sad mood
- Substantial loss of interest in things once considered important and pleasurable, or anhedonia
- Significant appetite and weight disturbances—increased appetite results in weight gain and the reverse occurs with poor appetite
- Sleep disturbances—difficulty staying asleep, waking up feeling tired, or increased sleep
- Fatigue
- Cognitive disturbances—difficulty concentrating, forgetfulness
- Feelings of worthlessness or excessive guilt
- Psychomotor agitation or retardation
- Thoughts of death or suicide

TREATMENT/MANAGEMENT

Pharmacologic interventions are first-line treatment for women who present in primary care settings with unipolar and bipolar major depression. Each disorder requires pharmacologic treatment unique to their symptoms and co-occurring psychiatric, substance use, anxiety, and/or personality disorders. Referral for CBT, mindfulness, and other psychotherapeutic interventions is also needed. CBT has proven efficacy as

sole or adjunct treatment to medication depending on severity of biological symptoms (e.g., psychomotor retardation, sleep disruption, and cognitive/concentration disturbances). Biological aspects of psychiatric symptoms must be stabilized prior to initiating psychotherapeutic interventions.

Complementary and Alternative Medicine

Regular exercise, yoga, meditation, and stress management activities are also useful in coping with depression. Over-the-counter herbal preparations are available (e.g., St. John's wort, SAMe), but most have side effects that interfere with the efficacy or safety of prescribed antidepressants. Queries about herbal preparations must be a part of the initial history and physical exam and include health teachings about serious and potentially fatal interactions, such as St. John's wort and SSRIs (e.g., serotonin syndrome).

Pharmacotherapeutics

Gender differences in responsivity and tolerability to SSRIs and tricyclic antidepressant medications have been identified. Researchers have identified that women are more likely to have a greater response to SSRIs and tricyclic antidepressants than men; this may be because of gender-related neurobiological differences (e.g., estrogen; Wu et al., 2020).

Premenstrual Dysphoric Disorder

SCOPE AND ETIOLOGY

PMDD is a distinct mood disorder that affects 3% to 8% of women of childbearing age (APA, 2013; Rapkin & Lewis, 2013). Mood disturbances emerge during the luteal phase of the menstrual cycle and cease shortly after the beginning of menses. Principal differences between major depressive episode and PMDD are its cyclic symptomatology and functional impairment. Although the precise cause of PMDD continues to be questioned, converging evidence links PMDD to a cyclic response to estrogen and progesterone and a heightened awareness of physical sensations and internal changes during this period (Casper & Yonkers, 2019). Increased incidence of subsequent depression during pregnancy, the postpartum period, and perimenopause also parallel PMDD with dysregulation of neuroendocrine processes including cortisol and hormonal levels and GABAergic and serotonergic neurocircuitry (Casper & Yonkers, 2019)).

EVALUATION/ASSESSMENT

Similar to other atypical depressive episodes, women with PMDD complain of a depressed mood, tension, anxiety, agitation, increased appetite, and sleep and concentration disturbances during the luteal phase of their menstrual cycle—core symptoms of PMDD. Headaches, muscle pain, bloating, and fatigue are also common.

DIFFERENTIAL DIAGNOSIS

A definite diagnosis can be made when at least five core major depressive symptoms occur a week before menses and diminish several days after menses that produce global functional impairment similar to major depression for at least two cycles (APA, 2013).

TREATMENT/MANAGEMENT

Early treatment initiation offers relief for women suffering from PMDD and reduces the risk of future depressive episodes during pregnancy, postpartum, and perimenopause.

Pharmacotherapeutics

Increasingly, SSRIs have become the mainstay treatment of PMDD and may be used during the luteal phase or limited to duration of symptoms. SNRIs and clomipramine also have proven efficacy in the treatment of PMDD (Casper & Yonkers, 2019).

Symptoms of PMDD respond to SSRIs when treatment is limited to 14 days of the menstrual cycle. Women with more severe PMDD may respond better to luteal-phase dosing than symptom-onset dosing (Casper & Yonkers, 2019). Although antidepressants are an integral part of treatment, mounting evidence indicates that a holistic approach, including dietary considerations, complementary therapies, CBTs, and exercise, may reduce symptoms and improve quality of life for women with PMDD.

Bipolar Disorders I and II

SCOPE AND ETIOLOGY

Bipolar disorder affects 0.5% to 1.5% of individuals in the United States (APA, 2013). Typically, the onset of bipolar disorders in females occurs during adolescence and the early 20s, placing them at greater risk of episodes during reproductive years (APA, 2013). The initial episode is more likely to be depressive in women compared with manic in men. Women are also more likely than men to have the rapid-cycling form of the illness and to display depressive characteristics (APA, 2013). Bipolar disorder presents special challenges to women of reproductive age as well as to their families and clinicians. Problems include lower fertility rates, strong genetic loading, and potential fetal teratogenic risks, as well as high risks of illness recurrence if treatment is discontinued abruptly (Sharma et al., 2020). Bipolar disorders are highly prevalent with other psychiatric disorders such as SUDs and personality disorders.

EVALUATION/ASSESSMENT

When evaluating women with major depressive symptoms, it is imperative to inquire about a past history of increased energy, decreased need for sleep, increased irritability, and engaging in pleasurable activities with a high risk of negative outcomes. This is important because an affirmative answer (Antai-Otong, 2009) may indicate either a manic or hypomanic episode that may or may not have been treated. Additional questions to elicit symptoms and to differentiate from major depression are listed in the following section as well as a comprehensive psychiatric and medical evaluation. Equally important is preconception counseling with women of reproductive age at least 3 months prior to a planned pregnancy who are currently being treated for bipolar disorders. Major components of the counseling include history of birth control, current stressors, and decision-making regarding whether to continue or discontinue medications during pregnancy (Barker et al., 2020).

DIFFERENTIAL DIAGNOSIS

This discussion is limited to manic and depressive episodes because of the difficulty in differentiating among rapid cycling, mixed type, and hypomania bipolar disorders. Women exhibiting bipolar disorder symptoms should be referred to a mental health clinician for diagnosis. *DSM-5* diagnostic criteria for major depression are noted earlier. *DSM-5* diagnostic criteria for manic and hypomanic episodes include each of the following, respectively (APA, 2013):

- Distinct period of abnormally and persistently elevated, expansive, or irritable mood, lasting at least 4 or more days for hypomanic and 1 week or more for manic
- Type I: At least one manic episode
- Type II: At least one hypomanic episode

Manic Episode Criteria

- During the period of mood disturbances *three or more* of the following occur:
- Overblown self-esteem
- Reduced need for sleep
- Racing thoughts
- Talkativeness; circumstantial, tangential, and pressured speech
- Increased involvement with pleasurable activities, especially that can cause harm (e.g., shopping sprees)
- Heightened goal-directed activity or agitation
- Easily distracted by unimportant external stimuli

Hypomanic Episode Criteria

- During the period of mood disturbances, *three or more* of the symptoms listed with a manic episode occur and are:
  - Less severe than manic episode
  - Observable by others
  - Normally not severe enough to cause marked impairment in social or occupational performance or necessitate hospitalization
- Mood disturbance significant enough to impair usual function, risk of violence to self and others, or psychotic characteristics
- Symptoms are severe enough to cause marked global impairment or necessitate hospitalization to prevent harm to self or others or there are psychotic features
- Symptoms are not caused by other medical illness or substances

TREATMENT/MANAGEMENT

Bipolar disorders are serious, chronic disorders that require referral for management by an interdisciplinary mental health team. High suicide risk is common in bipolar disorders and requires close follow-up. Results of a literature review of bipolar disorder and completed suicide (spanning the period 1970–2017) indicated that suicidal behaviors ranged from 4% to 19%, and 20% to 60% attempted suicide at least once in their lifetime (Plans et al., 2019). Individuals with bipolar II had the highest rate of completed suicide (Plans et al., 2019). They also concluded that major risk factors for suicide included early onset of illness, family history of suicide, previous attempts, and co-occurring psychiatric and medical conditions. Lithium was found to be the only medication with antisuicide properties. Treatment adherence is difficult with this disorder, making it difficult to reduce morbidity and mortality.

Pharmacotherapeutics

MANIC EPISODE

Management of bipolar disorder is determined by the clinical presentation. A manic episode may present a psychiatric emergency requiring immediate pharmacologic intervention. Early recognition and referral to psychiatric emergency services is critical to the safety of both the patient and the staff. Depending on the severity and nature of symptoms, first-line treatment of acute mania is aripiprazole and quetiapine in combination with lorazepam. These agents are administered intramuscularly (IM) to quickly manage agitation, delusions, hallucinations, paranoia, and intense anxiety. Haloperidol and lorazepam IM are considered second-line medications (Yatham et al., 2018). Inpatient psychiatric hospitalization or psychiatric ED admission is indicated to stabilize symptoms, ensure safety, and evaluate response to treatment and initiate atypical antipsychotics (e.g., lamotrigine, quetiapine) and mood stabilizers (e.g., lithium, valproate acid; Bai et al., 2020; Yatham et al., 2018). Typically, mood stabilizers and lithium require 10 to 14 days to reach therapeutic serum levels. Because of serious side effects unique to each agent, specifically teratogenic side effects, baseline laboratory studies, including a pregnancy test, are vital to ensure safe treatment for women.

BIPOLAR DEPRESSION (DEPRESSED EPISODE)

Bipolar depression is often misdiagnosed as unipolar depression and treated with monotherapy antidepressants. The distinction between unipolar depression and bipolar depression is that the former is synonymous to major depression without a history of manic or hypomanic episodes. Initial symptoms of bipolar depression manifest as switching to a manic episode with monotherapy antidepressants and failure to respond to treatment. Quality of life in terms of duration and recurrence is significantly worse in persons who suffer bipolar depression than bipolar-manic episodes. There is a paucity of research available for treatment of bipolar depression. Even more perplexing is a lack of data that monotherapy antidepressants are effective mood stabilizers in the treatment of bipolar depression. Ongoing controversy indicates that these agents need to be avoided to reduce the risk of mood-switching. First-line considerations must include conventional mood stabilizers, such as lithium and valproic acid, and newer agents, including lamotrigine, and atypical antipsychotics. Atypical antipsychotic agents continue to demonstrate efficacy in treating both bipolar-manic and depressive episodes (Bai et al., 2020; Yatham et al., 2018).

CONSIDERATIONS FOR SPECIAL POPULATIONS
Bipolar Disorder and Pregnancy

Management of bipolar illness in pregnancy is most difficult when the pregnancy is unplanned. Women with bipolar disorder are at high risk of symptom exacerbation during the immediate postpartum period and a recurrent episode after delivery (Sharma et al., 2020). Among women with bipolar disorder who decide to discontinue therapy during the postpartum period, the estimated risk of relapse is substantially higher than for nonpregnant, nonpuerperal women. Relapse occurs rapidly with acute symptoms emerging a few weeks after delivery (Sharma et al., 2020).

General guidelines for the treatment of bipolar disorder from the APA (2013) were discussed earlier; however, serious concerns arise when these guidelines are applied in the treatment of pregnant and postpartum women (APA, 2013). The decision to treat depression during pregnancy has to be guided by considerations of risks associated with untreated depression along with potential adverse effects on fetal exposure to specific medications. Taking antidepressants during pregnancy has risks and benefits. While several antidepressants, such as SSRIs (e.g., citalopram/escitalopram, fluoxetine, and sertraline) and SNRIs (e.g., duloxetine, venlafaxine) are unlikely to produce birth defects; paroxetine, another SSRI, is linked to fetal cardiac anomalies and should be avoided during pregnancy. No antidepressants are approved for use during pregnancy and all psychotropic medications cross the placenta and enter fetal circulation. Clinicians must carefully review all sources regarding medication side effects and adverse drug reactions in pregnant women, including the FDA category labeling, to determine risks and benefits of taking mood stabilizers, lithium, and other antimanic agents during pregnancy. Careful education of pregnant women and their significant others is needed.(Sharma et al., 2020).

Pregnancy and Mood Disorder

Despite the notion that pregnancy is a positive experience, many women experience tremendous stress and mood changes during this stage of life. Many are fearful of caring for a newborn and coping with the transition into parenting. Pregnancy, similar to other reproductive events, actually heightens the risk of emotional stress, risk of mental health problems, and new onset or relapse of depression (Yu et al., 2021). Depression in pregnant women is estimated to be 4% to 20% and higher in high-risk pregnancies (Yu et al., 2021). Women who have a history of depression during the nonpregnant period are at risk of relapse during pregnancy, even those currently euthymic (Yatham et al., 2018). Hormonal changes, significant stressors, and discontinuation of antidepressant medications increase the risk of depression during pregnancy. Other risk factors include past history of major depression, inadequate social support, discontinuation or reduction of antidepressant medication, marital/relationship discord, and uncertainty about pregnancy (Yu et al., 2021).

Pharmacotherapeutics During Pregnancy

Antidepressant medication should be considered during pregnancy if depressive symptoms are moderate to severe, or if withdrawal of maintenance medication is likely to result in recurrent depression. The potential benefits of using antidepressant medications in a pregnant or breastfeeding woman should be balanced against the potential risks to the newborn. Because of the risk of neonatal withdrawal syndrome, SSRIs should be used at the lowest effective dose during the third trimester of pregnancy and should be tapered before delivery (Yatham et al., 2018).

The primary goal of mental health treatment during pregnancy is full remission of depression to mitigate risk to the pregnant person and child during this period and the postpartum period. Early screening in those who are planning to get pregnant and those who are pregnant must be a priority to address the needs of both asymptomatic and symptomatic women to educate them about treatment options, including risk-benefits, and managing their illness during and after pregnancy.

Pharmacologic considerations for those with mood disorders during pregnancy necessitate an assessment and discussion with the patient and significant others about the risks and benefits of treatment for both the pregnant person and child. Although there is growing consensus among researchers concerning the risk:benefit of antidepressant use during pregnancy in those with severe depression, others caution the overstated analysis of data implicating the safety of antidepressants during gestation (Yatham et al., 2018). Risks associated with pharmacologic treatment should be compared with the risks of not treating depression, which may include poor parent–infant bonding, infanticide, lifelong social and developmental delays and adjustment problems, suicide, poor maternal and fetal nutrition, adverse neonatal obstetric outcomes, and the continuation of depression into the postpartum period (Yatham et al., 2018). As discussed earlier, poor medication management of psychiatric disorders during pregnancy and the postpartum period can have tragic consequences. Prevailing data indicate that most SSRIs are not major teratogens, except paroxetine (e.g., cardiac defects); the ultimate treatment decision lies with the pregnant person, partner/spouse, and/or significant others. Before prescribing these agents, the risk of harm to the developing fetus versus benefits to the pregnant person must be resolved case by case and requires careful discussion with the patient and her partner/spouse as part of the informed-consent process.

Agitation is a common cofeature of depression or mania and SUDs, which manifests as abnormal and excessive verbal or physical aggression, intense anxiety and arousal, restlessness and agitation, and marked negative effects on global functioning. Data from several studies indicated that benzodiazepines and haloperidol are the most commonly used drugs for acute agitation during psychiatric emergencies. Although, data failed to demonstrate efficacy in the long-term management of agitation and combativeness specifically during pregnancy. The advent of atypical antipsychotics with or without benzodiazepines are comparable with haloperidol and benzodiazepines and have a safer profile (Yatham et al., 2018). In the absence of evidence-based practice guidelines and demonstrated effective or safe treatment of agitation in women, primary care clinicians must learn and employ verbal deescalation and other means of security to manage potentially volatile situations with these patients.

Postpartum Depression

SCOPE AND ETIOLOGY

The incidence of PPD is relatively common and similar to rates of major depressive disorder in nonpregnant women, affecting 13.2% of women within 6 months of delivery (Bauman et al., 2020). Moreover, 50% to 80% will experience the "blues" lasting 4 to 10 days (Bauman et al., 2020.). Risks associated with PPD include a prior history of major depression or PPD; current stressors, such as transitioning into parenthood; and socioeconomic issues. Untreated PPD can have acute and long-term deleterious effects on the overall social, physiologic, and psychological well-being of the mother, newborn, and the entire family (Bauman et al., 2020).

RISK FACTORS

Risk factors for PPD include (Bauman et al., 2020

- Family or personal history of mood disorders (including PPD)
- Severe PMDD
- Psychosocial stressors, such as marital discord, financial problems, and so forth
- Limited or poor social support
- Mood instability during adolescence that caused severe distress
- Emotional reactivity to oral contraceptives leading to discontinuation
- Sadness, irritability, and mood disturbances during pregnancy
- Feelings of inadequacy as parent
- Sleep, appetite, and concentration disturbances

SYMPTOMS

Women with PPD often complain of fatigue, unexplained crying spells, irritability, sleep disturbances, anger, feelings of loss, and mild mood swings. Despite the high prevalence of PPD, many are unrecognized and untreated (Bauman et al., 2020; Yu et al., 2021). Normally, PPD is experienced after the first 2 weeks postpartum; for some it occurs sooner (Bauman et al., 2020). Symptoms usually begin during the third trimester. The incidence of PPD varies among cultures and ethnicities. Women with strong and quality social support and help with child care, meal preparation, feeding, and bathing tend to have a lower incidence of PPD (Bauman et al., 2020; Yu et al., 2021).

EVALUATION/ASSESSMENT

Symptoms and evaluation of PPD are similar to those for major depression. Postpartum "blues" are characterized by fluctuating mood, crying spells, irritability, anxiety, and sleep and appetite disturbances several weeks after delivery. Persistent symptoms that worsen during this period must be evaluated to distinguish a frank mood disorder from "postpartum blues." The Edinburgh Postnatal Depression Scale, a 10-item questionnaire, is a useful screening tool (Cox et al., 1987) for the early postpartum period. Women with PPD complain of mood, appetite, concentration, and sleep disturbances. Sleep problems involve difficulty sleeping even when the infant is asleep. A large number of women with PPD experience distressful and obsessional thoughts about harming their infants—although they are rarely acted on in the presence of nonpsychotic depression. Severe PPD concomitant with suicidal ideations heightens the risk of infanticide—not because of hatred of the infant, rather because of fears of abandonment with suicide (Yu et al., 2021). A history of PPD is associated with high prevalence and recurrence with subsequent pregnancies. Queries about previous PPD are critical for prevention, identification, and management of this highly recurrent condition (Bauman et al., 2020).

DIFFERENTIAL DIAGNOSIS

A comprehensive physical and psychiatric evaluation helps distinguish PPD from other mood disorders, including postpartum blues and postpartum psychosis (see the following section). When symptoms of postpartum blues persist more than several weeks, evaluation for PPD is needed. PPD is diagnosed when symptoms of major depression emerge within 4 weeks of delivery using *DSM-5* criteria, which includes each of the following (APA, 2013):

- Either depressed mood or lack of interest or pleasure plus at least four additional symptoms, including:
  - Marked weight loss
  - Activity disruptions—overactive or slowed actions
  - Frequent sense of worthlessness or unwarranted guilt
  - Sleep disturbances
  - Concentration disturbances, indecisiveness
  - Daily fatigue or lack of energy
  - Suicidal ideations, thoughts of death
- Symptoms are not consistent with mixed depression.
- Symptoms cause significant disruption in function and/or distress.
- Symptoms are not caused by other medical illness or substances.
- Symptoms are not caused by bereavement.

TREATMENT/MANAGEMENT

Early screening of PPD and prompt initiation of pharmacologic interventions are critical to symptom management to mitigate short- and long-term adverse consequences including functional deficits and newborn neglect that may negatively influence both parent–child bonding and the infant's mental and physical development (Yatham et al., 2018).

Complementary and Alternative Medicine

Health education and reassurance coupled with assuring home support for infant and self-care are usually adequate interventions for postpartum blues. These interventions are geared toward decreasing the likelihood of full-blown PPD, improving infant safety, and optimizing health for parent–infant bonding.

Pharmacotherapeutics

Most research indicates the safety of using several antidepressants during lactation or postpartum period. Fluoxetine, sertraline, paroxetine, and tricyclic antidepressants have been studied the most extensively (Sprague et al., 2020). When choosing an antidepressant or mood stabilizers, clinicians must consider the patient's previous response to medication, evidence-based data on efficacy, monotherapy, and flexible dosing.

First-line treatment for nonpsychotic PPD is based on the underlying psychiatric diagnosis. Unipolar PPD should be treated the same as any major depressive episode. Mainstay treatment for bipolar PPD should be the same as for bipolar I

and II depression, and follow what was used for the most recent episode (see previous section on bipolar disorders I and II).

Postpartum Psychosis

DEFINITION AND SCOPE

Postpartum psychosis is a rare disorder that is considered a psychiatric emergency. Care for women with postpartum psychosis extends beyond the scope of primary care clinicians. The role for clinicians in general obstetric, gynecologic, and primary care is accurate recognition of the major symptoms and prompt referral to psychiatric emergency services for evaluation and treatment. Psychosis is the most severe of the PPD symptoms.

SYMPTOMS

Psychosis can occur 2 to 3 days postpartum; most often symptoms appear within the first 2 weeks postpartum (APA, 2013). Psychosis may present as part of a continuum of major depression, bipolar disorder, or recurrent illness mood disorder. Delusions, hallucinations, depressed or elated mood, cognitive disturbances, and disorganized behavior and agitation are core symptoms of PPD with psychotic features.

TREATMENT/MANAGEMENT

Postpartum psychosis is considered a psychiatric emergency. It is often treated by using the same approach as with bipolar-manic psychosis (i.e., atypical antipsychotic medications, antimanic agents) and requires acute inpatient hospitalization. Untreated postpartum psychosis can have tragic consequences, including infanticide and suicide. Postpartum psychosis is recurrent and substantially worsens the risk of acting on homicidal thoughts toward the infant. When suspected, postpartum psychosis must be quickly evaluated and treated to reduce these potential outcomes.

Depression in Peri- and Postmenopause

ETIOLOGY

Although the role of estrogen deficiency and hormonal variance has been associated with depression during the transition to postmenopause, it remains unclear if there is an increased vulnerability to depression during this developmental stage. Findings from several community and clinic-based studies indicate that perimenopausal women reported more depressive complaints than either premenopausal or postmenopausal women, implicating biological changes during this transitional stage as a risk for depression (Wu et al., 2020). Vasomotor symptoms, vaginal dryness, decreased libido, night sweats, and irritability, especially severe symptoms, frequently cause insomnia and depression in women around menopause. Left unresolved or inadequately treated, these symptoms often diminish functional status, quality of life, and overall health, and become the basis for seeking medical attention.

EVALUATION/ASSESSMENT

Apart from routine diagnostic studies and physical and mental status evaluations, a history of symptoms and chief complaints guide the primary care provider in distinguishing symptoms unique to peri- and postmenopausal depression. A thorough history of mood changes during reproductive events across the life span must also be integrated in the diagnostic process.

DIFFERENTIAL DIAGNOSIS

Other diagnoses to consider in peri- and postmenopausal women who exhibit signs of depression are the same as for major depression (see previous discussion).

TREATMENT/MANAGEMENT

Mounting data support that monotherapy with SSRIs and SNRIs mitigate depressive symptoms, reduce baseline vasomotor symptoms, and improve quality of sleep, functional status, and quality of life in perimenopausal women (Wu et al., 2020). These agents are well tolerated and have a relatively safe side effect profile. The precise mechanisms of their actions are unknown, although vasomotor symptoms are linked to dysregulation of serotonin and norepinephrine and abrupt reduction in estrogen production (Wu et al., 2020). When prescribing short-term use of SSRIs and SNRIs to treat vasomotor symptoms, it is practical to start with a low dose (e.g., 10–20 mg escitalopram; 50–100 mg desvenlafaxine) and titrate based on response. When using for major depression, it is imperative to follow the APA (Gelenberg et al., 2010) practice guidelines on the Treatment of Patients with Major Depression to determine if continuation and maintenance treatment (e.g., 6–12 months) are indicated. Treatment must be periodically reassessed as vasomotor symptoms, a potential precursor to depression, are often time-limited and often subside over time (see Chapter 34, Menopause).

PSYCHOTIC DISORDERS

Schizophrenia

ETIOLOGY AND RISK FACTORS

Schizophrenia has genetic, neuroanatomic, neuroendocrine, and environmental underpinnings. Multiple factors are characteristic as the disorder has many subtypes with varying symptoms (APA, 2013; Keepers et al., 2020). Typical symptoms of schizophrenia encompass cognitive, emotional, psychosocial, and behavioral deficits. Collectively, these symptoms result in a lack of insight about the importance of treatment to manage symptoms. The prevalence of schizophrenia in women and men is similar; however, women are more likely to have mood symptoms than men. As mentioned, under normal and healthy circumstances, pregnancy is a very stressful experience. It is particularly stressful and often overwhelming to women with coexisting psychiatric conditions, such as depression, bipolar disorder, and schizophrenia.

EVALUATION/ASSESSMENT

Pesons with schizophrenia present with hallucinations, delusions, agitation, and disorganized thoughts and behaviors. A comprehensive physical and psychiatric evaluation is needed to determine the underlying etiology.

DIFFERENTIAL DIAGNOSIS

Acute psychosis must be differentiated from medical and other psychiatric conditions, substance intoxication, and withdrawal.

TREATMENT/MANAGEMENT

Acute psychosis is a psychiatric emergency requiring an immediate referral to the ED or psychiatric triage unit. Acute exacerbation of psychosis has been previously discussed and includes management of hallucinations, delusions, agitation, disorganized thinking, and risk of danger to self or others. Mainstay treatment for acute management involves administration of atypical antipsychotic agents IM such as aripiprazole or quetiapine as first-line medications, second-line medication such as haloperidol, and a benzodiazepine such as lorazepam. Patients are closely monitored for desired effect and side effects to ensure safe and effective symptom management. Explanations must occur before, during, and after medication administration to reduce anxiety and fear and ameliorate psychosis. Because of the complexity of schizophrenia, the importance of medications and a comprehensive treatment plan that includes psychotherapeutic interventions, and the high co-occurrence of psychiatric disorders, such as depression, SUD, and anxiety disorders, women with schizophrenia are managed by a mental health clinician and interdisciplinary team. Core elements of the interdisciplinary model include integrated symptom management, medication adherence, health education, and fostering hope and empowerment to optimize and attain positive treatment outcomes.

EATING DISORDERS

Eating disorders are severe, debilitating, and chronic conditions associated with co-occurring psychiatric conditions and medical complications. Eating disorders carry the highest mortality rate of all psychiatric disorders, with high suicidality and deaths from physiologic causes (APA, 2013). An estimated 2% to 4% of young adult females meet criteria for an eating disorder (APA, 2013). The peak age at onset is between 16 and 20 years of age, during which time women are leaving home and are faced with enormous psychosocial stressors (Resmark et al., 2019; Ruchkin et al., 2021; van Hoeken & Hoek, 2020). Eating disorders, especially anorexia nervosa, are psychiatric disorders depicted by an excessive fear of weight gain or persistent weight-avoidance behaviors. Collectively, these biological markers are associated with appetite regulatory hormones in women, which are highly heritable and familial. The incidence of eating disorders is similar among women from various cultures and ethnicities (Ruchkin et al., 2021; van Hoeken & Hoek, 2020). Demands for autonomy and social or sexual functioning may contribute to perception of eating, shape, and competence. Thus, other minoritized gender persons are also at increased risk for eating disorders. The two major eating disorders are anorexia nervosa and bulimia nervosa.

Anorexia Nervosa

ETIOLOGY

Anorexia nervosa (AN) is one of the most serious and potentially fatal of the eating disorders (Resmark et al., 2019; van Hoeken & Hoek, 2020). It is characterized by distorted body image and self-imposed nutritional limitations that result in serious malnutrition. Attitudes and behaviors in patients with eating disorders have costly psychological and physiologic consequences. Low self-esteem and confidence, disgust, and shame are common themes for those with eating disorders. AN is classified as restricted type or binge eating/purging type.

EVALUATION/ASSESSMENT

A comprehensive physical and psychiatric evaluation, including appropriate diagnostic studies and vital signs, is performed to make a diagnosis and rule out co-occurring psychiatric and/or medical conditions. This process is complicated by denial of symptoms, lack of insight into the illness, ritualistic behaviors, and resistance to treatment. Clinical findings often include low blood pressure, orthostatic hypotension, hypothermia, dependent edema, dental caries or erosion of enamel, and noticeable weight loss (Resmark et al., 2019; van Hoeken & Hoek, 2020). Patients with eating disorders often have a passion for preparing meals for others, while continuously restricting their own food intake. Binge eating tends to occur in secret, normally at night along with self-induced vomiting. Binge eating is associated with co-occurring SUD and borderline personality disorder. Denial is profound and withstands confrontation from others. Laxative and diuretic abuse and excessive exercising are used to maintain low body weight. Bizarre eating rituals are common such as cutting food into small pieces and spending enormous time rearranging it before eating. Medical attention tends to be sought when severe weight loss becomes obvious. A history of primary amenorrhea, hair loss, dry and brittle hair, fatigue, cold intolerance, bruising, and muscle weakness are common physical findings with eating disorders, especially AN. In suspected cases of eating disorders, queries about purging, diuretic and laxative use, dental integrity, and amenorrhea provide additional data to make a diagnosis (Resmark et al., 2019; van Hoeken & Hoek, 2020).

DIFFERENTIAL DIAGNOSIS

Early recognition and treatment of eating disorders may mitigate morbidity and mortality. *DSM-5* diagnostic criteria for AN (APA, 2013) include each of the following:

- Refusal to maintain body weight at or above minimal body weight for age and height (e.g., body weight less than 85% of that expected); BMI <15 kg/m^2
- Marked fear of gaining weight and becoming obese, although underweight
- Distortion in the way body weight is experienced—self-devaluation, negative self-image
- Amenorrhea—defined as the absence of menses 3 consecutive months (reproductive years)
- Restricted type: No regular purging or binge eating
- Binge eating/purging type: Regular purging or binge eating has occurred during current episode.

DIAGNOSTIC STUDIES

Based on the answers and physical findings concerning eating disorders, additional diagnostic studies may be indicated such as a comprehensive metabolic profile, bone density, and referral for a dental examination.

MANAGEMENT

Referral for psychiatric treatment is needed. Hospitalization is indicated for nutritional and medical stabilization, dehydration, electrolyte imbalance, and cardiovascular abnormalities. Common physical findings in patients with AN who require hospitalization include abnormal vital signs, specifically marked orthostatic hypotension with bradycardia; abnormal EKG; abnormal electrolytes, including hypokalemia; abnormal renal and liver function tests; inability to maintain normal body temperature; signs of malnourishment, such as generalized weakness, palpitations, shortness of breath, chest pain, cold extremities, and concentration and GI disturbances. These physiologic disturbances jeopardize health, and in severe cases, result in death. Parameters used to determine choice of treatment include current weight, rate of weight loss, cardiac function, metabolic status, suicidality, degree of denial, and impact on health (Resmark et al., 2019).

Those with a BMI <15 kg/m^2, rapid weight loss, or continuous weight loss >20% over a 6-month period and severe coexisting psychiatric vulnerabilities (e.g., suicide risk, self-injurious behaviors) should be referred for inpatient treatment. Length of inpatient treatment is based on individual responses to medical stabilization, psychiatric treatment, and family support (Resmark et al., 2019). An abundance of research indicates pharmacologic and psychotherapeutic interventions lack efficacy in the long-term treatment of AN, particularly when the woman denies her illness (Resmark et al., 2019; van Hoeken & Hoek, 2020).

Bulimia Nervosa

SCOPE AND ETIOLOGY

Bulimia nervosa (BN) is more prevalent than AN. Characteristics of BN include episodic, uncontrolled, compulsive, and rapid ingestion of large quantities of food within a short duration (binge eating) followed by self-induced vomiting, misuse of laxatives and fasting, and excessive exercise to reduce weight gain (APA, 2013). Similar to AN, the onset is from 16 to 18 years of age and there is a higher male/female ratio of 1:10 (APA, 2013; Ruchkin et al., 2021). Also similar to AN, BN has a chronic and recurring course and is associated with medical complications, such as electrolyte imbalance, dental caries, suicidality, and metabolic acidosis. BN is also more prevalent among other minoritized gender persons.

EVALUATION/ASSESSMENT

As with AN, assessment includes a thorough and comprehensive physical exam and psychiatric evaluation to identify coexisting medical and/or psychiatric conditions. Attitude about weight gain and food often provides the first clue of an eating disorder.

DIFFERENTIAL DIAGNOSIS

Differentiating between eating disorders and other possible medical and/or psychiatric causes is needed. *DSM-5* diagnostic criteria for BN (APA, 2013) include each of the following:

- Recurrent episodes of binge eating, which includes *both* consuming a larger than normal quantity of food in a short period of time *and* feeling no control over eating during the event
- Recurring episodes of inappropriate compensatory behavior to reduce weight gain
- Binge eating and compensatory behaviors to reduce weight gain occur at least two times a week on average for 3 months or more.
- Self-perception and evaluation are excessively affected by body weight and shape.
- The disturbance is not limited to episodes of anorexia nervosa.

TREATMENT/MANAGEMENT

Patients with BN require referral to a psychiatric clinician for management. Hospitalization is limited to medical and psychiatric stabilization, similar to AN. A comprehensive treatment plan to address underlying issues associated with an eating disorder is recommended. Psychotherapeutic interventions include psychotherapy, nutritional rehabilitation and counseling, and health education. Dissimilar to AN, pharmacologic interventions, such as mood stabilizers, antianxiety agents, SNRIs, and antipsychotic drugs, have proven efficacy in the treatment of BN (Svaldi et al., 2019).

SUBSTANCE USE DISORDERS

Scope and Etiology

The co-occurrence between specific mood and anxiety disorders and specific drug use disorders is pervasive in the U.S. population. SUDs are associated with increased morbidity, high risk of HIV or hepatitis infection, incarceration, and poor treatment outcomes. A recent national prospective study of psychiatric disorders and SUDs and risk of adverse outcomes found a higher incidence in women than men (Blanco et al., 2021). However, when data were adjusted for sociodemographics and adverse outcomes, researchers found few gender differences associated with psychiatric disorders and adverse outcomes (Blanco et al., 2021).

The high prevalence of depression in women also increases the incidence of women presenting with coexisting depression and SUD. Research findings (Pinedo et al., 2020) suggest substantial barriers to women with psychiatric disorders and co-occurring SUDs. Major barriers include lack of knowledge concerning how to access healthcare services, child care issues, stigma and shame of having an SUD problem, and a lack of support and encouragement to seek mental health services (Pinedo et al., 2020).

Evaluation/Assessment and Diagnostic Studies

Evaluating psychiatric complaints in patients with coexisting SUDs is challenging as substance use can mimic or complicate diagnosis of psychiatric symptoms. When these disorders occur simultaneously, patients may have difficulty maintaining abstinence, have a higher risk of suicide, and use substantial medical and psychiatric services. Those seeking help in primary care may initially present with physical complaints that require an extensive evaluation. Women metabolize alcohol differently than men. Women are more likely to suffer earlier onset of medical complications associated with alcoholism and other drug use and to acquire sexually transmitted infection (STI). Diagnostic studies provide evidence of these changes, especially disease that is associated with chronic drug use. Inquiring about active and past alcohol and other drug use is critical to identifying SUDs. Observing for signs of intoxication or withdrawal along with ordering drug screens and liver function tests can assist in making a diagnosis.

Differential Diagnosis

Differentiating between organic medical disease and sequelae of alcohol or other substance use is essential for appropriate management of both the medical problems and the substance abuse disorder. *DSM-5* diagnostic criteria for substance-related disorders (APA, 2013) are:

Dependence

- Maladaptive substance use pattern resulting in marked impairment or distress as demonstrated by three of more of the following, occurring during a given 12-month period:
  - Tolerance
  - Withdrawal
  - Larger amounts of substance use than intended
  - Persistent desire or unsuccessful effort to reduce use or control use
  - Increased substance-seeking behaviors
  - Global functional impairment (e.g., social, interpersonal, occupational)
  - continued use despite negative consequences

Abuse

- A maladaptive substance use pattern resulting in significant impairment or distress as demonstrated by one or more of the following, occurring during a given 12-month period:
  - Recurrent use resulting in functional impairment
  - Use when it is physically hazardous such as driving or operating equipment
  - Repeated legal problems because of substance use
  - Continued use despite negative consequences
- Use does not meet criteria for substance dependence.

Management

A referral to a mental health clinician for management of co-occurring psychiatric disorders and SUDs is critical to successful treatment outcomes. A gender-specific approach that addresses the needs of women and other minoritized gender persons is required as they frequently use drugs for different reasons than cisgender men. Gender-specific treatment requires an integration of biological, psychosocial, and spiritual needs that impact individual substance use. It must also focus on the patient's experiences, relationships, and overall health. Patients presenting with SUDs tend to experience guilt, shame, and anxiety about substance use and exhibit low self-esteem and self-worth along with greater depression than their cisgender male counterparts. Treatment approaches must focus on their strengths, uniqueness, and personal needs rather than confrontation, which is highly used with cisgender men with SUDs. In addition, treatment is guided by the specific active or past substance, patterns of abuse, quality of psychosocial support, current psychiatric symptoms, patient preferences and motivation for seeking treatment, and data from the medical and psychiatric evaluation. Health education about dangers of drug use during pregnancy must be an integral part of treatment planning.

Considerations for Special Populations

SUBSTANCE USE DISORDERS AND INCARCERATED WOMEN

Despite the high prevalence of co-occurring diagnosis in incarcerated women, symptoms are often unrecognized and untreated. The care of incarcerated women with co-occurring psychiatric and substance use problems must include a gender-specific approach that includes assessing mood and substance abuse problems; recognizing history of abuse, injury, or childhood trauma, and limited treatment choices; and determining if she has children and who is caring for them (Marotta, 2017; Salem et al., 2020). In addition, it is important to have pharmacologic interventions to treat specific psychiatric disorders, abstinence from substances, and psychotherapeutic interventions, including relational and interpersonal psychotherapy, trauma-focused therapies, peer support, personal safety, parenting classes, and life skills to engage healthy relationships and facilitate transition into the community. Pharmacologic and psychotherapeutic interventions and support of women with psychiatric disorders and SUDs can be effective (Marotta, 2017; Salem et al., 2020).

FUTURE DIRECTIONS

The prevalence of mental health problems among women and other minoritized gender persons challenges primary care clinicians to recognize these problems. These persons have unique presentations and needs and mental health problems often parallel traumas and reproductive transitions and are complicated by hormonal changes. As more and more women and other minoritized gender persons seek psychiatric help in primary care practices, it is imperative for clinicians to recognize the distinct risk factors among these patients associated with psychiatric disorders and initiate individualized treatment and referral to mental health services. More research is needed to address the needs of childbearing women and other minoritized gender persons during menses, pregnancy, and the postpartum period, as well as the unique needs of women and other minoritized gender persons during peri- and postmenopause.

REFERENCES

References for this chapter are online and available at https://connect.springerpub.com/content/book/978-0-8261-6722-4/part/part03/chapter/ch40

CHAPTER 41

Substance Abuse and Women*

ELIZABETH MAYERSON

Chapter Disclaimer. In the following discussion, the terms woman *and* women *are used to describe persons who have a female sex assigned at birth (persons with a cervix), including transgender men with cervix and gender diverse persons who have a cervix. Similarly, the terms* man *and* men *are used to describe persons who have male sex assigned a birth (persons with a penis), including transgender women with a penis and gender diverse persons who have a penis.*

Substance use affects the health of women, their children, and their families, often in profound ways, while also affecting workplace productivity and societal resources. Primary care providers (PCPs) see women more frequently than they do their male counterparts. The 2018 rate for physician office visits by women 15 to 64 years old exceeded that of male counterparts by 56% (Santo & Okeyode, 2018). Despite their more frequent use of primary care, women are approximately 50% less likely to be diagnosed with a substance use or dependence disorder or an alcohol misuse, abuse, or dependence disorder compared to men (Santo & Okeyode, 2018). Current trends also suggest increasing rates of substance use and abuse disorders in women with significant impact related to the COVID-19 pandemic (Brotto et al., 2021; Panchal et al., 2021; Reinert et al., 2021). Anxiety, depression, and loneliness related to the pandemic have had a disproportionately severe impact on women (Brotto et al., 2021). Women with substance use disorders (SUDs) often have symptoms of anxiety and depression and follow up with their PCPs due to these symptoms (Brahmbhatt et al., 2021; Ober et al., 2018).

PCPs are in an important position for engaging at-risk and substance-using women and identifying needs for intervention (John et al., 2021; Ober et al., 2018). Primary care represents a critical area in which tremendous health opportunity can be realized through providers' awareness, empathy, use of open-ended questions, reflective listening, and understanding of the process and the treatment of addictive disorders (Ober et al., 2018). Currently, identification and

treatment of SUDs in primary care are challenging (Brown et al., 2021; John et al., 2021). There is an ongoing shortage of behavioral health and SUD specialists, and many women do not have access to a provider other than their PCP (Brown et al., 2021; Chappell et al., 2021; Ober et al., 2018; Substance Abuse and Mental Health Services Administration [SAMHSA], 2021). Related to the increased need for PCPs to effectively identify and manage SUDs, the integration of treatment for SUDs in primary care along with collocated or integrated behavioral health has been advocated by multiple stakeholders including the National Academy of Medicine and *Healthy People 2030* (Brown et al., 2021; Chappell et al., 2021; Ober et al., 2018; Office of Disease Prevention and Health Promotion [ODPHP], n.d.).

This chapter addresses the scope of the problem of substance use among women and its causative, risk, and protective factors; diagnostic criteria; symptoms; evaluation process and screening for differential diagnoses; use of diagnostic studies; treatment and management, including risk reduction; and future directions. Additional resources, including web-based ones, will be recommended. As the field of substance use and care is evolving rapidly, the focus of this chapter is to provide a foundation for integrating new data and methods of care into practice as they become available.

DEFINITION AND SCOPE

The definition of *substance use* has changed with increasing understanding of how it is experienced as well as how it is caused. The *Diagnostic and Statistical Manual of Mental Disorders* (5th ed.; *DSM-5*; American Psychiatric Association, 2013) no longer includes use of the diagnostic labels' *substance abuse* and *substance dependence*. Instead, SUDs are described as mild, moderate, or severe depending on criteria for severity met by an individual (see Box 41.1 for symptoms

---

*This chapter is a revision of the chapter that appeared in the second edition of this textbook, authored by Susan Caverly, and we thank her for her original contribution.

Box 41.1 Common Substance Use Disorders in the United States

Alcohol Use Disorder (AUD): A diagnosis of AUD requires that certain diagnostic criteria are met, including problems controlling intake of alcohol, continued use of alcohol despite problems resulting from drinking, development of a tolerance, drinking that leads to risky situations, or the development of withdrawal symptoms. *Moderate drinking* is defined as up to one drink per day for women and up to two drinks per day for men; *binge drinking*, five or more alcoholic drinks on the same occasion on at least 1 day in the past 30 days. (Four drinks for women and five drinks for men over a 2-hour period produces blood alcohol concentrations greater than 0.08 g/dL.)

Tobacco Use Disorder: Symptoms of tobacco use disorder include consumption of larger quantities of tobacco over a longer period than intended; unsuccessful efforts to quit or reduce tobacco intake; use of an inordinate amount of time acquiring or using tobacco products; cravings for tobacco; failure to attend to responsibilities because of tobacco use; continued use despite adverse social or interpersonal consequences; forfeiture of social, occupational, or recreational activities in favor of tobacco use; use in hazardous situations; and continued use despite awareness of physical or psychological problems directly attributed to tobacco use.

Cannabis Use Disorder: Symptoms of cannabis use disorder include disruptions in functioning, development of tolerance, cravings for cannabis, and development of withdrawal symptoms, such as inability to sleep, restlessness, nervousness, anger, or depression within a week of ceasing heavy use.

Opioid Use Disorder: Symptoms of opioid use disorders include strong desire for opioids, inability to control or reduce use, continued use despite interference with major obligations or social functioning, use of larger amounts over time, development of tolerance, use of a great deal of time obtaining and using opioids, and withdrawal symptoms occurring after stopping or reducing use, such as negative mood, nausea or vomiting, muscle aches, diarrhea, fever, and insomnia.

Stimulant Use Disorder: Symptoms of this disorder include craving for stimulants, failure to control use when tempted, continued use despite interference with major obligations or social functioning, use of larger amounts over time, development of tolerance, use of a great deal of time obtaining and using stimulants, and withdrawal symptoms occurring after stopping or reducing use, including fatigue, vivid and unpleasant dreams, sleep problems, increased appetite, or irregular problems in controlling movement.

Hallucinogen Use Disorder: Symptoms of hallucinogen use disorder include craving for hallucinogens, failure to control use when attempted, continued use despite interference with major obligations or social functioning, use of larger amounts over time, use in risky situations such as driving, development of tolerance, and use of a great deal of time obtaining and using hallucinogens.

Source: Definitions abstracted from American Psychiatric Association. (2013). Diagnostic and statistical manual of mental disorders: DSM-5 *(5th ed.). American Psychiatric Publishing.*

associated with SUDs). The essential feature of an SUD is a cluster of cognitive, behavioral, and psychological symptoms indicating that the individual continues using the substance despite significant substance-related problems (American Psychiatric Association, 2013, *Substance Use Disorders, Features,* para. 1). SUDs occur when "recurrent use of drugs and/or alcohol causes impairment (clinical or functional), exemplified by health problems, disability, and failure to meet major responsibilities at work, school, or home." (American Psychiatric Association, 2013, *Substance Use Disorders, Features,* para. 4). The *DSM-5* guides the diagnosis of SUD, requiring that it be based on evidence of impaired control, social impairment, risky use, and pharmacologic criteria.

The *National Survey on Drug Use and Health* (NSDUH) reports that in 2020, 40.3 million adults had an SUD in the past year (SAMHSA, 2021). The *NSDUH: Women* reports 34.3 million women had a mental illness and/or SUD in 2019 (SAMHSA, 2020). In 2020, SAMHSA changed their data collection methodology to align with SUD criteria from the *DSM-5.* Due to this change, SAMHSA cautions against comparing data from 2020 to any other year (SAMHSA, 2021). Currently, the most common SUDs in the United States include alcohol use disorder (AUD), tobacco use disorder, cannabis use disorder, opioid use disorder, stimulant use disorder, and hallucinogen use disorder (SAMHSA, 2021). These are described in Box 41.1 and in later sections of this chapter.

INCIDENCE AND PREVALENCE

The use of *DSM-5* criteria for SUD diagnoses helps address stigma associated with an SUD diagnosis. However, this has created challenges when attempting to compare rates of SUD diagnoses over time, as demonstrated by SAMHSA's cautions regarding its 2020 survey data (SAMHSA, 2021).

Although clinicians and women themselves may search for clearer definitions of substance use and SUDs, there are multiple sources of definitions. The use and legality of some substances, such as nicotine, alcohol, and now cannabis, makes defining an SUD even more difficult. For example, identifying SUDs based on cannabis use has become increasingly difficult due to variation in legalization of cannabis and societal acceptance of cannabis use, both medicinal and recreational (Crawford et al., 2021). The *NSDUH* revealed that an estimated 14.2 million people age 12 and older met criteria for a cannabis use disorder in 2020 (SAMHSA, 2021). Substance use statistics are dynamic and complex to interpret. Changing patterns of substance use for one substance may result in changes in the use patterns for others. For instance, in states with legalized recreational cannabis, current data suggest individuals who either smoke or vape tobacco and/or binge drink alcohol are more likely to use cannabis as well (Crawford et al., 2021). Substance use statistical reports may reflect either current use (use within the prior month) and/or past year use. Thus, reporting practices can be confusing. Currently, *DSM-5* criteria are in place, making it somewhat challenging to compare data prior to 2016 in which differentiations between substance abuse and substance dependence were made.

The *NSDUH* revealed that the current use of all illicit substances was lower among women (12.1%) than men (14.9%) for respondents age 12 years and older (SAMHSA, 2021). Among those 12 to 17 years old, only 6.3% of females reported current use of illicit substances compared with 7.1% of males (SAMHSA, 2021). However, the misuse of prescription pain medications was higher for women (1.1%) than men (0.9%) in 2020 for those age 18 years and over (SAMHSA, 2021). Opioid deprescribing has been the standard of care in recent years due to the ongoing opioid epidemic (Centers for Disease Control and Prevention [CDC], 2018). This highlights the importance of recognizing how shifts in prescribing practices influence which substances are likely to be misused over time. The National Center for Health Statistics database shows that although death by overdose has remained lower for women than for men, from May 2020 through May 2021, death by overdose has risen by 21% (Ahmad et al., 2021).

The use and misuse of alcohol have significant impacts upon women. While men have higher rates of alcohol use compared to women, women have disproportionate rates of cardiovascular disease and liver disease related to alcohol use compared to men (National Institute on Drug Abuse [NIDA], 2020a, 2020b). This is in part due to hormonal, size, and body composition differences between men and women. Alcohol use in women is associated with an increased risk of breast cancer, and alcohol misuse in women is associated with increased risks of assault and sexual violence along with increased risk of suicide and motor vehicle accidents (NIDA, 2020a, 2020b). Women age 12 to 20 had higher rates of alcohol use and misuse in 2020 compared to men in the same age cohort (SAMHSA, 2021). Women age 21 and over had higher rates of lifetime alcohol use and past year alcohol use compared to men of the same age in 2020 (SAMHSA, 2021). Pregnant women who misuse alcohol risk fetal alcohol syndrome (FAS) in their babies (NIDA, 2020d).

Tobacco smoking has been reported to still be the greatest single cause of preventable deaths in the United States, and it is estimated that 57.3 million Americans ages 12 and over used tobacco or nicotine vaping in the past month in 2020 (SAMHSA, 2021). According to the Office on Smoking and Health (OSH), women who smoke tobacco have a 12 to 13 times greater risk of death associated with chronic obstructive pulmonary disease (COPD); a significantly greater risk of death related to tracheal, lung, or bronchial cancer; and

for middle-aged women, a greater risk of death resulting from coronary heart disease than women who do not smoke (CDC, n.d.-e). Currently, more women die from lung cancer than breast cancer (CDC, n.d.-e). Use of cigarettes has consistently decreased in the United States since the mid-1960s; however, disparities related to tobacco use remain based on race, level of education, ethnicity, and socioeconomic status (CDC, n.d.-d). For instance, Black Americans tend to smoke fewer cigarettes, start smoking at an older age, and yet are more likely to die due to tobacco-related illnesses compared to White Americans (CDC, n.d.-a). Native American and Native Alaskan peoples have the highest prevalence of cigarette smoking compared to all other racial and ethnic groups in the United States (CDC, n.d.-b). More Native American and Native Alaskan women smoke cigarettes in their third trimester of pregnancy compared to all other racial and ethnic groups in the United States (CDC, n.d.-b). Asian Americans, Native Hawaiians, and Pacific Islander peoples have the lowest prevalence of cigarette smoking compared to other racial groups, but there is ethnic variation within this group. Only 7.6% of Chinese Americans report cigarette smoking (lowest prevalence) compared to 20% of Korean American people (highest prevalence; CDC, n.d.-c). Hispanic and Latin American peoples have a higher prevalence of cigarette smoking compared to Asian Americans, but a lower prevalence compared to all other racial groups in the United States (CDC, n.d.-e). As with Asian Americans, there is ethnic variability in smoking prevalence among Hispanic/Latin Americans with Puerto Rican peoples having the highest prevalence of smoking (28.5%) in this group (CDC, n.d.-f). Additionally, the prevalence of cigarette smoking is higher in people who experience social, racial, and/or employment discrimination, unemployment, poverty, SUDs, mental health disorders, and chronic medical disorders (CDC, n.d.-d). Individuals who identify as LGBTQ+, veterans, homeless persons, and incarcerated individuals experience disproportionately more social disparities, which increases their risk for tobacco use disorders (CDC, n.d.-d).

Pregnant women who smoke face multiple risks. Tobacco impairs fertility in both men and women (CDC, n.d.-e). In addition to the health risks for the pregnant woman, there are risks to the fetus including preterm delivery, low birth weight, ectopic pregnancy, stillbirth, sudden infant death syndrome, and cleft lip and palate (NIDA, 2020d). For pregnant women who experience the social disparities described previously, their risk of tobacco use is increased along with their risk of additional SUDs and mental health disorders (Tsakiridis et al., 2021). Pregnant women ages 15 to 44 had a reported prevalence rate of substance use in 2019 as follows: tobacco 9.6%, alcohol 9.5%, cannabis 5.4%, opioids 0.4%, and cocaine 0.2% (SAMHSA, 2020). Neonatal abstinence syndrome (NAS) is a known risk associated with opioid use during pregnancy (NIDA, 2020d).

Mental health disorders are a risk factor for an SUD, may occur along with an SUD, or may be a symptom of an SUD (Reinert et al., 2021). Co-occurring mental health problems and SUDs are common. In 2019, the *NSDUH: Women* reported 4.6 million women age 18 and over met criteria for an SUD and a mental illness (SAMHSA, 2020). Also in 2019, 34.3 million adult women had a mental illness or SUD, representing a 6.8% increase compared to 2018 data, an increase that was due solely to increases in mental health disorders (SAMHSA, 2020). Severity of mental illness also appears to increase the risk of SUD. In 2020, illicit substance use among adults age 18 and over was highest among those with a severe mental illness (47.8%), followed by those with any mental illness (39.8%) and those without any mental illness (17%; SAMHSA, 2021). Use of cannabis, opioids, binge alcohol, and tobacco/nicotine products followed the same pattern among adults age 18 and over in 2020 with percentages of use highest among those with a severe mental illness (SAMHSA, 2021). Multiple sources report rates of SUD and mental health disorders have increased related to the COVID-19 pandemic (Brotto et al., 2021; Panchal et al., 2021; Reinert et al., 2021; SAMHSA, 2021).

The effects of the pandemic are multiple and far reaching. Most of the population in the United States, as well as around the world, have experienced trauma related to the pandemic, including illness, death of loved ones, isolation due to quarantine, loneliness, and loss of normal activities and routines (Brotto et al., 2021; Panchal et al., 2021). Individuals who experience discrimination due to race, ethnicity, financial status, and/or gender, or individuals in special populations such as veterans, LGBTQ+, homeless persons, and those who are incarcerated are disproportionately affected by COVID-19. These individuals experience poorer outcomes related to COVID-19 infection as well as an increased incidence of substance use and SUDs related to the pandemic (Brotto et al., 2021; NIDA, n.d.; Panchal et al., 2021; Reinert et al., 2021; SAMHSA, 2021). Women have experienced loss of employment and financial hardship at a rate greater than for men due to the pandemic (Brotto et al., 2021). These social determinants have in turn led to increases in SUDs and mental health disorders in women (Reinert et al., 2021; SAMHSA, 2020, 2021).

In addition to co-occurring mental health problems, other factors increase the risk for substance use by women. Trauma or adverse experiences in childhood, such as death of a parent or sibling or a history of child abuse or sexual abuse, increase the risk of SUD and mental health disorders (Gannon et al., 2021; Merrin et al., 2020). A family history of SUD and/or a mental health disorder is also a risk factor for an SUD (Brahmbhatt et al., 2021). In women age 18 or over, divorce, domestic violence, loss of child custody, or involvement with the legal system and/or with child protective services increase the risks of substance use, SUD, and mental health disorders or can exacerbate SUD and mental health disorders for women who have a preexisting diagnosis of an SUD and/or mental health disorder (NIDA, 2020a, 2020b). The risk is amplified for women who have a history as described earlier and are also members of a racial minority group, ethnic minority group, veterans, and/or the LGBTQ+ communities (NIDA, n.d.).

In summary, women who are compromised by factors such as abuse, racial and ethnic discrimination, homelessness, poverty, lack of education, criminal justice involvement, and mental illness or are members of groups such as veterans and LGBTQ+ individuals may be those most at risk for an SUD. Practitioners need to remain mindful of the myriad risk factors for SUDs that occur across patient populations and standardize a model to reduce biased selection into treatment, thereby ensuring that women are given access to respectful screening and/or evaluation for substance use.

ETIOLOGY OF SUBSTANCE USE DISORDERS

Substance use and other addictive disorders are complex biopsychosocial disorders, and the factors related to substance use among women of all ages and ethnicities are multifaceted. Increasingly, the biology of women places those who use substances more at risk for SUD and also more at risk for negative physical and psychiatric effects of substances (NIDA, 2020a, 2020b). This has been linked to the hormonal differences, including the impact of progesterone on certain neuroreceptors, something particularly evident regarding nicotine receptor upregulation (NIDA, 2020b). In addition, smaller body weight and lower fluid volume are thought to contribute to increased risk.

Generally, the areas of the brain that are thought to be most involved with the development and maintenance of SUDs are the ventral tegmental area (VTA), the nucleus accumbens (NAc), and the amygdala (American Psychiatric Association, 2013; Smith et al., 2019). Within these brain areas, multiple neurotransmitter receptor systems, including the gamma-aminobutyric acid (GABA), opioid, dopaminergic, serotonergic, endocannabinoid, nicotinic cholinergic, and N-methyl-D-asparatate (NMDA) glutamate systems, are implicated in SUDs (American Psychiatric Association, 2013; Smith et al., 2019). A pattern of binge/intoxication, withdrawal/negative affect, and preoccupation/anticipation is associated with SUDs and becomes more prominent with increases in the severity of the SUD (American Psychiatric Association, 2013; Smith et al., 2019). Rewarding neurotransmitter activity (dopamine in particular) has been found to increase during the intoxication phase of this cycle and to decrease during the withdrawal phase, whereas stress-related neurotransmitter activity, including dynorphin, corticotropin-releasing factor, and norepinephrine activity, is increased during withdrawal (American Psychiatric Association, 2013; Smith et al., 2019). Substances such as opioids and cannabis act as mimics for transmitters that are endogenous in the brain, whereas other substances, including stimulants, act by triggering the release of excess amounts of neurotransmitters into the neural synapses (American Psychiatric Association, 2013; Smith et al., 2019).

The craving state is associated with other brain regions including the amygdala and the orbitofrontal and prefrontal cortices and can be triggered by either cuing or internal distress. The term *salience* refers to the triggers that elicit increased attention or behavior-associated use of a particular substance (American Psychiatric Association, 2013; Smith et al., 2019). The plasticity of the neural network is affected through a variety of pathways creating changes that may be long lasting. At times this may be referred to as a *state of postacute withdrawal*, a phase during which the impact of salience and the experience of craving continue after sustained abstinence (American Psychiatric Association, 2013; Smith et al., 2019). Individuals may experience a response to salient cuing without full awareness, resulting in confusion as relapse occurs without their knowledge of when they decided to use. This distortion of the decision-making process represents a significant challenge to the maintenance of sobriety.

The nexus of genetics and environment is critical in the development of SUDs. Studies to identify genetic polymorphisms and risk genes for individual substance categories are underway. Specific genetic patterns have been discovered that appear to associate with either alcohol use disorder or nicotine use disorder (Iob et al., 2021). Researchers believe there may be a genetic sequence that is associated with all SUDs, based on observational studies demonstrating individuals who misuse one substance are likely to misuse multiple substances (Iob et al., 2021). A family history of SUDs is a key element of the psychosocial history necessary to adequately evaluate and understand the substance use risk for each individual. A positive family history yields both the potential for genetic predisposition to misuse substances and the increased probability of early exposure to substances, leading to enhanced opportunity for use at a young age. The environmental element may convey a normalization of substance overuse and a reduction in risk perspective related to substance use, thereby increasing the likelihood for early adoption of substance-using behavior. Evidence suggests that the earlier an individual initiates substance use, the greater the chance for developing a use disorder and the greater the risk for negative consequences (Weigard et al., 2020).

Risk Factors

A *risk factor* is defined by the American Psychological Association as, "a clearly defined behavior or constitutional (e.g., genetic) psychological, environmental, or other characteristic that is associated with an increased possibility or likelihood that a disease or disorder will subsequently develop in an individual" (American Psychological Association, 2020b). Conversely, a *protective factor* is defined as "a clearly defined behavior or constitutional (e.g., genetic), psychological, environmental, or other characteristic that is associated with a decreased probability that a particular disease or disorder will develop in an individual, that reduces the severity of an existing pathological condition, or that mitigates the effects of stress generally" (American Psychological Association, 2020a). For example, exercising regularly can serve as a protective factor by decreasing the likelihood or severity of coronary heart disease, hypertension, and depression. Likewise, supportive social networks and positive coping skills are examples of protective factors that reduce the effects of stressful life events and enhance mental health (American Psychological Association, 2020a). Three major types of risk and protective factors are biological, psychological, and social/environmental.

Biological risk factors include age, sex, ethnicity, genetic transmission, family history, personality disorders, and psychiatric disorders. Of these, genetic transmission, family history of disorders, and personal history of psychiatric disorders play a prominent role in the initiation and continuation of substance use (Green et al., 2021).

Psychological risk factors for substance use include personality, belief systems, and coping styles (e.g., sensation seeking and appraisal of substances as having no consequences, minor consequences, or positive benefits). In addition, low self-esteem, lack of resistance skills, prior experimentation, and negative life events such as child abuse, trauma, and deaths of significant others represent significant risk factors (Green et al., 2021). Young women who have experienced sexual assault are at increased risk for substance use (Gannon et al., 2021). The risk of lifetime alcohol dependence increased as a function of the number of lifetime assaults experienced (Gannon et al., 2021). The risk of SUD and mental health disorders has also increased across all ages of women related to the COVID-19 pandemic (Brotto et al., 2021; Panchal et al., 2021).

Social environmental risk factors include parental substance misuse, exposure to poor parenting practices, negative peer bonding, poor interpersonal relationships, lack of social support, negative educational experiences, easy access to substances, the changing of social and gender norms, economic and social incentives for drug trafficking, and exposure to drinking environments (Gannon et al., 2021; Green et al., 2021). A major risk factor for heterosexual women is their relationships with men who use substances (NIDA, 2020a, 2020b), whereas for lesbian women, going to gay bars and clubs is a major influence (NIDA, n.d.). Women who have sex with other women are predicted to have a higher use of injection drugs and a higher prevalence of sexually transmitted diseases and may be at heightened risk for consequences of drinking (NIDA, n.d.).

The initiation of substance use may involve all three types of risk factors: biological, psychological, and social/environmental. An early age of onset is one of the most important predictors of movement from smoking and alcohol use to illegal drug use. Prevalence rates of use and misuse of substances is higher in men than women in most age groups, but current data demonstrate this gap is narrowing (NIDA, 2020a, 2020b; SAMHSA, 2021). According to the *NSDUH*, in 2020 more women than men reported lifetime alcohol use (36.7% vs. 32.7%), past year alcohol use (31.6% vs. 27.9%), past month alcohol use (16.7% vs. 15.6%), and past month binge alcohol use (9.6% vs. 8.8%) in individuals age 12 to 20 years (SAMHSA, 2021). Young teenagers who use tobacco/nicotine products and/or alcohol are more likely to progress to use of additional, illegal substances (SAMHSA, 2021).

Findings suggest that gender differences for both the initiation and the heavy use of substances are associated with different perceptions of life problems and the drugs' effects on the individual. Women are more likely to use alcohol or other substances with the loss of a romantic relationship (Merrin et al., 2020), stress due to work or school obligations (NIDA, 2020a, 2020b), and loss of child custody (NIDA, 2020c) compared to men. The effects of the COVID-19 pandemic have exacerbated feelings of isolation, stress, and loneliness more so in women than men (Brotto et al., 2021; Panchal et al., 2021).

Protective Factors

Protective factors decrease the risk of SUDs by reducing exposure to risk factors, disrupting processes involved in the development of the disorder, and interacting with risk factors to reduce their effects (American Psychological Association, 2020a). Differences in gender roles may be protective factors that prevent women from using substances at the same rates as men. For example, there are social sanctions against women's substance use, and women tend to be more nurturing, less aggressive, and less sensation seeking than men (NIDA, 2020a, 2020b, 2020c).

Events along the life course, such as pregnancy, may be protective factors. In a qualitative study by Frazier et al. (2019), approximately 45% of pregnant women addicted to heroin reported that pregnancy led to cessation of drug use. The women had concerns about the development of their unborn babies and concerns regarding losing custody of their children (Frazer et al., 2019).

Linking Known Risk Factors With Prevention Programs

Outcome studies of prevention programs show reductions in substance use; that is, *prevention works* (Berger et al., 2021; Elms et al., 2018; Galanter, 2018; Martin et al., 2020; Martino et al., 2018; Meyer et al., 2019; Tsakiridis et al., 2021). Changing situational and environmental factors show *how programs work*.

The Institute of Medicine (IOM, 2014) identified three levels of prevention for alcohol, tobacco, and other drugs: universal, selective, and indicated. Universal prevention programs are analogous to universal precautions in healthcare settings; the prevention programs are applied to all members of a population or group without regard to specific risk factors. Universal prevention programs are either *direct*, meaning the programs serve a defined group of participants, or *indirect*, meaning the programs support population-based interventions (IOM, 2014).

Selective prevention programs target groups or populations considered to be at a greater risk for an SUD compared to the general population, for instance, a prevention program tailored to women with a history of domestic partner violence. Prevention programs are designed for the group as a whole, without regard to any specific individuals' risk. It is understood that risk will vary widely within the same group; some members will have no or low risk for an SUD while others may already have a diagnosis of an SUD (IOM, 2014).

Indicated prevention programs are designed to target individuals who are demonstrating behaviors consistent with warning signs of an SUD. For example, it may target a high school student whose grades have suddenly dropped, has become socially isolated, or has started skipping school or missing classes. Similarly, a college student may be referred to an indicated prevention program after episodes of binge alcohol use. The student may already be using substances but does not yet meet *DSM-5* criteria for an SUD. Referrals to indicated prevention programs can be made by family members, healthcare providers, mental healthcare specialists, educators, or the legal system (IOM, 2014).

Diagnostic Criteria

DSM-5 criteria is the gold standard for the diagnosis of SUDs and mental health disorders (American Psychiatric Association, 2013). Use of the diagnostic terms *substance abuse* and *substance dependence* has been eliminated from the *DSM-5*, and the term SUD is now used in place of *substance abuse* and *substance dependence* (American Psychiatric Association, 2013). The terminology change became effective in 2015. However, PCPs should be aware of this history, as retired terminology may still be used in clinical practice. *DSM-5* criteria now include language categorizing SUDs as either mild, moderate, or severe, depending upon the number of criteria that apply to an individual (American Psychiatric Association, 2013). The current diagnostic labels increase the specificity of the diagnosis and may assist in decreasing the stigma associated with an SUD diagnosis; however, stigma still exists (Witte et al., 2021). Use of the current terminology in the *DSM-5* has increased the number of persons with an SUD; this may aid the general public, as well as PCPs, to view SUDs as a serious medical problem, like the way diabetes or hypertension is diagnosed, managed, and treated. Criteria for remission in the *DSM-5* has extended the amount of time required for early remission (from 1 month to 3 months) as well as the amount of time required for sustained remission, which is defined as a substance-free time period of 12 or more months (American Psychiatric Association, 2013).

The *DSM-5* includes the following categories of drugs; alcohol, caffeine, cannabis, phencyclidine (PCP), other hallucinogens, inhalants, opioids, sedatives/hypnotics/anxiolytics, stimulants, tobacco, and other/unknown. There is some variation among the categories. For example, caffeine does not have an associated use disorder but is categorized as caffeine intoxication, caffeine withdrawal, or unspecified caffeine-related disorder. All remaining drug categories have an associated use disorder diagnosis (American Psychiatric Association, 2013). Severity is based upon the number of criteria met: two or three symptoms are diagnostic for a mild SUD; four to five symptoms, a moderate SUD; and six or more symptoms, a severe SUD. Symptoms must be present for at least 12 months (American Psychiatric Association, 2013). There are also SUD courses and features specifiers with corresponding ICD-11 (International Statistical Classification of Diseases and Related Health Problems, 11th rev.; World Health Organization, 2019) diagnosis codes: harmful patterns of use episodic or continuous, substance use dependence continuous episodic, early full remission, sustained partial remission, sustained full remission, and unspecified. The presence of tolerance and/or withdrawal is no longer required for any SUD diagnosis (American Psychiatric Association, 2013). Diagnostic criteria for all SUDs include the following:

A. A problematic pattern of use leading to clinically significant impairment or distress, as manifested by at least two of the following, occurring within a 12-month period:

1. Substance is often taken in larger amounts or over a longer period than intended.
2. There is a persistent desire or unsuccessful efforts to cut down or control use of the substance.
3. A great deal of time is spent in activities necessary to obtain, use, or recover from the effects of the substance.
4. Craving, or a strong desire to use or urge to use the substance.
5. Recurrent substance use resulting in a failure to fulfill major role obligations at work, school, or home.
6. Continued substance use despite having persistent or recurrent social or interpersonal problems caused or exacerbated by the effects of the substance.
7. Important social, occupational, or recreational activities are given up or reduced because of substance use.

8. Recurrent substance use in situations in which it is physically hazardous.
9. Substance use is continued despite knowledge of having a persistent or recurrent physical or psychological problem that is likely to have been caused or exacerbated by the substance.
10. Tolerance, as defined by either of the following:
    a. A need for markedly increased amounts of the substance to achieve intoxication or desired effect.
    b. Markedly diminished effect with continued use of the same amount of the substance.
11. Withdrawal, as manifested by either of the following:
    a. The characteristic withdrawal syndrome for the substance.
    b. The substance, or a closely related substance, is taken to relieve or avoid withdrawal symptoms.

Additionally, degree of remission, maintenance, or environment specifiers are applied (American Psychiatric Association, 2013).

The diagnostic process takes place over time. Although practitioners are pressed to establish a diagnosis after an initial interview, by their very nature these diagnoses are provisional. Moreover, accurate diagnosis is often not possible after a single encounter, especially for individuals for whom substance use is problematic.

Symptoms

The *DSM-5* criteria provide helpful descriptions of symptoms associated with each category of substances (see Box 41.1 for examples). Generally, there is a variety of emotional, behavioral, and physical symptoms and clinical presentations that warrant a more specific assessment for substance use. Impulsivity and uncharacteristic changes in performance of age- and role-appropriate behaviors may be associated with substance use. These include school or work absenteeism or diminished performance in those settings; financial irresponsibility; diminished self-care; frequent, poorly explained accidents or injuries; missed appointments; involvement with agencies such as Child Protective Services or courts; evidence of physical or emotional hyperarousal or hypoarousal; sleep dysregulation; and/or specific evidence of changes such as pupil size and reactivity, or abrupt changes in mental state characterized by emotional lability, cognitive clouding, psychosis or hypervigilance, and/or racing thoughts. Physical problems associated with liver or pancreatic illness, infection, skin erosions or lesions, dental erosion or extensive tooth pain, nasal excoriation, and sexually transmitted diseases warrant careful assessment for a SUD (Smith et al., 2019).

It is not uncommon for individuals engaged in substance use to experience symptoms of anxiety, depression, or a first episode of psychosis, with or without a prior episode of mental health treatment. Often, these individuals fail to respond as anticipated to interventions and historically may have been prescribed a variety of medications that were deemed ineffective or to have had untoward effects. At times the person who has an SUD presents with specific medication requests and compelling reasons why other medications are not acceptable options (Smith et al., 2019).

Women who have SUDs may report significant past or current trauma (possibly presenting with frequent accident-related injuries). They may struggle to bond with their children, and the children may have symptoms of failure to thrive or behavior that is disruptive and unresponsive to parenting recommendations (Martin et al., 2020; Tsakiridis et al., 2021).

EVALUATION AND ASSESSMENT

SUDs among women may go unnoticed for several reasons. Women are reluctant to report use or misuse and are more likely to seek healthcare for a substance-induced health problem rather than seeking treatment for substance abuse per se (Elms et al., 2018; Martin et al., 2020; Meyer et al., 2019; NIDA, 2020a, 2020b). For this reason, at-risk women drinkers are detected only about 10% of the time (Ober et al., 2018). Despite significant increases in substance abuse education over the past several decades, some healthcare providers have reported that they lack the assessment skills needed to work with this population; others have negative attitudes toward persons who misuse substances and hold a belief that individuals do not change substance use behavior; and still other clinicians wish to avoid involvement in situations that may entangle them legally to report incidents such as child abuse (Farhat et al., 2018; Mahmoud et al., 2021). Less than a third of PCPs report carefully screening their young adult patients for SUDs (Blevins et al., 2019). Older women are even less likely to be screened for SUDs by their PCPs, yet older women frequently use opioids on a long-term basis (Barbosa-Leiker et al., 2020).

Whether an artifact of true or perceived time constraints, knowledge or skill deficits, sociologic bias or stigma, and the reality that in years past there were no gender-specific treatments available, healthcare providers do not regularly assess female patients for substance use (Barbosa-Leiker et al., 2020; Mahmoud et al., 2021; NIDA, 2020a, 2020b). Integrating substance use assessment into routine and urgent healthcare encounters requires PCPs to develop the necessary skill set, an understanding of the disorder, the knowledge of treatment alternatives, and self-reflection regarding personal biases and stigmatizing language or behavior. A supportive, patient-centered approach more likely engages women who are using substances and allows them adequate comfort to reveal the struggles they are experiencing.

History

Inclusion of substance use questions in the health history requires specific questions in order to ascertain what substances have been used, the age at which the substances were first used, and the last episode of use. Context for the use, such as level of functioning before use and life events that occurred just before use or concurrent with initiation or exacerbation of use, help clarify the diagnosis and suggest treatment strategies. Often, asking specifically about the frequency and quantity of use for any substances used more than five times can focus the assessment (Smith et al., 2019). It is important to inquire about response to the use of each targeted substance, as well as the triggers for use after intervals of abstinence: This helps not only with understanding the substance use, but also with identifying potential co-occurring psychiatric diagnoses (Smith et al., 2019). Relapse is sometimes related to changes in hormone levels: Therefore, asking about menstrual cycles and postpartum experiences in association with other triggers can be helpful (NIDA, 2020a, 2020b). Asking about the person's own concerns regarding substance use, the benefits they perceive the substance provides, and explication of the negative impacts that substances may have had in their lives help the practitioner to formulate a functional analysis. As with any other disorder, it is important to ensure that women of childbearing age are asked if they are pregnant or planning to become pregnant (Tsakiridis et al., 2021). When feasible, the use of standardized assessment tools is recommended, as discussed later in this chapter.

Many individuals have prior experiences with substance use treatment. When this is the case, it is important to document both inpatient and outpatient treatment experiences, treatment completed or not completed, any past pharmacologic therapy for addiction, the person's perception of what had been helpful or problematic about the intervention or the program, and the length of sustained sobriety after each treatment encounter. This information is helpful for conceptualizing an individualized treatment approach and parsing intervention options (Smith et al., 2019).

Health history is most useful when it incorporates the following elements:

- Full psychosocial history (including resilience factors as well as risks, family relationships, peer relationships and influences, school experiences, work success, and stability)
- History of mental health symptoms and if applicable past interventions (including the person's assessment of benefit or detrimental impact of treatment)
- Developmental history (including fetal exposure to substances, birth challenges, and milestones)
- Family history of blood relatives who have experienced mental health and/or substance-use symptoms, clarifying the treatments they may have undertaken and the results (Smith et al., 2019)

Physical Examination

A routine physical examination usually includes the following systems likely to be affected by substance use. Attentiveness to abnormalities, especially in the areas noted, can help identify the possibility of an SUD and inform the practitioner as to the extent of physical compromise sustained from the substance use. The examples provided, while not an exhaustive listing, include many physical findings commonly occurring in consort with substance use. If a specific substance is suspected, it can also be useful to consult a reference that describes physical presentation common to that substance.

- Neurologic assessment targeting coordination, falls, head trauma, seizure history, pupillary reactivity and presentation, reflexes, gait, and temperature regulation
- Mental status assessment for orientation and alertness; memory and cognition; thought processing; and speech rate, pressure, and coherency

- Ear, nose, throat, and mouth assessment for dental health or damage, mucosal excoriation or erosion, and bleeding
- Integument assessment for evidence of needle tracks, skin picking, gooseflesh, abscess, cellulitis, or excoriation
- Respiratory assessment for evidence of infection, airway reactivity, and chronic pulmonary disease
- Cardiac assessment of heart rate and blood pressure and evidence of dependent edema and vascular insufficiency
- Gastrointestinal assessment of the liver, pancreas, stomach, and intestines, with emphasis on pain, hemorrhage, and inflammation
- Genitourinary assessment for evidence of pregnancy, trauma, infection, and renal impairment
- Musculoskeletal assessment for the presence of injuries resulting from substance use or possibly associated with chronic pain and therefore representing a barrier to sobriety (Smith et al., 2019)

Laboratory Testing

Point-of-care urine drug tests (UDTs) are commonly used in primary care (Dadiomov, 2020; Smith et al., 2019). Point-of-care UDTs are screening immunoassay tests and are easy to use, are available as test cups or test strips, are affordable, and will detect drugs or substances used within the past 5 to 7 days. The disadvantages of immunoassay tests are their reliability and validity. There are many false positives and false negatives, necessitating confirmatory testing (Dadiomov, 2020; Smith et al., 2019). For example, use of a quinolone antibiotic or diphenhydramine can produce a false positive result on UDT for opioids (Dadiomov, 2020).

Confirmatory UDTs are mass spectrometry tests and are available only in laboratories. Mass spectrometry has much greater reliability and validity than immunoassay testing. Mass spectrometry can specify which opioid a patient has taken, whether it is a synthetic or semisynthetic opioid, and can also detect drug metabolites that provide evidence of drug use (Dadiomov, 2020; Smith et al., 2019). The disadvantages of mass spectrometry testing include lack of point-of-care testing, increased cost, ability to detect substances used only within the past 1 to 2 days, and test results that take several days to obtain. Some laboratories perform mass spectrometry on site while others send specimens to another lab for analysis; this makes a difference in the cost of the testing. Costs will be increased if the laboratory is sending specimens to another facility for analysis (Dadiomov, 2020; Smith et al., 2019). There is debate about the expense of UDTs. Some argue immunoassay testing is not more cost effective if confirmatory mass spectrometry testing is required for each sample (Smith et al., 2019). Awareness of the population being tested is essential in determining which UDT to use. The ability to collect samples in a manner that prevents adulteration by patients is equally essential (Dadiomov, 2020; Smith et al., 2019).

There are additional tools that can be used in primary care for the detection of alcohol. A breathalyzer is an inexpensive tool that can be used to detect acute intoxication. Blood alcohol and serum gamma-glutamyl transferase (GGT) testing can be used to detect acute intoxication and chronic, heavy alcohol use, respectively. These blood tests require laboratory analysis with results available in 24 to 48 hours. GGT is also not specific for alcoholism; GGT can be elevated in liver diseases (Dadiomov, 2020). There is also the increased cost associated with blood testing. Blood testing is otherwise not useful in primary care to determine if a patient has an SUD. Aside from cost and invasiveness, blood testing cannot detect past substance use. Also impractical are nail and hair samples. Both must be sent to a lab for analysis, and neither can detect recent substance use (Dadiomov, 2020). Different labs and methods of screening have varying reference ranges. PCPs must be knowledgeable about the reference ranges for confirmatory UDTs in order to interpret the results correctly. Therefore, the best bet for the PCP is the UDT, either point-of-care or laboratory based, depending upon patient population and the ability to collect valid samples (Dadiomov, 2020; Smith et al., 2019).

PCPs should utilize UDTs in any patient who is being managed and treated for an SUD. Testing should be more frequent at the start of treatment and a schedule for testing can be negotiated depending upon patient stability and response to treatment. It is recommended unannounced UDTs should be performed periodically and as needed (Smith et al., 2019). Patients who are prescribed chronic controlled substances, demonstrating signs and symptoms of SUD, and requesting specific controlled substances should also be screened with a UDT (Smith et al., 2019). UDTs should also be included in prenatal testing. Current evidence suggests pregnant women who are screened for SUD early in pregnancy can be successfully managed with improved outcomes during pregnancy and delivery (CDC, 2018; Tsakiridis et al., 2021).

When working with women for whom substance use is suspected, it is important to note that the CDC recommends that women younger than 25 years who are sexually active be screened for chlamydia and that there be universal testing for gonorrhea and chlamydia infection among incarcerated adolescent and adult females up to the age of 35 years because of the potential for health impacts. It is also important to consider a pregnancy test for women of childbearing age (Workowski et al., 2021).

Laboratory studies to consider ordering when SUDs are being evaluated are those that assess for infection and liver, pancreas, renal, cardiac, and immune system compromise:

- CBC with differential and platelet count
- Aspartate aminotransferase (AST)
- Alanine aminotransferase (ALT)
- Serum GGT
- Hepatitis B and C screens
- HIV screen
- Amylase
- Blood urea nitrogen (BUN), creatinine, electrolytes
- UDTs
- EKG
- Sexually transmitted infections
- Pregnancy

The physiologic impact of SUD on the liver may be associated with abnormalities in laboratory results. Alkaline phosphatase, bilirubin, prothrombin time, ammonia, glucose, triglycerides, and AST/ALT ratio may be elevated. Mild macrocytic anemia may be present; phosphate, magnesium, and potassium levels may be low; and white blood cells may evidence abnormalities. Although an elevated serum GGT will

not be specific for excessive alcohol use, it can serve as both a screening tool and a means of monitoring use for individuals currently in treatment (Smith et al., 2019).

Differential Diagnosis

The symptoms related to the misuse of substances often co-occur with those of mental illness and commonly mimic psychiatric symptoms. This represents a challenge to practitioners to carefully evaluate for the possibility of a mental health diagnosis whenever considering the diagnosis of an SUD. Mood disorders are often misdiagnosed when individuals are not adequately assessed for substance use (Smith et al., 2019). It is critical to develop a timeline of symptom occurrence and comparatively a timeline of substance use. A UDT can be of help in the differential diagnosis of an acute-onset psychiatric disorder; however, if the symptoms have been present for more than a week, it is possible that the substance levels in the urine have diminished such that a drug screen will be negative (Dadiomov, 2020). For this reason, any diagnosis must be made utilizing the available history, considering not only symptoms and test results but also context for the symptom presentation. It is also necessary to nonjudgmentally consider the potential for secondary gain associated with the presentation of specific symptoms (Smith et al., 2019).

Substances that are stimulating in nature (including nicotine and caffeine) may cause hyperarousal, sleep interruption or restriction, cardiac stimulation with elevated heart rate and blood pressure, hypersexuality, and appetite suppression or weight loss. When the stimulant is chronically used or when it is depleted, exhaustion and depression can present (Smith et al., 2019). Emotional lability may vary from euphoric or mixed-state hypomania, anxiety, agitation, and confusion to psychosis. The use of stimulants may trigger a first episode of mood disorder or psychosis that may not resolve with sobriety. The dilation of pupils, bruxism, and skin picking may aid in the differential diagnosis (Smith et al., 2019).

Substances that are central nervous system depressants create symptoms of physiologic and mental sedation. Speech may be slurred, gait and coordination may be impaired (lots of dropping of belongings, bumps, and bruises), and complaints of constipation may be reported (Smith et al., 2019). An EKG may find changes in the QTc interval, and blood pressure and heart rate may be lowered during intoxication and elevated during withdrawal. When the substance is withdrawn, there is a risk of seizure (depending on the substance), gastrointestinal distress, temperature dysregulation, insomnia, emotional agitation, or anxiety. Pupillary constriction during the intoxication phase may be helpful in the differential diagnosis. In overdose or in combination with other depressant substances, respiratory depression can lead to coma or death (Smith et al., 2019).

Hallucinogenic or dissociative substances, including over-the-counter substances such as dextromethorphan, may present with either stimulant- or depressant-like effects, depending on the specific substance. These substances have the potential to cause mental distortions that mimic psychosis. Anabolic steroid use often presents with symptoms like those of excessive testosterone (enhanced muscle mass, acne, hypertension, and in women, masculinization). Impulsivity and mood dysregulation with rage episodes may lead to the diagnosis of intermittent explosive disorder or physical disorders such as pheochromocytoma (Smith et al., 2019).

When substance use is diminished or discontinued, psychiatric symptoms may present for the first time or exacerbate. This is especially the case when the individual has experienced trauma and the symptoms of posttraumatic stress disorder have been suppressed by substance use. Patients with mood disorders, anxiety disorders, and in particular, obsessive-compulsive disorder often become more acutely in need of psychiatric intervention with the onset of sobriety (Smith et al., 2019). Conversely, when these disorders are left untreated or unrecognized, patients' capacity to achieve or maintain sobriety is jeopardized. It is essential that both the psychiatric disorder and the SUD are adequately managed for stability to be achieved. Therefore, when established and patient accepted care is not helpful, it is necessary to reevaluate for additional psychiatric disorders or SUDs that have not been previously identified (Smith et al., 2019).

Screening

The goal of substance abuse screening is to identify individuals who have begun to develop problems or are at high risk for problems, as well as to accurately determine whether there is a problem (Smith et al., 2019). Good screening tools possess understandable directions, are quick to administer, and demonstrate sensitivity (accuracy in problem identification) and specificity (ruling out those not affected; Smith et al., 2019). It is important that the tools used for screening include an adequate number of questions regarding substance use and that these questions are framed in an open, nonjudgmental manner that encourages truthful responses.

Assessment Instruments

Tools recommended for SUD screening in primary care include the Opioid Risk Tool (ORT; Table 41.1; Smith et al., 2019; Webster & Webster, 2005) and the CAGE-AID Substance Abuse Screening Tool (Table 41.2; Brown & Rounds, 1995; Pautrat et al., 2022). An advantage to the ORT is gender-specific scoring. The ORT includes questions under three domains: family history of substance abuse (alcohol, illegal drugs, or prescription drugs), personal history of substance abuse (alcohol, illegal drugs, prescription drugs, age between 16 and 45 years, and history of preadolescent sexual abuse), and psychological disease (attention deficit disorder [ADD]/obsessive-compulsive disorder [OCD]/bipolar disorder/schizophrenia, and depression). The disadvantage to the ORT is its specificity for opioid abuse (Smith et al., 2019; Webster & Webster, 2005).

The CAGE-AID has been validated for use in primary care and screens for alcohol use as well as substance use (Brown & Rounds, 1995; Pautrat et al., 2022). The target

TABLE 41.1 The Opioid Risk Tool

MARK EACH BOX THAT APPLIES	FEMALE	MALE
Family history of substance abuse		
Alcohol	1	3
Illegal drugs	2	3
Prescription drugs	4	4
Personal history of substance abuse		
Alcohol	3	3
Illegal drugs	4	4
Prescription drugs	5	5
Age between 16 and 45 years	1	1
History of preadolescent sexual abuse	3	0
Psychological disease		
ADD, OCD, bipolar disorder, schizophrenia	2	2
Depression	1	1
Scoring totals		

Scoring: A score of 3 or lower indicates low risk for a future opioid abuse; 4–7 indicates moderate risk for opioid addiction; 8 or more indicates high risk for opioid addiction.
ADD, attention deficit disorder; OCD, obsessive compulsive disorder.
Source: Adapted from Webster, L. R., & Webster, R. M. (2005). Predicting aberrant behaviors in opioid-treated patients: Preliminary validation of the opioid risk tool. Pain Medicine, 6(6), 432–442. https://doi.org/10.1111/j.1526-4637.2005.00072.x

	TABLE 41.2 CAGE–AID Substance Abuse Screening Tool		
C	Have you ever felt the need to **cut** down on your drinking or drug use?	Yes	No
A	Have people **annoyed** you by criticizing your drinking or drug use?	Yes	No
G	Have you ever felt **guilty** about drinking or drug use?	Yes	No
E	Have you ever felt you needed a drink or used drugs first thing in the morning to steady your nerves or to get rid of a hangover (**eye-opener**)?	Yes	No

Scoring: A yes answer to one item indicates a possible substance use disorder (SUD) and a need for further testing.
Source: Adapted from Brown, R. L., & Rounds, L. A. (1995). Conjoint screening questionnaires for alcohol and other drug abuse: Criterion validity in a primary care practice. Wisconsin Medical Journal, 94(3), 135–140.

population for CAGE-AID is adults and adolescents but the tool does not discriminate between men and women. The CAGE-AID has four questions, one for each of the following: C (cutting down), A (annoyed), G (guilty), and E (eye-opener). See the complete tool in Table 41.2 (Brown & Rounds, 1995).

There is one in-depth assessment tool designed specifically for women: the female version of the Addiction Severity Index (ASI-F), which is based on the ASI (Brown et al., 1997) The ASI-F is very similar to the ASI except that it has a section pertaining to women's issues, albeit mostly reproductive. The ASI-F, like the ASI, is comprehensive. Items include medical, psychiatric, employment, and legal status; family and social relationships; family history of alcohol and other drug use; and current and past history of alcohol and other drug use. The assessment must be conducted in person the first time it is administered. Phone interviews can be conducted thereafter. The person being assessed responds verbally to items. At the end of each section, the clinician administering the ASI-F records what are referred to as *clinician confidence ratings*; that is, the clinician provides an opinion of the client's understanding of the questions in the section being completed and assesses the client's degree of distortion to each response (Brown et al., 1997). The ASI has an extensive history of psychometric development; however, the length of the instrument makes the use of the ASI-F impractical in primary care (Pautrat et al., 2022).

Screening Instruments for Varied Population Groups

There are several screening tools that might be used for screening for specific substances, general substance use, and symptoms of withdrawal. These are described in Box 41.2.

Another tool PCPs can use to detect substance use is the prescription drug monitoring program (PDMP). PDMPs are state-based electronic databases that collect controlled substance prescription information on all controlled substances dispensed in a particular state. All states and the District of Columbia have PDMPs (Smith et al., 2019). Some states mandate prescribers, or the prescribers' designated representative, to check the PDMP prior to any prescription for a controlled substance. This mandate is not consistent among all states. Likewise, some states' PDMPs can communicate with other states' PDMPs, but this too is not consistent. Checking PDMP data prior to prescribing a controlled substance

Box 41.2 Screening Tools for Substance Use Disorders

The Alcohol, Smoking, and Substance Involvement Screening Test (ASSIST) was developed by the World Health Organization (WHO) specifically for primary care. The tool has eight questions on lifetime and current substance use and has been found reliable and valid (Pautrat et al., 2022).

The Alcohol Use Disorders Identification Test (AUDIT; Smith et al., 2019) is a 10-item scale that can be self-administered or used in an interview. It requires 2 minutes for administration and 1 minute for scoring. A user's manual is available, and the tool has been translated into several non-English languages.

The Drug Abuse Screening Test (DAST), available from the Center for Addiction and Mental Health, is a 20-item instrument that can be self-administered or used as a structured interview and has been used for screening as well as determination of the level of treatment and goal planning. It has been validated with individuals who use psychoactive substances. The administration requires 5 minutes and yields a quantitative index score based on yes/no responses (Pautrat et al., 2022).

The Problem-Oriented Screening Instrument for Teenagers (POSIT; Pautrat et al., 2022) consists of 139 items with 10 subscales. It has a yes/no format and requires 20 minutes to administer. This scale has been determined to have adequate established validity and reliability.

The Substance Use Risk Profile-Pregnancy (SURP-P) may be useful in assessing women who are pregnant. The instrument queries about use of marijuana, number of alcoholic drinks consumed in the month preceding knowledge of pregnancy, and if the woman has ever felt the need to cut down on substance use. SURP-P has been found to be a highly sensitive screening tool that is easily administered (Coleman-Cowger et al., 2019).

For additional screening tools, the National Institute of Alcohol Abuse and Alcoholism (NIAAA; www.niaaa.nih.gov) and the National Institute of Drug Abuse (NIDA; www.drugabuse.gov) websites provide options for both brief and in-depth screening instruments and cite the literature supporting their use.

is considered a best practice endorsed by the CDC (2018). Preliminary evidence demonstrates a decrease in overdose deaths in states that mandate prescribers' use of the PDMP (Rhodes et al., 2019; Smith et al., 2019). It is worth noting that the PDMP databases, like the assessment/screening tools discussed, are not perfect but are, in conjunction with a thorough history and physical exam, useful in the detection of SUDs.

TREATMENT MANAGEMENT

Note that at each step in the management of substance abuse (screening, assessment, brief intervention, treatment, family interview or intervention, follow-up, and relapse prevention), motivational interviewing (MI) and efforts to promote engagement are critical aspects of the interaction that contribute to a successful outcome. Also note that the steps include ongoing assessment for factors that complicate the disorder or the treatment such as homelessness, health compromise, or mental illness, and integrate approaches for these disorders in further assessments or treatments.

The National Academy of Medicine report, *Educating Together, Improving Together: Harmonizing Interprofessional Approaches to Address the Opioid Epidemic* (Chappell et al., 2021), identifies five data-informed priorities: establishing minimum competencies in SUDs and pain management for healthcare professionals; fostering interprofessional collaboration among regulatory, licensing, and certifying organizations; providing on demand, learner-centered continuing professional education for healthcare professionals in SUD and pain management; standardization of accreditors' requirements for interprofessional education in pain management and SUDs; and improvements in collaborative efforts for practice improvements (Chappell et al., 2021). Central to all five priorities is the emphasis on multimodal treatment of SUDs including the patient as a partner in psychosocial and medication-assisted treatments for SUDs (Chappell et al., 2021).

Recommendations for the treatment or management of SUDs or co-occurring mental health and SUDs are commonly made after evaluation and diagnosis are completed but without having first engaged the individual and without factoring in their readiness for treatment, personal preferences, or needs. The consideration of treatment needs must include individual "fit" in order to promote the possibility of a successful outcome. Likewise, the goals for treatment must reflect the goals of the person the practitioner is striving to help rather than those of the care team or family. Readiness for change is often assessed using the transtheoretical, or stages of change, model first developed by Prochaska and DiClemente, which describes stages of precontemplation, contemplation, preparation, action, and maintenance. For engagement to occur, the practitioner needs to find ways of meeting the individual where they are and of matching communication and treatment recommendations to the individual's preparation for change (Prochaska et al., 1992).

Motivational Interviewing

MI represents one of the best practices for promoting engagement and helping move individuals toward the direction of healthy change. It is a purposeful model of communication that serves to activate a person's own motivation and resources for change. It is nondirective, yet mindfully directional (Miller & Rollnick, 2013). The spirit of MI conveys partnership and acceptance; it supports autonomy, affirms strength, and is evocative; and it does not strive to provide a remedy that may not have been requested. Rather than convincing or coercing the individual to comply with treatment recommendations, the communication and the context of the relationship promote the explication of participants' desire and goals for health. The use of MI has been found to be especially effective in work with individuals who have SUDs. The practitioner truly learns about the context and the goals of the patient, thereby allowing ultimate recommendations to be a good match for that individual. An added incentive for PCPs to learn and utilize MI in routine practice is the diffusion of conflict with patients and the increased probability that agreed-upon follow-up or homework will take place (Acquavita et al., 2021; Forray et al., 2019; Gonzalez et al., 2020; Miller & Rollnick, 2013).

Screening, Brief Intervention, and Referral to Treatment

The screening, brief intervention, and referral to treatment (SBIRT) process is grounded in MI and has been shown to be an effective means for identifying individuals who engage in substance misuse and for determining the severity of the disorder. SBIRT incorporates MI to provide brief intervention and to make referrals to treatment as indicated and accepted. This practice was initially implemented in the emergency care setting but is a natural fit for use in the primary care setting (Acquavita et al., 2021; Forray et al., 2019; Gonzalez et al., 2020; Moser et al., 2020).

Level of Care

The American Society of Addiction Medicine (ASAM) provides an algorithm for recommending placement in outpatient (once-a-week treatment), intensive outpatient (three-times-a-week treatment, including group as well as individual therapy), or inpatient treatment. The criteria reflect the severity of the substance use, as well as the social context of the individual. ASAM has created a national practice guideline, updated in 2020, that PCPs may access at www.asam.org/quality-care/clinical-guidelines/national-practice-guideline. ASAM has converted their guideline into a pocket guide containing updated assessment, diagnosis, and treatment recommendations in a readily accessible format for PCPs (ASAM, 2020). As with any guideline, the ASAM placement criteria are not proscriptive and do not replace clinical judgment.

For women and adolescent girls, the circumstances of substance use often demand the selection of treatment level be tailored to fit individual need. For example, a woman in an untenable living situation fraught with opportunity or pressure to use substances may require an inpatient episode of care to stabilize in a supportive environment. Other women who fear the loss of hard-to-replace jobs or have no one to care for their children may find outpatient treatment to be most beneficial (Dillaway et al., 2019). Some women will need a short inpatient treatment episode for medically supervised substance discontinuation. Women who are pregnant or postpartum may also have medical complications best served in an inpatient setting (LaPointe, 2019). However, individuals who are extremely anxious may find the ordeal of the inpatient setting impossible to tolerate. Women who are in the military or who have careers that would be severely limited by employer knowledge of their substance use may need both support and help to find adequate treatment that will not create more circumstantial problems. When barriers to seeking care are perceived to be too great to overcome, women will be less likely to engage in treatment. However, when it is possible to match care to patient need and capacity, thereby removing unnecessary stress, it allows the person to focus on participating in getting healthier rather than surviving an ordeal or awaiting the next crisis (LaPointe, 2019).

Psychotherapeutic Interventions

Multiple authors have identified psychotherapeutic interventions that are key in the management and treatment of women with SUDs (American Psychiatric Association, 2013; Berger et al., 2021; Brown et al., 2021; Elms et al., 2018; Galanter, 2018; Martin et al., 2020; Martino et al., 2018; Moser et al., 2020; Reinert et al., 2021; Smith et al., 2019). The NIDA (2018) has identified cognitive behavioral therapy (CBT), contingency management (CM), motivational enhancement therapy (MET), and family therapy as having particular benefits in the treatment of SUDs. McGovern et al. (2021), in their systematic review, found evidence of benefit for psychotherapeutic interventions but no evidence that one type of intervention is superior to another.

Some clinical practice guidelines explicitly indicate the number of sessions or weeks of therapy to be provided and for which outcomes have been determined. In substance use treatment as usual, a key measurement has often been retention in treatment rather than a specific treatment goal or outcome. Certainly, for psychotherapeutic interventions, it is widely held that the more "doses" of treatment provided, the greater the possibility of improved outcome; retention in treatment does allow more opportunity for doses of therapy to be received, but it does not indicate treatment benefit or change associated with treatment (McGovern et al., 2021; Smith et al., 2019).

Cognitive Behavioral Therapy

CBT is grounded in becoming aware of one's own automatic, possibly irrational thoughts and underlying assumptions that precede dysregulated emotional response and may result in behavior that is problematic, such as substance use. It is a skills-based learning therapy focused on developing replacement thoughts and a pattern of increased self-efficacy, but this does not diminish the importance of empathy and connection in the therapeutic relationship. CBT utilizes homework to practice skills and explores the role of beliefs, thoughts, and behaviors using tools such as functional analysis. CBT can be especially helpful for individuals who need to reframe traumatic experiences, manage anxiety or depressive symptoms, manage mood volatility and impulsiveness, and tolerate the discomfort of abstaining from substances and instead experience feelings (NIDA, 2018). For women who have SUDs, CBT can often be of tremendous value in enhancing self-worth and reinforcing capability while becoming free of substance use. It is well studied with models for use in substance use and in a myriad of mental health disorders (Elms et al., 2018; Green et al., 2021; NIDA, 2018b).

Contingency Management

CM is based on behavioral reinforcement theory. Nancy Petry developed a model for CM in which fishbowl draws are used in research studies as well as in the clinical setting and in drug courts to reward positive behaviors (Stitzer et al., 2010). Maintaining sobriety as evidenced by negative urine drug screens, completion of a CBT homework assignment, attendance at therapy sessions, or participation in a prosocial activity is rewarded by an opportunity to draw from the fishbowl. Often there is a perception that the use of CM represents bribery; however, the evidence is that it is a powerful tool found to have positive outcomes when used as an element of substance use treatment. Programs using CM may enlist participants to help determine what prizes might be made available. Whether the participant wins or not, the conveyance of affirmation for having earned the fishbowl draw represents a reinforcement (NIDA, 2018; Stitzer et al., 2010).

Motivational Enhancement Therapy

MET is therapy consistent with MI and SBIRT, as previously described. The emphasis is on guiding the individual toward positive health decisions that are grounded in their own goals and personal strengths (NIDA, 2018).

Family Therapy

Several family therapy approaches have been developed for use with families of young people who have behavioral disorders and substance use. Functional family therapy and multisystemic family therapy are among the most widely implemented, often among youth involved with the juvenile justice system. In these models, the work is designed to assist families in managing the communication and the environment in a way that diminishes conflict and reduces oppositional behaviors as well as substance use. When these therapies are funded through the juvenile justice system, the reduction of what is known as criminogenic behavior and recidivism is the key outcome measured (NIDA, 2018).

PSYCHOPHARMACOLOGIC INTERVENTIONS

The questions of when and what medication to prescribe for a woman known to have an SUD is always difficult. For women, decision-making about prescribing medication is further complicated by known pregnancy, the possibility of unplanned pregnancy, and lactation. The prescribing decision must often be based in a risk–benefit analysis: whether treating the SUD specifically using an opioid antagonist, partial agonist/antagonist, or full agonist or determining whether to provide medication to stabilize symptoms of mood, anxiety, or psychotic disorders (American Psychiatric Association, 2013). Often this is a very individualized clinical decision, rather than a blanket approach to treatment. There is always a potential for unintended consequences when prescribing a medication to a pregnant or nursing woman. The decision not to treat is also a treatment decision that has clinical consequences. Whenever possible, the decisions regarding a pharmacologic intervention will be most effective when arrived at in collaboration with the person seeking care. Communicating treatment recommendations and the limits of the treatment in a mutually respectful manner while acknowledging the woman's goals and strengths, without succumbing to demands that may be contrary to best practice or clinical judgment, is critical to maintaining a healthy and safe relationship that permits future care to be accessible (Elms et al., 2018; Martin et al., 2020; Smith et al., 2019).

The first step toward any pharmacologic treatment decision is to be clear as to the diagnosis (whether the symptoms are related to substance use or a co-occurring disorder), the goal (for any intervention but especially for a pharmacologic therapy), the plan for care, and most important, the plan for assessing response and potentially discontinuing medication not found helpful (American Psychiatric Association, 2013). The next step is a risk–benefit assessment considering factors such as general health status, risks associated with potential QTc interval changes, drug–drug interactions, the self-harm or safety status of the individual, the risk of the medication being diverted or not safely stored, the prospect of adherence to the recommended dosing regimen, and the potential for benefit (Smith et al., 2019).

Prescriptions that offer high potential for abuse or which have a known street value should be avoided whenever possible, whether or not it is clear that the patient has a substance use problem. When individuals are engaged in a methadone or buprenorphine (Suboxone) program, there are specific SAMHSA (2023) regulations specifying the management of these medications. Before providing a prescription or dispensing a take-home dose, it is necessary to assess whether the environment is stable enough for medication to be safely stored and administered. Safe storage is of particular importance when women have children in the home. When methadone is dispensed, take-home doses must be placed in a locked box before being taken from the provider agency dispensary (Smith et al., 2019).

Once determined that medication is indicated and a prescription is the best clinical action, there remain some challenges. SUDs vary over time in regard to preferred substance, severity of use or cravings, and symptoms manifested in association with the substance (American Psychiatric Association, 2013). It can be difficult to know whether an apparent medication response is due to the medication prescribed or to a change in illicit substance use. This can lead to repetitive changes in prescribed medications before an adequate trial has been accomplished. Prescription medications can and do interact with over-the-counter medications, herbal remedies, and illicit substances that the practitioner may not be aware the patient is using. Adherence to prescription regimens is universally difficult and far more so for individuals who are accustomed to self-prescribing. A conversation about the challenges of medication adherence prior to providing the first prescription can help both the practitioner and the patient to be mindful of this possibility and adds a layer of transparency that may result in greater sharing of information. It is also common for prescription medications to unmask disorders that had not been evident before the initiation of a medication or to cause an exacerbation of reported symptoms; this may be more likely the case if the medication is not taken as prescribed (Smith et al., 2019).

FOOD AND DRUG ADMINISTRATION–APPROVED MEDICATIONS FOR TREATING SUBSTANCE USE DISORDERS

Current recommendations include pharmacologic treatment for SUDs in conjunction with psychotherapeutic interventions when appropriate (ASAM, 2020; Galanter, 2018; Smith et al., 2019; Tsakiridis et al., 2021). The medications reviewed here act as antagonist, partial agonist, agonist, and replacement agents. The descriptions that follow are not intended as a full prescribing guide, but rather as a brief overview with a focus on use in pregnancy. NIDA (www.drugabuse.gov) and ASAM (www.asam.org) websites are valuable resources. The Department of Veterans Affairs (VA)/Department of Defense (DoD) guidelines (VA, 2021) recommend naltrexone and topiramate as first-line treatment for alcohol use disorder and suggest acamprosate and disulfiram or gabapentin as a second-line suggested medication for alcohol use disorder. The VA/DoD guidelines recommend buprenorphine/naloxone and methadone as first-line agents for opioid use disorder and extended-release naltrexone as a suggested second-line agent (VA, 2021). Buprenorphine without naloxone is Food and Drug Administration (FDA) approved for the treatment of opioid use disorder in pregnant women. FDA-approved medications for nicotine dependence are bupropion and varenicline. Currently, there are no other pharmacologic agents available for the treatment of SUDs (Smith et al., 2019). Research is ongoing and a vaccine for SUD as well as new medications continue to be investigated.

Alcohol

Disulfiram was approved in 1948 as an alcohol-sensitizing agent that inhibits the intermediate metabolism of alcohol, causing an elevation in serum acetaldehyde when alcohol is consumed. Alcohol use is an absolute contraindication with disulfiram and has been designated a black box warning for this drug. A cascade of physically uncomfortable symptoms known as the *disulfiram–ethanol reaction* arises, characterized by flushing, lowered blood pressure, elevated heart rate, nausea, vomiting, blurred vision, dizziness, or confusion. In some instances, psychotic symptoms may arise in susceptible individuals prescribed high doses. Common doses are 250 to 500 mg/day. Many cautions exist; caution is advised during pregnancy due to potential teratogenicity, and disulfiram should not be used during lactation. Drug–drug interactions and side effects limit the use of disulfiram (Prescribers' Digital Reference [PDR], 2023).

Acamprosate was approved in 2004 as an agent that affects glutamate and GABA neurotransmitter systems to reduce alcohol cravings, although it is not entirely clear how it accomplishes this. The dosing of this medication has been challenging, 666 mg (two tablets) three times daily. Acamprosate should be used with caution in pregnancy due to possible teratogenicity. Use of this drug during lactation may outweigh the risks of continued alcohol use but there is no human data on risk to the infant or effects on milk production (U. S. Food and Drug Administration [FDA], 2012).

Naltrexone (ReVia oral formulation as well as depot Vivitrol) was approved in 1984 as an opioid antagonist, blocking opioid receptors and thereby reducing the reward experienced in response to the use of alcohol. Vivitrol is the monthly injectable version of this medication. Both have been found to reduce cravings as well as use of alcohol. Naltrexone should be used with caution in pregnancy but may be used during lactation, based on limited human data available (FDA, 2013).

Opioids

Methadone was approved in the 1960s as a long-acting opioid agonist medication that blocks opioid receptors, thereby preventing intoxication from short-acting opioids and/or withdrawal symptoms. Methadone is approved as an opioid substitution therapy only when provided through programs regulated by SAMHSA and the Drug Enforcement Agency (DEA). Nurse practitioners are now among the licensed professionals with the authority to initiate therapy (methadone induction) in approved settings Methadone is used for opioid use disorder in pregnant women, less so since the introduction of buprenorphine. Both buprenorphine and methadone are present in breast milk. It is not uncommon for women to nurse while using methadone but the infant must be closely monitored for respiratory depression, and withdrawal could occur with abrupt cessation of breastfeeding (NIDA, 2020d). The management of care for pregnant women on methadone requires a team approach, and this team should include midwives or obstetric and pediatric practitioners, as well as chemical dependency professionals and social service providers. Doses may be given twice a day, and the dose requires adjustment over the course of the pregnancy and postpartum interval. The pregnant woman on methadone is a full participant in decisions regarding dosing and lactation after delivery and so must be given adequate information to make informed decisions and to follow recommendations for healthy infant outcomes. The inclusion of partners in this education and support process is highly recommended. Infants require monitoring for excessive sedation or for symptoms of withdrawal after birth and when nursing (FDA, 2018).

Buprenorphine was approved in 2002 as a partial mu-opioid agonist and kappa-opioid antagonist and was approved for the treatment of opioid dependence in 2002 in the United States. It is available in the form of Subutex (buprenorphine) as well as Suboxone (buprenorphine/naloxone). Both are available as sublingual tablets or sublingual dissolving strips. Suboxone was developed to reduce the potential for overdose resulting from the injection of buprenorphine, and the naloxone is not absorbed unless injected. It is generally recommended that pregnant women be given buprenorphine rather than the combination of buprenorphine/naloxone to avoid potential toxicity associated with the naloxone (Tsakiridis et al., 2021). Buprenorphine can be prescribed in office-based practices by eligible physicians, physician assistants, and certified APRNs who are state licensed and registered by the DEA to prescribe controlled substances (Becerra, 2021). Previous training requirements for eligible healthcare providers to prescribe buprenorphine were waived on April 28, 2021, in response to the lack of healthcare providers who can treat opioid use disorders with buprenorphine (Becerra, 2021). Individuals who are treated with buprenorphine usually fill prescriptions at a local pharmacy. The ability for women with SUD to obtain treatment with buprenorphine in the context of primary care along with obtaining the medication from a local pharmacy has enabled women with SUD to receive treatment without the stigma attached to receiving treatment at a methadone dispensary (ASAM, 2020; Frazer et al., 2019; Galanter, 2018; Ober et al., 2018; Smith et al., 2019; Tsakiridis et al., 2021; Witte et al., 2021; Zittleman et al., 2020).

Naltrexone (oral and depot) is an opioid antagonist, blocking opioid receptors. Vivitrol is the monthly injectable version of this medication, and is FDA approved for the treatment of opioid use disorder (FDA, 2013). Naltrexone implants are being studied in Europe and Australia. The implant is inserted subcutaneously into the abdomen under local anesthesia (Edinoff et al., 2021). Australian researchers have found naltrexone implants maintain adequate serum levels of naltrexone over 5 to 6 months in individuals who weigh 70 kg (154 lb; Edinoff et al., 2021). The implants dissolve and do not require removal. Research is ongoing on the safety and efficacy of naltrexone implants, and currently, naltrexone implants are not FDA approved for use in the United States (Edinoff et al., 2021).

Naltrexone should be used with caution during pregnancy but may be used during lactation as stated previously. Methadone and buprenorphine are better established treatments for pregnant and nursing women. It is important to educate individuals who achieve sobriety on naltrexone that if they do resume the use of opioid substances, they will have a lower tolerance and will be at risk of overdose if they resume their prior level of use immediately (FDA, 2013). This is somewhat different from individuals who have stabilized on an opioid agonist or on partial agonist medication. Still, for nonpregnant individuals with opioid use disorder, naltrexone may be used as a first-line pharmacologic agent, as it does not hold potential for escalating opioid dosages, which may occur with opioid agonist therapy (FDA, 2013).

Naloxone is an opioid antagonist that is administered by intravascular or intranasal methods to reverse opioid overdose. It has been available for medical use in emergency settings for years but was approved by the FDA in November 2015 for use as a nasal spray for opioid overdoses (PDR, 2022). Naloxone may be used in pregnancy and lactation as the risk of overdose far outweighs the risk of the drug, however, naloxone should not be used in pregnancy except in the case of an opioid overdose.

Limited access to naloxone in the community has been recognized as a risk factor for opioid overdose death (Evoy et al., 2021). Over the past 4 to 5 years, many states have implemented naloxone access laws (NALs) to increase naloxone access in the community (Evoy et al., 2021). These laws have enabled pharmacists to dispense naloxone without a prescription. However, as overdose deaths have continued to rise, in part due to the prevalence of illicit fentanyl as well as pandemic effects, a push to change naloxone to an over-the-counter (OTC) medication has been gaining traction (Evoy et al., 2021). OTC naloxone would aid in overcoming barriers to naloxone access such as confusion on the part of pharmacists regarding NALs and problems with obtaining and distributing naloxone in community settings (Evoy et al., 2021).

Nicotine

Nicotine replacement therapy (NRT) has been approved by the FDA in a variety of forms. Safety data during pregnancy are limited. Nicotine and NRT may be used during pregnancy and lactation as the benefits of the drug outweigh the risks of continued smoking. Nicotine replacement is available as an inhaler, gum, lozenge, or patch. A prescription is not required for nicotine replacement products. Dose and use of nicotine replacement products vary depending upon how much an individual smokes per day (American Cancer Society, n.d.).

Bupropion was FDA approved as Zyban for smoking cessation in 1997. It is classified as a norepinephrine-dopamine reuptake inhibitor antidepressant. Use of bupropion for smoking cessation is not recommended during pregnancy due to a potential risk of congenital heart defects, or during lactation due to seizure risk in infants. Bupropion can be very useful for nonpregnant women who have a diagnosis of depression and wish to stop smoking. Bupropion is dosed at 150 mg twice a day for sustained release preparations, 150 mg to 300 mg daily for extended-release preparations (FDA, 2017).

Varenicline is a nicotine partial agonist approved for smoking cessation in 2006. It should be used with caution in pregnancy and lactation as there is limited human data regarding risk. The dose of varenicline should be titrated up to 1 mg twice a day to minimize side effects. Depression is a potential adverse reaction associated with varenicline use, and the medication should be discontinued if depression develops or worsens due to therapy. Varenicline is often preferred by patients because it does not have the associated stigma of an antidepressant medication. Common side effects include nausea, vomiting, and vivid dreams (FDA, 2009).

Treatment Settings for Substance Use Disorders

Advances in technology have now enabled individuals with SUDs to receive diagnosis, management, and treatment, either with medication, counseling, or both through telehealth.

Telehealth office visits allow patients to "see" their healthcare provider using a computer with a webcam and microphone. Telehealth office visits eliminate the need to travel to a healthcare provider's office for care and offer patients the opportunity to receive care in their own homes, in a more comfortable, private setting. The COVID-19 pandemic ushered in the use of telehealth due to lockdown and quarantine. During the height of the pandemic, third-party payers started reimbursing healthcare providers for telehealth visits. Postpandemic, the use of telehealth continues to increase. Research on the efficacy of telehealth is ongoing. Current research indicates patient satisfaction with telehealth visits for counseling and medication management of individuals with SUDs (Kim & Tesmer, 2021; Mark et al., 2022; Sugarman et al., 2021; Torous et al., 2021). However, challenges in telehealth exist. Telehealth is available only if individuals have access to technology. In populations challenged with a lack of resources, and marginalized minoritized groups, access to telehealth services will continue to be limited (Kim & Tesmer, 2021; Mark et al., 2022; Sugarman et al., 2021; Torous et al., 2021). Healthcare policy is needed to address these barriers to improve telehealth access in communities with the greatest need (Chacon et al., 2021).

FUTURE DIRECTIONS

Women with SUDs continue to be a somewhat hidden population, regardless of other characteristics. Stigmatizing language and potential threats of job loss or loss of child custody, coupled with limited resource allocation, serve to encourage women to hide substance use (Berger et al., 2021; Elms et al., 2018). Greater emphasis must be placed on preparing healthcare providers to be knowledgeable about and comfortable in assessing women for substance use. Efforts to change stigmatizing language used by healthcare providers represents a meaningful step. Additional efforts include:

- Advocate for the development of a variety of gender-specific treatment modalities and ensure that they become available in an affordable, geographically distributed manner to enhance the possibility that women will access treatment. Child-friendly settings that offer family programs and day care if needed diminish barriers women experience in seeking help for substance use (NIDA, 2020c; SAMHSA, 2020).
- Strive to increase funding to address epigenomics and grow the understanding of gender differences in the development of SUDs (NIDA, 2020a, 2020b).
- Prioritize the evaluation of women who have co-occurring mental health disorders or SUDs, and when these are present, have a capacity for providing of integrated care at the most accessible location (SAMHSA, 2020).
- Focus on women veterans, determining the most acceptable and successful interventions by evaluating the outcomes of current programs and asking women what they need that is not currently available to them (VA, 2021).
- Incorporate evidence-based strategies in the development of any innovative models of care, evaluating

outcomes in a prospective manner and comparing them to care as usual (Chappell et al., 2021).

- Take action to press the pharmacology industry to gather the information that is lacking regarding the safety of pharmacologic therapies for use in adolescent girls, women, and pregnant and lactating women (Tsakiridis et al., 2021).
- Continue to investigate the use of telehealth in mental health and SUD treatment in an effort to improve access to services that have been limited during the COVID-19 pandemic or inaccessible to marginalized groups lacking resources and technology (Reinert et al., 2021).

REFERENCES

References for this chapter are online and available at https://connect.springerpub.com/content/book/978-0-8261-6722-4/part/part03/chapter/ch41

CHAPTER 42

Gender-Based Violence and Women's Health

ANGELA FREDERICK AMAR AND NECOLE LELAND

Gender-based violence, also known as violence against women, is a public health and societal concern. It denotes violence inflicted on women because of their subordinate status in society. It includes any act or threat by men or male-dominated institutions that inflicts harm on a woman or girl because of gender. Gender-based violence includes physical, sexual, and psychological violence such as domestic or intimate partner violence (IPV) and sexual abuse, including rape and sexual abuse of children by family members. Additional examples are sexual slavery and trafficking; traditional practices harmful to women, such as honor killings, burning or acid throwing, female genital mutilation, and dowry-related violence; violence in armed conflict; and sexual harassment and intimidation at work (World Health Organization [WHO], 2021a). Gender-based violence occurs in both the "public" or general community and in "private," or family, spheres. In most cultures, traditional beliefs, norms, and social institutions legitimize and therefore perpetuate violence against women. The state condones violence through policies or the actions of agents of the state, such as the police, military, or immigration authorities. Gender-based violence happens in all societies, across all social classes.

Gender-based violence is a major cause of injury that leads many survivors to seek care in the EDs of hospitals and clinics. However, long-term physical and mental health consequences cause survivors to seek healthcare in primary care, prenatal and postnatal areas, labor and delivery areas, pediatricians' offices, mental health services, and other areas within most hospitals and clinics (Ghandour et al., 2015; Keynejad et al., 2021). Each of these encounters gives nurses and other healthcare providers opportunities to identify and intervene for gender-based violence and health-related consequences (O'Gurek & Henke, 2018).

The purpose of this chapter is to orient the women's health nurse to IPV and sexual violence and their related behaviors such as stalking and strangulation. Limited aspects of perpetration, although not a focus of this chapter, are included to increase the clinician's awareness. Information is provided to assist the women's health nurse in the identification and

assessment of gender-based violence. Current evidence-based nursing responses and interventions are presented, as are resources useful to clinicians and to survivors of IPV and sexual violence and their families, friends, and other sources of social support. Because this book is geared toward women's health nurses, we refer primarily to the experiences of women in regard to IPV and sexual violence. Within the field, the term *victim* is used to connote victimization, and some feel that *survivor* should not be used until the process of healing is complete. However, in our society, the term *victim* is also identified with weakness. Others feel that the process of healing starts immediately and that living through a traumatic event confers survivor status. In this chapter, the term *survivor* is used in place of the term *victim*.

DEFINITION AND SCOPE (INCIDENCE/PREVALENCE)

IPV and sexual violence are both forms of gender-based violence that fall under the category of interpersonal violence. Both occur in the context of a social relationship that more often includes known perpetrators rather than strangers. IPV is a pattern of assaultive and coercive behaviors that adults or adolescents use against their intimate partners. Intimate partnerships include current or former dating, married, or cohabiting relationships of heterosexuals, lesbians, gay men, and anyone in the LGBTQIA community. Both men and women are identified as victims/survivors and perpetrators of IPV (Centers for Disease Control and Prevention [CDC], n.d.). However, women are often overrepresented in survivor status, and males are more likely to be identified as perpetrators (Breiding et al., 2014). Worldwide, 35% of women have experienced either physical and/or sexual IPV or nonpartner sexual violence (WHO, 2021b). A substantial proportion of U.S. female and male adults have experienced some form of sexual violence, stalking, or IPV during their lifetimes. The National Intimate Partner and Sexual Violence

Survey (NISVS) estimates that 142 million U.S. adults had some lifetime exposure to IPV, sexual violence, or stalking (Peterson et al., 2021). CDC data suggest that 23.6% of women and 11.5% of men reported experiencing physical or sexual IPV in their lifetimes. Severe physical violence is experienced by 22.3% of women and 12% of men (Breiding et al., 2015). IPV affects sexual and gender minorities in higher rates and potentially worse outcomes with increased vulnerability for transgender individuals as compared to cisgender (Decker et al., 2018; Peitzmeier et al., 2020).

IPV, also referred to as domestic violence, can take many forms. Physical IPV is inflicting physical pain or bodily harm against a partner. For example, physical IPV behaviors include hitting, punching, kicking, strangling, pushing, burning, and throwing things. Emotional abuse involves inflicting mental anguish and includes threatening, humiliating, intimidating, and degrading behaviors. It also includes coercive behaviors, such as jealousy and withholding financial support, that are used to maintain control. Sexual IPV is any form of sexual contact or exposure without consent or forced sexual activity. Most survivors experience multiple forms of violent behaviors in their relationships.

Sexual Violence

Sexual violence includes all sexual acts that occur against the wishes of the other person. It includes anal, vaginal, and oral sexual activities and intercourse. Sexual violence includes a range of behaviors from rape to a range of unwanted sexual behaviors with or without contact (Smith et al., 2018). Rape involves some form of sexual penetration of the survivor; sexual assault is a broader category that includes any type of unwanted or nonconsensual sexual activity. An estimated 19.3% of women and 1.7% of men have been raped, and 43.9% of women and 23.4% of men have experienced other forms of sexual violence during their lifetimes. Among female rape survivors, 78.7% were raped before age 25 and 40% before age 18 years (Breiding et al., 2015). Adolescents and young adults are at the highest risk of sexual victimization (Black et al., 2011). Although both men and women are victimized, survivors are more often women, and aggressors are more often male (Black et al., 2011; Breiding et al., 2015). In comparison with heterosexual women, bisexual women and lesbians experience more sexual violence and the same is true for men (Chen et al., 2020).

Rape is generally an underreported crime to law enforcement (Lurigio & Staton, 2020). Estimates of rape in general and victimization surveys are higher than actual crime reports from law enforcement. Societal stigma about sex, victim blaming, and the fact that most rapes are perpetrated by someone known to the survivor are all factors that make reporting to the police difficult (Hullenaar & Frisco, 2020; Wright et al., 2022). Furthermore, survivors are concerned that they will not be believed or will be blamed (Robinson et al., 2021). Barriers to not reporting or using services include shame, guilt, embarrassment, not wanting others to know, and thinking it was not serious enough to report (Stoner & Cramer, 2019). In fact, secondary victimization is often reported through experiences with healthcare providers and especially in the criminal justice system (Campbell et al., 2001). Men are particularly

vulnerable to the stigma of sexual assault, especially because of the societal belief that it cannot happen to men, which could account for the lower reporting. Homophobia and stigma also make it difficult for LGBTQIA individuals to report such crimes (Decker et al., 2018; Peitzmeier et al., 2020). Finally, the traumatic nature of experiencing violence could create a response involving high levels of psychological distress that may inhibit immediate reporting (Robinson et al., 2021).

Stalking

Stalking occurs when someone repeatedly harasses or threatens someone else, causing fear or safety concern (Smith et al., 2018). Specific behaviors include unwanted communication, watching or following from a distance, or showing up at places. Stalking can escalate to physical violence and is often a part of IPV (Morgan & Truman, 2022). Furthermore, the intrusive and persistent nature of stalking can cause individuals to fear for their safety, particularly when technology is involved.

The National Crime Victimization Survey (NCVS) and the 2019 Supplemental Victimization Survey (SVS) indicated that 1.3% (3.4 million) of all people ages 16 and older in the United States were stalked in 2019. Females were stalked twice as often as males, and less than a third of all stalking survivors reported it to the police (Morgan & Truman, 2022). The results from a recent three-sample cross-sectional study found rates of 13% to 47.9% (Nobles et al., 2018). In a 2016 sample, more participants reported stalking with technology than stalking using traditional means. Examples of stalking with technology are unwanted phone calls, voice messages, or text messages; spying using technology; tracking the survivor's whereabouts with an electronic tracking device or application; posting or threatening to post unwanted information on the internet; or monitoring activities using social media (Truman & Morgan, 2021).

Reproductive Coercion

Reproductive coercion is a more recently identified form of IPV. It is a behavior that interferes with the decision-making of a woman related to reproductive health and can include birth control sabotage or pregnancy coercion (Grace & Anderson, 2018). Tactics include promoting pregnancy in their female partners through verbal pressure and threats; direct interference with contraception or birth control sabotage; and threats and coercion related to pregnancy continuation or termination that aim to control pregnancy outcomes (Miller et al., 2014). Abusive male partners have been found to actively promote pregnancy via behaviors such as verbal pressure to become pregnant, condom manipulation, threats, or actual violence in response to condom requests and direct acts of birth control sabotage (e.g., removing a vaginal ring, throwing out birth control pills, and blocking women from seeking access to contraception; Fay & Yee, 2018). In addition, once a female partner is pregnant, an abusive male partner may initiate behaviors to control the outcome of pregnancy, including violent acts, attempts to induce miscarriage, and coercion to either continue or terminate the pregnancy. It is suspected that reproductive coercion provides the link between IPV and unintended pregnancy. WHO's Multi-country Study on Women's Health and Domestic Violence provides compelling evidence that IPV is a strong and consistent risk factor for unintended pregnancy (Pallitto et al., 2013).

Etiology

The cycle of violence is a common explanation of the dynamics of IPV relationships. Usually men are depicted as abusers and women as survivors; however, these roles can apply to both genders. The relationship usually begins without violence. The abuser presents as loving and caring. Tension builds gradually and eventually erupts in a violent episode. During the violent episode, the abuser is unpredictable, and the survivor feels helpless. After the violent episode, the abuser is contrite and attentive and tries to make amends. The couple returns to the first stage, a honeymoon period. The survivor feels uncertain while trying to reconcile the loving partner of the first and last stages with the abusive person of the middle stage. Soon, however, the tension builds to an eruption, and the same cycle repeats (Walker, 2009). This cycle of violence helps explain the dynamics of the relationship and each partner's behavior. Most outsiders see only the violence and have difficulty understanding and responding to the relationship. This framework, depicted in Figure 42.1, is a useful aid in understanding the dynamics of an abusive relationship.

Societal factors also affect conceptualizations of gender-based violence. Myths about violence and victims/survivors prevail. Many of these myths blame survivors for their victimization (Robinson et al., 2021). Discussions of sexual assault focus on what she was wearing, why she was there, and why she did not fight harder. We focus on why women stay in abusive relationships and ask why she does not leave rather than ask why he hits. These perceptions place the onus for preventing acts of interpersonal violence on the survivor rather than on the perpetrator. There is a large mismatch between the public perception of sexual assault and sexual assault offenders and the reality of sexual assault. The general public thinks of sexual assault as a very violent act, often involving extreme force or a weapon, between people who do not know each other and occurring in a public place. Most sexual assaults are committed by someone known to the survivor; force is not always used, and the locations are usually private (Reich et al., 2022). Furthermore, as a society, we place family and intimate and sexual relationships in a private zone that makes witnesses reluctant to intervene and prevents conversations regarding violence. This makes it difficult for those affected to recognize the problem and to seek help.

The gender-based violence movement provides a new context in which to examine and understand the phenomenon of violence against women. It shifts the focus from women as victims to gender and the unequal power relationships between women and men created and maintained by gender stereotypes as the basic underlying cause of violence against women. Institutions within society often lend support for violence through historical interpretations, various customs, and social mores. A historical patriarchal structure lends support to societal factors such as gender roles and equality, normalization of violence, and

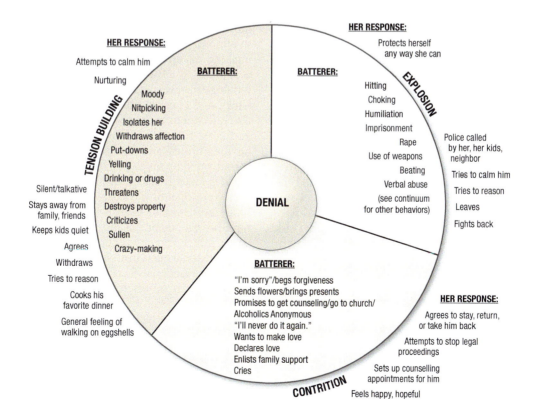

Figure 42.1 Cycle of violence.

objectification of women. Traditional gender role beliefs that support patriarchy and male dominance are associated with violence against women (WHO, 2019). It must be noted that not all men have violence-accepting attitudes or engage in violence against women. The term is not meant to suggest that all men are violent. Rather, it describes a context that normalizes violence and inequality with the institutions and structure of society.

One powerful societal institution used to support violence and to make it difficult to end violent relationships is organized religion. For example, the Bible is used to support husbands as in charge and wives as submissive. Popular media portrays violence and control as signs of a loving relationship that normalizes violence and makes it difficult for survivors to come forward. Misogynistic media that portray women as sexual objects negatively affect perceptions of gender equality. The objectification of women and their bodies is common. For example, women's bodies are used in advertisements for guns, alcohol, cars, and so on. Violence against women occurs in many countries in the world; however, the prevalence and severity of violence are higher in rural compared with industrialized areas (WHO, 2019). The cause of gender-based violence is complex and multifactorial. Causes exist at the individual, familial, institutional, and societal level. Identification of causes helps identify solutions. The involvement of multiple entities is necessary to make change.

Risk Factors

Understanding risk factors is important so that a behavior can be prevented. A consistent risk factor that predicts future violence is past violence (Conley et al., 2017). Individuals who experienced one form of violence are more likely to experience subsequent violence (Clare et al., 2021; Edwards & Banyard, 2022; Spencer et al., 2019). Individuals who experienced child abuse are more vulnerable to experiencing sexual assault and physical partner violence than children who were not abused (Basile & Smith, 2011).

Findings from WHO's Multi-country Study on Women's Health and Domestic Violence identified secondary education, high socioeconomic status (SES), and formal marriage as factors that offer protection from IPV. Alcohol abuse, cohabitation, young age, attitudes supportive of violence, outside sexual partners, and experience with or perpetration of other forms of violence in adulthood are factors that increased the risk for IPV (Clare et al., 2021; Yakubovich et al., 2018). A systematic review indicated that unplanned pregnancy and having parents with less than a high school education were risk factors and being older or married were protective (Yakubovich et al., 2018). People with disabilities have a greater risk of sexual violence than those without any (Mailhot Amborski et al., 2022). Women with disabilities are at greater risk for rape victimization and men with disabilities are at greater risk of being made to penetrate another (Basile et al., 2016). Women with disabilities are also at higher risk for IPV than women who do not have disabilities (García-Cuéllar et al., 2023). A woman's risk of being killed by an intimate partner is increased by the perpetrator's access to a gun or previous threat with a weapon, the perpetrator's stepchild in the household, perpetrator's previous and current estrangement from their partner (Milner et al., 2017; Spencer & Stith, 2020). Similarly, James

and colleagues (2013) found that abuse before pregnancy and lower education level were strong predictors of abuse during pregnancy. An association exists between abuse while pregnant and unintentional pregnancy, lower SES, and single marital status. A longitudinal study of women during pregnancy and for 6 weeks after birth found that partner alcohol misuse was a risk factor for women's IPV victimization during pregnancy and that stress may increase the risk for IPV (Hellmuth, 2013). For example, the abusive partner may discontinue violence while their partner is pregnant.

Reasons posited for why abusers are violent include violence in the family of origin, alcohol and drug use, and mental illness or character defects. Thus far, the science does not align with these hypotheses. A meta-analytic review noted that control, power, jealousy, and patriarchal beliefs were significantly stronger risk markers for IPV in clinical samples (Love et al., 2020). Risk factors for identifying perpetrators of partner homicide include having direct access to a gun, perpetrator's previous nonfatal strangulation, perpetrator's previous rape of the survivor, perpetrator's previous threat with a weapon, the perpetrator's demonstration of controlling behaviors, and the perpetrator's previous threats to harm the survivor (Aldridge & Browne, 2003; Spencer & Stith, 2020). Risk factors for male perpetration of IPV include substance abuse; growing up in a violent home/witnessing violence at an early age; gendered motivations to aggressive behavior, socioeconomic norms, and conditioning;, and access to firearms (Clare et al., 2021).

Females were more likely to experience dating violence as survivors and perpetrators with substance use and risky sexual behaviors as increased risk factors (Duval et al., 2020). Factors associated with increased risk for sexual assault included nonheterosexual identity, difficulty paying for basic necessities, fraternity/sorority membership, participation in more casual sexual encounters ("hook-ups") versus exclusive/monogamous or no sexual relationships, binge drinking, and experiencing sexual assault before college (Mellins et al., 2017, p. 2). The study of rapists has yielded four major typologies: power reassurance, power assertive, angry retaliatory, and anger excitation. The power reassurance rapist is also referred to as the gentleman rapist. He is the least violent and most common offender. He uses the assault to bolster his masculinity and self-esteem. The power assertive rapist is motivated by an ability to dominate another person. This rapist is sexually selfish and is not concerned about the survivor's emotional or physical well-being. The angry retaliatory rapist uses rape to punish women and express rage. These rapes are usually brutal and violent. The anger excitation rapist is a sadist who gets sexual gratification from inducing torture and suffering (Groth & Burgess, 1977; Hazelwood, 2017; Wojcik & Fisher, 2019). These typologies are useful for clinicians who care for offenders to understand their motivation.

HEALTH CONSEQUENCES OF INTIMATE PARTNER VIOLENCE

Violence against women is a significant public health issue costing society more than $4.1 billion in healthcare and mental health services for survivors (Smith et al., 2018). Injuries are common in IPV and sexual assault. The U.S. health-care community treats millions of intimate partner physical assaults and rapes annually, often unknown to the healthcare worker. Of the estimated 4.8 million intimate partner rapes and physical assaults perpetrated against women annually, approximately 2 million result in an injury to the survivor, and 552,192 result in some type of medical treatment for the survivor. Of the estimated 2.9 million intimate partner physical assaults perpetrated against men annually, 581,391 will result in an injury to the survivor, and 124,999 will result in some type of medical treatment for the survivor (Smith et al., 2018). Injury occurs in 36% of women who are raped, and in 41.5% of women and 19.9% of men who are physically assaulted by an intimate partner. Of those injured, most do not receive medical care.

The most common injuries received are minor, such as scratches, bruises, and welts. Common locations for genital injuries include tears or abrasions of the posterior fourchette, abrasion or bruising of the labia minora and fossa navicularis, and ecchymosis or tears of the hymen (Linden, 2011). A prospective study on sexual assault survivors presenting at an ED found that general body and genital trauma occurred in most cases (Keynejad et al., 2021). Finally, defensive injuries, such as lacerations, abrasions, and bruises, may be observed on the hands and the extensor surfaces of the arms and medial thighs.

Physical Health Consequences

The health consequences of experiencing physical, sexual, or psychological IPV can be found in every system of the body. A classic review by Campbell et al. (2003) reports that partner violence is associated with headache and back pain, vaginal infection and other gynecologic symptoms, and digestive problems. Common complaints of battered women include headaches, insomnia, choking sensations, hyperventilation, asthma, gastrointestinal symptoms, and chest, back, and pelvic pain (Keynejad et al., 2021). Many of the symptoms commonly seen are stress related. Other conditions are the result of the impact of IPV on the cardiovascular, gastrointestinal, endocrine, and immune systems through chronic stress or other mechanisms. Examples of health conditions associated with IPV include asthma, bladder and kidney infections, circulatory conditions, cardiovascular disease, fibromyalgia, irritable bowel syndrome, chronic pain syndromes, central nervous system disorders, gastrointestinal disorders, joint disease, migraines, and headaches (Basile et al., 2021; Black, 2011; Stubbs & Szoeke, 2022). Sexual assault is associated with a similar plethora of physical and mental health symptoms.

Strangulation is one of the most lethal forms of violence used against intimate partners. Asphyxia can induce loss of consciousness within about 10 seconds and death within 4 or 5 minutes. A person who was strangled can have substantial physical (dizziness, nausea, sore throat, voice changes, throat and neck injuries, breathing problems, ringing in ears, vision changes), neurologic (eyelid droop, facial droop, left- or right-side weakness, loss of sensation, loss of memory, paralysis), and psychological (posttraumatic stress disorder [PTSD], depression, insomnia) concerns (Sheridan & Nash,

2007). Strangulation is also a strong risk factor of homicide and an important factor to assess (Campbell, 2002).

Reproductive Health Consequences

Gynecologic problems are the most consistent, longest lasting, and largest physical health differences between women who experienced violence and those who did not. Women with abuse histories are more likely to report gynecologic problems, including abdominal pain, urinary problems, decreased sexual desire, and genital irritation (Musa, 2019). Differential symptoms and conditions include sexually transmitted infections (STIs), vaginal bleeding or infection, fibroids, decreased sexual desire, genital irritation, pain on intercourse, chronic pelvic pain, and urinary tract infections (Campbell, 2002). Sexual assault and rape are also associated with symptoms of vaginal itching, vaginal discharge, pain or discomfort, and fear of STIs and pregnancy.

Women who are abused during pregnancy are more likely to experience all forms of violence and to report injury, and are particularly likely to experience more severe forms of violence (Brownridge et al., 2011). Maternal exposure to IPV during pregnancy is associated with significantly increased risk of low birth weight and preterm birth (Shah & Shah, 2010). IPV coexisting with pregnancy is associated with late entry into prenatal care, low-birth-weight babies, premature labor, fetal trauma, and unhealthy maternal behavior (Jasinski, 2004; Shah & Shah, 2010). Adverse pregnancy outcomes, such as abortion, increased abortion rate, delayed prenatal care, fetal death, low birth weight, and preterm labor and delivery, are associated with IPV (Black, 2011). A systematic review identifies an association between experiencing IPV during pregnancy and perinatal death of the mother and fetus/neonate, specifically identified as outcomes such as low birth weight, miscarriage, perinatal death, and premature rupture of membranes (Pastor-Moreno et al., 2020). IPV is a strong risk factor for unintended pregnancy and abortion (Pallitto et al., 2013). Therefore, reducing IPV can significantly reduce risks to maternal and reproductive health. Sexual violence during pregnancy is significantly associated with increased reporting of pregnancy-related physical symptoms (Lukasse et al., 2012; Lutgendorf, 2019).

Mental Health

The experience of trauma triggers intense emotions and disintegrating effects on the mind. Myriad evidence suggests an association between IPV and depression, PTSD, and anxiety; the severity of mental health symptoms increases with the severity and extent of IPV exposure (Keynejad et al., 2021). Depression is the most common mental health symptom in response to violence. Anxiety is also a common consequence that often complicates the depression and continues for years after the traumatic experience. Lowered self-esteem often stems from self-blame. Substance use is common in survivors (Bacchus et al., 2018). Self-blame is influenced by society's victim-blaming regarding sexual violence (Ryan, 2019). Guilt and shame work to complicate the experience of depression. Substance use often starts as a way to self-medicate the pain of victimization (Ogden et al., 2022). Research on adolescents suggests an association of dating violence and substance abuse, unhealthy weight control, suicidality, depression, PTSD, general psychological distress, and low self-esteem (Amar & Gennaro, 2005; Bacchus et al., 2018).

DEPRESSION

The experience of violent victimization can bring about fear, uncertainty, vulnerability, and helplessness. Depression is a common psychological response to gender-based violence. Depressive symptoms include irritable or sad mood; lack of interest in or pleasure from most activities; significant changes in weight and/or appetite, activity, and sleep patterns; loss of energy and concentration; excessive feelings of guilt or worthlessness; and suicidality (American Psychiatric Association, 2013). The loss of energy, interest, and concentration may cause problems academically, socially, or professionally. Depression can result in suicidal ideation and suicide attempts. In women, IPV is associated with incident depressive symptoms and suicide attempts, and depressive symptoms with incident IPV. In men, few studies have been conducted, but evidence suggests that IPV is associated with incident depressive symptoms (Devries et al., 2013). A meta-analytic review found that women who were exposed to partner violence had greater risk of experiencing depressive symptoms and being diagnosed with a depressive disorder (Beydoun et al., 2012). Women with a history of sexual assault had a number of sleep difficulties, increased risk of depression, and overall poorer subjective well-being than their nonassaulted counterparts (Kendall-Tackett et al., 2013).

POSTTRAUMATIC STRESS DISORDER

PTSD may be an acute or chronic response to physical or sexual violence. To be diagnosed with PTSD an individual must have experienced, witnessed, or been confronted with a traumatic event and have characteristic resulting symptoms, usually within the subsequent 3 months. Resulting symptoms include (a) persistent reexperiencing of the event, (b) persistent avoidance of stimuli associated with the trauma, and (c) symptoms of increased arousal (American Psychiatric Association, 2013). Persistent reexperiencing of a traumatic event creates an intrusion to daily functioning. Survivors may experience flashbacks, nightmares, or other reenacting experiences. Avoidance behaviors are efforts to avoid feelings, thoughts, activities, places, and people associated with the traumatic event. Numbing behaviors, such as difficulty expressing feelings, lack of interest in pleasurable activities, or isolation from others, are another way to avoid the traumatic event. The restrictions may interfere with normal life functioning.

Other survivors may have symptoms of increased arousal. Hyperarousal symptoms include being extremely watchful of the environment, insomnia, and anger and rage. Individuals with increased arousal symptoms are constantly alert and on guard for signs of danger or trauma. Exposure to severe and uncontrollable stressors desensitizes a person to trauma; that is, the person is so used to being on edge that they may react to milder stressors with a major stress response. Intrusions, avoidance, and hyperarousal symptoms may persist for a long time after the attack and usually disrupt the individuals' interpersonal, social, or occupational function.

Many people who experience traumatic events do not develop PTSD. Lifetime prevalence estimates suggest that about 8% of the general population have PTSD, with women being twice as likely as men to have PTSD at some point during their lifetimes (Christiansen & Berke, 2020). Symptoms of PTSD often occur within 3 months of the stressor.

Acute stress disorder (ASD) is an immediate response to a traumatic event. ASD usually occurs within 1 month after the traumatic event. Individuals with ASD may experience dissociative symptoms, persistent reexperiencing of the event, marked avoidance, and marked arousal (American Psychiatric Association, 2013). Dissociative symptoms may occur during and after the trauma. They include numbing, detachment, reduced awareness of surroundings, depersonalization (feeling of lost identity), derealization (false perception that the environment is changed), and amnesia for important aspects of the trauma (American Psychiatric Association, 2013). These cognitive symptoms, during and after the trauma, provide an escape from the traumatic event by altering one's state of consciousness. The dissociative symptoms are not necessary for a diagnosis of PTSD. For a diagnosis of ASD, the symptoms must cause significant distress or impair functioning. Most people recover from ASD within a month; however, it is a significant predictor of PTSD (Garfin et al., 2018). If the symptoms are unresolved, then the diagnosis is changed to PTSD. The symptom profile of ASD is similar to that of PTSD. The main difference is that ASD has a shorter time of symptoms onset than PTSD. Past psychiatric history, peritraumatic dissociation, sexual assault with penetration, and ethnic background are risk factors of the development of ASD (Garcia-Esteve et al., 2021).

Interpersonal Difficulties

Interpersonal responses to violence include problems with intimacy. Violence with a known offender can lead to feelings of betrayal and difficulty trusting others (Hullenaar et al., 2022). Forced sex can lead to feelings of repulsion and lack of pleasure (Turchik & Hassija, 2014). Alternatively, forced sex has been associated with sexual risk taking such as promiscuity and unprotected sex (Johnson & Johnson, 2013; Turchik & Hassija, 2014). Social readjustment to the workplace seems to be the most difficult social impact of rape, and one study found productivity to suffer for up to 8 months after rape. Rape may be associated with deterioration of intimate relationships, which is often related to sexual problems or may stem from damage to beliefs such as those about the trustworthiness of others. Rape can also have a negative effect on the friends, family, and intimate partners of survivors, which further strains relationships (Basile & Smith, 2011).

HEALTHCARE USAGE AND PERCEPTIONS OF HEALTH

IPV and sexual violence have profound effects on the health of survivors that often translate to being heavy users of healthcare services. In a retrospective review of women who reported IPV in their lifetime, healthcare utilization was higher for all categories of service compared with women without IPV. Healthcare utilization decreased over time after the cessation of IPV; however, it was still 20% higher 5 years after the women's abuse ceased compared with women without IPV histories. It is estimated that the population economic burden from IPV is nearly $3.6 trillion over these survivors' lifetimes, based on 43 million U.S. adults with victimization histories (Peterson et al., 2018). This includes impaired health, lost productivity, and criminal justice costs. Additionally, the adjusted annual total healthcare costs were higher for women with a history of IPV compared with other women (Rivara et al., 2007). Higher heathcare costs among abused women were sustained for 3 years following the end of violence (Trabold et al., 2020).

In contrast, survivors of forced sex were less likely to have seen a physician for follow-up care than women who had not been sexually assaulted, and those who did seldom disclosed their assault to the provider (Short et al., 2021). However, rape creates additional costs to society. These include the direct costs of other services, including specialized nurse examiner programs in EDs, mental health services, criminal justice response, social services, and substance abuse treatment programs, as well as indirect costs such as estimates in dollars of the value of reduced quality of life for survivors (Basile & Smith, 2011).

EVALUATION/ASSESSMENT

Assessment Findings, Techniques, and Documentation

In clinical practice, clinicians routinely encounter survivors of gender-based violence. Providers should ask patients of all ages about current and past experiences of violence at every visit (Amar et al., 2013). Routine inquiry promotes and increases early identification of gender-based violence. Survivors may seek healthcare because of injuries; however, inquiries about violence should occur at every visit, regardless of the absence or presence of abuse indicators (Keynejad et al., 2021). The clinician should suspect abuse when the health visit is for ongoing emotional issues, drug or alcohol

misuse, repeated STIs, unexplained chronic pain, or repeated health consultations with no clear diagnosis (WHO, 2013). Screening can occur at annual visits, new patient visits, visits for new presenting complaints, prenatal and postnatal visits, and pediatric well- and sick-child visits (Amar et al., 2013; Keynejad et al., 2021). The interview should be conducted in private, and patients should be informed of any reporting requirements or limits to confidentiality. Patients are asked about current and lifetime exposure to IPV, including physical, emotional, and sexual abuse and sexual assault.

Building Rapport

The clinician must build rapport while assessing for violence. Verbal and nonverbal communication is a key component. It is important for the clinician to be direct, honest, and professional while using language that the patient understands. Table 42.1 provides communication tips. Survivors want someone who is sensitive, shows patience, respects their wishes, and supports their decision-making (Keynejad et al., 2021). Technical medical terms might be misinterpreted. For example, the clinician asks the survivor about choking rather than strangulation. Furthermore, individuals may answer affirmatively that they have experienced violent behaviors yet not identify themselves as abused, battered, or raped. Sample questions include, "Has your partner ever hit, shoved, or otherwise physically hurt you? Is your partner very jealous or controlling? Has your partner made you have sex when you didn't want to?" These questions are direct, gender neutral, and useful for identifying IPV (Heron & Eisma, 2021).

Verbal communication is important; however, nonverbal communication is equally important to assess. Behavioral clues from the survivor can be indicative of exposure to violence. For example, if a person cowers or flinches in response to touch, the clinician should suspect violence. Aspects of one's appearance can be used to conceal injuries. For example, hair in the face or makeup could be used to conceal bruises. Multiple injuries in various stages of healing should also raise suspicion and prompt the nurse to assess further. Another potential indicator of abuse is a mismatch between the injury and the story of how it happened (WHO, 2014; e.g., being told that multiple injuries to the chest and face resulted from a fall).

TABLE 42.1 Assessing for Violence: Communication Tips

DO	DON'T
Separate partners	Try to prove abuse by accusations or demands
Conduct the interview in private	Display horror, shock, anger, or disapproval
Be direct, honest, and professional	Place blame or make judgments
Use language the patient understands and ask about behaviors	Probe or press for answers that patient is not willing to give
Be understanding and attentive	Try to "prove" abuse using accusations or demands
Listen actively	Display horror, shock, anger, or disapproval

Safety Concerns

Because of the dynamics of abuse and concern for safety, it is important to interview the patient alone, separate from their partner. Interviews with an abusive partner present can result in the partner dominating the interview and the survivor being too fearful of retaliation to disclose. One large urban hospital evaluated the use of a computerized screening protocol for patients during the wait for services in the ED. Compared with face-to-face interviews, screening for IPV using the computerized tool has greater feasibility and acceptability in detection and disclosure of IPV along with the ability to integrate education and referrals (Anderson et al., 2021). Once a patient discloses violence, safety should be determined. Questions to assess immediate safety include:

- Are you in immediate danger?
- Do you have somewhere safe to go?
- Are you afraid your life is in danger?
- Has the violence gotten worse or scarier?
- Has your partner ever threatened to kill you, the children, or themself?

On receiving affirmative answers, the clinician should follow up with direct questions to determine the risk of danger. Safety assessments should be repeated at every follow-up visit (Groves et al., 2002).

Screening Tools

Several tools have been developed and tested for use in identifying gender-based violence in a variety of settings. Screening tools are available and clearly described on the Futures Without Violence website (www.futureswithoutviolence.org). The Abuse Assessment Screen (AAS) is a quick, easy-to-use measure that is effective in identifying IPV (Laughon et al., 2008). This widely used questionnaire contains four questions on a range of violent behaviors, one of which asks about abuse during pregnancy. Male and female body maps are available to document injuries. In addition to assessing for past-year IPV, it assesses for sexual violence from any person and asks about fear, which could include current stalking threats.

For women who screen positive for IPV, the danger assessment (DA) can help the provider to determine the woman's risk of being killed by IPV (Milner et al., 2017). The provider needs to know the risk of homicide to determine the urgency and types of referrals to make. There are four levels of danger: variable risk, increased danger, severe danger, and extreme danger. High DA scores are associated with a greater risk of lethal violence. However, low scores do not mean that there is no risk. Rather, low scores are indicative of unknown risk. The nurse and survivor should review the findings together. It is important that survivors be aware of and appreciate the lethal risk of their partner's behavior. Significant factors to consider in determining the patient's safety are any increases in frequency and severity of the violence, threats of homicide or suicide, presence of firearms or weapons in the home, increased drug or alcohol use, and attempts or separation from or plans to leave the partner (Campbell et al., 2017). Subsequent discussion with the woman should center on identifying resources and strategies for safety. If the woman

is ready, discussions can also address leaving the partner or ending the relationship. The clinician respects the woman's choice and works with her to support her wishes and keep her safe.

Clinical red flags for reproductive coercion include inconsistent or no contraception use, frequent requests for emergency contraception, and frequent visits for pregnancy and STI testing (Miller & McCaw, 2019). If reproductive coercion is suspected, the clinician should assess the women's pregnancy intention and ask direct questions regarding her partner's behavior. Assessing for other acts of violence is indicated for developing a comprehensive plan of action.

WHO recommends that providers should listen, inquire, validate, enhance safety, and support; the letters in the word LIVES can help providers remember (WHO, 2014). Listening is important for communicating positive regard, understanding, and attentiveness. The clinician inquires as necessary to determine and respond to emotional, physical, social, and practical needs. Inquiring does not mean probing and making the women recount details and unnecessarily relive the trauma. Rather, the clinician gathers only the information needed to plan care. Validation shows the survivor that the clinician understands and believes what is being said. Enhancing safety is done by discussing a plan to prevent harm in future violence, and support is provided by giving referrals to services, information, and support (WHO, 2013). Building rapport and a therapeutic relationship are the cornerstones that enable the clinician to work with the survivor to meet health and psychosocial needs.

Documentation

It is important to document the patient encounter. Documentation should include the patient's statements regarding the abuse, chief complaint, relevant history, results of physical examination, diagnostic procedures, and results of assessment, intervention, and referrals (Keynejad et al., 2021).

TREATMENT/MANAGEMENT

Focused Interventions

Focused intervention must follow routine screening. Patients who present for treatment after IPV episodes should receive immediate attention and care to treat their physical injuries. Once the medical or physical needs are attended to, the clinician can attend to safety and self-esteem needs. Abuse can erode the survivor's sense of self, and therefore the clinician is intentional in attempts to boost self-esteem. For example, the clinician can remind the survivor that it is not her fault. A critical area for assessment is determining the survivor's level of safety and planning strategies to maintain safety (Amar et al., 2013). Assessing and planning for safety is an ongoing process rather than a one-time event. Each visit represents an opportunity to reevaluate safety and to determine any immediate risk of harm. If it is not safe for a survivor to return home, the clinician should discuss options such as safe housing choices in domestic violence shelters or staying with friends and family. It is also useful to talk about legal resources such as the police and protective orders. Referrals to social workers can be helpful in identifying community resources. In addition, clinicians can contact the local hotline to learn of community resources. If the survivor does not wish to leave the relationship, the clinician respects her wishes and does not try to coerce her to leave. Rather, the clinician should help her think about her safety at home. A discussion of an escape plan to be used for rapid escape in a crisis is essential. Questions such as "If you need to leave your home in a hurry, where would you go?" can be helpful.

Safety plans are used to help a survivor plan to leave the abusive partner. These plans are important because leaving an abusive partner increases the risk of being killed by the partner (Campbell & Messing, 2017). The clinician would make sure that the survivor understands that the increased risk of injury necessitates careful planning before leaving an abusive relationship. All patients in violent relationships should be engaged in a discussion of options and creation of a safety plan. Together, the clinician and survivor might consider options of places and people she can go to for help. For example, the survivor might keep spare keys, clothes, money, and important papers in a safe place with easy access after leaving. The clinician could provide referrals, phone numbers, and websites for external services and information. Although face-to-face interviews can be effective in planning for safety, the use of a computerized aid can improve the safety decision-making process related to IPV (Glass et al., 2022; Hegarty et al., 2019).

Most women eventually leave a partner; however, some women make multiple attempts before they successfully leave (McKibbin & Gill-Hopple, 2018). Leaving is a process, and survivors need time to prepare emotionally for the ending of the relationship. Some women are not interested in leaving the partner; they only want the abuse to stop. It is important that the clinician respects the woman's choices and not assume she will leave. The clinician can ask direct questions to determine the woman's needs and perception of most useful forms of help. Providing information on domestic violence and resources with each visit helps prepare the woman. It is also important to be careful with handouts. Pamphlets and handouts related to IPV can alert the partner to the disclosure and prompt retaliatory violence and increased controlling behavior. A phone number on a prescription pad can be safe, effective, and nonthreatening.

Referrals

Experiencing violence creates multiple issues that require a multidisciplinary approach. Often, clinicians work with social services and the criminal justice system to ensure that survivors' needs are met. Referrals to advocacy and counseling are beneficial. These services can link survivors with resources and have documented results in decreasing reabuse and increasing quality of life (Wathen & MacMillan, 2003). Referrals are an important mechanism for connecting the survivor with resources for health, safety, and social support (WHO, 2013). Examples include crisis lines, shelters, support groups, legal aid, and mental health programs. From a legal perspective, good documentation of injuries using body maps, photographs, and descriptions help with a court case.

Referral to community resources includes notification of law enforcement and hospital social workers, as well as the provision of numbers to the domestic violence hotline, IPV shelter, and IPV legal advocate (Glass et al., 2001).

Nursing Care of Sexual Assault Survivors

When a sexual assault survivor reports to the ED, they are evaluated for any injuries or physical problems. Injuries are treated. Once the survivor has been cleared as medically stable, the sexual assault nurse examiner (SANE), sexual assault response team (SART), or other trained professional responds and is involved in collecting forensic evidence, documenting assessment findings, and connecting the survivor to resources and support (Linden, 2011). The gathering of forensic evidence is a critical element of postrape care for women who want to pursue legal action. Using a special kit, the healthcare worker collects, documents, and turns over to law enforcement the evidence for processing and legal action. The survivor is offered testing and prophylactic treatment for STIs and pregnancy. There is also a legal obligation to provide court testimony if the case goes to trial. The SANE is specifically trained to respond in a supportive and sensitive manner to individuals who have experienced trauma. The nurses who provide these services have undergone specialized training in the collection of forensic evidence, assessment and treatment of STIs and HIV, crisis intervention, and rape trauma syndrome (Adams & Hulton, 2016; Basile & Smith, 2011).

Crisis strategies, such as building rapport, encouraging verbalization of feelings, supporting existing coping strategies, helping mobilize social support systems, and providing referrals to resources, are used. It is important for all nurses to be aware of the available community resources. These include local and national hotlines, state coalitions, rape crisis centers, and web-based resources. The resources are designed primarily to support survivors. However, providers may call to get advice on ways to approach the survivor, resources available in the community, and management strategies.

Prevention/Intervention

An overarching consideration is the inclusion of trauma-informed care (TIC), which is a primary framework that emphasizes the effects of trauma and guides the entire organization and behavior of individuals in the system (Hopper et al., 2010). TIC services are those in which service delivery is influenced by an understanding of the impact of interpersonal violence and victimization on an individual's life and development. All staff of an organization, from the receptionist to direct care workers to the board of directors, must understand the influence of violence and trauma so that every interaction is consistent with the recovery process and reduces the possibility of retraumatization. Integrated services include core areas of outreach and engagement, screening and assessment, resource coordination and advocacy, crisis intervention, mental health and substance abuse services, trauma-specific services, parenting support, and healthcare.

Strategies for promoting a TIC system begin with education and training at all levels of the organization. Training helps the staff recognize that many of the problematic behaviors seen by survivors result from the trauma, often as means of coping with the abuse. This understanding shifts the focus from "What's wrong with you?" to "What happened to you?" The goal is to create a safe environment that minimizes the possibility of retraumatization. For example, when performing routine health assessments, the clinician recognizes the potential to trigger feelings of loss of control over one's body and provides detailed information on what will occur during the procedure. A TIC system is structured and organized to accommodate the vulnerabilities of trauma survivors and promotes service delivery in a manner that avoids inadvertent retraumatization and facilitates patient participation in treatment (Sperlich et al., 2021). Screening for and responding to IPV and sexual violence in primary care with a trauma-informed approach can promote health and healing for survivors (Palmieri & Valentine, 2021). Incorporating knowledge about trauma in all aspects of service delivery ensures that treatment minimizes revictimization while facilitating recovery and empowerment. Limited evidence is available on treatment and intervention for LGBTQ populations; more research is needed (MacGregor et al., 2021).

Interventions used for IPV take a psychoeducational approach coupled with referrals. Most programs teach women about the cycle of violence and safety-promoting behaviors. Referrals are provided for local community-based IPV services, as well as other agencies for additional services. However, a systematic review of interventions targeting IPV showed that most programs focus on empowerment, safety, and community referrals and demonstrate patient-level benefits (Bair-Merritt et al., 2014). The empowerment model provides a foundation for intervention that increases autonomy, reduces violence, decreases mental health issues, and increases well-being. This approach provides support from trained individuals, referrals to community resources, and engagement in harm reduction strategies (Trabold et al., 2020). Limited success is demonstrated from programs targeting women in decreasing partner violence and from programs targeting gender-based violence during pregnancy. A systematic review found that home visitation programs and multifaceted counseling interventions show promising effects for decreasing physical, sexual, and psychological violence and IPV during pregnancy (Van Parys et al., 2014). Cognitive behavioral couples' treatment has been found to reduce IPV (Stith et al., 2022). In addition, a Cochrane Review also found insufficient evidence to assess the effectiveness of interventions for domestic violence on pregnancy outcomes (Jahanfar et al., 2013). Limited research demonstrates evidence-based strategies for reproductive coercion. However, Miller et al. (2011) report that an intervention with a trained family planning specialist decreased pregnancy coercion.

Digital interventions may clinically reduce mental health symptoms and IPV (Emezue & Bloom, 2021). Jack and colleagues (2021) provided practical guidelines for telehealth that prioritize safety and promote privacy for IPV survivors along with assessment, planning, and intervention. Ford-Gilboe and colleagues (2020) found that a tailored online intervention showed promise for reducing barriers to support and improved outcomes. Mobile health technologies are commonly used for screening, education, and safety decision aids. A major strength is the ability to tailor interventions to individual needs within the mobile platform (Anderson et al., 2021).

Another intervention strategy is to target men who abuse. Court-mandated batterer intervention programs are the most commonly used option. Most programs use the Duluth model, which focuses on power and control (Paymar & Pence, 1993). Group therapy, psychoeducation, and a profeminist approach are common elements of most programs (Tarzia et al., 2020). Evidence supporting the effectiveness of batterer intervention programs is small from the perpetrator perspective and nonexistent when survivor perspective is considered (Feder & Wilson, 2005). Problems with these programs include the lack of non–English-language programs and a one-size-fits-all approach (Price & Rosenbaum, 2009). Limited benefit is seen for programs including substance abuse treatment as part of batterer intervention (Stephens-Lewis et al., 2021). One strategy that holds promise is the risk-need responsivity framework that provides treatment intensity focused on the individual risk (Travers et al., 2021). The court-mandated approach, while appropriate, does not ensure that perpetrators are emotionally committed to the effort required to make and sustain behavioral change.

Gender-based violence is violence directed atagainst a person because of their gender. IPV and sexual assault are two forms of gender-based violence that have significant health consequences for affected girls and women. Gender-based violence is an important public health and societal issue that requires major effort to eradicate. Because IPV and sexual violence affect the psychological and physical health of survivors, both increase the likelihood of contact with nurses in varied areas of healthcare. Clinicians' understanding of the societal norms and attitudes regarding violence and the dynamics of abuse is crucial for providing the needed care. Clinicians should screen for violence and its related consequences and provide counseling and referrals to survivors of gender-based violence.

REFERENCES

References for this chapter are online and available at https://connect.springerpub.com/content/book/978-0-8261-6722-4/part/part03/chapter/ch42

CHAPTER 43

Cardiovascular Disease in Women*

Kristin A. Bott, Sandra Biolo, Maria Cutrali, Annette Jakubisin-Konicki, and Joanne Thanavaro

All women face the threat of developing cardiovascular disease (CVD) regardless of race or ethnicity. CVD remains the leading cause of death in both men and women in the United States and is the leading global cause of death; 17.9 million people die each year from CVD (World Health Organization [WHO], 2021). In 2020, approximately 19 million deaths were attributed to CVD globally, which was an increase of 18.7% from 2010 (Tsao et al., 2022). In 2017, CVD accounted for 418,665 deaths in women in the United States, with more women than men dying each year of CVD (Elder et al., 2020).

Furthermore, CVD is associated with significant health and financial burden; the estimated direct and indirect cost was $363.4 billion in 2016–2017. The estimated direct costs of CVD increased from $103.5 billion in 1996–1997 to $216.0 billion in 2016–2017. Hospital inpatient stays accounted for the highest direct costs ($96.2 billion) in 2016 to 2017 (Virani et al., 2021).

In the United States, about 43 million women are living with some form of CVD or the aftereffects of stroke, and the population at risk is considerably larger (Mozaffarian et al., 2015). In addition to this significant number of women with known CVD, many women remain poorly informed or uninformed about their cardiovascular risk, particularly those who are either younger or of a minoritized ethnic group (Smith et al., 2018), leading to missed opportunities to prevent or minimize the effects of a major cardiac event. Despite an increase in awareness of heart disease as the leading cause of death in women, only 56% of women recognize it as a major health threat (Mosca et al., 2013). Among women in higher risk groups, specifically minoritized racial/ethnic groups, this lack of awareness was more profound, with only 36% of Black and 34% of Hispanic females aware of the significance of CVD in women (Mosca et al., 2013).

In response to the COVID-19 pandemic, the American Heart Association (AHA) temporarily set aside the 2030 Impact Goal of increasing life expectancy and commissioned a new goal with a shortened timeline of deliverables by 2024. The new goal specifically commits to giving special attention to the needs of those at greatest risk of poor health. To advance cardiovascular health in this short time frame, the AHA emphasized specific strategies that address health equity in blood pressure control and tobacco/nicotine exposure (Lloyd-Jones et al., 2021).

DEFINITION AND SCOPE OF CARDIOVASCULAR DISEASE

CVD is defined as a vascular disease affecting all blood vessels in the body, including those in the brain (cerebrovascular disease), kidneys (renal vascular disease), and extremities (peripheral vascular disease). Structural heart disease affects cardiac muscle and valves and can lead to other conditions of vascular dysfunction, such as hypertension (HTN) and conduction defects causing arrhythmias. In this chapter, the emphasis is on atherosclerosis, a disease process resulting in the formation of plaques typically composed of cholesterol, fat, calcium, and other substances building up on the endothelium, creating a thickening, hardening, and narrowing of the arteries. This narrowing results in a limitation of the flow of oxygen-rich blood to the body and leading to ischemic changes and infarction, or tissue death.

Since 1948, the Framingham Heart Study, funded by the National Institutes of Health, has supported the assessment of the epidemiology and risk factors for CVD. From these longitudinal data, investigators were able to identify major risk factors or general patterns that would suggest a likelihood of developing heart diseases (Andersson et al., 2021).

Although CVD was historically considered a "man's disease," it is now understood to be the leading cause of death in women. Women lag behind men by 10 to 12 years in CVD incidence (Mozaffarian et al., 2015). The lifetime risk at age 50 years of developing CVD is approximately 51.1% in men and 39.2% in

---

*This chapter is a revision of the chapter that appeared in the second edition of this textbook, authored by Tina M. Chasse Mulinski, Karin V. Nyström, and Catherine G. Winkler, and we thank them for their original contribution.

women, which nears a comparable risk between the genders with aging (Lloyd-Jones et al., 2006; Novella et al., 2012).

Although there has been progress in understanding the significance and difference in presentation of CVD in women, gender differences in pathobiology, clinical symptoms, medication management, risk identification and prevention, treatment, and prognosis are still not fully understood. Dramatic decreases in the mortality rate associated with heart disease has been observed in men and women, particularly those >65 years of age. Despite these decreases, morbidity and mortality data for women <55 years of age have stagnated (Wilmot et al., 2015).

While enrollment of women in cardiovascular clinical trials has increased, a systematic review demonstrated that there remains a predominance of men participants (Tsang et al., 2012) that potentially limit the generalizability of findings. Research on women is increasing with evaluation of female-predominant and female-specific risks (Elder et al., 2020); but, on average, mixed-gender trials represent women in less than a third of all participants (Saeed et al., 2017). Even fewer research studies include transgender persons; thus, there is a dearth of data regarding CVD and CVD risks among them. Due to this lack of data, the terms *woman* and *women* are used in this chapter to reflect evidence known about CVD in female persons. Whenever available, data regarding transgender persons are included. Further study is needed to uncover nuances of CVD among transgender men and transgender women and on effects related to gender-affirming hormone therapy (GAHT).

CARDIOVASCULAR RISK FACTORS

Recognizing the high burden of CVD among women, the AHA, the American College of Cardiology (ACC), and other organizations in 2004 sponsored an expert panel to develop guidelines for CVD prevention in women. These guidelines were subsequently updated in 2011 (Mosca et al., 2011) and were modified from evidence-based to effectiveness-based recommendations. This change acknowledged the benefits and risks observed in clinical practice or the *effectiveness* of preventive therapies, which is different from efficacy or *evidence* of benefits observed in clinical research alone (Mosca et al., 2011). Figure 43.1 shows CVD risk factors in women and Figure 43.2 depicts the flow diagram for evaluation of risks.

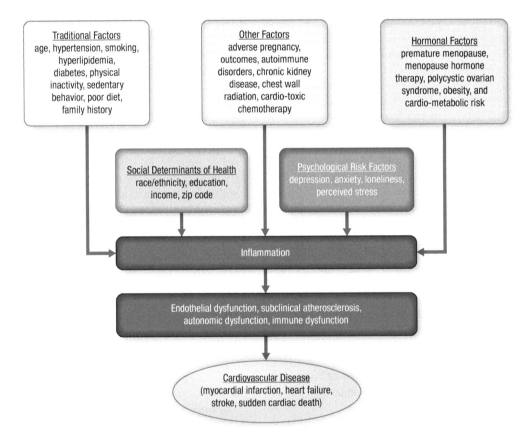

FIGURE 43.1 Cardiovascular disease (CVD) risk factors in women.
The factors shown in dark gray are incorporated in the atherosclerotic cardiovascular disease risk calculator. However, there are unique sex-specific factors as well as psychosocial factors that contribute to CVD risk and adverse outcomes.
Source: Cho, L., Davis, M., Elgendy, I., Epps, K., Lindley, K. J., Mehta, P. K., Michos, E. D., Minissian, M., Pepine, C., Vaccarino, V., Volgman, A. S., & ACC CVD Women's Committee Members. (2020). Summary of updated recommendations for primary prevention of cardiovascular disease in women: JACC state-of-the-art review. Journal of the American College of Cardiology, 75(20), 2602–2618. *https://doi .org/10.1016/j.jacc.2020.03.060*

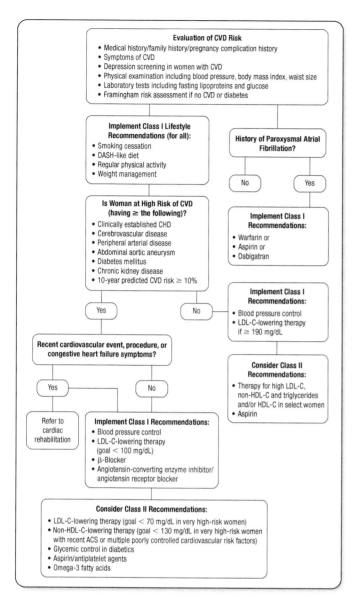

FIGURE 43.2 Evaluation of CVD risk.
ACS, acute coronary syndrome; CHD, coronary heart disease; CVD, cardiovascular disease; DASH, Dietary Approaches to Stop Hypertension; HDL-C, high-density lipoprotein cholesterol; LDL-C, low-density lipoprotein cholesterol.
Source: Mosca, L., Benin, E. J., Berra, K., Benzanon, J. L., Dolor, R. J., Lloyd-Jones, D. M., Newby, L. K., Piña, I. L., Roger, V. L., Shaw, L. J., Zhao, D., Beckie, T. M., Bushnell, C., D'Armiento, J., Kris-Etherton, P. M., Fang, J., Ganiats, T. G., Gomes, A. S., Gracia, C. R., . . . Wenger, N. K. (2011). Effectiveness-based guidelines for the prevention of cardiovascular disease in women—2011 update. Circulation, 123(11), 1243–1262. https://doi.org/10.1161/CIR.0b013e31820faaf8

In 2019 ACC/AHA primary prevention guidelines were updated for the general population. That same year the ACC CVD in Women Committee undertook a review of the 2019 primary prevention guidelines and major studies to summarize recommendations pertaining to women. In this update, topics were addressed that were specifically sex-related factors for CVD related to HTN, diabetes mellitus (DM), hyperlipidemia (HLD), anticoagulation in atrial fibrillation (AF), use of aspirin, menopausal hormone therapy, and psychosocial issues (Cho et al., 2020).

Cardiovascular risk factors can be categorized as traditional factors previously referred to as modifiable and nonmodifiable factors (age, HTN, smoking, HLD, DM, physical inactivity, sedentary behavior, poor diet, family history), other factors (adverse pregnancy outcomes, autoimmune disorders, chronic kidney disease [CKD], chest wall radiation, cardiotoxic chemotherapy), hormonal factors (premature menopause, menopause hormone therapy, polycystic ovary syndrome, obesity, and cardiometabolic risk), and psychosocial risk factors (depression, anxiety, loneliness, perceived stress). Psychological factors tend to be more of a risk for cardiometabolic disease in women than in men. Figure 43.1 depicts the most up-to-date assessment of CVD risk factors in women (Cho et al., 2020).

Classification of CVD in women is now based on the 2011 guidelines, with modifications that incorporate the new concept of "ideal cardiovascular health" as the baseline and two more categories listed as "at risk," defined as one or more major risk factors, and "high risk," or one or more high-risk states (Mosca et al., 2011). The new classification table includes the Framingham CVD risk profile and includes evolving factors that are unique to women and which may be associated with developing CVD (Table 43.1).

Traditional Risk Factors

AGE AND GENDER

The prevalence of heart disease in women rises sharply after menopause (Novella et al., 2012). Part of this increase is attributed to decreased endogenous estrogen (Novella et al., 2012). Other age-associated risk factors may also play a role. The onset of CVD at an older age is associated with a higher incidence of comorbid conditions, additional cardiovascular risk factors, and other disease states, including collagen vascular diseases or autoimmune problems (Gopalakrishnan et al., 2009).

Transgender persons are also at increased risk. As of 2016, there were approximately 1.4 million people in the United States identifying as transgender. The Behavioral Risk Factor Surveillance System data from 2014–2017 were used to evaluate the cross-sectional association between being transgender and the reported history of myocardial infarction (MI) and CVD risk factors. A regression model was constructed to study the association between being transgender and MI after adjusting for CVD risk factors including age, DM, HTN, HLD, CKD, smoking, and exercise. The transgender population had a higher rate of MI in comparison to the cisgender population overall; however, the increased risk did not occur in transgender women compared to cisgender men. Future studies among transgender persons are required to further address this increased risk (Alzahrani et al., 2019).

FAMILY HISTORY/GENETICS

A family history of premature CVD has been defined as the onset of CVD in a first-degree relative before the age of 55 years for men and 65 years for women (Mulders et al., 2011). These age-based cutoff points were selected based on the recommendations of the National Cholesterol Education Program (NCEP) Expert Panel on Detection, Evaluation, and Treatment of High Blood Cholesterol in Adults (2002) and Seventh Joint National Committee (JNC) on Prevention, Detection, Evaluation, and Treatment of High Blood Pressure

TABLE 43.1 Cardiovascular Disease Risk Classification for Women

RISK STATUS	CRITERIA
Ideal cardiovascular health (women who meet all criteria)	Total cholesterol <200 mg/dL (without treatment) Blood pressure <120/< 80 mmHg (without treatment) Fasting blood sugar <100 mg/dL (without treatment) Body mass index <25 kg/m² Smoking abstinence Goal physical activity for adults >20 years old: Moderate intensity ≥150 minutes/week Vigorous intensity >75 minutes/week or combination of moderate and vigorous Dietary Approaches to Stop Hypertension (DASH)–like, healthy diet
At risk (women with ≥1 major risk factor[s])	Advanced subclinical atherosclerosis (e.g., carotid plaque, thickened intima-media thickness, coronary calcifications) Blood pressure ≥120/≥80 mmHg Dyslipidemia, treated High-density lipoprotein cholesterol <50 mg/dL History of cardiovascular disease in a first-degree relative: Women <65 years of age Men <55 years of age Hypertension, treated Inactivity Metabolic syndrome Obesity (especially central adiposity) Poor diet Poor treadmill test exercise capacity and/or abnormal heart rate recovery after ceasing exercise Prior preeclampsia, gestational diabetes, or pregnancy-induced hypertension Smokes cigarettes Autoimmune collagen-vascular disease, systemic (e.g., rheumatoid arthritis or lupus) Total cholesterol ≥200 mg/dL
High risk (women with ≥1 high-risk states)	10-year predicted cardiovascular disease risk ≥10% Abdominal aortic aneurysm Cerebrovascular disease, clinically manifest Chronic or end-stage kidney disease Coronary heart disease, clinically manifest Diabetes mellitus Peripheral arterial disease, clinically manifest

Source: Adapted from Mosca, L., Benin, E. J., Berra, K., Benzanon, J. L., Dolor, R. J., Lloyd-Jones, D. M., Newby, L. K., Piña, I. L., Roger, V. L., Shaw, L. J., Zhao, D., Beckie, T. M., Bushnell, C., D'Armiento, J., Kris-Etherton, P. M., Fang, J., Ganiats, T. G., Gomes, A. S., Gracia, C. R., . . . Wenger, N. K. (2011). Effectiveness-based guidelines for the prevention of cardiovascular disease in women—2011 update. Circulation, 123(11), 1243–1262. https://doi.org/10.1161/CIR.0b013e31820faaf8

(JNC 7; Chobanian et al., 2003). Furthermore, a paternal history of premature heart attack has been shown to approximately double the risk of a heart attack in men and increase the risk in women by approximately 70% (Lloyd-Jones et al., 2004; Sesso et al., 2001). Premature CVD can also factor into some modifiable risk factors, including dyslipidemia, HTN, and DM. Therefore, it is difficult to assess exactly what percentage of CVD is directly related to the family history versus modifiable risk factors.

Other than markers for familial hypercholesterolemia (FH), genetic markers for CVD are still under investigation and have not been shown to add to cardiovascular risk predictions beyond the current models that include family history (Holmes et al., 2011). They have not been used yet to improve the prediction of subclinical atherosclerosis beyond the traditional risk factors (Hernesniemi et al., 2012). An association has been demonstrated between genetic markers and coronary artery calcification (Thanassoulis et al., 2012). Emerging evidence indicates a causal association between lipoprotein (a), a significantly genetic influenced proatherogenic low-density lipoprotein and atherosclerotic CVD (ASCVD) and thus an inherited cardiovascular risk factor (Cesaro et al., 2021).

SMOKING

Tobacco use continues to be the leading preventable risk factor for CVD in women. Over the past half century, the risk of death from cigarette smoking continued to rise among women, with an overall increase from all causes to include lung cancer, chronic obstructive pulmonary disease (COPD), stroke, and CVD; the risk is now nearly identical in men and women, compared with those who do not smoke (Huxley & Woodward, 2011). Smoking has been associated with half of all coronary events in women. Among adult women, those who smoke include White women (19%), Native American/Alaskan Native women (17%), Black women (15%), Hispanic women (7%), and Asian women (5%). There were approximately 6,300 new cigarette smokers every day based on an estimate in 2012 (Mozaffarian et al., 2015). Cigarette smoke affects not only smokers. Secondhand smoke can cause chronic respiratory conditions, cancer, and heart disease. Approximately 34,000 nonsmokers die from heart disease each year because of exposure to environmental tobacco smoke (U.S. Department of Health and Human Services, 2014).

Electronic cigarette products are another potential concern with respect to cardiovascular health. Since e-cigarettes are a relatively new product, data are still limited. Many e-cigarettes deliver larger dosages of nicotine and other by-products that are more detrimental to health than those of conventional cigarettes (Grana et al., 2014). Patterns of use need to be considered because e-cigarettes are often marketed as a smoking-cessation aid. However, many individuals use both e-cigarettes and conventional cigarettes, with no proven cessation benefits. Data do not demonstrate a lower disease burden for either CVD or lung disease with e-cigarette use, since dose delivery is inconsistent, use patterns vary, chemical substrates in the e-cigarette chamber are proving to cause significant lung disease, and nicotine addiction remains a public health problem.

Marijuana use has been associated with threefold greater mortality rate after acute MI; the risk increased with more frequent use (Mukamal et al., 2008). A more recent study followed 5,113 adults ages 18 to 30 for more than 25 years. Neither cumulative lifetime nor recent use of marijuana was associated with CVD incidence in middle age (Reis et al., 2017).

The combination of smoking with oral contraceptive use has a synergistic effect on risk of acute MI, stroke, and venous thromboembolism (Garcia et al., 2016). More cardiovascular data on the latest generation of contraceptive hormone formulations, including those that contain newer progestins that lower blood pressure and have nonoral routes (transdermal and vaginal), will need to be followed in the context of other cardiovascular risk factors, including smoking. More important, smoking cessation dramatically reduces mortality rates from all major smoking-related diseases, and it is never too late to quit.

OBESITY

More than two in three adults in the United States are overweight or obese, and the prevalence of obesity is higher among women than men. The effect of obesity on the risk of developing coronary artery disease (CAD) appears to be greater in women than in men. In the Framingham Heart Study, obesity increased the relative risk of CAD by 64% in women as compared to 46% in men. The recommended body mass index for women is to be less than 25 kg/m² to promote heart health (Mosca et al., 2011). Weight gain in the adult years is highly related to developing a greater CVD risk factor burden; this has been observed with relatively modest weight gain in prospective studies (Garcia et al., 2016).

Many comorbid conditions and CVD risk factors are associated with obesity, including DM, CAD, sleep apnea, some cancers, HTN, low high-density lipoprotein cholesterol (HDL-C), elevated triglycerides, and elevated levels of inflammatory markers. The combination of risk factors makes it imperative to treat obesity, which itself has become a chronic disease. The rise in the obesity rate is a significant contributor to the growing epidemic of type 2 DM. It is important that clinicians address risk-reducing interventions to prevent and treat obesity with patients early and often (see Chapter 13, Nutrition for Women).

DIABETES AND HYPERGLYCEMIA

More than 13.4 million U.S. women have a diagnosis of DM, and 90% to 95% of these women have type 2 DM (T2DM). The rate of T2DM in Hispanic women is more than double when compared with non-Hispanic White women (12.7% vs. 6.45%, respectively). In a meta-analysis of over 850,000 individuals the risk of CVD in persons with DM was 44% greater in women than in men. Additionally, the risk for fatal CAD is threefold higher in women with T2DM compared to women without T2DM (Garcia et al., 2016).

The American Diabetes Association (ADA, 2016) has set aggressive treatment goals for persons with DM regarding cardiovascular risk factors such as dyslipidemia and HTN and indications for antiplatelet therapies. The 2020 ADA guidelines for the diagnosis and classification of DM recognized women with impaired fasting glucose levels (i.e., 100–125 mg/dL) and impaired glucose tolerance (i.e., 2-hour post glucose load of 140–199 mg/dL) as having *prediabetes*; these women are at the highest risk for developing DM and CVD. Though not classified as a clinical entity, prediabetes is strongly associated with dyslipidemia, HTN, and obesity (ADA, 2020). Mechanisms influenced by increased blood glucose levels, which raise the CVD risk in women, include endothelial dysfunction, promotion of atheroma, and thrombus formation as a result of platelet overactivity and hypercoagulability (Bell, 1995). Women with DM require intensive cardiovascular screening. This is also the case among women who develop gestational DM and preeclampsia, who are further prone to develop subsequent DM along with adverse CVD profiles (Wenger, 1999).

METABOLIC SYNDROME

Metabolic syndrome is a combination of five cardiometabolic risk factors, which increase the risk for developing CVD and DM and of mortality. These five factors are elevated blood pressure (BP), increased waist circumference, elevated fasting triglycerides, low high-density lipoprotein, and elevated blood glucose, which create a prothrombotic and a proinflammatory state. This syndrome doubles the risk for CVD in those without DM and increases the risk for T2DM in those without DM. Various attempts at a clinical definition of metabolic syndrome have evolved over the years. The most recent international consensus definition is the presence of three or more of these risk factors with or without abdominal obesity (Alberti et al., 2009).

The metabolic syndrome criteria are fasting plasma glucose of at least 100 mg/dL or on hyperglycemic medication, serum triglycerides of at least 150 mg/dL, serum HDL-C of less than 50 mg/dL for women, and BP of at least 130/85 mmHg or on BP medication. In the United States, the cutoff points of waist circumference of ≥88 cm in females are also included in making this clinical diagnosis. This condition is estimated to be present in 47 million Americans, with a similar prevalence in men (24%) and women (23%). However, the gender equality is lost when comparing within ethnic groups. Although there were fewer White women with metabolic syndrome than White men, there are 57% more Black women with metabolic syndrome than Black men and 26% more Mexican American women than Mexican American men. In addition, the National Health and Nutrition Examination Survey (NHANES) data demonstrated an age-adjusted increase in metabolic syndrome of 23.5% in women (*p* = .021) and only 2.2% among men (*p* = .831) from 1988–1994 to 1999–2000 (Bentley-Lewis et al., 2007). Changes in levels of glucose and insulin, lipid patterns, and inflammatory and thrombotic process occurring during the transition to postmenopause and postmenopause increases the prevalence of metabolic syndrome in females (Cho et al., 2008).

Women also have the specific circumstances of pregnancy and conditions such as polycystic ovary syndrome that need to be factored into their clinical care because these factors increase the risk of weight gain and metabolic syndrome. In contrast, lactation or nursing decreased the incidence of metabolic syndrome by 22% (95% CI 1–39%) among women who breastfed for more than 1 month compared with women who did not breastfeed or who breastfed for less than 1 month (Bentley-Lewis et al., 2007). As it is with obesity, it is important to have a discussion early with patients to prevent and/or limit the progression of the condition through a proper diet and exercise plan. See Chapter 44, Endocrine-Related Problems.

PHYSICAL INACTIVITY

Evidence supports positive outcomes in several health indicators for those engaging in routine physical activity, many of which mitigate the impact of CVD (Jakubisin Konicki, 2019).

Despite this evidence, national health statistic data indicate that 80% of Americans do not participate in the minimum recommended level of physical activity (Lobelo et al., 2018). More women (46%) than men (37%) have higher rates of inactivity (National Center for Health Statistics, 2018). This is alarming since physical inactivity is responsible for 12.2% of the global burden for MI after controlling for CVD risk factors such as smoking, HTN, obesity, lipid profile, psychosocial causes, and DM (Yusef et al., 2004). See Chapter 14, Healthy Practices: Physical Activity.

PSYCHOSOCIAL FACTORS INCLUDING EMOTIONAL STRESS

Psychosocial stress tends to be a more important risk factor for cardiometabolic diseases in women than in men. Women generally have higher exposures to psychosocial stress and adversity than men and are more vulnerable to the effects of such exposure. Depression is twofold more common in women than men, and affects approximately 7% of the population each year. A diagnosis of clinical depression in a woman is associated with a doubling of risk of CVD as well as being a risk factor for incident MI and cardiac death (Cho et al., 2020). Stress-induced Takotsubo cardiomyopathy is a condition that is unique to women; it occurs after menopause when there has been exposure to sudden, unexpected emotional or physical stress (Garcia et al., 2016). Accordingly, screening for depression has been added to the effectiveness-based guidelines for the prevention of CVD in women (Mosca et al., 2011). See Chapter 40, Mental Health Challenges.

Nontraditional Risk Factors

AUTOIMMUNE AND INFLAMMATORY CONDITIONS/CHRONIC ILLNESSES

Multiple studies have recognized an association between inflammatory disease and increased mortality. Autoimmune diseases create an immune response to self-antigens that result in damage or dysfunction of tissues. The microvasculature in women plays an important role in their predisposition to developing CVD. Females develop rheumatoid arthritis (RA) 2.5 times more than men, and systemic lupus erythematous (SLE) nine times more than men. People with RA have a two to three times greater risk of MI and 50% higher risk of stroke. For those with SLE, the risk of MI is increased nine to 50 times over the risk in the general population (Garcia et al., 2016). The link between autoimmune diseases and CVD, whether direct or indirect, is thought to be related to inflammation and to the damaging effects on the vasculature. Further studies are needed to clarify this relationship.

PREMATURE MENOPAUSE

Defined as menopause occurring before 40 years of age, premature menopause is associated with increased CVD risk. The interaction between menopause and CVD is complex; it may be that women at increased risk for CVD experience menopause at an earlier age and the decrease in estrogens at an earlier age likely play a role (Cho et al., 2020). More studies are needed to further identify this risk. See Chapter 9, Midlife Women's Health, and Chapter 34, Menopause.

POLYCYSTIC OVARY SYNDROME

Polycystic ovary syndrome (PCOS) is an endocrine disorder characterized by ovulatory dysfunction (oligomenorrhea or amenorrhea), hyperandrogenism, infertility, and insulin resistance. Women with PCOS have increased risk of developing metabolic syndrome. Although the 2018 cholesterol guidelines do not include PCOS as a risk enhancer, the international guidelines for PCOS recommend that all women with PCOS should be closely monitored for CVD risk (Cho et al., 2020). See Chapter 44, Endocrine-Related Problems.

PREGNANCY-RELATED DISORDERS

An increased risk for CVD is associated with various pregnancy-related complications. Some pregnancy-related complications increase CVD risk among women <50 years of age, while others have greater effect after menopause. As with all risk factors, a careful history is needed. In parous women, evaluating for a history of various pregnancy-related complications can help identify those with increased risk of CVD in midlife (Charlton et al., 2014; Savitz et al., 2014; Smith et al., 2012; Timpka et al., 2018). CVD prediction tools currently do not account for the risk associated with pregnancy-related complications and thus underestimate the risk for CVD in parous females (Maffei et al., 2019; Sciomer et al., 2018).

Preterm Delivery

Defined as birth <37 weeks' gestation, preterm delivery (PTD) complicates 5% to 12.7% of deliveries worldwide. PTD is an independent risk factor for long-term CV morbidity and CV related hospitalizations. CVD risk is further increased in those with early PTD <34 weeks' gestation (Garcia et al., 2016).

Hypertensive Pregnancy Disorders

These disorders include gestational HTN, chronic HTN, and preeclampsia. *Gestational HTN* is defined as new-onset HTN (>140/90 mmHg) after 20 weeks' gestation in pregnant persons who are originally normotensive. *Preeclampsia* is new-onset HTN (>140/90 mmHg) with proteinuria (0.3 g/24 hours) and/or end organ dysfunction after 20 weeks' gestation. Having had preeclampsia carries a 3.7-fold relative risk of developing HTN 14 years after pregnancy, a 2.16 relative risk of ischemic heart disease (IHD) after 12 years, and 1.79 relative risk of venous thromboembolism after 5 years. The earlier presentation of preeclampsia in pregnancy is associated with poorer outcomes and the severity is correlated with the severity of CVD later in life (Garcia et al., 2016). See Chapter 39, Intrapartum and Postpartum Care.

Gestational Diabetes

Gestational diabetes mellitus (GDM) describes pregnant persons who are newly diagnosed with DM beyond the first trimester. GDM raises the risk of developing T2DM sevenfold, which is a major risk for CVD. It also raises CVD risk (twofold for stroke, fourfold for MI) independently of developing T2DM (Garcia et al., 2016). See Chapter 39, Intrapartum and Postpartum Care.

Persistence of Weight Gain After Pregnancy

Weight at 1 year postpartum is a strong predictor of the likelihood of being overweight 15 years later. An adverse cardiometabolic prolife emerges as early as 1 year postpartum in those who do not lose weight between 3 and 12 months after delivery (Garcia et al., 2016).

Pregnancy Loss

A meta-analysis of 10 studies identified miscarriage as having an associated 1.45-fold increase in CVD. Those who experience more than one miscarriage have an associated twofold increased risk of CVD (Cho et al., 2020).

Intrauterine Growth Restriction

Identified as a fetal weight below the 10th percentile for gestational age, intrauterine growth restriction (IUGR) pregnancy increases risk for HLD, hypertriglyceridemia, and insulin resistance (Cho et al., 2020).

OTHER RISK FACTORS TO CONSIDER
Radiation and Chemotherapy for Breast Cancer

Several treatments used for breast cancer can increase the risk for CVD. Advancements in breast cancer treatment have led to improved survival, along with an unintended elevated risk of CVD, specifically ischemic heart disease.

Migraine With Aura

Migraine headaches with aura have been identified as a potential risk factor for CVD in women. Research with female health professionals age 45 years or older noted that those experiencing migraine with aura had a higher adjusted incidence rate of CVD compared to women experiencing migraine without aura (Kurth et al., 2020). More research with an expanded population is needed.

Vitamin D Deficiency

Vitamin D deficiency has been established as an independent risk factor for CVD. It remains unclear if vitamin D supplementation significantly improves outcomes (Kienreich et al., 2013).

Elevated Homocysteine

Elevated plasma total homocysteine is possibly a modifiable risk factor for CVD and stroke, as well as other vascular conditions. Homocysteine, a sulfur-containing amino acid, has been linked to the development of atherosclerosis (Greenland et al., 2001). It promotes endothelial dysfunction and cell injury, enhances thromboxane A_2 and platelet aggregation, and has procoagulant effects (Harjai, 1999). The lack of controlled clinical intervention trials that demonstrate improved outcomes after treating elevated homocysteine levels in women with CVD has kept this possible risk factor from being recommended as part of routine screening.

Lipoprotein (a)

Lipoprotein (a) (Lp(a)) is produced in the liver and competes with plasminogen for binding sites, thereby inhibiting fibrinolysis (Scanu et al., 1991). Lp(a) has also been shown to increase cholesterol invasion into the arterial wall, enhance foam cell formation, generate free radicals in monocytes, and promote smooth muscle cell proliferation (Loscalzo et al., 1990), all of which are factors in the process of atherosclerosis. Lp(a) has a limited role in lower risk primary prevention in women.

C-Reactive Protein

CRP is a nonspecific marker of inflammation and has been established as an independent risk factor for CVD and stroke (Ridker et al., 2000, 2002). High-sensitivity CRP (hs-CRP) for the quantification of cardiovascular risk in women has been found to be a much better predictor of CVD risk than some traditional markers, such as the total cholesterol:HDL-C ratio (Ridker et al., 2002). The 2018 AHA/ACC cholesterol guidelines recommend using hs-CRP levels as a risk enhancer and encourage statin consideration in those at borderline or intermediate 10-year ASCVD risk with hsCRP ≥ 2 mg/L (Lawler et al., 2021).

Lack of Awareness of Significant Cardiovascular Risk and Delayed Treatment

A frequently overlooked problem is women's underestimation of their CVD risk factors and poor access to or use of health education materials. Targeted education that highlights the importance of knowledge about CVD in women, especially in racial/ethnic minorities, should be regularly updated and presented in a culturally sensitive format. Strategies for decreasing CVD have been developed to educate the public on traditional risk factors such as HTN, dyslipidemia, and smoking. Broader risk factor reduction has been recommended that includes cardiometabolic risks and metabolic syndrome in women. Opportunities exist for increasing knowledge and awareness of CVD as the leading cause of death, including further education on the symptoms of MI (often different in women than in men) and the most appropriate response to a CVD emergency (Giardina et al., 2011).

Women, unaware of their own cardiovascular risk, often defer making an emergency 911 call. Delays in care can result in extensions of myocardial damage and poorer clinical outcomes. In a study of 5,887 individuals with suspected cardiac symptoms, women were 50% more likely than men to receive delayed treatment (Concannon et al., 2009). In a study of 6,022 women who presented with STEMI (ST segment elevation myocardial infarction), the delay in seeking care was 30 minutes longer in women and was independently associated with a greater risk of 30-day mortality (Bugiardini et al., 2017). Although the reason for the delay was not specifically studied, research indicates that symptom presentation in women is often different and more diffuse than in men, and therefore may not be readily recognized as a cardiac event by the patient and the emergency medical service (EMS) staff. Clearly, the lack of appreciation by many women for the need of emergency care for CVD and the lack of recognition of CVD symptoms by clinicians are a threat to women's mortality and morbidity and should be addressed through ongoing public education.

Nonadherence to Medical Therapies

Nonadherence to medical therapies, including taking prescribed medications, can be considered a risk factor for

CVD. In the presence of ASCVD, medication nonadherence is associated with worse patient outcomes (Khera et al., 2019). Reasons for nonadherence to a prescribed medical therapy are multifactorial and recognizing them can provide opportunities to identify those at risk for nonadherence and the barriers to adherence (Gast & Mathes, 2019). The five identified principal categories associated with adherence are social, healthcare, patient, disease, and therapy (AlGhurair et al., 2012). In a meta-analysis of more than 100 medical adherence studies, women were as likely to be nonadherent to medical therapies as men (DiMatteo, 2004). Nonadherence to medications has been documented in more than 60% of patients with CVD (Kravitz et al., 1993). AHA reports that over 60% of patients with CVD are nonadherent to their medications, leading to poor control of risk factors and eventual progression of the disease. Medication nonadherence in chronic diseases results in up to $300 billion in avoidable healthcare costs in the United States. AHA recommendations to reduce the most common barriers for nonadherence—patient-level barriers, cost barriers, system barriers, and electronic health record barriers—are addressed in their medication adherence policy statement (AHA, n.d.). Self-reported adherence to cardiovascular medications in patients with CAD is less than 40% for the combination of aspirin, beta-blocker, and lipid-lowering agent in both isolated and long-term follow-up surveys (Newby et al., 2006). Moreover, the highest risk of nonadherence occurs during the immediate discharge period; 24% of patients with acute MI do not fill their medications within 7 days of discharge (Jackevicius, Ping, et al., 2008). Almost one in four patients is partially or completely nonadherent in filling prescriptions after discharge (Jackevicius, Ping, et al., 2008). This is because many patients have difficulty adjusting their lifestyle, if a change is warranted, as well as adding new medications that increase expenses and complicate daily schedules.

Some specific causes of medication nonadherence are fragmentation of the healthcare system, problems with accessing information, complexity of some medication regimens, poor communication between the clinician and patient, low functional/healthcare literacy of the patient, concerns about costs by the patient, and unintentional behaviors such as forgetting to take the medication. Healthcare providers should use multiple approaches to improve their patients' short- and long-term medication adherence (Baroletti & Dell'Orfano, 2010). Identifying methods to improve compliance begins with assessing why patients are not taking their medications. In some cases, it may help to change to a less expensive medication, offer samples, change to medications that require less frequent dosing, recommend systems for reminders (e.g., smartphone chime or pill organizers), or provide additional education to the patient and/or a support person on the importance of the medication regimen.

Clinicians make recommendations less often for preventive therapy in women (Mosca et al., 2005). This was thought to be a result of the lower perceived threat, despite the similar calculated risk for women and men. Educational interventions for clinicians and patients are needed to improve the quality of CVD preventive care, ensure adoption of CVD prevention guidelines, and lower CVD morbidity and mortality. CVD must be considered in all patients such that clinicians provide strategies for comprehensive health promotion and disease prevention and make both an early diagnosis and aggressive intervention plan when warranted.

DIAGNOSTIC STUDIES

Resting Electrocardiogram

Although the resting EKG is a routine component of many physical examinations, the sensitivity of resting abnormalities for the prediction of CVD events is overall rather low (Ashley et al., 2001). Thus, many women who experience their first cardiac event have a normal baseline EKG (Pignone et al., 2003). The resting EKG can be helpful for stratifying risk in women who have HTN because the presence of left ventricular hypertrophy (LVH) identified by EKG increases the risk of sudden cardiac death (Kannel & Abbott, 1986).

Exercise Electrocardiogram: Stress Testing

An exercise treadmill test (ETT) with EKG (or EKG stress test) is the recommended functional diagnostic test women should undergo if their pretest risk for CVD is intermediate and they have a normal resting EKG and are capable of maximum exercise. Despite sex-specific limitations in the accuracy of exercise EKG (false-positive EKG changes and the influence of submaximal exercise on sensitivity), guidelines note the evidence is insufficient to remove the EKG stress test as the initial test for symptomatic women with intermediate CVD risk (Garcia et al., 2016).

Stress testing is useful for diagnostic as well as prognostic information. Exercise capacity is a stress-test measure that has been found to be a potent predictor of all-cause mortality (Gulati et al., 2012). The metabolic equivalent of a task (MET) is a multiple of the resting rate of oxygen consumption. One MET represents the oxygen consumption of a seated individual at rest (American College of Sports Medicine, 1991). In addition, assessing the likelihood that the symptoms are cardiac in nature is also important. Women can present with more atypical symptoms than men. The U.S. Preventive Services Task Force (USPTF) recommends using available risk factor screening tools (e.g., the Framingham Heart Study score) and consider screening for CVD in those at intermediate risk for CVD, who could be reclassified as being high risk after additional testing and subsequently treated more aggressively for risk factor modification (Pignone et al., 2003).

It is generally accepted that if a woman can achieve 5 METs, exercise stress testing can be undertaken. Many household tasks (e.g., vacuuming, washing floors) are equivalent to approximately 4 to 5 METs. If the woman cannot adequately exercise for any reason, pharmacologic stress testing with an imaging modality is more appropriate.

Stress Testing With Imaging Modalities

The cardiac imaging modalities that are most widely studied and available are stress testing with nuclear imaging and stress echocardiography. Gated myocardial perfusion single-photon emission computed tomography (SPECT) is the most performed stress test. SPECT provides information about perfusion problems (e.g., ischemia) as well as about global and regional left ventricular function and left ventricular volumes (Klocke et al., 2003).

The American Society of Nuclear Cardiology (ASNC) Task Force on Women and Heart Disease (Mieres et al., 2003; Standbridge & Reyes, 2016) recommends stress testing with nuclear imaging for women with an intermediate to high pretest likelihood of CVD (Mieres et al., 2005). Stress testing with cardiac imaging is indicated for high- and intermediate-risk women who have symptoms of CVD, DM, and a baseline abnormal EKG (Mieres et al., 2005). For women with symptoms who cannot exercise at a level of at least 5 METs, pharmacologic stress testing is indicated (Mieres et al., 2005). Stress echocardiography, like nuclear myocardial perfusion imaging, is indicated for women who are at intermediate and high risk of CVD who have symptoms suggestive of myocardial ischemia (Mieres et al., 2005). Stress echocardiography can also provide useful information regarding left ventricular function, systolic and diastolic dysfunction, and valvular heart disease (Mieres et al., 2005).

Computed Tomography and Coronary Calcium Score

Coronary artery calcification (CAC) has emerged as the most predictive single CVD risk marker in asymptomatic persons, capable of adding predictive information beyond the traditional cardiovascular risk factors. CAC scoring appears to be useful for making decisions about preventive statin and/or aspirin use. In most studies, CAC testing has been shown to be cost effective compared with alternative approaches when factoring in patient preferences about taking preventive medications (Greenland et al., 2018).

CT of the coronary vasculature detects and quantifies the amount of calcium in the coronary arteries and signifies the presence of atherosclerotic disease. A CT-based CAC >300 Agatson units or a CAC score above the 75th percentile is the suggested threshold for initiating statin therapy in the ACC/AHA 2013 lipid guidelines (Saeed et al., 2017). The 2019 European Society of Cardiology/European Atherosclerosis Society Guidelines for management of dyslipidemia state that the measurement of carotid intima-media thickness (cIMT) is inferior to CAC score to predict cardiovascular events (Paraskevas et al., 2020).

Cardiovascular Magnetic Resonance Imaging

Cardiac magnetic resonance imaging (CMRI) allows for visualizing coronary arteries, determining flow within the coronary arteries, evaluating myocardial perfusion (similar to SPECT), assessing wall motion during stress, and identifying infarcted myocardium. CMR angiography is also a promising imaging modality. CMRI may be especially useful in women without obstructive CAD who instead have microvascular coronary dysfunction (MCD), since perfusion MRI,

together with ejection fraction (EF), has been found to predict prognosis (Shufelt et al., 2013).

Coronary Angiography and Cardiac Catheterization

In the event of a positive stress test, many women are referred for coronary angiography and cardiac catheterization. Women who present with acute coronary syndromes (ACSs) may also undergo cardiac catheterization. The term *angiography* refers to the visualization of the arteries with the use of contrast medium. Cardiac catheterization encompasses coronary angiography and the assessment of left ventricular function; it can also include hemodynamic measurements and the assessment of valvular regurgitation and stenosis. Women have been shown to have a higher rate of normal cardiac catheterizations than men (Rosengren & Hasdai, 2005). Gender bias regarding women and cardiac care in general, and to coronary angiography and cardiac catheterization specifically, has been researched and debated for decades (Rosengren & Hasdai, 2005). Golden et al. (2013) reported that women who presented to the ED with symptoms of ACS reported lower rates of referral for cardiovascular testing as well as lower rates of counseling regarding cardiac causes of their chest pain. These findings suggest that sex differences in cardiovascular testing may be partly explained by the discussions between women and their clinicians.

CARDIOVASCULAR DISEASE DIAGNOSES

Hypertension

DEFINITION AND SCOPE

HTN is both a diagnosis and a well-known major risk factor for cardiovascular, cerebrovascular, and renal disease. More CVD events are attributable to HTN than any other modifiable CVD risk factor (Goetsch et al., 2021). In the United States, 45% of adults in 2017–2018 had HTN and the prevalence increases with age. Three quarters of adults over age 60 had HTN. The prevalence is highest among non-Hispanic Black men and women. Among women HTN was higher among non-Hispanic Black (56.7%) than Hispanic White (36.7%) and Hispanic (36.8%) adults. In 1999–2000 and 2017–2018 the prevalence decreased and then increased among men, but no significant trend was observed among women. Prevalence was higher in men than women ages 18 to 39 (31.2% compared with 13%) and 40 to 59 (59.4% compared to 49.9%), but there was no significant difference between men and women age >60 (75.2% compared to 73.9%; Ostchega et al., 2020).

EVALUATION/ASSESSMENT

In 2017, the AHA/ACC published the Guideline for Prevention, Detection, Evaluation, and Management of High Blood Pressure, the first comprehensive update since the publication of the Joint National Committee (JNC) 7 in 2003 (McEvoy et al., 2020). One of the major changes was the elimination of pre-HTN, replacing it with *elevated BP*, which is defined as 120 to 129 mmHg systolic and less than 80 mmHg diastolic. Another major change was lowering the stage 1 HTN goal to 130 to 139 mmHg systolic and 80 to 89 mmHg diastolic, with no adjustment in the older adult. This resulted in a higher percentage of the population being categorized as having HTN (Basile & Bloch, 2023). The data supporting the changes in BP goals came from the SPRINT study, a multicenter, randomized, open label trial performed in the United States. Patients were randomly assigned to standard treatment (targeting systolic pressure to <140 mmHg) or intensive treatment (targeting systolic pressure to <120 mmHg); diastolic goal in both groups was <90 mmHg. The trial was halted early after median follow-up of 3.33 years because the intensive treatment group had significant benefit over standard. The key findings demonstrated that intensive compared to standard treatment significantly reduced the rate of primary end points (5.6% vs. 7.6%), including MI, ACS, stroke, heart failure, and cardiovascular death. Intensive treatment also significantly reduced mortality rate (3.5% vs. 4.6%; Mann & Hilgers, 2022).

Guidelines recommend diagnosing HTN with use of home or ambulatory BP monitoring (ABPM); measurements obtained in clinical settings should be used for detection (Whelton et al., 2017). Meeting one or more of the diagnostic criteria using ABPM qualifies as confirmation of HTN when using appropriate technique and with a device validated in the office (Box 43.1). Occasionally, out-of-office confirmation is not possible due to equipment availability, insurance, and cost. In these situations, a diagnosis can be confirmed by serial (at least three) office-based BP measurements spaced over a period of weeks to months with a mean systolic >140 mmHg or diastolic >80 mmHg. Home BP monitor criteria for diagnosing HTN, when using appropriate technique and with a deice validated in the office, is systolic >130 mmHg or diastolic >80 mmHg.

TREATMENT/MANAGEMENT

Guidelines for treating HTN are the same for men and women and the efficacy of pharmacologic agents is similar for both genders (see Figure 43.3).

Box 43.1 Ambulatory Blood Pressure Monitoring Criteria for Hypertension

24-hour mean systolic >125 mmHg or diastolic >75 mmHg

Daytime mean systolic >130 mmHg, diastolic >80 mmHg

Nighttime systolic mean >110 mmHg or diastolic >65 mmHg

Source: Basile, J., & Bloch, M. J. (2023). *Overview of hypertension in adults.* UpToDate. https://www.uptodate.com/contents/overview-of-hypertension-in-adults; Whelton, P., Carey, R., Aronow, W., Casey, D. E., Jr., Collins, K. J., Himmelfarb, C. D., DePalma, S. M., Gidding, S., Jamerson, K. A., Jones, D. W., MacLaughlin, E. J., Muntner, P., Ovbiagele, B., Smith, S. C. Jr., Spencer, C. C., Stafford, R. S., Taler, S. J., Thomas, R. J., Williams, K. A., Sr., . . . Wright, J. T., Jr. (2017). *ACC/AHA/AAPA/ABC/ACPM/AGS/APhA/ASH/ASPC/NMA/PCNA guideline for the prevention, detection, evaluation, and management of high blood pressure in adults.* Journal of the American College of Cardiology, 71(19), e127–e248. https://doi.org/10.1016/j.jacc.2017.11.006

Lifestyle Modifications

Lifestyle modifications should be prescribed for all patients with elevated BP or HTN. Not all patients require pharmacologic therapy. Routine exercise is recommended, consisting of three to four sessions per week or more of moderate-intensity aerobic activity for approximately 40 minutes. Limiting alcohol intake is recommended; women who consume two or more alcoholic beverages per day have a significantly increased incidence of HTN compared to nondrinkers. Women with a diagnosis of HTN should not consume more than one alcoholic drink daily.

Limited intake of sweets, sugar-sweetened beverages, and red meats is advised. Limiting sodium intake to an optimal goal of <1,500 mg/day is recommended; initially aim for at least a 1,000 mg/day reduction (Whelton et al., 2017).

Weight loss to ideal body weight is a core recommendation and should be achieved by a combination of reduced caloric intake and increased physical activity. Reducing body weight by 1 kg equates to 1 mmHg reduction in BP in most overweight adults.

Smoking cessation should also be encouraged as a part of overall cardiovascular risk reduction.

Pharmacotherapeutics

The ACC/AHA guideline on high blood pressure recommends selecting initial therapy for adults from these four classes: thiazide-like or thiazide-type diuretic, long-acting calcium channel blockers (most often a dihydropyridine such as amlodipine), angiotensin-converting enzyme (ACE) inhibitors, and angiotensin II receptor blockers (ARBs). Data published demonstrated no significant difference in cardiovascular mortality among patients with these four drug classes (Basile & Bloch, 2023; Whelton et al., 2017).

Additional consideration in initial therapy choice for Black patients should be a thiazide-like diuretic or long-acting dihydropyridine calcium channel blocker. Patients with diabetic nephropathy or nondiabetic CKD would benefit from ACE inhibitor or an ARB as initial therapy. Beta-blockers are no longer recommended as initial monotherapy in absence of a specific indication for their use such as ischemic heart disease or heart failure with reduced ejection fraction (Basile & Bloch, 2023; Whelton et al., 2017).

AHA/ACC guidelines stress the importance of attaining and maintaining blood pressure control by increasing the titration of the initial drug chosen or adding a second drug after 1 month of treatment. Other agents can be added in the same manner to achieve blood pressure goals. However, the use of ACE inhibitors with an ARB in the same patient is not recommended. Referral to a HTN specialist is recommended if adding a third agent fails to achieve blood pressure control (Whelton et al., 2017).

Dyslipidemia

ETIOLOGY AND RISK FACTORS

Dyslipidemia results from excessive production of lipoproteins, defective removal of lipoproteins, or both. Drugs such as oral contraceptive pills, corticosteroids, beta-blockers, diuretics, and alcohol can all cause and contribute to dyslipidemia.

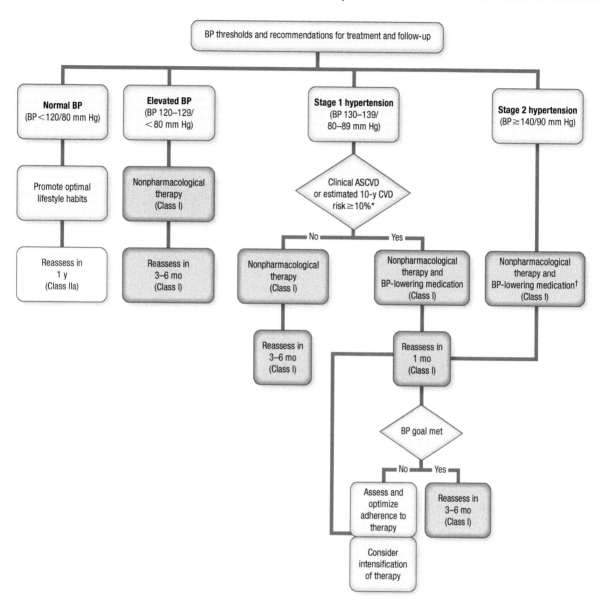

FIGURE 43.3 Blood pressure thresholds and recommendations for treatment and follow-up
*Using the ACC/AHA pooled cohort equations, note that patients with DM or CKD are automatically placed in the high-risk category. For initiation of RAS inhibitor or diuretic therapy, assess blood tests for electrolytes and renal function 2 to 4 weeks after initiating therapy.
†Consider initiation of pharmacologic therapy for stage 2 hypertension with two antihypertensive agents of different classes. Patients with stage 2 hypertension and BP ≥160/100 mmHg should be promptly treated, carefully monitored, and subject to upward medication dose adjustment as necessary to control BP. Reassessment includes BP measurement, detection of orthostatic hypotension in selected patients (e.g., older or with postural symptoms), identification of white coat hypertension or a white coat effect, documentation of adherence, monitoring of the response to therapy, reinforcement of the importance of adherence, reinforcement of the importance of treatment, and assistance with treatment to achieve BP target.
ACC, American College of Cardiology; AHA, American Heart Association; ASCVD, atherosclerotic cardiovascular disease; BP, blood pressure; CKD, chronic kidney disease; CVD, cardiovascular disease; DM, diabetes mellitus; RAS, renin–angiotensin system.
Source: Whelton, P., Carey, R., Aronow, W., Casey, D. E., Jr., Collins, K. J., Himmelfarb, C. D., DePalma, S. M., Gidding, S., Jamerson, K. A., Jones, D. W., MacLaughlin, E. J., Muntner, P., Ovbiagele, B., Smith, S. C., Jr., Spencer, C. C., Stafford, R. S., Taler, S. J., Thomas, R. J., Williams, K. A., Sr., . . . Wright, J. T., Jr. (2017). ACC/AHA/AAPA/ABC/ACPM/AGS/APhA/ASH/ASPC/NMA/PCNA guideline for the prevention, detection, evaluation, and management of high blood pressure in adults. Journal of the American College of Cardiology, 71(19), e127–e248. https://doi.org/10.1016/j.jacc.2017.11.006

Moreover, factors such as obesity and a high-fat diet and conditions such as DM, hypothyroidism, Addison disease, and Cushing disease can cause secondary dyslipidemia. Pregnancy can cause transient dyslipidemia, and lipid levels return to normal within 6 to 8 weeks after birth (Gotto & Pownall, 1999). Women who breastfed their infants had lower low-density lipoprotein cholesterol (LDL-C) and insulin levels than those who did not breastfeed (Gunderson et al., 2007). The long-term implications of the lower LDL-C levels in these women are not known (Gunderson et al., 2007).

Recent guidelines and major studies that were reviewed and summarized by the ACC CVD in Women committee

TABLE 43.2 Cardiovascular Disease Risk Factors in Women

RISK FACTOR TYPE	EXAMPLES
Traditional factors	Smoking, hypertension, age, hyperlipidemia, physical inactivity, diabetes, poor diet, sedentary behavior, family history
Hormonal factors	Premature menopause, polycystic ovary syndrome, menopause hormone therapy, cardiometabolic risk, and obesity
Other factors	Adverse pregnancy outcomes, chronic kidney disease, autoimmune disorders, cardiotoxic chemotherapy, chest wall radiation
Social determinants of health	Education, race/ethnicity, income, ZIP code
Psychological risk factors	Anxiety, depression, perceived stress, loneliness

Source: Adapted from Cho, L., Davis, M., Elgendy, I., Epps, K., Lindley, K. J., Mehta, P. K., Michos, E. D., Minissian, M., Pepine, C., Vaccarino, V., Volgman, A. S., & ACC CVD Women's Committee Members. (2020). Summary of updated recommendations for primary prevention of cardiovascular disease in women: JACC state-of-the-art review. Journal of the American College of Cardiology, 75(20), 2602–2618. https://doi.org/10.1016/j.jacc.2020.03.060

specify various CVD risk factors pertaining to women. These risk factors (Table 43.2) can result in inflammation, which can subsequently cause CVD (Cho et al., 2020).

Disorders of lipoprotein metabolism are well-established risk factors for CHD in both sexes. LDL appears to significantly affect men more than women. Women younger than 50 years old are at lower risk of having hypercholesterolemia than men, although, after menopause, LDL levels rise by 14% resulting in women having higher LDL levels than men over the age of 65. Therefore, a lipid profile should be assessed after menopause to determine a woman's CVD risk. A reduction in HDL in both younger and older years predicts coronary heart disease mortality more in women than men (Gao et al., 2019).

TREATMENT/MANAGEMENT

Guidelines for Dyslipidemia

Many clinical trials have demonstrated lower cardiac event rates with medical treatment of dyslipidemia. Women were underrepresented in earlier landmark clinical trials involving lipid-lowering drugs. However, the Heart Protection Study (HPS) included 5,082 women and 15,454 men with known vascular disease. The investigators found a 24% reduction in major vascular events at 5 years, independent of gender, in participants taking simvastatin (HPS Collaborative Group, 2002). More recently, the JUPITER Trial showed a significant reduction in ASCVD events compared with placebo among 6,801 women with elevated hs-CRP levels (>2 mg/L) and LDL-C levels <130 mg/dL treated with rosuvastatin (Mora et al., 2010). Current treatment guidelines do not differentiate between men and women; target goals for lipid profiles are the same (Stone et al., 2014).

Historically, the National Heart, Lung, and Blood Institute (NHLBI) and National Cholesterol Education Program (NCEP) developed guidelines for the treatment of dyslipidemia (NCEP Expert Panel, 2001). The guidelines for the treatment of blood cholesterol to reduce ASCVD in adults were revised in 2013 by the AHA and ACC, in collaboration with the NHLBI (Stone et al., 2014). With these guidelines, the focus of primary prevention shifted to evaluating absolute risk rather than treating to a specific cholesterol number. Individuals with established ASCVD are recommended for high-dose statin therapy (Stone et al., 2014). These guidelines recommend using a new Pooled Cohort Equation to estimate 10-year risk for ASCVD in White and Black men and women without known ASCVD (Stone et al., 2014). This risk calculator is available at www.cvriskcalculator.com and as an application for smartphones and tablets.

The risk calculator uses the cardiovascular risk factors of gender, age, race, total cholesterol, HDL-C, systolic blood pressure (mmHg), treatment of HTN, DM, and smoking to calculate a 10-year risk of developing ASCVD in individuals age 20 to 79 years. The application also calculates a lifetime risk score in persons age 20 to 59 years. In general, pharmacologic management of HLD is not considered beneficial for individuals with a 10-year ASCVD risk of <5%. The guidelines recommend treating HLD with 3-hydroxy-3-methylglutaryl-coenzyme A (HMG-CoA) reductase inhibitors, also known as statins. The presence of DM increases the risk substantially; at least moderate-intensity statin therapy is recommended for all adults ages 40 to 75 years with DM. Moderate-intensity statin therapy is recommended for individuals age 40 to 75 years without DM whose lifetime risk is 5% to 7.5% and for those with a 10-year risk >7.5% (Stone et al., 2014).

In the 2018 cholesterol clinical practice guidelines, recommendations for statins were delineated with respect to age, ASCVD risk factors/ASCVD risk enhancers, and 10-year ASCVD risk and focused on secondary prevention. There was a change from treating according to levels (total cholesterol, LDL, HDL, and triglycerides) to using ASCVD risk to determine which level of statin should be used.

Four groups were identified to benefit from initiation of statins (Table 43.3). The first group referred to secondary prevention in patients with clinical ASCVD. ASCVD was then further delineated to those with ASCVD who were not at very high risk and those with very high risk of ASCVD. ASCVD was defined as those patients with a history of MI, ACS, stable or unstable angina or other coronary arterial revascularization, transient ischemic attack (TIA) or stroke, and peripheral arterial disease (PAD) including aortic aneurysm, all of atherosclerotic origin. Very high risk ASCVD referred to those individuals with a history of one major ASCVD event and multiple high-risk conditions and those with multiple major ASCVD events (see Box 43.2). The second group identified recommendations for individuals with primary severe hypercholesterolemia (LDL-C ≥190 mg/dL). The third group identified DM-specific risk enhancers that were independent of other risk factors in individuals with DM, age 40 to 75 years with an LDL-C of 70 to 189 mg/dL (see Box 43.3). The fourth group benefited those for primary prevention (Grundy et al., 2019a).

TABLE 43.3 Statin Therapy: Categories of Intensity

INTENSITY	GOAL	DRUG EXAMPLES
High intensity	Aiming for at least 50% reduction in LDL	Atorvastatin 40–80 mg PO OD Rosuvastatin 2–40 mg PO OD
Moderate intensity	Aiming for 30%–49% reduction in LDL	Atorvastatin 10–20 mg PO OD Fluvastatin 80 mg PO OD Lovastatin 40–80 mg PO OD Pravastatin 40–80 mg PO OD Rosuvastatin 5–10 mg PO OD Simvastatin 20–40 mg PO OD
Low intensity	Aiming for LDL-C reduction of <30%	Fluvastatin 20–40 mg PO OD Lovastatin 20 mg PO OD Pravastatin 10–20 mg PO OD Simvastatin 10 mg PO OD
Nonstatins	Can be added to statin therapy and may improve cardiovascular outcomes	Ezetimibe PCSK9 inhibitors

LDL, low-density lipoprotein; LDC-C, low-density lipoprotein cholesterol; OD, once a day; PO, orally.
Source: Arnett, D. K., Blumenthal, R. S., Albert, M. A., Buroker, A. B., Goldberger, Z. D., Hahn, E. J., Himmelfarb, C. D., Khera, A., Lloyd-Jones, D., McEvoy, J. W., Michos, E. D., Miedema, M. D., Muñoz, D., Smith, S. C., Jr., Virani, S. S., Williams, K. A., Sr., Yeboah, J., & Ziaeian, B. (2019). 2019 ACC/AHA guideline on the primary prevention of cardiovascular disease: A report of the American College of Cardiology/American Heart Association Task Force on Clinical Practice Guidelines. Circulation, 140(11), e596–e646. https://doi.org/10.1161/CIR.0000000000000678

Box 43.2 Individuals at Very High Risk of Future ASCVD Events

High-Risk Conditions

Age ≥65 years

Diabetes mellitus

Hypertension

History of prior coronary artery bypass surgery

History of percutaneous coronary intervention outside of the major ASCVD event(s)

Heterozygous familial hypercholesterolemia

Current smoking

Persistently elevated LDL-C despite maximally tolerated statin therapy and ezetimibe (LDL ≥100 mg/dL)

Chronic kidney disease (eGFR 15–59 mL/minute)

History of CHF

Major ASCVD events

History of ischemic stroke

Recent ACS (in the past 12 months)

History of MI (other than recent ACS event listed above)

Peripheral arterial disease that is symptomatic (previous revascularization or amputation, history of claudication with ABI <0.85)

ABI, ankle-brachial index; ACS, acute coronary syndrome; ASCVD, atherosclerotic cardiovascular disease; CHF, congestive heart failure; eGFR, estimated glomerular filtration rate; LDL, low-density lipoprotein; LDL-C, low-density lipoprotein cholesterol; MI, myocardial infarction.
Source: Adapted from Grundy, S. M., Stone, N. J., Bailey, A. L., Beam, C., Birtcher, K. K., Blumenthal, R. S., Braun, L. T., de Ferranti, S., Faiella-Tommasino, J., Forman, D. E., Goldberg, R., Heidenreich, P. A., Hlatky, M. A., Jones, D. W., Lloyd-Jones, D., Lopez-Pajares, N., Ndumele, C. E., Orringer, C. E., Peralta, C. A., . . . Yeboah, J. (2019). 2018 AHA/ACC/AACVPR/AAPA/ABC/ACPM/ADA/AGS/APhA/ASPC/NLA/PCNA guideline on the management of blood cholesterol. Journal of the American College of Cardiology, 73(24), e285–e350. https://doi.org/10.1016/j.jacc.2018.11.003

A healthy lifestyle was encouraged for all ages to reduce ASCVD risk. In persons age 20 to 39 years, an assessment of lifetime risk is of importance and should be discussed with an emphasis placed on intensive lifestyle efforts. Lifestyle therapy is of the utmost importance in managing metabolic syndrome in all age groups. For individuals with known clinical ASCVD, reduction of LDL-C with high-intensity statin therapy is preferable or maximally tolerated statin therapy. The goal is to lower LDL–C levels by ≥50%.

In persons considered at very high risk of ASCVD, consider adding ezetimibe therapy to maximally tolerated statin if LDL-C remains ≥70 mg/dL. In the individual with very high risk ASCVD who is already on maximally tolerated statin and ezetimibe therapy, consider adding a PCSK9 (proprotein convertase subtilisin/kexin type 9) inhibitor, although long-term safety for more than 3 years is uncertain (Grundy et al., 2019a).

Individuals who have severe primary hypercholesterolemia, defined by an LDL-C of ≥190 mg/dL, begin high-intensity statin therapy (see Box 43.4) without calculating their 10-year ASCVD risk. If the LDL remains ≥100 mg/dL, ezetimibe is reasonable to add. If the LDL-C when taking a statin plus ezetimibe remains ≥100 mg/dL, consider adding a PCSK9 inhibitor, although long-term safety for more than 3 years is uncertain (Grundy et al., 2019a).

Individuals between the ages of 40 to 75 years with DM and an LDL-C ≥70 mg/dL, starting a moderate-intensity statin therapy is recommended without calculating a 10-year

ASCVD risk (see Box 43.4). In individuals with DM who are at higher risk, especially those with several risk factors or between the ages of 50 to 75 years, initiating high-intensity statin therapy should be considered to reduce the LDL-C level by ≥50% (Grundy et al., 2019a). If there are also risk-enhancing factors (see Box 43.3), treatment with a statin is recommended.

In individuals who are 40 to 75 years of age who have been evaluated for primary ASCVD prevention, a provider–patient risk discussion should occur before initiating statin therapy. This risk discussion should include a review of major risk factors (HTN, cigarette smoking, LDL-C, hemoglobin A1c [if appropriate], a calculated 10-year risk of ASCVD) and the presence of risk-enhancing factors: continued elevated LDL-C levels ≥160 mg/dL, family history of premature ASCVD, CKD, metabolic syndrome, history of premature

Box 43.3 Diabetes–Specific Risk Enhancers That Are Independent of Other Risk Factors in Diabetes Mellitus

Ankle-brachial index <0.9

Type 1 diabetes mellitus for ≥20 years

Type 2 diabetes mellitus ≥10 years

Retinopathy

Neuropathy

Albuminuria ≥30 mcg of albumin/mg creatinine

Estimated glomerular filtration rate <60 mL/min/1.73 m^2

Source: Adapted from Grundy, S. M., Stone, N. J., Bailey, A. L., Beam, C., Birt-cher, K. K., Blumenthal, R. S., Braun, L. T., de Ferranti, S., Faiella-Tommasino, J., Forman, D. E., Goldberg, R., Heidenreich, P. A., Hlatky, M. A., Jones, D. W., Lloyd-Jones, D., Lopez-Pajares, N., Ndumele, C. E., Orringer, C. E., Peralta, C. A., . . . Yeboah, J. (2019). 2018 AHA/ACC/AACVPR/AAPA/ABC/ACPM/ ADA/AGS/APhA/ASPC/NLA/PCNA guideline on the management of blood cholesterol. Journal of the American College of Cardiology, 73(24), e285–e350. *https://doi.org/10.1016/j.jacc.2018.11.003*

menopause (<40 years), preeclampsia, chronic inflammatory disorders (psoriasis, rheumatoid arthritis, or chronic HIV), high-risk ethnic groups (South Asian), triglycerides that are persistently ≥175 mg/dL, and in select individuals high-sensitivity C-reactive protein ≥2.0 mg/dL, apolipoprotein B ≥130 g/dL, ankle-brachial index <0.9, and Lp(a) ≥50 mg/dL or 125 nmol/L, especially when levels of Lp(a) are of higher values. These risk-enhancing factors may favor treatment with a statin in individuals with a 10-year risk of 5% to 7.5% (Grundy et al., 2019a; Figure 43.4).

In adults between the ages of 40 and 75 years who do not have DM but have LDL-C levels ≥70 mg/dL and a 10-year ASCVD risk of ≥7.5%, recommend a moderate intensity statin. Risk-enhancing factors would support initiation of statin therapy. If risk-enhancing factor status is uncertain, consider using a coronary calcium score (CAC) to further stratify the individual. If a statin is recommended, decrease LDL-C levels by ≥30%. If their 10-year risk is ≥20%, reduction in LDL-C levels by ≥50% is recommended (Grundy et al., 2019a).

Medication compliance, response to LDL-C lowering medications, and changes in lifestyle should be assessed. Repeat lipids in 4 to 12 weeks after initiating or adjusting a statin and then repeat lipids every 3 to 12 months as needed. In individuals with ASCVD at very high risk, if the LDL-C level is ≥70 mg/dL on maximally tolerated statin therapy, consider adding a nonstatin drug (Grundy et al., 2019a).

Pharmacotherapeutics

The first-line drug therapy for dyslipidemia is HMG-CoA reductase inhibitors, otherwise known as statins, which lower total cholesterol and LDL-C. Statins currently available are simvastatin, lovastatin, fluvastatin, atorvastatin, rosuvastatin, pravastatin, and pitavastatin. They vary in dosage and potency. Statins are the only lipid-lowering drugs that produce plaque stabilization and lower LDL-C. Patients with active liver

Box 43.4 Statin Therapy: Levels of Intensity

Low-intensity reduction: ≤30%

Fluvastatin 20 to 40 mg

Lovastatin 20 mg

Pravastatin 10 to 20 mg

Simvastatin 10 mg

Moderate-intensity reduction: 30% to 49%

Pitavastatin 1 to 4 mg

Fluvastatin XL 80 mg

Fluvastatin 40 mg twice daily

Lovastatin 40 mg (80 mg)

Pravastatin 40 mg (80 mg)

Simvastatin 20 to 40 mg

Rosuvastatin 5 mg (10 mg)

Atorvastatin 10 mg (20 mg)

High-intensity reduction: ≥50%

Atorvastatin (40 mg) 80 mg

Rosuvastatin 20 mg (40 mg)

The percentage of LDL-C reductions from the most common statin medications used in clinical practice were approximated using the median reduction in LDL-C from the VOYAGER database.

The percentage of LDL-C reductions for other statin medications were obtained according to FDA-approved product labeling in those adults with mixed dyslipidemia, hyperlipidemia, and primary hypercholesterolemia.

FDA, Food and Drug Administration; LDL-C, low-density lipoprotein cholesterol.
Source: Adapted from Grundy, S. M., Stone, N. J., Bailey, A. L., Beam, C., Birt-cher, K. K., Blumenthal, R. S., Braun, L. T., de Ferranti, S., Faiella-Tommasino, J., Forman, D. E., Goldberg, R., Heidenreich, P. A., Hlatky, M. A., Jones, D. W., Lloyd-Jones, D., Lopez-Pajares, N., Ndumele, C. E., Orringer, C. E., Peralta, C. A., . . . Yeboah, J. (2019). 2018 AHA/ACC/AACVPR/AAPA/ABC/ACPM/ ADA/AGS/APhA/ASPC/NLA/PCNA guideline on the management of blood cholesterol. Journal of the American College of Cardiology, 73(24), e285–e350. *https://doi.org/10.1016/j.jacc.2018.11.003*

disease or persons who are pregnant or may become pregnant are not candidates for statins (Grundy et al., 2019b).

Myopathy is a potential side effect of all statins, though the risk of myopathy is less than 1% in most individuals studied in large research trials. Sex- and age-specific research in the area of statin-induced myotoxicity is scarce (Bhardwaj et al., 2013). However, an incidence of approximately 5% has been observed (Pasternak et al., 2002). The risks of myositis or myopathy increase with high-intensity statin therapy and with concurrent use of medications such as niacin, verapamil, amiodarone, macrolide antibiotics, azole antifungals, fibric acid derivatives (especially gemfibrozil), and HIV protease inhibitors (Grundy et al., 2019b). In patients who have complaints of muscle

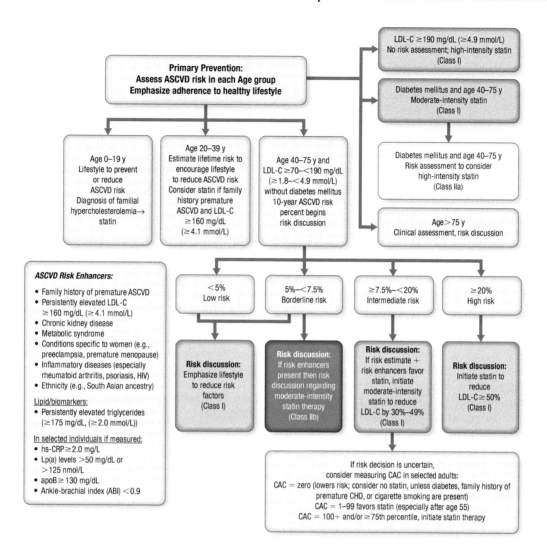

FIGURE 43.4 Primary prevention of ASCVD.
apoB, apolipoprotein B; ASCVD, atherosclerotic cardiovascular disease; CAC, coronary artery calcium; hsCRP, high-sensitivity C-reactive protein; LDL-C, low-density lipoprotein cholesterol; Lp(a), lipoprotein (a).
Source: Grundy, S. M., Stone, N. J., Bailey, A. L., Beam, C., Birtcher, K. K., Blumenthal, R. S., Braun, L. T., de Ferranti, S., Faiella-Tommasino, J., Forman, D. E., Goldberg, R., Heidenreich, P. A., Hlatky, M. A., Jones, D. W., Lloyd-Jones, D., Lopez-Pajares, N., Ndumele, C. E., Orringer, C. E., Peralta, C. A., . . . Yeboah, J. (2019). 2018 AHA/ACC/AACVPR/AAPA/ABC/ACPM/ADA/AGS/APhA/ASPC/NLA/PCNA guideline on the management of blood cholesterol. Journal of the American College of Cardiology, 73(24), e285–e350. https://doi.org/10.1016/j.jacc.2018.11.003

aches, creatine kinase (CK) level should be checked. However, routine monitoring of CK levels in patients without myositis symptoms is not recommended (Gotto & Pownall, 1999).

The cholesterol absorption inhibitor ezetimibe is approved for treating HLD. It lowers LDL-C modestly, has mild triglyceride-lowering capabilities, and works equally well in men and women (Ballantyne et al., 2005). Ezetimibe has a low incidence of side effects and only rarely causes an increase in liver transaminases. Clinical outcome studies with use of ezetimibe for the treatment of high LDL-C have been mixed. The ENHANCE trial investigated the effects of ezetimibe in combination with simvastatin versus simvastatin alone on cIMT in patients with heterozygous familial HLD (Kastelein et al., 2008). Despite significant decreases in

LDL-C in the ezetimibe–simvastatin group compared with the simvastatin group, the combination failed to demonstrate cIMT regression (Kastelein et al., 2008). However, the 2014 IMPROVE-IT study demonstrated improved outcomes in ACS patients treated with the combination ezetimibe–simvastatin over 7 years versus simvastatin alone. Individuals treated with ezetimibe had statistically significantly fewer CHD-related deaths, MIs, and urgent coronary revascularizations. The study validates the hypothesis that lowering LDL-C levels to below recommended targets in high-risk patients has benefit. Ezetimibe is a reasonable therapy in patients who cannot tolerate a statin or are not at goal on high-dose statin alone (Eisen et al., 2021).

PCSK9 is a proteolytic enzyme that originates mostly from the liver but is also produced by the kidney, central nervous system, and intestine, and possibly is involved in local regulation of LDL receptor expression. PCSK9 causes destruction of LDL receptors on the surface of liver hepatocytes. This causes more LDL to circulate in the bloodstream, raising the LDL level. PCSK9 inhibitors have emerged as an alternative or addition to statin therapy to achieve an LDL goal. PCSK9 inhibitors inhibit or bind the PCSK9 circulating in the bloodstream, thereby increasing the number of LDL receptors available for LDL adherence, subsequently decreasing LDL levels. Two PCSK9 inhibitors, both human monoclonal antibodies, alirocumab and evolocumab, are currently approved for use. Their efficacy in lowering LDL ranges from 45% to 65% and is derived from three variables: patient population, dose, and frequency (Roth & Davidson, 2018). Clinical trials evaluating PCSK9 inhibitors have shown a decrease in ASCVD events, especially in patients with recent ACS, peripheral arterial disease, or multivessel CAD (Rosenson et al., 2018). PCSK9 inhibitors are recommended for patients who are high risk with LDL levels ≥70 mg/dL who are on the maximally tolerated oral medications, which include statins and/or ezetimibe (Rosenson et al., 2018). The relationship between LDL-C and cardiovascular disease is well documented. Therefore, research continues to assess the benefits of lowering LDL-C and alternate pathways beyond the use of traditional medications such as statins, ezetimibe, and PCSK9 inhibitors. There is a significant role in researching nonstatin therapies for patients who develop statin intolerance.

Bempedoic acid (Nexletol) was Food and Drug Administration (FDA) approved in February 2020 for treatment of adults with established ASCVD or HeFH (heterozygous familial hypercholesterolemia) who need additional LDL-C lowering. It is a prodrug that, when activated, inhibits adenosine triphosphate citrate lyase (ACL) in the liver. By inhibiting ACL, bempedoic acid reduces conversion of citrate (mitochondrial derived) to cytosolic ACL, thereby reducing the substrate for fatty acid and cholesterol synthesis (Marrs & Anderson, 2020). A few days after bempedoic acid was approved, the FDA also approved bempedoic acid and ezetimibe (Nexlizet) for the treatment of adults with established ASCVD or HeFH who need additional reductions in LDL-C.

In 2022, the FDA approved Leqvio (inclisiran) for treating adults with HeFH and ASCVD who require additional reduction in their LDL-C. The drug inhibits PCSK9. It is a synthetic small interfering RNA (siRNA) that specifically targets inclisiran to hepatocytes. In the hepatocytes, its role is to bind to the RNA-induced silencing complex and block the translation of PCSK9 messenger RNA (mRNA) resulting in a reduction in PCSK9 synthesis and its secretion into the extracellular milieu. It is the first cholesterol-lowering therapy in its class approved for use in the United States (Cicero et al., 2022).

Nonpharmacologic Management

Treatment of dyslipidemia requires a multifaceted approach, which includes diet modification and exercise. The 2018 AHA/ACC guideline on the management of blood cholesterol states that individuals should consume a diet that emphasizes the consumption of fruits, vegetables, legumes, whole grains, healthy protein sources (low-fat poultry without the skin,

fish/seafood, nuts, and low-fat dairy products) and nontropical vegetable oils. Red meats, sugar-sweetened beverages, and sweets should be limited. The dietary pattern should be adjusted according to appropriate caloric requirements, nutritional therapies for medical conditions such as DM, and cultural and personal food preferences. The number of calories consumed should be adjusted to avoid weight gain or promote weight loss for those who are overweight or obese (Grundy et al., 2019a).

Dietary plans such as the AHA diet, the U.S. Department of Agriculture (USDA) Food Pattern, or the Dietary Approaches to Stop Hypertension (DASH) diet are specifically recommended by the 2018 AHA/ACC Guideline (Grundy et al., 2019a).

Physical activity has modest effects on lowering LDL-C (3–6 mg/dL) and non–HDL-C (6–9 mg/dL; Eckel et al., 2014). No consistent benefit of aerobic exercise alone has been demonstrated on either HDL-C or triglycerides (Eckel et al., 2014). The 2018 AHA/ACC Guideline on the Management of Blood Cholesterol strongly recommends engagement in aerobic physical activity, three to four exercise sessions per week of moderate to vigorous intensity, lasting an average of 40 minutes (Grundy et al., 2019a).

Complementary and Alternative Medicine Therapies

Omega-3 fish oil has been shown to be modestly effective in lowering triglycerides (20%–40%) and increasing HDL-C (5%–10%; Gotto & Pownall, 1999). Fish oil can be a useful add-on therapy for treating dyslipidemia. Unfortunately, because of a significant "first pass" effect by the liver, the dose of fish oil needs to be quite high to achieve benefits; 4,000 to 6,000 mg (four to six capsules, in divided doses, with meals) is needed. Newer formulations are "odorless" and "tasteless," making it more palatable, and fish oil is very safe in combination with other medications (Gotto & Pownall, 1999).

Fish oil is easily available and most frequently comprises about 1 g or less of docosahexaenoic acid (DHA) and eicosapentaenoic acid (EPA). Although posited to reduce inflammation, the mechanism by which fish oil reduces CV events is unknown. In 2018, the AHA conducted a large meta-analysis study that showed no benefit on primary prevention of CAD from fish oil. However, it was repeated the following year with three new trials and more participants. The 2019 analysis did show that fish oil supplementation decreased the risk of CAD, MI, and CAD death. In addition, greater risk reduction was related to higher doses of fish oil (Short et al., 2021).

Atherosclerotic Disease

ETIOLOGY

CVD and its root cause, atherosclerosis, are systemic disorders. As early as the 1960s, clinical experience, laboratory studies, and necropsy studies supported the concept that patients with disease in one vascular bed were likely to have disease in other vascular beds (Young et al., 1960). More recent studies have confirmed that patients who had peripheral vascular disease were more likely to have CAD and/or cerebrovascular disease than those who did not (Johnson et al., 2004). The pathogenesis of this chronic and progressive illness that leads to atherosclerotic plaque formation and cardiac events is multifactorial and explained by several mechanisms, leading clinicians to direct preventive strategies, acute treatments, and secondary interventions to prevent or delay future events.

Atherosclerosis is a result of interactions that occur between lipoprotein deposition in the subintimal space of the arterial wall and subsequent counterproductive inflammatory or immune responses. Coronary atheroma can progress over years resulting in calcifications, concentric arterial remodeling, and subsequent focal luminal stenoses, a process that can be hastened through a sequence of healed plaque rupture or erosion events (Joshi & de Lemos, 2021).

CAD is a vascular disease limited to the epicardial coronary arteries. Ischemic heart disease (IHD) is an ischemic disease that originates from microcirculation, from the coronary arteries, or from an imbalance in myocardial oxygen supply demand. In women, IHD terminology has advantages over CAD because women have a lower prevalence of anatomically obstructive CAD yet there is a greater rate of associated mortality and myocardial ischemia in females compared with males of similar age. The Women's Ischemia Syndrome Evaluation (WISE) and other similar studies have determined that microvascular dysfunction, plaque erosion/distal microembolization, and abnormal coronary reactivity are causative to the pathophysiology of IHD in females (Garcia et al., 2016).

IHD is the leading cause of death in women and is estimated to affect 67 million women globally. Although IHD was traditionally thought to be problematic for postmenopausal women, the yearly occurrence of acute MI hospitalizations among women under the age of 55 is increasing.

Traditional cardiovascular risk factors play an important role in the development of IHD in women as well as sex-specific IHD risk factors and pathophysiology. Therefore, female-specific risk stratification is necessary for IHD prevention, diagnosis, and treatment (Reynolds et al., 2022). Traditional ASCVD risk factors in women include smoking, overweight and obesity, physical inactivity, HTN, dyslipidemia, and DM (Garcia et al., 2016). Sex-specific IHD risk factors in women include autoimmune inflammatory diseases, premature menopause, and history of pregnancy-associated conditions such as preterm labor, GDM, hypertensive disorders of pregnancy (including preeclampsia), and small-for-gestational-age delivery (Reynolds et al., 2022). Breast cancer treatment and depression are additional ASCVD risk factors (Garcia et al., 2016).

Myocardial infarction with no obstructive CAD (MINOCA) and ischemia with no obstructive coronary arteries (INOCA) are mechanisms of IHD in women (Reynolds et al., 2022). INOCA can be described as ischemia with stable or unstable symptoms in individuals with normal or nonobstructive coronary arteries (defined as <50% stenosis). INOCA is a heterogeneous condition that corresponds with an elevated risk both for cardiovascular events and, after adjusting for traditional CV risk factors, for all-cause mortality in both sexes. Among symptomatic women with ischemic syndrome, cardiac mortality rates were 6% for no CAD and 11% for minimal CAD found within 10 years of their angiographic evaluation, demonstrating that INOCA is not benign (Reynolds et al., 2022).

In managing INOCA, guideline-indicated preventive pharmacologic therapies are recommended to control cardiovascular risk factors. For those patients who are symptomatic with nonobstructive CAD, it is recommended that preventive therapies be intensified. To improve microvascular function, statins and ACE inhibitor/ARB are recommended. Lifestyle modification and stress management should also be advised. Microvascular angina may be treated with lifestyle modification, nicorandil, calcium channel blockers, and beta-blockers. If vasospasm is suspected or diagnosed, a calcium channel blocker is preferred to a beta-blocker (Reynolds et al., 2022).

Calcium channel blockers are recommended for coronary artery spasm. The specific calcium channel blocker should be chosen for the patient with regard to their blood pressure, heart rate, and drug interactions. In those patients with persisting symptoms, dual calcium channel blocker therapy may provide some relief. A long-acting oral nitrate is also indicated, utilizing short-acting nitrates on demand for chest pain (Reynolds et al., 2022).

MINOCA is defined by <50% diameter stenosis in all the major epicardial coronary arteries, in the absence of an alternative cause for their clinical presentation such as myocarditis or a pulmonary embolism. In those women with MINOCA, 14% (relatively few) present with ST segment elevation MI, although ST segment elevation is associated with a higher risk of adverse outcomes. While MINOCA may appear a more favorable diagnosis than an MI with obstructive CAD (MI-CAD), it can result in fatality and prehospital deaths have been reported (Reynolds et al., 2022).

The pathogenesis of MINOCA is heterogeneous and may include plaque erosion, atherosclerotic plaque rupture, coronary spasm, coronary thromboembolism, and rarely coronary dissection. In those patients who have been diagnosed with Takotsubo syndrome, nonischemic cardiomyopathy, or acute myocarditis, they are not considered to have MINOCA once the alternative diagnosis has been determined. The optimal management of MINOCA may vary based on the etiology of the infarction; therefore, a systematic approach is critical to diagnosis. Clinical algorithms to aid in the diagnosis of MINOCA have been established to aid in the careful review of coronary angiographic findings for overlooked clinical diagnoses; contrast CMRI is now available to diagnose myocarditis or aid in the identification of the territory of acute infarction or injury, and left ventricular functional assessment is used to assess for wall motion abnormalities that are characteristic for Takotsubo syndrome. In addition, coronary functional assessments to aid in the diagnosis of epicardial microvascular coronary spasm and intracoronary imaging with optical coherence tomography or intravascular ultrasound to help identify atherosclerotic culprit lesions should be considered to enhance diagnostic sensitivity and define the treatment plan (Reynolds et al., 2022).

An MI that is due to a spontaneous coronary artery dissection (SCAD) has unique pathology in which an intramural hematoma develops spontaneously, with or without an intimal tear, and narrows the vessel lumen, limiting myocardial perfusion. The dissection may occur between any of the three layers of the arterial wall; specifically, the intima, media, or adventitia. SCAD is a nonatherosclerotic process but does cause narrowing that may be mistaken for an MI due to atherosclerosis and thrombosis. Among those patients with SCAD, 90% are women, the average age is approximately 50 years, and only a few have traditional cardiovascular risk factors. SCAD may account for nearly 35% of MI occurring in women 50 years old or younger. It is the leading cause of MI associated with pregnancy. The diagnosis of SCAD requires critical attention to the angiogram when there is a high index of suspicion, and intracoronary imaging may be considered when a definitive diagnosis cannot be established. Careful attention must be taken to avoid propagation of further dissection (Reynolds et al., 2022).

The preferred treatment of SCAD is conservative with close monitoring and medical therapy. This is because angiographic healing of SCAD occurs in 70% to 97% of cases in the weeks to months after the initial occurrence, and there is a higher rate of percutaneous coronary intervention (PCI) and bypass graft failure in the setting of SCAD as compared to those with MI due to CAD. Coronary revascularization for SCAD should be delineated to those patients with ongoing ischemia despite medical therapy or hemodynamic instability (Reynolds et al., 2022).

Myocarditis is an inflammatory disease of the heart and is included among secondary cardiomyopathies in the 1996 World Health Organization classification. It can occur because of exposure to toxic substances, immune system activation, and infections. It has a wide variety of clinical presentations and trajectories and is a common cause of sudden cardiac death in young people. In addition, the inflammation can result in extensive scarring that may subsequently lead to left ventricular remodeling, eventually leading to a dilated cardiomyopathy or possibly a predominant hypokinetic nondilated phenotype of cardiomyopathy. There are many different classifications for myocarditis depending on which cell types are affected by the inflammation (Ammirati et al., 2020).

Severe acute respiratory syndrome coronavirus 2 (SARS-CoV-2), also known as coronavirus disease 2019 (COVID-19), is a multisystem disease that resulted in acute respiratory illness. The majority of deaths were secondary to respiratory failure. However, some patients with COVID-19 did develop cardiovascular complications, especially myocarditis.

DIFFERENTIAL DIAGNOSIS
Angina Pectoris (Chronic Stable Angina)

ETIOLOGY, DEFINITION, SCOPE, AND DIAGNOSTIC STUDIES

Stable angina or stable ischemic heart disease occurs when the myocardial oxygen supply cannot meet its demand and subsequently results in myocardial ischemia. Ischemia occurs when there is an increase in oxygen demand (from psychosocial stress or exercise) in the setting of reduced coronary blood flow due to a fixed atherosclerotic coronary obstruction or when there is reduced perfusion due to abnormalities in the coronary microcirculation.

Angina has historically been described based on symptoms experienced by men including a recurrent type of discomfort in the retrosternal chest area that is provoked by exertion, stress, or anxiety; increases over a period of minutes; and

resolves with nitroglycerin treatment or rest within minutes. Usually described as tightening or squeezing that is hard to localize, it may radiate to the neck or jaw, down either arm but more frequently the left arm, or to the epigastric area. Other symptoms resulting from ischemia, also called anginal equivalents, may include indigestion and shortness of breath (Joshi & de Lemos, 2021).

Over the last decade, recognition has grown that women often present with unique symptoms of IHD. In women with INOCA, atypical angina may be more prevalent than typical angina. Therefore, when atypical angina is diagnosed, it is not recognized as ischemia, which delays treatment of ischemia in women (Reynolds et al., 2022). In view of this thought process, the updated chest pain guidelines in 2021 have discouraged the use of the word *atypical* as it could be a misleading descriptor of chest pain. They recommend using *noncardiac* if there is no suspicion of heart disease (Gulati et al., 2021).

Women have epicardial coronary arteries that are smaller than men even when adjusted for left ventricular mass and smaller body habitus. Women have a lower prevalence of obstructive coronary atherosclerosis compared with men even when the degree of ischemia is comparable. They are less likely to have adverse plaque characteristics and less atherosclerotic plaque of all subtypes when compared with men. The differences in CAD severity and plaque composition between males and females are more evident in populations among young adults and attenuated in older adults, which is thought to be due to the protective role of endogenous estrogen in premenopausal women (Reynolds et al., 2022).

Baseline and hyperemic myocardial blood flow, determined by PET, is usually higher in women compared to men, which results in similar global coronary flow reserve in women and men. Smaller diameter of female epicardial coronary arteries along with higher baseline myocardial blood flow are thought to result in a significant increase in endothelial shear stress conditions in women. However, the exact mechanisms of this are unknown. Low endothelial shear stress has been associated with pathologic remodeling, focal lipid accumulation, and plaque instability. For this reason, it is thought that higher shear stress conditions in female coronary arteries may contribute to sex differences and susceptibility to CAD (Reynolds et al., 2022).

The differences in women and men may be particularly evident during premenopausal ages due to estrogen-dependent effects on endothelial mediators, which include nitric oxide, endothelium-derived hyperpolarizing factor, and prostaglandins. The estrogen vascular actions are mediated by estrogen receptor α signaling promoting an anti-inflammatory, low vascular resistance phenotype that is protected from CVD. In the absence of estrogen, the estrogen receptor α–mediated effects are blunted and are consistent with variability seen in vascular stiffness throughout the lifespan of women. To note, more importantly, increased vascular stiffness is strongly associated with increased blood pressure, diastolic dysfunction, left ventricular remodeling, and ventricular coupling, which are thought to contribute to disease conditions that preferably affect postmenopausal women. These conditions include isolated systolic HTN and heart failure with preserved ejection fraction (HFpEF). In addition, distinct coronary plaque characteristics in women are noted, including reduced overall plaque burden, more diffuse and nonobstructive disease pattern, and calcium content as well as reduced signs of necrosis in the plaque core (Haider et al., 2019).

The primary mechanism responsible for MI in men is plaque rupture, while plaque erosion is the major cause of coronary thrombosis in women, especially in premenopausal women. Even though women overall have lower plaque burden, coronary artery calcium scoring has recently been identified to be a stronger risk predictor for future cardiovascular events in women as compared to men. Therefore, coronary artery calcium scoring has been recommended for evaluation of women who are asymptomatic with a 10-year CVD risk greater than 7.5% (Haider et al., 2019). These differences in coronary size and atherosclerosis development appear to favor the increased prevalence of INOCA in women (Reynolds et al., 2022).

While traditional risk factors for CVD are the same in men and women, the differences in impact and prevalence of these risk factors vary between them. This is particularly seen in acute coronary syndrome. Women who present with acute coronary syndrome have more comorbidities, including higher prevalence of HTN, DM, dyslipidemia, heart failure, and atrial fibrillation and are generally older. Women with type I and type II MI of early onset as a group have recently been noted to be affected by inequalities and adverse health outcomes. Data from the Variation in Recovery: Role of Gender and Outcomes of young AMI patients (VIRGO) study indicates that younger women have a poorer health status overall including mental health qualities of life than men prior to their event. Smoking and DM were shown to have a stronger effect on women. There is a 25% increased risk for fatal and nonfatal cardiovascular events in female smokers compared to male smokers independent of other risk factors. This risk factor was found to be highest among young and middle-aged women. Women with DM are at significantly higher risk of developing HFpEF or CAD than men. Lastly, a significant identifier in cases of younger women is family history, as women younger than 65 years of age with a maternal history of MI encounter a four times higher risk of ACS than same-age men and older women (Haider et al., 2019).

Two primary mechanisms of INOCA are coronary microvascular dysfunction (CMD) and coronary vasospasm. Suspicion should be raised for CMD when exertional or rest angina occurs in the absence of obstructive CAD (<50% diameter reduction or FFR [fractional flow reserve] >0.80), especially in the setting of definitive evidence of myocardial ischemia. Evidence of myocardial ischemia is demonstrated by dynamic ischemic electrocardiographic changes during an episode of angina or stress-induced angina and ischemic electrocardiographic changes in the setting of absence of transient/reversible abnormal myocardial perfusion and wall motion abnormality. CMD is diagnosed in the setting of impaired coronary flow reserve (CFR) <2.0 or 2.5, abnormal coronary microvascular resistance indices (index of microcirculatory resistance [IMR] <25 or hyperemic microvascular resistance [hMR] <2.0), coronary microvascular spasm, or coronary slow flow phenomenon. Traditional cardiovascular risk factors are associated with CMD but may account for less than 20% of the variability in CFR in women thought to possibly have CMD. The status of being postmenopausal does not appear to significantly contribute to CFR, although prior adverse pregnancy outcomes,

systemic inflammation, and prior breast cancer therapy may play a role (Reynolds et al., 2022).

Coronary microvascular dysfunction is characterized by functional as well as structural abnormalities. Functional abnormalities include smooth muscle dysfunction, autonomic dysfunction, and endothelial dysfunction. Structural abnormalities may include vascular wall infiltration (e.g., infiltrative heart disease such as Anderson-Fabry disease), vascular remodeling (e.g., arterial HTN and hypertrophic cardiomyopathy), perivascular fibrosis (e.g., aortic stenosis and arterial HTN), capillary rarefaction (e.g., aortic stenosis, heart failure, and arterial HTN), and luminal obstruction (e.g., microembolization during acute coronary syndrome or revascularization; Reynolds et al., 2022).

Epicardial coronary vasospasm is described as a subtotal coronary occlusion (>90% constriction) or transient total occlusion with angina and ischemic electrocardiographic changes. This can occur due to a provoking stressor or spontaneously. Women are approximately two times more likely to be found to have inducible coronary vasospasm compared with men as noted in a European study (Reynolds et al., 2022). However, in the Japanese population, coronary vasospasm was more common in men than women. Coronary vasospasm should be suspected when angina is nitrate responsive, occurs at rest between night and early morning, and is suppressed by calcium channel blockers. The mechanisms of coronary vasospasm include inflammation, oxidative stress, deficiency of endogenous nitric oxide activity, smooth muscle cell hyperreactivity, deficient variant aldehyde dehydrogenase genotype, and endothelial dysfunction. Vasospasm may be triggered in women with menstruation, and factors occurring in both sexes can include sympathetic activity, nonselective beta-blockers, allergic reactions, hyperventilation, muscarinic agonists, alcohol, ergot alkaloids, exposure to cold or to smoke, prostaglandins, and abnormal platelet activation (Reynolds et al., 2022).

In patients with coronary artery spasm on medical therapy, long-term prognosis is generally favorable (>95% survival over 5 years). However, if the patient has obstructive CAD, high incidence of MACE (major adverse cardiac events) has been noted in patients with coronary artery vasospasm even when under treatment with calcium channel blockade. Predictors of MACE include significant CAD, smoking, ST segment elevation, multivessel spasm, history of cardiac arrest, and reduction or withdrawal of antispasm medications (Reynolds et al., 2022).

The evaluation of ischemic heart disease in women can be very challenging to providers. The accuracy of standard noninvasive ischemia testing can vary significantly when compared with the definitive finding of anatomic obstructive CAD. The symptoms of female patients are less likely to be explained by invasive coronary angiography, and their abnormal stress tests in the absence of obstructive CAD are more likely to be interpreted as false-positive results when indeed they may be indicative of INOCA. The AHA/ACC chest pain guidelines provide clinical pathways that may start with functional or anatomic imaging, and either one of these pathways may subsequently lead to a diagnosis of INOCA (Reynolds et al., 2022).

All standard stress tests have a low sensitivity for detecting CMD; however, the presence of ischemic electrocardiographic changes, more specifically ST segment depression that persists for at least 1 minute into recovery, in the absence of obstructive CAD should prompt speculation for CMD. In women with myocardial bridging, exercise echocardiography is preferred to assess for end-systolic to early diastolic septal wall buckling with apical sparing. This occurrence is a sign of dynamic focal ischemia of a segment that is compressed. Women who have been diagnosed with INOCA should be evaluated for CMD. They should be referred for specialized testing such as stress CMRI and cardiac stress PET to confirm that ischemia in the setting of artifact or epicardial CAD is CMD. Assessing CFR in the left anterior descending artery in those with favorable anatomy by transthoracic Doppler echocardiography is not commonly performed. Additional assessments for atherosclerotic plaque burden using CT angiography (CTA) may help to further evaluate risk assessment and help guide preventive care strategies in those women with INOCA (Reynolds et al., 2022).

CFR defines the ratio between hyperemic coronary blood flow velocity and resting coronary flow velocity, which can be measured invasively using a coronary Doppler wire. Thermal dilution approach has also been validated using coronary pressures. Although initially designed to identify intermediate epicardial stenoses, CFR has now been adapted to assess for CMD as the entire coronary circulation including epicardial arteries and microvasculature can be assessed. CFR measurements in healthy asymptomatic individuals are usually >3.0, which indicates that when required, the coronary circulation can triple coronary blood flow. In comparison with men, CFR is generally lower in women, which may be due to sex differences in resting coronary flow. CFR <2.0 is significantly correlated with ischemia, which has been identified on SPECT imaging, with high specificity and sensitivity. Therefore, CFR is often considered the threshold for abnormal microcirculatory function. In those women suspected of having INOCA, CFR <2.32 was found to be the threshold for MACE (Reynolds et al., 2022).

EVALUATION/ASSESSMENT

HISTORY AND SYMPTOMS

Obtaining a complete history is the first step when evaluating the woman with chest pain. It is important to determine the nature of chest discomfort including location, description of pain, frequency, and duration. Women are more likely than men to present with stable angina as their first manifestation of CVD, whereas men more often present with infarction (Lerner & Kannel, 1986). Women have less exertional symptoms and instead are more likely to experience chest discomfort that occurs at rest or during sleep. Moreover, women experience other nonspecific symptoms of fatigue, nausea, and shortness of breath (Jackson, 2005).

Women are also less likely to describe their chest discomfort as substernal and crushing; rather, their symptoms are more often described as burning or squeezing or as a feeling of upper abdominal fullness (Jackson, 2005). As women age, there is a change in symptoms, and older women are more likely to present with a "typical" pattern of angina than younger women. Implications for practice included the following findings: (a) Older, White women without a history of DM or smoking were less likely to experience a cluster of prodromal symptoms but instead were likely to experience a single symptom, which

was profound fatigue; and (b) Black women younger than 50 years with multiple risk factors compared with other women were more likely to experience a cluster of symptoms composed of many distressing prodromal symptoms, and Black women who smoked, were younger, were obese, and were diabetic and had a history of CVD reported the largest cluster of acute MI symptoms (McSweeney et al., 2010). These data demonstrate the importance of a careful history to determine if the woman is experiencing a cluster of prodromal MI symptoms, which may help with a diagnosis of CVD to facilitate early treatment and a better clinical outcome.

PHYSICAL EXAMINATION AND DIAGNOSTIC STUDIES

The physical examination of women with angina is often benign. However, it may provide clues regarding the presence of cardiovascular risk factors or other vascular disease. During an episode of chest pain, a transient gallop or murmur of mitral regurgitation (MR) can be auscultated. Likewise, although the resting EKG of a woman with angina who is pain free is often normal, EKG changes may or may not be observed when the woman is having angina symptoms (Fraker & Fihn, 2007).

DIFFERENTIAL DIAGNOSIS

the differential diagnosis of angina pectoris includes angina, myocardial infarction, and cardiac syndrome X.

TREATMENT/MANAGEMENT

The initial medical management of stable angina should be coordinated by a cardiologist. The treatment for stable angina focuses on reducing the risk for myocardial infarction, death, and stroke through a reduction in episodes of angina, thereby improving quality of life. Lifestyle modifications regarding smoking cessation, diet (Mediterranean diet), physical activity, and weight loss are strongly encouraged. Optimal medical therapy should be initiated and includes antianginal medications such as beta-blockers, calcium channel blockers, or nitrates to improve quality of life in the setting of angina. Ranolazine can be used as a second-line therapy for refractory angina. Nitrates should be titrated based on symptoms, heart rate, blood pressure, and adverse effects. Consider sodium-glucose transporter-2 (SGLT2) inhibitors or glucagon-like peptide-1 (GLP-1) receptor agonists if the patient carries a diagnosis of DM. Secondary prevention medications should be utilized such as high potency statin and low-dose aspirin to decrease the risk for cardiovascular events. Lipid management can be controlled through the use of statins, ezetimibe, PCSK9 inhibitors, and icosapent ethyl for triglyceride levels. HTN should be well controlled. The aggressive target goal should be to achieve BP less than 130/80 mmHg (Joshi & de Lemos, 2021).

Management of refractory angina with coronary artery bypass graft (CABG) surgery and PCI as they relate to women are presented in the following sections.

Cardiac Syndrome X

ETIOLOGY

Cardiac syndrome X is identified by the presence of typical angina type symptoms and evidence of myocardial ischemia in the absence of flow-limiting stenosis noted on coronary angiography (Devabhaktuni, 2020). Microvascular angina (MVA) has largely replaced cardiac syndrome X. It is diagnosed when the pathogenesis is unknown (e.g., without abnormal flow reserve or without epicardial artery stenosis). Findings during diagnostic workup are compatible with coronary microvascular dysfunction/myocardial ischemia (Devabhaktuni, 2020).

Multiple mechanisms have been suggested to result in cardiac syndrome X (CSX). These mechanisms include endothelial dysfunction (MVA), which is currently the most prevailing theory, myocardial ischemia, abnormal autonomic control, altered cardiac sensitivity, insulin resistance, and estrogen deficiency. Cardiac syndrome X is seen more commonly in women than men and frequently occurs in perimenopausal and postmenopausal women (Devabhaktuni, 2020).

SCOPE

From 20% to 30% of patients who have a cardiac catheterization to assess chest pain symptoms may have nonobstructive CAD/cardiac syndrome X. Cardiac syndrome X occurs more often in women than in men. It occurs often in postmenopausal and perimenopausal women (Devabhaktuni, 2020).

The NHLBI's WISE study is the largest study of women with CVD to date (Johnson et al., 2004). In this study, nearly 60% of the 1,000 women referred for cardiac catheterization after an abnormal stress test did not have obstructive (flow-limiting) coronary lesions. Although women had lower angiographic disease burden and better left ventricular systolic function as determined by angiography, they had more symptoms and greater disability (Johnson et al., 2004). In addition, compared with age- and race-matched control subjects, women enrolled in the WISE study had higher cardiovascular event rates and mortality rates despite nonobstructive or angiographically normal coronary arteries (Kaski, 2006). Nearly 50% of women with normal coronary arteries in the WISE study had angiographic evidence of MCD as defined by reduced coronary flow velocity when injected with the vasodilator adenosine (Reis et al., 2001). These women had more cardiac events than women with normal microvascular vasodilator response. Moreover, MCD could not be predicted by traditional risk factors for heart disease (Reis et al., 2001). Patients with MCD have a 2.5% annual adverse cardiac event rate, which includes MI, congestive HF, stroke, and sudden cardiac death (Bugiardini & Bairey Merz, 2005). Data from the NHLBI-sponsored WISE study has shown that women with no obstructive CAD and evidence of myocardial ischemia have a poorer prognosis compared with women without obstructive CAD or myocardial ischemia (Johnson et al., 2004). Microvascular CAD is prevalent in women with signs and symptoms of ischemia and no obstructive CAD. The long-term prognosis is not benign, as previously thought; research findings suggest that these women are at increased risk for cardiac events. More research is needed to advance the understanding of MCD pathophysiology to guide diagnosis and therapy.

EVALUATION/ASSESSMENT

Workup for cardiac syndrome X includes routine laboratory studies, cholesterol levels, inflammatory markers, and levels of vitamin D. Vitamin D deficiency may be a risk factor as it may be related to increased inflammation, which can lead to the development of endothelial dysfunction and microvascular angina. Vitamin D levels of patients diagnosed with cardiac syndrome X appear to be significantly lower than levels in those who do not have this condition (Devabhaktuni, 2020).

Resting EKG findings may be normal although nonspecific ST-T wave abnormalities are often observed and at times associated with chest pain. Approximately 20% of patients with cardiac syndrome X have positive results on stress test, although many patients with this syndrome are unable to complete an exercise test because of mild chest discomfort or fatigue. Unlike obstructive CAD, left ventricular function is usually normal at rest and during stress. Particularly in young individuals with cardiac syndrome X, heart rate variability appears to be associated with exercise capacity (Devabhaktuni, 2020).

The standard test to evaluate for endothelial function is coronary flow reserve via Doppler guidewire in the cardiac catheterization laboratory (cath lab). This is done to assess the coronary blood flow and response to acetylcholine infusion and nitroglycerin. While myocardial ischemia secondary to abnormal coronary reactivity testing can be assessed noninvasively via SPECT, PET, and stress CMRI, the specificity and sensitivity of these measures has not been completely identified (Devabhaktuni, 2020).

TREATMENT/MANAGEMENT

The treatment of women with cardiac syndrome X or nonobstructive CAD is challenging. The goals of pharmacotherapy are to prevent complications and reduce morbidity. Beta-blockers appear to be most effective in decreasing the severity and frequency of angina and improving exercise tolerance. In low doses, metoprolol and atenolol selectively block beta-1-adrenergic receptors in the vascular smooth muscle and in the heart. This beta-1-receptor blockade decreases exercise and resting heart rate, systolic and diastolic blood pressure, and cardiac output.

ACE inhibitors are recommended, although the mechanism of action is not known. The thought is that there will be increased bioavailability of nitric oxide and, therefore, improvement in endothelial function. Statins are recommended, although the exact mechanism of benefit is unclear. Tricyclic antidepressants can be used and have been noted to be effective in the treatment of chronic pain and psychosomatic pain. Lastly, hormone therapy in postmenopausal women significantly reduces the frequency of anginal episodes, although hormonal therapy does carry significant cardiovascular risk as well. Therefore, the risks versus benefits must be weighed. The symptoms of patients with chest pain and normal angiograms appear to be improved with imipramine (Tofranil, Tofranil PM) possibly via a visceral analgesic effect (Devabhaktuni, 2020). Chest pain that is thought to be a result of cardiac syndrome X can be treated with nitrates and with the control of CVD risk factors including diet, smoking cessation, weight loss, and exercise (Devabhaktuni, 2020). The treatment of MCD can be challenging because of a current lack of uniform diagnostic criteria and multiple variables contributing to the pathophysiology. The goals of treatment are to control symptoms and improve quality of life, to reduce the incidence of hospitalization and repeated invasive testing, and to improve survival (Kothawade & Bairey Merz, 2011).

Acute Coronary Syndromes

Etiology

Approximately 70% to 80% of cases result from an unstable coronary plaque that fissures or ruptures and causes acute thrombosis (Morris, 2005). Further details of the process were presented in a review of vulnerable plaques (Finn et al., 2010) of more than 800 cases of sudden coronary death; at autopsy, 55% to 60% of subjects had underlying plaque rupture as the etiology, whereas 30% to 35% had erosion and 2% to 7% had thrombi attributed to calcified nodules.

ST segment elevation MI (STEMI) is caused by the acute and complete closure of a coronary artery, which results in myocardial necrosis and cell death; non-STEMI (NSTEMI) and unstable angina (UA) are caused by subtotal coronary occlusion, which results in varying amounts of myocardial damage.

Definition and Scope

ACSs include UA, non–Q-wave MI (also known as *NSTEMI*), and Q-wave MI (also known as *STEMI*). It is now understood that these conditions are not distinct, separate entities; rather, they exist on a continuum.

Acute MI is less likely to be the first presenting event in women, especially in younger women. Differences between men and women regarding morbidity and mortality decrease with advancing age (Lerner & Kannel, 1986). Autopsy studies revealed that plaque erosion is more common among women, particularly younger women, whereas plaque rupture is more common among men (Burke et al., 2003). This may explain why men experience greater prehospital acute MI mortality rates and why women have greater in-hospital mortality rates (Bairey Merz et al., 2006). Women generally present later during the course of MI because there is a delay in symptom recognition (Heer et al., 2002). One potential reason for the delay in treatment and poor outcomes is that women are more likely to experience a prodromal cluster of nonchest pain symptoms than men, which adds to the difficulty of securing a correct diagnosis (McSweeney et al., 2010).

Most deaths from acute MI occur outside of the hospital, with more men succumbing to sudden cardiac death than women; this may explain the disparity in mortality rates seen later in the course of the condition for women (Bairey Merz et al., 2006).

Evaluation/Assessment

Greater than 80% of women and men with ACS have chest pain or chest pressure as the presenting symptom. However, women present with more nonchest pain symptoms than men such as fatigue, dyspnea, neck pain, or nausea. Furthermore, women are more likely than men to present without chest pain, and they also attribute their symptoms to other conditions that are non–heart-related such as stress, anxiety, or acid reflux. Women tend to wait longer to seek medical attention and are less likely to have elevated troponin levels on admission or diagnostic EKG changes. Therefore, women

are at increased risk for delayed treatment or incorrect diagnosis. Women presenting with ACS tend to be older and have more comorbid conditions than men. Young age and the lack of chest discomfort at presentation were found to be the strongest predictors of misdiagnosis with regard to ACS and inappropriate discharge from the ED. Recently it has been noted that in younger demographic groups, there is a higher prevalence of comorbidities including DM, HTN, obesity, and depression in younger women with ACS as compared to men of equivalent age, suggesting that gender disparities in the management and outcome of ACS are not attributed to age alone (Haider et al., 2019).

Treatment/Management

Restoring coronary blood flow is the primary goal for a woman with STEMI (Kern, 2005), as it is with all patients per the 2013 American College of Cardiology Foundation (ACCF) and AHA Guideline for the Management of STEMI (O'Gara et al., 2013). For women with UA and NSTEMI, preventing further thrombosis and maintaining and improving existing coronary flow are the primary goals (Jneid et al., 2012; Morris, 2005).

Analysis of rhythm control trials involving conservative versus invasive revascularization in patients with NSTEMI between 1970 and 2008 demonstrated 33% reduced odds of death, MI, or rehospitalization for ACS when using an early invasive approach in women with high-risk features such as elevated troponin levels. In women without biomarker elevations, an early invasive approach demonstrated no substantial benefit and may have caused increased risk of MI or death. This was also noted in other studies such as TACTICS-TIMI 18 and in the 2014 AHA/ACC guidelines for management of patients with NSTEMI ACSs (Varghese & Wenger, 2018).

Despite guidelines, women are less likely than men to undergo revascularization with NSTEMI. The causes for this include atypical symptoms on presentation, inherent gender bias, underestimation of patient risk, conflicting data from post-hoc analysis of trials regarding the benefit of revascularization, and 1.5- to fourfold increase in vascular complications from the procedure (Varghese & Wenger, 2018).

THROMBOLYTICS FOR STEMI

Reperfusion therapy with thrombolytics benefits both genders and is indicated for women with chest pain symptoms of less than 12 hours' duration with ST segment elevation or new left bundle branch block (O'Gara et al., 2013). Women exhibit a higher incidence of cerebral bleeding complications related to thrombolytic therapy, which may affect decisions to forgo this therapy for women (Heer et al., 2002). Although findings of bleeding complications are controversial, factors such as an age older than 65 years, a low body weight (less than 70 kg), and HTN on admission all increase the risk of bleeding and are more prevalent among women (Rosengren & Hasdai, 2005).

PERCUTANEOUS CORONARY INTERVENTION FOR STEMI

In medical centers with appropriate resources immediately available, primary PCI (i.e., angioplasty with stenting) is preferred over intravenous thrombolytic therapy for the treatment of STEMI, and it is superior for decreasing mortality rates among both sexes (O'Gara et al., 2013). Meta-analyses and multiple rating control trials have demonstrated primary

PCI reduces MI, death, major bleeding, and stroke when compared with fibrinolysis particularly when treatment delays are minimized. This benefit is also seen among those patients transferred from non-PCI hospitals if their transfer times are within reason and ischemic and total ischemic time after presentation is less than 120 minutes (Lawton et al., 2022). In medical centers with PCI available, the standard of care is to expedite the process so that the time from medical contact to balloon or stent implantation is 90 minutes or less (O'Gara et al., 2013). Earlier studies comparing the outcomes utilizing bare-metal stents (BMS) and first-generation drug-eluting stents (DES) demonstrated an increased mortality rate with DES and increase in late stent thrombosis. The evolution of DES technology over the last 20 years, including polymer, optimization of drug, and stent design, has supported the efficacy and safety of the newer DES. Several large meta-analyses have been conducted and suggest the currently available DES have higher safety and efficacy and lower restenosis rates than both first-generation DES and BMS. Stents are ranked in safety from more to less as follows: durable-polymer DES > biodegradable-polymer DES > BMS. Newer generation DES have been recommended and are defined as any DES released after the original sirolimus-eluding or paclitaxel-eluding DES. Therefore, there is a limited role for the use of BMS as they are utilized only in particular circumstances such as unique patient circumstances that warrant extremely short duration of dual antiplatelet therapy (DAPT; e.g., <1 month) or lack of DES availability (Lawton et al., 2022).

Of particular importance to women is that stents appear to have favorable short-term and long-term results in smaller vessels as well as in larger vessels. Today, women remain at higher risk of in-hospital mortality and other complications. In contrast, long-term outcomes are similar or better in women and men. The use of a DES is associated with a similar benefit in both men and women (Anderson et al., 2012).

In the LEADERS FREE trial (December 2012 to May 2014), men and women had a similar 2-year occurrence of primary composite safety (including MI, stent thrombosis, and cardiac death) and success with respect to revascularization of the target lesion. In comparison to men, women had a greater major bleeding experience within the first 30 days of revascularization. In addition, women had greater major bleeding occurrences from vascular access sites (Mehran et al., 2020).

Studies have shown that women with ACS compared with men, especially after a STEMI, have less favorable short-term outcomes. This was felt to be related to women being older at presentation, longer system delays, prevalence of comorbid conditions, and underutilized guideline-directed therapies. Data regarding long-term morbidity and mortality following ACS were conflicting. In earlier studies, it was noted that long-term outcomes for women and men were similar. More recent data show that the long-term morbidity and mortality following ACS is higher in women than men, although once baseline variables were adjusted, these gender disparities no longer existed. However, short- and long-term outcomes in young and middle-aged women are worse compared to men at the same age. However, this group of women usually presents with worse health status, delays in the system, as well as inequities in diagnosis and treatment, which may be the etiology for high risk in this patient population (Haider et al., 2019).

PHARMACOTHERAPEUTICS

During the initial stages of ACS with or without PCI, aspirin has been the mainstay therapy. Women derive as much benefit as men do from aspirin therapy with ACS or MI (Antithrombotic Trialists Collaboration, 2002).

Women undergoing PCI for ACS should be given a loading dose of aspirin followed by daily dosing as well as a P2Y12 inhibitor followed by daily dosing. P2Y12 inhibitors that are available and currently utilized are clopidogrel, ticagrelor, and prasugrel. Per the guidelines, it is preferable that ticagrelor or prasugrel be utilized in preference to clopidogrel to reduce ischemic events. In patients whose history includes a transient ischemic attack or stroke, prasugrel should not be utilized. Unfractionated heparin had been the mainstay of pharmacologic management of ACS and MI. However, enoxaparin is now considered a safe alternative to unfractionated heparin (Lawton et al., 2022).

After PCI, DAPT is utilized to reduce ischemic events and prevent stent thrombosis. This is at the risk of increased bleeding. Data demonstrated decreased bleeding with shorter term DAPT (3 to 6 months) and decreased ischemic events (including stent thrombosis) with longer-term DAPT (greater than 12 months). In the 2016 focused update on duration of DAPT, the significance of assessing bleeding and ischemic risk when DAPT is considered was highlighted. Recommendations were provided for short and prolonged DAPT followed by aspirin monotherapy after revascularization. More recent trials have been published since the release of the 2016 guidelines. Five large trials were conducted and tested for a shorter duration DAPT followed by P2Y12 inhibitor monotherapy status post PCI. The duration of DAPT ranged from 1 to 3 months. The data supported a shorter course of DAPT followed by P2Y12 monotherapy. This strategy in comparison to standard DAPT therapy showed a reduction in bleeding events and the rates of ischemic events were equivalent. The trials largely supported ticagrelor and clopidogrel monotherapy, but one trial did include prasugrel monotherapy. A meta-analysis of the duration of DAPT utilizing these five trials demonstrated a 40% reduction in the rate of major bleeding events with shorter term DAPT followed by P2Y12 monotherapy and no significant difference in MACE was identified (Lawton et al., 2022).

Other treatment options for the patient with UA, NSTEMI, or STEMI include beta-blockers, nitrates, ACE inhibitors, and calcium channel blockers. Beta-blockers prevent recurrent MI and ischemia and are effective antianginal and antihypertensive agents. They are contraindicated for women with bronchospasm, hypotension, or advanced atrioventricular node block. The long-term use of ACE inhibitors helps with the prevention of recurrent ischemic events and the reduction of mortality, especially among women with left ventricular dysfunction. For women who are allergic to ACE inhibitors, ARBs are indicated (Krumholz et al., 2008). In addition to beta-blockers and ACE inhibitors, the Task Force on Performance Measures also reiterated the importance of the evaluation and treatment of risk factors during the inpatient care of the post-MI patient, especially checking lipid levels and providing smoking-cessation advice and counseling (Krumholz et al., 2008). Secondary prevention medications such as statins should be initiated as well as antithrombotic therapy. In the medical management of ACS, special attention should be paid to age-related change in formal kinetics, polypharmacy, teratogenic consequences in pregnancy and childbearing-age women, and drug–drug interactions in the older population (Varghese & Wenger, 2018).

CORONARY ARTERY BYPASS GRAFT SURGERY

The decision to treat women with PCI or CABG surgery is complex. In general, multivessel disease and left main CAD are indications for a surgical approach (Hillis et al., 2011). Fewer women are referred for CABG and PCI, with women making up only 33% of patients who have had PCI. Women have been reported to have worse outcomes than men after CABG surgery. However, results among various studies have been inconsistent. Observed differences may have been due to large differences in the baseline characteristics of males and females. To investigate this further, a systemic review and pooled analysis of patient data from large CABG trials was conducted to compare the adjusted outcomes of men and women (Gaudino et al., 2021).

The analysis of 13,193 patients (2,714 women) that had been followed for a mean of 5 years showed that after CABG, women have a higher occurrence of adverse cardiac and cerebrovascular events than men. Mortality rates were similar when compared with men. The higher incidence of MACCE (major adverse cardiac and cerebrovascular events) was determined to be due to a higher rate of repeat vascularization and MI (Gaudino et al., 2021).

Differences between males and females were found to be inversely associated with age and were not noted at 75 years old. CAD in young women has unique pathophysiologic characteristics and outcomes, which include microvascular dysfunction, spasm, myocardial bridging (occurring more often in women than men), coronary dissection (more common in women than men), and higher mortality rate after acute coronary events (Gaudino et al., 2021).

Vaccarino et al. (2014) found in a large registry of 51,187 patients (15,178 being women) that women under the age of 50 had double the higher adjusted operative mortality rate after CABG compared with men of the same age group. In addition, the operative outcomes between sexes decreased with increasing age (Guadino et al. 2021).

Also noted to be a significant modifier between males and females was the preoperative LVEF (left ventricular ejection fraction). Women who had a preoperative LVEF >30% were at increased risk of MACCE compared to men. However, in women with an LVEF <30%, the opposite was true.

Additionally, women were found to have a higher risk of perioperative MI after CABG. Women have native coronary arteries and bypass conduits that are generally smaller than men and in vitro evidence suggests that they may have a higher tendency to spasm when compared with men. The complication and propensity to spasm was thought to be increased in younger women, which may explain why age is a factor with differences in outcomes between males and females. Further investigation is necessary (Guadino, et al., 2021).

Alam et al. (2013) analyzed data from 20 studies and 966,492 patients (277,783 women) and discovered that female sex was associated with a higher risk of operative mortality when compared with men. In addition, they found that this higher risk of operative mortality was still prevalent at a 5-year follow-up. This was the only published meta-analysis at that time investigating the impact of sex and outcomes following CABG (Alam et al., 2013).

Analysis from Gaudino et al. (2021) suggests that variations in CABG surgical technique (off-pump vs. on-pump surgery and use of multiple arterial grafts [MAGs] vs. single arterial grafts [SAGs]) do not make the outcomes for women better and do not decrease the difference between sexes. Off-pump CABG did not result in any change in outcomes between women and men (Gaudino et al., 2021).

CARDIAC REHABILITATION

The leading cause of morbidity and death in females and males in the United States and globally is CVD. The development and diagnosis of CVD vary among males and females and foreshadow specific disparities in the clinical management and outcomes. One example of this is that females are often older, present with different symptomatology, and have more comorbidities when diagnosed with CAD. It has now been determined that female-specific risk factors such as preeclampsia and early menopause increase CVD risk for females. Despite this knowledge, a large proportion of cardiologists and primary care physicians lack knowledge/awareness with regard to CVD risk and management specifically of females. In addition, there is evidence that females who have CAD have worse short-term outcomes compared with males. Therefore, optimal secondary prevention strategies are vital to improve patient care and outcomes in those females with CVD (Smith et al., 2022).

The ACC/AHA guidelines recommend cardiac rehabilitation (CR) for secondary prevention for patients with CVD, which is a class I recommendation. The Centers for Medicare & Medicaid Services now provide coverage for CR for those patients following acute MI, coronary artery bypass surgery, heart valve replacement or repair, percutaneous transluminal coronary angioplasty or coronary stenting, heart–lung or heart transplant, as well as those with heart failure with reduced ejection fraction or stable angina (Smith et al., 2022).

Cardiac rehabilitation is a comprehensive multidisciplinary program focused on chronic disease management that encompasses core components including patient assessment, nutritional counseling, psychological management and counseling, exercise training, cardiovascular risk factor management, and physical activity counseling. There is significant evidence that indicates participation in cardiac rehabilitation is effective in improving CVD risk factor management, psychological management, quality of life, and exercise capacity. In addition, cardiac rehabilitation participation has also been associated with reduction in mortality rate and hospital readmissions. Sex disparities are present in outpatient phase 2 cardiac rehab programming despite these advantageous outcomes (Smith et al., 2022).

In 2016, approximately 24% of patients who were eligible Medicare beneficiaries participated in CR with approximately 57% and 27% of those beneficiaries completing greater than 24 and 36 CR sessions, respectively. To note, sex-specific disparities occur with referral to CR, enrollment, and completion. Females were 12% less likely to be referred to CR compared with males, noted by Li et al. (2018), using the AHA CAD registry data. Furthermore, it's been reported that females are less likely than males to enroll in CR, attend CR sessions, and finish the CR program. CR has been shown to elicit similar or greater mortality benefit in females compared with males despite the low CR participation rate in females (Smith et al., 2022).

Various CR delivery strategies may have the potential to alleviate sexual differences. One proposed example is hybrid CR, which, in addition to the conventional center CR, would provide the patient an opportunity to engage in CR programming outside the CR center such as in their home. Hybrid CR has the potential to resolve many of the CR participation barriers, specifically to females, such as family responsibilities and transportation. When hybrid CR is attended in another location other than a conventional center, it can be delivered in a synchronous or asynchronous manner such as communication (texting, telephone calls) versus audiovisual care during exercise (Smith et al., 2022).

The prescription for exercise in the outpatient phase 2 CR setting is not ideal for all patients, specifically females, which is evidenced by lower CR participation/adherence and blunted improvements in Vo_2 peak in females now in CR. Females more often feel that exercise is painful or tiring compared with males. Strategies for alternative approaches for intensity, modality, and frequency need to be further investigated. Alternative modalities such as dancing, Zumba, and group walking may be aerobic activities that are more viable for females to incorporate in the CR program (Vidal-Almela et al., 2021). In addition, it has now been determined that sex-specific risk-enhancing factors increase CVD risk. These enhancing factors include premature menopause, preeclampsia, adverse pregnancy outcomes (such as DM and gestational HTN), polycystic ovary syndrome, ovarian failure, inflammatory disorders, and certain hormone-based contraceptive methods (Smith et al., 2022).

Heart Failure

DEFINITION, SCOPE, AND ETIOLOGY

Heart failure (HF) is a complex syndrome that involves cardiac pump dysfunction (either systolic or diastolic) in combination with cardiac remodeling and the interaction of various hormonal and cytokine systems along with alterations in renal function, as well as activation of the rennin–angiotensin–aldosterone and sympathetic nervous systems that ultimately results in circulatory insufficiency (Koelling et al., 2004). HF can result from a structural or functional impairment of ventricular filling or ejection of blood (Heidenreich et al., 2022).

HF is identified as being in one of two categories: diastolic HF or systolic HF. In diastolic HF, also known as heart failure with preserved ejection fraction (HFpEF), there is inadequate filling of the heart with blood during diastole. The etiology for diastolic HF varies, although the usual cause, chronic HTN, is seen through hypertrophy (thickening of the walls of the heart), which results in a decreased ability for the chambers of the heart to fill with blood. This in turn decreases preload, resulting in a decreased amount of oxygenated blood being ejected and thereby decreasing blood supply to the tissues (Oberman & Bhardwaj, 2022). In systolic HF, also known as heart failure with reduced ejection fraction (HFrEF), there is an inability of the heart to pump blood effectively during

systole. The more common etiologies for systolic HF are HTN, CAD, dilated cardiomyopathy (DCM), and valvular disease. Other known etiologies are MI and aortic stenosis. There are many etiologies for DCM to develop causing dilatation of the heart chambers and a decreased ability to contract properly. Some etiologies are infections (such as Coxsackie B virus), toxins (such as ethanol), medications (e.g., trastuzumab), autoimmune/inflammatory disorders (e.g., sarcoidosis), and genetic conditions (Oberman & Bhardwaj, 2022).

HF is also categorized by the amount of blood that is moved through the left ventricle into the aorta over the total amount of blood that is available in the left side of the heart, which is known as LVEF (Oberman & Bhardwaj, 2022). Diastolic HF (HFpEF) is identified by an LVEF ≥50%. Systolic HF (HFrEF) is identified by an LVEF ≤40%. Other classifications of HF include heart failure with mildly reduced ejection fraction (HFmrEF), defined as LVEF 41% to 49%, and heart failure with improved EF (HFimpEF), with LVEF >40% when it was previously ≤40% (Heidenreich et al., 2022).

Etiologies for HF include MI, ischemic heart disease, valvular heart disease (VHD), genetic or familial cardiomyopathies, amyloidosis, cardiotoxicity with substance abuse (cocaine, alcohol, or methamphetamine) or with cancer or other treatments, tachycardia, stress-induced or right ventricular (RV) pacing cardiomyopathies, peripartum cardiomyopathy, myocarditis, autoimmune causes, sarcoidosis, iron overload (including hemochromatosis), thyroid disease, and other endocrine metabolic and nutritional causes (Heidenreich et al., 2022).

Many cardiomyopathies are unique to women and can result in HF. Peripartum cardiomyopathy presents with left ventricular diastolic dysfunction early after delivery but may also occur during pregnancy or after delivery (DeFilippis et al., 2021). Hypertropic cardiomyopathy is genetic and is usually diagnosed when clinical symptoms arise. Women, compared with men, are more likely to have obstructive physiology and a greater mortality rate (DeFilippis et al., 2021).

Cardiac sarcoidosis is identified by endomyocardial biopsy or a combination of clinical cardiac symptoms in the setting of a biopsy-confirmed extracardiac sarcoid (DeFilippis et al., 2021). Cardiac amyloidosis is an infiltrative myocardial disease that results in cardiomyopathy by the deposition of misfolded amyloid fibrils within the heart muscle (DeFillipis et al., 2021). The two most common types are monoclonal immunoglobulin amyloid light chain cardiomyopathy (AL-CM) and transthyretin amyloidosis (ATTR-CM; Heidenreich et al., 2022). AL cardiac amyloidosis has a slightly increased predominance in males and usually presents from the fifth to seventh decade of life.

ATTR-CM is no longer considered a rare disease entity. ATTR can result from pathogenic variants in the transthyretin gene *TTR* (variant transthyretin amyloidosis, ATTRv) or wild-type transthyretin (wild-type transthyretin amyloidosis, ATTRwt). Sex differences in ATTR-CM are most significant in ATTRwt, in which there is an 80% to 90% predominance of men versus women. Although in a prospective screening study in patients over 60 years of age, admitted with HFpEF and left ventricular wall thickness greater than 12 mm, it was found that there was an equal proportion of men and women who were identified as having ATTR-CM by scintigraphy. In addition, a prospective endomyocardial biopsy study that consisted of 108 patients with HFpEF (61% of these patients being women), 40% of the patients with ATTR-CM were women (DeFilippis et al., 2021).

HF is a major cause of death and morbidity in women. Women tend to develop HF at an older age compared with men. HFpEF is responsible for half the cases of HF in women. HFpEF is more prevalent in women than in men (Bozkurt & Khalaf, 2017). Women with HFpEF have more of a predisposition to HTN as opposed to CAD. However, once a woman develops CAD, the risk for HF development is high. In a Framingham cohort, after having an MI, women had an increased risk of symptomatic HF when compared to men. DM and HTN increase the risk for developing CAD more for women than for men, and this in turn can result in the development of HF in women (Bozkurt & Khalaf, 2017).

HFpEF (LVEF ≥55%) is twice as common in women than men. This is due to the physiologic differences in men and women (Eisenberg et al., 2018). Women have greater LV (left ventricular) contractility, lower LV mass, LV mass that is more preserved with aging, smaller coronary vessels, a lower rate of myocyte apoptosis, less catecholamine-mediated vasoconstriction, and a faster resting heart rate (Bozkurt & Khalaf, 2017).

In the United States, HF is a growing health and economic burden mostly due to the aging population. The total deaths caused by HF in the United States have increased from 275,000 in 2009 to 310,000 in 2014 (Heidenreich et al., 2022). Noted in the 2017 AHA Heart Disease and Stroke Statistics Update, HF prevalence has increased to 6.5 million among Americans who are ≥20 years old. It is estimated that by 2030, the incidence of HF will increase by 46%, which will affect more than 8 million individuals. HF equally affects both males and females and is the leading cause of morbidity and death (Bozkurt & Khalaf, 2017).

HF hospitalizations in the United States had decreased until about 2012. However, from 2013 to 2017, there has been a 26% increase in HF hospitalizations with 1.2 million hospitalizations among the 924,000 persons with HF (Heidenreich et al., 2022).

While the number of patients with HF has grown because of the increasing number of older adults, the incidence of HF has decreased. However, the incidence of HFpEF is increasing and the incidence of HFrEF is decreasing. Deaths due to cardiomyopathies have increased globally as a result of increased recognition, diagnosis, and documentation of specific cardiotoxicity and cardiomyopathies (Heidenreich et al., 2022).

EVALUATION/ASSESSMENT

The diagnosis of HF is made clinically and is based on one or more clinical symptoms of volume overload, including elevated jugular venous pressure, hepatojugular reflux, lung crackles, and lower-extremity edema (Box 43.5; Bristow & Lowes, 2005). Signs and symptoms of HF are similar for women and men (Box 43.5), although women have increased frequency with difficulty exercising, dyspnea upon exertion, and edema in comparison to men. Women also tend to have a worse quality of life than men for social activity and intermediate activities of daily living. In people who have HF, depression is more common in women than men. Women usually present with HF at an older age in comparison with men and develop a left bundle branch block on an EKG more

---

Box 43.5 Signs to Evaluate in Patients With Heart Failure

Elevated cardiac filling pressures and fluid overload

Elevated jugular venous pressure

S_3 gallop

Rales

Hepatojugular reflux

Ascites

Edema

Cardiac enlargement

Laterally displaced or prominent apical impulse

Murmurs that suggest valvular dysfunction

Reduced cardiac output

Narrow pulse pressure

Cool extremities

Tachycardia with pulsus alternans

Arrhythmia

Irregular pulse

Source: Adapted from Lindenfeld, J., Albert, N. M., Boehmer, J. P., Collins, S. P., Ezekowitz, J. A., Givertz, M. M., Katz, S. D., Klapholz, M., Moser, D. K., Rogers, J. G., Starling, R. C., Stevenson, W. G., Tang, W. H., Teerlink, J. R., & Walsh, M. N. (2010). HFSA 2010 comprehensive heart failure practice guideline. Journal of Cardiac Failure, 16(6), e46. *https://doi.org/10.1016/j.cardfail.2010.04.004*

---

frequently than men. In addition, women are less likely than men to be referred for diagnostic testing or specialty care, and they undergo fewer procedures including revascularization, cardiac resynchronization therapy (CRT), implantable cardioverter defibrillators (ICDs), and mechanical circulatory support (Bozkurt & Khalaf, 2017). Patients are classified based on functional capacity. The New York Heart Association (NYHA) classification system relates symptoms to everyday activities and to the woman's quality of life (Young & Mills, 2001). This system categorizes the severity of congestive HF by functional classes that depend on the degree of effort required to elicit symptoms. Class I patients have no limitation of physical activity: Ordinary activities do not produce symptoms of angina, dyspnea, or undue fatigue. Class II patients have a slight limitation of physical activity: Ordinary activities do produce cardiac symptoms. Class III patients have a marked limitation of physical activity: Although these patients are comfortable at rest, less-than-ordinary activities do produce cardiac symptoms. Those in Class IV have severe, persistent symptoms with any physical activity, and they can also have symptoms while at rest.

DIAGNOSTIC STUDIES

It is important that the specific cause of HF be identified because certain conditions require disease-specific therapies. Laboratory evaluation including urinalysis, serum electrolytes, blood urea nitrogen, serum creatinine, complete blood count, fasting lipid profile, thyroid-stimulating hormone levels, liver function tests, and iron studies including ferritin, serum iron, and transferrin saturation should be performed on initial evaluation of the patient to help provide information regarding the patient's comorbidities, potential causes of HF, eligibility for and adverse effects of treatments, and degree and prognosis of HF. Laboratory tests are repeated with changes in treatment or in clinical conditions (Heidenreich et al., 2022).

The measurement of B-type natriuretic peptide (BNP) or N-terminal prohormone of B-type natriuretic peptide (NT-proBNP) should be obtained and can be useful in supporting or excluding the diagnosis of HF in an individual. In patients with chronic HF, measurements of NT-proBNP or BNP levels are recommended to stratify risk. In hospitalized patients, BNP or NT-proBNP levels are recommended on admission to establish prognosis. In addition, a BNP or NT-proBNP level is useful predischarge in helping to plan the patient's course and postdischarge prognosis. It is important to note that obesity is associated with lower levels of BNP and NT-proBNP, which can decrease diagnostic sensitivity. There also needs to be consistency in obtaining either BNP or NT-proBNP; they are not interchangeable (Heidenreich et al., 2022).

An EKG should be obtained for the initial evaluation. It should be repeated when a clinical indication arises such as ischemia or myocardial injury, suspicion for an arrhythmia, conduction abnormality, or other cardiac abnormalities (Heidenreich et al., 2022). The EKG often reveals LVH. Tachycardia, rapid atrial fibrillation (AF), ischemic EKG changes, and evidence of atrioventricular and intraventricular conduction blocks and changes in voltage can be present (Madias, 2006).

A chest radiograph should be obtained to assess for pulmonary congestion, to determine heart size, and to detect an alternative pulmonary, cardiac, or other disease process that may be contributing to symptoms (Heidenreich et al., 2022). A chest radiograph often shows increased intravascular markings, frank pulmonary edema, or pleural effusions; cardiomegaly is a common finding as well (Madias, 2006).

DIFFERENTIAL DIAGNOSIS
Systolic Versus Diastolic Heart Failure

A transthoracic echocardiogram (TTE) has become an integral part of the evaluation of the woman with HF. It is helpful for making the diagnosis of diastolic HF by identifying LVH, which is the leading cause of diastolic HF (Jessup et al., 2009; Vasan & Levy, 2000). It provides important clues regarding the etiology of HF by assessing the cardiac structure and function of the heart and identifying abnormalities of the heart valves, myocardium, and pericardium (Heidenreich et al., 2022). The various etiologies of HF that may be found include ischemia, HTN, valvular disease, regurgitation, pericardial effusion, cardiomyopathy, cardiac amyloidosis, or a combination. Results of the TTE also help guide management because the test provides a measurement of the EF (Yancy et al., 2013).

At times, the TTE may not accurately evaluate the cardiac structure and function of the heart, or more information may be necessary to determine the cause for cardiac dysfunction.

TABLE 43.4 Heart Failure Classifications

CLASSIFICATION	DEFINITION
HFrEF (heart failure with reduced ejection fraction)	Ejection fraction ≤40%
HFimpEF (heart failure with improved EF [with an EF that had previously been ≤40%])	EF >40%
HFmrEF (heart failure with mildly reduced ejection fraction)	EF 41% to 49%
HFpEF (heart failure with preserved ejection fraction)	EF ≥50%

Source: Heidenreich, P. A., Bozkurt, B., Aguilar, D., Allen, L. A., Byun, J. J., Colvin, M. M., Deswal, A., Drazner, M. H., Dunlay, S. M., Evers, L. R., Fang, J. C., Fedson, S. E., Fonarow, G. C., Hayek, S. S., Hernandez, A. F., Khazanie, P., Kittleson, M. M., Lee, C. S., Link, M. S., . . . Yancy, C. W. (2022). 2022 AHA/ACC/HFSA guideline for the management of heart failure. Journal of the American College of Cardiology, 79(17), e263–e421. https://doi.org/10.1016/j.jacc.2021.12.012

Therefore, other imaging modalities are utilized to clarify the initial diagnosis of congestive HF and to provide a more accurate assessment of cardiac structure and function. These other imaging modalities may include stress echocardiography, SPECT imaging, CMR, cardiac CT, radionuclide ventriculography, invasive coronary angiography, or PET (Heidenreich et al., 2022).

HF is often separated into two diagnostic categories, depending on the left ventricular systolic function. Systolic HF refers to a LVEF <50%. Diastolic HF refers to a LVEF ≥50%; however, HF now includes a wide range of LV function (Heidenreich et al., 2022). Classification of HF defined by LVEF has been revised per the 2022 AHA/ACC/HFSA guidelines for HF management (Heidenreich et al., 2022). See Table 43.4 for HF classifications.

TREATMENT/MANAGEMENT

HF treatment continues to evolve, especially with the advent of new classes of medications and new indications for older medications. In addition, devices such as implantable defibrillators and biventricular pacemakers have been shown to improve morbidity and mortality rates among women with systolic HF (Agabiti-Rosei & Muiesan, 2002). Wilcox et al. (2014), in an analysis of data from the registry to Improve the Use of Evidence-Based Heart Failure Therapies in the Outpatient Setting (IMPROVE HF), found that cardiac resynchronization therapy (CRT) and implantable cardioverter defibrillator (ICD) therapy were equally effective in men and women with HF.

Another device, CardioMEMS, used to manage HF is an implantable wireless sensor placed through a catheter delivery system in the left lower lobe pulmonary artery and has the ability to measure pulmonary artery pressure (PAP) remotely. Using an external electronic system, patients obtain daily home measurements and transmit their PAP data wirelessly. Providers use the PAP reading to assess the patient's volume status to further guide their treatment regimen (Kotalczyk et al., 2022).

The CHAMPION (CardioMEMS Heart Center Allows Monitoring of Pressure to Improve Outcomes in New York Heart Association Class III Heart Failure Patients) trial was a randomized controlled trial conducted in 64 centers in the United States. CHAMPION participants had class III HF irrespective of LVEF and were randomized either to standard care or care guided by PAP readings. PAP-guided pharmacotherapy lowered the risk of hospitalizations. A subanalysis of CHAMPION patients with implanted CRTs showed that changes in medical therapy guided by PAP readings decreased HF symptoms as well as hospitalization (beyond the effective CRT) by 30% compared with standard therapy. Patients who received care guided by PAPs had increased medication titrations, a decrease in mean PAP, and improvement in quality of life (as noted by the Minnesota Living with Heart Failure Questionnaire). In addition, a subanalysis of patients with reduced LVEF and HF demonstrated that receiving optimal therapy guided by PAP readings had fewer hospitalizations and reduced mortality rate as compared with the control group (Kotalczyk et al., 2022).

In the CardioMEMS PAS (Post-Approval Study), sex differences were assessed in response to ambulatory hemodynamic monitoring. It was found that men and women who were enrolled in the CardioMEMS PAS had a similar decrease in PAPs over 1 year from their baseline. In addition, both sexes had a similar decrease in HF hospitalizations (DeFilippis et al., 2021).

Despite the benefits of telemetry medical monitoring, it remains underutilized in clinical practice. Challenges encountered in its use include adherence to therapeutic protocols by physicians and patients, lack of reimbursement, and the need for significant changes in hospitals' workflows or data overload. Telemedical monitoring can be advantageous in preventing hospitalizations and in the prevention of "face-to-face" follow-up, which became especially important during the era of the COVID-19 pandemic and efforts to maintain social distancing (Kotalczyk et al., 2022). It can also help those patients who cannot find transportation for frequent follow-ups.

According to the 2022 AHA/ACC/HFSA guideline for the management of HF, in those patients with NYHA class III HF, with an HF hospitalization within the previous year, it was felt that wireless monitoring of the PAP with an implantable device provided uncertain value (Heidenreich et al., 2022). There were methodologic concerns about bias that may have influenced the results of the CHampion study. Recently, there was a GUIDE-HF (Hemodynamic-Guided Management of Heart Failure) study that looked at hemodynamic guided management of patients with NYHA class II to IV. It was found that hemodynamic guided management did not significantly reduce the composite end point of total HF events and rate of mortality. The utility of noninvasive monitoring or remote monitoring of physiologic parameters (thoracic impedance, patient activity, and heart rate) obtained through implanted electrical devices such as ICDs or CRT defibrillators remains ambiguous. Further studies are recommended for this to become routine clinical care (Heidenreich et al., 2022).

Self-Management Measures

Patient education is a critical component of HF self-management. HF can be difficult to understand, and it requires complicated lifestyle and medication regimens for management. Deviating from the diet or medication plan can have disastrous consequences (Bristow & Lowes, 2005). Many clinics have implemented disease-management programs for women with HF, and these have been shown to decrease frequent hospitalizations (Chan et al., 2008; Sanghavi et al., 2014). APRN-run programs can be a cost-effective alternative to the traditional management of these women to improve health outcomes (Lowery et al., 2012; Stauffer et al., 2014).

Outpatient Emergency Department

In some parts of the United States, EDs have areas established exclusively to treat patients with HF who are volume overloaded with an intravenous diuretic or to assign the patient to observation for a few hours without admission. If patients in either program respond to treatment, they return home with continued outpatient management. Furthermore, in some extended-care facilities, patients with HF who require intravenous care may now receive the medication in place without transfer to the hospital. Home-care services can also assist with the monitoring of these women and with helping them to adhere to diet and medication regimens. Accordingly, home-monitoring programs appear to be the most effective in promoting long-term outcome benefit when they reinforce patient education toward medication adherence and patient self-efficacy (Konstam, 2012). In a review article Gandhi and Pinney (2014) have also found that a combination of biomarkers, monitoring devices, and disease-management programs together may work best for improving care for all patients with HF.

PHARMACOTHERAPEUTICS

LEFT VENTRICULAR DYSFUNCTION

The 2022 Guideline for the Management of Heart Failure (Heidenreich et al., 2022) addresses all classes of HF including HFrEF (LVEF ≤40%), HFimpEF (LVEF previously ≤40% and subsequent measurement shows LVEF >40%), HFmrEF (LVEF 41% to 49%), and HFpEF (LVEF ≥50%). All patients with prior HF history or current HF, despite measurement of LVEF, should be considered for guideline-directed medical therapy (GDMT; Colvin, 2022).

Diuretics are used to improve symptoms, relieve congestion, and prevent worsening HF. The goal is to use the lowest dose of diuretic to maintain euvolemia. The preferred diuretic medications in most HF patients are loop diuretics such as furosemide, torsemide, and bumetanide. Furosemide is most commonly used. In those patients with HTN, HF, and mild fluid retention, thiazide diuretics may be considered. In those patients who have persistent edema and are unresponsive to loop diuretics alone, metolazone or chlorothiazide may be added to the loop diuretic. However, these patients must be monitored closely as this combination can put patients at increased risk for hyponatremia, hypokalemia, worsening renal function, and death, whereas higher doses of loop diuretics alone did not adversely affect survival. There are limited randomized data that compare these two approaches, although the DOSE (Diuretic Optimization Strategies Evaluation) trial did favor the use of high-dose intravenous loop diuretics (Heidenreich et al., 2022).

The effects of diuretics on mortality and morbidity are uncertain with the exception of MRAs (mineralocorticoid receptor antagonists). Data obtained recently from the nonrandomized registry called Optimize-HF (Organized Program to Initiate Lifesaving Treatment in Hospitalized Patients with Heart Failure) showed reduced 30-day hospitalization for HF and a lower all-cause mortality rate with the use of diuretics compared with no diuretic use after a hospital discharge for HF (Heidenreich et al., 2022).

GDMT now consists of four classes of medications: (1) renin–angiotensin system inhibition (RASi) with the use of angiotensin receptor–neprilysin inhibitors (ARNi), ACE inhibitors (ACEi), or ARB alone; (2) beta-blockers; (3) MRAs; and (4) SGLT2 inhibitors (SGLT2i; Colvin, 2022).

ARNi is now recommended as the first-line RASi to reduce morbidity and mortality in HFrEF (class 1a recommendation; Colvin, 2022). When an ARNi is not appropriate, an ACEi is recommended. If an individual cannot tolerate an ACEi and an ARNi is not appropriate, an ARB is recommended. If an individual has been on an ACEi or ARB, it is recommended to discontinue the ACEi or ARB and initiate an ARNi for increased reduction in morbidity and mortality (Colvin, 2022). It is recommended that an ARNi be utilized before discharge as de novo treatment in patients hospitalized with acute HF if they have had a reduction in NT-proBNP, improvement in health status, and improvement of LV remodeling parameters compared with an ACEi or ARB (Heidenreich et al., 2022).

ARBs are indicated when women are intolerant to ACE inhibitors. For women who cannot take an ACE inhibitor or an ARB (e.g., women with renal disease), the combination of hydralazine and a nitrate is an acceptable alternative (Lindenfeld et al., 2010; Yancy et al., 2013).

Beta-blockers, which were formerly absolutely contraindicated for women with HF, have become one of the cornerstone therapies (Lindenfeld et al., 2010; Yancy et al., 2013). Because beta-blockers were a later addition to the treatment of congestive HF, women have not been adequately studied (Wenger, 2002). Beta-blockers are equally effective for reducing morbidity and mortality rates in both women and men (CIBIS-II Investigators and Committees, 1999; Ghali et al., 2002; Packer et al., 2001). In patients with HFrEF, with either previous or current symptoms, the use of one of three beta-blockers has been proved to reduce mortality (Heidenreich et al., 2022). These three beta-blockers are metoprolol (extended release, Toprol XL) and bisoprolol (Cardicor), which are both cardioselective agents, and carvedilol (Coreg), which is a noncardioselective beta-blocker with alpha-blocking properties. It is recommended that one of these beta-blockers be used to reduce hospitalizations and mortality risk. The benefits of beta-blockers were seen in patients with or without CAD, older patients, patients with or without DM, in women, and across ethnic and racial groups but not in those individuals with atrial fibrillation (Heidenreich et al., 2022). Moreover, these drugs are effective for the treatment of both ischemic and nonischemic forms of congestive HF (Yancy et al., 2013).

For Black individuals who remain symptomatic despite the use of beta-blockers, ACE inhibitors or ARB therapy, and MRAs, adding a combination of hydralazine (Unipres) and isosorbide dinitrate (Isordil) can be considered. This combination has been shown to improve symptoms and reduce morbidity and mortality among Black people. There are no significant data for the use of hydralazine and isosorbide dinitrate when taken with an ARNi. It is recommended as a part of standard therapy for Black people. It is unknown if there is any benefit in utilizing hydralazine and isosorbide dinitrate in non-Black people with HFrEF (Heidenreich et al., 2022).

MRAs, spironolactone (Aldactone) or eplerenone (Inspra), are recommended to reduce morbidity and mortality if the potassium is <5.0 mEq/L and glomerular filtration rate (GFR) is >30 mL/minute. This category of medications has shown improvements in HF hospitalizations, all-cause mortality rate, and sudden cardiac death in HFrEF patients (Heidenreich et al., 2022). Spironolactone and eplerenone have been found to improve mortality rates among women with class III and IV HF. This is primarily a result of these drugs' neurohormonal blockage effects and not because of their diuretic effects (Yancy et al., 2013).

For symptomatic chronic HFrEF, regardless of the presence or absence of type 2 DM, SGLT2 inhibitors are now a class 1A recommendation to decrease HF hospitalizations. In addition, SGLT2 inhibitors have also been found to be beneficial in HFpEF and HFmrEF (class 2a recommendation) in decreasing cardiovascular mortality risk and HF hospitalizations. In prespecified subgroup analyses, it was found that both men and women have similar benefits from SGLT2 inhibitors (Khan et al., 2022).

In patients with HFmrEF (LVEF 41%–49%), current or previously symptomatic, it is recommended to treat the patient with evidence-based GDMT (including beta-blockers for HFrEF, ARNi, ACEi, or ARB, and MRAs to reduce the risk of cardiovascular death and HF hospitalization, especially with those patients who have an LVEF on the lower end of the range. Data for this group of patients are either subsets of analyses or post hoc from previous HF trials with patients who would now be classified as HFmrEF. When the data were assessed, patients who were on the lower end of the LVEF spectrum seem to respond to medical therapies as patients with HFrEF. Thus, it was felt reasonable to treat these patients with the same GDMT (Heidenreich et al., 2022).

A small, randomized trial (TRED-HF) showed that there was a high rate of relapse of dilated cardiomyopathy (44%) within 6 months in patients who had discontinued GDMT. Therefore, it is now recommended that GDMT be continued in patients with HFimpEF even in those who are asymptomatic, to prevent LV dysfunction and relapse of heart failure (Colvin, 2022).

The 2022 AHA/ACC/HFSA guidelines for management of HF also made recommendations for other drug treatments in HF once GDMT has been optimized. In patients with class II to IV HF symptoms, it may be reasonable to add an omega-3 polyunsaturated fatty acid supplementation to a patient's medication regimen to reduce cardiovascular hospitalizations and mortality risk (class 2b recommendation). In those patients who are taking a renin–angiotensin–aldosterone system inhibitor (RAASi) who develop hyperkalemia, gastrointestinal potassium binders (patiromer [RLY5016] and sodium zirconium cyclosilicate [SZC]) may be an option for treatment to allow patients to continue/titrate their GDMT medications (class 2b recommendation). In those patients with symptomatic, NYHA class II to III, stable HFrEF, chronic, with LVEF ≤35%, receiving GDMT, inclusive of a beta-blocker at maximum tolerated dose, in normal sinus rhythm with a heart rate ≥70 bpm at rest, ivabradine may be a reasonable option to add to their medication regimen to reduce cardiovascular death and HF hospitalizations (class 2a recommendation). Vericiguat, an oral soluble guanylate cyclase stimulator, can be considered in high-risk patients with HFrEF with recent worsening HF, already on GDMT, and may reduce risks of cardiovascular death and HF hospitalization (class 2b recommendation). It can result in improvement in endothelial function, vasodilation, and decrease in fibrosis and remodeling of the heart (Heidenreich et al., 2022).

Digoxin (Lanoxin), which is one of the oldest pharmacologic agents available, is currently indicated only for women with systolic dysfunction who are still symptomatic despite conventional therapies (Lindenfeld et al., 2010; Yancy et al., 2013). One important caveat with digoxin use in women is the higher risk of digoxin toxicity at low doses. The Heart Failure Society of America (HFSA) guidelines of 2013 recommend digoxin levels of less than 1.0 ng/mL (Yancy et al., 2013). Digoxin can also help with the management of heart rate in women with AF (Lindenfeld et al., 2010; Yancy et al., 2013). In patients with symptomatic HFrEF despite being on GDMT or in those who are unable to tolerate GDMT, the utilization of digoxin can be considered to decrease hospitalizations for HF (class 2b recommendation; Heidenreich et al., 2022).

DIASTOLIC DYSFUNCTION

HFpEF (LVEF ≥50%) accounts for 50% of all patients with HF and is associated with significant mortality and morbidity rates. It is a disorder that is contributed to by comorbid conditions including DM, obesity, HTN, CAD, CKD, and specific causes such as cardiac amyloidosis. Therefore, treatment for these comorbid conditions is extremely important (Heidenreich et al., 2022).

HFpEF has a much greater prevalence in women than men. Before women present with HF, they are more likely to develop arterial stiffness, diastolic dysfunction, and coronary microvascular dysfunction with aging, all of which predispose them to HFpEF. A comparison of men and women found that women have higher LV filling pressures with exercise and poor diastolic reserve than men. Women also have a higher predisposition to coronary microvascular dysfunction than men (Khan et al., 2022).

Women with HFpEF have lower natriuretic peptide levels in comparison with men. This lower natriuretic peptide level plays an important role in the pathophysiologic mechanism in HFpEF in women, especially in those with obesity. Following menopause, the loss of estrogen as well as systemic inflammation caused by comorbidities such as obesity can lead to reduced signaling of cGMP (cyclic guanosine monophosphate)-protein kinase G. Sacubitril/valsartan (Entresto) increases cGMP-protein kinase G signaling, which is felt to possibly benefit postmenopausal women, especially those with metabolic comorbidities such as DM and obesity (Khan et al., 2022).

As with systolic HF, diuretics are used to control symptoms of fluid overload and reduce congestion (Heidenreich et al., 2022). However, managing fluid balance with diastolic HF can be more challenging. Patients with diastolic HF are more dependent on preload to maintain cardiac output as a result of the stiffened left ventricle (Barnard, 2005).

The 2022 ACC/AHA/HFSA guidelines regarding diastolic HF recommend the treatment of any underlying causative conditions (e.g., HTN). Patients with HFpEF and HTN should strive to keep BP well controlled in accordance with HTN guidelines to prevent morbidity. In addition, the guidelines recommend the following treatment options. SGLT2 inhibitors are useful in decreasing cardiovascular mortality and heart failure hospitalizations (class 2a recommendation). Management of AF in these patients can aid in the improvement of symptoms (class 2a recommendation). In select patients with HFpEF, especially those with an LVEF on the lower end of the spectrum, consideration for the use of MRAs, ARBs, and ARNi is recommended to decrease hospitalizations (class 2b recommendation; Heidenreich et al., 2022). Beta-blockers are important for the treatment of diastolic dysfunction to control HTN and tachycardia, thereby increasing diastolic LV filling time. Furthermore, measures to restore and maintain the sinus rhythm among women with AF who are symptomatic despite heart rate control can also be considered (Yancy et al., 2013).

ACE inhibitors and ARBs have been shown to reduce myocardial fibrosis and LVH; however, they have not been studied exclusively in the presence of diastolic HF. Even so, patients with diastolic dysfunction (as with systolic dysfunction) appear to have activation of the renin–angiotensin–aldosterone system, which makes these medications logical choices for the treatment of HF that results from diastolic dysfunction (Yancy et al., 2013).

Many cardiomyopathies are unique to women. These cardiomyopathies may be in either category of HFpEF or HFrEF. Peripartum cardiomyopathy is an idiopathic cardiomyopathy presenting with LV systolic dysfunction, usually early after delivery but can occur during pregnancy or up to a few months after the delivery (DeFilippis et al., 2021).

Hypertrophic cardiomyopathy is a genetic cardiomyopathy that is more likely to be diagnosed in women after they present with clinical symptoms. Women compared with men are more likely to have obstructive physiology and a higher mortality rate (DeFilippis et al., 2021).

Device Therapy for Heart Failure

Mortality rates among patients with HF and severely impaired LV systolic function (≤30%) are high (Yancy et al., 2013). Regrettably, HF represents a sentinel prognostic event in patients with a high risk for readmission (50% in 6 months) and a high 1-year mortality rate of 30% (Giamouzis et al., 2011; Kociol et al., 2010). Death is attributable to arrhythmia, MI, progressive HF, pulmonary or systemic emboli, electrolyte disturbances, and other vascular events (Lindenfeld et al., 2010). The risk of sudden cardiac death is decreased with appropriate pharmacologic therapy, as described previously. However, certain women may benefit from the implantation of an ICD.

The 2022 AHA/ACC/HFSA guidelines for device therapy recommend the implantation of an ICD in patients with an EF of 35% or less, who are NYHA class II or III, with nonischemic dilated cardiomyopathy or ischemic heart disease, at least 40 days post MI, on chronic GDMT, whose survival is anticipated to be greater than 1 year. In addition, ICD implantation is also recommended for primary prevention of sudden cardiac death to reduce mortality in patients with an EF ≤30%, who are at least 40 days post MI, with NYHA class I symptoms, currently on GDMT, whose survival is expected to be greater than 1 year (Heidenreich et al., 2022). These devices are not recommended or appropriate for the woman with end-stage (class D) disease with progressive and irreversible HF symptoms or with a limited life expectancy as a result of other disease states; such devices are unlikely to affect the overall prognosis of these women (Tracy et al., 2012; Yancy et al., 2013).

Sex differences in ICD implantation have been found. Based on many studies, women who are eligible for an ICD are less likely than men to have a device implanted. It remains questionable if an ICD prevents sudden death in women because landmark primary ICD trials included very few women. In meta-analyses, it was found that there was no survival benefit for women with an ICD. In addition, women were also less likely to receive appropriate ICD therapies in comparison to men. It is thought that the sex difference benefits of ICDs for primary prevention may be due to the cause of death. One study showed that there was 32% lower risk of sudden death in women than men and there was no sex difference in pump failure (DeFilippis et al., 2021).

CRT is another treatment option for patients with HF that can reduce hospitalizations, reduce total mortality, and improve symptoms and quality of life (Heidenreich et al., 2022). Biventricular pacing improves hemodynamic measurements such as cardiac index and systemic vascular resistance (Blanc et al., 1997). Furthermore, medication therapy using ACE inhibitors, ARBs, and beta-blockers along with CRT can slow and even partially reverse LV remodeling (Lindenfeld et al., 2010).

Criteria for CRT include symptomatic HF, NYHA class II to IV, with EF ≤35%, in normal sinus rhythm (NSR), left bundle branch block (LBBB) with a QRS complex ≥150 ms (class I indication). CRT may also be advantageous in (1) those individuals with an EF ≤35%, normal sinus rhythm, LBBB, QRS 120–149 ms, (2) individuals with an EF ≤35%, non-LBBB pattern, with QRS ≥150 ms, and (3) those individuals with significant pacemaker dependency despite what their underlying rhythm is. These three criteria are class IIa recommendations (DeFilippis et al., 2022).

CRT is underutilized in women compared to men even though women appear to have greater benefit. Women with HFrEF who are eligible for CRT are less likely than men to receive this therapy. This disparity has increased over time in United States. In the MASCOT (Management of Atrial Fibrillation Suppression in AF-HF Comorbidity Therapy) study, women with CRT in comparison to men had a greater decrease in LV end-diastolic dimension, increased improvement in quality of life, and fewer hospitalizations for HF. In another study, women had a greater increase in LVEF and greater reduction in LV end-diastolic dimension compared with men (DeFilippis et al., 2021). Wilcox et al. (2014) found that the use of guideline-directed CRT and ICD therapy was associated with substantially reduced 24-month mortality rate in eligible men and women with HF and reduced EF. Device therapies should be offered to all patients.

Critical to decision-making for device implantation is the woman's overall prognosis and her functional capacity at baseline. Women with HF have been found to have poorer health-related quality of life than men (Heo et al., 2007; Lesman-Leegte et al., 2009). In addition, many women need a great deal of psychological support because the implantation of such a device can be unnerving, impeding patient recovery and return to daily life—now with an ICD. Cultivation of social support networks can cushion the impact of stress through support and online chat groups.

Arrhythmias

Until recently, women have been underrepresented in electrophysiologic and most cardiovascular clinical trials. This underrepresentation has significant implications for understanding and treating female patients as guideline-directed therapies emerge from such clinical trials (Zeitler et al., 2022). The National Institutes of Health have taken aim at addressing this disparity more recently by adding a requirement to grant applications that they include sex differentiation (Legato et al., 2016).

Understanding that gender differences exist in the cardiac electrical system is paramount in guiding our assessment, treatment, and understanding the etiology behind cardiac electrical disturbances in women. In addition to understanding sex differences in the etiology of the electrophysiologic system, we must also address sex differences in device therapies and the effects of drugs and pregnancy (Zeitler et al., 2022).

In addition to sex differences, we also must take into consideration changes with aging and how that affects the heart and how it may be different in women. Aging is associated with many changes in the cardiovascular system that include decreased compliance of blood vessels, mild concentric LVH, increased atrial contraction contribution to LV filling, and a higher incidence of many cardiac arrhythmias and conduction disorders (Chow et al., 2012). Some alterations in cardiac rhythm do not produce symptoms, whereas others cause hemodynamic changes requiring treatment. The prognostic significance of any conduction abnormality or rhythm disturbance is dependent primarily on the presence and severity of any accompanying cardiac disease (Chow et al., 2012).

ETIOLOGY

Early research regarding the pharmacologic management of arrhythmias included few, if any, women. Recent studies have recognized this data gap and have described differences in electrophysiologic properties and cardiac substrate between men and women that can be attributed to several factors including circulating sex hormones, sex hormones affecting cell development, and autonomic function (Zeitler et al., 2022). The cardiac action potential is affected by sex hormone levels as they affect protein synthesis and affect the ion channels. This effect on ion channels changes the susceptibility to arrhythmias and EKG findings (such as the QT interval).

Differences in the conduction system between males and females are noted in several studies. The resting heart rate of a female is about 3.5 bpm higher than that of an age-matched male (Taneja et al., 2001). This difference by gender is thought to be a result of a known shorter sinus node recovery time in women (Connolly et al., 2009; Zeitler et al., 2022). Heart rate variability is a product of autonomic function and is thereby sensitive to hormonal changes (Brar et al., 2015). In an analysis of EKGs dating back to 1920, Bazett observed and documented that women have an inherently longer QT interval than men (Bazett, 1997). This difference occurs after males enter puberty due to the increasing testosterone levels and by the time the male reaches middle age and testosterone levels decrease, the difference in QT interval is no longer observed (Bidoggia et al., 2000).

The degree of autonomic variability in women, which suggests that women have a higher vagal tone, also contributes to the difference in how women may respond to certain therapies and medications (Ryan et al., 1994). Therefore, there may be more complexity in diagnosing and treating arrhythmias in women over the life cycle. Lastly, women may also respond differently to treatments for arrhythmias, especially pharmacologic management (Hongo & Scheinman, 2005).

DIFFERENTIAL DIAGNOSIS
Supraventricular Arrhythmias

DEFINITION AND ETIOLOGY

The term *supraventricular arrhythmia* (SVA) encompasses rhythms that originate at or above the sinoatrial (SA) node and includes arrhythmias such as atrioventricular nodal reentrant tachycardia (AVNRT), atrial tachycardia (AT), atrial fibrillation (AF), atrial flutter, and supraventricular tachycardia (SVT; DeSimone et al., 2018).

SYMPTOMS

Regardless of gender, these arrhythmias can cause patients uncomfortable symptoms. Women with SVA in addition to AF and ventricular arrhythmias can present with a variety of symptoms, including palpitations, heart racing, heart flutters, chest discomfort, lightheadedness, dizziness, presyncope, and fatigue. However, frank syncope is uncommon with SVA, occurring in only about 15% of patients (Blomström-Lundqvist et al., 2003).

DIAGNOSTIC STUDIES

A TTE may be used to evaluate structural heart disease, including valvular heart disease, that will increase the risk of arrhythmias. Twenty-four-hour Holter monitoring is helpful for evaluating the woman with frequent symptoms, but if the symptoms do not occur within that 24-hour time span, an alternative diagnostic monitoring device should be considered. An event recorder or loop recorder is indicated for less frequent symptoms and is used for longer than 24 hours. Implantable loop recorders are a third option for the patient whose symptoms may be less frequent or of short duration and are therefore difficult to capture on a loop recorder. Exercise testing can be helpful if the symptoms are brought on by stress or exercise. Laboratory examination of the woman with palpitations and a suspected arrhythmia includes electrolyte, magnesium, and thyroid function tests. A complete blood count may be indicated if anemia or infection is suspected because both conditions may precipitate tachyarrhythmias (Blomström-Lundqvist et al., 2003). Additionally, findings from these studies help the clinician to differentiate between SVA and ventricular tachycardia.

TREATMENT/MANAGEMENT

For women who have no evidence of preexcitation on the 12-lead EKG, who have normal LV function, and who tolerate the arrhythmia well, no specific therapy may be required, especially if the episodes are infrequent. Precipitating factors should be reviewed during the initial assessment, and if there is a history of excessive intake of alcohol, caffeine, or nicotine (which are stimulants); use of recreational drugs; or hyperthyroidism, these factors should be discussed and eliminated (Blomström-Lundqvist et al., 2003). Treatment of regular, stable SVT is aimed at symptom alleviation and prevention by utilizing agents to slow conduction through the AV node. Vagal manuevers can be attempted by the patient during an episode, but pharmacologic management is frequently required (DeSimone et al., 2018). Treatment with pharmacologic agents such as beta-blockers and calcium channel blockers are first-line medication therapy (Ahmad et al., 2021). Digoxin (Lanoxin) is less effective for the prevention of SVA. For women with SVT and no evidence of structural heart disease, propafenone (Rythmol), and flecainide (Tambocor) are effective for the prevention of recurrence, and they may be prescribed by cardiologists who specialize in arrhythmia management (Blomström-Lundqvist et al., 2003). Radiofrequency catheter ablation has also been very successful for the treatment of SVA (especially SVT) in both males and females. Success of ablation does not seem to differ by sex; however, what does appear to differ is the time to treatment. Women tend to have a longer time between symptoms onset to diagnosis and ablation of their SVT arrhythmia. This discrepancy is not due to referral pattern but is due to female preference for medication trials before invasive intervention. The major common theme in reasons for the delay is the female patients' perception or role as caregiver (Zeitler et al., 2022). Ablation is now considered first-line therapy (Page et al., 2016).

Atrial Flutter

ETIOLOGY, SYMPTOMS, AND EVALUATION/ASSESSMENT

Women with atrial flutter can present with symptoms similar to those of SVT, and the diagnostic workup is identical (Blomström-Lundqvist et al., 2003). However, these women often have more comorbidities and are more likely to have symptoms of fatigue, shortness of breath, and chest discomfort, as well as palpitations. HF and pulmonary disease are commonly seen among these women, who are typically older than women with SVT (Scheinman & Huang, 2003).

TREATMENT/MANAGEMENT

Guidelines regarding the pharmacologic management of atrial flutter are often combined with those of AF. Beta-blockers and nondihydropyridine calcium channel blockers can be used for initial rate control; this is a class I

TABLE 43.5 CHA₂DS₂–VASc Score

	CONDITION	POSSIBLE POINTS
C	Congestive heart failure	+ 1
H	Hypertension	+ 1
A	Age (older than 75 years)	+ 2
D	Diabetes mellitus	+ 1
S	Prior stroke or transient ischemic attack or thromboembolic event	+ 2
V	Vascular disease of any kind	+ 1
Sc	Sex category (female sex)	+ 1

Source: Lip, G. Y., Nieuwlaat, R., Pisters, R., Lane, D. A., & Crijns, H. J. (2010). Refining clinical risk stratification for predicting stroke and thromboembolism in atrial fibrillation using a novel risk factor-based approach: The Euro Heart Survey on Atrial Fibrillation. Chest, 137, 263–272. https://doi.org/10.1378/chest.09-1584

indication. However, the most common side effect is hypotension. Catheter ablation is also class I indication and considered first-line therapy for patients presenting with atrial flutter. Amiodarone, dofetilide, or sotalol are class IIa options for rhythm control strategy. Flecainide and propafenone are class IIb indicated for rhythm control in the absence of structural heart disease (Page et al., 2016). For atrial flutter stroke risk is assessed in the same manner as for AF. Although the mechanism is different than AF, the atrial flutter patient carries the risk of systemic embolization due to ineffective atrial squeeze and also carries a high coexistent prevalence of AF (January et al., 2019). CHA₂DS₂-VASc score (see Table 43.5) risk assessment and anticoagulation management recommendations should be followed. Patients who present with 48 hours or greater or unknown duration of atrial flutter can be considered for direct current cardioversion (DCCV) or pharmacologic cardioversion if a transesophageal echocardiogram is negative for thrombus or if the patient has been on uninterrupted anticoagulation for a minimum of 3 weeks prior to DCCV and will remain on anticoagulation for at least 4 weeks post cardioversion. Recommendations for anticoagulation of patients with nonvalvular AF include direct oral anticoagulants (DOACs) or vitamin K agonist (warfarin). DOACs are the preferred choice if not contraindicated as studies show superiority or lower bleeding risk compared to warfarin. For those patients requiring anticoagulation who have valvular atrial arrhythmia, vitamin K agonist (warfarin) is indicated (January, 2019).

Atrial Fibrillation

DEFINITION AND SCOPE, ETIOLOGY

AF is a common arrhythmia and the risk of developing AF increases with age. Obesity, DM, HTN, obstructive sleep apnea, European descent, ischemic heart disease, CKD, alcohol abuse/overuse, and smoking are among the list of additional risk factors for developing AF. AF is the primary diagnosis upon hospitalization in the United States in more than 454,000 cases per year. One out of every seven strokes is caused by AF, and these strokes tend to be more severe in nature in comparison to other stroke etiologies (Centers for Disease Control and Prevention [CDC], 2021). By the year 2030, it is estimated that 12.1 million people in the United States will be diagnosed with AF (CDC, 2021). Patients with AF are hospitalized twice as often as those without AF and are three times more likely to have multiple admissions. It is estimated that caring for patients with AF adds $26 billion to U.S. healthcare expenses (January et al., 2014). The increase in hospitalizations for AF occur for many reasons, including aging of the population, the rising prevalence of chronic heart disease, and more frequent diagnosis as a result of increased monitoring and awareness of the condition by practitioners and patients. The prevalence is higher among men than women (Feinberg et al., 1995); however, because the incidence of AF increases overwhelmingly with aging and because there are more women in the population older than 75 years, the total number of women and men with AF in this age group is equal (Humphries et al., 2001). Males have an overall larger left atrial size than females, which may partially account for the higher prevalence of AF in men; however, the etiology is not completely understood. In the landmark Women's Health Initiative program, those subjects who received hormone replacement therapy (HRT) had greater incidence of AF than those who received placebo. This indicates that postmenopausal HRT increases the woman's risk of developing AF and is important to consider in management (Perez et al., 2012). Women are more symptomatic than men, possibly because of faster heart rates and smaller body size, and unfortunately, women have experienced more problems when the heart rate is controlled (Michelena et al., 2010).

AF can occur in the presence or absence of heart disease. However, as with atrial flutter, individuals with AF often have HTN, valvular heart disease, and/or CVD. AF is associated with an increased risk of stroke, HF, and all-cause mortality, especially among women (Stewart et al., 2002). Furthermore, perioperative AF is associated with an increased long-term risk of ischemic stroke, especially after noncardiac surgery (Gialdini et al., 2014). The prognosis of those with AF is most benign among individuals who are younger than 60 years with no known heart disease; these patients are often referred to as having *lone AF*. Most individuals move out of this category over time as they age and develop other heart diseases and HTN (Alpert et al., 2014).

EVALUATION/ASSESSMENT AND DIAGNOSTIC STUDIES

Women who present with AF can have the same symptoms as previously mentioned for women with SVA. The initial diagnostic workup is similar as well. The hemodynamic consequences of AF include the loss of atrial kick, which can add up to 30% of cardiac output; this loss is particularly important to those with reduced heart function. In addition, the tachycardia itself can lead to a tachycardia-mediated cardiomyopathy (Fuster et al., 2006).

TREATMENT/MANAGEMENT

The first goal of AF management is rate control with either a beta-blocker or a calcium channel blocker. As with the other tachyarrhythmias, if hemodynamic instability exists, referral for electrical cardioversion is the preferred management strategy. As long as the patient is hemodynamically stable, the rate may be controlled with beta-blockers, nondihydropyridine calciumchannel blockers, or amiodarone (Pacerone). Digoxin can also be used to slow the ventricular rate in AF; however, it is rarely useful as monotherapy. Digoxin (Lanoxin) is not effective for controlling increased heart rate during times of exertion or exercise (Fuster et al., 2006).

Rate versus rhythm control is a difficult choice that most often requires referral to a cardiologist or an electrophysiology specialist. Most concerning with the diagnosis of AF is the risk of ischemic stroke, which averages 5% per year among patients with nonvalvular AF. Rates of ischemic stroke are two to seven times higher among women with AF than among those without AF (Cabin et al., 1990; Wolf et al., 1991) and in comparison to male patients, women have a greater overall stroke risk in AF, especially if they over age 75 years (Zeitler et al., 2022).

Some investigators have demonstrated a worse outcome and a higher rate of recurrence after cardioversion. The most effective treatment currently for the restoration of sinus rhythm in those with AF is catheter ablation. Females do tend to have higher recurrence of AF post ablation compared to males. This may be due to delayed ablation consultation referral, older age at time of referral relative to later age of onset, and less aggressive ablation technique by the operator for fear of increased procedural complication rate in women (Kummer et al., 2015).

AF affects the current risks and the long-term prognosis of women differently than of men. An analysis from the Euro Heart Survey on Atrial Fibrillation found that women with AF have more than double the thromboembolism risk of men with AF (Lip et al., 2010). In addition, a Swedish study found that the rate of ischemic stroke in AF patients younger than 65 years was 47% higher in women than men (Friberg et al., 2012). Last, women overall have a significantly higher risk of AF-related stroke than men and are more likely to live with stroke-related disability, which in turn leads to a significantly lower quality of life (Volgman et al., 2009). The diagnosis, symptoms, and treatments of AF can differ for women, too. A potential deadly difference in women 20 to 79 years old is that the risk of stroke is 4.6-fold greater in women than in men (Schnohr et al., 2006). In addition, mortality rate for women with AF is up to 2.5 times greater than that for men (Michelena et al., 2010).

The decision to place patients with AF on anticoagulation therapy is based on a number of factors. The choice of agent to use is dependent on balancing the risk of stroke or thromboembolic event with the risk of bleeding. Current guidelines recommend using the CHA_2DS_2-VASc score to determine the appropriateness of anticoagulation (January et al., 2014). It is a 10-point scale found to be a clinical predictor for estimating stroke risk in patients with nonrheumatic AF (Lip et al., 2010; Table 43.5). Individuals scoring 2 or higher on the CHA_2DS_2-VASc are considered at high risk for thromboembolic events and should have anticoagulation therapy, unless contraindicated (January et al., 2014). Those scoring less than 2 (0 or 1) are candidates for aspirin therapy with either 81 or 325 mg (January et al., 2014).

For many years, the standard of therapy for anticoagulation was vitamin K antagonists, namely, warfarin (Fuster et al., 2006). Warfarin therapy has been demonstrated to be superior to aspirin therapy (Fuster et al., 2006), alone or in combination with clopidogrel, for stroke prevention (Connolly et al., 2009). The risk of intracerebral hemorrhage (ICH) with the use of warfarin occurred in individuals with an international normalized ratio (INR) greater than 4.0. The advantages of warfarin include its ability to be quickly reversed by parenteral vitamin K or fresh frozen plasma (Mookadam et al., 2015). However, there are many disadvantages to warfarin therapy. INR monitoring is critical to the success of balancing this medication's anticoagulant effect with the risk for bleeding. It can take 5 days or longer for some individuals to reach the recommended therapeutic INR of 2.0 to 3.0. Warfarin's significant food and drug interactions affect the INR, and therefore, guidelines recommend monitoring at least every 30 days (Mookadam et al., 2015). These factors discourage providers from prescribing anticoagulation and patients accepting their recommendations (Hohnloser, 2011). Warfarin therapy is highly unpredictable (Macedo et al., 2015). A population-based data analysis of 140,078 patients with AF in their first year of warfarin therapy in the United Kingdom found that only 44% had optimal INRs more than 70% of the time (Macedo et al., 2015).

The search for more predictable anticoagulation has led to the development of DOACs. The four available agents are all indicated for use in patients with nonvalvular AF and cannot be used in patients with prosthetic heart valves. These agents have the advantage of fixed dosing and do not require blood test monitoring. In addition, they do not have dietary precautions, as they are not vitamin K antagonists. Most require adjustment for renal dysfunction (Mookadam et al., 2015).

Dabigatran is an oral direct thrombin inhibitor prescribed twice daily. It is superior to warfarin in the prevention of the primary outcomes of stroke or systemic embolism (Connolly et al., 2009). A lower dose is approved for use in patients with renal dysfunction, but it should be avoided in patients with severe renal dysfunction (Mookadam et al., 2015). A risk of major bleeding was found, similar to warfarin, in the analysis of all patients, and in subgroup analysis the risk of intracranial bleeding was lower in patients older than 75 years (Connolly et al., 2009). The main concern with direct thrombin inhibitors is the lack of a direct antidote. However, the FDA is currently reviewing the drug idarucizumab as an antidote to dabigatran, which showed good effect in the reversal of the anticoagulant effects of dabigatran in patients needing urgent surgery (Pollack et al., 2015).

Rivaroxaban, apixaban, and the newest approved edoxaban are factor Xa inhibitors approved for use in patients with nonvavular AF. All the factor Xa agents are fixed-dose agents that do not require blood testing of anticoagulation levels. Rivaroxaban is a direct factor Xa inhibitor approved in 2011. It is administered once daily and requires dose adjustment in patients with renal dysfunction. The ROCKET-AF trial demonstrated the noninferiority of rivaroxaban compared with warfarin in the prevention of stroke and embolism in patients with nonvalvular AF; rivaroxaban had no significant differences in rates of major bleeding and less risk of intracranial and fatal bleeding when compared with warfarin (Patel et al., 2011).

Apixaban is a direct factor Xa inhibitor that was approved for use in 2012. It is administered twice daily. The ARISTOTLE study compared apixaban to warfarin in patients with AF. Apixaban was found to be superior to warfarin ($p =.01$), and rates for major bleeding were found to be less than with warfarin therapy (Granger et al., 2011). Moreover, apixaban therapy reduced rates of all-cause mortality (Granger et al., 2011). Apixaban is approved in 2.5- and 5-mg doses. The 2.5-mg dose is recommended for patients with two of the three following factors: age more than 80 years, body weight less than 60 kg, and serum creatinine higher than 1.5 mg/dL (Granger et al., 2011).

Edoxaban is a direct factor Xa inhibitor approved for use in 2015 for anticoagulation in AF. It is a once-daily medication and has a dose adjustment with renal impairment. The ENGAGE-AF TIMI 48 trial studied edoxaban versus warfarin in the prevention of thromboembolic events in patients with nonvalvular AF (Giugliano et al., 2013). Edoxaban was found to be equal to warfarin in the prevention of stroke and embolism. There were lower rates of fatal bleeding and intracranial bleeding. However, significantly higher rates of gastrointestinal bleeding were noted (Giugliano et al., 2013).

The decision to withhold or stop anticoagulation therapy in women who are at high risk for bleeding can be difficult. The decision to initiate anticoagulation is individualized and discussed with the woman and her family as well as with all members of the healthcare team. Strategies to limit bleeding risk when prescribing anticoagulation have been studied. The European Society of Cardiology guidelines for the treatment of AF include utilization of a scoring system to assess patients at high risk for bleeding, called the HAS-BLED score (Lane & Lip, 2012). At the very least, patients at high bleeding risk require more frequent monitoring and follow-up (Mookadam et al., 2015).

Sinus Tachycardia

DEFINITION AND SCOPE

By definition, sinus tachycardia is a regular cardiac rhythm with rate faster than 100 bpm (Yusuf & Camm, 2005). Sinus tachycardia is a physiologic response to stress, anxiety, or exercise but is concerning or warrants further investigation when it occurs at rest. In many instances, women with symptoms of palpitations or heart racing will have a sinus tachycardia. Approximately 90% of patients with inappropriate sinus tachycardia are women (Blomström-Lundqvist et al., 2003; Krahn et al., 1995).

EVALUATION/ASSESSMENT

In the case of sinus tachycardia, it is most appropriate to find and treat the underlying disorder. Before medication is prescribed, a history is obtained to check for possible precipitating factors, such as excessive caffeine, alcohol, nicotine intake, recreational drugs, or hyperthyroidism. The condition, such as hyperthyroidism, is treated or the precipitating agents eliminated first before proceeding to medical management.

TREATMENT/MANAGEMENT

A beta-blocker is indicated for symptom management in many instances, especially in the case of hyperthyroidism. If a beta-blocker is contraindicated or not tolerated, a nondihydropyridine calcium channel blocker (e.g., diltiazem [Cardizem] or verapamil [Calan]) can be considered. Close monitoring is required because less rate-controlling medication is needed when the underlying condition has been successfully treated; often the medication can be tapered off completely (Blomström-Lundqvist et al., 2003).

Ventricular Arrhythmias

The presentation of ventricular arrhythmias ranges from single premature ventricular contractions (PVCs) of little or no hemodynamic significance to life-threatening ventricular tachycardia or ventricular fibrillation. These arrhythmias can occur in women with and without heart disease or cardiac disorders.

DIFFERENTIAL DIAGNOSIS AND TREATMENT/MANAGEMENT

The primary goal for managing life-threatening ventricular arrhythmias is the prevention of sudden cardiac death. Referral to an arrhythmia specialist is appropriate. Management is based on the etiology of arrhythmia. Possible treatments are medications, ablation, ICD placement, and sometimes a short-term intervention involving a wearable defibrillator in the form of a vest.

Long QT syndrome is a disorder that is more common in postpubertal women than in postpubertal men. In addition, women with long QT syndrome have an increased risk of arrhythmia for 9 to 12 months postpartum (Seth et al., 2006). Beta-blocker therapy should be continued during pregnancy and in the postpartum period. Long QT syndrome often goes undiagnosed, although 90% of these patients have experienced the condition by age 40 years. The problem arises from the ion channels in the heart muscle causing conduction defects, which predispose patients to torsades de pointes, which then can proceed to syncope and sudden cardiac death. A prolonged QT interval can be caused by some medications as well as hypokalemia and other nutritional and endocrine disorders. Long QT syndrome should be suspected in patients who have recurrent syncope during exertion and those with family histories of sudden, unexpected death (Meyer et al., 2003). A thorough history is key to protecting patients at risk.

Arrhythmias and Pregnancy

Pregnancy can predispose women to arrhythmias due to the many physiologic changes that the body undergoes during this time, including autonomic changes, systemic fluid variations, and systemic hemodynamic changes (Massari et al., 2018). Fortunately, most arrhythmias during pregnancy are benign. In addition, most arrhythmias in the pregnant woman arise in the setting of a structurally normal heart and are therefore tolerated well (Shotan et al., 1997). In women with a history of arrhythmia, ectopy may increase. Premature atrial contractions and PVCs are relatively common during pregnancy and generally do not require pharmacologic management. Often the heart rate increases by 25% in women who are pregnant; therefore, sinus tachycardia, especially in the third trimester is common. Ectopic beats and nonsustained arrhythmia are found in more than 50% of pregnant women assessed for palpitations, whereas sustained tachycardias are uncommon in 2 to 3/1,000 (Blomström-Lundqvist et al., 2003; Shotan et al.,

1997). The avoidance of triggers such as caffeine and emotional stress can be helpful.

SVT episodes may increase during pregnancy. Women with frequent SVT who are contemplating becoming pregnant may want to consider ablation therapy before conception to avoid medications while pregnant (Oakley et al., 2003). All antiarrhythmic medications cross the placenta, and pharmacokinetics can be altered during pregnancy, thereby necessitating more frequent monitoring of drug levels (Oakley et al., 2003). Therapeutic drug levels can be affected by an increase in intravascular volume requiring an increase in loading dose, a reduction of plasma proteins contributing to lower drug concentrations, increased renal blood flow with an increase in the clearance of drugs, increased hepatic metabolism of drug resulting from progesterone also increasing clearance, and changes in gastric absorption of medication, making serum drug concentrations variable (Perez-Silva & Merino, 2011).

For women who develop SVT during pregnancy, management is similar to that of the nonpregnant patient but does vary depending on the trimester of pregnancy (Ibetoh et al., 2021). Concerns related to treatment are related to potential pharmacotherapy contraindications and side effects and radiation to the unborn fetus (Kaspar et al., 2018). Regardless of trimester or pregnancy status, vagal maneuvers are attempted first to break the arrhythmia (Oakley et al., 2003). If vagal maneuvers are not successful, adenosine is the drug of choice for terminating a sustained SVT during all three trimesters and labor (Ibetoh et al., 2021). If the condition is recurrent and suppression is necessary, cardioselective beta-blockers (e.g., metoprolol) are recommended. Atenolol and verapamil are contraindicated during the first trimester; however, they can be used during the second and third trimesters (Ibetoh et al., 2021). Some experts recommend avoiding beta-blockers altogether during the first trimester, if possible; however, others contend that beta-blockers are acceptable during pregnancy (Hongo & Scheinman, 2005). Sotalol is more likely to cause fetal bradycardia because it more readily crosses the placenta (Oakley et al., 2003). Flecainide and propafenone have been safely used during pregnancy for the treatment of refractory SVT (Cox & Gardner, 1993). Direct current cardioversion with anesthesia can be performed safely for treatment of hemodynamically unstable or refractory SVT during all trimesters including labor, but it has triggered early preterm labor when performed during the third trimester (Ibetoh et al., 2021). Fluoroless radiofrequency catheter ablation with the use of echocardiography-guided catheters can be performed safely during pregnancy to treat SVT refractory to other treatment strategies (Curry & Quintana, 1970; Kaspar et al., 2018; Perez-Silva & Merino, 2011).

AF is relatively rare (2.2%) during pregnancy in patients with no known heart disease or dysfunction but, when present, poses a challenge not only for rhythm versus rate control management but from an anticoagulation perspective as well (Pachariyanon et al., 2019). Unfortunately, many of these women may be previously undiagnosed, and the increased intravascular volume of pregnancy triggers a symptomatic arrhythmia. These patients typically are discovered to have an undiagnosed underlying etiology driving the atrial fibrillation. This includes hyperthyroidism or hypothyroidism, structural anomalies, pulmonary embolism, drug toxicity, and electrolyte disturbances (DiCarlo-Meacham & Dahlke, 2011). Digoxin, beta-blockers, and calcium channel blockers are all appropriate for the rate control of AF during pregnancy; in women with underlying heart disease, beta-blockers or calcium channel blockers are safer in comparison to digoxin (Fuster et al., 2006; January et al., 2014; Oakley et al., 2003). Pregnancy induces a prothrombotic state for the patient but unfortunately data regarding stroke risk assessment and anticoagulation guidelines are lacking (Zeitler et al., 2022). Most women do not require anticoagulation during pregnancy unless they are at high risk for a thromboembolic event (e.g., women with valvular heart disease; Fuster et al., 2006).

Warfarin crosses the placenta and has been implicated in fetal hemorrhage and death; therefore, it is contraindicated during pregnancy. Low-molecular-weight heparin is the anticoagulant of choice in pregnancy (Fuster et al., 2006). Bradycardia that requires permanent pacemaker implantation is also uncommon during pregnancy; however, uterine compression of the inferior vena cava can rarely causes reflex bradycardia (Oakley et al., 2003). In addition, congenital heart block can become symptomatic during pregnancy. Permanent pacemaker implantation is safe during pregnancy if abdominal lead shielding is used (Oakley et al., 2003).

Ventricular tachycardia can occur during any term during pregnancy. It can present in women with congenital long QT interval syndrome or valvular heart disease, or it may be idiopathic. Most instances of ventricular tachycardia that occurs in pregnancy in the absence of structural heart disease are benign (Kotchetkov et al., 2010). If ventricular tachycardia presents during the last 6 weeks of pregnancy or after birth, postpartum cardiomyopathy must be ruled out. Because ventricular tachycardia during pregnancy can be exacerbated by increased catecholamines, beta-blockers are used as first-line therapy. Amiodarone is strictly reserved for emergent treatment of hemodynamically unstable and life-threatening ventricular arrhythmias secondary to its known fetal toxicity (Stec et al., 2013).

Any hemodynamically unstable rhythm can seriously compromise blood flow to the fetus and is considered a medical emergency. Electrical cardioversion can be used to convert any hemodynamically unstable tachyarrhythmia. Very little electrical energy reaches the fetus, and it is advisable to convert the rhythm quickly rather than to risk decreased blood flow to the fetus (Curry & Quintana, 1970; Ogburn et al., 1982; Zipes et al., 2006).

Valvular Heart Disease

DEFINITION AND SCOPE

In the United States, the prevalence of valvular heart disease is estimated at 2.5% (CDC, 2014).Valvular disease due to rheumatic fever has dramatically declined in the past few decades; however, age-related degenerative changes are becoming more common (DesJardin et al., 2022). Because of the increase in degenerative etiologies, the prevalence of valve disease increases after the age of 65 years, especially with aortic stenosis (AS) and mitral regurgitation (MR), which is responsible for three of four cases of valve disease (Iung & Vahanian, 2014). Valvular heart disease has contributed to increasing cardiac mortality and morbidity rates in the United States for the last several decades (Shoob et al., 2006). Despite these trends, there have been advances in noninvasive cardiac monitoring, minimally invasive surgical techniques, and appropriate timing of surgical interventions, along with sophisticated prosthetic valves; these have improved the overall prognosis for acute and chronic valvular disorders. The etiology and pathophysiologic consequences, evaluation, treatment, and continual care of women with valvular heart disease and consequent cardiac dysfunction necessitate a methodic approach to the efficient and practical use of a wide choice of diagnostic procedures, medical and surgical interventions, and long-term follow-up.

ETIOLOGY

The four heart valves normally regulate unidirectional blood flow through the heart's atria and ventricles and into the systemic circulation. Their structural and functional characteristics allow for efficient cardiac muscle contractility and relaxation and for optimal cardiac perfusion (Guyton & Hall, 2006).

Valvular diseases and the resultant changes in normal circulatory physiology are caused by either a forward flow through a narrow or irregular orifice (stenosis) or a regurgitant flow through an incompetent valve (insufficiency). Each of these structural abnormalities leads to hemodynamic changes that directly affect myocardial structure and function as well as coronary blood flow. With the widespread use of echocardiography to both diagnose and plot the trajectory of valve dysfunction, the guidelines for the management of specific valvular lesions have incorporated noninvasive and surgical interventions for patients with acute and chronic valve disease.

EVALUATION/ASSESSMENT

In general, patients with valve disease may present with a heart murmur, symptoms, or incidental findings of valvular abnormalities on chest imaging or noninvasive testing. Regardless, all patients with known or suspected valve disease should undergo an initial history and physical examination.

Cardiac auscultation as a screening method for valvular disease is an essential aspect of the cardiac evaluation. Murmurs are classified according to location, intensity, pitch, radiation, and duration on the basis of the timing of events during the cardiac cycle (Shipton & Wahba, 2001). Specific details of cardiac auscultation–associated physical examination findings that aid in the diagnosis of valvular dysfunction are provided in the ACC/AHA 2014 practice guidelines for the management of patients with valvular heart disease (Nishimura et al., 2014).

DIAGNOSTIC STUDIES

In evaluating patients with valvular heart disease, it is important to correlate the history and physical examination findings with the results of the EKG, chest radiograph, and TTE. Further testing, such as CT, CMRI, and stress testing, may be needed if there is a discrepancy between the physical examination findings and initial testing results. Invasive testing, including transesophageal echocardiography and cardiac catheterization, is often needed to determine an optimal treatment plan. There is a classification system to note the progression of valvular disease with four stages (A–D), similar to that

of the HF guidelines (see earlier section). The stages range from A (at risk) through B (progressive), C (asymptomatic severe), and D (symptomatic severe). These stages are based on valve anatomy, valve hemodynamics, the hemodynamic consequences, and symptoms (Nishimura et al., 2014, Otto et al. 2021).

DIFFERENTIAL DIAGNOSIS
Mitral Valve Prolapse

Definition, Scope, and Etiology

The term *mitral valve prolapse* (MVP) refers to the displacement of abnormally thickened redundant mitral valve leaflets that extend into the left atrium during systole and that may or may not be associated with MR. Other associated features of this syndrome may include left atrial dilatation, left ventricular enlargement, consequent SVA, and abnormalities that involve other valves as well.

It is estimated that 1% to 3% of the U.S. population is afflicted with MVP (Bonow et al., 2006), although the true prevalence is difficult to determine. MVP may have a much lower prevalence than previously estimated, and the prevalence may be similar among different ethnic groups (Theal et al., 2004). From a population perspective, the prevalence of serious cardiovascular complications associated with MVP is low. It is more commonly diagnosed in women than in men and is thought to be associated with either familial (e.g., Marfan syndrome or other connective tissue diseases) or acquired disorders (e.g., CAD). The health trajectory of a patient with MVP is variable, ranging from a benign hemodynamic state and a normal life expectancy to severe comorbid complications and the need for surgical intervention.

Evaluation/Assessment

Although a formal diagnosis is made with the use of echocardiography, a routine physical examination reveals an abnormal auscultatory sound that prompts further workup. The salient auscultatory characteristic of MVP is a high-pitched midsystolic "click" that is best heard at or medial to the apex of the heart. A subsequent late-systolic crescendo murmur indicates mild MR. Changes in the patient's body position, which affects ventricular blood volume, can alter auscultatory findings: Standing to decrease the end diastolic volume causes an earlier click during systole, whereas squatting to increase ventricular volume causes a delay in the click.

Diagnostic Studies

Noninvasive two-dimensional Doppler echocardiography provides the most specific and quantitative information to help define the degree of valve abnormality. For symptomatic women, TTE is performed to help with the determination of the need for cardiac catheterization; transesophageal echocardiography is performed when surgical repair is being considered (Bonow et al., 2006; Nishimura et al., 2014).

Treatment/Management

The ACC and AHA guidelines have approached the evaluation and management of women with MVP on the basis of the presence or absence of symptoms, although some indications overlap (Bonow et al., 2006; Nishimura et al., 2014). Surgical treatment is the intervention of choice when that patient has severe and symptomatic mitral stenosis, but not all patients will be a surgical candidate. In those cases, the patient may be a candidate for percutaneous balloon mitral valvuloplasty (PBMV; Yoon et al., 2017).

MONITORING AND SURGICAL MANAGEMENT

Most women with MVP have a benign course. However, potential associated complications include embolic events, infective endocarditis, and MR that eventually requires surgery. Symptomatic women who develop severe MR require valve repair or replacement to prevent complications such as HF, cerebrovascular events, arrhythmias, and death (Bonow et al., 2006). Mitral valve repair is preferred whenever possible over replacement (Nishimura et al., 2014).

Mitral Regurgitation

ETIOLOGY

MR is a dysfunction of the mitral valve causing retrograde blood flow from the left ventricle to the left atrium, which is the opposite of the proper direction. MR is characterized as either primary or secondary, which is categorized by the cause of the MR. Primary MR is also called degenerative or organic MR. This classification of MR results from a structural deformity or leaflet, chordae tendinea, or papillary muscle damage. Secondary MT is a result of left ventricular dysfunction with normal mitral valve leaflets and chords (Zhang et al., 2020). One of the initial hemodynamic changes that takes place with MR is an increase in the end-diastolic volume. An incompetent mitral valve allows for increased blood flow (and subsequent increased pressure) into the left atrium, which reduces afterload (thus decreasing the end-systolic volume). In a more chronic state, the heart compensates for changes in pressure and volume by increasing in size and becoming hypertrophied. A reduction in cardiac output with severe MR can result in pulmonary congestion, shock, and death (Chirillo et al., 2006).

EVALUATION/ASSESSMENT AND DIAGNOSTIC STUDIES

For the purpose of designing a treatment algorithm, the progression of MR can be categorized into three stages: (a) the asymptomatic patient with hemodynamically significant regurgitation, (b) the asymptomatic patient with decreased left ventricular function, and (c) the symptomatic patient with decreased left ventricular function (Carabello & Crawford, 1997; Nishimura et al., 2014). For women with chronic MR, cardiac enlargement with displacement of the left ventricular apical impulse can be appreciated during the physical examination. A holosystolic murmur can be auscultated and may also be accompanied by an S_3 or early diastolic flow rumble with or without the presence of HF. TTE provides a baseline evaluation of the severity of the MR.

TREATMENT/MANAGEMENT

Medical therapy is limited, although vasodilating agents such as nitroprusside are used to reduce afterload. For women who develop symptoms in the presence of acute and severe MR, surgery is recommended, particularly if left ventricular function is preserved. Surgical options include mitral valve repair, mitral valve replacement with the preservation of the valve apparatus, and mitral valve replacement with the removal of the valve apparatus (Bonow et al., 2006; Nishimura et al., 2014). Valve repair is preferred over valve replacement to avoid the need for chronic anticoagulation. The European Heart Survey showed that women with severe MR were referred for surgery at a more advanced clinical state than men were; also, MV repair was performed less often in women and conferred a higher mortality rate than it did in men (Carabello & Crawford, 1997).

Mitral Stenosis

ETIOLOGY

Mitral stenosis (MS) generally traces back to a case of rheumatic fever, although this presentation is becoming rarer as developing countries achieve access to healthcare. It is typically latent for an average of 20 years before symptoms appear, and it is the most common valvular disease discovered during pregnancy (Elkayam & Bitar, 2005). A funnel-shaped structure develops from both chordae and commissural fusions, and in conjunction with a thickening and calcification of the leaflets, it produces a narrowed orifice between the left atrium and the left ventricle. Other potential complications associated with MS are AF and embolization as a result of an increase in left atrial pressure and enlargement. MS affects women four times as often as men in developing countries. However, with the decline in the incidence of rheumatic fever in the United States and Europe, the ratio of women to men who present with MS is 2:1 (Bonow et al., 2006). Patients are generally 60 years old or older when they present with symptoms, and more than one third of patients who require surgical repair are more than 65 years old (Shoob et al., 2006).

SYMPTOMS, EVALUATION/ASSESSMENT, AND DIAGNOSTIC STUDIES

Women may present early during the course of MS with fatigue, dyspnea, orthopnea, new-onset AF, pulmonary edema, or an embolic event (e.g., stroke). Symptomatic women with MS require evaluation of the extent of their valve disease, as well as an assessment of their NYHA functional class status. The ACC/AHA guidelines categorize MS severity as mild, moderate, or severe on the basis of hemodynamic data and symptom history (Nishimura et al., 2014). Patient history, physical examination, and noninvasive studies, including chest radiography, EKG, and echocardiography, facilitate the diagnosis. During the cardiac examination, the characteristic "opening snap" during early diastole, a low-pitched rumbling diastolic murmur, and an accentuated S_1 are indicative of MS. Findings with worsening valve disease include signs of right ventricular overload, such as distended neck veins, a right ventricular heave, ascites, and peripheral edema. On chest radiography, left atrial enlargement may be noted. Both the pulmonary arterial and venous circulations may be distorted, and there may be evidence of interstitial edema that is consistent with congestion. Echocardiography is the most sensitive and specific noninvasive test used to assess the degree of restricted opening of the mitral valve leaflets; leaflet mobility, flexibility, thickness, and calcification; and suitability of valvotomy (Bonow et al., 2006; Nishimura et al., 2014). Because women with MS can remain clinically stable for years, there is generally no need for further immediate testing if the documented valve area is greater than 1.5 cm^2 and the mean gradient is less than 5 mmHg.

TREATMENT/MANAGEMENT

Medical therapy cannot correct mechanical obstruction of the mitral valve. Women who develop more severe MS can remain free of symptoms if they are educated to limit strenuous physical activity. Women are counseled to seek immediate evaluation if a sudden increase in shortness of breath occurs. Disease progression is monitored with an annual history and physical examination, EKG, and chest radiography. Surgical intervention generally correlates with clinical symptoms or with evidence of pulmonary HTN or ventricular dysfunction (Bonow et al., 2006; Nishimura et al., 2014).

Recommendations for the treatment of conditions associated with MS (e.g., AF) include anticoagulation, heart rate control, and chemical or electrical cardioversion. Long-term anticoagulation is warranted to prevent systemic embolic events. Without surgical intervention, mitral valve disease results in an 85% mortality rate at 20 years after symptom onset (Bonow et al., 2006).

Aortic Stenosis

DEFINITION, SCOPE, AND ETIOLOGY

Nonrheumatic AS has been described as a calcific disease in which there is an accumulation of lipids, smooth muscle cells, collagen inflammatory cells, and platelet adherence that produces plaque-laden areas along the leaflets and valve cusps; this imitates the atherosclerotic process that accompanies CAD (Carabello & Crawford, 1997). This generally idiopathic process results in the obstruction of blood flow through a narrowed orifice. Fewer women present with AS as a result of exposure to rheumatic fever. AS is the most common valvular lesion in the United States, affecting approximately 25% of individuals who are more than 65 years old, and it is associated with cardiovascular risk factors such as HTN, DM, gender, smoking, and dyslipidemia (Bonow et al., 2006). Furthermore, investigators pooled together databases and calculated an estimated prevalence of 12.4% for AS and 3.4% for severe AS as the burden of disease among older adults. Using these calculations, approximately 290,000 older patients with severe AS are potential candidates for transcatheter aortic valve replacement (TAVR; Osnabrugge et al., 2013).

EVALUATION/ASSESSMENT AND DIAGNOSTIC STUDIES

During the cardiac examination, the most common sign of AS is a late-systolic ejection murmur heard in the aortic area. The murmur can frequently be heard radiating to the neck. The murmur can mimic MR in that it may also be auscultated over the apex; it may also be associated with a thrill. As the AS worsens, pulsus parvus et tardus may be elicited; when this occurs, the carotid upstrokes diminish in amplitude and are delayed during the cardiac cycle, and the clinician may also detect a paradoxically split S$_2$ as a result of delayed ventricular emptying. The development of symptoms such as angina, HF, or syncope indicates a poor short-term prognosis with a high risk for sudden death within 2 to

3 years. Two-dimensional Doppler echocardiography is used to confirm the diagnosis.

TREATMENT/MANAGEMENT

Although the progression rate of AS is slow, the individual rate of progression to hemodynamic consequences varies, thus necessitating the close monitoring of both symptomatic and asymptomatic women by a specialist. No medical therapy has been shown to effectively treat AS. Lipid-lowering therapy may slow the progression of the mechanisms associated with atherosclerosis; however, because symptoms can quickly progress, surgical intervention is considered if diagnostic testing reveals moderate to severe AS (Bonow et al., 2006; Nishimura et al., 2014).

Aortic Regurgitation

ETIOLOGY

Aortic regurgitation (AR) is caused by disease that involves at least one of the aortic leaflets (e.g., infective endocarditis, rheumatic fever) or the aortic root (e.g., collagen vascular disease, annuloaortic ectasia). Acute AR, which is usually a complication of an invasive procedure, aortic dissection, or chest trauma, is a rare and life-threatening event. Chronic AR is more prevalent and imposes a cardiac trajectory with an initial compensatory increase in left ventricular mass, a low EF, and subsequent HF symptoms. The prevalence of AR increases with age and is detected more often in men than in women (Carabello & Crawford, 1997; DesJardin et al., 2022).

EVALUATION/ASSESSMENT

Multiple examination findings suggest regurgitant flow and increased systolic stroke volume. The classic murmur is a high-frequency decrescendo diastolic murmur heard at the left sternal border. An S$_3$ is sometimes noted, and S$_2$ may be absent altogether. With severe AR, women may present with bounding carotid pulses, head bobbing (de Musset sign), a pulsating uvula (Miller sign), and pistol-shot sounds heard over a compressed femoral artery (Traube sign).

TREATMENT/MANAGEMENT

Referral to a specialist is appropriate for women with AR to manage resultant HF or to provide surgical intervention. The guidelines recommend (class I) that the management of patients with severe heart valve disease is best achieved by a heart valve team composed minimally of a cardiologist and a cardiac surgeon but potentially including cardiologists, structural valve interventionalists, cardiovascular imaging specialists, cardiovascular surgeons, anesthesiologists, and nurses, all of whom have expertise in the management and outcome of patients with severe heart valve disease. Often, heart valve centers of excellence have a valve clinic with a valve team. The guidelines recommend (class IIa) that consultation with or referral to a heart valve center of excellence is reasonable for asymptomatic patients with severe valve disease. Surgical risk is evaluated through the Society of Thoracic Surgeons (STS), where surgeons predict the risk of death by assessing the patient's fragility (e.g., Katz Index of Independence in Activities of Daily Living; Bach, 2014).

Infective Endocarditis

PREVENTION

The ACC/AHA 2008 guideline update regarding valvular heart disease revised the recommendations for infective endocarditis prophylaxis (Wilson et al., 2007). Infective endocarditis is less likely to be caused by a procedure than by random exposure to bacteria, such as when brushing teeth, chewing gum, or other oral hygiene procedures, and it was also found that prophylactic antibiotic treatment prevents only a very small number of cases of infective endocarditis. Thus, prophylactic antibiotics are reserved for women who are at the highest risk of an adverse outcome from acquiring infective endocarditis (Wilson et al., 2007). The 2014 AHA/ACC Guideline for the Management of Patients with Valvular Heart Disease by Nishimura et al. (2014) recommends the same approach to care.

Considerations for Special Populations

The normal physiologic changes related to a woman's cardiovascular system during pregnancy become more critical in the setting of valvular disease. There is a 50% increase in blood volume and a consequent 25% increase in cardiac output that influences valvular function such that stenotic valve murmurs are accentuated and regurgitant murmurs may become nearly inaudible. Ideally, the management of women with known valvular lesions begins before conception. The 2006 ACC/AHA Guidelines for the Management of Patients with Valvular Heart Disease provide recommendations such as anticoagulation therapies, exercise restrictions, and prophylaxis endocarditis treatment for each specific valve condition (Bonow et al., 2006).

Cardiomyopathy

DEFINITION, SCOPE, AND ETIOLOGY

The AHA classified cardiomyopathies as primary (genetic, mixed, or acquired) or secondary (e.g., infiltrative, toxic, or inflammatory). The four major types are dilated cardiomyopathy, hypertrophic cardiomyopathy, restrictive cardiomyopathy, and arrhythmogenic right ventricular cardiomyopathy (Pelliccia et al., 2019).

Dilated cardiomyopathy, the most common form and affects 5 in 100,000 adults and 0.57 in 100,000 children. It is the third leading cause of HF in the United States after CAD and HTN (Wexler et al., 2009). The causes of cardiomyopathies are varied. Dilated cardiomyopathy in adults is most commonly caused by CAD (ischemic cardiomyopathy) and HTN, although viral myocarditis, valvular disease, and genetic predisposition may also play a role (Wexler et al., 2009).

Peripartum cardiomyopathy (PPCM) is associated with pregnancy; the heart dilates and weakens, leading to symptoms of HF. PPCM can be difficult to diagnose because symptoms of HF can mimic those of pregnancy. PPCM can be a major cause of maternal morbidity and mortality, especially in some minority groups such as Africans and African Americans (Givertz, 2013). Most affected women recover normal heart function; however, some will progress to severe HF requiring mechanical support or heart transplantation. Even when the heart recovers, another pregnancy may be associated with a risk of recurrent HF (Givertz, 2013). Additionally, women with significant left ventricular dysfunction are at increased risk for future cardiovascular events (McNamara et al., 2015).

Cardiomyopathies have a genetic component, and this is relevant to practice. Current practice guidelines include the use of genetic testing in patients with cardiomyopathies as part of our management strategy. Our evolving knowledge of cardiomyopathies provides evidence that understanding genetic testing will help to personalize care and risk stratify not only the patient but the patient's family members (Pelliccia et al., 2019).

DIFFERENTIAL DIAGNOSIS
Stroke

DEFINITION, SCOPE, AND ETIOLOGY

According to the 2015 AHA statistics, cardiovascular health encompasses several clinical conditions, including cerebrovascular disease and stroke. Stroke is currently the fifth leading cause of death and the leading cause of disability in adults in the United States; it is the third leading cause of death among women. Because of several important treatment modalities for acute stroke and because there has been a nationwide surge in establishing certified stroke centers, more patients are surviving their first stroke; there are currently 7 million stroke survivors, a majority of which are women. An additional 3.6 million people are projected to survive a stroke within the next two decades, and more than half of those individuals will be women. With a projected larger aging population, older women are expected to make up a majority of the stroke survivor population (Mozaffarian et al., 2015). The reasons for these statistics are multifold and include some of the following stark facts:

- Women live longer than men and therefore have a higher lifetime stroke risk than men.
- Women tend to have gaps in knowledge about stroke symptoms and stroke treatment options and therefore do not seek acute stroke care.
- Older women have a poorer functional recovery from stroke than men, as they frequently lack a support system to assist with rehabilitation and lifestyle and stroke-prevention strategies.
- Women have a higher rate of recurrent stroke compared with men.
- Stroke mortality rate is higher among women and is likely related to longer life expectancy.
- Women have been underrepresented in clinical trials related to stroke treatment and prevention and, as a result, may not be afforded gender-specific, evidence-based treatment.
- Women have sex-specific stroke risk factors, including pregnancy, gestational HTN, oral contraceptive pill use, menopause, and higher rates of other cardiovascular conditions.

In 2014, the AHA Stroke Association in collaboration with the Council on Cardiovascular and Stroke Nursing, the Council on Clinical Cardiology, the Council on Epidemiology and Prevention, and the Council for High Blood Pressure Research endorsed the first guideline dedicated to stroke risk and prevention in women. The AHA Science Advisory and Coordinating Committee approved a Healthcare Statement that summarized data on stroke risk factors unique to women and proposed a female-specific risk score to better capture adult women's stroke risk (Bushnell et al., 2014). Given that the majority of the population will be older women with multiple cardiovascular and cerebrovascular risk factors, this guideline provides an excellent reference for clinicians who prescribe both primary and secondary stroke-prevention strategies.

Stroke has been defined as a sudden death of brain cells due to the lack of oxygen caused by a blockage of blood flow (resulting in an ischemic stroke) or rupture of an artery in the brain (resulting in a hemorrhagic stroke). Approximately 87% of strokes are ischemic in nature, and 13% are hemorrhagic. Hemorrhagic stroke is further divided into intracerebral hemorrhage (ICH; 10%) and subarachnoid hemorrhage (SAH; 3%; Sacco et al., 2013).

Although women have an overall lower incidence of ischemic stroke than men, older women (older than 85 years) have a similar or higher incidence of ischemic stroke. Longevity and survival after their index stroke give women both a higher lifetime stroke risk and a higher stroke mortality rate.

RISK FACTORS

Table 43.6, taken from the 2014 AHA Guidelines, highlights stroke risk factors and the unique sex-specific factors, including those that are more prevalent in women than in men.

SYMPTOMS

Strokes usually present as a syndrome in which patients experience the sudden onset of neurologic deficits; the constellation of symptoms helps to localize the region in the central nervous system that has been injured. Public awareness campaigns have highlighted the most common symptoms by using the acronym F.A.S.T., which stands for *Facial* weakness or drooping, weakness in the *Arm*, *Speech* problems, and *Time*, emphasizing the importance of calling 911 and seeking medical help immediately. Clinicians are familiar with the five "suddens": unilateral numbness/weakness in face/arm/leg, confusion, trouble speaking, severe headache, trouble seeing

TABLE 43.6 Stroke Risk Factors, Categorized by Sex-Specific Features

RISK FACTOR	SEX-SPECIFIC RISK FACTORS	RISK FACTORS THAT ARE STRONGER OR MORE PREVALENT IN WOMEN	RISK FACTORS WITH SIMILAR PREVALENCE IN MEN AND WOMEN BUT UNKNOWN DIFFERENCE IN IMPACT
Pregnancy	X		
Preeclampsia	X		
Gestational diabetes	X		
Oral contraceptive use	X		
Postmenopausal hormone use	X		
Changes in hormonal status	X		
Migraine with aura		X	
Atrial fibrillation		X	
Diabetes mellitus		X	
Hypertension		X	
Physical inactivity			X
Age			X
Prior cardiovascular disease			X
Obesity			X
Diet			X
Smoking			X
Metabolic syndrome			X
Depression		X	
Psychosocial stress		X	

in one or both eyes, and trouble walking/lack of coordination. These "suddens" highlight symptoms that indicate further evaluation is needed.

Patients may also present with symptoms of sudden onset of vertigo with vomiting, unexplained syncope, or altered mental status that precedes the symptoms already discussed and heightens suspicion for a cerebrovascular event.

EVALUATION/ASSESSMENT

Although there are some common features to symptom presentation that may be indicative of stroke type, the diagnosis requires a detailed history, rapid imaging, and comprehensive neurologic exam.

DIFFERENTIAL DIAGNOSIS

ISCHEMIC STROKE

Definition, Scope, and Etiology

The classifications of ischemic stroke are generally divided into five subtypes. These classifications reflect a proposed etiology of ischemic stroke and serve as a guide for the appropriate treatments for secondary stroke prevention. Approximately 30% of patients who present with an ischemic stroke are diagnosed with large vessel disease, referring to atherosclerosis leading to stenosis or occlusion of a major artery in the brain or artery leading to the brain (including the carotid or vertebral arteries). An additional 20% of ischemic strokes are thought to be cardioembolic in nature, in which patients with vessel occlusions may have had an embolus travel from the heart (such as in AF). Approximately 15% of patients are diagnosed with small vessel disease, which refers to stenoses of the smaller vessels (deeper in the brain) typically related to long-standing DM or HLD. Stroke patients who fall into the category of "other" are patients for whom their stroke may result from vasculopathies or hypercoagulable states. Nearly 30% of patients have a final diagnosis of *cryptogenic stroke* such that despite a comprehensive diagnostic workup, there is no identified cause for their stroke.

Evaluation/Assessment and Diagnostic Studies

In addition to a careful medical history, diagnostic imaging (such as an MRI) and other studies (such as an echocardiogram) help to identify a suspected stroke etiology and guide secondary stroke prevention therapies.

TRANSIENT ISCHEMIC ATTACK

Definition

The term *transient ischemic attack* (TIA) is frequently used to describe stroke symptoms that are transient in nature and thus are too often mistakenly considered a less urgent medical issue. Traditionally, TIAs have been defined as events in which focal neurologic symptoms last less than 24 hours; however, the more routine use of neuroimaging studies such as a head CT scan or MRI have demonstrated that even patients with stroke symptoms lasting just several hours have evidence of infarction on CT or MRI. This has led to a more current definition of TIA, which is "a brief episode of neurological dysfunction caused by focal brain or retinal ischemia, with clinical symptoms typically lasting less than one hour, and without evidence of acute infarction" (Easton et al., 2009, p. 2277).

Evaluation/Assessment

A valuable risk assessment tool called the ABCD² score used to predict short-term stroke risk after a TIA was developed by Johnston et al. (2007) and considered five items that were assigned points to determine the 2-, 7-, 30-, and 90-day stroke risk. The seven-point scoring scale is based on age, blood pressure, clinical features, duration of symptoms, and history of DM. Based on the patient's score, practitioners can make clinical decisions regarding the benefit of recommending hospital admission for urgent workup and treatment (see Figure 43.5).

Intracerebral Hemorrhage. Spontaneous, nontraumatic ICH is the most common of the hemorrhages in which blood vessel rupture causes bleeding into the brain parenchyma. Uncontrolled HTN is the principal cause; other secondary causes include cerebral amyloid angiopathy (CAA), intracranial aneurysm rupture, vasculitis, and hemorrhagic transformation after an ischemic stroke. The incidence of ICH and mortality resulting from ICH in women is reportedly lower than in men, but after the age of 65 years, there were similar mortality risks.

Subarachnoid Hemorrhage. SAH occurs when an intracranial aneurysm ruptures and blood enters the spaces around the brain tissue. The incidence of SAH is higher in women and is noted after the age of 55 years. Women have a higher risk of SAH resulting primarily from the prevalence and location of cerebral aneurysms (Algra et al., 2012). These statistics underscore the fact that women in all age groups can be at risk for any one or more of these ischemic stroke subtypes, so a thorough health history and gender-specific risk factor profile help direct therapies for both primary and secondary ischemic stroke prevention.

Treatment/Management

In the primary care setting, it is critical to recognize the symptoms of stroke and quickly have the patient transported to an emergency care facility. In the emergency facility, the goal is to stabilize, assess, and image the patient within 60 minutes of presentation (Adams et al., 2007). Rapid identification, diagnosis, and initiation of treatment are the key to minimizing the residual effects of stroke.

After patient discharge from the acute care setting, management focuses on rehabilitation. Rehabilitation programs are interdisciplinary with physical therapy, speech therapy, and a number of others as needed to minimize an individual's residual effects.

Secondary Prevention

After a stroke that is not cardioembolic, the AHA and American Stroke Association recommend antiplatelet agents to decrease the risk for a second stroke or other cardiac events. Specifically, aspirin (50–325 mg/day) alone or in combination with dipyridamole extended release or clopidogrel alone (Adams et al., 2008) are prescribed. Consistent evaluation for adherence and encouragement to continue with therapy are important, as approximately 25% of patients stop taking their medications within 3 months after their stroke (Bushnell et al., 2010).

ABCD² Score

The ABCD² score is a risk-assessment tool designed to improve the prediction of short-term stroke risk after a TIA. The score is optimized to predict the risk of stroke within 2 days after a TIA but also predicts stroke risk within 90 days. The ABCD² score is calculated by summing up points for five independent factors.

RISK FACTOR	POINTS	SCORE
Age ≥ 60 years	1	☐
Blood pressure Systolic BP ≥ 140 mmHg *OR* Diastolic BP ≥ 90 mmHg	1	☐

Clinical features of TIA (*choose one*)
    Unilateral weakness with or without speech impairment *OR*
    Speech impairment without unilateral weakness
	2
	1
		☐

Duration
    TIA duration ≥ 60 minutos
    TIA duration 10–59 minutes
	2
	1
		☐

Diabetes	1	☐
Total ABCD² score	0–7	☐

Using the ABCD² Score

Higher ABCD² scores are associated with a greater risk of stroke during the 2, 7, 30, and 90 days after a TIA (figure). The authors of the ABCD² score made the following recommendations for hospital observation

ABCD² Score	2-Day Stroke Risk	Comment
0–3	1.0%	Hospital observation may be unnecessary without another indication (e.g., now atrial fibrillation)
4–5	4.1%	Hospital observation justified in most situations
6–7	8.1%	Hospital observation worthwhile

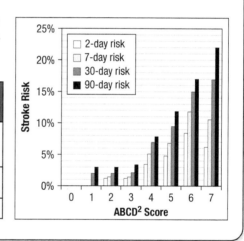

FIGURE 43.5 ABCD² risk assessment tool used to predict stroke risk after a transient ischemic attack (TIA): prognosis and key management considerations.
Source: Johnston, S. C., Rothwell, P. M., Nguyen-Huynh, M. N., Giles, M. F., Elkins, J. S., Bernstein, A. L., & Sidney, S. (2007). Validation and refinement of scores to predict very early stroke risk after transient ischemic attack. Lancet, 369, 283–292. https://doi.org/10.1016/S0140-6736(07)60150-0. Copyright © 2007, used with permission from Elsevier.

FUTURE DIRECTIONS

Much has been learned about women and heart disease during the past several years, and there is now clear evidence that CVD in women is indeed different from CVD in men. Clinicians need to continue to advocate for women who are at risk for heart disease and strive to provide best practices for preventing, identifying, and treating heart disease in women.

Future research will provide more data regarding unique symptoms and presentations among women, as well as treatment modalities that have superior outcomes for women. In the interim, aggressive preventive measures, early recognition, and aggressive management are critical.

REFERENCES

References for this chapter are online and available at https://connect.springerpub.com/content/book/978-0-8261-6722-4/part/part03/chapter/ch43

CHAPTER 44

Endocrine-Related Problems*

TRACI SHARKEY-WELLS

The endocrine system and nervous system control all physiologic processes in the body. The endocrine system acts as a chemical communication network that coordinates physiologic function through hormones that are released into the bloodstream from specific cells within ductless glands. Like other communication systems, the endocrine system is composed of transmitters (hormone-producing cells), signals (hormones), and receptors. Once in the circulation and extracellular fluid, hormones affect the function of target tissues. Hormonal mechanisms of action are generally described by the effects they have on target cells. Table 44.1 depicts the effects of common endocrine disorders on target organs. Endocrine hormones are secreted into the bloodstream and bind to distant target cells. Paracrine hormones are those that exert an effect on cells of the organ from which they are released. Autocrine hormones affect the same cells from which they are produced. Hormones can be peptides or proteins (e.g., prolactin, ACTH, insulin); steroids that are derived from cholesterol (e.g., sex hormones, adrenal steroids); amino acid derivatives (e.g., epinephrine, norepinephrine, thyroid hormones); or fatty acid derivatives (e.g., prostaglandins, leukotrienes).

All hormones bind selectively to receptors either in or on the surface of target cells. Intracellular receptors interact with hormones that modulate genetic function (e.g., corticosteroids, thyroid hormone). Hormones that bind with receptors on the target cell surface control enzyme activity or regulate ion channels (e.g., growth hormone, thyrotropin-releasing hormone).

Throughout this chapter the terms *woman* and *women* are used to refer to cisgender women and those born with a uterus, ovaries, and fallopian tubes. Due to limited research about endocrinologic health problems among nonbinary and transgender persons, the language used reflects the research available, generally done with women. Caring for transgender women and transgender men is not different and the use of gender-affirming hormone therapy (GAHT) is not known to change treatment guidelines.

HYPOTHALAMIC–PITUITARY RELATIONSHIPS

Endocrine organ functions within the body are modulated by pituitary hormones. An exception is secretion of insulin by the pancreas, which is primarily controlled by blood glucose level. Pituitary hormone secretion is controlled by the hypothalamus.

The hypothalamic–pituitary axis is the feedback system that controls interaction between the hypothalamus and pituitary gland. Input from all areas of the central nervous system is received by the hypothalamus to feed information back to the pituitary, which then releases specific hormones that stimulate endocrine glands throughout the body. The hypothalamus detects changes in circulating levels of hormones produced by these endocrine glands and either increases or decreases its stimulation of the pituitary to maintain homeostasis.

THYROID DISORDERS

The thyroid gland is one of the largest endocrine glands. It secretes thyroid hormone in response to signals received from the hypothalamus through the pituitary and functions through a negative feedback mechanism (Figure 44.1). Patients may present with signs of either thyroid excess or deficiency.

Hypothyroidism

DEFINITION AND SCOPE

Hypothyroidism results when the thyroid gland is unable to produce sufficient levels of thyroid hormone (triiodothyronine [T3] and thyroxine [T4]). Primary hypothyroidism

---

*This chapter is a revision of the chapter that appeared in the second edition of this textbook, authored by Adrienne Berarducci, and we thank her for her original contribution.

TABLE 44.1 Clinical Manifestations of Endocrine Disorders

SIGNS AND SYMPTOMS	POSSIBLE DISORDER
Anemia	Adrenal problems, thyroid problems
Anorexia/nausea	Adrenal problems, diabetes (DKA and HHS), thyroid disorders
Menstrual changes	Adrenal problems, PCOS, thyroid conditions, menopause, hyperprolactinemia
Nervousness	Adrenal and thyroid problems
Weakness/fatigue	Common with multiple endocrine problems
BOWEL CHANGES	
Constipation	Diabetic neuropathy, hypothyroidism
Hyperdefecation	Hyperthyroidism (frequent/increased bowel movements)
HAIR CHANGES	
Hirsutism	PCOS, Cushing syndrome
Hair loss	Hypothyroidism
THERMAL CHANGES	
Fever	Adrenal and thyroid problems
Decreased temperature	Diabetes, thyroid problems
WEIGHT CHANGES	
weight loss	Adrenal problems (AI), thyroid problems (hyperthyroidism), diabetes
weight gain	Cushing syndrome, thyroid problems (hypothyroidism), PCOS

AI, adrenal insufficiency; DKA, diabetic ketoacidosis; HHS, hyperosmolar hyperglycemia; PCOS, polycystic ovary syndrome.
Source: Data from Gardner, D., & Shoback, D. (2011). Greenspan's basic and clinical endocrinology (9th ed.). Lange Medical Books/McGraw-Hill.

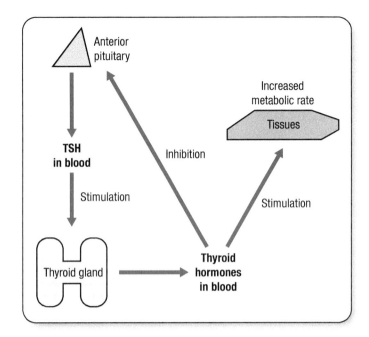

FIGURE 44.1 Thyroid negative feedback system.
TSH, thyroid-stimulating hormone.

due to loss of functional thyroid tissue or a defect in hormone synthesis. It may also occur in response to pathology of the pituitary gland or hypothalamus.

Autoimmune thyroid disease (Hashimoto thyroiditis) is the most common cause of hypothyroidism in the United States and other geographic areas where iodine intake is adequate. Worldwide, however, iodine deficiency remains the leading cause. Iatrogenic hypothyroidism can occur postpartum, following partial or complete surgical removal of the thyroid gland, or from radioactive iodine (RAI) ablation, or it may be drug-induced (e.g., lithium, alpha interferon, amiodarone, iodine). Secondary hypothyroidism is rare and occurs with disorders of the pituitary and hypothalamus that cause alterations in thyroid-stimulating hormone (TSH) production (e.g., pituitary adenoma). Congenital hypothyroidism occurs in infants born with a thyroid that is not fully developed or does not function properly. If untreated, congenital hypothyroidism can lead to mental dysfunction and growth failure. Newborns in the United States are generally screened for hypothyroidism as early detection and treatment can prevent these sequelae (Park & Chatterjee, 2005).

RISK FACTORS

Numerous risk factors are associated with hypothyroidism (Table 44.2). They include previous history of a thyroid disorder (e.g., goiter); partial or total thyroidectomy; radiation to the thyroid, neck, or chest; family history of thyroid disease; history of other autoimmune diseases (e.g., Sjögren syndrome, rheumatoid arthritis, lupus); pernicious anemia; type 1 diabetes; Turner syndrome; age greater than 60 years; or having been pregnant or delivered a baby within the past 6 months (Golden et al., 2009).

SYMPTOMS

Clinical manifestations of hypothyroidism result from reduced metabolic activity and metabolic rate (Bhuvana

is relatively common, with incidence increasing with age. About 4.6% of the United States population 12 years of age and older have hypothyroidism (Lee, 2015). The exact prevalence varies by causative factors and is influenced by both geographic location and environmental factors. The incidence of Hashimoto thyroiditis ranges from 0.3 to 5 per 1,000 and is 10 to 20 times more common in women than in men (Gardner & Shoback, 2011). Subclinical hypothyroidism is present in about 2% of the adult population and progresses to overt hypothyroidism in about 5% to 18% of patients (Baskin et al., 2002).

ETIOLOGY

Hypothyroidism is a common endocrine disorder resulting from thyroid hormone deficiency. Most commonly, this is

TABLE 44.2 Risk Factors for Primary and Secondary Hypothyroidism

TYPE OF HYPOTHYROIDISM	SELECT CAUSES AND RISK FACTORS
Primary	Older than 60 years Female History of hyperthyroidism or goiter (involving treatment with radioactive iodine) Family history of hypothyroidism History of radiation therapy to neck or chest Surgical removal of partial/complete thyroid Radioactive iodine ablation
Iatrogenic	Use of lithium Use of amiodarone Use of exogenous iodine Use of alpha interferon Interleukin 2, tyrosine kinase inhibitors, and checkpoint inhibitor immunotherapy (e.g., ipilimumab, pembrolizumab, and nivolumab)
Secondary	Pituitary adenoma Pituitary ablative therapy Peripheral thyroid hormone resistance
Congenital	Immature/underdeveloped thyroid gland

Source: Data from Gardner, D., & Shoback, D. (2011). Greenspan's basic and clinical endocrinology (9th ed.). Lange Medical Books/McGraw Hill; Park, S. M., & Chatterjee, V. K. (2005). Genetics of congenital hypothyroidism. Journal of Medical Genetics, 42(5), 379–389. https://doi.org/10.1136/jmg.2004.024158

Box 44.1 Common Symptoms Associated With Hypothyroidism

Fatigue

Weight gain

Puffy face and/or eyelids

Dull facial expression

Cold intolerance

Joint and muscle pain

Constipation

Dry skin and hair

Decreased sweating

Heavy or irregular menstrual periods

Impaired fertility

Hoarseness and/or slow speech

Blurred vision

Decreased hearing

Carpal tunnel syndrome

Depression

Confusion

Bradycardia

et al., 2002). Thyroid hormone deficiency can cause multiple symptoms that can vary greatly from person to person and affect several systems: central nervous, cardiovascular, musculoskeletal, and reproductive. Common symptoms include fatigue; weight gain; a puffy face and/or eyelids; dull facial expression; cold intolerance; joint and muscle pain; constipation; dry skin; dry, thinning hair and eyebrows, decreased sweating; heavy or irregular menstrual periods and impaired fertility; hoarseness; slow speech; blurred vision; decreased hearing; carpal tunnel syndrome; depression; confusion; and bradycardia (Box 44.1). However, hypothyroidism develops slowly, and many patients do not notice symptoms.

Symptoms more specific to Hashimoto disease are painless thyroid enlargement, subjective fullness in the throat, and exhaustion and transient neck pain with or without sore throat. Hypothyroidism is a contributor to hypercholesterolemia; therefore, individuals with hypercholesterolemia should be screened for hypothyroidism. In rare instances, severe, untreated hypothyroidism may lead to myxedema, an extreme form of hypothyroidism that results in altered mental status, hypothermia, bradycardia, hypercarbia, and hyponatremia. Ascites, pericardial effusion, and cardiomegaly may be present and can lead to cardiogenic shock. This life-threatening condition occurs most commonly in individuals with hypothyroidism in whom the condition has not been diagnosed and who are exposed to physical stress, such as hypothermia, infection, myocardial infarction, stroke, or medical intervention (e.g., surgery or hypnotic drugs). Myxedema requires immediate hospitalization and intensive treatment.

EVALUATION/ASSESSMENT
History

Symptoms of hypothyroidism are generally very subtle and gradual and may be mistaken for symptoms of depression and other illnesses. With suspected hypothyroidism and health maintenance encounters, providers need to take a detailed, deliberate approach in evaluating risk factors and symptoms as the obscure presentation may make them unnoticeable in some patients.

Physical Examination

Evaluation of the patient with hypothyroidism may reveal subtle changes, and detection requires careful physical assessment. Physical signs may include weight gain, slow speech and movements, xerosis, pallor, coarse and brittle hair, alopecia of varying degrees and patterns, dull and/or coarse facial expression, periorbital puffiness, macroglossia, simple or nodular goiter, bradycardia, hoarseness, edema, decreased systolic and increased diastolic blood pressure, and hyporeflexia with delayed relaxation phase. Other clinical manifestations can be related to different causes of hypothyroidism such as pituitary enlargement or adenoma and with diffuse or multinodular goiter (Garber et al., 2012).

DIFFERENTIAL DIAGNOSIS

Differential diagnosis can be extensive as many of the symptoms of hypothyroidism are nonspecific. Special consideration should be given to the possible presence of ischemic heart disease, liver abnormalities, and depression. Patients presenting with menstrual irregularity and/or infertility may also have underlying metabolic disease. Other possible causes of the symptoms include eating disorders, HIV infection, sepsis, diabetes, and renal failure (Gardner & Shoback, 2011).

DIAGNOSTIC STUDIES

Third-generation TSH serum assays are considered the most sensitive screening tool for primary hypothyroidism. In the presence of TSH levels elevated above the reference range, measurement of serum-free T4 or the free thyroxine index (FTI), which serves as a surrogate of the free hormone level, should be obtained. Measurement of T3 is not recommended.

Elevated TSH with decreased T4 or FTI indicates hypothyroidism. Elevated TSH (usually 4.5–10.0 mIU/L) with normal free T4 or FTI is considered mild disease or subclinical hypothyroidism (Garber et al., 2012). Symptoms of subclinical hypothyroidism are sometimes present after a patient has been acutely ill. In this situation it is referred to as euthyroid sick syndrome and usually resolves spontaneously without treatment in 6 weeks.

The complete blood count and metabolic profile may also exhibit abnormalities in patients with hypothyroidism, such as anemia, dilutional hyponatremia, hyperlipidemia, reversible increased creatinine, and elevated transaminases and creatinine kinase (Kreisman & Hennessey, 1999).

Although no universal screening guidelines exist for thyroid disease in adults, the American Thyroid Association (ATA) recommends screening at age 35 years and every 5 years thereafter, with closer attention to high-risk individuals, such as pregnant persons, persons older than 60 years, individuals with type 1 diabetes or other autoimmune disorders, and those with a history of neck irradiation (Ladenson et al., 2000).

TREATMENT/MANAGEMENT OF PRIMARY HYPOTHYROIDISM

The goal of hypothyroidism treatment is to restore a state of euthyroidism, accomplished with thyroid replacement therapy. As with all treatment, it should be tailored to the individual. Education should provide an understanding of the disease and its treatment. Referral to an endocrinologist is appropriate for those in whom euthyroidism is difficult to achieve (Box 44.2).

Self-Management Measures

Self-management measures are most often geared toward managing the many symptoms that patients can experience with hypothyroidism (Table 44.3). Patients who experience significant fatigue need to be cautioned to pace their activities and achieve adequate rest, especially until a euthyroid state is achieved. Measures for managing constipation may include increasing fluids, increasing dietary fiber, and using stool softeners.

Box 44.2 Patients With Hypothyroidism Who May Require Referral to Endocrinology

Patients younger than 18 years

Patients who are unresponsive to therapy

Patients who are pregnant

Patients with cardiovascular disease

Patients with other endocrine disorders

Patients with thyroid nodules

TABLE 44.3 Clinical Findings in Hypothyroidism

SYSTEM	SYMPTOMS	SIGNS
General	Fatigue/lethargy	Periorbital edema
	Weakness	Pallor
Endocrine	Swelling of thyroid	Goiter
	Menorrhagia	Galactorrhea
Metabolic	Cold intolerance	Hypothermia
	Weight gain	Obesity
Psychiatric	Depression	Depression
Musculoskeletal	Arthralgia, myalgia	
Skin	Decreased perspiration	Brittle nails
	Hair loss	Reduced skin turgor, alopecia/coarse hair, carotenemia
Gastrointestinal	Constipation	Megacolon
	Decreased appetite	
Respiratory	Snoring	Hypoventilation, sleep apnea
Cardiovascular	Dyspnea	Hypertension (diastolic), pericardial effusion, cardiomegaly/CHF, bradycardia
Nervous system	Paresthesia	Bradykinesia
	Numbness	Distal sensory loss
	Unsteadiness	Ataxia
	Reduced mentation	Dementia, hyporeflexia, pseudomyotonia, visual disturbances[a]

[a]Findings in secondary hypothyroidism.
CHF, congestive heart failure.
Source: Reprinted with permission from Guha, B., Krishnaswamy, G., & Peiris, A. (2002). The diagnosis and management of hypothyroidism. Southern Medical Journal, 95(5), 475–480.

Complementary and Alternative Medicine

The extant scientific literature does not recommend complementary and alternative medicine (CAM) modalities specifically for hypothyroidism. Some patients use CAM therapies to manage symptoms of the disorder such as fatigue, weight changes, and hair and skin changes; however, their use should be discussed with their clinician.

Pharmacotherapeutics

Updated guidelines from Jonklaas et al. (2014) indicate that levothyroxine (LT4) as monotherapy remains the treatment of choice for hypothyroidism. LT4 produces stable levels of both T3 and T4. The dosage is approximately 1.6 mcg/kg/day, taken every morning on an empty stomach. When initiating LT4, the patient's weight, lean body mass, pregnancy status, etiology of thyroid disorder, degree of TSH elevation, age, and comorbidities, including the presence of cardiac disease, are considered. Patients should avoid taking biotin 48 hours prior to having serum T4, T3, and TSH testing due to interference in the assay causing false elevations. Patients who are ingesting 5 to 10 mg of biotin (marketed over the counter to prevent hair loss) can have spurious results in these assays. Biotin may cause falsely low values in assays used to measure TSH, and falsely high values in competitive binding assays used to measure free T4, T3, free T3, and TSH receptor-binding inhibitor immunoglobulin.

Clinical benefits of LT4 replacement can begin to be appreciated in as little as 3 to 5 days and generally plateau at 6 weeks. Until TSH levels are within target range (1.0 to 2.0 U/mL), LT4 dosing changes are made every 6 to 8 weeks. Serum TSH levels within the normal reference range commonly require several months of monitoring and dose titration. Dosing aspects of LT4 treatment are depicted in Table 44.4.

Once the LT4 dose is stabilized, annual monitoring of serum TSH and clinical evaluation are maintained. Overtreatment must be monitored, and dose reductions initiated promptly. Patients need to be aware of symptoms of overtreatment to avoid potential health threats, such as tachycardia, palpitations, angina, increased sweating, nervousness, atrial fibrillation, increased nervousness, fatigue, headache, irritability, insomnia, and tremors. Excessive LT4 can also cause bone loss over time.

Consideration should be given to causes other than hypothyroidism in patients who remain symptomatic despite normalization of their TSH level. This may indicate dysfunctional conversion of T4 to T3 in the brain. Combination LT4/liothyronine (LT3) therapy may benefit these individuals; however, this is rarely observed.

Considerations for Special and Minoritized Populations

The bioequivalence of various brands of LT4 can also be problematic. Because bioequivalence has been based on total T4 measurements instead of TSH levels, bioequivalence does not equal therapeutic equivalence. Patients should be maintained on a consistent brand of LT4. If the brand is changed for any reason, then TSH levels should be repeated in 4 to 6 weeks and the dose adjusted as needed to maintain euthyroidism (Jonklaas et al., 2014).

Several conditions may require special dosing and monitoring of therapy for hypothyroidism. If dosage of LT4 is much higher than anticipated to maintain normal range TSH, consider evaluation for gastrointestinal disorders that may interfere with absorption. These include disorders such as *Helicobacter pylori*–related peptic ulcer disease and gastritis, gastroparesis, and celiac disease. Significant weight changes should also prompt closer patient monitoring.

TSH and LT4 monitoring requirements may increase when initiating or discontinuing estrogen because exogenous estrogen may affect LT4 requirements. Numerous other pharmacotherapeutics can interfere with thyroxine metabolism and require closer monitoring of symptoms and TSH levels upon initiation, maintenance, and discontinuation, such as calcium supplements, phenytoin, phenobarbital, sertraline, carbamazepine, rifampin, proton pump inhibitors, tyrosine kinase inhibitors, bile acid sequestrants, selective estrogen receptor modulators, and cytoprotective agents.

Untreated hypothyroidism in pregnancy increases maternal and fetal risks, such as hypertension, preeclampsia, anemia, cardiac dysfunction, spontaneous abortion, low birth weight, and fetal death (see Chapter 38, High-Risk Childbearing). Even mild, untreated maternal hypothyroidism has been associated with cognitive dysfunction in the child. Thyroid hormone demand increases by 30% to 50% during pregnancy and will likely require an increased dose of LT4. LT4 has been assigned pregnancy category A by the Food and Drug Administration and replacement, when warranted, should be maintained during pregnancy. A naturally occurring hormone, it is normally found in both maternal and fetal circulation. LT4 is excreted into human milk in small amounts. In replacement doses, it is not expected to cause adverse effects in the nursing infant. The manufacturer recommends that caution be used when administering LT4 to nursing persons. However, adequate replacement doses of LT4 are needed to maintain normal lactation.

Current recommendations indicate that pregnant persons should receive LT4 replacement therapy with the dose titrated to achieve a TSH concentration within the trimester-specific

TABLE 44.4 Dosing Aspects of Levothyroxine Treatment

POPULATION	DOSING OF LEVOTHYROXINE
Young, healthy patients	Start at anticipated full replacement dose
Older patients	One fourth to one half of the anticipated full replacement dose and titrate slowly after no less than 4 to 6 weeks
Known ischemic heart disease	One fourth to one half of the anticipated full replacement dose and titrate slowly after no less than 4 to 6 weeks
Mild to moderate hypothyroidism	Start at 50 to 75 mcg daily

Source: Data from Jonklaas, J., Bianco, A. C., Bauer, A. J., Burman K. D., Cappola, A. R., Celi, F., Cooper, D. S., Kim, B. W., Peeters, R. P., Rosenthal, M. S., & Sawka, A. M. (2014). Guidelines for the treatment of hypothyroidism: Prepared by the American Thyroid Association Task Force on Thyroid Hormone Replacement. Thyroid, 24(12), 1670–1751. https://doi.org/10.1089/thy.2014.0028

reference range. During the first half of pregnancy, serum TSH should be monitored every 4 months with LT4 dosing adjustments to maintain the trimester-specific TSH range. TSH should be reevaluated during the second half of pregnancy. For patients already taking LT4 for hypothyroidism, two additional doses of their current LT4 dose per week with several days' separation may be started as soon as pregnancy is confirmed (Stagnaro-Green et al., 2011).

Older adults with new-onset hypothyroidism should start at a dose of 25 to 50 mcg daily that is increased slowly by 12.5 to 25 mcg every 6 to 8 weeks. Reference ranges of serum TSH levels are higher in older populations (e.g., above 65 years), and so higher serum TSH targets may be appropriate for older people (Jonklaas et al., 2014).

TREATMENT/MANAGEMENT OF SUBCLINICAL HYPOTHYROIDISM

Significant controversy persists regarding the treatment of subclinical hypothyroidism (Cooper & Biondi, 2012). Studies have suggested that treatment of these patients reduces symptoms, prevents progression to overt hypothyroidism, and may be cardioprotective. However, an evidence-based consensus statement issued by the AACE, the ATA, and the Endocrine Society (Gharib et al., 2004) recommends against routine treatment if the TSH is between 4.5 and 10 mU/L. In a separate statement, they recommended measuring thyroid antibodies in the presence of elevated TSH without symptoms. If antibodies are present and the TSH is above 5 mU/L, treatment should be considered. Although patients are usually asymptomatic, there are potential associated risks. Thus, these patients should be followed every 3 months until they are stable, as evidenced by both clinical and laboratory evaluation. Individualized care was recommended in both statements (Gharib et al., 2005).

Hyperthyroidism

DEFINITION AND SCOPE

Hyperthyroidism is characterized by overproduction of T3 and/or T4. Symptoms develop in response to the effects of the excessive circulating thyroid hormone levels. The prevalence in the general population is low with peak incidence between the ages of 20 to 40 years (Baskin et al., 2002; Gardner & Shoback, 2011). Subclinical hyperthyroidism affects about 2% of the adult population and is thought to be related to oversensitivity of the pituitary gland in responding to minor elevations in T3 and T4. The clinical significance relates to progression to overt hyperthyroidism and possible effects on the cardiac and skeletal systems. In the older patient with subclinical hyperthyroidism, the risk of atrial fibrillation is increased threefold (Baskin et al., 2002; Gardner & Shoback, 2011).

ETIOLOGY

The most common causes include Graves disease (an autoimmune disorder, accounts for 70% to 80% of cases), toxic multinodular goiter, and toxic adenoma. A variety of other disorders can also cause hyperthyroidism (Box 44.3). More

Box 44.3 Causes of Hyperthyroidism

Graves disease (diffuse toxic goiter)

Plummer disease (toxic multinodular goiter)

Toxic adenoma

Subacute thyroiditis (s/p viral infection)

Subclinical thyroiditis

Excessive pituitary production of thyroid-stimulating hormone

Taking large amounts of tetraiodothyronine (through dietary supplements or medication)

Tumors of the ovaries

Tumors of the thyroid or pituitary gland

Drugs: amiodarone, potassium iodide, intravenous contrast agent

Source: Data from Gardner, D., & Shoback, D. (2011). Greenspan's basic and clinical endocrinology *(9th ed.). Lange Medical Books/McGraw-Hill.*

common in women than men, hyperthyroidism tends to run in families.

SYMPTOMS

Many of the presenting symptoms of hyperthyroidism are nonspecific; fatigue, nervousness, irritability, and heat intolerance with increased sweating are found in 80% to 96% of patients. Other symptoms may include weakness, weight loss, dyspnea, depression, alteration in appetite, menstrual irregularities, infertility, and increasing frequency of and changes in stool.

EVALUATION/ASSESSMENT

Physical examination includes a thorough assessment of the neck and thyroid gland. About 90% of patients with Graves disease who are younger than 50 years will have a firm, diffuse goiter, and about 75% will have a bruit noted with auscultation. Any thyroid nodule should be evaluated (see discussion under Thyroid Nodule). Thyroid tenderness may indicate the presence of thyroiditis and is not usually seen in uncomplicated Graves disease (Gharib et al., 2010; Gardner & Shoback, 2011).

On general inspection, the hair may be fine and silky. Nails may develop ridges and plates may have an irregular separation from the bed (onycholysis). Skin may be hyperpigmented, especially over the extensor surfaces of the elbows, knees, and small joints. Tachycardia (resting heart rate over 90 beats per minute) is found in about 96% of patients with hyperthyroidism and about 20% have atrial fibrillation, either of which may be experienced subjectively as palpitations. Increased cardiac output may be reflected by wide pulse pressure when measuring the blood pressure, and murmurs are common as well. A neurologic exam may reveal hand tremors, a fine tongue tremor, and/or hyperactive reflexes. If tremor is not readily seen, a piece of paper is placed on the outstretched hand; the tremors can then be seen easily (Bahn et al., 2011; Hueston, 2011; Ladenson, 2010; Mandel et al., 2011).

A detailed eye examination is needed as hyperthyroidism is associated with several ocular abnormalities. The patient should be evaluated for lid lag, stare, periorbital edema, and proptosis. Ophthalmic involvement in hyperthyroidism is due to lymphocyte and fluid infiltration into the periorbital tissues, causing an inflammatory response. This compresses the optic nerve and may lead to loss of vision (Hueston, 2011; Ladenson, 2010).

DIFFERENTIAL DIAGNOSIS

The main considerations in the differential diagnosis are TSH-induced hyperthyroidism, which can be caused by a pituitary adenoma secreting TSH or a problem in the feedback mechanism; euthyroid hyperthyroxinemia, caused by serum thyroid hormone-binding protein abnormalities; and low serum levels of TSH without hyperthyroidism, which may be seen in patients recovering from hyperthyroidism, and with central hypothyroidism.

Of note, suppressed or low TSH can also be seen with recent corticosteroid use such as cortisone injections, prednisone, decadron, or inhaled corticosteroids. Typically, these patients have normal free T4 and free T3 and therefore do not actually have hyperthyroidism.

DIAGNOSTIC STUDIES

As with hypothyroidism, laboratory evaluation of hyperthyroidism begins with TSH levels. Hyperthyroidism is suggested when TSH levels are lower than normal, Free T3 and T4 levels should then be measured to aid in diagnosis. Findings indicative of hyperthyroidism would show suppressed TSH with elevated free T4 and/or free T3. Thyroid-stimulating immunoglobulin (TSI) and TSH receptor antibodies are typically ordered to differentiate between the diagnosis of Graves disease and thyroiditis or toxic nodule. Ultrasonography (US) is sometimes performed to measure the size of the entire thyroid gland, as well as any masses within it. US may also distinguish if the mass is solid or cystic. CT or MRI of the head is done if a pituitary tumor is suspected. Thyroid radioiodine uptake and scan can help determine the cause. Subclinical hyperthyroidism is identified in the instance of low TSH with normal T3 and T4 levels in asymptomatic patients (Bahn et al., 2011).

TREATMENT/MANAGEMENT OF OVERT CLINICAL HYPERTHYROIDISM

Once diagnosed, three treatment options are available: surgery, antithyroid medications, and RAI. Treatment is determined based on the etiology and the patient's preference. Each option carries its own set of benefits and risks (Gardner & Shoback, 2011).

Several presentations require referral. Patients with ocular involvement in Graves disease require referral to an ophthalmologist for evaluation and long-term follow-up. Urgent referral is needed for those with eye pain, injected sclerae, or a change in vision. Radioactive sodium iodine-131 (^{131}I) may exacerbate Graves ophthalmopathy; these patients should be referred to an endocrinologist. If surgery is the best treatment option, referral to a surgeon is warranted. Thyroid storm (Box 44.4) is a medical emergency and requires immediate referral (Bahn et al., 2011; Gardner & Shoback, 2011).

Self-Management Measures

Self-management measures are designed to reduce symptoms. Patients should avoid caffeine and other stimulants as these may make palpitations and tremors worse. Once therapy has been initiated, careful balancing of diet and exercise is needed as weight gain is common.

Complementary and Alternative Medicine

Chinese herbal medicines are sometimes used instead of or in combination with antithyroid medications. These medicines generally include a combination of multiple plant and root products. The herbs are intended to weaken thyroxine's biological effects, reduce transformation of T4 to T3, and modulate the immune system or sympathetic nerve function (Chen, 2008). Although demonstrated to improve symptoms and reduce relapse rates and adverse effects (e.g., agranulocytosis) in one meta-analysis, strong evidence supporting the use of Chinese herbs for hyperthyroidism is lacking (Zeng et al., 2007).

Surgery

Surgical management may be the treatment of choice for patients with a very enlarged gland or multinodular goiter, especially in the presence of dysphagia. Surgery is the treatment of choice for those with Graves ophthalmopathy as ^{131}I often worsens the ophthalmopathy. Patients are treated first with antithyroid hormones to reach a euthyroid state.

Box 44.4 Signs of Thyroid Storm

Increased temperature up to 104°F

Unexplained jaundice

Tachycardia

CHF

Atrial fibrillation

CNS Symptoms

Agitation

Delirium

Seizure/coma

GI Symptoms

Nausea

Vomiting

Diarrhea

CHF, congestive heart failure; CNS, central nervous system; GI, gastrointestinal.
Source: Data from Gardner, D., & Shoback, D. (2011). Greenspan's basic and clinical endocrinology (9th ed.). Lange Medical Books/McGraw-Hill.

Potential complications include hypoparathyroidism and vocal cord injury and occur in about 1% of patients. Near total thyroidectomy is usually done and will induce hypothyroidism, requiring lifetime thyroid replacement. If too much of the thyroid gland is left behind, Graves disease can recur (Bahn et al., 2011).

Pharmacotherapeutics

ANTITHYROID MEDICATIONS

Antithyroid medications are given to lower the overall thyroid level by suppressing production of thyroid hormone. The most common medications used in managing hyperthyroidism are methimazole (MMI) and propylthiouracil (PTU). The starting dose depends on the severity of the hyperthyroidism. Prior to initiating antithyroid drug therapy, a baseline complete blood count, including white blood cell count with differential, and a liver profile including bilirubin and transaminases should be evaluated.

Currently, it is recommended that MMI be used for the treatment of Graves disease in most patients. PTU is not recommended for initial use except during the first trimester of pregnancy (when it is preferred), in the presence of thyroid storm, and in patients with minor reactions to MMI who refuse RAI therapy or surgery. At the initiation of MMI therapy, 10 to 20 mg daily will generally restore euthyroidism, following which the dose can be titrated to a maintenance level of 5 to 10 mg daily. Risks of major side effects are lower with MMI as compared with PTU, and MMI can be given as a single daily dose. Due to a shorter duration of action, PTU is generally administered two or three times daily. Depending on the severity of hyperthyroidism, starting doses generally range between 50 and 150 mg three times daily. Once clinical findings and thyroid function tests indicate euthyroid state, reduction of PTU dose to 50 mg two to three times daily is usually sufficient (Bahn et al., 2011).

Patients need to be monitored for adverse reactions. The most common side effect is a transient skin rash that can be managed with antihistamines. Although rare, agranulocytosis is a serious side effect requiring discontinuation of the medication. Symptoms of agranulocytosis include sore throat, fever, painful mouth ulcers, anal ulcerations, depressed immune response, and increased bacterial infections, and should be evaluated with complete blood count and red blood cell indices. The patient should stop the medication and call their clinician if these symptoms develop (Bahn et al., 2011).

RADIOACTIVE IODINE THERAPY

The goal of RAI (^{131}I) treatment is to ablate the thyroid tissue. Because it works quickly, RAI tends to minimize the morbidity associated with hyperthyroidism. As with surgery, pretreatment with antithyroid medications is frequently used to achieve a euthyroid state, especially in older patients. Because most patients (80%) become hypothyroid following ^{131}I treatment, thyroid replacement for life is generally needed. A pregnancy test must be obtained within 48 hours prior to treatment in any female of childbearing age who is to be treated with RAI; verification of a negative pregnancy test prior to RAI is mandatory. Patients choosing ^{131}I must be counseled to avoid close contact with children younger than 8 years of age and with pregnant persons. Breastfeeding is contraindicated for at least 2 weeks after receiving treatment (Bahn et al., 2011; Gardner & Shoback, 2011).

Beta-blockers may be used with ^{131}I as adjunctive therapy to provide symptomatic relief and help stabilize the patient. Nondihydropyridine calcium channel blockers are helpful if the patient cannot tolerate beta-blockers due to side effects such as lightheadedness or drowsiness. These medications are discontinued as soon as the patient is rendered euthyroid.

Considerations for Special and Minoritized Populations

Pregnancy presents some special concerns. ^{131}I is contraindicated in both pregnancy and breastfeeding. Antithyroid medications may cross the placenta and oversuppression can adversely affect the fetus. PTU is the medication of choice and is given in the lowest possible dose to maintain euthyroidism, which is important to both maternal and fetal well-being. The need for antithyroid medications usually decreases during pregnancy and so close monitoring of TSH, T3, and T4 is advised. Hyperthyroidism in pregnant persons is usually managed in collaboration with an endocrinologist.

TREATMENT/MANAGEMENT OF SUBCLINICAL HYPOTHYROIDISM

Management of subclinical hyperthyroidism is a widely debated subject as there is a paucity of long-term studies of subclinical hyperthyroidism treatment. Subclinical hyperthyroidism is defined by a low serum TSH level in the presence of normal range thyroid hormone levels. Management requires careful monitoring of thyroid function through clinical and laboratory evaluation. Treatment is currently recommended for patients 65 years of age and older, and in the presence of osteoporosis and atrial fibrillation. If treated, antithyroid drugs are usually used; however, ^{131}I is also an option (Palacios et al., 2012).

Thyroid Nodule

DEFINITION AND SCOPE

Thyroid nodules are a fairly common clinical finding in the United States. Based on palpation alone, current estimates suggest that prevalence is approximately 3% to 7% of adults (Popoveniuc & Jonklaas, 2012). Approximately 300,000 new thyroid nodules are diagnosed annually in the United States (Guo et al., 2017). It is usually found during routine physical examination or as an incidental finding during color doppler studies of the carotid artery or other imaging studies performed for unrelated reasons.

ETIOLOGY

Thyroid nodules can be either benign or malignant, and hence, the major reason for evaluation is to exclude a malignant nodule. Causes of thyroid nodules include benign nodular goiter, chronic lymphocytic thyroiditis, simple or hemorrhagic cysts, follicular adenomas, subacute thyroiditis, and various histologic primary and metastatic carcinomas (Gharib et al., 2010).

RISK FACTORS

A history of previous diseases or treatments involving the head and neck, recent pregnancy, and rapidity of onset and rate of growth of the neck mass should be documented. The malignancy rate is three- to fourfold higher for thyroid nodules found during childhood and adolescence as compared with adults. Thyroid cancer risk is also higher in males and in the older adult population.

SYMPTOMS

Although clinical signs help with risk assessment, most patients with thyroid nodules experience few or no symptoms.

EVALUATION/ASSESSMENT

A family history is important for the diagnosis, as both benign and malignant nodules can be familial. It is critical to ascertain family history of thyroid cancer, familial adenomatous polyposis, and multiple endocrine neoplasia syndrome as these disorders are associated with a very high risk of development of thyroid cancer.

DIAGNOSTIC STUDIES

High-resolution ultrasound imaging, third-generation serum thyrotropin (TSH) assay, and fine-needle aspiration (FNA) biopsy are the basis for evaluation and management of thyroid nodules.

TREATMENT/MANAGEMENT

All patients with new and/or changing nodules should be referred to an endocrinologist for further evaluation and FNA biopsy (Gharib et al., 2010).

PARATHYROID DISEASE

Parathyroid hormone (PTH) is secreted from four small glands adjacent to the thyroid gland. Secretion is based on a feedback loop. PTH aids in regulating serum calcium levels. Any disruption in PTH secretion can cause serum calcium concentrations to fluctuate outside the narrow normal range of 8.5 to 10.5 mg/dL (normal range may vary by laboratory; Shoback et al., 2011).

Maintaining this concentration requires the coordinated effects of multiple systems and organs such as the kidneys, intestines, and skeleton (Shoback et al., 2011). When plasma calcium levels fall, PTH secretion increases. PTH stimulates more efficient renal calcium reabsorption and intestinal calcium absorption. Excessive amounts of PTH activate bone remodeling to support extracellular fluid calcium at the expense of skeletal integrity (Moe, 2008).

Hyperparathyroidism

DEFINITION, SCOPE, AND ETIOLOGY

Hyperparathyroidism (HPT), overactivity of the parathyroid glands, is the most common cause of hypercalcemia. HPT is present in about 1% of the adult population and is more common in older postmenopausal persons. Women have a two- to fourfold increased likelihood of developing HPT

over men. The most common cause is a single adenoma of the parathyroid gland. Other causes of HPT include vitamin D deficiency, chronic kidney disease, hyperplasia of one or more of the parathyroid glands, and parathyroid cancer, although this is rare and accounts for less than 1% of all cases.

SYMPTOMS

The clinical manifestations of HPT involve multiple systems. The most common features are nephrolithiasis, bone fracture, constipation, abnormal cognitive function, depression, and hypertension (El-Hajj Fuleihan & Silverberg, 2023), hence the mnemonic "moans, groans, stones, bones, and thrones with psychic overtones."

EVALUATION/ASSESSMENT AND DIAGNOSTIC STUDIES

About 90% of those with HPT have an elevated PTH. Serum calcium levels are also abnormally high. Because low vitamin D levels are also associated with HPT, evaluating serum 25-hydroxyvitamin D is appropriate (Marcocci & Cetani, 2011).

TREATMENT/MANAGEMENT

The treatment of choice is surgical removal of the abnormal gland, which is curative 95% to 98% of the time. Surgical complications can include laryngeal nerve damage, recurrent HPT, or permanent hypoparathyroidism. Surgery is suggested if serum calcium levels are greater than 12 mg/dL on multiple occasions or if there is a 20% rise from baseline. Serum calcium and bone mineral density are evaluated annually after surgery. Medications are not typically used to treat HPT. However, in a nonsurgical candidate, cinacalcet (Sensipar) can be used in conjunction with close monitoring of calcium levels (Bilezikian et al., 2009; El-Hajj Fuleihan & Silverberg, 2023).

Hypoparathyroidism

DEFINITION AND ETIOLOGY

The most common cause of hypoparathyroidism, reduced function of the parathyroid glands, is neck surgery, such as surgery on the thyroid gland or neck neoplasms. Within hours of parathyroid gland removal, calcium concentration decreases while inorganic phosphorus increases. Urinary calcium excretion also increases. Although idiopathic disease is rare, if present, it is associated with autoimmune problems in multiple endocrine glands (Bilezikian et al., 2011; Gardner & Shoback, 2011).

SYMPTOMS, EVALUATION/ASSESSMENT, AND DIAGNOSTIC STUDIES

The history seeks information about risk factors and symptoms such as muscle cramps, dermatologic problems (dry skin, brittle nails, dermatitis), and cataract development. Clinical signs of hypoparathyroidism include neuromuscular irritability such as a positive Chvostek or Trousseau sign. Diagnosis is confirmed with a low or low-normal serum PTH (Gardner & Shoback, 2011).

TREATMENT/MANAGEMENT

Hypoparathyroidism is treated with calcium and vitamin D supplementation. If acute, 10% calcium gluconate can be given intravenously (Gardner & Shoback, 2011; Moe, 2008).

Long-term daily therapy is 1.5 to 3 g of oral elemental calcium with vitamin D (up to 1,000 IU). The goal is a serum calcium level between 8 and 9 mg/dL.

METABOLIC SYNDROME

Definition and Scope

Metabolic syndrome is a clustering of several cardiometabolic risk factors that greatly increase the risk of cardiovascular disease (CVD) and type 2 diabetes. The syndrome, as described by both the World Health Organization (WHO) and National Cholesterol Education Program (NCEP), includes a group of disorders: hyperinsulinemia/abnormal glucose tolerance, obesity, dyslipidemia, hypertension, and proinflammatory, prothrombotic state.

There are an estimated 47 million individuals (age adjusted U.S. persons older than 20 years; approximately 24%) with metabolic syndrome in the United States (Ford et al., 2002). The overall prevalence of 23.7% changes with age, affecting 6.7% of young adults (20–29 years), 43.5% of adults age 60 to 69 years, and 42% of those older than 70 years. Ethnicity is also a factor: more Hispanic American people are affected (31.9%) than non-Hispanic White people (23.8%) and Black people (21.6%). Gender differences place Black and Hispanic women at highest risk (Ford et al., 2002; Meigs, 2015).

Etiology

Several explanations have been suggested that describe the etiology of the metabolic syndrome. The American Association of Endocrinology (AAE) stresses the importance of insulin resistance; however, the AAE does not recognize obesity as a component of metabolic syndrome (Einhorn et al., 2003). Initial definition by WHO considered insulin resistance a major component of the metabolic syndrome (Alberti & Zimmet, 1998). The Expert Panel on Detection, Evaluation, and Treatment of High Blood Cholesterol in Adults (2001), which developed a widely accepted definition, suggested equal weight to any of the components of the syndrome: fasting blood glucose, glucose intolerance, obesity (measured as waist circumference), hypertension, and dyslipidemia. The International Diabetic Federation (IDF) considers central obesity, insulin resistance, and a proinflammatory/prothrombotic state as important causative factors in the metabolic syndrome (Nesto, 2003).

The underlying pathophysiology of metabolic syndrome is insulin resistance accompanying abnormal adipose deposition and function. Defined as a state in which the concentration of insulin is associated with an abnormal glucose response, this can lead to several pathogenic conditions (Freeman, 2006). Clinically, there is an imbalance of the amount of insulin required to maintain normal glucose levels, and the body is unable to control both hepatic glucose output and muscle glucose utilization (Masharani & German, 2011). Insulin regulation of protein and fat metabolism are disrupted.

Obesity and disorders of the adipose tissue play an important role in metabolic syndrome. Fat distribution and overall total body weight may be critical factors in pathogenesis. Obesity contributes to insulin resistance and to both hypertension and dyslipidemia. Excessive visceral adipose tissue releases several protein substances. Obesity also plays a role in endothelial dysfunction. The proinflammatory state is related to elevated C-reactive protein (CRP), fibrinogen, and other cytokines (Bentley-Lewis et al., 2007).

Hypertension is also related to insulin resistance, likely through sodium reabsorption pathways. The increase in sympathetic outflow and sodium reabsorption is thought to counter the vasodilatory effect, causing elevated blood pressure (Meigs, 2015). Insulin resistance causes an abnormality in the regulation of free fatty acids. This can lead to an increase in plasma lipid levels that may be diverted to the liver, promoting fatty liver disease or nonalcoholic steatohepatitis (NASH). Lipid levels increase, especially triglycerides (TG) and very low-density lipoprotein cholesterol (VLDL-C), while high-density lipoprotein cholesterol (HDL-C) levels remain low, promoting atherogenic dyslipidemia.

Several independent factors also play a role in the pathogenesis of metabolic syndrome, including age and ovarian failure. As estrogen levels decline in postmenopause, intra-abdominal fat increases, the lipid profile shifts in an atherogenic direction, and insulin resistance increases as observed by a rise in both glucose and insulin levels (Bentley-Lewis et al., 2007).

Risk Factors

Risk factors for metabolic syndrome are related to each of the components and to the syndrome overall. It remains unclear whether metabolic syndrome has a single cause, although it appears that multiple risk factors precipitate the syndrome. Insulin resistance and central obesity appear to be the most important precipitating factors. In most individuals, metabolic syndrome is lifestyle mediated, with greatest risk among those following a high fat, high concentrated sugar diet and having a sedentary lifestyle. Other risk factors include genetic predisposition, increased age, ethnicity, increased weight, postmenopausal status, low household income, smoking, and soft drink consumption (Alberti et al., 2009). Conflicting evidence exists regarding alcohol consumption and metabolic syndrome. Excessive alcohol intake is associated with numerous illnesses, although studies indicate that light to moderate drinking has a cardioprotective effect. There is a need for more prospective studies to determine the relationship between alcohol consumption and metabolic syndrome (Fujita & Takei, 2011).

Evaluation/Assessment and Diagnostic Studies

Several criteria have been proposed over the past decade to establish the diagnosis of metabolic syndrome. Diagnostic criteria developed by the NCEP Adult Treatment Panel III (Expert Panel on Detection, Evaluation, and Treatment of High Blood Cholesterol in Adults, 2001) based on common clinical measures, including waist circumference, TG, HDL-C, blood pressure, and fasting glucose level, continue to be used with minor modifications. Modifications to the original

TABLE 44.5 Metabolic Syndrome Diagnostic Criteria[a]

PARAMETER	DIAGNOSTIC THRESHOLD
Fasting blood sugar	≥ 100 mg/dL (or receiving medication for hyperglycemia)
Blood pressure	≥ 130/85 mmHg (or receiving medication for hypertension)
Triglycerides	≥ 150 mg/dL (or receiving medication for hypertriglyceridemia)
HDL-C	< 40 mg/dL in men or < 50 mg/dL in women (or receiving medication for reduced HDL-C)
Waist circumference	≥ 102 cm (40 in.) in men or ≥ 88 cm (35 in.) in women; if Asian American, ≥ 90 cm (35 in.) in men or ≥ 80 cm (32 in.) in women

[a]Three of the five diagnostic criteria must be met to establish a diagnosis of metabolic syndrome.
HDL-C, high-density lipoprotein cholesterol.
Source: Data from Grundy, S. M., Cleeman, J. I., Daniels, S. R., Donato, K. A., Eckel, R. H., Franklin, B. A., Gordon, D. J., Krauss, R. M., Savage, P. J., Smith, S. C., Jr., Spertus, J. A., & Costa, F. (2005). Diagnosis and management of the metabolic syndrome. An American Heart Association/National Heart, Lung, and Blood Institute scientific statement: Executive summary. Circulation, 112, 285–290. https://doi.org/10.1161/CIRCULATIONAHA.105.169405

diagnostic criteria include waist circumference adjustment to lower thresholds for individuals or ethnic groups predisposed to insulin resistance; designation of abnormal for the measures of TG, HDL-C, and blood pressure if an individual is taking pharmacotherapeutics to treat these factors; delineating a threshold for both systolic and diastolic hypertension; and in accordance with the American Diabetes Association (ADA), lowering the threshold for impaired fasting glucose level to 100 mg/dL. Metabolic syndrome is diagnosed when any three of the five diagnostic criteria exist, suggesting a multicausal etiology (Grundy et al., 2005). Diagnostic criteria for metabolic syndrome are depicted in Table 44.5.

Components of Metabolic Syndrome

OBESITY
Definition and Scope

Obesity, defined as a body mass index (BMI) of 30 kg/m² or greater, contributes to several conditions associated with metabolic syndrome. It is a common, serious, and costly disorder affecting more than one third of American adults (Bray, 2014). The presence of excessive weight is important, and the distribution of fat is critical to the metabolic syndrome diagnosis.

Etiology

Obesity is the accumulation of subcutaneous and visceral fat (Figure 44.2); it is the visceral fat (central obesity) that is problematic. Visceral fat is thought to be more predictive of metabolic syndrome than total body weight.

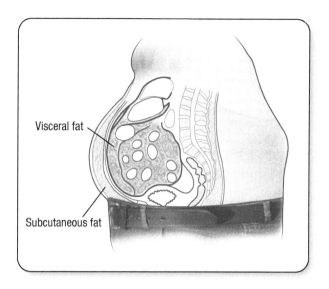

FIGURE 44.2 Subcutaneous versus visceral fat.

Evaluation/Assessment

Because the main concern is central obesity, measurement of waist circumference or calculation of the waist-to-hip ratio should be done. In women, central obesity is identified when waist circumference is greater than 35 inches or when the waist-to-hip ratio is greater than 0.85. To accurately measure the waist, the tape measure should be placed on the upper border of the iliac crest. Have the patient exhale and then measure without compressing the skin. The hips are measured at the widest point, again without compressing the skin. Data suggest that waist circumference is more reflective of CVD in women than is BMI and is also associated with higher risk for development of type 2 diabetes and all-cause mortality (American College of Cardiology [ACC] et al., 2014; Meigs, 2015). BMI and waist circumference are screening tools to be included in all health encounters. Decisions to treat obesity are determined by BMI, comorbidities, and waist circumference.

Treatment/Management

Weight loss should be encouraged at a BMI of 25 or greater with just one comorbidity, and elevated waist circumference is considered a comorbidity. Counseling regarding dietary factors, exercise requirements, and weight management programs should be incorporated into treatment plans for all patients who are overweight or obese or at high risk for obesity. It is critical that weight management programs include individual and/or group-based psychological/behavioral interventions.

PHARMACOTHERAPY

Pharmacologic treatment (orlistat, naltrexone-bupropion, phentermine-topiramate, liraglutide, semaglutide) should be considered in adults as an adjunct to lifestyle interventions in the management of obesity (see Chapter 13, Nutrition for Women). Current recommendations suggest that patients with a BMI of 28 kg/m² or more (with comorbidities) or BMI 30 kg/m² or more should be considered on an individual case basis following careful assessment of risk/benefit and patient willingness to accept pharmacologic intervention.

SURGERY

Bariatric surgery is an option for those in whom previous attempts at weight loss have failed or are physically unattainable when the following criteria are met: BMI 35 kg/m² or more and/or presence of one or more severe comorbidities that are expected to improve significantly with weight reduction (e.g., immobility, arthritis, type 2 diabetes; ACC et al., 2014).

ACANTHOSIS NIGRICANS

Definition and Scope

Acanthosis nigricans, which is caused by an increase in melanocytes and epidermal papillomatosis, is a common finding with metabolic syndrome. This skin change is characterized by hyperpigmented, hyperkeratotic plaque-like lesions found especially in intertriginous areas such as the axillae, neck, groin, under the breast, and the vulva. The skin is also hyperplastic and has a velvety or mossy appearance. It can occur in healthy individuals as well as in numerous health disorders and with exogenous hormone therapy including growth hormone and birth control pills. It is most commonly seen in individuals of African descent, partly because it is easier to visualize on darker skin.

Etiology and Risk Factors

When acanthosis nigricans develops in patients who are not obese, a diagnostic workup should be done. In rare instances, it is associated with lymphoma or malignancies of the gastrointestinal or genitourinary tract. In these cases, acanthosis nigricans may also appear on the lips, palms, and soles of feet and is generally severe. Occasionally, acanthosis nigricans is congenital or due to an endocrine disorder such as diabetes, gonadal disorders, and thyroid disease (Habif, 2009).

Evaluation/Assessment and Diagnostic Studies

Acanthosis nigricans is usually diagnosed by inspection of affected areas. Skin biopsies are occasionally required for atypical cases.

Treatment/Management

Treatment is cosmetic only and includes topical tretinoin, 20% urea, alpha-hydroxy acids, lactic or salicylic acid prescriptions, and laser resurfacing.

HYPERTENSION

Hypertension is a critical factor in the constellation of disorders that define the metabolic syndrome. Approximately 120 million US adults (48.1%) have hypertension. About 25% have their blood pressure under control (CDC, 2023). Additionally, it is estimated that one in three adults in the United States are prehypertensive (Nwankwo et al., 2013). For a comprehensive overview of hypertension, see Chapter 43, Cardiovascular Disease in Women.

IMPAIRED GLUCOSE TOLERANCE

While glucose levels may range from normal to elevated, hyperinsulinemia is always manifested. The ADA and AACE recognize the connection of diabetes to insulin resistance and the metabolic syndrome. An important part of metabolic syndrome

treatment is prevention of diabetes and CVD. The WHO criteria require glucose abnormalities to make a diagnosis of the metabolic syndrome, while the NCEP does not. In an 8-year Japanese study comparing these two definitions of metabolic syndrome, only the WHO criteria, which emphasized abnormal glucose tolerance, were predictive of developing CVD in women. These data support a link between diabetes and the metabolic syndrome; both are related to the development of CVD.

DYSLIPIDEMIA

Patients with metabolic syndrome have an abnormal, atherogenic lipid profile (see Chapter 43, Cardiovascular Disease in Women). TG levels are typically elevated, and serum HDL-C levels are low. Serum low-density lipoprotein cholesterol (LDL-C) levels are increased, and the size and density of the LDL particles are reduced. The reduced particle size can lead to further development of atherosclerosis; thus, treatment is aimed at restoring the lipid profile to normal.

PROINFLAMMATORY, PROTHROMBOTIC STATE

Proinflammatory, prothrombotic state abnormalities are derived largely from the secretory activity of adipose tissue, particularly visceral fat. Adipocytes release adipokines such as leptin, interleukin (IL) 6, and plasminogen activator inhibitor-1 (PAI-1), all markers for CVD risk. The clinical value of measuring these markers and CRP is unknown and should be considered for use in clinical practice only in settings that are assessing CVD risk. Both the American Heart Association (AHA) and Centers for Disease Control and Prevention (CDC) list CRP testing as optional; the decision to test is based on clinical judgment (Bray, 2015).

Differential Diagnosis

The differential diagnosis involves looking at the entire constellation of problems that make up metabolic syndrome. The clinician must consider whether other causes explain the presence of hypertension, glucose abnormalities, or dyslipidemia. Other potential causes must be identified and managed. For example, in hypertensive women, secondary causes such as renovascular disease, obstructive sleep apnea, and disorders of renin and aldosterone metabolism may need exploration (Tasali & Ip, 2008). In the presence of a strong family history of dyslipidemia, hereditary dyslipidemia may need to be excluded. Hyperglycemia can present with thyroid disorders and rare endocrinopathies including pheochromocytomas and glucagonomas and, if the situation warrants, may need extensive workup. If no other causes are present, then metabolic syndrome is identified as the primary diagnosis.

Diagnostic Studies

Preliminary laboratory studies in women suspected of having metabolic syndrome should include complete metabolic (chemistry) panels to evaluate serum glucose, renal function (creatinine, blood urea nitrogen [BUN], and estimated glomerular filtration rate [eGFR]), and lipid profile (TG, HDL-C, and LDL-C). In women with a family history of heart disease or other atherosclerotic disorder, consideration should be given for studies of lipoprotein(a), apolipoprotein-B100, high-sensitivity CRP, homocysteine, and fractionated LDL-C (Bray, 2015; Yaffe, 2007).

As previously discussed, factors associated with metabolic syndrome are found in other disorders and, as such, warrant assessment. Such assessment includes thyroid function tests, liver function tests, hemoglobin A1c, and uric acid. Extant data indicate that elevated TSH is associated with a higher prevalence of metabolic syndrome (Heima et al., 2012). Women with metabolic syndrome are more likely than the general population to have hyperuricemia, and this has been attributed to the proinflammatory nature of the syndrome (Puig & Martínez, 2008).

Imaging studies may be indicated for women with symptoms or signs of the many complications of the syndrome, including CVD. Complaints of chest pain, shortness of breath, significant fatigue, dyspnea, or claudication may necessitate additional diagnostic testing with EKG (rest/stress EKG), US (vascular or rest/stress echocardiography), stress single-photon emission computed tomography (SPECT), cardiac PET, or other imaging studies.

Exacerbating factors such as obstructive sleep apnea should also be investigated. Polysomnography (sleep study) should be considered in patients reporting snoring, periods of pauses in breathing, and/or daytime drowsiness (see Chapter 15, Healthy Practices: Sleep). This is critical in obese patients (Lam & Ip, 2007; Tasali & Ip, 2008).

Cardiovascular risk should be assessed using the ACC/AHA (Goff et al., 2014) calculator (available at tools.cardiosource.org/ASCVD-Risk-Estimator) to determine the risk of developing a first atherosclerotic cardiovascular disease (ASCVD) event. Risk factors used to assess the 10-year and lifetime risk of an ASCVD event are gender, age, race, total cholesterol level, HDL-C level, systolic blood pressure, treatment for hypertension, diabetes, and smoking status (see Chapter 43, Cardiovascular Disease in Women).

Treatment/Management

Metabolic syndrome is managed through focused treatment of each component. The primary goal is prevention of ASCVD and type 2 diabetes, achieved through risk reduction. The goals overlap as prevention of type 2 diabetes and treatment of other conditions are important factors in the prevention of ASCVD (Bray, 2015).

SELF-MANAGEMENT MEASURES

Lifestyle changes and management of obesity are the most important initial steps in treating metabolic syndrome. The major goal is lifestyle change to treat the underlying causes of obesity and physical inactivity and is essential for successful management of each metabolic syndrome component. For both long- and short-term risk reduction, therapeutic lifestyle changes (TLC) are first-line therapy for all patients with metabolic syndrome. TLC include both dietary and exercise modification and have been demonstrated to effectively reduce progression to diabetes and development of CVD. Reduction of some of the major risk factors such as smoking, stress, and sedentary lifestyle are important components of management goals and referral for appropriate intervention is indicated to support patients attempting TLC (Bray, 2015).

As with obesity, reduction in caloric intake and avoidance of high glycemic index foods and saturated fats are indicated. Not surprisingly, research indicates that the typical American diet is associated with a higher risk for developing metabolic syndrome; the opposite has been demonstrated in populations adhering to a typical Mediterranean diet (Yoneda et al., 2008). It is essential for diet modification programs to include a behavioral component as discussed in the obesity section, and referral for structured dietary modifications and weight loss may be warranted.

Exercise is an essential intervention in preventing and treating metabolic syndrome and obesity. Aerobic exercise, as opposed to resistance training, is recommended at least 5 days per week (Bateman et al., 2011; Roberts et al., 2013). Exercise programs should be tailored to the individual person to achieve the best outcomes. (See Chapter 13, Nutrition for Women, and Chapter 14, Healthy Practices: Physical Activity, for details about diet and exercise modifications used for metabolic syndrome, as well as information on supporting behavior change.)

PHARMACOTHERAPEUTICS

Medication therapies are used according to current authoritative guidelines for each component of the metabolic syndrome.

Dyslipidemia

Many patients will require lipid-modifying medications to control dyslipidemia, even those patients who achieve success in instituting and maintaining TLC. The goal for lipid management is threefold: to lower LDL-C, raise HDL-C, and lower TG, all of which help reduce CVD risk (Stone et al., 2014). As the goal is threefold, multiple medications may be needed. The use of multiple medications has been shown to achieve better lipid control. It is widely accepted to initiate statins (3-hydroxy-3-methylglutaryl coenzyme A [HMG-CoA] reductase inhibitors) in the presence of elevated LDL-C levels (Stone et al., 2014; Towne & Thara, 2008). Treatment of decreased HDL-C remains controversial, but may include niacin; however, careful monitoring is required as high doses may exacerbate hyperglycemia (Ito, 2004). Women with atherogenic dyslipidemia (elevated TG with low HDL-C), especially if overweight or obese, may benefit from fibrate medications; however, current recommendations for the treatment of cholesterol disorders emphasize statins over nonstatin medications (Stone et al., 2014).

Hypertriglyceridemia is amenable to both fibrates and niacin. Caution should be employed when prescribing fibrates due to well-documented drug interactions, especially when used in combination with statins. Omega-3 fatty acids may also help in lowering TG levels (see Chapter 43, Cardiovascular Disease in Women).

Hypertension

The goal of antihypertensive therapy in patients with metabolic syndrome is a blood pressure of less than 140/90 mmHg for most populations and 150/90 mmHg for patients age 60 years or older. Treatment guidelines follow the Eighth Joint National Committee on Prevention, Detection, Evaluation, and Treatment of High Blood Pressure (JNC 8; James et al., 2014; see Chapter 43, Cardiovascular Disease in Women).

Insulin Resistance

Insulin resistance is first managed with TLC. There is no set limit for how long TLC alone are tried to manage insulin resistance. The patient should be evaluated with fasting glucose every 3 months; TLC have been shown to prevent metabolic syndrome more effectively than metformin or placebo (cumulative incidence of metabolic syndrome at year 3 was 51% for placebo, 45% with metformin, and 34% for TLC). TLC should be the focus of initial and ongoing education about treatment for insulin resistance and should be maintained when pharmacotherapy is initiated.

The AACE recommends that clinicians use their judgment in making the decision to initiate pharmacotherapy and that pharmacotherapy should be considered when fasting blood glucose or A1c levels begin to rise. The goal of pharmacotherapy is to reduce insulin resistance, and this includes the use of metformin and/or thiazolidinediones (TZDs). Due to its proven safety record, metformin is used extensively. Titrating metformin from 500 mg once daily to 1,000 mg twice daily in increments of 500 mg every 3 to 5 days will help to avoid common gastrointestinal side effects such as abdominal discomfort, diarrhea, gas, and bloating. Liver and renal function are evaluated prior to initiating metformin and monitored at least yearly. Renal dysfunction, heart failure, current liver disease, metabolic acidosis, and current alcohol abuse are contraindications to the use of metformin (Bray, 2015).

TZDs, including rosiglitazone and pioglitazone, have also been investigated for controlling insulin resistance and preventing diabetes in patients with the metabolic syndrome; however, no outcome data are yet available for CVD prevention in those with either the metabolic syndrome or diabetes. As with any medication therapy, balancing the risks and side effects with the potential benefits must be considered (Grundy et al., 2005).

Proinflammatory, Prothrombotic State

No currently available pharmacotherapeutics are recommended for treatment of the proinflammatory/prothrombotic state.

Preventive Cardiovascular Treatment

Along with diet, exercise, and lifestyle behavior modifications, women age 40 to 70 years without increased risk for bleeding may benefit from low-dose aspirin therapy (75–100 mg/day) (see Chapter 43, Cardiovascular Disease in Women).

Surgical Considerations

Although surgical interventions for metabolic syndrome are not currently recommended, bariatric surgery referral may be considered for the morbidly obese when weight loss is not or cannot be achieved via diet and exercise (see Chapter 13, Nutrition for Women).

DIABETES

Definition and Scope

The ADA defines type 1 diabetes as an absolute insulin deficiency related to beta-cell dysfunction. Type 2 diabetes mellitus is defined as a progressive insulin secretory defect related to insulin resistance. Prediabetes exists when blood glucose levels are higher than normal but not high enough to be diagnosed as diabetes. The ADA (2014) defines "gestational diabetes" as the development of diabetes during pregnancy (see Chapter 38, High-Risk Childbearing).

In the United States, it is estimated that nearly 26 million Americans have diabetes and an additional 79 million are prediabetic. Diabetes affects over 8% of the U.S. population across their life span. The CDC (2011) reports that 11.3% of Americans 20 years of age and older are diabetic. In American adults 65 years of age and older, nearly 25% are affected. Alarmingly, approximately 27%, or 7 million Americans, are not aware that they have diabetes. In 2010, over 200,000 Americans 20 years of age or younger had either type 1 or type 2 diabetes. Diabetes was the seventh leading cause of death in the United States in 2013 and the leading cause of disabilities. The risk of death in people with diabetes is two times as great as in those who do not have the disease (CDC, 2015).

Type 2 diabetes accounts for approximately 90% to 95% of all diagnosed cases of diabetes. Current estimates suggest that approximately 40% of American adults will develop diabetes, primarily type 2. Recent data suggest that more than 50% of ethnic minorities will develop diabetes in their lifetime. The primary reason for the increased incidence of diabetes is the obesity epidemic in the United States (Gregg et al., 2014; Hackethal, 2014). Estimates suggest that 79 million or 35% of American adults age 20 years and older have prediabetes and will subsequently develop diabetes in their lifetime (CDC, 2011).

The most common metabolic disease of childhood, type 1 diabetes affects approximately one in every 400 to 600 children and adolescents and accounts for 5% of all diagnosed cases of diabetes in adults. According to the CDC, the total incidence of type 1 diabetes is approximately 1 million Americans. CDC estimates indicate that 15,600 new cases of type 1 diabetes were diagnosed each year from 2002 to 2005 in young people. In individuals younger than 10 years of age, the annual rate of new cases was 19.7 per 100,000 population. In those older than 10 years, the annual rate of newly diagnosed cases was 18.6 per 100,000 population (CDC, 2011).

In children, type 1 diabetes mellitus generally starts around age 4 years or older, with an abrupt onset. Peak incidence of onset in children is age 11 to 13 years. In adults, generally in their late 30s and early 40s, type 1 diabetes tends to present less aggressively. The slower onset form of type 1 diabetes seen in adults is referred to as latent autoimmune diabetes of the adult, or LADA (CDC, 2011).

Etiology

TYPE 1 DIABETES

Type 1 diabetes mellitus occurs due to lymphocytic infiltration and destruction of insulin-secreting beta cells in the islets of Langerhans in the pancreas. The resulting decline in beta-cell mass leads to reduced insulin secretion; over time, there is insufficient available insulin to maintain normal blood glucose levels. Generally, hyperglycemia develops after destruction of 80% to 90% of the beta cells and diabetes may then be diagnosed. Exogenous insulin is required to reverse this catabolic condition, prevent diabetic ketosis, decrease hyperglucagonemia, normalize the metabolism of lipids and proteins, and to sustain life.

Autoimmunity is currently considered the major factor in developing type 1 diabetes mellitus and may also be associated with other autoimmune diseases such as Addison disease, Hashimoto thyroiditis, and Graves disease (Borchers et al., 2010). Less common causes of type 1 diabetes mellitus include pancreatitis, pancreatic cancer, and pancreatic surgery.

TYPE 2 DIABETES

The pathophysiology of type 2 diabetes is a spectrum of metabolic process abnormalities affecting glucose metabolism; insulin resistance is central. As discussed previously (see Metabolic Syndrome), insulin resistance leads to higher levels of circulating insulin as well as hyperglycemia due to the inability of the body to use insulin in both muscle and adipose tissue. Over time, the pancreas cannot produce enough insulin to keep up with the demand, and a relative insufficiency of insulin is created, resulting in hyperglycemia. Just as with the metabolic syndrome, type 2 diabetes is usually associated with multiple metabolic comorbidities.

The etiology of type 2 diabetes is multifactorial and involves both environmental and genetic factors. Extant data suggest that type 2 diabetes develops in response to excessive calorie intake without sufficient caloric expenditure and/or obesity in individuals with a susceptible genetic type. Nearly 90% of persons with type 2 diabetes are obese; however, racial and ethnic factors influence the development of type 2 diabetes. Excess weight is a recognized risk factor for developing type 2 diabetes; however, individuals of Asian ancestry are at an increased risk for diabetes at lower weight levels when compared with persons of European ancestry. A greater risk for developing type 2 diabetes is also present in White people in the presence of hypertension and prehypertension as compared with Black people (WHO Expert Consultation, 2004). Genetic variants can be attributed to only about 10% of the inheritable component in type 2 diabetes (Billings & Florez, 2010). Secondary diabetes can develop in individuals due to glucocorticoid therapy and in insulin-antagonistic disorders such as Cushing syndrome, pheochromocytoma, and acromegaly.

Risk Factors

Risk factor assessment is an essential component of screening for diabetes and prediabetes. Women with any of the following risk factors should be screened at least every 3 years. In the presence of two or more risk factors, screening should occur annually (Handelsman et al., 2015).

- Family history of type 2 diabetes in a first-degree relative (such as parent or sibling)
- Age greater than 45 years, although type 2 diabetes is occurring with greater frequency in younger individuals
- Sedentary lifestyle
- BMI greater than or equal to 30 kg/m²
- BMI 25 to 29.9 kg/m² in the presence of other risk factors, such as ethnicity

- High-risk ethnicity including Hispanic, Native American, African American, Asian American, or Pacific Islander ancestry
- Prior history of impaired glucose tolerance (IGT) or impaired fasting glucose (IFG) or metabolic syndrome
- Hypertension (greater than 140/90 mmHg) or on antihypertensive therapy
- Dyslipidemia (HDL cholesterol level less than 35 mg/dL or TG level greater than 250 mg/dL)
- History of gestational diabetes or delivering a baby with a birth weight over 9 lb
- Polycystic ovary syndrome
- Nonalcoholic fatty liver disease
- Chronic or prolonged glucocorticoid therapy
- Antipsychotic drug therapy for schizophrenia or severe bipolar disorder
- Sleep disorders such as obstructive sleep apnea, chronic sleep deprivation, and night shift workers with glucose intolerance

Evaluation/Assessment

There are many differences between type 1 diabetes and type 2 diabetes (Table 44.6), and proper diagnosis is essential for management.

HISTORY

Many of the signs and symptoms of type 1 diabetes and type 2 diabetes are the same; however, their presentation is usually different (Table 44.6). Symptoms of type 1 diabetes have a rapid onset, while type 2 diabetes onset may be much slower, even insidious. In type 1 diabetes, polyuria and polydipsia are considered classic presenting signs; polyphagia with weight loss, blurred vision, and fatigue can also present. Type 2 diabetes can be largely asymptomatic; however, common presenting symptoms include fatigue, blurred vision, and *Candida* infections, as well as the classic symptoms of polydipsia, polyuria, polyphagia, weakness, and unexplained weight loss. Symptoms of autonomic neuropathy (dysphagia, bloating, change in bowel habits, and urinary and sexual dysfunction) as well as peripheral neuropathy (paresthesia of extremities) may be the first sign of type 2 diabetes. Chronic anovulation leading to oligomenorrhea or amenorrhea suggests an increase in the risk of type 2 diabetes, especially if accompanied by signs of hyperandrogenism. People with a history of gestational diabetes or a history of large babies (over 9 lb) are known to be at increased risk of developing type 2 diabetes (Wass et al., 2011).

PHYSICAL EXAMINATION

A thorough physical examination (Table 44.7) is performed to identify presenting signs of diabetes, rule out secondary diabetes, and evaluate other problems associated with the presenting signs and symptoms. Evaluation for signs of complications and target organ damage (Table 44.8), such as peripheral neuropathy and visual changes, is done at each visit.

Differential Diagnosis

The major diagnostic challenge is to differentiate between the possible causes of the patient's presenting symptoms.

TABLE 44.6 Comparison of Type 1 and Type 2 Diabetes

PARAMETER	TYPE 1	TYPE 2
Prevalence of each type	5%–10%	90%–95%
Age of diagnosis	Young, usually younger than 40 years	Older than 40 years usually
Condition in discovery	Mild to severe	Not ill, usually have mild symptoms
Cause	Absent or severely decreased insulin production	Insulin resistance or insulin secretory deficiency
Insulin levels	None to small amount	Markedly elevated early; later may see decrease

Source: Adapted from Beasler, R. S. (2014). Joslin's diabetes deskbook: A guide for primary care providers. *Joslin Diabetes Center.*

Fatigue and weakness can be presenting symptoms of thyroid disorders, anemia, chronic fatigue syndrome, diabetes, depression, and other conditions. Skin problems such as pruritus and dry skin also can present with several conditions. The urinary symptoms of diabetes can mimic the presence of a urinary tract infection (UTI).

Diagnostic Studies

Updated 2015 guidelines suggest differences in the diagnostic criteria for type 1 and type 2 diabetes (Handelsman et al., 2015). The criteria for diagnosing type 2 diabetes are summarized in Table 44.8 (American Diabetes Association, 2023).

The final differential between the two depends on the history, presentation of symptoms, physical examination, and plasma glucose studies. Routine screening for type 2 diabetes in adults older than 45 years is recommended because of the general lack of clinical symptoms in early hyperglycemia. While past experts recommended fasting plasma glucose as the initial screen, the 2-hour oral glucose tolerance test (OGTT) is a better predictor among patients with impaired fasting glucose. Patients who have a higher-than-normal glucose level that does not meet criteria for the diagnosis of diabetes are at particularly high risk for the development of diabetes and are frequently referred to as having prediabetes.

Once the diagnosis of type 2 diabetes is confirmed, several tests are done to guide management. Along with self-monitoring (see Self-Management Measures), a glycosylated hemoglobin A1c is assessed quarterly. The A1c measures the level of control during the previous 2- to 3-month period. The higher the A1c value, the poorer the glucose control. Maintaining an A1c of less than 6.5% is recommended; however, the closer to normal (5.5% or lesser) the levels are, the less likely individuals are to develop long-term sequelae. A1c results should be interpreted with caution in African Americans and in those with various anemias, hemoglobinopathies, and severe renal or hepatic disease (Handelsman et al., 2015).

TABLE 44.7 Physical Findings in Diabetes

EXAMINATION	FINDING	INTERPRETATION
General appearance	Altered level of consciousness	Suggest DKA
	Fruity breath	
	Loss of subcutaneous fat and muscle wasting	Suggest insulin deficiency
Height/weight BMI	BMI >25 kg/m²	Present in 80% of type 2 diabetes
Funduscopic examination (dilated)	Retinopathy	Suggest microvascular disease
	Microaneurysm	
	Exudate, hemorrhage, macular edema	
	Small, poorly responsive pupils	Suggest autonomic neuropathy
Oral examination	Gum disease	Suggest poor glycemic control
Thyroid examination	Wide range of findings from normal to abnormal	If abnormal, can suggest thyroid-caused symptoms or type 1 diabetes as it is associated with increased autoimmune disease
Skin	Acanthosis nigricans	Suggest type 2 diabetes
Cardiac examination	Cardiomegaly or gallop rhythm, little variation in rhythm with deep inspiration	CHF Autonomic neuropathy
Abdominal	Hepatomegaly	CHF
Pulses	Bruit (carotid/femoral) decrease/absent peripheral pulse	PVD
	Atrophy of subcutaneous skin and hair loss—legs and ankle–brachial blood pressure index 0.9	
Feet	Foot ulcer, unrecognized trauma, infection, neuropathic arthropathy	PVD Sensory neuropathy Neuropathy disorders
CNS	Abnormalities suggest neuropathic disease	Place and type can suggest sensory peripheral or autonomic neuropathy

BMI, body mass index; CHF, congestive heart failure; CNS, central nervous system; DKA, diabetic ketoacidosis; PVD, peripheral vascular disease.
Source: Data from American Diabetes Association. (2023). Standards of care in diabetes—2023. https://professional.diabetes.org/content-page/practice-guidelines-resources.

TABLE 44.8 Prediabetes and Diabetes Diagnostic Criteria for Nonpregnant Adults

NORMAL	PREDIABETES	DIABETES[a]
FPG <100 mg/dL	Impaired fasting glucose FPG ≥100–125 mg/dL	FPG >126 mg/dL
2-hour PG <140 mg/dL	Impaired glucose tolerance 2-hour PG ≥140 to 199 mg/dL	2-hour PG ≥200 mg/dL Random PG ≥200 mg/dL in the presence of clinical symptoms
Hb A$_1$c <5.5%	Hb A$_1$c 5.5%–6.4%	Hb A$_1$c ≥6.5%

[a]Diagnosis of diabetes is confirmed when a repeated serum test again demonstrates elevated levels.
FPG, fasting plasma glucose; Hb A1c, hemoglobin A1c; PG, plasma glucose; 2-hour PG, plasma glucose performed 2 hours after 75-g oral glucose load.
Source: Adapted from Handelsman, Y., Bloomgarden, Z. T., Grunberger, G., Umpierrez, G., Zimmerman, R. S., Bailey, T. S., Blonde, L., Bray, G. A., Cohen, A. J., Dago-go-Jack, S., Davidson, J. A., Einhorn, D., Ganda, O. P., Garber, A. J., Garvey, W. T., Henry, R. R., Hirsch, I. B., Horton, E. S., Hurley, D. L., . . . Zangeneh, F. (2015). American Association of Clinical Endocrinologists and American College of Endocrinology—Clinical practice guidelines for developing a diabetes mellitus comprehensive care plan, 2015. Endocrine Practice, 21(Suppl. 1), 1–87. https://doi.org/10.4158/EP15672.GL

Microalbumin is generally assessed at the time of diagnosis to identify microalbuminuria, which is present with early renal disease and may require treatment. Serum creatinine is also done yearly, and the eGFR is calculated in all adults. An EKG should be performed on all adults as a baseline. Diabetes is one of the greatest risk factors for CVD and congestive heart failure (CHF), and routine screening is needed. Dyslipidemia is also frequently seen with diabetes and should be screened for annually. Aggressive management of dyslipidemia is recommended by both the ADA and the AACE. An exercise stress test is considered in patients older than 35 years, or older than 25 years if they have had diabetes for 15 years or more. Liver function studies are often needed as a baseline before starting medication (Handelsman et al., 2015).

Screening for gestational diabetes should occur between 24 and 28 weeks of gestation via 2-hour OGTT. Gestational diabetes is diagnosed if any of the three criteria are met with 2-hour OGTT: fasting plasma glucose greater than 92 mg/dL and/or 1-hour plasma glucose (PG) 180 mg/dL or more and/or 2-hour PG 153 mg/dL or more (Handelsman et al., 2015).

Type 1 diabetes may be present in both lean and overweight patients. As it is generally characterized by insufficient endogenous insulin and exogenous insulin dependence, diagnosis requires documentation of C-peptide and insulin levels in addition to assessment of autoantibodies (islet cell and glutamic acid decarboxylase antibodies).

Treatment/Management

The goals for management are threefold: restore and maintain normal blood glucose levels, prevent target organ damage, and control and/or prevent comorbidities. Meeting these goals requires a partnership between the clinician and patient. Diabetes cannot be adequately controlled without systematic intensive therapy that is monitored by the patient. The best approach to management is a multidisciplinary team that includes the patient, an endocrinologist, primary care provider, diabetes educator, and nutritionist. For any treatment to succeed, the patient must understand the disease, treatment, and her role in management.

Along with diet, exercise, and glycemic control, it is important to address other lifestyle behaviors and comorbidities. To obtain optimal outcomes, aggressive treatment is needed. It is important to address the issues of smoking, dyslipidemia, and hypertension. Patients should be encouraged to stop smoking and referral for smoking cessation assistance may be warranted. Intensive hypertension management to reduce blood pressure to less than 140/90 mmHg should be started (ADA, 2016). LDL should be treated to reach the target of less than 100 mg/dL. If CVD diagnosis is already established, the goal for blood pressure is less than 120/80 mmHg if this can be safely achieved, and the LDL target is less than 70 mg/dL (see Chapter 43, Cardiovascular Disease in Women). These therapies, along with good glycemic control (A1c less than 6.5%), help to prevent the long-term problems associated with diabetes (Garber et al., 2020).

Referral to specialty clinicians may be needed when caring for patients with diabetes. Consider referral to nephrology if the eGFR is abnormal. Referral to cardiology is warranted if evidence of CVD is identified. Annual ophthalmologic evaluation is recommended. Most patients are referred to podiatry for foot care, and referral to neurology may be needed if peripheral neuropathy develops. Other referrals are initiated as needed for management of sequelae.

SELF-MANAGEMENT MEASURES
Self-Monitoring of Blood Glucose

A large part of patient education focuses on self-management. One of the most critical techniques is self-monitoring of blood glucose (SMBG). SMBG provides immediate feedback on current glucose levels, which can help determine any actions needed. SMBG together with the periodic A1c directs the glycemia treatment modalities: diet, exercise, and medication. SMBG should be done before and after each meal and at bedtime until good control is accomplished; then the timing and frequency of SMBG is determined by the patient's needs. Pre- and postprandial goals recommended for capillary blood by the ADA are 80 to 130 mg/dL preprandial and less than 180 mg/dL at peak postprandial (ElSayed et al., 2023). Continuous glucose monitors are now becoming more widely available and can obtain 288 glucose readings per day, allowing patients to better understand how diet and exercise affect their overall blood glucose control. They also improve compliance with data collection since they require minimal to no finger sticks. Available options include Dexcom G6, Freestyle Libre 2, Medtronic guardian sensor, and Eversense.

Hyperglycemia and Hypoglycemia

Once SMBG is established, patients need to know how to manage the results. Education includes managing hyper- and hypoglycemia, medication use, changes in response to illness, and when to contact her clinician. Hypoglycemia can develop with treatment and is more common in those with very tight control. Patients are taught to recognize and manage hypoglycemia (glucose less than 60 mg/dL). The symptoms of hypoglycemia vary and are additive

(Table 44.9). If the patient is conscious and able to follow commands, hypoglycemia is treated by administering oral carbohydrates (e.g., glucose tablets, 2 tablespoons of raisins, 4 oz. of a full sugar soda beverage, or 1 cup of milk). Blood glucose levels are rechecked within 30 to 60 minutes; if the patient is still hypoglycemic, further intake of carbohydrates is needed. Once stabilized, the patient should consume a snack or meal to avoid recurrence. Severe hypoglycemia can be an emergency requiring ED treatment with parenteral glucagon. Severe hyperglycemia can be managed with insulin; the patient should call her clinician or go to the ED if she is experiencing symptoms of diabetic ketoacidosis. Illness can precipitate elevations in blood glucose; however, the only medication that can be altered to meet these needs is insulin. The patient should contact her clinician if she is experiencing persistent hyperglycemia of more than 250 mg/dL (Garber et al., 2020; ADA, 2020).

Exercise

Another vital part of diabetes management is physical activity. Exercise has been shown to lower blood glucose, reduce A1c, increase insulin sensitivity, decrease the need for insulin, and increase the number of insulin receptors. Physical activity, including moderate intensity aerobic exercise (59%–70% of maximum heart rate), flexibility exercises, and resistance training, should be done for a minimum of 150 minutes/week. Careful balance between insulin and glucose needs to be maintained for safe exercise in patients with type 1 diabetes. Patients with type 1 diabetes should have a readily available source of carbohydrate when exercising in case of hypoglycemia. With repeated exercise, patients can determine their individual reaction and learn to adjust food and insulin to meet their needs. Exercise helps to reduce insulin resistance and can help with weight management, especially when combined with dietary modifications. Exercise for patients with diabetes should include three components: aerobic exercise, flexibility training, and resistance training. One hour of moderate intensity aerobic exercise provides the same benefit as a 700-calorie reduction in food intake. While many patients cannot exercise for 150 minutes each week, any exercise helps to improve glycemic control. Resistance training improves insulin sensitivity at about the same rate as aerobic exercise and increases both metabolic rate and muscle mass. High-intensity resistance training (three sets, three times per week) can reduce A1c by 1.1% to 1.2% (Handelsman et al., 2015).

MEDICAL NUTRITION THERAPY

Medical nutrition therapy (MNT) is an integral part of diabetes management and plays a critical role in controlling the metabolic parameters of the disease. The same types of dietary changes used with TLC apply to MNT for patients with diabetes. Weight loss of 5% to 10% should be encouraged in all overweight and obese patients. In type 2 diabetes, weight management to reduce insulin resistance is recommended. A moderate decrease in caloric intake (250–500 kcal/day) can result in a slow and consistent weight loss. Fasting should be avoided as a method to reduce weight, and meals and snacks should be eaten on a regular schedule. Current recommendations suggest a plant-based diet consisting of fresh fruits and vegetables, low-glycemic-index carbohydrates, and low saturated fats. Meats should be lean, and processed meats should be avoided. Making healthier choices can help reduce caloric intake and provide a starting point for quantity reduction. For example, fruit or raw vegetables for a snack instead of crackers and cheese may reduce caloric intake by 150 calories per day. Micronutrient and vitamin supplementation is not recommended in the absence of insufficiency or deficiency (Handelsman et al., 2015).

COMPLEMENTARY AND ALTERNATIVE MEDICINE

Cinnamon may aid in a modest reduction of blood sugar levels (0.1–0.2% decrease in A1c); however, research is limited and it should be avoided in patients with liver disorders.

PHARMACOTHERAPEUTICS
Medication Therapy for Type 2 Diabetes

As the pathophysiology of type 2 diabetes is multifactorial, treatment is likely to require multiple therapies. The choice for oral therapy can be complex. If glycemic control is not achieved after 3 to 6 months of lifestyle management, a

---

TABLE 44.9 Symptoms of Mild, Moderate, and Severe Hypoglycemia

MILD	MODERATE	SEVERE
• Pallor • Diaphoresis • Tachycardia • Palpitations • Hunger • Paresthesias • Shakiness/tremor	Symptoms of mild plus: • Inability to concentrate • Confusion • Slurred speech • Irrational or uncontrolled behavior • Slowed reaction time • Blurred vision • Somnolence • Extreme fatigue	Symptoms of mild and moderate plus: • Disoriented behavior • Loss of consciousness • Inability to wake up • Seizures • Impaired neurologic function

Source: Adapted from Handelsman, Y., Bloomgarden, Z. T., Grunberger, G., Umpierrez, G., Zimmerman, R. S., Bailey, T. S., Blonde, L., Bray, G. A., Cohen, A. J., Dagogo-Jack, S., Davidson, J. A., Einhorn, D., Ganda, O. P., Garber, A. J., Garvey, W. T., Henry, R. R., Hirsch, I. B., Horton, E. S., Hurley, D. L., . . . Zangeneh, F. (2015). American Association of Clinical Endocrinologists and American College of Endocrinology—Clinical practice guidelines for developing a diabetes mellitus comprehensive care plan, 2015. Endocrine Practice, 21(Suppl. 1), 1–87. https://doi.org/10.4158/EP15672.GL

program of medication therapy should be initiated. This clinical decision is usually based on glucose level as well as evidence of target organ damage. Many noninsulin and insulin medications, which provide an opportunity to truly tailor a regimen and individualize care, are available.

There are several considerations in selecting a treatment regimen. First, the underlying pathology must be considered. How severe is the hyperglycemia? Are both insulin resistance and insulin deficiency present? Is glucose toxicity (glucose more than 600 mg/dL) present? The age and weight of the patient and comorbidities also need to be considered. Each class of medication carries its own set of side effects and precautions that must be weighed. Medication therapy usually involves multiple medications from different classes and both noninsulin medications and insulin are considered first-line therapy. Clinicians should refer to full prescribing information when selecting and initiating diabetes medication for dosing, precautions, contraindications, and interactions. Agents used in diabetic therapy include insulin and the following noninsulin medications: biguanides (metformin), sulfonylureas (SU), meglitinide derivatives, alpha-glucosidase inhibitors (AGi), thiazolidinediones (TZDs), glucagon-like peptide-1 (GLP-1) agonists, dipeptidyl peptidase IV (DPP-4) inhibitors, selective sodium-glucose transporter-2 (SGLT-2) inhibitors, amylinomimetics, bile acid sequestrants, and dopamine agonists. Table 44.10 summarizes critical factors to be considered when prescribing noninsulin diabetes agents.

Weight loss in the presence of poorly controlled blood glucose suggests insulin deficiency. The pattern of SMBG levels throughout the day is most helpful in determining which medication to use because medications are used to target hyperglycemia occurring at different times. Additionally, the A1c level at the time of initiation of a medication regimen guides the selection of pharmacologic agents. In patients who begin pharmacologic treatment for type 2 diabetes with a baseline A1c level less than 7.5%, monotherapy is recommended. If the glycemic goal is not met after 3 months, a second agent should be added. With a baseline A1c level greater than or equal to 7.5%, metformin or another first-line agent should be augmented with a second noninsulin or insulin agent. If glycemic control is not achieved in 3 months, a third agent should be added. For patients with a baseline A1c level greater than or equal to 9.0%, in the absence of overt symptoms, dual or triple therapy should be employed. If overt symptoms are present, insulin and possibly noninsulin therapy should be used. Lifestyle modifications along with medically assisted weight loss should be incorporated in all therapeutic plans to achieve and maintain glycemic control. Table 44.11 summarizes pharmacologic agent choices for glycemic control based on baseline A1c level.

Noninsulin Agents

When lifestyle changes are not sufficient to achieve glycemic control, typically patients are started on noninsulin agents. For patients who are overweight, metformin is usually the first agent prescribed. If single therapy does not work, or if the A1c is 7.5% or greater, additional agents are added. Many patients require treatment with two, three, or more different medicines. If oral-agent combinations are ineffective, an injected medicine such as a GLP-1, amylin analog, or insulin may be prescribed. Combinations of noninsulin and insulin agents are used because different drugs target different parts of the glycemic regulation system. Table 44.10 summarizes critical factors to be considered when prescribing noninsulin diabetes agents.

Insulin Therapy

TYPE 1 DIABETES MELLITUS

With type 1 diabetes, insulin therapy is required for survival and must be started at diagnosis. As intensive therapy is recommended, the clinician may choose to refer these patients for management by a clinician specializing in endocrinology. For most patients with type 1 diabetes, physiologic regimens using insulin analogs should be prescribed. Patients should be started on multiple daily injections of one to two doses of basal insulin to most closely approximate normal pancreatic function. Basal insulin is used in combination with rapid-acting prandial insulin before each meal. The insulin dose is determined by the patients weight, blood glucose level, activity, and food intake, and thus requires intensive self-monitoring. Alternatively, insulin may be administered via continuous subcutaneous infusion (insulin pump) using rapid-acting insulin analog. A clear understanding by the patient of the treatment and how it works is critical to success. Insulins differ in their onset, peak, and duration, and they are selected to meet individual metabolic needs.

The initial insulin dose for type 1 diabetes is based on body weight with a recommended starting dosage of 0.4 to 0.5 unit/kg daily. Daily basal dosing should represent 40% to 50% of the daily insulin dose administered as either a daily injection of a basal analog or to doses of NPH insulin. Prandial insulin dosage should represent 50% to 60% of total daily insulin dose and should be administered in divided doses 15 minutes prior to each meal based on estimating the carbohydrate content of each meal.

TYPE 2 DIABETES MELLITUS

In some patients with type 2 diabetes, the beta cells cannot meet the demand for insulin. When glycemic control cannot be achieved with TLC and noninsulin agents, insulin is started. Because insulin resistance is a major factor in type 2 diabetes, treatment with an agent that lowers insulin resistance (Table 44.10) may be needed in addition to insulin. Insulin may be needed initially to help control hyperglycemia; if the patient is able to modify other factors, such as obesity, she may be able to discontinue the insulin in the future.

Complications

Complications related to diabetes are of special concern for women (Table 44.12). Two factors increase the risks associated with heart disease in women with diabetes. First, she loses the natural protection to CVD that is seen in other premenopausal women. Second, among people with diabetes who have a cardiac event, women have a lower survival rate. Of the women who do survive, the quality of life is poorer than that of men. Mortality rates are higher in women with

TABLE 44.10 Noninsulin Agents

CLASS	ACTION	FASTING GLUCOSE LOWERING	POSTPRANDIAL GLUCOSE LOWERING	NAFLD BENEFIT	HYPOGLYCEMIA	WEIGHT	RENAL/GU EFFECTS	GI ADVERSE EFFECTS
Alpha-glucosidase inhibitors	Delay carbohydrate absorption from intestine	Neutral	Moderate	Neutral	Neutral	Neutral	Neutral	Moderate
Amylin analog	Decrease glucagon secretion Slow gastric emptying Increase satiety	Mild	Moderate-marked	Neutral	Neutral	Loss	Neutral	Moderate
Biguanide	Decrease hepatic glucose production Increase muscle uptake of glucose	Moderate	Mild	Mild	Neutral	Slight loss	Contraindicated in moderate to severe chronic kidney disease	Moderate
Bile acid sequestrant	Possibly decrease hepatic glucose production and increase incretin levels	Mild	Mild	Neutral	Neutral	Neutral	Neutral	Moderate
DPP-4 inhibitors	Increase glucose-dependent insulin secretion Decrease secretion of glucagon	Mild	Moderate	Neutral	Neutral	Neutral	Dose adjustment necessary if renal impairment present (except linagliptin)	Neutral
Dopamine-2 agonist	Activates dopaminergic receptors	Neutral	Mild	Neutral	Neutral	Neutral	Neutral	Moderate
Glinides	Increase insulin secretion	Mild	Moderate	Neutral	Mild-moderate	Gain	Increased risk of hypoglycemia	Neutral
GLP-1 receptor agonists	Increase glucose-dependent insulin secretion Decrease glucagon secretion Slow gastric emptying Increase satiety	Mild-moderate	Moderate-marked	Mild	Neutral	Loss	Contraindicated if creatinine clearance <30 mg/mL	Moderate
SGLT-2 inhibitors	Increase urinary excretion of glucose	Moderate	Mild	Neutral	Neutral	Loss	GU infection risk	Neutral
Sulfonylureas	Increase insulin secretion	Moderate	Moderate	Neutral	Moderate to severe	Gain	Increased risk of hypoglycemia	Neutral
Thiazolidinediones	Increase glucose uptake in muscle and fat Decrease hepatic glucose production	Moderate	Mild	Moderate	Neutral	Gain	Potential to worsen fluid retention	Neutral

DPP-4, dipeptidyl peptidase IV; GI, gastrointestinal; GLP-1, glucagon-like peptide-1; GU, genitourinary; NAFLD, nonalcoholic fatty liver disease; SGLT-2, sodium-glucose transporter-2.
Source: Adapted from Handelsman, Y., Bloomgarden, Z. T., Grunberger, G., Umpierrez, G., Zimmerman, R. S., Bailey, T. S., Blonde, L., Bray, G. A., Cohen, A. J., Dagogo-Jack, S., Davidson, J. A., Einhorn, D., Ganda, O. P., Garber, A. J., Garvey, W. T., Henry, R. R., Hirsch, I. B., Horton, E. S., Hurley, D. L., . . . Zangeneh, F. (2015). American Association of Clinical Endocrinologists and American College of Endocrinology—Clinical practice guidelines for developing a diabetes mellitus comprehensive care plan, 2015. Endocrine Practice, 21(Suppl. 1), 1–87. https://doi.org/10.4158/EP15672.GL

TABLE 44.11 Pharmacologic Interventions for Glycemic Control

A1C LEVEL <7.5%	A1C LEVEL ≥7.5%		A1C LEVEL ≥9.0%	
Monotherapy	Dual Therapy	Triple Therapy	Asymptomatic	Symptomatic
Metformin GLP-1RA SGLT-2i DPP-4i AGi TZD SU/GLP	Metformin or other first-line agent plus one of the following: GLP-1RA SGLT-2i DPP-4i AGi TZD SU/GLP Basal insulin Colesevelam Bromocriptine-QR	Metformin or other first-line agent and second-line agent plus one of the following: GLP-1RA SGLT-2i DPP-4i AGi TZD SU/GLP Basal insulin Colesevelam Bromocriptine-QR	Dual or triple therapy	Insulin and possibly noninsulin agents
If glycemic control not achieved in 3 months, advance to dual therapy	If glycemic control not achieved in 3 months, advance to triple therapy	If glycemic control not achieved in 3 months, add or intensify insulin therapy	If glycemic control not achieved in 3 months, add or intensify insulin therapy	If glycemic control not achieved in 3 months, intensify insulin therapy

AGi, alpha-glucosidase inhibitor; DPP-4i, dipeptidyl peptidase IV inhibitor; GLP-1 RA, glucagon-like peptide-1 receptor agonist; QR, quick release; SGLT-2i, selective sodium-glucose transporter-2 inhibitor; SU/GLP, sulfonylureas/glucagon-like peptide; TZD, thiazolidinedione.
Source: Adapted from Garber, A. J., Handelsman, Y., Grunberger, G., Einhorn, D., Abrahamson, M. J., Barzilay, J. I., Blonde, L., Bush, M. A., DeFronzo, R. A., Garber, J. R., Garvey, W. T., Hirsch, I. B., Jellinger, P. S., McGill, J. B., Mechanick, J. I., Perreault, L., Rosenblit, P. D., Samson, S., & Umpierrez, G. E. (2020). Consensus statement by the American Association of Clinical Endocrinologists and American College of Endocrinology on the comprehensive type 2 diabetes management algorithm—2020 executive summary. Endocrine Practice, 26(1), 107–139. https://doi.org/10.4158/CS-2019-0472

diabetes. While diabetic retinopathy is a problem for all patients with diabetes, women are more likely to develop the proliferative form of the disease and more likely to lose their sight. Aggressive management is important to prevent these complications.

Large-scale clinical trials of SGLT-2 inhibitors have shown an impact on cardiovascular outcomes, including heart failure hospitalization and cardiovascular death, which appears to be independent of their glucose-lowering efficacy.

Considerations for Special and Minoritized Populations

PERSONS OF CHILDBEARING AGE

There is a unique burden with diabetes because of the progression of the disease as well as its effect on pregnancy. Diabetes can cause difficulties in pregnancy such as increased risk of pregnancy loss at all stages and increased birth defects (see Chapter 38, High-Risk Childbearing). Gestational diabetes (see Chapter 38, High-Risk Childbearing), which increases the mother's risk of developing diabetes later in life, complicates 2% to 5% of all pregnancies (Beckles & Thompson-Reid, 2001).

OLDER PERSONS

Close monitoring is especially important for older persons. As older persons are more likely to have other existing health conditions, the likelihood of medication interactions is increased. Concerns with hyper- and hypoglycemia are higher in older persons, who may have increased risks for falls or other medical conditions that can cause similar symptoms. Furthermore, poor glucose control can act

TABLE 44.12 Complications of Diabetes

COMPLICATION	STATISTICS
Death	68% of the deaths in diabetics are related to CVD 16% of the deaths in diabetics are related to stroke
CVD	Risk two to four times higher
Stroke	Risk two to four times higher
Hypertension	67% of diabetics have BP 140/90 mmHg or greater
Eyes (blindness)	Leading cause of blindness in adults, 28.5% of adults with diabetes older than 40 years have diabetic retinopathy
Kidney disease	Leading cause of end-stage renal disease
Nervous system disease	60%–70% of diabetics have CNS damage (peripheral neuropathy, sexual dysfunction, gastroparesis, carpal tunnel syndrome)
Amputation	Leading cause of lower limb amputations (nontraumatic)
Dental disease	One third of diabetics have severe periodontal disease with tooth loss
Complications of pregnancy	Increased incidence of birth defects Spontaneous abortion in up to 20% of pregnancies Large babies

BP, blood pressure; CNS, central nervous system; CVD, cardiovascular disease.
Source: Data from Centers for Disease Control and Prevention. (2011). National diabetes fact sheet: National estimates and general information on diabetes and prediabetes in the United States. U.S. Department of Health and Human Services. http://www.cdc.gov/diabetes/pubs/pdf/ndfs_2011.pdf

synergistically with other health problems to accelerate complications (Beckles & Thompson-Reid, 2001).

PRISON POPULATIONS

In 2021, 83,000 women and 1.1 million men were incarcerated in state and federal facilities in the United States compared with 1.5 million male inmates (Carson, 2022). An estimated 4.8% of the total incarcerated population, or around 80,000 people, have diabetes. Patient advocacy and diligence are required to assure that the same standard of care for diabetes is applied and met for incarcerated persons as has been proved effective for all people with diabetes (ADA, 2014).

HYPOTHALAMUS AND PITUITARY GLAND DISORDERS

Many consider the pituitary the "master gland." The hypothalamus and pituitary gland form a unit that controls many endocrine system functions. Thyroid, adrenal, and gonadal functions are controlled by this unit as well as a wide range of physiologic activities. Additionally, neuroendocrinologic function, which includes regulation of the endocrine system and modulation of nervous system activity, is dependent on this unit (Carroll et al., 2011).

Hyperprolactinemia

DEFINITION AND SCOPE

Hyperprolactinemia is a condition of elevated serum prolactin, an amino acid protein produced in the lactotroph cells of the anterior pituitary gland. Dopamine has the predominant inhibitory influence in the regulation of prolactin secretion. Prolactinemia may occur as a physiologic, pharmacologic, or pathologic response.

In the United States, hyperprolactinemia occurs in less than 1% of the general population and in 5% to 14% of persons with secondary amenorrhea. Nearly 75% of those who present with galactorrhea and amenorrhea are found to have hyperprolactinemia. Prolactin-secreting tumors are found in nearly one third of these patients (Lee et al., 2012).

ETIOLOGY

Physiologic hyperprolactinemia generally produces mild to moderate symptoms and most commonly occurs due to nipple stimulation and lactation in the first 4 to 6 weeks postpartum. With pregnancy, there is a steady increase in prolactin that peaks at the time of delivery. Nipple stimulation further increases the levels of prolactin, allowing for breastfeeding. Without nipple stimulation, levels return to normal in 4 to 6 weeks. Physiologic hyperprolactinemia can also be mediated by stress, such as myocardial infarction, hypoglycemia, or surgery. Other causes include sleep, food ingestion, and physical exercise. Pharmacologic agents that affect the hypothalamic dopamine system and/or pituitary dopamine receptors can also stimulate prolactin release, resulting in hyperprolactinemia. Serum levels of prolactin increase within hours of medication dosing and will return to normal within 4 days

TABLE 44.13 Selected Drugs Known to Cause Hyperprolactinemia and/or Galactorrhea[a]

DRUG CLASS	DRUG
Antipsychotic	Haldol
	Orap
	Zyprexa
	Risperdal
Antidepressant	Anafranil
	Norpramin
Gastrointestinal	Tagamet (IV)
	Reglan
Antihypertensives	Aldomet
	Reserpine
	Verapamil
Opiates	Codeine
	Morphine

[a]A selected sample of drugs. List not comprehensive.
Source: Data from Snyder, P. J. (2014). *Clinical manifestations and evaluation of hyperprolactinemia.* UpToDate. *https://www.uptodate.com/contents/clinical -manifestations-and-evaluation-of-hyperprolactinemia.*

of discontinuation. Several classes of medications (Table 44.13) can lead to this disorder. Withdrawal from the medication is curative. Not all medications in any one class cause hypersecretion, so changing agents may resolve the problem (Melmed et al., 2011; Serri et al., 2006; Snyder, 2014).

The major pathological causes of hyperprolactinemia are pituitary tumor, decreased dopamine inhibition of prolactin, hypothyroidism, chronic renal disease, or hypothalamic or pituitary disorders (e.g., head trauma, pituitary adenoma, or sarcoidosis). Hyperprolactinemia is also associated with insulin resistance and may be seen with the metabolic syndrome, polycystic ovarian syndrome (PCOS), or diabetes. This may be related to the proinflammatory state thought to be present in these conditions, which seems to be independent of BMI (Melmed et al., 2011; Snyder, 2014).

SYMPTOMS AND EVALUATION/ASSESSMENT

Galactorrhea, defined as milk or milk-like secretion from the breast, is the most common presenting symptom. Eighty percent of nonpregnant or lactating persons with galactorrhea have hyperprolactinemia. Oligomenorrhea or amenorrhea leading to suboptimal fertility is another common symptom. The suboptimal fertility can be in the form of either difficulty getting pregnant or recurrent spontaneous abortion. Symptoms such as headache, visual changes, and cranial neuropathies may indicate a mass and need to be evaluated accordingly. In patients experiencing increased intracranial pressure due to a mass, the presenting symptom may be seizures. A complete breast and pelvic exam should be completed (Snyder, 2014).

DIFFERENTIAL DIAGNOSIS

All causes of oligomenorrhea, amenorrhea, and infertility, including PCOS, are part of the differential diagnosis. Acute inflammatory diseases (e.g., sarcoidosis, histiocytosis) can also be the cause. Medications, benign and malignant tumors, hypothyroidism, chronic liver and renal disease, and normal physiologic changes (e.g., pregnancy and increased breast stimulation) must be considered as well (Melmed et al., 2011).

DIAGNOSTIC STUDIES

The primary diagnostic test is serum prolactin. The diagnosis of hyperprolactinemia is made when serum prolactin levels are found on two separate occasions to be above the norm established for the laboratory used. Prolactin secretion is pulsatile; it increases with sleep, stress, pregnancy, and chest wall stimulation or trauma, and therefore must be drawn after fasting. Serum prolactin levels between 20 and 200 mcg/L can be found in persons with hyperprolactinemia due to any cause. Serum prolactin levels above 200 mcg/L generally indicate the presence of a pituitary (lactotroph) adenoma. Dedicated pituitary MRI should be obtained if pituitary adenoma is suspected. Mammogram should be considered.

TREATMENT/MANAGEMENT

Management of drug-induced hyperprolactinemia includes discontinuation of the medication or substitution of an alternative medication and estrogen replacement in women with long-term hypogonadism. Dopamine agonists are often used for treatment of prolactinomas and require endocrinology referral. Oral contraceptives are used for those with amenorrhea due to prolactinomas. Resistant and malignant prolactinomas generally require increasing doses of dopamine agonists and/or transsphenoidal surgery, radiation therapy, as well as other chemotherapeutics (Melmed et al., 2011).

Self-Management Measures

For those with physiologic causes of hyperprolactinemia, the condition will remit once the cause is removed. In the case of increased nipple stimulation, if it is self- or partner-induced, counseling or referral for evaluation of the behavior may be warranted. Referral may also be warranted in patients with excess stress and limited coping skills.

Pharmacotherapeutics

When possible, the treatment of choice is medical management with a dopamine agonist. The two most common medications are bromocriptine (Parlodel) and cabergoline (Dostinex). Treatment may not need to be continued indefinitely. If medications are withdrawn, monitoring for recurrence is warranted.

CONSIDERATIONS FOR SPECIAL AND MINORITIZED POPULATIONS

The issues for pregnant persons are mainly related to the effect of dopamine agonists in pregnancy. Bromocriptine has been studied and does not seem to cause fetal damage. Few data are available on the other medications currently used. Patients should be monitored for worsening symptoms. There is approximately a 25% chance that a tumor will increase in size. Periodic checks of prolactin levels are not useful as levels normally increase during pregnancy. The signs and symptoms the patient is experiencing at each prenatal visit can be used to follow the disease course. As abnormalities of the visual field and/or severe headaches can signify an increase in tumor size, assessment for both is critical. If present, neuroimaging (MRI) without gadolinium is indicated (Melmed et al., 2011).

Polycystic Ovary Syndrome

DEFINITION AND SCOPE

PCOS is one of the most common endocrine disorders of reproductive-age women in the United States, presenting as menstrual irregularity and evidence of androgen excess. With a prevalence of 4% to 12% among premenopausal women, it is responsible for 75% of anovulatory infertility. Incidence is higher in Native American and Hispanic women when compared with White and Black women (Ehrmann, 2005). While PCOS has always been associated with infertility and increased risk of endometrial and ovarian cancer, it is also recognized as a significant risk factor for metabolic diseases, such as diabetes, dyslipidemia, and CVD (Azziz et al., 2004; Ovalle & Azziz, 2002). Although some studies have suggested an increased risk for breast cancer in women with PCOS, findings from a recent meta-analysis refute this (Barry et al., 2014).

ETIOLOGY

PCOS develops in the context of abnormalities of the hypothalamic–pituitary–ovarian axis, insulin resistance, and altered adipocyte function (Sachdeva, 2010). Together these factors and perhaps genetic abnormalities cause increased androgen levels, decreased ovulatory function, and increased metabolic risk.

PCOS is associated with abnormal androgen and estrogen metabolism and in the control of androgen production. Women with PCOS may have high serum male sex steroid levels including testosterone, androstenedione, and dehydroepiandrosterone sulfate (DHEA-S). However, normal levels of the hormones may be encountered in these patients.

Women with PCOS often have insulin resistance and hyperinsulinemia, both of which are markedly increased in the presence of obesity. Defects in insulin receptor signaling pathways are thought to promote insulin resistance in PCOS patients, and elevated insulin levels may have gonadotropin-augmenting effects on ovarian function. Increased androgenicity is thought to occur from suppression of hormone-binding globulins in the liver due to hyperinsulinemia (Barber et al., 2006).

Insulin resistance in PCOS has been associated with low levels of adiponectin, a hormone secreted by adipocytes that help regulate glucose levels and metabolism of lipids. Interestingly, both obese and nonobese women with PCOS have lower levels of adiponectin than women who do not have PCOS (Toulis et al., 2009).

Although controversial, one proposed mechanism for anovulation and elevated androgen levels suggests that oversecretion of luteinizing hormone (LH) may lead to changes in the LH to follicle-stimulating hormone (FSH) ratio (LH:FSH). This, in turn, causes abnormal gonado-tropic releasing hormone (GnRH) levels. As a result, the ovaries cannot aromatize androgens to estrogens, which leads to decreased estrogen levels and consequent anovula-tion. Anovulation results in a lack of progesterone needed to protect the endometrium. With high LH levels and steady-state FSH, follicles may start to develop but do not reach maturity. This can account for the typical polycystic ovary seen on ultrasound imaging (Barbieri & Ehrmann, 2022).

RISK FACTORS

PCOS is a genetically heterogeneous syndrome in which the genetic contributions remain incompletely described; how-ever, studies of family members with PCOS indicate that an autosomal dominant mode of inheritance occurs. Fathers of PCOS patients may be abnormally hairy. Mothers may have oligomenorrhea and siblings may have oligomenorrhea and hirsutism. Family history of type 2 diabetes in a first-degree relative has also been indicated as a risk factor for PCOS, impaired glucose tolerance, type 2 diabetes, and metabolic abnormalities (Ehrmann, 2005).

SYMPTOMS AND EVALUATION/ASSESSMENT

Women with PCOS usually present with multiple symptoms, although not all are present in any one person.

History

Thorough investigation of a patient's personal and family health history is warranted to determine significant risk fac-tors for PCOS. Family history may include menstrual dis-orders, adrenal enzyme deficiencies, infertility, hirsutism, obesity, metabolic syndrome, and diabetes. A comprehensive menstrual history is needed to identify the most common presenting symptom: menstrual irregularities. These irreg-ularities typically begin at menarche. Oligomenorrhea and secondary amenorrhea are the most common. Some women also experience abnormal uterine bleeding. Infertility is com-mon with PCOS; thus, asking about attempts at conception is important. Other symptoms to discuss are hirsutism, acne, and alopecia (American College of Obstetricians and Gyne-cologists [ACOG], 2018).

Physical Examination

The goal of the physical exam is twofold: to exclude other causes of the symptoms and to identify risk factors for chronic disease. AACE advocates using the Rotterdam criteria to establish the diagnosis of PCOS in the presence of two of the following criteria: androgen excess, ovulatory dysfunction, or polycystic ovaries. Note that the presence of polycystic ovary is not needed for diagnosis (Legro et al., 2013).

Women suspected of having PCOS should be evaluated for hypertension, obesity, dermatologic changes, virilization, and pelvic masses. Obesity with central adiposity is present in approximately 50% of women with PCOS. The obesity is thought to be related to both androgen excess and insulin resistance (Moran et al., 2011).

Enlarged ovaries are present in 50% to 75% of women with PCOS. This enlargement is due to the formation of cysts that give the syndrome its name as well as an increase in the ovar-ian stroma. The ovarian changes are a result of the disease and are not a cause of the syndrome. While polycystic ovaries are present in many women, irregular menstrual patterns and signs of androgen excess are more common and better pre-dictors of the disorder (Legro et al., 2013).

Skin and hair changes are also common. Alopecia or male pattern balding occurs in up to 25% of women and can be distressing. This symptom is related to the excessive level of androgens. Insulin resistance can lead to the development of acanthosis nigricans, as is seen with metabolic syndrome (Moran et al., 2011; Norman et al., 2007).

Differential Diagnoses

The differential diagnoses to be considered depend on the presenting symptoms. PCOS should be assessed in any patient with an abnormal menstrual pattern that is coupled with signs and symptoms of excessive androgens. In women of all ages, other causes of hyperandrogenism need to be ruled out, such as medication-induced issues, hyperprolactinemia, adrenal hyperplasia (Cushing's syndrome), and androgen-producing tumors. Virilization is not usually seen with PCOS; if pres-ent, it may suggest adrenal hyperplasia or androgen-secreting tumor. Thyroid dysfunction can mimic some of the symp-toms and should be ruled out (ACOG, 2018).

Diagnostic Studies

Current AACE guidelines do not recommend routine hor-monal laboratory studies or US to establish the diagnosis of PCOS in adult women if frank symptoms are present. The guidelines advise that an adult can be diagnosed with PCOS if they have at least two of the following symptoms: excess androgen, ovulatory dysfunction, or polycystic ova-ries. During the perimenopausal transition and postmeno-pause, diagnosis should be based on documented, chronic oligomenorrhea, as well as hyperandrogenism during the reproductive years. Polycystic ovaries visualized on US may provide supportive evidence although this is not likely in postmenopausal persons. In addition, any diagnosis of PCOS must rule out other androgen-excess disorders. Cli-nicians should screen patients for endometrial cancer, mood disorders, obstructive sleep apnea if obese, diabetes, and CVD. In adolescents with persistent oligomenorrhea, diag-nosis of PCOS should be based on clinical presentation and hormonal analysis once other possible etiologies have been excluded (Legro et al., 2013).

When indicated, laboratory tests are used to rule out other causes of the symptoms and to document PCOS abnormal-ities. Measurement of serum 17-hydroxyprogesterone levels after a cosyntropin stimulation test can be used to exclude late-onset adrenal hyperplasia. If Cushing syndrome is sus-pected, 24-hour urine sample for free cortisol and creatinine should be obtained. A dexamethasone suppression test is also useful in assessing for Cushing syndrome. Serum insulin-like growth factor (IGF)-1 is a highly sensitive and specific bio-marker of growth hormone excess and is used to rule out acromegaly only if there is a clinical suspicion of this disorder. Hyperprolactinemia can be excluded by obtaining a fasting serum prolactin level. OGTT (2-hour OGTT) is recommended to evaluate for type 2 diabetes. Thyroid function tests, specifically third-generation TSH and free T4, should be obtained to exclude hypothyroidism (Barbieri & Ehrmann, 2022).

Elevated levels of total or free testosterone can confirm the androgen excess; however, they do not diagnose the cause. The typical range for elevated testosterone levels with PCOS is more than 50 ng/dL of total testosterone or more than 0.9 ng/dL of free testosterone. Levels are much higher in the presence of an androgen-secreting ovarian tumor (Legro et al., 2013). Depending on the androgen measured, up to 90% of women with PCOS will have elevated blood levels. LH and FSH levels may also be useful. An LH:FSH ratio greater than 3 is often present in PCOS. Serum estradiol levels are usually normal, while serum estrone is elevated due to the conversion of androgen to estrone in the adipose tissue. Sex hormone–binding globulin (SHBG) is usually decreased. Currently, the SHBG test is performed as a baseline study to determine the free androgen index (FAI), especially when ovarian mass or tumor is suspected. Several tests are available to determine insulin levels; however, the results of these tests are not well defined and as such are not recommended (Legro et al., 2013; Royal College of Obstetricians and Gynaecologists, 2007). Current, accepted guidelines should be used to screen for hyperlipidemia and hypertension. In obese women, the same screening measures used in metabolic syndrome should be employed. Frequency of rescreening depends on the initial results. If the results are abnormal, then rescreening may be indicated in 3 to 6 months, as opposed to 1 to 5 years or at the usual age for general screening.

Imaging studies such as transvaginal pelvic/ovarian US are performed when the manual pelvic examination is inadequate, in the presence of abdominal and/or pelvic pain, when testosterone levels are excessively elevated (greater than 200 ng/dL), and to assess for endometrial thickness or anatomic etiology in the presence of amenorrhea. If a solid mass or tumor is suspected, CT or MRI should be obtained to assess the adrenal glands and ovaries. MRI is preferred for imaging the ovaries in very obese patients (the ovaries may not always be visualized with transvaginal US), adolescents, and those in whom transvaginal US may be inappropriate (Lalwani et al., 2012; Trivax & Azziz, 2007).

Treatment/Management

Goals for the management of PCOS are to decrease androgen levels; control symptoms; prevent long-term problems; reduce BMI; decrease cardiovascular risk, including dyslipidemia; protect the endometrium; delay or prevent diabetes; decrease blood pressure; and induce ovulation if pregnancy is desired.

Self-Management Measures

First-line treatment modalities include TLC. Although the role of exercise, healthy diet, and weight reduction in improving PCOS is unclear, it is recommended for overweight and obese patients for other health benefits, primarily reduction of cardiovascular and diabetes risk (Legro et al., 2013). Setting

realistic goals that are acceptable to the patient is important to the success of TLC.

Pharmacotherapeutics

An Endocrine Society task force developed evidence-based guidelines for the treatment of PCOS in 2013 using the Grading of Recommendations, Assessment, Development, and Evaluation (GRADE) system to rate the strength and quality of recommendations. These guidelines are summarized in the following text (Legro et al., 2013).

HORMONAL CONTRACEPTIVES

Current guidelines recommend hormonal contraceptives (including pill, patch, vaginal ring) as first-line therapy for patients with menstrual abnormalities and PCOS-related hirsutism and/or acne. As with use of hormonal contraceptives for prevention of pregnancy, screening for contraindications using established guidelines (CDC, 2010) is imperative.

METFORMIN

Use of metformin is indicated for people with PCOS with an established diagnosis of type 2 diabetes or impaired glucose tolerance who have been unsuccessful with lifestyle modifications. It is also recommended as second-line therapy for people with PCOS who have menstrual irregularities and cannot tolerate hormonal contraceptives or in whom hormonal contraceptives are contraindicated. Current guidelines do not recommend metformin as first-line therapy for people with PCOS for treatment of hirsutism and/or acne, for prevention of pregnancy complications, or for treatment of obesity.

TREATMENT OF INFERTILITY

Clomiphene citrate or comparable estrogen modulators (e.g., letrozole) is the recommended first-line therapy for anovulatory infertility. People with PCOS having in vitro fertilization should be prescribed metformin as adjuvant therapy for infertility to prevent ovarian hyperstimulation syndrome.

OTHER PHARMACOTHERAPEUTICS

Treatment of PCOS should not include insulin sensitizers such as inositols due to lack of documented benefit or thiazolidinediones owing to safety concerns. Current expert opinion does not recommend the use of statin therapy for hyperandrogenism and anovulation in women with PCOS as sufficient risk–benefit data are lacking. Statins are recommended for people with PCOS who meet indications of current evidence-based recommendations for statin therapy (Stone et al., 2014; see Chapter 43, Cardiovascular Disease in Women).

Treatment/Management of Adolescents

When the goal of treatment is to relieve anovulatory symptoms, treat hirsutism and/or acne, or prevent pregnancy in adolescents with suspected PCOS, hormonal contraceptives are considered first-line therapy. However, optimal duration of contraceptive use has not been established for this population.

If the adolescent has impaired glucose tolerance and/or metabolic syndrome, metformin may be considered, although optimal duration of this therapy has not been established.

Treatment/Management of Premenarchal Girls

For adolescents with advanced pubertal development (Tanner stage IV or above of breast development) accompanied by clinical and biochemical indicators of hyperandrogenism, initiation of hormonal contraceptives is suggested.

ADRENAL DISORDERS

The major function of the adrenal gland is the biosynthesis of steroids. As with the reproductive system, the regulation of these steroids is by a feedback mechanism. Aldosterone, the major mineralocorticoid, influences ion transport and plays a role in controlling blood pressure. Cortisol, the major glucocorticoid, is important in the regulation of many body systems including fetal lung maturity, bone remodeling, and calcium absorption. The third major group of steroids released from the adrenal gland is androgens. Dehydroepiandrosterone (DHEA), androstenedione, and testosterone are all released into circulation. Excess androgen can originate from either ovarian (PCOS) or adrenal sources.

Addison Disease

DEFINITION

The most common cause of primary adrenal insufficiency is Addison disease.

SYMPTOMS

The signs and symptoms related to the underproduction of cortisol seen in Addison disease are outlined in Table 44.14. Of these, the most common presenting symptoms are fatigue, weakness, and skin hyperpigmentation.

DIAGNOSTIC STUDIES

Initial testing for adrenal insufficiency is a fasting early morning serum cortisol.

TREATMENT/MANAGEMENT

All forms of adrenal insufficiency are treated with glucocorticoid replacement with prednisone, hydrocortisone, or dexamethasone. In addition, fludrocortisones are used to replace mineralocorticoid deficiency (Nieman, 2023a).

Cushing Syndrome

DEFINITION, SCOPE, AND ETIOLOGY

Oversecretion of glucocorticoids is known as Cushing syndrome. The most common presentation (65%–70%) is due to oversecretion of ACTH by a pituitary adenoma and is eight times more likely to occur in women. The increased amplitude and duration of ACTH secretion usually results in bilateral hyperplasia of the adrenal gland, leading to increased secretion of adrenocortical hormones and androgens.

TABLE 44.14 Comparison of Addison Disease and Cushing Syndrome

TARGET	ADDISON DISEASE	CUSHING SYNDROME
Liver	↓ Hepatic glucose output and glycogen storage	↑ Hepatic glucose output ↑ Hepatic glycogen stores
Adipose tissue	↓ Adipose tissue ↓ Lipolysis	Central obesity Moon facies, buffalo hump
Muscle	Weakness ↓ Muscle glycogen ↓ Urinary nitrogen excretion	Weakness and wasting ↑ Urinary nitrogen excretion
Plasma glucose	Hypoglycemia ↑ Insulin sensitivity	↓ Insulin sensitivity → diabetes IGT
Hypothalamus, pituitary	Oligomenorrhea	Oligomenorrhea
Kidney Calcium homeostasis Sodium, potassium, ECF	Retardation of bone growth ↓ Growth hormone, ↓ ECF volume Hyponatremia Hyperkalemia	Hypercalciuria, hypokalemic acidosis, secondary hyperthyroidism, retardation of bone growth
Pancreas	Hypoinsulinemia	Hyperinsulinemia
Carrier protein		↓ in total T4
Skin	Hyperpigmentation	Easy bruising, dermal atrophy
Breast		Galactorrhea
Heart	↓ Peripheral resistance Orthostatic hypotension	Hypertension
CNS	Depression ↓ Appetite ↓ Intraocular pressure	Euphoria → Depression ↑ Appetite Sleep disturbance Impaired memory Cataracts, ↑ ocular pressure

↓ = decreased; ↑ = increased; → = leads to; CNS, central nervous system; ECF, extracellular fluid; IGT, impaired glucose tolerance; T4, thyroxine.
Source: Data from Nieman, L. K. (2023a). *Epidemiology and clinical manifestations of Cushing's syndrome. UpToDate. http://www.uptodate.com/contents/epidemiology-and-clinical-manifestations-of-cushings-syndrome;* Nieman, L. K. (2023b). *Treatment of adrenal insufficiency. UpToDate. https://www.uptodate.com/contents/treatment-of-adrenal-insufficiency-in-adults*

SYMPTOMS

As with Addison disease, the effects of Cushing syndrome are manifested throughout the body (Table 44.14). The clinical signs and symptoms depend on the degree and duration of excess of all three steroids secreted in the adrenal gland and vary according to the increases in the different hormones.

Presenting symptoms vary depending on the system involved. Most patients experience fatigue. Changes in menstrual patterns (oligomenorrhea, amenorrhea) often prompt patients to seek evaluation. Over time, problems such as osteoporosis, diabetes, hypertension, and CVD develop.

DIAGNOSTIC STUDIES

The two tests most often used to diagnose Cushing syndrome are 24-hour urine test for free cortisol and the overnight dexamethasone suppression test (Nieman, 2023a).

TREATMENT/MANAGEMENT

Treatment of Cushing syndrome is aimed at the primary cause of the disease and can involve medication, surgery, or irradiation. Treatment goals are threefold: reversal of clinical signs and symptoms, removal of tumors, and avoidance of dependence on medication. While all three goals are important, the first goal takes priority (Nieman, 2023a). Untreated Cushing syndrome is fatal, caused by the hypercortisol state and its complications. Any patient with symptoms suggestive of adrenal disorders requires referral to an endocrine specialist.

HIRSUTISM

Definition, Scope, Etiology, and Risk Factors

Hirsutism, the development of excess body hair in women, can be associated with several disease processes and is present in 5% to 10% of women (Sachdeva, 2010). Of particular interest is its association with PCOS, hyperprolactinemia, and insulin resistance, with PCOS accounting for 80% to 90% of all cases (Talaei et al., 2013). It is most often caused by an increase in secreted or converted free androgens in circulation. It may also be related to certain medications including testosterone, progestin, phenobarbital, phenytoin, and minoxidil. Between 5% and 10% of cases of hirsutism may be due to racial/ethnic differences and is considered normal. Those of Mediterranean descent tend to have more body hair than other ethnic groups.

Symptoms and Evaluation/Assessment

The hair appears in androgen-dependent areas such as the upper lip, chin, chest, lower abdomen, back, and thighs. Assessment is aimed at identifying the reason for the androgen excess. The basic approach is to document the degree of androgen excess as well as exclude any rare yet serious causes such as an androgen-secreting tumor. Abrupt, rapid onset, usually over less than 1 year, as well as onset later in life may be signs of an androgen-secreting tumor. Signs of virilization can signal not only an ovarian tumor but also developing Cushing syndrome. A complete menstrual history that includes age of menarche, regularity of cycle, symptoms of ovulation, and pregnancy history can indicate underlying causes. A complete medication history, including current and past use of medications known to cause hirsutism, is also important.

The physical exam includes evaluation for other signs of hyperandrogenism such as seborrhea, alopecia, and acne. Any signs of virilization are noted and described (Bode et al., 2012; Sachdeva, 2010).

Diagnostic Studies

Several laboratory tests are ordered to help establish the cause and rule out various syndromes associated with hyperandrogenism (Table 44.15). Total and bioavailable testosterone levels are usually elevated and provide a diagnosis of androgen excess. Serum 17-hydroxyprogesterone should be evaluated if congenital adrenal hyperplasia is suspected. If the patient presents with signs of Cushing syndrome, 24-hour urine free cortisol should be measured. An elevated DHEA-S level suggests an adrenal source and can signal an adrenal tumor; if present, evaluation for a tumor is done using CT, MRI, and/or US. Pelvic US should be performed if ovarian mass or PCOS is suspected. Serum TSH should be measured and will be elevated in hirsutism (Bode et al., 2012; Sachdeva, 2010).

Treatment/Management

Management of the disorders that cause hirsutism is discussed in the pertaining chapter sections. The focus of management is cosmetic and encompasses two approaches: hair removal and suppression of hair growth. Shaving, topical depilatories, waxing, laser treatment, and electrolysis are options for reducing hair growth. Medications, including eflornithine hydrochloride cream 13.9% (Vaniqa cream) and oral spironolactone, can also be used. There is some evidence

TABLE 44.15 Laboratory Findings With Hyperandrogenism

CAUSE	FINDING
Cushing syndrome	↑ Cortisol level Dexamethasone suppression: negative
Adrenal tumor	↑ Testosterone and DHEA level
Ovarian tumor	↑ Testosterone level DHEA level low
Hyperprolactinemia	↑ Prolactin level
Insulin resistance	↑ Glucose ↑ Lipids ↑ Insulin
PCOS	LH/FSH ratio ↑ 3 ↑ Insulin
Idiopathic	Normal laboratory findings

↓ = decreased; ↑ = increased; DHEA, dehydroepiandrosterone; FSH, follicle-stimulating hormone; LH, luteinizing hormone; PCOS, polycystic ovary syndrome.
Source: Data from Sachdeva, S. (2010). Hirsutism evaluation and treatment. Indian Journal of Dermatology, 55(1), 3–7. https://doi.org/10.4103/0019-5154.60342; Talaei, A., Adgi, Z., & Mohamadi Kelishadi, M. (2013). Idiopathic hirsutism and insulin resistance. International Journal of Endocrinology, 2013, 593197. https://doi .org/10.1155/2013/593197

that hormonal contraception can suppress adrenal production of androgens.

FUTURE DIRECTIONS

The endocrine system is complex and affects multiple other body systems. Problems can affect patients in multiple ways, and often the presentation for a single problem varies from one patient to another. A careful history and physical exam coupled with appropriate diagnostic studies assist with identifying the most likely diagnosis and developing an appropriate evidence-based management plan. Future research will provide additional information for identification and treatment of these problems in patients across a variety of orientations.

REFERENCES

References for this chapter are online and available at https://connect.springerpub.com/content/book/978-0-8261-6722-4/part/part03/chapter/ch44

CHAPTER 45

Chronic Illness and Women

Tara Fernandez Bertulfo, Annette Jakubisin-Konicki, Jennifer Wright, and Versie Johnson-Mallard

Six in ten Americans live with at least one chronic disease, heart disease and stroke, cancer, or diabetes. These and other chronic diseases are the leading causes of death and disability in America, and they are also a leading driver of health care costs.

—Centers for Disease Control and Prevention
(CDC, n.d.-c, para. 1).

Several chronic diseases disproportionately affect women. It is important to monitor for chronic health concerns and follow current best practices for managing chronic conditions. With careful management, the negative effects of chronic conditions can be reduced. Assisting women to attend to their health and maximize their wellness requires skill as many women put their own health needs after those of their family members (see Chapter 11, Well Women's Health).

DEFINITION AND SCOPE

Chronic disease is defined broadly as a condition that lasts 1 year or longer and requires ongoing medical care or limits activities of daily living (CDC, n.d.-a). Chronic diseases are prevalent in the United States and are a significant cause of death and disability. This trend is a dramatic break from the past when infectious disease and trauma were the primary causes of death and disease. In 2018, 51.8% of U.S. adults (or 129 million) had at least one chronic condition, and 27.2% (68 million) had multiple chronic conditions. Prevalence was highest among women, non-Hispanic White adults, adults age 65 or older, and those living in rural areas (Boersma et al., 2020). Seven of the top 10 causes of death in 2010 were chronic diseases (CDC, 2012). Two of these chronic diseases—heart disease and cancer—together accounted for nearly 48% of all deaths (CDC, 2014).

The risk of chronic disease increases in women of child-bearing age who have certain pregnancy complications. Gestational diabetes increases a woman's risk of cardiovascular disease by 68% and increases the risk of type 2 diabetes after pregnancy by 10-fold. Hypertension in pregnancy increases the risk of cardiovascular disease later in life by 67% and increases the odds of a stroke by 83% (American Heart Association, 2021). The risk of developing a chronic disease also increases with age. Thus, increased longevity has resulted in the increased prevalence of many chronic diseases (Atella et al., 2019). Chronic conditions such as diabetes, obesity, osteoporosis, osteoarthritis (OA), and cardiovascular disease can affect all aspects of a woman's life.

According to data from the 2018 National Health Interview Survey (NHIS), women are more likely than men to have two or more chronic conditions. These data (shown in Table 45.1) are categorized by sex, ethnicity, age, and insurance status. The possible chronic conditions were arthritis, cancer, chronic obstructive pulmonary disease (COPD), coronary heart disease, current asthma, diabetes, hepatitis, hypertension, stroke, and weak/failing kidneys.

The National Center for Health Statistics (NCHS) most recent report in *Morbidity Mortality Weekly Report*, published in 2022, tracks the prevalence of selected chronic conditions; the 2019 data regarding women 18 years of age and older are presented in Table 45.2. Among common conditions are obesity, arthritis, high blood pressure, high cholesterol, and asthma (Watson et al., 2022).

The NCHS is the principal source of information on the health of the civilian noninstitutionalized population of the United States and is one of the major data collection programs of the Centers for Disease Control and Prevention (CDC). A wide range of questions about health and health practices are asked in the survey, which is available on the CDC website.

ETIOLOGY

The cause, or etiology, of a chronic disease is typically multifactorial. These factors might be the physical, social, and psychological environment; biology and genetics, including sex; lifestyle and associated risks; or a combination of the factors (Fish, 2008; Pennell et al., 2012). There may also be a long stage of subclinical disease during which the disease process has begun yet symptoms have not yet appeared.

Multiple factors may interact and combine in specific ways to place the individual at higher risk for developing disease than if a single factor were present alone. For example, an obese woman who smokes is at greater risk for developing

TABLE 45.1 Percentage and Number of U.S. Adults Ages 18 Years or Older With Chronic Conditions, by Select Characteristics, 2018

CHARACTERISTIC	1 CHRONIC CONDITION		≥2 CHRONIC CONDITIONS	
	% POPULATION (95% CI)	*N*	% POPULATION (95% CI)	*N*
TOTAL 249 MILLION PEOPLE				
Male	24.6 (23.9–25.3)	61,371	27.2 (26.5–27.9)	67,854
Female	24.8 (23.9–25.7)	32,025	28.4 (27.5–29.4)	36,679
Non-Hispanic White	25.6 (24.8–26.4)	40,248	30.6 (29.7–31.6)	48,202
Non-Hispanic Black	25.4 (23.3–27.6)	7,390	27.0 (25.0–29.1)	7,855
Other	21.6 (19.0–24.4)	3,280	16.4 (14.0–19.0)	2,486
Age				
18–44 years	20.7 (19.7–21.8)	23,841	6.7 (6.1–7.3)	7,723
45–64 years	30.4 (29.2–31.6)	25,250	33.0 (31.7–34.3)	27,383
≥65 years	23.9 (22.7–25.1)	12,280	63.7 (62.3–65.1)	32,748
AGE 18–64 YRS			**INSURANCE STATUS**	
Private	25.7 (24.7–26.7)	35,065	15.7 (14.9–16.5)	21,418
Public	23.4 (21.4–25.5)	5,830	27.6 (25.5–29.9)	6,886
Uninsured	21.6 (19.4–23.9)	5,511	11.6 (10.1–13.2)	2,995
AGES 65 YRS AND OLDER			**INSURANCE STATUS**	
Private	24.4 (22.6–26.3)	5,190	63.2 (61.2–65.3)	13,451
Dual eligible	16.4 (13.0–20.1)	577	76.9 (72.5–80.8)	2,713
Medicare Advantage and Medicare only	25.2 (22.9–28.9)	5,320	58.5 (54.8–62.1)	12,902
Urban	24.5 (23.7–25.2)	53,125	26.1 (25.3–26.9)	56,577
Rural	25.5 (23.8–27.2)	8,246	34.8 (32.8–37.0)	11,277

Note: Numbers may not sum to group totals because of rounding.
Source: Adapted from Boersma, P., Black, L. I., & Ward, B. W. (2020). Prevalence of multiple chronic conditions among US adults, 2018. Preventing Chronic Disease, 17, E106. https://doi.org/10.5888/pcd17.200130

cardiovascular disease than an obese woman who is not a smoker. The cumulative effect of these factors increases the individual's risk for developing a chronic disease.

Chronic illness trajectory refers to the overall course of a person's experience because of the illness over time. This trajectory can describe not only pathologic changes but also other aspects of the disease such as symptom experience, physical functioning, quality of life, social or role performance, and other variables (CDC, 2021a, 2021b). Each aspect of the disease progression is considered an outcome; its trajectory can be monitored.

Unlike acute conditions, which are often self-limiting, chronic conditions are generally not easily curable or self-limiting. A chronic disease can vary over time, sometimes transiently improving, often worsening. Chronic diseases can be ongoing such as diabetes, or they can be recurring, such as

with depression. The course of a specific illness depends on the characteristics of the condition (e.g., relapsing, episodic), characteristics of the individual (e.g., age, gender), and psychological, family, and sociocultural factors.

Healthcare providers can use the concept of illness trajectory to identify and understand the specific needs of patients and families as the patient moves along the continuum of chronic illness. It is useful for providers to have a general understanding of the usual course of a disease. The patient and provider can then compare the patient's course of the disease with the usual progression. If the disease is characterized by general deterioration, then slowing the progression of the disease represents a major therapeutic success. On the other hand, if the patient's disease is progressing faster than is typical, this could invoke analysis and redesign of the treatment plan. More data are needed regarding the typical progression

TABLE 45.2 Number and Percent of Any and Specific Chronic Conditions Reported by Adults Ages 18–34 Years, by Selected Characteristics—Behavioral Risk Factor Surveillance System, United States, 2019

CHARACTERISTICS	NO.	CHRONIC CONDITIONS, % POPULATION (95% CI)								
		ANY CHRONIC CONDITION	OBESITY	DEPRESSION	HIGH BLOOD PRESSURE	HIGH CHOLESTEROL	ASTHMA	ARTHRITIS	OTHER
Overall	67,104	53.8 (53.1–54.5)	25.5 (24.9–26.1)	21.3 (20.8–21.8)	10.7 (10.3–11.1)	9.8 (9.3–10.2)	9.2 (8.9–9.6)	5.9 (5.6–6.2)	7.4 (7.1–7.8)
Age group, years									
18–24	24,411	48.7 (47.6–49.8)	19.4 (18.5–20.3)	22.0 (21.2–22.9)	7.9 (7.3–8.4)	7.2 (6.6–7.9)	10.3 (9.7–10.9)	3.5 (3.2–3.9)	5.5 (5.0–6.1)
25–34	42,693	57.3 (56.5–58.2)	29.8 (29.0–30.5)	20.8 (20.2–21.4)	12.7 (12.2–13.2)	11.6 (11.0–12.2)	8.5 (8.1–9.0)	7.5 (7.1–7.9)	8.7 (8.2–9.2)
Women	31,973	57.7 (56.7–58.7)	27.9 (27.0–28.8)	27.0 (26.2–27.9)	7.8 (7.4–8.3)	9.6 (8.9–10.3)	11.5 (11.0–12.1)	6.9 (6.5–7.4)	8.4 (7.9–9.0)

Source: Adapted from Watson, K. B., Carlson, S. A., Loustalot, F., Town, M., Eke, P. I., Thomas, C. W., & Greenlund, K. J. (2022). Chronic conditions among adults aged 18–34 years—United States, 2019. MMWR Morbidity and Mortality Weekly Report, 71, 964–970. https://doi.org/10.15585/mmwr.mm7130a3

of the multiple outcomes of common chronic diseases so that providers and patients can evaluate the success of the treatment regimen.

TREATMENT/MANAGEMENT OF CHRONIC ILLNESS

Unlike acute care, in which the goal of treatment is typically to cure, in chronic care, the goal is to manage the disease and help the patient cope with its effects. In chronic care, an ideal outcome might be that the disease stabilizes, and the patient achieves a "new normal." Often this is a state of being in which the patient learns to function at a new normal and to accept the illness as a part of their life.

The effects of chronic disease on the individual are often substantial, affecting physical health, physical functioning, symptom experience, quality of life, and social and role performance. Chronic diseases such as diabetes, heart failure, hypertension, arthritis, and lung disease are associated with significant underlying pathology. Factors related to the disease itself, such as the type of organ damage, disease severity, treatment regimen, personal factors (such as individual coping ability), and social support, can influence whether the chronic disease is associated with altered physical functioning or disability. Chronic conditions frequently cause disabling symptoms such as pain and fatigue and may have a profound influence on the individual and their family. These factors are considered in managing the patient.

The term *chronic disease* invokes the pathologic manifestations of the disease. However, because the effects of the disease are generally much broader, the term *chronic illness* is used to refer to the individual's experience with the disease. Clinicians and researchers are increasingly aware of the influence of the individual's experience with the disease on its course and outcomes. Therefore, in this chapter, aspects of both the chronic disease and the experience of having this disease are addressed. For similar reasons, treatment is referred to as *chronic care*, not chronic disease care.

Goals of chronic care include slowing the rate of decline due to the disease, reducing the frequency of disease exacerbations or complications, mitigating the functional impairment, maximizing the quality of life, reducing hospitalizations, and maintaining a sense of normalcy. Chronic care services also address the woman's experience of the disease, the impact of the disease on her daily life and functioning, and the suffering caused by the disease. Chronic care requires significant emphasis on health promotion, to slow or reverse the progression of the disease.

The care paradigm for chronic disease is very different from that for an acute medical problem. When a patient presents with an acute problem such as a fractured bone, the clinician, the expert, provides direct and immediate interventions to correct or cure the underlying problem and treat the related symptoms. The patient receives the care, often somewhat passively. With chronic care, the ideal circumstance involves the patient partnering with her clinician to design and implement a plan of care. This plan incorporates biological disease management with health promotion to slow disease progression.

The plan of care includes supportive services such as counseling related to diet, exercise, lifestyle, and self-care. Psychological care services may be required to assist in the adjustment to the condition. In addition, women frequently use complementary and alternative approaches to healthcare, and these approaches should be integrated into the plan of care.

In individuals who are well, self-care focuses on self-improvement. In chronic illness, self-care is a fundamental and integral part of treatment and women who engage in self-care have significantly improved clinical outcomes, with better quality of life, fewer hospitalizations, and longer survival (Jonkman et al., 2016). The patient lives with her illness and sees the clinician only occasionally and then typically for brief visits. The patient must monitor her condition on a day-to-day basis and recognize deterioration or improvement. It is important to educate patients on how to prepare for the clinician encounter, so that they can take an active role in monitoring, managing, and decision-making. Patient-centered care mandates that the patient be the primary decision-maker in managing the disease and its effects. Therefore, chronic care requires developing skills in decision counseling and decision support. The clinician can make recommendations based on science and experience regarding surgical or medical and pharmaceutical treatments; the well-informed patient will be able to choose among the options based on her own analysis.

Women with chronic illness live with symptoms and disabilities that they often must manage for their lifetime and that require collaborative partnerships with clinicians to assist them in integrating self-care into their daily activities. This requires that clinicians are not only knowledgeable about managing medical treatment regimens but also able to provide emotional and intangible support, including ongoing patient and family education and counseling.

Caring for a woman with a chronic illness necessitates caring for her family as well. Chronic illness changes family members' roles, responsibilities, and boundaries, especially when the traditional caregiver, the woman, is the one who is ill. It can disrupt her self-image and self-esteem. It can result in uncertain and unpredictable futures. Moreover, it can trigger distressing emotions—anxiety, depression, resentment, and feelings of helplessness, as well as illness-related factors such as permanent changes in physical appearance or bodily functioning.

A woman who is chronically ill may feel guilty about the demands that her illness makes on the family. She may resent the change in roles and responsibilities caused by the limitations imposed by the illness, and she must deal with the threat to her role autonomy (Lawrence, 2012).

The management of symptoms and prognosis is the focus of individuals living with chronic disease. However, supporting families with chronic illness is a critical concern for all healthcare providers. While the care of the individual with the illness is essential, the care of the family must be simultaneously addressed. To support the struggle that families experience, simply recognizing the issues openly may be what is needed. In this manner, the woman's family can use their own interactions to situate the illness within the evolving family and best identify their own strategies for accomplishing family goals (Eggenberger et al., 2011). Including care directed at family processes may have profound effects on individual and family outcomes because individual health and family health are interdependent (Eggenberger et al., 2011). To facilitate women's coping with chronic illness, clinicians need to consider the various types, sources, and benefits of support available. The COVID-19 pandemic was profound for individuals with chronic conditions. It is unknown at the time of publication of this chapter how COVID-19 exacerbates chronic disease (Hacker et al., 2021).

SELECTED CHRONIC ILLNESSES

Chronic Obstructive Pulmonary Disease

DEFINITION AND SCOPE

COPD is often referred to as a man's disease. However, COPD is among the leading causes of death in the United States. The number of women who die from COPD exceeds that of men. In the United States about 15 million people report having been diagnosed with COPD (CDC, 2021a, 2021b).

ETIOLOGY, RISK FACTORS

COPD is a common, preventable, and treatable disease characterized by persistent airflow limitation that is usually progressive and associated with an enhanced chronic inflammatory response in the airways and the lungs to noxious particles or gases (CDC, 2021a, 2021b; Global Initiative for Chronic Obstructive Lung Disease [GOLD], 2015; Watson et al., 2022). Risk factors associated with COPD include tobacco smoke, indoor and outdoor pollution, and occupational dusts and chemicals.

SYMPTOMS

Symptoms of COPD include dyspnea, chronic cough, and chronic sputum production.

EVALUATION/ASSESSMENT

Clinical physical findings in COPD may include the following: prolonged forced expiratory time, tachypnea, cyanosis, tachycardia, end-expiratory wheezes on forced expiration, decreased breath sounds, and/or inspiratory crackles, hyperresonance on percussion, and signs of cor pulmonale.

DIAGNOSTIC TESTING

To make a clinical diagnosis of COPD, spirometry is required. To diagnose COPD, the ratio between forced expiratory volume (FEV_1) and forced vital capacity (FVC) is determined; $FEV_1/$FVC <0.70 confirms the presence of persistent airflow limitation.

TREATMENT/MANAGEMENT

With the growing burden of COPD among women, understanding the clinical presentation and providing access to care are important (Aryal et al., 2014; Martinez et al., 2012). Smoking cessation is one of the most important interventions that can potentially slow COPD disease progression. FEV_1 decreases by approximately 25 to 30 mL/year starting at age 35 years; however, the rate of decline is faster (threefold to fourfold) in smokers.

Pharmacologic treatment is used to reduce symptoms and the frequency and severity of exacerbations. Medications include bronchodilators, inhaled corticosteroids, or combination inhaled corticosteroid/bronchodilator therapy and preventive vaccines. Nonpharmacologic treatments include oxygen therapy and pulmonary rehabilitation. Oxygen therapy has been shown to improve survival and quality of life in patients with COPD and chronic hypoxemia. Pulmonary rehabilitation improves functional status and quality of life.

Asthma

DEFINITION AND SCOPE, ETIOLOGY

Asthma refers to a disorder of variable expiratory airflow obstruction that arises in association with symptoms of wheezing, cough, and dyspnea. Inflammation of the airways may increase airway responsiveness that allows triggers to initiate bronchoconstriction. Asthma causes increased mucus secretions that can occlude the airway.

Asthma is one of the leading chronic conditions in the United States. It has marked health disparities, especially in older women, in whom the highest mortality rate is seen (Pate et al., 2021). In women above 65 years of age, the death rate is approximately four times higher than the overall mean rate (Pate et al., 2021).

RISK FACTORS

Hormones may explain the increased risk for asthma among women. Estrogen and progesterone affect airway caliber and asthma exacerbations. Postmenopausal women taking hormone therapy (HT) have a 2.24-fold increase in asthma diagnosis as compared with women not taking HT (Barr et al., 2004).

EVALUATION/ASSESSMENT

Patients presenting with asthma may have the following clinical findings: tachypnea, nasal flaring, tachycardia, hyperresonance, prolonged expiration, wheezing, diminished lung sounds, sputum production, and nocturnal cough and wheezing. The lung exam often reveals diminished airflow with wheezing as a major characteristic. Diagnosis is made based on recurrence of symptoms, and the severity of disease is determined based on symptoms.

DIFFERENTIAL DIAGNOSES

Asthma is differentiated from other chronic restrictive airway diseases such as reactive airway, COPD, and chronic bronchitis.

DIAGNOSTIC TESTING

Pulmonary function studies, pre- and postbronchodilator, are the main diagnostic tests used to identify asthma. Women also use peak flow meters to monitor their respiratory function and guide self-care (see Treatment/Management section).

TREATMENT/MANAGEMENT

During the initial visit for asthma, severity is determined, and a treatment/action plan is established. Follow-up visits include reassessment of symptoms and adjustment of the management plan as needed (Figure 45.1). Medications used to manage asthma include rescue inhalers and inhaled corticosteroids. Identification and avoidance of triggers that cause

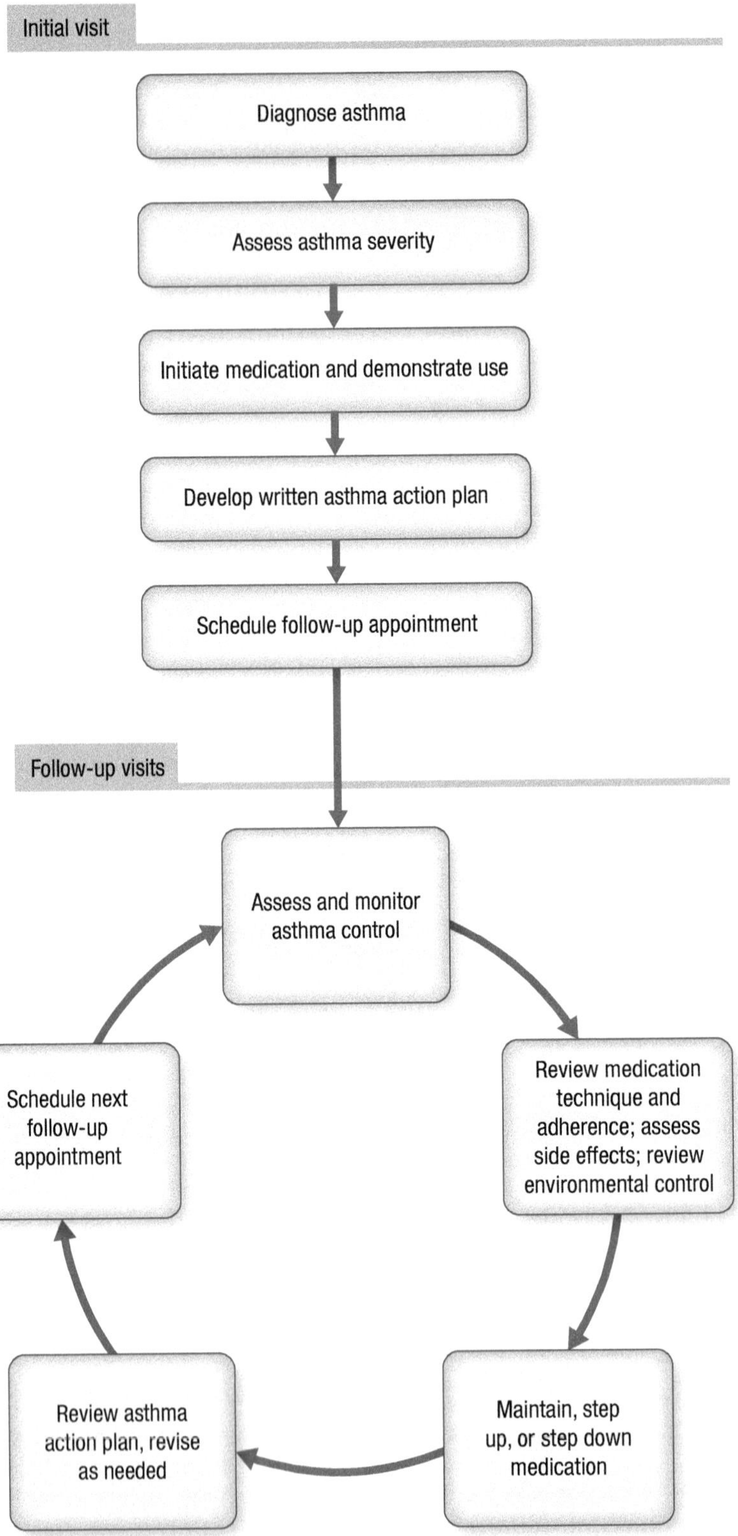

Initial visit

Diagnose asthma

Assess asthma severity

Initiate medication and demonstrate use

Develop written asthma action plan

Schedule follow-up appointment

Follow-up visits

Assess and monitor asthma control

Review medication technique and adherence; assess side effects; review environmental control

Maintain, step up, or step down medication

Review asthma action plan, revise as needed

Schedule next follow-up appointment

FIGURE 45.1 Asthma management.
Source: Adapted from National Heart, Lung, and Blood Institute. (2012). Asthma care quick reference: Diagnosing and managing asthma. National Institutes of Health. https://www.nhlbi.nih.gov /files/docs/guidelines/asthma_qrg.pdf

Level of severity (Columns 2–5) is determined by events listed in Column 1 for both impairment (frequency and intensity of symptoms and functional limitations) and risk (of exacerbations). Assess impairment by patient's or caregiver's recall of events during the previous 2–4 weeks; assess risk over the last year. Recommendations for initiating therapy based on level of severity are presented in the last row.

Components of Severity	Intermittent Ages 0–4 years	Intermittent Ages 5–11 years	Intermittent Ages ≥12 years	Mild Ages 0–4 years	Mild Ages 5–11 years	Mild Ages ≥12 years	Moderate Ages 0–4 years	Moderate Ages 5–11 years	Moderate Ages ≥12 years	Severe Ages 0–4 years	Severe Ages 5–11 years	Severe Ages ≥12 years
Impairment												
Symptoms	≤2 days/week	≤2 days/week	≤2 days/week	>2 days/week but not daily	>2 days/week but not daily	>2 days/week but not daily	Daily	Daily	Daily	Throughout the day	Throughout the day	Throughout the day
Nighttime awakenings	0	≤2x/month	≤2x/month	1–2x/month	3–4x/month	3–4x/month	3–4x/month	>1x/week	>1x/week but not nightly	>1x/week	Often 7x/week	Often 7x/week
SABA* use for symptom control (not to prevent EIB*)	≤2 days/week	≤2 days/week	≤2 days/week	>2 days/week but not daily	>2 days/week but not daily and not more than once on any day	>2 days/week but not daily and not more than once on any day	Daily	Daily	Daily	Several times per day	Several times per day	Several times per day
Interference with normal activity	None	None	None	Minor limitation	Minor limitation	Minor limitation	Some limitation	Some limitation	Some limitation	Extremely limited	Extremely limited	Extremely limited
Lung function ↑ FEV₁* (% predicted)	Not applicable	>80%	Normal FEV₁ between exacerbations >80%	Not applicable	>80%	>80%	Not applicable	60–80%	60–80%	Not applicable	<60%	<60%
↑ FEV₁/FVC*		>85%	Normal†		>80%	Normal†		75–80%	Reduced 5%†		<75%	Reduced >5%†
Risk												
Asthma exacerbations requiring oral systemic corticosteroids‡	0–1/year	0–1/year	0–1/year	≥2 exacerb. in 6 months, or wheezing ≥4x per year lasting >1 day AND risk factors for persistent asthma	≥2/year	≥2/year						
Recommended Step for Initiating Therapy (See "Stepwise Approach for Managing Asthma Long Term," page 7)	Step 1	Step 1	Step 1	Step 2	Step 2	Step 2	Step 3	Step 3 medium-dose ICS* option	Step 3	Step 3	Step 3 medium-dose ICS* option or Step 4	Step 4 or 5

Generally, more frequent and intense events indicate greater severity.

Generally, more frequent and intense events indicate greater severity. Frequency and severity may fluctuate over time for patients in any severity category.

Relative annual risk of exacerbations may be related to FEV₁*.

Consider severity and interval since last asthma exacerbation.

Consider short course of oral systemic corticosteroids.

The stepwise approach is meant to help, not replace, the clinical decisionmaking needed to meet individual patient needs.

In 2–6 weeks, depending on severity, assess level of asthma control achieved and adjust therapy as needed. For children 0–4 years old, if no clear benefit is observed in 4–6 weeks, consider adjusting therapy or alternate diagnoses.

FIGURE 45.2 Classification of asthma severity.

*EIB, exercise-induced bronchospam; FEV, forced expiratory volume in 1 second; FVC, forced vital capacity; ICS, inhaled corticosteroid; SABA, short-acting beta₂-agonist.

†Normal FEV₁/FVC by age: 8–19 years, 85%; 20–39 years, 80%; 40–59 years, 75%; 60–80 years, 70%.

‡Data are insufficient to link frequencies of exacerbations with different levels of asthma severity. Generally, more frequent and intense exacerbations (e.g., requiring urgent care, hospital or intensive care admission, and/or oral corticosteroids) indicate greater underlying disease severity. For treatment purposes, patients with ≥2 exacerbations may be considered to have persistent asthma, even in the absence of impairment levels consistent with persistent asthma.

Source: National Heart, Lung, and Blood Institute. (2012). Asthma care quick reference: Diagnosing and managing asthma. National Institutes of Health. http://www.nhlbi.nih.gov/files/docs/guidelines/asthma_qrg.pdf

exacerbations are important, such as smoking cessation. Medications are prescribed in a stepwise manner based on symptom severity (see Figure 45.2). When symptoms are increasing, the woman uses a peak flow meter to determine how limited her airflow has become (Willems et al., 2006). Short-acting bronchodilators are used, preferably with a spacer, to relieve symptoms and to reopen her airways. If home care is unsuccessful, she is educated to seek clinical care. Women are encouraged during pregnancy to continue use of medication even though safety data is limited (Pate et al., 2021).

Celiac Disease

DEFINITION, ETIOLOGY, AND SYMPTOMS

Celiac disease (CD), also called celiac sprue, nontropical sprue, and gluten-sensitive enteropathy, is a common chronic condition caused by an inflammatory response to ingestion of gluten proteins. In CD, the effect of gluten causes atrophy of the villi of the small intestine, which may lead to nutrient malabsorption. The presenting symptoms are a wide array of gastrointestinal (GI) manifestations including diarrhea, weight loss, and malabsorption.

CD occurs at the same frequency in both sexes; however, women are diagnosed more frequently than men (2:1). Unfortunately, women report a lower quality of life (Choung et al., 2017; Lebwohl et al., 2018). The prevalence of CD was as high in first- and second-degree relatives without symptoms as in relatives with symptoms, highlighting the importance of genetic predisposition as a risk factor for CD (Choung et al., 2017; Lebwohl et al., 2018). Black patients are less frequently diagnosed.

DIFFERENTIAL DIAGNOSIS

Differential diagnosis for CD includes Crohn disease, ulcerative colitis (UC), tropical sprue, Zollinger–Ellison syndrome, autoimmune enteropathy, T-cell lymphoma, and combined immunodeficiency states.

DIAGNOSTIC STUDIES

Initial diagnostic testing for CD includes serologic studies while the woman is on a gluten-containing diet. The two initial tests are immunoglobulin A (IgA) and anti-tissue transglutaminase (tTG). If CD is the primary working diagnosis, an endoscopy with intestinal biopsy should be performed regardless of the serologic test results. Although genetic testing may be performed, it should be saved for patients with atypical presentation of the disease (Choung et al., 2017; Lebwohl et al., 2018).

TREATMENT/MANAGEMENT

The gold standard of treatment for CD is nutritional consultation to guide the complete elimination of gluten from the diet. Glutens are the components found in rye, wheat, and barley grains. Patients are taught how to read food labels and to request gluten-free options when dining out (Choung et al., 2017; Lebwohl et al., 2018). Table 45.3 lists common gluten-free and gluten-containing foods.

Inflammatory Bowel Disease

DEFINITION AND SCOPE

Inflammatory bowel disease (IBD), not to be confused with irritable bowel syndrome (IBS), describes chronic autoimmune diseases that cause inflammation of the GI tract. The two chronic diseases in this category are UC and Crohn disease. IBD is commonly diagnosed during women's reproductive years.

ETIOLOGY

While ongoing inflammation in the GI tract occurs in both Crohn disease and UC, there are important differences between the two diseases (Crohn's & Colitis Foundation, n.d.). UC is a chronic, recurrent disease characterized by diffuse mucosal inflammation of the colon. Crohn disease is a chronic, recurrent disease characterized by patchy, transmural inflammation of any part of the GI mucosa from the mouth to the anus. IBD is a lifelong illness with profound psychosocial, emotional, and economic impacts.

RISK FACTORS

Use of hormonal contraceptives by women with IBD may increase disease relapse and risk of other adverse health outcomes, including thrombosis. Additionally, IBD-related malabsorption might interfere with the effectiveness of oral contraceptives. Women should consider highly effective, first-line contraceptive methods, such as an IUD or implant, to avoid contraceptive failure and an unintended pregnancy when their disease may be more active (Gawron, 2018).

TABLE 45.3 Gluten-Containing and Gluten-Free Foods

GLUTEN–FREE FOODS		FOODS CONTAINING GLUTEN		CHECK THE LABEL
Amaranth	Glucose syrup	Barley	Malt	Dextrin made from wheat
Arrowroot	Herbs	Some flavorings added to foods	Seitan	Tofu
Buckwheat	Lecithin	Gluten	Teriyaki sauce	
Citric acid	Maltodextrin	Guar gum	Triticale	
Corn	Millet Montina Quinoa Yeast	Hydrolyzed vegetable protein	Wheat—bulgur, durum, einkorn, farina, graham, kamut, semolina, and spelt	

Source: Adapted from Gluten-Free Living. (2013). Ingredients index. https://www.glutenfreeliving.com/ingredient.php

SYMPTOMS, EVALUATION/ASSESSMENT

Patients with IBD can present with a variety of symptoms that need to be differentiated from other GI diseases as well as differentiated between UC and Crohn disease. Patients with mild UC present with frequent loose bowel movements associated with cramping; often there is blood and mucus in the stool. With more severe UC, the patient experiences more frequent stools (more than 10 per day and often at night) and more blood and mucus in the stool. The patient could have tachycardia, fever, weight loss, and signs of undernutrition such as hypoproteinemia and peripheral edema.

The patient with Crohn disease commonly presents with abdominal cramping and tenderness, fever, anorexia, weight loss, and pain. There may be intermittent blood loss in the stool. The loss of mucosa could be sufficient to interfere with bile salt absorption, producing steatorrhea. If the bowel perforates, peritonitis will occur.

TREATMENT/MANAGEMENT

Treatment for IBD is multifaceted and includes the use of medication, alterations in diet and nutrition, and sometimes surgical procedures to repair or remove affected portions of the GI tract. Aminosalicylates (5-ASA) and corticosteroids are usually the first line of treatment for IBD. If these treatments are unsuccessful, an immunomodulator or biological treatment such as a tumor necrosis factor (TNF) blocker may be indicated as an ongoing treatment to decrease the inflammatory response and ideally achieve remission. In addition, because stress is often associated with IBD "flares," methods of stress reduction and relaxation such as meditation or yoga are often prescribed.

RHEUMATIC DISORDERS

Osteoarthritis

DEFINITION AND SCOPE

OA is the most common form of arthritis and is a common cause of disability among older people. Women have higher rates of OA, and it is more prominent after age 50 years. The presentation may range from incidental asymptomatic findings to a progressively disabling joint disorder.

ETIOLOGY, RISK FACTORS, AND SYMPTOMS

OA of the knee is characterized by degeneration of the articular cartilage, morphologic changes to the subchondral bone, and damage to the surrounding soft tissue (Felson, 2004). These structural changes lead to joint pain, quadriceps muscle weakness, reduced range of motion, joint instability, and poor balance (Baert et al., 2014). As a result, most individuals with symptomatic knee OA report difficulty with walking, stair climbing, rising from a car, or carrying heavy loads. Early in the disease, patients may experience stiffness upon arising, which recedes with activity. As the disease progresses, stiffness and joint pain with movement become more constant. Incidence of OA increases with aging and is more common in those who have family members with the disease.

EVALUATION/ASSESSMENT

The physical exam may reveal joint erythema, warmth, and edema as well as limited range of motion and crepitus. Heberden nodes may be present at the distal interphalangeal joints. Bouchard nodes may be present at the middle interphalangeal joints. In more advanced disease muscle weakness and muscle wasting of the affected joint are apparent (Shorter et al., 2019).

DIFFERENTIAL DIAGNOSIS

The differential diagnosis for joint pain, joint edema, and fatigue includes:

- Infection
- Other connective tissue disorders (e.g., lupus, scleroderma)
- Fibromyalgia
- Rheumatoid arthritis (RA)
- Psoriatic arthritis
- Gout (crystalline arthritis)

DIAGNOSTIC TESTING

OA is usually diagnosed on the clinical presentation of age greater than 45 years, morning stiffness lasting less than 30 minutes, and usage-related persistent joint pain in one or a few joints. X-ray imaging is used when the diagnosis is unclear or other diagnoses or comorbid conditions are being considered (Sakellariou et al., 2017). The x-ray images typically reveal:

- Cartilage loss, joint space narrowing
- Increased bone density at narrowed joint spaces (in response to increased friction with cartilage loss)
- Osteophytes
- Bone erosion

TREATMENT/MANAGEMENT

Management goals for patients with OA are to optimize function, minimize pain, and if possible, to modify the process resulting in joint damage associated with the disease (Nelson et al., 2014). Chronic pain and disability are often associated with OA. Treatment encompasses both nonpharmacologic and pharmacologic approaches. Nonpharmacologic treatment may include weight loss, rest, physical therapy and structured exercise programs, assistive devices (canes, raised toilet seats, and walkers), heat and cold therapy, supportive orthotic shoes, and use of transcutaneous electrical stimulation. Other nonpharmacologic treatments may include participation in non-weight-bearing or low-impact exercise and tai chi programs and treatment with traditional Chinese acupuncture. Pharmacologic recommendations may include the following: topical capsaicin, topical nonsteroidal anti-inflammatory drugs (NSAIDs), and oral NSAIDs, including cyclooxygenase-2 (COX-2) selective inhibitors. Evaluation of intra-articular platelet-rich plasma injections have not been shown to be beneficial in the reduction of pain or altered joint structure for individuals with knee arthritis (Bennell et al., 2021).

Rheumatoid Arthritis

DEFINITION AND SCOPE

RA is a chronic, inflammatory autoimmune disease and is the most common chronic inflammatory polyarticular arthritis,

TABLE 45.4 Classification Criteria for Rheumatoid Arthritis

Target population to be tested should have at least one joint with definite clinical swelling[a] and with the synovitis not better explained by another disease.

CRITERIA	SCORE
A. THE NUMBER AND SIZE OF JOINTS THAT ARE SWOLLEN	
1 Large joint	0
2–10 Large joints	1
1–3 Small joints (with or without involvement of large joints)	2
4–10 Small joints (with or without involvement of large joints)	3
>10 Joints (at least 1 small joint)	5
B. SEROLOGY	
Negative RF and negative ACPA	0
Low-positive RF or low-positive ACPA	2
High-positive RF or high-positive ACPA	3
C. ACUTE PHASE REACTANTS	
Normal CRP and normal ESR	0
Abnormal CRP or abnormal ESR	1
D. DURATION OF SYMPTOMS	
<6 weeks	0
<6 weeks	1

Scoring: Add score of categories A–D; a score of ≥6/10 is needed for classification of a patient as having definite RA.
[a]The criteria are aimed at classification of newly presenting patients. In addition, patients with erosive disease typical of RA with a history compatible with prior fulfillment of the 2010 criteria should be classified as having RA. Patients with long-standing disease, including those whose disease is inactive (with or without treatment) and who, based on retrospectively available data, have previously fulfilled the 2010 criteria should be classified as having RA.
ACPA, antibodies to citrullinated protein antigens; CRP, C-reactive protein; ESR, erythrocyte sedimentation rate; RA, rheumatoid arthritis; RF, rheumatoid factor.
Source: Republished with permission from John Wiley & Sons, Inc., from Arthritis & Rheumatism *by American College of Rheumatology; American Rheumatism Association; Arthritis Foundation; permission conveyed through Copyright Clearance Center, Inc.*

with a preferential involvement of the small joints. It is a systemic illness and if insufficiently treatment may evolve to include extra-articular manifestations and may involve other organ systems of the body (Aletaha & Smolen, 2018). RA is two times more common in women than in men (Hunter et al., 2017).

ETIOLOGY

The exact cause of RA is unknown. It is thought to be a process involving the influence of complex environmental, genetic, immunologic factors that trigger adaptive responses associated with autoimmunity, resulting the development and expression of the disease (Aletaha & Smolen, 2018). The microbiome is also thought to be a potential trigger, driving autoimmune joint disease processes (Manfredo Vieira et al., 2018; Pianta et al., 2017).

RISK FACTORS

Risk factors for RA include female gender, middle age (onset usually occurs between 40 and 60 years of age), family history of RA, smoking, environmental exposures, obesity,

geographic area, and race/ethnicity (Aletaha & Smolen, 2018; Cross et al., 2014).

SYMPTOMS

The most common symptoms of arthritis include pain, fatigue, joint deformity, stiffness, and swelling. Symptoms of pain, joint swelling, and fatigue are intermittent and can be severe, debilitating, and unpredictable, and often curb function and limit daily life (De Cock et al., 2014).

Women with arthritis must deal with an uncertain prognosis, medical regimen, and multiple losses—a loss in mobility, the inability to work, and an altered self-identity due in part to a changed bodily appearance; changes in leisure activities frequently accompany RA.

DIAGNOSIS OF RHEUMATOID ARTHRITIS: CLASSIFICATION CRITERIA

The American College of Rheumatology (ACR) and the European League Against Rheumatism (EULAR) worked together to develop the 2010 Rheumatoid Arthritis Classification Criteria for RA (Aletaha et al., 2010; Table 45.4).

TREATMENT/MANAGEMENT

RA treatment is focused on timely, early use of therapeutic interventions to arrest disease progression and reduce disability. Ongoing care coordination by a rheumatologist has shown better outcomes in those with RA (Smolen et al., 2020). As with OA, both nonpharmacologic and pharmacologic approaches are important. Nonpharmacologic approaches may include occupational therapy, physical therapy, modifying the home environment, and so forth. Pharmacologic management includes disease-modifying antirheumatic drugs (DMARDs) and medications to manage pain.

Systemic Lupus Erythematosus

DEFINITION AND SCOPE

Systemic lupus erythematosus (SLE) is an autoimmune disease affecting virtually any organ with immunologic and clinical manifestations. The disease affects the skin, joints, kidneys, blood cells, and nervous system (Cervera et al., 2009). Greater than 90% of patients with SLE will present with arthralgias and arthritis as one of the earliest manifestations (Corzo et al., 2020). Once thought to be a disease striking reproductive age women, the onset has been noted to be diagnosed in women older 50 years of age. The later age of onset affects the clinical presentation, disease course, response to treatment, and prognosis of SLE. Newly diagnosed patients have increased anxieties about fatal chronic illness with unpredictable flares and potential disability.

SYMPTOMS AND EVALUATION/ASSESSMENT

There is heterogeneity to the clinical presentations of SLE requiring a comprehensive initial evaluation of both the history and physical examination. SLE may present with a butterfly-shaped rash on the face at onset in approximately 30% of the cases, whereas fatigue and arthritis or arthralgia is present at onset in greater than 50% (Corzo et al., 2020). Other presentations can be nonspecific (e.g., fatigue, hair loss, or hematuria), and the diagnosis of SLE requires the healthcare provider to take a thorough history, a complete physical examination, and interpretation of diagnostic tests.

The guidelines for diagnosis include both a clinical and an immunologic group. Criteria need not be present simultaneously. The clinical domains and criteria include constitutional (fever), hematologic (leukopenia, thrombocytopenia, autoimmune hemolysis), neuropsychiatric (delirium, psychosis, seizure), mucocutaneous (acute cutaneous lupus, chronic cutaneous lupus, oral ulcers, nonscarring alopecia), serosal (pleural or pericardial effusion, acute pericarditis), musculoskeletal (synovitis, serositis), and renal (proteinuria, renal biopsy class II, III, IV, or V [lupus nephritis]). The immunologic criteria include elevated antinuclear antibodies (ANA), elevated anti-double-stranded DNA (anti-ds-DNA), anti-Smith antibodies, antiphospholipid antibodies, low complement proteins, and anticardiolipin antibodies or anti-beta-2 glycoprotein 1 antibodies (Ma et al., 2020; Petri et al., 2021).

Three different classification criteria for the diagnosis of SLE exist. The 1997 ACR criteria note a diagnosis of SLE is made if (a) a patient satisfies four of the SLICC criteria (including at least one immunologic criterion and at least one clinical criterion); or (b) a patient has biopsy-proven nephritis (inflammation of the kidney) compatible with SLE in the presence of either ANA or anti-ds-DNA (Hochberg, 1997).

TREATMENT/MANAGEMENT

The overarching goals for the treatment of SLE are to achieve the lowest level of disease activity, minimize the effect on organs, ensure long-term survival, and improve the quality of life. Evidence-based treatment guidelines have been established by professional organizations based on organs involved, disease severity, and comorbid conditions. Treatment for SLE may include NSAIDs for less severe symptoms, local or systemic corticosteroids for acute exacerbations, and systemic corticosteroids for severe manifestations. It is usually managed primarily by a clinician with rheumatology expertise to optimize pharmacologic and nonpharmacologic interventions and achieve treatment goals.

HEADACHES/MIGRAINES

Definition and Scope

Migraines and other recurrent headache disorders cause personal suffering and decreased economic productivity (Burch et al., 2015). The frequency of occurrence of headache is two to three times more common in women than in men, and migraines and other severe or frequent headaches are more prevalent in women than in men, especially during the reproductive years (Loder et al., 2015). The prevalence ratio is consistent across all racial and ethnic groups (Smitherman et al., 2013). Interestingly, U.S. military personnel have lower headache rates than the general population.

Etiology

The cause of headaches, in particular, migraine, is multifactorial. Migraine is a complex brain event. Headache can typically be accompanied by sensory and language dysfunction, visual aura, mood change, fatigue, yawning, neck stiffness, polyurea, and GI disturbance, and a variety of visual, somatic sensory, and cognitive phenomena are among the clinical features that may precede, accompany, or follow the headache (Charles, 2009). While migraine causes are not fully understood, genetics and environmental factors along with pathophysiology of the trigeminal nerve and changes in the brainstem could all contribute to the etiology of headache.

Risk Factors

Risk factors for migraine headaches can be categorized into triggers like wine (red or white), alcoholic beverages in general, strong cheese, processed meats, caffeine, and noxious gases. Other risk factors include female gender, obesity, depression, stressful life events, low education, and social determinants of health. Health disparities also exist related to diagnosis and treatment of headaches among Black and Hispanic individuals (Loder et al., 2015).

Symptoms

Common presenting symptoms include severe headache, bilateral or unilateral; photophobia; photophonia; and nausea. The following symptoms increase the odds of finding a pathologic abnormality on neuroimaging: worst headache of her life, rapidly increasing headache frequency, history of lack of coordination, history of localized neurologic signs or a history of subjective numbness or tingling, and history of headache causing awakening from sleep (Burch et al., 2018).

Evaluation/Assessment

A careful history is needed to identify possible triggers, patterns, and associated symptoms. The physical examination focuses on identifying any neurologic deficits.

Differential Diagnosis

When a woman first presents with a headache, it is classified (migraine, tension, etc.). In the differential diagnosis the following need to be ruled out: central lesions, cerebral mass, trigeminal neuralgias, cluster headaches, and increased intracranial pressure.

Diagnostic Studies

A diagnosis of migraine headache is usually made based on clinical history and physical exam. For women with worrisome symptoms (see the preceding Symptoms section) or findings of neurologic abnormalities, head CT or MRI/MRA is warranted.

Treatment/Management

Treatment for acute headaches includes migraine-aborting agents such as triptans (sumatriptan and zolmitriptan), frovatriptan for short-term menstrual associated migraine (MAM) prevention, and pain medications. Antiemetics are also used due to the concomitant presentation of nausea with migraine. Preventive strategies include avoiding triggers, which can effectively be identified through documenting a headache diary. Preventive medications are useful for women who experience moderate to severe migraines frequently and include beta-blockers (e.g., metoprolol, propranolol) and antiepileptic drugs (AEDs), such as sodium valproate and topiramate

(Silberstein et al., 2012). Lamotrigine has been found ineffective for migraine prevention (Silberstein et al., 2012). Newer migraine preventive treatments are available in the form of CGRP (calcitonin gene-related peptide) inhibitors. This is the first category of pharmaceuticals developed as targeted therapy for migraine prevention. CGRP is a neuropeptide discovered over 3 decades ago. CGRP is a pain modulator located centrally and peripherally in the nervous system. Specifically, monoclonal antibodies act as an antagonism of the CGRP molecule (eptinezumab, galcanezumab, and fremanezumab) or the CCRP receptor (erenumab; Mohanty & Lippmann, 2020). CGRPs can decrease intensity and frequency of migraines, offering a better quality of life.

FUTURE DIRECTIONS

Chronic diseases are very common among women, affecting not only physical health but also physical functioning, symptom experience, quality of life, and role performance. The U.S. healthcare system is designed to respond promptly and effectively to cure and manage acute problems. However, in chronic disease, a different paradigm is needed. The goals of chronic treatment are to mitigate the disease progression and limit the effects of the disease on the woman's day-to-day life. These goals are best accomplished when the woman partners with her clinician to make treatment decisions and to monitor disease and symptom progression. Clinicians need to be sensitive to the long-term implications of chronic disease, and to approach each individual's situation from a holistic standpoint.

As research on the Human Genome Project continues, some chronic diseases may be identifiable earlier, thus reducing overall disability. However, patient responses to knowing they carry a genetic risk for developing a disease, or that they have a disease that is subclinical, will need to be carefully monitored. The stress related to knowing a disease is coming may have negative consequences on physical and mental health.

REFERENCES

References for this chapter are online and available at https://connect.springerpub.com/content/book/978-0-8261-6722-4/part/part03/chapter/ch45

CHAPTER 46

Care of Women With Disabilities

Tracie Harrison and Janiece L. Taylor

By midlife, few women can say that disability has not profoundly affected their lives. According to the American Community Survey, 13% of the U.S. noninstitutionalized population have a disability (U.S. Census Bureau, 2022). Women have higher rates of disability when compared with men, which are 13.2% and 12.8%, respectively (U.S. Census Bureau, 2022). This equates to over 42 million people. According to the 2019 and 2021 American Community Survey, women have higher rates of self-care difficulty, independent living difficulty, and ambulation difficulty when compared to men (U.S. Census Bureau, 2020). Moreover, 61% of people who provide support to people with disabilities are female (National Alliance for Caregiving [NAC], 2020).

It is now time for women's health APRNs to be well prepared in providing care to women aging with and into disability; aspects of care once reserved for specialists in rehabilitation therapies are now in the domain of the APRN in primary care. Along with the increased expectations for providing more expansive primary care to women with disabilities, primary care visits now require APRNs to be judicious with their time. They need to be knowledgeable, focused, pragmatic, and organized with a bountiful set of resources for the health benefit of women with a growing number of disabling conditions, circumstances, and environments. APRNs are called upon to provide not only primary care, but disability healthcare for women, incorporating anticipatory guidance regarding the health-related concerns and needs of women with varying degrees of functional limitations (FLs).

This chapter begins with definitions that facilitate understanding of the problems facing women aging with or into disability, including the process of disablement. Next, social determinants of health confronting women with disabilities are discussed. Racial and ethnic considerations are provided for women with disabilities. Finally, the evidential basis for an assessment to guide preemptive primary care for women living with disability is proposed.

BACKGROUND

Several standpoints on aging and disability form an essential foundation for APRNs providing care for women with disabilities (Thurman & Harrison, 2020). Disability does not mean poor health. Illness may progress over time to a state of poor function and loss of social roles, often called disablement (Verbrugge & Jette, 1994). Disablement is the progression from pathologic change in cellular function to impaired organ function, to experiencing limitations in physical function, and finally to losing social roles. Impairments, such as diabetes and congestive heart failure, and FL, such as paralysis and shortness of breath, have a way of weaving their way through all domains of women's health, leaving a profound effect on the female body. Disability, which is the inability to carry out relevant roles due to the social impact of either a physical impairment or an FL, may be the result of quickly advancing or even mismanaged impairment and FL. The progression from a state of poor cellular or organ function to the point at which the body is no longer able to walk or stand is considered an organ system impairment; this condition has often been the focus of medical providers concerned with providing billable services over the years. The movement from disease to disability has not traditionally been a primary concern of medicine; for example, a woman's loss of employment due to her inability to lift boxes at work, manage bills at home, or go to the park with her dog are each an example of how disease may become a disability but may not be under the purview of the APRN. Yet, within this view of the disablement process, these physical, mental, and social states of being are all intertwined, and treatment is incomplete if all areas are not addressed.

In providing care to women with disabilities, it may be helpful to understand the differences that occur between women who were born with or who acquired an FL early in life, and those who acquired an FL later in life, such as after age 65. This distinction can clarify women's physiology, psychology, and social responses/needs. This distinction extends beyond the fact that both groups of women live with disabilities for a considerable amount of time, sometimes referred to by many in medicine and nursing as disease or "abnormality." Another distinction that may be helpful is between those who have a condition that is *age related* and those with a condition that is *aging related* (Li et al., 2021). This categorization reflects how pathology and impairment conditions accumulate and evolve with age. The mean age of onset may show that the disease is one that is *aged* into; for instance, men and women may develop a cardiomyopathy on average by age 65 years. There is beginning evidence that women's physiology as compared with men's physiology may put them at increased risk with aging (Mellor et al., 2014). A condition is age related when it occurs within a comparatively older age range and is aging related when it is due to the changes that occur with age.

The comparison between women with early onset disability, such as cerebral palsy and spinal muscle atrophy, and those with later onset disability, such as stroke and osteoarthritis, may or may not create a substantial difference in the types of services they need. Comparison of the two groups of women may, however, create an understanding of how they respond to the type and timing of services offered. For instance, in a grounded theory study of 45 women with an FL, timing, resources, and meaning of impairment, along with exposure to an accessible environment post-FL, made a difference in how women with a disability promoted health over time (Harrison et al., 2010). Timing of onset made a difference in which skills were developed for adapting to an environment. Timing of impairment, which may not only predefine a woman's identity and status in society as being disabled but also give her the time and confirm the absolute necessity for crafting unique skills for performing her roles, makes a difference in women's health. Although researchers often define aging as a slow process (Bauer et al., 2015), women with early onset disabilities frequently describe the aging process as short and unpredictable (Harrison, 2006). These include women with spinal cord injury, multiple sclerosis, paralytic polio with or without postpolio syndrome, and spinal muscle atrophy. Differences between women who are aging with a disability and women who age into them later in life are critical considerations for APRNs working collaboratively to plan the best course of action, which is often a challenge due to limited resources.

Due to the high prevalence of disability among women, this group, in general, is often faced with disability, associated poverty, and inequity. Once a limitation occurs, women have historically been without economic support that could help them transition into a new role, gain needed disability resources, or carry them through to old age with housing and food. In part, this occurs because once FL is part of women's lives, they tend to have very low employment rates. For instance, overall labor participation rates are lower for people with FL than for people without; the unemployment rate for people with a disability was more than twice that

of people with no disability in the third quarter of 2021, 10.6% compared with 4.9% (U.S. Bureau of Labor Statistics, 2021, April). In 2019, 17.8% of women with disabilities were employed (U.S. Bureau of Labor Statistics, 2021, April). To demonstrate that women are not to be blamed for this inequity, but instead considered survivors of it, the system-level inequities that lead to the employment distribution are discussed. Awareness of the social determinants of disablement is essential to ensure that women receive needed support.

In the context of COVID-19, it is clear that people with disability are at high risk for contracting COVID-19 and other contagious diseases due to their high exposure to attendant care and personal assistance from other people who may have been exposed to viruses or bacteria. The exposure to contagious disease due to high contact with other people who help with dressing, grooming, hygiene, home cleaning, and dietary needs is magnified by a lack of emergency care that acknowledges the dire consequences for people with cognitive disabilities who may not be able to recognize the symptoms, screening tools, or needed responses to the COVID-19 crisis (Sabatello et al., 2020). Further, people with disability who also live with a level of lung function that requires oxygen or whose lung function provides diminished respiratory exchange may also be at high mortality risk if exposed to COVID-19 (Scully, 2020).

Without stereotyping or assuming the exposures, illness level, function, or needs of people with disability it is unclear if they have a high degree of susceptibility to COVID-19. There have been studies that demonstrate a correlation between use of personal protective equipment among women and among those with a chronic condition being higher than among men and those without a chronic condition (Gamsizkan et al., 2021). Never assuming a biased stance toward those with disabilities requires a high level of communication engagement that gathers the information needed to make critical joint decisions.

SOCIAL DETERMINANTS OF HEALTH POLICIES, AND SOCIOECONOMIC HARDSHIP

According to Hirschman (2013), the "able-bodied man" was the center of political thought when the foundation of political freedom was established in this country; equality and justice were defined for our nation by our forefathers on the basis of equality of right, thereby leaving women with disabilities out of the discourse among human beings who are "in a state of perfect freedom to order their actions, and dispose of their possessions, and persons as they think fit" (p. 167). Understanding that women living with disability have the right to services that enable their freedom within our society requires consideration in order to ensure social justice in health and healthcare (Hirschman, 2012).

Hirschman (2013) argues that women with disabilities were without an equality of right as originally conceived; instead, they had the equality of right to envision a life and to achieve that through the combined rights of a community of people functioning with them and on their behalf. It is the belief of the authors of this chapter that a woman may have an FL in any domain of life but if she is able to achieve her will through combined action, she is not disabled. In other words, women may suffer from our society's view that individuals bear sole responsibility for their independent ability to perform all aspects of a job, working for their own long-term benefit in this country. However, these authors posit that the community may benefit from the unique knowledge and standpoint of a woman with an FL concentrating her work in a specific domain, like a social assembly line. If we act on each other's behalf, we might come to create a more sustainable environment for all workers in the community, improving productivity, enhancing the well-being of all. Policies related to illness and injury in the United States relegate the individual woman to a state of poverty, then blame her for her insufficiencies. APRNs must negotiate on behalf of women living with disability or risk being of little benefit to women and society. Policies related to work are discussed here due to their high significance in the lives of women and women with disabilities. The ability to turn capacity into productive income and compete within the free market is as essential to women's well-being as it is to men's.

Injuries and illnesses that occur early in women's lives may lead to lasting FL and result in disability, which is of considerable concern to gerontologists, epidemiologists, political and administrative leaders, economists, and demographers, as well as the APRN. Early onset injuries and illnesses increase the risk for loss of benefits, income, and health over the life course through two major mechanisms: injuries may result in the loss of work incentive and/or ability, and injuries may exacerbate a preexisting condition. Both mechanisms push people out of the job market earlier than needed (Harrison et al., 2013).

APRNs are often needed to assist with the paperwork that can make a difference in the lives of women with severe FL, whether that was gained on the job or not. Most important to realize is that policies that support the injured workers on the state or federal level in the event they are unable to work are in the domain of the APRN. First, worker compensation benefits cover only injuries arising out of and during employment that are approved as work related by the employer, depending on the state's unique set of laws. Quite the reverse, Social Security Disability Insurance (SSDI) benefits are federally managed and paid to workers with permanent impairments rendering them unable to maintain gainful employment; it does not matter if the employee can prove the injury occurred on the job or not (Social Security Administration, 2021). Both workers' compensation and SSDI programs are designed to ensure that workers do not accrue more than 80% of a capped wage so that people do not profit or benefit from FL and unemployment.

Work-related injury is a major cause of FL and permanent job loss in the United States for those without early onset FL (see Chapter 17, Women and the Workplace). A significant portion of the U.S. population experiences permanent economic loss, as well as pain and suffering, due to occupational injuries. In 2020, private industry reported a decline of injury cases compared to 2019, a rate of 2.2 cases per full time employment (FTE) compared to 2.6 FTE cases in 2019 (U.S. Bureau of Labor Statistics, 2021, November 3). Illnesses increased from 12.4 cases per 100 FTE to 55.9 cases per 100 FTE, driven by COVID-19 respiratory infections (U.S. Bureau of Labor Statistics, 2021, November 3).

The median number of days away from work in all private industry occupations increased from 8 days in 2019 to 12 days in 2020. Ten occupations accounted for almost 40% of all private industry days away from work (U.S. Bureau of Labor Statistics, 2021, November 3). Nursing assistants (who represent a higher number of women and minorities) had the highest number of days away from work (an increase of 249.7% from 2019) with cases for RNs increasing 290.8% since 2019. The effect of the pandemic particularly affected caregivers. Heavy and tractor-trailer truck drivers had a decrease of 9.4% with laborers and freight, stock, and material movers essentially unchanged in 2020 (U.S. Bureau of Labor Statistics, 2021, November 3). These injuries are only those reported as meeting the definition for work-related injuries. They do not cover those injuries that may occur and result in an exacerbation of mental or physical illness causing worsened FL.

In our nation's social safety net in place for the injured worker, the SSDI is to be the last rung available to prevent the suffering of our disabled workforce, which is tied to their payments into the system over their lifetime of working. It is provided under the Old-Age, Survivors, and Disability Insurance program and administered through the Social Security Administration. Kaye (2010) asserted that people with FLs exit the job market during times of economic stress due to a push from work conditions and life circumstances that generate internal and physical surroundings that exacerbate a preexisting condition. Kaye noted that job losses between 2008 and 2010 (time of economic recession) were greater among workers with FL than among those without, which caused the portion of U.S. workers with FL to decrease significantly. Kaye suggested that despite the Americans with Disabilities Act (1990), FL does not provide protection from unemployment; in fact, it is a risk factor for job loss. Long-term joblessness, defined as being without employment for more than 1 year, can have a negative impact on health (Couch et al., 2014). During the pandemic, White and Black women with disabilities experienced greater employment losses compared to white men without disabilities (Schur et al., 2021).

Provider documentation of the person with a disability's diagnosis code is important for social benefits. Looking further into these reasons for exiting the job market and the variations in outcomes once people do exit, Meseguer (2013) reported that despite the federal guidelines for SSDI being the same across the states, the outcomes vary by state. In his analysis, the primary provider's recording of diagnosis code was the largest contributor to being selected initially for benefits. The persons' requests for reevaluation of paperwork applications were seldom overturned, but their requests for a hearing quite often resulted in SSDI acceptance. This indicates the need for careful documentation that accurately reflects the ongoing condition of the person with the FL. It is costly to society for the state to hold judicial hearings to truly understand the state of FL the person is living with at the time.

RACE AND ETHNICITY FACTORS AMONG WOMEN WITH DISABILITIES

Just getting to the [appointment]—down the steps in here and then down the steps there. I mean they had a lift for me when I got to the shuttle bus. But my pain was trying to get out of the house. Just the part of getting up, getting my clothes on, getting down the steps.

—A Black woman with a physical disability

In this section, these authors are asking for a commitment from the APRN to provide equitable care that will overcome imbalances in social determinants to women with disabilities. To assist the APRN in achieving this, a background is provided on groups of women who may have heightened needs that, if not investigated, could be overlooked in primary or specialty care. These are Black women with disability, Indigenous women with disability, Asian American women with disability, and Mexican American women with disability The trends reported represent risk factors for women who occupy a sociocultural space that could place them at an elevated chance of worsening health and function, and this section is meant to inspire understanding of potential population needs. Although race and ethnicity are social constructs that do not have a basis in discriminating against people based upon biological deterministic thinking, the categories do help to locate possible barriers and risk factors in society (Kanakamedala & Haga, 2012). Further, these categories have helped scientists to realize that the participation of people within minority populations remains low (Turner et al., 2022).

Black Women

Black people have the worst health profiles in the United States in comparison to all other racial ethnic groups (Thorpe et al., 2016), which has significant implications for the care of Black women with disabilities. Black women have a higher prevalence of disability than White or Hispanic women (Ross & Bateman, 2018; Varadaraj et al., 2021). The social determinants of health that lead to poor health profiles in Black people are only further complicated and exemplified when a Black woman has a disability. Membership in multiple marginalized groups (e.g., race, gender, and disability status) presents more barriers to receiving healthcare than being in only one marginalized group (Gkiouleka et al., 2018). In the preceding quote, the woman experienced barriers to getting to her appointments that arguably could exist for any woman with a disability; however, additional barriers such as difficulty accessing health insurance, segregated education, and segregated neighborhoods are often experienced by women with disability from underrepresented race/ethnic groups and may impede their access to healthcare and healthcare information (Goodman et al., 2017; Samuel et al., 2021; Taylor et al., 2020). In addition to social determinants of health, Black women may have cultural or societal expectations placed on them that may influence their health. For example, some Black women with disabilities may experience the "Strong Black Woman Schema," which may negatively affect their psychological well-being (Abrams et al., 2019; Miles, 2019). The expectation

to be strong or physically to keep pushing can lead to physical decline and negatively affect the psychological well-being of Black women with disability (Harrison, 2009; Miles, 2019). Social determinants of health and societal and cultural expectations of Black women with disability strongly impact their health outcomes and should inform the healthcare we provide to this population.

When providing care for Black women with disabilities it is important to understand their health risk profiles and potential cultural influences, and use a person-centered holistic approach to providing care. It is crucial to conduct baseline assessments with both objective and subjective measures to identify any early risk factors or warning signs. For example, asking about pain and/or depression and discussing treatment preferences are important because the women may not always remember or feel comfortable bringing up these symptoms unless asked (Booker et al., 2019; Drazich et al., 2022). In addition, it is important for providers to identify any barriers that Black women with disabilities face individually, structurally, or financially before making recommendations about treatments or follow-ups. For example, a provider recommending physical therapy may not have identified the physical, environmental, and financial barriers presented to a patient attempting to participate in physical therapy. Black women with disabilities may have trouble with transportation, physical limitations, or financial concerns surrounding copays or taking time off work that make getting access to physical therapy very difficult. Furthermore, it is important for APRNs to be culturally aware when providing care for Black women with disabilities. To provide quality healthcare, it is essential that clinicians avoid comments and behaviors that further perpetuate ideas such as the "Strong Black Woman Schema" or other expectations of the women to fulfill certain roles (Jefferies, 2020).

As APRNs caring for Black women with disabilities it is important to be aware of the multiple intersections that can influence their health; however, it is equally important to avoid stereotypes and address any unconscious biases that exist when providing care (Beach et al., 2021; Narayan, 2019; Persaud, 2019). Treating the women as individuals and working with them to build on their own strengths and values can lead to the best outcomes. Nurses caring for Black women with disabilities are uniquely positioned to work with the women to promote health and thrive as they age with or into disabilities.

Indigenous Women

There is evidence that Indigenous women are at high risk for FLs when compared to other groups. An example of this work with the disability population of Indigenous women was done by Dias Junior and Verona (2018). The authors studied an Indigenous group of both men and women in Brazil with visual, hearing, and motor impairments comparing them to other groups of people. They found the Indigenous population of women to have the highest severity of visual impairment, and regardless of type and degree of severity, they had the highest degree of severity in hearing and mobility limitations.

Some of the disparities in disablement outcomes found in the Indigenous populations of women may be related to social determinants of health. The placement of women and girls at risk for violence, organ removal, forced prostitution, and forced labor put them at risk for long-term physical and mental injury. With most human trafficking victims being women for sexual slave labor, these women are placed in situations that expose them to prolonged and repeated trauma. Human trafficking of Indigenous women in Monterrey City, Mexico was studied by Acharya (2019). After interviewing 68 Indigenous women who had been human trafficked in Mexico, the author reported that women entered into the high-risk situations due to poverty, dysfunctional families, and unemployment. The majority worked 7 days/week and many experienced physical and/or sexual violence, 45.6% and 42.6%, respectively. Due to their work, the majority report skin damage, eye injuries, mouth and teeth injuries, ear damage, back injury, head injuries, broken bones, and finger injuries. Further, 90% had depression and 72% could not control emotions. This led the researcher to surmise that 33.8% had mobility limitations, 60% had hearing limitations, and 16% had visual limitations. All the women were limited socially due to discrimination and perceived stigma.

Noting the disparity for women with intellectual and/or developmental disability (IDD), Williamson et al. (2021) worked with Indigenous women with IDD using self-determination from within an intersectionality perspective. They theorized that the lower rates of cervical and mammography screenings were due to the intersections of oppression experienced by the women. They formed a community advisory board that helped steer the group to create a framework built on local knowledge that honored their self-determination in both the IDD and Indigenous groups.

Asian American Women

The Asian American population is representative of a very diverse group of women. The prevalence, significance, and implication of disablement in the Asian American population is less well studied than it is in groups of non-Hispanic White, Hispanics, and Black women. According to Sharma (2020), estimating using a national U.S. sample from the National Health Interview Survey, Chinese American women have an increased risk for FLs after age 75 compared to Chinese American men. Asian Indian men and women in the United States have the relatively highest probability of FLs across age ranges when compared to Filipino and Chinese Americans. This continues until age 85, when the Chinese Americans have a leading rate. Being married and having higher levels of education were protective factors for both genders.

Hispanic/Latina Women

For women over the age of 80, Cené et al. (2016) reported that racial and ethnic variations in function were not clear in their analysis of the women's health initiative data. Importantly, there were differences, a survival variant, in how many women in each racial and ethnic group lived to be included. Hispanic women had worse mean physical functioning scores as their age increased. Importantly, physical functioning improved with physical activity in the Latina women over age 80 group. Depression was an issue in Hispanic women

with disability who reported better self-reported health and being happy most of the time. They also reported better quality of life when they reported being happy most of the time.

It is difficult to always know the risk factors for different groups of women based upon race/ethnicity. It is not suggested that the APRN memorize those at greatest disadvantage and then single them out for intensive visits. It is advised that the APRN prepare to have a dialogue with patients to understand their baseline needs, barriers, and facilitators (Shen et al., 2018). To provide person-centered care, the APRN must conduct an accurate assessment of each person's sociocultural background, which includes racial/ethnic background, and elicit how the person believes it affects their ability to live with a disability.

RISK FOR HEALTH DECLINE AMONG WOMEN WITH DISABILITIES

The United Nations (UN) published a brief on gender, age, and disability (UN, 2018). In it, the UN authors emphasize the importance of older women to society, worldwide, with and without disabilities. The women who maintain and spread our cultural heritage to future generations; the women who nurture multiple generations of their children and their neighbor's children, and the women who work to ensure their families are fed, clothed, and nurtured are an essential part of the fabric of every society. When also experiencing a disability, they become the "systematically overlooked and under-represented in development policies, programs, initiatives, legislation, as well as humanitarian efforts" (UN, 2018, p. 1). Women with disability are the most at-risk group known worldwide.

Published tools validated for the classification of disability for work-eligibility-related purposes include those developed by Oyeleye (2019). The purpose of the assessment guide (Box 46.1) is to focus understanding of the needs for ongoing disability-related care and possible risk factor assessment of women living with disabilities. The factors included in this guide are grounded in the assumption that women with disabilities should receive preemptive primary care that works to eliminate modifiable factors that worsen health with age.

Despite the association between poor health and limitations, people who live with a physical, mental, intellectual, and/or sensory limitation are at higher risk for the accumulation of a greater number of chronic illnesses over time than those who do not have limitations (Dixon-Ibarra & Horner-Johnson, 2014). This is called accelerated aging among people with disabilities. Risk factors for a decline in health among women with disabilities have been identified in published literature. There is, however, an exception for women with disabilities and women without disabilities who report current pregnancy; they tend to have better health risk profiles, such as less tobacco use and fewer mental health issues (Iezzoni et al., 2015). The tool presented here is intended to begin a conversation about women living with disability and how we can assist them with risk factors specific to them. Nine risk factors defined at this time are age, menopausal status, muscular fitness, oral health,

Box 46.1 Assessment Guide for Women Aging With Disabilities: Risk Factors for Health Decline

Age

- 60+ years with later onset disability
- 40+ years with early onset disability
- Age since onset of functional limitation changes the risk for mortality; alter health promotion activities in response

Age of Menopause

- Postmenopausal musculoskeletal changes
- Time since ovulation
- Oophorectomy early in life

Oral Health

- Yearly oral evaluations by dentist
- Goal: no ongoing periodontal disease
- Risk factor: loss of teeth
- Risk factor: fewer than nine teeth left

Physical Activity and Health Promotion

- Planned physical activity at least 3 days/week
- The ability to maintain support in this goal diminishes during exacerbations

Cognitive Decline

- Mild cognitive impairment with age
- Dementia onset
- Consider interventions to address decline

Long-Term Use of Accommodations

- Manual wheelchair use is a risk factor
- History of painful injuries in arms and shoulders
- Lack of mobility
- Never dismiss musculoskeletal complaints
- May need to address pain management routine as aging and wear/tear continue

Musculoskeletal Health

- Notable decline in strength
- May need to change accommodations to something less risky for injury or decline

Mental Health

- History of depression
- History of posttraumatic stress disorder
- History of multiple mood disorders

Sensory Ability

- Notable loss of vision with accommodation
- Notable loss of hearing with accommodation
- Refer for evaluations and provide specific and detailed notes

physical activity, long-term use of accommodations, cognitive decline, mental health, and sensory ability. These factors are discussed in the following sections of this chapter.

Age

Age is the springboard for the risk assessment of health outcomes in all women, including women with disabilities. As women at any age may have disabilities and this discussion is focused on women with an already notable disability, age is an important consideration due to both age-related and aging-dependent changes in the body that occur over time.

Some authors define *aging* using a series of notable demarcations of damage in cells, organs, tissues, and so on (Huang et al., 2015). Others view aging as growth in personality, wit, and wisdom. Within this model of risk factors, age will be described as a complex process of variable rates of change in numerous domains of life, each leading to positive and/or negative consequences for the function and performance of the woman. This definition allows for multiple interpretations of the impact of age on the health of women with a disability.

First, within any developmental age group, an APRN should attend to both the psychosocial risk factors for the loss of social roles and the biological risk factors for physical loss. Allowing these possible developmental roles to guide the conversation, an APRN can assess whether a woman is able to meet the role expectations important to her at that age or during that time, which serves as an approach to assessing levels of disability. Because a woman's roles shift over time, her perspective on her ability to meet valued role expectations should be reassessed periodically. In a study of women with multiple sclerosis followed for 7 years, Harrison et al. (2008) found that high levels of FL and fast rates of decline in function predicted negative attitudes toward aging. They also found that women with high levels of FLs had low levels of social support, which is when they may have needed it most.

Age may also potentiate the effect of gender, placing older women at higher risk than younger women for illnesses or impairments, such as cancer. For instance, in the case of cancer, there are six common hallmarks of aging along with the disease: genomic instability, epigenetic alteration, aberrant telomeres, reprogrammed metabolism, impaired degradation, and impaired immune-inflammatory response (Huang et al., 2015). Without going into each of these processes, suffice it to say that aging women are at higher risk for aging-related diseases such as those cancers unique to women. These include breast, vaginal, and cervical cancers. Women with disabilities bear the same risk. Maintaining an attitude of awareness of risk for women with disabilities is essential in primary disability healthcare.

Women with early onset disabilities have reported being told by physicians that their life expectancy would be shorter than for those without disabilities and that they should plan their lives accordingly (Iezzoni et al., 2021). This experience is commonly reported by women with early onset disabilities, such as spinal muscle atrophy or spinal cord injuries, who on average live shorter periods of time. The need for them to plan for the changes occurring with aging was not part of their life plan, due to the fact that they did not anticipate a long life span. Nonetheless, many women who experience disability early in life do age into their later years. Consequently, a part of the APRN primary care visit is assessment of women's readiness for retirement, shift in accommodations, and the loss of family members, providers, and attendants over time.

In an important review article by Karvonen-Gutierrez (2015), the author reported that midlife women may be at the most high-risk period of their lives. This is the time when women accumulate mobility disability at a higher rate than in previous years and that rate of mobility disability affects their ability to perform necessary and socially important roles. For women with a long-standing disability, accelerated aging is often noted during midlife. Hence, it is important for the practitioner to look at women in middle age as being at a critical period for intervention; this refers to women who are both aging into and aging with a disability.

Awareness that life may be shortened or at heightened risk given the differences in the women's bodies at a common social and developmental period, midlife, is not without merit. Women with early onset disabilities may not have the same life span as someone without a disability. Women without disabilities may be at higher risk during periods of high developmental role performance. Campbell et al. (1999) expressed concern that those with early onset conditions may have accelerated aging. This is because they may have been exposed to excessive (a) environmental barriers (e.g., slick floors and no elevators), (b) pathologic conditions (e.g., tuberculosis), (c) medical-exposure risk (e.g., excessive x-rays), (d) general wear and tear of the body (e.g., straining with pain to carry heavy objects), and (e) high levels of endogenous stressors for a long period of time due to the aforementioned, all of which contribute to shortening their life expectancy. These excessive exposures may wear all women down with heightened effects at midlife.

Age of Menopause

As women complete the transition to menopause, previous function may worsen due to common symptoms of menopause such as hot flushes, fatigue, poor concentration, palpitations, anxiety attacks, urinary problems, heavy periods, sleep disturbance, irritability, and mood disturbance. After menopause, women may have a decrease in overall muscle mass and an increase in adipose tissue. For women with long-standing FLs, such as those with spinal cord injuries, an increase in adipose tissue with decreasing muscle can alter the ability to remain agile and to transfer without assistance. Loss of muscle mass may decrease women's activity level, contributing to weight gain and diminishing socialization. It may also place them at risk for injury as transfers, with or without assistance, become more difficult. The period after menopause is a good time to reassess women's use of appropriate accommodations for their ambulatory and other needs.

The actual experience of menopause is similar for women with and without disabilities (de Almeida & Greguol, 2015). There is, however, concern that treatments for problems experienced during or around that period might cause women with disabilities to forgo needed care. For example, access to incontinence therapy or bladder repair surgeries might be a challenge, depending on the nature of the woman's disabling physical condition, her financial resources, other resources in her area. and her access to support after surgery.

Oral Health

Oral health reflects a complex attitude toward teeth, appearance, oral hygiene, dental practices, and availability, as well as socioeconomic access to dental care. First, periodontal disease has been associated with coronary disease, diabetes, stroke, and rheumatoid arthritis (Hoyuela et al., 2015). Studies linking worsening of multiple sclerosis and dental pathology have been mixed (Dulamea et al., 2015). The risk for the spread of infection from the mouth to other areas in the body is a concern, especially during operative procedures. Lampley et al. (2014) indicated that periodontal disease has been considered a possible link to infection in people who have artificial joint replacement, culminating in lengthy operative and convalescent periods. The need for dental clearance preoperatively is often a matter of provider preference and is currently being debated (Lampley et al., 2014).

Periodontal disease can be painful, disabling, and life threatening, thus increasing risk for poor health among women living with disability. Finally, Holm-Pedersen et al. (2008) found that disability was significantly associated with tooth loss. These researchers set out to follow 573 nondisabled people for 20 years, which dwindled down to a total of 78 people by the end. They found that having one to nine teeth (e.g., edentulous) was associated with disability onset at age 75 and 80 years. They also found that being edentulous at 70 years was predictive of a higher risk for mortality than for women who were not edentulous. Ensuring that women take care of their teeth as part of their health promotion is essential, and it may provide lasting health protection.

Physical Activity

Physical activity is an important dimension in the lives of women with disabilities. It affects how women view their potential for action and their views regarding their body. Rolfe et al. (2009) conducted a qualitative study on exercise in women with disabilities. The researchers reported that "women described how exercise improves their psychosocial health and well-being, fosters a sense of independence and accomplishment, and increases their awareness of their body's abilities and limitations" (Rolfe et al., 2009, p. 748).

More recent research with a feminist disability lens has built on the earlier work, suggesting that healthcare providers consider women's disability sports as an "expansionary opportunity" (Hammond & Macdougall, 2020, p. 57).

Cognitive Decline

There are studies that demonstrate a relationship between FLs and cognitive ability. As suggested by Gothe et al. (2014), despite the reports that cognitive and physical function tend to decline together with age, there are new reports that cognitive decline may be a precursor to functional decline. The positive aspect of this work is the focus on strategies to improve cognitive function, which might possibly stave off functional decline as well. Monitoring for cognitive decline and its root cause may help with understanding a woman's risk for problems and her ability to adapt. Women with disabilities have routinely reported that their ability to maintain activity in their communities has been dependent on their ability to solve problems, to identify threats to their current functional routine, and to think of new ways to overcome structural, emotional, and interpersonal barriers (Harrison et al., 2010, 2013).

Long-Term Use of Accommodations

As women use accommodations in their daily mobility routine, injury, strain, and/or chronic pain often happen (Nawoczenski et al., 2012). This is especially true of women who use a manual wheelchair for mobility: the regular push and pull of the wheel can lead to painful strain. The most commonly reported problem among those using manual wheelchairs is shoulder impingement syndrome, which might be further differentiated as either subacromial or internal impingement (Nawoczenski et al., 2012). Furthermore, transfers from seat to seat with arms instead of the lower body can lead to wear and tear on the upper arm joints and soft tissues. This is often seen in women with spinal cord injury for various reasons, which include (a) vascular occlusion, progressive resorption of the clavicle at the end region, (b) clavicle malalignment during movement of the wheelchair, (c) a bent posture while sitting in the wheelchair, and finally, (d) altered muscle growth due to variations in muscle development related to how the muscles are used (Giner-Pascual et al., 2011). Giner-Pascual et al. (2011) reported that if men and women used a wheelchair seat positioned parallel to the ground, as compared with a seat tilted at an angle, they were at an increased risk for structural injury in their shoulders and subsequent pain.

The use of accommodations, such as canes and wheelchairs, can have a positive effect on the body. For instance, in a study of older adults with hemiparesis, one-sided paralysis, adults were significantly faster with a stronger gait if they used a cane for sit-to-stand transfers than if they did not (Hu et al., 2013). The person with hemiparesis was able to extend their paralyzed knee more and balance the load in movement. It is suggested that the strategy of using a cane during sit-to-stand transfer from seat to wheelchair and afterward during movement can help prevent falls as well. This is because the cane keeps the body from swaying; for example, it keeps the load balanced. It is important that the provider balance their understanding of negative outcomes with accommodations with that of good outcomes, and make the most appropriate person-centered recommendations they can over time.

Musculoskeletal Health

Changes in the musculoskeletal system can evolve into pathologic conditions, such as osteoarthritis or osteoporosis. These aging-related disease shifts are most notable in the movement from osteopenia to osteoporosis (Freemont & Hoyland, 2007). The age-related changes we all face include (a) losses in bone tissues with subsequent weakness; (b) lack of cushioning effects of water between the joints, which results in osteoarthritis; (c) loss of elasticity in the ligaments that stretch and return to prior shape; (d) losses of muscle mass and power, often partly due to denervation; (e) redistribution of fat; (f) stiffening of collagen and elastin; and (g) change in humoral factors that mediate growth, development, and life span (Freemont & Hoyland, 2007).

For women with disabilities, the loss of strength can make a difference in their being independent. For instance, losses of muscle strength may prevent a woman from transferring from her wheelchair to her car seat. Further, sarcopenia with loss in muscle strength tends to be more common in postmenopausal women (Anagnostis et al., 2015). This is consistent with a study by Andrews et al. (2014), who wrote that muscle strength was strongly associated with physical disability in women with lupus, even after adjustment for covariates.

Women with a disability enter into postmenopausal musculoskeletal changes with varying degrees of muscle strength due to earlier onset FLs. There is a need to prepare the woman and her family for changes in her ability that come with age, as well as the changes that occur in people who are aging alongside her. Of people who provide support to people with disabilities, 61% are female (NAC, 2020) who may not be able to physically provide care over time. The type of accommodation that worked at age 35 years to lift a woman from her wheelchair to her bed might not work at age 60 years.

According to the American Community Survey, women have higher rates of self-care difficulty, independent living difficulty, and ambulation difficulty when compared to men (U.S. Census Bureau, 2022). Women with disabilities will have increased difficulties with self-care compared to nondisabled women. A thorough musculoskeletal assessment at baseline and a periodical assessment over time are warranted. A change of equipment might be needed through occupational or physical therapy. This is important given the evidence that overall happiness among people with polio-related disability was significantly related to their assistive technology (Spiliotopoulou et al., 2012).

Mental Health

In a study of predictive factors of increasing functional decline among 1,187 men and women (63% women) age 60 years or older with multiple disabling conditions, investigators found that among older women mental health was the main outcome predictor of activities of daily living (Laan et al., 2013). For men, the predictors were transient ischemic attacks and myocardial infarction. Women tended to respond physically to their mental state. In a study of early aging among people with posttraumatic stress disorder (PTSD), Lohr et al. (2015) reported that seven of 10 studies reported higher mortality rate for those with PTSD. They also found higher proinflammatory markers in those with PTSD. Although this finding was not specific to women, the relationship of mental health to physical disability in aging women is noteworthy. Therefore, assessment for mental health issues such as depression and PTSD is important as a basis for mental health treatment when warranted. Further, treating conditions such as migraine headaches can be difficult in the care of women with disabilities due to the number of associated comorbid conditions requiring special attention to treatment selection (Minen et al., 2016).

Sensory Ability

FLs of vision (3.1%) and hearing (5.2%) occur in the adult general population ages 65 and older (Federal Interagency Forum on Aging-Related Statistics, 2020). Vision impairment is associated with more cognitive impairment and decline among the population of older adults (Nagarajan et al., 2022). In the aforementioned study by Laan et al. (2013), vision was an independent predictor of decline among older women with chronic illnesses and/or disabilities. Individuals with age-related hearing loss have a greater chance of developing dementia (Livingston et al., 2020). When a woman with a disability loses her hearing or vision, the changes can result in institutionalization if accommodations are not planned for and made.

Health Promotion

There are studies that address our clinical need for an overall healthy lifestyle guide/program for women with disabilities. For instance, as early as 2003, Stuifbergen et al. tested in a randomized control trial the wellness intervention they created for women with multiple sclerosis. They integrated an educational and skill-building lifestyle change program, along with a supportive telephone follow-up. The lifestyle change program consisted of eight sessions over an 8-week period; it guided participants in self-assessment of behaviors, resources, and barriers and supported specific strategies aimed at building self-efficacy for health behaviors. This program has also been tested in low-income cancer survivors (Meraviglia et al., 2015). It might supplement the care that is provided in the clinical setting to ensure that the provider and the woman with the disability are working together in the best direction. This includes ensuring that all staff members are trained in providing accessible care to people with disabilities and being culturally aware of how their actions might affect others. Looking at the trajectory of disability (Kim et al., 2020), engaging a midlife group of women in health promotion activities might be an excellent way to prepare women for the future. Starting earlier with women who have early onset disabilities, for example, young adulthood, might be best for this group. In this way, the possibility of midlife mortality might be diminished.

SUMMARY

This chapter begins with consideration of definitions that facilitate understanding of the problems faced by women who are aging with or into disability. Socioeconomic conditions confronting women with disabilities are discussed. The multitude of factors and subgroups of women that can influence outcomes after the onset of a FL due to any known cause are vast. This chapter begins a conversation that requires an ongoing dialogue. The impact the APRN has on the outcomes of the woman with the disability cannot be understated. The APRN can write a referral that helps to support her work role, facilitate interactions within multiple domains of her life, and prevent her continuation without services.

Finally, the chapter proposes the evidential basis for an assessment tool to guide preemptive care for women living with disability. To support APRNs providing primary healthcare to women with disabilities, an assessment tool incorporating nine risk factors salient for decline among women with physical disabilities is provided. The tool is intended as a guide for assessment, not as a predictive measure, and is designed to support APRNs as they venture beyond the disease-central focus they have been prepared to address and assist women with managing aging, disability, and any relevant barriers set before them. Nevertheless, few providers currently have the requisite knowledge of disability-related healthcare (Iezzoni et al., 2021). APRNs are being called upon to provide disability-related healthcare focusing on health promotion in the context of FL for the prevention of exacerbations and comorbidities. In addition, APRNs can provide access to the appropriate consultations and services and provide for the elimination of social and cultural barriers to health over the life course (Smeltzer, 2021). Again, it is expected that women with disabilities have issues related to bowel movements and pain care on an ongoing basis. The need to treat the pain reported with a supportive, essentially stable approach to their pain management regimen must go without saying.

REFERENCES

References for this chapter are online and available at https://connect.springerpub.com/content/book/978-0-8261-6722-4/part/part03/chapter/ch46